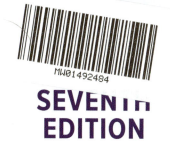
SEVENTH EDITION

Rodak's

HEMATOLOGY

Clinical Principles and Applications

SEVENTH EDITION

Rodak's HEMATOLOGY

Clinical Principles and Applications

Elaine M. Keohane, PhD, MLS(ASCP) SH^CM

Professor Emeritus, Clinical Laboratory and Medical Imaging Sciences
School of Health Professions
Rutgers, The State University of New Jersey
Newark, New Jersey

Michelle Montgomery Butina, PhD, MLS(ASCP)^CM

Associate Professor, Pathology, Anatomy, and Laboratory Medicine
Vice Chair, Biomedical Laboratory Diagnostics
Program Director, Medical Laboratory Science
School of Medicine
West Virginia University
Morgantown, West Virginia

Kamran M. Mirza, MD, PhD, FCAP, FASCP, MLS(ASCP)

Godfrey D. Stobbe Professor of Pathology Education
Clinical Professor of Pathology
Assistant Chair for Education
Director, Division of Education Programs
Pathology
Michigan Medicine
Ann Arbor, Michigan

Jeanine M. Walenga, PhD, MLS(ASCP)H^CM

Professor, Thoracic-Cardiovascular Surgery, Pathology, and Physiology
Co-Director, Hemostasis and Thrombosis Research Unit
Stritch School of Medicine
Loyola University Chicago
Laboratory Director, Clinical Coagulation
Laboratory Director, Urinalysis and Medical Microscopy
Associate Director, Point of Care & Referred Testing
Pathology and Laboratory Medicine
Loyola University Health System
Maywood, Illinois

ELSEVIER

Elsevier
3251 Riverport Lane
St. Louis, Missouri 63043

Senior Content Strategist: Kelly Skelton
Senior Content Development Specialist: Sarah Vora
Publishing Services Manager: Julie Eddy
Senior Project Manager: Rachel E. McMullen
Design Direction: Patrick Ferguson

Printed in India

Last digit is the print number: 9 8 7 6 5 4 3 2 1

Working together
to grow libraries in
developing countries

www.elsevier.com • www.bookaid.org

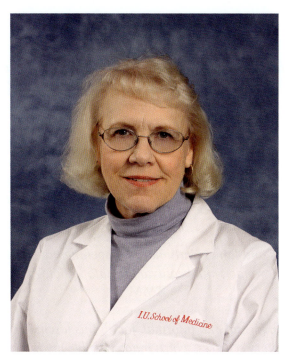

Bernadette "Bunny" Beales Rodak, MS, MLS(ASCP)SH, Professor Emeritus of Pathology at Indiana University School of Medicine, died at the age of 70 on March 22, 2016. Bunny was the founding author and editor of *Hematology: Clinical Principles and Applications*, renamed *Rodak's Hematology: Clinical Principles and Applications* in 2016. For over 20 years and through five editions, she dedicated countless hours to this indispensable text while mentoring five coeditors and more than 50 authors. Bunny considered the combination of this textbook and the *Clinical Hematology Atlas,* coauthored with friend and colleague **Jacqueline Carr** through five editions, to be her greatest contribution to medical laboratory hematology. Bunny's work continues to inform and inspire a generation of medical laboratory practitioners and scholars as her textbook now offers its seventh edition.

Bunny authored numerous influential publications and conducted countless professional presentations. She chaired the American Society for Clinical Laboratory Science (ASCLS)

Hematology and Hemostasis Scientific Assembly and went on to coordinate all of the ASCLS Scientific Assemblies. She was editor-in-chief of the ASCLS *Clinical Laboratory Science* journal and led an online expert team to answer consumer laboratory-related questions. She was a member of the ASCLS Education and Research Fund, which in 2016, endowed the Bernadette "Bunny" Rodak Memorial Scholarship. In 2013, the ASCLS awarded her their coveted Robin H. Mendelson Memorial Award, recognizing her achievements and contributions to medical laboratory science worldwide.

While an acknowledged innovator and role model, Bunny was readily available to students and colleagues. She put everyone at ease and, being humble, never revealed her long history of community service. All her acquaintances attest to her kind and helpful spirit. Bunny's colleagues miss her gracious smile and are honored to continue her work.

The Former and Current Editors

To my students for being great teachers, to my mentors for their guidance and support, and to Camryn, Riley, Harper, Stella, Jackie, Alana, Ken, and Jake for grounding me in the important things in life.
EMK

To my mentors, Kathryn Doig and Lynn Maedel, for sharing your inquisitiveness, enthusiasm, and vast knowledge of blood cells; your support and encouragement inspired me to take this exciting journey, and I am eternally grateful.
MMB

To John Anastasi and James Vardiman, for opening my eyes to the mystery, wonder, and beauty of hematopathology.
KMM

To my teachers, both formal and informal, for all this fascinating knowledge in the clinical laboratory sciences, which made possible my interesting career.
JMW

David Alter, MD, DABCC, MPH
Director of Clinical Chemistry
Associate Professor
Pathology and Laboratory Medicine
Emory University
School of Medicine
Atlanta, Georgia

C. L. Freeman, PhD, MLS(ASCP)BB
Program Director
Medical Laboratory Technology
Fayetteville Technical Community College
Fayetteville, North Carolina

Amy Kapanka, MS, MLS(ASCP)SC
Program Director
Medical Laboratory Technology
Professor
Hawkeye Community College
Waterloo, Iowa

Emily Kaufman, MLS(ASCP)^{CM}
Generalist Medical Laboratory Scientist
Formerly at Cleveland Clinic Akron General
Akron, Ohio

Angela Njoku, MS, MLS(ASCP)
Adjunct Professor
Clinical Laboratory Technology
St. Louis Community College
St. Louis, Missouri

Malissa S. Norfolk, MBA, MLS(ASCP)^{CM} SH^{CM}
Medical Laboratory Science
College of Nursing and Health Science
University of Massachusetts Dartmouth
Dartmouth, Massachusetts

CONTRIBUTORS

Nicholas C. Brehl, MEd, MLS(ASCP)^{CM}
Assistant Professor of Clinical Pathology and
  Laboratory Medicine
Director, Health Professions Programs,
  Medical Laboratory Science Program
Indiana University School of Medicine
Indianapolis, Indiana

Michelle Montgomery Butina, PhD, MLS(ASCP)^{CM}
Associate Professor, Pathology, Anatomy,
  and Laboratory Medicine
Vice Chair, Biomedical Laboratory
  Diagnostics
Program Director, Medical Laboratory
  Science
School of Medicine
West Virginia University
Morgantown, West Virginia

Karen S. Clark, BS, MLS(ASCP)SH
POC Supervisor, Pathology
Baptist Memorial Hospital Memphis
Memphis, Tennessee

Stephanie B. Cochrane, EdD, MS, MLS(ASCP)^{CM}
Lecturer, Clinical Laboratory and Medical
  Imaging Sciences;
Clinical Coordinator, Medical Laboratory
  Science Program
School of Health Professions
Rutgers University
Newark, New Jersey

Magdalena Czader, MD, PhD
Professor, Pathology and Laboratory
  Medicine
Indiana University School of Medicine
Indianapolis, Indiana

Phillip J. DeChristopher, MD, PhD
Medical Director, Transfusion Medicine
Professor, Pathology and Laboratory
  Medicine
Loyola University Health System
Maywood, Illinois

Kathryn Doig, PhD, MLS(ASCP)^{CM}SH^{CM}
Professor Emeritus, Biomedical Laboratory
  Diagnostics
Michigan State University
East Lansing, Michigan

George A. Fritsma, MS, MLS
Proprietor, The Fritsma Factor, Your
  Interactive Hemostasis Resource
Precision BioLogic Inc.
Dartmouth, Nova Scotia, Canada
Clinical Associate Professor, Laboratory
  Medicine
University of Alabama at Birmingham
Birmingham, Alabama
Clinical Associate Professor, Biomedical
  Laboratory Diagnostics
Michigan State University
East Lansing, Michigan
Clinical Associate Professor, Clinical
  Laboratory and Medical Imaging
  Sciences
School of Health Professions
Rutgers University
Newark, New Jersey

Bertil Glader, MD, PhD
Professor, Pediatric Hematology/Oncology
Professor, Pathology
Stanford University
Stanford, California

Kathryn E. Golab, MLS(ASCP)^{CM}SH^{CM}
Clinical Laboratory Utilization Specialist
Wisconsin Diagnostic Laboratories
Milwaukee, Wisconsin;
Resident, Doctor of Clinical Laboratory
  Science Program
School of Health Professions
Rutgers University
Newark, New Jersey

Karen Golemboski, PhD, MLS(ASCP)
Professor, Medical Laboratory Science
Bellarmine University
Louisville, Kentucky

Brandy Gunsolus, DCLS, MLS(ASCP)^{CM}
Pathology Utilization, Pathology
Augusta University Medical Center
Augusta, Georgia
Adjunct Associate Professor, Clinical
  Laboratory and Medical Imaging
  Sciences
School of Health Professions
Rutgers University
Newark, New Jersey

Teresa G. Hippel, BS, MLS(ASCP)SH
Quality Reviewer, Diagnostic Laboratories
Vanderbilt University Medical Center
Nashville, Tennessee

S. Renee Hodgkins, PhD, MLS(ASCP)
Clinical Associate Professor, Clinical
  Laboratory Sciences
Director, Doctorate in Clinical Laboratory
  Science Program
University of Kansas Medical Center
Kansas City, Kansas

Debra A. Hoppensteadt, PhD, MLS(ASCP)SH
Professor, Pathology, and Pharmacology
Loyola University Chicago
Maywood, Illinois

Cynthia L. Jackson, PhD, HCLD(ABB)
Director, Molecular Genomic Pathology
  Laboratory
Lifespan Academic Medical Center
Professor, Pathology
Warren Alpert School of Medicine at Brown
  University
Providence, Rhode Island

Walter P. Jeske, PhD
Professor, Cardiovascular Research Institute
Stritch School of Medicine
Health Sciences Division
Loyola University Chicago
Maywood, Illinois

Constantine E. Kanakis, MD, MSc, MLS(ASCP)
Resident Physician, Pathology and
  Laboratory Medicine
Loyola University Medical Center
Adjunct Instructor
Medical Laboratory Science Graduate
  Program
Loyola Parkinson School of Health Sciences
  and Public Health
Maywood, Illinois

Elaine M. Keohane, PhD, MLS(ASCP) SH^{CM}
Professor Emeritus, Clinical Laboratory and
  Medical Imaging Sciences
School of Health Professions
Rutgers University
Newark, New Jersey

Ameet R. Kini, MD, PhD
Professor, Pathology and Laboratory
  Medicine
Stritch School of Medicine
Loyola University Chicago
Maywood, Illinois

Kristen N. Krum, MD, MS
Assistant Professor, Pathology
Loyola University Medical Center
Maywood, Illinois

Clara Lo, MD
Clinical Associate Professor, Pediatric
 Hematology-Oncology
Stanford University
Palo Alto, California

Naveen Manchanda, MD
Associate Professor of Clinical Medicine
Internal Medicine
Indiana University School of Medicine
Indianapolis, Indiana

Steven Marionneaux, PhD, MLS(ASCP)
Medical and Scientific Affairs Adviser
Cellavision, Inc.
Lund, Sweden
Adjunct Assistant Professor, Clinical
 Laboratory and Medical Imaging
 Sciences
School of Health Professions
Rutgers University
Newark, New Jersey

Peter Maslak, MD
Chief, Immunology Laboratory Service
Laboratory Medicine
Attending Physician, Leukemia Service
Internal Medicine
Memorial Sloan Kettering Cancer Center
Professor of Clinical Medicine
Internal Medicine
Weill Cornell Medical College
New York, New York

Susan A. McQuiston, MS, JD
Instructor, Biomedical Laboratory
 Diagnostics
Michigan State University
East Lansing, Michigan

Shashi Mehta, PhD
Associate Professor, Clinical Laboratory and
 Medical Imaging Sciences
School of Health Professions
Rutgers University
Newark, New Jersey

**Kamran M. Mirza, MD, PhD, FCAP,
FASCP, MLS(ASCP)**
Godfrey D. Stobbe Professor of Pathology
 Education
Clinical Professor of Pathology,
Assistant Chair for Education,
Director, Division of Education Programs
Pathology
Michigan Medicine
Ann Arbor, Michigan

Tara Cothran Moon, PhD, MLS(ASCP)^{CM}
Professor, Clinical Laboratory Science
University of North Carolina at Chapel Hill
Chapel Hill, North Carolina

**Yukari Nishizawa-Brennen, PhD,
MLS(ASCP)^{CM}SC^{CM}, MT(Japan)**
Assistant Professor, Biomedical Laboratory
 Diagnosis Program
Michigan State University
East Lansing, Michigan

**Catherine N. Otto, PhD, MBA,
MLS(ASCP)^{CM}SH^{CM}, DLM^{CM}**
Professor (Retired), Clinical Laboratory and
 Medical Imaging Sciences
School of Health Professions
Rutgers University
Newark, New Jersey

Ruth Perez, MS, MLS(ASCP)
Program Director, Medical Laboratory
 Science
Clinical Laboratory and Medical Imaging
 Sciences
School of Health Professions
Rutgers University
Newark, New Jersey

Tim R. Randolph, PhD, MLS(ASCP)
Professor, Clinical Health Sciences
Doisy College of Health Sciences
Saint Louis University
St. Louis, Missouri

Mark A. Russell, MD
Hematopathology Fellow, Pathology and
 Laboratory Medicine
Loyola University Medical Center
Maywood, Illinois

Kathleen M. Sakamoto, MD, PhD
Professor, Pediatrics
Stanford University
Stanford, California

Mayukh Kanti Sarkar, PhD, MLS(ASCP)
Project Manager, Regulatory Affairs –
 Hemostasis
Sysmex America Inc.
Lincolnshire, Illinois

Natasha Marie Savage, MD
Associate Professor, Pathology
Medical College of Georgia at Augusta
 University
Augusta, Georgia

Gail H. Vance, MD
Sutphin Professor of Cancer Genetics,
 Medical and Molecular Genetics
Professor, Pathology and Laboratory
 Medicine
Indiana University School of Medicine
Indianapolis, Indiana

Carolina Vilchez, MS, MLS(ASCP)H
Clinical Educator, William O. Green, Jr. M.D.
 Medical Laboratory Science Program
The Valley Hospital
Ridgewood, New Jersey

Jeanine M. Walenga, PhD, MLS(ASCP)H^{CM}
Professor, Thoracic-Cardiovascular Surgery,
 Pathology, and Physiology
Co-Director, Hemostasis and Thrombosis
 Research Unit
Stritch School of Medicine
Loyola University Chicago
Laboratory Director, Clinical Coagulation,
 Urinalysis and Medical Microscopy
Associate Director, Point of Care & Referred
 Testing
Pathology and Laboratory Medicine
Loyola University Health System
Maywood, Illinois

PREFACE

The science of *clinical laboratory hematology* involves the analysis of normal and pathologic peripheral blood cells, hematopoietic (blood-producing) tissue, and hematopoietic cells in nonvascular body cavities such as cerebrospinal and serous fluids. Laboratory hematology also includes the analysis of the cells and coagulation proteins essential to clinical hemostasis. Hematology laboratory assay results are critical for diagnosis, prognosis, and monitoring treatment of primary and secondary hematologic and hemostatic disorders. Similarly, hematology and hemostasis test results are used to establish safety in the perioperative period, monitor treatments during surgical procedures, and monitor transfusion needs in trauma patients.

Rodak's Hematology: Clinical Principles and Applications systematically presents basic to advanced concepts to provide a solid foundation of healthy and pathologic states upon which readers can develop their skills in interpreting and correlating laboratory findings in anemias, hematologic malignancies, benign leukocyte disorders, and hemorrhagic and thrombotic conditions. It provides key features for accurate identification of normal and pathologic cells in blood, bone marrow, and body fluids. The focus, level, and detail of hematology, hematopathology, and hemostasis procedures, including their sources of error, along with the related clinical applications, interpretations, and testing algorithms are a highlight of this text.

The current practice of clinical laboratory hematology has been enhanced by profound changes as reflected in the numerous updates in the seventh edition of *Rodak's Hematology: Clinical Principles and Applications*. The seventh edition includes many improvements in the figures, tables, and boxes; significant updating of all chapters to include state-of-the-art content; major revisions in the chapters on automated blood cell analysis, acute leukemias, and hematology and hemostasis in selected populations (the last-mentioned including a new section on transgender populations); addition of a new chapter on patient safety; and addition of the thromboinflammatory reaction induced by COVID-19. Further, Michelle Montgomery Butina and Kamran M. Mirza are new coeditors, joining continuing editors, Elaine M. Keohane and Jeanine M. Walenga. Meticulous editing and attention to overall presentation of the material in the book add to the value of the seventh edition. Chapter highlights and new content are described below.

ORGANIZATION

Rodak's Hematology: Clinical Principles and Applications, seventh edition, is organized into 7 parts, 43 printed chapters, 4 e-chapters, and reference intervals for common laboratory assays conveniently located after the Index at the end of the book. Expanded appendices can be downloaded from the Evolve website allowing for easy access and searches of key abbreviations, formulas, glossary terms, and answers to case studies and review questions.

PART I: INTRODUCTION TO HEMATOLOGY

Chapter 1 previews the science of clinical laboratory hematology. Chapter 2 is new to the seventh edition and provides an overview of patient safety in hematology and hemostasis to ensure that the total testing process is safe, timely, efficient, equitable, patient centered, and effective. Chapter 3 provides comprehensive, updated coverage of quality assurance for laboratory testing, with enhanced sections on method evaluation, assay validation, multisite validation, and system-wide comparability.

PART II: BLOOD CELL PRODUCTION, STRUCTURE, AND FUNCTION

Chapters 4 and 5 include photomicrographs and figures to describe general cell structure and an updated section on selected cell processes, along with the morphologic and molecular details of hematopoiesis. Chapters 6, 10, and 11 discuss erythropoiesis, leukopoiesis, and megakaryopoiesis using numerous photomicrographs to demonstrate ultrastructure and microscopic morphology. Chapters 7 and 8 examine mature red blood cell metabolism, membrane and hemoglobin structure and function, and red blood cell senescence and destruction. Discussion of iron kinetics and laboratory assessment in Chapter 9 has been updated with new figures and coverage of systemic and cellular regulation of iron. Chapter 11 also includes a description of the function of platelets, detailing the primary hemostatic mechanisms of platelet adhesion, aggregation, and activation with updated information on the platelet proteome and the role of platelets in the inflammatory response.

PART III: LABORATORY EVALUATION OF BLOOD CELLS

Chapter 12 describes traditional (manual) clinical hematology laboratory procedures such as microscopy-based cell counts and hemoglobin and hematocrit determinations as well as point-of-care technology. Chapter 13 includes updated descriptions, principles of operation, and figures of the major, state-of-the-art automated blood cell analyzers. It also describes new analyzer parameters and their clinical use. The digital data management capabilities of these analyzers have revolutionized the way blood specimens for the complete blood count, differential count, and morphology assessment are analyzed and how test results are reported and interpreted. Chapter 14 describes peripheral blood film examination and the differential cell count correlation to the complete blood count. Chapter 15 follows up with bone marrow aspirate and biopsy collection, preparation, examination, and reporting.

PART IV: ERYTHROCYTE DISORDERS

Chapter 16 provides an overview of the anemias and describes cost-effective diagnostic approaches that integrate patient history, physical examination, and symptoms, with laboratory results for hemoglobin, red blood cell indices, reticulocyte count, and abnormal red blood cell morphology. Chapters 17 to 19 describe disorders of iron and DNA metabolism and bone marrow failure. Algorithms help the reader to distinguish types of microcytic and macrocytic anemias. Chapters 20 to 23 discuss hemolytic anemias due to intrinsic or extrinsic defects. Chapter 20 also includes detailed figures that explain extravascular and intravascular hemolysis and hemoglobin catabolism. Chapters 24 and 25 provide updates in pathophysiology, diagnosis, and treatment of the hemoglobinopathies and thalassemias, including the use of Clustered Regularly Interspaced Short Palindromic Repeats (CRISPR) technology.

PART V: LEUKOCYTE DISORDERS

The chapters in this section begin with nonmalignant disorders, followed by an introduction to hematologic neoplasms, three chapters discussing diagnostic methodologies, and finally chapters discussing the major categories of hematologic neoplasms.

Chapter 26 is updated with many excellent photomicrographs and summary boxes of nonmalignant leukocyte disorders manifested by the abnormal distribution or morphology of white blood cells. These include bacterial and viral infections, various systemic disorders, and benign lymphoproliferative disorders. Chapter 27 provides an introduction to hematologic neoplasms, including sections on classification, molecular pathogenesis, and general categories of treatment options. Chapter 28 describes flow cytometry and its diagnostic applications, including numerous scatterplots of normal and leukemic conditions. Chapter 29 covers molecular diagnostics, with many figures on basic molecular biology, real-time polymerase chain reaction (PCR), microarrays, and DNA sequencing, including next-generation sequencing. Molecular diagnosis has augmented or in many instances replaced long-indispensable laboratory assays. Chapter 30 provides details on traditional cytogenetic procedures for detection of quantitative and qualitative chromosome abnormalities and more sensitive methods such as fluorescence in situ hybridization (FISH) and genomic hybridization arrays. Chapters 31 to 34, with significant updating according to the 2022 World Health Organization classification, provide the latest pathophysiologic models for acute lymphoblastic and myeloid leukemias and myeloproliferative, myelodysplastic, and mature lymphoid neoplasms, with numerous full-color photomicrographs and illustrations. The chapters discuss traditional monitoring of leukemias and lymphomas at the cellular level; detection of minimal residual disease at the molecular level; and new targeted molecular, immunologic, and cellular therapies, which have dramatically improved survival.

PART VI: HEMOSTASIS AND THROMBOSIS

The chapters of this section begin with the mechanisms of normal hemostasis followed by the hemorrhagic disorders, thrombotic disorders, and anticoagulant therapies. Disorder-specific laboratory testing accompanies the clinical discussion of the disorder in each chapter. Routine coagulation tests and instrumentation are discussed in the chapters at the end of this section.

Chapter 35 describes in detail the plasma- and cell-based coagulation models including the interactions between primary hemostasis, secondary hemostasis, and fibrinolysis. Chapters 36 to 38 detail the hemorrhagic disorders including the diagnosis, management, and current therapies of acquired coagulopathies such as the acute coagulopathy of trauma and shock and inherited coagulopathies such as the hemophilias with a significant update on von Willebrand disease. Two chapters are devoted to quantitative and qualitative platelet defects as the cause of bleeding, with new and revised tables and figures. Chapter 39 describes the known mechanisms associated with venous thrombosis, pulmonary embolism, and arterial thrombosis. Detailed discussions of antiphopsholipid syndrome, disseminated intravascular coagulation, and heparin-induced thrombocytopenia, with its related vaccine-induced thrombocytopenia-thrombosis, are also provided. Thrombosis management in terms of prophylaxis and treatment, with current updates, is discussed in Chapter 40. The classical anticoagulants warfarin, heparin, and low-molecular-weight heparins are covered, along with new intravenous and oral thrombin and factor Xa inhibitor anticoagulants. Methods for monitoring each anticoagulant as used in various clinical settings as well as methods for monitoring the different classes of antiplatelet drugs are provided. Chapter 41 details coagulation specimen collection and handling and covers the traditional coagulation laboratory assays that assess platelet function, coagulation factors, and fibrinolytic parameters, including clot-based and chromogenic assays. Updates for new thrombin generation and viscoelastometry (VET) tests are included. Chapter 42 reviews the latest coagulation analyzers and point-of-care instrumentation for coagulation testing.

PART VII: HEMATOLOGY AND HEMOSTASIS IN SELECTED POPULATIONS

Chapter 43 underwent a major revision and provides valuable information on the hematology and hemostasis laboratory findings in the pediatric, pregnant, and geriatric populations as well as a new section on transgender populations, all correlated with information from previous chapters.

E-CHAPTERS

Four chapters that round out the details of good laboratory practice particular to hematology and hemostasis testing are provided in an online format. Chapter E1 provides the laboratory safety requirements to maintain a safe working environment to prevent accidents and mitigate exposure to biological, chemical, electrical, and fire hazards. Chapter E2 describes the most up-to-date requirements for blood specimen collection from venipuncture and skin puncture. Chapter E3 describes the principles, care, and use of microscopes, including light, phase contrast, polarized light, darkfield, and fluorescent microscopy. Chapter E4 describes methods for analyzing normal and pathologic cells of cerebrospinal fluid, joint fluid, transudates, and exudates.

READERS

Rodak's Hematology: Clinical Principles and Applications is designed for medical laboratory scientists, medical laboratory technicians, and students and faculty of undergraduate and graduate educational programs in the clinical laboratory sciences and pathology. This text is also a helpful study guide for pathology and hematology-oncology residents and fellows and a valuable shelf reference for hematologists, pathologists, and hematology and hemostasis laboratory managers.

TEXTBOOK FEATURES

The outstanding value and quality of *Rodak's Hematology: Clinical Principles and Applications* reflect the educational and clinical expertise of its current and previous editors and authors who are each well known nationally, experienced, and respected in their field of expertise. The text is enhanced by nearly 700 full-color digital photomicrographs, figures, and line art. Detailed text boxes and tables clearly summarize important information. Reference intervals for common hematology, body fluid, and hemostasis laboratory assays are conveniently located after the Index at the end of the book.

Each chapter contains the following for enhanced pedagogical features:

- **Learning objectives** at all taxonomy levels in the cognitive domain
- One or two **case studies**, with open-ended discussion questions at the beginning of the chapter that stimulate interest and provide opportunities for application of chapter content in real-life scenarios
- A bulleted **summary** at the end of each chapter that provides a comprehensive review of essential material
- **Review questions** at the end of each chapter that correlate to chapter objectives and are in the multiple-choice format used by certification examinations

The Evolve website has multiple features **for the instructor**:

- A **test bank** that contains multiple-choice questions with rationales and cognitive levels
- **Instructor's manuals** for every chapter that contain key terms, objectives, outlines, and study questions
- **Learning objectives with taxonomy levels** to supplement lesson plans
- **Case studies** that have been updated and feature discussion questions and photomicrographs when applicable

- **PowerPoint presentations** for every chapter that can be used "as is" or as a template to prepare lectures
- An **image collection** that provides electronic files of all the chapter figures that can be downloaded into PowerPoint presentations

The Evolve website has important features for **the student and instructor**:

- **E-Chapters** on safety in the hematology laboratory, blood specimen collection, care and use of the microscope, and body fluid analysis
- **Appendices** that include an updated list of major abbreviations, commonly used formulas, answers to case studies and review questions, and an expanded glossary
- **Animations**

ACKNOWLEDGMENTS

The editors express their immense gratitude to Bernadette ("Bunny") Rodak, who laid the foundation for *Rodak's Hematology: Clinical Principles and Applications* with her expert writing, editing, detailed figures, and especially her contribution of almost 300 outstanding digital photomicrographs. Now in its seventh edition, we are honored to continue her work on this exceptional textbook. We sincerely thank George A. Fritsma for his significant contribution to this text as a coeditor in two editions and author of 10 chapters in previous editions, for coauthoring five chapters in the seventh edition, for sharing his immense expertise in hemostasis, and for his constant support and encouragement. We thank Kathryn Doig for her contributions as coeditor for the third edition and author of seven chapters in previous editions and for her tenaciousness, creativity, and care in updating three chapters coauthored in the seventh edition. We thank Larry J. Smith for his expertise and diligence as coeditor of the fifth edition and for authoring a chapter in previous editions. We thank Catherine N. Otto for her expertise and diligence as coeditor of the sixth edition and author of two chapters in previous editions, and authoring three chapters in the seventh edition. The editors also thank the many authors who have made and continue to make significant contributions to this work. All of these outstanding professionals have generously shared their time and expertise to make *Rodak's Hematology: Clinical Principles and Applications* into a worldwide educational resource and premier reference textbook for medical laboratory scientists and technicians as well as pathology and hematology practitioners, residents, and fellows.

We also express our appreciation to Elsevier, especially Sarah Vora, Rachel McMullen, and Kelly Skelton, whose professional support and reminders kept the project on track.

Finally, and with the utmost gratitude, we acknowledge our families, friends, and professional colleagues who have supported and encouraged us through this project.

Elaine M. Keohane
Michelle Montgomery Butina
Kamran M. Mirza
Jeanine M. Walenga

CONTENTS

PART I Introduction to Hematology

1 An Overview of Clinical Laboratory Hematology, 1
Elaine M. Keohane

2 Patient Safety in Hematology and Hemostasis, 8
Catherine N. Otto and Karen Golemboski

3 Quality Assurance in Hematology and Hemostasis Testing, 18
Mayukh Kanti Sarkar and George A. Fritsma

PART II Blood Cell Production, Structure, and Function

4 Cell Structure and Function, 43
Elaine M. Keohane

5 Hematopoiesis, 59
Kamran M. Mirza

6 Erythrocyte Production and Destruction, 78
Michelle Montgomery Butina

7 Erythrocyte Metabolism and Membrane Structure and Function, 95
S. Renee Hodgkins

8 Hemoglobin Metabolism, 109
Catherine N. Otto

9 Iron Kinetics and Laboratory Assessment, 122
Kathryn Doig and Yukari Nishizawa-Brennen

10 Leukocyte Development, Kinetics, and Functions, 139
Mark A. Russell and Ameet R. Kini

11 Platelet Production, Structure, and Function, 159
Walter P. Jeske

PART III Laboratory Evaluation of Blood Cells

12 Manual, Semiautomated, and Point-of-Care Testing in Hematology, 178
Karen S. Clark and Teresa G. Hippel

13 Automated Blood Cell Analysis, 198
Elaine M. Keohane

14 Examination of the Peripheral Blood Film and Correlation with the Complete Blood Count, 225
Carolina Vilchez

15 Bone Marrow Examination, 244
Kamran M. Mirza

PART IV Erythrocyte Disorders

16 Anemias: Red Blood Cell Morphology and Approach to Diagnosis, 262
Naveen Manchanda

17 Disorders of Iron Kinetics and Heme Metabolism, 275
Tara Cothran Moon and Kathryn Doig

18 Anemias Caused by Defects of DNA Metabolism, 296
Tara Cothran Moon

19 Bone Marrow Failure, 313
Clara Lo, Bertil Glader, and Kathleen M. Sakamoto

20 Introduction to Increased Destruction of Erythrocytes, 330
Kathryn Doig and Susan A. McQuiston

21 Intrinsic Defects Leading to Increased Erythrocyte Destruction, 352
S. Renee Hodgkins

22 Extrinsic Defects Leading to Increased Erythrocyte Destruction—Nonimmune Causes, 379
Catherine N. Otto

23 Extrinsic Defects Leading to Increased Erythrocyte Destruction—Immune Causes, 392
Ruth Perez

24 Hemoglobinopathies (Structural Defects in Hemoglobin), 408
Tim R. Randolph

25 Thalassemias, 440
S. Renee Hodgkins

PART V Leukocyte Disorders

26 Nonmalignant Leukocyte Disorders, 464
Steven Marionneaux

27 Introduction to Hematologic Neoplasms, 489
Constantine E. Kanakis and Kamran M. Mirza

28 Flow Cytometric Analysis in Hematologic Disorders, 500
Magdalena Czader

29 Molecular Diagnostics in Hematopathology, 519
Cynthia L. Jackson and Shashi Mehta

30 Cytogenetics, 550
Gail H. Vance

31 Acute Leukemias, 566
Mark A. Russell and Ameet R. Kini

32 Myeloproliferative Neoplasms, 583
Tim R. Randolph

33 Myelodysplastic Neoplasms, 618
Nicholas C. Brehl

34 Mature Lymphoid Neoplasms, 634
Steven Marionneaux and Peter Maslak

PART VI Hemostasis and Thrombosis

35 Normal Hemostasis, 661
Jeanine M. Walenga and Kristen N. Krum

36 Hemorrhagic Disorders and Laboratory Assessment, 686
Mayukh Kanti Sarkar and George A. Fritsma

37 Qualitative Disorders of Platelets and Vasculature, 713
Walter P. Jeske and Phillip J. DeChristopher

38 **Quantitative Disorders of Platelets: Thrombocytopenia and Thrombocytosis,** 734

Phillip J. DeChristopher and Walter P. Jeske

39 **Thrombotic Disorders and Laboratory Assessment,** 761

Mayukh Kanti Sarkar, George A. Fritsma, and Jeanine M. Walenga

40 **Antithrombotic Therapies and Laboratory Assessment,** 789

Mayukh Kanti Sarkar and George A. Fritsma

41 **Laboratory Evaluation of Hemostasis,** 811

Mayukh Kanti Sarkar and George A. Fritsma

42 **Hemostasis and Coagulation Instrumentation,** 841

Debra A. Hoppensteadt

PART VII Hematology and Hemostasis in Selected Populations

43 **Hematology and Hemostasis in the Pediatric, Pregnant, Geriatric, and Transgender Populations,** 862

Brandy Gunsolus and Natasha Marie Savage

Hematology/Body Fluids/Hemostasis Reference Intervals, 912

ECHAPTERS (EVOLVE)

E1 **Safety in the Hematology Laboratory**

Kathryn E. Golab

E2 **Blood Specimen Collection**

Stephanie B. Cochrane

E3 **Care and Use of the Microscope**

Elaine M. Keohane

E4 **Body Fluid Analysis in the Hematology Laboratory**

Michelle Montgomery Butina

APPENDICES (EVOLVE)

Appendix A: Abbreviations
Appendix B: List of Formulas
Appendix C: Answers
Appendix D: Glossary

An Overview of Clinical Laboratory Hematology

*Elaine M. Keohane**

OUTLINE

History
Red Blood Cells
   Hemoglobin, Hematocrit, and Red Blood Cell Indices
   Reticulocytes
White Blood Cells
Platelets
Complete Blood Count

Blood Film Examination
Endothelial Cells
Coagulation
Advanced Hematology Procedures
Additional Hematology Procedures
Quality Assurance and Quality Control
Safety

The average human possesses 5 liters of blood. Blood transports oxygen from lungs to tissues; clears tissues of carbon dioxide; transports glucose, proteins, and lipids; and moves wastes to the liver and kidneys. The liquid portion is plasma, which, among many components, provides coagulation enzymes that protect vessels from trauma and maintain the circulation.

Plasma transports and nourishes blood cells. There are three categories of blood cells: red blood cells (RBCs), or *erythrocytes*; white blood cells (WBCs), or *leukocytes*; and platelets (PLTs), or *thrombocytes*.[1] Hematology is the study of these blood cells. By expertly staining, counting, analyzing, and recording the appearance, phenotype, and genotype of all three types of cells, the medical laboratory professional is able to predict, detect, and diagnose blood diseases and many systemic diseases that affect blood cells. Physicians rely on hematology laboratory test results to select and monitor therapy for these disorders; consequently, a complete blood count (CBC) is ordered on nearly everyone who visits a provider or is admitted to a hospital.

HISTORY

The first scientists, such as Athanasius Kircher in 1657, described "worms" in the blood, and Anton van Leeuwenhoek in 1674 gave an account of RBCs,[2] but it was not until the late 1800s that Giulio Bizzozero described platelets as "petite plaques."[3] The development of the Wright stain by James Homer Wright in 1902 opened a new world of visual blood film examination through the microscope. Although automated analyzers now differentiate and enumerate blood cells, Wright's Romanowsky-type stain (polychromatic, a mixture of acidic and basic dyes), and refinements thereof, remains the foundation of blood cell identification.[4]

In the present-day hematology laboratory, RBC, WBC, and platelet appearance is analyzed through automation or visually using 500× to 1000× light microscopy examination of cells fixed to a glass microscope slide and stained with *Wright* or *Wright-Giemsa stain* (Chapters 4, 13, 14, and E3). The scientific term for cell appearance is *morphology,* which encompasses cell color, size, shape, cytoplasmic inclusions, and nuclear condensation.

RED BLOOD CELLS

RBCs are anucleate, biconcave, discoid cells filled with a reddish protein, hemoglobin, which transports oxygen and carbon dioxide (Chapters 8 and 9). RBCs appear salmon pink and measure 7 to 8 μm in diameter with a zone of pallor that occupies one-third of their center (Figure 1.1A), reflecting their biconcavity (Chapters 6 and 7).

Since before 1900, physicians and medical laboratory professionals counted RBCs in measured volumes to detect anemia or polycythemia. *Anemia* means loss of oxygen-carrying capacity and is often reflected in a reduced RBC count or decreased RBC hemoglobin concentration (Chapters 16–25). *Polycythemia* means an increased RBC count reflecting increased circulating RBC mass, a condition that leads to hyperviscosity (Chapter 32).

---

*The author extends appreciation to George A. Fritsma, whose work in prior editions provided the foundation for this chapter.

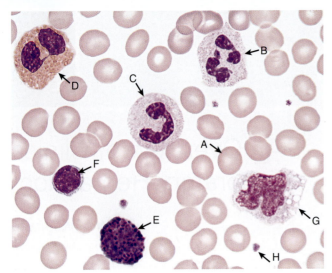

Figure 1.1 Composite of Cells Found in Peripheral Blood of Healthy Individuals. Erythrocyte (red blood cell, RBC) *(A)*; neutrophil (segmented neutrophil, NEUT, SEG, polymorphonuclear neutrophil, PMN) *(B)*; band (band neutrophil, BAND) *(C)*; eosinophil (EO) *(D)*; basophil (BASO) *(E)*; lymphocyte (LYMPH) *(F)*; monocyte (MONO) *(G)*; platelet (PLT) *(H)*. (Wright-Giemsa stain, ×1000.)

Historically, microscopists counted RBCs by carefully pipetting a tiny aliquot of whole blood and mixing it with 0.85% (normal) saline. Normal saline matches the osmolality of blood; consequently, the suspended RBCs retained their intrinsic morphology, neither swelling nor shrinking. A 1:200 dilution was typical for RBC counts, and a glass pipette designed to provide this dilution, the Thoma pipette, was used routinely until the advent of automation.

The diluted blood was transferred to a glass counting chamber called a hemacytometer (Figure 12.1). The microscopist observed and counted RBCs in selected areas of the hemacytometer, applied a mathematical formula based on the dilution and on the area of the hemacytometer counted (Chapter 12), and reported the RBC count in cells per microliter (μL, mcL; also called *cubic millimeter* [mm³]), milliliter (mL; also called *cubic centimeter* [cc]), or liter (L).

Visual RBC counting was developed before 1900 and, although inaccurate, was the only way to count RBCs until the late 1950s, when automated particle counters became available in the clinical laboratory. The first electronic counter was patented in 1953 by Joseph and Wallace Coulter of Chicago, Illinois,[5] and today many high-quality automated blood cell analyzers exist using multiple complex technologies (Chapter 13). However, the Coulter principle of direct current electrical impedance is still used to count RBCs in many modern analyzers. Fortunately, the widespread availability of automated cell analysis has replaced visual RBC counting, although visual counting skills remain useful where automated analyzers are unavailable.

Hemoglobin, Hematocrit, and Red Blood Cell Indices

RBCs also are assayed for hemoglobin (HGB) concentration and hematocrit (HCT) (Chapter 12). Hemoglobin measurement relies on a weak solution of potassium cyanide and potassium ferricyanide (historically known as *Drabkin reagent)*. An aliquot of whole blood is mixed with a measured volume of reagent, hemoglobin is converted to stable *cyanmethemoglobin* (hemiglobincyanide), and the absorbance or color intensity of the solution is measured in a spectrophotometer at 540 nm wavelength.[6] The color intensity is compared with that of a known standard and is mathematically converted to hemoglobin concentration. Modifications of the cyanmethemoglobin method are used in most automated applications, although some automated blood cell analyzers replace it with a formulation of the ionic surfactant (detergent) *sodium lauryl sulfate* to reduce environmental cyanide.

Hematocrit is the ratio of the volume of packed RBCs to the volume of whole blood and is manually determined by transferring blood to a plastic tube with a uniform bore, centrifuging, measuring the column of RBCs, and dividing by the total length of the column of RBCs plus plasma.[7] The normal ratio approaches 50%. Hematocrit is also called *packed cell volume* (PCV), the packed cells referring to RBCs. Often one can see a light-colored layer between the RBCs and plasma. This is the *buffy coat* and contains WBCs and platelets, and it is excluded from the hematocrit determination. The medical laboratory professional may use the three numerical results, RBC count, HGB, and HCT, to compute the RBC indices *mean cell volume* (MCV), *mean cell hemoglobin* (MCH), and *mean cell hemoglobin concentration* (MCHC) (Chapter 12). The MCV, although a volume measurement recorded in femtoliters (fL), reflects RBC diameter on a Wright-stained blood film. The MCHC, expressed in grams per deciliter (g/dL), reflects RBC staining intensity and amount of central pallor. The MCH in picograms (pg) expresses the mass of hemoglobin per cell and parallels the MCHC. A fourth RBC index, *red cell distribution width* (RDW), expresses the degree of *variation* in RBC volume. Extreme RBC volume variability is visible on the Wright-stained blood film as variation in diameter and is called *anisocytosis*. The RDW is based on the standard deviation of RBC volume and is routinely reported by automated blood cell analyzers (Chapter 13). In addition to aiding in diagnosis of anemia, RBC indices provide stable measurements for internal quality control of automated blood cell analyzers (Chapter 3). Sample reference intervals for RBC parameters can be found after the Index at the end of the book; these vary by age and sex (Chapter 43).

Medical laboratory professionals routinely use light microscopy at 500× or 1000× magnification to visually review RBC morphology, commenting on RBC diameter, color or hemoglobinization, and shape and the presence of cytoplasmic inclusions (Chapters 14 and 16). All these parameters—RBC count, HGB, HCT, indices, and RBC morphology—are employed to detect, diagnose, assess the severity of, and monitor the treatment of anemia, polycythemia, and the numerous systemic conditions that affect RBCs (Chapters 17–25 and Chapter 32). Automated blood cell analyzers are used in nearly all clinical laboratories to generate these data, although visual examination of the Wright-stained blood film is still essential to verify abnormal results.[8]

Reticulocytes

On the Wright-stained blood film, 0.5% to 2.5% of RBCs exceed the 7- to 8-μm average diameter and stain slightly blue-gray. These are *polychromatic (polychromatophilic) erythrocytes,* newly released from the RBC production site: the bone marrow (Chapters 5 and 6). Polychromatic erythrocytes are closely observed because they indicate the ability of the bone marrow to increase RBC production in anemia caused by blood loss or excessive RBC destruction (Chapters 20–24).

Methylene blue dyes, called *nucleic acid stains* or *vital stains,* are used to differentiate and count these young RBCs. Vital (or supravital) stains are dyes absorbed by live cells.[9] Young RBCs contain ribonucleic acid (RNA) and are called *reticulocytes* when the RNA is visualized using vital stains (Chapter 12). Counting reticulocytes visually by microscopy was (and remains) a tedious and imprecise procedure until the development of automated reticulocyte counting by the TOA Corporation (presently Sysmex) in the 1990s. Now all fully automated blood cell analyzers provide a relative reticulocyte percentage, an *absolute reticulocyte count,* and an especially sensitive measure of RBC production, the *immature reticulocyte fraction* (Chapter 13). However, it is still necessary to confirm automated analyzer counts visually from time to time, so medical laboratory professionals must retain this skill.

WHITE BLOOD CELLS

WBCs, or leukocytes, are a loosely related category of cell types dedicated to protecting their host from infection and injury (Chapters 5 and 10). WBCs are transported in the blood from their source, usually bone marrow or lymphoid tissue, to their tissue or body cavity destination. WBCs are so named because they are nearly colorless in an unstained cell suspension.

WBCs may be counted visually using a microscope and hemacytometer (Chapter 12). The technique is the same as RBC counting, but the typical dilution is 1:20, and the diluent is a dilute acid solution. The acid causes RBCs to *lyse* or rupture; without it, RBCs, which are 500 to 1000 times more numerous than WBCs, would obscure the WBCs. The WBC count reference intervals can be found after the Index at the end of the book. Visual WBC counting has been largely replaced by automated blood cell analyzers, but it is accurate and useful in situations in which no automation is available. Medical laboratory professionals who analyze body fluids such as cerebrospinal fluid or pleural fluid may employ visual WBC counting (Chapter E4).

A decreased WBC count is called *leukopenia,* and an increased WBC count is called *leukocytosis,* but the WBC count alone has modest clinical value. The microscopist must differentiate the categories of WBCs in the blood by using a Wright-stained blood film and light microscopy (Chapters 10 and 14). The types of WBCs found in peripheral blood in healthy individuals are as follows:

- Neutrophils (NEUTs, segmented neutrophils [SEGs], polymorphonuclear neutrophils [PMNs]) (Figure 1.1B). Neutrophils are phagocytic cells whose major purpose is to engulf and destroy microorganisms and foreign material,

either directly or after they have been labeled for destruction by the immune system. The term *segmented* refers to their multilobed nuclei. The cytoplasm of neutrophils contains pink- or lavender-staining granules filled with bactericidal substances. An increase in neutrophils is called *neutrophilia* and often signals bacterial infection. A decrease is called *neutropenia* and has many causes, but it is often caused by certain medications or viral infections.

- Bands (BANDS, band neutrophils) (Figure 1.1C). Bands are slightly less mature neutrophils with a nonsegmented nucleus in a U or S shape. An increase in bands also signals bacterial infection and is customarily called a *left shift.*
- Eosinophils (EOs) (Figure 1.1D). Eosinophils are cells with round, bright orange-red cytoplasmic granules filled with proteins involved in immune system regulation. An elevated eosinophil count is called *eosinophilia* and often signals a response to allergy or parasitic infection.
- Basophils (BASOs) (Figure 1.1E). Basophils are cells with dark purple, irregular cytoplasmic granules that obscure the nucleus. The basophil granules contain histamines and various other proteins. An elevated basophil count is called *basophilia.* Basophilia is rare and often signals a hematologic disease.

  The distribution of eosinophils and basophils in blood is so small compared with that of neutrophils that the terms *eosinopenia* and *basopenia* are theoretical and not used. Neutrophils, bands, eosinophils, and basophils are collectively called *granulocytes* because of their prominent cytoplasmic granules, although their functions differ.
- Lymphocytes (LYMPHs) (Figure 1.1F). Lymphocytes comprise a complex system of cells that provide for host immunity. Lymphocytes recognize foreign antigens and mount *humoral* (antibody) and *cell-mediated* immune responses. On the Wright-stained blood film, most lymphocytes are nearly round, are slightly larger than RBCs, and have a round, condensed nucleus and a thin rim of nongranular cytoplasm. An increase in the lymphocyte count is called *lymphocytosis* and often is associated with viral infections. Reactive lymphocytes with characteristic morphology often accompany lymphocytosis (Chapter 26). An abnormally low lymphocyte count is called *lymphopenia* or *lymphocytopenia* and is often associated with drug therapy or immunodeficiency.
- Monocytes (MONOs) (Figure 1.1G). Monocytes are immature *macrophages* passing through the blood from their point of origin, usually the bone marrow, to a targeted tissue location. Macrophages are the most abundant cell type in the body, although monocytes comprise a minor component of peripheral blood WBCs. Macrophages occupy every body cavity; some are motile and some are immobilized. Their tasks are to identify and *phagocytize* (engulf and consume) foreign particles and assist the lymphocytes in mounting an immune response through the assembly and presentation of antigen *epitopes.* On the Wright-stained blood film, monocytes have a slightly larger diameter than other WBCs, blue-gray cytoplasm with fine azure granules, and a nucleus that is usually indented or folded. An increase in the number of

monocytes is called *monocytosis*. Benign monocytosis may be found in certain infections or in inflammation (Chapter 26). Medical laboratory professionals seldom document a decreased monocyte count, so the theoretical term *monocytopenia* is seldom used.

Leukemia is an uncontrolled proliferation of a clone of malignant WBCs. Leukemia may be chronic, for example, chronic myeloid leukemia or chronic lymphocytic leukemia, or acute, for example, acute myeloid leukemia or acute lymphoblastic leukemia (Chapter 27 and Chapters 31–34). Leukemias may involve any of the cell lines and are categorized by their respective immunophenotypes and genetic aberrations (Chapters 28–30). Some leukemias are more common in a specific age group; chronic lymphocytic leukemia is more prevalent in people older than 65 years, whereas acute lymphoblastic leukemia is the most common form of childhood leukemia (Chapters 31 and 34). Medical laboratory scientists participate in characterization of leukemias using Wright-stained bone marrow smears, flow cytometric immunophenotyping, molecular diagnostic technology, cytogenetics, and, occasionally, cytochemical staining (Chapter 15 and Chapters 28–30).

PLATELETS

Platelets, or thrombocytes, are true blood cells that maintain blood vessel integrity by initiating vessel wall repairs (Chapter 11). Platelets rapidly adhere to the surfaces of damaged blood vessels and form aggregates with neighboring platelets to plug the hole in the damaged vessels. Platelets are the major cells that control *hemostasis*, a series of cellular and plasma-based mechanisms that seal wounds, repair vessel walls, and maintain vascular patency (unimpeded blood flow) (Chapter 35). Platelets are only 2 to 4 μm in diameter, round or oval, anucleate, and slightly granular (Figure 1.1H). Their small size makes them appear insignificant, but they are essential to life and are extensively studied for their complex physiology. Uncontrolled platelet and hemostatic activation is responsible for deep vein thrombosis, pulmonary emboli, acute myocardial infarctions (heart attacks), cerebrovascular accidents (strokes), peripheral artery disease, and repeated spontaneous abortions (miscarriages) (Chapter 39).

The microscopist counts platelets employing the same technique used in counting WBCs on a hemacytometer, although a different counting area, diluent, and dilution are usually used (Chapter 12). Owing to their small volume, platelets are hard to distinguish visually in a hemacytometer, and phase microscopy provides for easier identification. Automated blood cell analyzers have largely replaced visual platelet counting and provide greater accuracy (Chapter 13). The reference interval for the platelet count can be found after the Index at the end of the book.

One advantage of automated blood cell analyzers is their ability to generate a mean platelet volume (MPV), which is unavailable through visual methods. The presence of predominantly larger platelets generates an elevated MPV value, which sometimes signals a regenerative bone marrow response to platelet consumption (Chapters 11 and 38).

Elevated platelet counts, called *thrombocytosis*, signal inflammation or trauma but convey modest intrinsic significance. *Essential thrombocythemia* is a rare malignant condition characterized by extremely high platelet counts and uncontrolled platelet production. Essential thrombocythemia is a life-threatening hematologic disorder (Chapters 32 and 38).

A low platelet count, called *thrombocytopenia*, is a common consequence of drug treatment and may be life-threatening. Because the platelet is responsible for normal blood vessel maintenance and repair, thrombocytopenia is usually accompanied by easy bruising and uncontrolled hemorrhage (Chapter 38). Thrombocytopenia accounts for many hemorrhage-related emergency department visits. Accurate platelet counting contributes to patient safety because it provides for the diagnosis of thrombocytopenia in many disorders or therapeutic regimens.

COMPLETE BLOOD COUNT

A CBC is performed on automated blood cell analyzers and includes the RBC, WBC, and platelet measurements indicated in Box 1.1. The medical laboratory professional may collect a blood specimen for the CBC, but a phlebotomist, nurse, physician assistant, physician, or patient care technician may also collect the specimen (Chapters 12, 41, and E2). No matter who collects a blood specimen, the medical laboratory professional is responsible for the integrity of the specimen and ensures that it is submitted in the appropriate anticoagulant and tube and is free of clots and hemolysis (red-tinted plasma indicating RBC damage). The specimen must be of sufficient volume because "short draws" result in incorrect anticoagulant-to-blood ratios. The specimen must be tested or prepared for storage within the appropriate time frame to ensure accurate analysis (Chapter 3) and must be accurately registered in the work list, a process known as specimen *accession*. Accession may be automated, relying on bar code or radiofrequency identification technology, thus reducing instances of identification error.

BOX 1.1 Basic Complete Blood Count Measurements Generated by Automated Blood Cell Analyzers

RBC Parameters	WBC Parameters
RBC count	WBC count
HGB	NEUT count: % and absolute
HCT	LYMPH count: % and absolute
MCV	MONO count: % and absolute
MCH	EO and BASO counts: % and absolute
MCHC	
RDW	**Platelet Parameters**
RETIC count	PLT count
	MPV

BASO, Basophil; *EO*, eosinophil; *HCT*, hematocrit; *HGB*, hemoglobin; *LYMPH*, lymphocyte; *MCH*, mean cell hemoglobin; *MCHC*, mean cell hemoglobin concentration; *MCV*, mean cell volume; *MONO*, monocyte; *MPV*, mean platelet volume; *NEUT*, segmented neutrophil; *PLT*, platelet; *RBC*, red blood cell; *RDW*, red cell distribution width; *RETIC*, reticulocyte; *WBC*, white blood cell.

Although all laboratory scientists and technicians are equipped to perform visual RBC, WBC, and platelet counts using dilution pipettes, hemacytometers, and microscopes, most laboratories employ automated blood cell analyzers to generate the CBC. Many blood cell analyzers also provide comments on RBC, WBC, and platelet morphology (Chapter 13). When one of the results from the blood cell analyzer is abnormal, the instrument provides an indication of this, sometimes called a *flag*. In this case, a reflex *blood film examination* is performed (Chapter 14).

The blood film examination (described next) is a specialized, demanding, and fundamental CBC activity. Nevertheless, if all blood cell analyzer results are within reference intervals, the blood film examination is usually omitted from the CBC. However, providers may request a blood film examination on the basis of clinical suspicion even when the analyzer results fall within their respective reference intervals.

BLOOD FILM EXAMINATION

To complete a blood film examination, the microscopist prepares a "wedge-prep" blood film on a glass microscope slide, allows it to dry, and fixes and stains it using Wright or Wright-Giemsa stain (Chapter 14). The microscopist visually performs an estimate of the WBC count (with the 40× or 50× objective at 400× or 500× magnification) and platelet count (with the 100× oil immersion objective at 1000× magnification) for comparison with their respective analyzer counts and investigates discrepancies. Next, the microscopist systematically reviews, identifies, and tabulates 100 (or more) WBCs to determine their percent distribution. This process is referred to as determining the *WBC differential* ("diff"). The WBC differential relies on the microscopist's skill, visual acuity, and integrity, and it provides extensive diagnostic information. Finally, the microscopist examines the morphology of WBCs, RBCs, and platelets by light microscopy for abnormalities of shape, diameter, color, or inclusions using 1000× magnification. Digital morphology recognition systems such as the CellaVision DM9600 (Chapter 14) automate the WBC, RBC, and platelet morphology assessment and WBC differential processes, but the medical laboratory professional or the hematopathologist is the final arbiter for all cell identification. Results of the CBC, including all automated blood cell analysis and blood film examination parameters and interpretive comments, are provided in paper or digital format for the provider's review, with abnormal results highlighted.

ENDOTHELIAL CELLS

Because they are structural and do not flow in the bloodstream, endothelial cells, the endodermal cells that form the inner surface of the blood vessel, are seldom studied in the hematology laboratory. Nevertheless, endothelial cells are important in maintaining normal blood flow, in tethering (decelerating) platelets during times of injury, and in enabling WBCs to escape from the vessel to the surrounding tissue when needed (Chapter 35). Increasingly refined laboratory methods are becoming available to assay and characterize the secretions of these important cells.

COAGULATION

Most hematology laboratories include a blood coagulation-testing department (Chapters 41 and 42). Platelets are a key component of hemostasis, as previously described; plasma coagulation is the second component (Chapter 35). The coagulation system employs a complex sequence of plasma proteins, some enzymes, and some enzyme cofactors to produce clot formation after blood vessel injury. Another six to eight enzymes exert control over the coagulation mechanism, and a third system of enzymes and cofactors digests clots to restore vessel patency, a process called *fibrinolysis*. Bleeding (Chapters 36–38) and clotting (Chapter 39) disorders are numerous and complex, and the coagulation section of the hematology laboratory provides a series of plasma-based and whole blood laboratory assays that assess these plasma proteins and their interactions with hematologic cells.

The medical laboratory professional focuses especially on blood specimen integrity for the coagulation laboratory because minor blood specimen defects, including clots, hemolysis, lipemia, plasma bilirubin, and short draws, render the specimen useless (Chapter 41). High-volume coagulation tests suited to the acute care facility include the platelet count and MPV as described earlier, *prothrombin time* and *partial thromboplastin time* (or activated partial thromboplastin time), *thrombin time* (or thrombin clotting time), *fibrinogen assay,* and *D-dimer* assay (Chapter 41). The prothrombin time and partial thromboplastin time are particularly high-volume assays used in screening profiles. These tests assess each portion of the coagulation pathway for deficiencies and are used to monitor anticoagulant therapy (Chapter 40). In addition to these high-volume screening assays, moderate-volume assays for specific hemostatic parameters, including clot-based assays, chromogenic substrate assays, and immunoassays, are available in specialized or tertiary care facilities. The specialized or tertiary care coagulation laboratory with its interpretive complexities attracts advanced medical laboratory scientists with specialized knowledge and communication skills.

ADVANCED HEMATOLOGY PROCEDURES

Besides performing the CBC, the hematology laboratory provides *bone marrow examinations, flow cytometry immunophenotyping, cytogenetic analysis,* and *molecular diagnostic assays.* Performing these tests may require advanced preparation or particular dedication by medical laboratory scientists with a desire to specialize.

Medical laboratory scientists assist physicians with bedside *bone marrow* collection, then prepare, stain, and microscopically review bone marrow smears (Chapter 15). Bone marrow *aspirates* and *biopsy specimens* are collected and stained to analyze nucleated cells that are the immature precursors to blood cells (Chapter 5). Cells of the *erythroid* series are precursors to RBCs (Chapter 6); *myeloid* series cells mature to form bands and neutrophils, eosinophils, basophils, and monocytes (Chapter 10); and *megakaryocytes* produce platelets (Chapter 11). Medical laboratory scientists, clinical pathologists, and hematologists review Wright-stained aspirate smears for morphologic abnormalities, high or low bone marrow cell concentration, and inappropriate cell line distributions. For instance, an increase in the erythroid cell line may indicate bone marrow compensation for excessive RBC destruction or blood loss (Chapter 16 and Chapters 20–24). The biopsy specimen, enhanced by *hematoxylin and eosin* (H&E) staining, may reveal abnormalities in bone marrow architecture indicating leukemia, bone marrow failure, or one of a host of additional hematologic disorders. Results of examination of bone marrow aspirates and biopsy specimens are compared with CBC results generated from the peripheral blood to correlate findings and develop pattern-based diagnoses.

In the bone marrow laboratory, cytochemical stains may occasionally be employed to differentiate abnormal myeloid, erythroid, and lymphoid cells. These stains include *myeloperoxidase, Sudan black B, nonspecific and specific esterase, periodic acid-Schiff, tartrate-resistant acid phosphatase,* and *alkaline phosphatase* (Chapters 31 and 32). The cytochemical stains are time-honored tests that in most laboratories have been replaced by flow cytometry immunophenotyping, molecular diagnostic, and cytogenetic techniques (Chapters 28–30). Since 1980, however, *immunostaining* methods have enabled identification of cell lines by detecting lineage-specific antigens on the surface or in the cytoplasm of leukemia and lymphoma cells. An example of immunostaining is a visible dye that is bound to antibodies to CD42b, a membrane protein that is present in the megakaryocytic lineage and may be diagnostic for megakaryoblastic leukemia (Chapter 31).

Flow cytometers may be *quantitative,* such as clinical flow cytometers that have grown from the original Coulter principle, or *qualitative,* including laser-based instruments that have migrated from research applications to the clinical laboratory (Chapters 13 and 28). The former devices are automated clinical blood cell analyzers that generate the quantitative parameters of the CBC through application of electrical impedance and laser or light beam interruption. Qualitative laser-based flow cytometers are mechanically simpler but technically more demanding. Both qualitative and quantitative flow cytometers are employed to analyze cell populations by measuring the effects of individual cells on laser light, such as *forward-angle fluorescent light scatter* and *right-angle fluorescent light scatter,* and by *immunophenotyping* for cell membrane epitopes using monoclonal antibodies labeled with fluorescent dyes. The qualitative flow cytometry laboratory is indispensable to leukemia and lymphoma diagnosis.

Cytogenetics (Chapter 30), a time-honored form of chromosome analysis, examines hematopoietic cells in bone marrow aspirate to identify large numerical or structural abnormalities in chromosomes at the microscopic level of resolution, such as the Philadelphia chromosome, a reciprocal translocation between chromosomes 9 and 22 that is diagnostic in chronic myeloid leukemia, and t(15;17), a translocation between chromosomes 15 and 17 that is diagnostic in acute promyelocytic leukemia. Cytogenomic techniques evaluate whole genome DNA to identify small numerical or structural abnormalities in chromosomes at the submicroscopic level of resolution, such as gains or losses of minute amounts of DNA. Cytogenetic and cytogenomic analysis remains essential to the diagnosis and treatment of leukemia.

Molecular diagnostic techniques (Chapter 29), the fastest-growing area of laboratory medicine, enhance and even replace some of the advanced hematologic methods. Real-time polymerase chain reaction, microarray analysis, fluorescence in situ hybridization, and next-generation DNA sequencing systems are highly sensitive and specific methods that enable medical laboratory scientists to detect various chromosome abnormalities and gene mutations that confirm specific types of leukemia and lymphoma, establish their therapeutic profile and prognosis, and monitor the effectiveness of treatment.

ADDITIONAL HEMATOLOGY PROCEDURES

Medical laboratory professionals provide several time-honored whole blood methods to support hematologic diagnosis. The *glucose-6-phosphate dehydrogenase assay* phenotypically detects an inherited RBC enzyme deficiency causing episodic hemolytic anemia (Chapter 21). The sickle cell solubility screening assay and its follow-up tests, hemoglobin electrophoresis and high-performance liquid chromatography, are used to detect and diagnose sickle cell anemia and other inherited qualitative hemoglobin abnormalities and thalassemias (Chapters 24 and 25). One of the oldest hematology tests, the *erythrocyte sedimentation rate,* detects inflammation and roughly estimates its intensity (Chapter 12).

Finally, the medical laboratory professional reviews the cell counts, distribution, and morphology in body fluids other than blood (Chapter E4). These include cerebrospinal fluid, synovial (joint) fluid, pericardial fluid, pleural fluid, and peritoneal fluid, in which RBCs and WBCs may be present in disease and in which malignant cells that require specialized detection skills may be present. Analysis of nonblood body fluids is always performed with a rapid turnaround because cells in these environments rapidly lose their integrity. The conditions leading to a need for body fluid analysis are invariably acute.

QUALITY ASSURANCE AND QUALITY CONTROL

Medical laboratory professionals employ particularly complex quality control systems in the hematology laboratory (Chapter 3). Because of the unavailability of weighed standards, the measurement of cells and biological systems defies chemical standardization and requires elaborate calibration, validation, matrix effect examination, linearity, and reference interval determinations. An internal standard methodology known as the *moving average* also supports hematology laboratory applications.[10] Medical laboratory professionals in all disciplines compare methods through clinical efficacy calculations that produce clinical sensitivity, specificity, and positive and negative predictive values for each assay. They must monitor specimen integrity and test ordering patterns and ensure the integrity and delivery of reports, including numerical and narrative statements and reference interval comparisons. As in most branches of laboratory science, the hematology laboratory places an enormous responsibility for accuracy, integrity, judgment, and timeliness on the medical laboratory professional.

SAFETY

Safety can be discussed in two contexts—laboratory safety and patient safety. *Laboratory safety* requires all medical laboratory professionals to maintain a safe working environment to prevent accidents and mitigate exposure to biological, chemical, electrical, and fire hazards (Chapter E1). Written safety plans, training programs, emergency management plans, and use of appropriate personal protective equipment (PPE) are critical in maintaining a safe laboratory environment.

Patient safety requires all health care professionals to work with each other and their patients and caregivers to improve the delivery of health care and reduce medical errors (Chapter 2). In 2001 the Institute of Medicine (IOM), now the National Academy of Medicine, specified six aims to improve health care delivery to ensure that it is safe, timely, efficient, equitable, patient-centered, and effective.[11] Further, in 2003 the IOM specified five core competencies for all health care professionals to achieve those aims: provide patient-centered care, work in interdisciplinary teams, employ evidence-based practice, apply quality improvement, and utilize informatics.[12] Medical laboratory professionals play a vital role in collaborating with other health care providers to improve the delivery of laboratory services and ensure that laboratory tests are appropriately ordered, accurately performed in a timely manner, appropriately interpreted by health care providers, and accurately applied to the individual patient in a clear, timely, equitable, and effective manner.

REFERENCES

1. Smock, K. J. (2019). Examination of the blood and bone marrow. In Greer, J. P., Rodgers, G. M., Glader, B., et al. (Eds.), *Wintrobe's Clinical Hematology.* (14th ed., p. 1–16). Philadelphia: Lippincott Williams and Wilkins.
2. Wintrobe, M. M. (1985). *Hematology, the Blossoming of a Science: A Story of Inspiration and Effort.* Philadelphia: Lea & Febiger.
3. Bizzozero, J. (1882). Über einem neuen formbestandtheil des blutes und dessen rolle bei der thrombose und der blutgerinnung. *Virchows Arch Pathol Anat Physiol Klin Med, 90,* 261–332.
4. Woronzoff-Dashkoff, K. K. (2002). The Wright-Giemsa stain. Secrets revealed. *Clin Lab Med, 22,* 15–23.
5. Coulter, W. H. (1956). High speed automatic blood cell counter and cell size analyzer. National Electronics Conference, Chicago; and (1957) *Proc Natl Electron Conf, 12,* 1034–1042.
6. Klungsöyr, L., & Stöa, K. F. (1954). Spectrophotometric determination of hemoglobin oxygen saturation: the method of Drabkin & Schmidt as modified for its use in clinical routine analysis. *Scand J Clin Lab Invest, 6,* 270–276.
7. Mann, L. S. (1948). A rapid method of filling and cleaning Wintrobe hematocrit tubes. *Am J Clin Pathol, 18,* 916.
8. Barth, D. (2012). Approach to peripheral blood film assessment for pathologists. *Semin Diagn Pathol, 29,* 31–48.
9. Biggs, R. (1948). Error in counting reticulocytes. *Nature, 162,* 457.
10. Gulati, G. L., & Hyun, B. H. (1986). Quality control in hematology. *Clin Lab Med, 6,* 675–688.
11. Institute of Medicine. Committee on Quality of Health Care in America. (2001). *Crossing the Quality Chasm: A New Health System for the 21st Century.* Washington, DC: The National Academies Press.
12. Institute of Medicine. (2003). *Health Professions Education: A Bridge to Quality.* Washington, DC: The National Academies Press.

Patient Safety in Hematology and Hemostasis

Catherine N. Otto and Karen Golemboski

OBJECTIVES

After completion of this chapter, the reader will be able to:

1. Define patient safety.
2. Summarize the content of the National Academy of Medicine reports on health care quality.
3. Define each of the six quality aims for patient safety in health care.
4. Give examples of each of the six quality aims in medical laboratory professional practice in hematology and hemostasis.
5. List the five essential competencies for health care professionals.
6. Give examples of use for each of the five health care professional competencies in medical laboratory practice in hematology and hemostasis.

OUTLINE

Definition of Patient Safety
Definition of Health Care Quality
Total Testing Process in the Clinical Laboratory
Six Aims of Health Care Quality
  Safe Hematology and Hemostasis Testing
  Effective Hematology and Hemostasis Testing
  Efficient Hematology and Hemostasis Testing
  Timely Hematology and Hemostasis Testing
  Patient-Centered Hematology and Hemostasis Testing
  Equitable Hematology and Hemostasis Testing
Essential Competencies for Health Care Professionals
  Interprofessional Teamwork
  Evidence-Based Practice and Patient-Centered Care
  Informatics and Quality Improvement Processes

Applications in the Hematology and Hemostasis Laboratory
  Interprofessional Teamwork in the Hematology and Hemostasis Laboratory
  Evidence-Based Practice in the Hematology and Hemostasis Laboratory
  Patient-Centered Care in the Hematology and Hemostasis Laboratory
  Informatics in the Hematology and Hemostasis Laboratory
  Quality Improvement in the Hematology and Hemostasis Laboratory
  How Can Medical Laboratory Professionals Achieve Competency in These Areas?

CASE STUDY

After studying the material in this chapter, the reader should be able to respond to the following case study. Answers can be found in Appendix C.

Several values were flagged on the complete blood count (CBC) as being below the reference interval from a patient identified as L.M. The CBC results were released to the electronic medical record and to the provider who ordered the CBC. After reviewing the test results, the provider called the clinical laboratory to ask why the CBC report did not include reference intervals for transgender individuals who are transitioning or who have completed their transition.

1. Identify which CBC parameters need separate reference intervals for transgender individuals.
2. Explain how this may impact treatment for this patient.
3. Identify the dimensions of patient safety affected in this situation.
4. Describe solutions (recommendations) to improve dimensions of patient safety.

Patient safety and its importance in providing quality health care and improving patient outcomes came to the forefront in 2000 when the Institute of Medicine (a component of the National Academies of Sciences, Engineering, and Medicine) published *To Err Is Human*, reporting that up to 98,000 people die each year as a result of an adverse event while hospitalized.[1] Since 2000 the Institute of Medicine, now referred to as the National Academy of Medicine (NAM), has published multiple reports in their Quality Chasm Series, defining health care quality and its dimensions, identifying competencies for all health care practitioners (including medical laboratory professionals), and providing recommendations for improving diagnoses.[1-3] Although health care delivery systems have adopted quality improvement and other processes to reduce errors in delivery, and health care professional educational programs have incorporated curricula in patient safety competencies, medical errors still occur every day in every delivery setting in the United States.[3] The importance of professionals (medical laboratory professionals) involved in the health care diagnostic process was a key outcome of the 2015 NAM report *Improving Diagnosis in Health Care*.[3] This chapter introduces the reader to critical patient safety concepts needed for effective medical laboratory science practice.

DEFINITION OF PATIENT SAFETY

The term *patient safety* is an all-encompassing term that includes all aspects of delivering health care; it is more than just ensuring that a patient does not fall while in the hospital. Patient safety is defined by the NAM as "freedom from accidental injury: avoidance, prevention, and amelioration of adverse outcomes or injuries stemming from the process of care."[1] Adverse outcomes that may result from the laboratory testing process include false-positive and false-negative test results; missed and delayed diagnoses; or missed, delayed, or inappropriate treatment. Injuries from the laboratory testing process can include hematomas or nerve damage following venipuncture. From a broader perspective, though, patient safety is related to many more aspects of laboratory practice.

DEFINITION OF HEALTH CARE QUALITY

Following *To Err Is Human*, the subsequent NAM report (*Crossing the Quality Chasm*) detailed the gap between the current US health care system and a system delivering ideal health care, suggesting how health care professionals might move "across the chasm" from a flawed system to a high-quality system. This report defines health care quality as "the degree to which health services for individuals and populations increase the likelihood of desired health outcomes and are consistent with current professional knowledge."[2] Based on this definition, the NAM focuses on both *safety* and *quality* in the outcome of health care for the patient. This may seem intuitive in the 21st century; however, until the early 2000s, evaluation of health care quality focused on meeting accreditation standards such as those from The Joint Commission (for health care organizations) and the College of American Pathologists (for clinical laboratories), which placed a significant focus on the analytical phase of the Total Testing Process in the clinical laboratory (detailed in the following section). Medical laboratory professionals have used quality control and proficiency testing to evaluate analytical quality since the middle of the 20th century. With the changing focus on the patient and the outcome of their care, medical laboratory professionals are now obligated to evaluate and improve the quality of the entire testing process.

TOTAL TESTING PROCESS IN THE CLINICAL LABORATORY

The Total Testing Process in the clinical laboratory is a 3-phase, 11-step process (Figure 2.1). The process begins with the *preanalytical* (also called *preexamination*) *phase* that includes a clinical question ("Does the patient have this or that condition?"), followed by identifying the laboratory test to order, and then ordering it.[4] The next step involves collecting the specimen and transporting it to the medical laboratory.[4] The *analytical* (*examination*) *phase* begins with preparing the specimen for analysis, followed by analysis of the specimen, and then verification of the test results.[4] The *postanalytical* (*postexamination*) *phase* begins with reporting the test results to the provider, who then answers the clinical question and takes action that influences patient care.[4] Examples of outcomes of clinical laboratory testing include accurate, inaccurate, delayed, or no diagnosis achieved, or accurate, inaccurate, delayed, or no treatment employed. A key element of the Total Testing Process is the importance of *thinking* by the provider (to order the laboratory test and interpret the results within the context of the patient's symptoms) and the medical laboratory professional (to consult with providers on test selection and test result interpretation), described as the brain-to-brain loop.[5,6]

SIX AIMS OF HEALTH CARE QUALITY

The second report in the NAM Quality Chasm Collection, *Crossing the Quality Chasm*, identified *six aims or dimensions of health care quality*: safe, effective, efficient, timely, patient-centered, and equitable (Table 2.1).[2] These six dimensions of health care quality are important because they apply to all aspects of the health care delivery system, and their definitions identify a standard to measure quality. Each of the quality aims can be applied to medical laboratory professional practice in general and to the hematology and hemostasis laboratory specifically, as will be discussed in this chapter. When medical laboratory professionals focus on patient safety and health care quality goals, patients are more likely to avoid adverse outcomes of health care delivery, including errors in diagnosis; delays in treatment; unnecessary testing; and adverse events, such as death, misdiagnosis, mistreatment, and disability. Patient safety and reducing harm to patients requires attention to all six quality aims.

Safe Hematology and Hemostasis Testing

Safe health care is defined as "avoiding harm to patients from the care that is intended to help them."[2] Adverse events and medical errors are serious events that result in harm to patients and care that is unsafe. Laboratory testing services are not immune to errors or adverse events. One outcome of a delay in test results is a delay in diagnosis that leads to delay in treatment, lack of treatment, impairment, or death. Best practices in medical laboratory patient safety ensure that each patient receives the right test for their condition, at the right time, with accurate test results that provide information for the best outcome.

Errors or defects in the other five dimensions of health care affect safe laboratory testing. Patients incur harm if the wrong laboratory test is ordered, if the venipuncture to collect their blood specimen is performed inaccurately, or if the provider does not accurately interpret the test results or makes an inaccurate diagnosis based on the test results. Patients may incur harm if unnecessary laboratory tests are ordered and performed, laboratory test results are not available in a timely manner to

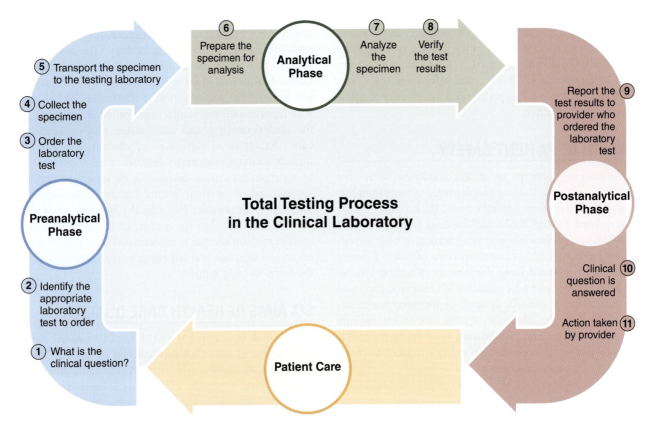

Figure 2.1 **Total Testing Process in the Clinical Laboratory.** Three phases and 11 steps in the Total Testing Process are depicted. The process begins with the preanalytical phase and flows through the analytical and then postanalytical phases to provide patient care. (Modified from Schumacher, G. E., & Barr, J. T. [1998]. Total testing process applied to therapeutic drug monitoring: impact on patient outcomes and economics. *Clin Chem, 44,* 370–374.)

TABLE 2.1	Quality Aims to Evaluate and Improve Patient Safety in Health Care
Quality Aim	**Definition**
Safe	"avoiding injuries to patients from the care that is intended to help them."
Effective	"providing services based on scientific knowledge to all who could benefit and refraining from providing services to those not likely to benefit (avoiding underuse and overuse, respectively)."
Efficient	"avoiding waste, including waste of equipment, supplies, ideas, and energy."
Timely	"reducing waits and sometimes harmful delays for both those who receive care and those who give care."
Patient-centered	"providing care that is respectful and responsive to individual patient preferences, needs, and values and ensuring that patient values guide all clinical decisions."
Equitable	"providing care that does not vary in quality because of personal characteristics such as gender, ethnicity, geographic location, and socioeconomic status."

From Institute of Medicine Committee on Quality of Health Care in America. (2001). *Crossing the Quality Chasm: A New Health System for the 21st Century.* Washington, DC, The National Academy Press, pp. 5–6.

diagnose or treat a condition, the patient's input is not considered, or the patient does not have access to clinical laboratory testing.

In the preanalytical phase of testing, specimens for hematology and hemostasis testing must be appropriately collected from an accurately identified patient (Chapter E2). It is standard practice in all aspects of health care delivery to require two patient identifiers (e.g., first and last name and birth date) before any interaction or procedure, yet specimens are still collected from incorrectly identified patients, and specimens that were collected properly are mislabeled. This can lead directly to patient harm if test results from misidentified specimens are reported using the wrong patient's name.

Defects in specimen integrity (clotted, hemolyzed, incorrect anticoagulant, or insufficient quantity) affect the ability to analyze hematology and hemostasis specimens. Given that hematology and hemostasis tests require anticoagulated whole blood specimens, a clotted specimen cannot be tested, and it must be recollected (Chapters 12 and 41). An unacceptable specimen submitted for analysis is an inefficiency requiring recollection of the specimen at the minimum and no diagnosis or treatment if the specimen is not recollected and analyzed at the worst. Thus

TABLE 2.2 Recommendations From *Choosing Wisely**	
Recommendation	**Source**
"Don't perform repetitive CBC and chemistry testing in the face of clinical and lab stability."	SHM-AHM
"Don't order an erythrocyte sedimentation rate (ESR) to look for inflammation in patients with undiagnosed conditions. Order a C-reactive protein (CRP) to detect acute phase inflammation."	ASCP
"Avoid using hemoglobin to evaluate patients for iron deficiency in susceptible populations. Instead use ferritin."	ASCLS
"Do not order red blood cell folate levels at all. In adults, consider folate supplementation instead of serum folate testing in patients with macrocytic anemia."	ASCP
"Do not perform peripheral blood flow cytometry to screen for hematological malignancy in the settings of mature neutrophilia, basophilia, erythrocytosis, thrombocytosis, isolated anemia, or isolated thrombocytopenia."	ASCP
"Avoid routine prothrombin time (PT) and partial thromboplastin time (PTT, APTT) pre-operative screens on asymptomatic patients, use instead a history-based bleeding assessment test."	ASCLS
"Don't test vitamin K levels unless the patient has an abnormal international normalized ratio (INR) and does not respond to vitamin K therapy."	ASCP
"Don't test or treat for suspected heparin-induced thrombocytopenia (HIT) in patients with a low pre-test probability of HIT."	ASH
"Don't treat patients with immune thrombocytopenic purpura (ITP) in the absence of bleeding or a very low platelet count."	ASH
"Don't order a factor V Leiden (FVL) mutation assay as the initial test to identify a congenital cause for a thrombotic event. First, order a phenotypic activated protein C resistance (APCR) ratio assay."	ASCLS
"Do not test for protein C, protein S, or antithrombin (ATIII) levels during an active clotting event to diagnose a hereditary deficiency because these tests are not analytically accurate during an active clotting event."	ASCP
"Do not order a protein S activity assay for measuring protein S function. Instead order free protein S antigen."	ASCLS

*These tests and their clinical applications are discussed in the chapters of this text.
ASCLS, American Society for Clinical Laboratory Science; *ASCP,* American Society for Clinical Pathology; *ASH,* American Society of Hematology; *CBC,* complete blood count; *SHM-AHM,* Society of Hospital Medicine-Adult Hospital Medicine.
Data from ABIM Foundation: *Choosing Wisely.* https://www.choosingwisely.org/. Accessed October 14, 2022.

it is important to ensure that specimens are recollected for those situations in which the original specimen was inadequate.

Effective Hematology and Hemostasis Testing

Effective health care is defined as "providing services based on scientific knowledge to all who could benefit and refraining from providing services to those not likely to benefit."[2] This means that medical laboratory professionals focus on providing appropriate laboratory tests and limit the use of laboratory tests that are not beneficial to the patient's condition. Effective laboratory testing requires understanding which laboratory tests are appropriate for specific diseases and their sequential use, communicating that information to providers, and incorporating test ordering guidelines into laboratory information systems. Ensuring that laboratory tests are used effectively requires employing evidence-based laboratory medicine and working with other health care professionals to incorporate and use the best laboratory tests for each disease process.

Identifying appropriate use of laboratory testing is a critical component of providing effective laboratory testing services. An example of a program that lists recommendations for both providers and patients is *Choosing Wisely*, sponsored by the American Board of Internal Medicine (ABIM) Foundation and supported by numerous professional organizations (Table 2.2). *Choosing Wisely* publishes peer-reviewed recommendations for testing supported by evidence.[7] Two examples related to hematology and hemostasis submitted by the American Society for Clinical Laboratory Science (ASCLS) recommend ordering a free protein S antigen to measure protein S function instead of a protein S assay (Chapter 39) and using ferritin to evaluate susceptible patients for iron deficiency instead of a hemoglobin level (Chapter 17).[8]

Efficient Hematology and Hemostasis Testing

Efficient laboratory testing is defined as "avoiding waste, including waste of equipment, supplies, ideas and energy."[2] An efficient laboratory testing process is one that has no defects: the specimen is appropriately collected, it is transported to the medical laboratory in a timely manner, the analysis is accurately performed, and the test results are sent to the provider in a timely manner. There is waste and inefficiency any time there is a problem with specimen integrity (clotted ethylenediaminetetraacetic acid specimen for a CBC or an inadequately filled sodium citrate tube for a prothrombin time) (Chapters 12 and 41). The integrity of each specimen is the responsibility of medical laboratory professionals, regardless of which member of the health care team collects the specimen. Thus the medical laboratory professional is responsible for educating other health care professionals on specimen collection methods and how defects in specimen collection affect patient care.

Beyond analyzing each specimen in an efficient manner, appropriate test utilization is an important goal for medical laboratory professionals. Inappropriate laboratory testing includes overuse, underuse, and misuse. In the hematology laboratory, a common example of overuse is a daily CBC for inpatients with no sign of bleeding or other hemodynamic instability. Overuse is both inefficient and ineffective, as well as unpleasant for the patient. Underuse is equally ineffective; ordering a test that provides diagnostic clarity, for example, allows correct treatment to be started more quickly. Testing misuse might be an order for the wrong test, for example, a factor X assay instead of anti-factor Xa (Chapters 40 and 41), or the misinterpretation of results from a correctly ordered test, for example, ordering iron studies for a patient with a mean cell volume of 125 fL (Chapters 17 and 18).

Timely Hematology and Hemostasis Testing

Timely laboratory testing is defined as "reducing waits and sometimes harmful delays for both those who receive and those who give care."[2] Medical laboratory professionals have been measuring the turnaround time for many laboratory test results since the inception of the profession. Turnaround time is generally considered to be the time elapsed from the test order to the test report, but there is little consistency as to the specifics: Should the measured time start when the test order is placed or when the specimen reaches the laboratory? What is the end of the process—when the result is released or when action is taken with the patient? If only analytical time is tracked, then other phases of the Total Testing Process are not considered. This approach can overlook factors that are important for patients who are waiting in the emergency department or for other health care professionals who need information about the patient. Even though the preanalytical and postanalytical phases of testing involve nonlaboratory personnel, oversight of these phases is still a responsibility of the medical laboratory professional. In the hematology laboratory in particular, results of the CBC are often used with other tests as the basis for decisions about diagnosis, treatment, and hospital admission.

Patient-Centered Hematology and Hemostasis Testing

The definition of patient-centered laboratory testing services is "providing care that is respectful of and responsive to individual preferences, needs, and values and ensuring that patient values guide all clinical decisions."[2] Information is a critical component of delivering patient-centered care. Medical laboratory professionals should provide patients with information to prepare for laboratory tests (such as instructions for collecting fasting blood specimens or an explanation of the venipuncture procedure with information for care afterward) and to understand testing (e.g., reasons for genetic testing). Information should be written at an appropriate reading level for patients and available in multiple languages for patients who are not literate in English. Information may be provided as a document distributed to the patient in the phlebotomy waiting area or on the laboratory's website. Patient-centered service also requires communicating in a manner that meets individual preferences, such as addressing patients using their preferred pronouns and name.

Equitable Hematology and Hemostasis Testing

The definition of equitable laboratory testing services is "providing care that does not vary in quality because of personal characteristics such as gender, ethnicity, geographic location, and socioeconomic status."[2] Equitable health care, including laboratory testing, is influenced by social determinants of health. Social determinants of health are "conditions in the places where people live, learn, work, and play that affect a wide range of health and quality of life risks and outcomes."[9] Social

determinants of health play a significant role in the differences in individual health status.[10] Examples of social determinants of health include access to health care (e.g., access to health insurance, living in a rural or urban location, availability of transportation), quality of health care (e.g., disparities in the delivery of care, lack of health literacy, language barriers), social and economic factors (e.g., degree of trust in the health care system, cultural beliefs regarding medical care, employment, and education level), physical environment (e.g., air and water quality, community safety, type of housing), and individual behaviors (e.g., use of tobacco, alcohol, or illicit drugs, diet, and exercise).[11]

Increasing equitable laboratory testing services for hematology and hemostasis testing (in fact, all laboratory testing) requires focusing on improving testing from the patient's perspective instead of the provider's habit or convenience. The hours of operation for phlebotomy services are one system perspective to consider for improving equitable access to laboratory testing services. Expanding the hours that phlebotomy services are available to include early morning and evening hours as well as weekends increases access to laboratory testing services to individuals who cannot take time off from work during the day or do not have child care. Medical laboratory professionals can improve the patient experience by providing information about testing in languages other than English to support individuals for whom English is not their first language. If written patient information (e.g., ASCLS Patient Safety Tips[12]) is distributed to patients in English, it is also equitable to provide it in the predominant non-English language of individuals in the community. Equitable testing services are combined with effective testing services when reference intervals are available for parameters that have a sex-based difference (e.g., red blood cell count and hemoglobin level for individuals who are transgender) (Chapter 43). Both laboratory and hospital information systems should allow inclusion of gender identity for patients, not just listing the sex assigned at birth.

ESSENTIAL COMPETENCIES FOR HEALTH CARE PROFESSIONALS

Health Professions Education: A Bridge to Quality, published in 2003 by the Institute of Medicine, provides a blueprint to achieve quality health care.[13] It identifies the need to prepare future health care professionals with competencies to ensure health care quality. This report identifies *five competencies* considered essential for all health care professionals[13]: practice in interprofessional teams, employ evidence-based practice, provide patient-centered care, use information technology, and apply quality improvement processes. The following sections discuss why these competencies are important for medical laboratory professionals.

Interprofessional Teamwork

Students in different health care professional programs generally learn in separate programs; however, in practice, health care works best when professionals from different disciplines work as a team.[13] Communication with others is crucial, including providers who need information about test selection, nurses who are preparing patients for testing, and clerical assistants who are entering test orders. It is important to apply expertise in all aspects of care, and for medical laboratory professionals, that often means where laboratory operations interface with non-laboratorians who order, facilitate, or interpret laboratory tests. Working in interprofessional teams is rooted in the understanding of and respect for the scopes of practice and importance of other health care professionals. Teamwork requires a willingness to share information, to avoid and to resolve conflicts, and to approach situations with an openness to other viewpoints and priorities.[13]

Evidence-Based Practice and Patient-Centered Care

The competencies of evidence-based practice and patient-centered care create a framework on which interprofessional cooperation can be built. First, it is critical to remember that the patient should be at the center of every practice decision. If health care workers focus on the patient and their well-being, different viewpoints become an asset rather than grounds for disagreement. Additionally, when it is agreed that high-quality evidence (such as practice guidelines and peer-reviewed publications) is the basis for practice, each professional can contribute the best evidence from their own scope of practice to create a well-designed approach to patient care. Providing the best evidence to patients in a format they can understand increases shared decision making, which leads to better patient outcomes.[14]

Informatics and Quality Improvement Processes

The remaining two competencies are learned skills with significant overlap, which allow professionals to assess and improve systems. Information technology, in addition to facilitating care directly via test ordering and reporting of test results, allows health care professionals to access information and to evaluate data, for example, to locate high-quality evidence and to monitor the state of operations in their own facility.

Health care must be a continuous learning environment: as new evidence becomes available, as practice guidelines are introduced and updated, as benchmarks and outcomes are evaluated, health care professionals should strive to improve systems and processes to achieve high-quality health care. Quality improvement processes such as the Plan-Do-Study-Act (PDSA) method help to structure and monitor interventions for improvement.[15]

APPLICATIONS IN THE HEMATOLOGY AND HEMOSTASIS LABORATORY

Interprofessional Teamwork in the Hematology and Hemostasis Laboratory

Teamwork is a skill that is applicable to both the preanalytical and the postanalytical phases of testing. Uncertainty and questions often arise with test selection and specimen collection (preanalytical phase) and then again with test interpretation (postanalytical phase). Decisions on appropriate molecular testing to diagnose leukemias requires teamwork among many health care professionals in various departments such as hematology,

flow cytometry, and cytogenetics (Chapters 28–34). In addition to responding to questions about tests, specimens, and results, medical laboratory professionals should be proactive with educational offerings for other health care professionals on topics that have generated repeated questions from those outside the laboratory. Providers might appreciate information about the effect of pretest probability on test interpretation (Chapter 3), for example, or the application of new parameters reported by the hematology analyzer (Chapter 13). It is important for medical laboratory professionals to maintain an attitude of availability for consultation, recognizing that neither providers nor nurses receive extensive education in these topics.[3]

Medical laboratory professionals should also be respectful of the expertise available to them from other health care professionals. Nurses may be able to provide insight about a patient's condition that impacts specimen collection, or perhaps providers can consult about unusual results or emerging diseases that relate to hematology testing.

Laboratory expertise that is shared only with other medical laboratory professionals does not always improve patient outcomes. Interpretation of complex laboratory testing may benefit from regularly scheduled, combined efforts from providers and medical laboratory professionals. In some hospitals, diagnostic management teams comprising care providers and medical laboratory professionals (pathologists, laboratory managers, and medical laboratory scientists, including those with a doctorate in clinical laboratory science [DCLS]) work together to evaluate test results from specific patients and provide patient-specific interpretive reports.[16]

Evidence-Based Practice in the Hematology and Hemostasis Laboratory

Because it can be difficult to keep up with the pace of new publications in medicine, many professional groups have joined forces to provide widely disseminated guidelines through the *Choosing Wisely* campaign.[7,8] These recommendations offer a starting point to introduce evidence-based practice into laboratory operations. For example, the *Choosing Wisely* list of the Society of Hospital Medicine-Adult Hospital Medicine (SHM-AHM) includes no repetitive CBC or chemistry testing for patients who are clinically stable (see Table 2.2). A laboratory manager could monitor tests ordered to determine if some providers regularly order repeat testing without obvious evidence of need; if so, an educational initiative may help to reduce unnecessary daily CBC orders. Alternatively, recently reported test results can be displayed within the electronic test ordering system to alert the ordering provider. Appropriate laboratory test utilization can save resources (efficiency) and improve diagnosis (effectiveness), and benefits the patient in terms of fewer specimen collections. A significant percentage of patients in intensive care units and neonatal intensive care units develop anemia during hospitalization, with phlebotomy performed for numerous specimen collections a contributing factor.[17,18] In addition, the *Choosing Wisely* statements are short and simple enough to provide patient-friendly information, allowing patients to engage in their own care planning through conversations with providers.

Patient-Centered Care in the Hematology and Hemostasis Laboratory

The importance of patient-centered care is emphasized by its inclusion in both the six health care quality aims and the five essential competencies described earlier in "Six Aims of Health Care Quality" and "Essential Competencies for Health Care Professionals," respectively. The NAM endorses a model of patient-centered care that specifies care and communication that respect patient values and preferences, coordinated care with well-managed transitions, provision of adequate information and education, attention to physical comfort, emotional support, and involvement of family and friends of the patient.[14]

Coordinated care includes interprofessional communication, establishment of responsibility and accountability, and anticipating and meeting patients' needs.[19] Proactively providing information about community transportation options for patients who need to schedule additional laboratory procedures can increase compliance with their treatment plan. Creating a procedure to establish which office will transmit results from emergency department visits to primary care providers will help to ensure continuity of care. Communication with patients by medical laboratory professionals can improve patient compliance with recommended medication-related testing.[20] Medical laboratory professionals generally have limited patient interaction and therefore little communication with the patient directly, but attention to communication among professionals can improve care coordination. For example, coordinating results between a hematology laboratory and cytology department regarding body fluid specimens (Chapter E4) increased the detection of malignancies and helped to define the educational interventions required to maintain the improvement.[21]

Medical laboratory professionals can directly affect patient care by helping patients (and those close to them) understand their laboratory test results. Patient portals provide increased access to results, but this is unlikely to help patients engage in their care if the information is not meaningful for nonmedical professionals. In a study piloting a user-centered design for laboratory test results, Zhang and colleagues[22] determined that patients found many laboratory reports difficult to read and interpret, with desired information missing or not understandable (such as the implications of abnormal results and next steps). Additionally, providers may find it difficult to extract useful information from reports of complex testing, such as molecular diagnostics.[23] A good starting point would be to track questions received in the laboratory and provide education about the most common inquiries. Providing reports that meet users' needs will require a joint effort between medical laboratory professionals and providers or patients because only the end users (that is, patients or providers) can determine if the information is usable for them.[24]

Informatics in the Hematology and Hemostasis Laboratory

The value of informatics in the laboratory, as in other applications of big data, lies in the ability to draw conclusions from large quantities of available data. The process of data analytics may not be required for laboratory practice, but understanding the potential questions to ask and application of the answers are essential. Data analyses provide a base on which to build each of the other competencies. In a particular facility, questions could include the following:

- What testing patterns indicate a need for clinical decision support systems (e.g., diagnostic algorithms or test bundles)?
- What is the current best evidence for interpretation of a particular analytical procedure?
- How can patients and families access the information they need to participate in shared decision making about their care plan?
- Does the outcome of a particular system meet criteria from benchmark institutions?

Informatics can also move the overall function of the laboratory forward in a more holistic manner. For example, extensive harmonization of laboratory testing and reporting can ensure that patient results for the same analyte from different laboratories are directly comparable.[25] Future models suggest a more extensive integration of disciplines, such as radiology and pathology, to improve diagnosis and therapeutic decisions.[26] Each of these advances requires laboratory data to be widely available and consistently mined for information.

Quality Improvement in the Hematology and Hemostasis Laboratory

Quality improvement, also known as process improvement, involves monitoring the results of a system or process to determine if the system is functioning optimally. If data show that the results could be improved, a structured plan is developed to sequentially apply changes to the system (interventions), with continued monitoring to identify changes that may result.[27] Systems thinking and quality improvement concepts initially proved useful in other industries, such as aviation and manufacturing, and their incorporation into health care has resulted in significant improvement for many patient safety indicators.[28]

In the hematology and hemostasis laboratory, potential quality improvement projects span all phases of the Total Testing Process. Preanalytical outcomes might include the rate of specimen rejection due to defects in specimen quality (e.g., clots or inadequate blood volume in sodium citrate tubes). Analytical indicators could include failures to recognize an interfering substance (e.g., lipemia causing an erroneously high hemoglobin value). Projects evaluating the postanalytical phase could monitor stat turnaround times or rate of failure to report critical values correctly.[27]

How Can Medical Laboratory Professionals Achieve Competency in These Areas?

Each of the essential competencies requires intentional preparation and specific learning methods. Few people will enter the medical laboratory profession with an intuitive understanding of quality improvement processes, and simply participating in group projects does not necessarily develop teamwork skills. The education of medical laboratory professionals is always challenging, with an ever-growing body of knowledge and limited time or opportunity for interprofessional activities. New professionals may need to investigate individual opportunities to acquire one or more of these skills, but the effort will pay off in improved patient outcomes.[29]

SUMMARY

- Patient safety encompasses all aspects of each patient's experience with the health care system.
- It is the responsibility of every health care professional to ensure that patients receive care that is safe, effective, timely, efficient, patient centered, and equitable.
- Improving medical laboratory testing requires that medical laboratory professionals develop skills in each of the five patient safety competencies: practicing in interprofessional

teams, employing evidence-based practice, using information technology, applying quality improvement processes, and providing patient-centered care.

Now that you have completed this chapter, go back and read again the case study at the beginning and respond to the questions presented. Answers can be found in Appendix C.

REVIEW QUESTIONS

Answers can be found in Appendix C.

1. Which one of the following is an example of improving patient safety for patients who require a laboratory test as part of their health care?
   a. Counting the number of clotted specimens for a CBC received by the laboratory
   b. Measuring the amount of time it takes for a CBC to be reported to the provider
   c. Ensuring that the correct laboratory test is performed for the patient's condition
   d. Wearing a laboratory coat and gloves while analyzing specimens

2. What is the focus of the National Academy of Medicine's definition of health care quality?
   a. Meeting College of American Pathologists accreditation requirements
   b. Improving patients' health outcomes
   c. Meeting The Joint Commission accreditation requirements
   d. Improving laboratory proficiency testing outcomes

3. Which one of the following examples of collected data is needed for a medical laboratory professional to improve the efficiency of the preanalytical phase of the Total Testing Process in the clinical laboratory?
   a. The number of underfilled sodium citrate tubes for prothrombin time procedures
   b. The number of times the quality control specimens are outside ± 2 SD
   c. The number of times the proficiency testing does not meet requirements
   d. The number of times a prothrombin time procedure needs to be repeated

4. Which one of the following actions can lead to harm for a patient who needs laboratory testing?
   a. Asking the patient their name and birth date before performing venipuncture for a CBC
   b. Reviewing the results of the quality control specimens before analyzing the patient's specimen
   c. Sending an abnormally low platelet count result to a provider without completing the required confirmation checks
   d. Daily maintenance on the coagulation analyzer before analyzing quality control specimens

5. Which one of the following is an example of improving the effectiveness of hematology laboratory testing?
   a. Following the guidelines promoted by *Choosing Wisely* for inpatients
   b. Counting the number of clotted CBC specimens received in the laboratory
   c. Measuring the amount of time it takes for a CBC to be completed after it is collected
   d. Performing quality control on the hematology analyzer before analyzing patient specimens

6. Which one of the following statements accurately characterizes the subject of *Crossing the Quality Chasm*?
   a. Certain competencies are essential for all health care professionals.
   b. Good health care can be described using six different dimensions of care.
   c. Laboratory records should include quality control and proficiency testing results.
   d. Many Americans experience harm as a result of health care procedures.

7. Which one of the following is an example of interprofessional teamwork?
   a. An interpreter was hired by the laboratory director to translate patient venipuncture preparation instructions into Vietnamese to accommodate a large immigrant population.
   b. Medical laboratory scientists in the hematology laboratory discuss an unusual abnormal cell found on a slide.
   c. The charge nurse on one floor asks the medical laboratory scientist in hematology to create an educational presentation about anticoagulants and phlebotomy.
   d. The *Choosing Wisely* campaign recommends a C-reactive protein level to detect inflammation instead of the erythrocyte sedimentation rate.

8. Which one of the following illustrates evidence-based practice?
   a. Good health care can be described using six different dimensions of care.
   b. Many Americans experience harm as a result of health care procedures.
   c. Medical laboratory scientists in the hematology laboratory discuss an unusual abnormal cell found on a slide.
   d. The *Choosing Wisely* campaign recommends a C-reactive protein level to detect inflammation instead of the erythrocyte sedimentation rate.

9. Which one of the following laboratory projects would NOT require the use of informatics?
   a. Comparing patient safety indicators with benchmark information from regional laboratories
   b. Demonstrating competency in abnormal cell identification among hematology personnel
   c. Determining the change in turnaround time for CBCs after installing a new instrument
   d. Determining the number of anti-factor Xa tests ordered inappropriately in the last 2 years

10. Which one of the following situations illustrates patient-centered care?
    a. Hiring an interpreter to translate patient venipuncture preparation instructions into Vietnamese to accommodate a large immigrant population
    b. Asking the patient their name and birth date before performing venipuncture for a CBC
    c. Improving laboratory proficiency testing outcomes
    d. Reviewing the results of the quality control specimens before analyzing the patient's specimen

ADDITIONAL RESOURCES

Agency for Healthcare Quality and Research. TeamSTEPPS. https://www.ahrq.gov/teamstepps/index.html

American Society for Clinical Laboratory Science Patient Safety Committee. Patient Safety Resources. https://ascls.org/patient-safety-resources/

Institute for Healthcare Improvement. https://www.ihi.org/

National Academies Press. Quality Chasm Series. https://nap.nationalacademies.org/search/?rpp=20&ft=1&term=quality+-chasm+series

National Quality Foundation. Advancing Anticoagulation Stewardship: A Playbook. https://acforum-excellence.org/Resource-Center/resource_files/1977-2022-08-24-063128.pdf

REFERENCES

1. Committee on Quality Health Care in America, Kohn, L. T., Corrigan, J. M., & Donaldson M. S. (Eds.), (2000). *To Err is Human: Building a Safe Health System*. Washington, DC: The National Academy Press.
2. Committee on Quality of Health Care in America. (2001). *Crossing the Quality Chasm: A New Health System for the 21st Century*. Institute of Medicine. Washington, DC: The National Academy Press.
3. National Academies of Sciences, Engineering and Medicine. (2015). *Improving Diagnosis in Health Care*. Washington, DC: The National Academies Press.
4. Schumacher, G. E., & Barr, J. T. (1998). Total testing process applied to therapeutic drug monitoring: impact on patient outcomes and economics. *Clin Chem, 44*, 370–374.
5. Lundberg, G. D. (1981). Acting on significant laboratory results. *JAMA, 245*, 1762–1763.
6. Plebani, M., Laposata, M., & Lundberg, G. D. (2011). The brain-to-brain loop concept for laboratory testing 40 years after its introduction. *Am J Clin Pathol, 136*, 829–833.
7. ABIM Foundation. *Choosing Wisely*. https://www.choosingwisely.org/. Accessed October 14, 2022.
8. ABIM Foundation. *Choosing Wisely*. Clinician Lists. https://www.choosingwisely.org/clinician-lists/#parentSociety=American_Society_for_Clinical_Laboratory_Science. Accessed October 14, 2022.
9. Centers for Disease Control and Prevention. *Social Determinants of Health: Know What Affects Health*. https://www.cdc.gov/socialdeterminants/. Accessed October 21, 2022.
10. World Health Organization. *Social Determinants of Health*. https://www.who.int/health-topics/social-determinants-of-health#tab=tab_1. Accessed October 21, 2022.
11. University of Wisconsin Population Health Institute. County Health Rankings Model. https://www.countyhealthrankings.org/explore-health-rankings/measures-data-sources/county-health-rankings-model. Accessed October 21, 2022.
12. American Society for Clinical Laboratory Science. *Laboratory Patient Safety Tips: Blood Specimen Collection (Venipuncture)*. https://ascls.org/wp-content/uploads/2012/11/Brochure_Venipuncture_2017.pdf. Accessed October 21, 2022.
13. Institute of Medicine of the National Academies. (2003). *Health Professions Education: A Bridge to Quality*. Washington, DC: The National Academy Press.
14. Barry, M., & Edgman-Levitan, S. (2012). Shared decision making — the pinnacle of patient centered care. *N Engl J Med, 366*, 780–781.
15. Leis, J. A., & Shojania, K. G. (2017). A primer on PDSA: executing plan-do-study-act cycles in practice, not just in name. *BMJ Qual Saf, 26*, 572–577.
16. Seegmiller, A., Kim, A., Mosse, C., et al. (2013). Optimizing personalized bone marrow testing using an evidence-based, interdisciplinary team approach. *Am J Clin Pathol, 140*, 643–650.
17. Bodley, T., Chan, M., Levi, O., et al. (2021). Patient harm associated with serial phlebotomy and blood waste in the intensive care unit: a retrospective cohort study. *PLoS ONE, 16*, e0243782. https://doi.org/10.1371/journal.pone.0243782.
18. Capalletti, P. (2016). Appropriateness of diagnostics tests. *Intl J Lab Haematol, 38*(Suppl 1), 91–99.
19. Agency for Healthcare Research and Quality. *Care Coordination*. https://www.ahrq.gov/ncepcr/care/coordination.html. Accessed October 31, 2022.
20. Raebel, M., Shetterly, A., Bhardwaja, B., et al. (2020). Technology-enabled outreach to patients taking high-risk medications reduces a quality gap in completion of clinical laboratory testing. *Popul Health Manag, 23*, 3–11.
21. Zhang, M., Maglantay, R., Jr., Cunningham, V., et al. (2021). Improving malignancy detection rates in body fluids submitted to the hematology laboratory for nucleated cell count and differential: a quality improvement study. *Arch Pathol Lab Med, 145*, 201–207.
22. Zhang, Z., Kmoth, L., Xiao, L., et al. (2021). User-centered system design for communicating clinical laboratory test results: design

and evaluation study. *JMIR Hum Factors*, 8(4), e26017. https://doi.org/10.2196/26017.

23. Sharma, V., Fong, A., Beckman, R., et al. (2018). Eye-tracking study to enhance usability of molecular diagnostics reports in cancer precision medicine. *JCO Precision Oncology*, 2, 1–11.

24. Tzelepis, F., Sanson-Fisher, R., Zucca, A., et al. (2015). Measuring the quality of patient-centered care: why patient-reported measures are critical to reliable assessment. *Patient Pref and Adherence*, 9, 831–835.

25. Plebani, M. (2016). Harmonization in laboratory medicine: requests, samples, measurements and reports. *Crit Rev Clin Lab Sci*, 53, 184–196.

26. Lippi, G., & Plebani, M. (2020). Integrated diagnostics: the future of laboratory medicine? *Biochem Med (Zagreb)*, 30(1). https://doi.org/10.11613/BM.2020.010501.

27. Howanitz, P., Lehman, C., Jones, B., et al. (2015). Clinical laboratory quality practices when hemolysis occurs. *Arch Pathol Lab Med*, 139, 901–906.

28. Golemboski, K. (2011). Improving patient safety: lessons from other disciplines. *Clin Lab Sci*, 24, 114–119.

29. Morris, S., Otto, C. N., & Golemboski, K. (2013). Improving patient safety and healthcare quality in the 21st century: competencies required of future medical laboratory science practitioners. *Clin Lab Sci*, 16, 200–204.

3

Quality Assurance in Hematology and Hemostasis Testing

*Mayukh Kanti Sarkar and George A. Fritsma**

OBJECTIVES

After completion of this chapter, the reader will be able to:

1. Describe the procedures to validate and document a new or modified laboratory assay.
2. Compare a new or modified assay with a reference using statistical tests to establish accuracy.
3. Select appropriate statistical tests for a given application and interpret the results.
4. Define and compute precision using standard deviation and coefficient of variation.
5. Determine assay linearity using graphical representations and transformations.
6. Discuss analytical limits and analytical sensitivity and specificity.
7. Prepare multisite validation protocols.
8. Explain Food and Drug Administration clearance levels for laboratory assays.
9. Compute a reference interval and a therapeutic range for a new or modified assay.
10. Interpret internal quality control using controls and moving averages.
11. Explain the benefits of participation in periodic external quality assessment.
12. Measure and describe assay clinical efficacy.
13. Interpret relative and absolute risk ratios.
14. Interpret receiver operating characteristic curves.
15. Describe methods to enhance and assess laboratory staff competence.
16. Describe a quality assurance plan to control for preanalytical and postanalytical variables.
17. List the agencies that regulate hematology and hemostasis quality.

OUTLINE

Statistical Significance and Expressions of Central Tendency and Dispersion
　Statistical Significance
　Computing the Mean
　Determining the Median
　Determining the Mode
　Computing the Variance
　Computing the Standard Deviation
　Computing the Coefficient of Variation
Method Validation
　Accuracy
　Statistical Tests
　Precision
　Linearity and the Analytical Measurement Range
　Analytical Sensitivity (Lower Limit of Detection)
　Analytical Specificity
　Levels of Laboratory Assay Approval
　Documentation and Reliability
Multisite Validation
　System-Wide Comparability
　Multisite Reference Interval and Therapeutic Range

Lot-to-Lot Comparisons
Reference Interval and Therapeutic Range Development
　Direct Reference Interval Determination
　Indirect Reference Interval Determination
　Therapeutic Target Range
Internal Quality Control
　Controls
　Moving Average ($\overline{X}_B$) of Red Blood Cell Indices
　Delta Checks
External Quality Assessment
Assessing Diagnostic Efficacy
　Effects of Population Incidence and Odds Ratios on Diagnostic Efficacy
Receiver Operating Characteristic Curve
Assay Feasibility
Laboratory Staff Competence
　Proficiency Systems
　Continuing Education
Quality Assurance Plan: Preanalytical and Postanalytical
Agencies that Address Hematology and Hemostasis Quality

*The authors extend appreciation to Heather DeVries, David McGlasson, and Milo Schield for sharing their expertise in the preparation of this chapter.

CASE STUDY

After studying the material in this chapter, the reader should be able to respond to the following case study. Answers can be found in Appendix C.

On an 0800 assay run, the results for three levels of a preserved hemoglobin control specimen were 2 g/dL higher than the upper reference limit. The medical laboratory professional reviewed delta check data on the hemoglobin results for the last 10 patients in sequence and noticed that the day's results were consistently 1.8 to 2.2 g/dL higher than results generated the previous day.

1. What do you call the type of error detected in this case?
2. Can you continue to analyze specimens if you subtract 2 g/dL from the results?
3. What aspect of the assay should you first investigate in troubleshooting this problem?

BOX 3.1 Examples of Components of Quality Assurance

1. *Preanalytical* variables: assay selection based on patient indication; implementation of assay selection; patient identification and preparation; specimen collection equipment and technique; specimen transport, preparation, and storage; monitoring of specimen condition
2. *Analytical* variables: laboratory staff competence; assay and instrument selection; assay and instrument validation, including linearity, accuracy, precision, analytical measurement range (AMR), and specificity; internal quality control; external quality assessment
3. *Postanalytical* variables: accurate transcription and posting of results; content and format of laboratory report, narrative report; reference interval (RI) and therapeutic range; timeliness in communicating critical values; patient and provider satisfaction; turnaround time; cost analysis; provider application of laboratory results; patient outcome

In medical laboratory science, *quality* implies the ability to provide *accurate, reproducible* assay results that offer clinically useful information.[1] Because providers base clinical decision making on laboratory results, assay results must be *reliable*.[2] Reliability requires vigilance and effort on the part of all laboratory professionals.[3] An experienced medical laboratory scientist who is a quality assurance (QA) and quality control (QC) specialist often directs this effort.

Of the terms *quality control* and *quality assurance*, QA is the broader concept, encompassing *preanalytical, analytical,* and *postanalytical* variables (Box 3.1). QC processes are employed to document assay validity, accuracy, and precision, including external quality assessment, publication of *reference intervals* (RIs) and *therapeutic ranges* (when applicable), and *lot-to-lot validation*.

Preanalytical variables (Table 3.1) are addressed in blood specimen collection texts and in Chapter 41 and Chapter E2, which include sections on coagulation specimen management.[4,5] Postanalytical variables are discussed briefly at the end of this chapter and are listed in Table 3.2. QA further encompasses laboratory assay utilization and provider test ordering patterns, known as "pre-pre" analytical variables, and the appropriate application of laboratory assay results, known as "post-post" analytical variables.[6] A combined 17% medical error rate is associated with the pre-pre and post-post analytical phases of laboratory test utilization and application, prompting laboratory directors and scientists to develop *clinical query systems* that guide providers in laboratory assay selection.[7] Clinical query systems are enhanced by *reflex assay algorithms* developed in collaboration with the affiliated medical and surgical staff.[8] Equally important, a system of *narrative reports* that accompany and augment numerical laboratory assay output, authored by medical laboratory professionals and directors, is designed to assist providers with case management. A discussion of pre-pre and post-post analytical variables extends beyond the scope of this textbook but may be found in the references listed at the end of this chapter.[9,10] QC relies on the initial computation of central tendency and dispersion.

STATISTICAL SIGNIFICANCE AND EXPRESSIONS OF CENTRAL TENDENCY AND DISPERSION

Statistical Significance

When applying a statistical test such as the *Student t-test* of means or the *analysis of variance* (ANOVA), the statistician

TABLE 3.1 Preanalytical Quality Assurance Components and Laboratory Staff Responsibility

Preanalytical Component	Laboratory Staff Responsibility
Test orders	Conduct systematic utilization reviews to ensure that provider-generated orders are comprehensive and appropriate to patient indications. Inform provider about laboratory test availability and ways to avoid unnecessary orders. Ensure repeat testing is necessary.
Test request forms	Are requisition forms legible? Can the phlebotomist confirm patient identity? Are provider orders promptly and correctly interpreted and transcribed? Is adequate diagnostic, treatment, and patient preparation information provided to assist the laboratory staff to check test relevance and interpret results?
Stat orders and timeliness	Do turnaround time expectations match clinical necessity and ensure that stat orders are reserved for medical emergencies? Does laboratory management meet established turnaround time requirements?
Specimen collection	Is the patient correctly identified, prepared, and available for specimen collection? Is fasting and therapy status appropriate for the assay? Is the tourniquet correctly applied and released within 1 minute? Are venipuncture sites appropriately cleansed? Are timed specimens collected at the specified intervals? Are specimen tubes collected in the specified order of draw? Are additive tubes properly mixed? Are specimen tubes labeled after blood collection, and are the labels confirmed by patient identification band or with the patient?
Specimen transport	Are specimens delivered intact, sealed, and within specified time limits? Are specimens maintained at the correct temperature?
Specimen management	Are specimens centrifuged correctly? Are tests begun within specified time intervals? Are specimens and aliquots stored properly? Are coagulation specimens consistently platelet-poor?

TABLE 3.2 Postanalytical Quality Assurance and Laboratory Staff Responsibility

Postanalytical Component	Laboratory Staff Responsibility
Publication of reports	Are results accurately transcribed into the information system? Are they reviewed for errors by other laboratory staff? If autoverification is in effect, are the correct parameters employed? Do reports provide RIs? Do they flag abnormal results? Are result narratives appended when necessary? Does the laboratory staff conduct in-service education to support test result interpretation? Are critical values provided to applicable providers? Are verbal reports confirmed with feedback? Are inconsistent findings resolved?
Timeliness	Are turnaround times recorded and analyzed? Are laboratory reports being posted to patient medical records in a timely fashion?
Patient satisfaction	Does the facility include laboratory care in patient surveys? Was specimen collection explained to the patient?

RI, Reference interval.

TABLE 3.3 Typical Student *t*-Test Results*

Example 1	Reference Method	New or Modified Method
n	10	10
$\overline{X}$	0.45	0.46
SD	0.01	0.02
Null hypothesis	$\overline{X}$ of control = $\overline{X}$ of test	
Selected *P*-value	0.01	
Computed *P*-value	0.085	
Computed two-tailed *t*-value	0.99	
Critical two-tailed *t*-value	2.88	

Null hypothesis is supported, means are not unequal

Example 2	Reference Method	New or Modified Method
n	10	10
$\overline{X}$	0.40	0.44
SD	0.07	0.07
Null hypothesis	$\overline{X}$ of control = $\overline{X}$ of test	
Selected *P*-value	0.01	
Computed *P*-value	0.008	
Computed two-tailed *t*-value	3.89	
Critical two-tailed *t*-value	2.88	

Null hypothesis is rejected, means are unequal

*In the first example of a two-tailed Student *t*-test, the difference in the means does not rise to statistical significance; the computed *P*-value exceeds the selected *P*-value, the computed *t*-value is smaller than the critical *t*-value, and the means are "not unequal." In the second example, the computed *P*-value is smaller than the selected *P*-value, the computed *t*-value exceeds the critical *t*-value, the means are unequal, and the result is statistically significant.
$\overline{X}$, Mean; *n*, number of data points; *SD*, standard deviation.

begins with a *null hypothesis*. The null hypothesis states that there is no difference between or among the means or variances of the populations being compared.[11] The *alternative (research) hypothesis* is the logical opposite of the null hypothesis.[12] For example, the null hypothesis may state that there is no difference between the population means using the *t*-test, but the alternative hypothesis states that the null hypothesis is rejected and a statistical difference between the population means does exist (Table 3.3). In medical research, the null and alternative hypotheses may go unstated but are always implied.[13]

The power of a statistical test is defined as its ability to reject the null hypothesis when the null hypothesis is false. Power is expressed as *P*, which stands for the *probability* that the test can detect an effect. The *P* scale ranges from 0 to 1. Power is determined by the sample size (number of data points, *n*), the design of the research study, and the study's ability to control for extraneous variables.

The conventional levels for significance, or for rejecting the null hypothesis, are $P \leq 0.05$ (5%) or $P \leq 0.01$ (1%). In the former instance, a 5% chance exists that the effect has occurred by chance alone; in the latter instance, a more stringent 1% chance exists. Often researchers combine the statistical results, and thus the powers of several studies, to compute a common, more robust *P*-value, a process called *meta-analysis*.

The term *significant* has a specific meaning based on the *P*-value, and it should not be generalised to imply *practical* or *clinical* significance.[14] A statistical test result may indicate a statistically significant difference that is based on a selected study condition and power, but the difference may not possess practical importance because the clinical difference may be inconsequential. Experience and clinical judgment help when analyzing data, as does asking the question "Will this result generate a change in the prognosis, diagnosis, or treatment plan?"

Computing the Mean

The arithmetic mean ($\overline{X}$), or average, of a data set is the sum ($\sum$) of the individual data values divided by the number (*n*) of data points. A data set that represents a single population, for instance, a series of prothrombin time results from a defined cohort, is called a *sample*. Often, clinical laboratory professionals apply the terms *sample* and *specimen* interchangeably. A specimen may be defined as a single data point within a data set (sample). In the clinical laboratory, a specimen often means a tube of blood or a fragment of tissue collected from a patient, which provides a single data point. The sum of sample data values above the mean is equal to the sum of the data values below the mean; however, the actual number of points above and below the mean are not necessarily equal.[15] The mean is a standard expression of central tendency employed in most scientific applications; however, it is profoundly affected by outliers and is unreliable in a skewed population. The formula for computing the arithmetic mean is:

$$\text{Mean}\left(\overline{X}\right) = \frac{\left(\Sigma x\right)}{n},$$

where $\overline{X}$ = mean; $\sum x$ = sum of data point values; and n = number of data points.

The geometric mean is the n root of the product of n individual data points and is used to compute means of unlike data sets. The geometric mean of the prothrombin time RI is used to compute the prothrombin time international normalized ratio (INR) (Chapter 41). The formula for computing the geometric mean is:

Geometric mean of n instances of $a = \sqrt[n]{a_1 a_2 \dots a_n}$.

In the clinical laboratory, the QA specialist employs a spreadsheet to calculate the arithmetic and geometric mean. For example, using Microsoft Excel, the specialist employs the function "Average" to compute arithmetic mean and the function "Geometric Mean" for the prothrombin time mean.

Determining the Median

The median is the data point that separates the upper half from the lower half of a data set (sample). To find the median, the data set is arranged in numerical order and the central data point is selected. If the data set has an even number of data points, the median is the mean of the two central points. The median is a robust expression of central tendency in a skewed distribution because it minimizes the effects of outliers.

Determining the Mode

The mode of a data set (sample) is the data point that appears most often in the sample. The mode is not a true measure of central tendency because there is often more than one mode in a data set. For instance, a typical white blood cell histogram may be trimodal, with three modes, one each for lymphocytes, monocytes, and neutrophils. Conversely, in a Gaussian, or normal, sample, in which the data points are distributed symmetrically, the mean, median, and mode coincide at a single data point.

Computing the Variance

Variance (σ^2) expresses the deviation of each data point from its expected value, usually the mean of the data set (sample) from which the data point is drawn. The difference between each data point from the mean is squared, the squared differences are summed, and the sum of squares is divided by $n - 1$. Variance is expressed in the units of the variable squared as follows:

$$\sigma^2 = \frac{\sum \left(x_i - \overline{X}\right)^2}{(n-1)},$$

where σ^2 = sample variance; x_i = value of each data point; $\overline{X}$ = mean; and n = number of data points.

Computing the Standard Deviation

Standard deviation (SD), a commonly used measure of dispersion, is the square root of the variance and is the mean distance of all the data points in a sample from the sample mean (Figure 3.1). The larger the SD of a sample, the greater the deviation from the

mean. In clinical analyses, the SD of an assay is an expression of its quality based on its inherent dispersion or variability. The formula for SD is:

$$SD = \sqrt{\left[\frac{\sum \left(x_i - \overline{X}\right)^2}{(n-1)}\right]},$$

where SD = standard deviation; x_i = each data point value; $\overline{X}$ = mean; and n = number of data points.

SD states the confidence, or degree of *random error*, for statistical conclusions. Dispersion is typically expressed as $\overline{X}$ ± 2 SD or the 95.5% *prediction interval*, commonly termed the *confidence interval* (CI) in laboratory science. Data points that are more than 2 SD from the mean are outside the 95.5% CI and may be considered abnormal. The dispersion of data points within $\overline{X}$ ± 2 SD is considered the expression of random or chance variation. Typically, $\overline{X}$ ± 2 SD is used to establish biological RIs (reference or normal ranges), provided that the frequency of the data points is Gaussian, or normally distributed, meaning symmetrically distributed about the mean.

Computing the Coefficient of Variation

The coefficient of variation (CV) is the *normalized expression* of the SD, ordinarily articulated as a percentage (CV%). CV% is the most used measure of dispersion in laboratory medicine. It assesses method performance and is extensively used in evaluation of processes such as monthly QC reviews and lot-to-lot reagent and control changes. CV% is expressed without units (except percentage), thus making it possible to compare data sets that use different units. The computation formula is:

$$CV\% = 100\frac{SD}{\overline{X}},$$

where $CV\%$ = coefficient of variation expressed as a percentage; SD = standard deviation; and $\overline{X}$ = mean.

METHOD VALIDATION

Before patient testing can begin, each new instrument, new assay, assay modification, or instrument-assay combination must be validated, confirming the intended results. This includes multiple instruments of the same make and model as well as loaner instruments. Method validation includes proof of accuracy, precision, reportable ranges including the *analytical measurement range* (AMR), and detection of interfering substances (analytical specificity). Modifications to US Food and Drug Administration (FDA)-approved assays and laboratory-developed tests (LDTs) have additional requirements, including but not limited to analytical sensitivity and specificity, specimen and reagent stability, and carryover. The results of these validation procedures are faithfully recorded and summarized in an evaluation that is signed by the laboratory director or designee before implementation. Multiple identical instruments and test systems require individual evaluation and approval. If an instrument in a series of instruments fails validation, based on

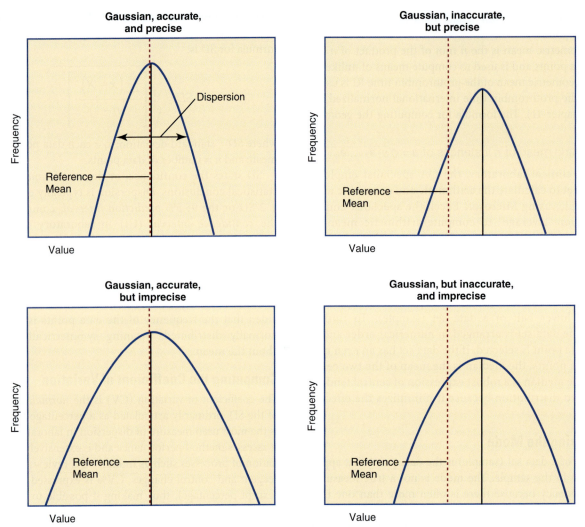

Figure 3.1 Frequency Distribution Graphs (Histograms) Generated From Repeated Assays of an Analyte. Incremental values are plotted on the horizontal *(x)* scale, and number of times each value was obtained (frequency) is plotted on the vertical *(y)* scale. In this example, the values are normally distributed about their mean (symmetric, Gaussian distribution). Results from an accurate assay generate a mean that closely duplicates the reference mean. Results from a precise assay generate small dispersion about the mean, whereas imprecision is reflected in a broad curve. The ideal assay is both accurate and precise.

an unacceptably large CV% or out-of-limit bias, the instrument is quarantined for troubleshooting. Documentation must be made available to laboratory assessors during periodic laboratory inspections required to maintain laboratory accreditation and licensure.[16]

Accuracy

Accuracy is the measure of agreement between an assay value and the theoretical true value of its analyte (Figure 3.1). Some statisticians prefer to define accuracy as the magnitude of error separating the assay result from the true value. In hematology testing, the concept of a true value is often not applicable. *Comparability* may take the place of accuracy in these situations. To test for comparability, the laboratory professional employs the laboratory's current reagent-instrument system as the reference assay for comparison with a new reagent-instrument system. Alternatively, the operator compares a reagent-instrument system with a previously validated external reference method.

By comparison, *precision* is the expression of reproducibility or dispersion about the mean, often expressed as SD or CV%, as discussed in the previous section. Accuracy is easy to define but difficult to establish and maintain; precision is relatively easy to measure and maintain.

For many analytes, laboratory professionals employ *primary standards* to establish accuracy. A primary standard is a material of known, fixed composition that is prepared in pure form, often by determining its dry mass on an analytical balance. The laboratory professional dissolves the weighed standard in an aqueous solute, prepares suitable dilutions, calculates the anticipated concentration for each dilution, and assigns the calculated concentrations to assay outcomes. For example, the laboratory professional may obtain pure glucose, weigh 100 mg, dilute it in 100 mL (1 dL) of buffer, and assay an aliquot of the solution using photometry. The resulting absorbance would then be assigned the value of 100 mg/dL. The laboratory professional may repeat this procedure using a series of four additional glucose solutions at 20, 60, 120, and 160 mg/dL to produce a five-point *standard curve*. The curve may be reassayed several times to generate means for each concentration. Standard curve generation is automated; however, laboratory professionals retain the option of generating curves manually when necessary. The assay is then used on human serum or plasma, with absorbance compared with the standard curve to generate a result. The matrix of a primary standard need not match the matrix of the patient specimen; the standard may be dissolved in an aqueous buffer, whereas the test specimen may be human serum or plasma.

To save time and resources, the laboratory professional may employ a secondary standard, perhaps purchased, that the vendor has previously calibrated to a primary standard. The secondary standard may be a preserved plasma preparation at a certified known concentration. The laboratory professional merely thaws or reconstitutes the secondary standard and incorporates it into the test series during validation or revalidation. Manufacturers often match secondary standards as closely as possible to the test specimen's matrix, for instance, serum to serum, plasma to plasma, and whole blood to whole blood. Primary and secondary standards are seldom assayed during routine patient specimen testing, only during calibration or when the assay tends to be unstable.

In hematology and hemostasis, where the analytes are often cell suspensions or enzymes, there are just a handful of primary standards: cyanmethemoglobin, fibrinogen, factor VIII, protein C, antithrombin, and von Willebrand factor.[17] For scores of analytes, the hematology and hemostasis professional relies on *calibrators*. Calibrators for hematology may be preserved human blood cell suspensions, sometimes supplemented with microlatex particles, or nucleated avian red blood cells (RBCs) as surrogates for hard-to-preserve human white blood cells (WBCs). In hemostasis, most calibrators may be frozen or lyophilized plasma from a pool of healthy human donors. For most of these analytes, it is impossible to prepare weighed-in standards; instead, calibrators are assayed using *reference methods* (gold standards) at selected independent expert laboratories. For instance, a vendor may prepare a 1000-L lot of preserved human blood cell suspension, assay for the desired analytes within their laboratory (in-house) and send aliquots to five laboratories that employ well-controlled reference instrumentation and methods. The vendor obtains analyte results from all five laboratories, averages the results, compares them with their in-house values, and publishes the averages as the reference calibrator values. The vendor then distributes sealed aliquots to customer laboratories with the calibrator values published in the accompanying package inserts. Vendors may market calibrators in sets of three or five, spanning the range of assay linearity (analytical measurement range, AMR) or the range of potential clinical results; alternatively, one calibrator can be diluted into multiple concentrations.

As with secondary standards, vendors attempt to match their calibrators as closely as possible to the physical properties of the test specimen. For instance, human preserved blood used to calibrate complete blood count (CBC) analytes

generated by an automated blood cell analyzer is prepared to closely match the matrix of fresh anticoagulated patient blood specimens, despite the need for preservatives, refrigeration, and sealed packaging. Vendors undergo rigorous certification processes by governmental or voluntary standards agencies to verify and maintain the validity of their products.[18]

The laboratory professional assays the calibration material using the new or modified assay and compares results with the vendor's published results. When new results parallel published results within a selected range, for example ±10%, the results are recorded, and the assay is validated for accuracy. If they fail to match, the new assay is modified or a new RI (and therapeutic range when applicable) is prepared.

Medical laboratory professionals may employ locally collected fresh blood from a healthy subject as a calibrator; however, the process for validation and certification is laborious, so few attempt it. The selected specimens are assayed using reference instrumentation and methods, calibration values are assigned, and the new or modified assay is calibrated (adjusted) from these values. Routine QC materials are not suitable for local calibration.

New or modified assays may also be compared with reference methods. A reference method may be a previously employed, well-controlled assay or an assay currently being used by an alternate laboratory. Several statistics are available to compare results of the new or modified assay with a reference method, including the Student *t*-test, analysis of variance (ANOVA), linear regression, the Pearson correlation coefficient, and the Bland-Altman plot.

Statistical Tests
Comparing the Means of Two Data Sets Using the Student *t*-Test

The Student *t*-test compares the mean of a data set (sample) of a new or modified assay with the sample mean of a reference assay. In the *unpaired Student t-test,* the operator assumes that population distributions are normal (Gaussian), the SDs are equal, and the assays are independent. Often laboratory professionals use the more robust *paired Student t-test,* in which the new and reference assays are performed using specimens (aliquots) from the same subjects. Laboratory professionals also choose between the *one-tailed* and *two-tailed t-test,* depending on whether the population being sampled has one (high *or* low) versus two (high *and* low) reference limits. For instance, when assaying plasma for glucose, providers are concerned about both elevated and reduced glucose values, so the laboratory professional would use the two-tailed *t*-test; however, when assaying for bilirubin, clinical concern focuses only on elevated bilirubin concentrations, so the laboratory professional would apply the more robust one-tailed *t*-test in method comparison studies.

The laboratory professional generates *t*-test data by entering the paired data sets side by side into columns of a spreadsheet such as Microsoft Excel and applying an automated *t*-test formula. The program generates the number, mean, and variance for each data set (sample; n_1, n_2; $\overline{X}_1$, $\overline{X}_2$; σ^2_1, σ^2_2), and the degrees of freedom (*df*) for the test: $df = n_1 + n_2 - 2$. The operator selects the appropriate critical value (*P*), often $P \leq 0.05$. The program uses *df* and *P* to compare the computed *t*-value with the *standard table of critical t-values* (Table 3.4) and reports a computed *P*-value. For instance, if the two assays are performed on aliquots from each of 10 subjects, the *df* is 18. If the computed *t*-value is higher than 2.10 (critical *t*-value at $P \leq 0.05$), the means of the two data sets are unequal. Applying a stricter critical *t*-value at $P \leq 0.01$, the computed *t*-value would have to be 2.88 or higher for the means to be considered unequal.[19] To provide a more precise indication of significance, the program reports the actual computed *P*-value. If the computed *P*-value is smaller than a selected *P*-value (e.g., 0.05 or 0.01, depending on desired stringency), the means of the two data sets are unequal and the difference is statistically significant. If the computed *P*-value is larger than the selected *P*-value, the means of the two data sets are not unequal. Table 3.3 illustrates a typical *t*-test result.

When the *t*-test indicates that two sample means are *not unequal,* the operator may choose to implement the new or modified assay. However, statistically, if two means are judged not unequal, that is not the same as *equal.* To increase the power of the validation, the laboratory professional often chooses to compute the *Pearson correlation coefficient* and to apply *linear regression* and the *Bland-Altman plot.*[20]

Using Analysis of Variance to Compare Variances of More Than Two Data Sets

ANOVA accomplishes the same outcomes as the Student *t*-test; however, ANOVA may be applied to more than two sets of data. A laboratory professional may choose to compare two, three, or four new methods with a reference method. ANOVA computes variance (σ^2) within each group (within-group σ^2), an overall σ^2 (between-group σ^2), and an *F*-statistic (similar to the *t*-statistic) based on dividing the between-group σ^2 by the within-group σ^2. The *F*-statistic is compared with a table of critical *F*-statistic values to determine significance analogous to the *t*-statistic as shown in Table 3.4.

Similar to the Student *t*-test, ANOVA is available on computer spreadsheets. The operator enters the data in one column per data set (group or sample) and applies the ANOVA formula. The test reports *between-groups df* (the number of groups – 1) and the *within-group df* (total of data points – 1 per group). The test also computes and reports the sum of squares within and between groups, the total sum of squares, the mean squares within and between groups, and the *F*-statistic. Spreadsheet programs compare the *F*-statistic with the table of critical *F*-values and report the *P*-value, which the operator then compares with the selected *P*-value limit to determine significance. Table 3.5 illustrates typical ANOVA results.

Comparing Data Sets Using the Pearson Correlation Coefficient

In addition to comparing means by the Student *t*-test or variances by ANOVA, the laboratory professional compares a set

TABLE 3.4   Excerpt From the Standard Table of Critical *t*-Values for a Two-Tailed Test*

df	P ≤ 0.05	P ≤ 0.01	df	P ≤ 0.05	P ≤ 0.01	df	P ≤ 0.05	P ≤ 0.01
2	t = 4.30	t = 9.93	12	2.18	3.06	22	2.07	2.82
4	2.78	4.60	14	2.15	2.98	24	2.06	2.80
6	2.45	3.71	16	2.12	2.92	26	2.06	2.78
8	2.31	3.36	18	2.10	2.88	28	2.05	2.76
10	2.23	3.17	20	2.09	2.85	30	2.04	2.75

*The quality control specialist matches the *df* with the test and looks up the critical *t*-value at the selected level of significance, often $P \leq 0.05$ or $P \leq 0.01$. If the computed *t*-value exceeds the critical *t*-value from the table, the null hypothesis is rejected, the means of the data sets are unequal, and the difference between the means is statistically significant.
df, Degrees of freedom.

TABLE 3.5   Typical Analysis of Variance Results*

SUMMARY OF DESCRIPTIVE STATISTICS PROVIDED WITH AUTOMATED ANOVA

Group	n	Σ	$\overline{X}$	σ^2
Reference	25	63.74	2.55	1.07
Test 1	25	61.17	2.45	0.60
Test 2	25	65.08	2.60	0.68

ANOVA EXAMPLE

Variation Source	df	SS	MS	F	Critical F-value, P ≤ 0.05	P-value
Between groups	2	0.32	0.17	0.20	3.12	0.82
Within groups	72	56.37	0.78			
Total	74	56.69				

*The computed *F*-value does not exceed the critical *F*-value from the table of critical values. The computed *P*-value exceeds the selected *P*-value of 0.05. This test fails statistical significance at $P \leq 0.05$; the null hypothesis is supported, and there is no significant difference among the groups.
$\overline{X}$, Mean; *ANOVA,* analysis of variance; *df,* degrees of freedom; *MS,* mean squares; *SS,* sum of squares.

of paired data to learn if the data points agree with adequate precision throughout the AMR. For instance, to validate a new prothrombin time reagent, the laboratory professional assembles 100 plasma aliquots, assays them in sequence using first the new and then the current reagents, and records the paired data points in two spreadsheet columns, *x* and *y*. The laboratory professional then applies the spreadsheet's *Pearson correlation coefficient* formula to generate a Pearson *r*, or *correlation coefficient,* which may range from −1.0 to +1.0. The spreadsheet uses this formula:

$$r = \frac{\left(\Sigma xy / n - \overline{XY} \right)}{SD_X SD_Y},$$

where r = Pearson correlation coefficient; Σxy = sum of the products of each pair of scores; n = number of values; $\bar{X}$ = mean of the x distribution; $\bar{Y}$ = mean of the y distribution; SD_X = standard deviation of the x distribution; and SD_Y = standard deviation of the y distribution.

Pearson r-values from 0 to +1.0 represent positive correlation; 1.0 equals perfect correlation. Laboratory professionals employ the Pearson formula to assess the range of values from two like assays or to compare assay results with previously assigned standard or calibrator results. Most operators set an r-value of 0.975 (or r^2-value of 0.95) as the lower limit of correlation; any Pearson r-value less than 0.975 is considered invalid because it indicates unacceptable variation from the reference method.

When the Pearson r-value result indicates the adequacy of the range of values, the linear regression r-value equation described in the next section is applied. Linear regression finds the line that best predicts x from y, but the equation for linear regression does not account for dispersion. The Pearson correlation coefficient formula quantifies how x and y vary together while documenting dispersion.

Comparing Data Sets Using Linear Regression

If a set of five calibrator dilutions is tested by both a new and a reference assay, results may be analyzed by the following regression equation:

$$y = a + bx$$
$$\text{slope}(b) = \left[n\,\Sigma XY - (\Sigma X)(\Sigma Y) \right] / \left[n\,\Sigma X^2 - (\Sigma X)^2 \right]$$
$$\text{Intercept}(a) = \left[\Sigma Y - b(\Sigma X) \right] / n,$$

where x and y are the variables; a = the intercept between the regression line and the y-axis; b = the slope of the regression line; n = number of values or data points; X = first calibrator value; Y = second calibrator value; ΣXY = sum of the product of first and second calibrator values; ΣX = sum of first calibrator values; ΣY = sum of second calibrator values; and ΣX^2 = sum of squared first calibrator values.

Perfect correlation generates a *slope* of 1 and a *y intercept* of 0 and is illustrated as a *line of identity* on a graph when plotting the values (data points) of the new versus the reference assay (Figure 3.2). Local policy based on total error calculation establishes limits for slope and y intercept; for example, many laboratory directors reject a slope of <0.9 or >1.10, or an intercept of more than 10% above or below zero.

Slope measures *proportional systematic error*; the higher the analyte value, the greater the deviation from the line of identity. Proportional errors are caused by malfunctioning instrument components or a failure of some part of the testing process. The magnitude of the error increases with the concentration or activity of the analyte. An assay with proportional error may be invalid.

Intercept measures *constant systematic error* (or *bias,* in laboratory vernacular), a constant difference between the new assay and reference assay regardless of assay result magnitude. A laboratory director may choose to adopt a new assay with constant systematic error but must modify the published RI.

Regression analysis gains sufficient power when 40 or more patient specimens are tested using both the new assay and the reference assay in place of or in addition to calibrators. Data may be entered into a spreadsheet program that offers an automatic regression equation.

Comparing Data Sets Using the Bland-Altman Difference Plot

Linear regression and the Pearson correlation coefficient are essential tests of accuracy and performance; however, both are influenced by dispersion. The Bland-Altman difference plot, also known as the Tukey mean-difference plot, provides a graphical representation of agreement between two assays.[21] Similar to the t-test, the Pearson correlation, and linear regression, paired assay results are tabled in automated spreadsheet columns. This formula is applied:

$$S(x,y) = (S_1 + S_2)/2, \text{ and } S_1 - S_2,$$

where S = individual coordinates.

The operator computes the mean value of each specimen by the two assays and the signed difference between the values. A chart is prepared with the means plotted on the x-axis and the numerical or percentage differences on the y-axis. Reference limits (cut points, thresholds, decision limits, decision points, target points) are provided, characteristically at $\bar{X} \pm 2$ SD (Figure 3.3). The plot visually illustrates the magnitude of the differences. In a normal (Gaussian) distribution, 95.5% of the values are expected to fall within the reference limits; when more than 5% of the data points fall outside the reference limits, the assay is rejected.

Precision

In contrast to accuracy, the assessment of precision (dispersion, reproducibility, variation, random error) is a simple validation effort because it merely requires performing a series of assays on a single specimen or lot of reference material (Figure 3.1).[22] Precision studies always assess both *within-day* and *day-to-day* variation (random error) about the mean.[23] Unlike accuracy, precision studies are usually performed on three to five calibration specimens or QC material, although they may also be performed using a set of patient specimens. Managers of smaller laboratories may choose to test only two specimens or more typically QC material. To establish within-day precision reference limits using two specimens, the QC specialist selects one specimen within the RI and the other outside the RI of the analyte. They are assayed 20 consecutive times using the same reagent batch and one test run. For identical instruments, the same method is also followed for the second instrument. For day-to-day precision, 20 assays are required on at least 5 runs on 5 consecutive days. The day-to-day precision study employs the same source specimen and instrument but separate aliquots and is performed using the QC material. If patient specimens are used in coagulation precision studies, aliquots should be prepared and frozen until ready for each run. Day-to-day precision accounts for the effects of different operators, reagents, and environmental conditions such as

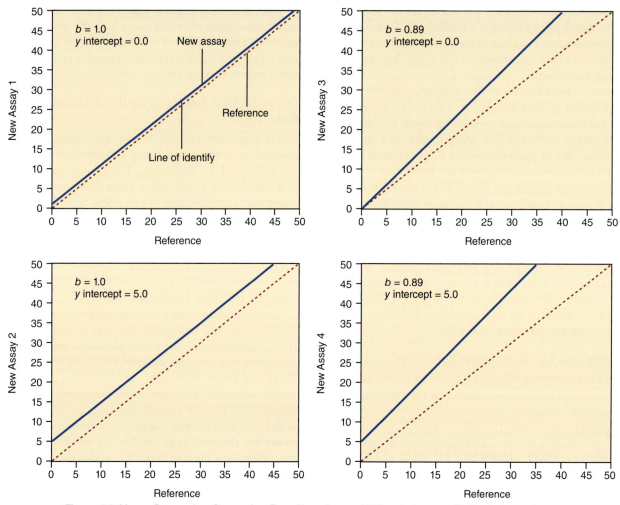

Figure 3.2 Linear Regression Comparing Four New Assays With a Reference Method. Assay 1 correlates perfectly with the reference method and generates a line of identity in which the slope *(b)* is 1.0 and the *y* intercept is 0.0. The *y* intercept of assay 2 is 5.0, which illustrates a constant systematic error, or bias. The slope *(b)* value for assay 3 is 0.89, which illustrates a proportional systematic error. Assay 4 has both bias and proportional error. Regression analysis gains sufficient power when 40 or more specimens (calibrators and/or patients) are tested using both the new and the reference assay.

temperature and barometric pressure. No matter what materials are used in precision studies, their levels should be close to clinically significant decision points.

The collected data from within-day and day-to-day sequences are reduced by formulas to the mean and a measure of dispersion such as SD or, most often, coefficient of variation in percent (CV%), as described before in "Statistical Significance and Expressions of Central Tendency and Dispersion." The CV% documents the degree of dispersion or random error generated by an assay, a function of assay stability.

The CV% limits are established locally. For analytes based on primary standards, the within-run CV% limit may be 5% or less, and for hematology assays, it may be 10% or less. For hemostasis assays, the CV% limits are defined in the reagent package insert or application sheets and can range from 5% to 20%; however, the day-to-day run CV% limits may be as high as 30%, depending on the stability and complexity of the assay. Although accuracy, linearity, AMR,

and interferences are just as important, laboratory professionals often equate the quality of an assay with its CV%. The best assay is one that combines the smallest CV% with the greatest accuracy.

Precision for visual light microscopy leukocyte differential counts on stained blood films is broad, particularly for low-frequency eosinophils and basophils.[24] Most visual differential counts are performed by reviewing 100 to 200 leukocytes. Although impractical, it would take differential counts of 800 or more leukocytes to improve precision to measurable, though inadequate levels. Differential counts generated by automated blood cell analyzers, however, provide CV% levels of 5% or lower because these instruments count thousands of cells.

Linearity and the Analytical Measurement Range

Linearity is the ability to generate results proportional to the calculated concentration or activity of the analyte.[25] The QC

Specimen	PTT 1	PTT 2	(S1+S2)/2	S1-S2	Difference, %
1	31.5	31.1	31.3	−0.4	−1.3
2	30.0	29.9	30.0	−0.1	−0.3
3	34.3	33.5	33.9	−0.8	−2.4
4	35.6	34.7	35.2	−0.9	−2.6
5	28.6	28.2	28.4	−0.4	−1.4
6	30.8	30.3	30.6	−0.5	−1.6
7	28.1	28.4	28.3	0.3	1.1
8	28.0	28.0	28.0	0.0	0.0
9	28.6	28.1	28.4	−0.5	−1.8
10	29.4	29.2	29.3	−0.2	−0.7

There was a total of 31 data points, 10 of which are shown.

A

Parameter	Value
n	31 (see table A for 10 of the data points)
r^2	0.999 (target ≥ 0.95)
Slope	1.05 (target = 0.9–1.1)
Intercept	1.08
$\overline{X}$ PTT 1 (reference assay)	48.09
$\overline{X}$ PTT 2	47.73
$\overline{X}$ of means (used for Bland-Altman correlation)	47.91
$\overline{X}$ difference	0.36
$\overline{X}$ difference, %	0.98
$\overline{X}$ difference, %/A versus B	0.8 (target = ±8%)
Minimum difference, %	3.92
Maximum difference, %	3.95
Maximum PTT result in seconds	110.02

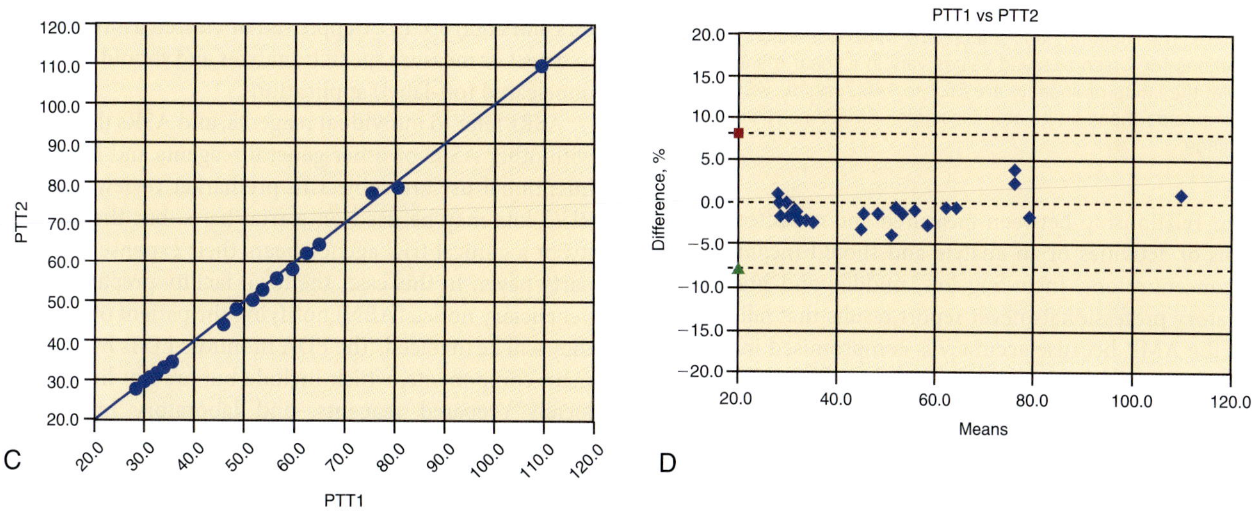

B

C

D

Figure 3.3 Bland-Altman Data and Plot. (A), Excerpt illustrating 10 of the 31 PTT result data points from a current and new reagent. (B), Preliminary correlation data. (C), Identity line. (D), Bland-Altman plot based on the 31 PTT result data points. The differences between the results from each assay are within the reference limits; the new PTT assay is validated. *PTT,* Partial thromboplastin time.

specialist dilutes a high-level calibrator to produce at least five dilutions spanning the full range of the assay. Many analyzers are programmed to make these dilutions as part of the calibration process. The instrument assays each dilution at least twice, sometimes in triplicate. The computed values and assayed results for each dilution are paired and plotted on a linear graph—x-scale and y-scale, respectively. The line is inspected visually for nonlinearity at the highest and lowest dilutions (Figure 3.4). The acceptable range of linearity is established just above the low value and below the high value at which linearity loss is evident. Although formulas exist for computing the limits of linearity, visual inspection is an accepted practice. Nonlinear results may be transformed using semilog or log-log graphs when necessary. Current coagulation analyzers provide computed results with a pass or fail result after calibration.

During assay runs, patient specimens with results above the linear range must be diluted and reassayed. Coagulation analyzers perform this operation automatically, for example, for fibrinogen and D-dimer. Results from diluted specimens that fall within the linear range are valid; however, they must be multiplied by the dilution factor (reciprocal of the dilution) to produce the final concentration. Lower limits are especially important when counting platelets or assaying coagulation factors. For example, the difference between <1% and 3% coagulation factor VIII activity affects treatment options and the potential for predicting coagulation factor inhibitor formation. Likewise, the difference between a platelet count of 10,000/μL and 5000/μL affects the decision to treat with platelet concentrate.

Whereas linearity is the ability to generate a result that is proportional to the expected value, the AMR defines the upper and lower limits of those values. Verification of the AMR proves

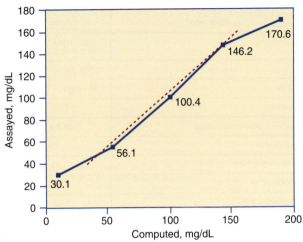

Figure 3.4 Linearity Determination. The operator or instrument prepares at least five dilutions of standard or calibrator. Dilutions must span the AMR. The concentration of the analyte for each of the five dilutions is calculated and expressed as a unit such as mg/dL. The assayed values are plotted on the *y* scale, and the computed values are plotted on the *x* scale. The linear range is selected by visual inspection, containing the dilutions for which assayed values vary in a linear manner. In this example, the limits of linearity are 56.1 to 146.2 mg/dL. Assay results that fall outside these limits are inaccurate. *AMR,* Analytical measurement range.

a linear relationship between measured and expected concentrations or activities of an analyte and should include at least four concentrations, including low, middle, and high values. Laboratory professionals never report results that fall below or above the AMR because accuracy is compromised in the nonlinear regions of the assay.

Analytical Sensitivity (Lower Limit of Detection)

Analytical sensitivity (lower limit of detection [LLD]) assays are coupled with linearity and AMR studies and are required of local laboratory professionals when modifying an FDA-approved assay or developing an LDT.[26] A *zero calibrator,* or blank, is assayed 10 to 20 times, and the mean and SD are computed from the results. The LLD is computed as 3 SD above the mean of blank assay results. This limit prevents false-positive results generated by low-end assay interference, commonly called *noise.* The manufacturer or distributor typically performs limit assays in compliance with the FDA and provides the results in the package insert; however, local policies may require that results of the manufacturer's limit studies be confirmed.

Analytical Specificity

Analytical specificity is the ability of an assay to distinguish the analyte of interest from anticipated interfering substances within the specimen matrix. The laboratory professional employs a subject's specimens known to contain potential interferences (pending subject consent) or spiked specimens with potential interfering substances and measures the effects of each on the assay results. Except for laboratory-developed tests (LDTs) or modifications of FDA-approved assays, analytical specificity is determined by the manufacturer and need not be confirmed at the local laboratory unless there is suspicion

of interference from a particular substance not assayed by the manufacturer. Common interferences include hemolysis, lipemia, and icterus. Manufacturer specificity data are transferred from the package insert to the laboratory validation report. QC specialists publish procedures on how to address the results of a specimen known to contain an interfering substance. Interference studies allow the laboratory director to intervene when a form of interference may compromise a laboratory result, for instance, when hemolysis affects the results of a chromogenic assay.

Levels of Laboratory Assay Approval

The FDA categorizes assays as *approved, cleared, modified-cleared, analyte-specific reagent* (ASR), *research use only* (RUO), and *laboratory-developed test* ("home-brew" tests).[27] When a local laboratory professional modifies an approved or cleared assay, the assay becomes categorized as modified-cleared. For instance, some facilities employ chromogenic anti-factor Xa heparin assays for rivaroxaban and apixaban using ASR calibrators and controls. FDA-approved or cleared assays are approved to detect or measure specific analytes and should not be used for noncleared (off-label) applications.

ASRs refer to individual reagents, and ASRs that are bundled with other ASRs or other general reagents and labeled with an intentional use are subject to premarket review requirements. RUO kits may be used on a trial basis, but the patient, facility, or a clinical trial agency bears their expense, not the third-party payer. In this case, the local facility prepares an advance beneficiary notice (ABN) notifying the patient of the possibility they will be invoiced. The FDA monitors LDTs by regulating the main components, which include but are not limited to ASRs, locally prepared reagents, and laboratory instrumentation. Details are given in Table 3.6.

Documentation and Reliability

Validation is recorded on standard forms available from commercial sources, such as the Data Innovations EP Evaluator. Requirements established in the Clinical Laboratory Improvement Amendments of 1988 (CLIA) include that validation records are stored for at least 2 years in readily accessible databases and made available to laboratory assessors on request.[28,29]

Precision and accuracy records document assay reliability over specified periods. The recalibration interval may be once every 6 months or in accordance with operators' manual recommendations. Recalibration is necessary whenever reagent lots are updated unless the laboratory professional can demonstrate that the reportable range is unchanged using lot-to-lot comparison. When control results demonstrate a shift or consistently fall outside reference limits, or when an instrument is repaired, the laboratory professional repeats the validation procedure and maintains the records.

Regularly scheduled validity rechecks, lot-to-lot comparisons, instrument preventive maintenance, staff competence, and scheduled performance of internal QC and external quality assessment procedures ensure continued reliability and enhance the value of a laboratory assay to the patient and provider.

TABLE 3.6 **Categories of Assay Approval by the US Food and Drug Administration**

Laboratory Assay Category	Comment
FDA-approved or cleared assay	Local facility may use package insert data for linearity, interferences, and specificity, but must establish clinical accuracy and precision.
Modified-cleared assay	Local facility modifies FDA-approved or cleared assay.
ASR	Manufacturer may provide individual reagents but not in kit form and may not provide package insert validation data. Reagents are not promoted for use on specific instruments or in specific assays. Local facility performs all validation steps.
RUO	Local facility performs all validation steps. RUO assays are intended for clinical trials and third-party payers are not required to pay. Local facility prepares an ABN to indicate patient may be required to pay.
Laboratory-developed assay	Assay is devised locally ("home-brew"). FDA evaluates using criteria developed for FDA-approved or cleared assay kits.

ABN, Advance Beneficiary Notice; *ASR*, analyte-specific reagent; *FDA*, Food and Drug Administration; *RUO*, research use only.

MULTISITE VALIDATION

Many US health care systems operate multiple laboratories under a single CLIA license. These systems combine high-volume and low-volume laboratories, ranging from reference and medical center laboratories to acute care facilities, satellite clinics, and physicians' group offices. One facility, presumably the busiest and staffed with a QC specialist, serves as a central laboratory. Patients inevitably choose to have their work done at a variety of facilities, depending on provider availability or convenience.[30]

Although the QC specialist tries to achieve uniformity, the various sites may be equipped using instruments with different technologies from competing suppliers. Ideally, reagent manufacturers sequester single reagent lots to be shared among the laboratories; in many systems, however, individual facilities may employ variant sole-source reagents and kits. Nevertheless, providers at satellite sites prefer to rely on system-wide RIs that are uniformly interpretable at their individual locations.

System-Wide Comparability

Each site validates its instrument-reagent systems, perhaps relying on central laboratory support. Subsequently, the system is validated as a whole. The QC specialist verifies performance across the system with comparability studies that resemble proficiency surveys. These are required at least twice a year, reflecting proficiency survey agency schedules. Typically, the central laboratory QC specialist prepares subject specimens to distribute to satellite facility personnel. For coagulation, although fresh plasma would be ideal, volume requirements may necessitate the use of frozen or preserved pooled plasma, preserved aliquots from proficiency agencies, or QC materials. QC material is acceptable only if all the sites' reagents and QC materials share the same lot number, which may not apply if the coagulometers are different. For hematology, patient anticoagulated whole blood specimens or preserved QC materials may be used. System-wide comparison efforts are most effective when all facilities are using the same reagent lots and identical or at least similar equipment. In any event, the QC specialist compares satellite facility specimen results to analyze the accuracy of each location. Outliers trigger troubleshooting and remedial modifications.

Multisite Reference Interval and Therapeutic Range

Once an assay is validated, each facility develops an RI and, when applicable, a therapeutic range, using the principles described subsequently in "Reference Interval and Therapeutic Range Development." Specimen collection from 20 healthy subjects is a challenge for low-volume facilities, so laboratory professionals enlist the help of larger satellites, provided that both institutions serve similar population demographics. Practice guidelines discourage central laboratories from supplying healthy subject specimen aliquots to the entire system on the principle that their aliquots may not match local demographics. To reduce the inevitable confusion generated from multiple RIs, the central laboratory may develop and publish a system-wide RI from individual facility intervals, presuming the individual RIs are similar. For this purpose, the QC specialist employs a statistical program such as the Data Innovations EP Evaluator, which the specialist may choose to make available throughout the system for data collection. The computed central RI is distributed throughout the system and replaces individual RIs.

LOT-TO-LOT COMPARISONS

Laboratory managers reach agreements with vendors to sequester kit and reagent lots, thereby ensuring infrequent lot changes, optimistically no more than once a year.[31] The new reagent lot must arrive approximately 1 month before the laboratory runs out of the old lot so that *lot-to-lot comparisons* may be completed and differences resolved, if necessary. The QC specialist uses control or patient specimens and prepares a range of analyte dilutions, typically five, spanning the limits of linearity. If the reagent kits provide controls, these are also included, and all are assayed using the old and new reagent lots. Results are charted as illustrated in Table 3.7.

Reference limits vary by laboratory, but many QC specialists reject the new lot when more than one specimen data point pair generates a variance greater than 10% or when all variances are positive or negative. In the latter case, the new lot may be rejected, or it may be necessary to use the new lot but develop a new RI and therapeutic range. For several analytes, lot-to-lot comparisons include revalidation of the AMR.

REFERENCE INTERVAL AND THERAPEUTIC RANGE DEVELOPMENT

Once an assay is validated, the QC specialist develops the RI (previously called reference range). Some laboratory professionals use the vernacular phrase *normal range*; however,

TABLE 3.7 **Example of a Reagent Lot-to-Lot Comparison**

Specimen	Old Lot Value	New Lot Value	% Difference*
Low value	7	13	85.7
Low middle value	12	12	0
Middle value	20.5	19.4	−5.4
High middle value	31	19	−38.7
High value	48	48	0
Old kit control 1	9	11	22.2
Old kit control 2	22	24	9.1
New kit control 1	10	10	0
New kit control 2	24	24	0

*Negative % difference indicates the new lot value is below the old lot (reference) value. The new lot is rejected because the low and high middle value results differ by more than 10%.

statisticians prefer RI. Using strict mathematical definitions, *range* encompasses all assay results from largest to smallest, whereas *interval* is a statistic that trims outliers. The therapeutic range is correctly named because therapeutic ranges may not be computed with the same statistical rigor as the RI.

Direct Reference Interval Determination

To develop an RI using the direct computation method, the QC specialist carefully defines the desired healthy population and recruits representative subjects to provide blood specimens. The definition may, for example, exclude smokers, women taking oral contraceptives, and people using specified over-the-counter or prescription medications. Subjects may be paid. The number of male and female subjects should be approximately equal, and the eligible subjects should match the institution's population demographics. When practical, large-volume blood specimens are collected, aliquoted, and placed in long-term storage. For instance, plasma aliquots for coagulation RI development are stored for up to 12 months at or below −70° C. Laboratory directors may choose to purchase healthy subject specimen sets from plasma distributors, such as the frozen CRYO*check* Normal Donor Set (Precision BioLogic), which provides 25 carefully selected healthy subject plasmas for use in the hemostasis laboratory. These sets may be particularly useful for specialty coagulation testing when validated before implementation. For prothrombin times (PTs) and partial thromboplastin times (PTTs), healthy subject sets may generate narrow RIs that are impractical for daily application. It may also be impractical to develop local RIs for infants, children, or elderly adults such as those over 80 (Chapter 43).[32] In these cases, the laboratory director may choose to use published (textbook) RIs.[33] In general, although published RIs are available for educational and general discussion purposes, local laboratories must generate their own RIs for adults to most closely match the demographics of the area served by their institution.

The minimum number of healthy subject specimens (data points) required to develop an RI may be determined using statistical power computations; however, practical limitations prevail.[34] For a new assay with no currently established RI, a minimum of 120 data points is necessary. In most cases, however, the assay

manufacturer provides an RI in the package insert, and the local laboratory professionals need only assay 30 specimens, approximately 15 male and 15 female, to validate the manufacturer's RI, a process called *transference*. Likewise, the laboratory professional may refer to published RIs and, once they are locally validated, transfer them to the institution's report form.

QC specialists assume that the population specimens employed to generate RIs will produce frequency distributions (in laboratory vernacular, *histograms*) that are normal, bell-shaped (Gaussian) curves (Figure 3.5). In a Gaussian frequency distribution, the mean is at the center and coincides with the median, and the dispersion about the mean is identical in both directions. In many instances, however, biologic frequency distributions are log-normal with a tail on one end. For example, laboratory professionals assumed for years that the visual reticulocyte percentage RI in adults was 0.5% to 1.5%; however, repeated analysis of healthy populations in several locations has established the interval to be 0.5% to 2%, owing to a subset of healthy subjects whose reticulocyte counts fall at the high end of the interval.[35] QC specialists may employ a log-normal distribution, or they may transform the data and replot the curve using a semilog or log-log graphic display. The decision to transform may arise locally but eventually may become adopted as a national practice standard.

In a normal (Gaussian) distribution, the mean ($\overline{X}$) is computed by dividing the sum of the observed values by the number of data points, *n*, as shown in the equation provided in "Statistical Significance and Expressions of Central Tendency and Dispersion." The SD is calculated using the formula provided in the same section. A typical RI is computed as mean ±2 SD and assumes that the distribution is normal (Gaussian). Some laboratory directors prefer to set the reference limits using ±3 SD when the distribution is especially narrow. Reference limits at mean ±2 SD encompass 95.46% of results from healthy individuals, known as the *95.5% CI*. This implies that 4.54% of results from theoretically healthy individuals fall outside the interval by chance alone. An SD computed from a non-Gaussian distribution may turn out to be too narrow to reflect the true RI and may thus encompass less than 95.5% of results from presumed healthy subjects and generate an excess of false-positive results. Assays with high CV% values have high levels of random error reflected in a broad curve; low CV% assays with tight dispersion have smaller random error and generate a narrow curve, as illustrated in Figure 3.1. The breadth of the curve may also reflect biologic variation in analyte values.

Indirect Reference Interval Determination

Indirect RIs may be derived from stored patient data. The QC specialist mines the laboratory database to compute the mean and confidence interval. Indirect RI computation removes the need to identify, collect, assay, aliquot, and store representative specimens, while providing for a much larger sample size. The indirect RI may more closely represent facility demographics and permits for partition by age, sex, or physical condition. To eliminate presumed abnormal data points, the QC specialist applies robust statistical tests to exclude outliers and to sequester disease-related results in the final computation.[36]

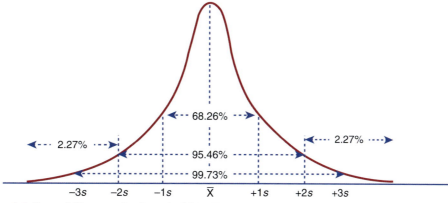

Figure 3.5 Normal (Symmetric, Gaussian) Distribution. When the test values obtained for a given subject population are normally distributed, the mean locates at the peak and the mean and median coincide. Segments of the population distribution representing ±1, ±2, and ±3 standard deviations are illustrated. In developing the reference interval (RI), laboratory directors often use ±2 standard deviations to establish the 95.5% confidence interval or, when the precision is constricted, ±3 standard deviations. The selection of ±2 standard deviations means that 95.46% of the test values from the healthy population are included within the reference interval. Consequently, 4.54%, or approximately 1 in 20 test results from theoretically healthy subjects, fall outside the interval, half (2.27%) above and half below. *s,* Standard deviation.

Therapeutic Target Range

A few hematology and hemostasis assays are used to monitor drug therapy. For instance, the INR for PT is used to monitor the effects of oral warfarin therapy, and the therapeutic range is universally established at an INR of 2 to 3. Conversely, the therapeutic range for monitoring unfractionated heparin treatment using the PTT assay must be established locally by graphically comparing a regression of the PTT results in seconds against the results of the *chromogenic anti-Xa heparin assay,* whose therapeutic range is established empirically as 0.3 to 0.7 international heparin units. The PTT therapeutic range is called the ex vivo *Brill-Edwards curve* and is described in Chapter 40.

If assay revalidation or lot-to-lot comparison reveals a systematic change caused by reagent or kit modifications, a new RI (and therapeutic range, when applicable) is established. The laboratory director must advise the hospital staff of RI and therapeutic range changes because failure to observe new intervals and ranges may result in diagnosis and treatment errors.

INTERNAL QUALITY CONTROL

Controls

Laboratory QC specialists prepare, or more often purchase, assay *controls*. Although it may appear similar, a control is wholly distinct from a calibrator. Indeed, cautious laboratory directors may insist that controls be purchased from distributors other than from those who supply their calibrators. As discussed previously in "Method Validation," calibrators are used to adjust or revalidate instrumentation or to develop a calibration curve. Calibrators are assayed by a reference method in expert laboratories, and their assigned value is certified. Controls are used independently of the calibration process so that systematic errors caused by deterioration of the calibrator or a change in the analytical process are detected through internal QC. This process is continuous and is called *calibration*

verification. Compared with calibrators, control materials are inexpensive and are prepared from the same matrix as patient specimens, except for preservatives, lyophilization, or freezing necessary to prolong shelf life. Controls provide known values and are assayed alongside patient specimens to accomplish within-run assay validation. In nearly all instances, two controls are required per test run: one within the RI and one above or below the RI. For some assays, there is reason to select controls whose values are just outside the upper or lower reference limits, or slightly abnormal. In institutions that perform continuous runs, the controls should be run at least once per shift, for instance, at 0700, 1300, and 2300. In laboratories where assay runs are discrete events, two controls are assayed with each run.

Control results must fall within predetermined reference limits, typically ±2 SD. Control manufacturers provide reference limits; however, local QC specialists must validate and transfer manufacturer reference limits or establish their own, usually by computing SD from the first 20 control assays, during which time the previous control lot remains in service. Whenever the result for a control is outside the established reference limits, the run is rejected, and the cause is found and corrected. The steps for correction are listed in Table 3.8.

Control results are plotted on a Levey-Jennings chart that displays each data point compared with the mean and reference limits (Figure 3.6).[37] The Levey-Jennings chart assumes that the control results distribute in a Gaussian manner and imprints reference limits at 1, 2, and 3 SD above and below the mean. In addition to being analyzed for single-run errors, the data points are examined for sequential errors over time (Figure 3.7). Both single-run and long-term control variation are a function of assay dispersion or random error and reflect the CV% of an assay.

Westgard established a series of internal QC rules that are routinely applied to long-term deviations, called the Westgard rules.[38] The rules were developed for assays that

TABLE 3.8   Steps Used to Correct an Out-of-Control Assay Run

Step	Description
1. Reassay	When a reference limit of ±2 SD is used, 5% of expected assay results fall above or below the limit.
2. Prepare new control and reassay	Controls may deteriorate over time when exposed to adverse temperatures or subjected to conditions causing evaporation.
3. Prepare fresh reagents and reassay	Reagents may have evaporated or become contaminated.
4. Recalibrate instrument	Instrument may require repair.

SD, Standard deviation.

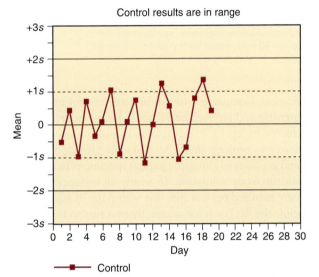

Figure 3.6 **Levey-Jennings Chart Illustrating Acceptable Control Results.** Control results from 19 runs in 19 days fall within the reference limits established as ±2 standard deviations. Results distribute evenly about the mean. *s*, Standard deviation.

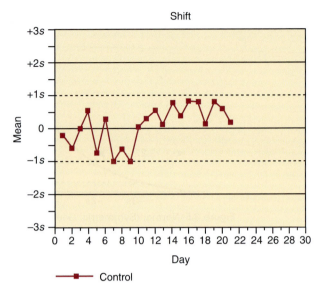

Figure 3.7 **Levey-Jennings Chart Illustrating a Systematic Error.** Control results from 21 runs in 21 days fall within the reference limits established as ±2 standard deviations; however, the final 11 control results locate above the mean. When 10 consecutive control results fall on one side of the mean, the assay has been affected by a systematic error, in this case a *Westgard 10$_X$* condition, also called a *shift* (Table 3.9). The operator troubleshoots and recalibrates the assay. *s*, Standard deviation.

TABLE 3.9   Westgard Rules Employed in Hematology and Hemostasis*

1$_{3S}$	A single control value is outside the ±3 SD reference limit.
2$_{2S}$	Two control values are outside the ±2 SD reference limit.
R$_{4S}$	Two consecutive control values within a run are more than 4 SD apart.
4$_{1S}$	Four consecutive control values within a run exceed the mean by ±1 SD.
10$_X$	Also called a *shift*. A series of 10 consecutive control values remain within the reference limits but are consistently above or below the mean.
7$_T$	Also called a *trend*. A series of at least 7 control values trends in a consistent direction.

10$_X$ or 7$_T$ may indicate an instrument calibration issue that has introduced a constant systematic error (bias). Shifts or trends may be caused by deterioration of reagents, pump fittings, or light sources. Abrupt shifts may reflect a reagent or instrument fitting change.

*In all cases, assay results are rejected, and the error is identified using the steps in Table 3.8.
SD, Standard deviation.

employ primary standards, but a few Westgard rules that are the most useful in hematology and hemostasis laboratories are provided in Table 3.9, along with the appropriate actions to be taken.

Moving Average ($\overline{X}_B$) of Red Blood Cell Indices

In 1974 Bull and colleagues[39] proposed a method of employing *patient* RBC indices to monitor the stability of automated blood cell analyzers, recognizing that the RBC indices mean cell volume (MCV), mean cell hemoglobin (MCH), and mean cell hemoglobin concentration (MCHC) remain consistent on average despite individual patient variations. Each consecutive sequence of 20 patient RBC index assay results is collected and treated by the moving average formula (in reference), which accumulates, "smooths," and "trims" data to reduce the effects of outliers. Each trimmed 20-specimen mean, $\overline{X}_B$, is plotted on a Levey-Jennings chart and tracked for trends and shifts using Westgard rules. The formula has been automated and embedded in the circuitry of automated blood cell analyzers, which provide Levey-Jennings charts for MCV, MCH, and MCHC.

The moving average concept has been generalised to WBC and platelet counts and to some clinical chemistry analytes, albeit with moderate success.

To begin, 500 consecutive specimens are analyzed for the mean MCV, MCH, and MCHC. A Levey-Jennings chart is prepared using ±3% of the mean or 1 SD as the reference limits, and subsequent data accumulation commences in groups of 20.

The moving average method requires a computer to calculate the averages, does not detect within-run errors, and is less sensitive than the use of commercial controls in detecting systematic shifts and trends. It works well in institutions that assay specimens from generalised populations that contain minimal numbers of sickle cell or oncology patients. A population that has a high percentage of abnormal hematologic results, as may be seen in a tertiary care facility, may generate a preponderance of moving average outliers.[40] Moving average systems do not replace the use of control specimens but rather, provide additional means to detect shifts and trends.

Delta Checks

The delta check system compares a current analyte result with the result from the most recent previous analysis for the same patient.[41] Certain patient values remain relatively consistent over time unless there is an intervention. A result that fails a delta check, often defined as a 20% deviation, is investigated for an intervention such as a transfusion or surgery or for a profound change in the patient's condition since the previous analysis. If there is no ready clinical explanation, the failed delta check may indicate an analytical error or mislabeled specimen. In hemostasis, failed delta checks should also encompass a review of specimen collection errors. Results that fail a delta check are sequestered until the cause is found. Laboratory directors may require delta checks on MCV, red cell distribution width (RDW), HGB, platelet count (PLT), PT, INR, and PTT. Reference limits for delta checks are based on clinical impression and are assigned by hematology and hemostasis laboratory directors in collaboration with providers and laboratory staff. Computerization is essential, and delta checks are designed only to identify gross errors, not changes in random error, or shifts or trends. There is no regulatory requirement for delta checks.

EXTERNAL QUALITY ASSESSMENT

External quality assessment further validates the accuracy of hematology and hemostasis assays by comparing results from identical aliquots of specimens distributed at regular intervals among laboratories nationwide or worldwide. The aliquots are often called *survey* or *proficiency testing* specimens and include preserved human subject plasma and whole blood, stained peripheral blood films and bone marrow smears, and photomicrographs of cells or tissues.

In most proficiency testing systems, reference limits for the test specimens are established in-house by their manufacturer or distributor and are then further validated by preliminary distribution to a handful of "expert" laboratories. Separate reference limits may be assigned for various assay methods and instruments, as feasible.

Laboratories that participate in external quality assessment are directed to manage the survey specimens using the same procedures as those employed for patient specimens—that is, survey specimens should not receive special attention. Turnaround is swift, and results are sent electronically to the proficiency testing agency.

In addition to establishing an RI and reference limits, agencies that administer surveys reduce the returned data to statistics, including the mean, median, and SD of all participant results. Provided that the survey is large enough, the statistics may also be computed individually for the various instruments and assay methods. The statistics collected from participants should match the predetermined RIs. If they do not, the agency troubleshoots the assay and assigns the most reliable statistics, usually the group mean and SD.

The agency provides a report to each laboratory, illustrating its results in comparison with the RIs and limits and appending a comment if the laboratory result exceeds the established reference limits, usually ±2 SD from the mean. For example, survey results are attached with "acceptable" or "not acceptable" comments or result codes with detailed explanations. If the specimen is a blood film or bone marrow smear, a photomicrograph, or a problem that requires a binary (positive/negative, yes/no) response, the local laboratory comment is compared with expert opinion and consensus.

Although a certain level of error is tolerated, error rates that exceed established reference limits result in corrective recommendations or, in extreme circumstances, loss of laboratory accreditation or licensure.

There are several external quality assessment agencies; however, in the United States the College of American Pathologists (CAP; https://www.cap.org/) and the American Proficiency Institute (API; https://api-pt.com/) provide the largest survey systems. Survey packages are provided for laboratories offering all levels of service. The API and CAP are nongovernmental agencies; however, survey participation is necessary to meet the accreditation requirements of The Joint Commission (https://www.jointcommission.org/) and to qualify for Medicare reimbursement. The North American Specialized Coagulation Laboratory Association (NASCOLA; https://www.nascola.com/) provides survey systems for specialty coagulation laboratories in the United States and Canada, and is affiliated with the External Quality Control of Diagnostic Assays and Tests (ECAT; https://www.ecat.nl/) Foundation External Quality Assessment Program of The Netherlands, which provides survey materials throughout Europe. Many state health agencies provide proficiency testing surveys, requiring laboratories to participate as a condition of licensure.

ASSESSING DIAGNOSTIC EFFICACY

Since the 1930s, surgeons have required the *bleeding time* test to predict the risk of intraoperative hemorrhage. The laboratory professional activates an automated lancet to make a 5-mm long, 1-mm deep incision in the volar surface of the forearm and uses a clean piece of filter paper to meticulously absorb drops of blood in 30-second intervals. The time interval from initial incision to bleeding cessation is recorded, typically 2 to 9 minutes. The test is simple and logical, and experts have claimed for more than 50 years that if the incision bleeds for longer than 9 minutes, there is a risk of surgical bleeding. In the 1990s clinical researchers compared within-range and prolonged bleeding times with instances of intraoperative bleeding and found to their surprise that prolonged bleeding time results predicted less than 50% of intraoperative bleeds.[42,43] Often, bleeds occurred despite a bleeding time shorter than 9 minutes.

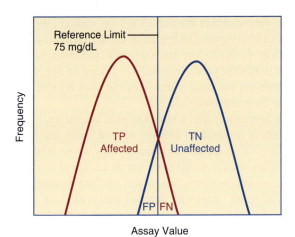

Figure 3.8 Typical Bimodal Clinical Efficacy Frequency Distribution. The intersection between a disease-affected and a healthy (unaffected) population with an assay reference limit of 75 mg/dL is illustrated. To the left of the reference limit is the segment of 45 true-positives *(TP)* in the disease (affected) arm and 10 false-positives *(FP)* in the healthy (unaffected) arm. To the right of the reference limit is the segment of 40 true-negatives *(TN)* in the healthy (unaffected) arm and 5 false-negatives *(FN)* in the disease (affected) arm. The goal for a new assay is to establish the limit at the point that generates the smallest false-positive and false-negative results.

Thus the positive predictive value of the bleeding time for intraoperative bleeding was less than 50%, which is the probability of turning up heads in a coin toss. Today the bleeding time test is widely agreed to have no clinical efficacy and is obsolete, though still available.

Similar to the bleeding time test, many time-honored hematology and hemostasis assays gained credibility based on logic and expert opinion. Now, however, besides being valid, accurate, linear, and precise, a new or modified assay must be diagnostically effective.[44] To compute diagnostic efficacy, the QC specialist obtains a series of specimens from healthy subjects, volunteers who do not have the disease or condition being measured, called *controls,* and from patients who *conclusively possess a disease or condition.* The diagnosis in patients is based on downstream clinical outcomes, discharge notes, or the results of valid existing laboratory tests, excluding the new assay. The new assay is then applied to specimens from both the healthy control and the disease patient groups to assess its efficacy.

In a perfect world, the laboratory scientist sets the reference limit at the 95.5% CI limit (±2 SD) of the mean. When the reference limit is used, the test hopefully yields a positive result, meaning a level elevated beyond the upper reference limit or reduced to less than the lower reference limit, in every instance of disease and a negative result, within the RI, in all subjects (controls) without the disease. In reality, there is always some overlap: a gray area in which some positive test results are generated from nondisease specimens (*false-positives*) and some negative results are generated from specimens taken from patients with proven disease (*false-negatives*) (Figure 3.8). False-positives cause unnecessary anxiety, follow-up expense, and erroneous diagnostic leads—worrisome, expensive, and time-consuming, but seldom fatal. False-negatives fail to detect the disease and may delay treatment, a potentially life-threatening circumstance. The QC specialist

employs diagnostic efficacy computations to establish the effectiveness of laboratory assays and to minimize both false-positive and false-negative results (Table 3.10). Diagnostic efficacy testing includes determination of diagnostic sensitivity and specificity, positive and negative *predictive value,* and *receiver operating characteristic* (ROC) analysis.

To start a diagnostic efficacy study, the QC specialist or researcher selects control specimens from healthy subjects and specimens from patients proven to have the disease or condition addressed by the assay. To make this discussion simple, assume that 50 specimens of each are chosen. All are assayed and the results are shown in Table 3.11. The QC specialist next computes diagnostic sensitivity and specificity and positive and negative predictive value as shown in Table 3.12. These values are then used to consider the conditions in which the assay may be effectively employed.

Effects of Population Incidence and Odds Ratios on Diagnostic Efficacy

Epidemiologists describe population events using the terms *prevalence* and *incidence. Prevalence* describes the total number of events or conditions in a broadly defined population, for instance, the total number of patients with chronic heart disease in the United States. Prevalence quantitates the burden of a disease on society but is not qualified by time intervals and does not predict disease risk.

Incidence describes the number of events occurring within a randomly selected number of subjects representing a population over a defined time, for instance, the number of new cases of heart disease per 100,000 US residents per year. Incidence numbers are noncumulative. Incidence can be further defined, for instance, by the number of heart disease cases per 100,000 nonsmokers, 100,000 women, or 100,000 people ages 40 to 50. Medical laboratory professionals and QC specialists use incidence, not prevalence, to select laboratory assays for specific applications such as screening or confirmation.

For all assays, as diagnostic sensitivity increases, specificity decreases. A *screening* test is an assay that is applied to many subjects within a convenience sample where the participant's condition is unknown, for example, lipid profiles offered in a shopping mall. Assays that possess high sensitivity and low specificity make effective screening tests, although they produce many false-positives. For instance, if the condition being studied has an incidence of 0.0001 (1 in 10,000 per year) and the false-positive rate is a modest 1%, the assay will produce 99 false-positive results for every true-positive result. Clearly, such a test is useful only when the consequence of a false-positive result is minimal and follow-up confirmation is readily available.

Conversely, as specificity increases, sensitivity decreases. Assays with high specificity provide effective confirmation when used in follow-up to positive results on screening assays. High-specificity assays produce some false-negatives and should not be used as initial screening assays. A positive result on both a screening assay and a confirmatory assay provides a definitive conclusion. A positive screening result followed by a negative confirmatory test result generates a search for alternative diagnoses.

Laboratory assays are most effective when chosen to assess patients with high clinical pretest probability. In such instances, the incidence of the condition is high enough to mitigate the effects of false-positives and false-negatives. For instance, when a provider orders hemostasis testing for patients who are experiencing easy bruising, there is a high pretest probability, which raises the diagnostic efficacy of the assays. Conversely, ordering hemostasis assays as screens of healthy individuals before elective surgery introduces a low pretest probability and reduces the efficacy of the test profile, raising the relative rate of false-positives.

Epidemiologists further assist laboratory professionals by designing prospective randomized controlled trials to predict the relative odds ratio (or relative risk ratio [RRR]) and the absolute odds ratio (or absolute risk ratio [ARR]) of an intervention that is designed to modify the incidence of an event within a selected population. This is illustrated in the following example.[45]

You design a 5-year study in which you select 2000 obese smokers ages 40 to 60 who have no heart disease. You randomly select 1000 for intervention: periodic laboratory assays for inflammatory markers, with follow-up aspirin for those who have positive assay results. The 1000 controls are tested with the same laboratory assays but are given a placebo that resembles aspirin. The primary end point is acute myocardial infarction (AMI). No one dies or drops out, and at the end of 5 years, 100 of the 1000 control subjects and 50 of the 1000 subjects in the intervention arm have experienced AMIs. The control arm ratio is $100/1000 = 0.1$, the intervention arm ratio is $50/1000 = 0.05$, and the RRR is $0.05/0.1 = 0.5$ (50%). You predict from your study that the odds (RRR) of having a heart attack are cut in half by the intervention. You repeat the study using 2000 slim nonsmokers ages 20 to 40. In this sample, 10 of the 1000 control subjects and 5 subjects in the intervention group experience AMIs; the computation is $0.005/0.01 = 0.5$, the same as in the obese smoker group, thus enabling you to generalie your obese smoker results to slim nonsmokers. RRR has been used extensively to support widespread medical interventions, often without regard to control arm incidence or the risks associated with generalizing to nonstudied populations.

TABLE 3.10 Diagnostic Efficacy Definitions and Binary Display

True-positive	Assay correctly identifies a disease or condition in patients who have the disease or condition.
True-negative	Assay correctly excludes a disease or condition in patients without it.
False-positive	Assay incorrectly identifies a disease or condition when none is present.
False-negative	Assay incorrectly excludes a disease or condition when it is present.

	Individuals Unaffected by Disease or Condition	Individuals Affected by Disease or Condition
Assay is negative	True-negative	False-negative
Assay is positive	False-positive	True-positive

TABLE 3.11 Diagnostic Efficacy Study*

	Unaffected by Disease or Condition	Affected by Disease or Condition
Assay is negative	True-negative: 40	False-negative: 5
Assay is positive	False-positive: 10	True-positive: 45

*These are data on specimens from 50 individuals who are unaffected by a disease or condition and 50 individuals who are affected by a disease or condition. These data are used in the calculations in Table 3.12.

TABLE 3.12 Diagnostic Efficacy Computations*

Statistic	Definition	Formula	Example
Diagnostic sensitivity	Proportion with a disease who have a positive test result	Sensitivity (%) = TP/(TP + FN) × 100	$45/(45 + 5) \times 100 = 90\%$
	Distinguish diagnostic sensitivity from analytical sensitivity. Analytical sensitivity is a measure of the smallest increment of the analyte that can be distinguished by the assay.		
Diagnostic specificity	Proportion without a disease who have a negative test result	Specificity (%) = TN/(TN + FP) × 100	$40/(40 + 10) \times 100 = 80\%$
	Distinguish diagnostic specificity from analytical specificity. Analytical specificity is the ability of the assay to distinguish the analyte from interfering substances.		
PPV	Proportion with a disease who have a positive test result compared with all individuals who have a positive test result	PPV (%) = TP/(TP + FP) × 100	$45/(45 + 10) \times 100 = 82\%$
	PPV predicts the probability that an individual with a positive assay result has the disease or condition.		
NPV	Proportion without a disease who have a negative test result compared with all individuals who have a negative test result	NPV (%) = TN/(TN + FN) × 100	$40/(40 + 5) \times 100 = 89\%$
	NPV predicts the probability that an individual with a negative assay result does not have the disease or condition.		

*Using data from Table 3.11.

FN, False-negative; *FP*, false-positive; *NPV*, negative predictive value; *PPV*, positive predictive value; *TN*, true-negative; *TP*, true-positive.

You go on to compute the ARR, which is the absolute value of the arithmetic *difference* in the event rates of the control and intervention arms. In our example using the obese smokers group, the ARR = 0.1 − 0.05 = 0.05, or 5% (not 50%, as reported in the above example using RRR). The ARR is often expressed as the number necessary to treat (NNT), the inverse of ARR. In our example, for every subject whose AMI is prevented by the laboratory test and subsequent treatment, you would have to treat 20 total subjects over a 5-year period. Further, if you reduce the ARR to an annual rate, 0.05/5 years = 0.01, or a 1% annual reduction. You conclude from your study that 100 interventions per year are required to prevent 1 AMI.

Finally, your RRR and ARR are not discrete integers but means computed from samples of 1000, so they must include an expression of dispersion, usually ±2 SD or a 95.5% CI. Suppose the 95.5% CI for the RRR turns out to be relatively broad: −0.1 to +1.1. A ratio of 1 implies no effect from the intervention; that is, the rate of change in the intervention arm is equal to the rate of change in the control arm. Given that the 95.5% CI embraces the number 1, the intervention has failed to provide any benefit.

In summary, once a laboratory assay is verified to be accurate and precise, it must then be determined to possess diagnostic efficacy and to provide for effective intervention as determined by favorable RRR and ARR or NNT values. Application of the ROC curve may help achieve these goals.

RECEIVER OPERATING CHARACTERISTIC CURVE

An ROC curve is a further refinement of diagnostic efficacy testing that may be employed to determine the reference limit for an assay when the assay generates a *continuous variable*. In diagnostic efficacy testing as described in the previous section, the ±2 SD limits of the RI are used as the reference limits for discriminating a positive from a negative test result. Often, the "true" reference limit varies from the ±2 SD limit. Using ROC analysis, the reference limit is adjusted by increments of 1 (or other increments depending on the analytical range), and the true-positive (sensitivity) and false-positive (1 − specificity) rates are recomputed for each new reference limit using the same formulas provided previously in "Assessing Diagnostic Efficacy." The reference limit that is finally selected is the one that provides the largest true-positive and smallest false-positive rate (Figure 3.9). The operator generates a line graph plotting true-positive rates on the y-axis and false-positive rates on the x-axis. Measuring the *area under the curve* (a computer-based calculus function) assesses the overall efficacy of the assay. If the area under the curve is 0.5, the curve is at the line of identity between false- and true-positives and the assay provides no discrimination. Most experts agree that a clinically useful assay should have an area under the curve of 0.85 or higher.[46,47]

ASSAY FEASIBILITY

Most laboratory managers and directors review assay feasibility before launching complex validation, efficacy, RI, and QC initiatives. Feasibility studies include a review of assay throughput (number of assays per unit time), dwell time (length of assay interval from specimen sampling to report), cost per test, cost/benefit ratio, turnaround time, and technical skill required to perform the assay. To select a new instrument, the manager reviews issues of operator safety, footprint, overhead, compatibility with laboratory utilities and information system, need for middleware, frequency and duration of breakdowns, and distributor support and service.

LABORATORY STAFF COMPETENCE

Staff integrity and professional staff competence are the keys to assay reliability. In the United States, California, Florida, Georgia, Hawaii, Louisiana, Montana, Nevada, New York, North Dakota, Tennessee, West Virginia, and Puerto Rico enforce laboratory personnel licensure laws.[48] In these states, only licensed laboratory professionals may be employed in medical center or reference laboratories. Legislatures in other states have considered and rejected licensure bills, the bills having been opposed by competing health care specialty associations and for-profit entities. In nonlicensure states, conscientious laboratory directors employ only nationally certified professionals. Certification is available worldwide from the Board of Certification of the American Society for Clinical Pathology. Studies of laboratory errors and outcomes demonstrate that laboratories that employ only licensed or certified professionals produce the most reliable assay results.[49]

Competent laboratory professionals continuously watch for and document errors by inspecting the results of internal validation and QC programs and external quality assessment. Error is inevitable, and incidents should be documented and highlighted for quality improvement and remedial instruction. When error is associated with reprimand, the opportunity for improvement may be lost to cover-up. Except in cases of negligence, the analysis of error without blame is consistently practiced to improve the quality of laboratory services.

Proficiency Systems

Laboratory managers and directors assess and document professional staff skills using proficiency systems. The hematology laboratory manager may, for instance, maintain and secure a collection of normal and abnormal blood films, case studies, or laboratory assay reports that medical laboratory technicians and scientists are required to examine at regular intervals. Medical laboratory professionals who fail to reproduce results within the reference limits on examination of the blood film are provided remedial instruction. The proficiency set may also be used to assess applicants for laboratory positions. Proficiency testing systems are available from external quality assessment agencies, and proficiency reports are made accessible to laboratory assessors.

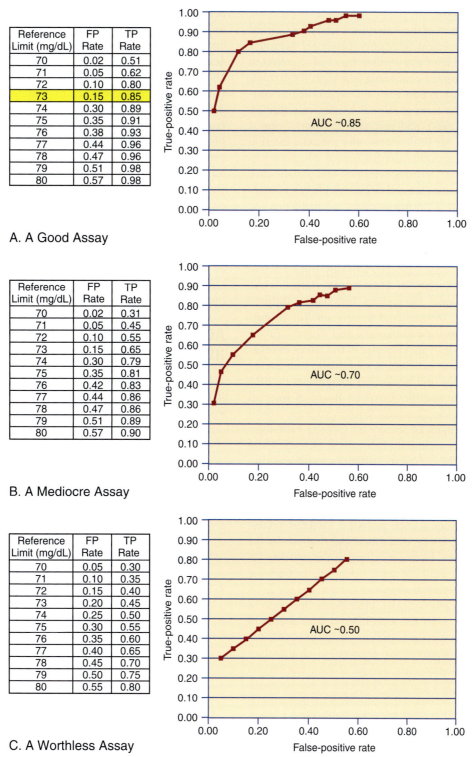

A. A Good Assay

Reference Limit (mg/dL)	FP Rate	TP Rate
70	0.02	0.51
71	0.05	0.62
72	0.10	0.80
73	0.15	0.85
74	0.30	0.89
75	0.35	0.91
76	0.38	0.93
77	0.44	0.96
78	0.47	0.96
79	0.51	0.98
80	0.57	0.98

B. A Mediocre Assay

Reference Limit (mg/dL)	FP Rate	TP Rate
70	0.02	0.31
71	0.05	0.45
72	0.10	0.55
73	0.15	0.65
74	0.30	0.79
75	0.35	0.81
76	0.42	0.83
77	0.44	0.86
78	0.47	0.86
79	0.51	0.89
80	0.57	0.90

C. A Worthless Assay

Reference Limit (mg/dL)	FP Rate	TP Rate
70	0.05	0.30
71	0.10	0.35
72	0.15	0.40
73	0.20	0.45
74	0.25	0.50
75	0.30	0.55
76	0.35	0.60
77	0.40	0.65
78	0.45	0.70
79	0.50	0.75
80	0.55	0.80

Figure 3.9 Receiver Operating Characteristic Curves for a Typical Assay Using Reference Limits Between 70 and 80 mg/dL. **(A)**, The true-positive and false-positive rates for each reference limit from 70 to 80 mg/dL are computed and graphed as paired variables on a linear scale, with true-positive rate on the vertical *(y)* scale and false-positive rate on the horizontal *(x)* scale. The assay provides acceptable discrimination between individuals affected by the disease or condition and nonaffected individuals, with an area under the curve *(AUC)* of 0.85, and 73 mg/dL is the reference limit that produces the most desirable false-positive and true-positive rates. **(B)**, This assay has unacceptable discrimination between individuals affected by the disease or condition and unaffected individuals, with an AUC of 0.70. No reference limit produces a desirable false-positive and true-positive rate. **(C)**, This assay, with an AUC of 0.50, has no ability to discriminate. *FP,* False-positive; *TP,* true-positive.

Continuing Education

The Board of Certification of the American Society for Clinical Pathology and state medical laboratory personnel licensure boards require medical laboratory technicians and scientists to participate in and document continuing education for *periodic recertification* or *relicensure*. Educators and experts deliver continuing education in the form of journal articles, case studies, online seminars (webinars), and seminars and workshops at professional meetings. Medical centers offer periodic internal continuing education opportunities (in-service education) in the form of grand rounds, lectures, seminars, and participative educational events. Presentation and discussion of current cases are particularly effective. Continuing education maintains the critical skills of laboratory professionals and provides opportunities to learn about new clinical and technical approaches. The American Society for Clinical Laboratory Science (https://ascls.org/), American Society for Clinical Pathology (https://www.ascp.org/), American Society of Hematology (https://www.hematology.org/), National Hemophilia Foundation (https://www.hemophilia.org/), International Society on Thrombosis and Haemostasis (https://www.isth.org/), and Fritsma Factor (https://fritsmafactor.com/) are examples of the scores of organizations that direct their activities toward quality continuing education in hematology and hemostasis. Originated in 2012 by Consumers Reports and the American Board of Internal Medicine Foundation, the Choosing Wisely program, now a collaboration of the American Society for Clinical Pathology, American Society for Clinical Laboratory Science, and American Society for Microbiology, advances a national dialogue on avoiding wasteful or unnecessary diagnostic laboratory procedures (https://www.ascp.org/content/get-involved/choosing-wisely/choosing-wisely-ascp#).

The medical laboratory science profession stratifies professional staff responsibilities by educational preparation. In the United States, professional levels are defined as the associate (2-year) degree level, or *medical laboratory technician*; the bachelor (4-year) degree level, or *medical laboratory scientist*; and the levels of advanced degrees: master's degree, professional doctorate in clinical laboratory science (DCLS), and PhD in clinical laboratory and related sciences. Many colleges and universities offer articulation programs that enable professional personnel to advance their education and responsibility levels. Several of these institutions provide undergraduate and graduate distance-learning opportunities. A current list is maintained by the National Accrediting Agency for Clinical Laboratory Sciences (https://naacls.org/), and the American Society for Clinical Laboratory Science publishes the *Directory of Graduate Programs for Clinical Laboratory Practitioners*. Enlightened employers encourage their laboratory professionals to participate in advanced educational programs, and many provide resources for this purpose. Education contributes to quality laboratory services.

QUALITY ASSURANCE PLAN: PREANALYTICAL AND POSTANALYTICAL

In addition to keeping analytical QC records, US regulatory agencies such as the Centers for Medicare and Medicaid Services (https://www.cms.gov/) require laboratory directors to maintain records of preanalytical and postanalytical QA and quality improvement efforts.[50] When epidemics or emergent conditions trigger the FDA to implement Emergency Use Authorization (EUA) requirements, temporary rules may require laboratory directors to maintain all QA records.[51] Although not exhaustive, Table 3.1 lists and characterizes several examples of preanalytical quality efforts, and Table 3.2 provides a review of postanalytical components. All QA plans provide objectives, sources of authority, scope of services, an activity calendar, corrective action, periodic evaluation, standard protocol, personnel involvement, and methods of communication.[52]

API Paperless Proficiency Testing and CAP Q-PROBES are subscription services that provide model QA programs. Experts in QA continuously refine the consensus of appropriate indicators of laboratory medicine quality. QA programs search for events that provide improvement opportunities.

AGENCIES THAT ADDRESS HEMATOLOGY AND HEMOSTASIS QUALITY

Following are representative agencies that provide QA services in hematology and hemostasis laboratory testing:

- Data Innovations North America (https://datainnovations.com/). QA management software including instrument management middleware, laboratory production management software, EP Evaluator, RI tables, and allowable total error tables.
- Clinical and Laboratory Standards Institute (CLSI) (https://clsi.org/). International guidelines and standards for laboratory practice that include method evaluation and assessment of diagnostic accuracy, EP-prefix standards, and QA and quality management systems, QMS-prefix standards.
- Centers for Medicare and Medicaid Services (CMS) (https://www.cms.gov/). Administers the laws and rules developed from the *Clinical Laboratory Improvement Amendments of 1988*. Establishes *Current Procedural Terminology* (CPT) codes, reimbursement rules, and classifies assay complexity.
- American Proficiency Institute (API) (https://api-pt.com/). Laboratory proficiency testing and QA programs, continuing education programs and summaries, tutorials, and special topics library.
- College of American Pathologists (CAP) (https://www.cap.org/). Laboratory accreditation, proficiency testing, and QA programs; laboratory education, reference resources, and e-lab solutions.
- The Joint Commission (https://www.jointcommission.org/). Medical center-wide accreditation and certification programs.
- Laboratory Medicine Quality Improvement (cdc.gov/osels/lspppo/Laboratory_Medicine_Quality_Improvement/index.html). An initiative of the US Centers for Disease Control and Prevention.

SUMMARY

- Hematology and hemostasis laboratory quality control (QC) relies on descriptive statistics that provide measures of central tendency, measures of dispersion, and significance.
- Each new assay or assay modification must be validated for accuracy, precision, linearity, analytical measurement range (AMR), specificity, and lower limit of detection (LLD).
- In the hematology and hemostasis laboratory, accuracy validation usually requires a series of calibrators. Accuracy is established using the Student *t*-test, analysis of variance (ANOVA), Pearson correlation, linear regression, and Bland-Altman distribution.
- Precision is established by using repeated within-day and day-to-day assays, then computing the mean, standard deviation (SD), and coefficient of variation (CV) of the results.
- Vendors usually provide assay linearity, specificity, and LLD; however, laboratory managers may require that these parameters be revalidated locally. These parameters must be validated when a Food and Drug Administration (FDA)-approved assay is modified or when the laboratory professional develops a local laboratory-developed test.
- Internal QC is accomplished by assaying controls with each test run. Control results are compared with reference limits, usually the mean of the control assay ±2 SD. When a specified number of control values are outside the reference limits, the assay is suspended, and the laboratory professional begins troubleshooting. Control results are plotted on Levey-Jennings charts and examined for shifts and trends. Internal QC is enhanced using the moving average algorithm and delta checks.
- Conscientious laboratory directors subscribe to an external quality assessment system, also known as *proficiency testing* or *proficiency surveys*. External quality assessment enables the director to compare selected assay results with other laboratory results, nationally and internationally, as a further check of accuracy. Maintaining a good external quality assessment record is essential to laboratory accreditation. Most states require external quality assessment for laboratory licensure.
- Laboratory assays are analyzed for diagnostic efficacy, including diagnostic sensitivity and specificity, true-positive and true-negative rates, and positive and negative predictive values. Highly sensitive assays may be used for population screening but may discriminate poorly between healthy and diseased populations. Specific assays may be used to confirm a condition but generate numerous false-negatives. Assays are chosen based on the value of their intervention, measured by relative or absolute risk ratios. Diagnostic efficacy computations expand to include receiver operating characteristic (ROC) curve analysis.
- Meticulous laboratory managers hire only certified or licensed medical laboratory scientists and technicians and provide regular individual proficiency tests that are correlated with in-service education. They encourage staff members to participate in continuing education activities and in-house discussion of cases. Quality laboratories provide resources for staff to pursue higher education.
- The laboratory director maintains a protocol for assessing and improving on preanalytical and postanalytical variables and finds means to communicate enhancements to other members of the health care team.

Now that you have completed this chapter, go back and read again the case study at the beginning and respond to the questions presented. Answers can be found in Appendix C.

REVIEW QUESTIONS

Answers can be found in Appendix C.

1. What procedure is NOT employed to validate a new assay?
   a. Comparison of assay results with a reference method
   b. Test for assay precision
   c. Test for assay linearity
   d. Moving average algorithm
2. You validate a new assay using linear regression to compare assay calibrator results with the distributor's published calibrator results. The slope is 0.99 and the *y* intercept is +10%. What type of error is present?
   a. No error
   b. Random error
   c. Constant systematic error
   d. Proportional systematic error
3. Which one of the following is a statistical test that compares means?
   a. Bland-Altman
   b. Student *t*-test
   c. ANOVA
   d. Pearson
4. The acceptable hemoglobin control value range is 13 ± 0.4 g/dL. The control is assayed five times and produces the following five results:

   12.0 g/dL   12.3 g/dL   12.0 g/dL   12.2 g/dL   12.1 g/dL

   These results are:
   a. Accurate but not precise
   b. Precise but not accurate
   c. Both accurate and precise
   d. Neither accurate nor precise

5. A WBC count control has a mean value of 6000/μL and an SD of 300/μL. What is the 95.5% confidence interval?
   a. 3000 to 9000/μL
   b. 5400 to 6600/μL
   c. 5500 to 6500/μL
   d. 5700 to 6300/μL

6. The ability of an assay to distinguish the targeted analyte from interfering substances within the specimen matrix is called:
   a. Analytical specificity
   b. Analytical sensitivity
   c. Clinical specificity
   d. Clinical sensitivity

7. The laboratory purchases reagents from a manufacturer and develops an assay using a protocol published in a volume of the *Methods in Molecular Biology* series. How would the FDA classify this assay?
   a. Cleared
   b. Research use only
   c. Analyte-specific reagent
   d. Laboratory-developed test

8. What process ensures comparability in multisite validation?
   a. Distribution of proficiency materials to all sites
   b. Publication of individual site reference intervals
   c. Clinical sensitivity and specificity computations
   d. ROC analysis

9. A laboratory scientist measures prothrombin time for plasma aliquots from 15 healthy men and 15 healthy women. The scientist computes the mean and 95.5% confidence interval and notes that they duplicate the manufacturer's statistics within 5%. This procedure is known as:
   a. Setting the RI
   b. Confirming linearity
   c. Determining the therapeutic range
   d. Establishing the RI by transference

10. You purchase a preserved whole blood specimen from a distributor who provides the mean values for several complete blood count analytes. What is this specimen called?
    a. Normal specimen
    b. Calibrator
    c. Control
    d. Blank

11. You perform a clinical efficacy test and get the following results:

	Unaffected by Disease	Affected by Disease
Assay is negative	40	5
Assay is positive	10	45

What is the number of false-negative results?
    a. 45
    b. 40
    c. 10
    d. 5

12. What agency provides external quality assurance (proficiency) surveys and laboratory accreditation?
    a. Clinical Laboratory Improvement Advisory Committee (CLIAC)
    b. Centers for Medicare and Medicaid Services (CMS)
    c. College of American Pathologists (CAP)
    d. The Joint Commission

13. What agency provides continuing medical laboratory education?
    a. Clinical Laboratory Improvement Advisory Committee (CLIAC)
    b. American Society for Clinical Laboratory Science (ASCLS)
    c. Centers for Medicare and Medicaid Services (CMS)
    d. College of American Pathologists (CAP)

14. Regular review of blood specimen collection quality is an example of:
    a. Postanalytical quality assurance
    b. Preanalytical quality assurance
    c. Analytical quality control
    d. External quality assurance

15. Review of laboratory report integrity is an example of:
    a. Postanalytical quality assurance
    b. Preanalytical quality assurance
    c. Analytical quality control
    d. External quality assurance

16. When performing an ROC analysis, what parameter assesses the overall efficacy of an assay?
    a. Area under the curve
    b. Reference limit
    c. Positive predictive value
    d. Negative predictive value

17. You require your laboratory staff to annually perform manual lupus anticoagulant profiles on a set of plasmas with known values. This exercise is known as:
    a. Assay validation
    b. Proficiency testing
    c. External quality assessment
    d. Pre-preanalytical variable assay

REFERENCES

1. Westgard, J. O. (2016). *Basic QC Practices: Training in Statistical Quality Control for Medical Laboratories.* (4th ed.). Madison, WI: Westgard QC.
2. Westgard, J. O. (2017). A total quality-control plan with right-sized statistical quality-control. *Clin Lab Med, 37,* 137–150.
3. CLSI. (2011). *Quality Management System: Continual Improvement.* (3rd ed., CLSI guideline QMS06-A3). Wayne, PA: Clinical and Laboratory Standards Institute.
4. Ernst, D. J., & Ernst, C. (2017). *The Lab Draw Answer Book.* Orem, UT: Center for Phlebotomy Education.
5. CLSI. (2017). *Collection of Diagnostic Venous Blood Specimens.* (7th ed., CLSI standard GP41). Wayne, PA: Clinical and Laboratory Standards Institute.
6. Plebani, M. (2012). Quality indicators to detect pre-analytical errors in laboratory testing. *Clin Biochem Rev, 33,* 85–88.
7. Can Çubukçu, H., Vanstapel, F., Thelen, M., et al. (2021). Improving the laboratory result release process in the light of ISO 15189:2012 standard. *Clin Chim Acta, 522,* 167–173.
8. Ducatman, B. S., Ducatman, A. M., Crawford, J. M., et al. (2020). The value proposition for pathologists: a population health approach. *Acad Pathol, 14,* 7.
9. Hickner, J., Graham, D. G., Elder, N. C., et al. (2008). Testing practices: a study of the American Academy of Family Physicians National Research Network. *Qual Saf Health Care, 17,* 194–200.
10. Laposata, M., & Dighe, A. (2007). "Pre-pre" and "post-post" analytical error: high-incidence patient safety hazards involving the clinical laboratory. *Clin Chem Lab Med, 45,* 712–719.
11. Stunt, J., van Grootel, L., Bouter, L., et al. (2021). Why we habitually engage in null-hypothesis significance testing: a qualitative study. *PLoS One, 16*(10):e0258330. https://doi.org/10.1371/journal.pone.0258330.
12. Huck, S. W. (2011). *Reading Statistics and Research.* (6th ed.). New York: Pearson.
13. Fritsma, G. A., & McGlasson, D. L. (2012). *Quick Guide to Laboratory Statistics and Quality Control.* Washington, DC: AACC Press.
14. Carobene, A., Banfi, G., Locatelli, M., et al. (2022). Personalized reference intervals: from the statistical significance to the clinical usefulness. *Clin Chim Acta, 524,* 203–204.
15. Chaudhary, D., Hussain, K., Semwal, N., et al. (2021). A review on analytical method validation. *J Advancement Pharmacol, 1,* 38–45.
16. College of American Pathologists. (2021). *Why CAP Accreditation.* https://www.cap.org/laboratory-improvement/accreditation/why-cap-accreditation. Accessed August 2, 2022.
17. CLSI. (2018). *Measurement Procedure Comparison and Bias Estimation using Patient Samples.* (3rd ed., CLSI guideline EP09c). Wayne, PA: Clinical and Laboratory Standards Institute.
18. Clinical Laboratory Improvement Amendments. (2003). *Calibration and Calibration Verification.* http://www.cms.gov/Regulations-and-Guidance/Legislation/CLIA/CLIA_Brochures.html. Accessed August 2, 2022.
19. CLSI. (2009). *Laboratory Instrument Implementation, Verification, and Maintenance.* (CLSI guideline GP31-A). Wayne, PA: Clinical and Laboratory Standards Institute.
20. Jan, S.-L., & Shieh, G. (2018). The Bland-Altman range of agreement: exact interval procedure and sample size determination. *Comput Biol Med, 100,* 247–252.
21. Bland, J. M., & Altman, D. G. (1986). Statistical methods for assessing agreement between two methods of clinical measurement. *Lancet, 327,* 307–310.
22. Westgard, J. O., Quam, E. F., Barry, P. L., et al. (2016). *Basic QC Practices.* (4th ed.). Madison, WI: Westgard QC.
23. CLSI. (2008). *Protocol for the Evaluation, Validation, and Implementation of Coagulometers.* (CLSI guideline H57-A). Wayne, PA: Clinical and Laboratory Standards Institute.
24. CLSI. (2007). *Reference Leukocyte (WBC) Differential Count (Proportional) and Evaluation of Instrumental Methods.* (2nd ed., CLSI guideline H20-A2). Wayne, PA: Clinical and Laboratory Standards Institute.
25. Rogers, M. W., Letsos, C. B., Henderson, M. P. A., et al. (2018). Method evaluation and quality control. In Bishop, M. L., Fody, E. P., & Schoeff, L. E. (Eds.), *Clinical Chemistry: Principles, Techniques, and Correlations.* (8th ed., pp. 49–86). Philadelphia: Wolters Kluwer.
26. Christenson, R. H., & Duh, S.-H. (2012). Methodological and analytic considerations for blood biomarkers. *Prog Cardiovasc Dis, 55,* 25–33.
27. *Regulation of Clinical Tests: In Vitro Diagnostic (IVD) Devices, Laboratory Developed Tests (LDTs), and Genetic Tests.* (2017). Congressional Research Service. https://www.everycrsreport.com/files/20170411_R43438_73b86dc30fca1703aa59bfe65161c32b5b48a9ae.html. Accessed August 2, 2022.
28. *Data Innovations EP Evaluator.* (2021). https://www.datainnovations.com/ep-evaluator-0. Accessed August 2, 2022.
29. Clinical Laboratories Improvement Act program; granting and withdrawal of deeming authority to private nonprofit accreditation organizations and of CLIA exemption under state laboratory programs—HCFA. Final rule. (1992). *Fed Regist, 57,* 33992–34021. https://pubed.ncbi.nlm.nih.gov/10120445/. Accessed August 2, 2022.
30. CLSI. (2012). *Verification of Comparability of Patient Results Within One Health Care System.* (CLSI guideline, interim revision EP31-A-IR). Wayne, PA: Clinical and Laboratory Standards Institute.
31. CLSI. (2010). *Defining, Establishing and Verifying Reference Intervals in the Clinical Laboratory.* (3rd ed., CLSI guideline EP28-A3C). Wayne, PA: Clinical and Laboratory Standards Institute.
32. Wong, E. C. C., Brugnara, C., Straseski, J., et al. (2020). *Pediatric Reference Intervals.* (8th ed.). San Diego: Academic Press Elsevier.
33. Malone, B. (2012). The quest for pediatric reference ranges: why the national children's study promises answers. *Clin Lab News, 38,* 3–4.
34. Krejcie, R. V., & Morgan, D. W. (1970). Determining sample size for research activities. *Educ Psychol Meas, 30,* 607–610.
35. Pagana, K. D., Pagana, T. J., & Pagana, T. N. (2022). Reticulocyte count. In Pagana, K. D., Pagana, T. J., & Pagana, T. N., (Eds.), *Mosby's Manual of Diagnostic and Laboratory Tests.* (7th ed., p. 430). St. Louis, MO: Elsevier.
36. Jones, G. R. D., Haeckel, R., Loh, T. P., et al, on behalf of the IFCC Committee on Reference Intervals and Decision Limits. (2019). Indirect methods for reference interval determination – review and recommendations. *Clin Chem Lab Med, 57,* 20–29.
37. Levey, S., & Jennings, E. R. (1950). The use of control charts in the clinical laboratory. *Am J Clin Pathol, 20,* 1059–1066.
38. Westgard, J. O., Barry, P. L., Hunt, M. R., et al. (1981). A multi-rule Shewhart chart for quality control in clinical chemistry. *Clin Chem, 27,* 493–501.
39. Bull, B. S., Elashoff, R. M., Heilbron, D. C., et al. (1974). A study of various estimators for the derivation of quality control

procedures from patient erythrocyte indices. *Am J Clin Pathol*, *61*, 473–481.

40. Vis, J. Y., & Huisman, A. (2016). Verification and quality control of routine hematology analyzers. *Int J Lab Hematol*, *38*(Suppl. 1), 100–109.

41. Randell, E. W., & Yenice, S. (2019). Delta checks in the clinical laboratory. *Crit Rev Clin Lab Sci*, *56*, 75–97.

42. Lind, S. E. (1991). The bleeding time does not predict surgical bleeding. *Blood*, *77*, 2547–2552.

43. Gewirtz, A. S., Miller, M. L., & Keys, T. F. (1996). The clinical usefulness of the preoperative bleeding time. *Arch Pathol Lab Med*, *120*, 353–356.

44. Tripepi, G., Jager, K. J., Dekker, F. W., et al. (2010). Measures of effect in epidemiological research. *Clin Practice*, *115*, 91–93.

45. Replogle, W. H., & Johnson, W. D. (2007). Interpretation of absolute measures of disease risk in comparative research. *Fam Med*, *39*, 432–435.

46. Søreide, K. (2009). Receiver-operating characteristic curve analysis in diagnostic, prognostic and predictive biomarker research. *J Clin Pathol*, *62*, 1–5.

47. Hajian-Tilaki, K. (2013). Receiver operating characteristic (ROC) curve analysis for medical diagnostic test evaluation. *Caspian J Intl Med*, *4*, 627–635.

48. Rohde, R. E., Falleur, D. M., & Ellis, J. R. (2015). Almost anyone can perform your medical laboratory tests - wait, what? *Elsevier Connect*. https://www.elsevier.com/connect/almost-anyone-can-perform-your-medical-laboratory-tests-wait-what. Accessed August 2, 2022.

49. Delost, M. D., Miller, W. G., Chang, G. A., et al. (2009). Influence of credentials of clinical laboratory professionals on proficiency testing performance. *Am J Clin Pathol*, *132*, 550–554.

50. Westgard, J. O., Ehrmeyer, S. S., & Darcy, T. P. (2004). *CLIA Final Rule for Quality Systems, Quality Assessment Issues and Answers*. Madison, WI: Westgard QC.

51. Ehrmeyer, S. (2021). *The New Poor Lab's Guide to the Regulations*. Madison, WI: Westgard QC.

52. Blaetz, M. (2020). Diagnostic preparedness - getting on track with quality assessments. *Today's Clin Lab*. https://www.clinicallabmanager.com/regulatory/getting-on-track-with-quality-assessments-22550. Accessed August 2, 2022.

4

Cell Structure and Function

Elaine M. Keohane*

OBJECTIVES

After completion of this chapter, the reader will be able to:

1. Describe the structure, composition, and general function of cell membranes.
2. Describe the structure, composition, and function of components of the nucleus, including staining qualities visible by light microscopy.
3. Describe the structure, composition, and general function of cytoplasmic organelles, including staining qualities visible by light microscopy, if applicable.
4. Describe various mechanisms in which molecules are transported across the plasma membrane.
5. Describe the processes of cell communication and signal transduction, including the various types of receptors and ligands.
6. Associate the stages of the cell cycle with activities of the cell, including the location and function of checkpoints in the cycle.
7. Describe the role of cyclins and cyclin-dependent kinases in cell cycle regulation.
8. Differentiate between apoptosis and necrosis.
9. Describe the general structure and function of the hematopoietic microenvironment and the effect of growth factors.

OUTLINE

Cell Organization
Plasma Membrane
  Membrane Proteins
  Membrane Carbohydrates
Nucleus
  Chromatin
  Nuclear Envelope
  Nucleoli
Cytoplasm
  Ribosomes
  Endoplasmic Reticulum
  Golgi Apparatus

Mitochondria
Lysosomes
Microfilaments and Intermediate Filaments
Microtubules
Centrosomes
Selected Cell Processes
  Plasma Membrane Transport
  Cell Communication and Signal Transduction
  Cell Cycle and its Regulation
  Cell Death by Necrosis and Apoptosis
Hematopoietic Microenvironment

Knowledge of the normal structure, composition, and function of cells is fundamental to the understanding of blood cell pathophysiology covered in later chapters. From the invention of the microscope and the discovery of cells in the 1600s to the present-day highly sophisticated analysis of cell ultrastructure with electron microscopy and other technologies, a remarkable body of knowledge is available about the structure of cells and their varied organelles. Complementing these discoveries were other advances in technology that enabled detailed understanding of the biochemistry, metabolism, and genetics of cells at the molecular level. Today, highly sophisticated analysis of cells using flow cytometry, molecular genetic testing, and cytogenetics (Chapters 28–30) has become the standard of care in diagnosis and management of many malignant and nonmalignant blood cell diseases. This new and ever-expanding knowledge has revolutionized the diagnosis and treatment of hematologic diseases, resulting in a dramatic improvement in patient survival for many conditions that previously had a dismal prognosis. With all these advances, however, the visual examination of blood cells on a peripheral blood film by light microscopy still

*The author extends appreciation to Keila B. Poulsen, whose work in prior editions provided the foundation for this chapter.

remains the hallmark for the initial evaluation of hematologic abnormalities.

This chapter provides an overview of the structure, composition, and function of the components of the cell; selected cell processes including membrane transport, cell communication and signal transduction, the cell cycle and its regulation, and cell death by apoptosis and necrosis; and the hematopoietic microenvironment.

CELL ORGANIZATION

Cells are the structural units that constitute living organisms. Cells have specialized functions and contain the components necessary to perform and perpetuate these functions (Figures 4.1 and 4.2). Regardless of shape, size, or function, human cells contain:

- A *plasma membrane* that separates the *cytoplasm* and cellular components from the extracellular environment;
- A membrane-bound *nucleus* (with the exception of mature red blood cells (RBCs) and platelets); and
- Other unique subcellular structures and organelles that support various cellular functions.[1,2]

Table 4.1 summarizes the cellular components and their functions, which are explained in more detail further on in the chapter.

PLASMA MEMBRANE

The plasma membrane serves as a semipermeable outer boundary separating the cellular components from their surrounding environment. The cell membrane serves four basic functions: (1) it provides a physical but flexible barrier to contain and protect cell components

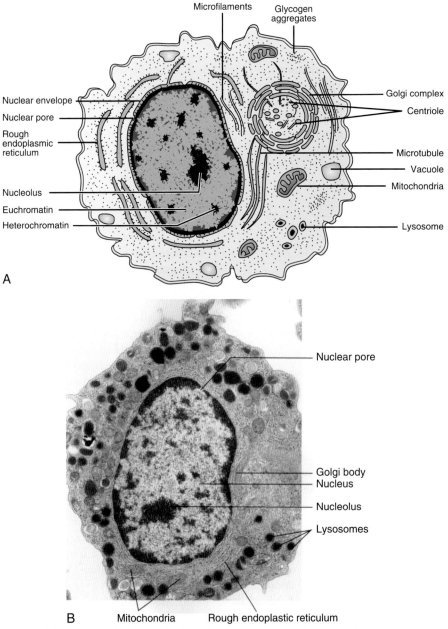

Figure 4.1 Cell Structure. **(A),** Schematic of an electron micrograph of cell organization and components. **(B),** Electron micrograph of a cell with labeled organelles. (B from Carr, J. H. [2022]. *Clinical Hematology Atlas.* [6th ed., Figure 2.3B]. St. Louis: Elsevier.)

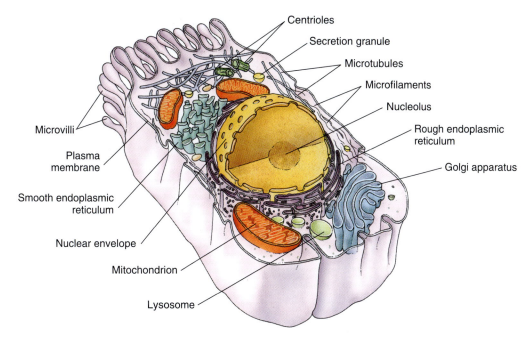

Centrioles
Secretion granule
Microtubules
Microfilaments
Nucleolus
Rough endoplasmic reticulum
Golgi apparatus
Microvilli
Plasma membrane
Smooth endoplasmic reticulum
Nuclear envelope
Mitochondrion
Lysosome

Figure 4.2 Three-Dimensional Schematic Diagram of an Idealized Cell, as Visualized by Transmission Electron Microscopy. Various organelles and cytoskeletal elements are displayed. (From Gartner, L. P. [2021]. Cytoplasm. In *Textbook of Histology*. [5th ed., Figure 2.5]. Philadelphia: Elsevier.)

from the extracellular environment; (2) it regulates and facilitates the interchange of substances with the environment by endocytosis, exocytosis, and selective permeability (using various membrane channels and transporters); (3) it establishes electrochemical gradients between the interior and exterior of the cell; and (4) it has receptors that allow the cell to respond to other cells and to a multitude of signaling molecules through signal transduction pathways.[2,3]

Relevant to hematology, the membrane is also the location of cell surface glycoprotein and glycolipid molecules (surface markers or antigens) used for blood cell identity. Each type of blood cell expresses a unique repertoire of surface antigens at different stages of differentiation.[4] Antigen-specific monoclonal antibodies enable identification of these antigens using flow cytometry (Chapter 28). An international nomenclature was developed, called the *cluster of differentiation,* or *CD,* system, in which a CD number was assigned to each identified blood cell antigen.[4] More than 400 CD antigens have been identified on blood cells.[4] The CD nomenclature allows scientists, providers, and laboratory practitioners to communicate in a universal language for hematology research and diagnostic and therapeutic practice.

In addition to the plasma membrane, many components found within the cell (e.g., mitochondria, Golgi apparatus, nucleus, and endoplasmic reticulum) have similarly constructed membrane systems. The RBC membrane has been the most widely studied, and its structure and function is described in detail in Chapter 7.

To accomplish its many requirements, the cell membrane must be resilient and elastic. It achieves these qualities by being a fluid structure of proteins floating in lipids. The lipids are phospholipids and cholesterol, arranged in two layers. The phosphate end of the phospholipid and the hydroxyl radical of cholesterol are polar-charged hydrophilic (water-soluble) structures that orient toward the extracellular and cytoplasmic surfaces of the cell membrane. Fatty acid chains of the phospholipids and the steroid nucleus of cholesterol are nonpolar-charged hydrophobic (water-insoluble) structures and are directed toward each other in the center of the bilayer (Figure 7.2).[3] Phospholipids are distributed asymmetrically in the membrane with mostly phosphatidylserine and phosphatidylethanolamine in the inner layer and sphingomyelin and phosphatidylcholine in the outer layer (Chapters 7 and 11). In the outer layer, carbohydrates (oligosaccharides) are covalently linked to some membrane phospholipids, forming glycolipids.[3]

Membrane Proteins

Cell membranes contain two types of proteins: transmembrane and cytoskeletal. Transmembrane proteins traverse the entirety of the lipid bilayer in one or more passes and penetrate the plasma and cytoplasmic layers of the membrane. A transmembrane protein may have carbohydrate chains covalently linked to its plasma component, forming a glycoprotein.[2] The transmembrane proteins serve as channels and transporters of water, ions, and other molecules between the cytoplasm and the external environment. They also function as receptors and adhesion molecules. Cytoskeletal proteins are found only on the cytoplasmic side of the membrane and form the lattice of the cytoskeleton. The cytoplasmic ends of transmembrane proteins attach to the cytoskeletal proteins at junctional complexes to provide structural integrity to the cell and vertical support in linking the membrane to the cytoskeleton (Figure 7.4).[5] Inherited mutations in genes coding for transmembrane or cytoskeletal proteins can disrupt membrane integrity, decrease the life span of RBCs, and lead to a hemolytic anemia. An example is hereditary spherocytosis (Chapter 21).

Membrane Carbohydrates

The carbohydrate chains of glycoproteins and glycolipids extend beyond the outer cell surface, providing an external protective carbohydrate coating called the *glycocalyx*.[2,3] Substances adsorbed from the extracellular matrix (ECM) also contribute to this coating. The carbohydrate moieties function in cell-to-cell recognition and adhesion and provide a negative surface charge to repel adjacent cells in circulation.

TABLE 4.1   Summary of Cellular Components and Functions

Organelle	Location	Appearance and Size	Function
Plasma membrane	Outer boundary of cell	Lipid bilayer consisting of phospholipids, cholesterol, proteins; glycolipids and glycoproteins form a glycocalyx	Provides physical barrier for cell; facilitates and restricts interchange of substances with environment; maintains electrochemical gradient; has receptors for signal transduction
Nucleus	Within cell	Round or oval; varies in diameter; composed of DNA and proteins; surrounded by inner and outer membranes	Controls cell division and functions; contains genetic code
Nucleolus	Within nucleus	Usually round or irregular in shape; composed of ribosomal RNA and the genes coding it and accessory proteins; may have one to several within the nucleus	Synthesizes ribosomal RNA and assembles ribosome subunits
Ribosomes	Free in cytoplasm and on outer surface of rough endoplasmic reticulum	Macromolecular complex composed of protein and ribosomal RNA; composed of large and small subunits	Synthesizes proteins
Rough endoplasmic reticulum	Membranous network throughout cytoplasm	Branching, membrane-lined tubules and sacs; studded with ribosomes on outer surface; membrane continuous with nuclear membrane	Synthesizes membrane-bound and secreted proteins
Smooth endoplasmic reticulum	Membranous network throughout cytoplasm	Membrane-lined tubules lacking ribosomes; continuous with rough endoplasmic reticulum	Synthesizes phospholipids and steroids; detoxifies drugs; stores calcium
Golgi apparatus	Next to nucleus and rough endoplasmic reticulum	System of stacked, membrane-bound, flattened sacs	Modifies and packages macromolecules for other organelles and for secretion
Mitochondria	Randomly distributed in cytoplasm	Elliptical or oval structures surrounded by inner and outer membranes; inner membrane has infoldings called *cristae*	Produces most of the ATP for the cell by aerobic respiration/oxidative phosphorylation
Lysosomes	Randomly distributed in cytoplasm	Membrane-bound sacs; diameter varies	Contains hydrolytic enzymes that degrade unwanted material in the cell
Microfilaments	Near nuclear envelope, plasma membrane, and mitotic processes	Double-stranded, intertwined solid structures of actin; 5–7 nm in diameter	Supports cytoskeleton and motility
Intermediate filaments	Cytoskeleton	Solid structures 8–10 nm in diameter; self-assemble into larger bundles	Provides strong structural support
Microtubules	Cytoskeleton and centrioles near nucleus	Hollow cylinder 25 nm in diameter; consists of 13 protofilaments formed from α- and β-tubulin	Maintains cell shape; involved in cell and organelle motility and mitotic process
Centrosome	Near nucleus	Composed of two cylinder-shaped centrioles, each with nine bundles of three microtubules; centrioles oriented at right angles to each other	Contains centrioles that serve as insertion points for mitotic spindle fibers

ATP, Adenosine triphosphate; *DNA*, deoxyribonucleic acid; *RNA*, ribonucleic acid.

NUCLEUS

The nucleus is composed of three components: chromatin, nuclear envelope, and nucleoli. It is the control center of the cell and the largest organelle within the cell. The nucleus is composed largely of deoxyribonucleic acid (DNA) and is the site of DNA replication and transcription (Chapter 29). It controls the chemical reactions within the cell and directs its reproductive process. The nucleus has an affinity for basic dyes because of the nucleic acids contained within it; it stains deep purple with Wright stain (Chapters 6 and 10).

Chromatin

The chromatin consists of one long molecule of double-stranded DNA in each chromosome that is tightly folded, with histone and nonhistone proteins. The first level of folding is the formation of *nucleosomes* along the length of the DNA molecule. Each nucleosome is 11 nm in length and consists of approximately 150 base pairs of DNA wrapped around a histone protein core.[6] The positive charge of the histones facilitates binding with the negatively charged phosphate groups of DNA. The nucleosomes are folded into 30 nm chromatin fibers, and these fibers are further folded into loops, then supercoiled chromatin fibers that greatly condense the DNA (Figure 30.3). This highly structured folding allows the long strands of DNA to be tightly condensed in the nucleus when inactive and enables segments of the DNA to be rapidly unfolded for active transcription when needed. This complex process of gene expression is controlled by transcription factors and other regulatory proteins and processes. Inappropriate silencing of genes needed for blood cell maturation contributes to the molecular pathophysiology of acute leukemias and myelodysplastic neoplasms (Chapters 31 and 33).

Morphologically, chromatin is divided into two types: (1) *heterochromatin,* which has a more darkly stained, condensed clumping pattern and is the transcriptionally inactive area of the nucleus, and (2) *euchromatin,* which has a diffuse, uncondensed, open chromatin pattern and is the genetically active area of the nucleus where DNA transcription into messenger RNA (mRNA) occurs. The euchromatin is loosely coiled and turns a pale blue when stained with Wright stain. More mature cells have more heterochromatin because they are less transcriptionally active.

Nuclear Envelope

Surrounding the nucleus is a nuclear envelope consisting of two phospholipid bilayer membranes. The inner membrane surrounds the nucleus, and the outer membrane is continuous with the membrane of the rough endoplasmic reticulum (RER).[1,6] Between the two nuclear membranes is a 30- to 50-nm perinuclear space that is also continuous with the lumen of the RER.[6] Nuclear pore complexes penetrate the nuclear envelope, which allows passage of molecules between the nucleus and the cytoplasm.

Nucleoli

The nucleus contains one to several nucleoli. The nucleolus is the site of ribosomal RNA (rRNA) production and assembly into ribosome subunits. Because ribosomes synthesize proteins, the number of nucleoli in the nucleus is proportional to the amount of protein synthesis that occurs in the cell. As blood cells mature, protein synthesis decreases, and the nucleoli eventually disassemble.

Nucleoli contain a large amount of rRNA, the genes that code for rRNA (or rDNA), and ribosomal proteins. In ribosome biogenesis, rDNA is first transcribed to rRNA precursors. The rRNA precursors are processed into smaller RNA molecules and subsequently complexed with proteins forming the small and large ribosome subunits.[6] Ribosomal proteins enter the nucleus through the nuclear pores after being synthesized in the cytoplasm. After the ribosome subunits are synthesized and assembled, they are transported out of the nucleus through the nuclear pores. Once in the cytoplasm, large and small ribosome subunits self-assemble into a functional ribosome during protein synthesis (Chapter 29).[6]

CYTOPLASM

The cytoplasmic matrix is a homogeneous, continuous, aqueous solution called the *cytosol.* It is the environment in which the organelles exist and function. These organelles are discussed individually next.

Ribosomes

Ribosomes are macromolecular complexes composed of a small and large subunit of rRNA and many accessory ribosomal proteins. Ribosomes are found free in the cytoplasm or on the surface of RER. In the cytoplasm, they may exist singly or form chains (polyribosomes). Ribosomes serve as the site of protein synthesis. This is accomplished with transfer RNA (tRNA) for amino acid transport to the ribosome and specific mRNA molecules. The mRNA provides the genetic code for the sequence of amino acids for the protein being synthesized (Chapter 29). Cells that actively produce proteins have many ribosomes in the cytoplasm, which give it a dark blue color (basophilia) when stained with Wright stain. Cytoplasmic basophilia is particularly prominent in erythroid precursor cells when hemoglobin and other cell components are actively synthesized (Chapter 6).

Endoplasmic Reticulum

The endoplasmic reticulum (Figure 4.2) is a membrane-bound, interconnected network of flattened sacs and tubes located adjacent to the nucleus and extending throughout the cytoplasm. The channels within the endoplasmic reticulum are called *cisternae.*[3] Its membrane is continuous with the outer membrane of the nucleus, and its lumen is continuous with the perinuclear space between the outer and inner nuclear membranes. This arrangement provides a pathway for the flow of molecules between the nucleus and the cytoplasm.

RER has a studded look on its outer surface because of the presence of ribosomes. RER synthesizes and processes membrane-bound proteins and proteins that will be secreted from the cell.[2,3] Smooth endoplasmic reticulum (SER) is continuous with the RER but does not have ribosomes. SER is involved in synthesis of phospholipids and steroids, detoxification or inactivation of harmful compounds or drugs, and calcium storage and release.[2,3]

Golgi Apparatus

The Golgi apparatus (Figure 4.2) is a system of membrane-bound, stacked, flattened sacs called *cisternae* that are involved in modifying, sorting, and packaging macromolecules for secretion or delivery to other organelles. It contains numerous enzymes for these activities. The Golgi apparatus locates in close proximity to the RER and the nucleus. In Wright-stained bone marrow smears of developing white blood cell precursors, the Golgi area may be observed as an unstained region next to the nucleus (Chapter 10).

Vesicles containing membrane-bound and soluble proteins from the RER enter the Golgi network on the "cis face" and are directed through the stacks where the proteins are modified, as needed, by enzymes for glycosylation, sulfation, or phosphorylation.[1–3] Vesicles with processed proteins exit the Golgi on the "trans face" to form lysosomes or secretory vesicles bound for the plasma membrane.[1–3]

Mitochondria

Mitochondria (Figure 4.3) have an outer and inner membrane separated by an intermembrane space. The inner membrane is

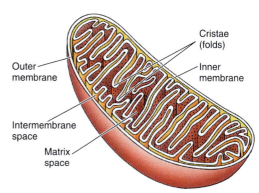

Figure 4.3 Mitochondrion Sectioned Longitudinally to Demonstrate Its Outer Membrane and Folded Inner Membrane Forming Cristae. (Modified from Gartner, L. P. [2021]. Cytoplasm. In *Textbook of Histology.* [5th ed., Figure 2.29A]. Philadelphia: Elsevier.)

highly convoluted, forming many infoldings called *cristae.* The interior of the mitochondrion, called *mitochondrial matrix,* is surrounded by the inner membrane and contains mitochondrial DNA, ribosomes, and various enzymes and proteins.

Mitochondria generate most of the adenosine triphosphate (ATP) for the cell by aerobic respiration. In the matrix, mitochondrial enzymes oxidize pyruvate and fatty acids to acetyl coenzyme A (CoA), which is then oxidized in the citric acid cycle producing nicotinamide adenine dinucleotide (NADH) and flavin adenine dinucleotide ($FADH_2$) for the electron-transport pathway. This pathway efficiently generates ATP through oxidative phosphorylation using proteins embedded in the inner membrane.[2] The convoluted structure of the inner membrane dramatically increases its surface area and thus increases the ATP-producing capability of the cell. A component of heme biosynthesis also occurs in the mitochondrial matrix (Chapter 8).

The mitochondria are capable of self-replication. This organelle has its own circular DNA for the mitochondrial division cycle and RNA for protein synthesis. There may be fewer than 100 or up to several thousand mitochondria per cell. The number is directly related to the amount of energy required by the cell.

Lysosomes

Lysosomes contain hydrolytic enzymes (acid hydrolases) bound within a membrane and are involved in the intracellular digestive process. These acid hydrolases are active only at a pH of about 5.0, so the lysosome membrane has proton pumps to transport hydrogen ion into the lysosome to maintain the acidic pH.[2] The lysosome membrane is also important in preventing the acid hydrolases from entering the cytoplasm and digesting cellular components and macromolecules. In addition, the acid hydrolases are inactivated at the higher pH of the cytosol, which protects the cell in case they are inappropriately released into the cytoplasm. Lysosomes fuse with endosomes and phagosomes (Chapter 10); this allows the lysosome hydrolytic enzymes to safely digest their contents.[1] With Wright stain, lysosomes are visualized as granules in white blood cells and platelets (Chapters 10 and 11). Lysosomal lipid storage diseases result from inherited mutations in genes for enzymes that catabolize certain lipids. Gaucher and Neimann-Pick diseases are examples of these disorders (Chapter 26).

Microfilaments and Intermediate Filaments

Actin microfilaments are double-stranded, intertwined solid structures approximately 5 to 7 nm in diameter.[3] They associate with myosin to enable cell motility, contraction, and intracellular transport. They locate near the nucleus and assist in cell division. They also locate near the plasma membrane and provide cytoskeletal support.

Intermediate filaments, with a diameter of approximately 8 to 10 nm, self-assemble into larger bundles.[3] They are the most durable element of the cytoskeleton and provide structural stability for the cells, especially cells subjected to more physical stress, such as the epidermal layer of skin.[1] Examples include the keratins and lamins.

Microtubules

Microtubules are hollow, cylindrical structures that are approximately 25 nm in diameter and vary in length. They consist of α- and β-tubulin heterodimers that self-assemble into protofilaments; 13 parallel protofilaments form each microtubule.[1,2] This arrangement gives the microtubules structural strength. Tubulins can rapidly polymerize, forming microtubules, and then rapidly depolymerize when no longer needed by the cell.

Microtubules help support the cytoskeleton to maintain cell shape and are involved in cell motility (e.g., cilia and flagella) and the intracellular movement of some organelles.[2] Microtubules also form the mitotic spindle fibers during mitosis and are the major component of centrioles.

Centrosomes

The centrosome consists of two cylinder-shaped centrioles that are typically oriented at right angles to each other (Figure 4.2). A centriole consists of nine bundles of three microtubules each.[2] They serve as insertion points for the mitotic spindle fibers during mitosis.

SELECTED CELL PROCESSES

Plasma Membrane Transport

The plasma membrane forms a semipermeable barrier between the intracellular and extracellular environments. Because of its phospholipid bilayer structure, hydrophilic ions and polar molecules have limited ability to pass through the membrane without specialized transmembrane proteins. It is essential for cellular function and survival that the membrane allows movement of the appropriate molecules in and out of the cell. There are two general mechanisms in which molecules pass through the plasma membrane: passive transport and active transport (Box 4.1).

Passive transport involves the movement of molecules across the plasma membrane *along* their concentration gradients without requiring the expenditure of energy. Passive transport includes simple diffusion, facilitated diffusion, and osmosis.

BOX 4.1 Mechanisms for Transport Across the Plasma Membrane

Passive Transport (*Along* the Concentration Gradient; Does Not Require Energy Expenditure)
Simple diffusion
Facilitated diffusion (channels and carriers)
Osmosis

Active Transport (*Against* the Concentration Gradient; Requires Energy Expenditure)
Primary: transmembrane protein pumps, channels, ATPases (uses ATP for energy)
Secondary: transmembrane protein symports and antiports (uses energy from electrochemical gradients)
Vesicular: vesicles transport molecules and particles into and out of cell
  Exocytosis
  Endocytosis
    Pinocytosis
    Phagocytosis
    Receptor-mediated endocytosis

ATP, Adenosine triphosphate.

Simple diffusion involves the gradient-driven movement of small nonpolar (hydrophobic) molecules across the membrane, such as oxygen and carbon dioxide.[2,3] *Facilitated diffusion* uses channels or carriers, consisting of transmembrane proteins, that allow ions (such as Na^+, K^+, Ca^{2+}) and small polar molecules (such as glucose) to selectively pass through the membrane. Carriers differ from channels in that they change conformation in the transport process.[3] *Aquaporins* are a special type of membrane channel that transport water across the plasma membrane at a faster rate than osmosis.[3] *Osmosis* involves the movement of water across the selectively permeable plasma membrane from the low solute concentration side of the membrane to the high solute concentration side. The osmotic movement of water continues until an equilibrium of solute concentration is reached on each side of the membrane.[3] This process is demonstrated in RBCs in the osmotic fragility test (Chapter 21).

Active transport involves the movement of small molecules or ions across a membrane *against* their concentration gradients and requires the expenditure of energy to overcome the gradient. In *primary active transport,* transmembrane proteins (transport pumps, channels, and ATPases) move ions across the membrane using energy from the hydrolysis of adenosine triphosphate (ATP).[3] These pumps mainly involve the movement of Na^+, K^+, Ca^{2+}, and Mg^{2+} across membranes against their concentration gradient to support a cellular function. For example, RBCs use the transport pump, *sodium-potassium ATPase,* to maintain higher intracellular levels of K^+ and lower intracellular levels of Na^+. This helps to maintain their volume and shape (Chapter 7).

In *secondary active transport,* a small molecule or ion is transported *against* its concentration gradient, coupled with the transport of a second molecule moving *along* its concentration gradient. This type of transport uses an electrochemical gradient for energy. In *symports,* the transported molecules move in the same direction, while in *antiports,* the transported molecules move in the opposite direction. Symports and antiports often use Na^+ moving along its concentration gradient to transport another molecule (such as glucose or H^+) against its concentration gradient.[3]

Vesicular transport is another type of active transport that uses membrane coated sacs (vesicles) to bring in or expel macromolecules and other substances from the cell. *Exocytosis* is the transport of substances (usually secretory proteins) out of the cell through cytoplasmic vesicles that fuse with the plasma membrane and discharge their contents outside the cell. *Endocytosis* is the transport of substances into the cell by engulfing them in a vesicle formed by the plasma membrane. There are three types of endocytosis: pinocytosis, phagocytosis, and receptor-mediated endocytosis.

In *pinocytosis,* the plasma membrane invaginates (folds inward), creating a small pit with extracellular contents.[3] The pit pinches off and disconnects from the plasma membrane, forming a fluid-filled vesicle inside the cell.[2,3] This process also helps to recycle membrane components.[2]

In *phagocytosis,* the plasma membrane extends out into the extracellular environment, forming pseudopods to engulf particulate matter and bring the particles into the cell in a phagosome.[3] Neutrophils and monocytes/macrophages are *phagocytes* with receptors that either directly bind to a particle (such as a bacterium, foreign antigen, or a senescent RBC) or bind to antibodies or complement coating the particle. The receptor binding activates the cell to form pseudopods to engulf the particle, bring it into the cell as a phagosome, and then digest it (Chapter 10 and Box 10.2).[2]

In *receptor-mediated endocytosis,* protein receptors in the plasma membrane bind with high affinity to specific molecules or ligands, causing the receptors to cluster and the membrane to invaginate forming a clathrin-coated pit. The pit pinches off, forming a membrane-bound *endosome* that contains the membrane receptors and their bound ligands. This process allows the cell to bring in and concentrate specific molecules needed by the cell.[2] The ligand releases from the receptor in the endosome and can be transported into the cytosol for use by the cell. The empty receptors may be recycled to the cell surface by fusion of the endosome membrane with the plasma membrane, thus enabling the receptors to bind additional ligands if needed by the cell.[2] Iron (bound to its transport protein, transferrin) enters cells by this process by binding to transferrin receptor 1 on the plasma membrane (Chapter 9 and Figure 9.8).

Cell Communication and Signal Transduction

Communication between cells is essential for survival, and it is critical that the communication is specific, coordinated, and regulated. Adjacent cells can communicate with each other directly through intercellular pores or *gap junctions,* which connect the cytoplasm between two cells, enabling the rapid exchange of molecules. In this case, only very small molecules can pass through the gap junctions, such as cyclic adenosine monophosphate (cAMP) and Ca^{2+}.[7] When cells are not adjacent, cell communication involves a signaling cell that produces a signaling molecule, or *ligand,* and a target cell with a specific *receptor* for the ligand. The ligand may be brought to the receptor on the target cell by the signaling cell (*contact-dependent* or *juxtacrine signaling*).[3,7] For example, in the immune response, antigen epitopes (the ligand) on a macrophage (signaling cell) membrane are presented to antigen receptors on B or T lymphocytes (target cells), resulting in their activation (Chapter 10). Some cells secrete ligands that can bind to their own surface receptors, thus serving as signaling and target cells (*autocrine signaling*).[3,7] Other ligands are rapidly degraded after secretion and can activate nearby target cells only (*paracrine signaling*).[3,7] Often, however, the ligand (such as a hormone) is secreted by the signaling cell in one location and is carried to target cells throughout the body, usually through the bloodstream (*endocrine signaling*).[3,7] Hematopoietic cells in the bone marrow use all types of these signaling mechanisms.

Ligands may be hormones, neurotransmitters (such as norepinephrine and histamine), peptides, or small molecules (amino acids, nucleotides, ions). Receptors may be located in the plasma membrane, cytoplasm, or nucleus. Hydrophobic ligands (such as steroid hormones or nitric acid) can pass through the plasma membrane and bind and activate cytoplasmic receptors. Some of these activated receptors can bind to specific DNA sequences in the nucleus to increase or suppress gene expression.[3,7] However, if the ligand is hydrophilic, it cannot readily pass through the plasma membrane and requires a transmembrane protein receptor to bind the ligand in its extracellular domain and transmit the signal into the cell through its cytoplasmic domain.[3]

The signal transduction pathway is a very complex, multistep process that begins with the ligand (first messenger) binding to its specific receptor on or in the target cell. That binding results in activation of a cascade of various intermediate signaling proteins (usually effector enzymes such as kinases, phosphodiesterases, phospholipases, adenylyl cyclase, or guanosine triphosphate (GTP) coupled proteins or G-proteins) to amplify the signal.[3,7] The effector enzymes may generate second messengers, small molecules such as Ca^{2+}, cAMP, cyclic guanosine monophosphate (cGMP), diacetylglycerol (DAG), and inositol triphosphate (IP_3).[3,7] The second messengers further amplify the signal. A detailed explanation of the reactions in signal transduction pathways is beyond the scope of this chapter. Ultimately, specific target proteins in the cell are altered, and cellular functions are modified. The target proteins may be transport proteins, metabolic enzymes, gene regulatory proteins, cytoskeletal proteins, or cell cycle proteins, which then modify ion transport, cell metabolism, gene expression, cell shape or movement, and cell growth and division, respectively (Figure 4.4).[7] In addition, the cell modification could be an activation or inhibition of various cellular processes with or without changes in gene expression.[7]

There are approximately 25 families of receptors. Most plasma membrane receptors involved in signal transduction fall

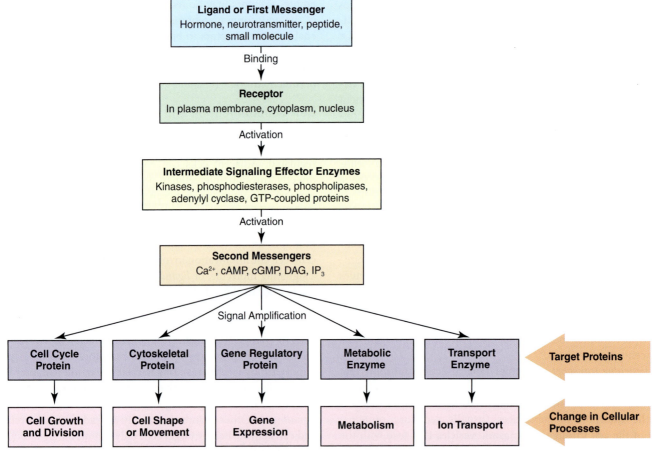

Figure 4.4 Overview of Signal Transduction. A ligand or first messenger (hormone, neurotransmitter, peptide, small molecule) binds to a receptor, which may be in the plasma membrane, cytoplasm, or nucleus. The binding activates intracellular signaling effector enzymes (kinases, phosphodiesterases, phospholipases, adenylyl cyclase, guanosine triphosphate coupled proteins or G proteins), which activate second messengers (calcium, cyclic adenosine monophosphate, cyclic guanosine monophosphate, diacetylglycerol, inositol triphosphate) to amplify the signal. The amplified signal regulates the activity of one or more target proteins (transport proteins, metabolic enzymes, gene regulatory proteins, cytoskeletal proteins, cell cycle proteins), which results in a change in ion transport, cell metabolism, gene expression, cell shape or movement, and cell growth and division. The signal can activate or inhibit the cellular process with or without changes in gene expression. *Ca2+,* Calcium; *cAMP,* cyclic adenosine monophosphate; *cGMP,* cyclic guanosine monophosphate; *DAG,* diacetylglycerol; *GTP,* guanosine triphosphate; *IP3,* inositol triphosphate. (Adapted from Koeppen, B. M., & Stanton, B. A. [2018]. Signal transduction, membrane receptors, second messengers, and regulation of gene expression. In Koeppen, B. M. & Stanton, B. A. [Eds.], *Berne and Levy Physiology.* [10th ed., Figure 3.1]. Philadelphia: Elsevier. Redrawn from Alberts, B., Johnson, A., Lewis, J., et al: *Molecular Biology of the Cell.* 6th ed. New York: Garland Science; 2015.)

into three main types: ion channel-linked, G-protein coupled, and enzyme-linked receptors (Figure 4.5).[2,3,7]

When a ligand binds to the extracellular component of an ion channel-linked receptor, it opens a channel in the receptor to allow certain ions to pass through the membrane (Figure 4.5A).[3]

In this case, the receptor accomplishes both the ligand binding and signal transduction functions. This type of signaling converts a chemical signal to an electrical signal by rapidly altering the membrane potential between cells.[3,7] This is important for the function of neurons and muscle cells.

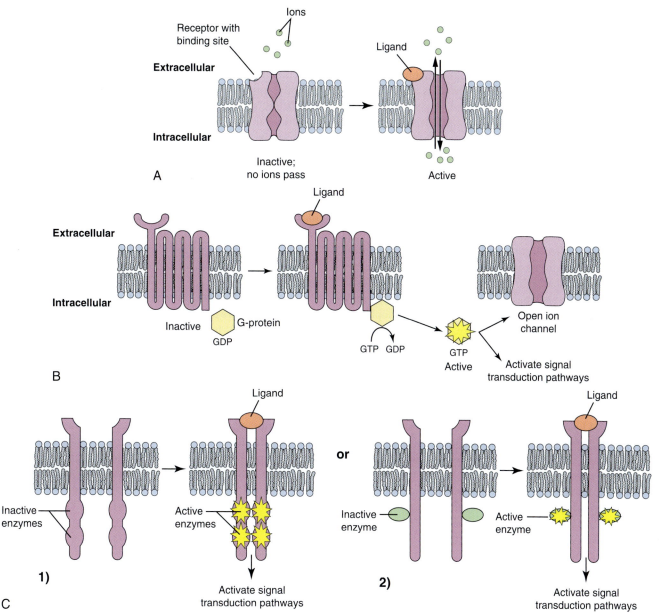

Figure 4.5 General Types of Plasma Membrane Receptors Involved in Signal Transduction. **(A),** Ion channel-linked receptor. When ligand binds to the extracellular component of an ion channel-linked receptor, it opens a channel in the receptor to allow certain ions to pass through the membrane. **(B),** G-protein coupled receptor. When ligand binds to the extracellular component of the receptor, it undergoes a conformational change, causing the guanosine diphosphate to be replaced by guanosine triphosphate on the G-protein associated with its cytoplasmic component. This activates and releases the G-protein from the receptor. The activated G-protein can then interact with ion channels to change membrane permeability or activate signal transduction pathways to amplify the signal, which alters various cell functions and/or gene expression. The G-protein may be monomeric (single protein) or may be heterotrimeric, consisting of α, β, and γ subunits. **(C),** Enzyme-linked receptor. When ligand binds to the extracellular component of the receptor, it forms a dimer and undergoes a change in conformation. This can either activate an enzymatic domain in its cytoplasmic component *(1)* or activate an enzyme associated with its cytoplasmic component *(2)*. The enzyme, usually a protein kinase, is activated by phosphorylation and subsequently activates signal transduction pathways to amplify the signal, which alters various cell functions and/or gene expression. *GDP,* Guanosine diphosphate; *GTP,* guanosine triphosphate.

G-protein coupled receptors are multipass transmembrane proteins (seven transmembrane repeats) associated with a G-protein on the cytoplasmic side of the membrane.[3] The G-protein may be monomeric (single protein) or may be heterotrimeric, consisting of α, β, and γ subunits.[7] Inactive G-proteins have bound guanosine diphosphate (GDP).[7] When ligand binds to the receptor, there is a conformational change, causing the G-protein to bind to the receptor and its GDP to be replaced by guanosine triphosphate (GTP). This activates and releases the G-protein from the receptor.[3,7] The activated G-protein can then interact with ion channels to change membrane permeability or activate intermediate effector proteins that work with second messengers to amplify the signal to alter various cell processes (Figure 4.5B).[3,7] For example, platelets have at least eight different G-protein coupled receptors that bind to their specific ligands to promote platelet aggregation and secretion in the platelet activation process (Chapter 11 and Figures 11.8 and 11.11).

Enzyme-linked receptors are single-pass transmembrane proteins with an extracellular ligand-binding domain, a transmembrane domain, and a cytoplasmic component that extends into the cytosol. When ligand binds to the extracellular component, the receptor forms a dimer and undergoes a change in conformation. The change in conformation of the receptor can either (1) activate an enzymatic domain in its cytoplasmic component, or (2) activate an enzyme associated with its cytoplasmic component.[3] The associated enzyme, usually a protein kinase, is activated by phosphorylation (adding a phosphate ion) and subsequently activates other proteins and second messengers in the cytosol to alter a cell function or gene expression (Figure 4.5C).[3] An example of the first type is FLT3, a receptor tyrosine kinase present on hematopoietic stem and progenitor cells. When activated by FLT3 ligand, the receptor forms a dimer and changes conformation, which activates the kinase domains in its cytoplasmic component. The activated kinases then activate various downstream pathways to promote expression of genes required for cell differentiation, proliferation, and survival.[8] An example of the second type is the erythropoietin receptor on early erythroid cells and its associated tyrosine kinase enzyme, Janus kinase 2 (JAK2). When erythropoietin binds to the receptor, it forms a dimer, the JAK2 kinases associated with its cytoplasmic domain are activated, and they subsequently activate additional downstream pathways, promoting the expression of genes that cause an increased number of RBCs to enter the circulation (Chapters 6 and 32 and Figure 32.9).[8] Mutations in these receptors can lead to hematologic malignancies (Chapters 31 and 32).

A special class of membrane receptors are cell adhesion molecules (CAMs), which are important for cell-to-cell signaling and for the binding of cells to ligands in the ECM. CAMs are a large group of transmembrane receptors with an large extracellular component, a single-pass transmembrane domain, and a short cytoplasmic component.[9] Their cytoplasmic domains are linked to actin or intermediate filaments in the cytoskeleton, either directly or indirectly through accessory proteins.[9,10] Their cytoplasmic components can also link to kinases to initiate signal transduction pathways in the same manner as the enzyme-linked receptors described in the preceding paragraph.[9,10]

Activation of cell membrane CAMs can affect cell shape, motility, and the ability of its other CAMs to bind ligands.[9] CAM activation can also promote cell proliferation and increased synthesis and secretion of specific proteins by altering gene expression.[9] Examples of CAMs include integrins, selectins, mucins, immunoglobulin-type CAMs, and leucine-rich-type CAMs.[9,10] CAMs bind to ligands in the ECM such as collagen, laminin, vitronectin, and fibronectin, and to proteins in circulation such as fibrinogen and von Willebrand factor.[9,10]

Integrins are a type of CAM and comprise a family of 24 transmembrane proteins that are important for cell adhesion, motility, growth, and survival.[10,11] They are heterodimers consisting of α and β chains that can transmit signals in two directions through the membrane. When a ligand binds to the extracellular domains, there is a clustering and change in conformation in the cytoplasmic domain that interacts with the cytoskeleton causing actin polymerization (*outside-in signaling*).[11] This can result in changes in cell shape and motility as well as activate kinases in the enzyme-linked receptor manner discussed earlier.[11] The cytoplasmic component of the receptor can also be activated by stimuli in the cytosol such as phosphorylation (*inside-out signaling*). This causes a change in conformation in the extracellular component of the receptor, allowing ligands to bind.[11]

Integrins and other CAM receptors are present in the platelet membrane and are important for platelet activation (Chapter 11 and Figure 11.8). Integrins are also present on hematopoietic cells in the bone marrow, where they are important for hematopoietic cell adhesion to the bone marrow stroma and for cell-to-cell interaction (Chapter 5).

In these examples, signal transduction usually begins with an extracellular ligand transmitting a signal into the cell through a transmembrane receptor. The receptor is activated and subsequently activates a series of enzymes and second messengers in downstream reactions. Ultimately, target proteins in the cell are modified, causing a change in cell behavior, gene expression, or both.[3,7] Signal transduction is highly regulated, with feedback mechanisms to deactivate the receptor once the desired cell effect is achieved.[7]

Cell Cycle and its Regulation
Stages
The purpose of the cell cycle is to replicate DNA once and distribute identical chromosome copies equally to two daughter cells during mitosis.[12] The cell cycle is a biochemical and morphologic four-stage process through which a cell passes when it is stimulated to divide (Figure 4.6). These stages are G_1 (gap 1), S (DNA synthesis), G_2 (gap 2), and M (mitosis). The G_1 stage is a period of cell growth and synthesis of components necessary for replication.[12] In the S stage, DNA replication takes place (Chapter 29). An exact copy of each chromosome is produced, and they pair together as *sister chromatids*. The centrosome is also duplicated during the S stage.[12] In the G_2 stage, the tetraploid DNA is checked for proper replication and damage (discussed in "Regulation of the Cell Cycle"). The time spent in each stage can be variable, but mitosis takes approximately 1 hour.[12] During G_0 (quiescence), the cell is not actively in the cell cycle.

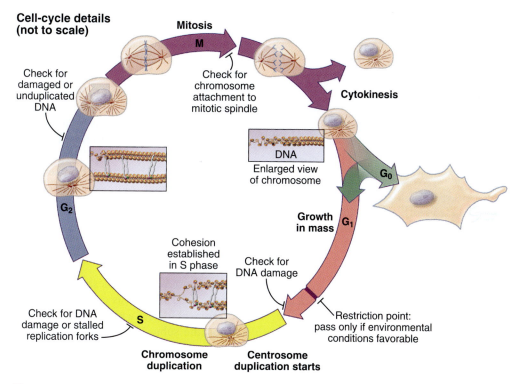

Figure 4.6 Stages of the Cell Cycle. Diagrams of cellular morphology and chromosome structure across the cell cycle. (Modified from Pollard, T. D., Earnshaw, W. C., Lippincott-Schwartz, J., et al. [2017]. Introduction to the cell cycle. In *Cell Biology*. [3rd ed., Figure 40.2]. Philadelphia: Elsevier.)

Mitosis or M stage involves the division of chromosomes and cytoplasm into two daughter cells. It is divided into six phases (Figure 4.6) as follows:[12]

1. *Prophase:* the chromosomes condense, the duplicated centrosomes begin to separate, and mitotic spindle fibers appear.
2. *Prometaphase:* the nuclear envelope disassembles, the centrosomes move to opposite poles of the cell and serve as a point of origin of the mitotic spindle fibers; the sister chromatids (chromosome pairs) attach to the mitotic spindle fibers.
3. *Metaphase:* the sister chromatids align on the mitotic spindle fibers at a location equidistant from the centrosome poles.
4. *Anaphase:* the sister chromatids separate and move on the mitotic spindles toward the centrosomes on opposite poles.
5. *Telophase:* the nuclear membrane reassembles around each set of chromosomes, and the mitotic spindle fibers disappear.
6. *Cytokinesis:* the cell divides into two identical daughter cells.

Interphase is a term used for the nonmitosis stages of the cell cycle, that is, G_1, S, and G_2.

Regulation of the Cell Cycle

The cell cycle is a highly complex process that can malfunction. To prevent abnormal or mutated cells from going through the cell cycle and producing an abnormal clone, checkpoints occur in the cycle to detect abnormalities (Figure 4.6).[1,12] A restriction point in late G_1 checks for adequate nutrients and appropriate cell volume. The *G_1 checkpoint* at the end of G_1 checks the DNA for damage and either makes the cell wait for DNA repair or initiates apoptosis. The *S phase checkpoint* checks DNA for

damage and completion of replication. The *G_2 checkpoint* takes place after DNA synthesis at the end of G_2, and it verifies that replication took place without error or damage. If damaged or unduplicated DNA is detected, mitosis is blocked. The last checkpoint, the *metaphase checkpoint,* takes place during mitosis at the time of metaphase. The attachment and alignment of chromosomes on the mitotic spindle and the integrity of the spindle apparatus are checked.[1,12] Anaphase will be blocked if any defects are detected.

Progression through the cell cycle is regulated by cyclin and cyclin-dependent kinases (CDKs). A cyclin activates a specific CDK, forms a cyclin/CDK complex, and directs the CDK to phosphorylate key substrates that drive the cell through a specific transition in the cell cycle. Cyclin is named appropriately because the concentrations of specific cyclins increase and decrease at designated times in the cell cycle, and cyclin/CDK complexes drive the cycle through its successive, orderly stages. The G_1 stage begins when external stimuli, such as growth factors, cause an increase in one or more of the D cyclins (D1, D2, D3), which then complex with CDK4 or CDK6.[12] To transition the cell from G_1 to S, cyclin E increases and binds to CDK2, forming the cyclin E/CDK2 complex. In the S stage, cyclin E degrades and cyclin A increases and complexes with CDK2, forming cyclin A/CDK2. This complex is required for progression through the S stage. Cyclin A also partners with CDK1, forming the cyclin A/CDK1 complex, which is needed for completion of the S stage and the G_2 to M transition. For mitosis to occur, cyclin B must replace cyclin A and bind to CDK1, forming the cyclin B/CDK1 complex. This complex takes the

TABLE 4.2　Cyclins and Cyclin-Dependent Kinases in Cell Cycle Progression

Stage	Major Activities and Complexes Required
G_1	External stimuli (e.g., growth factor) and ↑ D cyclins (D1, D2, D3) *Complex:* Cyclin D/CDK4, 6
G_1/S	↑ Cyclin E *Complex:* Cyclin E/CDK2 required for G1 to S transition
S	↓ Cyclin E ↑ Cyclin A *Complex:* Cyclin A/CDK2 required for progression through S stage
G_2/M	CDK1 signals end of S stage *Complex:* Cyclin A/CDK1 required for completion of S stage and G2 to M transition
M	↓ Cyclin A ↑ Cyclin B *Complex:* Cyclin B/CDK1 required for mitosis ↓ Cyclin B signals end of mitosis

cell through the intricate process of mitosis.[12,13] Degradation of cyclin B triggers the end of mitosis and initiates cytokinesis. Inhibitors of the cyclin/CDK complexes also play a primary role in cell cycle regulation.[13] Table 4.2 summarizes the actions of the major cyclins and CDKs in the cell cycle.

Tumor suppressor proteins are needed for the proper function of the checkpoints (Chapter 27). One of the first tumor suppressor genes recognized was *TP53*, which codes for the TP53 protein that detects DNA damage during the G_1 stage. It can also assist in triggering apoptosis. Many tumor suppressor genes have been described.[13] When these genes are mutated or deleted, cells with abnormal or deleted DNA/chromosomes are allowed to go through the cell cycle and replicate. Some of these cells simply malfunction, but others form malignant neoplasms, often with aggressive characteristics. For example, patients with chronic lymphocytic leukemia have a more aggressive disease with a shorter survival time when their leukemic cells lose TP53 activity, either through gene mutation or deletion (Chapter 34).

Cell Death by Necrosis and Apoptosis

Cell death occurs as a normal physiologic process in the body or as a response to injury. Events that injure cells include ischemia (oxygen deprivation), mechanical trauma, toxins, drugs, infectious agents, autoimmune reactions, genetic defects including acquired and inherited mutations, and improper nutrition.[14] There are two major mechanisms for cell death: necrosis and apoptosis.[15] *Necrosis* is a pathologic process caused by direct external injury to cells, such as from ischemia, infections, trauma, or toxins.[14] *Apoptosis* is a self-inflicted cell death originating from the activation signals within the cell itself.[15] Most apoptosis occurs as a normal physiologic process to eliminate potentially harmful cells (e.g., self-reacting lymphocytes [Chapter 5]), cells that are no longer needed (e.g., excess erythroid progenitors in oxygen-replete states [Chapter 6] or neutrophils after phagocytosis), and aging cells.[14,15] Apoptosis of older, terminally differentiated cells balances with new cell growth to maintain needed numbers of functional cells in organs, hematopoietic tissue, and epithelial cell barriers, particularly in skin

and intestines. On the other hand, apoptosis also initiates in response to internal or external pathologic injury to a cell. For example, if DNA damage occurred during the replication phase of the cell cycle and the damage is beyond the capability of the DNA repair mechanisms, the cell will activate apoptosis to prevent its further progression through the cell cycle. Apoptosis can also be triggered in virally infected cells by the virus itself or by the body's immune response.[14] This is one of the mechanisms to remove virally infected cells from the body.

The first morphologic manifestation of necrosis is a swelling of the cell.[15] The cell may be able to recover from minor injury at that point. More severe damage, however, disrupts organelles and membranes; enzymes leak out of lysosomes that denature and digest DNA, RNA, and intracellular proteins; and ultimately, the cell lyses.[14] An inflammatory response usually accompanies necrosis because of the release of cell contents into the extracellular space.

The morphologic manifestation of apoptosis is shrinkage of the cell.[15] The nucleus condenses and undergoes systematic fragmentation as a result of cleavage of the DNA between nucleosome subunits (multiples of 180 to 200 base pairs). The plasma membrane remains intact, but the phospholipids lose their asymmetric distribution and "flip" phosphatidylserine from the inner to the outer leaflet.[16] The cytoplasm and nuclear fragments bud off in membrane-bound vesicles. Macrophages, recognizing the phosphatidylserine and other signals on the membranes, rapidly phagocytize the vesicles. Thus cellular products are not released into the extracellular space, and an inflammatory response is not elicited.[14] Figure 4.7 and Table 4.3 summarize the differences between necrosis and apoptosis.

Activation of apoptosis occurs through extrinsic and intrinsic pathways. Both pathways involve the activation of proteins called *caspases*. The extrinsic pathway, also called the *death receptor pathway,* initiates with the binding of ligand to a death receptor on the cell membrane. Examples of death receptors and their ligands include Fas and Fas ligand and tumor necrosis factor receptor 1 (TNFR1) and tumor necrosis factor.[14,17] The binding recruits various adapter proteins that bind and activate caspase-8 (or sometimes caspase-10).[15,16] The intrinsic pathway is initiated by intracellular stressors (such as hypoxia, DNA damage, or membrane disruption) that stimulate the release of cytochrome *c* from mitochondria.[17] Cytochrome *c* binds to apoptotic protease-activating factor-1 (APAF-1) and caspase-9, forming an *apoptosome,* which activates caspase-9. Both pathways converge when the initiator caspases (8, 9, or 10) activate effector/executioner caspases (3, 6, and 7), which leads to apoptosis.[15,17]

Various cellular proapoptotic and antiapoptotic proteins tightly regulate apoptosis. Examples of antiapoptotic proteins include some members of the Bcl-2 family of proteins (such as Bcl-2, Bcl-X_L) as well as various growth factors such as erythropoietin.[15,16] BAX and BAK are examples of proapoptotic proteins.[15,17] The ratio of these intracellular proteins plays a primary role in regulating apoptosis. Any dysregulation, mutation, or translocation can cause inhibition or overexpression of apoptotic proteins, which can lead to hematologic neoplasms or cell malfunctions.[14,16]

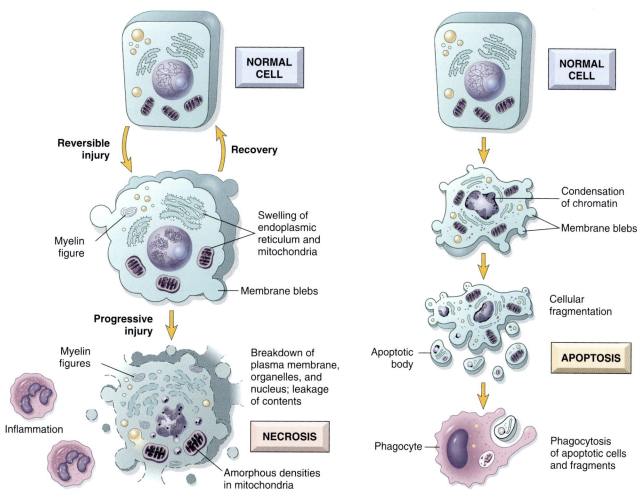

Figure 4.7 Schematic Illustration of the Morphologic Changes in Cell Injury Culminating in Necrosis or Apoptosis. (From Oakes, S. A. [2021]. Cell injury, cell death, and adaptations. In Kumar, V., Abbas, A. K., & Aster, J. C. [Eds.], *Robbins and Cotran Pathologic Basis of Disease.* [10th ed., Figure 2.4]. Philadelphia: Elsevier.)

TABLE 4.3   Comparison of Necrosis and Apoptosis

	Necrosis	Apoptosis
Cell size	Enlarged as a result of swelling	Reduced as a result of shrinkage
Nucleus	Random breaks and lysis (karyolysis)	Condensation and fragmentation between nucleosomes
Plasma membrane	Disrupted with loss of integrity	Intact with loss of phospholipid asymmetry
Inflammation	Enzyme digestion and leakage of cell contents; inflammatory response occurs	Release of cell contents in membrane-bound apoptotic bodies, which are phagocytized by macrophages; no inflammation occurs
Physiologic or pathologic function	Pathologic; results from cell injury	Mostly physiologic to remove unwanted cells; pathologic in response to cell injury

HEMATOPOIETIC MICROENVIRONMENT

Hematopoiesis occurs predominantly in the bone marrow from the third trimester of fetal life through adulthood (Chapter 5). The bone marrow microenvironment must provide for hematopoietic stem cell self-renewal, proliferation, differentiation, and apoptosis and support the developing progenitor and precursor blood cells. This protective environment is provided by stromal cells, such as endothelial cells, fibroblasts, specialized adventitial reticular cells, adipocytes (fat cells), chondrocytes, osteoblasts, and osteoclasts.[18,19] Stromal cells secrete substances that form an ECM, including collagen, fibronectin, thrombospondin, laminins, tenascin, and proteoglycans (such as hyaluronate, chondroitin sulfate, and heparan sulfate).[18,19] The ECM is critical for cell growth and for anchoring developing blood cells in the bone marrow. Hematopoietic cells have various receptors for growth factors and adhesion molecules. Adhesion receptors provide a mechanism for attachment to ECM in bone marrow. These receptors also provide a means of cell-cell interaction, which is essential for regulated hematopoiesis.[9]

Stromal cells secrete various growth factors that participate in complex processes to regulate the proliferation and differentiation of progenitor and precursor blood cells (Chapter 5). Growth factors must bind to specific receptors on their target cells to exert their effect. Most growth factors are produced by cells in the hematopoietic microenvironment and exert their effects in local cell interactions. One growth factor, erythropoietin, has a hormone-type stimulation in that it is produced in another location (kidney) and exerts its effect on erythroid progenitors in the bone marrow (Chapters 5 and 6). An important feature of growth factors is their use of synergism to stimulate a cell to proliferate or differentiate. In other words, several different growth factors work together to generate a more effective response.[8] Growth factors are specific for their corresponding receptors on target cells.

Growth factor receptors are transmembrane proteins.[8] When the growth factor (or ligand) binds the extracellular domain of the receptor, a signal is transmitted to the nucleus in the cell through the cytoplasmic domain, which subsequently activates a signal transduction cascade that influences the differentiation, proliferation, and survival of hematopoietic cells. The receptors comprise multiple receptor families including enzyme-linked and G-protein coupled receptors.[8] Mutations in growth factor receptors and signal transduction proteins may lead to hematologic neoplasms (Chapter 27).

SUMMARY

- The cell contains cytoplasm that is separated from the extracellular environment by a plasma membrane, a membrane-bound nucleus (with the exception of mature red blood cells and platelets), and other unique subcellular structures and organelles.
- The plasma membrane is a bilayer of phospholipids, cholesterol, and proteins. Glycolipids and glycoproteins on the outer surface form the glycocalyx.
- The cytoplasm contains ribosomes for protein synthesis, which can be free in the cytoplasm or located on rough endoplasmic reticulum (RER). The RER makes most of the membrane proteins and proteins for secretion from the cell. Smooth endoplasmic reticulum (SER) lacks ribosomes; SER is involved in synthesis of phospholipids and steroids, detoxification or inactivation of harmful compounds or drugs, and calcium storage and release.
- The Golgi apparatus modifies and packages macromolecules for secretion and for transport to other cell organelles. Mitochondria make adenosine triphosphate (ATP) to supply energy for the cell. Lysosomes contain hydrolytic enzymes involved in the cell's intracellular digestive process.
- Molecules can enter the cell through passive or active transport. Passive transport, in which molecules cross a membrane along their concentration gradients without the expenditure of energy, includes simple diffusion, facilitated diffusion, and osmosis. Active transport, in which molecules cross a membrane against their concentration gradients, requires the expenditure of energy. Active transport can be primary, secondary, or vesicular.
- Cells have complex mechanisms for communication. Adjacent cells can communicate directly with each other through gap junctions. When cells are not adjacent, communication involves a signaling cell that produces a ligand and a target cell with a specific receptor for the ligand. The signal transduction pathway is a very complex, multistep process that begins with the ligand (first messenger) binding to its specific receptor on or in the target cell. That binding results in activation of a cascade of various intermediate signaling proteins and second messengers to amplify the signal. Ultimately, a target protein in the cell is modified, causing a change in cell behavior, gene expression, or both.
- The cell cycle involves four active stages: G_1 (gap 1), S (DNA synthesis), G_2 (gap 2), and M (mitosis). Cell cycle progression is regulated by cyclins and cyclin-dependent kinases. Checkpoints in the cell cycle recognize abnormalities and initiate apoptosis.
- Two major mechanisms for cell death are necrosis and apoptosis. Necrosis is a pathologic process caused by direct external injury to cells, whereas apoptosis is a self-inflicted cell death originating from the activation signals within the cell itself. Most apoptosis occurs as a normal physiologic process to eliminate unwanted cells, but it can also be initiated in response to internal or external pathologic injury to a cell.
- The bone marrow provides a suitable microenvironment for hematopoietic stem cell self-renewal, proliferation, differentiation, and apoptosis. Stromal cells secrete substances that form an extracellular matrix to support hematopoietic cell growth and function and help to anchor developing cells in the bone marrow. Growth factors participate in complex processes to regulate the proliferation and differentiation of hematopoietic stem and progenitor cells.

REVIEW QUESTIONS

Answers can be found in Appendix C.

1. The organelle involved in packaging and trafficking of cellular products is the:
   a. Nucleus
   b. Golgi apparatus
   c. Mitochondria
   d. Rough endoplasmic reticulum

2. The glycocalyx is composed of membrane:
   a. Phospholipids and cholesterol
   b. Glycoproteins and glycolipids
   c. Transmembrane and cytoskeletal proteins
   d. Rough and smooth endoplasmic reticulum

3. The "control center" of the cell is the:
   a. Nucleus
   b. Cytoplasm
   c. Membrane
   d. Microtubular system
4. The nucleus is composed largely of:
   a. RNA
   b. DNA
   c. Ribosomes
   d. Glycoproteins
5. The site of protein synthesis is the:
   a. Nucleus
   b. Mitochondria
   c. Ribosomes
   d. Golgi apparatus
6. The shape of a cell is maintained by which of the following?
   a. Microtubules
   b. Spindle fibers
   c. Ribosomes
   d. Centrioles
7. Functions of the cell membrane include all of the following EXCEPT:
   a. Regulation of molecules entering or leaving the cell
   b. Receptor recognition of extracellular signals
   c. Maintenance of electrochemical gradients
   d. Lipid production and oxidation
8. The energy source for cells is the:
   a. Golgi apparatus
   b. Endoplasmic reticulum
   c. Nucleolus
   d. Mitochondrion
9. Ribosomes are synthesized by the:
   a. Endoplasmic reticulum
   b. Mitochondrion
   c. Nucleolus
   d. Golgi apparatus
10. Euchromatin functions as the:
    a. Site of microtubule production
    b. Transcriptionally active DNA
    c. Support structure for nucleoli
    d. Attachment site for centrioles

11. The sodium-potassium ATPase in the red blood cell membrane is an example of:
    a. Passive transport
    b. Facilitative transport
    c. Active transport
    d. Vesicular transport
12. Which one of the following statements concerning cellular signal transduction is FALSE?
    a. Membrane-permeable ligands can directly bind to intracellular receptors.
    b. A transmembrane receptor can transmit a signal into the cell through its cytoplasmic domain when ligand binds its extracellular domain.
    c. The binding of membrane receptors to fixed ligands such as extracellular matrix can transmit intracellular signals.
    d. The binding of ligands to membrane receptors is not able to induce changes in gene expression.
13. The cell cycle is regulated by:
    a. Cyclins and cyclin-dependent kinases
    b. Protooncogenes
    c. Apoptosis
    d. Growth factors
14. The transition from the G_1 to S stage of the cell cycle is regulated by:
    a. Cyclin B/CDK1 complex
    b. Cyclin A/CDK2 complex
    c. Cyclin D1
    d. Cyclin E/CDK2 complex
15. Apoptosis is morphologically identified by:
    a. Cellular swelling
    b. Nuclear condensation
    c. Rupture of the cytoplasm
    d. Rupture of the nucleus
16. Regulation of the hematopoietic microenvironment is provided by the:
    a. Stromal cells and growth factors
    b. Hematopoietic stem cells
    c. Liver and spleen
    d. Cyclins and caspases

REFERENCES

1. Pollard, T. D., Earnshaw, W. C., Lippincott-Schwartz, J., et al. (2017). Introduction to cells. In *Cell Biology*. (3rd ed., pp. 3–14). Philadelphia: Elsevier.
2. Gartner, L. P. (2022). Cytoplasm. In *Textbook of Histology*. (5th ed., pp. 11–43). Philadelphia: Elsevier.
3. Mescher, A. L. (2021). The cytoplasm. In *Junqueira's Basic Histology Text and Atlas*. (16th ed., Chapter 2). New York: McGraw-Hill.
4. Engel, P., Boumsell L., Balderas, R., et al. (2015). CD nomenclature 2015: human leukocyte differentiation antigen workshops as a driving force in immunology. *J Immunol, 195*, 4555–4563.
5. Mohandas, N., & Gallagher, P. G. (2008). Red cell membrane: past, present, and future. *Blood, 112*, 3939–3948.
6. Mescher, A. L. (2021). The nucleus. In *Junqueira's Basic Histology Text and Atlas*. (16th ed., Chapter 3). New York: McGraw-Hill.
7. Koeppen, B. M., & Stanton, B. A. (2018). Signal transduction, membrane receptors, second messengers, and regulation of gene expression. In Koeppen, B. M. & Stanton, B. A. (Eds.), *Berne and Levy Physiology*. (10th ed., pp. 35–50). Philadelphia: Elsevier.
8. Kaushansky, K. (2021). Signal transduction pathways. In Kaushansky, K., Lichtman, M. A., Prchal, J. T., et al. (Eds.), *Williams Hematology*. (10th ed., pp. 263–272). New York: McGraw-Hill.
9. McEver, R. P., Alcaide, P., & Luscinskas, F. W. (2023). Cell adhesion. In Hoffman, R., Benz, E. J., Silberstein, L. E., et al. (Eds.), *Hematology: Basic Principles and Practice*. (8th ed., pp. 165–173). Philadelphia: Elsevier.
10. Pollard, T. D., Earnshaw, W. C., Lippincott-Schwartz, J., et al. (2017). Cellular adhesion. In *Cell Biology*. (3rd ed., pp. 525–541). Philadelphia: Elsevier.

11. Puigserver, P. (2023). Signaling transduction and metabolomics. In Hoffman, R., Benz, E. J., Silberstein, L. E., et al. (Eds.), *Hematology: Basic Principles and Practice.* (8th ed., pp. 59–70). Philadelphia: Elsevier.

12. Pollard, T. D., Earnshaw, W. C., Lippincott-Schwartz, J., et al. (2017). Introduction to the cell cycle. In *Cell Biology.* (3rd ed., pp. 697–711). Philadelphia: Elsevier.

13. Zhou, L., & Grant, S. (2021). Cell-cycle regulation and hematologic disorders. In Kaushansky, K., Lichtman, M. A., Prchal, J. T., et al. (Eds.), *Williams Hematology.* (10th ed., pp. 229–262). New York: McGraw-Hill.

14. Oakes, S.A. (2021). Cell injury, cell death, and adaptations. In Kumar, V., Abbas, A. K., & Aster, J. C. (Eds.), *Robbins and Cotran Pathologic Basis of Disease.* (10th ed., pp. 33–69). Philadelphia: Elsevier.

15. Strati, P., Konopleva, M., & Wierda, W. (2023). Cell death. In Hoffman, R., Benz, E. J., Silberstein, L. E., et al. (Eds.), *Hematology: Basic Principles and Practice.* (8th ed., pp. 191–200). Philadelphia: Elsevier.

16. Glennon, E. K. K., Vijayan, K., & Kaushansky, A. (2021). Cell death. In Kaushansky, K., Lichtman, M. A., Prchal, J. T., et al. (Eds.), *Williams Hematology.* (10th ed., pp. 221–228). New York: McGraw-Hill.

17. McIlwain, D. R., Berger, T., & Mak, T. W. (2013). Caspase functions in cell death and disease. *Cold Spring Harb Perspect Biol*, 5.a008656.

18. Dave, U. P., & Koury, M. J. (2021). Structure of the marrow and the hematopoietic microenvironment. In Kaushansky, K., Lichtman, M. A., Prchal, J. T., et al. (Eds.), *Williams Hematology.* (10th ed., pp. 47–78). New York: McGraw-Hill.

19. Kaushansky, K. (2021). Hematopoietic stem cells, progenitors, and cytokines. In Kaushansky, K., Lichtman, M. A., Prchal, J. T., et al. (Eds.), *Williams Hematology.* (10th ed., pp. 273–294). New York: McGraw-Hill.

5

Hematopoiesis

*Kamran M. Mirza**

OBJECTIVES

After completion of this chapter, the reader will be able to:

1. Define *hematopoiesis*.
2. Describe the evolution and formation of blood cells from embryo to fetus to adult, including anatomic sites and cells produced.
3. Predict the likelihood of encountering active marrow from biopsy sites when given the patient's age.
4. Relate normal and abnormal hematopoiesis to the various organs involved in the hematopoietic process.
5. Explain the stem cell theory of hematopoiesis, including the characteristics of hematopoietic stem cells, the names of various progenitor cells, and their lineage associations.

6. Discuss the roles of various cytokines and hematopoietic growth factors in differentiation and maturation of hematopoietic progenitor cells, including nonspecific and lineage-specific factors.
7. Describe general morphologic changes that occur during blood cell maturation.
8. Define *apoptosis* and discuss the relationships among apoptosis, growth factors, and hematopoietic stem cell differentiation.
9. Discuss therapeutic applications of cytokines and hematopoietic growth factors.

OUTLINE

Hematopoietic Development
 Mesoblastic Phase
 Hepatic Phase
 Medullary (Myeloid) Phase
Adult Hematopoietic Tissue
 Bone Marrow
 Liver
 Spleen
 Lymph Nodes
 Thymus

Hematopoietic Stem Cells and Cytokines
 Stem Cell Theory
 Stem Cell Cycle Kinetics
 Stem Cell Phenotypic and Functional Characterization
 Cytokines and Growth Factors
Lineage-Specific Hematopoiesis
 Erythropoiesis
 Leukopoiesis
 Megakaryocytopoiesis
Therapeutic Applications

CASE STUDY

After studying the material in this chapter, the reader should be able to respond to the following case study. Answers can be found in Appendix C.

 A 22-year-old patient visits her physician with symptoms of fatigue, fever, and frequent bruising. Specimens collected for testing included peripheral blood and bone marrow. Results of the CBC were WBC, 2.5×10^9/L; HGB, 8.3 g/dL; and PLT, 50×10^9/L. Reference intervals can be found after the Index at the end of the book. Bone marrow testing confirms the unexplained decrease in WBCs, RBCs, and platelets.

1. Identify the best site for collection of the bone marrow specimen. Explain.
2. Compare and contrast sites for hematopoiesis for the fetus, infant, and adult.
3. What do you expect this patient's bone marrow to look like in this situation?

HEMATOPOIETIC DEVELOPMENT

Hematopoiesis is the continuous, regulated process of renewal, proliferation, differentiation, and maturation of all blood cell lines. These processes result in the formation, development, and specialization of all functional blood cells that are released from the bone marrow into the circulation. Mature blood cells have a limited life span (e.g., 120 days for red blood cells [RBCs]), and a cell population capable of self-renewal sustains the system. A hematopoietic stem cell (HSC) is capable of self-renewal (i.e., replenishment) and directed differentiation into all required cell lineages.[1] Thus the hematopoietic system serves as a functional model to study stem cell biology, proliferation, and maturation and their contribution to disease and tissue repair.

---

*The author extends appreciation to Larry Smith and Richard C. Meagher, whose work in previous editions provided the foundation for this chapter.

Hematopoiesis in the developing human can be characterized as a select distribution of embryonic cells in specific sites that rapidly change during development.[2] In contrast, hematopoiesis in healthy adults is restricted primarily to the bone marrow. During fetal development, the restricted sequential distribution of cells is initiated in the yolk sac, then progresses to the aorta-gonad-mesonephros (AGM) region *(mesoblastic phase)* and to the fetal liver *(hepatic phase)*, and finally resides in the bone marrow *(medullary phase)*. Because of the different locations and resulting microenvironmental conditions (i.e., niches) encountered, each of these locations has distinct but related populations of cells.

Mesoblastic Phase

Hematopoiesis is considered to begin around the 19th day of embryonic development after fertilization.[3] Early in embryonic development, cells from the mesoderm migrate to the yolk sac. Some of these cells form primitive erythroblasts in the central cavity of the yolk sac, and others *(angioblasts)* surround the cavity of the yolk sac and eventually form blood vessels.[4-7] These primitive but transient yolk sac erythroblasts are important in early embryogenesis to produce hemoglobin (Gower-1, Gower-2, and Portland) needed for delivery of oxygen to rapidly developing embryonic tissues (Chapter 8).[8] Yolk sac hematopoiesis differs from hematopoiesis that occurs later in the fetus and adult in that it occurs intravascularly (or within developing blood vessels).[8]

Cells of mesodermal origin migrate to the AGM region and give rise to HSCs for definitive or permanent adult hematopoiesis.[4,7] The AGM region was previously considered to be the only site of definitive hematopoiesis; however, subsequent studies clearly demonstrated that the yolk sac was the major site of adult blood formation in the embryo.[9] There is evidence to support this view via transplant experiments in murine populations demonstrating T cell recovery after transplantation of yolk sac into fetuses.[10] However, other studies have theorized that de novo production of HSCs could occur at different times or locations.[11] Reports indicate that Flk1+ HSCs separated from human umbilical cord blood could generate hematopoietic and endothelial cells in vitro.[12] Some reports indicate that purified murine HSCs generate endothelial cells after in vivo transplantation.[13] More recently, researchers have challenged the AGM origin of HSCs based on transgenic mouse data demonstrating that yolk sac hematopoietic cells in 7.5-day embryos express *RUNX1* regulatory elements needed for definitive hematopoiesis.[14] Overall, these findings suggest that the yolk sac contains either definitive HSCs or cells that can give rise to HSCs.[14] The precise origin of adult HSCs remains unresolved.

Hepatic Phase

The hepatic phase of hematopoiesis begins at 5 to 7 gestational weeks and is characterized by recognizable clusters of developing erythroblasts, granulocytes, and monocytes colonizing the fetal liver, thymus, spleen, placenta, and ultimately the bone marrow space in the final medullary phase.[8] These varied niches support development of HSCs that migrate to them. However, the contribution of each site to the final composition of the adult HSC pool remains unknown.[15,16] Developing erythroblasts signal the beginning of definitive hematopoiesis with a decline in primitive hematopoiesis of the yolk sac. In addition, lymphoid cells begin to appear.[17,18] Hematopoiesis during this phase occurs extravascularly, with the liver remaining the major site of hematopoiesis during the second trimester of fetal life.[8] Hematopoiesis in the AGM region and the yolk sac disappears during this stage. Hematopoiesis in the fetal liver reaches its peak by the third month of fetal development, then gradually declines after the sixth month, retaining minimal activity until 1 to 2 weeks after birth (Figure 5.1).[8] The developing spleen, kidney, thymus, and lymph nodes contribute to the hematopoietic process during this phase. The thymus, the first fully developed organ in the fetus, becomes the major site of T cell production, whereas the kidney and spleen produce B cells.

Production of megakaryocytes begins during the hepatic phase. The spleen gradually decreases granulocytic production and subsequently contributes solely to lymphopoiesis. During the hepatic phase, fetal hemoglobin (Hb F) is the predominant hemoglobin, but detectable levels of adult hemoglobin (Hb A) may be present (Chapter 8).[8]

Medullary (Myeloid) Phase

Hematopoiesis in the bone marrow (termed *medullary hematopoiesis* because it occurs in the medulla or inner part of the bone cavity) begins between the fourth and fifth month of fetal development.[3] During the medullary phase, HSCs and mesenchymal cells migrate into the core of the bone.[8] Mesenchymal cells, a type of embryonic tissue, differentiate into structural elements (e.g., stromal cells such as endothelial cells and reticular adventitial cells) that support developing hematopoietic elements.[19] Hematopoietic activity, especially myeloid activity, is apparent during this stage of development, and the myeloid-to-erythroid ratio gradually approaches 3:1 to 4:1 (healthy adult levels).[8] By the end of 24 weeks' gestation, the bone marrow becomes the *primary* site of hematopoiesis.[8] Measurable levels of erythropoietin (EPO), granulocyte colony-stimulating factor (G-CSF), granulocyte-macrophage colony-stimulating factor (GM-CSF), and Hb F and Hb A can be detected.[8] In addition, cells at various stages of maturation can be seen in all blood cell lineages.

ADULT HEMATOPOIETIC TISSUE

In adults, hematopoietic tissue is located in the bone marrow, lymph nodes, spleen, liver, and thymus. The bone marrow contains developing erythroid, myeloid, megakaryocytic, and lymphoid cells. Lymphoid development occurs in both primary and secondary lymphoid tissue. Primary lymphoid tissue consists of the bone marrow and thymus and is where T and B lymphocytes are derived. Secondary lymphoid tissue, where lymphoid cells respond to foreign antigens, consists of the spleen, lymph nodes, and mucosa-associated lymphoid tissue.

Bone Marrow

Bone marrow, one of the largest organs in the body, is located within the cavities of the cortical bones. Resorption of cartilage and endosteal bone creates a central space within the bone.

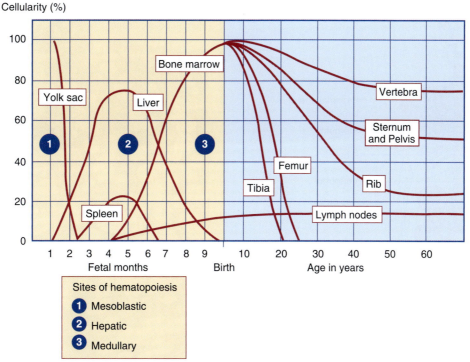

Figure 5.1 Sites of Hematopoiesis by Age. In fetal development (left side of graph), the major sites of hematopoiesis are the yolk sac during the first month of gestation (mesoblastic phase), the liver in the second trimester (hepatic phase), and the bone marrow in the third trimester (medullary phase). After birth (right side of graph) and during infancy and early childhood, all the bones of the body are filled with active hematopoietic tissue (red marrow). Between 5 and 7 years, adipocytes (fat cells or yellow marrow) begin to replace hematopoietic cells, and the marrow cellularity (proportion of red marrow to yellow marrow) decreases with age. In the adult, active hematopoietic tissue (red marrow) is limited to the vertebrae, sternum, pelvis, and ribs as well as scapulae, skull, and proximal portion of the long bones (not shown).

Projections of calcified bone, called *trabeculae,* radiate out from the bone cortex into the central space, forming a three-dimensional matrix resembling a honeycomb. The trabeculae provide structural support for the developing blood cells that mature within a sea of interposed mature adipocytes (fat cells).

Normal bone marrow contains two major components: *red marrow,* hematopoietically active marrow that is composed of developing blood cells and their progenitors, and *yellow marrow,* hematopoietically inactive marrow composed primarily of adipocytes, with undifferentiated mesenchymal cells and macrophages. During infancy and early childhood, all the bones in the body contain primarily red (active) marrow. Between 5 and 7 years, adipocytes become more abundant and begin to occupy the spaces in the long bones previously dominated by active marrow. The process of replacing the active marrow by adipocytes (yellow marrow) during development is called *retrogression* and eventually results in restriction of the active marrow in the adult to the sternum, vertebrae, scapulae, pelvis, ribs, skull, and proximal portion of the long bones (Figure 5.2). Hematopoietically inactive yellow marrow is scattered throughout the red marrow so that, in adults, there are approximately equal amounts of red and yellow marrow in these areas (Figure 5.3). The ratio of the red marrow to the yellow marrow (i.e., the hematopoietic cells to the adipocytes), often termed *marrow cellularity,* typically decreases with age. Yellow marrow is capable of reverting back to active marrow in cases of increased demand on the bone marrow, such as in excessive blood loss or hemolysis.[3]

The bone marrow contains hematopoietic cells, stromal cells, and blood vessels (arteries, veins, and vascular sinuses). Stromal cells originate from mesenchymal cells that migrate into the central cavity of the bone. *Stromal cells* include endothelial cells, adipocytes, osteoblasts, osteoclasts, and fibroblasts.[3] *Endothelial cells* are broad, flat cells that form a single continuous layer along the inner surface of the arteries, veins, and vascular sinuses.[20] Endothelial cells regulate the flow of particles entering and leaving hematopoietic spaces in the vascular sinuses. *Adipocytes* are large cells with a single fat vacuole; they play a role in regulating the volume of the marrow in which active hematopoiesis occurs. They also secrete cytokines or growth factors that positively stimulate HSC numbers and bone homeostasis.[21,22] Macrophages function in phagocytosis, and both macrophages and lymphocytes secrete various cytokines that regulate hematopoiesis; they are located throughout the marrow space.[3,23] Other cells involved in cytokine production include endothelial cells and adventitial reticular cells. *Osteoblasts* are bone-forming cells, and *osteoclasts* are bone-resorbing cells. *Adventitial reticular cells* form an incomplete layer of cells on the abluminal surface of the vascular sinuses.[3] They extend long, reticular fibers into the perivascular space that form a supporting lattice for the developing hematopoietic cells.[3] Stromal cells secrete a semifluid extracellular matrix

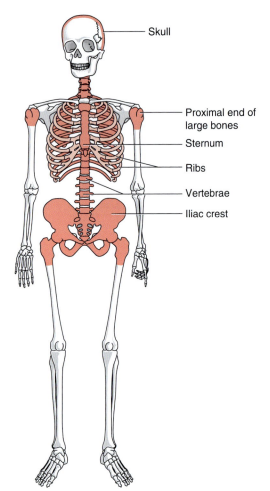

Figure 5.2 Adult Skeleton. Darkened areas depict sites of active hematopoiesis (red marrow).

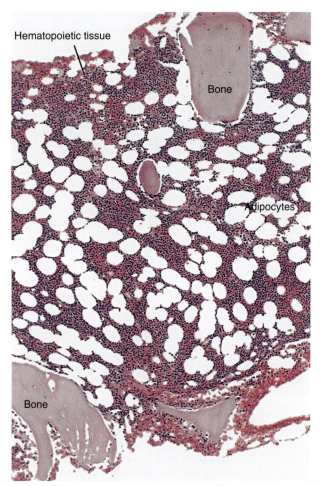

Figure 5.3 Fixed and Stained Bone Marrow Biopsy Specimen. The extravascular tissue consists of blood cell precursors and various tissue cells with scattered fat tissue. A normal adult bone marrow specimen displays 50% hematopoietic cells and 50% fat. (Hematoxylin and eosin stain, ×100.)

that serves to anchor developing hematopoietic cells in the bone cavity. The extracellular matrix contains substances such as *fibronectin, collagen, laminin, thrombospondin, tenascin,* and *proteoglycans* (such as *hyaluronate, heparan sulfate, chondroitin sulfate,* and *dermatan*).[3,24] Stromal cells play a critical role in the regulation of hematopoietic stem and progenitor cell survival and differentiation.

Red Marrow

The red marrow is composed of hematopoietic cells arranged in *extravascular cords.* Cords are located in spaces between vascular sinuses and are supported by trabeculae of spongy bone.[3] The cords are separated from the lumen of the vascular sinuses by endothelial and adventitial reticular cells (Figure 5.4). Hematopoietic cells develop in specific *niches* within the cords. *Erythroid precursors* or *erythroblasts* develop in small clusters, and the more mature forms are located adjacent to the outer surfaces of the vascular sinuses (Figures 5.4 and 5.5)[3]; in addition, erythroblasts are found surrounding iron-laden macrophages (Figure 5.6). *Megakaryocytes* are located adjacent to the walls of the vascular sinuses, which facilitates the release of platelets into the lumen of the sinus.[3] Immature *myeloid (granulocytic) cells* are evenly spaced throughout the bone marrow near specialized stromal cells and the vascular sinuses, and away

from arterioles and the *endosteum* (the inner lining of the cortical bone).[25]

The mature blood cells of the bone marrow eventually enter the peripheral circulation by a process that is not completely understood. Through a highly complex interaction between the maturing blood cells and the vascular sinus wall, blood cells pass between layers of adventitial cells that form a discontinuous layer along the abluminal side of the sinus. Under the layer of adventitial cells is a *basement membrane,* followed by a continuous layer of *endothelial cells* on the luminal side of the vascular sinus. The adventitial cells are capable of contracting, which allows mature blood cells to pass through the basement membrane and interact with the endothelial layer.

As blood cells come in contact with endothelial cells, they bind to the surface through a receptor-mediated process. Nucleated cells and mature red blood cells pass through pores in the endothelial cytoplasm, are released into the vascular sinus, and then move into the peripheral circulation.[3,26]

Marrow Circulation

The nutrient and oxygen requirements of the marrow are fulfilled by the *nutrient* and *periosteal arteries,* which enter via the

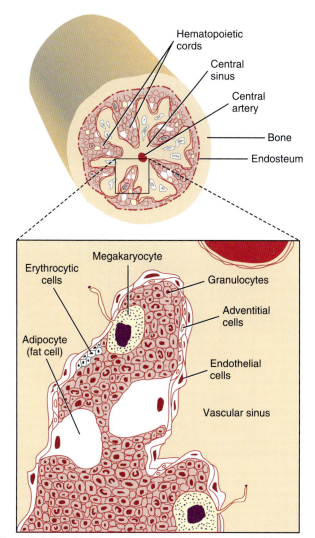

Figure 5.4 Graphic Illustration of the Arrangement of a Hematopoietic Cord and Vascular Sinus in Bone Marrow.

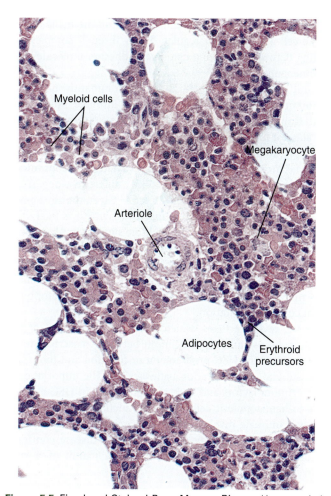

Figure 5.5 Fixed and Stained Bone Marrow Biopsy. Hematopoietic tissue reveals areas of granulopoiesis (lighter-staining cells), erythropoiesis (with darker-staining nuclei), and adipocytes (unstained areas). (Hematoxylin and eosin stain, ×400.)

bone *foramina.* The nutrient artery supplies blood only to the marrow. It coils around the central longitudinal vein, which passes along the bone canal. In the marrow cavity, the nutrient artery divides into ascending and descending branches that also coil around the central longitudinal vein. The arteriole branches that enter the endosteum form *sinusoids* (endosteal beds), which connect to periosteal capillaries that extend from the periosteal artery.[3] The *periosteal arteries* provide nutrients for the osseous bone and the marrow. Their capillaries connect to the venous sinuses located in the endosteal bed, which empty into a larger collecting sinus that opens into the central longitudinal vein.[3] Blood exits the marrow via the central longitudinal vein, which runs the length of the marrow. The central longitudinal vein exits the marrow through the same foramen where the nutrient artery enters. Hematopoietic cells located in the endosteal bed receive their nutrients from the nutrient artery.[3]

Hematopoietic Microenvironment

The *hematopoietic inductive microenvironment,* or *niche,* plays an important role in nurturing and protecting HSCs and regulating their quiescence, self-renewal, and differentiation.[20,27] As

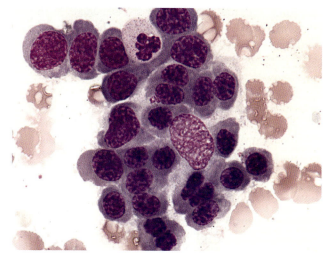

Figure 5.6 Bone Marrow Aspirate. Macrophage surrounded by developing erythroid precursors. (Wright-Giemsa stain, ×1000.) (Courtesy Peter Maslak, Memorial Sloan Kettering Cancer Center, New York, NY.)

the site of hematopoiesis transitions from yolk sac to liver to bone marrow, so must the microenvironmental niche for HSCs. The adult bone marrow HSC niche has received the most attention, although its complex nature makes studying it difficult.

Stromal cells form an extracellular matrix in the niche to promote cell adhesion and regulate HSCs through complex signaling networks involving cytokines, adhesion molecules, and maintenance proteins.[28,29]

Studies suggest that HSCs are predominantly quiescent, maintained in a nondividing state by intimate interactions with thrombopoietin-producing osteoblasts.[30] Opposing studies suggest that vascular cells are critical to HSC maintenance through CXCL12, which regulates migration of HSCs to the vascular niche.[31] These studies suggest a heterogeneous microenvironment that may affect the HSC differently, depending on location and cell type encountered.[32] Given the close proximity of cells within the bone marrow cavity, it is likely that niches may overlap, providing multiple signals simultaneously and thus ensuring tight regulation of HSCs.[32] Although the cell-cell interactions are complex and multifactorial, understanding these relationships is critical to the advancement of cell therapies based on HSCs such as clinical hematopoietic stem cell transplantation.

Some review articles, which are beyond the scope of this chapter, discuss and help to delineate between transcription factors required for HSC proliferation or function and those that regulate HSC differentiation pathways.[33,34] The importance of transcription factors and their regulatory role in HSC maturation in hematopoietic cell lineage production is demonstrated by their intimate involvement in disease evolution, such as in leukemia. Ongoing study of hematopoietic disease continues to demonstrate the complex and delicate nature of normal hematopoiesis.

Liver

The liver consists of two lobes situated beneath the diaphragm in the abdominal cavity. The position of the liver with regard to the circulatory system is optimal for gathering, transferring, and eliminating substances through the bile duct.[35,36] The liver serves as the major site of blood cell production during the second trimester of fetal development. In adults, hepatocytes have many functions, including protein synthesis and degradation, coagulation factor synthesis, carbohydrate and lipid metabolism, drug and toxin clearance, iron recycling and storage, and hemoglobin degradation, in which bilirubin is conjugated and transported to the small intestine for eventual excretion.

Anatomically, hepatocytes are arranged in radiating plates emanating from a central vein (Figure 5.7). Adjacent to the longitudinal plates of hepatocytes are vascular sinusoids lined with endothelial cells. A small noncellular space separates the endothelial cells of the sinusoids from the plates of hepatocytes. This spatial arrangement allows plasma to have direct access to the hepatocytes for two-directional flow of solutes and fluids.

The lumen of the sinusoids contains *Kupffer cells* that maintain contact with the endothelial cell lining. Kupffer cells are macrophages that remove senescent cells and foreign debris from the blood that circulates through the liver; they also secrete mediators that regulate protein synthesis in the hepatocytes.[37] The particular anatomy, cellular components, and location in the body enable the liver to carry out many varied functions.

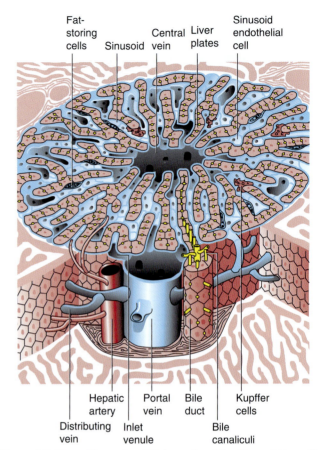

Figure 5.7 Three-Dimensional Schematic of the Normal Liver. The portal vein and hepatic artery bring blood to the liver sinusoids. Passage through the hepatic sinusoids allows blood content to be accessed by liver plates and Kupffer cells. Efferent flow out of the liver is via the central vein.

Liver Pathophysiology

The liver can maintain hematopoietic stem and progenitor cells to produce various blood cells (called *extramedullary hematopoiesis*) as a response to infectious agents or in pathologic myelofibrosis of the bone marrow.[38] It is directly affected by storage diseases of the monocyte/macrophage (Kupffer) cells as a result of enzyme deficiencies that cause hepatomegaly with ultimate dysfunction of the liver (Gaucher disease, Niemann-Pick disease) (Chapter 26). In severe hemolytic anemias, the liver increases the conjugation of *bilirubin* and the storage of iron (Chapter 17). The liver sequesters membrane-damaged RBCs and removes them from the circulation. In *porphyrias,* hereditary or acquired defects in the enzymes involved in heme biosynthesis result in the accumulation of the various intermediary *porphyrins* that damage hepatocytes, erythrocyte precursors, and other tissues (Chapter 17).

Spleen

The spleen, the largest lymphoid organ in the body, lies beneath the diaphragm behind the fundus of the stomach in the upper left quadrant of the abdomen. It is vital but not essential for life and functions as an indiscriminate filter of the circulating blood. In a healthy individual, the spleen contains about 20 to 40 mL of blood.[39] The exterior surface of the spleen is surrounded by

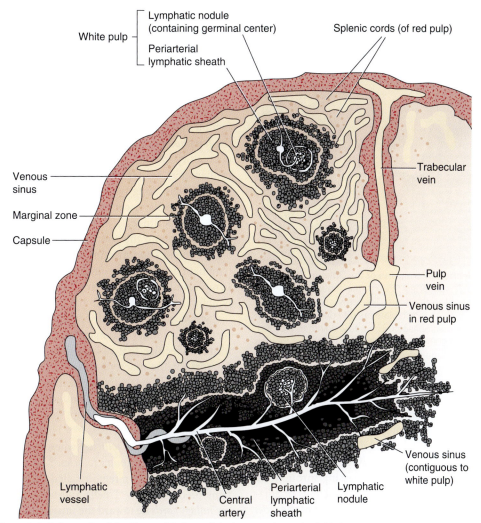

White pulp
- Lymphatic nodule (containing germinal center)
- Periarterial lymphatic sheath

Splenic cords (of red pulp)

Venous sinus

Marginal zone

Capsule

Trabecular vein

Pulp vein

Venous sinus in red pulp

Venous sinus (contiguous to white pulp)

Lymphatic vessel

Central artery

Periarterial lymphatic sheath

Lymphatic nodule

Figure 5.8 Schematic of the Normal Spleen. Splenic parenchyma is divided into white pulp and red pulp. The white pulp contains mature lymphocytes in periarterial lymphatic sheaths. (From Weiss, L., & Tavossoli, M. [1970]. Anatomical hazards to the passage of erythrocytes through the spleen. *Semin Hematol, 7,* 372–380.)

a layer of *peritoneum* covering a connective tissue capsule. The capsule projects inwardly, forming trabeculae that divide the spleen into discrete regions. Located within these regions are three types of splenic tissue: *white pulp, red pulp,* and a *marginal zone.*[39] The white pulp consists of scattered follicles with germinal centers containing lymphocytes, macrophages, and dendritic cells. Aggregates of T lymphocytes surround arteries that pass through these germinal centers, forming a region called the *periarteriolar lymphatic sheath (PALS).* Interspersed along the periphery of the PALS are lymphoid nodules containing primarily B lymphocytes. Activated B lymphocytes are found in the germinal centers.[37]

The marginal zone surrounds the white pulp and forms a reticular meshwork containing blood vessels, macrophages, memory B cells, and CD4+ T cells.[40] The red pulp is composed primarily of vascular sinuses separated by cords of reticular cell meshwork *(cords of Billroth)* containing loosely connected specialized macrophages. This creates a spongelike matrix that functions as a filter for blood passing through the region.[37] As RBCs pass through the cords of Billroth, there is a decrease in the flow of blood, which leads to stagnation

and depletion of the glucose supply of RBCs. These cells are subject to increased damage and stress that may lead to their removal from the spleen. The spleen uses two methods for removing senescent or abnormal RBCs from the circulation: *culling,* in which the cells are phagocytized with subsequent degradation of cell organelles, and *pitting,* in which splenic macrophages remove inclusions or damaged surface membrane from the circulating RBCs.[39] The spleen also serves as a storage site for platelets. In a healthy individual, approximately 30% of the total platelet count is sequestered in the spleen.[41]

The spleen is highly vascular with a rich supply of blood. Blood enters the spleen through the *central splenic artery* located at the *hilum* on the surface of the spleen and branches outward through the trabeculae.[42] The branches enter all three regions of the spleen: the white pulp, with its dense accumulation of lymphocytes; the marginal zone; and the red pulp. In the red pulp, blood flows into venous sinuses, which merge into the trabecular veins.[42] The trabecular veins converge into the splenic vein, which exits the spleen at the hilum (Figure 5.8).[42]

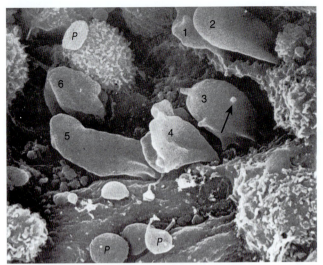

Figure 5.9 Scanning Electron Micrograph of the Spleen. Note erythrocytes (numbered *1* to *6*) squeezing through the fenestrated wall in transit from the splenic cord to the sinus. The view shows the endothelial lining of the sinus wall, to which platelets (*P*) adhere, along with white blood cells, probably macrophages. The *arrow* points to a protrusion on a red blood cell (×5000). (From Weiss, L. [1974]. A scanning electron microscopic study of the spleen. *Blood, 43,* 665.)

Spleen Pathophysiology

As blood enters the spleen, it may follow one of two routes. The first is a slow-transit pathway through the red pulp in which the RBCs pass circuitously through the macrophage-lined cords before reaching the sinuses. Plasma freely enters the sinuses, but the RBCs have a more difficult time passing through the tiny openings created by the *interendothelial junctions* of adjacent endothelial cells (Figure 5.9). The combination of the slow passage and the continued RBC metabolism creates an environment that is acidic, hypoglycemic, and hypoxic. The increased environmental stress on the RBCs circulating through the spleen leads to possible hemolysis.

In the rapid-transit pathway, blood cells enter the splenic artery and pass directly to the sinuses in the red pulp and continue to the venous system to exit the spleen. When *splenomegaly* occurs, the spleen becomes enlarged and often palpable. This occurs as a result of many conditions including but not limited to chronic leukemias, inherited membrane or enzyme defects in RBCs, hemoglobinopathies, Hodgkin disease, thalassemia, malaria, and myeloproliferative neoplasms. *Splenectomy* may be beneficial in cases of excessive destruction of RBCs, such as in severe hereditary spherocytosis (Chapter 21) or in autoimmune hemolytic anemia when treatment with corticosteroids does not effectively suppress hemolysis (Chapter 23).[39,43] Splenectomy may also be indicated in severe refractory immune thrombocytopenic purpura or in storage disorders, with portal hypertension and splenomegaly resulting in peripheral cytopenias.[39] After splenectomy, platelet and leukocyte counts increase transiently.[39] In sickle cell anemia, repeated splenic infarcts caused by sickled RBCs trapped in the small vessel circulation of the spleen cause tissue damage and necrosis, which often results in *autosplenectomy* (Chapter 24).

Hypersplenism is an enlargement of the spleen resulting in some degree of pancytopenia despite the presence of a hyperactive bone marrow. The most common cause is congestive splenomegaly secondary to cirrhosis of the liver and portal hypertension. Other causes include thrombosis, vascular stenosis, other vascular deformities such as aneurysm of the splenic artery, and cysts.[44]

Lymph Nodes

Lymph nodes are organs of the lymphatic system located along the *lymphatic capillaries* that are parallel to, but not part of, the circulatory system. These bean-shaped structures (1 to 5 mm in diameter) are typically present in groups or chains at various intervals along lymphatic vessels. They may be superficial (inguinal, axillary, cervical, supratrochlear) or deep (mesenteric, retroperitoneal). Lymph is the fluid portion of blood that escapes into the connective tissue and is characterized by a low protein concentration and the absence of RBCs. *Afferent* lymphatic vessels carry circulating lymph *to* the lymph nodes. Lymph is filtered by the lymph nodes and exits via the *efferent* lymphatic vessels located in the hilus of the lymph node.[40]

Lymph nodes can be divided into an outer region called the *cortex* and an inner region called the *medulla.* An outer capsule forms trabeculae that radiate through the cortex and provide support for the macrophages and lymphocytes located in the node. The trabeculae divide the interior of the lymph node into follicles (Figure 5.10). After antigenic stimulation, the cortical region of some follicles develops foci of activated B cell proliferation called *germinal centers.*[40,45] Follicles with germinal centers are called *secondary follicles,* whereas those without germinal centers are called *primary follicles.*[40] Located between the cortex and the medulla is a region called the *paracortex,* which contains predominantly T cells and numerous macrophages. The *medullary cords* lie toward the interior of the lymph node. These cords consist primarily of plasma cells and B cells.[40] Lymph nodes have three main functions: they are a site of lymphocyte proliferation; they are involved in the initiation of the specific immune response to foreign antigens; and they filter particulate matter, debris, and bacteria entering the lymph node via the lymph.

Lymph Node Pathophysiology

Lymph nodes, by their nature, are vulnerable to the same organisms that circulate through the tissue. Sometimes increased numbers of microorganisms enter the nodes, overwhelming the macrophages and causing *adenitis* (infection or inflammation of the lymph node). More serious is the common entry into the lymph nodes of malignant cells that have broken loose from malignant tumors. These malignant cells may grow and metastasize to other lymph nodes in the same group.

Thymus

To understand the role of the thymus in adults, certain formative intrauterine processes that affect function must be considered. First, the thymus tissue originates from endodermal and mesenchymal tissue. Second, the thymus is populated initially by primitive lymphoid cells from the yolk sac and the liver. This increased population of lymphoid cells physically pushes the epithelial cells of the thymus apart; however, their long

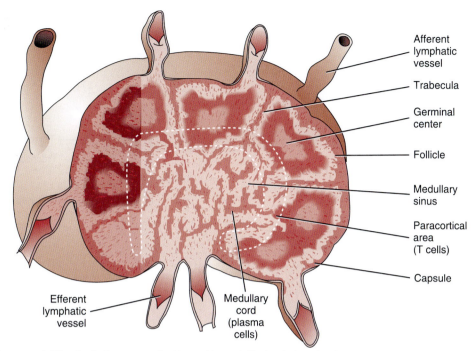

Figure 5.10 Histologic Structure of a Normal Lymph Node. Trabeculae divide the lymph node into follicles with an outer cortex (predominantly B cells) and a deeper paracortical zone (predominantly T cells). A central medulla is rich in plasma cells. After antigenic stimulation, secondary follicles develop germinal centers consisting of activated B cells. Primary follicles (not shown) lack germinal centers.

processes remain attached to one another by desmosomes. In adults, T cell progenitors migrate to the thymus from the bone marrow for further maturation.

At birth, the thymus is an efficient, well-developed organ. It consists of two lobes, each measuring 0.5 to 2 cm in diameter, and is further divided into lobules. The thymus is located in the upper part of the anterior mediastinum at about the level of the great vessels of the heart. It resembles other lymphoid tissue in that the lobules are subdivided into two areas: the cortex (a peripheral zone) and the medulla (a central zone) (Figure 5.11). Both areas are populated with the same cellular components—lymphoid cells, reticular cells, epithelial cells, dendritic cells, and many macrophages—although in different proportions.[40] The cortex is characterized by a blood supply system that is unique in that it consists only of capillaries. Its function seems to be that of a "waiting zone" densely populated with progenitor T cells. When these progenitor T cells migrate from the bone marrow and first enter the thymus, they have no identifiable CD4 and CD8 surface markers *(double-negative T cells),* and they locate to the corticomedullary junction.[45,46] Under the influence of chemokines, cytokines, and receptors, these cells move to the cortex and express both CD4 and CD8 *(double-positive T cells).*[39,45,46] Subsequently they give rise to mature T cells that express either CD4 or CD8 surface antigen as they move toward the medulla.[45] Eventually the mature T cells leave the thymus to populate specific regions of other lymphoid tissue, such as the T cell-dependent areas of the spleen, lymph nodes, and other lymphoid tissues. The lymphoid cells that do not express the appropriate antigens and receptors, or are self-reactive, die in the cortex or medulla as a result of apoptosis

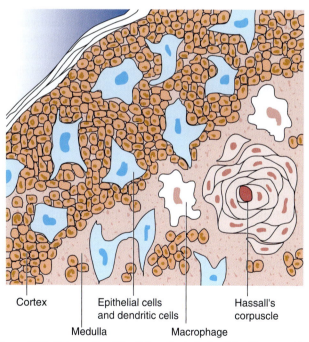

Figure 5.11 Schematic of the Edge of a Lobule of the Thymus. Note cells of the cortex and medulla. Similar to other lymphoid organs, the thymus is divided into cortical and medullary zones. A unique feature of the thymus is the presence of epithelial structures and characteristic Hassall's corpuscles, which are formed by concentric arrangements of type VI epithelial reticular cells. (From Abbas, A. K., Lichtman, A. H., & Pober, J. S. [1991]. *Cellular and Molecular Immunology.* Philadelphia: Saunders.)

and are phagocytized by macrophages.[40,45,46] The medulla seems to be a holding zone for mature T cells until they are needed by the peripheral lymphoid tissues. The thymus also

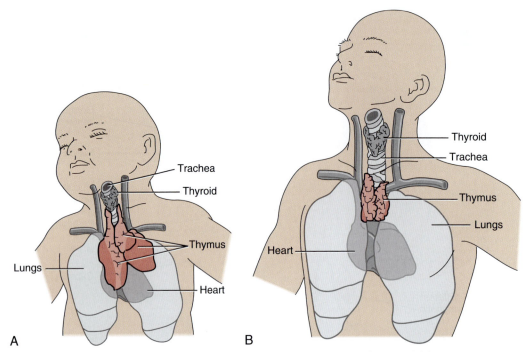

Figure 5.12 Differences in the Size of the Thymus. (A), Infant. (B), Adult.

contains other cell types, including B cells, eosinophils, neutrophils, and other myeloid cells.[37]

Gross examination indicates that the size of the thymus is related to age. The thymus weighs 12 to 15 g at birth, increases to 30 to 40 g at puberty, and decreases to 10 to 15 g at later ages. It is hardly recognizable in old age because of atrophy (Figure 5.12). However, the thymus retains the ability to produce new T cells even when atrophic, as evidenced by its ability to do so after irradiation treatment in patients undergoing bone marrow transplantation.

Thymus Pathophysiology

Nondevelopment of the thymus during gestation results in the lack of formation of T lymphocytes. Related manifestations seen in patients with this condition are failure to thrive, uncontrollable infections, and death in infancy. Adults with thymic disturbance are not affected because they have developed and maintained a pool of T lymphocytes for life.

HEMATOPOIETIC STEM CELLS AND CYTOKINES

Stem Cell Theory

In 1961, Till and McCulloch[47] conducted a series of experiments in which they irradiated spleens and bone marrow of mice, creating a state of aplasia. These aplastic mice were given an intravenous injection of marrow cells. Colonies of HSCs were seen 7 to 8 days later in the spleens of the irradiated (recipient) mice. These colonies were called *colony-forming unit-spleen* (CFU-S). These investigators later found that these colonies were capable of self-renewal and the production of differentiated progeny. CFU-S represent what we now refer to as *committed myeloid progenitors* or *colony-forming unit-granulocyte, erythrocyte,*

monocyte, and megakaryocyte (CFU-GEMM).[47,48] These cells are capable of giving rise to multiple lineages of blood cells.

Morphologically unrecognizable hematopoietic progenitor cells can be divided into two major types: noncommitted or undifferentiated HSCs and committed progenitor cells. These two groups give rise to all mature blood cells. Initially, there were two theories describing the origin of hematopoietic progenitor cells. The *monophyletic theory* suggests that all blood cells are derived from a single progenitor stem cell called a *pluripotent hematopoietic stem cell*. The *polyphyletic theory* suggests that each of the blood cell lineages is derived from its own unique stem cell. The monophyletic theory is the most widely accepted theory among experimental hematologists.

By definition, HSCs are capable of self-renewal, are pluripotent, and give rise to differentiated progeny and are able to reconstitute the hematopoietic system of a lethally irradiated host. The undifferentiated HSCs can differentiate into progenitor cells committed to either lymphoid or myeloid lineages. These lineage-specific progenitor cells are the *common lymphoid progenitor*, which proliferates and differentiates into T, B, and natural killer lymphocyte and dendritic lineages, and the *common myeloid progenitor*, which proliferates and differentiates into individual granulocytic, erythrocytic, monocytic, and megakaryocytic lineages. The resulting limited lineage-specific progenitors give rise to morphologically recognizable, lineage-specific precursor cells (Figure 5.13 and Table 5.1). Despite the limited numbers of HSCs in the bone marrow, 6 billion blood cells per kilogram of body weight are produced each day for the entire life span of an individual.[3] Most of the cells in normal bone marrow are precursor cells at various stages of maturation.

HSCs are directed to one of three possible fates: self-renewal, differentiation, or apoptosis.[49] When the HSC divides, it gives

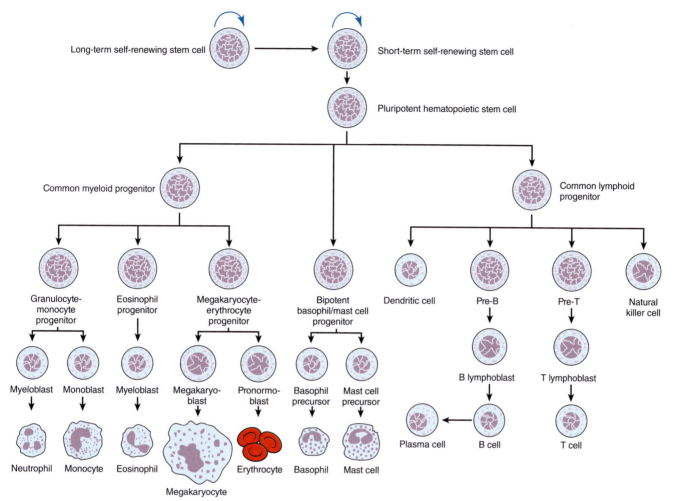

Figure 5.13 Diagram of Hematopoiesis. Note derivation of cells from the pluripotent hematopoietic stem cell.

TABLE 5.1	Culture-Derived Colony-Forming Units
Abbreviation	**Cell Line**
CFU-GEMM	Granulocyte, erythrocyte, megakaryocyte, monocyte
CFU-E	Erythrocyte
CFU-Meg	Megakaryocyte
CFU-M	Monocyte
CFU-GM	Granulocyte, monocyte
CFU-BASO	Myeloid to basophil
CFU-EO	Myeloid to eosinophil
CFU-G	Myeloid to neutrophil
CFU-pre-T	T lymphocyte
CFU-pre-B	B lymphocyte

rise to two identical daughter cells. Both daughter cells may follow the path of differentiation, leaving the stem cell pool (*symmetric division*), or one daughter cell may return to the stem cell pool and the other daughter cell may follow the path of differentiation (*asymmetric division*) or undergo apoptosis. Many theories have been proposed to describe the mechanisms that determine the fate of the stem cell. Till and McCulloch[47] proposed that hematopoiesis is a random process whereby the HSC randomly commits to self-renewal or differentiation. This model is also called the *stochastic* model of hematopoiesis. Later

studies suggested that the microenvironment in the bone marrow determines whether the HSC will self-renew or differentiate (*instructive* model of hematopoiesis).[49] Researchers believe that the ultimate decision made by the HSC can be described by both the stochastic and the instructive models of hematopoiesis. The initial decision to self-renew or differentiate is probably stochastic, whereas lineage differentiation that occurs later is determined by various signals from the hematopoietic inductive microenvironment in response to specific requirements of the body.

The multilineage priming model suggests that HSCs receive low-level signals from the *hematopoietic inductive microenvironment* to amplify or repress genes associated with commitment to multiple lineages. The implication is that the cell's fate is determined by intrinsic and extrinsic factors. Extrinsic regulation involves proliferation and differentiation signals from specialized niches located in the hematopoietic inductive microenvironment via direct cell-to-cell or cellular-extracellular signaling molecules.[49] Some of the cytokines released from the hematopoietic inductive microenvironment include factors that regulate proliferation and differentiation, such as KIT ligand, thrombopoietin (TPO), and FLT3 ligand. Intrinsic regulation involves genes such as *TAL1*, which is expressed in cells in the *hemangioblast*, a bipotential progenitor cell of mesodermal origin that gives rise to hematopoietic and endothelial lineages, and *GATA2,* which is expressed in later-appearing HSCs. Both these genes are essential for primitive and definitive hematopoiesis.[49] In addition to factors involved in differentiation and regulation, there are regulatory signaling factors, such as Notch-1 and Notch-2, that allow HSCs to respond to hematopoietic inductive microenvironment factors, altering cell fate.[50]

As hematopoietic cells differentiate, they take on various morphologic features associated with maturation. These include an overall decrease in cell volume and a decrease in the nucleus-to-cytoplasm ratio. Additional changes that take place during maturation occur in the cytoplasm and nucleus. Changes in the nucleus include loss of nucleoli, decrease in the diameter of the nucleus, condensation of nuclear chromatin, possible change in the shape of the nucleus, and possible loss of the nucleus. Changes occurring in the cytoplasm include decrease in basophilia, increase in the proportion of cytoplasm, and possible appearance of granules in the cytoplasm. Specific changes in each lineage are discussed in subsequent chapters.

Stem Cell Cycle Kinetics

The bone marrow is estimated to be capable of producing approximately 2.5 billion erythrocytes, 2.5 billion platelets, and 1 billion granulocytes per kilogram of body weight daily.[3] The determining factor controlling the rate of production is physiologic need. HSCs exist in the marrow in the ratio of 1 per 1000 nucleated blood cells.[4] They are capable of many mitotic divisions when stimulated by appropriate cytokines. When mitosis has occurred, the cell may reenter the cycle or go into a resting phase, termed G_0. Some cells in the resting phase reenter the active cell cycle and divide, whereas other cells are directed to terminal differentiation (Figure 5.14).

From these data, a mitotic index can be calculated to establish the percentage of cells in mitosis in relation to the total number of cells. Factors affecting the mitotic index include the duration of mitosis and the length of the resting state. Normally, the mitotic index is approximately 1% to 2%. An increased

mitotic index implies increased proliferation. An exception to this rule is in the case of megaloblastic anemia (Chapter 18), in which mitosis is prolonged.[51] An understanding of the mechanism of the cell cycle aids in understanding the mode of action of specific drugs used in the treatment and management of proliferative disorders.

Stem Cell Phenotypic and Functional Characterization

The identification and origin of HSCs can be determined by immunophenotypic analysis using flow cytometry. The earliest identifiable human HSCs capable of initiating long-term cultures are CD34+, CD38−, HLA-DR^low, Thy_1^low, and Lin−.[50] This population of marrow cells is enriched in primitive progenitors. The expression of CD38 and HLA-DR is associated with a loss of *stemness.* The acquisition of CD33 and CD38 is seen on committed myeloid progenitors, and the expression of CD10 and CD38 is seen on committed lymphoid progenitors.[50] The expression of CD7 is seen on T lymphoid progenitor cells and natural killer cells, and the expression of CD19 is seen on B lymphoid progenitor cells (Chapter 28).

Functional characterization of HSCs can be accomplished through in vitro techniques using long-term culture assays. These involve the enumeration of colony-forming units (e.g., CFU-GEMM) on semisolid media, such as methylcellulose. Primitive progenitor cells, such as the *high proliferative potential colony-forming cell* and the *long-term colony initiating cell,* have also been identified. These hematopoietic precursor cells give rise to colonies that can survive for 5 to 8 weeks but can be replated.[50] In vivo functional assays also are available and require transplantation of cells into syngeneic, lethally irradiated animals, followed by transference of the engrafted bone marrow cells into a secondary recipient.[50] These systems promote the proliferation and differentiation of HSCs, thus allowing them to be characterized; they may serve as models for developing clinically applicable techniques for gene therapy and HSC transplantation.

From our rudimentary knowledge of stem cell biology, it has been possible to move from the bench to the bedside with amazing speed and success. Hematopoietic stem cell transplantation (HSCT) is more than a half-century old, and we have witnessed tremendous growth in the field as a result of the reproducibility of clinical procedures to produce similar outcomes. However, caution must be exercised because the cells capable of these remarkable clinical events are still not well defined, the niche that they inhabit is still not completely understood, and the signals that they potentially respond to are plentiful and diverse in action. Treatment of hematologic disorders is based on fundamental understanding of the biologic principles of HSC proliferation and maturation. The control mechanisms that regulate HSCs and the requisite processes necessary to manipulate them to generate sufficient numbers for clinical use remain largely unknown.

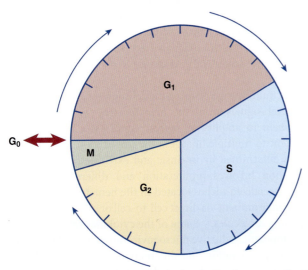

Figure 5.14 Schematic of the Cell Cycle. G_0, Resting stage; G_1, cell growth and synthesis of components necessary for cell division; G_2, premitotic phase; *M*, mitosis; *S*, DNA replication.

Cytokines and Growth Factors

A group of specific glycoproteins called *hematopoietic growth factors* or *cytokines* regulate the proliferation, differentiation,

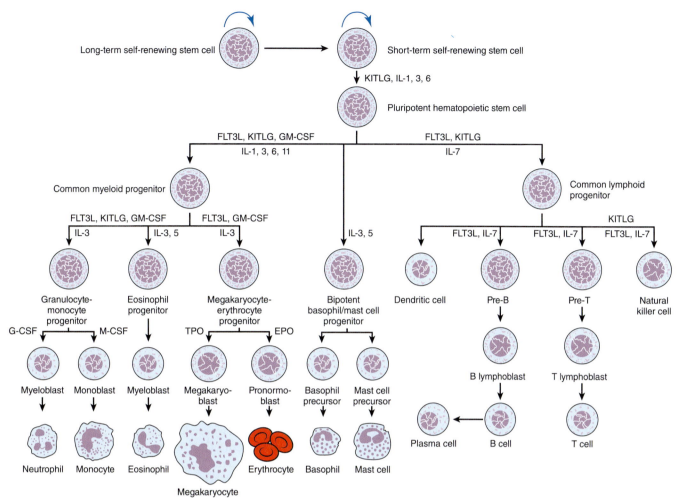

Figure 5.15 Diagram of Derivation of Hematopoietic Cells. Note sites of action of cytokines. *EPO,* Erythropoietin; *FLT3L,* FLT3 ligand; *G-CSF,* granulocyte colony-stimulating factor; *GM-CSF,* granulocyte-macrophage colony-stimulating factor; *IL-1,* interleukin-1; *IL-3,* interleukin-3; *IL-5,* interleukin-5; *IL-6,* interleukin-6; *IL-7,* interleukin-7; *IL-11,* interleukin-11; *KITLG,* KIT ligand; *M-CSF,* macrophage colony-stimulating factor; *TPO,* thrombopoietin.

and maturation of hematopoietic precursor cells.[52] Figure 5.15 illustrates the hematopoietic system and the sites of action of some of the cytokines. These factors are discussed in more detail in subsequent chapters.

Cytokines are a diverse group of soluble proteins that have direct and indirect effects on hematopoietic cells. Classification of cytokines has been difficult because of their overlapping and redundant properties. The terms *cytokine* and *growth factor* are often used synonymously; cytokines include *interleukins (ILs), lymphokines, monokines, interferons, chemokines,* and *colony-stimulating factors (CSFs).*[52] Cytokines are responsible for stimulation or inhibition of production, differentiation, and trafficking of mature blood cells and their precursors. Many of these cytokines exert a positive influence on HSCs and progenitor cells with multilineage potential (e.g., KIT ligand, FLT3 ligand, GM-CSF, IL-1, IL-3, IL-6, and IL-11).[53] Cytokines that exert a negative influence on hematopoiesis include transforming growth factor-β, tumor necrosis factor-α, and the interferons.[50]

Hematopoietic progenitor cells require cytokines on a continual basis for their growth and survival. Cytokines prevent hematopoietic precursor cells from dying by inhibiting apoptosis; they stimulate hematopoietic precursor cells to divide by decreasing the transit time from G_0 to G_1 of the cell cycle; and they regulate cell differentiation into the various cell lineages.

Apoptosis refers to programmed cell death, a normal physiologic process that eliminates unwanted, abnormal, or harmful cells. Apoptosis differs from necrosis, which is accidental death from trauma (Chapter 4). When cells do not receive the appropriate cytokines necessary to prevent cell death, apoptosis is initiated. In some disease states, apoptosis is turned on, which results in early cell death, whereas in other states, apoptosis is inhibited, which allows uncontrolled proliferation of cells.[54]

Research techniques have accomplished the purification of many cytokines and the cloning of pure recombinant growth factors, some of which are discussed later in "Therapeutic Applications." The number of cytokines identified has expanded greatly in recent years and is expected to further increase as research continues. This chapter focuses primarily on CSFs, KIT ligand, FLT3 ligand, and IL-3. A detailed discussion is beyond the scope of this text, and the reader is encouraged to consult current literature for further details.

Colony-Stimulating Factors

CSFs are produced by many different cells. They have a high specificity for their target cells and are active at low concentrations.[52] The names of the individual factors indicate the predominant cell lines that respond to their presence. The primary target of G-CSF is the granulocytic cell line, and GM-CSF targets the granulocytic-monocytic cell line. The biologic activity of CSFs was first identified by their ability to induce hematopoietic colony formation in semisolid media. In addition, it was found in cell culture experiments that although a particular CSF may have specificity for one cell lineage, it is often capable of influencing other cell lineages as well. This is particularly true when multiple growth factors are combined.[55] Although GM-CSF stimulates the proliferation of granulocyte and monocyte progenitors, it also works synergistically with IL-3 to enhance megakaryocyte colony formation.[55]

Early-Acting Multilineage Growth Factors

Ogawa[56] described early-acting growth factors (multilineage), intermediate-acting growth factors (multilineage), and late-acting growth factors (lineage restricted). KIT ligand, also known as *stem cell factor,* is an early-acting growth factor; its receptor is the transmembrane protein, KIT. KIT is a receptor-type tyrosine-protein kinase that is expressed on HSCs and is downregulated with differentiation. The binding of KIT ligand to the extracellular domain of the KIT receptor triggers its cytoplasmic domain to induce a series of signals that are sent via signal transduction pathways (Chapter 4) to the nucleus of the HSC, stimulating the cell to proliferate. As HSCs differentiate and mature, the expression of KIT receptor decreases. Activation of the KIT receptor by KIT ligand is essential in the early stages of hematopoiesis.[53]

FLT3 is also a receptor-type tyrosine-protein kinase. KIT ligand and FLT3 ligand work synergistically with IL-3, GM-CSF, and other cytokines to promote early HSC proliferation and differentiation. In addition, IL-3 regulates blood cell production by controlling the production, differentiation, and function of granulocytes and macrophages.[57] GM-CSF induces expression of specific genes that stimulate HSC differentiation to the common myeloid progenitor.[58]

Interleukins

Cytokines originally were named according to their specific function, such as lymphocyte-activating factor (now called IL-1), but continued research found that a particular cytokine may have multiple actions. A group of scientists began calling some of the cytokines *interleukins,* numbering them in the order in which they were identified (e.g., IL-1, IL-2). Characteristics shared by interleukins include the following:

- They are proteins that exhibit multiple biologic activities, such as the regulation of autoimmune and inflammatory reactions and hematopoiesis.
- They have synergistic interactions with other cytokines.
- They are part of interacting systems with amplification potential.
- They are effective at very low concentrations.

LINEAGE-SPECIFIC HEMATOPOIESIS

Erythropoiesis

Erythropoiesis occurs in the bone marrow and is a complex, regulated process for maintaining adequate numbers of erythrocytes in the peripheral blood. CFU-GEMM gives rise to the earliest identifiable colony of RBCs, called the *burst-forming unit-erythroid* (BFU-E). The BFU-E produces a large multi-clustered colony that resembles a cluster of grapes containing brightly colored hemoglobin. These colonies range from a single large cluster to 16 or more clusters. BFU-Es contain only a few receptors for EPO, and their cell cycle activity is not influenced significantly by the presence of exogenous EPO. BFU-Es under the influence of IL-3, GM-CSF, TPO, and KIT ligand develop into *colony-forming unit-erythroid* (CFU-E) colonies.[47] The CFU-E has many EPO receptors and has an absolute requirement for EPO. Some CFU-Es are responsive to low levels of EPO and do not have the proliferative capacity of the BFU-E.[24] EPO serves as a differentiation factor that causes the CFU-E to differentiate into pronormoblasts, the earliest visually recognized erythrocyte precursors in the bone marrow.[59]

EPO is a lineage-specific glycoprotein produced in the *renal peritubular interstitial cells.*[24] In addition, a small amount of EPO is produced by the liver.[53] Oxygen availability in the kidney is the stimulus that activates production and secretion of EPO.[60] EPO exerts its effects by binding to the EPO transmembrane receptors expressed by erythroid progenitors and precursors.[60] EPO serves to recruit CFU-E from the more primitive BFU-E compartment, prevents apoptosis of erythroid progenitors, and induces hemoglobin synthesis.[59,61] Erythropoiesis and actions of EPO are discussed in detail in Chapter 6.

Leukopoiesis

Leukopoiesis can be divided into two major categories: *myelopoiesis* and *lymphopoiesis.* Factors that promote differentiation of the CFU-GEMM into neutrophils, monocytes, eosinophils, and basophils include GM-CSF, G-CSF, macrophage colony-stimulating factor (M-CSF), IL-3, IL-5, IL-6, IL-11, and KIT ligand. GM-CSF stimulates the proliferation and differentiation of neutrophil and macrophage colonies from the colony-forming unit-granulocyte-monocyte. G-CSF and M-CSF stimulate neutrophil differentiation and monocyte differentiation from the colony-forming unit-granulocyte and colony-forming unit-monocyte.[24] IL-3 is a multilineage stimulating factor that stimulates the growth of granulocytes, monocytes, megakaryocytes, and erythroid cells. Eosinophils require GM-CSF, IL-5, and IL-3 for differentiation. The requirements for basophil differentiation are less clear, but it seems to depend on the presence of IL-3 and KIT ligand. Growth factors promoting lymphoid differentiation include IL-2, IL-7, IL-12, and IL-15 and to some extent, IL-4, IL-10, IL-13, IL-14, and IL-16.[54] Leukopoiesis is discussed further in Chapter 10.

Megakaryocytopoiesis

Earlier influences on megakaryocytopoiesis include GM-CSF, IL-3, IL-6, IL-11, KIT ligand, and TPO.[54] The stimulating hormonal factor TPO (also known as MPL ligand), along with

IL-11, controls the production and release of platelets. The liver is the main site of production of TPO.[62,63] Megakaryocytopoiesis is discussed in Chapter 11.

THERAPEUTIC APPLICATIONS

Clinical use of growth factors approved by the US Food and Drug Administration has contributed numerous options in the treatment of hematologic malignancies and solid tumors. In addition, growth factors can be used as priming agents to increase the yield of HSCs during apheresis for transplantation protocols. Advances in molecular biology have resulted in cloning of the genes that are responsible for the synthesis of various growth factors and the recombinant production of large quantities of these proteins. Table 5.2 provides an overview of selected cytokines and their major functions and clinical applications. Many more examples can be found in the literature.

In addition to the cytokines previously mentioned, it is important to recognize another family of low-molecular-weight proteins known as chemokines (chemotactic cytokines), which complement cytokine function and help to regulate the adaptive and innate immune system. These interacting biologic mediators have remarkable capabilities, such as controlling growth and differentiation, hematopoiesis, and

a number of lymphocyte functions including recruitment, differentiation, and inflammation.[64-66] The chemokine field has developed rapidly and is beyond the scope of this chapter. Nevertheless, a classification system has been developed based on the positions of the first two cysteine residues in the primary structure of these molecules, and the classification system divides the chemokine family into four groups. References provide a starting point for further investigation of chemokines.[64-67]

Several chemokine-related discoveries have led to a successful transplantation-based HSC collection strategy targeting the HSC-microenvironment niche interaction to cause release of HSCs from the bone marrow compartment (referred to as *stem cell mobilization*) into the peripheral circulation so that they may be harvested by apheresis techniques.[68] Experimental studies conducted in the 1990s identified a critical role for CXCL12 and its receptor CXCR4 in the migration of HSCs during early development.[69] Further investigation in adult bone marrow demonstrated that CXCL12 is a key factor in the retention of HSCs within the stem cell niche. It was also found that inhibiting the CXCL12-CXCR4 interaction permitted release of HSCs into the peripheral circulation for harvesting by apheresis.[69] Plerixafor (a CXCR4 antagonist) is used as a single agent and in conjunction with G-CSF in novel mobilization strategies to optimize donor stem cell collection.[68,69]

TABLE 5.2 Selected Cytokines, Characteristics, and Current and Potential Therapeutic Applications

Cytokine	Primary Cell Source	Primary Target Cell	Biologic Activity	Current/Potential Therapeutic Applications
EPO	Kidney (peritubular interstitial cell)	Bone marrow erythroid progenitors (BFU-E and CFU-E)	Simulates proliferation of erythroid progenitors and prevents apoptosis of CFU-E	Anemia of chronic renal disease (in predialysis, dialysis-dependent, and chronic anemia patients) Treatment of anemia in cancer patients on chemotherapy Autologous predonation blood collection Post autologous hematopoietic stem cell transplant
G-CSF	Endothelial cells Placenta Monocytes Macrophages	Neutrophil precursors Fibroblasts Leukemic myeloblasts	Stimulates granulocyte colonies Promotes differentiation of progenitors toward neutrophil lineage Stimulates neutrophil maturation	Chemotherapy-induced neutropenia Stem cell mobilization Hematopoietic stem cell transplantation Congenital neutropenia Idiopathic neutropenia Cyclic neutropenia
GM-CSF	T cells Macrophages Endothelial cells Fibroblasts Mast cells	Bone marrow progenitor cells Dendritic cells Macrophages NKT cells	Promotes antigen presentation Promotes T cell homeostasis Acts as hematopoietic cell growth factor	Chemotherapy-induced neutropenia Stem cell mobilization Hematopoietic stem cell transplantation Leukemia treatment
IL-2	CD4+ T cells NK cells B cells	T cells NK cells B cells Monocytes	Promotes cell growth/activation of CD4+ and CD8+ T cells Suppresses T_{reg} responses Mediates immune tolerance	Metastatic melanoma Renal cell carcinoma Non-Hodgkin lymphoma Asthma
IL-3	Activated T cells NK cells	Hematopoietic stem cells and progenitors	Promotes proliferation of hematopoietic progenitors	Stem cell mobilization Postchemotherapy/transplantation Bone marrow failure states

Continued

TABLE 5.2   Selected Cytokines, Characteristics, and Current and Potential Therapeutic Applications—cont'd

Cytokine	Primary Cell Source	Primary Target Cell	Biologic Activity	Current/Potential Therapeutic Applications
IL-6	T cells Macrophages Fibroblasts	T cells B cells Liver	Costimulates hematopoietic cells with other cytokines Promotes cell growth/activation of T cells and B cells Promotes megakayocyte maturation Promotes neural differentiation Acts as acute phase reactant	Stimulation of platelet production but not at tolerable doses Melanoma Renal cell carcinoma IL-6 inhibitors may be promising
IL-10	CD4+, Th2 T cells CD8+ T cells Monocytes Macrophages	T cells Macrophages	Inhibits cytokine production Inhibits macrophages	Target lymphokines in prevention of B cell lymphoma and Epstein-Barr virus lymphomagenesis HIV infection
IL-12	Macrophages	T cells	Promotes T cell, Th1 differentiation	Allergy treatment Adjuvant for infectious disease therapy Asthma Possible role for use in vaccines
IL-15	Activated CD4+ T cells	CD4+ T cells CD8+ T cells NK cells	Promotes CD4+/CD8+ T cell proliferation Promotes CD8+/NK cell cytotoxicity	Melanoma Rheumatoid arthritis Adoptive cell therapy Generation of antigen-specific T cells
IFN-α	Dendritic cells NK cells T cells B cells Macrophages Fibroblasts Endothelial cells Osteoblasts	Macrophages NK cells	Exhibits antiviral properties Enhances MHC expression	Adjuvant treatment for stage II/III melanoma Hematologic malignancies: Kaposi sarcoma, hairy cell leukemia, and chronic myeloid leukemia

BFU-E, Burst-forming unit-erythroid; *CFU-E,* colony-forming unit-erythroid; *EPO,* erythropoietin; *G-CSF,* granulocyte colony-stimulating factor; *GM-CSF,* granulocyte-macrophage colony-stimulating factor; *HIV,* human immunodeficiency virus; *IFN,* interferon; *IL,* interleukin; *MHC,* major histocompatibility complex; *NK,* natural killer; *NKT,* natural killer T cells; *Th1,* T helper, type 1; *Th2,* T helper, type 2; *T reg,* regulatory T cells.
Data from Waldmann, T. A. (2018). Cytokines in cancer immunotherapy. *Cold Spring Harb Perspect Biol, 10,* 224–235; Bossi, P., Gurizzan, C., Lorini, L., et al. (2021). Not all hematopoietic growth factors are created equal: should we gain information for their use with immunotherapy? *J Immunother Cancer, 9,* e003154; Gout, D. Y., Groen, L. S., & van Egmond, M. (2022). The present and future of immunocytokines for cancer treatment. *Cell Mol Life Sci, 10,* 509–521; and Ahlqvist-Rastad, J., Albertsson, M., Bergh, J., et al. (2007). Erythropoietin therapy and cancer related anaemia: updated Swedish recommendations. *Med Oncol, 3,* 267–272.

▌ S U M M A R Y

- Hematopoiesis is a continuous, regulated process of blood cell production that includes cell renewal, proliferation, differentiation, and maturation. These processes result in the formation, development, and specialization of all the functional blood cells.
- During fetal development, hematopoiesis progresses through the mesoblastic, hepatic, and medullary phases.
- Organs that function at some point in hematopoiesis include the liver, spleen, lymph nodes, thymus, and bone marrow.
- The bone marrow is the primary site of hematopoiesis at birth and throughout life. In certain situations, blood cell production may occur outside the bone marrow; such production is termed *extramedullary.*
- The *hematopoietic inductive microenvironment* in the bone marrow is essential for regulating hematopoietic stem cell (HSC) maintenance, self-renewal, and differentiation.

- Monophyletic theory suggests that all blood cells arise from a single stem cell called a *pluripotent hematopoietic stem cell.*
- HSCs are capable of self-renewal. They are pluripotent and can differentiate into all the different types of blood cells. One HSC can reconstitute the entire hematopoietic system of a lethally irradiated host.
- As cells mature, certain morphologic characteristics of maturation allow specific lineages to be recognized. General characteristics of maturation include decreased cell diameter, decreased nuclear diameter, loss of nucleoli, condensation of nuclear chromatin, and decreased basophilia in cytoplasm. Some morphologic changes are unique to specific lineages (e.g., loss of the nucleus in red blood cells).
- Cytokines and growth factors play a major role in the maintenance, proliferation, and differentiation of HSCs

and progenitor cells; they are also necessary to prevent premature apoptosis. Cytokines include interleukins, colony-stimulating factors, chemokines, interferons, and others.

• Cytokines can exert a positive or negative influence on HSCs and blood cell progenitors; some are lineage specific, and some function only in combination with other cytokines.

• Cytokines have provided new options in the treatment of hematologic malignancies and solid tumors. They are also used as priming agents to increase the yield of HSCs during apheresis for transplantation protocols.

Now that you have completed this chapter, go back and read again the case study at the beginning and respond to the questions presented. Answers can be found in Appendix C.

REVIEW QUESTIONS

Answers can be found in Appendix C.

1. The process of formation and development of blood cells is termed:
   a. Hematopoiesis
   b. Hematemesis
   c. Hematocytometry
   d. Hematorrhea

2. During the second trimester of fetal development, the primary site of blood cell production is the:
   a. Bone marrow
   b. Spleen
   c. Lymph nodes
   d. Liver

3. Which one of the following organs is responsible for the maturation of T lymphocytes and regulation of their expression of CD4 and CD8?
   a. Spleen
   b. Liver
   c. Thymus
   d. Bone marrow

4. The best source of active bone marrow from a 20-year-old would be:
   a. Iliac crest
   b. Femur
   c. Distal radius
   d. Tibia

5. Physiologic programmed cell death is termed:
   a. Angiogenesis
   b. Apoptosis
   c. Aneurysm
   d. Apohematics

6. Which organ is the site of sequestration of platelets?
   a. Liver
   b. Thymus
   c. Spleen
   d. Bone marrow

7. Which one of the following morphologic changes occurs during normal blood cell maturation?
   a. Increase in cell diameter
   b. Development of cytoplasm basophilia
   c. Condensation of nuclear chromatin
   d. Appearance of nucleoli

8. Which one of the following cells is a product of the common lymphoid progenitor?
   a. Megakaryocyte
   b. T lymphocyte
   c. Erythrocyte
   d. Granulocyte

9. What growth factor is produced in the kidneys and is used to treat anemia associated with kidney disease?
   a. EPO
   b. TPO
   c. G-CSF
   d. KIT ligand

10. Which one of the following cytokines is required very early in the differentiation of a hematopoietic stem cell?
    a. IL-2
    b. IL-8
    c. EPO
    d. FLT3 ligand

11. When a patient has severe anemia and the bone marrow is unable to effectively produce RBCs to meet the increased demand, one of the body's responses is:
    a. Extramedullary hematopoiesis in the liver and spleen
    b. Decreased production of erythropoietin by the kidney
    c. Increased apoptosis of erythrocyte progenitor cells
    d. Increased proportion of yellow marrow in the long bones

12. Hematopoietic stem cells produce all lineages of blood cells in sufficient quantities over the lifetime of an individual because they:
    a. Are unipotent
    b. Have the ability of self-renewal by asymmetric division
    c. Are present in large numbers in the bone marrow niches
    d. Have a low mitotic potential in response to growth factors

REFERENCES

1. Weijts, B., Yvernogeau, L., & Robin, C. (2021). Recent advances in developmental hematopoiesis: diving deeper with new technologies. *Front Immunol, 12,* 1–16.

2. Zhang, Y., Huang, Y., Hu, L., et al. (2022). New insights into human hematopoietic stem and progenitor cells via single-cell omics. *Stem Cell Rev Rep, 4,* 1322–1336.

3. Dave, U. P., & Koury, M. J. (2021). Structure of the marrow and the hematopoietic microenvironment. In Kaushansky, K., Lichtman, M. A., Prchal, J. T., et al. (Eds.), *Williams Hematology.* (10th ed., pp. 47–78). New York: McGraw-Hill.

4. Rossmann, M. P., & Chute, J. P. (2023). Hematopoietic stem cell biology. In Hoffman, R., Benz, E. J., Silberstein, L. E., et al. (Eds.), *Hematology Basic Principles and Practice.* (8th ed., pp. 95–114). Philadelphia: Elsevier.

5. Peault, B. (1996). Hematopoietic stem cell emergence in embryonic life: developmental hematology revisited. *J Hematother, 5,* 369–378.

6. Tavian, M., Coulombel, L., Luton, D., et al. (1996). Aorta-associated CD34+ hematopoietic cells in the early human embryo. *Blood, 87,* 67–72.

7. Ivanovs, A., Rybtsov, S., Welch, L., et al. (2011). Highly potent human hematopoietic stem cells first emerge in the intraembryonic aorta-gonad-mesonephros region. *J Exp Med, 208,* 2417–2427.

8. Palis, J., & Segal, G. B. (2021). Hematology of the fetus and newborn. In Kaushansky, K., Lichtman, M. A., Prchal, J. T., et al. (Eds.), *Williams Hematology.* (10th ed., pp. 93–110). New York: McGraw-Hill.

9. Baron, M. H., Isern, J., & Fraser, S. T. (2012). The embryonic origins of erythropoiesis in mammals. *Blood, 119,* 4828–4837.

10. Yoder, M. C., Hiatt, K., & Mukherjee, P. (1997). In vivo repopulating hematopoietic stem cells are present in the murine yolk sac at day 9.0 postcoitus. *Proc Natl Acad Sci, 94,* 6776–6780.

11. Bailey, A. S., & Fleming, W. H. (2003). Converging roads: evidence for an adult hemangioblast. *Exp Hematol, 31,* 987–993.

12. Pelosi, E., Valtieri, M., Coppola, S., et al. (2002). Identification of the hemangioblast in postnatal life. *Blood, 100,* 3203–3208.

13. Bailey, A. S., Jiang, S., Afentoulis, M., et al. (2004). Transplanted adult hematopoietic stems cells differentiate into functional endothelial cells. *Blood, 103,* 13–19.

14. Frame, J. M., Fegan, K. H., Conwa, S. J., et al. (2016). Definitive hematopoiesis in the yolk sac emerges from Wnt-responsive hemogenic endothelium independently of circulation and arterial identity. *Stem Cells, 34,* 431–444.

15. Patel, S. H., Christodoulou, C., Weinreb, C., et al. (2022). Lifelong multilineage contribution by embryonic-born blood progenitors. *Nature, 606,* 747–753.

16. DeWitt, N. (2007). Rewriting in blood: blood stem cells may have a surprising origin. *Nat Rep Stem Cells* 10.1038/stem-cells.2007.42.

17. Bertrand, J., Chi, N., Santoso, B., et al. (2010). Haematopoietic stem cells derive directly from aortic endothelium during development. *Nature, 464,* 108–111.

18. Yokomizo, T., & Dzierzak, E. (2010). Three-dimensional cartography of hematopoietic clusters in the vasculature of whole mouse embryos. *Development, 137,* 3651–3661.

19. Charbord, P. (2010). Bone marrow mesenchymal stem cells: historical overview and concepts. *Hum Gene Ther, 21,* 1045–1056.

20. Gupta, P., Blazar, B., Gupta, K., et al. (1998). Human CD34+ bone marrow cells regulate stromal production of interleukin-6 and granulocyte colony-stimulating factor and increase the colony-stimulating activity of stroma. *Blood, 91,* 3724–3733.

21. Rosen, C. J., Ackert-Bicknell, C., Rodriguez, J. P., et al. (2009). Marrow fat and bone marrow microenvironment: developmental, functional, and pathological implications. *Crit Rev Eukaryot Gene Expr, 19,* 109–124.

22. Scadden, D., & Silberstein, L. (2023). Hematopoietic microenvironment. In Hoffman, R., Benz, E. J., Silberstein, L. E., et al. (Eds.), *Hematology Basic Principles and Practice.* (8th ed., pp. 157–164). Philadelphia: Elsevier.

23. Jacobsen, R. N., Perkins, A. C., & Levesque, J. P. (2015). Macrophages and regulation of erythropoiesis. *Curr Opin Hematol, 22,* 212–219.

24. Kaushansky, K. (2021). Hematopoietic stem cells, progenitors, and cytokines. In Kaushansky, K., Lichtman, M. A., Prchal, J. T., et al. (Eds.), *Williams Hematology.* (10th ed., pp. 273–294). New York: McGraw-Hill.

25. Wu, Q., Zhang, J., & Lucas, D. (2021). Anatomy of hematopoiesis and local microenvironments in the bone marrow. Where to? *Front Immunol, 12,* 768439.

26. Levi, M. (2021). The inflammatory response. In Kaushansky, K., Lichtman, M. A., Prchal, J. T., et al. (Eds.), *Williams Hematology.* (10th ed., pp. 295–308). New York: McGraw-Hill.

27. Klein, G. (1995). The extracellular matrix of the hematopoietic microenvironment. *Experientia, 51,* 914–926.

28. Ehninger, A., & Trumpp, A. (2011). The bone marrow stem cell niche grows up: mesenchymal stem cells and macrophages move in. *J Exp Med, 208,* 421–428.

29. Smith, J. N. P., & Calvi, L. M. (2013). Current concepts in bone marrow microenvironmental regulation of hematopoietic stem and progenitor cells. *Stem Cells, 31,* 1044–1050.

30. Yoshihara, H., Arai, F., Hosokawa, K., et al. (2007). The niche regulation of quiescent hematopoietic stem cells through thrombopoietin/Mpl signaling. *Cell Stem Cell, 1,* 685–697.

31. Morrison, S. J., & Spradling, A. C. (2008). Stem cells and niches: mechanisms that promote stem cell maintenance throughout life. *Cell, 132,* 598–611.

32. Ema, H., & Suda, T. (2012). Anatomically distinct niches regulate stem cell activity. *Blood, 120,* 2174–2181.

33. Iwasaki, H., & Akashi, K. (2007). Myeloid lineage commitment from the hematopoietic stem cell. *Immunity, 26,* 726–740.

34. Kim, S. I., & Bresnick, E. H. (2007). Transcriptional control of erythropoiesis: emerging mechanisms and principles. *Oncogene, 26,* 6777–6794.

35. Abdel-Misih, S. R. Z., & Bloomston, M. (2010). Liver anatomy. *Surg Clin North Am, 90,* 643–653.

36. Roy-Chowdhury, N., & Roy-Chowdhury, J. (2021). Liver physiology and energy metabolism. In Feldman, M., Friedman, L. S., & Brandt, L. J. (Eds.), *Sleisenger and Fordtran's Gastrointestinal and Liver Disease.* (11th ed., pp. 1135–1153). Philadelphia: Elsevier.

37. Collin, M., & Hill, G. R. (2019). Monocytes, macrophages, and dendritic cells. In Greer, J. P., Rodgers, G. M., Glader, B., et al. (Eds.), *Wintrobe's Clinical Hematology.* (14th ed., pp. 203–225). Philadelphia: Wolters Kluwer Health/Lippincott Williams & Wilkins.

38. Kim, C. H. (2010). Homeostatic and pathogenic extramedullary hematopoiesis. *J Blood Med, 1,* 13–19.

39. Ollila, T. A., Zayac, A. S., & Schiffman, F. J. (2023). The spleen and its disorders. In Hoffman, R., Benz, E. J., Silberstein, L. E., et al. (Eds.), *Hematology Basic Principles and Practice.* (8th ed., pp. 2378–2393). Philadelphia: Elsevier.

40. Scoville, S., & Caligiuri, M. A. (2021). The organization and structure of lymphoid tissues. In Kaushansky, K., Lichtman, M. A., Prchal, J. T., et al. (Eds.), *Williams Hematology*. (10th ed., pp. 79–92). New York: McGraw-Hill.

41. Warkentin, T. E. (2023). Thrombocytopenia caused by hypersplenism, platelet destruction, or surgery/hemodilution. In Hoffman, R., Benz, E. J., Silberstein, L. E., et al. (Eds.), *Hematology Basic Principles and Practice*. (8th ed., pp. 2033–2048). Philadelphia: Elsevier.

42. Cesta, M. F. (2006). Normal structure, function, and histology of the spleen. *Toxicol Pathol, 34*, 455–465.

43. Chou, S. T., & Schreiber, A. D. (2015). Autoimmune hemolytic anemia. In Orkin, S. H., Fisher, D. E., Ginsburg, D., et al. (Eds.), *Nathan and Oski's Hematology and Oncology of Infancy and Childhood*. (8th ed., pp. 411–430). Philadelphia: Elsevier.

44. Chapman, W. C., Jr., & Chapman, W. C. (2019). Disorders of the spleen. In Greer, J. P., Rodgers, G. M., Glader, B., et al. (Eds.), *Wintrobe's Clinical Hematology*. (14th ed., pp. 1394–1407). Philadelphia: Wolters Kluwer Health/Lippincott Williams & Wilkins.

45. Park, C. (2019). Lymphocytes and lymphatic organs. In Greer, J. P., Rodgers, G. M., Glader, B., et al. (Eds.), *Wintrobe's Clinical Hematology*. (14th ed., pp. 226–259). Philadelphia: Wolters Kluwer Health/Lippincott Williams & Wilkins.

46. Carty, S. A., Riese, M. J., & Koretzky, G. A. (2023). T-cell immunity. In Hoffman, R., Benz, Jr., E. J., Silberstein, L. E., et al. (Eds.), *Hematology Basic Principles and Practice*. (8th ed., pp. 271–288). Philadelphia: Elsevier.

47. Till, T. E., & McCulloch, E. A. (1961). A direct measurement of the radiation sensitivity of normal mouse marrow cells. *Radiat Res, 14*, 213–222.

48. Quigley, J. G., Means, R. T., Jr., & Glader, B. (2019). The birth, life, and death of red blood cells: erythropoiesis, the mature red blood cell, and cell destruction. In Greer, J. P., Rodgers, G. M., Glader, B., et al. (Eds.), *Wintrobe's Clinical Hematology*. (14th ed., pp. 90–130). Philadelphia: Wolters Kluwer Health/Lippincott Williams & Wilkins.

49. Metcalf, D. (2007). On hematopoietic stem cell fate. *Immunity, 26*, 669–673.

50. Verfaillie, C. (2003). Regulation of hematopoiesis. In Wickramasinghe, S. N., & McCullough, J. (Eds.), *Blood and Bone Marrow Pathology*. New York: Churchill Livingstone.

51. Antony, A. C. (2023). Megaloblastic anemias. In Hoffman, R., Benz, Jr., E. J., Silberstein, L. E., et al. (Eds.), *Hematology Basic Principles and Practice*. (8th ed., pp. 524–554). Philadelphia: Elsevier.

52. Horst Ibelfault's, C. O. P. E. (2016). *Cytokines Online Pathfinder Encyclopedia*. version 45.1 http://www.cells-talk.com. Accessed August 30, 2022.

53. Chow, A., & Frenette, P. S. (2019). Origin and development of blood cells. In Greer, J. P., Rodgers, G. M., Glader, B., et al. (Eds.), *Wintrobe's Clinical Hematology*. (14th ed., pp. 67–89).

54. Rot, A., Hub, E., Massberg, S., et al. (2023). Role of chemokines in leukocyte trafficking. In Hoffman, R., Benz, Jr., E. J., Silberstein, L. E., et al. (Eds.), *Hematology Basic Principles and Practice*. (8th ed., pp. 137–148). Philadelphia: Elsevier.

55. Sieff, C., Daley, G. Q., & Zon, L. I. (2015). Anatomy and physiology of hematopoiesis. In Orkin, S. H., Fisher, D. E., Ginsburg, D., et al. (Eds.), *Nathan and Oski's Hematology and Oncology of Infancy and Childhood*. (8th ed., pp. 3–51). Philadelphia: Elsevier.

56. Ogawa, M. (1993). Differentiation and proliferation of hematopoietic stem cells. *Blood, 81*, 2844–2853.

57. Dougan, M., Dranoff, G., & Dougan, S. K. (2019). GM-CSF, IL-3, and IL-5 family of cytokines: regulators of inflammation. *Immunity, 50*, 796–811.

58. Broughton, S. E., Dhagat, U., Hercus, T. R., et al. (2012). The GM-CSF/IL-3/IL-5 cytokine receptor family: from ligand recognition to initiation of signaling. *Immunol Rev, 250*, 277–302.

59. Sawada, K., Krantz, S. B., & Dai, C. H. (1990). Purification of human burst-forming units-erythroid and demonstration of the evolution of erythropoietin receptors. *J Cell Physiol, 142*, 219–230.

60. Rizzo, J. D., Seidenfield, J., Piper, M., et al. (2001). Erythropoietin: a paradigm for the development of practice guidelines. *Haematology, 1*, 10–30.

61. Cazzola, M., Mercuriall, F., & Bruguara, C. (1997). Use of recombinant human erythropoietin outside the setting of uremia. *Blood, 89*, 4248–4267.

62. Wolber, E. M., Ganschow, R., Burdelski, M., et al. (1999). Hepatic thrombopoietin mRNA levels in acute and chronic liver failure of childhood. *Hepatol, 29*, 1739–1742.

63. Wolber, E. M., Dame, C., Fahnenstich, H., et al. (1999). Expression of the thrombopoietin gene in human fetal and neonatal tissues. *Blood, 94*, 97–105.

64. Fields, J. K., Günther, S., & Sundberg, E. J. (2019). Structural basis of IL-1 family cytokine signaling. *Front Immunol, 10*, 1412.

65. Raza, S., Rajak, S., Tewari, A., et al. (2022). Multifaceted role of chemokines in solid tumors: from biology to therapy. *Semin Cancer Biol, 86*, 1105–1121.

66. Do, H. T. T., Lee, C. H., & Cho, J. (2020). Chemokines and their receptors: multifaceted roles in cancer progression and potential value as cancer prognostic markers. *Cancers, 12*, 287.

67. Bachelerie, F., Ben-Baruch, A., Burkhardt, A. M., et al. (2013). International union of basic and clinical pharmacology. LXXXIX. Update on the extended family of chemokine receptors and introducing a new nomenclature for atypical chemokine receptors. *Pharmacol Rev, 66*, 1–79.

68. Luster, A. D. (1998). Chemokines—chemotactic cytokines that mediate inflammation. *N Engl J Med, 338*, 436–445.

69. Chang, H. H., Liou, Y. S., & Sun, D. S. (2021). Hematopoietic stem cell mobilization. *Tzu Chi Med J, 34*, 270–275.

6

Erythrocyte Production and Destruction

Michelle Montgomery Butina*

OBJECTIVES

After completion of this chapter, the reader will be able to:

1. Correlate the erythroblast, normoblast, and rubriblast nomenclatures for red blood cell (RBC) stages.
2. Name the erythrocyte progenitors and distinguish them from precursors.
3. List and describe erythroid precursors in order of maturity, including the morphologic characteristics, cellular activities, normal location, and length of time in the stage for each.
4. Name the stage of erythroid development when given a written description of the morphology of a cell in a Wright-stained bone marrow preparation.
5. Explain the nucleus-to-cytoplasm (N:C) ratio, describe the appearance of a cell when given the N:C ratio, and estimate the N:C ratio from the appearance of a cell.
6. List and compare the cellular organelles of immature and mature erythrocytes and describe their specific functions.
7. Explain how reticulocytes can be recognized in a Wright-stained peripheral blood film.
8. Define and differentiate the terms *polychromasia, diffuse basophilia, punctate basophilia,* and *basophilic stippling.*
9. Define and differentiate *erythron* and *RBC* mass.
10. Explain how hypoxia stimulates RBC production.
11. Describe the general chemical composition of erythropoietin (EPO) and name the site of production.
12. Discuss various mechanisms by which EPO contributes to erythropoiesis.
13. Explain the processes by which EPO promotes early release of reticulocytes.
14. Explain how erythroid progenitors and precursors evade apoptosis.
15. Explain the ways in which EPO reduces bone marrow transit time.
16. Describe features of the bone marrow that contribute to establishing the microenvironment necessary for the proliferation of RBCs, including location and arrangement relative to other cells.
17. Discuss the various roles bone marrow macrophages have in RBC development.
18. Explain how RBCs enter the bloodstream.
19. Describe characteristics of senescent RBCs and explain why RBCs age.
20. Explain and differentiate the two normal mechanisms of erythrocyte destruction, including location and process.

OUTLINE

Erythropoiesis
  Maturation Process
  Criteria Used in Identification of Erythroid Precursors
  Maturation Sequence
Dynamics of Red Blood Cell Production and Destruction
  Hypoxia—the Stimulus to Red Blood Cell Production
  Erythropoietin

  Other Stimuli to Erythropoiesis
Microenvironment of the Bone Marrow
  Role of Bone Marrow Macrophages
Erythrocyte Destruction
  Macrophage-Mediated Hemolysis (Extravascular Hemolysis)
  Fragmentation Hemolysis (Intravascular Hemolysis)

CASE STUDY

After studying the material in this chapter, the reader should be able to respond to the following case study. Answers can be found in Appendix C.

A 42-year-old premenopausal woman had emphysema. This lung disease impairs the ability to oxygenate the blood, so patients experience significant fatigue and shortness of breath. To alleviate these symptoms, oxygen is typically prescribed, and this patient had a portable oxygen tank she carried with her at all times, breathing through a nasal cannula. Before she began using oxygen, her RBC count was 5.8×10^{12}/L. The reference interval can be found after the Index at the end of the book. After oxygen therapy for several months, her RBC count dropped to 5.0×10^{12}/L.

1. What physiologic response explains the elevation of the first RBC count?
2. What hormone is responsible? How is its production stimulated? What is the major way in which it acts?
3. What explains the decline in RBC count with oxygen therapy for this patient?

*The author extends appreciation to Kathryn Doig, whose work in prior editions provided the foundation for this chapter.

The red blood cell (RBC), or erythrocyte, provides a classic example of the biologic principle that cells have specialized functions and that their structures are specific for those functions. The erythrocyte has one true function: to carry oxygen from the lung to the tissues, where the oxygen is released. This is accomplished by the attachment of the oxygen to hemoglobin, the major cytoplasmic component of mature RBCs. The role of the RBC in returning carbon dioxide to the lungs and buffering the pH of the blood is important but is secondary to its oxygen-carrying function. To protect this essential life function, the mechanisms controlling the development, production, and normal destruction of RBCs are fine-tuned to avoid interruptions in oxygen delivery, even under adverse conditions such as blood loss with hemorrhage. This chapter and subsequent chapters discussing RBC metabolism, membrane structure, hemoglobin, and iron establish the foundation for understanding the body's response to diminished oxygen-carrying capacity of the blood, called *anemia*.

The mammalian erythrocyte is unique among animal cells in that in its mature, functional state, it does not have a nucleus. Although amphibians and birds possess RBCs, their nonmammalian RBCs retain the nuclei throughout the cells' lives. The implications of this unique mammalian adaptation are significant for cell function and life span.

ERYTHROPOIESIS

RBCs are formally called *erythrocytes*. *Erythropoiesis* is the process of differentiation and maturation of erythrocytes in the bone marrow.[1] Nucleated RBC precursors, normally restricted to the bone marrow, are called *normoblasts* (such as pronormoblast or basophilic normoblast) or *erythroblasts*. These terms refer to developing nucleated RBC precursors with normal morphology. Three nomenclatures are used for naming erythroid precursors (Table 6.1). The normoblastic terminology is commonly used in the United States and is descriptive of the appearance of the cells. Some prefer the rubriblast terminology because it parallels the nomenclature used for granulocyte development (Chapter 10). The erythroblast terminology is used primarily in Europe. Normoblastic terminology is used in this chapter.

Maturation Process
Erythroid Progenitors
As described in Chapter 5, erythrocytes develop from the megakaryocyte-erythroid progenitor (MEP), which develops from hematopoietic stem cells. The morphologically identifiable lineage-specific erythrocyte progenitor cells from the MEP is the *burst-forming unit-erythroid* (BFU-E), followed by the *colony-forming unit-erythroid* (CFU-E).[2] These erythroid progenitors are named for their ability to form colonies on semisolid media in tissue culture experiments that enable the study of their characteristics and development.[3,4] The earliest committed progenitor, the BFU-E, gives rise to large colonies, as BFU-Es are capable of multisubunit colonies (called *bursts*), whereas the CFU-E gives rise to smaller colonies.[3]

Estimates of time spent at each stage suggest that it takes about 1 week for the BFU-E to mature to the CFU-E and another week for the CFU-E to become a pronormoblast,[5] which is the first morphologically identifiable RBC precursor. While at the CFU-E stage, the cell completes approximately three to five divisions before maturing further.[5] As seen in "Maturation Sequence," it takes approximately another 6 to 7 days for the precursors to become mature enough to enter the circulation, so approximately 18 to 21 days are required to produce a mature RBC from the BFU-E.

Erythroid Precursors
Normoblastic proliferation, similar to the proliferation of other blood cell lines, is a process encompassing replication (i.e., division) to increase cell numbers and development from immature to mature cell stages (Figure 6.1). The earliest morphologically recognizable erythrocyte precursor, the pronormoblast, is derived via the BFU-E and CFU-E from hematopoietic stem cells, as discussed in Chapter 5. The pronormoblast is able to divide, with each daughter cell maturing to the next stage of development, the basophilic normoblast. Each of these cells can divide, with each of its daughter cells maturing to the next stage, the polychromatic normoblast. Each of these cells also can divide and mature. In the erythrocyte cell line, there are typically three and occasionally as many as five divisions,[6] with subsequent nuclear and cytoplasmic maturation of the daughter cells; therefore, from a single pronormoblast, 8 to 32 mature RBCs usually result. The conditions under which the number of divisions can be increased or reduced are discussed in "Dynamics of Red Blood Cell Production and Destruction." The changes and cellular activities at each stage described here occur in an orderly and sequential erythroid developmental process.

TABLE 6.1	Three Erythroid Precursor Nomenclature Systems	
Normoblastic	**Rubriblastic**	**Erythroblastic**
Pronormoblast	Rubriblast	Proerythroblast
Basophilic normoblast	Prorubricyte	Basophilic erythroblast
Polychromatic (polychromatophilic) normoblast	Rubricyte	Polychromatic (polychromatophilic) erythroblast
Orthochromic normoblast	Metarubricyte	Orthochromic erythroblast
Polychromatic (polychromatophilic) erythrocyte*	Polychromatic (polychromatophilic) erythrocyte*	Polychromatic (polychromatophilic) erythrocyte*
Erythrocyte	Erythrocyte	Erythrocyte

*Polychromatic erythrocytes are called reticulocytes when observed with vital stains.

Criteria Used in Identification of Erythroid Precursors

Morphologic identification of blood cells depends on a well-stained peripheral blood film or bone marrow smear (Chapters 14 and 15). In hematology, a modified Romanowsky stain, such as Wright or Wright-Giemsa, is commonly used. The descriptions that follow are based on the use of these types of stains.

The stage of maturation of any blood cell is determined by careful examination of the nucleus and the cytoplasm. The most important features in the identification of RBCs include the nuclear diameter, nucleus-to-cytoplasm (N:C) ratio (Box 6.1), nuclear chromatin pattern (texture, density, homogeneity), presence or absence of nucleoli, and cytoplasmic color.

As erythroid precursors mature, several general trends affect their appearance. Figure 6.2 graphically represents these trends.

1. Overall diameter of the cell decreases.
2. Diameter of the nucleus decreases more rapidly than the diameter of the cell. As a result, the N:C ratio also decreases.
3. Nuclear chromatin pattern becomes coarser, clumped, and condensed. The nuclear chromatin of erythroid precursors is inherently coarser than that of myeloid precursors. It becomes even coarser and more clumped as the cell matures, developing a raspberry-like appearance, in which the dark staining of the chromatin is distinct from the

almost white appearance of the parachromatin. This chromatin/parachromatin distinction is more dramatic than in other cell lines. Ultimately, the nucleus becomes quite condensed, with no parachromatin evident at all, and the nucleus is said to be *pyknotic*. Condensation of the chromatin is important for the extrusion (expulsion) of the pyknotic nuclei in the polychromatic erythrocyte or reticulocyte stage.[2,7]

4. Nucleoli disappear. Nucleoli represent areas where the ribosomes are formed and are seen early in cell development as cells begin actively synthesizing proteins (Chapter 4). As erythroid precursors mature, nucleoli disappear, which precedes the ultimate cessation of protein synthesis.
5. Cytoplasm color changes from blue to gray-blue to salmon pink. Blueness or *basophilia* is due to acidic components that attract basic stains, such as methylene blue. The degree of cytoplasmic basophilia correlates with the amount of ribosomal ribonucleic acid (RNA). The ribosomes and other organelles decline over the life of the developing erythroid precursor, and the blueness fades. Pinkness, called *eosinophilia* or *acidophilia*, is due to accumulation of more basic components that attract acid stains, such as eosin. Eosinophilia of erythrocyte cytoplasm correlates with the accumulation of hemoglobin as the cell matures. Thus the cell starts out being active in protein production

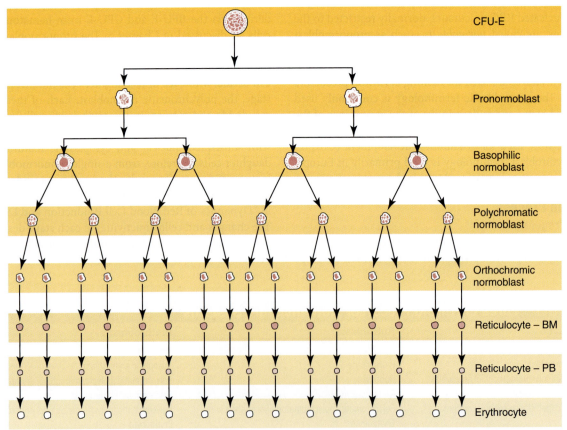

Figure 6.1 Typical Production of Erythrocytes From Two Pronormoblasts Illustrating Three Mitotic Divisions Among Precursors. *BM,* Bone marrow; *CFU-E,* colony-forming unit-erythroid; *PB,* peripheral blood.

on the ribosomes that make the cytoplasm basophilic, transitions through a period in which the red of hemoglobin begins to mix with that blue, and ultimately ends with a thoroughly salmon pink color when the ribosomes are gone and only hemoglobin remains.

Maturation Sequence

Table 6.2 lists the stages of erythroid development in order and compares them. The listing makes it appear that these stages are clearly distinct and easily identifiable. Cell maturation is a gradual process, however, with changes occurring in a generally predictable sequence but with some variation for each individual cell. The identification of the stage of a given cell depends on the preponderance of characteristics, although the cell may not possess all the features of the archetypal descriptions that follow. Essential features of each stage are in italics in the following descriptions. The cellular functions described subsequently are also summarized in Figure 6.3.

Pronormoblast (Rubriblast)

Figure 6.4 shows the pronormoblast.

Nucleus. The nucleus takes up much of the cell, with an N:C ratio of 8:1. The nucleus is round to oval, *containing one or two nucleoli. The purple-red chromatin is open* and contains few, if any, fine clumps.

Cytoplasm. The cytoplasm is dark blue because of the concentration of ribosomes and RNA. The Golgi complex may be visible next to the nucleus as a pale, unstained area. Pronormoblasts may show small tufts of irregular cytoplasm along the periphery of the membrane.

Division. The pronormoblast undergoes mitosis and gives rise to two daughter pronormoblasts. More than one division is possible before maturation into basophilic normoblasts.

BOX 6.1 Nucleus-to-Cytoplasm Ratio

The nucleus-to-cytoplasm (N:C) ratio is a morphologic feature used to identify and stage red blood cell (RBC) and white blood cell precursors. The ratio is a visual estimate of the area of the cell occupied by the nucleus compared with that of the cytoplasm. If the areas of each are approximately equal, the N:C ratio is 1:1. Although not mathematically proper, it is common for ratios other than 1:1 to be referred to as if they were fractions. If the nucleus takes up less than 50% of the area of the cell, the proportion of nucleus is lower and the ratio is lower (e.g., 1:5 or less than 1). If the nucleus takes up more than 50% of the area of the cell, the ratio is higher (e.g., 3:1 or 3). In the RBC line, the proportion of nucleus shrinks as the cell matures and the cytoplasm increases proportionately, although the overall cell diameter grows smaller. In short, the N:C ratio decreases.

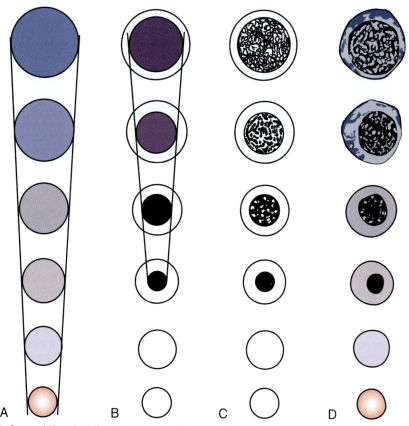

Figure 6.2 General Trends Affecting the Morphology of Erythroid Precursors During the Developmental Process. (A), Cell diameter decreases and cytoplasm changes from blue to salmon pink. (B), Nuclear diameter decreases and color changes from purplish-red to a very dark purple-blue. (C), Nuclear chromatin becomes coarser, clumped, and condensed. (D), Composite of changes during the developmental process. (Modified from Diggs, L. W., Sturm, D., & Bell, A. [1985]. *The Morphology of Human Blood Cells.* [5th ed.]. Abbott Park, IL: Abbott Laboratories.)

TABLE 6.2	Normoblastic Series: Summary of Stage Morphology				
Cell or Stage	**Diameter (μm)**	**Nucleus-to-Cytoplasm Ratio**	**Nucleoli**	**Nucleated Cells in Bone Marrow (%)**	**Bone Marrow Transit Time (h)**
Pronormoblast	12–20	8:1	1–2	1	24
Basophilic normoblast	10–15	6:1	0–1	1–4	24
Polychromatic normoblast	10–12	4:1	0	10–20	30
Orthochromic normoblast	8–10	1:2	0	5–10	48
Bone marrow polychromatic erythrocyte*	8–10	No nucleus	0	1	24–48

*Also called *reticulocyte.*

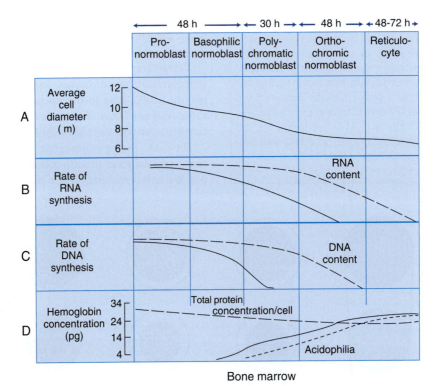

Figure 6.3 Changes in Cellular Diameter, RNA Synthesis and Content, DNA Synthesis and Content, and Protein and Hemoglobin Content During Erythroid Development. (A), Cell diameter (*solid line*) shrinks from the pronormoblast to the reticulocyte stage. (B), The rate of ribonucleic acid *(RNA)* synthesis (*solid line*) for protein production is at its peak at the pronormoblast stage and ends in the orthochromic normoblast stage. RNA accumulates so that the RNA content (*dashed line*) remains relatively constant into the orthochromic normoblast stage when it begins to degrade, being eliminated by the end of the reticulocyte stage. (C), The rate of deoxyribonucleic acid *(DNA)* synthesis (*solid line*) correlates to the stages of development that are able to divide: pronormoblast, basophilic normoblast, and early polychromatic normoblast stages. DNA content (*dashed line*) of a given cell remains relatively constant until the nucleus begins to break up and is extruded during the orthochromic normoblast stage. There is no DNA (i.e., no nucleus) in reticulocytes. (D), The *dashed line* represents the total protein concentration, which declines slightly during maturation. Proteins other than hemoglobin predominate in early stages. The hemoglobin concentration (*solid line*) begins to rise in the basophilic normoblast stage, reaching its peak in reticulocytes and representing most of the protein in more mature cells. Hemoglobin synthesis is visible as acidophilia (*dotted line*) that parallels hemoglobin accumulation but is delayed because the earliest production of hemoglobin in basophilic normoblasts is not visible microscopically. (Modified from Granick, S., & Levere, R. D. [1964]. Heme synthesis in erythroid cells. In Moore, C. V., & Brown, E. B. [Eds.], *Progress in Hematology.* New York: Grune & Stratton.)

Location. The pronormoblast is present only in the bone marrow in healthy states.

Cellular activity. The pronormoblast begins to accumulate the components necessary for hemoglobin production. The proteins and enzymes necessary for iron uptake and protoporphyrin synthesis are produced. Globin production begins.[8]

Length of time in this stage. This stage lasts slightly more than 24 hours.[8]

Basophilic Normoblast (Prorubricyte)

Figure 6.5 shows the basophilic normoblast.

Nucleus. *The chromatin begins to condense,* revealing clumps along the periphery of the nuclear membrane and a few in the interior. As the chromatin condenses, the parachromatin areas become larger and sharper, and the N:C ratio decreases to about 6:1. The chromatin stains deep purple-red. Nucleoli may be present early in the stage but disappear later.

Cytoplasm. *The cytoplasm may be a deeper, richer blue* than in the pronormoblast, hence the name *basophilic* (dark blue) for this stage.

Division. The basophilic normoblast undergoes mitosis, giving rise to two daughter cells. More than one division is possible before the daughter cells mature into polychromatic normoblasts.

Location. The basophilic normoblast is present only in the bone marrow in healthy states.

Cellular activity. Detectable hemoglobin synthesis occurs,[8] but the many cytoplasmic organelles, including ribosomes and a substantial amount of messenger RNA (chiefly for hemoglobin production), completely mask the minute amount of hemoglobin pigmentation.

Length of time in this stage. This stage lasts slightly more than 24 hours.[8]

Polychromatic (Polychromatophilic) Normoblast (Rubricyte)

Figure 6.6 shows the polychromatic normoblast.

Nucleus. The chromatin pattern varies during this stage of development, showing some openness early in the stage but becoming condensed by the end. *The condensation of chromatin* reduces the diameter of the nucleus considerably, so the N:C ratio decreases from 4:1 to about 1:1 by the end of the stage. Notably, *no nucleoli are present.*

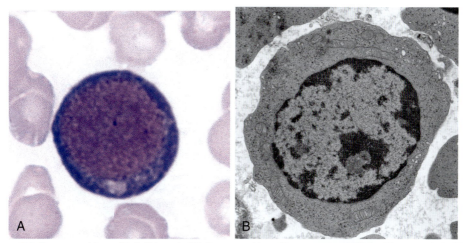

Figure 6.4 Pronormoblasts (Rubriblasts). **(A)**, Pronormoblast. (Bone marrow, Wright-Giemsa stain, ×1000.) **(B)**, Electron micrograph of a pronormoblast (×15,575). (B from Carr, J. H. [2022]. *Clinical Hematology Atlas.* [6th ed.]. St. Louis: Elsevier.)

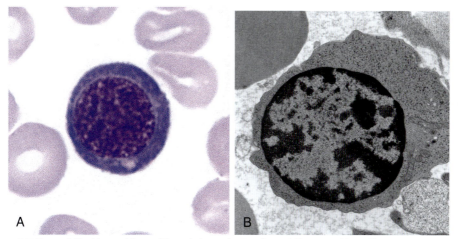

Figure 6.5 Basophilic Normoblasts (Prorubricytes). **(A)**, Basophilic normoblast. (Bone marrow, Wright-Giemsa stain, ×1000.) **(B)**, Electron micrograph of a basophilic normoblast (×15,575). (B from Carr, J. H. [2022]. *Clinical Hematology Atlas.* [6th ed.]. St. Louis: Elsevier.)

Cytoplasm. This is the first stage in which the pink color associated with stained hemoglobin can be seen. The stained color reflects the accumulation of hemoglobin pigmentation over time and concurrent decreasing amounts of RNA. The color produced is a mixture of pink and blue, resulting in a *murky gray-blue.* The name of this stage refers to this combination of multiple colors, as *polychromatophilic* means "loving several colors."[1]

Division. This is the last stage in which the cell is capable of undergoing mitosis, although likely only early in the stage. The polychromatic normoblast goes through mitosis, producing daughter cells that mature and develop into orthochromic normoblasts.

Location. The polychromatic normoblast is present only in the bone marrow in healthy states.

Cellular activity. Hemoglobin synthesis increases, and the accumulation begins to be visible as a pinkish color in the cytoplasm. Cellular RNA and organelles are still present, particularly ribosomes, which contribute a blue color to the cytoplasm. The progressive condensation of the nucleus and disappearance of nucleoli are evidence of progressive decline in transcription of deoxyribonucleic acid (DNA).

Length of time in this stage. This stage lasts approximately 30 hours.[8]

Orthochromic Normoblast (Metarubricyte)

Figure 6.7 shows the orthochromic normoblast.

Nucleus. *The nucleus is completely condensed* (i.e., pyknotic) or nearly so. As a result, the N:C ratio is low or approximately 1:2.

Cytoplasm. The increase in the *salmon pink color* of the cytoplasm reflects nearly complete hemoglobin production. The residual ribosomes and RNA react with the basic component of the stain and contribute a slightly bluish hue to the cell, but that fades toward the end of the stage as the RNA and organelles are degraded.

Division. The orthochromic normoblast is not capable of division because of the condensation of the chromatin.

Location. The orthochromic normoblast is present only in the bone marrow in healthy states.

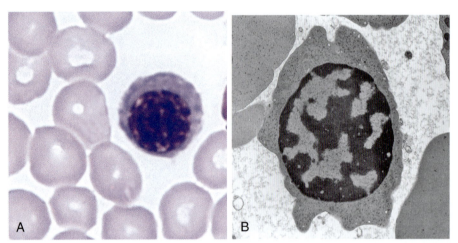

Figure 6.6 **Polychromatic Normoblasts (Rubricytes).** **(A)**, Polychromatic normoblast. (Bone marrow, Wright-Giemsa stain, ×1000.) **(B)**, Electron micrograph of a polychromatic normoblast (×15,575). (B from Carr, J. H. [2022]. *Clinical Hematology Atlas.* [6th ed.]. St. Louis: Elsevier.)

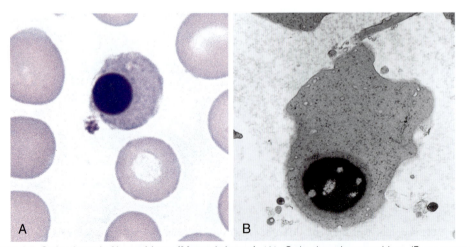

Figure 6.7 **Orthochromic Normoblasts (Metarubricytes).** **(A)**, Orthochromic normoblast. (Bone marrow, Wright-Giemsa stain, ×1000.) **(B)**, Electron micrograph of an orthochromic normoblast (×20,125). (B from Carr, J. H. [2022]. *Clinical Hematology Atlas.* [6th ed.]. St. Louis: Elsevier.)

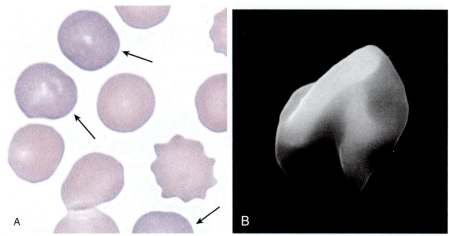

Figure 6.8 Polychromatic Erythrocytes (Shift Reticulocytes). **(A)**, Polychromatic erythrocytes (*arrows*). (Peripheral blood, Wright-Giemsa stain, ×1000.) **(B)**, Scanning electron micrograph of a polychromatic erythrocyte (×5000). (B from Carr, J. H. [2022]. *Clinical Hematology Atlas.* [6th ed.]. St. Louis: Elsevier.)

Cellular activity. Hemoglobin production continues on the remaining ribosomes using messenger RNA produced earlier. Late in this stage, the nucleus is removed from the cell by extrusion or expulsion, known as enucleation.[1] The process of enucleation is believed to be similar to cytoplasmic division (cytokinesis), as many of the cytokinesis principles are similar. Enucleation and chromatin condensation are complex processes controlled by several mechanisms/regulators, including histone modification, transcription factors, noncoding RNAs, and cytoskeletal elements.[2,7]

The nucleus moves to the cell membrane and into a pseudopod-like projection. The nucleus-containing projection separates from the cell by having the membrane seal and pinch off the projection; therefore the nucleus is enveloped by cell membrane.[9] The enveloped extruded nucleus, called a *pyrenocyte,*[5] is then engulfed by bone marrow *macrophages.*[1] The macrophages recognize "eat me" signals expressed by the pyrenocyte surface. Phosphatidylserine (erythrocyte cell membrane phospholipid) is believed to be the primary signal.[10,11] The bone marrow macrophages that engulf the pyrenocyte are known as erythroblastic island macrophages and are discussed further in "Microenvironment of the Bone Marrow."[12,13] Often, small fragments of nucleus are left behind if the projection is pinched off before the entire nucleus is enveloped. These fragments are called *Howell-Jolly bodies* when seen in peripheral RBCs (Table 16.3 and Figure 16.1) and are typically removed from the cells by the splenic macrophage pitting process once the cell enters the circulation.

Length of time in this stage. This stage lasts approximately 48 hours.[8]

Polychromatic (Polychromatophilic) Erythrocyte or Reticulocyte

Figure 6.8 shows the polychromatic erythrocyte.

Nucleus. Beginning at the polychromatic erythrocyte stage, there is *no nucleus.* The polychromatic erythrocyte is a good example of the prior statement that a cell may not have all the classic features described but may be staged by the majority of features. In particular, when a cell loses its nucleus, regardless of cytoplasmic appearance, it is a polychromatic erythrocyte.

Cytoplasm. The cytoplasm can be compared with that of the late orthochromic normoblast in that the predominant color is that of hemoglobin, yet with a bluish tinge due to some residual ribosomes and RNA. By the end of the polychromatic erythrocyte stage, *the cell is the same color as a mature RBC, salmon pink.* It remains *larger than a mature cell with a larger cell volume.*[14] The shape of the cell is not the mature biconcave disc but is *irregular* in electron micrographs (Figure 6.8B).

Division. Lacking a nucleus, the polychromatic erythrocyte cannot divide.

Location. The polychromatic erythrocyte resides in the bone marrow for about 1 to 2 days and then moves into the peripheral blood for about 1 day before reaching maturity. During the first several days after exiting the marrow, the polychromatic erythrocyte is retained in the spleen for pitting of inclusions and membrane polishing by splenic macrophages, which results in the biconcave discoid mature RBC.[15]

Cellular activity. The polychromatic erythrocyte completes production of hemoglobin from a small amount of residual messenger RNA using the remaining ribosomes.[16,17] The cytoplasmic protein production machinery is simultaneously being dismantled. Degradation of the mitochondria and clearance of the other organelles (e.g., Golgi apparatus, endoplasmic reticulum, peroxisomes) start upon enucleation through a process known as autophagy and contributes to a decrease in cell diameter.[18] Autophagy is a cellular process that normally occurs during stress conditions or aging in which unnecessary or damaged cellular components are degraded or lysed.[2,7,19] Mitochondrial clearance occurs through a specific type of autophagy known as *mitophagy,* in which the mitochondria are delivered to lysosomes for degradation.[1,2,7,20] Other maturation activities include membrane remodeling to eventually produce biconcave discs.[1,14]

The acidic components that attract the basophilic stain decline during this stage to the point that the polychromatophilia is only slightly evident in the polychromatic erythrocytes on a peripheral blood film stained with Wright stain. A small amount of residual ribosomal RNA is present, however, and can

BOX 6.2 Cellular Basophilia: Diffuse and Punctate

The *reticulum* of a polychromatic erythrocyte (reticulocyte) is not seen using Wright stain; however, the residual RNA imparts a bluish tinge to the cytoplasm, as seen in Figure 6.8A. Based on the Wright-stained appearance, the reticulocyte is called a *polychromatic erythrocyte* because it lacks a nucleus and is no longer an erythroblast but still has a bluish tinge. When polychromatic erythrocytes are prominent on a peripheral blood film, the examiner uses the comment *polychromasia* or *polychromatophilia*. Wright-stained polychromatic erythrocytes are also called *diffusely basophilic erythrocytes* for their regular bluish tinge. This term distinguishes polychromatic erythrocytes from red blood cells with *punctate basophilia,* in which the blue appears in distinct dots throughout the cytoplasm. More commonly known as *basophilic stippling* (Table 16.3 and Figure 16.1), punctate basophilia is associated with some anemias. Similar to the basophilia of polychromatic erythrocytes, punctate basophilia is due to residual ribosomal RNA, but the RNA is degenerate and stains deeply with Wright stain.

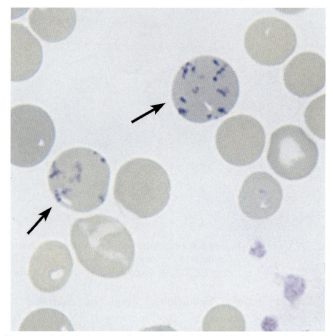

Figure 6.9 Reticulocytes (*arrows*). (Peripheral blood, new methylene blue stain, ×1000.)

be visualized with a vital stain such as new methylene blue (so called because the cells are stained while alive in suspension, i.e., vital) before the blood film is made (Box 6.2). The residual ribosomes appear as a mesh of small blue strands, a reticulum, or, when more fully digested, merely blue dots (Figure 6.9). When so stained, the polychromatic erythrocyte is called a *reticulocyte*. However, the name reticulocyte is often used to refer to the stage immediately preceding the mature erythrocyte, even when stained with Wright stain and without demonstrating the reticulum.

Length of time in this stage. The cell typically remains a polychromatic erythrocyte for about 3 days,[8] with the first 2 days spent in the bone marrow and the third spent in the peripheral blood, although possibly sequestered in the spleen.

Erythrocyte

Figure 6.10 shows the erythrocyte.

Nucleus. *No nucleus* is present in mature RBCs.

Cytoplasm. The mature circulating erythrocyte is a biconcave disc measuring 7 to 8 μm in diameter, with a thickness of about 1.5 to 2.5 μm. On a Wright-stained blood film, it appears as a *salmon pink–stained cell* with a *central pale area* that corresponds to the concavity. The central pallor is about one-third the diameter of the cell.

Division. The erythrocyte cannot divide.

Location and length of time in this stage. Mature RBCs remain active in the circulation for approximately 120 days.[21] Aging leads to their removal by the spleen as described in "Macrophage-Mediated Hemolysis (Extravascular Hemolysis)."

Cellular activity. The mature erythrocyte delivers oxygen to tissues, releases it, and returns to the lung to be reoxygenated. The dynamics of this process are discussed in detail in Chapter 8. The interior of the erythrocyte contains mostly hemoglobin, the oxygen-carrying component. It has a surface area-to-volume ratio and shape that enable optimal gas exchange to occur. If the cell was spherical, it would have hemoglobin at the center of the cell that would be relatively distant from the membrane and

would not be readily oxygenated and deoxygenated. With the biconcave shape, even hemoglobin molecules that are toward the center of the cell are not distant from the membrane and are able to exchange oxygen.

The cell's main function of oxygen delivery throughout the body requires a membrane that is flexible and deformable, that is, able to flex but return to its original shape. The interaction of various membrane components described in Chapter 7 creates these properties. RBCs must squeeze through small spaces such as the basement membrane of the bone marrow venous sinus. Similarly, when a cell enters the red pulp of the spleen, it must squeeze between epithelial cells to move into the venous outflow. Membrane flexibility is crucial for RBCs to enter and subsequently remain in the circulation.

DYNAMICS OF RED BLOOD CELL PRODUCTION AND DESTRUCTION

The dynamics of RBC production and destruction is termed *erythrokinetics*.[22] To understand erythrokinetics, it is helpful to appreciate the concept of the *erythron*. *Erythron* is the name given to the collection of all stages of erythrocytes throughout the body: the developing precursors in the bone marrow and the circulating erythrocytes in the peripheral blood and vascular spaces within organs, such as the spleen. The erythron is distinguished from the RBC *mass*. The erythron is the entirety of erythroid cells in the body, whereas the RBC mass refers only to the cells in circulation. This discussion of erythrokinetics begins with the kidneys detecting too little tissue oxygen, thus promoting them to produce erythropoietin (EPO). Through various mechanisms, the production of EPO ultimately leads to more RBCs entering into circulation.

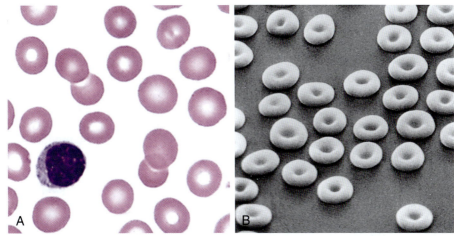

Figure 6.10 Mature Erythrocytes. (A), Mature erythrocytes and one lymphocyte. (Peripheral blood, Wright-Giemsa stain, ×1000.) **(B),** Scanning electron micrograph of mature erythrocytes (×2000). (A modified from Carr, J. H. [2022]. *Clinical Hematology Atlas.* [6th ed.]. St. Louis: Elsevier.)

Hypoxia—the Stimulus to Red Blood Cell Production

As mentioned previously, the role of RBCs is to carry oxygen. To regulate the production of RBCs for that purpose, the body requires a mechanism for sensing whether there is adequate oxygen being carried to the tissues. If tissue oxygen is inadequate, RBC production and the functional efficiency of existing cells must be enhanced. Thus a second feature of the oxygen-sensing system must be a mechanism for influencing the production of RBCs.

The primary oxygen-sensing system of the body is located in peritubular fibroblasts of the kidney.[23,24] Hypoxia, too little tissue oxygen, is detected by the peritubular fibroblasts, which then produce EPO, the major stimulatory cytokine for RBCs. Under normal circumstances, the amount of EPO produced fluctuates very little, maintaining a level of RBC production that is sufficient to replace the approximately 1% of RBCs that normally die each day (discussed in "Erythrocyte Destruction"). When there is hemorrhage, increased RBC destruction, or other factors that diminish the oxygen-carrying capacity of the blood, the production of EPO is increased in the kidneys.

Increased EPO production, caused by hypoxia, is regulated by a family of transcription factor proteins, called *hypoxia-inducible factors* (HIFs). HIFs respond to hypoxia by binding to kidney hypoxia responsive elements of the EPO gene.[25] This results in increased EPO gene transcription and EPO production. EPO will then bind to its receptor (EPOR) on erythroid progenitors and early erythroid precursors, thereby triggering multiple signaling pathways, which ultimately leads to increased cell division and maturation, increased intestinal iron absorption and hemoglobin synthesis, and more RBCs entering the circulation (Box 6.3).[25-27]

Erythropoietin

EPO is a glycoprotein hormone consisting of approximately 165 amino acids.[28-30] It consists of a *carbohydrate unit* and a *terminal sialic acid unit,* both of which play a role in the biologic activity of the hormone.[24]

BOX 6.3 Hypoxia and Red Blood Cell Production

Steady-state hematopoiesis, occurring in healthy individuals, provides red blood cells (RBCs) at a constant rate, and erythropoiesis occurs in the linear fashion described in "Maturation Sequence." However, during times of stress erythropoiesis when there is a rapid need for more RBCs, such as in anemia, erythropoiesis occurs in a more adaptable manner, as described next.

The kidney is the body's hypoxia sensor and provides early detection when oxygen levels decline. Regardless of the cause of hypoxia (e.g., decreased RBC number, defective hemoglobin, poor lung function), stimulation of RBC production is warranted because the number of RBCs present is not meeting the oxygen need. The physiologic response to hypoxia is regulated by hypoxia-inducible factors (HIFs) that result in gene expression changes, which ultimately lead to promotion of erythropoiesis. HIFs are a family of proteins that are continually produced and degraded in nonhypoxic conditions. Fundamentally, in hypoxic conditions, the proteins build up and activate the transcription of genes that will promote adaptation to the hypoxic condition. This promotion of erythropoiesis, regulated by HIFs, includes increased production of renal erythropoietin (EPO), enhanced iron uptake and intestinal absorption, and stimulation of erythroid progenitor maturation and proliferation.

Erythropoietin binds to its receptors on erythroid progenitors and early precursors, ultimately increasing the production of RBCs by (1) allowing early release of reticulocytes from the bone marrow, (2) preventing apoptotic cell death, and (3) reducing the time needed for cells to mature in the bone marrow. In severe anemia, EPO production can be increased by up to 1000-fold.

A physiologic adaptation to hypoxia occurs in the fetus and newborn as a result of the predominance of fetal hemoglobin (Hb F), which has a higher affinity for oxygen and releases oxygen less readily to the tissues compared with adult hemoglobin (Hb A). To compensate for this hypoxia, more RBCs are produced, mediated by the action of erythropoietin. Thus a normal newborn has a relatively higher concentration of RBCs and hemoglobin compared with most adults.

Mei, Y., Liu, Y., & Ji, P. (2021). Understanding terminal erythropoiesis: an update on chromatin condensation, enucleation, and reticulocyte maturation. *Blood Rev, 46,* 100740; Song, S. H., & Groom, A. C. (1972). Sequestration and possible maturation of reticulocytes in the normal spleen. *Can J Physiol Pharmacol, 50,* 400–406; Lee, E., Choi, H. S., Hwang, J. H., et al. (2014). The RNA in reticulocytes is not just debris: it is necessary for the final stages of erythrocyte formation. *Blood Cell Mol Dis, 53,* 1–10; Mills, E. W., Wangen, J., Green, R., et al. (2016). Dynamic regulation of a ribosome rescue pathway in erythroid cells and platelets. *Cell Rep, 17,* 1–10.

Action

EPO is a true hormone, being produced at one location (kidney) and secreted into circulation and acting at a distant location (bone marrow). It is a growth factor (or cytokine) that stimulates erythropoiesis by first binding to its receptor (EPOR) on the surface of EPO-responsive erythroid progenitor cells. CFU-Es are extremely sensitive to EPO. The interaction of EPO with its receptor triggers multiple signaling pathways.

The EPO receptor is a protein cell surface receptor consisting of a single carbohydrate chain with extracellular and cytoplasmic domains.[5,28] The binding of EPO to the extracellular domain of the EPO receptor (on CFU-Es and pronormoblasts) results in a change in the conformation and dimerization of the receptor chains thereby activating it.[5] This in turn activates *Janus-activated tyrosine kinase 2* (JAK2) signal transducers associated with the cytoplasmic domains of the EPO receptor (Figure 32.9).[5,27] JAK2 then activates downstream intracellular signaling pathways, such as signal transduction and activator of transcription 5 (STAT5), which ultimately promotes erythroid survival, proliferation, or differentiation (Figure 32.9).[19,27] Other signaling pathways involved include PI3 kinase, MAP kinase, and protein kinase C.[19,25]

EPO has three major effects: (1) allowing early release of reticulocytes from the bone marrow, (2) inhibiting apoptotic cell death, and (3) reducing the time needed for cells to mature in the bone marrow. These processes are described in detail in the following sections. The essence is that EPO puts more RBCs into the circulation at a faster rate than occurs without its stimulation.

Early release of reticulocytes. EPO promotes early release of reticulocytes from the bone marrow by two mechanisms. EPO induces changes in the adventitial cell layer of the bone marrow/sinus barrier that increase the width of the spaces for RBC egress into the sinus.[31] This mechanism alone, however, is insufficient for cells to leave the marrow. RBCs are held in the marrow because they express surface membrane receptors for adhesive molecules located on the bone marrow stroma, such as fibronectin (discussed in "Microenvironment of the Bone Marrow"). EPO downregulates the expression of these receptors so that cells can exit the marrow earlier than they normally would.[32-34]

The result is the presence in the circulation of reticulocytes that are still very basophilic because they have not spent as much time degrading their ribosomes and RNA or making hemoglobin as they normally would before entering the bloodstream. These are called *shift reticulocytes* because they have been shifted from the bone marrow early (Figure 6.8A). Their bluish cytoplasm with Wright stain is evident, so the overall blood picture is said to have polychromasia. Even nucleated RBCs (i.e., erythroblasts or normoblasts) can be released early in cases of extreme anemia when the demand for RBCs in the peripheral circulation is great. Releasing cells from the bone marrow early is a quick fix, so to speak; it is limited in effectiveness because the available precursors in the marrow are depleted within several days and still may not be enough to meet the need in the peripheral blood for more cells. A more sustained response is required in times of increased need for RBCs in the circulation.

Inhibition of apoptosis. A second, and probably more important, mechanism by which EPO increases the number of circulating RBCs is by increasing the number of cells that will be able to mature into circulating erythrocytes. It does this by decreasing apoptosis, the programmed death of RBC progenitors.[35,36] To understand this process, an overview of apoptosis in general is helpful.

Apoptosis: programmed cell death. As noted previously, it takes about 18 to 21 days to produce an RBC from stimulation of the earliest erythroid progenitor cell (BFU-E) to release from the bone marrow. In times of increased need for RBCs, such as when there is loss from the circulation during hemorrhage, this time lag would be a significant problem. One way to prepare for such a need would be to maintain a store of mature RBCs in the body for emergencies. However, mature RBCs cannot be indefinitely stored because they have a limited life span. Therefore instead of storing RBCs for emergencies, the body constantly produces more CFU-Es than needed. In healthy states, the extra progenitors are allowed to die (undergo apoptosis). When there is an increased demand for RBCs, however, the erythroid progenitors have about an 8- to 10-day head start in the production process. This process of intentional wastage of cells occurs by apoptosis, and it is part of the cell's genetic program.

Process of apoptosis. During the process of apoptosis, the following morphologic changes can be seen: condensation of the nucleus, causing increased basophilic staining of the chromatin; nucleolar disintegration; and shrinkage of cell volume, with concomitant increase in cell density and compaction of cytoplasmic organelles, while mitochondria remain normal.[37] This is followed by a partition of cytoplasm and nucleus into membrane-bound apoptotic bodies that contain varying amounts of ribosomes, organelles, and nuclear material. The last stage of degradation produces nuclear DNA fragments consisting of multimers of 180- to 185-base pair segments. Characteristic blebbing of the plasma membrane is observed. The apoptotic cell contents remain membrane bound and are ingested by macrophages, which prevents an inflammatory reaction. The membrane-bound vesicles display "eat me" signals on the membrane surface (discussed in "Macrophage-Mediated Hemolysis [Extravascular Hemolysis]"), which promote macrophage ingestion (Chapter 4).[38]

Evasion of apoptosis by erythroid progenitors and precursors. Under normal circumstances, many erythroid progenitors will undergo apoptosis because they are not needed. However, when increased numbers of RBCs are needed, apoptosis can be avoided. One effect of EPO is an indirect avoidance of apoptosis by removing an apoptosis induction signal. Among the crucial molecules in the messaging system is the death receptor Fas on the membrane of the earliest erythroid precursors, while its ligand, FasL, is expressed by more mature erythroid precursors.[37,39] When EPO levels are low, cell production should be at a low rate because hypoxia is not present; thus excess early erythroid precursors should undergo apoptosis. This occurs when the older FasL-bearing erythroid precursors, such as polychromatic normoblasts, cross link with Fas-marked immature erythroid precursors, such as pronormoblasts and basophilic normoblasts, which are then stimulated to undergo apoptosis.[37] As long as the more mature erythroid precursors with FasL are present in the marrow, erythropoiesis is subdued. If the FasL-bearing cells are depleted, as when EPO stimulates early bone marrow release, the younger Fas-positive precursors are allowed to develop, which increases the overall output of RBCs from the marrow.

A second mechanism for escaping apoptosis exists for erythroid progenitors: direct EPO rescue from apoptosis. This is the major way in which EPO is able to increase RBC production. When EPO binds to its receptor on the CFU-E, one of the effects is to reduce production of Fas ligand.[40] Thus the younger cells avoid the apoptotic signal from the older cells. Additionally, EPO is able to stimulate production of various antiapoptotic molecules, which allows the cell to survive and mature.[41,42] The cell that has the most EPO receptors and is most sensitive to EPO rescue is the CFU-E, although the late BFU-E and early pronormoblast have some receptors.[42] Without EPO, the CFU-E does not survive.[43]

As discussed previously, binding of EPO to its receptors on erythroid progenitors and precursors activates JAK2 protein associated with its cytoplasmic domain (Figure 32.9). Activated JAK2 then phosphorylates (activates) the STAT5 pathway, leading to the production of the antiapoptotic molecule Bcl-XL (now called *Bcl-2-like protein 1*).[40,41] EPO-stimulated cells develop this molecule on their mitochondrial membrane, which in turn prevents release of cytochrome *c*. Cytochrome *c* is an apoptosis initiator, and thus by preventing its release, apoptosis is not initiated.[44] The effect of EPO is mediated by the transcription factor GATA1, which is essential to RBC survival.[45]

Reduced bone marrow transit time. Apoptosis rescue (in "Dynamics of Red Blood Cell Production and Destruction") is the major way in which EPO increases RBC mass, that is, by increasing the number of erythroid cells that survive and mature to enter the circulation. Yet, another effect of EPO is to reduce bone marrow transit time by increasing the rate at which the surviving precursors can enter the circulation. This is accomplished by two means: increased rate of cellular processes and decreased cell cycle times.

Increased rate of cellular processes. EPO stimulates the synthesis of RNA in erythroid precursors and effectively increases the rate of the developmental process. Among the processes that are accelerated is hemoglobin production.[24] In addition, EPO induces erythroid precursors to secrete erythroferrone, which acts on hepatocytes to decrease hepcidin production.[46] This allows more iron to be absorbed from the intestines to support the increased hemoglobin synthesis (Chapter 9).[46] As mentioned earlier, another accelerated process is bone marrow egress as a result of the loss of adhesive receptors (such as the fibronectin receptor discussed in "Microenvironment of the Bone Marrow") and the acquisition of egress-promoting surface molecules.[47]

The other process that is accelerated is the cessation of division. Cell division takes time and would delay entry of cells into the circulation, so cells enter cell cycle arrest sooner. As a result,

the cells spend less time maturing in the bone marrow. In the circulation, such cells are larger because of lost mitotic divisions, and they do not have time before entering the circulation to dismantle the protein production machinery that gives the bluish tinge to the cytoplasm. These cells are true shift reticulocytes similar to those in Figure 6.8A, recognizable in the Wright-stained peripheral blood film as especially large, bluish cells typically lacking central pallor. These shift reticulocytes are also called *stress reticulocytes* because they exit the marrow early during conditions of bone marrow "stress," such as in certain anemias.

Decreased cell cycle times. EPO also can reduce the time it takes for cells to mature in the bone marrow by reducing individual cell cycle time, specifically the length of time that cells spend between mitoses.[48] This effect is only about a 20% reduction, however, so that the normal transit time in the marrow of approximately 6 days from pronormoblast to erythrocyte can be shortened by only about 1 day by this effect.

With the decreased cell cycle time and fewer mitotic divisions, the time it takes from pronormoblast to reticulocyte can be shortened by about 2 days total. If the reticulocyte leaves the marrow early, another day can be saved, and the typical 6-day transit time is reduced to less than 4 days under the influence of increased EPO.

Measurement of Erythropoietin

Quantitative measurements of EPO are performed on plasma and other body fluids. EPO can be measured by chemiluminescence. Although the reference interval for each laboratory varies, 10 to 30 U/L is sufficient to maintain steady-state erythropoiesis in a healthy adult.[43] Increased amounts of EPO in the urine are expected in most patients with anemia, with the exception of patients with anemia caused by renal disease.

Therapeutic Uses of Erythropoietin

Recombinant EPO became commercially available in 1989 as a therapeutic agent for certain anemias such as those associated with chronic kidney disease and chemotherapy.[29] First- and second-generation recombinant EPO required multiple administrations per week, whereas third-generation recombinant EPO has a longer half-life, reducing its administration to monthly or less frequently.[29,49] It is also used to stimulate RBC production before autologous blood donation and after bone marrow transplantation. The indications for EPO therapy are summarized in Table 5.2.

More recent research on EPO has revealed that it has more effects in addition to promoting erythropoiesis. EPO receptors have been found on other cell types such as heart, nerve, and skeletal muscle cells. Studies suggest that EPO promotes bone modeling (repair and healing), aids in tissue protection, and plays a role in immunity.[28,30]

Some athletes illicitly use EPO injections to enhance endurance and stamina, especially in long-distance running and cycling. The use of EPO is one method of blood doping that increases oxygen-carrying capacity, thereby increasing performance in endurance sports.[49] Recombinant EPO was placed on the list of banned substances in 1990 by the International

Olympic Committee.[29] Today, there are other erythropoiesis-stimulating agents (ESAs) used in blood doping such as HIF stabilizers and synthetic oxygen carriers.[29,49] Numerous adverse effects are associated with using ESAs, including myocardial infarction, arrhythmia, congestive heart failure, and arterial and venous thrombosis.[29]

Other Stimuli to Erythropoiesis

In addition to tissue hypoxia, other factors influence RBC production to a modest extent. It is well documented that testosterone directly stimulates erythropoiesis, which partially explains the higher hemoglobin concentration in men than in women.[50] Also, pituitary[51] and thyroid[52] hormones have been found to affect the production of EPO and so have indirect effects on erythropoiesis.

MICROENVIRONMENT OF THE BONE MARROW

The microenvironment of the bone marrow is described in Chapter 5, and the cytokines essential to hematopoiesis are discussed there. In this chapter, the details pertinent to erythropoiesis (i.e., the erythropoietic microenvironment) are emphasized, including the role of bone marrow macrophages and fibronectin (anchoring molecule).

Hematopoiesis occurs in bone marrow cords, essentially a loose arrangement of cells outside a dilated sinus area between the arterioles that feed the bone and the central vein that returns blood to efferent veins. Erythropoiesis typically occurs in niches known as *erythroblastic islands* (EBI) within the bone marrow (Figure 5.6). These islands consist of a central macrophage surrounded by erythroid precursors in various stages of development. The central EBI macrophage is rich in ferritin and has 5 to 30 developing erythroid cells rosetting around it.[11,12,53] These central macrophages are often described as nurse cells due to the various supporting roles they play in erythropoiesis.[13,54]

Role of Bone Marrow Macrophages

Bone marrow macrophages promote erythropoiesis via the following: 1) interactions between central macrophage and developing erythroid cells, 2) secretion of growth factors, 3) providing iron, and 4) engulfing nuclei during the orthochromic normoblast stage of maturation.[2,13] The role bone marrow macrophages play in engulfing and digesting extruded nuclei is discussed in detail in "Maturation Sequence."

Interactions between the central or nurse macrophage and the developing erythroid cells occur via a number of adhesion molecules. Adhesion molecules are expressed by both macrophages and the developing erythroid cells. These molecules aid in island formation, specifically clustering and tethering of cells.[1,11] The major adhesion molecules expressed by macrophages include CD163, CD169, Vcam1 (vascular cell adhesion molecule 1), and Emp (erythroid macrophage protein).[1,13,53] The above-mentioned adhesive molecules tie the developing erythroid cells to the macrophages, yet developing erythroid cells are also anchored to the extracellular matrix of the bone

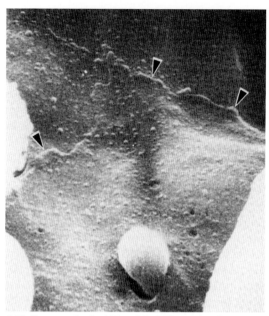

Figure 6.11 Egress of a Red Blood Cell Through a Pore in an Endothelial Cell of the Bone Marrow Venous Sinus. *Arrowheads* indicate the endothelial cell junctions. (From De Bruyn, P. P. H. [1981]. Structural substrates of bone marrow function. *Semin Hematol, 18,* 182.)

marrow, chiefly by fibronectin.[33] Studies suggest that these adhesion molecules aid not only in island formation but also regulation of erythropoiesis.[11,13]

When it comes time for RBCs to leave the marrow, they cease production of the receptors for adhesive molecules.[33] Without the receptor, cells are free to move from the marrow into the venous sinus. Entering the venous sinus requires the RBC to traverse the barrier created by the adventitial cells on the cord side, the basement membrane, and the endothelial cells lining the sinus. Egress through this barrier occurs between adventitial cells, through holes (fenestrations) in the basement membrane, and through pores in the endothelial cells (Figure 6.11).[31,55,56]

Studies have shown that EBI macrophages also secrete growth factors such as insulin-like growth factor 1 (IGF-1) and bone morphogenetic protein 4 (BMP-4) that stimulate proliferation.[11,13,53] Hemoglobin produced during erythropoiesis requires iron that is primarily derived through splenic degradation of senescent RBCs (approximately 120 days old), thus recycling the iron in RBCs. Additional iron requirements are met through dietary intake. Both processes are described in detail in Chapter 9. The iron is transported in the blood to EBI macrophages and normoblasts in the bone marrow.[12,13] Excess iron is stored in EBI macrophages as ferritin. Several studies suggest that these nurse macrophages also supply maturing erythroid cells with iron.[12,13,57,58]

ERYTHROCYTE DESTRUCTION

All cells experience deterioration of their enzymes over time because of natural catabolism. Most cells are able to replenish needed enzymes and continue their cellular processes. As a nonnucleated cell, however, the mature erythrocyte is unable to generate new enzymes, so as its cellular functions decline, the cell ultimately approaches death. The average RBC has sufficient enzyme function to live 120 days. Because RBCs lack mitochondria, they rely on glycolysis for production of adenosine triphosphate (ATP). The loss of glycolytic enzymes is central to this process of cellular aging, called *senescence,* which culminates in phagocytosis by macrophages in the spleen. This is the major method by which RBCs die normally.

Macrophage-Mediated Hemolysis (Extravascular Hemolysis)

Hemolysis is the disruption of RBC membrane integrity that destroys the cell and releases hemoglobin and other cell contents. *Extravascular hemolysis* refers to hemolysis of RBCs outside of the blood vessels, such as in the spleen or liver. As an RBC reaches the end of its life span, a cumulative cascade of events serve as aging markers for splenic clearance of the aged/senescent RBC.[4]

At any given time, a substantial volume of blood is in the spleen, which generates an environment that is inherently stressful on cells. Movement through the splenic red pulp is sluggish. The available glucose in the surrounding blood is depleted quickly as cell flow stagnates, so glycolysis slows. The pH is low, which promotes iron oxidation. Maintaining reduced iron is an energy-dependent process, so factors that promote iron oxidation cause the RBC to expend more energy and accelerate the catabolism of enzymes.

In this hostile environment, senescent RBCs succumb to various stresses. Their deteriorating glycolytic processes lead to reduced ATP production, which is complicated further by diminished amounts of available glucose. Membrane systems that rely on ATP begin to fail. Among these are enzymes that maintain the location and reduction of phospholipids of the membrane. Lack of ATP leads to oxidation of membrane lipids and proteins. Other ATP-dependent enzymes are responsible for maintaining the high level of intracellular potassium while pumping sodium out of the cells. As this system fails, intracellular sodium increases, and potassium decreases. The effect is that the selective permeability of the membrane is lost, and water enters the cell. The discoid shape is lost, and the cell becomes a sphere.

RBCs must remain highly flexible to exit the spleen by squeezing through the so-called splenic sieve formed by the endothelial cells lining the venous sinuses and the basement membrane. Spherical RBCs are rigid and are not able to squeeze through the narrow spaces; they become trapped against the endothelial cells and basement membrane. These physiochemical changes promote ingestion by splenic macrophages that patrol along the sinusoidal lining.[11,59] Essentially, when senescent RBCs fail the physical fitness test, they are destroyed by macrophages in the spleen.[4]

In addition to the aging changes that serve as recognition tags for clearance, there are changes in the RBC membrane that may also signal phagocytosis by splenic macrophages.[60,61]

It is highly likely that there is no single signal but rather, that macrophages recognize several "eat me" signals expressed on senescent RBCs.[57] Examples of the signals that are being further investigated include band 3 and phosphatidylserine. Band 3 is an integral protein of the RBC membrane that acts as an antigen for immunoglobulin G autoantibodies tagging it for macrophage clearance.[11,59,62] Phosphatidylserine is a membrane phospholipid normally located on the inner leaflet of the RBC membrane. However, in senescent RBCs, due to the breakdown of membrane phospholipids, phosphatidylserine is on the outer leaflet of the RBC and serves as an "eat me" signal.[11,59,63]

When an RBC lyses within a macrophage, the major components are catabolized. Iron is removed from the heme. It can be stored in the macrophage as ferritin until transported out. The globin of hemoglobin is degraded and returned to the metabolic amino acid pool. The protoporphyrin component of heme is degraded through several intermediaries to bilirubin, which is released into the blood and ultimately excreted by the liver in bile. The details of bilirubin metabolism are discussed in Chapter 20.

Some researchers propose that an erythrocyte can die as a nonnucleated cell version of apoptosis, termed *eryptosis,* a form of suicidal cell death. Eryptosis is characterized by cell membrane blebbing, cell shrinkage, and exposure of phosphatidylserine, as described previously.[63-65] Supposedly, this process occurs when an RBC is damaged or injured before senescence.[60,61,63,64] Clearance of senescent RBCs and eryptosis share some of the same characteristics; whether these are two different mechanisms of death or the same is still being investigated.[65]

Fragmentation Hemolysis (Intravascular Hemolysis)

Although most natural RBC deaths occur in the spleen, a small portion of RBCs (nonsenescent or senescent) rupture *intravascularly* (within the lumen of blood vessels). The vascular system can be traumatic to RBCs, with turbulence occurring in the chambers of the heart or at points of bifurcation (division) of vessels. Small breaks in blood vessels and resulting clots can also trap and rupture cells. The intravascular rupture of RBCs from turbulence or anatomic restrictions in the vasculature results in fragmentation and release of the cell contents into the blood; this is called *fragmentation* or *intravascular hemolysis.* Fragmentation hemolysis is discussed in Chapter 20.

When the membrane of the RBC has been breached, regardless of where the cell is located when it happens, the cell contents enter the surrounding blood. Although fragmentation lysis is a relatively small contributor to RBC demise under normal circumstances, the body still has a system of plasma proteins, including haptoglobin and hemopexin, to salvage the released hemoglobin so that its iron is not lost in the urine. Hemolysis and the functions of haptoglobin and hemopexin are discussed in Chapter 20.

SUMMARY

- Red blood cells (RBCs) develop from committed erythroid progenitor cells in the bone marrow, the burst-forming unit-erythroid (BFU-E) and the colony-forming unit-erythroid (CFU-E).
- The morphologically identifiable precursors of mature RBCs, in order from youngest to oldest, are the pronormoblast, basophilic normoblast, polychromatic normoblast, orthochromic normoblast, and polychromatic erythrocyte or reticulocyte.
- As erythroid precursors age, the nucleus becomes condensed and ultimately is expelled from the cell, which produces the polychromatic erythrocyte or reticulocyte stage. The cytoplasm changes color from blue, reflecting abundant ribosomal RNA, to salmon pink as hemoglobin accumulates and the RNA is degraded. Each stage can be identified by the extent of these nuclear and cytoplasmic changes.
- It takes approximately 18 to 21 days for the BFU-E to mature to an RBC, of which about 6 days are spent as identifiable precursors in the bone marrow. The mature erythrocyte has a life span of 120 days in the circulation.
- Hypoxia of peripheral blood is detected by the peritubular fibroblasts of the kidney, which upregulates transcription of the *EPO* gene to increase the production of erythropoietin (EPO).
- EPO, the primary hormone that stimulates the production of erythrocytes, is able to rescue the CFU-E from apoptosis, shorten the time between mitoses in precursors, release reticulocytes from the marrow early, and reduce the number of mitoses of precursors.
- Apoptosis is the mechanism by which an appropriate normal production level of RBCs is controlled. Fas, the death receptor, is expressed by young erythroid precursors, and FasL,

the ligand, is expressed by older erythroid precursors. As long as older cells mature slowly in the marrow, they induce the death of unneeded younger cells.
- EPO rescues CFU-E cells from apoptosis by stimulating the production of antiapoptotic molecules that counteract the effects of Fas and FasL, and simultaneously decreases Fas production by young erythroid precursors.
- Erythroid precursors in various stages of maturation are found in erythroblastic islands where they surround a central macrophage. Survival of erythroid precursors in the bone marrow depends on adhesive molecules that tether developing cells to the central macrophage and anchor them to extracellular matrix of bone marrow.
- As erythroid cells mature, they lose adhesive molecule receptors, which allows their egress from the bone marrow. Egress occurs between adventitial cells but through pores in the endothelial cells of the venous sinus.
- Extravascular or macrophage-mediated hemolysis accounts for most normal RBC death. Aged RBCs, or senescent cells, become trapped in the splenic sieve, where they are readily phagocytized by macrophages. In addition, RBC membrane changes also serve as "eat me" signals that promote phagocytosis by splenic macrophages.
- Intravascular or fragmentation hemolysis results when mechanical factors rupture the cell membrane while the cell is in the peripheral circulation. This form of hemolysis accounts for a small percentage of normal RBC death.

Now that you have completed this chapter, go back and read again the case study at the beginning and respond to the questions presented. Answers can be found in Appendix C.

REVIEW QUESTIONS

Answers can be found in Appendix C.

1. Which of the following is an erythroid progenitor?
   a. Pronormoblast
   b. Reticulocyte
   c. CFU-E
   d. Orthochromic normoblast
2. Which of the following is the most mature normoblast?
   a. Orthochromic normoblast
   b. Basophilic normoblast
   c. Pronormoblast
   d. Polychromatic normoblast
3. Which erythroid precursor can be described as follows? The cell is of medium diameter compared with other normoblasts, with an N:C ratio of 1:1. The nuclear chromatin is condensed and chunky throughout the nucleus. No nucleoli are seen. The cytoplasm is gray-blue.
   a. Reticulocyte
   b. Pronormoblast
   c. Orthochromic normoblast
   d. Polychromatic normoblast

4. At which normoblastic stage does globin production begin?
   a. Orthochromic normoblast
   b. Pronormoblast
   c. Polychromatic normoblast
   d. Basophilic normoblast
5. Hypoxia stimulates RBC production by:
   a. Inducing more pluripotent stem cells into the erythroid lineage
   b. Stimulating EPO production by the kidney
   c. Increasing the number of RBC mitoses
   d. Stimulating the production of fibronectin by macrophages of the bone marrow
6. Erythropoietin can increase the production of RBCs by:
   a. Promoting apoptosis of erythroid progenitors
   b. Decreasing intravascular hemolysis
   c. Increasing EPO receptor sites
   d. Promoting early release of reticulocytes from bone marrow

7. In the bone marrow, erythroid precursors are located:
   a. Surrounding central macrophages in erythroblastic islands
   b. Adjacent to megakaryocytes along the adventitial cell lining
   c. Surrounding central fat cells in apoptotic islands
   d. In the center of the hematopoietic cords
8. Which of the following determines the timing of egress of RBCs from the bone marrow?
   a. Stromal cells decrease production of adhesive molecules over time as RBCs mature.
   b. Endothelial cells of the venous sinus form pores at specified intervals of time, allowing egress of free cells.
   c. Periodic apoptosis of pronormoblasts in the marrow cords occurs.
   d. Maturing erythroid cells lose receptors for adhesive molecules that bind them to bone marrow.
9. What single feature of normal RBCs is most responsible for limiting their life span?
   a. Loss of the nucleus
   b. Increased flexibility of the cell membrane
   c. Reduction of hemoglobin iron
   d. Loss of mitochondria
10. Extravascular hemolysis occurs when:
    a. RBCs are mechanically ruptured
    b. RBCs extravasate from blood vessels into the tissues
    c. Splenic macrophages ingest senescent RBCs
    d. RBCs are trapped in blood clots outside the blood vessels

REFERENCES

1. Yeo, J. H., Lam, Y. W., & Fraser, S. T. (2019). Cellular dynamics of mammalian red blood cell production in the erythroblastic island niche. *Biophys Rev, 11*(6), 873–894.
2. Mei, Y., Liu, Y., & Ji, P. (2021). Understanding terminal erythropoiesis: an update on chromatin condensation, enucleation, and reticulocyte maturation. *Blood Rev, 46*, 100740.
3. Nandakumar, S. K., Ulirsch, J. C., & Sankaran, V. G. (2016). Advances in understanding erythropoiesis: evolving perspectives. *Br J Haematol, 173*, 206–218.
4. Corrons, J., Casafont, L. B., & Frasnedo, E. F. (2021). Concise review: how are red blood cells born, how do they live and die? *Ann Hematol, 100*(10), 2425–2433.
5. Papayannopoulou, T., & Migliaccio, A. R. (2023). Biology of erythropoiesis, erythroid differentiation, and maturation. In Hoffman, R., Benz, E. J., Silberstein, L. E., et al. (Eds.), *Hematology: Basic Principles and Practice.* (8th ed., pp. 303–321). Philadelphia: Elsevier.
6. Szirmani, E. H. R., & Erslev, A. J. (1956.). Bone marrow kinetics. In Szirmani, E. (Ed.), *Nuclear Hematology.* (pp. 89–132). New York: Academic Press.
7. Moras, M., Lefevre, S. D., & Ostuni, M. A. (2017). From erythroblasts to mature red blood cells: organelle clearance in mammals. *Front Physiol, 8*, 1076.
8. Granick, S., & Levere, R. D. (1964). Heme synthesis in erythroid cells. In Moore, C. V., & Brown, E. B. (Eds.), *Progress in Hematology* (vol 4). (pp. 1–47). New York: Grune & Stratton.
9. Skutelsky, E., & Danon, D. (1967). An electron microscopic study of nuclear elimination from the late erythroblast. *J Cell Biol, 33*, 625–635.
10. Vahedi, A., Bigdelou, P., & Farnoud, A. M. (2020). Quantitative analysis of red blood cell membrane phospholipids and modulation of cell-macrophage interactions using cyclodextrins. *Sci Rep, 10*(1), 15111.
11. Klei, T. R., Meinderts, S. M., van den Berg, T. K., et al. (2017). From the cradle to the grave: the role of macrophages in erythropoiesis and erythrophagocytosis. *Front Immunol, 8*, 73.
12. Lévesque, J. P., Summers, K. M., Bisht, K., et al. (2021). Macrophages form erythropoietic niches and regulate iron homeostasis to adapt erythropoiesis in response to infections and inflammation. *Exp Hematol, 103*, 1–14.

13. Li, W., Guo, R., Song, Y., et al. (2021). Erythroblastic island macrophages shape normal erythropoiesis and drive associated disorders in erythroid hematopoietic diseases. *Front Cell Dev Biol, 8*, 613885.
14. Ovchynnikova, E., Aglialoro, F., von Lindern, M., et al. (2018). The shape shifting story of reticulocyte maturation. *Front Physiol, 9*, 829.
15. Song, S. H., & Groom, A. C. (1972). Sequestration and possible maturation of reticulocytes in the normal spleen. *Can J Physiol Pharmacol, 50*, 400–406.
16. Lee, E., Choi, H. S., Hwang, J. H., et al. (2014). The RNA in reticulocytes is not just debris: it is necessary for the final stages of erythrocyte formation. *Blood Cell Mol Dis, 53*, 1–10.
17. Mills, E. W., Wangen, J., Green, R., et al. (2016). Dynamic regulation of a ribosome rescue pathway in erythroid cells and platelets. *Cell Rep, 17*, 1–10.
18. Rhodes, M. M., Koury, S. T., Kopsombut, P., et al. (2016). Stress reticulocytes lose transferrin receptors by an extrinsic process involving spleen and macrophages. *Am J Hematol, 91*(9), 875–882.
19. Jafari, M., Ghadami, E., Dadkhah, T., et al. (2019). PI3k/AKT signaling pathway: erythropoiesis and beyond. *J Cell Physiol, 234*(3), 2373–2385.
20. Yoo, S.-M., & Jung, Y.-K. (2018). A molecular approach to mitophagy and mitochondrial dynamics. *Mol Cells, 41*(1), 18–26.
21. Ashby, W. (1919). The determination of the length of life of transfused blood corpuscles in man. *J Exp Med, 29*, 268–282.
22. Giblett, E. R., Coleman, D. H., Pirzio-Biroli, G., et al. (1956). Erythrokinetics: quantitative measurements of red cell production and destruction in normal subjects and patients with anemia. *Blood, 11*(4), 291–309.
23. Jacobson, L. O., Goldwasser, E., Fried, W., et al. (1957). Role of the kidney in erythropoiesis. *Nature, 179*, 633–634.
24. Kurtz, A., Wenger, R. H., & Eckardt, K. (2013). Hematopoiesis and the kidney. In Alpern, R. J., Caplan, M. J., & Moe, O. W. (Eds.), *Seldin, Giebisch's The Kidney: Physiology and Pathophysiology.* (5th ed., pp. 3087–3124). San Diego: Elsevier.
25. Haase, V. H. (2013). Regulation of erythropoiesis by hypoxia-inducible factors. *Blood Rev, 27*(1), 41–53.
26. Liang, R., & Ghaffari, S. (2016). Advances in understanding the mechanisms of erythropoiesis in homeostasis and disease. *Br J Haematol, 174*(5), 661–673.

27. Bhoopalan, S. V., Huang, L. J., & Weiss, M. J. (2020). Erythropoietin regulation of red blood cell production: from bench to bedside and back. *F1000Research*, 9, F1000 Faculty Rev-1153.

28. Tsiftsoglou, A. S. (2021). Erythropoietin (EPO) as a key regulator of erythropoiesis, bone remodeling and endothelial transdifferentiation of multipotent mesenchymal stem cells (MSCs): implications in regenerative medicine. *Cells*, 10(8), 2140.

29. Salamin, O., Kuuranne, T., Saugy, M., et al. (2018). Erythropoietin as a performance-enhancing drug: its mechanistic basis, detection, and potential adverse effects. *Mol Cell Endocrinol*, 464, 75–87.

30. Peng, B., Kong, G., Yang, C., et al. (2020). Erythropoietin and its derivatives: from tissue protection to immune regulation. *Cell Death Dis*, 11(2), 79.

31. Chamberlain, J. K., Leblond, P. F., & Weed, R. I. (1975). Reduction of adventitial cell cover: an early direct effect of erythropoietin on bone marrow ultrastructure. *Blood Cells*, 1, 655–674.

32. Patel, V. P., & Lodish, H. F. (1986). The fibronectin receptor on mammalian erythroid precursor cells: characterization and developmental regulation. *J Cell Biol*, 102, 449–456.

33. Vuillet-Gaugler, M. H., Breton-Gorius, J., Vainchenker, W., et al. (1990). Loss of attachment to fibronectin with terminal human erythroid differentiation. *Blood*, 75, 865–873.

34. Goltry, K. L., & Patel, V. P. (1997). Specific domains of fibronectin mediate adhesion and migration of early murine erythroid progenitors. *Blood*, 90, 138–147.

35. Sieff, C. A., Emerson, S. G., Mufson, A., et al. (1986). Dependence of highly enriched human bone marrow progenitors on hemopoietic growth factors and their response to recombinant erythropoietin. *J Clin Invest*, 77, 74–81.

36. Eaves, C. J., & Eaves, A. C. (1978). Erythropoietin (Ep) dose-response curves for three classes of erythroid progenitors in normal human marrow and in patients with polycythemia vera. *Blood*, 52, 1196–1210.

37. DeMaria, R., Testa, U., Luchetti, L., et al. (1999). Apoptotic role of Fas/Fas ligand system in the regulation of erythropoiesis. *Blood*, 93, 796–803.

38. Martin, S. J., Reutelingsperger, C. P., McGahon, A. J., et al. (1995). Early redistribution of plasma membrane phosphatidylserine is a general feature of apoptosis regardless of the initiating stimulus: inhibition by overexpression of Bcl-2 and Abl. *J Exp Med*, 182, 1545–1556.

39. Zamai, L., Burattini, S., Luchetti, F., et al. (2004). In vitro apoptotic cell death during erythroid differentiation. *Apoptosis*, 9, 235–246.

40. Elliott, S., Pham, E., & Mcdougall, I. C. (2008). Erythropoietins: a common mechanism of action. *Exp Hematol*, 36, 1573–1584.

41. Dolznig, H., Habermann, B., Stangl, K., et al. (2002). Apoptosis protection by the Epo target Bcl-X(L) allows factor-independent differentiation of primary erythroblasts. *Curr Biol*, 12, 1076–1085.

42. Sawada, K., Krantz, S. B., Dai, C. H., et al. (1990). Purification of human blood burst-forming units-erythroid and demonstration of the evolution of erythropoietin receptors. *J Cell Physiol*, 142, 219–230.

43. Brugnara, C., & Eckardt, K. (2020). Hematologic aspects of kidney disease. In Yu, A. S. L., Chertow, G. M., Luyckx, V. A., et al. (Eds.), *Brenner & Rector's The Kidney* (11th ed., pp 1861–1900). Philadelphia: Elsevier.

44. Basanez, G., Soane, L., & Hardwick, J. M. (2012). A new view of the lethal apoptotic pore. *PLoS Biol*, 10(9), e100139.

45. Gregory, T., Yu, C., Ma, A., et al. (1999). GATA-1 and erythropoietin cooperate to promote erythroid cell survival by regulating bcl-xL expression. *Blood*, 94, 87–96.

46. Kautz, L., Jung, G., Valore, E. V., et al. (2014). Identification of erythroferrone as an erythroid regulator of iron metabolism. *Nat Genet*, 46(7), 678–684.

47. Sathyanarayana, P., Menon, M. P., Bogacheva, O., et al. (2007). Erythropoietin modulation of podocalyxin and a proposed erythroblast niche. *Blood*, 110(2), 509–518.

48. Hanna, I. R., Tarbutt, R. O., & Lamerton, L. F. (1969). Shortening of the cell-cycle time of erythroid precursors in response to anaemia. *Br J Haematol*, 16, 381–387.

49. Atkinson, T. S., & Kahn, M. J. (2020). Blood doping: then and now. A narrative review of the history, science and efficacy of blood doping in elite sport. *Blood Rev*, 39, 100632.

50. Jacobson, W., Siegman, R. L., & Diamond, L. K. (1968). Effect of testosterone on the uptake of tritiated thymidine in bone marrow of children. *Ann N Y Acad Sci*, 149, 389–405.

51. Golde, D. W., Bersch, N., & Li, C. H. (1977). Growth hormone: species-specific stimulation of in vitro erythropoiesis. *Science*, 196, 1112–1113.

52. Popovic, W. J., Brown, J. E., & Adamson, J. W. (1977). The influence of thyroid hormones on in vitro erythropoiesis: mediation by a receptor with beta adrenergic properties. *J Clin Invest*, 60, 908–913.

53. Eggold, J. T., & Rankin, E. B. (2019). Erythropoiesis, EPO, macrophages, and bone. *Bone*, 119, 36–41.

54. May, A., & Forrester, L. M. (2020). The erythroblastic island niche: modeling in health, stress, and disease. *Exp Hematol*, 91, 10–21.

55. Chamberlain, J. K., & Lichtman, M. A. (1978). Marrow cell egress: specificity of the site of penetration into the sinus. *Blood*, 52, 959–968.

56. DeBruyn, P. P. H. (1981). Structural substrates of bone marrow function. *Semin Hematol*, 18, 179–193.

57. Sukhbaatar, N., & Weichhart, T. (2018). Iron regulation: macrophages in control. *Pharmaceuticals (Basel)*, 11(4), 137.

58. Li, W., Wang, Y., Zhao, H., et al. (2019). Identification and transcriptome analysis of erythroblastic island macrophages. *Blood*, 134(5), 480–491.

59. Thiagarajan, P., Parker, C. J., & Prchal, J. T. (2021). How do red blood cells die? *Front Physiol*, 12, 655393.

60. Dreischer, P., Duszenko, M., Stein, J., et al. (2022). Eryptosis: programmed death of nucleus-free, iron-filled blood cells. *Cells*, 11(3), 503.

61. Föller, M., & Lang, F. (2020). Ion transport in eryptosis, the suicidal death of erythrocytes. *Front Cell Dev Biol*, 8, 597.

62. Badior, K. E., & Casey, J. R. (2018). Molecular mechanism for the red blood cell senescence clock. *IUBMB Life*, 70(1), 32–40.

63. Qadri, S. M., Bissinger, R., Solh, Z., et al. (2017). Eryptosis in health and disease: a paradigm shift towards understanding the (patho) physiological implications of programmed cell death of erythrocytes. *Blood Rev*, 31(6), 349–361.

64. Lang, E., Qadri, S. M., & Lang, F. (2012). Killing me softly - suicidal erythrocyte death. *Int J Biochem Cell Biol*, 44(8), 1236–1243.

65. Repsold, L., & Joubert, A. M. (2018). Eryptosis: an erythrocyte's suicidal type of cell death. *Biomed Res Int*, 9405617.

7

Erythrocyte Metabolism and Membrane Structure and Function

S. Renee Hodgkins*

OBJECTIVES

After completion of this chapter, the reader will be able to:

1. List the erythrocyte metabolic processes that require energy.
2. Diagram the Embden-Meyerhof anaerobic glycolytic pathway in the red blood cell (RBC), highlighting adenosine triphosphate (ATP) consumption and generation.
3. Describe the process of detoxifying peroxide through the hexose monophosphate pathway.
4. Diagram the methemoglobin reductase pathway and explain its importance in maintaining functional hemoglobin.
5. Describe the Rapoport-Luebering pathway that generates 2,3-bisphosphoglycerate, state the effect of its formation on ATP production, and explain its importance in oxygen transport.
6. Describe the arrangement and function of lipids in the RBC membrane and the role of enzymes in maintaining the asymmetric balance of the phospholipids in each layer.
7. Explain cholesterol exchange between the RBC membrane and plasma, including factors that affect the exchange and the impact on the RBC shape when the cholesterol-to-phospholipid ratio is disrupted.
8. Explain the role of RBC transmembrane proteins in maintaining membrane stability and provide examples of these proteins.
9. Discuss the two major macromolecular complexes responsible for cytoskeletal anchoring and structural integrity, including the proteins involved (e.g., α-spectrin and β-spectrin, ankyrin, protein 4.2, protein 4.1, actin, adducin, tropomodulin, dematin, and band 3).
10. Name conditions caused by mutations in transmembrane and cytoskeletal proteins that disrupt vertical and horizontal (lateral) linkages in the RBC membrane.
11. Explain the importance of the semipermeable RBC membrane.
12. Cite the relative concentrations of RBC cytoplasmic potassium, sodium, and calcium, and name the structures that maintain those concentrations.

OUTLINE

Erythrocyte Metabolism (Energy Production Through Anaerobic Glycolysis)
Glycolysis Diversion Pathways (Shunts)
  Hexose Monophosphate Pathway
  Methemoglobin Reductase Pathway
  Rapoport-Luebering Pathway

Red Blood Cell Membrane Structure and Function
  Red Blood Cell Membrane Deformability
  Red Blood Cell Membrane Lipids
  Red Blood Cell Membrane Proteins
  Osmotic Balance and Permeability

CASE STUDY

After studying the material in this chapter, the reader should be able to respond to the following case study. Answers can be found in Appendix C.

Cyanosis is a blue skin coloration that occurs when the blood does not deliver enough oxygen to the tissues. It is a common sign of heart or lung disease, in which the blood fails to become oxygenated or is distributed improperly throughout the body. In the 1940s, Dr. James Deeny, an Irish provider, was experimenting with the use of vitamin C (ascorbic acid), which is a potent reducing agent, as a treatment for heart disease.[1] Unfortunately, it was ineffective for nearly all patients. However, he discovered two brothers with cyanosis, neither of whom was diagnosed with heart or lung disease. When he treated them with vitamin C, the skin of each brother returned to a normal, healthy pink color.[1] It was later determined that they had familial idiopathic methemoglobinemia.

1. What is the significance of finding this condition in brothers?
2. How is methemoglobin formed?
3. Which pathway is responsible for reducing methemoglobin?
4. What role does vitamin C (ascorbic acid) play as a reducing agent?
5. How was vitamin C able to reverse the cyanosis?

---

*The author extends appreciation to Kathryn Doig and George A. Fritsma, whose work in prior editions provided the foundation for this chapter.

There are approximately 5 million erythrocytes, or red blood cells (RBCs), per microliter of circulating blood, making the RBC the primary cell in the blood. The mature RBC lacks a nucleus, has a biconcave shape, and has an average volume of 90 fL (Chapter 6). The biconcave shape supports deformation, enabling the circulating cell to pass smoothly through capillaries, where it readily exchanges oxygen (O_2) and carbon dioxide (CO_2) while contacting the vessel wall.[2,3] The cytoplasm of the RBC contains abundant hemoglobin (a complex of globin, protoporphyrin, and iron), which transports O_2 from the lungs to the tissues. Hemoglobin has four globin chains, and each chain contains a heme molecule with an iron in the ferrous state. This allows each hemoglobin molecule to carry four O_2 molecules (Chapter 8). The RBC also transports CO_2 and bicarbonate (HCO_3^-) from the tissues back to the lungs.

RBCs are produced through normoblastic proliferation and mature in the bone marrow (Chapter 6). The nucleus, present in maturing normoblasts, is extruded as part of the RBC maturation process, typically as the RBC moves from the bone marrow to circulation. Cytoplasmic ribosomes and mitochondria also are degraded and cleared 24 to 48 hours after bone marrow release, eliminating the cells' ability to produce proteins or support oxidative metabolism.[2,3] Without mitochondria for aerobic respiration via oxidative phosphorylation, adenosine triphosphate (ATP) is produced within the cytoplasm through *anaerobic glycolysis* (Embden-Meyerhof pathway [EMP]) for the lifetime of the cell. ATP is necessary as it drives mechanisms that slow the oxidation of proteins and iron by environmental peroxides and superoxide anions, maintaining hemoglobin's function and membrane integrity. Oxidation, however, eventually takes a toll, limiting the RBC circulating life span to 120 days, whereupon it is disassembled into its reusable components: globin chains and iron from hemoglobin, and phospholipids and proteins from the cell membrane. The protoporphyrin ring of hemoglobin is not reusable and is excreted as bilirubin (Chapters 6 and 20).

This chapter is one of four chapters that present the physiology of normal RBC production, structure, function, and senescence. The other chapters include Chapter 6, "Erythrocyte Production and Destruction," Chapter 8, "Hemoglobin Metabolism," and Chapter 9, "Iron Kinetics and Laboratory Assessment." Taken as a unit, these four chapters form the basis for understanding RBC disorders (anemias), as described in Chapters 16 through 25. This chapter describes RBC energy production through anaerobic glycolysis; glycolysis diversion pathways that provide protective mechanisms for the RBC; and RBC membrane structure and function, including composition, shape stabilization, and osmotic balance and permeability.

ERYTHROCYTE METABOLISM (ENERGY PRODUCTION THROUGH ANAEROBIC GLYCOLYSIS)

Lacking mitochondria, the RBC relies on anaerobic glycolysis for its energy.[4] Exchange of O_2 and CO_2 is a passive function from high partial pressure to low partial pressure; however, the cells' metabolic processes listed in Box 7.1 require energy.

BOX 7.1   Erythrocyte Metabolic Processes Requiring Energy

Intracellular cationic gradient maintenance
Maintenance of membrane phospholipid distribution
Maintenance of skeletal protein deformability
Maintenance of functional hemoglobin with ferrous iron
Protecting cell proteins from oxidative denaturation
Glycolysis initiation and maintenance
Glutathione synthesis
Nucleotide salvage reactions

As energy production slows, the RBC grows senescent and is removed from the circulation (Chapter 6).

Anaerobic glycolysis (or EMP) (Figure 7.1) requires glucose to generate ATP, a high-energy phosphate source. RBCs lack internal energy stores and rely on plasma glucose to enter the cell to generate ATP. Glucose enters the RBC through facilitated diffusion via the transmembrane protein *Glut-1*.[5] Glucose is then catabolized to pyruvate (pyruvic acid) in the EMP, generating four molecules of ATP per molecule of glucose, for a net gain of two molecules of ATP. The sequential list of biochemical intermediates involved in glucose catabolism, with corresponding glycolytic enzymes, is given in Figure 7.1. Glycolysis is organized into three phases as seen in Figure 7.1 and in Tables 7.1 through 7.3.

The first phase of glycolysis employs glucose phosphorylation, isomerization, and diphosphorylation to yield fructose 1,6-bisphosphate (F1,6-BP). Intermediate stages employ the enzymes *hexokinase, glucose-6-phosphate isomerase,* and *6-phosphofructokinase.* The initial hexokinase and 6-phosphofructokinase steps consume a total of two ATP molecules and limit the rate of glycolysis. *Fructose-bisphosphate aldolase* then cleaves F1,6-BP to produce glyceraldehyde-3-phosphate (G3P) (see Figure 7.1 and Table 7.1).

The second phase of anaerobic glycolysis converts G3P to 3-phosphoglycerate (3-PG). The substrates, enzymes, and products for this phase of glycolytic metabolism are summarized in Table 7.2. In the first step, G3P is oxidized to 1,3-bisphosphoglycerate (1,3-BPG) through the action of *glyceraldehyde-3-phosphate dehydrogenase* (G3PD), with the reduction of nicotinamide adenine dinucleotide (NAD) to NADH. 1,3-BPG is dephosphorylated by *phosphoglycerate kinase,* which generates two ATP molecules and 3-PG (see Figure 7.1).

The third phase of glycolysis converts 3-PG to pyruvate and generates ATP. Substrates, enzymes, and products are listed in Table 7.3. The 3-PG is isomerized by *phosphoglycerate mutase* to 2-phosphoglycerate (2-PG). *Enolase (phosphopyruvate hydratase)* then converts 2-PG to phosphoenolpyruvate (PEP). *Pyruvate kinase* (PK) splits off the phosphates, forming two ATP molecules and pyruvate. PK activity is allosterically modulated by increased concentrations of F1,6-BP, which enhances the affinity of PK for PEP.[4] Thus when F1,6-BP is plentiful, increased activity of PK favors pyruvate production. Pyruvate may diffuse from the RBC or may become a substrate for *lactate dehydrogenase,* with regeneration of the oxidized form of

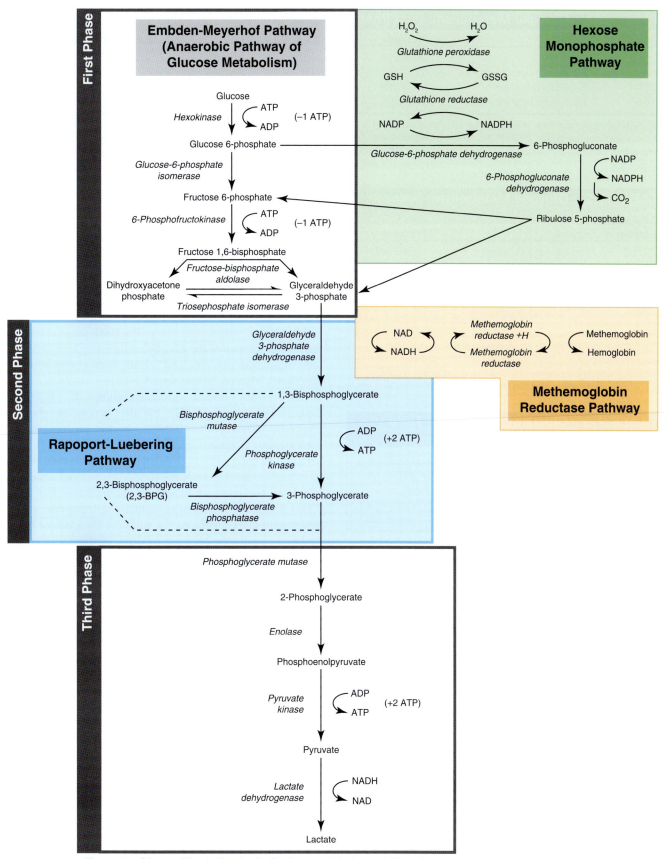

Figure 7.1 Glucose Metabolism in the Erythrocyte. Methemoglobin reductase is also called cytochrome-b_5 reductase. *ADP,* Adenosine diphosphate; *ATP,* adenosine triphosphate; *GSH,* reduced glutathione; *GSSG,* oxidized glutathione; *NAD,* nicotinamide adenine dinucleotide (oxidized form); *NADH,* nicotinamide adenine dinucleotide (reduced form); *NADP,* nicotinamide adenine dinucleotide phosphate (oxidized form); *NADPH,* nicotinamide adenine dinucleotide phosphate (reduced form).

TABLE 7.1 Glucose Metabolism: First Phase

Substrates	Enzyme	Products
Glucose, ATP	Hexokinase	G6P, ADP
G6P	Glucose-6-phosphate isomerase	F6P
F6P, ATP	6-phosphofructokinase	F1,6-BP, ADP
F1,6-BP	Fructose-bisphosphate adolase	DHAP, G3P

ADP, Adenosine diphosphate; *ATP*, adenosine triphosphate; *DHAP*, dihydroxyacetone phosphate; *F1,6-BP*, fructose-1,6-bisphosphate; *F6P*, fructose-6-phosphate; *G3P*, glyceraldehyde-3-phosphate; *G6P*, glucose-6-phosphate.

TABLE 7.2 Glucose Metabolism: Second Phase

Substrates	Enzyme	Products
G3P, NAD	Glyceraldehyde-3-phosphate dehydrogenase	1,3-BPG, NADH
1,3-BPG, ADP	Phosphoglycerate kinase	3PG, ATP
1,3-BPG	Bisphosphoglycerate mutase	2,3-BPG
2,3-BPG	Bisphosphoglycerate phosphatase	3-PG

1,3-BPG, 1,3-bisphosphoglycerate; *2,3-BPG*, 2,3-bisphosphoglycerate; *3-PG*, 3-phosphoglycerate; *ADP*, adenosine diphosphate; *ATP*, adenosine triphosphate; *G3P*, glyceraldehyde-3-phosphate; *NAD*, nicotinamide adenine dinucleotide (oxidized form); *NADH*, nicotinamide adenine dinucleotide (reduced form).

TABLE 7.3 Glucose Metabolism: Third Phase

Substrates	Enzyme	Products
3-PG	Phosphoglycerate mutase	2-PG
2-PG	Enolase (phosphopyruvate hydratase)	PEP
PEP, ADP	Pyruvate kinase	Pyruvate, ATP
Pyruvate, NADH	Lactate dehydrogenase*	Lactate, NAD

*The activity of lactate dehydrogenase to convert pyruvate to lactate is modulated by the ratio of NAD to NADH.
2-PG, 2-phosphoglycerate; *3-PG*, 3-phosphoglycerate; *ADP*, adenosine diphosphate; *ATP*, adenosine triphosphate; *NAD*, nicotinamide adenine dinucleotide (oxidized form); *NADH*, nicotinamide adenine dinucleotide (reduced form); *PEP*, phosphoenolpyruvate.

nicotinamide adenine dinucleotide (NAD^+). The ratio of NAD^+ to the reduced form (NADH) modulates the activity of lactate dehydrogenase (see Figure 7.1).

Hematologists have identified hereditary deficiencies of nearly every glycolytic enzyme. Their common result is shortened RBC survival, known collectively as *hereditary nonspherocytic hemolytic anemia* (Chapter 21).

GLYCOLYSIS DIVERSION PATHWAYS (SHUNTS)

Three alternative pathways, called *diversions or shunts*, branch from the glycolytic pathway. The three diversions are the *hexose monophosphate pathway* (HMP), the *methemoglobin reductase pathway*, and the *Rapoport-Luebering pathway*.

Hexose Monophosphate Pathway

Oxidative glycolysis occurs through a diversion of glucose catabolism into the HMP, also known as the *pentose phosphate*

TABLE 7.4 Glucose Metabolism: Hexose Monophosphate Pathway

Substrates	Enzyme	Products
G6P, NADP	Glucose-6-phosphate dehydrogenase and 6-phosphogluconolactonase	6-PG, NADPH
6-PG, NADP	6-phosphogluconate dehydrogenase	R5P, NADPH, CO₂

6-PG, 6-phosphogluconate; *G6P*, glucose-6-phosphate; *NADP*, nicotinamide adenine dinucleotide phosphate (oxidized form); *NADPH*, nicotinamide adenine dinucleotide phosphate (reduced form); *R5P*, ribulose 5-phosphate.

shunt (see Figure 7.1). The HMP detoxifies hydrogen peroxide (H_2O_2), other organic hydroperoxides (ROOH), hydroxyl radicals (OH-), and superoxide anions (O_2^-) which arise from O_2 reduction in the cell's aqueous environment. HMP neutralizes these oxidants through reduced glutathione and NADPH. H_2O_2 oxidizes heme iron to the nonfunctional ferric state and oxidizes and denatures proteins and lipids. The HMP shunt extends the functional life span of the RBC by maintaining membrane proteins, lipids, and enzymes, and keeping hemoglobin iron in the functional, reduced, ferrous state.[4]

The HMP diverts glucose-6-phosphate (G6P) to 6-phosphogluconate (6-PG) by the action of *glucose-6-phosphate dehydrogenase* (G6PD). In the process, oxidized nicotinamide adenine dinucleotide phosphate (NADP) is converted to its reduced form (NADPH). NADPH is then available to reduce oxidized glutathione (GSSG) to reduced glutathione (GSH) in the presence of *glutathione reductase* (see Figure 7.1). Glutathione is a cysteine-containing tripeptide, and the designation GSH highlights the sulfur in the cysteine moiety. Reduced glutathione becomes oxidized as it reduces H_2O_2 to water and O_2 via *glutathione peroxidase*.

During steady-state glycolysis, 5% to 10% of G6P is diverted to the HMP. After oxidative challenge, HMP activity may increase up to 30-fold.[6] The HMP further catabolizes 6-PG to ribulose 5-phosphate, CO_2, and NADPH by the action of *6-phosphogluconate dehydrogenase*. The substrates, enzymes, and products of the HMP are listed in Table 7.4.

G6PD provides the only means of generating NADPH for glutathione reduction, and in its absence, RBCs are particularly vulnerable to oxidative damage (Chapter 21).[7] With normal G6PD activity, the HMP detoxifies oxidative compounds and safeguards hemoglobin, sulfhydryl-containing enzymes, and membrane thiols, allowing RBCs to safely carry O_2. However, in G6PD deficiency, the most common inherited RBC enzyme deficiency worldwide, the ability to detoxify is hampered, resulting in hereditary nonspherocytic anemia.

Methemoglobin Reductase Pathway

Heme iron is constantly exposed to O_2 and H_2O_2.[8] H_2O_2 oxidizes heme iron from the ferrous (2^+) to the ferric (3^+) state. When the iron state is ferric, the affected hemoglobin molecule is called *methemoglobin* and cannot carry O_2. Although the HMP prevents hemoglobin oxidation by reducing H_2O_2, it is not able to reduce methemoglobin once it forms. NADPH is able to do so but only slowly. The reduction of methemoglobin by NADPH is rendered more efficient in the presence of *methemoglobin reductase,* also called cytochrome-b_5 reductase. Using H^+ from NADH formed when G3P is converted to 1,3-BPG, cytochrome-b_5 reductase acts as an intermediate electron carrier, returning the oxidized ferric iron to its ferrous, O_2-carrying state (see Figure 7.1). This enzyme accounts for more than 65% of the methemoglobin-reducing capacity within the RBC.[8] Returning to the case study at the beginning of the chapter, vitamin C (ascorbic acid) was able to directly reduce the ferric iron to ferrous iron as a reducing agent or electron donor in the brothers with familial idiopathic methemoglobinemia (or cytochrome-b_5 reductase deficiency).[1]

Rapoport-Luebering Pathway

A third metabolic shunt generates *2,3-bisphosphoglycerate* (2,3-BPG), also called 2,3-diphosphoglycerate. 1,3-BPG is diverted by *bisphosphoglycerate mutase* to form 2,3-BPG (see Figure 7.1). 2,3-BPG binds between the globin chains in the interior cavity of the hemoglobin tetramer to stabilize it in the deoxygenated state (tense or low O_2 affinity state). This binding shifts the hemoglobin-O_2 dissociation curve to the right, which enhances delivery of O_2 to the tissues (Chapter 8).

2,3-BPG forms 3-PG by the action of *bisphosphoglycerate phosphatase.* This diversion of 1,3-BPG to form 2,3-BPG sacrifices the production of two ATP molecules. There is further loss of two ATP molecules at the level of PK because fewer molecules of PEP are formed. Because two ATP molecules were used to generate 1,3-BPG and production of 2,3-BPG eliminates the production of four ATP molecules, the cell is put into ATP deficit by this diversion. There is a delicate balance between ATP generation to support the energy requirements of cell metabolism and the need to maintain the appropriate oxygenation and deoxygenation status of hemoglobin. Acidic pH and low concentrations of 3-PG and 2-PG inhibit the activity of *bisphosphoglycerate mutase,* thus inhibiting the shunt and retaining 1,3-BPG in the EMP. These conditions and decreased ATP activate *bisphosphoglycerate phosphatase,* which returns 2,3-BPG to the glycolysis mainstream. In summary, these conditions favor generation of ATP by causing the conversion of 1,3-BPG directly to 3-PG and returning 2,3-BPG to 3-PG for ATP generation downstream by PK.

RED BLOOD CELL MEMBRANE STRUCTURE AND FUNCTION

Red Blood Cell Membrane Deformability

RBCs are biconcave, 7 to 8 μM in diameter, with a volume range of 80 to 100 fL and a mean volume of 90 fL. Their average surface area is 140 μm^2, which is a 40% excess of surface area compared with a sphere of 7 to 8 μm in diameter.[9] This excess surface area-to-volume ratio enables RBCs to stretch undamaged up to 2.5 times their resting diameter as they pass through narrow capillaries and through splenic pores 2 μm in diameter.[10] This property is called RBC *deformability.* The RBC plasma membrane is 100 times more elastic than a comparable latex membrane, yet it has tensile (lateral) strength greater than that of steel.[9] The deformable RBC membrane provides the broad surface area and close tissue contact necessary to support the delivery of O_2 from the lungs to body tissues and to transport CO_2 from body tissues to the lungs.

RBC deformability depends not only on RBC geometry but also on relative cytoplasmic (hemoglobin) viscosity. The normal mean cell hemoglobin concentration (MCHC) ranges from 32 to 36 g/dL (Chapter 12 and after the Index at the end of the book) and as MCHC rises, internal viscosity rises.[11] MCHCs greater than 36 g/dL compromise deformability and shorten the RBC life span because viscous cells become damaged as they stretch to pass through narrow capillaries or splenic pores. As RBCs age, they lose membrane surface area while retaining hemoglobin. As the MCHC rises, the RBC becomes unable to deform and pass through the small splenic pores, becoming trapped in the splenic cords. Consequently, the RBC is phagocytized and destroyed by splenic macrophages (Chapter 6).

Red Blood Cell Membrane Lipids

Besides geometry and viscosity, membrane elasticity (pliancy) also contributes to deformability. The RBC membrane consists of approximately 8% carbohydrates, 40% lipids, and 52% proteins.[12] The lipid portion is equal parts of cholesterol and phospholipids and forms a bilayer universal to all animal cells (Figure 7.2). Phospholipids form an impenetrable fluid barrier as their hydrophilic polar head groups are arrayed on the membrane's surfaces, oriented toward both the aqueous plasma and the cytoplasm, respectively, as described in the fluid mosaic membrane model (FMMM).[13] Their hydrophobic nonpolar acyl tails arrange themselves to form a central layer sequestered (hidden) from the aqueous plasma and cytoplasm.[13] The phospholipids provide a dynamic fluidity to the membrane; if a portion of the lipid bilayer is lost, the membrane can self-seal to retain the cytoplasmic contents. The membrane also maintains extreme differences in osmotic pressure, cation concentrations, and gas concentrations between external plasma and the cytoplasm through the dynamic interaction of the lipids and proteins.[14]

Free cholesterol, or *un*esterified cholesterol, is equally distributed between the outer and inner layers of the phospholipid bilayer and evenly dispersed within each layer, approximately one cholesterol molecule per phospholipid molecule. The β-hydroxyl group of cholesterol, the only hydrophilic domain of the molecule, anchors within the phospholipid polar heads, while the rest of the molecule becomes *intercalated* among and parallel to the acyl tails. Cholesterol confers *tensile strength* to the lipid bilayer.[15] As cholesterol concentration rises, the membrane gains strength but loses elasticity. Because of the large quantity of free cholesterol in the RBC, the erythrocyte membrane may play an active role in cholesterol metabolism through reverse cholesterol transport, allowing cholesterol exchange with lipoproteins (high-density lipoprotein).[16]

The ratio of cholesterol to phospholipids remains relatively constant to maintain the balance of deformability, elasticity, and strength. Membrane enzymes maintain the cholesterol concentration by regularly exchanging membrane and plasma

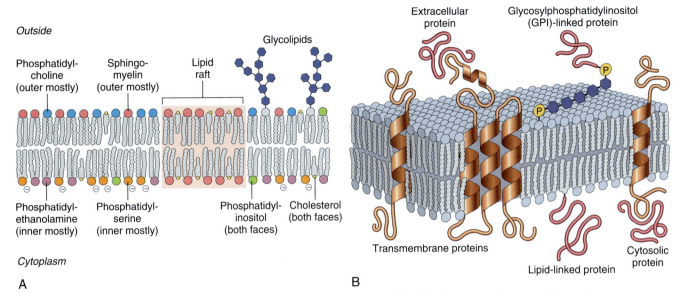

Outside

Phosphatidyl-
choline
(outer mostly)

Sphingo-
myelin
(outer mostly)

Lipid
raft

Glycolipids

Phosphatidyl-
ethanolamine
(inner mostly)

Phosphatidyl-
serine
(inner mostly)

Phosphatidyl-
inositol
(both faces)

Cholesterol
(both faces)

Cytoplasm

A

Extracellular
protein

Glycosylphosphatidylinositol
(GPI)-linked protein

Transmembrane proteins

Lipid-linked protein

Cytosolic
protein

B

Figure 7.2 Plasma Membrane Organization and Asymmetry. **(A),** The plasma membrane is a bilayer of phospholipids, cholesterol, and associated proteins. The phospholipid distribution within the membrane is asymmetric; phosphatidylcholine and sphingomyelin are overrepresented in the outer leaflet, and phosphatidylserine (negative charge) and phosphatidylethanolamine are predominantly found on the inner leaflet; glycolipids occur only on the outer face, where they contribute to the extracellular glycocalyx. Nonrandom concentration of certain membrane components such as cholesterol creates membrane domains known as lipid rafts. **(B),** Transmembrane proteins may traverse the membrane once or multiple times. Proteins may be linked to transmembrane proteins on their extracellular or intracellular domains, linked to glycosylphosphatidylinositol *(GPI)* anchors, or bound directly to phospholipids. Transmembrane proteins can transduce signals across the membrane. (From Mitchell, R. N. [2018]. The cell as a unit of health and disease. In Kumar, V., Abbas, A. K., & Aster, J. C. [Eds.], *Robbins Basic Pathology.* [10th ed., p. 8, Figure 1.7]. Philadelphia: Elsevier.)

cholesterol. Deficiencies in these enzymes are associated with RBC membrane abnormalities such as *acanthocytes* and *target cells (codocytes).*[15] For example, lecithin cholesterol acyltransferase converts free cholesterol to esterified cholesterol. This conversion prevents the cholesterol exchange between the plasma and the membrane. Deficiencies of this enzyme result in increased free cholesterol and increased RBC membrane cholesterol. Acanthocytes are formed when the cholesterol-to-phospholipid ratio increases. When the cholesterol-to-phospholipid ratio remains equal despite increased levels of cholesterol, target cell formation occurs.[12,15]

The *phospholipids* are asymmetrically distributed in the FMMM of the RBC membrane. Phosphatidylcholine (PC) and sphingomyelin (SP) predominate in the outer layer; phosphatidylserine (PS) and phosphatidylethanolamine (PE) form most of the inner layer (see Figure 7.2A). Distribution of these four phospholipids is energy dependent, relying on a number of membrane-associated lipid transport proteins, termed *flippases, floppases,* and *scramblases* for their functions.[9,17] Flippases and floppases work unidirectionally "flipping in" PE and PS and "flopping out" PC and SP, respectively. Scramblase redistributes the phospholipids bidirectionally. Small amounts of phosphatidylinositol (PI) are also limited to the inner leaflet.[9,17] When phospholipid distribution is disrupted, as in sickle cell anemia and thalassemia (Chapters 24 and 25) or in aging RBCs (energy depletion), PS, the only negatively charged phospholipid, redistributes from the inner to the outer layer. Splenic

macrophages possess receptors that bind to the PS displayed on *senescent* and damaged RBCs and remove them from circulation.[17] C-reactive protein and inflammatory conditions increase the PS distribution in the outer layer of the RBC membrane leading to increased RBC death (also called *eryptosis*) (Chapter 6).[18]

Membrane phospholipids and cholesterol may also *redistribute laterally* so that the RBC membrane may respond to stresses and deform within 100 ms of being challenged by the presence of a narrow passage, such as a capillary.[9] Cholesterol and SP may also form lipid rafts, which are clusters of lipids grouped together, rather than asymmetrically distributed throughout the membrane, that are involved in receptor signaling.[9] As the proportion of cholesterol increases, the RBC becomes more rigid and is unable to deform as readily. In liver disease, membrane cholesterol concentration becomes increased because of an increased plasma bile salt concentration.[19] As a result, the cell membrane surface area-to-volume ratio increases, giving the RBC a target cell appearance (Figure 16.1).

Glycolipids (sugar-bearing lipids) make up 5% of the external half of the RBC membrane (see Figure 7.2A).[20] They associate in clumps or rafts and support carbohydrate side chains that extend into the aqueous plasma to anchor the *glycocalyx.*[14] The glycocalyx is a layer of carbohydrates whose net negative charge prevents microbial attack and mechanical damage by preventing adhesion to neighboring RBCs or to the endothelium. Glycolipids may bear copies of carbohydrate-based blood group antigens, such as antigens of the ABH and the Lewis blood group systems.

Red Blood Cell Membrane Proteins

Although cholesterol and phospholipids constitute the principal RBC membrane structure, *transmembrane (integral)* and *cytoskeletal (skeletal, peripheral)* proteins make up 52% of the membrane structure by mass.[21] A proteomic study revealed that there are at least 300 RBC membrane proteins, including 105 transmembrane proteins.[22] Some proteins have a few hundred copies per cell and others have more than 1 million copies per cell. Of the purported 300 membrane proteins, about 50 have been characterized and named.[22]

Nomenclature

RBC membrane proteins have both numerical naming and conventional naming. Numerical naming, for instance, band 3, protein 4.1, and protein 4.2, derives from historical (preproteomics) protein identification techniques that distinguished membrane proteins using *sodium dodecyl sulfate-polyacrylamide gel electrophoresis* (SDS-PAGE), as illustrated in Figure 7.3.[25] The protein names corresponded to their location on the SDS-PAGE separation, a property of their molecular weight and net charge, and are identified using Coomassie blue dye. The glycophorins, with abundant carbohydrate side chains, must be stained using periodic acid-Schiff dye to be visualized. These methods can still be used to separate RBC membrane proteins; however, other methods are used for diagnosing membrane protein disorders (Chapter 21).

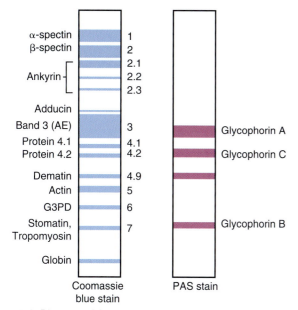

Figure 7.3 Diagram of Sodium Dodecyl Sulfate-Polyacrylamide Gel Electrophoresis of Red Blood Cell Membrane Proteins Stained With Coomassie Blue *(Left)* and Periodic Acid-Schiff *(Right)*. Note the positions of some of the major red blood cell membrane proteins. *AE,* Anion exchanger; *G3PD,* glyceraldehyde-3-phosphate dehydrogenase; *PAS,* periodic acid-Schiff. (Adapted from Beck, W. S., & Tepper, R. I. [1991]. Hemolytic anemias III: Membrane disorders. In Beck, W. S. [Ed.], *Hematology* [5th ed., Figure 14.1]. Cambridge, MA: The MIT Press.)

Band 3 and protein 4.2 are the major components of the ankyrin complex and link their associated proteins and the lipid bilayer membrane to the spectrin cytoskeleton through ankyrin (Figure 7.4).[26,27] Likewise, band 3, protein 4.2, adducin, and actin are the major components of the actin junctional (4.1) complex and link the lipid membrane to the spectrin cytoskeleton through protein 4.1.[24,28–30] The 4.1 anchorage also includes the protein *dematin,* which links with transmembrane protein Glut-1.[31] Band 3 is found in the ankyrin complex, in the actin junctional complex, and as a singular transmembrane protein. Band 3 serves as a structural protein and as a regulator of the EMP pathway (glucose metabolism) by binding deoxyhemoglobin, demonstrating the interplay between the RBC membrane structure and RBC metabolism.[32]

Transmembrane Proteins

The *transmembrane* proteins serve many functions including *transport* sites, *adhesion* sites, and *signaling receptors.* Any disruption in transport protein function changes the osmotic tension of the cytoplasm, which leads to a rise in viscosity and loss of deformability. Any change affecting adhesion proteins permits RBCs to adhere to one another and to the vessel walls, promoting fragmentation (vesiculation), reducing membrane flexibility, and shortening the RBC life span. Signaling receptors bind plasma ligands and trigger activation of intracellular signaling proteins, which then initiate various energy-dependent cellular activities, a process called *signal transduction.* Through *glycosylation,* the transmembrane proteins also support *surface carbohydrates,* which join with glycolipids to make up the protective glycocalyx. A summary of selected transmembrane proteins and RBC functions is listed in Table 7.5.[23,24]

Most transmembrane proteins assemble into one of two major macromolecular complexes named by their respective cytoskeletal anchorages: the *ankyrin complex* and the *actin junctional complex,* also called *protein 4.1 complex* (see Figure 7.4).[24,28] The major components of the ankyrin complex are band 3 multimers and protein 4.2, which anchor the lipid bilayer to the spectrin cytoskeleton through ankyrin. Major components of the actin junctional complex (4.1 complex) are band 3 dimers, protein 4.2, and adducin, which anchor the lipid bilayer to the spectrin cytoskeleton through protein 4.1. Actin, dematin, tropomyosin, and tropomodulin are additional proteins that help link the junctional complex to the ends of the spectrin tetramers to form a hexagonal cytoskeletal lattice adjacent to the inner (cytoplasmic) lipid bilayer. The actin protofilament is drawn perpendicular to the plane of the lipid bilayer; however, it actually lies parallel to the membrane. Band 3 dimers also float untethered within the lipid bilayer. The anchoring of the transmembrane complexes through protein 4.2 to cytoskeletal proteins (adjacent to the inner or cytoplasmic side of the membrane) prevents loss of the lipid bilayer. In addition, the linking of cytoskeletal proteins by the actin junctional complex provides membrane structural integrity because the cell relies on an intact cytoskeleton to maintain its biconcave shape despite deformability. Transmembrane proteins also provide vertical membrane structure.

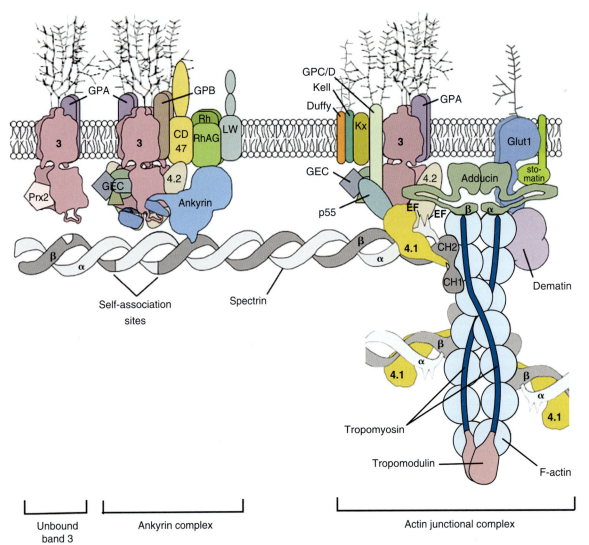

Figure 7.4 **Schematic Model of the Red Blood Cell Membrane.** α-spectrin and β-spectrin are the most abundant cytoskeletal proteins. Band 3 is the most abundant transmembrane protein and is found unbound, in the ankyrin complex, and in the actin junctional complex. The transmembrane proteins assemble into one of two complexes defined by their anchorage to either the cytoskeletal protein ankyrin or to cytoskeletal proteins actin and 4.1. Protein 4.2 connects the actin junctional complex to α-spectrin. The major proteins may not be drawn to the actual shape of the protein; however, they are roughly to scale. *CH1* and *CH2*, Actin-binding domains of β spectrin; *Duffy,* Duffy blood group system protein; *EF,* Ca^{2+}-binding EF hand domain of α spectrin; *GEC,* glycolytic enzyme complex (G3PD, phosphofructokinase, and aldolase); *GPA,* glycophorin A; *GPB,* glycophorin B; *GPC/D,* glycophorin C/D; *Kell,* Kell blood group system protein; *Kx,* X-linked Kell antigen expression protein; *LW,* Landsteiner-Weiner blood group system protein; *Prx2,* peroxiredoxin-2; *Rh,* Rh blood group system protein; *RhAG,* Rh-associated glycoprotein. (Modified from Korsgren, C., Peters, L. L., Lux, S. E. [2010]. Protein 4.2 binds to the carboxyl-terminal EF-hands of erythroid alpha-spectrin in a calcium- and calmodulin-dependent manner. *J Biol Chem, 285,* 4757–4770.)

Blood group antigens. The carbohydrate-defined *blood group antigens* are supported in the RBC membrane by transmembrane proteins (see Figures 7.2B and 7.4 and Table 7.5).[29] The blood group antigens are located in membrane macromolecular complexes that serve as transporters, structural components, enzymes, receptors, and adhesion molecules. Half of the known transmembrane proteins (approximately 25) are involved in the macromolecular complexes that define blood antigen group such as Band 3 (anion transport) and Glut-1 (glucose transport), which support the majority of

ABH system carbohydrate determinants (i.e., blood type).[9,33] Several transmembrane proteins provide peptide epitopes. For instance, glycophorin A carries the peptide-defined M and N determinants, and glycophorin B carries the Ss determinants, which together comprise the MNSs system, whereas the minor glycophorins C and D carry the Gerbich system antigens.[34,35]

The Rh system employs two transmembrane lipoproteins and one multipass glycoprotein, each of which crosses the membrane 12 times.[36] The two lipoproteins present the D and CcEe epitopes, respectively. The expression of the D and CcEe antigens requires

TABLE 7.5   Names and Properties of Selected Transmembrane RBC Proteins

Transmembrane Protein	Gene	Band	MW (kD)	Copies/Cell (×10³)	% of TP	Function
Aquaporin 1	AQP1		28	120–160		Water transporter, Colton antigen
Band 3 (anion exchanger, AE1)	SLC4A1	3	90–102	1200	27%	Anion transporter, location of ABH antigens
Ca²⁺-ATPase	ATP2B1		110			Ca²⁺ transporter
Duffy	FY, DARC, ACKR1		35–43	6–13		G protein-coupled receptor, chemokine receptor, Duffy antigens, receptor for malarial parasites
Glut-1	SLC2A1	4.5	45–75	200–700	5%	Glucose transporter, location of ABH blood group antigens
Glycophorin A	GYPA	PAS-1	36	1000	85% of GP	Sialic acid transporter, location of MN blood group antigens
Glycophorin B	GYPB	PAS-4	20	250	10% of GP	Sialic acid transporter, location of Ss blood group antigens
Glycophorin C	GYPC	PAS-2	14–32	135	4% of GP	Sialic acid transporter, location of Gerbich system antigens
ICAM-4	ICAM4					Integrin adhesion
K⁺-Cl⁻ cotransporter						Transports K⁺, Cl⁻
Kell	KEL		93	3–18		Zn²⁺-binding endopeptidase, Kell antigens
Kidd	SLC14A1		43	14		Urea transporter, Kidd (Jk) antigens
Na⁺, K⁺-ATPase	ATP1A2		140	0.5		Na⁺, K⁺ transporter
Na⁺-K⁺-2Cl⁻ cotransporter						Na⁺, K⁺, Cl⁻ transporter
Rh	RHCE, RHD		30–45	200		D and CcEe antigens; stabilizes band 3 and Rh macrocomplexes[36]
RhAG	RHAG		45–100	100–200		D and CcEe antigen component; CO_2, cation, and ammonium transporter[36]

ATPase, Adenosine triphosphatase; *Duffy,* Duffy blood group system protein; *GP,* glycophorin; *ICAM,* intracellular adhesion molecule; *Kell,* Kell blood group system protein; *MW,* molecular weight; *PAS,* periodic acid-Schiff dye; *RBC,* red blood cell; *Rh,* Rh blood group system protein; *RhAG,* Rh antigen expression protein; *TP,* total protein.
Data from references 23, 24, 28, 29, and 33–39.

the separately inherited glycoprotein RhAG, which localizes near the Rh lipoproteins in the ankyrin complex. Loss of the RhAG glycoprotein prevents expression of both the D and the CcEe antigens (Rh-null) and is associated with RBC morphologic abnormalities (Chapter 21). Additional blood group antigens (such as Duffy, Kell, and Kidd) localize to the actin junctional (4.1) complex or specialized proteins (e.g., protein 4.1R).[37–39]

Glycosylphosphatidylinositol anchor and paroxysmal nocturnal hemoglobinuria. A few copies of the phospholipid PI reside in the outer, plasma-side layer of the membrane. PI serves as a base on which a glycan core of sugar molecules is synthesized, forming the transmembrane glycosylphosphatidylinositol (GPI) anchor (see Figure 7.2B). More than 30 proteins bind to the GPI anchor and appear to float on the surface of the membrane. Two of these proteins that appear extracellularly and are bound to the transmembrane GPI anchor, *decay-accelerating factor* (DAF, or CD55) and *membrane inhibitor of reactive lysis* (MIRL, or CD59), protect the RBC membrane from lysis by complement.[40]

The phosphatidylinositol glycan anchor biosynthesis class A *(PIGA)* gene codes for a glycosyltransferase required to add *N*-acetylglucosamine to the PI base early in the biosynthesis of the GPI anchor on the membrane. In paroxysmal nocturnal hemoglobinuria (Chapter 21), an acquired mutation in the *PIGA* gene affects the cells' ability to synthesize the GPI anchor. Without the transmembrane GPI anchor, the cell membrane becomes deficient in CD55 and CD59, and the cells are susceptible to complement-mediated hemolysis.[40]

Cytoskeletal Proteins

The principal cytoskeletal proteins are the filamentous α-spectrin and β-spectrin (Table 7.6 and see Figure 7.4), which assemble to form an *antiparallel* heterodimer held together with a series of lateral bonds.[28,41] Antiparallel means that the carboxyl (COOH) end of one strand associates with the amino (NH₃) end of the other, and the two heterodimers self-associate head to head to form a tetramer. The ends of the spectrin tetramers are linked in the actin junctional complex, forming a hexagonal cytoskeletal lattice adjacent to the inner (cytoplasmic) lipid bilayer. This provides *lateral* or *horizontal* membrane stability.[42] Because the cytoskeletal proteins do not penetrate the bilayer, they are also called *peripheral* proteins.

Spectrin stabilization. Essential to RBC membrane cytoskeleton stabilization are the ankyrin complex and actin junctional complex proteins: ankyrin, protein 4.1, adducin,

TABLE 7.6   **Names and Properties of Selected Cytoskeletal Red Blood Cell Proteins**

Skeletal Protein	Gene	Band	MW (kD)	Copies/Cell (×10³)	% of TP	Function
α-Spectrin	SPTA1	1	240–280	242	16%	Filamentous antiparallel heterodimer, primary cytoskeletal proteins
β-Spectrin	SPTB	2	220–246	242	14%	
Adducin	ADD1 ADD2	2.9	80–103	60	4%	Caps actin filament, binds Ca²⁺/calmodulin
Ankyrin	ANK1	2.1	206–210	124	4.5%	Anchor band 3, protein 4.2, and other proteins in the ankyrin complex to spectrin
Dematin	EPB49	4.9	43–52	140	1%	Actin bundling protein
β-Actin	ACTB	5	42–43	500	5.5%	Binds β-spectrin
G3PD	GAPD	6	35–37	500	3.5%	Carbohydrate metabolism, phosphorylates G3P
Protein 4.1	EPB41	4.1	66–80	200	5%	Anchors the actin junctional complex to spectrin tetramers, RBC cytoskeleton shape
Protein 4.2 (protein kinase)	EPB42	4.2	72–77	250	5%	Part of ankyrin complex, ATP binding protein
Tropomodulin	TMOD1	5	41–43	30	—	Caps actin filament
Tropomyosin	TPM3	7	27–38	70	1%	Stabilizes and regulates actin polymerization

ATP, Adenosine triphosphate; *G3PD,* glyceraldehyde-3-phosphate dehydrogenase; *MW,* molecular weight; *RBC,* red blood cell; *TP,* total protein.
Data from references 23, 24, and 28.

dematin, *actin, tropomyosin,* and *tropomodulin* (see Figure 7.4 and Table 7.6).[24,27,28] The secondary structure of both α-spectrin and β-spectrin features triple-helical repeats of 106 amino acids each; 20 such repeats make up α-spectrin, and 16 make up β-spectrin.[43] The α-spectrin and β-spectrin form heterodimers in an antiparallel fashion. Two heterodimers associate head to head to form spectrin tetramers. A single helix at the amino terminus of α-spectrin consistently binds a pair of helices at the carboxyl terminus of the β-spectrin chain, forming a stable triple helix that holds together the ends of the heterodimers.[28] Joining these ends are actin and protein 4.1 in the actin junctional complex. Actin forms short filaments of 14 to 16 monomers whose length is regulated by tropomyosin. Adducin and tropomodulin cap the ends of actin. Dematin appears to stabilize the actin junctional complex and helps maintain the RBC shape.[44] The spectrin cytoskeleton functions as a coil to allow for the RBC to resume its shape after deformation.

Membrane Deformation and Associated Disorders

Spectrin dimer bonds that appear along the length of the molecules disassociate and reassociate (open and close) during RBC deformation. Likewise, the 20 α-spectrin and 16 β-spectrin repeated helices unfold and refold.[45] These flexible interactions, plus the spectrin-protein 4.1 junctions in the actin junctional complexes between the tetramers, are key regulators of membrane elasticity and mechanical stability. Abnormalities in any of these proteins result in deformation-induced membrane fragmentation. For instance, *hereditary elliptocytosis* (Chapter 21) arises from one of several autosomal dominant mutations affecting the spectrin dimer-to-dimer lateral bonds or the spectrin-protein 4.1 junction (see Table 7.6).[46] These *horizontal* interaction defects inhibit the membrane's ability to rebound from deformation (Figure 7.5). Ultimately, the RBCs progressively elongate to form visible elliptocytes, which causes a mild to severe hemolytic anemia.[46–48] Conversely,

autosomal dominant mutations that affect the integrity of band 3, ankyrin, protein 4.2, or α-spectrin or β-spectrin are associated with *hereditary spherocytosis* (Chapter 21).[46–48] In these cases, there are too few *vertical anchorages* to maintain membrane stability (see Figure 7.5). The lipid membrane peels off in small fragments called *blebs,* or *vesicles,* and immediately reseals, keeping the cytoplasmic volume intact. This results in a reduced surface area-to-volume ratio and the formation of spherocytes.

Osmotic Balance and Permeability

The RBC membrane is semipermeable. It is impermeable to cations Na⁺, K⁺, and Ca²⁺ and permeable to water and the anions bicarbonate (HCO_3^-) and chloride (Cl^-), which freely exchange between plasma and RBC cytoplasm. *Aquaporin-1* regulates the influx of water into the RBC in response to osmotic changes. Aquaporin 1 (see Table 7.5) is a transmembrane protein that forms pores or channels whose surface charges create inward water flow in response to internal osmotic changes and allows this free exchange. Decreases in *aquaporin 1* expression have been linked with *hereditary* spherocytosis (Chapter 21) and conditions where there is loss of RBC membrane.[49]

The ATP-dependent cation pumps *Na⁺-ATPase* and *K⁺-ATPase* (see Table 7.5) regulate the concentrations of Na⁺ and K⁺, maintaining intracellular-to-extracellular ratios of 1:12 and 25:1, respectively.[50,51] *Ca²⁺-ATPase* expels calcium from the cell, maintaining low intracellular levels of 30 to 60 nM compared with 1.8 mM in the plasma.[52] Calmodulin, a cytoplasmic Ca²⁺-binding protein, controls the function of Ca²⁺-ATPase. These pumps, in addition to aquaporin 1, maintain osmotic balance in the RBC.

The cation pumps consume a significant portion of RBC ATP production. ATP loss or pump damage permits Ca²⁺ and Na⁺ influx, with water following osmotically. The cell swells, becomes spheroid, and eventually ruptures. This phenomenon

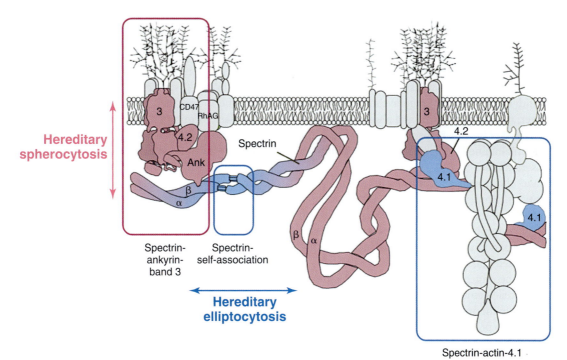

Figure 7.5 Membrane Defects in Hereditary Spherocytosis and Elliptocytosis. Hereditary spherocytosis is caused by a quantitative deficiency of spectrin, ankyrin, band 3, or protein 4.2, proteins involved in the vertical interactions that attach the membrane cytoskeleton to the overlying lipid bilayer with its transmembrane proteins. Hereditary elliptocytosis is caused by functional defects in the horizontal protein interactions that hold the cytoskeleton together. These are either defects near the head end of spectrin that impair self-association of spectrin dimers or deficiency of protein 4.1, a protein that bolsters the attachment of spectrin to actin. (From Lux, S. E. [2015]. Disorders of the red cell membrane. In Orkin, S. H., Fisher, D. E., Ginsburg, D., et al., [Eds.], *Nathan and Oski's Hematology and Oncology of Infancy and Childhood* [8th ed., p. 521, Figure 16.4]. Philadelphia: Elsevier.)

is called *colloid osmotic hemolysis*. The concentration of K^+ is higher in RBCs than plasma K^+, whereas Na^+ and Ca^{2+} cytoplasmic concentrations are lower. Disequilibria are maintained by the energy-dependent membrane enzymes: K^+-ATPase, Na^+-ATPase, and Ca^{2+}-ATPase. Pump failure leads to cation imbalance, water influx, cell swelling, and hemolysis. Hemolysis can cause falsely increased levels of plasma K^+.

Defects in the ion channels result in RBC volume disorders, such as *overhydrated stomatocytosis (hereditary hydrocytosis)*, in which the membrane is excessively permeable to sodium and potassium, and *dehydrated stomatocytosis (hereditary xerocytosis)*, in which the RBC membrane is excessively permeable to potassium (Chapter 21).[53]

Sickle cell disease also provides an example of increased cation permeability. When hemoglobin S polymerizes upon deoxygenation, the cell deforms into a sickle shape and the membrane becomes more permeable to Ca^{2+}. This causes a downstream effect of increased Na^+ and K^+, eventually resulting in hemolysis.[52] Over time the increased Ca^{2+} leads to decrease in deformability and irreversibly sickled shape (Chapter 24).

SUMMARY

- Red blood cells (RBCs) lack mitochondria, the cellular adenosine triphosphate (ATP) powerhouse. Instead, ATP is produced in the RBC cytoplasm through anaerobic glycolysis using the Embden-Meyerhof pathway (EMP).
- Glucose is required to generate ATP and enters the RBC by facilitated diffusion via the transmembrane protein Glut-1.
- The EMP metabolizes glucose to pyruvate, consuming two ATP molecules. The EMP subsequently generates four ATP molecules per glucose molecule, a net gain of two. Within the EMP, there are three diversion pathways (shunts): the hexose-monophosphate pathway (HMP), methemoglobin reductase pathway, and Rapoport-Luebering pathway.

- The HMP converts glucose to pentose and generates the reduced form of nicotinamide adenine dinucleotide phosphate (NADPH). NADPH reduces oxidized glutathione. Reduced glutathione reduces peroxides and protects proteins, lipids, and heme iron from oxidation.
- The methemoglobin reductase pathway converts ferric heme iron (Fe^{3+}, methemoglobin) that is unable to bind oxygen (O_2) to the reduced ferrous (Fe^{2+}) form, which allows for O_2 binding.
- The Rapoport-Luebering pathway generates 2,3-bisphosphoglycerate and enhances O_2 delivery to tissues.
- The RBC membrane is a lipid bilayer whose hydrophobic components are sequestered from aqueous plasma and cytoplasm. The membrane provides a semipermeable barrier, separating plasma from cytoplasm and maintaining an osmotic differential.

- Deformability of the RBC is determined by the geometric shape, viscosity, and cell membrane composition. Inability to deform and pass through the small splenic pores results in the removal of the RBC from circulation.
- RBC membrane phospholipids are asymmetrically distributed. Phosphatidylcholine and sphingomyelin predominate in the outer layer; phosphatidylserine and phosphatidylethanolamine form most of the inner layer. The asymmetry of the phospholipids is maintained by membrane enzymes flippase, floppase, and scramblase.
- RBC membrane cholesterol and phospholipids are found in equal quantities. Abnormalities in the concentration of membrane cholesterol and phospholipids are associated with changes in RBC morphology: acanthocytosis (increased cholesterol to phospholipids) and target cells (increased cholesterol and increased phospholipid).
- RBC transmembrane proteins transport ions, water, and glucose and anchor cell membrane receptors. Transmembrane proteins are critical in the ankyrin complex and the actin junctional (4.1) complex to provide the vertical membrane support and to connect the lipid bilayer to the underlying cytoskeleton to maintain membrane integrity and prevent membrane loss.

- Shape and flexibility of the RBC, which are essential to its function, depend on the cytoskeleton. The cytoskeleton is derived from peripheral proteins on the cytoplasmic side of the lipid membrane. The major cytoskeletal proteins are α-spectrin and β-spectrin heterodimers, which associate with tetramers, and their ends connect to the actin junctional complex, forming a hexagonal cytoskeletal lattice adjacent to the cytoplasmic side of the lipid bilayer. Cytoskeletal proteins provide the horizontal or lateral support for the membrane.
- Hereditary spherocytosis arises from defects in spectrin or proteins forming the ankyrin complex that provide vertical support for the membrane. Hereditary elliptocytosis is due to defects in cytoskeletal proteins that provide horizontal support for the membrane.
- Osmotic balance of the RBC is maintained through ATP-dependent pumps to maintain high RBC cytoplasmic K^+ concentration. Pump failure leads to cation imbalance, water influx, and hemolysis.

Now that you have completed this chapter, go back and read again the case study at the beginning and respond to the questions presented. Answers can be found in Appendix C.

REVIEW QUESTIONS

Answers can be found in Appendix C.

1. Which RBC process does NOT require energy?
   a. Cytoskeletal protein deformability
   b. Maintaining cytoplasm cationic electrochemical gradients
   c. Oxygen transport
   d. Preventing the peroxidation of proteins and lipids
2. What pathway anaerobically generates energy in the form of ATP?
   a. 2,3-BPG pathway
   b. Embden-Meyerhof pathway
   c. Hexose monophosphate pathway
   d. Rapoport-Luebering pathway
3. Which of the following hexose-monophosphate shunt products participate in the detoxification of peroxides?
   a. 2,3-BPG and 3-phosphoglycerate
   b. ATP and NADH
   c. NADPH and reduced glutathione
   d. Pyruvate and lactate
4. What is the role of 2,3-BPG in the RBC?
   a. Enhances O_2 release from hemoglobin
   b. Increases the production of ATP in the RBC
   c. Protects hemoglobin from oxidation
   d. Provides glucose to the EMP
5. Hemoglobin iron may become oxidized to ferric iron (Fe^{3+}) by several pathologic mechanisms. What portion of the Embden-Meyerhof pathway reduces iron to the ferrous form (Fe^{2+})?
   a. Hexose monophosphate pathway
   b. Methemoglobin reductase pathway
   c. Rapoport-Luebering pathway
   d. 2,3-BPG shunt

6. RBC membranes block passage of most large molecules such as proteins but allow passage of small molecules such as water and the anions bicarbonate (HCO_3^-) and chloride (Cl^-). What is the term for this membrane property?
   a. Deformable
   b. Flexible
   c. Intangible
   d. Semipermeable
7. How are the RBC membrane phospholipids arranged?
   a. In a hexagonal lattice
   b. In chains beneath a protein cytoskeleton
   c. With two layers whose composition is asymmetric
   d. With hydrophobic portions facing the plasma
8. RBC membrane cholesterol is replenished from the:
   a. Cytoplasm
   b. EMB pathway
   c. Mitochondria
   d. Plasma
9. Which of the following is an example of a transmembrane or integral membrane protein?
   a. Actin
   b. Ankyrin
   c. Band 3
   d. Spectrin
10. What is one of the roles of aquaporin-1 in the RBC membrane?
    a. Attach the cytoskeleton to the lipid layer and prevent membrane loss
    b. Create water influx in response to osmotic gradient changes
    c. Initiate the production of 2,3-BPG in response to hypoxia
    d. Provide strength and flexibility to the RBC

11. Defects in vertical linkages in the RBC membrane are associated with which of the following conditions?
   a. Hereditary elliptocytosis
   b. Hereditary spherocytosis
   c. Hereditary xerocytosis
   d. Overhydrated stomatocytosis

12. Abnormalities in the horizontal and vertical linkages of the transmembrane and cytoskeletal RBC membrane proteins may be seen as:
   a. Enzyme pathway deficiencies
   b. Methemoglobin increase
   c. Reduced hemoglobin content
   d. Shape changes

REFERENCES

1. Percy, M. J., & Lappin, T. R. (2008). Recessive congenital methaemoglobinaemia: cytochrome b5 reductase deficiency. *Brit J Haematol, 141*, 298–308.
2. Mohandas, N. (2021). Structure and composition of the erythrocyte. In K. Kaushansky, J. T. Prchal, L. J. Burns, et al. (Eds.), *Williams Hematology*. (10th ed., pp 513–528). New York: McGraw-Hill.
3. Quigley, J. G., Means, R. T., & Glader, B. (2018). The birth, life, and death of red blood cells, erythropoiesis, the mature red blood cell, and cell destruction. In Greer, J. P., Arber, D. A., Glader, B., et al. (Eds.), *Wintrobe's Clinical Hematology*. (14th ed., pp. 83–124). Philadelphia: Wolters Kluwer Health/Lippincott Williams & Wilkins.
4. Bartels M, Van Beer, E., & Wijk, R. (2021). Erythrocyte enzyme disorders. In K. Kaushansky, J. T. Prchal, L. J. Burns, et al. (Eds.), *Williams Hematology*. (10th ed., pp. 749–784). New York: McGraw-Hill.
5. Zhang, J. Z., & Ismail-Beigi, F. (1998). Activation of glut1 glucose transporter in human erythrocytes. *Arch Biochem Biophys, 356*(1), 86–92.
6. Gregg, X. T., & Prchal, J. T. (2023). Red blood cell enzymopathies. In Hoffman, R., Benz, E. J., Silberstein, L. E., et al. (Eds.), *Hematology, Basic Principles and Practice*. (8th ed., pp. 638–649). Philadelphia: Elsevier.
7. Beutler, E. (1990). Disorders of red cells resulting from enzyme abnormalities. *Semin Hematol, 27*, 137–167.
8. Prchal, J. T. (2021). Methemoglobinemia and other dyshemoglobinemias. In K. Kaushansky, J. T. Prchal, L. J. Burns, et al. (Eds.), *Williams Hematology*. (10th ed., pp. 859–870). New York: McGraw-Hill.
9. Mohandas, N., & Gallagher, P. G. (2008). Red cell membrane: past, present, and future. *Blood, 112*, 3939–3948.
10. Kim, J., Lee, H., & Shin, S. (2015). Advances in the measurement of red blood cell deformability: a brief review. *J Cell Biotechnology, 1*, 63–79.
11. Mohandas, N., & Chasis, J. A. (1993). Red blood cell deformability, membrane material properties, and shape: regulation by transmembrane, skeletal and cytosolic proteins and lipids. *Semin Hematol, 30*, 171–192.
12. Cooper, R. A. (1970). Lipids of human red cell membrane: normal composition and variability in disease. *Semin Hematol, 7*, 296–322.
13. Singer, S. J., & Nicolson, G. L. (1972). The fluid mosaic model of the structure of cell membranes. *Science, 175*, 720–731.
14. Nicolson, G. L. (2014). The fluid mosaic model of membrane structure: still relevant to understanding the structure, function and dynamics of biological membranes after more than 40 years. *Biochim Biophys Acta, 1838*, 1451–1466.
15. Cooper, R. A. (1978). Influence of the increased membrane cholesterol on membrane fluidity and cell function in human red blood cells. *J Supramol Struct, 8*, 413–430.

16. Ohkawa, R., Low, H., Mukhamedova, N., et al (2020). Cholesterol transport between red blood cells and lipoproteins contributes to cholesterol metabolism in blood. *J Lipid Res, 61*(12), 1577–1588.
17. Zhou, Q., Zhao, J., Stout, J. G., et al. (1997). Molecular cloning of human plasma membrane phospholipid scramblase. A protein mediating transbilayer movement of plasma membrane phospholipids. *J Biol Chem, 272*, 18240–18244.
18. Abed, M., Thiel, C., Towhid, S. T., et al. (2017). Simulation of erythrocyte cell membrane scrambling by C-reactive protein. *Cell Physiol Biochem, 41*, 806–818.
19. Cooper, R. A., & Jandl, J. H. (1968). Bile salts and cholesterol in the pathogenesis of target cells in obstructive jaundice. *J Clin Invest, 47*, 809–822.
20. Alberts, B., Johnson, A., Lewis, J., et al. (2015). Membrane structure. In *Molecular Biology of the Cell*. (6th ed., pp. 565–596). New York: Garland Science.
21. Steck, T. (1974). The organization of proteins in the human red blood cell membrane. *J Cell Biol, 62*, 1–19.
22. Pasini, E. M., Kirkegaard, M., Mortensen, P., et al. (2006). In-depth analysis of the membrane and cytosolic proteome of red blood cells. *Blood, 108*, 791–801.
23. Bennett, V. (1985). The membrane skeleton of human erythrocytes and its implications for more complex cells. *Annu Rev Biochem, 54*, 273–304.
24. Burton, N. M., & Bruce, L. J. (2011) Modeling the structure of the red cell membrane. *Biochem Cell Biol, 89*, 200–215.
25. Fairbanks, G., Steck, T. L., & Wallach, D. F. (1971). Electrophoretic analysis of the major polypeptides of the human erythrocyte membrane. *Biochemistry, 10*, 2606–2617.
26. Reinhart, A. F., Casey, J. C., Kalli, A. C., et al. (2016). Band 3, the human red cell chloride/bicarbonate anion exchanger (AE1, SLC4A1), in a structural context. *Biochimica et biophysica acta, 1858*, 1507–1532.
27. Bennett, V. (1983). Proteins involved in membrane-cytoskeleton association in human erythrocytes: spectrin, ankyrin, and band 3. *Methods Enzymol, 96*, 313–324.
28. Mankelow, T. J., Satchwell, T. J., & Burton, N. M. (2012). Refined views of multi-protein complexes in the erythrocyte membrane. *Blood Cells Mol Dis, 49*, 1–10.
29. Reid, M. E., & Mohandas, N. (2004). Red blood cell blood group antigens: structure and function. *Semin Hematol, 41*, 93–117.
30. Giger, K., Habib, I. Ritchie, K., et al. (2016). Diffusion of glycophorin A in human erythrocytes. *Biochim Biophys Acta, 1858*, 2839–2845.
31. Khan, A. A., Hanada, T., Mohseni, M., et al. (2008). Dematin and adducin provide a novel link between the spectrin cytoskeleton and human erythrocyte membrane by directly interacting with glucose transporter-1. *J Biol Chem, 283*, 14600–14609.
32. Wang, Y., Zhao, N., Xiong, et al. (2020). Downregulated recycling process but not de novo synthesis of glutathione limits antioxidant capacity of erythrocytes in hypoxia. *Oxid Med Cell Longev, 2020*, 7834252.

33. Daniels, G. (2013). ABO, H, and Lewis systems. In *Human Blood Groups*. (3rd ed., pp. 11–95). West Sussex, UK: Wiley-Blackwell.

34. Daniels, G. (2013). MNS blood group system. In *Human Blood Groups*. (3rd ed., pp. 96–161). West Sussex, UK: Wiley-Blackwell.

35. Daniels, G. (2013). Gerbich blood group system. In *Human Blood Groups*. (3rd ed., pp. 410–426). West Sussex, UK: Wiley-Blackwell.

36. Daniels, G. (2013). Rh and RHAG blood group systems. In *Human Blood Groups*. (3rd ed., pp. 182–258). West Sussex, UK: Wiley-Blackwell.

37. Daniels, G. (2013). Duffy blood group system. In *Human Blood Groups*. (3rd ed., pp. 306–324). West Sussex, UK: Wiley-Blackwell.

38. Azouzi, S., Collec, E., Mohandas, N., et al. (2015). The human Kell blood group binds the erythroid 4.1R protein: new insights into the 4.1R-dependent red cell membrane complex. *Br J Haematol*, *171*(5), 862–871.

39. Daniels, G. (2013). Kidd blood group system. In *Human Blood Groups*. (3rd ed., pp. 325–335). West Sussex, UK: Wiley-Blackwell.

40. Parker, C. J. (2021). Paroxysmal nocturnal hemoglobinuria. In K. Kaushansky, J. T. Prchal, L. J. Burns, et al. (Eds.), *Williams Hematology*. (10th ed., pp. 625–638). New York: McGraw-Hill.

41. Shotton, D. M., Burke, B. E., & Branton, D. (1979). The molecular structure of human erythrocyte spectrin: biophysical and electron microscope studies. *J Mol Biol*, *131*, 303–329.

42. Liu, S. C., Drick, L. H., & Palek, J. (1987). Visualization of the hexagonal lattice in the erythrocyte membrane skeleton. *J Cell Biol*, *104*, 527–536.

43. Speicher, D. W., & Marchesi, V. T. (1984). Erythrocyte spectrin is composed of many homologous triple helical segments. *Nature*, *311*, 177–180.

44. Lu, Y., Hanada, T., Fujiwara, Y., et al. (2016). Gene disruption of dematin causes precipitous loss of erythrocyte membrane stability and severe hemolytic anemia. *Blood*, *128*, 93–103.

45. An, X., Guo, X., Zhang, X., et al. (2006). Conformational stabilities of the structural repeats of erythroid spectrin and their functional implications. *J Biol Chem*, *281*, 10527–10532.

46. Da Costa, L., Galimand, J., Fenneteau, O., et al. (2013). Hereditary spherocytosis, elliptocytosis, and other red cell membrane disorders. *Blood Reviews*, *27*, 167–178.

47. Andolfo, I., Russo, R., Gambale, A., et al. (2016). New insights on hereditary erythrocyte membrane defects. *Haematologica*, *101*, 1284–1294.

48. Gallagher, P. G. (2013). Abnormalities of the erythrocyte membrane. *Pediatr Clin North Am*, *60*, 1349–1362.

49. Crisp, R. L., Maltaneri, R. E., Vittori, D. C., et al. (2016). Red blood cell aquaporin-1 expression is decreased in hereditary spherocytosis. *Ann Hematol*, *95*, 1595–1601.

50. Brugnara, C. (1997). Erythrocyte membrane transport physiology. *Curr Opin Hematol*, *4*, 122–127.

51. Chu, H., Puchulu-Campanella, E., Galan, J. A., et al. (2012). Identification of cytoskeletal elements enclosing the ATP pools that fuel human red blood cell membrane cation pumps. *Proc Natl Acad Sci*, *109*, 12794–12799.

52. Bogdanova, A., Makhro, A., Wang, J., et al. (2013) Calcium in red blood cells – a perilous balance. *Int J Mol Sci*, *14*, 9848–9872.

53. Badens, C., & Guizouarn, H. (2016). Advances in understanding the pathogenesis of the red cell volume disorders. *Br J Haematol*, *174*, 674–685.

8

Hemoglobin Metabolism

*Catherine N. Otto**

OBJECTIVES

After completion of this chapter, the reader will be able to:

1. Describe the components and structure of hemoglobin.
2. Describe steps in heme synthesis that occur in the mitochondria and the cytoplasm.
3. Name the genes and the chromosome location and arrangement for the various polypeptide chains of hemoglobin.
4. Describe the polypeptide chains produced and the hemoglobins they form in the embryo, fetus, newborn, and adult.
5. List the three types of normal hemoglobin in adults and their reference intervals.
6. Describe mechanisms that regulate hemoglobin synthesis.
7. Describe the mechanism by which hemoglobin transports oxygen to the tissues and transports carbon dioxide to the lungs.
8. Explain the importance of maintaining hemoglobin iron in the ferrous state (Fe^{2+}).
9. Explain the significance of the sigmoid shape of the oxygen dissociation curve.
10. Correlate right and left shifts in the hemoglobin-oxygen dissociation curve with conditions that can cause shifts in the curve.
11. Differentiate T and R forms of hemoglobin and the effect of oxygen and 2,3-bisphosphoglycerate on those forms.
12. Explain the difference between adult hemoglobin (Hb A) and fetal hemoglobin (Hb F) and how that difference affects oxygen affinity.
13. Compare and contrast the composition and the effect on oxygen binding of methemoglobin, carboxyhemoglobin, and sulfhemoglobin.

OUTLINE

Hemoglobin Structure
  Heme Structure
  Globin Structure
  Complete Hemoglobin Molecule
Hemoglobin Biosynthesis
  Heme Biosynthesis
  Globin Biosynthesis
  Hemoglobin Assembly
Hemoglobin Ontogeny
Regulation of Hemoglobin Production
  Heme Regulation

  Globin Regulation
  Systemic Regulation of Erythropoiesis
Hemoglobin Function
  Oxygen Transport
  Carbon Dioxide Transport
  Nitric Oxide Transport
Dyshemoglobins
  Methemoglobin
  Sulfhemoglobin
  Carboxyhemoglobin
Hemoglobin Measurement

CASE STUDY

After studying the material in this chapter, the reader should be able to respond to the following case study. Answers can be found in Appendix C.

Hemoglobin and hemoglobin fractionation and quantification using high-performance liquid chromatography (HPLC) were performed on a mother and her newborn infant, both presumed to be healthy. The assays were part of a screening program to establish reference intervals. The mother's HGB was 14 g/dL, and the newborn's HGB was 20 g/dL. Reference intervals can be found after the Index at the end of the book. The mother's hemoglobin fractions were quantified as 97% Hb A, 2% Hb A2, and 1% Hb F by HPLC. The newborn's results were 88% Hb F and 12% Hb A.

1. Were these hemoglobin results within expected reference intervals?
2. Why were the mother's and the newborn's hemoglobin concentration so different?
3. What is the difference between the test to determine the hemoglobin concentration and the test to analyze hemoglobin by HPLC?
4. Why were the mother's and newborn's hemoglobin fractions so different?

*The author extends appreciation to Mary Coleman and Elaine M. Keohane, whose work in prior editions provided the foundation for this chapter.

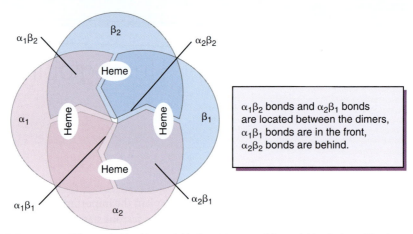

Figure 8.1 Structure of Hemoglobin. Hemoglobin is a tetramer of four globin chains with a heme attached to each globin chain.

Hemoglobin is one of the most studied proteins in the body because of the ability to easily isolate it from red blood cells (RBCs). It comprises approximately 95% of the cytoplasmic content of RBCs.[1] The body efficiently carries hemoglobin in RBCs, which provides protection from denaturation in the plasma and loss through the kidneys. Free (non-RBC) hemoglobin, generated from RBCs through hemolysis, has a short half-life outside of RBCs. When released into the plasma, it is rapidly salvaged to preserve its iron and amino acid components; when salvage capacity is exceeded, it is excreted by the kidneys (Chapter 20). The concentration of hemoglobin within RBCs is approximately 34 g/dL, and its molecular weight is approximately 64,000 Daltons.[2] The main function of hemoglobin is to transport oxygen from the lungs to tissues and transport carbon dioxide from tissues to the lungs for exhalation. Hemoglobin also contributes to acid-base balance by binding and releasing hydrogen ions and transporting nitric oxide, a regulator of vascular tone.[1,3]

This chapter discusses the structure, biosynthesis, ontogeny, regulation, and function of hemoglobin. The formation, composition, and characteristics of several dyshemoglobins, namely methemoglobin, carboxyhemoglobin, and sulfhemoglobin, and hemoglobin measurement, are also discussed at the end of the chapter.

HEMOGLOBIN STRUCTURE

Hemoglobin is the first protein whose structure was described using x-ray crystallography.[4] The hemoglobin molecule is a globular protein consisting of two different pairs of polypeptide chains and four heme groups, with one heme group embedded in each of the four polypeptide chains (Figure 8.1).

Heme Structure

Heme consists of a ring of carbon, hydrogen, and nitrogen atoms called *protoporphyrin IX,* with a central atom of divalent ferrous iron (Fe^{2+}) (Figure 8.2). Each of the four heme groups is positioned in a pocket of the polypeptide chain near the surface of the hemoglobin molecule. The ferrous iron in each heme molecule reversibly combines with one oxygen molecule. When the ferrous irons are oxidized to the ferric

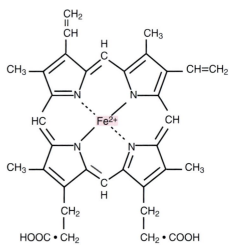

Figure 8.2 Structure of Heme. Heme consists of protoporphyrin IX with a central ferrous iron atom.

TABLE 8.1	**Globin Chains**	
Symbol	**Name**	**Number of Amino Acids**
α	Alpha	141
β	Beta	146
γ_A	Gamma A	146 (position 136: alanine)
γ_G	Gamma G	146 (position 136: glycine)
δ	Delta	146
ϵ	Epsilon	146
ζ	Zeta	141
ϑ	Theta	Unknown

state (Fe^{3+}), they no longer can bind oxygen. Oxidized hemoglobin is also called *methemoglobin* and is discussed later in "Methemoglobin."

Globin Structure

The four globin chains comprising each hemoglobin molecule consist of two identical pairs of unlike polypeptide chains, 141 to 146 amino acids each. Variations in amino acid sequences give rise to different types of polypeptide chains. Each chain is designated by a Greek letter (Table 8.1).[1,3]

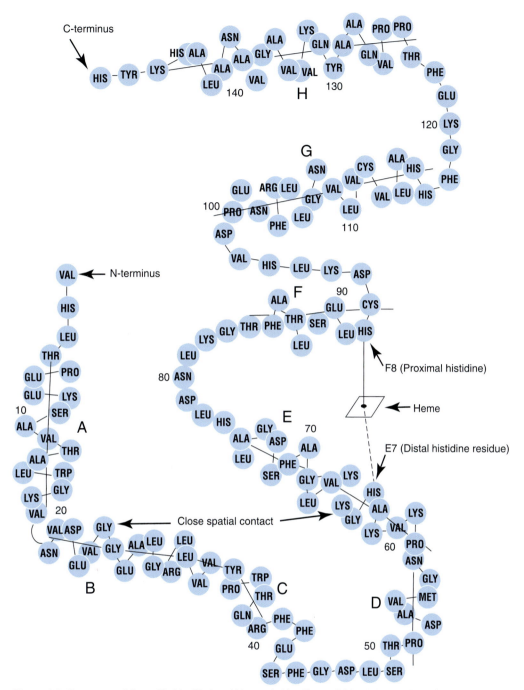

Figure 8.3 Structure of the β-Globin Chain of Hemoglobin. The β-globin chain consists of helical (labeled *A* through *H*) and nonhelical segments. Heme (protoporphyrin IX with a central iron atom) is suspended in a pocket between the *E* and *F* helices. The iron atom of heme is linked to the F8 proximal histidine on one side of the heme plane *(solid line)*. Oxygen binds to the iron atom on the other side of the plane and is close (but not linked) to the E7 distal histidine *(dotted line)*. (Modified from Huisman, T. H., Schroder, W. A. [1971]. *New Aspects of the Structure, Function, and Synthesis of Hemoglobins*. Boca Raton: CRC Press; and Stamatoyan-nopoulos, G. [1994]. *The Molecular Basis of Blood Diseases.* [2nd ed.]. Philadelphia: Saunders.)

Each globin chain is divided into eight helices separated by seven nonhelical segments (Figure 8.3).[3] The helices, designated A to H, contain subgroup numberings for the sequence of the amino acids in each helix and are relatively rigid and linear. Flexible nonhelical segments connect the helices, as reflected by their designations: NA for the sequence between the N-terminus and the A helix, AB for the sequence between the A and B helices, and so forth, with BC, CD, DE, EF, FG, GH, and finally HC between the H helix and the C-terminus.[3]

Complete Hemoglobin Molecule

The hemoglobin molecule can be described by its primary, secondary, tertiary, and quaternary protein structures. The *primary structure* refers to the amino acid sequence of the

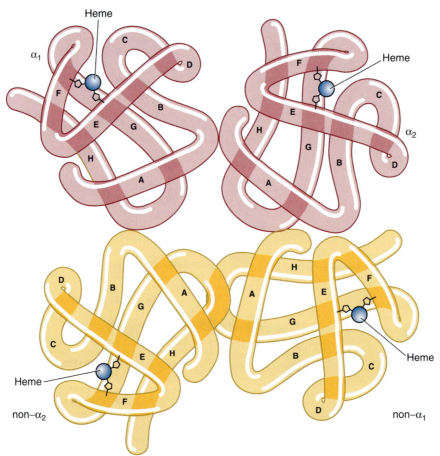

Figure 8.4 Hemoglobin Molecule Illustrating Tertiary Folding of the Four Polypeptide Chains. Heme is suspended between the *E* and *F* helices of each polypeptide chain. Pink represents α_1 *(left)* and α_2 *(right)*; yellow represents non-α_2 *(left)* and non-α_1 *(right)*. The polypeptide chains first form α_1-non-α_1 and α_2-non-α_2 dimers and then assemble into a tetramer (quaternary structure), with α_1-non-α_2 and α_2-non-α_1 bonds.

polypeptide chains. The *secondary structure* refers to chain arrangements in helices and nonhelices. The *tertiary structure* refers to the arrangement of the helices into a pretzel-like configuration.

Globin chains loop to form a cleft pocket for heme. Each chain contains a heme group that is suspended between the E and F helices of the polypeptide chain (Figure 8.3).[2,3] The iron atom at the center of the protoporphyrin IX ring of heme is positioned between two histidine radicals, forming a proximal histidine bond within F8 and, through the linked oxygen, a close association with the distal histidine residue in E7.[3] Globin chain amino acids in the cleft are hydrophobic, whereas amino acids on the outside are hydrophilic, which renders the molecule water soluble. This arrangement also helps iron remain in its divalent ferrous form regardless of whether it is oxygenated (carrying an oxygen molecule) or deoxygenated (not carrying an oxygen molecule).

The *quaternary structure* of hemoglobin, also called a *tetramer,* describes the complete hemoglobin molecule. The complete hemoglobin molecule is spherical, has four heme groups attached to four polypeptide chains, and may carry up to four molecules of oxygen (Figure 8.4). The predominant adult hemoglobin, Hb A, is composed of two α-globin chains and two β-globin chains. Strong α_1-β_1 and α_2-β_2 bonds hold the dimers in a stable form. The α_1-β_2 and α_2-β_1 bonds are important for

the stability of the quaternary structure in the oxygenated and deoxygenated forms (Figure 8.1).[1,2]

A small percentage of Hb A is *glycated*. Glycation is a posttranslational modification formed by the nonenzymatic binding of various sugars to globin chain amino groups over the life span of the RBC. The most characterized of the glycated hemoglobins is Hb A_{1c}, in which glucose attaches to the N-terminal valine of the β chain.[1] Normally, about 4% to 6% of Hb A circulates in the A_{1c} form. In uncontrolled diabetes mellitus, the amount of A_{1c} is increased proportionally to the mean blood glucose level over the preceding 2 to 3 months.

HEMOGLOBIN BIOSYNTHESIS

Heme Biosynthesis

Heme biosynthesis occurs in the mitochondria and cytoplasm of bone marrow erythroid precursors, beginning with the pronormoblast through the circulating polychromatic (also known as polychromatophilic) erythrocyte (Chapter 6). As they lose their ribosomes and mitochondria, mature erythrocytes can no longer make hemoglobin.[1]

Heme biosynthesis begins in the mitochondria with the condensation of *glycine* and *succinyl coenzyme A* (CoA) catalyzed by *aminolevulinate synthase* to form *aminolevulinic acid* (ALA)

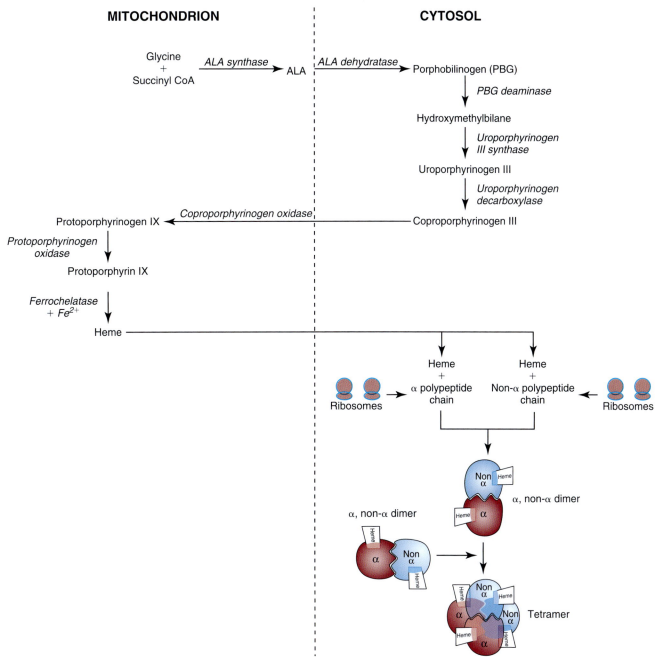

Figure 8.5 Heme Biosynthesis and Hemoglobin Assembly. Heme biosynthesis begins with the condensation of glycine and succinyl coenzyme A *(CoA)* forming aminolevulinic acid *(ALA)* in a reaction catalyzed by aminolevulinate synthase. In the cytoplasm, ALA undergoes several transformations from porphobilinogen *(PBG)* to coproporphyrinogen III which, catalyzed by coproporphyrinogen oxidase, becomes protoporphyrinogen IX. In the mitochondria, protoporphyrinogen IX is converted to protoporphyrin IX by protoporphyrinogen oxidase. Ferrous *(Fe²⁺)* ion is added, catalyzed by ferrochelatase to form heme. In the cytoplasm, heme assembles with an α chain and non-α chain, forming a dimer, and ultimately, two dimers join to form the hemoglobin tetramer.

(Figure 8.5).[1] In the cytoplasm, *aminolevulinic acid dehydratase* (also known as *porphobilinogen synthase*) converts ALA to *porphobilinogen* (PBG). PBG undergoes several transformations in the cytoplasm from *hydroxymethylbilane* to *coproporphyrinogen III.* This pathway then continues in the mitochondria until, in the final step of production of heme, Fe^{2+} combines with *protoporphyrin IX* in the presence of *ferrochelatase (heme synthase)* to make heme.[1]

Transferrin, a plasma protein, carries iron in the ferric (Fe^{3+}) form to developing erythroid cells (Chapter 9). Transferrin binds to transferrin receptors on erythroid precursor cell membranes, and the receptors and transferrin (with bound iron) are brought into the cell in an endosome (Figure 9.8). Acidification of the endosome releases iron from transferrin. Iron is transported out of the endosome and into the mitochondria, where it is reduced to the ferrous state and is united with protoporphyrin

IX to make heme. Heme leaves the mitochondria and is joined to the globin chains in the cytoplasm.

Globin Biosynthesis

Six structural genes code for six globin chains. The α- and ζ-globin genes are on the short arm of chromosome 16; the $\in$-, γ-, δ-, and β-globin gene cluster is on the short arm of chromosome 11 (Figure 25.1). In the human genome, there is one copy of each globin gene per chromatid for a total of two genes per diploid cell, with the exception of α and γ. There are two copies of the α- and γ-globin genes per chromatid for a total of four genes per diploid cell.

Production of globin chains takes place in erythroid precursors from the pronormoblast through the circulating polychromatic erythrocyte but not in mature erythrocytes.[1] Transcription of the globin genes to messenger ribonucleic acid (mRNA) occurs in the nucleus, and translation of mRNA to the globin polypeptide chain occurs on ribosomes in the cytoplasm. Although transcription of α-globin genes produces more mRNA than the β-globin gene, there is less efficient translation of the α-globin mRNA.[2] Therefore the α and β chains are produced in approximately equal amounts. After translation is complete, chains are released from the ribosomes in the cytoplasm.

Hemoglobin Assembly

After their release from ribosomes, each globin chain binds to a heme molecule and then forms a heterodimer (Figure 8.5). The non-α chains have a charge difference that determines their affinity to bind to α chains. The α chain has a positive charge and has the highest affinity for a β chain because of its negative charge.[1,2] The γ-globin chain has the next highest affinity, followed by the δ-globin chain.[2] Two heterodimers then combine to form a tetramer. This completes the hemoglobin molecule.

Two α and two β chains form Hb A, the major hemoglobin present from 6 months of age through adulthood. Hb A_2 contains two α and two δ chains. Owing to a mutation in the promoter region of the δ-globin gene, production of the δ chain polypeptide is very low.[5] Consequently, Hb A_2 comprises less than 3.5% of total hemoglobin in adults. Fetal hemoglobin (Hb F) contains two α and two γ chains. In healthy adults, Hb F comprises 1% to 2% of total hemoglobin, and it is present only in a small proportion of the RBCs (uneven distribution). These RBCs with Hb F are called F or A/F cells.[1,2]

The various amino acids that comprise the globin chains affect the net charge of the hemoglobin tetramer. Electrophoresis and high-performance liquid chromatography (HPLC) are used for fractionation, presumptive identification, and quantification of normal hemoglobins and hemoglobin variants (Chapter 24). Molecular genetic testing of globin gene DNA provides definitive identification of variant hemoglobins.

HEMOGLOBIN ONTOGENY

Hemoglobin composition differs with prenatal gestation time and postnatal age. Hemoglobin changes reflect the sequential activation and inactivation (or switching) of the globin genes,

progressing from the ζ- to the α-globin gene on chromosome 16 and from the $\in$- to the γ-, δ-, and β-globin genes on chromosome 11. The ζ- and $\in$-globin chains normally appear only during the first 3 months of embryonic development. These two chains, when paired with the α and γ chains, form the embryonic hemoglobins (Figure 8.6). During the second and third trimesters of fetal life and at birth, Hb F ($\alpha_2\gamma_2$) is the predominant hemoglobin. By 6 months of age and through adulthood, Hb A ($\alpha_2\beta_2$) is the predominant hemoglobin, with small amounts of Hb A_2 ($\alpha_2\delta_2$) and Hb F.[2] Table 8.2 presents the reference intervals for the normal hemoglobin fractions at various ages.

REGULATION OF HEMOGLOBIN PRODUCTION

Heme Regulation

The key rate-limiting step in heme synthesis is the initial reaction of glycine and succinyl CoA to form ALA, catalyzed by ALA synthase (Figure 8.5). Heme inhibits the transcription of the ALA synthase gene, which leads to a decrease in heme production (a negative feedback mechanism). Heme inhibits other enzymes in the biosynthesis pathway, including ALA dehydrase and PBG deaminase. A negative feedback mechanism by heme or substrate inhibition by protoporphyrin IX is believed to inhibit the ferrochelatase enzyme.[1] Conversely, an increased demand for heme induces an increased synthesis of ALA synthase.[1]

Globin Regulation

Globin synthesis is highly regulated so that there is a balanced production of globin and heme. This is critical because an excess of globin chains, protoporphyrin IX, or iron can accumulate and damage the cell, reducing its life span.

Globin production is mainly controlled at the transcription level by a complex interaction of DNA sequences (cis-acting promoters, enhancers, and silencers) and soluble transcription factors (trans-acting factors) that bind to DNA or to one another to promote or suppress transcription.[2] Initiation of transcription of a particular globin gene requires (1) the promoter DNA sequences immediately before the 5′ end or the beginning of the gene; (2) a key transcription factor called Krüppel-like factor 1 (KLF1); (3) a number of other transcription factors (such as GATA1, Ikaros, TAL1, p45-NF-E2, and LDB1); and (4) an enhancer region of DNAse 1 hypersensitive nucleic acid sequences located more than 20 kilobases upstream (before the 5′ start site of the gene) from the globin gene called the locus control region (LCR).[6] For example, to activate transcription of the β-globin gene in the β-globin gene cluster on chromosome 11, the LCR, the promoter for the β-globin gene, and various transcription factors join together to form a three-dimensional active chromosome hub (ACH), with KLF1 playing a key role in connecting the complex.[6,7] Because the LCR is located a distance upstream from the β-globin gene complex, a loop of DNA is formed when the LCR and β-globin gene promoter join together in the chromosome hub.[7] The other globin genes in the cluster ($\in$-, γ-, and δ-globin) are maintained in the inactive state in the DNA loop, so only the β-globin gene is transcribed.[6,7]

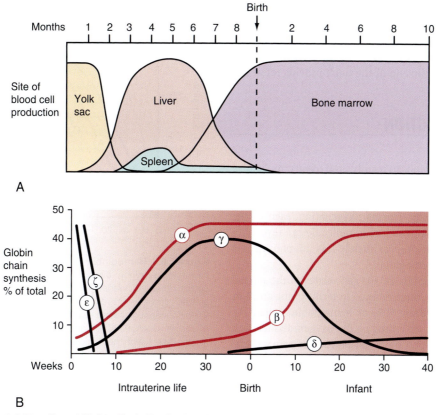

Figure 8.6 Timeline of Globin Chain Production From Intrauterine Life to Adulthood. See also Table 8.2.

TABLE 8.2	Normal Hemoglobins	
Stage	**Globin Chain**	**Hemoglobin**
Intrauterine		
Early embryogenesis (product of yolk sac erythroblasts)	$\zeta_2 + \epsilon_2$	Gower-1
	$\alpha_2 + \epsilon_2$	Gower-2
	$\zeta_2 + \gamma_2$	Portland
Begins in early embryogenesis; peaks during third trimester and begins to decline just before birth	$\alpha_2 + \gamma_2$	F
Birth		
	$\alpha_2 + \gamma_2$	F, 60%–90%
	$\alpha_2 + \beta_2$	A, 10%–40%
Two Years Through Adulthood		
	$\alpha_2 + \gamma_2$	F, 1%–2%
	$\alpha_2 + \delta_2$	A2, <3.5%
	$\alpha_2 + \beta_2$	A, >95%

KLF1 also plays a key regulatory role in the switch from γ chain to β chain production (γ-β switching) that begins in late fetal life and continues through adulthood. KLF1 is an exact match for binding to the DNA promoter sequences of the β-globin gene, whereas the γ-globin gene promoter has a slightly different sequence.[6] This results in a preferential binding to and subsequent activation of transcription of the β-globin gene.[7] KLF1 also regulates the expression of repressors of γ-globin gene transcription, such as BCL11A and MYB.[6,8]

Globin synthesis is also regulated during translation when mRNA coding for the globin chains associates with ribosomes to produce the polypeptide. Many protein factors are required to control initiation, elongation, and termination steps of translation. Heme is an important regulator of globin mRNA translation at the initiation step by promoting activation of a translation initiation factor and inactivating its repressor.[1] Conversely, when the heme level is low, the repressor accumulates and inactivates the initiation factor, thus blocking translation of the globin mRNA.[1,2]

Systemic Regulation of Erythropoiesis

When there is an insufficient quantity of hemoglobin or if the hemoglobin molecule is defective in transporting oxygen, tissue hypoxia occurs. Hypoxia is detected by the peritubular cells of the kidney, which respond by increasing production of erythropoietin (EPO). EPO increases the number of erythrocytes produced and released into the periphery; it also accelerates the rate of synthesis of erythrocyte components, including hemoglobin (Chapter 6).

Although each laboratory establishes its own reference intervals based on their instrumentation, methodology, and patient population, in general, reference intervals for hemoglobin concentration are as follows:

Men:	13.5–18.0 g/dL (135–180 g/L)
Women:	12.0–16.0 g/dL (120–160 g/L)
Newborns:	16.5–21.5 g/dL (165–215 g/L)

Reference intervals for infants and children vary according to age group. Individuals living at high altitudes have slightly higher levels of hemoglobin as a compensatory mechanism to provide more oxygen to the tissues in the oxygen-thin air. Tables after the Index at the end of the book provide reference intervals for all age groups.

HEMOGLOBIN FUNCTION

Oxygen Transport

The function of hemoglobin is to readily bind oxygen molecules in the lung, which requires high oxygen affinity; to transport oxygen; and to efficiently unload oxygen to the tissues, which requires low oxygen affinity. During oxygenation, each of the four heme iron atoms in a hemoglobin molecule can reversibly bind one oxygen molecule. Approximately 1.34 mL of oxygen is bound by each gram of hemoglobin.[1]

The affinity of hemoglobin for oxygen relates to the partial pressure of oxygen (PO_2), often defined in terms of the amount of oxygen needed to saturate 50% of hemoglobin, called P_{50} *value.* The relationship is described by the oxygen dissociation curve of hemoglobin, which plots the percent oxygen saturation of hemoglobin versus the PO_2 (Figure 8.7). The curve is *sigmoidal,* which indicates low hemoglobin affinity for oxygen at low oxygen tension and high affinity for oxygen at high oxygen tension.

Cooperation among hemoglobin subunits contributes to the shape of the curve. Hemoglobin that is completely deoxygenated has little affinity for oxygen. However, with each oxygen molecule that is bound, there is a change in the conformation of the tetramer that progressively increases the oxygen affinity of the other heme subunits. Once one oxygen molecule binds, the remainder of the hemoglobin molecule quickly becomes fully oxygenated.[2] Therefore with high oxygen tension in the lungs, the affinity of hemoglobin for oxygen is high, and hemoglobin becomes rapidly saturated with oxygen. Conversely, with relatively low oxygen tension in the tissues, the affinity of hemoglobin for oxygen is low, and hemoglobin rapidly releases oxygen.

Normally, a PO_2 of approximately 27 mm Hg results in 50% oxygen saturation of the hemoglobin molecule. If there is a shift of the curve to the left, 50% oxygen saturation of hemoglobin occurs at a PO_2 of less than 27 mm Hg. If there is a shift of the curve to the right, 50% oxygen saturation of hemoglobin occurs at a PO_2 higher than 27 mm Hg.

The reference interval for arterial oxygen saturation is 96% to 100%. If the oxygen dissociation curve shifts to the left, a patient with arterial and venous PO_2 levels in the reference intervals (80 to 100 mm Hg arterial and 30 to 50 mm Hg venous) will have a higher percent oxygen saturation and a higher affinity for oxygen than a patient for whom the curve is normal. With a shift in the curve to the right, a lower oxygen affinity is seen.

In addition to the PO_2, shifts of the curve to the left or right occur if there are changes in the pH of the blood. In the tissues, a lower pH shifts the curve to the right and reduces the affinity of hemoglobin for oxygen, and the hemoglobin more readily releases oxygen. A shift in the curve because of a change in pH (or hydrogen ion concentration) is termed the *Bohr effect.*

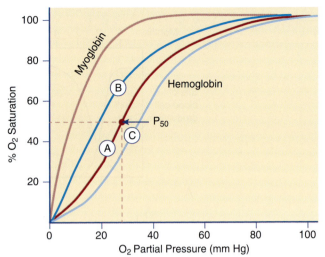

Figure 8.7 Hemoglobin-Oxygen Dissociation Curves. Normal hemoglobin-oxygen dissociation curve *(A)*. P_{50} is the oxygen *(O_2)* partial pressure needed for 50% O_2 saturation of hemoglobin. Left-shifted curve with reduced P_{50} can be caused by decreases in 2,3-bisphosphoglycerate (2,3-BPG), H^+ ions (raised pH), partial pressure of carbon dioxide (PCO_2), and/or temperature *(B)*. A left-shifted curve is also seen with hemoglobin F and hemoglobin variants that have increased oxygen affinity. A right-shifted curve with increased P_{50} can be caused by elevations in 2,3-BPG; H^+ ions (lowered pH); PCO_2; and/or temperature *(C)*. A right-shifted curve is also seen with hemoglobin variants that have decreased oxygen affinity. Myoglobin, a muscle protein, produces a markedly left-shifted curve, indicating a very high oxygen affinity. It is not effective in releasing oxygen at physiologic oxygen tensions.

It facilitates the ability of hemoglobin to exchange oxygen and carbon dioxide (CO_2).

The concentration of 2,3-bisphosphoglycerate (2,3-BPG, formerly 2,3-diphosphoglycerate) also has an effect on oxygen affinity. In the deoxygenated state, the hemoglobin tetramer assumes a *tense* or *T* conformation that is stabilized by the binding of 2,3-BPG between the β-globin chains (Figure 8.8). The formation of salt bridges between the phosphates of 2,3-BPG and positively charged groups on the globin chains further stabilizes the tetramer in the T conformation.[1] The binding of 2,3-BPG shifts the oxygen dissociation curve to the right, favoring the release of oxygen.[1] In addition, a lower pH and higher partial pressure of carbon dioxide (PCO_2) in the tissues further shifts the curve to the right, favoring the release of oxygen.[1]

As hemoglobin binds oxygen molecules, a change in conformation of the hemoglobin tetramer occurs, with a change in hydrophobic interactions at the $\alpha_1\beta_2$ contact point, a disruption of the salt bridges, and release of 2,3-BPG.[1] A 15-degree rotation of the $\alpha_1\beta_1$ dimer relative to the $\alpha_2\beta_2$ dimer occurs along the $\alpha_1\beta_2$ contact point.[2] When the hemoglobin tetramer is fully oxygenated, it assumes a *relaxed* or *R* state (Figure 8.8).

Clinical conditions that produce a shift of the oxygen dissociation curve to the left include a lowered body temperature as a result of external causes; multiple transfusions of stored blood with depleted 2,3-BPG; alkalosis; and presence of hemoglobin variants with a high affinity for oxygen. Conditions producing a shift of the curve to the right include increased body

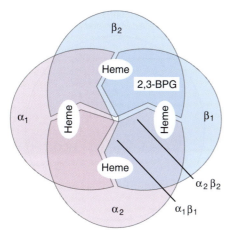 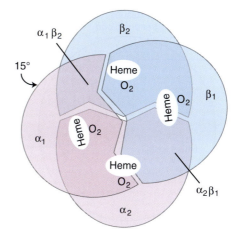

Deoxygenated (tense, "T") state　　　　　　Oxygenated (relaxed, "R") state

Figure 8.8 Tense *(T)* and Relaxed *(R)* Forms of Hemoglobin. The tense form incorporates one 2,3-bisphosphoglycerate *(2,3-BPG)* molecule, bound between the β-globin chains with salt bridges. It is unable to transport oxygen. As hemoglobin binds oxygen molecules, the $\alpha_1\beta_1$ and $\alpha_2\beta_2$ dimers rotate 15° relative to each other as a result of the change in hydrophobic interactions at the $\alpha_1\beta_2$ contact point, salt bridges are disrupted, and 2,3-BPG is released.

temperature; acidosis; presence of hemoglobin variants with a low affinity for oxygen; and an increased 2,3-BPG concentration in response to hypoxic conditions such as high altitude, pulmonary insufficiency, congestive heart failure, and severe anemia (Chapter 16).

The sigmoidal oxygen dissociation curve generated by normal hemoglobin contrasts with myoglobin's hyperbolic curve (Figure 8.7). Myoglobin, present in cardiac and skeletal muscle, is a 17,000-Dalton, monomeric, oxygen-binding heme protein. It binds oxygen with greater affinity than hemoglobin. Its hyperbolic curve indicates that it releases oxygen only at very low partial pressures, which means it is not as effective as hemoglobin in releasing oxygen to the tissues at physiologic oxygen tensions. Myoglobin is released into the plasma when there is damage to the muscle in myocardial infarction, trauma, or severe muscle injury, called *rhabdomyolysis*. Myoglobin is normally excreted by the kidney, but levels may become elevated in renal failure. Serum myoglobin levels aid in diagnosis of myocardial infarction in patients who have no underlying trauma, rhabdomyolysis, or renal failure. Myoglobin in the urine produces a positive result on urine biochemical analysis (by reagent test strip) for blood; this must be differentiated from a positive result caused by hemoglobin.

Hb F (the primary hemoglobin in newborns) has a P_{50} of 19 to 21 mm Hg, which results in a left shift of the oxygen dissociation curve and increased affinity for oxygen relative to that of Hb A. This increased affinity for oxygen is due to its weakened ability to bind 2,3-BPG.[2] There is only one amino acid difference in a critical 2,3-BPG binding site between the γ chain and the β chain that accounts for this difference in binding.[2]

In fetal life, the high oxygen affinity of Hb F provides an advantage by allowing more effective oxygen withdrawal from the maternal circulation. At the same time, Hb F has a disadvantage in that it delivers oxygen less readily to tissues. The bone marrow in the fetus and newborn compensates by producing more RBCs to ensure adequate oxygenation of the tissues. This response is mediated by EPO (Chapter 6). Consequently, the RBC count, hemoglobin concentration, and hematocrit of a newborn are higher than adult values, but they gradually decrease to normal physiologic levels by 6 months of age as the γ-β switching is completed and most of the Hb F is replaced by Hb A.

Carbon Dioxide Transport

A second crucial function of hemoglobin is the transport of carbon dioxide. In venous blood, the carbon dioxide diffuses into the RBCs and combines with water to form carbonic acid (H_2CO_3). This reaction is facilitated by the RBC enzyme carbonic anhydrase. Carbonic acid then dissociates to release H^+ and bicarbonate (HCO_3^-) (Figure 8.9).

The H^+ from the second reaction binds oxygenated hemoglobin (HbO_2), and the oxygen is released from the hemoglobin because of the Bohr effect. The oxygen then diffuses out of the cell into the tissues. As the concentration of the negatively charged bicarbonate increases, it diffuses across the RBC membrane into the plasma. Chloride (Cl^-), also negatively charged, diffuses from the plasma into the cell to maintain electroneutrality across the membrane; this is called the *chloride shift* (Figure 8.9).

In the lungs, oxygen diffuses into the cell and binds to deoxygenated hemoglobin (HHb) because of the high oxygen tension. H^+ is released from hemoglobin and combines with bicarbonate to form carbonic acid. Carbonic acid is converted to water and CO_2; the latter diffuses out of the cells and is expelled by the lungs. As more bicarbonate diffuses into the cell to produce carbonic acid, chloride diffuses back out into the plasma. Approximately 85% of the CO_2 produced in the tissues is transported by hemoglobin as H^+.[1] In this capacity, hemoglobin provides a buffering effect by binding and releasing H^+.[1] A small percentage of CO_2 remains in the cytoplasm, and the remainder binds to the globin chains as a carbamino group.

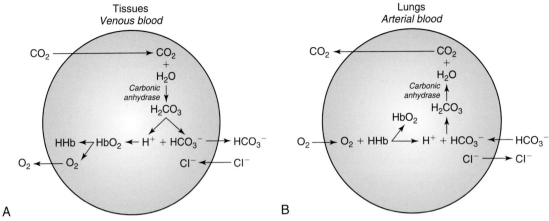

Figure 8.9 Transport and Release of Oxygen (O_2) and Carbon Dioxide (CO_2) in the Tissues and Lungs. **(A)**, In the tissues, CO_2 diffuses into the red blood cell and combines with water (H_2O) to form carbonic acid (H_2CO_3). This reaction is catalyzed by carbonic anhydrase. H_2CO_3 disassociates to hydrogen (H^+) and bicarbonate (HCO_3^-) ions. H^+ binds to oxyhemoglobin (HbO_2), resulting in the release of O_2 as a result of the Bohr effect. O_2 diffuses out of the cell into the tissues. HCO_3^- diffuses out of the cell as its concentration increases and is replaced by chloride (Cl^-) to maintain electroneutrality (chloride shift). Some CO_2 directly binds to the globin chains of hemoglobin. **(B)**, In the lungs, O_2 binds to deoxygenated hemoglobin (HHb) because of the high oxygen tension. H^+ dissociates from HbO_2 and combines with HCO_3^- to form H_2CO_3, which then dissociates into CO_2 and H_2O. The CO_2 diffuses out of the red blood cells and is exhaled by the lungs.

Nitric Oxide Transport

A third function of hemoglobin involves the binding, inactivation, and transport of nitric oxide.[1,9] Nitric oxide is secreted by vascular endothelial cells and causes relaxation of vascular wall smooth muscle and vasodilation.[1] When released, free nitric oxide has a very short half-life, but some enters RBCs and can bind to cysteine in the β chain of hemoglobin, forming S-nitrosohemoglobin.[1,9,10] Some investigators propose that hemoglobin preserves and transports nitric oxide to hypoxic microvascular areas, which stimulates vasodilation and increases blood flow (hypoxic vasodilation).[9] In this way, hemoglobin may work with other systems in regulating local blood flow to microvascular areas by binding and inactivating nitric oxide (causing vasoconstriction and decreased blood flow) when oxygen tension is high and releasing nitric oxide (causing vasodilation and increased blood flow) when oxygen tension is low.[9] This theory is not universally accepted, and the roles of hemoglobin, endothelial cells, and nitric oxide in regulating blood flow and oxygenation of the microcirculation are still being investigated.[10]

DYSHEMOGLOBINS

Dyshemoglobins (dysfunctional hemoglobins that are unable to transport oxygen) include methemoglobin, sulfhemoglobin, and carboxyhemoglobin. Dyshemoglobins form and may accumulate to toxic levels after exposure to certain drugs or environmental chemicals or gases. The offending agent modifies the structure of the hemoglobin molecule, preventing it from binding oxygen. Most cases of dyshemoglobinemia are acquired; a small fraction of methemoglobinemia cases are hereditary.

Methemoglobin

Methemoglobin (MetHb) is formed by the reversible oxidation of heme iron to the ferric state (Fe^{3+}). Normally, a small amount of methemoglobin is continuously formed by oxidation of iron during normal oxygenation and deoxygenation of hemoglobin.[10,11] However, methemoglobin reduction systems, predominantly the NADH-cytochrome b5 reductase 3 (NADH-methemoglobin reductase) pathway, normally limit its accumulation to only 1% of total hemoglobin (Chapter 7 and Figure 7.1).[10-12]

Methemoglobin cannot carry oxygen because oxidized ferric iron cannot bind it. An increase in methemoglobin level results in decreased delivery of oxygen to the tissues. Individuals with methemoglobin levels less than 25% are generally asymptomatic.[13] If the methemoglobin level increases to more than 30% of total hemoglobin, cyanosis (bluish discoloration of skin and mucous membranes) and symptoms of hypoxia (dyspnea, headache, vertigo, change in mental status) occur.[11,12] Levels of methemoglobin greater than 50% can lead to coma and death.[11,12]

An increase in methemoglobin, called *methemoglobinemia,* can be acquired or hereditary. The acquired form, also called *toxic methemoglobinemia,* occurs in individuals after exposure to an exogenous oxidant, such as nitrites, primaquine, dapsone, or benzocaine.[11,13] As the oxidant overwhelms the hemoglobin reduction systems, the level of methemoglobin increases, and the patient may exhibit cyanosis and symptoms of hypoxia.[10] In many cases, withdrawal of the offending oxidant is sufficient for a recovery, but if the level of methemoglobin increases to 30% or more of total hemoglobin, intravenous methylene blue is administered. Methylene blue reduces methemoglobin ferric iron to the ferrous state through NADPH-methemoglobin reductase and NADPH produced by glucose-6-phosphate dehydrogenase in the hexose monophosphate shunt (Figure 7.1).[10] In life-threatening cases, exchange transfusion may be required.[11]

Hereditary causes of methemoglobinemia are rare and include mutations in the gene for NADH-cytochrome b_5 reductase 3 *(CYB5R3)*, resulting in a diminished capacity to reduce methemoglobin, and mutations in the α-, β-, or γ-globin gene, resulting in a structurally abnormal polypeptide chain that favors the oxidized ferric form of iron and prevents its reduction.[10,11] The methemoglobin produced by the latter group is called *hemoglobin M (Hb M)* (Chapter 24). Hb M is inherited in an autosomal dominant pattern, with methemoglobin comprising 30% to 50% of total hemoglobin.[11] There is no effective treatment for this form of methemoglobinemia.[10,11] Cytochrome b_5 reductase deficiency is an autosomal recessive disorder, and methemoglobin elevations occur in individuals who are homozygous or compound heterozygous for a *CYB5R3* mutation.[10,11] Most individuals with Hb M or homozygous cytochrome b_5 reductase deficiency maintain methemoglobin levels less than 50%; they have cyanosis but only mild symptoms of hypoxia that do not require treatment.[10-12] Individuals heterozygous for the *CYB5R3* mutation have normal levels of methemoglobin but develop methemoglobinemia, cyanosis, and hypoxia when exposed to an oxidant drug or chemical.[11,13]

Methemoglobin is assayed by spectral absorption analysis instruments such as the CO-oximeter. Methemoglobin shows an absorption peak at 630 nm.[11] With high levels of methemoglobin, the blood takes on a chocolate brown color and does not revert back to normal red color after oxygen exposure.[11,12] The methemoglobin in Hb M disease has different absorption peaks, depending on the variant.[10] Hemoglobin electrophoresis, HPLC, and DNA mutation testing are used for identification of Hb M variants. Cytochrome b_5 reductase 3 deficiency is diagnosed by enzyme assays and DNA mutation testing.[10]

Sulfhemoglobin

Sulfhemoglobin is formed by irreversible oxidation of hemoglobin by drugs (such as sulfanilamides, phenacetin, nitrites, and phenylhydrazine) or exposure to sulfur chemicals in industrial or environmental settings.[10,11] It is formed by the addition of a sulfur atom to the pyrrole ring of heme and has a greenish pigment.[10] Sulfhemoglobin is ineffective for oxygen transport, and patients with elevated levels present with cyanosis. Sulfhemoglobin cannot be converted to normal Hb A; it persists for the life of the cell. Treatment consists of prevention by avoidance of the offending agent.

Sulfhemoglobin has a similar peak to methemoglobin on a spectral absorption instrument. The sulfhemoglobin spectral curve, however, does not shift when cyanide is added, a feature that distinguishes it from methemoglobin.[10]

Carboxyhemoglobin

Carboxyhemoglobin (COHb) results from the combination of carbon monoxide (CO) with heme iron. The affinity of carbon monoxide for hemoglobin is 240 times that of oxygen.[10] Once one molecule of carbon monoxide binds to hemoglobin, it shifts the hemoglobin-oxygen dissociation curve to the left, further increasing its affinity and severely impairing release of oxygen to the tissues.[10,14] Carbon monoxide has been termed the *silent killer* because it is an odorless and colorless gas, and victims may quickly become hypoxic.[14]

Some carboxyhemoglobin is produced endogenously, but it normally comprises less than 2% of total hemoglobin.[10] Exogenous carbon monoxide is derived from the exhaust of automobiles; tobacco smoke; and industrial pollutants such as coal, gas, and charcoal burning. In smokers, COHb levels may be as high as 15%.[13] As a result, smokers may have a higher hematocrit and polycythemia to compensate for the hypoxia.[10,13]

Exposure to carbon monoxide may be coincidental, accidental, or intentional (suicidal). Many deaths from house fires are the result of inhaling smoke, fumes, or carbon monoxide.[14] Even when heating systems in homes are properly maintained, accidental poisoning with carbon monoxide may occur. Toxic effects, such as headache, dizziness, and disorientation, begin to appear at blood levels of 20% to 30% COHb.[10,13] Levels of more than 40% of total hemoglobin may cause coma, seizure, hypotension, cardiac arrhythmias, pulmonary edema, and death.[10,14]

Carboxyhemoglobin may be detected by spectral absorption instruments at 540 nm.[11] It gives blood a cherry red color, which is sometimes imparted to the skin of victims.[14] A diagnosis of carbon monoxide poisoning is made if the COHb level is greater than 3% in nonsmokers and greater than 10% in smokers.[14] Treatment involves removing the carbon monoxide source and administration of 100% oxygen.[10] Use of hyperbaric oxygen therapy is controversial;[14] it is primarily used to prevent neurologic and cognitive impairment after acute carbon monoxide exposure in patients whose COHb level exceeds 25%.[14]

HEMOGLOBIN MEASUREMENT

The *cyanmethemoglobin* method is the reference method for hemoglobin assay.[15] A lysing agent present in the cyanmethemoglobin reagent frees hemoglobin from RBCs. Free hemoglobin combines with potassium ferricyanide contained in the cyanmethemoglobin reagent, which converts hemoglobin iron from the ferrous to the ferric state to form methemoglobin. Methemoglobin combines with potassium cyanide to form the stable pigment cyanmethemoglobin. The cyanmethemoglobin color intensity, which is proportional to hemoglobin concentration, is measured at 540 nm spectrophotometrically and compared with a standard (Chapter 12). The cyanmethemoglobin method is performed manually but has been adapted for use in automated blood cell analyzers.

Many instruments now use sodium lauryl sulfate (SLS) to convert hemoglobin to SLS-methemoglobin. This method does not generate toxic wastes (Chapter 13).

Hemoglobin electrophoresis and HPLC are used to separate the different types of hemoglobins such as Hb A, A_2, and F (Chapters 24 and 25).

SUMMARY

- The hemoglobin molecule is a tetramer composed of two pairs of unlike polypeptide chains. A heme group (protoporphyrin IX + Fe^{2+}) is bound to each of the four polypeptide chains.
- Hemoglobin, contained in red blood cells (RBCs), carries oxygen from the lungs to the tissues. Oxygen binds to ferrous iron in heme. Each hemoglobin tetramer can bind four oxygen molecules.
- Six structural genes code for the six globin chains of hemoglobin. The α- and ζ-globin genes are on chromosome 16; the $\in$-, γ-, δ-, and β-globin gene cluster is on chromosome 11. There is one copy of the δ-globin gene and one β-globin gene per chromosome, for a total of two genes per diploid cell. There are two copies of the α- and γ-globin genes per chromosome, for a total of four genes per diploid cell.
- Three hemoglobins found in healthy adults are Hb A, Hb A_2, and Hb F. Hb A ($\alpha_2\beta_2$), composed of two $\alpha\beta$ heterodimers, is the predominant hemoglobin of adults. Hb F ($\alpha_2\gamma_2$) is the predominant hemoglobin in the fetus and newborn. Hb A_2 ($\alpha_2\delta_2$) is present from birth through adulthood but at low levels.
- Hemoglobin ontogeny describes which hemoglobins are produced by the erythroid precursor cells from the fetal period through birth to adulthood.
- Complex genetic mechanisms regulate the sequential expression of the polypeptide chains in the embryo, fetus, and adult. Heme provides negative feedback regulation on protoporphyrin and globin chain production.

- The hemoglobin-oxygen dissociation curve is sigmoid because of cooperativity among the hemoglobin subunits in binding and releasing oxygen.
- 2,3-bisphosphoglycerate (2,3-BPG) produced by the glycolytic pathway facilitates the delivery of oxygen from hemoglobin to the tissues. The Bohr effect is the influence of pH on the release of oxygen from hemoglobin.
- In tissues, carbon dioxide diffuses into RBCs and combines with water to form carbonic acid (H_2CO_3). Carbonic acid is then converted to bicarbonate and hydrogen ions (HCO_3^- and H^+). Most of the carbon dioxide is carried by hemoglobin as H^+.
- Methemoglobin, sulfhemoglobin, and carboxyhemoglobin cannot transport oxygen. These dyshemoglobins can accumulate to toxic levels as a result of exposure to certain drugs, industrial or environmental chemicals, or gases. A small fraction of methemoglobinemia cases are hereditary. Cyanosis occurs in patients with increased levels of methemoglobin or sulfhemoglobin.
- Although the *cyanmethemoglobin* method is the reference method for hemoglobin assay, many instruments use sodium lauryl sulfate (SLS) to convert hemoglobin to SLS-methemoglobin, which does not generate toxic waste.

Now that you have completed this chapter, go back and read again the case study at the beginning and respond to the questions presented. Answers can be found in Appendix C.

REVIEW QUESTIONS

Answers can be found in Appendix C.

1. A hemoglobin molecule is composed of:
   a. One heme molecule and four globin chains
   b. Ferrous iron, protoporphyrin IX, and a globin chain
   c. Protoporphyrin IX and four globin chains
   d. Four heme molecules and four globin chains
2. Normal adult Hb A contains which polypeptide chains?
   a. α and β
   b. α and δ
   c. α and γ
   d. α and $\in$
3. A key rate-limiting step in heme synthesis is suppression of:
   a. Aminolevulinate synthase
   b. Carbonic anhydrase
   c. Protoporphyrin IX reductase
   d. Glucose-6-phosphate dehydrogenase
4. Which of the following forms of hemoglobin molecule has the lowest affinity for oxygen?
   a. Tense
   b. Relaxed

5. Using the normal hemoglobin-oxygen dissociation curve in Figure 8.7 for reference, predict the position of the curve when there is a decrease in pH.
   a. Shifted to the right of normal with decreased oxygen affinity
   b. Shifted to the left of normal with increased oxygen affinity
   c. Shifted to the right of normal with increased oxygen affinity
   d. Shifted to the left of normal with decreased oxygen affinity
6. The predominant hemoglobin found in a healthy newborn is:
   a. Gower-1
   b. Gower-2
   c. A
   d. F
7. What is the normal distribution of hemoglobins in healthy adults?
   a. 80% to 90% Hb A, 5% to 10% Hb A_2, 1% to 5% Hb F
   b. 80% to 90% Hb A_2, 5% to 10% Hb A, 1% to 5% Hb F
   c. >95% Hb A, <3.5% Hb A_2, 1% to 2% Hb F
   d. >90% Hb A, 5% Hb F, <5% Hb A_2

8. Which of the following is a description of the structure of oxidized hemoglobin?
   a. Hemoglobin carrying oxygen on heme; synonymous with oxygenated hemoglobin
   b. Hemoglobin with iron in the ferric state (methemoglobin) and not able to carry oxygen
   c. Hemoglobin with iron in the ferric state so that carbon dioxide replaces oxygen in the heme structure
   d. Hemoglobin carrying carbon monoxide; hence *oxidized* refers to the single oxygen

9. In the quaternary structure of hemoglobin, the globin chains associate into:
   a. α tetramers in some cells and β tetramers in others
   b. A mixture of α tetramers and β tetramers
   c. α dimers and β dimers
   d. Two αβ dimers

10. How are the globin chain genes arranged?
    a. With α genes and β genes on the same chromosome, including two α genes and two β genes
    b. With α genes and β genes on separate chromosomes, including two α genes on one chromosome and one β gene on a different chromosome
    c. With α genes and β genes on the same chromosome, including four α genes and four β genes
    d. With α genes and β genes on separate chromosomes, including four α genes on one chromosome and two β genes on a different chromosome

11. The nature of the interaction between 2,3-BPG and hemoglobin is that 2,3-BPG:
    a. Binds to the heme moiety, blocking the binding of oxygen
    b. Binds simultaneously with oxygen to ensure that it stays bound until it reaches the tissues, when both molecules are released from hemoglobin
    c. Binds to amino acids of the globin chain, contributing to a conformational change that inhibits oxygen from binding to heme
    d. Oxidizes hemoglobin iron, diminishing oxygen binding and promoting oxygen delivery to the tissues

REFERENCES

1. Quigly, J. G., Means, R. T., Jr., & Glader, B. (2019). The birth, life, and death of red blood cells: erythropoiesis, the mature red blood cell and cell destruction. In Greer, J. P., Arber, D. A., Glader, B. et al. (Eds.), *Wintrobe's Clinical Hematology.* (14th ed., pp. 319–330). Philadelphia: Wolters Kluwer.

2. Steinberg, M. H., Benz, E. J., Jr., & Ebert, B. L. (2023). Pathobiology of the human erythrocyte and its hemoglobins. In Hoffman, R., Benz, E. J., Silberstein, L. E., et al. (Eds.), *Hematology Basic Principles and Practice.* (8th ed., pp. 451–462). Philadelphia: Elsevier.

3. Sheehan, V. A., Gordeuk, V. R., & Kutlar, A. (2021). Disorders of hemoglobin structure: sickle cell anemia and related abnormalities. In Kaushansky, K., Prchal, J. T., Burns, L. J., et al. (Eds.), *Williams' Hematology.* (10th ed., pp. 825–827). New York: McGraw-Hill.

4. Perutz, M. F., Rossmann, M. G., Cullis, A. F., et al. (1960). Structure of hemoglobin: a three dimensional Fourier synthesis at 5.5A resolution obtained by x-ray analysis. *Nature, 185,* 416–422.

5. Donze, D., Jeancake, P. H., & Townes, T. M. (1996). Activation of delta-globin gene expression by erythroid Krüpple-like factor: a potential approach for gene therapy of sickle cell disease. *Blood, 88,* 4051–4057.

6. Tallack, M. R., & Perkins, A. C. (2013). Three fingers on the switch: Krüppel-like factor 1 regulation of a-globin to β-globin gene switching. *Curr Opin Hematol, 20,* 193–200.

7. Tolhuis, B., Palstra, R.-J., Splinter, E., et al. (2002). Looping and interaction between hypersensitive sites in the active β-globin locus. *Molecular Cell, 10,* 1453–1465.

8. Zhou, D., Liu, K., Sun, C. W., et al. (2010). KLF1 regulates BCL11A expression and gamma to beta-globin switching. *Nat Genet, 42,* 742–744.

9. Allen, B. W., Stamler, J. S., & Piantadosi, C. A. (2009). Hemoglobin, nitric oxide and molecular mechanisms of hypoxic vasodilation. *Trends Mol Med, 15,* 452–460.

10. Verhovsek, M., & Steinberg, M. H. (2019). Hemoglobins with altered oxygen affinity, unstable hemoglobins, M-hemoglobins, and dyshemoglobinemias. In Greer, J. P., Arber, D. A., Glader, B. et al. (Eds.), *Wintrobe's Clinical Hematology.* (14th ed., pp. 2646–2665). Philadelphia: Wolters Kluwer.

11. Benz, E. J., Jr., & Ebert, B. L. (2023). Hemoglobin variants associated with hemolytic anemia altered oxygen affinity, and methemoglobinemias. In Hoffman, R., Benz, E. J., Silberstein, L. E., et al. (Eds.), *Hematology: Basic Principles and Practice.* (8th ed., pp. 630–637). Philadelphia: Elsevier.

12. Skold, A., Cosco, D. I., & Klein, R. (2011). Methemoglobinemia: pathogenesis, diagnosis, and management. *South Med J, 104,* 757–761.

13. Vajpayee, N., Graham, S. S., & Bem, S. (2022). Basic examination of blood and bone marrow. In McPherson, R. A., & Pincus, M. R. (Eds.), *Henry's Clinical Diagnosis and Management by Laboratory Methods.* (24th ed., pp.540–542). Philadelphia: Elsevier Inc.

14. Guzman, J. A. (2012). Carbon monoxide poisoning. *Crit Care Clin, 28,* 537–548.

15. CLSI. (2000). *Reference and Selected Procedures for the Quantitative Determination of Hemoglobin in Blood* (3rd ed., CLSI guideline H15-A3). Wayne, PA: Clinical and Laboratory Standards Institute.

Iron Kinetics and Laboratory Assessment

Kathryn Doig and Yukari Nishizawa-Brennen

OBJECTIVES

After completion of this chapter, the reader will be able to:

1. Describe the essential metabolic processes in which iron participates.
2. Correlate the terms *ferric* and *ferrous* to oxidation state (reduced/oxidized) and ionic forms of iron.
3. State whether body iron is regulated by excretion or absorption.
4. Describe the compartments in which body iron is distributed, including the relative amounts in each site.
5. Trace a molecule of iron from its absorption through the enterocyte to transport into mitochondria and then recycling via macrophages, including the names of all proteins with which it interacts and that control its kinetics.
6. Name the ionic form and number of molecules of iron that bind to one molecule of apotransferrin.
7. Explain how hepcidin regulates body iron levels.
8. Explain how individual cells acquire iron.
9. Explain how individual cells regulate the amount of iron they absorb.
10. Describe the role of each of the following in the kinetics of iron, including its location or source tissue:
    a. Divalent metal transporter 1
    b. Ferroportin
    c. Transferrin
    d. Transferrin receptor 1
    e. Transferrin receptor 2
    f. Hepcidin
    g. Erythroferrone
    h. Ferritin
11. For the proteins listed in objective 10, distinguish those that are involved in the kinetics of iron within individual cells versus those involved in systemic body iron regulation.

12. Discuss how hepatocytes sense circulating and tissue levels of iron and modulate hepcidin production.
13. Discuss how erythroblasts are able to impact hepcidin production.
14. List factors that increase and decrease the bioavailability of iron.
15. Name foods high in ionic or heme-containing iron.
16. For each of the following assays, describe the principle of the assay and the iron compartment assessed:
    a. Serum iron (SI)
    b. Total iron-binding capacity (TIBC)
    c. Percent transferrin saturation
    d. Prussian blue staining
    e. Ferritin
    f. Soluble transferrin receptor (sTfR)
    g. Hemoglobin content of reticulocytes
    h. Soluble transferrin receptor/log ferritin
    i. Thomas plot
    j. Zinc protoporphyrin
17. Plot given patient values on a Thomas plot and interpret the patient's iron status.
18. Calculate the percent transferrin saturation when given total SI and TIBC.
19. When given reference intervals, interpret the results of each of the assays in objective 16 plus a Thomas plot and sTfR/log ferritin and recognize results consistent with decreased, normal, and increased iron status.
20. Identify instances in which sTfR, hemoglobin content of reticulocytes, sTfR/log ferritin, and Thomas plots may be needed to improve diagnosis of iron-restricted erythropoiesis.

OUTLINE

Iron Chemistry
Iron Kinetics
  Systemic (Body) Iron Kinetics
  Body Iron Recycling and Salvage
  Cellular Iron Kinetics
Dietary Iron, Bioavailability, and Demand
Laboratory Assessment of Body Iron Status
  Serum Iron
  Total Iron-Binding Capacity

Percent Transferrin Saturation
Prussian Blue Staining
Ferritin
Soluble Transferrin Receptor
Hemoglobin Content of Reticulocytes
Soluble Transferrin Receptor/Log Ferritin
Thomas Plot
Zinc Protoporphyrin

CASE STUDY

After studying the material in this chapter, the reader should be able to respond to the following case study. Answers can be found in Appendix C.

In 1995, Garry and colleagues[1] assessed changes in stored iron in 16 female and 20 male regular blood donors aged 64 to 71. They measured hemoglobin (HGB), hematocrit (HCT), serum ferritin concentration, and percent transferrin saturation in specimens from the donors, who gave an average of 15 units (approximately 485 mL/unit) of blood over 3.5 years. The investigators collected comparable data from nondonors. Of the donors, 10 females and 6 males took a dietary supplement providing approximately 20 mg of iron per day. In addition, mean dietary iron intake was 18 mg/day for the females and 20 mg/day for the males. Over the period of the study, mean iron stores in female donors decreased from 12.53 to 1.14 mg/kg of body weight. Mean iron stores in male donors declined from 12.45 to 1.92 mg/kg. Iron stores of nondonors remained unchanged. Based on HGB and HCT results, no donors became anemic. As iron stores decreased, the calculated iron absorption rose to 3.55 mg/day for the females and 4.10 mg/day for the males—more than double the normal rate for both females and males.

1. Why did the donors' iron stores decrease?
2. Why did the donors' iron absorption rate increase? Explain using the names of all proteins involved.
3. Name the laboratory test(s) performed in the study used to evaluate directly the iron storage compartment.
4. What is the diagnostic value of the percent transferrin saturation?

Among the metals that are required for metabolic processes, none is more important than iron. It is critical to energy production in all cells, being at the center of the cytochromes of mitochondria. Oxygen needed for energy production is carried by iron in the hemoglobin molecule in red blood cells (RBCs). Iron is so critical to the body that there is no mechanism for active excretion, just minimal daily loss with exfoliated skin and hair and sloughed intestinal epithelia. Iron is even recycled to conserve as much as possible in the body. To ensure against times when iron may be scarce in the diet, the body stores iron as well.

A man harbors more than 2.5 g of iron,[2] with 4 g as a typical amount. The largest percentage of body iron, nearly 65%, is held within hemoglobin in RBCs of various stages (Table 9.1), whereas almost 25% of body iron is in storage.[2] The remaining approximately 10% is divided among the myoglobin in muscles, the cytochromes, various iron-containing enzymes, iron-sulfur clusters in iron-sulfur proteins, and an important but nearly negligible amount in the plasma.

A more functional approach to thinking about body iron distribution conceives of the iron as distributed in three compartments (see Table 9.1). The *functional compartment* contains all iron that is functioning within cells, including iron in hemoglobin, myoglobin (in muscles), sulfur-iron clusters, some enzymes, and cytochromes (in all cells other than mature RBCs). The *storage compartment* is the iron that is not currently functioning but is available when needed. The major repositories of this stored iron are hepatocytes and macrophages of the spleen and bone marrow, but every cell except for mature RBCs stores some iron for its own use. The third compartment is the *transport compartment* of iron that is in transit from one body site to another in the plasma.

Although the reactivity of iron ions makes them central to energy production processes, it also makes them dangerous to the stability of cells. Thus the body regulates iron carefully at the level of the whole body as well as within individual cells, maintaining levels that are necessary for critical metabolic processes while avoiding the dangers of excess iron accumulation. The conditions that develop when this balance is perturbed are described in Chapter 17. The routine tests used to assess body iron status are discussed in this chapter.

IRON CHEMISTRY

The metabolic functions of iron depend on its ability to change its valence state from reduced ferrous (Fe^{2+}) iron to the oxidized ferric (Fe^{3+}) state. Thus it is involved in oxidation and reduction reactions such as the electron transport within mitochondrial cytochromes. Ferrous iron (Fe^{2+}) can react with peroxide via the Fenton reaction, forming highly reactive oxygen molecules.

$$Fe^{2+} + HO\text{-}OH \rightarrow \bullet Fe^{3+} + HO^- + \bullet OH$$

The resulting hydroxyl radical ($\bullet OH$), also known as a free radical, is especially reactive as a short-lived but potent oxidizing agent, able to damage proteins, lipids, and nucleic acids. As will be described in the section on iron kinetics, there are various mechanisms within the body and individual cells to reduce the potential for this type of damage.

TABLE 9.1 Iron Compartments in Normal Humans, Relative Iron Distribution, and Iron Oxidation State

Compartment	Form and Anatomic Site	Approximate Percent of Total Body Iron	Oxidation state
Functional	Hemoglobin iron in RBCs of all stages of development	65	2+
	Myoglobin iron in muscles	6	2+
	Peroxidase, catalase, cytochromes, iron-sulfur clusters, enzymes in all cells	4	2+/3+
Storage	Ferritin and hemosiderin mostly in macrophages and hepatocytes; small amounts in all cells except mature RBCs	25	3+
Transport	Transferrin in plasma	0.1	3+

RBCs, Red blood cells.
Adapted from Theil, E., Raymond, K. (1994). Transition-metal storage, transport, and biomineralization. In Bertini, I., Gray, H. B., Lippard, S. J., Valentine, J. S., (Eds.), *Bioinorganic chemistry*. Mill Valley, CA: University Science Books, p 611.

IRON KINETICS

Acquiring iron from the diet is the first step in an intricate process of trafficking iron to mitochondria in cells. Some mechanisms are unique to erythroblasts synthesizing heme for hemoglobin, and they will be the focus of this discussion. The iron must traverse a myriad of environments and cross multiple membranes before final insertion into protoporphyrin. Under normal circumstances, iron is rarely allowed to move independently as an ion in body fluids, through membranes, or in cytosol. Rather, it is chaperoned by proteins that protect cells from its oxidizing effects by holding the iron inside the protein away from aqueous surroundings. This is analogous to how the heme of hemoglobin is sequestered inside hydrophobic pockets in the globin structure (Chapter 8). The oxidation state in such chaperone proteins is often Fe^{3+}, but transfer across membranes usually requires the Fe^{2+} form. Therefore specialized proteins are typically located on membranes to reduce iron before membrane transit and then oxidize it afterwards. These generalities regarding iron trafficking will be evident in the discussion of both systemic iron kinetics and individual cell iron kinetics.

Systemic (Body) Iron Kinetics

Figure 9.1 provides an overview of systemic (body) iron regulation that can be a reference throughout the section on iron kinetics. The total amount of iron available to all body cells, systemic iron, is regulated by absorption of dietary iron into the body because there is no mechanism for active excretion.

Absorption of Dietary Iron in the Intestines

Iron can be absorbed in the small intestines as ferritin from either animal or vegetable sources, as heme from animal sources, or as ionic iron, mostly from vegetable sources. As ferritin contributes the least to dietary iron, heme and ionic iron will be the focus of the following discussion. However, for completeness, mention of ferritin is included.

Ferritin absorption. Ferritin is the storage form of iron found in both animal and plant cells. Intestinal cells, *enterocytes,* can absorb ferritin from either source via both *endocytosis* (Chapter 4) and *macropinocytosis* (Chapter 4).[3,4] Identifying the receptor for enterocyte endocytic absorption is an area of research, though the transferrin-1 receptor (TfR1) is likely, as other cells have been shown to rely on it.[5] While it is not a major source of dietary iron, increasing the ferritin content of plant staples could help prevent iron deficiency in many parts of the world.[6]

Heme absorption. Heme carrier protein 1 (HCP1) in the luminal membrane of enterocytes permits heme absorption by receptor mediated endocytosis,[7,8] even though it is actually more efficient at carrying folic acid.[9,10] When the endosome fuses with a lysosome, heme regulatory gene-1 (HRG-1), a carrier protein in the lysosome membrane, is able to transfer the heme into the cytosol.[11] Once the heme enters the enterocyte cytoplasm, the iron is freed from protoporphyrin by heme oxygenase, likely on the surface of the smooth endoplasmic reticulum (Figure 9.2).[8] Its fate is then the same as ionic iron as described next.

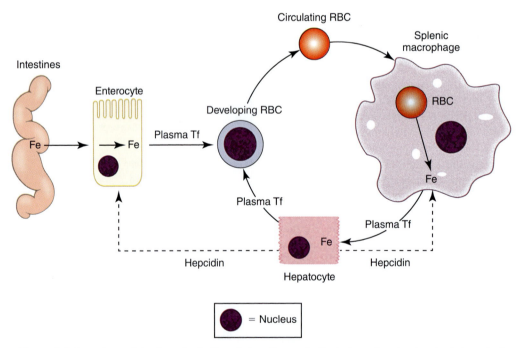

Figure 9.1 Overview of the Iron Cycle Regulating Systemic Body Iron. Iron is absorbed through the enterocyte of the duodenum and into the plasma via the portal circulation. There it binds to apotransferrin to form transferrin *(Tf)* for transport to cells, such as the developing red blood cells *(RBCs)*. In RBCs, the iron is used in hemoglobin that circulates with the cell until it becomes aged and is ingested by a macrophage. There the iron is removed from the hemoglobin and can be recycled into the blood for use by other cells. The level of stored and circulating body iron is detected by the hepatocyte, which is able to produce a protein, hepcidin, when iron levels get too high. Hepcidin will inhibit the absorption and recycling of iron by acting on enterocytes, macrophages, and hepatocytes. When body iron decreases, hepcidin will also decrease so that absorption and recycling are again activated. (From Doig, K. [2013]. *Iron: The Body's Most Precious Metal.* [p. 1]. McLean, VA: American Society for Clinical Laboratory Science.)

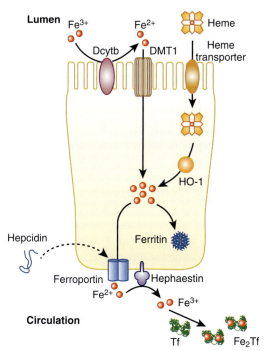

Figure 9.2 Absorption of Iron in the Small Intestine. Ferric iron *(Fe³⁺)* in the intestinal lumen is reduced *(Fe²⁺)* before transport across the luminal membrane of the enterocyte by the ferrireductase, duodenal cytochrome *b (Dcytb)*. It is then transported through the luminal membrane into the enterocyte cytoplasm by divalent metal transporter 1 *(DMT1)*. Iron can also be absorbed as heme by an enterocyte membrane heme transporter. The iron is removed from heme by heme oxygenase-1 *(HO-1)*. Ferritin, not shown, can also be absorbed. Some absorbed iron may be stored as ferritin. Most is chaperoned as Fe²⁺ to the opposite membrane by poly(rC) binding proteins and carried into the blood by ferroportin. It is reoxidized to Fe³⁺ by hephaestin as it exits the enterocyte for transport in the blood by transferrin *(Tf)*. Each Tf molecule can carry two (Fe³⁺) ions *(Fe₂Tf)*. Hepcidin is a hepatic protein that degrades ferroportin, preventing iron transport out of the enterocyte. (Modified from Ganz, T. [2023]. Iron homeostasis and its disorders. In: Hoffman, R., Benz, E. J., Silberstein, L. E., et al. [Eds.], *Hematology: Basic Principles and Practice.* [8th ed., p. 482, Figure 36.8]. Philadelphia: Elsevier; and Anderson, G. J., Frazer, D. M., & McLaren, G. D. [2009]. Iron absorption and metabolism. *Curr Opin Gastroenterol, 25,* p. 130, Figure 1.)

Ionic iron absorption. For many people, most dietary iron is nonheme ionic iron in the Fe^{3+} form and must be reduced by duodenal cytochrome *b* on the luminal side of the enterocyte membrane before it can enter the enterocyte (see Figure 9.2). Once the iron is in reduced form (Fe^{2+}), it is carried across the luminal membrane of the enterocyte by divalent metal transporter 1 (DMT1) (see Figure 9.2).

Whether derived from absorbed heme or absorbed as an ion, the iron can be stored as ferritin (discussed in "Cellular Iron Storage") within the enterocyte and used for its needs. However, most of the iron will be chaperoned through the cytoplasm to the basolaminal side of the enterocyte for transport into the plasma. The chaperone molecules are poly(rC) binding proteins (PCBP). Cytosolic PCBP2 docks with DMT1 for a handoff of the iron.[12] PCBP2 then carries Fe^{2+} iron through the aqueous cytosol, protecting the cell from the oxidizing effects of the Fenton reaction. The chaperone then docks to a transmembrane protein on the basolaminal side of the cell for a handoff [13] that will allow the iron to be exported from the cell and into the blood, thus truly absorbing it into the body. Any iron that is not transferred out of the enterocyte before the cell is sloughed off is not truly absorbed and is lost in the stool.

The protein on the basolaminal side of the enterocyte that exports Fe^{2+} iron into the blood is ferroportin. Ferroportin is the only known protein that exports iron across cell membranes. When the body has adequate stores of iron, the hepatocytes sense that and will increase production of *hepcidin*, a protein able to bind to ferroportin, leading to its inactivation[14,15] As a result, iron absorption into the body via enterocyte ferroportin decreases. When the body iron begins to decrease, the liver senses that change and decreases hepcidin production. As a result, ferroportin is again active and able to transport iron into the blood. This is often called the *hepcidin-ferroportin axis*. Thus homeostasis of body iron is maintained by modest fluctuations in liver hepcidin production in response to body iron status. The regulation of systemic body iron is summarized in Figure 9.3 and discussed in "Absorption of Dietary Iron in the Intestines."

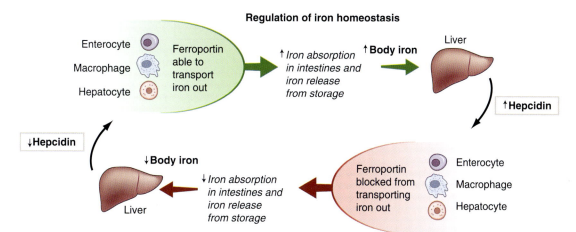

Regulation of iron homeostasis

Figure 9.3 Regulation of Iron Homeostasis. When body iron levels rise *(upper center)*, the liver is able to detect it. Production of hepcidin is upregulated and secreted into the blood, where it travels to the iron-regulating cells: enterocytes, macrophages, and hepatocytes. Hepcidin will react with ferroportin in their membranes and prevent iron from exiting those cells into the blood. As a result, body iron will decline and the liver will sense it. Hepcidin production will be curtailed. Ferroportin in the membranes of the iron-regulating cells will then be active and transport iron into the plasma. The cycle then repeats.

While not part of dietary iron absorption, it is appropriate to mention here that two other cell types are critical to supplying daily iron, macrophages and hepatocytes. They recycle iron (see "Body Iron Recycling and Salvage") from dying cells and possess ferroportin in their membranes to export salvaged iron (see Figure 9.3). They are also sensitive to the effects of hepcidin and it restricts their iron recycling. Regulation of hepcidin production is important to understanding iron kinetics, particularly in the disease states discussed in Chapter 17, but it first requires an understanding of iron transport by transferrin.

Iron Transport in the Blood

Iron exported from the enterocyte via ferroportin is Fe^{2+} and must be converted to the Fe^{3+} form for transport in the blood. Hephaestin, a protein on the exterior of the basolaminal enterocyte membrane, is able to oxidize iron as it exits the enterocyte. Once oxidized, the iron is ready for plasma transport, carried by a specific liver-produced protein, apotransferrin (ApoTf) (see

Figure 9.2). When iron binds, the molecule is known as *transferrin* (Tf). Apotransferrin binds up to two ferric (Fe^{3+}) ions and thus when fully loaded is often referred to as *diferric transferrin* or *holotransferrin,* as the convention of using the prefix "holo" indicates that the protein is carrying its ligand.

Regulation of Body Iron

The mechanisms by which the body senses iron levels and responds with hepcidin adjustments have been an area of intense research because they may hold the key to treatments for iron-related anemias and hemochromatoses (Chapter 17). Liver and erythrocyte iron sensing systems have been identified.

Liver iron sensing and hepcidin production. The hepatic system for sensing and regulating hepcidin production has two pathways that are modeled in Figure 9.4. One can detect plasma iron levels, while the other detects the amount of tissue (i.e., stored) iron (Figure 9.4). Table 9.2 lists the major proteins involved and their functions. The importance of the proteins in

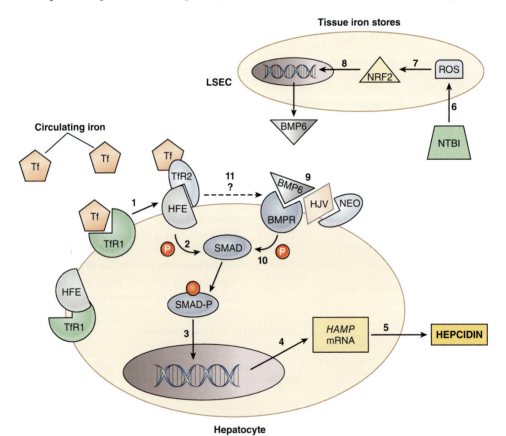

Figure 9.4 Hepatocyte Hepcidin Regulation Under Conditions of Plentiful Body Iron. The hepatocyte has two sensing pathways for iron leading to hepcidin production: circulating iron and stored tissue iron. In the hepatocyte membrane, transferrin receptor 1 *(TfR1)* is associated with hemochromatosis protein *(HFE)*. When TfR1 binds transferrin *(Tf)*, HFE is released and binds to transferrin receptor 2 *(TfR2)*, which also binds Tf *(1)*. This complex is able to add a phosphate *(P)* to sons of mothers against decapentaplegic *(SMAD)* *(2)*. SMAD transfers to the nucleus *(3)*. There it upregulates hepcidin antimicrobial peptide gene *(HAMP)*, the hepcidin gene *(4)*. This leads to hepatocyte secretion of hepcidin *(5)*. When Tf is highly saturated, excess plasma iron in the form of nontransferrin-bound iron *(NTBI)* will enter cells including the liver sinusoidal endothelial cells *(LSEC)* *(6)*. There the production of reactive oxygen species *(ROS)* by NTBI leads to activation of nuclear factor erythroid 2-related factor 2 *(NRF2)* *(7)*. NRF2 upregulates bone morphogenetic protein 6 *(BMP6)* production *(8)*. BMP6 secreted from the LSEC then binds to bone morphogenetic protein receptor *(BMPR)* and coreceptor hemojuvelin *(HJV)* on the hepatocyte membrane *(9)*. This complex is stabilized by neogenin *(NEO)*. The complex is able to add a phosphate to SMAD, leading to hepcidin production as described in 3, 4, and 5 *(10)*. The HFE-TfR2 complex may associate with BMP-HJV complex to phosphorylate SMAD *(11)*. The production of hepcidin inactivates ferroportin in enterocytes to reduce iron absorption.

TABLE 9.2 Functions and Locations of Proteins Involved in Body Iron Sensing and Hepcidin Production

Protein	Location	Function
Transferrin receptor 1 (TfR1)	Hepatocyte membrane	Binds circulating diferric transferrin, thus releasing hemochromatosis protein (HFE) for hepcidin signal transduction
Hemochromatosis protein (HFE)	Hepatocyte membrane	Once released from TfR1, binds to transferrin receptor 2 (TfR2). Associates with bone morphogenetic protein receptor (BMPR) to initiate the signal to upregulate hepcidin production.
Transferrin receptor 2 (TfR2)	Hepatocyte membrane	With freed HFE, associates with BMPR to initiate the signal to upregulate hepcidin production
Bone morphogenetic protein (BMP)	Secreted product from liver sinusoidal endothelial cells	The ligand that initiates hepcidin signal transduction when it binds to its receptor on the hepatocyte membrane
Bone morphogenetic protein receptor (BMPR)	Hepatocyte (and other cells) membrane	A common membrane receptor initiating signal transduction within a cell when its ligand (BMP) binds
Hemojuvelin (HJV)	Hepatocyte membrane	A coreceptor acting with BMPR for signal transduction leading to hepcidin production
Neogenin (NEO)	Hepatocyte membrane	Provides structural support to the BMPR-HJV complex
Sons of mothers against decapentaplegic (SMAD)	Hepatocyte (and other cells) cytoplasm	A second messenger of signal transduction, phosphorylated by the BMPR-HJV complex and able to migrate to the nucleus and upregulate hepcidin gene expression
Matriptase-2 (MT2)	Hepatocyte membrane	Cleaves hemojuvelin to downregulate hepcidin production
Transferrin receptor 2 (TfR2)	Erythroblast membrane	Stabilizes the erythropoietin receptor (EPOR) unless it binds Tf and is internalized
Erythropoietin receptor (EPOR)	Erythroblast membrane	Binds erythropoietin to prevent apoptosis of early erythroblasts and upregulates production of erythroferrone in polychromatic erythroblasts
Erythroferrone (ERFE)	Secreted by polychromatic erythroblasts	Able to bind BMP to downregulate hepcidin production in the liver

Table 9.2 to hepcidin production has been demonstrated via mutations, both natural in humans and induced in mice, which lead to either iron overload or iron deficiency. Testing for these mutations is increasing in molecular diagnostic laboratories. The diseases associated with some of the known human mutations are described in Chapter 17.

Liver sensing of circulating iron. When body iron is plentiful and plasma transferrin is well saturated, there is more diferric transferrin available to bind to the TfR1 and transferrin receptor 2 (TfR2) on hepatocytes. This binding contributes to a sequence of *signal transduction* (Chapter 4) events involving Tf-TfR-hemochromatosis protein (HFE) and other proteins in Table 9.2 that results in the secretion of hepcidin (see Figure 9.4, *1–5*).[16] Conversely, when body iron is low, there is less diferric transferrin to trigger this pathway. In this case, hepcidin production declines, ferroportin is more active, and more iron enters the blood from enterocytes, macrophages, and hepatocytes (Figure 9.5).

Liver sensing of stored iron. The liver's second iron-sensing branch is sensitive to tissue iron levels. Previously, it was emphasized that iron is rarely unchaperoned. Most plasma iron is bound to Tf, but when Tf is highly saturated, non-transferrin-bound iron (NTBI) rises in the plasma. NTBI is iron that is nonspecifically attached to proteins such as albumin or combined with compounds such as citrate, from which it can easily be dislodged.[17] Most cells can take up NTBI by multiple

mechanisms including DMT-1, as enterocytes do.[18] This less-regulated cellular acquisition of iron can generate reactive oxygen species via the Fenton reaction. When this occurs in liver sinusoidal endothelial cells, the endothelial cell increases production and secretion of bone morphogenetic protein 6 (BMP6) (see Figure 9.4, *6–10*).[19,20,21] BMP6 from the endothelial cells forms a complex with hemojuvelin (HJV) and other proteins on the hepatocyte surface to initiate the signal to increase hepcidin production, which will reduce iron absorption and recycling.[22] Thus the liver monitors and responds to transient circulating iron fluctuations via the Tf-TfR2-HFE complex on the hepatocyte membrane, but changes to stored iron levels are detected by the sinusoidal endothelial cells that then regulate hepatocyte hepcidin production via BMP-HJV.

Erythrocyte iron sensing and hepcidin production. An erythroid mechanism of hepcidin regulation was mentioned earlier in addition to the hepatic ones just described. Erythroblasts secrete a hormone, *erythroferrone* (ERFE),[23] that sequesters BMPs,[24] making them unavailable to stimulate hepcidin production. As a result, iron absorption and recycling increases (Figure 9.6). Hence by ERFE production, developing RBCs promote the availability of iron for their hemoglobin production. Erythroblasts must reach the polychromatophilic stage to secrete ERFE. Erythropoietin (EPO) is necessary to prevent apoptosis of the colony-forming-unit-erythroid and

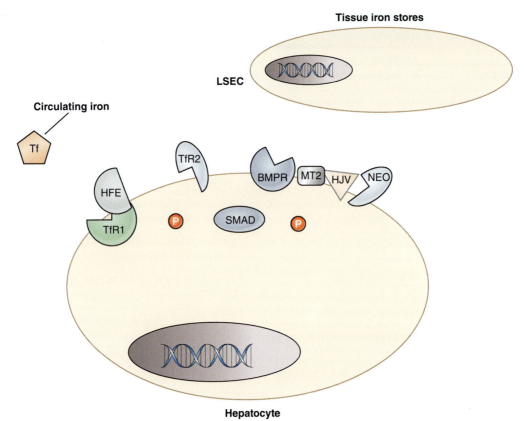

Figure 9.5 Hepatocyte Hepcidin Regulation Under Conditions of Scarce Body Iron. When body iron is scarce, there is little transferrin *(Tf)* to associate with transferrin receptor 1 *(TfR1)* or transferrin receptor 2 *(TfR2)*. Hemochromatosis protein *(HFE)* remains bound to TfR1. TfR2 without Tf or HFE is unable to phosphorylate *(P)* sons of mothers against decapentaplegic *(SMAD)*; therefore there is no signal to the nucleus to initiate hepcidin production. Tissue iron is also low, so liver sinusoidal endothelial cells *(LSEC)* do not secrete bone morphogenetic protein 6. Hemojuvelin *(HJV)* is cleaved by matriptase 2 *(MT2)*, which prevents HJV binding to bone morphogenetic protein receptor *(BMPR)*. Phosphorylation of SMAD is prevented and there is no signal to hepcidin production. As a result, ferroportin is active in enterocytes to increase body iron.

allow cells to mature to the polychromatophilic stage (Chapter 6) (Figure 9.7).[25–27] Additionally, EPO is able to upregulate ERFE production in individual erythroblasts.[23] In anemias with ineffective erythropoiesis, hyperplasia (i.e., increased numbers) of erythroblasts, mainly polychromatic normoblasts,[23] leads to even higher levels of ERFE. This mechanism appears to explain the excess absorption of iron in anemias, such as β-thalassemia, in which ineffective erythropoiesis leads to iron overload (Chapter 17).[28] Although two other products of erythroblasts, growth differentiation factor-15 (GDF-15) and twisted gastrulation protein homolog 1 (TWSG1), have been found to affect hepcidin production, their in vivo effect in humans appears to be minimal.[29]

To summarize body iron kinetics, iron is absorbed in the cells of the small intestine and chaperoned to the other side of the cell where it is carried through the cell membrane by ferroportin. Once outside the enterocyte, the iron binds to Tf to be carried to cells, such as erythroblasts. Ferroportin activity is reduced by hepcidin secretion by the liver and also affects iron recycling from macrophages and hepatocytes. The liver senses circulating and tissue iron levels to adjust hepcidin production. Erythroblasts sense iron also and produce EFRE to inhibit hepcidin production when they need iron.

Body Iron Recycling and Salvage

When cells die, their iron is recycled. Multiple mechanisms salvage iron from dying cells. The largest percentage of recycled iron comes from RBCs. When senescent (aging) RBCs are ingested by macrophages in the spleen, the hemoglobin is degraded and the iron is held by the macrophages as ferritin. Ferroportin in macrophage membranes[30] allows macrophages to be iron exporters so that the salvaged iron can be used by other cells. The exported Fe^{2+} is oxidized by plasma ceruloplasmin for transport in the blood.[2] The Fe^{3+} is then bound to plasma apoTf, just as if it were newly absorbed from the intestine. Macrophages also export iron as ferritin, which is the source of plasma ferritin.[31]

Haptoglobin and hemopexin are plasma proteins that salvage plasma hemoglobin or heme, respectively, freed during fragmentation hemolysis. Macrophages carry a receptor for the haptoglobin-hemoglobin complex, whereas hepatocytes have a hemopexin-heme receptor, making them both important cells in iron salvage. Hepatocytes also possess ferroportin[30] so that the salvaged iron can be exported to apoTf and ultimately to other body cells. In fact, the recycling of iron by macrophages and hepatocytes is the largest source of iron daily for cell production. These salvage pathways are described in greater detail in Chapter 20.

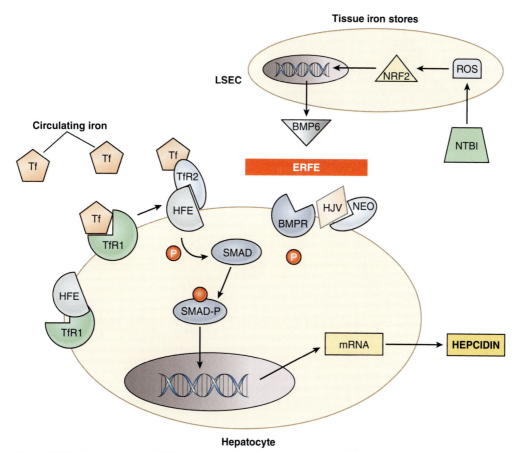

Figure 9.6 Erythroferrone Inhibition of Hepcidin Production. In conditions with ineffective erythropoiesis, erythroblasts secrete erythroferrone *(ERFE)*, which blocks bone morphogenetic protein 6 *(BMP6)* and prevents it from binding to the bone morphogenetic protein receptor *(BMPR)* on the hepatocyte membrane. Phosphorylation *(P)* of sons of mothers against decapentaplegic *(SMAD)* is diminished, and hepcidin production is reduced. More iron can be absorbed by enterocytes even though body iron is already plentiful.

The kidney is also an important organ in the maintenance of body iron. Iron-containing plasma proteins like Tf and ferritin appear in the urinary filtrate. They are reabsorbed by the kidney nephron, principally the proximal tubule cell. Without reabsorption of these proteins and subsequent salvage of their iron, iron deficiency can develop. The role of the kidney in iron handling is described in detail in Chapter 20.

Cellular Iron Kinetics

Cellular Iron Acquisition and Intracellular Trafficking

To this point, the discussion has focused on absorption of iron from the diet into the body and its regulation. The focus now shifts to how individual cells are able to acquire, store, and regulate the iron they need for their metabolic processes. Erythroblasts that have the greatest iron demand of any body cell will be the emphasis.

Cellular iron acquisition. Individual cells tightly regulate the amount of iron they absorb to minimize the adverse effects of free radicals. This is accomplished by relying on specific carriers to move iron into the cell by *receptor-mediated endocytosis* (Chapter 4) (Figure 9.8).[32] Cell membranes, including those of developing erythroblasts, possess TfR1. TfR1 has the highest affinity for diferric Tf at the physiologic pH of the plasma and extracellular fluid. When TfR1 molecules bind Tf, they move within the membrane and

cluster together. Once a critical mass accumulates, the membrane begins to invaginate (i.e., indent), progressing until the invagination pinches off as an *endosome*. Protons are pumped into the endosome. The resulting drop in pH changes the affinity of Tf for iron, so the iron releases. Simultaneously, the affinity of TfR1 for apoTf at that pH increases so the apoTf remains bound to the receptor. The iron is reduced by six-transmembrane epithelial antigen of the prostate 3 (STEAP3)[33] and exported from the endosome by DMT1.[34]

After export of the endosomal iron, the endosome returns to the cell membrane, where its membrane fuses with the cell membrane, opening the endosome and essentially reversing its formation.[32] At the pH of the extracellular fluid, TfR1 has a very low affinity for apoTf, so the apoTf releases into the plasma, available to bind iron once again. The TfR1 is also available again to carry new molecules of iron-loaded Tf into the cell.

A secondary method for entry of Tf to erythrocytes is via TfR2. While the function of TfR2 on the erythroblast membrane is mainly as an iron sensor. TfR2 is internalized when Tf binds and the iron is processed for the cell's use. In the case of Tf binding to TfR2, the endosome is not recycled like TfR1 but is channeled to a lysosome for release of the iron.[35] Transfer of the iron out of the lysosome appears to occur via direct lysosomal-mitochondrial contact.[35] The proteins involved are still being researched.

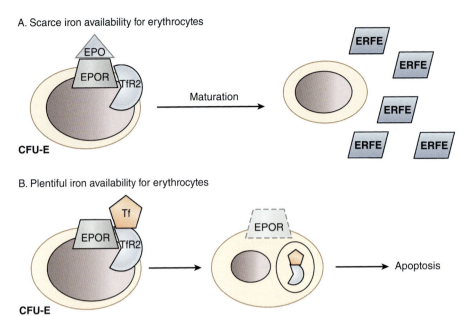

Figure 9.7 Erythrocyte Iron Sensing and Erythroferrone Production. (A) The erythropoietin receptor *(EPOR)* on the membrane of the colony-forming-unit-erythroid *(CFU-E)* is stabilized by transferrin receptor 2 *(TfR2)*. This allows the CFU-E to bind erythropoietin *(EPO)*, which prevents apoptosis and allows the cell to mature. At the polychromatic normoblast stage, the erythrocyte can secrete erythroferrone *(ERFE)*, which blocks hepcidin production and promotes intestinal iron absorption, providing iron to the erythroblasts for hemoglobin production. **(B)** When iron is plentiful, TfR2 binds transferrin *(Tf)* and the complex is internalized into a lysosome. This leaves the EPOR unstable and unable to bind EPO effectively. The cell undergoes apoptosis and does not mature to produce ERFE.

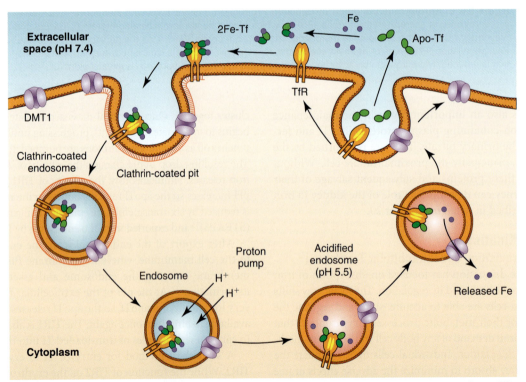

Figure 9.8 Cellular Iron Regulation. A critical mass of transferrin receptor 1 *(TfR)* with bound transferrin *(Tf)* will initiate an invagination of the membrane that ultimately fuses to form an endosome. Protons *(H⁺)* inside the endosome lower the pH, and the iron releases from Tf and is reduced to Fe^{2+}. Once reduced, it is transported into the cytosol by divalent metal transporter 1 *(DMT1)*. In the cytosol, iron may be stored as ferritin or transferred to the mitochondria, where it is transported across the membrane by mitoferrin (not shown). The TfR with apotransferrin *(apoTf)* is returned to the cell membrane, where the apoTf releases and the TfR is available to bind more Tf for iron transport into the cell. (Courtesy Thomas Walz, PhD.)

Extracellular ferritin is likely another source of iron for cells, especially developing RBCs in the erythropoietic islands of the bone marrow as the central macrophages secrete ferritin.[36] Electron microscopy revealed a process by which ferritin appeared to be directly absorbed into erythroblasts.[37] Gelvan and colleagues[38] demonstrated that erythroblasts absorb ferritin via endocytosis, but the receptor was not identified. TfR1 may be the receptor when a critical mass accumulates on the erythrocyte surface during periods of cellular iron scarcity[39] and the large load of iron carried by ferritin would be valuable to the cell. Tf and ferritin bind to different portions of the TfR1 receptor.[5] Absorbed ferritin is delivered to the lysosome for digestion and release of the iron as described more fully below. As with iron from TfR2, the means by which iron from the lysosome is transferred to the mitochondria is not fully elucidated.

Intracellular iron trafficking. Cytoplasmic trafficking of iron is still not fully understood despite significant research efforts. Multiple avenues are likely, with some perhaps unique to erythroblasts, allowing them to acquire more iron than other cells. Some of the iron clearly finds its way to storage as ferritin, likely via a PCBP chaperone.[40] There is evidence that other iron ions are transferred directly into the mitochondria from the endosome[41] or lysosome.[35] The process whereby the endosome and the mitochondria touch during iron transfer has been called "kiss and run," because the encounter is brief. However the iron arrives at the mitochondrial membrane, mitoferrin-1 is the carrier protein that moves iron through the membrane in erythroblasts.[42] It appears to hand the Fe^{2+} iron off directly to ferrochelatase for incorporation into protoporphyrin for heme production,[43] finally completing the journey to functionality that began with dietary iron ingestion.

In summary, cellular iron kinetics is characterized chiefly by the endocytic absorption of Tf via TfR1, though Tf may also be absorbed via TfR2. Ferritin may also be absorbed via TfR1 to provide iron to erythroblasts. Iron is channeled efficiently from the endosome or lysosome to the mitochondria for incorporation into protoporphyrin and formation of heme.

Cellular Iron Storage

Cells are able to store iron so they have a reserve if supplies of new iron decline. Although all cells store iron except mature erythrocytes, macrophages and hepatocytes that are central to recycling systemic body iron contain the most.

Ferric (Fe^{3+}) iron is stored in a cagelike protein called *apoferritin*. The apoferritin molecule typically receives Fe^{2+} iron from PCBP, but stores it as Fe^{3+}.[44] The heavy chain of ferritin (H-ferritin) possesses ferrioxidase activity to make the conversion.[44] Once iron binds, it is known as *holoferritin*. One ferritin molecule can bind more than 4000 iron ions in conditions of iron overload but binds about 2000 with normal iron levels.[45] Although ferritin is typically considered a cytoplasmic protein, it has been established that mitochondria contain ferritin as well.[46]

Ferritin iron can be mobilized for use during times of iron need by proteosomal or lysosomal degradation of the protein,[45,47] a process that has recently been termed ferritinophagy.[48,49] The iron is then channeled to the mitochondria as

described previously. Partially degraded ferritin in organelles is known as *hemosiderin*.[45,50,51]

Intracellular Iron Regulation

To regulate the amount of iron inside the cell and avoid free radicals, cells are able to control the amount of TfR1 on their surface. The process depends on an elegant system of iron-sensitive cytoplasmic proteins that are able to affect the posttranscriptional function of the messenger ribonucleic acid (mRNA) for TfR1.[52] The result is that when iron stores inside the cell are sufficient, production of TfR1 declines, thus reducing cellular iron absorption. Conversely, when iron stores inside the cell are low, TfR1 production increases to acquire more iron. The change in the amount of TfR1 in response to available iron is useful in diagnosis of iron-restricted anemias (discussed in "Intracellular Iron Regulation").

Ferritin production is also controlled by iron-sensitive cytoplasmic proteins, but production is counter to TfR1.[53,54] When iron is plentiful, ferritin production increases as TfR1 decreases. Ferritin production will decrease when iron is scarce, while TfR1 increases.

DIETARY IRON, BIOAVAILABILITY, AND DEMAND

Under normal circumstances, the majority of iron for cellular processes, including hemoglobin production, derives from the recycling process described earlier. A small amount of new iron is needed daily and is acquired from the diet. Foods containing high levels of iron include red meats, legumes, and dark green leafy vegetables.[55] Although some foods may be high in iron, that iron may not be readily absorbed and thus is not bioavailable. As mentioned earlier in "Absorption of Dietary Iron in the Intestines," iron can be absorbed as either ionic iron or nonionic iron in the form of heme or ferritin. Ionic iron must be in the Fe^{2+} form for absorption into the enterocyte via the luminal membrane carrier, DMT1. However, most dietary ionic iron is Fe^{3+}, especially from plant sources. As a result, it is not readily absorbed. Furthermore, other dietary compounds can bind ionic iron and inhibit its absorption. These include oxalates, phytates, and phosphates.[55] Release from these binders and reduction to the Fe^{2+} form are enhanced by gastric acid, acidic foods (e.g., citrus), and the enterocyte luminal membrane ferrireductase, duodenal cytochrome *b*.[56] Nevertheless, absorption of ionic iron is limited, and although the US diet contains on the order of 10 to 20 mg of iron per day, only 1 to 2 mg is absorbed.[55] This amount is adequate for most males, but menstruating females pregnant females, lactating females, and growing children usually need additional iron supplementation to meet their increased need for iron. Chapter 17 discusses this further.

Heme, with its bound iron, is more readily absorbed than ionic iron.[57] Thus meat, with heme in both myoglobin of muscle and hemoglobin of blood, is the most bioavailable source of dietary iron. As mentioned earlier in "Absorption of Dietary Iron in the Intestines," ferritin can also be absorbed, though it is not typically a substantial source of dietary iron.

LABORATORY ASSESSMENT OF BODY IRON STATUS

Disease occurs when body iron levels are either too low or too high (Chapter 17). The tests used to assess body iron status are able to detect both conditions. The screening tests for iron status include serum iron (SI), total iron-binding capacity (TIBC), percent transferrin saturation, and serum ferritin. When the results of screening assays are equivocal, additional tests include Prussian blue staining of tissues, soluble transferrin receptor (sTfR), and hemoglobin content of reticulocytes. The results of measured parameters can be combined to calculate an sTfR/log ferritin ratio or graph a Thomas plot. Zinc protoporphyrin (ZPP) and free erythrocyte protoporphyrin (FEP) are other assays with special application in sideroblastic anemia and iron deficiency anemia. Diagnostically, the tests can be organized to assess each of the iron compartments as indicated in Table 9.3.

Serum Iron

SI can be measured colorimetrically using any of several reagents such as ferrozine. Fe^{3+} is first released from Tf by acid, followed by reduction to Fe^{2+}, and then the reagent is allowed to react with this Fe^{2+}, forming a colored complex that can be detected spectrophotometrically. Reference intervals are reported separately for males, females, and children, and will vary from laboratory to laboratory and from method to method. Low SI is expected in iron-restricted anemias (Chapter 17), while high levels are seen in iron overload conditions (Chapter 17). The SI level has limited utility on its own because of its high within-day and between-day variability; it also increases after recent ingestion of iron-containing foods and supplements. To avoid the apparent diurnal variation, standard practice has been to collect the specimen fasting and early in the morning, when levels are expected to be highest. However, this practice has recently been questioned.[58] A diurnal variation in hepcidin has been detected that may explain some of the SI variability and may still support the early morning phlebotomy practice.[59,60] A typical reference interval is provided in Table 9.3.

Total Iron-Binding Capacity

The amount of iron in plasma or serum will be limited by the amount of apoTf that is available to carry it. As a traditional method to assess this, Tf is maximally saturated by addition of excess Fe^{3+} to the specimen. Any unbound iron is removed by precipitation with magnesium carbonate powder. Then the basic iron method as described in the previous section is performed on the absorbed serum, beginning with the release of the iron from Tf. The amount of iron detected represents all the binding sites available on apoTf, that is, the TIBC. Even though many common methods use addition of excess iron to saturate apoTf, they do not require the step separating unbound iron from bound iron, thus allowing fully automated analysis. In one example method (Figure 9.9), the initial reaction is performed by adding a known amount of iron at a basic pH that saturates the apoTf, and then light absorption for unbound $[Fe^{3+}]$ is measured at a wavelength selected between 530 and 560 nm. In the second step, the pH of the solution is lowered, which releases the iron from Tf. The light absorption of this solution includes the total $[Fe^{3+}]$ of SI (i.e., transferrin-bound iron) and the added reagent iron. TIBC can be calculated from the difference in light absorption of the two steps.[61] TIBC is expressed as an iron value, although it is actually an indirect measure of apoTf. A typical reference interval is provided in Table 9.3. TIBC will rise in iron deficiency. TIBC can drop when liver disease impairs protein production.

Percent Transferrin Saturation

Because the SI represents the number of Tf sites bound with iron and the TIBC represents the total number of TF sites for iron binding, the degree to which the available sites are occupied by iron can be calculated. The percent of TF saturated with iron is calculated as:

$$SI / TIBC \times 100\% = \% \text{ transferrin saturation}$$

TABLE 9.3   Assessment of Body Iron Status

Laboratory Assay	Typical Adult Male Reference Interval	Diagnostic Use and Compartment Assessed
Serum iron level	50–160 μg/dL	Indicator of available transport iron
Total iron-binding capacity	250–400 μg/dL	Total amount of iron that could be transported in the plasma; indirect indicator of transferrin level
Transferrin saturation	20%–55%	Percentage of transferrin iron-binding sites that are occupied by iron; indirect indicator of transport iron and transferrin level
Serum ferritin level	40–400 ng/mL	Indicator of iron stores
Bone marrow or liver biopsy with Prussian blue staining	Normal iron stores visualized	Visual qualitative assessment of tissue iron stores
sTfR level	1.15–2.75 mg/L	Indicator of functional iron available in cells
sTfR/log ferritin index	0.63–1.8	Indicator of functional iron available in cells
RBC zinc protoporphyrin level	<80 μg/dL of RBCs	Indicator of functional iron available in RBCs
Hemoglobin content of reticulocytes	27–34 pg/cell	Indicator of functional iron available in developing RBCs

RBC, Red blood cell; *sTfR,* soluble transferrin receptor.

Step 1. Saturating transferrin at high pH with known amount of iron

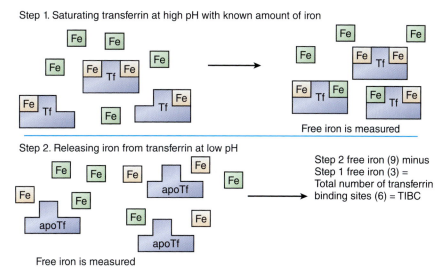

Free iron is measured

Step 2. Releasing iron from transferrin at low pH

Step 2 free iron (9) minus
Step 1 free iron (3) =
Total number of transferrin
binding sites (6) = TIBC

Free iron is measured

Figure 9.9 Principle of Automated Assays for Total Iron-Binding Capacity. In step 1, the patient specimen contains transferrin *(Tf)*, with some sites occupied by iron *(Fe)* and others empty. In this diagram, three transferrin molecules are carrying four iron ions. A known amount of iron is added to the specimen at a high pH to saturate the transferrin, that is, five ions of iron in the diagram. The amount of free iron after Tf saturation is measured. Two ions have bound to the open sites on Tf, leaving three ions free. In step 2, the specimen is acidified to release all iron from Tf. The free iron in the acidified specimen equals the patient specimen iron plus the added iron. The iron value from step 1 *(3)* is subtracted from the value in step 2 *(9)* to provide the total number of iron-binding sites on the apotransferrin *(6)*, which is the total iron-binding capacity.

It is important that both SI and TIBC be expressed in the same units, but it does not matter which units are used in the calculation. A typical reference interval is provided in Table 9.3. A convenient rule of thumb evident from the table is that about one-third of Tf is typically saturated with iron. The percent saturation is expected to be low in iron deficiency and increased in conditions of iron overload.

Prussian Blue Staining

Prussian blue is actually a chemical compound with the formula $Fe_4[Fe(CN)_6]_3$.[62] The compound forms in tissues and cells during the staining process, which uses acidic potassium ferrocyanide ($K_4[Fe(CN)_6]$) as the reagent/stain. The Fe^{3+} in the tissue reacts with the reagent, forming the Prussian blue compound that is easily seen microscopically. Hemosiderin, an insoluble form of iron in lysosomes, stains readily, forming distinct dark blue granules, while soluble ferritin produces a diffuse cytoplasmic blueness.[63] Tissues can be graded or scored semiquantitatively by the amount of stain that is observed. The location of the iron is also important, in macrophages versus parenchymal cells of the liver or erythroblasts in bone marrow.

Prussian blue stain is considered the gold standard for assessment of body iron stores. Staining is conducted routinely when bone marrow or liver biopsy specimens are collected for other purposes. Increased amounts of stainable iron are expected in iron overload conditions (Chapter 17), while decreased amounts are expected in iron deficiencies (Chapter 17). In the bone marrow, iron in macrophages but not erythroblasts is consistent with anemia of inflammation (Chapter 17).

Ferritin

Ferritin is the iron-storage protein that functions mainly within cells, though the role for plasma ferritin as an iron transporter,

particularly to erythroblasts, was described earlier. Macrophages are the source of plasma ferritin.[31]

Until the development of serum ferritin assays, the only way to truly assess body iron stores was to collect a bone marrow specimen and stain it with Prussian blue. Such an invasive procedure prevented regular assessment of body iron. The development of the serum immunoassay for ferritin has provided a convenient, minimally invasive, quantitative assessment of body iron stores. The level of serum ferritin has been found to correlate highly with stored iron as assessed by Prussian blue stains of bone marrow.[64] Thus values are expected to decrease with iron deficiency and increase with iron overload. Typical reference intervals are provided in Table 9.3.

There is a significant drawback in the interpretation of serum ferritin results. Ferritin is an acute phase protein or acute phase reactant.[65] The acute phase reactants are proteins that are produced, mostly by the liver, during the acute (or initial) phase of inflammation, especially during infections. They include cytokines that are nonspecific, but also other proteins with the apparent intent to suppress bacteria. Because bacteria need iron, the body's production of ferritin during an infection seems to be an attempt to sequester the iron away from the bacteria, which may be the role for plasma ferritin. Thus increases in ferritin can be induced without an increase in the amount of systemic body iron (a falsely increased result). These rises may not exceed the reference interval but may still be high enough to elevate a patient's ferritin to greater than what it would otherwise be. Ferritin values between 30 and 100 ng/mL are most equivocal, making it difficult to recognize true iron deficiency when an inflammatory condition is also present.[66] Therefore the predictive value of a ferritin result within the reference interval is weak. However, only a decreased level of stored body iron can lower ferritin levels to less than the reference interval, so the predictive value of a low ferritin result is high for iron deficiency.

Soluble Transferrin Receptor

As described previously, cells regulate the amount of TfR1 on their membrane based on the amount of intracellular iron. When the intracellular iron decreases, the cell expresses more TfR1 on the membrane. A truncated form of the receptor is shed into the plasma and can be detected by immunoassay.[67] Thus increases in the soluble receptor, sTfR, reflect either increases in the amounts of TfR1 on individual cells, as in iron deficiency, or an increase in the number of cells, each with a normal amount of TfR1. The latter occurs during instances of rapid erythropoiesis, such as a response to hemolytic anemia. Typical reference intervals are provided in Table 9.3.

Hemoglobin Content of Reticulocytes

Chapter 13 describes how some automated blood cell analyzers are able to report a value for the amount of hemoglobin in reticulocytes; it is analogous to the mean cell hemoglobin, but just for reticulocytes. Because under normal conditions the number of circulating reticulocytes represents the status of erythropoiesis in the prior 24-hour period, the amount of hemoglobin in reticulocytes provides a near real-time, though indirect, assessment of iron available for hemoglobin production.[68] The hemoglobin content of reticulocytes will decrease when iron for erythropoiesis is restricted. A representative adult reference interval is provided in Table 9.3. Separate reference intervals may be provided for children and infants. Instrument assessment of this parameter is proprietary, and each manufacturer refers to their parameter with a different name (Chapter 13).

Soluble Transferrin Receptor/Log Ferritin

Although ferritin and sTfR values alone can point to iron deficiency, the ratio of sTfR to ferritin or sTfR to log ferritin improves the identification of iron deficiency when individual assay values are equivocal.[69,70] Because the sTfR rises in iron deficiency and the ferritin (and its log) drops, these ratios are especially useful to amplify changes when one of the parameters has changed but is not outside the reference interval. A typical reference interval is provided in Table 9.3.

Thomas Plot

Thomas and Thomas[71] demonstrated that when the sTfR/log ferritin is plotted against the hemoglobin content of reticulocytes, a four-quadrant plot results that can improve the identification of iron deficiency (Figure 9.10).[72] In instances where there is *true iron deficiency*, the sTfR will rise and the ferritin will drop so that the sTfR/log ferritin will be high and the hemoglobin content of reticulocytes will be low; patient results will plot to the lower right quadrant. In instances where the ferritin may be falsely elevated by

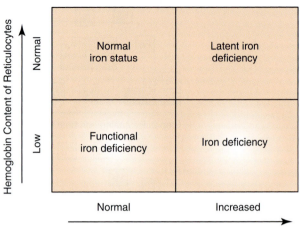

THOMAS PLOT

Figure 9.10 Thomas Plot. Plotting the ratio of soluble transferrin receptor *(sTfR)* to log ferritin (sTfR/log ferritin) against the hemoglobin content of reticulocytes produces a graph with four quadrants. Patients with values within the reference intervals for each assay will cluster in the upper left quadrant. Patients with functional iron deficiency, such as the anemia of chronic inflammation, will cluster at the lower left. Latent iron deficiency, before anemia develops, will cluster at the upper right, and frank iron deficiency will cluster in the lower right quadrant. (Modified from Doig, K. [2013]. *Iron: The Body's Most Precious Metal.* [p. 24]. McLean, VA: American Society for Clinical Laboratory Science.)

inflammation, the sTfR/log ferritin will be normal despite reduced availability of iron for hemoglobin production, resulting in low hemoglobin content in reticulocytes. In this instance, patient values will plot to the lower left quadrant, called *functional iron deficiency*, because the systemic body stores are adequate but not available for transport and use by cells. As iron deficiency develops, other cells are starved for iron before erythrocytes; production of hemoglobin in reticulocytes remains at a normal level for as long as possible. However, the body's other iron-starved cells will increase sTfR production and systemic iron stores of ferritin will be depleted, thus elevating the sTfR/log ferritin value. Results in these early iron-deficient patients will plot to the upper right quadrant, called *latent iron deficiency*, which is the preanemic iron deficiency state. By incorporating several different assessments of iron status, the use of the *Thomas plot*, as it is called, can improve the identification of iron deficiency in instances when other tests are equivocal. Chapter 17 elucidates further the impact of various diseases on the parameters of the Thomas plot.

Zinc Protoporphyrin

Protoporphyrin accumulates in RBCs when the enzymatic incorporation of iron into protoporphyrin IX is inhibited. The majority of protoporphyrin binds to zinc nonenzymatically, called *zinc protoporphyrin* (ZPP), while the remaining protoporphyrin is called *free erythrocyte protoporphyrin* (FEP). Both ZPP and FEP are easily measured by fluorescence. Although ZPP will rise during iron-deficient erythropoiesis, the value of this test is greatest when the activity of the ferrochelatase is impaired, as in lead poisoning (Chapter 17).[73]

SUMMARY

- Iron kinetics encompasses all processes, cells, locations, and carriers involved in trafficking iron from intestinal absorption to insertion into protoporphyrin in the mitochondria of cells. Kinetics of total body iron differs from kinetics of iron in individual cells.

- Most body iron is found in hemoglobin or stored as ferritin.

- Iron is so critical for transport and use of oxygen that the body conserves and recycles it, and it does not have a mechanism for its active excretion. Free radical production by iron ions severely damages cells and thus demands regulation at the body and cellular levels. The body adjusts its iron levels by intestinal absorption, depending on need.

- Macrophages and hepatocytes are responsible for distributing iron to other body cells and are the source for most iron used daily. Macrophages salvage iron when they ingest senescent (aging) red blood cells (RBCs). Hepatocytes and macrophages both salvage iron from fragmented RBCs. Macrophages also release ferritin into plasma, which can be used as an iron source by some cells, such as erythroblasts.

- A small amount of dietary iron is required daily to replace iron lost with sloughed skin and intestinal cells. Dietary iron is absorbed into enterocytes as Fe^{2+} iron by the divalent metal transporter 1 (DMT1) on the luminal side of the cells. Heme and ferritin can also be absorbed and the iron extracted by the enterocyte. Iron is chaperoned through the cytoplasm by polycytosine-binding proteins and exported into the plasma via ferroportin, a protein carrier in the enterocyte basolaminal membrane.

- Iron, exported from enterocytes, is carried in the plasma in Fe^{3+} form attached to apotransferrin (apoTf). Each molecule of apoTf can bind two Fe^{3+} ions. apoTf with two bound iron ions is called transferrin (Tf), diferric transferrin, or holotransferrin.

- Individual cells absorb the majority of iron when diferric Tf binds to transferrin receptor 1 (TfR1) on their surfaces. Bound receptors cluster and indent the membrane to form an endosome. Iron released by acid within the endosome is exported into the cytosol, or perhaps directly into mitochondria, for incorporation into cytochromes and heme. Alternatively, it can also be stored as ferritin in the cytosol. The iron-depleted endosome fuses with the cell membrane, releasing the apoTf and thus allowing the TfR1 on the cell membrane to bind more diferric Tf.

- Individual cells adjust the amount of TfR1 on their surface to regulate the amount of iron they absorb; receptor numbers rise when the cell needs additional iron but decrease when the iron in the cell is adequate. Truncated soluble transferrin receptors (sTfRs) are shed into the plasma in proportion to their number on cells.

- Cells store iron as ferritin when they have an excess. Iron can be released from ferritin when needed by degradation of the protein by lysosomes. Partially degraded ferritin can be detected in cells as stainable hemosiderin. Ferritin is secreted into the plasma by macrophages in proportion to the amount of iron that is in storage. Ferritin is elevated in plasma by the acute phase response, unrelated to amounts of stored iron.

- Body iron is regulated by a liver-produced hormone, hepcidin. Hepcidin can bind to ferroportin, a membrane iron exporter on enterocytes, macrophages, and hepatocytes. When hepcidin binds to ferroportin, the ferroportin is inactivated and iron export from the cell is blocked. When body iron is adequate, the liver produces hepcidin to decrease enterocyte iron absorption and recycling. When body iron is low, hepcidin production decreases allowing more iron to be absorbed into the body and recycled.

- Hepcidin production is regulated chiefly by the liver, which is able to sense the amount of iron in circulation and the amount of iron in storage. Erythroblasts also sense iron availability. When iron levels are low, erythroblasts secrete a hormone, erythroferrone, which reduces hepcidin production, providing more iron for hemoglobin production.

- Dietary iron is most bioavailable as heme from meat sources. Plant sources typically supply Fe^{3+} iron that must be released from iron-binding compounds and reduced before absorption. This occurs with gastric acidity and a luminal ferrireductase.

- Laboratory tests for assessment of iron status include total serum iron (SI), total iron-binding capacity (TIBC), percent Tf saturation, Prussian blue staining for iron in tissues, serum ferritin, sTfR, hemoglobin content of reticulocytes, and zinc protoporphyrin (ZPP). Additional parameters derived from these, sTfR/log ferritin and the Thomas plot, are particularly useful for the recognition of iron deficiency when other test results are equivocal.

- SI is measured using a colorimetric reaction after being released from Tf and reduced to Fe^{2+}.

- The TIBC assay requires saturating apoTf with reagent iron. It is followed by using the SI procedure on the saturated specimen.

- The percent Tf saturation can be calculated by dividing the SI by the TIBC and expressing as a percentage.

- The total SI result becomes more useful when it is interpreted with TIBC and percent transferrin saturation.

- Prussian blue staining allows assessment of body iron stores in tissues but is highly invasive. The reagent reacts with Fe^{3+} in hemosiderin producing a dark precipitate that is evaluated microscopically and reported semiquantitatively.

- Immunoassay for serum ferritin can assess levels of body iron stores without an invasive biopsy. Levels are falsely elevated in inflammatory conditions, but a low ferritin value is highly predictive of iron deficiency.

- sTfRs in serum increase during iron deficiency or rapid erythropoiesis. They are measured by immunoassay.

- Hemoglobin content of reticulocytes can provide a near real-time assessment of iron availability for hemoglobin production. Iron deficiency can be detected before anemia develops. Hematology analyzers use varying methods to identify reticulocytes and measure their hemoglobin.

- Increased ZPP or free erythrocyte protoporphyrin will be observed whenever iron incorporation into protoporphyrin is inhibited. Levels rise in iron deficiency, yet it is more useful in detecting lead poisoning. Both analytes are measured with fluorescence.

Now that you have completed this chapter, go back and read again the case study at the beginning and respond to the questions presented. Answers can be found in Appendix C.

REVIEW QUESTIONS

Answers can be found in Appendix C.

1. Iron is transported in plasma via:
   a. Hemosiderin
   b. Ferritin
   c. Transferrin
   d. Hemoglobin

2. What is the major metabolically available storage form of iron in the body?
   a. Ferroportin
   b. Ferritin
   c. Transferrin
   d. Hemoglobin

3. The total iron-binding capacity (TIBC) of the serum is an indirect measure of which iron-related protein?
   a. Hemosiderin
   b. Ferritin
   c. Transferrin
   d. Haptoglobin

4. Which of the following sets of test results would indicate iron deficiency?
   a. Increased soluble transferrin receptor (sTfR), increased log ferritin, increased sTfR/log ferritin ratio
   b. Increased sTfR, decreased log ferritin, decreased sTfR/log ferritin ratio
   c. Increased sTfR, decreased log ferritin, increased sTfR/log ferritin ratio
   d. Decreased sTfR, decreased log ferritin, decreased sTfR/log ferritin ratio

5. What membrane-associated protein in enterocytes transports iron from the intestinal lumen into the enterocyte?
   a. Divalent metal transporter 1
   b. Ferroportin
   c. Transferrin
   d. Hephaestin

6. Iron is transported out of macrophages, hepatocytes, and enterocytes by what membrane protein?
   a. Transferrin
   b. Ferroportin
   c. Divalent metal transporter 1
   d. Ferrochelatase

7. Following are several of the many steps in the process from absorption and transport of iron to incorporation into heme. Place them in the proper order.
   i. Transferrin picks up ferric iron.
   ii. Iron is transferred to the mitochondria.
   iii. DMT1 transports ferrous iron into the enterocyte.
   iv. Ferroportin transports iron from enterocyte to plasma.
   v. The transferrin receptor transports iron into the cell.
   a. v, iv, i, ii, iii
   b. iii, ii, iv, i, v
   c. ii, i, v, iii, iv
   d. iii, iv, i, v, ii

8. What is the fate of the transferrin receptor when it has completed its role in the delivery of iron into a cell?
   a. It is recycled to the plasma membrane and released into the plasma.
   b. It is recycled to the plasma membrane, where it can bind its ligand again.
   c. It is catabolized and the amino acids are returned to the metabolic pool.
   d. It is retained in the endosome for the life span of the cell.

9. The transfer of iron from the enterocyte into the plasma is REGULATED by:
   a. Transferrin
   b. Ferroportin
   c. Hephaestin
   d. Hepcidin

10. What is the percent transferrin saturation for a patient with total serum iron of 63 µg/dL and TIBC of 420 µg/dL?
    a. 6.7%
    b. 12%
    c. 15%
    d. 80%

11. Referring to Figure 9.10, into which quadrant of a Thomas plot would a patient's results fall with the following test results?
    Soluble transferrin receptor: increased above reference interval
    Ferritin: decreased below reference interval
    Hemoglobin content of reticulocytes: within the reference interval
    a. Normal iron status
    b. Latent iron deficiency
    c. Functional iron deficiency
    d. Iron deficiency

12. Which of the following would be the most helpful information to differentiate iron deficiency anemia from anemia caused by functional iron deficiency?
    a. Hemoglobin content of reticulocyte
    b. Soluble transferrin receptor (sTfR)
    c. Ferritin
    d. Total iron-binding capacity

13. Developing erythroblasts in the bone marrow affect the supply of body iron by secreting which of the following hormones?
    a. Erythropoietin
    b. Erythroferrone
    c. Hepcidin
    d. Haptoglobin

14. Which of the following is secreted by hepatocytes to regulate iron absorption and recycling?
    a. Hepcidin
    b. Bone morphogenetic protein 6
    c. Ferritin
    d. Ferroportin

15. Which of the following plays a role in body iron SENSING so as to adjust iron absorption and recycling?
    a. Hepcidin
    b. Transferrin receptor 2
    c. Ferroportin
    d. Divalent metal transporter 1

REFERENCES

1. Garry, P. J., Koehler, K. M., & Simon, T. L. (1995). Iron stores and iron absorption: effects of repeated blood donations. *Am J Clin Nutr, 62*(3), 611–620.
2. Goodnough, L. T., & Nemeth, E. (2019). Iron deficiency and related disorders. In Greer, J. P., Rodgers, G. M., Glader, B., et al. (Eds.), *Wintrobe's Clinical Hematology*. (14th ed., pp. 615–643). Philadelphia: Lippincott Williams and Wilkins.
3. Theil, E. C., Chen, H., Miranda, C., et al. (2012). Absorption of iron from ferritin is independent of heme iron and ferrous salts in women and rat intestinal segments. *J Nutr, 142*(3), 478–483.
4. Kalgaonkar, S., & Lönnerdal, B. (2009). Receptor-mediated uptake of ferritin-bound iron by human intestinal Caco-2 cells. *J Nutr Biochem, 20*(4), 304–311.
5. Li, L., Fang, C. J., Ryan, J. C., et al. (2010). Binding and uptake of H-ferritin are mediated by human transferrin receptor-1. *Proc Natl Acad Sci USA, 107*(8), 3505–3510.
6. Lönnerdal, B. (2007). The importance and bioavailability of phytoferritin-bound iron in cereals and legume foods. *Int J Vitam Nutr Res, 77*(3), 152–157.
7. Shayeghi, M., Latunde-Dada, G. O., Oakhill, J. S., et al. (2005). Identification of an intestinal heme transporter. *Cell, 122*(5), 789–801.
8. Yanatori, I., Tabuchi, M., Kawai, Y., et al. (2010). Heme and non-heme iron transporters in non-polarized and polarized cells. *BMC Cell Biol, 11*, 39.
9. Le Blanc, S., Garrick, M. D., & Arredondo, M. (2012). Heme carrier protein 1 transports heme and is involved in heme-Fe metabolism. *Am J Physiol Cell Physiol, 302*, C1780–C1785.
10. Laftah, A. H., Latunde-Dada, G. O., Fakih, S., et al. (2009). Haem and folate transport by proton-coupled folate transporter/haem carrier protein 1 (SLC46A1). *Br J Nutr, 101*(8), 1150–1156.
11. Rajagopal, A., Rao, A. U., Amigo, J., et al. (2008). Haem homeostasis is regulated by the conserved and concerted functions of HRG-1 proteins. *Nature, 453*(7198), 1127–1131.
12. Yanatori, I., Yasui, Y., Tabuchi, M., et al. (2014). Chaperone protein involved in transmembrane transport of iron. *Biochem J, 462*(1), 25–37.
13. Yanatori, I., Richardson, D. R., Imada, I., et al. (2016). Iron export through the transporter ferroportin 1 is modulated by the iron chaperone PCBP2. *J Biol Chem, 291*(33), 17303–17318.
14. Nemeth, E., Tuttle, M. S., Powelson, J., et al. (2004). Hepcidin regulates cellular iron efflux by binding to ferroportin and inducing its internalization. *Science, 306*(5704), 2090–2093.
15. Aschemeyer, S., Qiao, B., Stefanova, D., et al. (2018). Structure-function analysis of ferroportin defines the binding site and an alternative mechanism of action of hepcidin. *Blood, 131*(8), 899–910.
16. Wang, C., & Babitt, J. L. (2019). Liver iron sensing and body iron homeostasis. *Blood, 133*(1), 18–29.
17. Anderson, G. J. (1999). Non-transferrin-bound iron and cellular toxicity. *J Gastroenterol Hepatol, 14*(2), 105–108.
18. Sherman, H. G., Jovanovic, C., Stolnik, S., et al. (2018). New perspectives on iron uptake in eukaryotes. *Front Mol Biosci, 19*(5), 97.
19. Duarte, T. L., Talbot, N. P., & Drakesmith, H. (2021). NRF2 and hypoxia-inducible factors: key players in the redox control of systemic iron homeostasis. *Antioxid Redox Signal, 35*(6), 433–452.
20. Lim, P. J., Duarte, T. L., Arezes, J., et al. (2019). Nrf2 controls iron homeostasis in haemochromatosis and thalassaemia via Bmp6 and hepcidin. *Nat Metab, 1*(5), 519–531.
21. Canali, S., Zumbrennen-Bullough, K. B., Core, A. B., et al. (2017). Endothelial cells produce bone morphogenetic protein 6 required for iron homeostasis in mice. *Blood, 129*(4), 405–414.
22. Andriopoulos, B., Corradini, E., Xia, Y., et al. (2009). BMP6 is a key endogenous regulator of hepcidin expression and iron metabolism. *Nat Genet, 41*(4), 482–487.
23. Kautz, L, Jung, G., Valore, E. V., et al. (2014). Identification of erythroferrone as an erythroid regulator of iron metabolism. *Nat Genet, 46*(7), 678–684.
24. Arezes, J., Foy, N., McHugh, K., et al. (2018). Erythroferrone inhibits the induction of hepcidin by BMP6. *Blood, 132*(14), 1473–1477.
25. Kawabata, H., Germain, R. S., Vuong, P. T., et al. (2000). Transferrin receptor 2-alpha supports cell growth both in iron-chelated cultured cells and in vivo. *J Biol Chem, 275*(22), 16618–16625.
26. Nai, A., Lindonnici, M. R., Rausa, M., et al. (2015). The second transferrin receptor regulates red blood cell production in mice. *Blood, 125*(7), 1170–1179.
27. Richard, C., & Verdier, F. (2020). Transferrin receptors in erythropoiesis. *Int J Mol Sci, 21*(24), 9713.
28. Kautz, L., Jung, G., Du, X., et al. (2015). Erythroferrone contributes to hepcidin suppression and iron overload in a mouse model of β-thalassemia. *Blood, 126*(17), 231–237.
29. Kim, A., & Nemeth, E. (2015). New insights into iron regulation and erythropoiesis. *Curr Opin Hematol, 22*(3), 199–205.
30. Le, N. T., & Richardson, D. R. (2002). Ferroportin1: a new iron export molecule? *Int J Biochem Cell Biol, 34*(2), 103–108.
31. Cohen, L. A., Gutierrez, L., Weiss, A., et al. (2010). Serum ferritin is derived primarily from macrophages through a nonclassical secretory pathway. *Blood, 116*(9), 1574–1584.
32. Harding, C., Heuser, J., & Stahl, P. (1983). Receptor-mediated endocytosis of transferrin and recycling of the transferrin receptor in rat reticulocytes. *J Cell Biol, 97*(2), 329–339.
33. Ohgami, R. S., Campagna, D. R., Greer, E. L., et al. (2005). Identification of a ferrireductase required for efficient transferrin-dependent iron uptake in erythroid cells. *Nat Genet, 37*(11), 1264–1269.
34. Fleming, M. D., Romano, M. A., Su, M. A., et al. (1998). Nramp2 is mutated in the anemic Belgrade (b) rat: evidence of a role for Nramp2 in endosomal iron transport. *Proc Natl Acad Sci U S A, 95*(3), 1148–1153.
35. Khalil, S., Holy, M., Grado, S., et al. (2017). A specialized pathway for erythroid iron delivery through lysosomal trafficking of transferrin receptor 2. *Blood Adv, 1*(15), 1181–1194.
36. Leimberg, M. J., Prus, E., Konijn, A. M., et al. (2008). Macrophages function as a ferritin iron source for cultured human erythroid precursors. *Cell Biochem, 103*(4), 1211–1218.
37. Policard, A., & Bessis, M. (1962). Micropinocytosis and rhopheocytosis. *Nature, 194* (4823), 110–111.
38. Gelvan, D., Fibach, E., Meyron-Holtz, E. G., et al. (1996). Ferritin uptake by human erythroid precursors is a regulated iron uptake pathway. *Blood, 88*(8), 3200–3207.
39. Sakamoto, S., Kawabata, H., Masuda, T., et al. (2015). H-ferritin is preferentially incorporated by human erythroid cells through

transferrin receptor 1 in a threshold dependent manner. *PLoS One, 10*(10), e0139915.

40. Leidgens, S., Bullough, K. Z., Shi, H., et al. (2013). Each member of the poly-r(C)-binding protein 1 (PCBP) family exhibits iron chaperone activity toward ferritin. *J Biol Chem, 288*(24), 17791–17802.

41. Sheftel, A. D., Zhang, A., Brown, C., et al. (2007). Direct interorganellar transfer of iron from endosome to mitochondrion. *Blood, 110*(1), 125–132.

42. Shaw, G. C., Cope, J. J., Li, L., et al. (2006). Mitoferrin is essential for erythroid iron assimilation. *Nature, 440*(2), 96–100.

43. Chen, W., Dailey, H. A., & Paw, B. H. (2010). Ferrochelatase forms an oligomeric complex with mitoferrin-1 and Abcb10 for erythroid heme biosynthesis. *Blood, 116*(4), 628–630.

44. Ebrahimi, K. H., Bill, E., Hagedoorn, P. L., et al. (2012). The catalytic center of ferritin regulates iron storage via Fe(II)-Fe(III) displacement. *Nat Chem Bio, 8*, 941–948.

45. Theil, E. C. (2013). Ferritin: the protein nanocage and iron biomineral in health and in disease. *Inorg Chem, 52*, 12223–12233.

46. Levi, S., Corsi, B., Bosisio, M., et al. (2001). A human mitochondrial ferritin encoded by an intronless gene. *J Biol Chem, 276*(27), 24437–24440.

47. Zhang, Y., Mikhael, M., Xu, D., et al. (2010). Lysosomal proteolysis is the primary degradation pathway for cytosolic ferritin and cytosolic ferritin degradation is necessary for iron exit. *Antioxid Redox Signal, 13*(7), 999–1009.

48. Santana-Codina, N., & Mancias, J. D. (2018). The role of NCOA4-mediated ferritinophagy in health and disease. *Pharmaceuticals (Basel), 11*(4), 114.

49. Mancias, J. D., Wang, X., Gygi, S. P., et al. (2014). Quantitative proteomics identifies NCOA4 as the cargo receptor mediating ferritinophagy. *Nature, 509*(7498), 105–109.

50. Miyazaki, E., Kato, J., Kobune, M., et al. (2002). Denatured H-ferritin subunit is a major constituent of haemosiderin in the liver of patients with iron overload. *Gut, 50*(3), 413–419.

51. Weir, M. P., Gibson, J. F., & Peters, T. J. (1984). Haemosiderin and tissue damage. *Cell Biochem Funct, 2*(4), 186–194.

52. Casey, J. L., Hentze, M. W., Koeller, D. M., et al. (1988). Iron-responsive elements: regulatory RNA sequences that control mRNA levels and translation. *Science, 240*(4854), 924–928.

53. Hentzes, M. W., Caughman, W., Rouault, T. A., et al. (1987). Identification of the iron-responsive element for the translational regulation of human ferritin mRNA. *Science, 238*(4833), 1570–1573.

54. Thomson, A. M., Rogers, J. T., & Leedman, P. J. (1999). Iron-regulatory proteins, iron-responsive elements and ferritin mRNA translation. *Int J Biochem Cell Biol, 31*(10), 1139–1152.

55. Hallberg, L. (1981). Bioavailability of dietary iron in man. *Annu Rev Nutr, 1*, 123–147.

56. McKie, A. T., Barrow, D., Latunde-Dada, G. O., et al. (2001). An iron-regulated ferric reductase associated with the absorption of dietary iron. *Science, 291*(5509), 1755–1759.

57. Layrisse, M., Cook, J. D., Martinez, C., et al. (1969). Food iron absorption: a comparison of vegetable and animal foods. *Blood, 33*, 430–443.

58. Dale, J. C., Burritt, M. F., & Zinsmeister, A. R. (2002). Diurnal variation of serum iron, iron-binding capacity, transferrin saturation, and ferritin levels. *Am J Clin Pathol, 117*, 802–808.

59. Schaap, C. C., Hendriks, J. C., Kortman, G. A., et al. (2013). Diurnal rhythm rather than dietary iron mediates daily hepcidin variations. *Clin Chem, 59*(3), 527–535.

60. Kroot, J. J., Hendriks. J. C., Laarakkers, C. M., et al. (2009). (Pre) analytical imprecision, between-subject variability, and daily variations in serum and urine hepcidin: implications for clinical studies. *Anal Biochem, 389*(2), 124–129.

61. Yamanashi, H., Kimura, S., Iyama, S., et al. (1997). Fully automated measurement of total iron-binding capacity in serum. *Clin Chem, 43*(12), 2413–2417.

62. American Chemical Society. (2017). Molecule of the week: Prussian blue. January 23, 2017. https://www.acs.org/content/acs/en/molecule-of-the-week/archive/p/prussian-blue.html. Accessed March 24, 2022.

63. Guindi, M. (2018). Liver disease in iron overload. In Saxena, R. (Ed.), *Practical Hepatic Pathology: A Diagnostic Approach.* (2nd ed., pp. 151–165). Philadelphia: Elsevier.

64. Lipschitz, D. A., Cook, J. D., & Finch, C. A. (1974). A clinical evaluation of serum ferritin as an index of iron stores. *N Engl J Med, 290*(22), 1213–1216.

65. Konijn, A. M., & Hershko, C. (1977). Ferritin synthesis in inflammation. I. Pathogenesis of impaired iron release. *Br J Haematol, 37*(1), 7–16.

66. Munoz, M., Garcia-Erce, J. A., & Remacha, A. F. (2011). Disorders of iron metabolism. Part II: iron deficiency and iron overload. *J Clin Pathol, 64*, 287–296.

67. Shih, Y. J., Baynes, R. D., Hudson, B. G., et al. (1990). Serum transferrin receptor is a truncated form of tissue receptor. *J Biol Chem, 265*, 19077–19081.

68. Brugnara, C., Zurakowski, D., DiCanzio, J., et al. (1999). Reticulocyte hemoglobin content to diagnose iron deficiency in children. *JAMA, 281*(23), 2225–2230.

69. Punnonen, K., Irjala, K., & Rajamaki, A. (1997). Serum transferrin receptor and its ratio to serum ferritin in the diagnosis of iron deficiency. *Blood, 89*(3), 1052–1057.

70. Castel, R., Tax, M. G., Droogendijk, J., et al. (2012). The transferrin/log(ferritin) ratio: a new tool for the diagnosis of iron deficiency anemia. *Clin Chem Lab Med, 50*(8), 1343–1349.

71. Thomas, C., & Thomas, L. (2002). Biochemical markers and hematologic indices in the diagnosis of functional iron deficiency. *Clin Chem, 48*(7), 1066–1076.

72. Leers, M. P. G., Keuren, J. F. W., & Oosterhuis, W. P. (2010). The value of the Thomas-plot in the diagnostic work up of anemic patients referred by general practitioners. *Int J Lab Hemat, 32*, 572–581.

73. Piomelli, S. (1987). The diagnostic utility of measurements of erythrocyte porphyrins. *Hematol Oncol Clin North Am, 1*(3), 419–430.

10

Leukocyte Development, Kinetics, and Functions

*Mark A. Russell and Ameet R. Kini**

OBJECTIVES

After completion of this chapter, the reader will be able to:

1. Describe the pathways and progenitor cells involved in the derivation of leukocytes from the hematopoietic stem cell to mature forms.
2. Name the different stages of neutrophil, eosinophil, and basophil development and describe the morphology of each stage.
3. Discuss the important functions of neutrophils, eosinophils, and basophils.
4. Describe the morphology of promonocytes, monocytes, macrophages, T and B lymphocytes, and immature B cells (hematogones).
5. Discuss the functions of monocytes, macrophages, T cells, B cells, and natural killer cells in the immune response.
6. Compare the kinetics of neutrophils and monocytes.
7. Discuss in general terms how the various types of lymphocytes are produced.

OUTLINE

Granulocytes
  Neutrophils
  Eosinophils
  Basophils
  Mast Cells

Mononuclear Cells
  Monocytes
  Lymphocytes

CASE STUDY

After studying the material in this chapter, the reader should be able to respond to the following case study. Answers can be found in Appendix C.

A 5-year-old female presented with shortness of breath and wheezing. The patient gave a history of similar symptoms in the last 6 months. After the patient was given albuterol to control her acute symptoms, long-term control of her disease was achieved through the use of corticosteroids along with monoclonal antibodies to interleukin-5 (IL-5).

1. Which leukocytes are important in mediating the clinical symptoms in this patient?
2. A complete blood count with differential was performed on this patient. What are the typical findings in such patients?
3. How did monoclonal antibodies to IL-5 help in controlling her disease?

Leukocytes, also known as *white blood cells* (*WBCs*), are so named because they are relatively colorless compared to red blood cells (RBCs). The number of different types of leukocytes varies, depending on whether they are being viewed with a light microscope after staining with a Romanowsky stain (5 or 6 types) or are identified according to their surface antigens using flow cytometry (at least 10 different types). For the purposes of this chapter, the classical light microscope classification of leukocytes will be used.

Granulocytes are a group of leukocytes whose cytoplasm is filled with granules with differing staining characteristics and whose nuclei are segmented or lobulated. Individually, they include *eosinophils,* with granules containing basic proteins that stain pink/orange with acid stains such as eosin; *basophils,*

---

*The authors extend appreciation to Reeba Omman, Woodlyne Roquiz, Sameer Al Daffalha, and Anne Stiene-Martin, whose work in prior editions provided the foundation for this chapter.

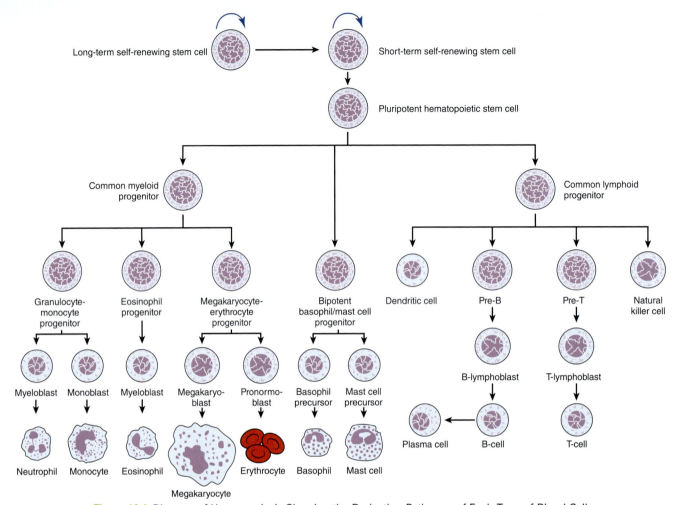

Figure 10.1 Diagram of Hematopoiesis Showing the Derivation Pathways of Each Type of Blood Cell from a Hematopoietic Stem Cell.

with granules that are acidic and stain blue with basic stains such as methylene blue; and *neutrophils*, with granules that react with both acid and basic stains, which gives them a lavender color. Because nuclear segmentation is quite prominent in mature neutrophils, they also have been called *polymorphonuclear cells (PMNs)*.

Mononuclear cells are categorized into *monocytes* and *lymphocytes*. These cells have nuclei that are not segmented but are round, oval, indented, or folded. Leukocytes develop from hematopoietic stem cells (HSCs) in the bone marrow, where most undergo differentiation and maturation (Figure 10.1), and are then released into the circulation. The number of circulating leukocytes varies with sex, age, activity, and time of day. This number also differs according to whether or not the leukocytes are reacting to stress, being consumed, or being destroyed, and whether or not they are being produced by the bone marrow in sufficient numbers.[1] Reference intervals for the total leukocyte count can be found after the Index at the end of the book, and they vary among laboratories, depending on the patient population and the type of instrumentation used.

The overall function of leukocytes is in mediating *immunity*, either innate (nonspecific), as in phagocytosis by neutrophils, or specific (adaptive), as in the production of antibodies by lymphocytes and plasma cells. The term *kinetics* refers to the movement of cells through developmental stages, into the circulation, and from the circulation to the tissues and includes the time spent in each phase of the cell's life. As each cell type is discussed in this chapter, developmental stages, kinetics, and specific functions will be addressed.

GRANULOCYTES

Neutrophils

Neutrophils are present in the peripheral blood in two forms according to whether the nucleus is segmented or still in a band shape. Segmented neutrophils make up the vast majority of circulating leukocytes.

Neutrophil Development

Neutrophil development occurs in the bone marrow. Neutrophils share a common progenitor with monocytes and distinct from

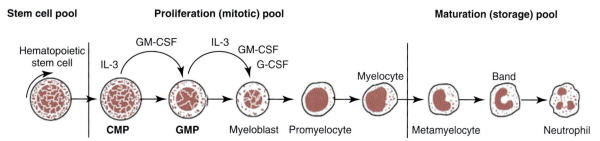

Figure 10.2 Neutrophil Development Showing Stimulating Cytokines and the Three Bone Marrow Pools. *CMP*, Common myeloid progenitor; *G-CSF*, granulocyte colony-stimulating factor; *GM-CSG*, granulocyte-macrophage colony-stimulating factor; *GMP*, granulocyte-monocyte progenitor; *IL-3*, interleukin-3.

eosinophils and basophils, known as the granulocyte-monocyte progenitor (GMP).[2] The major cytokine responsible for the stimulation of neutrophil production is granulocyte colony-stimulating factor (G-CSF).[3,4]

There are three pools of developing neutrophils in the bone marrow (Figure 10.2): the stem cell pool, the proliferation pool, and the maturation pool.[5-8] The stem cell pool consists of HSCs that are capable of self-renewal and differentiation.[9] The proliferation (mitotic) pool consists of cells that are dividing and includes (listed in the order of maturation) common myeloid progenitors (CMPs), also known as colony-forming units–granulocyte, erythrocyte, monocyte, and megakaryocyte (CFU-GEMMs); GMPs; myeloblasts; promyelocytes; and myelocytes. The third marrow pool is the maturation (storage) pool consisting of cells undergoing nuclear maturation that form the marrow reserve and are available for release: metamyelocytes, band neutrophils, and segmented neutrophils.

HSCs, CMPs, and GMPs are not distinguishable with the light microscope and Romanowsky staining and may resemble early type I myeloblasts or lymphoid cells. They can, however, be identified through surface antigen detection by flow cytometry.

Myeloblasts make up 0% to 3% of the nucleated cells in the bone marrow and measure 14 to 20 μm in diameter. They are often subdivided into type I, type II, and type III myeloblasts. The type I myeloblast has a high nucleus-to-cytoplasm (N:C) ratio of 8:1 to 4:1 (the nucleus occupies most of the cell, with very little cytoplasm), slightly basophilic cytoplasm, fine nuclear chromatin, and two to four visible nucleoli. Type I blasts have no visible granules when observed under light microscopy with Romanowsky stains. The type II myeloblast shows the presence of dispersed *primary (azurophilic) granules* in the cytoplasm; the number of granules does not exceed 20 per cell (Figure 10.3). Type III myeloblasts have a darker chromatin and a more purple cytoplasm, and they contain more than 20 granules that do not obscure the nucleus. Type III myeloblasts are rare in normal bone marrow, but they can be seen in certain types of acute myeloid leukemias. Combining type II and type III blasts into a single category of "granular blasts" has been proposed because of the difficulty in distinguishing type II blasts from type III blasts.[10]

Promyelocytes make up 1% to 5% of the nucleated cells in the bone marrow. They are relatively larger than the myeloblast cells and measure 16 to 25 μm in diameter. The nucleus is round

to oval and is often eccentric. A paranuclear halo or "hof" is usually seen in normal promyelocytes but not in the malignant promyelocytes of acute promyelocytic leukemia (described in Chapter 31). The cytoplasm is evenly basophilic and full of primary (azurophilic) granules. These granules are the first in a series of granules to be produced during neutrophil maturation (Box 10.1).[11] The nucleus is similar to that described earlier for myeloblasts except that chromatin clumping (heterochromatin) may be visible, especially around the edges of the nucleus. One to three nucleoli can be seen but may be obscured by the granules (Figure 10.4).

Myelocytes make up 6% to 17% of the nucleated cells in the bone marrow and are the final stage in which cell division (mitosis) occurs. During this stage, the production of primary granules ceases and the cell begins to manufacture secondary (specific) neutrophil granules. This stage of neutrophil development is sometimes divided into early and late myelocytes. Early myelocytes may look very similar to the promyelocytes (described earlier) in size and nuclear characteristics except that patches of grainy pale pink cytoplasm representing secondary granules begin to be evident in the area of the Golgi apparatus. This has been referred to as the *dawn of neutrophilia*. Secondary neutrophilic granules slowly spread through the cell until its cytoplasm is more lavender-pink than blue. As the cell divides, the number of primary granules per cell is decreased and their membrane chemistry changes so that they are much less visible. Late myelocytes are somewhat smaller than promyelocytes (15 to 18 μm), and the nucleus has considerably more heterochromatin. Nucleoli are difficult to see by light microscopy (Figure 10.5).

Metamyelocytes constitute 3% to 20% of nucleated marrow cells. From this stage forward, the cells are no longer capable of division and the major morphologic change is in the shape of the nucleus. The nucleus is indented (kidney bean shaped or peanut shaped), and the chromatin is increasingly clumped. Nucleoli are absent. Synthesis of tertiary granules (also known as *gelatinase granules*) may begin during this stage. The size of the metamyelocyte is slightly smaller than that of the myelocyte (14 to 16 μm). The cytoplasm contains very little residual ribonucleic acid (RNA) and therefore little or no basophilia (Figure 10.6).

Bands make up 9% to 32% of nucleated marrow cells and 0% to 5% of the nucleated peripheral blood cells. All evidence of RNA (cytoplasmic basophilia) is absent, and tertiary granules

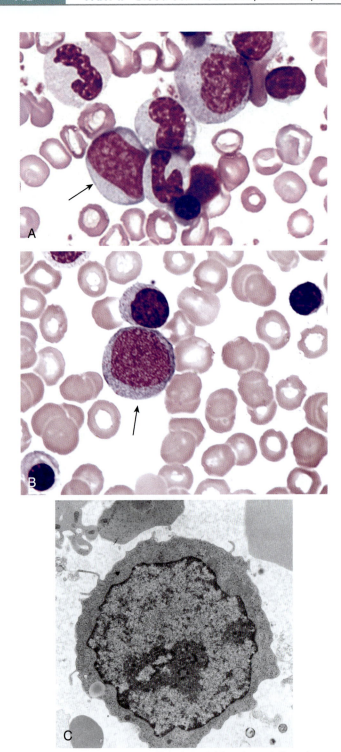

Figure 10.3 Myeloblasts. **(A)**, Type I myeloblast *(arrow)*. Note that no granules are visible in the cytoplasm. **(B)**, Type II myeloblast *(arrow)*, with a few azure granules in the cytoplasm. (A, B, Bone marrow, Wright-Giemsa stain, ×1000.) **(C)**, Electron micrograph of a myeloblast (×16,500). (C from Carr, J. H. [2022]. *Clinical Hematology Atlas.* [6th ed.]. St. Louis: Elsevier.)

continue to be formed during this stage. Secretory granules (also known as *secretory vesicles*) may begin to be formed during this stage. The nucleus is highly clumped and the nuclear indentation that began in the metamyelocyte stage now exceeds half the diameter of the nucleus, but actual segmentation has not

yet occurred (Figure 10.7). Over the past 70 years, there has been considerable controversy over the definition of a band and the differentiation between bands and segmented forms. There have been three schools of thought concerning identification of bands, from the most conservative—holding that the nucleus in a band must have the same diameter throughout its length—to the most liberal—requiring that a filament between segments be visible before a band becomes a segmented neutrophil. The middle ground states that when doubt exists, the cell should be called a *segmented neutrophil.* An elevated band count was thought to be useful in the diagnosis of patients with infection. However, the clinical utility of band counts has been called into

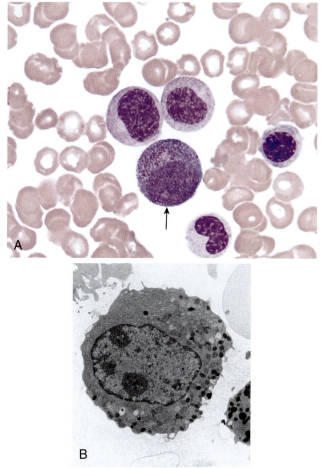

Figure 10.4 Promyelocytes. **(A)**, Promyelocyte *(arrow)* with nucleoli and a large number of azure granules. (Bone marrow, Wright-Giemsa stain, × 1000.) **(B)**, Electron micrograph of a promyelocyte (×13,000). (B from Carr, J. H. [2022]. *Clinical Hematology Atlas.* [6th ed.]. St. Louis: Elsevier.)

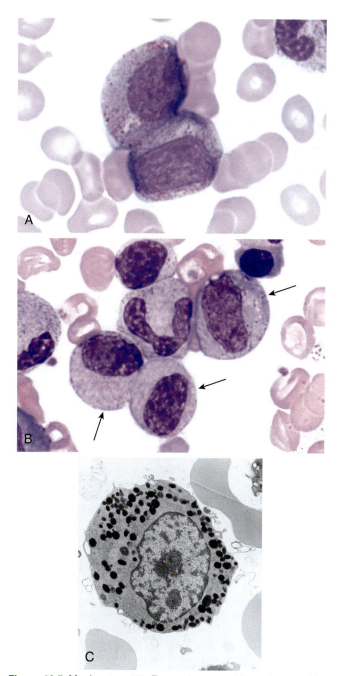

Figure 10.5 Myelocytes. **(A)**, Two early neutrophil myelocytes. Note that they are very similar to the promyelocyte except for several light areas in their cytoplasm where specific granules are beginning to appear. **(B)**, *Arrows* are pointing to three late myelocytes in the field. Their cytoplasm has few if any primary granules, and the lavender secondary granules are easily seen. (A, B, Bone marrow, Wright-Giemsa stain, ×1000.) **(C)**, Electron micrograph of a late neutrophil myelocyte (×16,500). (C from Carr, J. H. [2022]. *Clinical Hematology Atlas.* [6th ed.]. St. Louis: Elsevier.)

question,[12] and most laboratories no longer perform routine band counts. The Clinical and Laboratory Standards Institute (CLSI) recommends that bands should be included within the neutrophil count and not reported as a separate category because of the difficulty in reliably distinguishing bands from segmented neutrophils.[13]

Segmented neutrophils make up 7% to 30% of nucleated cells in the bone marrow. Secretory granules continue to be formed during this stage. The only morphologic difference between segmented neutrophils and bands is the presence of two to five nuclear lobes connected by threadlike filaments (Figure 10.8). Reference intervals for the relative and absolute counts of segmented neutrophils in the peripheral blood may be found after the Index at the end of the book. They are present in the highest numbers in the peripheral blood of adults. Pediatric values vary with age and do not begin to increase to adult values until after 4 to 7 years of age.

Neutrophil Kinetics

Neutrophil kinetics involves the movement of neutrophils and neutrophil precursors between the different pools in the bone marrow, the peripheral blood, and tissues. Neutrophil production has been calculated to be on the order of 0.9 to 1.0 × 10⁹ cells/kg per day.[14]

The proliferative pool contains approximately 2.1×10^9 cells/kg, whereas the maturation pool contains roughly 5.6×10^9 cells/kg, or a 5-day supply.[14] The transit time from the HSC to

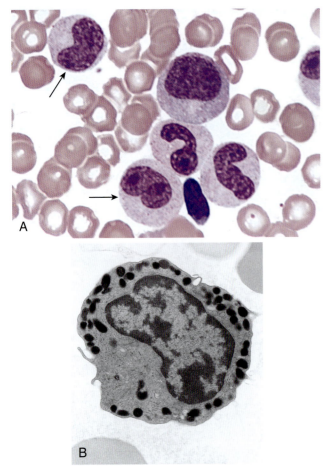

Figure 10.6 Metamyelocytes. (A), Two neutrophil metamyelocytes *(arrows).* Note that there is no remaining basophilia in the cytoplasm, and the nucleus is indented. (Bone marrow, Wright-Giemsa stain, ×1000.) **(B),** Electron micrograph of a neutrophil metamyelocyte (×22,250). (B from Carr, J. H. [2022]. *Clinical Hematology Atlas.* [6th ed.]. St. Louis: Elsevier.)

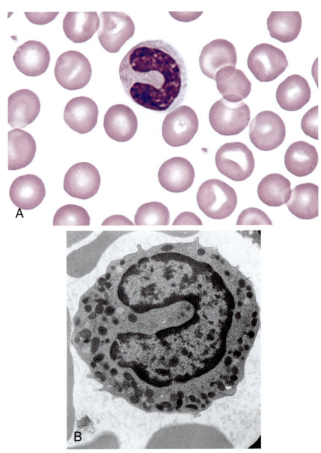

Figure 10.7 Neutrophil Bands. (A), Neutrophil band; note the nucleus is indented more than 50% of the width of the nucleus. (Peripheral blood, Wright-Giemsa stain, ×1000.) **(B),** Electron micrograph of a band neutrophil (×22,250). (B from Carr, J. H. [2022]. *Clinical Hematology Atlas.* [6th ed.]. St. Louis: Elsevier.)

the myeloblast has not been measured. The transit time from myeloblast through myelocyte has been estimated to be roughly 6 days, and the transit time through the maturation pool is approximately 4 to 6 days.[7,14,15] Granulocyte release from the bone marrow is stimulated by G-CSF.[3,4]

Once in the peripheral blood, neutrophils are divided randomly into a circulating neutrophil pool (CNP) and a marginated neutrophil pool (MNP). The neutrophils in the MNP are loosely localized to the walls of capillaries in tissues such as the liver, spleen, and lung. There does not appear to be any functional differences between neutrophils of either the CNP or the MNP, and cells move freely between the two peripheral pools.[16] The ratio of these two pools is roughly equal overall[7,17]; however, marginated neutrophils in the capillaries of the lungs make up a considerably larger portion of peripheral neutrophils.[18] The half-life of neutrophils in the blood is relatively short at approximately 7 hours.[7,19]

Integrins and selectins are of significant importance in allowing neutrophils to marginate and exit the blood and enter the tissues by a process known as *diapedesis.*[20,21] Those neutrophils that do not migrate into the tissues eventually undergo programmed cell death or apoptosis and are removed by macrophages in the spleen, bone marrow, and liver.[22]

Once neutrophils are in the tissues, their life span is variable, depending on whether or not they are responding to infectious or inflammatory agents. In the absence of infectious or inflammatory agents, the neutrophil's life span is measured in hours. Spontaneous neutrophil apoptosis is regulated by proapoptotic and antiapoptotic members of the Bcl-2 family. Some products of inflammation and infection such as Mcl-1 and myeloperoxidase (MPO) tend to prolong the neutrophil's life span through antiapoptotic signals, whereas others such as MAC-1 trigger the death and phagocytosis of neutrophils.[23]

Neutrophil Functions

Neutrophils are part of the innate immune system. Characteristics of innate immunity include destruction of foreign organisms that is not antigen specific; no protection against reexposure to the same pathogen; reliance on the barriers provided by skin and mucous membranes, as well as phagocytes such as neutrophils and monocytes; and inclusion of a humoral component known as the *complement system.*

The major function of neutrophils is phagocytosis and destruction of foreign material and microorganisms. The

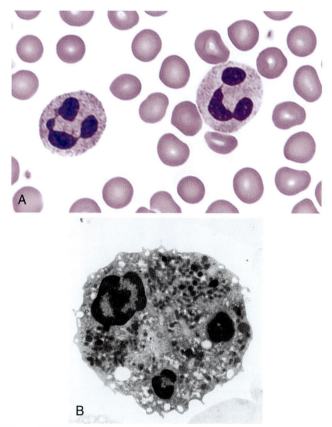

Figure 10.8 Neutrophils. **(A)**, Segmented neutrophils, also known as a *polymorphonuclear cell (PMN)*. (Peripheral blood, Wright-Giemsa stain, ×1000.) **(B)**, Electron micrograph of a segmented neutrophil (×22,250). (B from Carr, J. H. [2022]. *Clinical Hematology Atlas.* [6th ed.]. St. Louis: Elsevier.)

BOX 10.2 Phagocytosis

Recognition and Attachment
Phagocyte receptors recognize and bind to certain foreign molecular patterns and opsonins such as antibodies and complement components.

Ingestion
Pseudopodia are extended around the foreign particle and enclose it within a "phagosome" (engulfment).
The phagosome is pulled toward the center of the cell by polymerization of actin and myosin and by microtubules.

Killing and Digestion
Oxygen Dependent
Respiratory burst through the activation of NADPH oxidase. H_2O_2 and hypochlorite are produced.

Oxygen Independent
The pH within the phagosome becomes alkaline and then neutral, the pH at which digestive enzymes work.
Primary and secondary lysosomes (granules) fuse to the phagosome and empty hydrolytic enzymes and other bactericidal molecules into the phagosome.

Formation of Neutrophil Extracellular Traps
Nuclear and organelle membranes dissolve, and activated cytoplasmic enzymes attach to DNA.
The cytoplasmic membrane ruptures, and DNA with attached enzymes is expelled so that the bacteria are digested in the external environment.

NADPH, Nicotinamide adenine dinucleotide phosphate (reduced form).

---

process involves seeking (chemotaxis, motility, and diapedesis) and destruction (phagocytosis and digestion).

Neutrophil extravasation involves rolling, adhesion, crawling, and finally, transmigration.[24] Neutrophil recruitment to an inflammatory site begins when chemotactic agents bind to neutrophil receptors. Chemotactic agents may be produced by microorganisms, damaged cells, or other leukocytes such as lymphocytes or other phagocytes. The first neutrophil response is to roll along endothelial cells of the blood vessels using stronger adhesive molecules than those used by nonstimulated marginated neutrophils. Rolling consists of transient adhesive contacts between neutrophil selectins and adhesive molecules on the surface of endothelial cells (P selectins and E selectins). Activation is facilitated by the rolling of neutrophils on endothelium surfaces by chemokines. When integrins bind to ligands on the neutrophil surface, an outside-in signaling activates signaling pathways, stabilizes adhesion, and initiates cell motility.[20,25] Once adhesion occurs, the neutrophil scans the region while tightly attached and does not always transmigrate at the location of adhesion.[26] Active crawling depends on signaling between intercellular adhesion molecule-1 (ICAM-1) (expressed by endothelial cells) and macrophage-1 antigen (MAC-1, expressed by neutrophils).[27] Neutrophils then transmigrate in a directional manner either between endothelial cells

(paracellular) or through endothelial cells (transcellular) toward the area of greatest concentration of chemotactic agents.[24]

Once at the site of infection or inflammation, neutrophils begin the process of phagocytosis (Box 10.2). They use their enormous inventory of surface receptors either to recognize directly the pathogen, apoptotic cell, or particle or to recognize opsonic molecules attached to the foreign particle such as antibodies or complement components. Surface cell receptors are primed when neutrophils are exposed to lipopolysaccharide, tumor necrosis factor-α or granulocyte-macrophage colony-stimulating factor (GM-CSF), which are recognized by Toll-like receptors (TLRs).[28] With recognition comes attachment and engulfment, in which cytoplasmic pseudopodia surround the particle, forming a phagosome within the neutrophil cytoplasm.[23] Formation of the phagosome allows the reduced nicotinamide adenine dinucleotide (NADH) oxidase complex (NOX2) within the phagosome membrane to assemble; this leads to the generation of reactive oxygen species (ROS) such as hydrogen peroxide, which is converted to hypochlorite by MPO.[29] Likewise, a series of metabolic changes culminate in the fusion of primary (e.g., MPO, defensins) and/or secondary (e.g., phagocytic receptors, nicotinamide adenine dinucleotide phosphate [reduced form, NADPH] oxidase) granules to the phagosome and the release of numerous bactericidal molecules into the phagosome.[30] This combination of ROS and nonoxygen-dependent mechanisms is generally able to destroy most pathogens.

In addition to emptying their contents into phagosomes, tertiary granules degrade the extracellular matrix and act as chemotactic agents for extravasation and migration of additional neutrophils to the site of inflammation.[11,24]

A second function of neutrophils is the generation of neutrophil extracellular traps, or NETs.[31,32] NETs are extracellular threadlike structures believed to represent chains of nucleosomes from unfolded nuclear chromatin material (DNA). These structures have enzymes from neutrophil granules attached to them and have been shown to be able to trap and kill gram-positive and gram-negative bacteria, as well as fungi. NETs are generated at the time that neutrophils die as a result of antibacterial activity. The term *NETosis* has been used to describe this unique form of neutrophil cell death that results in the release of NETs.

A third and final function of neutrophils is their secretory function. Neutrophils are a source of transcobalamin I or R binder protein, which is necessary for the proper absorption of vitamin B_{12}. In addition, they are a source of a variety of cytokines.

Eosinophils

Eosinophils make up 1% to 3% of nucleated cells in the bone marrow. Of these, slightly more than a third are mature, a quarter are eosinophilic metamyelocytes, and the remainder are eosinophilic promyelocytes or eosinophilic myelocytes. Reference intervals for the relative and absolute counts of eosinophils in the peripheral blood may be found after the Index at the end of the book.

Eosinophil Development

Eosinophil development is similar to that described earlier for neutrophils, and evidence indicates that eosinophils arise from the CMP.[33,34] Eosinophil lineage is established through signaling via cytokines interleukin-3 (IL-3), IL-5 (induced by IL-33), and GM-CSF, leading to activation of three transcription factors: GATA-1, PU.1, and c/EBP. IL-5 and IL-33 are critical for eosinophil growth and survival.[35,36] Eosinophilic promyelocytes can be identified cytochemically because of the presence of Charcot-Leyden crystal protein in their primary granules. The first maturation phase that can be identified as eosinophilic using light microscopy and Romanowsky staining is the early myelocyte.

Eosinophil myelocytes are characterized by the presence of large (resolvable at the light microscope level), pale, reddish-orange secondary granules, along with azure granules in blue cytoplasm. The nucleus is similar to that described for neutrophil myelocytes. Transmission electron micrographs of eosinophils reveal that many secondary eosinophil granules contain an electron-dense crystalline core (Figure 10.9).[37]

Eosinophil metamyelocytes and bands resemble their neutrophil counterparts with respect to their nuclear shape. Secondary granules increase in number, and a third type of granule is generated called the *secretory granule* or *secretory vesicle*. The secondary granules become more distinct and refractory. Electron microscopy indicates the presence of two other organelles: lipid bodies and small granules (Box 10.3).[38]

Mature eosinophils usually display a bilobed nucleus. Their cytoplasm contains characteristic refractile, orange-red

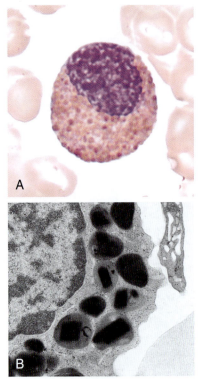

Figure 10.9 Immature Eosinophils. **(A)**, Eosinophilic myelocyte. Note the rounded nucleus and the cytoplasm in which there are numerous large, pale, orange-red secondary eosinophil granules. (Bone marrow, Wright-Giemsa stain, ×1000.) **(B)**, Electron micrograph of eosinophil granules showing the central crystalline core in some of the granules. (From Carr, J. H. [2022]. *Clinical Hematology Atlas.* [6th ed.]. St. Louis: Elsevier.)

secondary granules (Figure 10.10). Electron microscopy of mature eosinophils reveals extensive secretory vesicles, and their number increases considerably when the eosinophil is stimulated or activated.[37]

Eosinophil Kinetics

The time from the last myelocyte mitotic division to the emergence of mature eosinophils from the marrow is about 3.5 days. The mean turnover of eosinophils is approximately 2.2×10^8 cells/kg per day. There is a large storage pool of eosinophils in the marrow consisting of between 9 and 14×10^8 cells/kg.[38]

Once in the circulation, eosinophils have a circulating half-life of roughly 18 hours[39]; however, the half-life of eosinophils is prolonged when eosinophilia occurs. The tissue destinations of eosinophils under normal circumstances appear to be underlying columnar epithelial surfaces in the respiratory, gastrointestinal, and genitourinary tracts. Survival time of eosinophils in human tissues ranges from 2 to 5 days.[40]

Eosinophil Functions

Eosinophils have multiple functions. Eosinophil granules are full of a large number of previously synthesized proteins, including cytokines, chemokines, growth factors, and cationic proteins. There is more than one way for eosinophils to degranulate in an inflammatory process. By classical exocytosis, granules move to the plasma membrane, fuse with the plasma membrane, and empty their contents into the extracellular

BOX 10.3 Eosinophil Granules

Primary Granules

Formed during promyelocyte stage
Contain:
  Charcot-Leyden crystal protein

Secondary Granules

Formed throughout remaining maturation
Contain:
  Major basic protein (core)
  Eosinophil cationic protein (matrix)
  Eosinophil-derived neurotoxin (matrix)
  Eosinophil peroxidase (matrix)
  Lysozyme (matrix)
  Catalase (core and matrix)
  β-Glucuronidase (core and matrix)
  Cathepsin D (core and matrix)
  Interleukin-2, -4, and -5 (core)
  Interleukin-6 (matrix)
  Granulocyte-macrophage colony-stimulating factor (core)
  Others

Small Lysosomal Granules

Acid phosphatase
Arylsulfatase B
Catalase
Cytochrome b_{558}
Elastase
Eosinophil cationic protein

Lipid Bodies

Cyclooxygenase
5-Lipoxygenase
15-Lipoxygenase
Leukotriene C_4 synthase
Eosinophil peroxidase
Esterase

Storage Vesicles

Carry proteins from secondary granules to be released into the extracellular medium

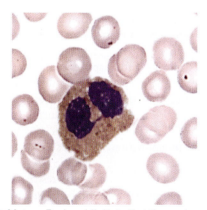

Figure 10.10 Mature Eosinophil. Note that the nucleus has only two segments, which is usual for these cells. The background cytoplasm is colorless and filled with orange-red secondary eosinophil granules. (Peripheral blood, Wright-Giemsa stain, ×1000.)

space. Compound exocytosis is a second mechanism in which granules fuse together within the eosinophil before fusing with the plasma membrane. A third method is known as *piecemeal degranulation,* in which secretory vesicles remove specific proteins from the secondary granules. These vesicles then migrate to the plasma membrane and fuse to empty the specific proteins into the extracellular space.[37] A fourth method of degranulation is cytolysis that occurs when extracellular intact granules are deposited during cell lysis.[41]

Eosinophils play important roles in immune regulation. They transmigrate into the thymus of the newborn and are thought to be involved in the deletion of double-positive thymocytes.[42] Eosinophils are capable of acting as antigen-presenting cells and promoting the proliferation of effector T cells.[43] They are also implicated in the initiation of either type 1 or type 2 immune responses because of their ability to rapidly secrete preformed cytokines in a stimulus-specific manner. They are also important factors in acute and chronic allograft rejection.[44] Eosinophils regulate mast cell function through the release of *major basic protein* (MBP), which causes mast cell degranulation and cytokine production, and they also produce nerve growth factor that promotes mast cell survival and activation.

Eosinophil production is increased in infection by parasitic helminths, and in vitro studies have found that the eosinophil is capable of destroying tissue-invading helminths through the secretion of MBP and eosinophil cationic protein and the production of ROS.[43] There is also a suggestion that eosinophils play a role in preventing reinfection.[45]

Finally, eosinophilia is a hallmark of allergic disorders, of which asthma has been the best studied. The number of eosinophils in blood and sputum correlates with disease severity. This has led to the suggestion that the eosinophil is one of the causes of airway inflammation and mucosal cell damage through secretion or production of a combination of basic proteins, lipid mediators, ROS, and cytokines such as IL-5.[43] Eosinophils also have been implicated in airway remodeling (increase in thickness of the airway wall) through eosinophil-derived fibrogenic growth factors, especially in steroid-resistant asthma.[46–48] Treatment with an anti–IL-5 monoclonal antibody has been found to reduce exacerbations in certain asthmatic patients.[49] Eosinophil accumulation in the gastrointestinal tract occurs in allergic disorders such as food allergy, allergic colitis, and inflammatory bowel disease such as Crohn's disease and ulcerative colitis.[50,51]

Basophils

Basophils and mast cells are two cells with morphologic and functional similarities and have been shown to be derived from a common basophil/mast cell progenitor (BMCP) in the bone marrow[52]; however, basophils are true leukocytes because they mature in the bone marrow and circulate in the blood as mature cells with granules, whereas mast cell precursors leave the bone marrow and use the blood as a transit system to gain access to the tissues where they mature. This common BMCP has been found in the bone marrow and additionally in the peritoneal cavity in a mouse model.[53] Basophils are discussed first. Basophils are the

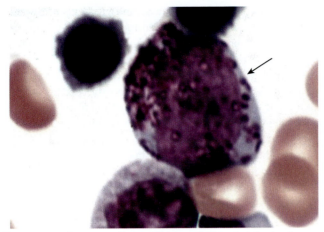

Figure 10.11 Immature Basophil *(arrow).* Note that the background cytoplasm is deeply basophilic, with few large basophilic granules and there appears to be a nucleolus. (Bone marrow, Wright-Giemsa stain, ×1000.)

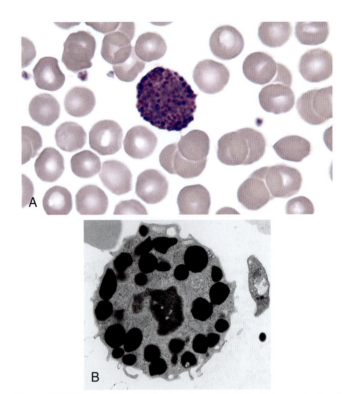

Figure 10.12 Basophils. **(A)**, Mature basophil. Note that granules tend to obscure the nucleus and the background cytoplasm is only slightly basophilic. (Peripheral blood, Wright-Giemsa stain, ×1000.) **(B)**, Electron micrograph of a basophil (×28,750). (B from Carr, J. H. [2020]. *Clinical Hematology Atlas.* [6th ed.]. St. Louis: Elsevier.)

least numerous of the WBCs in the bone marrow and peripheral blood. They make up less than 1% of nucleated cells in the bone marrow. Reference intervals for the relative and absolute counts of basophils in the peripheral blood may be found after the Index at the end of the book.

Basophil Development

Basophils are derived from progenitors in the bone marrow and spleen, where they differentiate under the influence of a number of cytokines, including IL-3 and thymic stromal lymphopoietin (TSLP).[54] Two basophil populations are identified: IL-3-elicited basophils that are immunoglobulin E (IgE) dependent and non-IgE dependent TSLP-elicited basophils.[55–57] The type of mediator response is determined by the balance between these two populations.[56] Because of their very small numbers, the stages of basophil maturation are very difficult to observe and have not been well characterized. Basophils will therefore be described simply as immature basophils and mature basophils.

Immature basophils have round to somewhat lobulated nuclei with only slightly condensed chromatin. Nucleoli may or may not be apparent. The cytoplasm is blue and contains large blue-black secondary granules (Figure 10.11). Primary azure granules may or may not be seen. Basophil granules are water soluble and therefore may be dissolved if the blood film is washed too much during the staining process.

Mature basophils contain a lobulated nucleus that is often obscured by its granules. The chromatin pattern, if visible, is clumped. Actual nuclear segmentation with visible filaments occurs rarely. The cytoplasm is colorless and contains large numbers of the characteristic large blue-black granules. If any granules have been dissolved during the staining process, they often leave a reddish-purple rim surrounding what appears to be a vacuole (Figure 10.12).

Basophil Kinetics

Basophil kinetics is poorly understood because of their very small numbers.[58] The life span of basophils is relatively longer than that of the other granulocytes, at 60 hours.[58] This has been

attributed to the fact that when they are activated by IL-3 and IL-25, antiapoptotic pathways are initiated that prolong the basophil life span.[59]

Basophil Functions

Basophil functions are also poorly understood because of the small numbers of these cells and the lack of animal models such as basophil-deficient animals. However, the recent development of a conditional basophil-deficient mouse model promises to enhance the understanding of basophil function.[60] Previously, basophils were regarded as "poor relatives" of mast cells and minor players in allergic inflammation because, like mast cells, they have IgE receptors on their surface membranes that when cross-linked by antigen, result in granule release.[61] Basophils function in both innate and adaptive immunity. Basophils are capable of releasing large quantities of subtype 2 helper T cell (T_H2) cytokines such as IL-4 and IL-13 that regulate the T_H2 immune response.[62,63] Basophils also induce B cells to synthesize IgE.[64] Whereas mast cells are the effectors of IgE-mediated chronic allergic inflammation, basophils function as *initiators* of the allergic inflammation through the release of preformed cytokines.[61] Basophil activation is not restricted to antigen-specific IgE cross linking, but it can be triggered in nonsensitized individuals by a growing list of parasitic antigens, lectins, viral superantigens, cytokines, chemokines, growth factors, proteases, and components of the complement system.[64]

The contents of basophil granules are not well known. Box 10.4 provides a short list of some of the substances released by

BOX 10.4 Basophil Granules

Secondary Granules
Histamine
Platelet-activating factor
Leukotriene C_4
Interleukin-4
Interleukin-13
Vascular endothelial growth factor A
Vascular endothelial growth factor B
Heparan sulfate

activated basophils. Moreover, mature basophils are evidently capable of synthesizing granule proteins based on activation signals. For example, basophils can be induced to produce a mediator of allergic inflammation known as *granzyme B*.[65] Mast cells can induce basophils to produce and release retinoic acid, a regulator of immune and resident cells in allergic diseases.[66] Basophils also play a role in angiogenesis through the expression of vascular endothelial growth factor (VEGF) and its receptors.[67]

Along with eosinophils, basophils are involved in the control of helminth infections by enclosing toxic egg products with granulomas and preventing tissue damage.[68] They promote eosinophilia, are associated with hindering migration of larvae to other organs, and contribute to efficient worm expulsion.[69,70] Finally, data from the basophil-deficient mouse model indicate that basophils play a nonredundant role in mediating acquired immunity against ticks.[60]

Mast Cells

Mast cells are not considered to be leukocytes. They are tissue effector cells of allergic responses and inflammatory reactions. A brief description of their development and function is included here because (1) their precursors circulate in the peripheral blood for a brief period on their way to their tissue destinations,[71] and (2) mast cells have several phenotypic and functional similarities with both basophils and eosinophils.[72]

BMCPs originate from the bone marrow and spleen.[52,53] Mast cell progenitors (MCPs) are released into the blood before reaching tissues such as the intestine and lung, where they mediate their actions.[73] The major cytokine responsible for mast cell maturation and differentiation is KIT ligand (stem cell factor).[73] Once the MCP reaches its tissue destination, complete maturation into mature mast cells occurs under the control of the local microenvironment (Figure 10.13).[74]

Mast cells function as effector cells in allergic reactions through the release of a wide variety of lipid mediators, proteases, proteoglycans, and cytokines as a result of cross linking of IgE on the mast cell surface by specific allergens. Mast cells also can be activated independently of IgE, which leads to inflammatory reactions. They can function as antigen-presenting cells to induce the differentiation of T_H2 cells[75]; therefore mast cells act as mediators in both innate and adaptive immunity.[73] Mast cells can have antiinflammatory and immunosuppressive functions, and thus they can both enhance and suppress features of

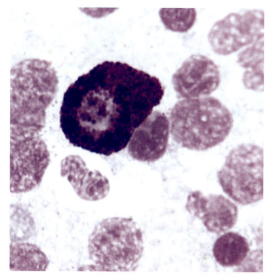

Figure 10.13 Tissue Mast Cell in Bone Marrow. Note that the nucleus is rounded and the cell is packed with large basophilic granules. Mast cells tend to be a little larger than basophils (12 to 25 μm). (Wright-Giemsa stain, ×1000.). (From Carr, J. H. [2022]. *Clinical Hematology Atlas*. [6th ed.]. St. Louis: Elsevier.)

the immune response.[76] Finally, they may act as immunologic "gatekeepers" because of their location in mucosal surfaces and their role in barrier function.[73]

MONONUCLEAR CELLS

Monocytes

Reference intervals for monocytes in the peripheral blood can be found after the Index at the end of the book.

Monocyte Development

Monocyte development is similar to neutrophil development because both cell types are derived from the GMP (see Figure 10.1). Macrophage colony-stimulating factor (M-CSF) is the major cytokine responsible for the growth and differentiation of monocytes. The morphologic stages of monocyte development are monoblasts, promonocytes, and monocytes. Monoblasts in normal bone marrow are very rare and are difficult to distinguish from myeloblasts based on morphology. Malignant monoblasts in acute monoblastic leukemia are described in Chapter 31. Therefore only promonocytes and monocytes are described here.

Promonocytes are 12 to 18 μm in diameter, and their nucleus is slightly indented or folded. The chromatin pattern is delicate, and at least one nucleolus is apparent. The cytoplasm is blue and contains scattered azure granules that are fewer and smaller than those seen in promyelocytes (Figure 10.14). Electron microscopic and cytochemical studies have found that monocyte azure granules are heterogeneous with regard to their content of lysosomal enzymes, peroxidase, nonspecific esterases, and lysozyme.[77]

Monocytes appear to be larger than neutrophils (diameter of 15 to 20 μm) because they tend to stick to and spread out on glass or plastic. Monocytes are slightly immature cells whose

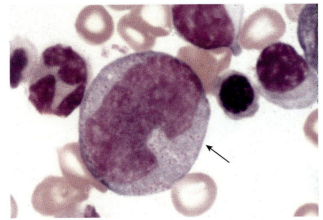

Figure 10.14 Promonocyte *(arrow)*. Note that the nucleus is deeply indented and should not be confused with a neutrophil band form (compare the chromatin patterns of the two). The cytoplasm is basophilic with azure granules that are much smaller than those seen in promyelocytes. The azure granules in this cell are difficult to see and give the cytoplasm a slightly grainy appearance. (Bone marrow, Wright-Giemsa stain, ×1000.)

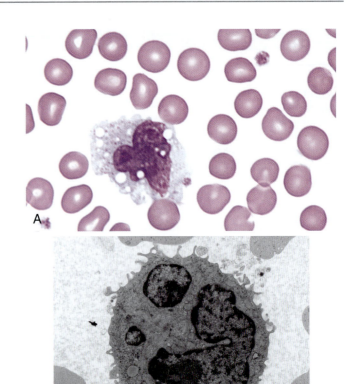

Figure 10.15 Monocytes. **(A)**, Typical monocyte. Note the vacuolated cytoplasm, a contorted nucleus that folds on itself, the loose or lacelike chromatin pattern, and very fine azure granules. (Peripheral blood, Wright-Giemsa stain, ×1000.) **(B)**, Electron micrograph of a monocyte. Note that the villi on the surface are much greater in number than is seen on neutrophils (×16,500). (B from Carr, J. H. [2022]. *Clinical Hematology Atlas.* [6th ed.]. St. Louis: Elsevier.)

ultimate goal is to enter the tissues and mature into macrophages, osteoclasts, or dendritic cells.

The nucleus may be round, oval, or kidney shaped but more often is deeply indented (horseshoe shaped) or folded on itself. The chromatin pattern is looser than in the other leukocytes and has sometimes been described as lacelike or stringy. Nucleoli are generally not seen with the light microscope; however, electron microscopy reveals nucleoli in roughly half of circulating monocytes. Their cytoplasm is blue-gray, with fine azure granules often referred to as *azure dust* or a ground-glass appearance. Small cytoplasmic pseudopods or blebs may be seen. Cytoplasmic and nuclear vacuoles also may be present (Figure 10.15). Based on flow cytometry immunophenotyping, three subsets of human monocytes have been described: the classical, intermediate, and nonclassical monocytes.[78] Studies have found that certain subsets of monocytes expand with infections and inflammatory and autoimmune conditions.[79] It is not clear whether the expansion is a cause or consequence of these conditions. For example, in atherosclerosis, it has been found that classical monocytes advance inflammation and sift through necrotic debris, whereas nonclassical and possibly intermediate monocyte cells reduce inflammation to support healing.[80] The exact role of monocytes in health and disease needs further exploration.

Monocyte/Macrophage Kinetics

The promonocyte pool consists of approximately 6×10^8 cells/kg, and they produce 7×10^6 monocytes/kg per hour. Under normal circumstances, promonocytes undergo two mitotic divisions in 60 hours to produce a total of four monocytes. Under conditions of increased demand for monocytes, promonocytes undergo four divisions to yield a total of 16 monocytes in 60 hours. There is no storage pool of mature monocytes in the bone marrow[81] and unlike neutrophils, monocytes are released immediately into the circulation upon maturation. Therefore, when the bone marrow recovers from marrow

failure, monocytes are seen in the peripheral blood before neutrophils and a relative monocytosis may occur. There is recent evidence, however, that a relatively large reservoir of immature monocytes resides in the subcapsular red pulp of the spleen. Monocytes in this splenic reservoir appear to respond to tissue injury such as myocardial infarction by migrating to the site of tissue injury to participate in wound healing.[82]

Like neutrophils, monocytes in the peripheral blood can be found in a marginal pool and a circulating pool. Unlike with neutrophils, the marginal pool of monocytes is 3.5 times the circulating pool.[83] Monocytes remain in the circulation approximately 3 days.[84] Monocytes with different patterns of chemokine receptors have different target tissues and different functions. Box 10.5 contains a list of the various tissue destinations of monocytes.[85] Once in tissues, monocytes differentiate into macrophages, osteoclasts (Figure 10.16), or dendritic cells, depending on the microenvironment of the local tissues. Macrophages can be as large as 40 to 50 μm in diameter. They usually have an oval nucleus with a netlike (reticulated) chromatin pattern. Their cytoplasm is pale, often vacuolated, and often filled with debris of phagocytized cells or organisms.

The life span of macrophages in the tissues depends on whether they are responding to inflammation or infection, or

BOX 10.5 Monocyte Destinations

Differentiation into Macrophages

In areas of inflammation or infection (inflammatory macrophages)
As "resident" macrophages in:
    Liver (Kupffer cells)
    Lungs (alveolar macrophages)
    Brain (microglia)
    Skin (Langerhans cells)
    Spleen (splenic macrophages)
    Intestines (intestinal macrophages)
    Peritoneum (peritoneal macrophages)
    Bone (osteoclasts)
    Synovial macrophages (type A cell)
    Kidneys (renal macrophages)
    Reproductive organ macrophages
    Lymph nodes (dendritic cells)

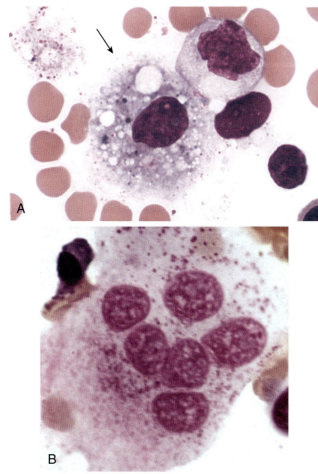

Figure 10.16 Bone Marrow Cells. **(A)**, Active marrow macrophage *(arrow)*. **(B)**, Osteoclast with six nuclei. Both these cells are derived from monocytes. (A, B, Wright-Giemsa stain, ×1000.)

they are "resident" macrophages such as Kupffer cells or alveolar macrophages. Resident macrophages survive far longer than tissue neutrophils. For example, Kupffer cells have a life span of approximately 21 days.[86] Inflammatory macrophages, on the other hand, have a life span measured in hours.

Monocyte/Macrophage Functions

Functions of monocytes/macrophages are numerous and varied. They can be subdivided into innate immunity, adaptive immunity, and housekeeping functions.

- *Innate immunity:* Monocytes/macrophages recognize a wide range of bacterial pathogens by means of pattern recognition receptors (TLRs) that stimulate inflammatory cytokine production and phagocytosis. Macrophages can synthesize nitric oxide, which is cytotoxic against viruses, bacteria, fungi, protozoa, helminths, and tumor cells.[30] Monocytes and macrophages also have Fc receptors and complement receptors. Hence they can phagocytize foreign organisms or materials that have been coated with antibodies or complement components.

- *Adaptive immunity:* Both macrophages and dendritic cells degrade antigen and present antigen fragments on their surfaces (antigen-presenting cells). Because of this, they interact with and activate both T lymphocytes and B lymphocytes to initiate the adaptive immune response. Dendritic cells are the most efficient and potent of the antigen-presenting cells.

- *Housekeeping functions:* These include removal of debris and dead cells at sites of infection or tissue damage, destruction of senescent RBCs and maintenance of a storage pool of iron for erythropoiesis, and synthesis of a wide variety of proteins, including coagulation factors, complement components, interleukins, growth factors, and enzymes.[87]

Lymphocytes

Lymphocytes are divided into three major groups: T cells, B cells, and natural killer (NK) cells. T and B cells are major players in adaptive immunity. NK cells make up a small percentage of lymphocytes and are part of innate immunity. Adaptive immunity has three characteristics. It relies on an enormous number of distinct lymphocytes, each having surface receptors for a different specific molecular structure on a foreign antigen; after an encounter with a particular antigen, memory cells are produced that will react faster and more vigorously to that same antigen on reexposure; and self-antigens are "ignored" under normal circumstances (referred to as *tolerance*).

Lymphocytes can be subdivided into two major categories: those that participate in humoral immunity by producing antibodies and those that participate in cellular immunity by attacking foreign organisms or cells directly. Antibody-producing lymphocytes are called *B lymphocytes* or simply *B cells* because they develop in the bone marrow. Cellular immunity is accomplished by two types of lymphocytes: T cells, so named because they develop in the thymus, and NK cells, which develop in both the bone marrow and the thymus.[88–90]

Lymphocytes are different from the other leukocytes in several ways, including the following:

1. Lymphocytes are not end cells. They are resting cells and, when stimulated, undergo mitosis to produce both memory and effector cells.
2. Unlike other leukocytes, lymphocytes recirculate from the blood to the tissues and back to the blood.

3. B and T lymphocytes are capable of rearranging antigen receptor gene segments to produce a wide variety of antibodies and surface receptors.
4. Although early lymphocyte progenitors such as the common lymphoid progenitor originate in the bone marrow, T and NK lymphocytes develop and mature outside the bone marrow.

For these reasons, lymphocyte kinetics are extremely complicated, not well understood, and beyond the scope of this chapter.

Reference intervals for lymphocytes in the peripheral blood can be found after the Index at the end of the book.

Lymphocyte Development

For both B and T cells, development can be subdivided into antigen-independent and antigen-dependent phases. Antigen-independent lymphocyte development occurs in the bone marrow and thymus (sometimes referred to as *central* or *primary lymphatic organs*), whereas antigen-dependent lymphocyte development occurs in the spleen, lymph nodes, tonsils, and mucosa-associated lymphoid tissue such as the Peyer patches in the intestinal wall (sometimes referred to as *peripheral* or *secondary lymphatic organs*).

B lymphocytes develop initially in the bone marrow and go through three stages known as *pro-B, pre-B,* and *immature B cells* (Figure 10.17). It is during these stages that immunoglobulin gene rearrangement occurs so that each B cell produces a unique immunoglobulin antigen receptor. The immature B cells, which have not yet been exposed to antigen *(antigen-naïve B cells),* leave the bone marrow to migrate to secondary lymphatic organs, where they take up residence in specific zones such as lymph node follicles. These immature B cells, also known as *hematogones,*[91] have a homogeneous nuclear chromatin pattern and extremely scanty cytoplasm (Figure 10.18). These cells are normally found in newborn peripheral blood and bone marrow and in regenerative bone marrows. Leukemic cells from patients with acute lymphoblastic leukemia (ALL) can sometimes resemble hematogones, but the leukemic cells can be distinguished from hematogones by flow cytometry immunophenotyping.[92]

It is in the secondary lymphatic organs or in the blood where B cells may come in contact with antigen, which results in cell division and the production of memory cells and effector cells. Effector B cells are antibody-producing cells known as *plasma cells* and *plasmacytoid lymphocytes* (Figure 10.19).

Approximately 3% to 21% of circulating lymphocytes are B cells. Resting B lymphocytes cannot be distinguished

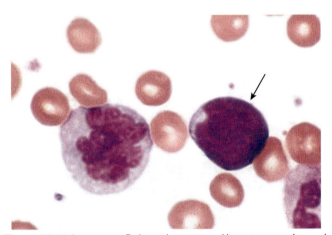

Figure 10.18 Immature B Lymphocyte or Hematogone *(arrow).* Note the extremely scanty cytoplasm. This was taken from the bone marrow of a newborn infant. (Wright-Giemsa stain, ×1000.)

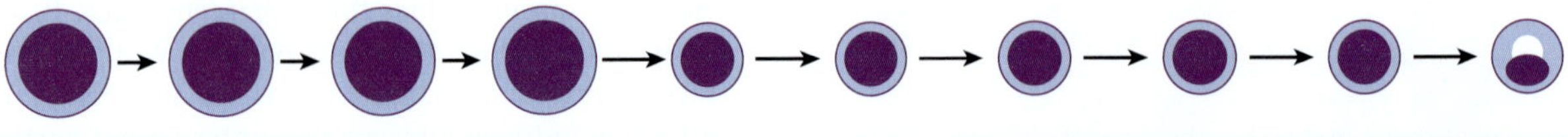

	Stage 1 Hematogones (Pre-pro-B Cells)	Stage 2 Hematogones (Pro-B and Pre-B Cells)	Stage 3 Hematogones (Immature B Cells)	Stage 3 Hematogones (Transitional B Cells)	Naïve B Cells	Germinal Center B Cells	Natural Memory B Cells	IgM+ Post-Germinal Center Memory B Cells	Switched Post-Germinal Center Memory B Cells	Plasma Cells
TdT	+	−	−	−	−	−	−	−	−	−
CD34	+/−	−	−	−	−	−	−	−	−	−
CD19	++	++	++	++	++	++	++	++	++	++
CD20	−	−	+	+	+	+	+	+	+	−
CD38	++	++	++	++	+/−	++	+/−	+/−	+/−	+++
CD10	++	+	+	+	+	+	−	−	−	−
CD5	−	−	−	+	−	−	−	−	−	−
CD27	−	−	−	−	−	+	+	+	+	+
CD45	dim +	dim +	+	+	+	+	+	+	+	+/−
IgM	−	−	+				+	+		
IgD	−	−	−				+	−	−	

Figure 10.17 Maturation of B Lymphocytes. B-cell development and selected immunophenotypic markers. +, Positive (expressed); ++, strongly positive; +++, very strongly positive; −, negative (not expressed); +/−, may be positive or negative; dim +, weakly positive. (Data from Clavarino, G., Delouche, N., Vettier, C., et al. [2016]. Novel strategy for phenotypic characterization of human B lymphocytes from precursors to effector cells by flow cytometry. *PLoS One, 11,* 9, e0162209.)

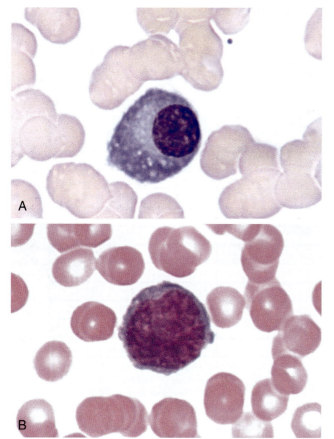

Figure 10.19 Plasma Cell Versus Plasmacytoid Lymphocyte. **(A)**, Plasma cell. **(B)**, Plasmacytoid lymphocyte. These are effector cells of the B lymphocyte lineage. (A, B, Peripheral blood, Wright-Giemsa stain, ×1000.)

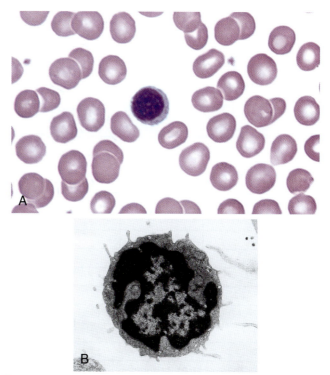

Figure 10.20 Lymphocytes. **(A)**, Small resting lymphocyte. (Peripheral blood, Wright-Giemsa stain, ×1000.) **(B)**, Electron micrograph of a small lymphocyte (×30,000). (B from Carr, J. H. [2022]. *Clinical Hematology Atlas.* [6th ed.]. St. Louis: Elsevier.)

morphologically from resting T lymphocytes. Resting lymphocytes are small (around 9 μm in diameter), and the N:C ratio ranges from 5:1 to 2:1. The chromatin is arranged in blocks, and the nucleolus is rarely seen, although it is present (Figure 10.20).

T lymphocytes develop initially in the thymus—a lymphoepithelial organ located in the upper mediastinum.[93] Lymphoid progenitor cells migrate from the bone marrow to the thymic cortex where, under the regulation of cytokines produced by thymic epithelial cells, they progress through stages known as *pro-T, pre-T,* and *immature T cells* (Figure 10.21). During these phases, they undergo antigen receptor gene rearrangement to produce T cell receptors that are unique to each T cell. T cells whose receptors react with self-antigens are allowed to undergo apoptosis.[94] In addition, T cells are subdivided into two major categories, depending on whether or not they have CD4 or CD8 antigen on their surfaces. Immature T cells then proceed to the thymic medulla, where further apoptosis of self-reactive T cells occurs. The remaining immature T cells (or *antigen-naïve T cells*) then leave the thymus and migrate to secondary lymphatic organs, where they take up residence in specific zones such as the paracortical areas. T cells comprise 51% to 88% of circulating lymphocytes.

T cells in secondary lymphatic organs or in the circulating blood eventually come in contact with antigens. This results in cell activation and the production of either memory cells

or effector T cells, or both (Figure 10.22). The transformation of resting lymphocytes into activated forms is the source of so-called medium and large lymphocytes that have increased amounts of cytoplasm and usually make up only about 10% of circulating lymphocytes. The morphology of effector T cells varies with the subtype of T cell involved, and they are often referred to as *reactive lymphocytes.*

NK cells are a heterogeneous group of cells with respect to their surface antigens. The majority are large granular lymphocytes that are positive for CD56, CD16, CD7, and negative for CD3 (Figure 10.23).[95] The mature NK cell is relatively large compared with other resting lymphocytes because of an increased amount of cytoplasm. Its cytoplasm contains azurophilic granules that are peroxidase negative. Approximately 4% to 29% of circulating lymphocytes are NK cells.

Lymphocyte Functions

Functions can be addressed according to the type of lymphocyte. *B lymphocytes* are essential for antibody production. In addition, they have a role in antigen presentation to T cells and may be necessary for optimal CD4 activation. B cells also produce cytokines that regulate a variety of T cell and antigen-presenting cell functions.[96]

T lymphocytes can be divided into CD4+ T cells and CD8+ T cells. CD4+ effector lymphocytes are further subdivided into T_H1, T_H2, T_H17, and T_{reg} (CD4+CD25+ regulatory T) cells. T_H1 cells mediate immune responses against intracellular pathogens. T_H2 cells mediate host defense against extracellular parasites, including helminths. They are also important in the induction

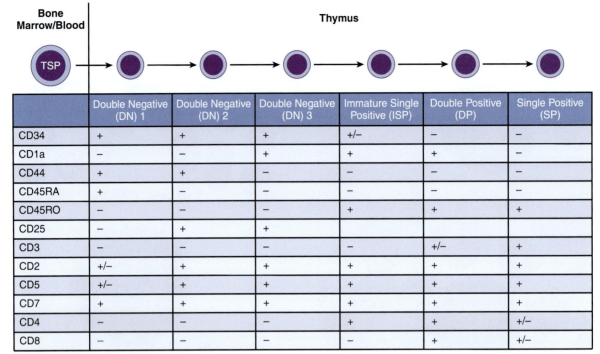

	Double Negative (DN) 1	Double Negative (DN) 2	Double Negative (DN) 3	Immature Single Positive (ISP)	Double Positive (DP)	Single Positive (SP)
CD34	+	+	+	+/–	–	–
CD1a	–	–	+	+	+	–
CD44	+	+	–	–	–	–
CD45RA	+	–	–	–	–	–
CD45RO	–	–	–	+	+	+
CD25	–	+	+			
CD3	–	–	–	–	+/–	+
CD2	+/–	+	+	+	+	+
CD5	+/–	+	+	+	+	+
CD7	+	+	+	+	+	+
CD4	–	–	–	+	+	+/–
CD8	–	–	–	–	+	+/–

Figure 10.21 Maturation of T Lymphocytes. T-cell development in humans and selected immunophenotypic markers. +, Positive (expressed); –, negative (not expressed); +/–, may be positive or negative; *TSP*, thymus seeing progenitor. (Data from Famili, F., Wiekmeijer, A. S., & Staal, F. J. [2017]. The development of T cells from stem cells in mice and humans. *Future Sci, 3*, 1–21.)

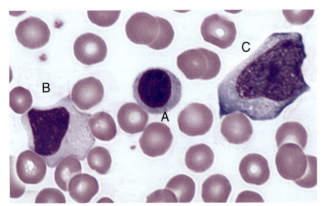

Figure 10.22 Three Cells Representing Lymphocyte Activation. A small resting lymphocyte *(A)* is stimulated by antigen and begins to enlarge to form a medium to large lymphocyte *(B)*. The nucleus reverts from a clumped to a delicate chromatin pattern with nucleoli *(C)*. The cell is capable of dividing to form effector cells or memory cells. (A-C, Peripheral blood, Wright-Giemsa stain, ×1000.)

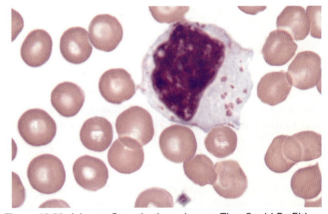

Figure 10.23 A Large Granular Lymphocyte That Could Be Either a Cytotoxic T Lymphocyte or a Natural Killer Lymphocyte. (Peripheral blood, Wright-Giemsa stain, ×1000.)

of asthma and other allergic diseases. T_H17 cells are involved in the immune responses against extracellular bacteria and fungi. T_{reg} cells play a role in maintaining self-tolerance by regulating immune responses.[97,98]

CD8+ effector lymphocytes are capable of killing target cells by secreting granules containing granzyme and perforin or by activating apoptotic pathways in the target cell.[99] These cells are sometimes referred to as *cytotoxic T lymphocytes.*

NK lymphocytes function as part of innate immunity and are capable of killing certain tumor cells and virus-infected cells without prior sensitization. In addition, NK cells modulate the functions of other cells, including macrophages and T cells.[100]

SUMMARY

- Granulocytes are classified according to their staining characteristics and the shape of their nuclei. Neutrophils are a major component of innate immunity as phagocytes; eosinophils are involved in allergic reactions and helminth destruction; and basophils function as initiators of allergic reactions, helminth destruction, and immunity against ticks.
- Neutrophil development can be subdivided into specific stages, with cells at each stage having specific morphologic characteristics (myeloblast, promyelocyte, myelocyte, metamyelocyte, band, and segmented neutrophil). Various granule types are produced during neutrophil development, each with specific contents.
- Eosinophil development also can be subdivided into specific stages, although eosinophilic myeloblasts are not recognizable and eosinophil promyelocytes are rare.
- Basophil development is difficult to describe, and basophils have been divided simply into immature and mature basophils.
- Mononuclear cells consist of monocytes and lymphocytes. Monocytes are precursors to tissue cells such as osteoclasts, macrophages, and dendritic cells. As a group, they perform several functions as phagocytes.

- Monocyte development can be subdivided into the promonocyte, monocyte, and macrophage stages, each with specific morphologic characteristics.
- The majority of lymphocytes are involved in adaptive immunity. B lymphocytes and plasma cells produce antibodies against foreign organisms or cells, and T lymphocytes mediate the immune response against intracellular and extracellular invaders. Both B and T lymphocytes produce memory cells for specific antigens so that the immune response is faster if the same antigen is encountered again.
- Lymphocyte development is complex, and morphologic divisions are not practical because a large number of lymphocytes develop in the thymus. Benign B-lymphocyte precursors (hematogones) as well as B-lymphocyte effector cells (plasma cells and plasmacytoid lymphocytes) have been described. NK lymphocytes and cytotoxic T cells also have a distinct and similar morphology.

Now that you have completed this chapter, go back and read again the case study at the beginning and respond to the questions presented. Answers can be found in Appendix C.

REVIEW QUESTIONS

Answers can be found in Appendix C.

1. Neutrophils and monocytes are direct descendants of a common progenitor known as:
   - **a.** CLP
   - **b.** GMP
   - **c.** MEP
   - **d.** HSC
2. The stage in neutrophilic development in which the nucleus is indented in a kidney bean shape and the cytoplasm has secondary granules that are lavender in color is the:
   - **a.** Band
   - **b.** Myelocyte
   - **c.** Promyelocyte
   - **d.** Metamyelocyte
3. Type II myeloblasts are characterized by:
   - **a.** The presence of fewer than 20 primary granules per cell
   - **b.** Basophilic cytoplasm with many secondary granules
   - **c.** The absence of granules
   - **d.** The presence of a folded nucleus
4. Which one of the following is a function of neutrophils?
   - **a.** Presentation of antigen to T and B lymphocytes
   - **b.** Protection against reexposure by same antigen
   - **c.** Nonspecific destruction of foreign organisms
   - **d.** Initiation of delayed hypersensitivity response
5. Which of the following cells are important in immune regulation, allergic inflammation, and destruction of tissue invading helminths?
   - **a.** Neutrophils and monocytes
   - **b.** Eosinophils and basophils
   - **c.** T and B lymphocytes
   - **d.** Macrophages and dendritic cells

6. Basophils and mast cells have high-affinity surface receptors for which immunoglobulin?
   - **a.** A
   - **b.** D
   - **c.** E
   - **d.** G
7. Which of the following cell types is capable of differentiating into osteoclasts, macrophages, or dendritic cells?
   - **a.** Neutrophils
   - **b.** Lymphocytes
   - **c.** Monocytes
   - **d.** Eosinophils
8. Macrophages aid in adaptive immunity by:
   - **a.** Degrading antigen and presenting it to lymphocytes
   - **b.** Ingesting and digesting organisms that neutrophils cannot
   - **c.** Synthesizing complement components
   - **d.** Storing iron from senescent red cells
9. Which of the following is the final stage of B-cell maturation after activation by antigen?
   - **a.** Large, granular lymphocyte
   - **b.** Plasma cell
   - **c.** Reactive lymphocyte
   - **d.** Immunoblast
10. The following is unique to both B and T lymphocytes and occurs during their early development:
    - **a.** Expression of surface antigens CD4 and CD8
    - **b.** Maturation in the thymus
    - **c.** Synthesis of immunoglobulins
    - **d.** Rearrangement of antigen receptor genes

REFERENCES

1. Lee, M., Lee, S. Y., & Bae, Y. S. (2022). Emerging roles of neutrophils in immune homeostasis. *BMB Rep, 55*, 473–480.

2. Gorgens, A., Radtke, S., Horn, P. A., et al. (2013). New relationships of human hematopoietic lineages facilitate detection of multipotent hematopoietic stem and progenitor cells. *Cell Cycle, 12*, 3478–3482.

3. Chaiworapongsa, T., Romero, R., Berry, S. M., et al. (2011). The role of granulocyte colony-stimulating factor in the neutrophilia observed in the fetal inflammatory response syndrome. *J Perinatal Med, 39*, 653–666.

4. Price, T. H., Chatta, G. S., & Dale, D. C. (1996). Effect of recombinant granulocyte colony-stimulating factor on neutrophil kinetics in normal young and elderly humans. *Blood, 88*, 335–340.

5. Iwasaki, H., & Akashi, K. (2007). Hematopoietic developmental pathways: on cellular basis. *Oncogene, 26*, 6687–6696.

6. Manz, M. G., Miyamoto, T., Akashi, K., et al. (2002). Prospective isolation of human clonogenic common myeloid progenitors. *Proc Natl Acad Sci U S A, 99*, 11872–11877.

7. Bongers, S. H, Chen, N., van Grinsven, E., at al. (2021). Kinetics of neutrophil subsets in acute, subacute, and chronic inflammation. *Front Immunol, 12*, 1–12.

8. Terstappen, L. W., Huang, S., Safford, M., et al. (1991). Sequential generations of hematopoietic colonies derived from single nonlineage-committed CD34+CD38- progenitor cells. *Blood, 77*, 1218–1227.

9. Adams, G. B., & Scadden, D. T. (2006). The hematopoietic stem cell in its place. *Nat Immunol, 7*(4), 333–337.

10. Goasguen, J. E., Bennett, J. M., Bain, B. J., et al. (2014). Proposal for refining the definition of dysgranulopoiesis in acute myeloid leukemia and myelodysplastic syndromes. *Leuk Res, 38*, 447–453.

11. Faurschou, M., & Borregaard, N. (2003). Neutrophil granules and secretory vesicles in inflammation. *Microbes Infect, 5*(14), 1317–1327.

12. Cornbleet, P. J. (2002). Clinical utility of the band count. *Clin Lab Med, 22*(1), 101–136.

13. Clinical and Laboratory Standards Institute. (2007). *Reference Leukocyte (WBC) Differential Count (Proportional) and Evaluation of Instrumental Methods.* (2nd ed., CLSI approved standard, H20-A2). Wayne, PA: Clinical and Laboratory Standards Institute.

14. Dancey, J. T., Deubelbeiss, K. A., Harker, L. A., et al. (1976). Neutrophil kinetics in man. *J Clin Invest, 58*(3), 705–715.

15. Athens, J. W. (1963). Blood: leukocytes. *Annu Rev Physiol, 25*, 195–212.

16. Hetherington, S. V., & Quie, P. G. (1985). Human polymorphonuclear leukocytes of the bone marrow, circulation, and marginated pool: function and granule protein content. *Am J Hematol, 20*(3), 235–246.

17. Cartwright, G. E., Athens, J. W., & Wintrobe, M. M. (1964). The kinetics of granulopoiesis in normal man. *Blood, 24*, 780–803.

18. Liu, J., Pang, Z., Wang, P., et al. (2017). Advanced role of neutrophils in common respiratory diseases. *J Immunol Res, 2017*, 1–12.

19. Saverymuttu, S. H., Peters, A. M., Keshavarzian, A., et al. (1985). The kinetics of 111indium distribution following injection of 111indium labelled autologous granulocytes in man. *Br J Haematol, 61*(4), 675–685.

20. Ley, K., Laudanna, C., Cybulsky, M. I., et al. (2007). Getting to the site of inflammation: the leukocyte adhesion cascade updated. *Nat Rev Immunol, 7*(9), 678–689.

21. Zarbock, A., Ley, K., McEver, R. P., et al. (2011). Leukocyte ligands for endothelial selectins: specialized glycoconjugates that mediate rolling and signaling under flow. *Blood, 118*(26), 6743–6751.

22. Furze, R. C., & Rankin, S. M. (2008). The role of the bone marrow in neutrophil clearance under homeostatic conditions in the mouse. *FASEB J, 22*(9), 3111–3119.

23. Stuart, L. M., & Ezekowitz, R. A. (2005). Phagocytosis: elegant complexity. *Immunity, 22*(5), 539–550.

24. Kolaczkowska, E., & Kubes, P. (2013). Neutrophil recruitment and function in health and inflammation. *Nat Rev Immunol, 13*(3), 159–175.

25. Cicchetti, G., Allen, P. G., & Glogauer, M. (2002). Chemotactic signaling pathways in neutrophils: from receptor to actin assembly. *Crit Rev Oral Biol Med, 13*(3), 220–228.

26. Jenne, C. N., Wong, C. H., Zemp, F. J., et al. (2013). Neutrophils recruited to sites of infection protect from virus challenge by releasing neutrophil extracellular traps. *Cell Host Microbe, 13*(2), 169–180.

27. Phillipson, M., Heit, B., Colarusso, P., et al. (2006). Intraluminal crawling of neutrophils to emigration sites: a molecularly distinct process from adhesion in the recruitment cascade. *J Exp Med, 203*(12), 2569–2575.

28. Lim, J. J., Grinstein, S., & Roth, Z. (2017). Diversity and versatility of phagocytosis: roles in innate immunity, tissue remodeling, and homeostasis. *Front Cell Infect Microbiol, 7*, 191.

29. Winterbourn, C. C., Kettle, A. J., & Hampton, M. B. (2016). Reactive oxygen species and neutrophil function. *Annu Rev Biochem, 85*, 765–792.

30. Dale, D. C., Boxer, L., & Liles, W. C. (2008). The phagocytes: neutrophils and monocytes. *Blood, 112*(4), 935–945.

31. Zhang, H., Wang, Y., Qu, M., et al. (2023). Neutrophil, neutrophil extracellular traps and endothelial cell dysfunction in sepsis. *Clin Transl Med, 13*, 1–19.

32. Brinkmann, V., & Zychlinsky, A. (2012). Neutrophil extracellular traps: is immunity the second function of chromatin? *J Cell Biol, 198*(5), 773–783.

33. Mori, Y., Iwasaki, H., Kohno, K., et al. (2009). Identification of the human eosinophil lineage-committed progenitor: revision of phenotypic definition of the human common myeloid progenitor. *J Exp Med, 206*(1), 183–193.

34. Uhm, T. G., Kim, B. S., & Chung, I. Y. (2012). Eosinophil development, regulation of eosinophil-specific genes, and role of eosinophils in the pathogenesis of asthma. *Allergy Asthma Immunol Res, 4*(2), 68–79.

35. Johnston, L. K., & Bryce, P. J. (2017). Understanding interleukin 33 and its roles in eosinophil development. *Front Med (Lausanne), 4*, 51.

36. Johnston, L. K., Hsu, C. L., Krier-Burris, R. A., et al. (2016). IL-33 precedes IL-5 in regulating eosinophil commitment and is required for eosinophil homeostasis. *J Immunol, 197*(9), 3445–3453.

37. Melo, R. C., Spencer, L. A., Perez, S. A., et al. (2009). Vesicle-mediated secretion of human eosinophil granule-derived major basic protein. *Lab Invest, 89*(7), 769–781.

38. Giembycz, M. A., & Lindsay, M. A. (1999). Pharmacology of the eosinophil. *Pharmacol Rev, 51*(2), 213–340.

39. Steinbach, K. H., Schick, P., Trepel, F., et al. (1979). Estimation of kinetic parameters of neutrophilic, eosinophilic, and basophilic granulocytes in human blood. *Blut, 39*(1), 27–38.

40. Park, Y. M., & Bochner, B. S. (2010). Eosinophil survival and apoptosis in health and disease. *Allergy Asthma Immunol Res, 2*(2), 87–101.

41. Spencer, L. A., Bonjour, K., Melo, R. C., et al. (2014). Eosinophil secretion of granule-derived cytokines. *Front Immunol,* https://doi.org/10.3389/fimmu.2014.00496.

42. Throsby, M., Herbelin, A., Pleau, J. M., et al. (2000). CD11c1 eosinophils in the murine thymus: developmental regulation and recruitment upon MHC class I-restricted thymocyte deletion. *J Immunol, 165*(4), 1965–1975.

43. Hogan, S. P., Rosenberg, H. F., Moqbel, R., et al. (2008). Eosinophils: biological properties and role in health and disease. *Clin Exp Allergy, 38*(5), 709–750.

44. Long, H., Liao, W., Wang, L., et al. (2016). A player and coordinator: the versatile roles of eosinophils in the immune system. *Transfus Med Hemother, 43*(2), 96–108.

45. Hagan, P., Wilkins, H. A., Blumenthal, U. J., et al. (1985). Eosinophilia and resistance to *Schistosoma haematobium* in man. *Parasite Immunol, 7*(6), 625–632.

46. Isgro, M., Bianchetti, L., Marini, M. A., et al. (2013). The C-C motif chemokine ligands CCL5, CCL11, and CCL24 induce the migration of circulating fibrocytes from patients with severe asthma. *Mucosal Immunol, 6*(4), 718–727.

47. Mattoli, S. (2015). Involvement of fibrocytes in asthma and clinical implications. *Clin Exp Allergy, 45*(10), 1497–1509.

48. Saunders, R., Siddiqui, S., Kaur, D., et al. (2009). Fibrocyte localization to the airway smooth muscle is a feature of asthma. *J Allergy Clin Immunol, 123*(2), 376–384.

49. Robinson, D. S. (2013). Mepolizumab for severe eosinophilic asthma. *Expert Rev Respir Med, 7*(1), 13–17.

50. Hogan, S. P., Waddell, A., & Fulkerson, P. C. (2013). Eosinophils in infection and intestinal immunity. *Curr Opin Gastroenterol, 29*(1), 7–14.

51. Walsh, R. E., & Gaginella, T. S. (1991). The eosinophil in inflammatory bowel disease. *Scand J Gastroenterol, 26*(12), 1217–1224.

52. Dahlin, J. S., Hamey, F. K., Pijuan-Sala, B., et al. (2018). A single-cell hematopoietic landscape resolves 8 lineage trajectories and defects in Kit mutant mice. *Blood, 131*(21), e1–e11.

53. Hamey, F. K., Lau, W., Kucinski, I., et al. (2021). Single-cell molecular profiling provides a high-resolution map of basophil and mast cell development. *Allergy, 76*(6), 1731–1742.

54. Oetjen, L. K., Noti, M., & Kim, B. S. (2016). New insights into basophil heterogeneity. *Semin Immunopathol, 38*(5), 549–561.

55. Siracusa, M. C., Saenz, S. A., Wojno, E. D., et al. (2013). Thymic stromal lymphopoietin-mediated extramedullary hematopoiesis promotes allergic inflammation. *Immunity, 39*(6), 1158–1170.

56. Siracusa, M. C., Saenz, S. A., Hill, D. A., et al. (2011). TSLP promotes interleukin-3-independent basophil haematopoiesis and type 2 inflammation. *Nature, 477*(7363), 229–233.

57. Siracusa, M. C., Kim, B. S., Spergel, J. M., et al. (2013). Basophils and allergic inflammation. *J Allergy Clin Immunol, 132*(4), 789–801; quiz 788.

58. Ohnmacht, C., & Voehringer, D. (2009). Basophil effector function and homeostasis during helminth infection. *Blood, 113*(12), 2816–2825.

59. Wang, H., Mobini, R., Fang, Y., et al. (2010). Allergen challenge of peripheral blood mononuclear cells from patients with seasonal allergic rhinitis increases IL-17RB, which regulates basophil apoptosis and degranulation. *Clin Exp Allergy, 40*(8), 1194–1202.

60. Wada, T., Ishiwata, K., Koseki, H., et al. (2010). Selective ablation of basophils in mice reveals their nonredundant role in acquired immunity against ticks. *J Clin Invest, 120*(8), 2867–2875.

61. Obata, K., Mukai, K., Tsujimura, Y., et al. (2007). Basophils are essential initiators of a novel type of chronic allergic inflammation. *Blood, 110*(3), 913–920.

62. Schroeder, J. T., MacGlashan, D. W., Jr., & Lichtenstein, L. M. (2001). Human basophils: mediator release and cytokine production. *Adv Immunol, 77*, 93–122.

63. Sullivan, B. M., & Locksley, R. M. (2009). Basophils: a nonredundant contributor to host immunity. *Immunity, 30*(1), 12–20.

64. Steiner, M., Huber, S., Harrer, A., et al. (2016). The evolution of human basophil biology from neglect towards understanding of their immune functions. *Biomed Res Int,* Article ID 8232830. https://doi.org/10.1155/2016/8232830.

65. Tschopp, C. M., Spiegl, N., Didichenko, S., et al. (2006). Granzyme B, a novel mediator of allergic inflammation: its induction and release in blood basophils and human asthma. *Blood, 108*(7), 2290–2299.

66. Spiegl, N., Didichenko, S., McCaffery, P., et al. (2008). Human basophils activated by mast cell-derived IL-3 express retinaldehyde dehydrogenase-II and produce the immunoregulatory mediator retinoic acid. *Blood, 112*(9), 3762–3771.

67. de Paulis, A., Prevete, N., Fiorentino, I., et al. (2006). Expression and functions of the vascular endothelial growth factors and their receptors in human basophils. *J Immunol, 177*(10), 7322–7331.

68. Eberle, J. U., & Voehringer, D. (2016). Role of basophils in protective immunity to parasitic infections. *Semin Immunopathol, 38*(5), 605–613.

69. Obata-Ninomiya, K., Ishiwata, K., Tsutsui, H., et al. (2013). The skin is an important bulwark of acquired immunity against intestinal helminths. *J Exp Med, 210*(12), 2583–2595.

70. Schwartz, C., Turqueti-Neves, A., Hartmann, S., et al. (2014). Basophil-mediated protection against gastrointestinal helminths requires IgE-induced cytokine secretion. *Proc Natl Acad Sci U S A, 111*(48), E5169–E5177. https://doi.org/10.1073/pnas.1412663111.

71. Hallgren, J., & Gurish, M. F. (2011). Mast cell progenitor trafficking and maturation. *Adv Exp Med Biol, 716*, 14–28.

72. Valent, P. (1994). The phenotype of human eosinophils, basophils, and mast cells. *J Allergy Clin Immunol, 94*(6 Pt 2), 1177–1183.

73. Shea-Donohue, T., Stiltz, J., Zhao, A., et al. (2010). Mast cells. *Curr Gastroenterol Rep, 12*(5), 349–357.

74. Kambe, N., Hiramatsu, H., Shimonaka, M., et al. (2004). Development of both human connective tissue-type and mucosal-type mast cells in mice from hematopoietic stem cells with identical distribution pattern to human body. *Blood, 103*(3), 860–867.

75. Nakano, N., Nishiyama, C., Yagita, H., et al. (2009). Notch signaling confers antigen-presenting cell functions on mast cells. *J Allergy Clin Immunol, 123*(1), 74–81.e1.

76. Galli, S. J., Grimbaldeston, M., & Tsai, M. (2008). Immunomodulatory mast cells: negative, as well as positive, regulators of immunity. *Nat Rev Immunol, 8*(6), 478–486.

77. Nichols, B. A., Bainton, D. F., & Farquhar, M. G. (1971). Differentiation of monocytes. Origin, nature, and fate of their azurophil granules. *J Cell Biol, 50*(2), 498–515.

78. Ziegler-Heitbrock, L., Ancuta, P., Crowe, S., et al. (2010). Nomenclature of monocytes and dendritic cells in blood. *Blood, 116*(16), e74–80.

79. Wong, K. L., Yeap, W. H., Tai, J. J., et al. (2012). The three human monocyte subsets: implications for health and disease. *Immunol Res, 53*(1–3), 41–57.

80. Idzkowska, E., Eljaszewicz, A., Miklasz, P., et al. (2015). The role of different monocyte subsets in the pathogenesis of atherosclerosis and acute coronary syndromes. *Scand J Immunol, 82*(3), 163–173.

81. Meuret, G., Bammert, J., & Hoffmann, G. (1974). Kinetics of human monocytopoiesis. *Blood, 44*(6), 801–816.

82. Swirski, F. K., Nahrendorf, M., Etzrodt, M., et al. (2009). Identification of splenic reservoir monocytes and their deployment to inflammatory sites. *Science, 325*(5940), 612–616.

83. Meuret, G., Batara, E., & Furste, H. O. (1975). Monocytopoiesis in normal man: pool size, proliferation activity and DNA synthesis time of promonocytes. *Acta Haematol, 54*(5), 261–270.

84. Whitelaw, D. M. (1972). Observations on human monocyte kinetics after pulse labeling. *Cell Tissue Kinet, 5*(4), 311–317.

85. Kumar, S., & Jack, R. (2006). Origin of monocytes and their differentiation to macrophages and dendritic cells. *J Endotoxin Res, 12*(5), 278–284.

86. Crofton, R. W., Diesselhoff-den Dulk, M. M., & van Furth, R. (1978). The origin, kinetics, and characteristics of the Kupffer cells in the normal steady state. *J Exp Med, 148*(1), 1–17.

87. Nathan, C. F. (1987). Secretory products of macrophages. *J Clin Invest, 79*(2), 319–326.

88. Di Santo, J. P., & Vosshenrich, C. A. (2006). Bone marrow versus thymic pathways of natural killer cell development. *Immunol Rev, 214*, 35–46.

89. Lotzova, E., Savary, C. A., & Champlin, R. E. (1993). Genesis of human oncolytic natural killer cells from primitive CD34+CD33- bone marrow progenitors. *J Immunol, 150*(12), 5263–5269.

90. Res, P., Martinez-Caceres, E., Cristina Jaleco, A., et al. (1996). CD34+CD38dim cells in the human thymus can differentiate into T, natural killer, and dendritic cells but are distinct from pluripotent stem cells. *Blood, 87*(12), 5196–5206.

91. Sevilla, D. W., Colovai, A. I., Emmons, F. N., et al. (2010). Hematogones: a review and update. *Leuk Lymphoma, 51*(1), 10–19.

92. McKenna, R. W., Washington, L. T., Aquino, D. B., et al. (2001). Immunophenotypic analysis of hematogones (B-lymphocyte precursors) in 662 consecutive bone marrow specimens by 4-color flow cytometry. *Blood, 98*(8), 2498–2507.

93. Haynes, B. F. (1984). The human thymic microenvironment. *Adv Immunol, 36*, 87–142.

94. von Boehmer, H., Teh, H. S., & Kisielow, P. (1989). The thymus selects the useful, neglects the useless and destroys the harmful. *Immunol Today, 10*(2), 57–61.

95. Grossi, C. E., Cadoni, A., Zicca, A., et al. (1982). Large granular lymphocytes in human peripheral blood: ultrastructural and cytochemical characterization of the granules. *Blood, 59*(2), 277–283.

96. LeBien, T. W., & Tedder, T. F. (2008). B lymphocytes: how they develop and function. *Blood, 112*(5), 1570–1580.

97. Vignali, D. A., Collison, L. W., & Workman, C. J. (2008). How regulatory T cells work. *Nat Rev Immunol, 8*(7), 523–532.

98. Zhu, J., & Paul, W. E. (2008). CD4 T cells: fates, functions, and faults. *Blood, 112*(5), 1557–1569.

99. Rufer, N., Zippelius, A., Batard, P., et al. (2003). Ex vivo characterization of human CD8+ T subsets with distinct replicative history and partial effector functions. *Blood, 102*(5), 1779–1787.

100. Vivier, E., Tomasello, E., Baratin, M., et al. (2008). Functions of natural killer cells. *Nat Immunol, 9*(5), 503–510.

11

Platelet Production, Structure, and Function

Walter P. Jeske*

OBJECTIVES

After completion of this chapter, the reader will be able to:

1. Diagram megakaryocyte localization in bone marrow.
2. List the transcription products that trigger and control megakaryocytopoiesis and endomitosis.
3. Diagram terminal megakaryocyte differentiation, the proplatelet process, and thrombocytopoiesis.
4. Describe the ultrastructure of resting platelets in the circulation, including the plasma membrane, tubules, microfibrils, and granules.
5. List the important platelet receptors and their ligands.

6. Characterize platelet function, including adhesion, aggregation, and secretion.
7. Explain the biochemical pathways of platelet activation including integrins, G-proteins, and the eicosanoid and the inositol triphosphate-diacylglycerol pathways.
8. Summarize mechanisms by which platelets contribute to an inflammatory response.
9. Summarize the components within a platelet used for protein synthesis including its transcriptome.

OUTLINE

Megakaryocytopoiesis
  Megakaryocyte Differentiation and Progenitors
  Endomitosis
  Terminal Megakaryocyte Differentiation
  Thrombocytopoiesis (Platelet Shedding)
  Megakaryocyte Membrane Receptors and Markers
  Hormones and Cytokines of Megakaryocytopoiesis
Platelets
Platelet Ultrastructure
  Resting Platelet Plasma Membrane
  Surface-Connected Canalicular System
  Dense Tubular System
  Cytoskeleton: Microfilaments and Microtubules
  Platelet Granules: α-Granules, Dense Granules, and
    Lysosomes

  Plasma Membrane Receptors That Provide for Adhesion
  Seven-Transmembrane Repeat Receptors
  Additional Membrane Receptors
Platelet Function
  Adhesion: Platelets Bind Elements of the Vascular Matrix
  Aggregation: Platelets Irreversibly Cohere
  Secretion: Activated Platelets Release Granular Contents
  Generation of Platelet Microparticles
Platelet Signaling Pathways
  G-Proteins
  Eicosanoid Synthesis
  Inositol Triphosphate-Diacylglycerol Activation Pathway
Platelets and Inflammation
Platelet Proteome

CASE STUDY

After studying the material in this chapter, the reader should be able to respond to the following case study. Answers can be found in Appendix C.

A 35-year-old woman noticed multiple pinpoint red spots and bruises on her arms and legs. The hematologist confirmed the presence of petechiae, purpura, and ecchymoses on her extremities and ordered a CBC, PT, and PTT. The PLT was 35×10^9/L, the MPV was 13.2 fL, and the diameter of platelets on the Wright-stained peripheral blood film appeared to exceed 6 μm. Other CBC parameters and the coagulation parameters were within reference intervals. Reference intervals can be found after the Index at the end of the book. A Wright-stained

bone marrow aspirate smear revealed 10 to 12 small unlobulated megakaryocytes/low-power microscopic field.

1. Do these signs and symptoms indicate mucocutaneous (systemic) or anatomic bleeding?
2. What is the probable cause of the bleeding?
3. Does the patient's bleeding result from altered platelet production in the bone marrow?
4. List the growth factors involved in recruiting megakaryocyte progenitors.

*The author extends appreciation to George A. Fritsma, whose work in prior editions provided the foundation for this chapter.

Platelets are nonnucleated blood cells that circulate at a concentration of 150 to 450 × 10^9/L, with average platelet counts slightly higher in women than in men and slightly lower in members of both sexes who are older than 65 years.[1] Platelets trigger primary hemostasis on exposure to subendothelial collagen or endothelial cell inflammatory proteins at the time of blood vessel injury (Chapter 35).

MEGAKARYOCYTOPOIESIS

Platelets arise from unique bone marrow cells called *megakaryocytes*. Megakaryocytes are the largest cells in the bone marrow and possess multiple chromosome copies (polyploid). On a Wright-stained bone marrow aspirate smear, each megakaryocyte is 30 to 50 μm in diameter with a multilobulated nucleus and abundant granular cytoplasm. Megakaryocytes account for less than 0.5% of all bone marrow cells; on a normal Wright-stained bone marrow aspirate smear, two to four megakaryocytes per 10× low-power field may be identified (Chapter 15).[2]

In healthy, intact bone marrow tissue, megakaryocytes, under the influence of an array of stromal cell cytokines, cluster with hematopoietic stem cells in vascular niches adjacent to venous sinusoid endothelial cells (Figure 11.1).[3] Responding to the growth factor *thrombopoietin* (TPO), megakaryocyte progenitors are recruited from *common myeloid progenitors* (Chapter 5) and subsequently differentiate through several maturation stages. Megakaryocytes can also be found in the lungs and may contribute to the overall platelet production.[4,5]

Megakaryocyte Differentiation and Progenitors

Megakaryocyte progenitors arise from the common myeloid progenitor under the influence of the transcription gene product, GATA-1, regulated by cofactor FOG1 (Box 11.1).[3] Megakaryocyte differentiation is suppressed by another transcription gene product, MYB, so GATA-1 and MYB act in opposition to balance megakaryocytopoiesis with erythropoiesis, where the same progenitor cell can be differentiated into the platelet cell line or the red blood cell (RBC) line. Three megakaryocyte lineage-committed progenitor stages, defined by their in vitro culture colony characteristics, arise from the common myeloid progenitor (Figure 5.13). In order of differentiation, these are the least mature *burst-forming unit megakaryocyte* (BFU-Meg); the intermediate *colony-forming unit megakaryocyte* (CFU-Meg); and the more mature progenitor, the *light-density colony-forming unit megakaryocyte* (LD-CFU-Meg).[6] All three progenitor stages resemble lymphocytes and cannot be distinguished by Wright-stained light microscopy. The BFU-Meg and CFU-Meg are diploid and undergo normal mitosis to maintain a viable pool of megakaryocyte progenitors. Their proliferative properties are reflected in their ability to form hundreds (BFU-Megs) or dozens (CFU-Megs) of colonies in culture (Figure 11.2).[7] The third stage, LD-CFU-Meg, undergoes *endomitosis*, a form of mitosis unique to megakaryocytes in which DNA replication and cytoplasmic maturation are normal, but cells lose their capacity to divide.

Endomitosis

Endomitosis is a form of mitosis that lacks telophase and cytokinesis (separation into daughter cells). As GATA-1 and FOG1-driven transcription slows, another transcription factor, RUNX1, mediates the switch from mitosis to endomitosis by suppressing the Rho/ROCK signaling pathway. In response to the reduced Rho/ROCK signal, inadequate levels of actin and myosin (muscle fiber like molecules) assemble in the cytoplasmic constrictions where separation would otherwise occur, preventing cytokinesis.[8] Subsequently, under the influence of transcription factor NF-E2, DNA replication proceeds to the production of 8N, 16N, or even 32N ploidy.[3] Although some megakaryocytes reach 128N, this level of ploidy is unusual and may signal hematologic disease. Megakaryocytes employ their multiple DNA copies to synthesize abundant cytoplasm, which ultimately is incorporated into platelets.

Terminal Megakaryocyte Differentiation

As endomitosis proceeds, megakaryocyte progenitors leave the proliferative phase and enter *terminal differentiation*, a series of stages exhibiting unique Wright-stained morphology in bone marrow

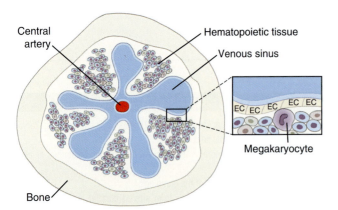

Figure 11.1 Cross Section of Bone Marrow Hematopoietic Tissue. The nerve, artery, and vein run longitudinally through the center of the marrow. Venous sinuses extend laterally from the central vein throughout the hematopoietic tissue. Differentiating and mature megakaryocytes localize to the abluminal (nonblood) surface of sinusoid-lining endothelial cells in preparation for movement into the bloodstream. *EC,* Endothelial cell.

BOX 11.1   Endomitosis

Endomitosis is no longer a mystery to the molecular biologists who mapped its translational control genes, but it may seem mysterious to those who do not work daily with gene, gene product, and mutation abbreviations. The abbreviations have antecedents; for instance, GATA-1 stands for "globin transcription factor-1," a protein product of the X chromosome gene *GATA1*. FOG1 stands for "friend of GATA," a product of the *ZFPM1* (zinc finger protein multitype 1) gene. Laboratory scientists rarely refer to gene names, only their abbreviations, though they are familiar with their characteristics and functions. The abbreviations have moved rapidly into clinical laboratory jargon as they are becoming key diagnostic markers. In this chapter, we use gene product abbreviations without reference to their antecedents.

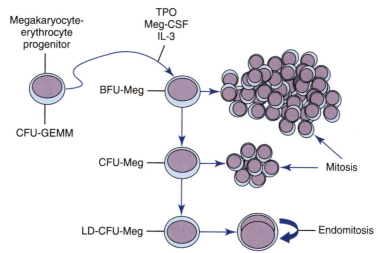

Figure 11.2 Three Stages of Megakaryocyte Progenitors. The BFU-Meg clones hundreds of daughter cells through mitosis. The CFU-Meg clones dozens of daughter cells through mitosis. The LD-CFU-Meg undergoes the first stage of endomitosis. *BFU-Meg,* Burst-forming unit megakaryocyte; *CFU-Meg,* colony-forming unit megakaryocyte; *CFU-GEMM,* colony-forming unit, granulocyte, erythrocyte, monocyte, megakaryocyte; *IL-3,* interleukin-3; *LD-CFU-Meg,* low-density colony-forming unit megakaryocyte; *Meg-CSF,* megakaryocyte colony-stimulating factor; *TPO,* thrombopoietin.

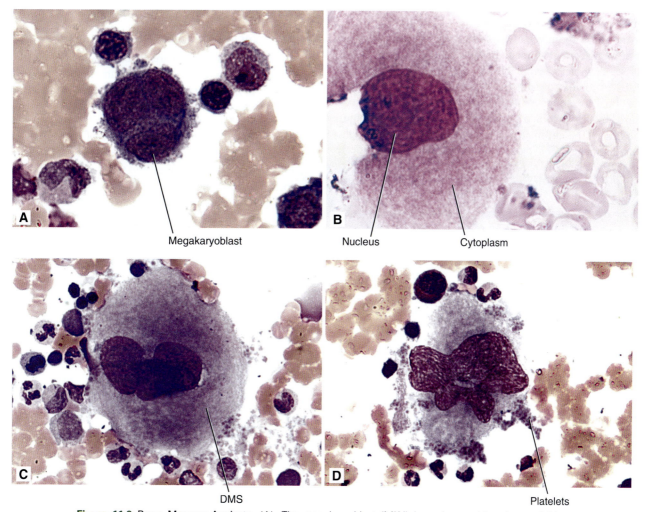

Figure 11.3 Bone Marrow Aspirate. (A), The megakaryoblast (MK-I) (arrow) resembles the myeloblast and pronormoblast (rubriblast); identification by morphology alone is inadvisable. This megakaryoblast has cytoplasmic blebs that resemble platelets. **(B),** Promegakaryocyte (MK-II). Cytoplasm is abundant, and the nucleus has minimal lobularity. **(C),** Megakaryocyte (MK-III). The nucleus is lobulated, with basophilic chromatin. The cytoplasm is azurophilic and granular, with evidence of the demarcation membrane system. **(D),** Terminal megakaryocyte shedding platelets from the proplatelet process. (A–D, Wright-Giemsa stain, ×1000.) *DMS,* Demarcation membrane system.

aspirate smears (Figure 11.3) or hematoxylin and eosin-stained bone marrow biopsy sections (Table 11.1). However, there is seldom a clinical need to distinguish MK-I, MK-II, and MK-III stages during a routine examination of a bone marrow aspirate smear.

The least differentiated megakaryocyte precursor is called the *MK-I stage* or *megakaryoblast*. Although megakaryoblasts no longer look like lymphocytes, they cannot be reliably distinguished from bone marrow myeloblasts or pronormoblasts (also named rubriblasts) using light microscopy (Figure 11.3A). Occasionally, plasma membrane *blebs* that resemble platelets may project from the margin of the megakaryoblast. Development of α-granules, dense granules, and the demarcation membrane system (DMS) occurs during the megakaryoblast phase.[9]

The DMS is a series of membrane-lined channels that grow inward from the plasma membrane to subdivide the entire cytoplasm. The DMS is biologically identical to the megakaryocyte plasma membrane and ultimately delineates individual platelets during thrombocytopoiesis.

Nuclear lobularity first becomes apparent as an indentation at the 4N replication stage, rendering the cell identifiable by light microscopy as an *MK-II stage*, or *promegakaryocyte*. The promegakaryocyte reaches its full ploidy level by the end of the MK-II stage (Figure 11.3B).

At the most abundant *MK-III stage*, the *megakaryocyte* is easily recognized at 10× magnification on the basis of its 30- to 50-µm diameter (Figure 11.3C). The nucleus is intensely indented or lobulated, with the degree of lobulation roughly proportional to ploidy. When necessary, ploidy levels can be measured by flow cytometry using the nucleic acid dye propidium iodide.[10] The chromatin is variably condensed with light and dark patches. The cytoplasm is azurophilic (lavender), granular, and plateletlike. At full maturation platelet shedding, or *thrombocytopoiesis,* proceeds.

Thrombocytopoiesis (Platelet Shedding)

Figure 11.3D illustrates the process of platelet shedding, termed *thrombocytopoiesis*. During thrombocytopoiesis, a single megakaryocyte may shed 2000 to 4000 platelets. In an average-size healthy human, 10^8 megakaryocytes produce 10^{11} platelets per day. The total platelet population turns over in 8 to 9 days, with the platelet life span being governed by the relative amounts of proapoptotic Bak and antiapoptotic Bcl-xL proteins.[11] In instances of high platelet consumption, such as immune thrombocytopenic purpura (Chapter 38), platelet production may increase by as much as 10-fold.

Evaluation of bone marrow biopsy preparations rarely shows evidence of platelet budding or shedding. However, in megakaryocyte cultures examined by transmission electron microscopy, DMS dilation, the formation of longitudinal bundles of tubules, the development of proplatelet processes, and the appearance of transverse constrictions can be observed. In the bone marrow environment, proplatelet processes are believed to pierce through or between sinusoid-lining endothelial cells, extend into the venous blood, and shed platelets (Figure 11.4). Thrombocytopoiesis leaves behind naked megakaryocyte nuclei that are consumed by marrow macrophages.[12]

Megakaryocyte Membrane Receptors and Markers

In specialty and tertiary care laboratories, immunostaining of fixed tissue, flow cytometry with immunologic probes, and fluorescent in situ hybridization with genetic probes are techniques used to identify visually indistinguishable megakaryocyte progenitors in hematologic disease. There are several megakaryocyte membrane markers that can be measured by flow cytometry, including MPL, which is the TPO receptor present at all maturation stages, and the stem cell and common myeloid progenitor marker CD34. CD34 expression disappears as differentiation proceeds. The platelet membrane glycoprotein (GP) IIb/IIIa (CD41/CD61) first appears on megakaryocyte progenitors and remains present throughout maturation, along with immunologic markers CD36 (platelet GPIV), CD42 (GPIb), and CD62 (P-selectin). Cytoplasmic coagulation factor VIII, von Willebrand factor (VWF), and fibrinogen may be detected in the fully developed megakaryocyte by immunostaining (Table 11.2).[13-15]

TABLE 11.1 Features of the Three Terminal Megakaryocyte Differentiation Stages

	MK-I	MK-II	MK-III
Precursors (%)	20	25	55
Diameter (µm)	14–18	15–40	30–50
Nucleus	Round	Indented	Multilobed
Nucleoli	2–6	Variable	Not visible
Chromatin	Homogeneous	Moderately condensed	Deeply and variably condensed
Nucleus-to- cytoplasm ratio	3:1	1:2	1:4
Mitosis	Absent	Absent	Absent
Endomitosis	Present	Ends	Absent
Cytoplasm	Basophilic	Basophilic and granular	Azurophilic and granular
α-Granules	Present	Present	Present
Dense granules	Present	Present	Present
Demarcation system	Present	Present	Present

MK-I, Megakaryoblast; *MK-II,* promegakaryocyte; *MK-III,* megakaryocyte.

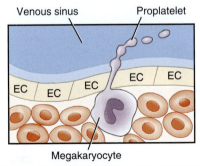

Figure 11.4 Platelet Shedding. Megakaryocyte is adjacent to the abluminal (nonblood) membrane of the sinusoid-lining endothelial cell of the bone marrow hematopoietic tissue and extends a proplatelet process through or between the endothelial cells into the vascular sinus. *EC,* Endothelial cell.

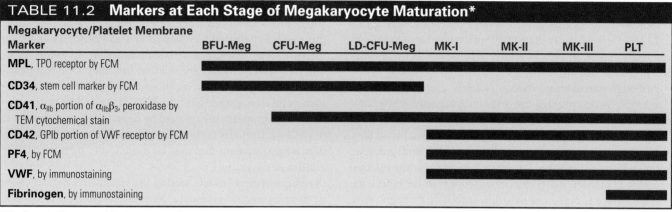

Megakaryocyte/Platelet Membrane Marker	BFU-Meg	CFU-Meg	LD-CFU-Meg	MK-I	MK-II	MK-III	PLT
MPL, TPO receptor by FCM	████████████████████████████████████
CD34, stem cell marker by FCM	████████████████████						
CD41, α_IIb portion of α_IIbβ_3, peroxidase by TEM cytochemical stain		████████████████████████████					
CD42, GPIb portion of VWF receptor by FCM				████████████████████
PF4, by FCM				████████████████████
VWF, by immunostaining				████████████████████
Fibrinogen, by immunostaining							████

*The bars indicate at which stage of differentiation the marker appears and at which stage it disappears.

BFU-Meg, Burst-forming unit-megakaryocyte; *CFU-Meg*, colony-forming unit-megakaryocyte; *FCM*, flow cytometry; *GP*, glycoprotein; *LD-CFU-Meg*, low-density colony-forming unit-megakaryocyte; *MK-I*, megakaryoblast; *MK-II*, promegakaryocyte; *MK-III*, megakaryocyte; *PF4*, platelet factor 4; *PLT*, platelets; *TEM*, transmission electron microscopy; *TPO*, thrombopoietin; *VWF*, von Willebrand factor.

TABLE 11.3 Hormones and Cytokines That Control Megakaryocytopoiesis

Cytokine/Hormone	Differentiation to Progenitors	Differentiation to Megakaryocytes	Late Maturation	Thrombocytopoiesis	Therapeutic Agent
TPO	+	+	+	0	Available
IL-3	+	+	0		
IL-6	0	0	+	+	
IL-11	0	+	+	+	Available

IL, Interleukin; *TPO*, thrombopoietin; +, present; 0, absent.

Hormones and Cytokines of Megakaryocytopoiesis

The growth factor TPO is a 70,000-Dalton molecule that possesses 23% homology with erythropoietin, the hormone that stimulates RBC production.[16] Messenger ribonucleic acid (RNA) for TPO has been found in the kidney, liver, stromal cells, and smooth muscle cells, though the liver has the most copies and is considered the primary source. TPO circulates as a hormone in plasma and is the ligand that binds the megakaryocyte and platelet membrane receptor protein, MPL, named for v-mpl, a viral oncogene associated with murine myeloproliferative leukemia. The plasma concentration of TPO is inversely proportional to platelet and megakaryocyte mass, implying that membrane binding and consequent removal of TPO by platelets is the primary mechanism for controlling platelet count.[17] Both in vitro and in vivo experiments have shown that TPO, in synergy with other cytokines, induces stem cells to differentiate into megakaryocyte progenitors and that it further induces the differentiation of megakaryocyte progenitors into megakaryoblasts and megakaryocytes. TPO also induces the proliferation and maturation of megakaryocytes and induces thrombocytopoiesis (Table 11.3).

Synthetic TPO receptor agonists such as avatrombopag, eltrombopag, lusutrombopag, and romiplostim activate the TPO receptor and are approved for raising platelet counts in patients with immune thrombocytopenia, aplastic anemia, and chronic liver disease.[18] Increasing evidence suggests that romiplostim may also be beneficial in the treatment of chemotherapy-induced thrombocytopenia.[19]

Other cytokines that function with TPO to stimulate megakaryocytopoiesis include interleukin-3 (IL-3), IL-6, and IL-11

(Table 11.3). IL-3 acts in synergy with TPO to induce the early differentiation of stem cells, whereas IL-6 and IL-11 act in the presence of TPO to enhance endomitosis, megakaryocyte maturation, and thrombocytopoiesis. An IL-11 polypeptide mimetic, oprelvekin, stimulates platelet production in patients with chemotherapy-induced thrombocytopenia.[20] Other cytokines and hormones that participate synergistically with TPO and the interleukins are stem cell factor, also called kit ligand or mast cell growth factor; granulocyte-macrophage colony-stimulating factor (GM-CSF); granulocyte colony-stimulating factor (G-CSF); and acetylcholinesterase-derived megakaryocyte growth-stimulating peptide.[21]

Platelet factor 4 (PF4), β-thromboglobulin, neutrophil-activating peptide 2, IL-8, and other factors inhibit in vitro megakaryocyte growth. Limited data are available, however, to define their role in controlling megakaryocytopoiesis in vivo.[22] Reduction in levels of the transcription factors FOG1, GATA-1, and NF-E2 diminish megakaryocytopoiesis at the progenitor, endomitotic, and terminal maturation phases.[23]

PLATELETS

The megakaryocyte proplatelet process sheds platelets, anuclear cells containing granular cytoplasm, into the venous sinus of the bone marrow. On a Wright-stained wedge-preparation blood film, platelets, averaging 2.5 μm in diameter, are distributed throughout the RBC monolayer at 7 to 21 cells per 100× field (Figure 1.1).[24] Mean platelet volume (MPV), as measured by a clinical profiling instrument (Chapter 13), ranges from 7 to 12 fL, and a frequency distribution of platelet volume is able to indicate subpopulations such as large platelets (Figures 13.6 and 13.9). Heterogeneity in the MPV of healthy humans reflects random variation in platelet release volume and is not a function of platelet age or vitality.[25]

Although circulating, resting platelets are biconvex, the platelets in blood collected using the anticoagulant ethylenediaminetetraacetic acid (EDTA) (lavender closure tubes) tend to "round up." On a Wright-stained wedge-preparation blood film, platelets appear circular to irregular, lavender, and granular. Because of their small size, it is difficult to examine the internal structure of platelets using light microscopy.[26] In the blood, the platelet surface is even, and they flow smoothly through veins, arteries, and capillaries. In contrast to leukocytes, which tend to roll along the vascular endothelium, platelets cluster with the erythrocytes near the center of the blood vessel. In contrast to erythrocytes, however, platelets move back and forth with the leukocytes from venules into the white pulp of the spleen, where both become sequestered in dynamic equilibrium.

The normal peripheral blood platelet count ranges from 150 to 450×10^9/L. The platelet count decreases with increasing age, such that after 65 years, platelet counts of 122 to 350×10^9/L and 140 to 379×10^9/L are seen in men and women, respectively. This count represents only two-thirds of total body platelets; the remaining one-third is sequestered within the spleen. Sequestered platelets are immediately available in times of demand such as in acute inflammation or after an injury, after major surgery, or during plateletpheresis. In hypersplenism or splenomegaly, increased sequestration may cause a relative thrombocytopenia.

Reticulated platelets, sometimes known as *stress platelets,* appear in compensation for thrombocytopenia (Figure 11.5).[25] Reticulated platelets are markedly larger than ordinary mature circulating platelets; their diameter in peripheral blood films exceeds 6 µm, and their MPV reaches 12 to 14 fL.[26] Similar to ordinary platelets, they round up in EDTA, but in *citrated* (blue

closure tubes) whole blood, reticulated platelets are cylindrical and beaded, resembling fragments of megakaryocyte proplatelet processes. Reticulated platelets carry free ribosomes and fragments of rough endoplasmic reticulum, analogous to RBC reticulocytes, which triggers speculation that they arise from early and rapid proplatelet extension and release. Nucleic acid dyes such as thiazole orange bind the RNA of the endoplasmic reticulum. This property is exploited by hematology instruments to provide a quantitative evaluation of reticulated platelet production, a measurement that may be more useful than the MPV.[24] Platelet-dense granule nucleotides, however, may interfere with this measurement, falsely raising the reticulated platelet count by binding nucleic acid dyes. Reticulated platelets are potentially prothrombotic and may be associated with increased risk of adverse events in a variety of disease states, including infection/sepsis, coronary artery disease, liver disease, preeclampsia, and hematologic disorders.[27-32]

PLATELET ULTRASTRUCTURE

Platelets, although anucleate, are strikingly complex and are metabolically active. Their ultrastructure has been studied using scanning and transmission electron microscopy, flow cytometry, and molecular sequencing.

Resting Platelet Plasma Membrane

The platelet *plasma membrane* resembles any biologic membrane (Chapter 4): a bilayer composed of proteins and lipids, as diagrammed in Figure 11.6. The predominant lipids are phospholipids, which form the basic structure, and cholesterol, which distributes asymmetrically throughout the phospholipids. The phospholipids form a bilayer with their polar heads oriented toward aqueous environments, toward the blood plasma

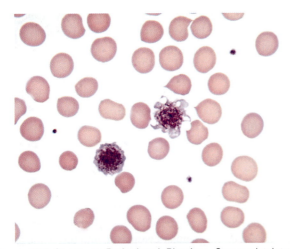

Figure 11.5 Stress or Reticulated Platelets. Stress platelets may appear in blood circulation in compensation for thrombocytopenia. The diameter of reticulated platelets exceeds 6 µm. Reticulated platelets carry free ribosomes and fragments of rough endoplasmic reticulum, detectable in flow cytometry using nucleic acid dyes. (Peripheral blood, Wright-Giemsa stain, ×500.)

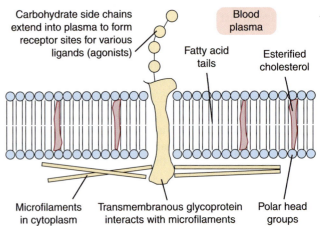

Figure 11.6 Platelet Plasma Membrane. The platelet possesses a standard biologic membrane composed of a phospholipid bilayer with polar head groups oriented toward the aqueous blood plasma (neutral phospholipids) and platelet cytoplasm (charged phospholipids) and nonpolar fatty acid tails that orient toward the center. The phospholipid backbone is interspersed with esterified cholesterol that maintains membrane integrity and function. A series of transmembranous proteins communicate with microfilaments (shown here), G-proteins, and enzymes. The transmembranous proteins support carbohydrate side chains (receptors) that extend into the plasma.

externally and the cytoplasm internally. Their fatty acid chains, esterified to carbons 1 and 2 of the phospholipid triglyceride backbone, orient toward each other, perpendicular to the plane of the membrane, to form a hydrophobic barrier sandwiched within the hydrophilic layers.

The neutral phospholipids phosphatidylcholine and sphingomyelin predominate in the outer blood plasma layer; the anionic or polar phospholipids phosphatidylinositol, phosphatidylethanolamine, and phosphatidylserine predominate in the inner cytoplasmic layer. During platelet activation, these phospholipids, especially phosphatidylinositol, support platelet activation by supplying arachidonic acid, an unsaturated fatty acid, which becomes converted to eicosanoids including thromboxane A_2 (TXA_2) (detailed in the "Eicosanoid Synthesis" section).

Esterified cholesterol moves freely throughout the hydrophobic internal layer, exchanging with unesterified cholesterol from the surrounding plasma. Cholesterol stabilizes the membrane, promotes membrane fluidity, and helps control the transmembranous passage of materials through the selectively permeable plasma membrane.

Anchored within the membrane are glycoproteins and proteoglycans that support surface glycosaminoglycans, oligosaccharides, glycolipids, and essential plasma surface-oriented glycosylated receptors that respond to cellular and humoral stimuli called *ligands* or *agonists*. *Ligand binding* transmits a stimulus through the membrane to organelles internal to the platelet. The platelet membrane surface, called the *glycocalyx,* is 20 to 30 nm thick, which is thicker than the analogous surface layer of leukocytes or erythrocytes. This thick layer is also adhesive due to adsorption of albumin, fibrinogen, and other plasma proteins, allowing a ready response to hemostatic demands. In many instances, the glycocalyx facilitates transport of adherent proteins to internal storage organelles using a process called *endocytosis.* The platelet carries its functional environment with it while maintaining a negative surface charge that repels other platelets, other blood cells, and the endothelial cells that line the blood vessels.

Surface-Connected Canalicular System

The plasma membrane invaginates, producing a unique *surface-connected canalicular system* (SCCS) (Figure 11.7). The SCCS twists spongelike throughout the platelet, enabling the platelet to store additional quantities of many of the hemostatic proteins found on the glycocalyx. The glycocalyx is less developed in the SCCS, however, and lacks some of the glycoprotein receptors present on the platelet surface. The SCCS also allows for enhanced interaction of the platelet with its environment, increasing access to the platelet interior as well as increasing egress of platelet release products. The SCCS is the route for endocytosis and for secretion of α-granule contents upon platelet activation.

Dense Tubular System

Closely aligned to the SCCS is the *dense tubular system* (DTS) (Figure 11.7), a condensed remnant of the rough endoplasmic reticulum. The DTS sequesters Ca^{2+} and bears a number of enzymes important for platelet activation including phospholipase A_2, cyclooxygenase, and thromboxane synthase, all of which participate in the production of TXA_2 and phospholipase C that support production of the signaling molecules inositol triphosphate (IP_3) and diacylglycerol (DAG).

Cytoskeleton: Microfilaments and Microtubules

A thick, circumferential bundle of microtubules maintains the platelet's discoid shape (Figure 11.7). The *circumferential microtubules* parallel the plane of the outer surface of the platelet and reside just within, although not touching, the plasma membrane. There are 8 to 20 tubules composed of multiple subunits of tubulin that disassemble at refrigerator temperature or when platelets are treated with colchicine. When microtubules disassemble in the cold, platelets become round, but on warming to 37° C, they recover their original disc shape. On cross section, microtubules are cylindrical, with a diameter of 25 nm. The circumferential microtubules could be a single spiral tubule.[33] In addition to maintaining the shape of resting platelets, microtubules move inward on platelet activation to enable release of α-granule

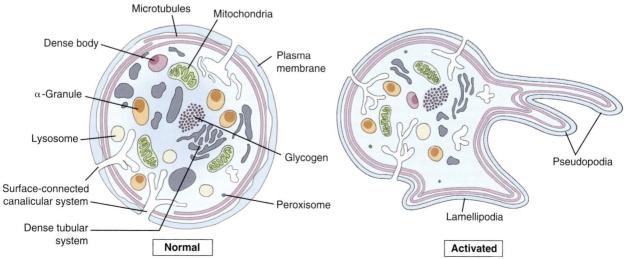

Figure 11.7 Diagram of Platelet Subcellular Organelles.

contents and subsequently reassemble in long parallel bundles during platelet shape change to provide rigidity to pseudopods.

In the narrow area between the microtubules and the membrane lies a thick meshwork of *microfilaments* composed of actin. *Actin* is contractile in platelets (as in muscle) and anchors the plasma membrane glycoproteins and proteoglycans. Actin also is present throughout the platelet cytoplasm, constituting 20% to 30% of platelet protein. In the resting platelet, actin is globular and amorphous, but as the cytoplasmic calcium concentration rises, actin becomes filamentous and contractile.

The cytoplasm also contains intermediate filaments, ropelike polymers 8 to 12 nm in diameter, of desmin and vimentin. The intermediate filaments connect with actin and the tubules, maintaining the platelet shape. Microtubules, actin microfilaments, and intermediate microfilaments control platelet shape change, extension of pseudopods, and secretion of granule contents.

Platelet Granules: α-Granules, Dense Granules, and Lysosomes

There are 50 to 80 *α-granules* (sometimes called light granules) in each platelet, which stain medium gray in osmium-dye transmission electron microscopy preparations (Figure 11.7). The proteins within α-granules are endocytosed from the surrounding environment or synthesized within the megakaryocyte and stored in platelets (Table 11.4). Several α-granule proteins are membrane

bound. As part of the platelet activation process, α-granule membranes fuse with the SCCS. Their contents flow to the nearby microenvironment, where they participate in platelet adhesion and aggregation and support plasma coagulation.[34]

There are two to seven *dense granules* per platelet (Figure 11.7). These granules appear later than α-granules during megakaryocyte differentiation and stain black (opaque) when treated with osmium in transmission electron microscopy. Small molecules are probably endocytosed and are stored in the dense granules; these are listed in Table 11.5. In contrast to the α-granules, which employ the SCCS, dense granules migrate to the plasma membrane and release their contents directly into the plasma upon platelet activation. Membranes of dense granules contain many of the same integral proteins as the α-granules—P-selectin, $\alpha_{IIb}\beta_3$, and a complex of glycoproteins Ib, IX, and V (GPIb/IX/V), for instance—which implies a common source for the membranes of both types of granules.[35]

Platelets also contain a few *lysosomes* that are similar to those in neutrophils (300-nm diameter granules that stain positive for arylsulfatase, β-glucuronidase, acid phosphatase, and catalase). The contents of lysosomes likely digest vessel wall matrix components during in vivo aggregation and may also digest autophagic debris.

Plasma Membrane Receptors That Provide for Adhesion

The platelet membrane contains more than 50 distinct receptors, including members of the cell adhesion molecule (CAM) *integrin* family (the CAM *leucine-rich repeat* family, the CAM *immunoglobulin gene* family, the CAM *selectin* family), the *seven-transmembrane receptor* family, and some miscellaneous receptors (Figure 11.8).[36] Table 11.6 lists the receptors that support the initial phases of platelet adhesion and aggregation.

Integrins are heterodimeric proteins that integrate their ligands, which they bind on the outside of the cell, with the internal cytoskeleton triggering cellular activation. Several platelet *integrins* bind subendothelial proteins, enabling the platelet to adhere to the injured blood vessel lining. GPIa/IIa, or, using integrin terminology, $\alpha_2\beta_1$, is an integrin that binds the subendothelial collagen that becomes exposed in the damaged blood vessel wall, promoting adhesion of the platelet to the

TABLE 11.4 Representative Platelet α-Granule Proteins

	Coagulation Proteins	Noncoagulation Proteins
Proteins Present in Platelet Cytoplasm and α-Granules		
Endocytosed	Fibronectin Fibrinogen	Albumin Immunoglobulins
Megakaryocyte synthesized	Factor V Thrombospondin VWF	
Proteins Present in α-Granules but Not Cytoplasm		
Megakaryocyte synthesized	β-thromboglobulin HMWK PAI-1 Plasminogen PF4 Protein C inhibitor	EGF Multimerin PDCI PDGF TGF-β VEGF/VPF
Platelet Membrane-Bound Proteins		
Restricted to α-granule membrane	P-selectin	GMP-33 Osteonectin
In α-granule and plasma membrane	GPIIb/IIIa GPIV GPIb/IX/V GPVI	cap1 CD9 PECAM-1

cap1, Adenyl cyclase-associated protein; *CD*, cluster of differentiation; *EGF*, endothelial growth factor; *GMP*, guanidine monophosphate; *GP*, glycoprotein; *HMWK*, high-molecular-weight kininogen; *PAI-1*, plasminogen activator inhibitor; *PDCI*, platelet-derived collagenase inhibitor; *PDGF*, platelet-derived growth factor; *PECAM-1*, platelet endothelial cell adhesion molecule-1; *PF4*, platelet factor 4; *TGF-β*, transforming growth factor-β; *VEGF/VPF*, vascular endothelial growth factor/vascular permeability factor; *VWF*, von Willebrand factor.

TABLE 11.5 Platelet-Dense Granule Contents

Small Molecule	Property
ADP	Nonmetabolic; supports neighboring platelet aggregation by binding to P2Y$_1$ and P2Y$_{12}$ ADP receptors
ATP	Function unknown, but ATP release is detectable on platelet activation
Serotonin	Vasoconstrictor that binds endothelial cells and platelet membranes; supports procoagulant protein binding to COAT platelets
Ca^{2+} and Mg^{2+}	Divalent cations support platelet activation and coagulation

ADP, Adenosine diphosphate; *ATP*, adenosine triphosphate.

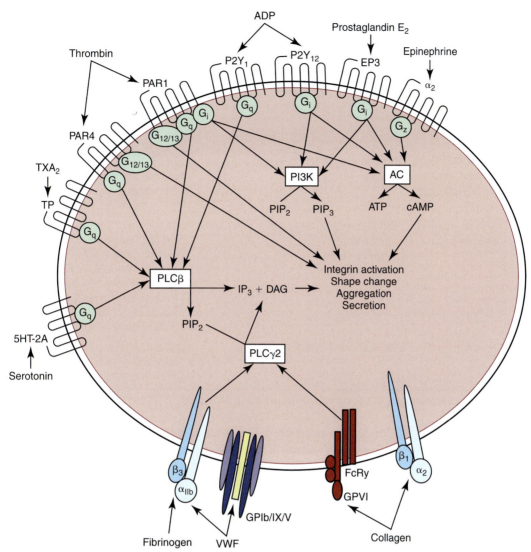

Figure 11.8 Diagram of the Platelet Membrane Receptors and Associated Activation Pathways. The seven-transmembrane repeat receptors for serotonin, thromboxane, thrombin, ADP, prostaglandin E₂, and epinephrine are coupled to G-proteins, which become stimulated when agonists bind their respective receptors to subsequently activate phospholipase enzymes (PLCβ, PI3K), and adenyl cyclase. Integrins include collagen receptor α₂β₁ and fibrinogen/VWF receptor α₁₁bβ₃. The integrins and glycoproteins activate PLCγ2, which also activates the PIP₂ pathway. The key collagen receptor is *GPVI*, and the key VWF receptor is GPIb/IX/V. *AC,* Adenyl cyclase; *ADP,* adenosine diphosphate; *DAG,* diacylglycerol; *GPIb/IX/V,* glycoproteins Ib, IX, and V complex; *GPVI,* glycoprotein VI; *IP₃,* inositol-1,4,5-triphosphate; *PAR1,* protease-activated receptor 1; *PAR4,* protease-activated receptor 4; *PI3K,* phosphoinositide 3-kinase; *PIP₂,* phosphatidylinositol-4,5-bisphosphate; *PIP₃,* phosphatidylinositol-3,4,5-triphosphate; *PLCγ2,* phospholipase Cγ2; *PLCβ,* phospholipase Cβ; *TP,* TXA₂ receptor; *TXA₂,* thromboxane A₂; *VWF,* von Willebrand factor.

vessel wall (Table 11.6). Likewise, α₅β₁ and α₆β₁ bind the adhesive endothelial cell proteins laminin and fibronectin, which further promotes platelet adhesion. Another collagen-binding receptor is GPVI, a member of the immunoglobulin gene family, so named because the genes of its members have multiple immunoglobulin-like domains. The unclassified platelet receptor GPIV is a key collagen receptor that also binds the adhesive protein thrombospondin.[37]

GPIb/IX/V is a *leucine-rich-repeat* family CAM, named for its members' multiple leucine-rich domains. GPIb/IX/V arises from the genes *GP1BA, GP1BB, GP5,* and *GP9*. It is composed of two molecules each of GPIbα, GPIbβ, and GPIX and

one molecule of GPV, which are bound noncovalently.[38] The two copies of subunit GPIbα bind VWF and support platelet *tethering* (deceleration or slowing of platelet movement in the bloodstream). Platelet deceleration is necessary in capillaries and arterioles where blood flow is rapid and shear rates exceed 1000 s⁻¹. The accompanying GPIbβ molecules cross the platelet membrane and interact with actin-binding protein to provide "outside-in" signaling. Two molecules of GPIX and one of GPV help assemble the four GPIb molecules.

The subunits of the integrin GPIIb/IIIa (α₁₁bβ₃), are in a low-affinity conformation (α₁₁b and β₃) as they are distributed across the plasma membrane, the SCCS, and the internal layer of

TABLE 11.6 Glycoprotein Platelet Membrane Receptors That Participate in Adhesion and Initiation of Aggregation by Binding Specific Ligands

Electrophoresis Nomenclature	Current Nomenclature	Ligand	Cluster Designation	Comments
GPIa/IIa	Integrin: $\alpha_2\beta_1$	Collagen	CD29, CD49b	Avidity is upregulated via inside-out activation that depends on collagen binding to GPVI.
	Integrin: $\alpha_v\beta_1$	Vitronectin		
	Integrin: $\alpha_5\beta_1$	Laminin	CD29, CD49e	
	Integrin: $\alpha_6\beta_1$	Fibronectin	CD29, CD49f	
GPVI	CAM of the immunoglobulin gene family	Collagen		Key collagen receptor, triggers activation, release of agonists that increase the avidity of integrins $\alpha_2\beta_1$ and $\alpha_{IIb}\beta_3$.
GPIb/IX/V	CAM of the leucine-rich repeat family	VWF and thrombin bind GPIbα; thrombin cleaves a site on GPV	CD42a, CD42b, CD42c, CD42d	GPIb/IX/V is a 2:2:2:1 complex of GPIbα and Ibβ, GPIX, and GPV. There are 25,000 copies on the resting platelet membrane surface, 5%–10% on the α-granule membrane, but few on the SCCS membrane. GPIbα is the VWF-specific site. On activation, 50% of GPIbα/Ibβ is cleared from the membrane. Bernard-Soulier syndrome mutations are identified for all but GPV. Bound to subsurface actin-binding protein.
GPIIb/IIIa	Integrin: $\alpha_{IIb}\beta_3$	Fibrinogen, VWF	CD41, CD61	GPIIb and GPIIIa are distributed on the surface membrane, SCCS, and α-granule membranes (30%). A heterodimer forms on activation.

CAM, Cell adhesion molecule; *GP,* glycoprotein; *SCCS,* surface-connected canalicular system; *VWF,* von Willebrand factor.

α-granule membranes of resting platelets. These form an active heterodimer, $\alpha_{IIb}\beta_3$, after initiation of an "inside-out" signaling mechanism triggered by an agonist binding to its receptor. Although various agonists may activate the platelet, $\alpha_{IIb}\beta_3$ is a physiologic requisite because it binds soluble fibrinogen, leading to interplatelet cohesion, called platelet aggregation. The $\alpha_{IIb}\beta_3$ integrin also binds other adhesive proteins that contain the target *arginine-glycine-aspartate* (RGD) amino acid sequence such as VWF, vitronectin, and fibronectin.[39]

Seven-Transmembrane Repeat Receptors

Thrombin, thrombin receptor activation peptide (TRAP), adenosine diphosphate (ADP), epinephrine, serotonin, and TXA_2 (and other prostaglandins) can function individually or in combination to activate platelets (Figure 11.8). These platelet agonists are ligands for *seven-transmembrane repeat receptors* (STRs), so named for their unique membrane-anchoring structure. The STRs have seven hydrophobic anchoring domains supporting an external binding site and an internal terminus that interacts with G-proteins to mediate outside-in platelet signaling. The STRs expressed on the platelet surface are listed in Table 11.7.[40]

Thrombin cleaves two STRs, protease-activated receptor 1 (PAR1) and PAR4, that together have a total of 1800 membrane copies on an average platelet. Thrombin cleavage of either of these two receptors activates the platelet through G-proteins that in turn activate at least two internal physiologic pathways. Thrombin also interacts with platelets by binding or digesting two CAMs in the leucine-rich repeat family, GPIbα and GPV, both of which are parts of the GPIb/IX/V VWF adhesion receptor.[40]

There are about 600 copies of the high-affinity ADP receptors P2Y$_1$ and P2Y$_{12}$ per platelet.[41] These receptors are linked to different G-proteins and produce distinct intracellular signals that have

complementary effects on platelet aggregation.[42] P2Y$_1$ signaling leads to an increase in intracellular calcium levels and contributes to initial platelet activation, shape change, and the formation of small reversible aggregates, whereas P2Y$_{12}$ signaling leads to a decrease in cyclic adenosine monophosphate (cAMP) levels and supports the formation of irreversible platelet aggregates.

TPα and TPβ receptors bind TXA_2. This interaction leads to increased TXA_2 production from the platelet, a G-protein-based autocrine (self-perpetuating) system that activates neighboring platelets. Epinephrine binds α_2-adrenergic sites that couple to G-proteins and open membrane calcium channels. The α_2-adrenergic sites function similarly to those located on heart muscle. The receptor site IP binds *prostacyclin* (prostaglandin I_2 [PGI_2]), a prostaglandin produced by endothelial cells (detailed in the "Eicosanoid Synthesis" section). Prostacyclin binding results in an increase in the internal cAMP concentration of the platelet and an inhibition of platelet activation. The platelet membrane also contains STRs for serotonin, adenosine, and vasopressin.[43]

Additional Membrane Receptors

The platelet contains many additional receptors (Chapter 4) beyond those with known clinical relevance discussed in the preceding paragraphs. The CAM immunoglobulin family includes the intercellular adhesion molecules, or ICAMs (CD50, CD54, CD102), which play a role in inflammation and the immune reaction; platelet endothelial cell adhesion molecule-1 (PECAM-1), or CD31, which mediates platelet-to-leukocyte and platelet-to-endothelial cell adhesion; and FcγRIIa (CD32), a low-affinity receptor for the immunoglobulin Fc portion that plays a role in a dangerous condition called heparin-induced thrombocytopenia (Chapter 39).[44] P-selectin (CD62) is a CAM that facilitates platelet binding to endothelial cells, leukocytes, and

TABLE 11.7 **Platelet Seven-Transmembrane Repeat Receptor-Ligand Interactions, G-Protein Activation, and Effect on Platelets**

Receptor	Ligand	G-Protein	Effect
PAR1	Thrombin	G_i	Deceleration of adenylate cyclase and reduction in cAMP
		G_q	Activation of phospholipase C and increase of IP_3-DAG
		G_{12}	Activation of protein kinase C and actin microfilaments
PAR4	Thrombin	G_q	Activation of phospholipase C and increase of IP_3-DAG
		G_{12}	Activation of protein kinase C and actin microfilaments
$P2Y_1$	ADP	G_q	Activation of phospholipase C and increase of IP_3-DAG
		G_{12}	Activation of protein kinase C and actin microfilaments
$P2Y_{12}$	ADP	G_i	Deceleration of adenylate cyclase and reduction in cAMP
TPα and TPβ	TXA_2	G_q	Activation of phospholipase C and increase of IP_3-DAG
		G_{12}	Deceleration of adenylate cyclase and reduction in cAMP
α_2-Adrenergic	Epinephrine	G_i	Deceleration of adenylate cyclase and reduction in cAMP
IP	PGI_2	G_s	Acceleration of adenylate cyclase and increase in cAMP (pathway is in endothelial cells not platelets, but prostacyclin affects platelet function)
5HT-2A	Serotonin	G_q	Activation of phospholipase C and increase of IP_3-DAG

ADP, Adenosine diphosphate; *cAMP*, cyclic adenosine monophosphate; *DAG*, diacylglycerol; *IP*, PGI_2 receptor; IP_3, inositol-1,4,5- triphosphate; *PAR*, protease-activated receptor; PGI_2, prostaglandin I_2 (prostacyclin); TXA_2, thromboxane A_2; *5HT*, 5-hydroxytryptamine (serotonin).

one another.[45] P-selectin is found on the α-granule membranes of the resting platelet but migrates via the SCCS to the surface of activated platelets. P-selectin quantification by flow cytometry is a common means for measuring in vivo platelet activation.

PLATELET FUNCTION

Platelet activation is key to preventing blood loss and is integral to both primary and secondary hemostasis. Platelet function includes platelet adhesion, aggregation, and secretion.[46,47] Although the following discussion implies a linear and stepwise process, these activities often occur simultaneously.

Adhesion: Platelets Bind Elements of the Vascular Matrix

As blood flows, it creates stress, or *shear force*, measured in units labeled s^{-1}, on the vessel wall. Shear forces range from $500\ s^{-1}$ in venules and veins to $5000\ s^{-1}$ in arterioles and capillaries and up to $40,000\ s^{-1}$ in stenosed (hardened) arteries. In vessels where the shear rate is more than $1000\ s^{-1}$, platelet adhesion and aggregation require a defined sequence of events that involves collagen; tissue factor; phospholipid; VWF; and a number of platelet CAMs, ligands, and activators (Figure 11.9).[48]

Injury to the blood vessel wall disrupts the continuity of the endothelium, exposing the collagen of the extracellular matrix (ECM) to flowing blood (Figure 11.9A and B).[49] Damaged endothelial cells release VWF from cytoplasmic storage organelles. This VWF adheres to sites of blood vessel injury by binding to the ECM collagen (Figure 11.9C).[50] VWF, whose molecular weight ranges from 500,000 to 20,000,000 Daltons, also circulates as a globular protein (Chapter 36). Under shear stress, VWF becomes threadlike as it unrolls and exposes sites that weakly bind the GPIbα portion of the platelet membrane GPIb/IX/V leucine-rich receptor. This reversible binding process "tethers,"

and thereby decelerates, the forward motion of the platelet. Secure adherence of platelets to the site of endothelial damage is promoted by the ECM collagen and by thrombin generated from the coagulation cascade (Chapter 35).[51] Platelet adhesion to the site of injury remains consolidated by the plasma enzyme *ADAMTS13*, also called *VWF-cleaving protease*, which digests large VWF multimers, leaving only the VWF and platelets that are securely bound to the ECM collagen.

The VWF-GPIbα tethering reaction allows platelets to roll along the surface of the endothelium until the platelet GPVI receptor comes in contact with the exposed ECM collagen.[51] Type I fibrillar collagen binding to platelet GPVI, anchored in the platelet membrane by an Fc receptor-like molecule (see Figure 11.8), triggers internal platelet activation pathways releasing TXA_2 and ADP, an outside-in reaction.[52] These agonists attach to their respective receptors: TPα and TPβ for TXA_2, and $P2Y_1$ and $P2Y_{12}$ for ADP, triggering an inside-out reaction that raises the affinity of integrin $\alpha_2\beta_1$ for collagen. The combined effect of GPIb/IX/V, GPVI, and $\alpha_2\beta_1$ causes the platelet to become firmly affixed to the damaged surface, where it subsequently loses its discoid shape and spreads.[53]

Aggregation: Platelets Irreversibly Cohere

In addition to collagen exposure and VWF secretion, blood vessel injury exposes *tissue factor* expressed on subendothelial smooth muscle cells and fibroblasts. Tissue factor triggers the production of thrombin, which cleaves platelet PAR1 and PAR4. This further activation generates the *collagen and thrombin activated (COAT)* platelet (Figure 11.10), which is integral to the cell-based coagulation model described in Chapter 35.

TXA_2 and ADP secreted from the platelet granules to the microenvironment also trigger inside-out activation of the integrin $\alpha_{IIb}\beta_3$ (GPIIb/IIIa receptor), enabling it to bind the RGD sequences within fibrinogen and VWF and support

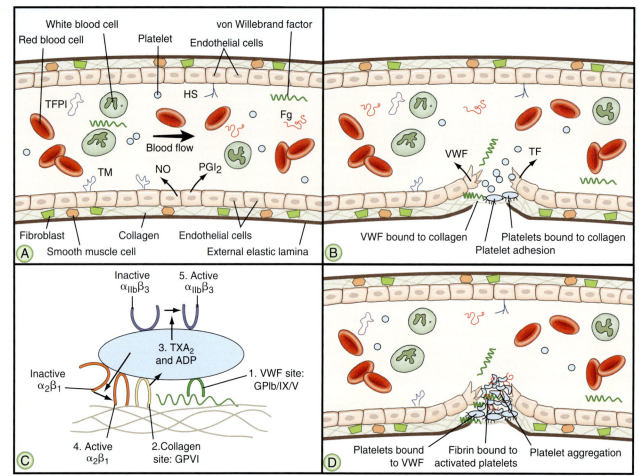

Figure 11.9 Primary Hemostasis: The Process of Platelet Response to Blood Vessel Injury. **(A)**, Normal blood flow in intact vessels. Red blood cells and platelets flow near the center, and white blood cells marginate and roll evenly along the smooth endothelium. Endothelial cells and the subendothelial matrix, which contains collagen, smooth muscle cells (in arteries), and collagen-producing fibroblasts, have several mechanisms by which they can limit blood clotting (TM, TFPI, HS) and platelet activation (NO, PGI$_2$). **(B)**, Trauma to the blood vessel wall exposes subendothelial collagen and tissue factor, triggering platelet adhesion. **(C)**, VWF serves as a bridge between subendothelial collagen and the platelet receptor GPIb/IX/V. Platelet interaction with collagen via $\alpha_2\beta_1$ and GPVI receptors triggers release of TXA$_2$ and ADP and subsequent activation of the $\alpha_{IIb}\beta_3$ receptor. **(D)**, Activation of $\alpha_{IIb}\beta_3$ supports platelet-platelet aggregation through binding of arginine-glycine-aspartate (RGD)-containing ligands such as fibrinogen and VWF. This forms a platelet plug that closes off the site of injury. *ADP*, Adenosine diphosphate; *Fg*, fibrinogen; *GPIb/IX/V*, glycoprotein Ib, IX, and V complex; *GPVI*, glycoprotein VI; *HS*, heparan sulfate; *NO*, nitric oxide; *PGI$_2$*, prostacyclin; *TF*, tissue factor; *TFPI*, tissue factor pathway inhibitor; *TM*, thrombomodulin; *TXA$_2$*, thromboxane A$_2$; *VWF*, von Willebrand factor.

platelet-to-platelet binding, referred to as *platelet aggregation.* P-selectin from the α-granule membranes moves to the surface membrane to promote binding of platelets with leukocytes.

On activation, in conjunction with aggregation, platelets *change shape* from discoid to round and extend pseudopods. This allows platelets to cover more surface area, and it enhances platelet binding to other platelets and foreign surfaces. Membrane phospholipid asymmetry is lost, with the more polar molecules, especially phosphatidylserine, flipping to the outer layer. As platelet aggregation continues, membrane integrity is lost, platelets exhaust internal energy sources, and a syncytium or massive clump of platelets forms.

Platelet aggregation is a key part of primary hemostasis, which in arteries may end with the formation of a "white clot," a clot composed primarily of platelets and VWF (see Figure 11.9D). Although aggregation is a normal part of vessel repair,

the presence of white clots often implies inappropriate platelet activation in seemingly uninjured arterioles and arteries and is the pathologic basis for arterial thrombotic events such as acute myocardial infarction, peripheral artery disease, and ischemic stroke (Chapters 39 and 40). The risk of these cardiovascular events rises in proportion to the number and avidity of platelet membrane $\alpha_2\beta_1$ and GPVI receptors.[54]

The combination of polar phospholipid exposure on activated platelets, platelet fragmentation with cellular microparticle release, and secretion of the platelet's α-granule and dense granule contents triggers secondary hemostasis, called *coagulation* (Chapter 35). Fibrin and RBCs deposit around and within the platelet syncytium to form a bulky "red clot." The red clot is essential to wound repair, but it may also be characteristic of inappropriate coagulation in venules and veins, resulting in deep vein thrombosis and pulmonary embolism (Chapters 39 and 40).

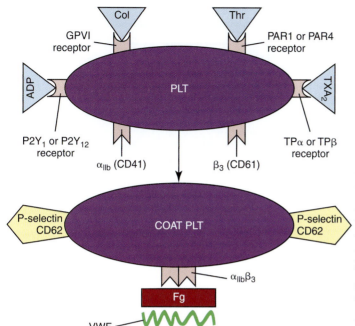

Figure 11.10 Illustration of a COAT Platelet. Platelets become activated by agonists, for example, ADP, TXA$_2$, collagen, or thrombin. P-selectin (CD62) moves from the α-granules to the platelet membrane to support platelet adhesion to surfaces "foreign" to platelets such as collagen or implanted medical devices. The inactive α$_{IIb}$ and β$_3$ units assemble to form the active arginine-glycine-aspartate (RGD) receptor α$_{IIb}$β$_3$, which binds fibrinogen and VWF. Further activation of the platelet by a combination of collagen and thrombin yields the *collagen and thrombin activated* (COAT) platelet, a highly efficient procoagulant platelet that aids in stabilizing the fibrin clot. *ADP,* Adenosine diphosphate; *Col,* collagen; *Fg,* fibrinogen; *PLT,* platelet; *Thr,* thrombin; *TXA$_2$,* thromboxane A$_2$; *VWF,* von Willebrand factor.

Secretion: Activated Platelets Release Granular Contents

Outside-in activation of the platelet through STRs (such as ADP binding to P2Y$_{12}$) and collagen binding to GPVI triggers actin microfilament contraction. Intermediate filaments also contract, moving the circumferential microtubules inward compressing the granules. Contents of α-granules and lysosomes flow through the SCCS, while dense granules migrate to the plasma membrane where their contents are secreted. The dense granule contents are small-molecule vasoconstrictors and platelet agonists that amplify primary hemostasis; most of the α-granule contents are large-molecule coagulation proteins that participate in secondary hemostasis (see Tables 11.4 and 11.5).

By presenting polar phospholipids on their membrane surfaces, platelets provide a localized cellular milieu that supports coagulation. *Phosphatidylserine* is the polar phospholipid on which the *factor IX/VIII (tenase)* and factor *X/V (prothrombinase)* complexes assemble. The formation of both complexes is supported by ionic calcium secreted from the dense granules.[55,56] The α-granule contents fibrinogen, factors V and VIII, and VWF (which binds and stabilizes factor VIII) are secreted and increase the localized concentrations of these essential coagulation proteins, further supporting the action of tenase and prothrombinase. Thrombin that is generated from

coagulation activation is a key component of both primary and secondary hemostasis. Platelet secretions provide for cell-based, controlled, localized coagulation. Table 11.8 lists some additional α-granule secretion products that, although not proteins of the coagulation pathway, indirectly support hemostasis.

Generation of Platelet Microparticles

Microparticles are membrane-derived vesicles that form in response to an activating stimulus. Activation of a platelet increases the intracellular concentration of calcium, which causes an inhibition of the enzymes responsible for maintaining the asymmetric distribution of phospholipids in the plasma membrane. Further, it activates intracellular calpain that cleaves the platelet cytoskeleton. Together, these effects lead to the outward blebbing of the plasma membrane and the formation of platelet microparticles. Platelet microparticles, believed to be the most abundant microparticles in the circulation, are formed after exposure of platelets to strong agonists or shear stress. These vesicles are made up of the plasma membrane and cytosolic material of the parent cell from which they are derived and retain the cell surface proteins found on the parent cell. As such, microparticles have been found to modulate inflammation, oxidative stress, angiogenesis, and thrombosis.[57] The promotion of coagulation is the most studied platelet microparticle function and results from the expression of phosphatidylserine on the surface of the microparticles. Elevated levels of platelet microparticles in patients with hypercoagulable conditions have been shown to be predictive of adverse outcomes in some settings.[58]

PLATELET SIGNALING PATHWAYS

During the processes of platelet adhesion, aggregation, and secretion described in the previous section, platelet activation is enhanced by additional signaling pathways as described in the following.

G-Proteins

G-proteins control cellular activation for all cells at the inner membrane surface (Figure 11.11; Table 11.7). G-proteins are αβγ heterotrimers (proteins composed of three dissimilar peptides) that bind guanosine diphosphate (GDP) when inactive. For the STRs, membrane receptor-ligand (agonist) binding promotes GDP release and its replacement with guanosine triphosphate (GTP). The Gα portion of the three-part G molecule briefly disassociates, exerts enzymatic guanosine triphosphatase activity, and hydrolyzes the bound GTP to GDP. The G-protein resumes its resting state, but the hydrolysis step provides the necessary phosphorylation to trigger eicosanoid synthesis or the IP$_3$-DAG pathway to promote platelet activation.

Eicosanoid Synthesis

The eicosanoid synthesis pathway, alternatively called the *prostaglandin, cyclooxygenase,* or *thromboxane* pathway, is one of two essential platelet activation pathways triggered by G-proteins (Figure 11.12). The platelet membrane's inner leaflet is rich in phosphatidylinositol, a phospholipid whose number 2 carbon binds numerous types of unsaturated fatty acids, but especially 5,8,11,14-eicosatetraenoic acid, commonly called *arachidonic*

TABLE 11.8 Selected Platelet α-Granule Proteins and Their Properties

α-Granule Protein	Properties
Platelet-derived growth factor	Supports mitosis of vascular fibroblasts and smooth muscle cells
Endothelial growth factor	Supports mitosis of vascular fibroblasts and smooth muscle cells
Transforming growth factor-β	Supports mitosis of vascular fibroblasts and smooth muscle cells
Fibronectin	Adhesion molecule
Thrombospondin	Adhesion molecule
Platelet factor 4	Heparin neutralization, suppresses megakaryocytopoiesis
β-thromboglobulin	Found nowhere but platelet α-granules
Plasminogen	Fibrinolysis promotion
Plasminogen activator inhibitor-1	Fibrinolysis control
α₂-antiplasmin	Fibrinolysis control
Protein C inhibitor	Coagulation control

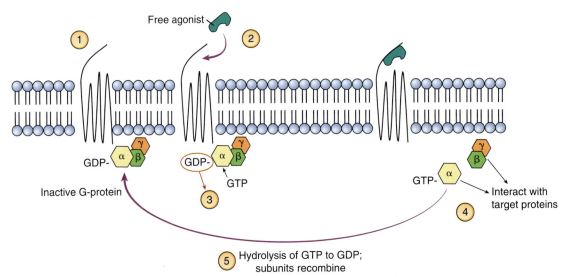

Figure 11.11 G-Protein Coupled Mechanism of Platelet Activation. In the absence of a platelet activating substance (agonist), G-proteins are in a resting state bound to GDP *(1)*. When an agonist binds its corresponding receptor on the platelet *(2)*, it triggers a G-protein to swap GDP for GTP *(3)*. The GTP-bound α-subunit of the G-protein dissociates from the βγ-subunit, and both the α-subunit and the βγ-subunit interact with second messengers, such as cAMP and others listed in Table 11.7 to mediate signal transduction within the platelet *(4)*. On GTP hydrolysis, the α-subunit and βγ-subunit reunite, and the G-protein returns to a resting state bound to GDP *(5)*. *cAMP,* Cyclic adenosine monophosphate; *GDP,* guanosine diphosphate; *GTP,* guanosine triphosphate.

acid. Membrane receptor-ligand binding and the consequent G-protein activation triggers phospholipase A_2, a membrane enzyme that cleaves the ester bond connecting the number 2 carbon of the triglyceride backbone with arachidonic acid. Cleavage releases arachidonic acid to the platelet cytoplasm, where it becomes the substrate for *cyclooxygenase,* anchored in the DTS. Cyclooxygenase converts arachidonic acid to prostaglandin G_2 and prostaglandin H_2, and then *thromboxane synthase* acts on prostaglandin H_2 to produce TXA_2. TXA_2 binds membrane receptors TPα or TPβ, inhibiting adenylate cyclase activity and reducing cAMP concentrations, which mobilizes ionic calcium from the DTS. The rising cytoplasmic calcium level causes contraction of actin microfilaments producing platelet shape change and further platelet activation. When reagent arachidonic acid is used as an agonist in laboratory assays (Chapter 41), it bypasses the membrane and directly enters the eicosanoid synthesis pathway.

The cyclooxygenase pathway in endothelial cells incorporates the enzyme *prostacyclin synthase* in place of the thromboxane synthase found in platelets (Figure 11.12). The eicosanoid pathway endpoint for the endothelial cell is prostaglandin I_2, or *prostacyclin,* which binds the IP receptor activating the IP_3-DAG pathway, leading to an acceleration of adenylate cyclase, an increase in cAMP, and a sequestration of ionic calcium to the DTS. The lack of ionic calcium shuts down platelet function. Thus the endothelial cell eicosanoid pathway suppresses platelet activation in the intact blood vessel, creating a dynamic equilibrium with the eicosanoid pathway within the platelet where platelet activation occurs.

TXA_2 has a half-life of 30 seconds, diffuses from the platelet, and is spontaneously reduced to thromboxane B_2, a stable, measurable plasma metabolite. Efforts to produce a clinical assay for plasma thromboxane B_2 as a measure of platelet activity have been unsuccessful because special specimen management is required to prevent ex vivo platelet activation with unregulated

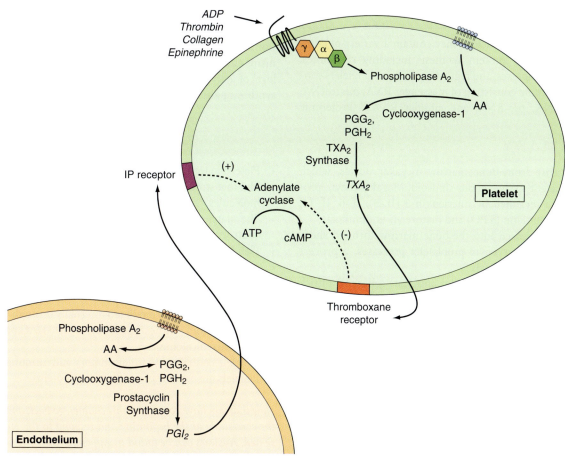

Figure 11.12 Eicosanoid Synthesis. Ligands (agonists) ADP, thrombin, collagen, and epinephrine bind their respective platelet membrane receptors. The binding activates phospholipase A_2 through the G-protein mechanism described in Figure 11.11. Phospholipase A_2 releases arachidonic acid from the platelet membrane phosphatidylinositol. AA is acted on by cyclooxygenase, peroxidase, and thromboxane synthase to produce TXA_2, which activates the platelet by reducing cAMP production, thus mobilizing ionized calcium (Ca^{2+}) from the dense tubules. In the endothelial cell, the eicosanoid pathway is nearly identical except that prostacyclin synthase replaces thromboxane synthase. The resulting prostacyclin acts to reduce platelet function by increasing cAMP levels. *AA,* Arachidonic acid; *ADP,* adenosine diphosphate; *ATP,* adenosine triphosphate; *cAMP,* cyclic adenosine monophosphate; *IP,* prostacyclin (PGI_2); *PGG₂,* prostaglandin G_2; *PGH₂,* prostaglandin H_2; *PGI₂,* prostacyclin; *TXA₂,* thromboxane A_2.

release of thromboxane B_2 subsequent to specimen collection. Thromboxane B_2 is acted on by a variety of liver enzymes to produce an array of soluble urine metabolites, including 11-dehydrothromboxane B_2, which is stable and measurable.[59,60]

Inositol Triphosphate-Diacylglycerol Activation Pathway

The *IP₃-DAG pathway* is the second G-protein-dependent platelet activation pathway. G-protein activation triggers the enzyme *phospholipase C*. Phospholipase C cleaves membrane phosphatidylinositol 4,5-bisphosphate (PIP_2) to form IP_3 and DAG, both second messengers for intracellular activation. IP_3 promotes release of ionic calcium from the DTS, which triggers actin microfilament contraction. IP_3 may also activate phospholipase A_2. DAG triggers a multistep process: activation of phosphokinase C, which triggers phosphorylation of the protein pleckstrin, which regulates actin microfilament contraction.

PLATELETS AND INFLAMMATION

Beyond their established role in hemostasis, platelets may contribute to inflammatory and immune responses through a variety of mechanisms.[61,62] Platelets express FcγIIa and FcγIIIa receptors as well as multiple toll-like receptors on their surface, allowing them to interact with a variety of immune complexes and pathogens.[63] Additionally, on their activation, platelets release from their granules, or can be induced to produce, a number of inflammatory mediators such as RANTES, PF4, and IL-1β. Platelets can form heterotypic aggregates via P-selectin binding to P-selectin glycoprotein ligand-1 (PSGL-1) found on leukocytes, CD40L binding to CD40 found on antigen-presenting cells, or fibrinogen-mediated cross-linking of $\alpha_{IIb}\beta_3$ on platelets and $\alpha_M\beta_2$ on monocytes.[64] Binding of platelets to leukocytes initiates signaling leading to enhanced expression of thrombotic and inflammatory mediators.[64,65]

PLATELET PROTEOME

Although platelets are anuclear, they contain a variety of components required for protein synthesis including ribosomes, polyribosome complexes, and regulatory factors.[66] Platelets contain a transcriptome consisting of messenger RNA, microRNA, noncoding RNA, pre-RNA, and circular RNA.[67] Proteomic analysis has indicated that platelets contain thousands of unique transcripts that can be translated in response to platelet activation and ligand binding to the GPIIb/IIIa receptor. Such mechanisms allow platelets to alter their phenotype in response to the level of activation. Additionally, it is suggested that the protein synthesis pattern of platelets can be altered by disease state.[68]

SUMMARY

- Platelets arise from bone marrow megakaryocytes, which reside adjacent to the venous sinusoid. Megakaryocyte progenitors are recruited by interleukin-3 (IL-3), IL-6, IL-11, and thrombopoietin (TPO) and mature via endomitosis.
- Platelets are released into the bone marrow through shedding from megakaryocyte proplatelet processes, a process called thrombocytopoiesis.
- Circulating platelets are complex anucleate cells with a thick surface glycocalyx bearing an assortment of coagulation factors and plasma proteins.
- The surface-connected canalicular system (SCCS) and closely aligned dense tubular system (DTS) of the platelet facilitate the storage and release of hemostatic proteins, Ca^{2+}, and enzymes.
- Platelet cytoplasm contains a system of cytoplasmic microfibrils and microtubules that are involved in platelet shape change through membrane contraction and pseudopod extension.

- Platelet cytoplasm also contains α-granules and dense granules that store and secrete coagulation factors and vasoactive molecules.
- The platelet membrane contains an array of receptors that control platelet activation on binding their respective ligands.
- Platelet adhesion to VWF and exposed collagen, platelet-platelet aggregation, and secretion of substances stored within platelet granules are the three key functions of an activated platelet.
- Platelet activation is mediated internally through G-proteins, the eicosanoid synthesis pathway, the IP_3-DAG pathway, and free ionized calcium.
- Platelets contribute to inflammatory and immune responses.
- Platelets are capable of synthesizing proteins.

Now that you have completed this chapter, go back and read again the case study at the beginning and respond to the questions presented. Answers can be found in Appendix C.

REVIEW QUESTIONS

Answers can be found in Appendix C.

1. The megakaryocyte progenitor that undergoes endomitosis is:
   a. MK-I
   b. LD-CFU-Meg
   c. CFU-Meg
   d. BFU-Meg
2. The growth factor that is produced in the kidney and induces growth and differentiation of committed megakaryocyte progenitors is:
   a. PDGF
   b. VEGF
   c. Thrombopoietin
   d. Erythropoietin
3. What platelet organelle sequesters ionic calcium and binds a series of enzymes of the eicosanoid pathway?
   a. Dense tubular system
   b. Dense granules
   c. Surface-connected canalicular system
   d. Glycocalyx
4. What plasma protein binds GPIIb/IIIa and supports platelet aggregation?
   a. Albumin
   b. Fibrin
   c. Thrombin
   d. Fibrinogen

5. What platelet membrane phospholipid flips from the inner surface to the plasma surface on activation and serves as the assembly point for coagulation factors?
   a. Phosphatidylethanolamine
   b. Phosphatidylinositol
   c. Phosphatidylcholine
   d. Phosphatidylserine
6. What is the name of the eicosanoid metabolite produced by endothelial cells that suppresses platelet activity?
   a. Thromboxane A_2
   b. Arachidonic acid
   c. Cyclooxygenase
   d. Prostacyclin
7. Which of the following molecules is stored in platelet α-granules?
   a. Serotonin
   b. ADP
   c. Platelet factor 4
   d. Thrombopoietin
8. What plasma protein is essential for platelet adhesion under high shear stress conditions?
   a. VWF
   b. Factor VIII
   c. Fibrinogen
   d. P-selectin

9. Reticulated platelets can be enumerated in peripheral blood to detect:
   a. The extent of platelet activation
   b. Abnormal organelles associated with diseases such as leukemia
   c. Increased platelet production in response to need
   d. Inadequate rates of membrane cholesterol exchange with the plasma

10. White clots:
    a. Are largely composed of platelets and von Willebrand factor
    b. Form normally in response to vascular injury and are completely harmless
    c. Are characteristic of the secondary hemostatic process
    d. Occur primarily in the deep veins of the leg

11. On activation, platelets secrete their α-granule contents via:
    a. The dense tubule system
    b. The surface-connected canalicular system
    c. The glycocalyx
    d. Microtubules

12. Microparticles:
    a. Are stored in platelet-dense granules
    b. Bud off of platelets after their exposure to strong agonists
    c. Are immature platelets
    d. Exhibit no biologic activity

REFERENCES

1. Butkiewicz, A. M., Kemona, H., Dymicka-Piekarska, V., et al. (2006). Platelet count, mean platelet volume and thrombocytopoietic indices in healthy women and men. *Thromb Res, 118,* 199–204.
2. Reddy, V., Marques, M. B., & Fritsma, G. A. (2013). *Quick Guide to Hematology Testing.* (2nd Ed.). Washington, DC: AACC Press.
3. Deutsch, V. R., & Tomer, A. (2013). Advances in megakaryocytopoiesis and thrombopoiesis: from bench to bedside. *Br J Haematol, 161,* 778–793.
4. Lefrancais, E., Ortiz-Munoz, G., Caudrillier, A., et al. (2017). The lung is a site of platelet biogenesis and a reservoir for haematopoietic progenitors. *Nature, 544,* 105–109.
5. Lefrancais, E., & Looney, M. R. (2019). Platelet biogenesis in the lung circulation. *Physiology, 34,* 392–401.
6. Chang, Y., Bluteau, D., Bebili, N., et al. (2007). From hematopoietic stem cells to platelets. *J Thromb Haemost, 5*(Suppl. 1), 318–327.
7. Italiano, J. E., Jr., & Hartwig, J. H. (2012). Megakaryocyte structure and platelet biogenesis. In Marder, V. J., Aird, W. C., Bennett, J. S., et al. (Eds.), *Hemostasis and Thrombosis: Basic Principles and Clinical Practice.* (6th ed., pp. 365–372). Philadelphia: Lippincott Williams & Wilkins.
8. Lordier, L., Jalil, A., Aurade, F., et al. (2008). Megakaryocyte endomitosis is a failure of late cytokinesis related to defects in the contractile ring and Rho/Rock signaling. *Blood, 112,* 3164–3174.
9. Machlus, K. R., & Italiano, J. E. (2023). Megakaryocyte and platelet structure. In Hoffman, R., Benz, E. J., Silberstein, L. E., et al. (Eds.), *Hematology: Basic Principles and Practice.* (8th ed., pp 1937–1949). Philadelphia: Elsevier.
10. Tomer, A., Harker, L. A., & Burstein, S. A. (1988). Flow cytometric analysis of normal human megakaryocytes. *Blood, 71*(5), 1244–1252.
11. Josefsson, E. C., Vainchenker, W., & James, C. (2020). Regulation of platelet production and life span: role of Bcl-xL and potential implications for human platelet diseases. *Int J Mol Sci.* doi:10.3390/ijms21207591.
12. Junt, T., Schulze, H., Chen, Z., et al. (2007). Dynamic visualization of thrombopoiesis within bone marrow. *Science, 317,* 1767–1770.
13. Della Porta, M. G., Lanza, F., Del Vecchio, L., & Italian Society of Cytometry (GIC). (2011). Flow cytometry immunophenotyping for the evaluation of bone marrow dysplasia. *Cytometry B Clin Cytom, 80,* 201–211.
14. Berndt, M. C., & Andrews, R. K. (2012). Major platelet glycoproteins: platelet glycoprotein Ib-IX-V. In Marder, V. J., Aird, W. C., Bennett, J. S., et al. (Eds.), *Hemostasis and Thrombosis: Basic Principles and Clinical Practice.* (6th ed., pp. 382–385). Philadelphia: Lippincott Williams & Wilkins.
15. Yee, F., & Ginsberg, M. H. (2012). Major platelet glycoproteins: integrin aIIbb3 (GP IIb-IIIa). In Marder, V. J., Aird, W. C., Bennett, J. S., et al. (Eds.), *Hemostasis and Thrombosis: Basic Principles and Clinical Practice.* (6th ed., pp. 386–392). Philadelphia: Lippincott Williams & Wilkins.
16. Kuter, D. J. (2010). Biology and chemistry of thrombopoietic agents. *Semin Hematol, 47,* 243–248.
17. Kaushansky, K. (2005). The molecular mechanisms that control thrombopoiesis. *J Clin Invest, 115,* 3339–3347.
18. Deng, J., Hu, H., Huang, F., et al. (2021). Comparative efficacy and safety of thrombopoietin receptor agonists in adults with thrombocytopenia: a systematic review and network meta-analysis of randomized controlled trial. Frontiers in *Pharmacology, 12,* doi.org/10.3389/fphar.2021.704093.
19. Wilkins, C. R., Ortiz, J., Gilbert, L. J., et al. (2022). Romiplostim for chemotherapy-induced thrombocytopenia: efficacy and safety of extended use. *Res Pract Thromb Haemost, 6,* e12701.
20. Sitaraman, S. V., & Gewirtz, A. T. (2001). Oprelvekin. Genetics Institute. *Curr Opin Investig Drugs, 2,* 1395–1400.
21. Stasi, R. (2009). Therapeutic strategies for hepatitis - and other infection-related immune thrombocytopenias. *Semin Hematol, 46*(Suppl. 2), S15–S25.
22. Lambert, M. P., Rauova, L., Bailey, M., et al. (2007). Platelet factor 4 is a negative autocrine in vivo regulator of megakaryopoiesis: clinical and therapeutic implications. *Blood, 110,* 1153–1160.
23. Yu, M., & Cantor, A. B. (2012). Megakaryopoiesis and thrombopoiesis: an update on cytokines and lineage surface markers. *Methods Mol Biol, 788,* 291–303.
24. Lance, M. D., Sloep, M., Henskens, Y. M., et al. (2012). Mean platelet volume as a diagnostic marker for cardiovascular disease: drawbacks of preanalytical conditions and measuring techniques. *Clin Appl Thromb Hemost, 18,* 561–568.
25. Leader, A., Pereg, D., & Lishner, M. (2012). Are platelet volume indices of clinical use? A multidisciplinary review. *Ann Med, 44,* 805–816.

26. Carr, J. H. (2021). *Clinical Hematology Atlas.* (6th ed.). St. Louis: Elsevier.

27. Michur, H., Maslanka, K., Szczepinski, A., et al. (2008). Reticulated platelets as a marker of platelet recovery after allogeneic stem cell transplantation. *Int J Lab Hematol, 30,* 519–525.

28. Liu, Q., Song, M., Yang, B., et al. (2017). Clinical significance of measuring reticulated platelets in infectious diseases. *Medicine, 96,* 52(e9424).

29. Buttarello, M., Mezzapelle, G., Freguglia, F., et al. (2020). Reticulated platelets and immature platelet fraction: clinical applications and method limitations. *Int J Lab Hematol, 42,* 363–370.

30. Corpataux, N., Franke, K., Kille, A., et al. (2020). Reticulated platelets in medicine: current evidence and further perspectives. *J Clin Med, 9.* https://doi.org/10.3390/jcm9113737.

31. Zhao, Y., Lai, R., Zhang, Y., et al. (2020). The prognostic value of reticulated platelets in patients with coronary artery disease: a systematic review and meta-analysis. *Front Cardiovasc Med, 23.* https://doi.org/10.3389/fcvm.2020.578041.

32. Cesari, F., Marcucci, R., Gori, A. M., et al. (2013). Reticulated platelets predict cardiovascular death in acute coronary syndrome patients. Insights from the AMI-Florence 2 Study. *Thromb Haemost, 109,* 846–853.

33. White, J. G., & Rao, G. H. (1998). Microtubule coils versus the surface membrane cytoskeleton in maintenance and restoration of platelet discoid shape. *Am J Pathol, 152,* 597–609.

34. Smith, C.W. (2021). Release of alpha-granule contents during platelet activation. *Platelets, 33*(4), 491–502.

35. Rand, M. L., & Israels, S. J. (2023). Molecular basis of platelet function. In Hoffman, R. H., Benz, E. J., Silberstein, L. E., et al. (Eds.), *Hematology: Basic Principles and Practice.* (8th ed., pp 1950–1967), Philadelphia: Elsevier.

36. Savage, B., & Ruggeri, Z. V. (2012). The basis for platelet adhesion. In Marder, V. J., Aird, W. C., Bennett, J. S., et al. (Eds.), *Hemostasis and Thrombosis: Basic Principles and Clinical Practice.* (6th ed., pp. 400–449), Philadelphia: Lippincott Williams & Wilkins.

37. Tandon, N. N., Kraslisz, U., & Jamieson, G. A. (1989). Identification of glycoprotein IV (CD36) as a primary receptor for platelet-collagen adhesion. *J Biol Chem, 264,* 7576–7583.

38. Li, R., & Emsley, J. (2013). The organizing principle of platelet glycoprotein Ib-IX-V complex. *J Thromb Haemost, 11*(4), 605–614.

39. Giordano, A., Musumeci, G., D'Angelillo, A., et al. (2016). Effects of glycoprotein IIb/IIIa antagonists: anti platelet aggregation and beyond. *Curr Drug Metab, 17*(2), 194–203.

40. De Candia, E. (2012). Mechanisms of platelet activation by thrombin: a short history. *Thromb Res, 129,* 250–256.

41. Moliterno, D. J. (2008). Advances in antiplatelet therapy for ACS and PCI. *J Interven Cardiol, 21*(Suppl. 1), S18–S24.

42. Gurbel, P. A., Kuliopulos, A., & Tantry, U. S. (2015). G-protein-coupled receptor signaling pathways in new antiplatelet drug development. *Arterioscler Thromb Vasc Biol, 35,* 500–512.

43. Thibeault, P. E., Ramachandran, R. (2021). Biased signaling in platelet G-protein coupled receptors. *Can J Physiol Pharmacol, 99,* 255–269.

44. Greinacher, A. (2015). Heparin-induced thrombocytopenia. *New Eng J Med, 373*(3), 252–261.

45. Keating, F. K., Dauerman, H. L., Whitaker, D. A., et al. (2006). Increased expression of platelet P-selectin and formation of platelet-leukocyte aggregates in blood from patients treated with unfractionated heparin plus eptifibatide compared with bivalirudin. *Thromb Res, 118,* 361–369.

46. Ye, S., & Whiteheart, S. W. (2012). Molecular basis for platelet secretion. In Marder, V. J., Aird, W. C., Bennett, J. S., et al. (Eds.), *Hemostasis and Thrombosis: Basic Principles and Clinical Practice.* (6th ed., pp. 441–449). Philadelphia: Lippincott Williams & Wilkins.

47. Stalker, T. J., Newman, D. K., Ma, P., et al. (2012). Platelet signaling. *Handb Exp Pharmacol, 210,* 59–85.

48. Stegner, D., & Nieswandt, B. (2011). Platelet receptor signaling in thrombus formation. *J Mol Med, 89,* 109–121.

49. Twarock, S., Bagheri, S., Bagheri, S., et al. (2016). Platelet-vessel wall interactions and drug effects. *Pharmacology & Therapeutics 167,* 74–84.

50. Zhou, Z., Nguyen, T. C., Guchhait, P., et al. (2010). Von Willebrand factor, ADAMTS-13, and thrombotic thrombocytopenic purpura. *Semin Thromb Hemost, 36,* 71–81.

51. Ruggeri, Z. M., & Mendolicchio, G. L. (2007). Adhesion mechanisms in platelet function. *Circ Res, 100,* 1673–1685.

52. Varga-Szabo, D., Pleines, I., & Nieswandt, B. (2008). Cell adhesion mechanisms in platelets. *Arterioscler Thromb Vasc Biol, 28,* 403–412.

53. Jung, S. M., Moroi, M., Soejima, K., et al. (2012). Constitutive dimerization of glycoprotein VI (GPVI) in resting platelets is essential for binding to collagen and activation in flowing blood. *J Biol Chemistry, 287,* 30000–30013.

54. Furihata, K., Nugent, D. J., & Kunicki, T. J. (2002). Influence of platelet collagen receptor polymorphisms on risk for arterial thrombosis. *Arch Pathol Lab Med, 126,* 305–309.

55. Kunicki, T. J., & Nugent, D. J. (2012). Platelet glycoprotein polymorphisms and relationship to function, immunogenicity, and disease. In Marder, V. J., Aird, W. C., Bennett, J. S., et al. (Eds.), *Hemostasis and Thrombosis: Basic Principles and Clinical Practice.* (6th ed., pp. 393–399), Philadelphia: Lippincott Williams & Wilkins.

56. Zieseniss, S., Zahler, S., Muller, I., et al. (2001). Modified phosphatidylethanolamine as the active component of oxidized low density lipoprotein promoting platelet prothrombinase activity. *J Biol Chem, 276,* 19828–19835.

57. Puhm, F., Boilard, E., & Machlus, K. R. (2021). Platelet extracellular vesicles. Beyond the blood. *Arterioscler Thromb Vasc Biol, 41,* 87–96.

58. Jeske, W. P., Walenga, J. M., Menapace, B., et al. (2016). Blood cell microparticles as biomarkers of hemostatic abnormalities in patients with implanted cardiac assist devices. *Biomarkers in Medicine, 10*(10), 1095–1104.

59. Carroll, R. C., Craft, R. M., Snider, C. C., et al. (2013). A comparison of VerifyNow with Platelet Mapping – detected aspirin resistance and correlation with urinary thromboxane. *Anesth Analg, 116,* 282–286.

60. Eikelboom, J. W., & Hankey, G. J. (2004). Failure of aspirin to prevent atherothrombosis: potential mechanisms and implications for clinical practice. *Am J Cardiovasc Drugs, 4,* 57–67.

61. Portier, I., & Campbell, R.A. (2021). Role of platelets in detection and regulation of infection. *Arterioscler Thromb Vasc Biol, 41,* 70–78.

62. Koupenova, M., Livada, A. C., & Morrell, C. N. (2022). Platelet and megakaryocyte roles in innate and adaptive immunity. *Circ Res, 130,* 288–308.

63. Guo, L., & Rondina, M. T. (2019). The era of thromboinflammation: platelets are dynamic sensors and effector cells during infectious diseases. *Front Immunol.* https://doi.org/10.3389/fimmu.2019.02204.

64. Oyarzun, C. P. M., & Heller, P. G. (2019). Platelets as mediators of thromboinflammation in chronic myeloproliferative neoplasms. *Front Immunol.* https://doi.org/10.3389/fimmu.2019.01373.

65. Gawaz, M., Langer, H., & May, A. E. (2005). Platelets in inflammation and atherogenesis. *J Clin Invest, 115,* 3378–3384.

66. Zimmerman, G. A., & Weyrich, A. S. (2008). Signal-dependent protein synthesis by activated platelets. New pathways to altered phenotype and function. *Arterioscler Thromb Vasc Biol, 28,* s17–s24.

67. Davizon-Castillo, P., Rowley, J. W., & Rondina, M. T. (2020). Megakaryocyte and platelet transcriptomics for discoveries in human health and disease. *Arterioscler Thromb Vasc Biol, 40,* 1432–1440.

68. Middleton, E. A., Rowley, J. W., Campbell, R. A., et al. (2019). Sepsis alters the transcriptional and translational landscape of human and murine platelets. *Blood, 134*(12), 911–923.

12

Manual, Semiautomated, and Point-of-Care Testing in Hematology

Karen S. Clark and Teresa G. Hippel

OBJECTIVES

After completion of this chapter, the reader will be able to:

1. List the anticoagulant used for collection of blood specimens for routine hematology tests and describe general handling and processing requirements.
2. State the dimensions of the counting area of a Neubauer ruled hemacytometer.
3. Describe the performance of manual cell counts for white blood cells, red blood cells, and platelets, including types of diluting fluids, typical dilutions and their calculations, and typical areas counted in the hemacytometer.
4. Calculate hemacytometer cell counts when given numbers of cells, area counted, and dilution.
5. Correct white blood cell counts for the presence of nucleated red blood cells.
6. Describe the principle and procedure of the cyanmethemoglobin assay for determination of hemoglobin including construction and use of the cyanmethemoglobin standard curve.
7. Describe the principle and procedure for performing a microhematocrit.

8. Compare hemoglobin and hematocrit values using the rule of three.
9. Calculate red blood cell indices when given appropriate data, and interpret the results relative to the volume, hemoglobin content, and hemoglobin concentration in the red blood cells.
10. Describe the principle and procedure for performing a manual reticulocyte count and the clinical value of the test.
11. Given the appropriate data, calculate the relative, absolute, and corrected reticulocyte counts and the reticulocyte production index; interpret results to determine the adequacy of the bone marrow erythropoietic response in an anemia.
12. Describe the principle and procedures for performing the erythrocyte sedimentation rate and state its clinical utility.
13. Identify sources of error in routine manual procedures discussed in this chapter and recognize written scenarios describing such errors.
14. Discuss the advantages and disadvantages of point-of-care testing as they apply to hematology tests.

OUTLINE

Specimen Collection
Manual Cell Counts
  Principle
  Equipment
  Calculations
  White Blood Cell Count
  Platelet Count
  Red Blood Cell Count
  Disposable Blood Cell Count Dilution Systems
  Body Fluid Cell Counts
Hemoglobin Determination
  Principle

Microhematocrit
  Principle
Rule of Three
Red Blood Cell Indices
  Mean Cell Volume
  Mean Cell Hemoglobin
  Mean Cell Hemoglobin Concentration
Reticulocyte Count
  Principle
  Absolute Reticulocyte Count
  Corrected Reticulocyte Count
  Reticulocyte Production Index
  Automated Reticulocyte Counts

Erythrocyte Sedimentation Rate
  Principle
  Modified Westergren Erythrocyte Sedimentation Rate
  Wintrobe Erythrocyte Sedimentation Rate
  Disposable Kits
  Automated Erythrocyte Sedimentation Rate

Additional Tests for Red Blood Cells
Point-of-Care Testing
  Point-of-Care Tests

CASE STUDIES

After studying the material in this chapter, the reader should be able to respond to the following case studies. Answers can be found in Appendix C. Hematology reference intervals can be found after the Index at the end of the book.

Case 1

The following results were obtained for a patient with normocytic, normochromic RBCs on a peripheral blood film.

RBC	4.63×10^{12}/L	HCT	40% (0.40 L/L)
HGB	15 g/dL		

1. Using the rule of three, given the hemoglobin concentration here, what is the expected value for the hematocrit?
2. What could cause the hemoglobin to be falsely elevated or the hematocrit to be falsely low?
3. What would you do to correct for the interferences you listed in question 2?

Case 2

For another patient, the following results were obtained.

RBC	3.20×10^{12}/L	HCT	18.9% (0.19 L/L)
HGB	5.8 g/dL		

1. Calculate the RBC indices.
2. How would you describe the RBC volume and hemoglobin concentration based on these indices?
3. How should you verify this?

Case 3

The following results were obtained for a patient using a point-of-care device that employs the conductivity method to measure the hematocrit.

Sodium	160 mmol/L (Reference interval: 135–145 mmol/L)
Potassium	3.6 mmol/L (Reference interval: 3.5–5.5 mmol/L)
HCT	17.0% (0.17 L/L)
HGB	6.0 g/dL

1. Which electrolyte concentration could affect the hematocrit?
2. What other factors can falsely decrease the hematocrit value using this point-of-care device?

Clinical laboratory hematology has evolved from simple observation and description of blood and its components to a highly automated, extremely technical science including examination at the molecular level. However, some of the more basic tests have not changed significantly over the years. This chapter provides an overview of these basic tests and presents the manual and semiautomated methods that can be used in lieu of automated blood cell analysis. A discussion of point-of-care (POC) testing in hematology is included.

SPECIMEN COLLECTION

Most routine hematology tests require a whole blood specimen collected by venipuncture or skin puncture into tubes with an anticoagulant to prevent clotting. Ethylenediaminetetraacetic acid (EDTA, usually as K_2EDTA) is the most common anticoagulant for routine hematology testing, including the complete blood count (CBC) and differential count (Chapters 13 and 14), because of its minimal effects on blood cell morphology. EDTA prevents clotting in the specimen by binding (chelating) calcium required for fibrin clot formation. EDTA collection tubes for hematology are recognized by their lavender stoppers. Established protocols must be followed, including accurate

patient identification, proper patient preparation, and use of the appropriate body sites for venipuncture and skin puncture. Collection tubes must be filled to the proper level to maintain an appropriate blood-to-anticoagulant ratio and mixed by inversion according to tube manufacturer requirements. Ideally specimens for CBC testing should be analyzed within 6 hours of collection if stored at room temperature and 24 hours if stored at 4° C to minimize spurious results.[1] In addition, peripheral blood films prepared within 4 hours of collection reduce cell deterioration and morphology artifacts. Before testing, the specimen must be well mixed and inspected to ensure it is free of clots. Standard precautions and appropriate safety protocols for specimen collection and handling and discarding of contaminated equipment and supplies must be followed to prevent transmission of bloodborne pathogens (Chapter E1).[2]

Following published protocols for specimen collection is a critically important step in providing accurate laboratory test information for patients, regardless of whether the analytical method is performed at the patient's bedside in an inpatient setting, an outpatient physician's office, or a clinical laboratory. Procedures published by the Clinical and Laboratory Standards Institute (CLSI) describe state-of-the-art methods for collecting and processing blood specimens and should be followed by all health care professionals who collect blood specimens.[3,4] Important components of specimen collection that influence testing include the equipment employed to obtain the specimen, the site used and technique for venipuncture or skin puncture, and handling of the specimen after collection. Further details regarding collecting blood specimens can be found in Chapter E2.

MANUAL CELL COUNTS

Although most routine cell-counting procedures in the hematology laboratory are automated, it may be necessary to use manual methods when counts exceed the linearity of an instrument, when an instrument is nonfunctional and there is no backup, in remote laboratories in developing countries, or in a disaster situation when testing is done in the field. Although the discussion in this chapter concerns whole blood, body fluid cell counts are also often performed using manual methods. Chapter E4 discusses the specific diluents and dilutions used for body fluid cell counts. Chapter 13 discusses automated cell-counting instrumentation in detail.

Principle

Manual cell counts determine the number of cells per microliter (μL) or per liter (L) of whole blood. They are performed using a hemacytometer, or counting chamber, and manual dilutions made with calibrated, automated pipettes and diluents (commercially available or prepared in the laboratory). The procedure for the performance of manual cell counts is essentially the same for white blood cells (WBCs), red blood cells (RBCs), and platelets; only the dilution, diluting fluid, and area counted vary. Any particle (e.g., sperm) can be counted using this system.

Equipment

Hemacytometer

The manual cell count uses a hemacytometer or counting chamber. The most common one is the Levy chamber with improved Neubauer ruling. It is composed of two raised surfaces, each with a 3 mm × 3 mm square counting area or grid (total area 9 mm^2), separated by an H-shaped moat. As shown in Figure 12.1, this grid is made up of nine 1 mm × 1 mm squares. Each of the four corner (WBC) squares is subdivided further into 16 squares, and the center square subdivided into 25 smaller squares. Each of these smallest squares is 0.2 mm × 0.2 mm, which is $\frac{1}{25}$ of the center square, or 0.04 mm^2. A coverslip is placed on top of the counting surfaces. The distance between each counting surface and the coverslip is 0.1 mm; thus the total *volume* of one entire grid or counting area on one side of the hemacytometer is 0.9 mm^3. Hemacytometers and coverslips must meet the specifications of the National Bureau of Standards, as indicated by "NBS" on the chamber. When the dimensions of the hemacytometer are thoroughly understood, the area counted can be changed to facilitate the counting of specimens with extremely low or high counts.

Calculations

The general formula for manual cell counts is as follows and can be used to calculate any type of cell count:

$$\text{Total count} = \frac{\text{cells counted} \times \text{dilution factor}}{\text{area (mm}^2) \times \text{depth (0.1)}}$$

or

$$\text{Total count} = \frac{\text{cells counted} \times \text{dilution factor} \times 10^*}{\text{area (mm}^2)}$$

*Reciprocal of depth.

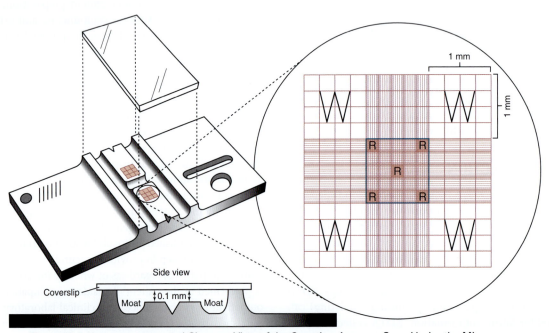

Figure 12.1 Hemacytometer and Close-up View of the Counting Areas as Seen Under the Microscope. The areas for the standard white blood cell count are labeled *W*, and the areas for the standard red blood cell count are labeled *R*. The entire center square, outlined in blue, is used for counting platelets. The side view of the hemacytometer shows a depth of 0.1 mm from the surface of the counting grid to the coverslip.

The calculation yields the number of cells per mm^3. One mm^3 is equivalent to 1 μL. The count per μL is converted to the count per L by multiplying by a factor of 10^6.

White Blood Cell Count

Whole blood anticoagulated with EDTA or blood from a skin puncture is diluted with 1% buffered ammonium oxalate or a weak acid solution (3% acetic acid or 1% hydrochloric acid). The diluting fluid lyses the nonnucleated RBCs in the specimen to prevent their interference in the count. The typical dilution of blood for the WBC count is 1:20. A hemacytometer is charged (filled) with the well-mixed dilution and placed under a microscope and the number of cells in the four large corner squares (4 mm^2) is counted.

PROCEDURE

1. Clean the hemacytometer and coverslip with alcohol and dry thoroughly with a lint-free tissue. Place the coverslip on the hemacytometer.
2. Make a 1:20 dilution by placing 25 μL of well-mixed blood into 475 μL of WBC diluting fluid in a small test tube.
3. Cover the tube and mix by inversion.
4. Allow the dilution to sit for 10 minutes to ensure that the RBCs have lysed. The solution will be clear once lysis has occurred. WBC counts should be performed within 3 hours of dilution.
5. Mix again by inversion and fill a plain microhematocrit tube with the dilution.
6. Charge both sides of the hemacytometer by holding the microhematocrit tube at a 45-degree angle and touching the tip to the coverslip edge where it meets the V-shape indentation in the counting surface. The dilution should flow evenly under the coverslip and cover the entire counting surface without flowing into the moat.
7. After charging the hemacytometer, place it in a moist chamber (Box 12.1) for 10 minutes before counting the cells to give them time to settle. Care should be taken not to disturb the coverslip.
8. While keeping the hemacytometer in a horizontal position, place it on the microscope stage.
9. Lower the condenser on the microscope and focus by using the low-power (10×) objective lens (100× total magnification). The cells should be distributed evenly in all of the squares.
10. For a 1:20 dilution, count all of the cells in the four corner squares, starting with the square in the upper left-hand corner (see Figure 12.1). Cells that touch the top and left lines should be counted; cells that touch the bottom and right lines should be ignored (Figure 12.2). Figure 12.3 depicts the appearance of WBCs in the hemacytometer using the low-power objective lens of a microscope.
11. Repeat the count on the other side of the counting chamber. The difference between the total cells counted on each side should be less than 10%. A greater variation could indicate an uneven distribution, which requires that the procedure be repeated.
12. Average the number of WBCs counted on the two sides. Using the average, calculate the WBC count using one of the equations given earlier.

Example Using the First Equation

When a 1:20 dilution is used, the four large squares on one side of the chamber yield counts of 23, 26, 22, and 21. The total count is 92. The four large squares on the other side of the chamber yield counts of 28, 24, 22, and 26. The total count is 100. The difference between sides is less than 10%.

The average number of cells of the two sides of the chamber is 96. Using the average in the formula:

$$\text{WBC count} = \frac{\text{cells counted} \times \text{dilution factor}}{\text{area counted (mm}^2) \times \text{depth}}$$

$$= \frac{96 \times 20}{4 \times 0.1}$$

$$= 4800/\text{mm}^3 \text{ or } 4800/\mu L \text{ or}$$

$$4.8 \times 10^3/\mu L \text{ or } 4.8 \times 10^9/L$$

Alternatively, a 1:100 dilution may be used counting the number of cells in the entire counting area (nine large squares, 9 mm^2) on both sides of the chamber. As an example, if an average of 54 cells were counted in the entire counting area on both sides of the chamber:

$$\text{WBC count} = \frac{\text{cells counted} \times \text{dilution factor}}{\text{area counted (mm}^2) \times \text{depth}}$$

$$= \frac{54 \times 100}{9 \times 0.1}$$

$$= 6000/\text{mm}^3 \text{ or } 6000/\mu L \text{ or}$$

$$6.0 \times 10^3/\mu L \text{ or } 6.0 \times 10^9/L$$

Reference Intervals

Adult and pediatric reference intervals can be found after the Index at the end of the book.

Sources of Error and Comments

1. The hemacytometer and coverslip should be cleaned properly before they are used. Dust and fingerprints may cause difficulty in distinguishing the cells.
2. The diluting fluid should be free of contaminants.
3. If the count is low, a greater area may be counted (e.g., 9 mm^2) to improve accuracy.
4. The chamber must be charged properly to ensure an accurate count. Uneven flow of the diluted blood into the chamber or bubbles in the dilution result in an irregular distribution of cells. If the chamber is overfilled or underfilled, the chamber must be cleaned and recharged.
5. After the chamber is filled, allow the cells to settle for 10 minutes before counting.
6. Any nucleated red blood cells (NRBCs) present in the specimen are not lysed by the diluting fluid. The NRBCs are counted as WBCs because they are indistinguishable when seen on the hemacytometer. If five or more NRBCs per 100 WBCs are observed on the differential count on a stained peripheral blood film, the WBC count must be corrected for these cells. This is accomplished by using the following formula:

$$\frac{\text{Uncorrected WBC count} \times 100}{\text{Number of NRBCs per 100 WBCs} + 100}$$

Report the result as the "corrected" WBC count.
7. The accuracy of the manual WBC count can be assessed by performing a WBC estimate on a Wright-stained peripheral blood film made from the same specimen (Chapter 14).

BOX 12.1 How to Make a Moist Chamber

A moist chamber may be made by placing a piece of damp filter paper in the bottom of a Petri dish. An applicator stick broken in half can serve as a support for the hemacytometer.

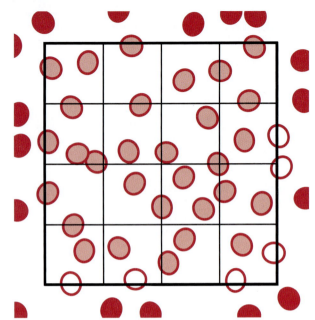

Figure 12.2 Counting rule for One Large Corner Square of a Hemacytometer. Cells touching the left and top lines *(solid circles)* are counted. Cells touching bottom and right lines *(open circles)* are not counted.

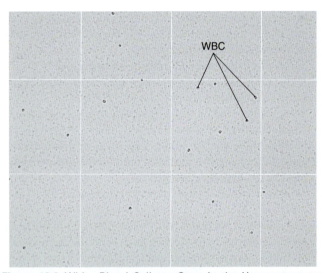

Figure 12.3 White Blood Cells as Seen in the Hemacytometer. Low power (10× objective) 100× total magnification. *WBC,* White blood cell.

Platelet Count

Platelets adhere to foreign objects and to each other, which makes them difficult to count. They also are small and can be confused easily with dirt or debris. In this procedure, whole blood, with EDTA as the anticoagulant, is diluted 1:100 with 1% ammonium oxalate to lyse the nonnucleated RBCs. The platelets are counted in the 25 small squares in the large center square (1 mm²) of the hemacytometer using a phase-contrast microscope in the reference method described by Brecher and Cronkite.[5] A light microscope can also be used, but visualizing the platelets may be more difficult.

PROCEDURE

1. Make a 1:100 dilution by placing 20 μL of well-mixed blood into 1980 μL of 1% ammonium oxalate in a small test tube.
2. Mix the dilution thoroughly and charge the chamber. (Note: A special thin, flat-bottomed counting chamber is used for phase-contrast microscopy platelet counts.)
3. Place the charged hemacytometer in a moist chamber (see Box 12.1) for 15 minutes to allow the platelets to settle.
4. Platelets are counted using the 40× objective lens (400× total magnification). The platelets have a diameter of 2 to 4 μm and appear round or oval, displaying a light purple sheen when phase-contrast microscopy is used. The shape and color help distinguish the platelets from highly refractile dirt and debris. "Ghost" RBCs often are seen in the background.
5. Count the number of platelets in the 25 small squares in the center square of the grid (see Figure 12.1). The area of this center square is 1 mm². Platelets should be counted on each side of the hemacytometer, and the difference between the totals should be less than 10%.
6. Calculate the platelet count by using one of the equations given earlier. Using the first equation as an example, if 200 platelets were counted in the entire center square,

$$\frac{200 \times 100}{1 \times 0.1}$$

$$= 200,000/mm^3 \text{ or } 200,000/\mu L$$

$$\text{or } 200 \times 10^3/\mu L \text{ or } 200 \times 10^9/\mu L$$

7. The accuracy of the manual platelet count should be verified by performing a platelet estimate on a Wright-stained peripheral blood film made from the same specimen (Chapter 14).

Reference Intervals

Adult and pediatric reference intervals can be found after the Index at the end of the book.

Sources of Error and Comments

1. Inadequate mixing and poor collection of the specimen can cause the platelets to clump on the hemacytometer. If the problem persists after redilution, a new specimen is needed. A skin puncture specimen is less desirable because of the tendency of the platelets to aggregate or form clumps.
2. Dirt in the pipette, hemacytometer, or diluting fluid may cause the counts to be inaccurate.
3. If fewer than 50 platelets are counted on each side, the procedure should be repeated by diluting the blood to 1:20. If more than 500 platelets are counted on each side, a 1:200 dilution should be made. The appropriate dilution factor should be used in calculating the results.
4. If the patient has an elevated platelet count, the five small RBC squares (see Figure 12.1) may be counted. Then the area is 0.2 mm² on each side.
5. The phenomenon of "platelet satellitosis" may occur when EDTA anticoagulant is used. This refers to the adherence of platelets around neutrophils, producing a ring or satellite effect (Figure 14.1). Using sodium citrate as the anticoagulant should correct this problem. Because of the dilution in the citrate evacuated tubes, it is necessary to multiply the obtained platelet count by 1.1 for accuracy (Chapter 14).

Red Blood Cell Count

Manual RBC counts are rarely performed because of the inaccuracy of the count and questionable necessity. Use of other, more accurate manual RBC procedures, such as the microhematocrit and hemoglobin concentration, is desirable when automation is not available.

Table 12.1 contains the most common dilutions and counting areas for performing manual WBC, platelet, and RBC counts.

Disposable Blood Cell Count Dilution Systems

Capillary pipette and diluent systems are commercially available for WBC counts. One such product is the Leuko-TIC 1:20 "blue" (Bioanalytic) test system for counting WBCs (Figure 12.4).[6] It consists of a vial containing 380 µL of an acetate buffer (pH 3.0) and detergent to lyse the RBCs and a gentian violet stain (0.1 g/L) to visualize the WBCs. Two types of capillary pipettes are provided: one specimen sampling pipette (calibrated to accept 20 µL of blood) and another chamber-filling pipette for charging the hemacytometer. A capillary holder can be used to hold the sampling pipette in the blood collection process. Blood from a well-mixed EDTA-anticoagulated specimen or from a skin puncture is allowed to enter the sampling pipette by capillary action to the fill volume. After removing any blood from the outside of the pipette, the specimen-filled pipette is added to the vial. The vial is then capped and mixed until all the blood is flushed out of the pipette, thus making a 1:20 dilution. After mixing and allowing at least 30 seconds for lysis of the RBCs, the hemacytometer is charged using the chamber-filling capillary pipette.

WBCs are counted in the 4 large corner squares of the hemacytometer (4 mm^2) using low power (100× total magnification). The standard formula is used to calculate the cell count per µL or L.

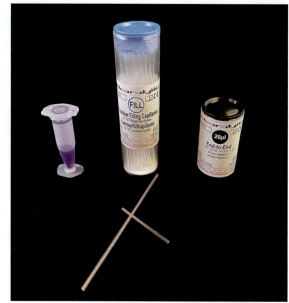

Figure 12.4 Leuko-TIC 1:20 "Blue" Test System for Manual White Blood Cell Counts. The system consists of a vial containing 380 µL of an acetate buffer (pH 3.0) and detergent to lyse the red blood cells and a gentian violet stain (0.1 g/L) to visualize the white blood cells. Two types of capillary pipettes are provided, one specimen sampling pipette (end-to-end capillary) calibrated to accept 20 µL of blood to make a 1:20 dilution and another chamber-filling pipette for charging the hemacytometer. A capillary holder can be used to handle the sampling pipette in the blood collection process (not shown). (Courtesy Fredrik Skarstedt, Indiana University School of Medicine.)

Body Fluid Cell Counts

Body fluid cell counts are discussed in detail in Chapter E4.

HEMOGLOBIN DETERMINATION

Principle

The cyanmethemoglobin (hemiglobincyanide) method for hemoglobin determination is the reference method approved by the CLSI.[7] In the cyanmethemoglobin method, blood is diluted in an alkaline Drabkin solution of potassium ferricyanide, potassium cyanide, sodium bicarbonate, and a surfactant. The hemoglobin is oxidized to methemoglobin (Fe^{3+}) by the potassium ferricyanide, $K_3Fe(CN)_6$. The potassium cyanide (KCN) then converts the methemoglobin to cyanmethemoglobin:

$$\text{Hemoglobin}(Fe^{2+}) + K_3Fe(CN)_6 \rightarrow \text{methemoglobin}(Fe^{3+})$$
$$+ KCN \rightarrow \text{cyanmethemoglobin}$$

The absorbance of the cyanmethemoglobin at 540 nm is directly proportional to the hemoglobin concentration. Sulfhemoglobin is not converted to cyanmethemoglobin; it cannot be measured by this method. Sulfhemoglobin fractions of more than 0.05 g/dL are seldom encountered in clinical practice, however.[8]

TABLE 12.1 Manual Cell Counts With Most Common Dilutions and Counting Areas				
Cells Counted	**Diluting Fluid**	**Dilution**	**Objective**	**Area Counted**
White blood cells	1% ammonium oxalate or 3% acetic acid or 1% hydrochloric acid	1:20 1:100	10× 10×	4 mm^2 9 mm^2
Red blood cells	Isotonic saline	1:100	40×	0.2 mm^2 (5 small squares of center square)
Platelets	1% ammonium oxalate	1:100	40× phase	1 mm^2

PROCEDURE

1. Create a standard curve, using a commercially available cyanmethemoglobin standard.
   a. When a standard containing 80 mg/dL of hemoglobin is used, the following dilutions should be made:

Hemoglobin Concentration (g/dL)	Blank	5	10	15	20
Cyanmethemoglobin standard (mL)	0	1.5	3	4.5	6
Cyanmethemoglobin reagent (mL)	6	4.5	3	1.5	0

   b. Transfer the dilutions to cuvettes. Set the wavelength on the spectrophotometer to 540 nm and use the blank to set to 100% transmittance.
   c. Using semilogarithmic paper, plot percent transmittance on the y-axis and the hemoglobin concentration on the x-axis. The hemoglobin concentrations of the control and patient specimens can be read from the standard curve (Figure 12.5).
   d. A standard curve should be set up with each new lot of reagents. It also should be checked when alterations are made to the spectrophotometer (e.g., bulb change).
2. Controls should be analyzed with each batch of specimens. Commercial controls are available.
3. Using the patient's whole blood anticoagulated with EDTA or heparin or blood from a capillary puncture, make a 1:251 dilution by adding 0.02 mL (20 µL) of blood to 5 mL of cyanmethemoglobin reagent. The pipette should be rinsed thoroughly with the reagent to ensure that no blood remains. Follow the same procedure for the control specimens.
4. Cover and mix well by inversion or use a vortex mixer. Let stand for 10 minutes at room temperature to allow full conversion of hemoglobin to cyanmethemoglobin.
5. Transfer all the solutions to cuvettes. Set the spectrophotometer to 100% transmittance at the wavelength of 540 nm, using cyanmethemoglobin reagent as a blank.
6. Using a matched cuvette, continue reading the percent transmittance of the patient specimens and record the values.
7. Determine the hemoglobin concentration of the control specimens and the patient specimens from the standard curve.

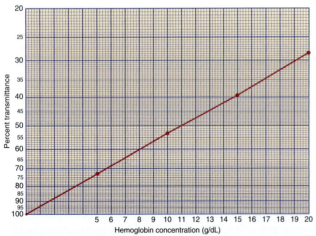

Figure 12.5 Standard Curve for Cyanmethemoglobin Standard of 80 mg/dL. A blank (100% transmittance) and four dilutions were made: 5 g/dL (72.9% transmittance), 10 g/dL (53.2% transmittance), 15 g/dL (39.1% transmittance), and 20 g/dL (28.7% transmittance).

Reference Intervals

Adult and pediatric reference intervals can be found after the Index at the end of the book.

Sources of Error and Comments

1. Cyanmethemoglobin reagent is sensitive to light. It should be stored in a brown bottle or in a dark place.
2. A high WBC count (greater than 20×10^9/L) or a high platelet count (greater than 700×10^9/L) can cause turbidity and a falsely high result. In this case, the reagent-specimen solution can be centrifuged and the supernatant measured.
3. Lipemia also can cause turbidity and a falsely high result. It can be corrected by adding 0.01 mL of the patient's plasma to 5 mL of the cyanmethemoglobin reagent and using this solution as the reagent blank.
4. Cells containing hemoglobin S (Hb S) and hemoglobin C (Hb C) may be resistant to hemolysis, causing turbidity; this can be corrected by making a 1:2 dilution with distilled water (1 part diluted specimen plus 1 part water) and multiplying the results from the standard curve by 2.
5. Abnormal globulins, such as those found in patients with plasma cell myeloma or Waldenström macroglobulinemia, may precipitate in the reagent. If this occurs, add 0.1 g of potassium carbonate to the cyanmethemoglobin reagent. Commercially available cyanmethemoglobin reagent has been modified to contain KH_2PO_4 salt, so this problem is not likely to occur.
6. Carboxyhemoglobin takes 1 hour to convert to cyanmethemoglobin and, theoretically, could cause erroneous results in specimens from heavy smokers. The degree of error is probably not clinically significant, however.
7. Because the hemoglobin reagent contains cyanide, it is highly toxic and must be used cautiously. Consult the safety data sheet supplied by the manufacturer. Acidification of cyanide in the reagent releases highly toxic hydrogen cyanide gas. A licensed waste disposal service should be contracted to discard the reagent; reagent-specimen solutions should not be discarded into sinks.
8. Commercial absorbance standards kits are available to calibrate spectrophotometers.
9. Handheld systems are commercially available to measure the hemoglobin concentration. An example is the HemoCue,[9,10] in which hemoglobin is converted to azide methemoglobin and is read photometrically at two wavelengths (570 nm and 880 nm). This method avoids the necessity of specimen dilution and interference from turbidity. It is discussed later in "Point-of-Care Testing." Another method that has been used in some automated instruments involves the use of sodium lauryl sulfate (SLS) to convert hemoglobin to SLS-methemoglobin. This method does not generate toxic wastes.[11,12]

MICROHEMATOCRIT

Principle

The hematocrit is the volume of packed RBCs that occupies a given volume of whole blood. This is sometimes referred to as the *packed cell volume* (PCV). It is reported either as a percentage (e.g., 36%) or in liters per liter (0.36 L/L).

PROCEDURE

1. Fill two plain capillary tubes approximately three-quarters full with blood anticoagulated with EDTA or heparin. Mylar-wrapped tubes are recommended by the National Institute for Occupational Safety and Health to reduce the risk of capillary tube injuries.[13] Alternatively, blood may be collected into heparinized capillary tubes by skin puncture. Wipe any excess blood from the outside of the tube.
2. Seal the end of the tube with the colored ring using nonabsorbent clay. Hold the filled tube horizontally and seal by placing the dry end into the tray with sealing compound at a 90-degree angle. Rotate the tube slightly and remove it from the tray. The plug should be at least 4 mm long.[13]
3. Balance the tubes in a microhematocrit centrifuge with the clay ends facing the outside away from the center, touching the rubber gasket.
4. Tighten the head cover on the centrifuge and close the top. Centrifuge the tubes at 10,000g to 15,000g for the time that has been determined to obtain maximum packing of RBCs, as detailed in Box 12.2. Do not use the brake to stop the centrifuge.
5. Determine the hematocrit by using a microhematocrit reading device (Figure 12.6). Read the level of RBC packing; do not include the buffy coat (WBCs and platelets) when taking the reading (Figure 12.7).
6. The values of the duplicate hematocrits should agree within 1% (0.01 L/L).[13]

BOX 12.2 Determining Maximum Packing Time for Microhematocrit

The time to obtain maximum packing of red blood cells should be determined for each centrifuge. Duplicate microhematocrit determinations should be made using fresh, well-mixed blood anticoagulated with ethylenediaminetetraacetic acid (EDTA). Two specimens should be used, with one of the specimens having a known hematocrit of 50% or higher. Starting at 2 minutes, centrifuge duplicates at 30-second intervals and record results. When the hematocrit has remained at the same value for two consecutive readings, optimum packing has been achieved, and the second time interval should be used for microhematocrit determinations.[13]

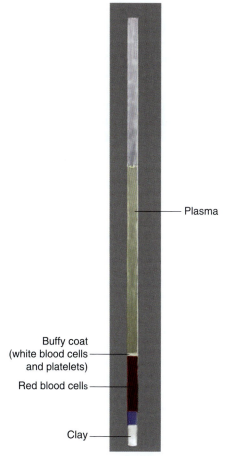

Figure 12.7 Capillary Tube With Anticoagulated Whole Blood After Centrifugation. Note the layers containing plasma, the buffy coat (white blood cells and platelets), and the red blood cells.

Reference Intervals

Adult and pediatric reference intervals can be found after the Index at the end of the book.

Sources of Error and Comments

1. Improper sealing of the capillary tube causes a decreased hematocrit reading as a result of leakage of blood during centrifugation. A higher number of RBCs are lost compared with plasma because of the packing of the cells in the lower part of the tube during centrifugation.
2. An increased concentration of anticoagulant (short draw in an evacuated tube) decreases the hematocrit reading as a result of RBC shrinkage.
3. A decreased or increased result may occur if the specimen was not mixed properly.
4. The time and speed of the centrifugation and the time when the results are read are important. Insufficient centrifugation or a delay in reading results after centrifugation causes hematocrit readings to increase. Time for complete packing should be determined for each centrifuge and rechecked at regular intervals. When the microhematocrit centrifuge is calibrated, one of the specimens used must have a hematocrit of 50% or higher.[13]

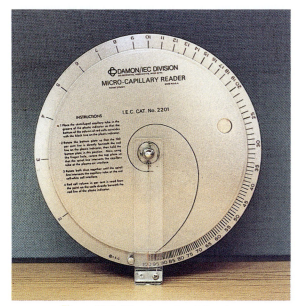

Figure 12.6 Microhematocrit Reader.

5. The buffy coat of the specimen should not be included in the hematocrit reading because this falsely elevates the result.

6. A decrease or increase in the readings may be seen if the microhematocrit reader is not used properly.

7. Many disorders, such as sickle cell anemia, macrocytic anemias, hypochromic anemias, spherocytosis, and thalassemia, may cause plasma to be trapped in the RBC layer even if the procedure is performed properly. The trapping of the plasma causes the microhematocrit to be 1% to 3% (0.01 to 0.03 L/L) higher than the value obtained using automated blood cell analyzers that calculate or directly measure the hematocrit and are unaffected by the trapped plasma.

8. A temporarily low hematocrit reading may result immediately after a blood loss because plasma is replaced faster than the RBCs.

9. The fluid loss associated with dehydration causes a decrease in plasma volume and falsely increases the hematocrit reading.

10. Proper specimen collection is an important consideration. The introduction of interstitial fluid from a skin puncture or the improper flushing of an intravenous catheter causes decreased hematocrit readings.

11. The READACRIT centrifuge (Becton Dickinson) uses precalibrated capillary tubes and has built-in hematocrit scales, which eliminates the need for separate reading devices (Figure 12.8). The use of BD SurePrep Capillary Tubes (Becton Dickinson) eliminates the use of sealants. They have a factory-inserted plug that seals automatically when the blood touches the plug.

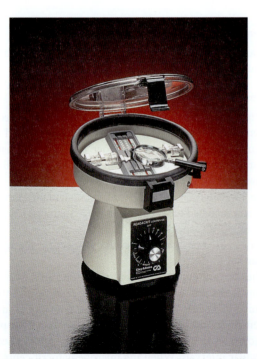

Figure 12.8 READACRIT Centrifuge with Built-in Capillary Tube Compartments and Scales to Read Hematocrit. (Courtesy and © Becton, Dickinson and Company, Franklin Lakes, NJ.)

RULE OF THREE

When specimens are analyzed by automated or manual methods, a quick visual check of the results of the hemoglobin and hematocrit can be done by applying the "rule of three." This rule applies only to specimens that have normocytic, normochromic RBCs. The value of the hematocrit should be three times the value of the hemoglobin plus or minus 3: Hemoglobin (HGB) × 3 = hematocrit (HCT) ± 3 (%) or 0.03 (L/L). It should become habit for the analyst to multiply the hemoglobin by 3 mentally for every specimen; a value discrepant with this rule may indicate abnormal RBCs, or it may be the first indication of error.

For example, the following results are obtained from patients:

Case 1

HGB = 12 g/dL   HCT = 36% (0.36 L/L)
According to the rule of three,

$$HGB(12) \times 3 = HCT(36)$$

An acceptable range for the hematocrit would be 33% to 39%. These values conform to the rule of three.

Case 2

HGB = 9 g/dL   HCT = 32%
According to the rule of three,

$$HGB(9) \times 3 = HCT(27 \text{ versus actual value of } 32)$$

An acceptable range for hematocrit would be 24% to 30%, so these values do not conform to the rule of three.

Case 3

HGB = 15 g/dL   HCT = 36%
According to the rule of three,

$$HGB(15) \times 3 = HCT(45 \text{ versus actual value of } 36)$$

An acceptable range for hematocrit would be 42% to 48%, so these values do not conform to the rule of three.

If values do not agree, the peripheral blood film should be examined for abnormal RBCs; causes of false increases and decreases in hemoglobin or hematocrit values should also be investigated. In the second case, the peripheral blood film had RBCs that were low in hemoglobin concentration (hypochromic) and were smaller in volume (microcytic), so the rule of three cannot be applied. If RBCs do appear normal, possible causes of a falsely low hemoglobin concentration or a falsely elevated hematocrit should be investigated. In the third case, the specimen had lipemic plasma causing a falsely elevated hemoglobin concentration, and a correction must be made to obtain an accurate hemoglobin value ("Sources of Error and Comments" in "Hemoglobin Determination").

When an unexplained discrepancy is found, the specimens analyzed before and after the specimen in question should be checked to determine whether their results conform to the rule. If they do not conform, further investigation should be done to identify the problem. Control specimens should be checked when such a discrepancy is found. If appropriate results are obtained for the control, random error may have occurred (Chapter 3).

RED BLOOD CELL INDICES

The mean cell volume (MCV), mean cell hemoglobin (MCH), and mean cell hemoglobin concentration (MCHC) are the RBC indices. These are calculated to determine the average volume and hemoglobin content and concentration of the RBCs in the specimen. In addition to serving as a quality control check, the indices may be used for initial classification of anemias. Table 12.2 provides a summary of the RBC indices, morphology, and correlation with various anemias. The morphologic classification of anemia on the basis of MCV is discussed in detail in Chapter 16.

Mean Cell Volume

The MCV is the average volume of the RBC, expressed in femtoliters (fL), or 10^{-15} L:

$$MCV = \frac{HCT\,(\%) \times 10}{RBC\ count\,(\times 10^{12}/L)}$$

For example, if the HCT = 45% and the RBC count = 5×10^{12}/L, the MCV = 90 fL.

The reference interval for adults is 80 to 100 fL. RBCs with an MCV of less than 80 fL are microcytic, and RBCs with an MCV of more than 100 fL are macrocytic.

Mean Cell Hemoglobin

The MCH is the average weight of hemoglobin in an RBC, expressed in picograms (pg), or 10^{-12} g:

$$MCH = \frac{HGB\,(g/dL) \times 10}{RBC\ count\,(\times 10^{12}/L)}$$

For example, if the hemoglobin = 16 g/dL and the RBC count = 5×10^{12}/L, the MCH = 32 pg.

The reference interval for adults is 26 to 34 pg. The MCH generally is not considered in the classification of anemias.

Mean Cell Hemoglobin Concentration

The MCHC is the average concentration of hemoglobin in each individual RBC. The units used are grams per deciliter (formerly given as a percentage):

$$MCHC = \frac{HGB\,(g/dL) \times 100}{HCT\,(\%)}$$

For example, if the HGB = 16 g/dL and the HCT = 48%, the MCHC = 33.3 g/dL.

Values of normochromic RBCs range from 32 to 36 g/dL; values of hypochromic cells are less than 32 g/dL, and values of "hyperchromic" cells are greater than 36 g/dL. The term *hyperchromic* is a misnomer. A cell does not really contain more than 36 g/dL of hemoglobin, but its shape may have become spherocytic, which makes the cell appear full. An MCHC between 36 and 38 g/dL should be checked for spherocytes. An MCHC greater than 38 g/dL should be investigated for a falsely elevated hemoglobin concentration or falsely low hematocrit. Another cause for a markedly increased MCHC could be the presence of a cold agglutinin. Incubating the specimen at 37° C for 10 to 15 minutes before analysis usually produces accurate results (Table 13.2).

RETICULOCYTE COUNT

The reticulocyte is the last immature RBC stage. Normally, a reticulocyte spends 1 to 2 days in the bone marrow and 1 day in the peripheral blood before developing into a mature RBC. The reticulocyte contains remnant cytoplasmic ribonucleic acid (RNA) and organelles such as mitochondria and ribosomes (Chapter 6). The reticulocyte count is used to assess the erythropoietic activity of the bone marrow.

Principle

Whole blood, anticoagulated with EDTA, is stained with a supravital stain, such as new methylene blue. Any nonnucleated RBC that contains two or more particles of blue-stained granulofilamentous material after new methylene blue staining is defined as a *reticulocyte* (Figure 12.9).

TABLE 12.2 Red Blood Cell Indices, Red Blood Cell Morphology, and Disease States			
MCV (fL)	MCHC (g/dL)	Red Blood Cell Morphology	Found in
<80	<32	Microcytic; hypochromic	Iron deficiency anemia, anemia of inflammation, thalassemia, Hb E disease and trait, sideroblastic anemia
80–100	32–36	Normocytic; normochromic	Hemolytic anemia, myelophthisic anemia, bone marrow failure, chronic renal disease
>100	32–36	Macrocytic; normochromic	Megaloblastic anemia, chronic liver disease, bone marrow failure, myelodysplastic neoplasms

Hb, Hemoglobin; *MCHC*, mean cell hemoglobin concentration; *MCV*, mean cell volume.

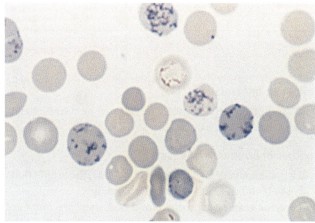

Figure 12.9 Reticulocytes. Reticulocytes are nonnucleated red blood cells with two or more blue-stained filaments or particles. (Peripheral blood, new methylene blue vital stain, ×1000.)

PROCEDURE

1. Mix equal amounts of blood and new methylene blue stain (2 to 3 drops, or approximately 50 μL each), and allow to incubate at room temperature for 3 to 10 minutes.[14]
2. Remix the preparation.
3. Prepare two wedge films (Chapter 14).
4. In an area in which cells are close together but not touching, count 1000 RBCs under the oil immersion objective lens (1000× total magnification) and simultaneously, count the number of reticulocytes among the 1000 RBCs. Reticulocytes are included in the total RBC count (i.e., a reticulocyte counts as both an RBC and a reticulocyte).
5. To improve accuracy, another laboratorian should count the other film; counts should agree within 20%.
6. Calculate the % reticulocyte count:

$$\text{Reticulocytes } (\%) = \frac{\text{number of reticulocytes} \times 100}{1000 \,(\text{RBCs Counted})}$$

For example, if 15 reticulocytes are counted,

$$\text{Reticulocytes } (\%) = \frac{15 \times 100}{1000} = 1.5\%$$

Or the number of reticulocytes counted can be multiplied by 0.1 (100/1000) to obtain the result.

Miller Disc

Because large numbers of RBCs should be counted to obtain a more precise reticulocyte count, the Miller disc was designed to reduce this labor-intensive process. The disc is composed of two squares, with the area of the smaller square measuring one-ninth the area of the larger square. The disc is inserted into the eyepiece of the microscope, and the grid in Figure 12.10 is seen. RBCs are counted in the smaller square, and reticulocytes are counted in the larger square. Selection of the counting area is the same as described earlier. A minimum of 112 cells should be counted in the small square because this is equivalent to 1008 RBCs in the large square and satisfies the College of American Pathologists (CAP) hematology standard for a manual reticulocyte count based on at least 1000 RBCs counted.[15]

The calculation formula for percent reticulocytes is:

$$\text{Reticulocytes } \% = \frac{\substack{\text{number of reticulocytes in square A} \\ (\text{large square}) \times 100}}{\text{number RBCs in square B} (\text{small square}) \times 9}$$

For example, if 15 reticulocytes are counted in the large square and 112 RBCs are counted in the small square,

$$\text{Reticulocytes } (\%) = \frac{15 \times 100}{112 \times 9} = 1.5\%$$

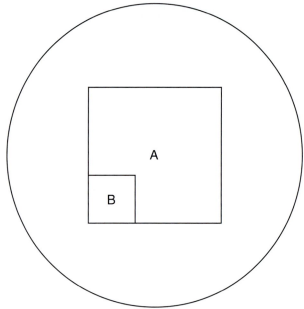

Figure 12.10 Miller Ocular Disc Counting Grid as Viewed Through a Microscope. The area of square *B* is one-ninth the area of square *A*. Alternatively, square *B* may be in the center of square *A*.

3. Moisture in the air, poor drying of the slide, or both may cause areas of the slide to appear refractile, and these areas could be confused with reticulocytes. The RNA remnants in a reticulocyte are not refractile.
4. Other RBC inclusions that stain supravitally include Heinz, Howell-Jolly, and Pappenheimer bodies (Table 16.3). Heinz bodies are precipitated hemoglobin, usually appear round or oval, and tend to adhere to the cell membrane (Figure 12.11). Howell-Jolly bodies are round nuclear fragments and are usually singular. Pappenheimer bodies are iron in the mitochondria whose presence can be confirmed with an iron stain, such as Prussian blue. This stain is discussed in Chapter 15.
5. If a Miller disc is used, it is important to heed the "edge rule" as described in the WBC count procedure and illustrated in Figure 12.2; significant bias is observed if the rule is ignored.[14]

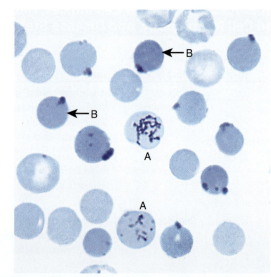

Figure 12.11 Reticulocytes and Heinz Bodies. Reticulocytes *(A)*; Heinz bodies *(B)*. (Peripheral blood, new methylene blue vital stain, ×1000.)

Reference Intervals

Adult and pediatric reference intervals can be found after the Index at the end of the book.

Sources of Error and Comments

1. If a patient is very anemic or polycythemic, the proportion of dye to blood should be adjusted accordingly.
2. An error may occur if the blood and stain are not mixed before the films are made. The specific gravity of the reticulocytes is lower than that of mature RBCs, and reticulocytes settle at the top of the mixture during incubation.

Absolute Reticulocyte Count

Principle

The absolute reticulocyte count (ARC) is the actual number of reticulocytes in 1 L or 1 μL of blood.

Calculation

$$ARC = \frac{reticulocytes(\%) \times RBC\,count(\times 10^{12}/L)}{100}$$

For example, if a patient's reticulocyte count is 2% and the RBC count is $2.20 \times 10^{12}/L$, the ARC is calculated as follows (note that the calculated result has to be converted from $10^{12}/L$ to $10^9/L$):

$$ARC = \frac{2 \times (2.20 \times 10^{12}/L)}{100} = 0.044 \times 10^{12}/L = 44 \times 10^9/L$$

The ARC can also be reported as the number of cells per μL. Using the example just given, the RBC count in μL ($2.20 \times 10^6/\mu L$) is used in the formula, and the ARC result is $44 \times 10^3/\mu L$.

Reference Intervals

Adult and pediatric reference intervals can be found after the Index at the end of the book.

Corrected Reticulocyte Count

Principle

In specimens with a low hematocrit, the percentage of reticulocytes may be falsely elevated because the whole blood contains fewer RBCs. A correction factor is used, with the average normal hematocrit considered to be 45%.

Calculation

Corrected reticulocyte count (%) =

$$reticulocyte(\%) \times \frac{patient\,HCT(\%)}{45}$$

Reference Interval

Patients with a hematocrit of 35% should have an elevated corrected reticulocyte count of 2% to 3% to compensate for the mild anemia. In patients with a hematocrit of less than 25%, the count should increase to 3% to 5% to compensate for the moderate anemia. The corrected reticulocyte count depends on the degree of anemia.

Reticulocyte Production Index

Principle

Reticulocytes that are released from the bone marrow prematurely are called *shift reticulocytes*. These reticulocytes are "shifted" from the bone marrow to the peripheral blood earlier than usual to compensate for anemia. Instead of losing their reticulum in 1 day, as do most normal circulating reticulocytes, these cells take 2 to 3 days to lose their reticula. When erythropoiesis is evaluated, a correction should be made for

the presence of shift reticulocytes if polychromasia is reported in the RBC morphology on the peripheral blood film. Most normal (nonshift) reticulocytes become mature RBCs within 1 day after entering the bloodstream and thus represent 1 day's production of RBCs in the bone marrow. Cells shifted to the peripheral blood prematurely stay longer as reticulocytes and contribute to the reticulocyte count for more than 1 day. For this reason, the reticulocyte count is falsely increased when polychromasia is present because the count no longer represents the cells maturing in just 1 day. On many automated blood cell analyzers, this mathematical adjustment of the reticulocyte count has been replaced by the measurement of immature reticulocyte fraction (Chapter 13).[14]

The patient's hematocrit is used to determine the appropriate correction factor (reticulocyte maturation time in days):

Patient's Hematocrit (%)	Correction Factor (Maturation Time, Days)
40–45	1
35–39	1.5
25–34	2
15–24	2.5
<15	3

Calculation

The reticulocyte production index (RPI) is calculated as follows:

$$RPI = \frac{reticulocyte(\%) \times [HCT(\%)/45\%]}{maturation\,time}$$

or

$$RPI = \frac{Corrected\,reticulocyte\,count}{maturation\,time}$$

For example, for a patient with a reticulocyte count of 7.8% and an HCT of 30%, and with polychromasia noted on the peripheral blood film, the previous table indicates a maturation time of 2 days. Thus:

$$RPI = \frac{7.8 \times [30/45]}{2}$$

$$RPI = 2.6$$

Reference Interval

An adequate bone marrow response usually is indicated by an RPI that is greater than 3. An inadequate erythropoietic response is seen when the RPI is less than 2.[16]

Reticulocyte Controls

Commercial controls are available for monitoring manual and automated reticulocyte counts. Examples include Retic-Chex II (Streck) and Liquichek Reticulocyte Control (Bio-Rad Laboratories). Most of the controls are available at three levels. Control specimens are treated in the same manner as patient specimens. The control can be used to verify the laboratorian's accuracy and precision when manual counts are performed.

Automated Reticulocyte Counts

All major automated blood cell analyzers perform automated reticulocyte counts using optical scatter or fluorescence after the RBCs are treated with fluorescent dyes or nucleic acid stains to stain residual RNA in the reticulocytes. The percentage and the absolute count are provided. These results are statistically more valid because of the large number of cells counted. Other reticulocyte parameters that are offered on automated analyzers include a maturation index/immature reticulocyte fraction (IRF) (reflecting the proportion of the more immature reticulocytes in the specimen), the reticulocyte hemoglobin concentration, and reticulocyte indices (such as the mean reticulocyte volume and distribution width). The IRF may be especially useful in detecting early erythropoietic activity after chemotherapy or hematopoietic stem cell transplantation. The reticulocyte hemoglobin is useful to detect early iron deficiency (Chapter 17). Automated reticulocyte counting is discussed in Chapter 13.

ERYTHROCYTE SEDIMENTATION RATE

The erythrocyte sedimentation rate (ESR) is ordered with other tests to detect and monitor the course of inflammatory diseases such as rheumatoid arthritis and other inflammatory arthropathies, infections, or certain malignancies. It is also useful in the diagnosis of giant cell (temporal) arteritis and polymyalgia rheumatica.[17] The ESR, however, is not a specific test for inflammatory diseases and is elevated in many other conditions such as plasma cell myeloma, pregnancy, anemia, and older age. It is also prone to technical errors that can falsely elevate or decrease the sedimentation rate, although newer automated methods reduce these errors. Because of its low specificity and sensitivity, the ESR is not recommended as a screening test to detect inflammatory conditions in asymptomatic individuals.[17] Other tests for inflammation, such as the C-reactive protein (CRP) level, may be a more predictable and reliable alternative to monitor inflammation.[18,19] However, a meta-analysis published in 2020 found that the diagnostic accuracy of the ESR and CRP are similar when used to assess inflammation, particularly in orthopedic patients.[20]

Principle

When anticoagulated blood is allowed to stand at room temperature undisturbed for a period of time, the RBCs settle toward the bottom of the tube. The ESR is the distance in millimeters that the RBCs fall in 1 hour. The ESR is affected by RBCs, plasma, and mechanical and technical factors. RBCs have a net negative surface charge and tend to repel one another. The repulsive forces are partially or totally counteracted if there are increased quantities of positively charged plasma proteins. Under these conditions the RBCs settle more rapidly as a result of the formation of rouleaux (stacking of RBCs). Examples of macromolecules that can produce this reaction are elevated levels of acute phase reactants (particularly fibrinogen) and immunoglobulins.[19,20]

Normal RBCs have a relatively small mass and settle slowly. Certain diseases can cause rouleaux formation, in which the plasma fibrinogen and globulins are altered. This alteration changes the RBC surface, which leads to stacking of the RBCs, increased RBC mass, and a more rapid ESR. The ESR is directly proportional to the RBC mass and inversely proportional to plasma viscosity. Several methods, both manual and automated, are available for measuring the ESR. Only the most commonly used methods are discussed here.

Modified Westergren Erythrocyte Sedimentation Rate

The modified Westergren method is the most commonly used manual method. One advantage of this method is that the taller column height allows the detection of highly elevated ESRs. It is the method recommended by the International Council for Standardization in Hematology (ISCH) and the CLSI.[17,21]

PROCEDURE

1. Use well-mixed blood collected in EDTA and dilute at four parts blood to one part 3.8% sodium citrate or 0.85% sodium chloride (e.g., 2 mL blood and 0.5 mL diluent). Alternatively, blood can be collected directly into special sedimentation test tubes containing sodium citrate. Standard coagulation test tubes are not acceptable because the dilution is nine parts blood to one part sodium citrate.[17]
2. Fill a 200-mm Westergren tube with the diluted specimen to the 0 mm mark.
3. Place the tube into an ESR rack (tube holder) and allow to stand undisturbed for exactly 1 hour at room temperature (18° to 25° C). Ensure that the rack is level.
4. Record the number of millimeters the RBCs have fallen in 1 hour. The buffy coat should not be included in the reading. Read the tube from the bottom of the plasma layer to the top of the sedimented RBCs (Figure 12.12). Report the result in mm per 1 hour.[17]

Reference Intervals

Reference intervals according to sex and age can be found after the Index at the end of the book. The ESR increases with age and is higher in females compared with males.

Wintrobe Erythrocyte Sedimentation Rate

When the Wintrobe method was first introduced, oxalated whole blood was used, but now either EDTA or citrated whole blood is acceptable. The blood is placed in a 100-mm column (compared with the 200-mm column used in the Westergren method). The shorter column height increases the sensitivity in detecting a slightly elevated ESR.

PROCEDURE

1. Use fresh blood collected in EDTA anticoagulant. A minimum of 2 mL of whole blood is needed.
2. After mixing the blood thoroughly, fill a Pasteur pipette using a rubber pipette bulb.
3. Place the filled pipette into the Wintrobe tube until the tip reaches the bottom of the tube.
4. Carefully squeeze the bulb and expel the blood into the Wintrobe tube while pulling the Pasteur pipette up from the bottom of the tube. There must be steady, even pressure on the bulb to expel blood into the tube as well as continuous movement of the pipette up the tube to prevent the introduction of air bubbles into the column of blood.
5. Fill the Wintrobe tube to the 0 mm mark.
6. Place the tube into a Wintrobe rack (tube holder) and allow to stand undisturbed for exactly 1 hour at room temperature. The rack must be perfectly level and placed in a draft-free room.
7. Record the number of millimeters the RBCs have fallen in 1 hour. Read the tube from the bottom of the plasma layer to the top of the sedimented RBCs. Report the result in mm per 1 hour.

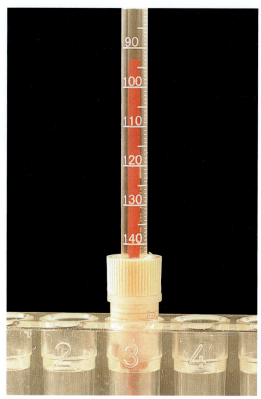

Figure 12.12 Erythrocyte Sedimentation Rate. Reading at 1 hour = 93 mm, which is elevated above the reference interval.

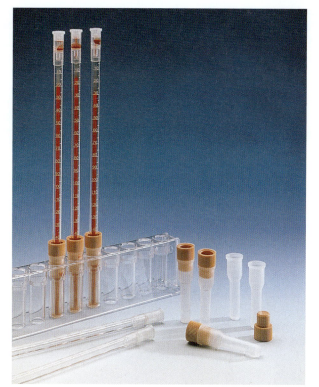

Figure 12.13 Sediplast Disposable Sedimentation Rate System. (Courtesy Polymedco, Cortlandt Manor, NY.)

Sources of Error and Comments

1. If the concentration of anticoagulant is increased, the ESR will be falsely low.
2. The anticoagulants sodium or potassium oxalate and heparin cause the RBCs to shrink and falsely elevate the ESR.
3. A significant change in the temperature of the room alters the ESR.
4. Even a slight tilt of the pipette causes the ESR to increase.
5. Blood specimens must be analyzed within 4 hours of collection if kept at room temperature (18° to 25° C).[17] If the specimen is allowed to sit at room temperature for more than 4 hours, the RBCs start to become spherical, which may inhibit the formation of rouleaux. Blood specimens may be stored at 4° C up to 24 hours, but must be rewarmed by holding the specimen at ambient room temperature for at least 15 minutes before testing.[17]
6. Bubbles in the column of blood invalidate the test results.
7. The blood must be filled properly to the zero mark at the beginning of the test.
8. A clotted specimen cannot be used.
9. The tubes must not be subjected to vibrations on the laboratory bench, which can falsely increase the ESR.
10. Hematologic disorders that prevent the formation of rouleaux (e.g., the presence of sickle cells and spherocytes) decrease the ESR.
11. The ESR of patients with severe anemia is of little diagnostic value because it will be falsely elevated.

Table 12.3 is a summary of some of the factors that influence the ESR.

Disposable Kits

Disposable commercial kits are available for ESR testing (Figure 12.13). Several kits include safety caps for the columns that allow the blood to fill precisely to the zero mark. This safety cap makes the column a closed system and eliminates the error involved in manually setting the blood to the 0 mm mark.

Automated Erythrocyte Sedimentation Rate

Automated ESR systems use a modified Westergren method involving centrifugation or an alternative method such as photometry. For example in the automated quantimetric photometry method used by iSED (Alcor Scientific), a small amount of specimen is automatically withdrawn from a standard EDTA blood collection tube, and RBC rouleaux formation is measured in a microflow cell. The size of the rouleaux aggregates is directly proportional to the ESR.[22]

Automated ESR systems have many advantages, such as specimen identification capability, smaller sample volume requirements, automated sampling and mixing to minimize handling of blood specimens, and a shorter turnaround time. They also incorporate a quality control system and can interface with the laboratory information system. Examples of automated ESR analyzers and their features are listed in Table 12.4. The ICSH recommends that manufacturers of automated ESR instruments validate their new technologies against the gold standard Westergren method, including accuracy, precision, interferences, analytical measurement range, carryover, age- and sex-specific reference intervals, and sensitivity to fibrinogen.[23]

TABLE 12.3   Factors Affecting Erythrocyte Sedimentation Rate

Category	Increased ESR	Decreased ESR
Inflammatory diseases	Giant cell (temporal) arteritis Infections Malignancies Polymyalgia rheumatica Rheumatoid arthritis and other inflammatory arthropathies	
Blood proteins and lipids	Hypercholesterolemia Hyperfibrinogenemia Increased IgM Increased alpha$_2$-macroglobulin Markedly increased IgG	Afibrinogenemia Dysfibrinogenemia Hypofibrinogenemia Increased fatty acids Increased lysolecithin Markedly increased bile salts
Red blood cells	Anemia Macrocytosis RBC agglutination	Anisocytosis (marked) Microcytosis Poikilocytosis (including acanthocytosis, Hb C crystals, sickle cells, spherocytosis) Polycythemia Thalassemia
White blood cells	Plasma cell myeloma	Leukocytosis (marked)
Drugs		Low-molecular-weight dextran Phenylbutazone Sodium salicylate Thiosemicarbazone Valproic acid
Clinical conditions	Acute tissue damage Advanced age Extreme obesity Female sex Pregnancy Renal failure	Cachexia Congestive heart failure
Specimen handling	Heparin or oxalate anticoagulant	Delay in testing over 4 h at RT Increased anticoagulant to blood ratio Refrigerated specimen not returned to room temperature for 15 minutes before testing
Technique*	High RT Tilted ESR tube Vibration during procedure	Low room temperature

*Results are invalidated by clotted blood specimens, bubbles in the ESR column, and errors in specimen dilution, filling the tube, timing, and reading the RBC column
ESR, Erythrocyte sedimentation rate; *h,* hours; *Hb,* hemoglobin; *Ig,* immunoglobulin; *RBC,* red blood cell; *RT,* room temperature.
Data from: CLSI. (2011). *Procedures for the Erythrocyte Sedimentation Rate (ESR) Test.* (5th ed., CLSI approved standard, H2-A5). Wayne, PA: Clinical and Laboratory Standards Institute, and Jerado, R. L. (2001). Why shouldn't we determine the erythrocyte sedimentation rate? *Clin Infect Dis, 33,* 548–549.

Some features to consider when selecting an automated ESR system include size of the analyzer, required sample volume, specimen identification, walkaway and continuous process flow, testing time, quality control program, and interface capabilities.

ADDITIONAL TESTS FOR RED BLOOD CELLS

Additional manual and semiautomated methods are included in other chapters that are relevant to their clinical application. Examples include Chapter 21 for the osmotic fragility test and qualitative and quantitative assays for glucose-6-phosphate dehydrogenase and pyruvate kinase activity; Chapter 24 for the solubility test for Hb S, hemoglobin electrophoresis (alkaline and acid pH), high-performance liquid chromatography, and unstable hemoglobin test; and Chapter 25 for the vital stain for Hb H inclusions and the Kleihauer-Betke acid elution test for Hb F distribution in the RBCs.

POINT-OF-CARE TESTING

POC testing offers the ability to produce rapid and accurate results that facilitate faster treatment, which can decrease hospital length of stay. POC testing is rarely performed by laboratory personnel; it is carried out most often by nurses. Manufacturers

TABLE 12.4 Comparison of Selected Automated Erythrocyte Sedimentation Rate Analyzers

Instrument	Principle of Measurement	Capacity	Tube/Specimen Requirements	Throughput	Delivery to Result Time	Features
iSED, miniiSED (Alcor Scientific)	Quantimetric photometry	20 positions (iSED);1 position (miniiSED)	100 μL drawn from standard (13 × 75 mm) EDTA blood collection tube (iSED and miniiSED); or 100 μL drawn from BD Microtainer MAP ETDA tube (miniiSED)	180 specimens/h	20 seconds (iSED) 15 seconds (MiniiSED)	Internal barcode reader, mixer, printer; unaffected by variables such as hematocrit, mean cell volume, temperature; barcoded Seditrol controls; interfaces with LIS
Diesse CUBE 30 Touch, Diesse MINI-CUBE (Streck)	Modified Westergren sedimentation method	30 positions (CUBE 30); 4 positions (MINI-CUBE)	Standard (13 × 75 mm) EDTA blood collection tube placed in instrument (CUBE 30 and MINI-CUBE; can also use BD Microtainer ETDA tube or BD Microtainer MAP microtube (MINI CUBE); specimen is not consumed	90 specimens/h (CUBE 30); 12 specimens/h (MINICUBE)	20 minutes	Internal (CUBE 30) or external (MINI-CUBE) barcode scanner and printer; internal mixing function; barcoded ESR-Chex Plus bilevel controls; interfaces with LIS
Excyte Mini, Excyte 20, Excyte 40 (ELITech Group)	Modified Westergren sedimentation method	10, 20, or 40 position instruments	Uses special Excyte glass or plastic collection tubes prefilled with sodium citrate	40–80 specimens/h depending on instrument capacity	15–30 minutes	Barcode scanning, printer, mixer; Accu-Sed Plus ESR bilevel controls

EDTA, Ethylenediaminetetraacetate; *ESR,* erythrocyte sedimentation rate; *h,* hour; *LIS,* laboratory information system.
Data from Alcor Scientific. iSED. https://alcorscientific.com/clinical-laboratory/ised/; Streck. Diesse CUBE. https://www.streck.com/products/sed-rate/; ELITech. Excyte. https://www.elitechgroup.com/north-america/products/hematology/erythrocyte-sedimentation-rate/excyte-analyzers/. Accessed September 3, 2022.

have created analyzers with nonlaboratory operators in mind, but results obtained using these systems are still affected by preanalytical and analytical variables. The laboratory professional's partnership with nursing is the key to success in any hospital's POC program.

Point-of-care testing is defined as diagnostic testing at or near the site of patient care. The Clinical Laboratory Improvement Amendments of 1988 (CLIA) introduced the concept of "testing site neutrality," which means that regardless of where the diagnostic testing is performed or who performs the test, all testing sites must follow the same regulatory requirements based on the "complexity" of the test. Under CLIA, POC testing (including physician-performed microscopy) is classified as "waived" or "moderately complex." Tests are classified as waived if they are determined to be "simple tests with an insignificant risk of an erroneous result." POC testing is commonly performed in hospital inpatient units, outpatient clinics, surgery centers, emergency departments, long-term care facilities, and dialysis units. For waived POC testing, facilities are required to obtain a certificate of waiver, pay the appropriate fees, and follow the manufacturers' testing instructions.[24] For any POC program to be successful, certain key elements must be present. Clear administrative responsibility, well-written procedures, a training program, quality control, proficiency testing, and equipment maintenance are essential for success. The first step is appointing a laboratory POC testing coordinator. This person not only is the "go-to" person but is also an important liaison between the laboratory and nursing staff. The second step to ensuring a successful program

is to create a multidisciplinary team with authority to affect all aspects of the POC program. This committee has the authority to oversee the integrity and quality of the existing POC program and institute changes or new testing as needed. It is also important to have administrative support to help remove barriers.

A POC testing program must include a written policy that defines the program and outlines who is responsible for each part of the program. The policy indicates where testing is performed and who performs the testing. Testing procedures should clearly state how to perform the tests and address how to handle critical values and discrepant results. The program must be monitored. An ongoing evaluation of the POC testing is vital for success.

When selecting an instrument to be used in the POC testing program, it is helpful to invite vendors to demonstrate their equipment. An equipment display available for hands-on use by the operators can be very helpful in selection of the appropriate instrumentation. Patient correlation studies are useful in selecting equipment that best covers the patient population for the institution. POC operators need handheld analyzers that are lightweight, accurate, and fast and require low specimen volume. The POC testing system should also address the following laboratory concerns:

- What is the analytical measurement range?
- How well does the test system correlate with laboratory instrumentation?
- Can it be interfaced to the laboratory information system?
- Does it provide reliable results?

- Does the company supply excellent technical support?
- Is it affordable?

Paramount to POC testing is patient safety. It is important to maintain good laboratory practices, which include use of appropriate procedures for specimen collection, identification of the patient and specimen, storage of reagents, instrument maintenance, and accurate documentation of patient test results (use of POC interfaces to the laboratory information system and electronic medical record is beneficial). Laboratory oversight is sometimes absent, and basic safety precautions necessary for waived tests can be easily overlooked, often as a result of a lack of understanding, lack of training, and high personnel turnover rates.[25]

Point-of-Care Tests

POC instruments are available to measure parameters such as hemoglobin and hematocrit; some are capable of performing a CBC.

Hematocrit

The most common methods for determining the hematocrit include the microhematocrit centrifuge, conductometric methods, and determination by automated blood cell analyzers (Chapter 13). Centrifuge-based microhematocrit systems have been available for years, and the results obtained correlate well with the results produced by standard automated blood cell analyzers. Nonlaboratorians and inexperienced operators, however, may be unaware of the error that can be introduced by insufficient centrifugation time and inaccurate reading of the microhematocrit tube ("Sources of Error and Comments" in "Microhematocrit"). One example of a centrifuge-based device is the HemataStat II (Separation Technology). The i-STAT 1 (Abbott Laboratories) (Figure 12.14)[26] and the epoc Blood Analysis System (Siemens Healthineers) (Figure 12.15)[27] use the conductivity method to determine the hematocrit along with

other analytes. Plasma conducts electrical current, whereas WBCs act as insulators. In the i-STAT system, before the measured conductance is converted into the hematocrit value, corrections are applied for temperature of the specimen, size of the fluid segment being measured, and relative conductivity of the plasma component. The first two corrections are determined from the measured value of the calibrant conductance, and the last correction is determined from the measured concentrations of sodium and potassium in the specimen.[26]

Sources of error and comments. Conductivity of a whole blood specimen is dependent on the amount of electrolytes in the plasma portion. Conductivity does not distinguish RBCs from other nonconductive elements such as proteins, lipids, and WBCs that may be present in the specimen.

A low total protein level will falsely decrease the hematocrit. The presence of lipids can interfere with the hematocrit measurement. An increased WBC count will falsely increase the hematocrit. The presence of cold agglutinins can falsely decrease the hematocrit.[26]

Other instruments. Some other instruments that measure hematocrit along with other analytes include the ABL 77 (Radiometer), IRMA TRUPOINT (LifeHealth), and Gem Premier (Instrumentation Laboratory) (Figure 12.16).

Hemoglobin Concentration

In POC testing, hemoglobin concentration is measured by modified hemoglobinometers or by oximeters integrated with a blood gas analyzer. The HemoCue hemoglobinometer (HemoCue) uses a small cuvette that contains a lysing agent and reagents to form a hemoglobin azide, which is measured by a photometer at two wavelengths (570 nm and 880 nm) (Figure 12.17).[10] The 880 nm measurement serves as a blank and eliminates interference from turbidity in the specimen. Results obtained with the instrument compare well with results produced by reference methods, but a major source of error is mixing of blood with tissue fluid during skin puncture collection. The Avoximeter 4000 (Werfen) is a co-oximeter that measures total hemoglobin in addition to other analytes (such as blood gases and some electrolytes) by a spectrophotometric method.

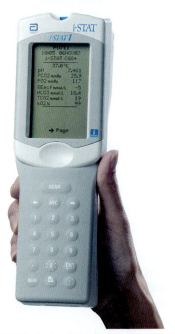

Figure 12.14 i-STAT Instrument for Measuring Hematocrit. (Courtesy Abbott Laboratories, Abbott Park, IL.)

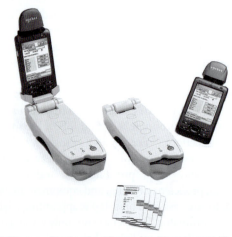

Figure 12.15 epoc Device for Measuring Hematocrit. (Courtesy Siemens Healthineers, Malvern, PA.)

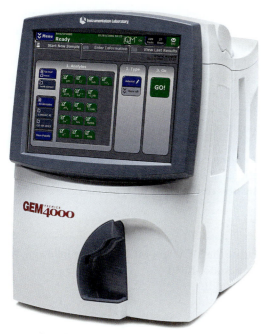

Figure 12.16 Gem Premier Instrument for Measuring Hematocrit. (Courtesy Instrumentation Laboratory, Lexington, MA.)

Cell Counts

Traditional cell-counting methods can be employed at the point of care for the analysis of WBCs, RBCs, and platelets. The ICHOR Hematology Analyzer (Helena Laboratories) performs a CBC along with platelet aggregation. Another option for cell

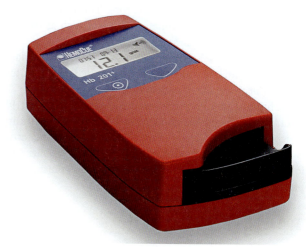

Figure 12.17 The HemoCue Hb 201+ System for Measuring Hemoglobin. (Courtesy HemoCue, Inc., Brea, CA.)

quantitation and differentiation employs a buffy coat analysis method. Quantitative buffy coat analysis (QBC STAR, Drucker Diagnostics) involves centrifugation in a specialized blood collection capillary tube coated with dry reagents and anticoagulant and contains a mechanical float designed to expand the buffy coat layer. The components (platelets, mononuclear cells, and granulocytes) can be measured with the assistance of fluorescent dyes and a measuring device.[28] Hemoglobin and hematocrit are also measured.

SUMMARY

- Although most laboratories are highly automated, manual tests discussed in this chapter, such as the cyanmethemoglobin method of hemoglobin determination and centrifuge-based measurement of the microhematocrit, are used as a part of quality control and backup methods of analysis in many laboratories.

- A manual count of white blood cells (WBCs) and platelets determines the number of cells per microliter (μL) or liter (L) of whole blood using special diluents and a hemacytometer or counting chamber. After anticoagulated whole blood is mixed with the diluent, the hemacytometer is charged and cells are counted under a microscope. A standard formula is used to calculate the number of cells per μL or L. Manual red blood cell (RBC) counts are rarely performed because of the inaccuracy of the count.

- The reference method for hemoglobin determination is based on the absorbance of cyanmethemoglobin at 540 nm. In the manual method, anticoagulated whole blood is mixed with the cyanmethemoglobin reagent and measured in a spectrophotometer. A standard curve is employed to obtain the results in grams per deciliter (g/dL).

- The microhematocrit is a measure of the packed RBC volume. In the manual method, a capillary tube is filled with anticoagulated whole blood and centrifuged, and the volume of the packed RBCs is measured compared with the volume of whole blood in a microhematocrit reader. The microhematocrit is

reported either as a percentage (e.g., 36%) or in liters per liter (0.36 L/L).

- The rule of three specifies that the value of the hematocrit should be three times the value of the hemoglobin plus or minus 3 (%) or 0.03 (L/L). A value discrepant with this rule may indicate abnormal RBCs, or it may be the first indication of error.

- RBC indices, the mean cell volume (MCV), mean cell hemoglobin (MCH), and mean cell hemoglobin concentration (MCHC), are calculated to determine the average volume, hemoglobin content, and hemoglobin concentration of RBCs. The indices provide an indication of possible causes of an anemia.

- The manual reticulocyte count, which is used to assess the erythropoietic activity of the bone marrow, is accomplished by mixing anticoagulated whole blood with a supravital stain (e.g., new methylene blue), preparing a blood film of the mixture on a slide, and using a microscope to count the number of reticulocytes compared with the total number of RBCs. Reticulocytes contain two or more particles of blue-stained granulofilamentous material. The result is reported in a percentage (%). A corrected reticulocyte count and a reticulocyte production index (RPI) may be calculated.

- The manual erythrocyte sedimentation rate (ESR), a measure of the settling of RBCs in a 1-hour period, depends on the ability of RBCs to form rouleaux. It is subject to many physiologic and technical errors. Automated methods are available that minimize these errors. The ESR is used to detect and monitor inflammatory diseases such as rheumatoid arthritis, infections, and some malignancies.

- Point-of-care (POC) testing is often performed by nonlaboratory personnel. It is defined as diagnostic laboratory testing at or near the site of patient care.
- The Clinical Laboratory Improvement Amendments of 1988 (CLIA) introduced the concept of "testing site neutrality," which means that it does not matter where diagnostic testing is performed or who performs the test; all testing sites must follow the same regulatory requirements based on the "complexity" of the test.

- Tests are classified as waived if they are determined to be "simple tests with an insignificant risk of an erroneous result." Most but not all POC testing is waived.
- For a POC testing program to be successful, key elements such as clear administrative responsibility, well-written procedures, quality control, proficiency testing, and equipment maintenance must be present.
- Paramount to POC testing is patient safety.

Now that you have completed this chapter, go back and read again the case studies at the beginning and respond to the questions presented. Answers can be found in Appendix C.

REVIEW QUESTIONS

Answers can be found in Appendix C.

1. A 1:20 dilution of blood is made with 3% glacial acetic acid as the diluent. The four large corner squares on both sides of the hemacytometer are counted, for a total of 100 cells. What is the total WBC count ($\times 10^9$/L)?
   a. 0.25
   b. 2.5
   c. 5
   d. 10

2. The total WBC count is 20×10^9/L. On the peripheral blood film, 25 NRBCs per 100 WBCs are observed. What is the corrected WBC count ($\times 10^9$/L)?
   a. 0.8
   b. 8
   c. 16
   d. 19

3. If potassium cyanide and potassium ferricyanide are used in the manual method for hemoglobin determination, the final product is:
   a. Methemoglobin
   b. Azide methemoglobin
   c. Cyanmethemoglobin
   d. Myoglobin

4. Which of the following would NOT interfere with the result when hemoglobin determination is performed by the cyanmethemoglobin method?
   a. Increased lipids
   b. Elevated WBC count
   c. Lyse-resistant RBCs
   d. Fetal hemoglobin

5. A patient has a hemoglobin level of 8.0 g/dL. According to the rule of three, what is the expected range for the hematocrit?
   a. 21% to 24%
   b. 23.7% to 24.3%
   c. 24% to 27%
   d. 21% to 27%

6. Calculate the MCV and MCHC for the following values:
   RBCs = 5.00×10^{12}/L
   HGB = 9 g/dL
   HCT = 30%

	MCV (fL)	MCHC (g/dL)
a.	30	18
b.	60	30
c.	65	33
d.	85	35

7. What does the reticulocyte count assess?
   a. Inflammation
   b. Response to infection
   c. Erythropoietic activity of the bone marrow
   d. Ability of RBCs to form rouleaux

8. For a patient with the following test results, which measure of bone marrow RBC production provides the most accurate information?
   Observed reticulocyte count = 5.3%
   HCT = 35%
   Morphology—moderate polychromasia
   a. Observed reticulocyte count
   b. Corrected reticulocyte count
   c. RPI
   d. ARC

9. Given the following values, calculate the RPI:
   Observed reticulocyte count = 6%
   HCT = 30%
   a. 2
   b. 3
   c. 4
   d. 5

10. Which of the following would be associated with an elevated ESR value?
    a. Microcytosis
    b. Polycythemia
    c. Decreased globulins
    d. Inflammation

REFERENCES

1. Cornet, E., Behier, C., & Troussard, X. (2012). Guidance for storing blood samples in laboratories performing complete blood count with differential. *Int J Lab Hematol, 34*, 655–660.

2. Department of Labor OSHA. (1991). Occupational exposure to bloodborne pathogens; final rule. *Fed Reg, 56*, 64175–64182.

3. CLSI. (2017). *Collection of Diagnostic Venous Blood Specimens.* (7th ed., CLSI approved standard, GP41). Wayne, PA: Clinical and Laboratory Standards Institute.

4. CLSI. (2020). *Collection of Capillary Blood Specimens.* (7th ed., CLSI approved standard, GP42). Wayne, PA: Clinical and Laboratory Standards Institute.

5. Brecher, G., & Cronkite, E. P. (1950). Morphology and enumeration of human blood platelets. *J Appl Physiol, 3*, 365–377.

6. Leuko-TIC 1:20 Blue Test Kit Insert. Bioanalytic GmbH. Umkirch/Freiburg, Germany. http://www.bioanalytic.de/en/product/article/leuko-tic-120-blue-plus.html. Accessed September 15, 2022.

7. CLSI. (2000). *Reference and Selected Procedures for the Quantitative Determination of Hemoglobin in Blood.* (3rd ed., CLSI approved standard, H15-A3). Wayne, PA: Clinical and Laboratory Standards Institute.

8. Zwart, A., van Assendelft, O. W., Bull, B. S., et al. (1996). Recommendations for reference method for haemoglobinometry in human blood (ICSH Standard 1995) and specifications for international haemiglobincyanide reference preparation (4th ed.). *J Clin Pathol, 49*, 271–274.

9. von Schenck, H., Falkensson, M., & Lundberg, B. (1986). Evaluation of "HemoCue," a new device for determining hemoglobin. *Clin Chem, 32*, 526–529.

10. HemoCue. https://www.hemocue.us/hb-201/. Accessed September 3, 2022.

11. Lewis, S. M., Garvey, B., Manning, R., et al. (1991). Lauryl sulphate haemoglobin: a non-hazardous substitute for HiCN in haemoglobinometry. *Clin Lab Haematol, 13*, 279–290.

12. Karsan, A., MacLaren, I., Conn, D., et al. (1993). An evaluation of hemoglobin determination using sodium lauryl sulfate. *Am J Clin Pathol, 100*, 123–126.

13. CLSI. (2000). *Procedure for Determining Packed Cell Volume by the Microhematocrit Method.* (3rd ed., CLSI approved standard, H07-A3). Wayne, PA: Clinical and Laboratory Standards Institute.

14. CLSI. (2004). *Methods for Reticulocyte Counting (Automated Blood Cell Counters, Flow Cytometry, and Supravital Dyes).* (2nd ed., CLSI approved standard, H44-A2). Wayne, PA: Clinical and Laboratory Standards Institute.

15. College of American Pathologists. (2001). Q & A Miller disk clarification. *CAP Today, 95.* http://www.captodayonline.com/Archives/q_and_a/qa_04_04.html. Accessed September 3, 2022.

16. Koepke, J. F., & Koepke, J. A. (1986). Reticulocytes. *Clin Lab Haematol, 8*, 169–179.

17. CLSI. (2011). *Procedures for the Erythrocyte Sedimentation Rate (ESR) Test.* (5th ed., CLSI approved standard, H2-A5). Wayne, PA: Clinical and Laboratory Standards Institute.

18. Colombet, I., Pouchot, J., Kronz, V., et al. (2010). Agreement between the erythrocyte sedimentation rate and C-reactive protein in hospital practice. *Am J Med, 123*, 863.e7–863.e13.

19. Jurado, R. L. (2001). Why shouldn't we determine the erythrocyte sedimentation rate? *Clin Infect Dis, 33*, 548–549.

20. Lapic, I., Padoan, A., Bozzato, D., et al. (2020). Erythrocyte sedimentation rate and C-reactive protein in acute inflammation. Meta-analysis of diagnostic accuracy studies. *Am J Clin Path, 153*, 14–29.

21. Jou, J. M., Lewis, S. M., Briggs, C., et al. (2011). International Council for Standardization in Haematology: ICSH review of the measurement of the erythrocyte sedimentation rate. *Int J Lab Hematol, 33*, 125–132.

22. Alcor Scientific. iSED instrument. https://alcorscientific.com/clinical-laboratory/ised/. Accessed September 3, 2022.

23. Kratz, A., Plebani, M., Peng, M., et al. on behalf of the International Council for Standardization in Haematology (ICSH). (2017). ICSH recommendations for modified and alternate methods measuring the erythrocyte sedimentation rate. *Int J Lab Hem, 39*, 448–457.

24. Centers for Medicare and Medicaid Services. Clinical Laboratory Improvement Amendments (CLIA 1988): overview. http://www.cms.hhs.gov/clia/. Accessed September 3, 2022.

25. Good Laboratory Practices. (12.17.2002). https://www.cms.gov/Regulations-and-Guidance/Legislation/CLIA/Downloads/wgoodlab.pdf. Accessed September 3, 2022.

26. Abbott Point of Care Cartridge and Hematocrit/HCT and Calculated Hemoglobin/HB information sheets, in i-STAT 1 system manual (revised June 11, 2008). Abbott Park, Ill, Abbott Laboratories.

27. Epoc Blood Analysis System Resource Guide, Siemens Healthineers. https://www.manualslib.com/manual/2170749/Siemens-Healthcare-Epoc.html. Accessed 9/7/2022.

28. QBC Dry Hematology Analyzers. https://druckerdiagnostics.com/products/dry-hematology-analyzers/. Accessed September 3, 2022.

ADDITIONAL RESOURCES

College of American Pathologists. https://www.cap.org/.

Point of Care.net. http://www.pointofcare.net.

Howerton, D., Anderson, N., Bosse, D., et al. (2005). Good laboratory practices for waived testing sites. Survey findings from testing sites holding a certificate of waiver under the Clinical Laboratory Improvement Amendments of 1988 and recommendations for promoting quality testing. *MMWR, 54*(RR13), 1–25. https://www.cdc.gov/mmwr/preview/mmwrhtml/rr5413a1.htm. Accessed September 3, 2022.

13

Automated Blood Cell Analysis

*Elaine M. Keohane**

OBJECTIVES

After completion of this chapter, the reader will be able to:

1. Explain the different principles and methodologies used in automated blood cell analysis.
2. Compare and contrast how the principles and methodologies are implemented in the four major analyzers for the measurement of the complete blood count, including the white blood cell count and differential, red blood cell count, hemoglobin concentration, hematocrit, red blood cell indices, red cell distribution width, nucleated red blood cell count, reticulocyte count, reticulocyte hemoglobin content, immature reticulocyte fraction, platelet count, mean platelet volume, and immature platelet fraction.
3. Identify the parameters directly measured on the four analyzers and explain how the remainder of the parameters are derived.
4. Explain how the various analyzers use histograms, scattergrams, dataplots, scatterplots, and cytograms to visually display blood cell analysis data.
5. Identify limitations and interferences in automated blood cell analysis and describe appropriate corrective actions.
6. Discuss the clinical utility of automated blood cell analysis parameters.

OUTLINE

General Principles of Automated Blood Cell Analysis
    Electrical Impedance
    Radiofrequency Conductivity
    Optical Light Scatter
    Cytochemical and Fluorescent Staining
    Spectrophotometry for Hemoglobin Determination
Principal Analyzers
    Overview
    Beckman Coulter
    Sysmex
    Abbott
    Siemens Healthineers
Validation and Calibration of Automated Analyzers

Limitations and Interferences
    Limitations of Impedance Technology
    Errors in Hemoglobin Determination
    Effects of Red Blood Cell Agglutination
    Spurious Thrombocytopenia
    Errors in Reticulocyte Counting
    Specimen Integrity and Stability
    Data Suppression and Flagging
Clinical Utility of Automated Blood Cell Analysis
    Traditional Complete Blood Count
    Red Cell Distribution Width
    Reticulocyte Analysis
    Platelet Analysis
    Nucleated Red Blood Cells
Analyzer Selection

CASE STUDY

After studying the material in this chapter, the reader should be able to respond to the following case study. Answers can be found in Appendix C.

Review the following results from a complete blood count (CBC) performed on an automated blood cell analyzer on a 44-year-old woman. Reference intervals can be found after the Index at the end of the book.

WBC	9.5×10^9/L	HGB	12.2 g/dL
RBC	2.25×10^{12}/L	HCT	30.4%
MCV	135.1 fL	MCHC	40.1 g/dL
MCH	54.2 pg	RDW	26%
		PLT	195×10^9/L

1. Which parameter(s) are not within reference intervals?
2. What is the possible interference that is causing these CBC results?
3. Explain the corrective action to be taken for this specimen.

*The author extends appreciation to Sharral Longanbach and Martha K. Miers, whose work in prior editions provided the foundation for this chapter.

Since the 1980s, automated blood cell analysis has virtually replaced manual hemoglobin (HGB), hematocrit (HCT), and cell counting because of its greater accuracy and precision. Automated blood cell analyzers are marketed by multiple analyzer manufacturers. Modern analyzers provide the parameters of a complete blood count (CBC), reticulocyte and platelet analysis, nucleated red blood cell (NRBC) count, and a five- or six-part white blood cell (WBC) differential listed in Box 13.1. In addition to greater accuracy and precision, automation allows more efficient workload management and more timely diagnosis and treatment of disease.

GENERAL PRINCIPLES OF AUTOMATED BLOOD CELL ANALYSIS

Despite the number of blood cell analyzers available from different manufacturers and their varying levels of sophistication and complexity, they rely on various combinations of the same technologies, including electrical impedance, radiofrequency (RF) conductivity, optical light scatter, staining with cytochemical and fluorescent dyes, and spectrophotometry (for the measurement of hemoglobin concentration). Electrical impedance, or low-voltage direct current (DC) resistance, was developed by Coulter in the 1950s.[1] The first multiparameter automated blood cell analyzer (Coulter Model S) was released in the late 1960s.[2] RF resistance/conductivity is a modification introduced by TOA Medical Electronics Company and is used in conjunction with DC electrical impedance in some analyzers. Optical light scatter and cytochemistry was introduced by Technicon Instruments Corporation in the 1970s, and Ortho Clinical Diagnostics followed with laser-based optical analyzers. Fluorescence technology was introduced in the 1990s to assist in the identification and counting of WBCs and NRBCs,

and to determine the platelet and reticulocyte counts with an assessment of their immature fraction.

Electrical Impedance

The impedance principle of cell analysis is based on the measurement of changes in electrical resistance produced by cells as they traverse a small aperture. Cells suspended in an electrically conductive diluent such as isotonic saline are pulled through an aperture in an aperture tube. Low-voltage DC is applied between an external electrode (suspended in the cell dilution in the aperture bath) and an internal electrode (housed inside the aperture tube). Electrical resistance between the two electrodes, or impedance in the current, occurs as the cells pass through the aperture, causing voltage pulses that are measurable (Figure 13.1).[1,2] The number of pulses is proportional to the number of cells counted. The amplitude (height) of the pulses is proportional to the cell volume. Upper and lower *electronic volume thresholds,* designated for each cell type, allows discrimination of cells based on their volume. All particles producing pulses within the volume thresholds of each cell type are identified, counted, and sized as that specific cell population.

Pulse height analyzers collect and sort the pulses according to their amplitude. The data are plotted on a frequency distribution graph, or *volume distribution histogram,* with cell volume on the x-axis and relative number of cells on the y-axis. Figure 13.2 illustrates the construction of a frequency distribution graph for a red blood cell (RBC) population. In addition to

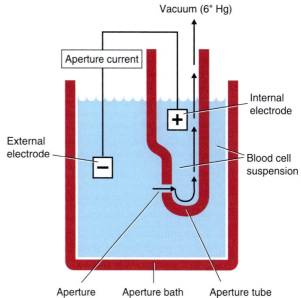

Figure 13.1 Coulter (Impedance) Principle of Cell Counting. Cells suspended in an electrically conductive diluent are pulled through an aperture in an aperture tube. Low-voltage direct current (DC) is applied between an external electrode (suspended in the cell dilution in the aperture bath) and an internal electrode (housed inside the aperture tube). Electrical resistance between the two electrodes, or impedance in the current, occurs as the cells pass through the aperture, causing voltage pulses that are measurable. The number of pulses is proportional to the number of cells counted. The height of the pulses is proportional to cell volume. (From Coulter Electronics. [1988]. *Coulter STKR Product Reference Manual,* PN 4235547. Hialeah, FL: Coulter Electronics.)

BOX 13.1 Complete Blood Count Parameters Available on Automated Blood Cell Analyzers

Red Blood Cell Parameters
Red blood cell count (RBC)
Hemoglobin (HGB)
Hematocrit (HCT)
Mean cell volume (MCV)
Mean cell hemoglobin (MCH)
Mean cell hemoglobin concentration (MCHC)
Red cell distribution width (RDW-CV and RDW-SD)
Nucleated red blood cells (NRBC)
Reticulocytes (RETIC/RETC/RET)*
Immature reticulocyte fraction (IRF)
Mean reticulocyte volume (MRV)
Reticulocyte hemoglobin content (RET-He/CHr)

White Blood Cell Parameters
White blood cell count (WBC)
Differential
Neutrophils (NEUT/NE/NEU)*
Lymphocytes (LYMPH/LY/LYM)*
Monocytes (MONO/MO)*
Eosinophils (EO/EOS)*
Basophils (BASO/BA)*
Immature granulocytes (IG)*

Platelet Parameters
Platelet count (PLT)
Mean platelet volume (MPV)
Immature platelet fraction (IPF)

---

* Reported in % (relative count) and cells per microliter or liter (absolute count).

Oscilloscope

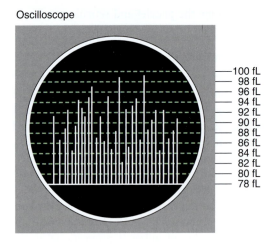

— 100 fL
— 98 fL
— 96 fL
— 94 fL
— 92 fL
— 90 fL
— 88 fL
— 86 fL
— 84 fL
— 82 fL
— 80 fL
— 78 fL

Histogram

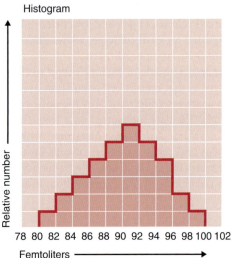

Relative number

78 80 82 84 86 88 90 92 94 96 98 100 102

Femtoliters

Figure 13.2 Red Blood Cell Oscilloscope Display and Histogram. The oscilloscope shows voltage pulses of red blood cells. They are counted within the electronic thresholds established for the analyzer. The amplitude of the pulse is proportional to cell volume. The pulse signals are converted to a frequency distribution graph in which cell volume in femtoliters is plotted on the *x*-axis and relative number or frequency of cells by their volume is plotted on the *y*-axis. (Modified from Coulter Electronics. [1983]. *Significant Advances in Hematology: Hematology Education Series*, PN 4206115A. Hialeah, FL: Coulter Electronics.)

the RBC count, histogram analysis enables the determination of the mean cell volume (MCV) of the RBC population. The RBC count and MCV, in conjunction with a direct spectrophotometric measurement of hemoglobin, allows calculation of the hematocrit, mean cell hemoglobin (MCH), and mean cell hemoglobin concentration (MCHC).[3]

Volume distribution histograms also can be used for the evaluation of subgroups within a population.[4–6] Figure 13.3 depicts histograms of WBC, RBC, and platelet populations based only on impedance on an older Coulter analyzer.[6] Particles with volumes between 2 and 20 femtoliters (fL) were counted as platelets, and particles greater than 36 fL were counted as RBCs. Interpretation of RBC and platelet histograms is discussed in Chapter 14. For the WBCs, the use of lytic reagents to lyse RBCs and control WBC shrinkage allowed for the separation and counting of WBCs into three populations (lymphocytes,

mononuclear cells, and granulocytes) in one volume histogram, for a *three-part differential*.[6] A WBC histogram was constructed from the data by counting particles with volumes between 35 and 90 fL as lymphocytes, particles between 90 and 160 fL as mononuclears (monocytes, blasts, immature granulocytes, and reactive lymphocytes), and particles between 160 and 450 fL as granulocytes. This also allowed the calculation of relative and absolute counts for the three populations. Computerized algorithms flagged results for increased eosinophils or basophils, abnormal cells (e.g., reactive lymphocytes and blasts), cell population overlaps, or interferences from NRBCs, clumped platelets, unlysed RBCs, or electronic noise.[6]

Several factors may affect volume measurements in impedance technology. Aperture diameter is crucial, and the RBC/platelet aperture is smaller than the WBC aperture to increase platelet counting sensitivity. On earlier systems, protein buildup occurred, decreasing the diameter of the orifice, slowing the flow of cells, and increasing their relative electrical resistance. Protein buildup results in lower cell counts and falsely elevated cell volumes. Impedance analyzers once required frequent manual aperture cleaning, but modern analyzers incorporate *burn circuits* or other internal cleaning systems to prevent or slow protein buildup.[4,6] Carryover of cells from one specimen to the next is also minimized by these internal cleaning systems. Coincident passage of more than one cell at a time through the aperture causes artificially large pulses, which results in falsely increased cell volumes and falsely decreased cell counts. This count reduction, or *coincident passage loss*, is statistically predictable (and mathematically correctable) because of its direct relationship to cell concentration and the effective volume of the aperture.[4,6] Coincidence correction is completed by the analyzer computer before final printout of the cell counts. Recirculation of cells back into the sensing zone causes erroneous pulses and falsely elevates cell counts. A backwash or sweep-flow mechanism prevents recirculation of cells back into the sensing zone.[4,6] In addition, the biconcave shape of the RBCs results in their bending, deforming, and misaligning as they pass through the aperture causing erroneous pulse heights. This error can be minimized by using a reagent to sphere the RBCs without changing their volume, called *isovolumetric sphering*.[7]

Other factors affecting pulse height measurements include orientation of cells along the inner opening of the aperture instead of the center causing pulse height irregularities. To minimize this error, an outer sheath fluid surrounds and narrows the specimen stream by *laminar flow* and directs the cells to pass through the central axis of the aperture. Laminar flow also narrows the specimen stream so the cells align in single file, passing through the aperture one at a time in a process called *hydrodynamic focusing*.[6] The outer sheath fluid also minimizes protein buildup and prevents recirculation of cells back into the sensing zone. Coincident passage loss is also reduced because cells line up one after another in the direction of the flow.[6] Laminar flow and hydrodynamic focusing are discussed further in Chapter 28.

Although the development of impedance technology was the first major step toward automated analysis, it was limited in that it was only able to discriminate cells based on their

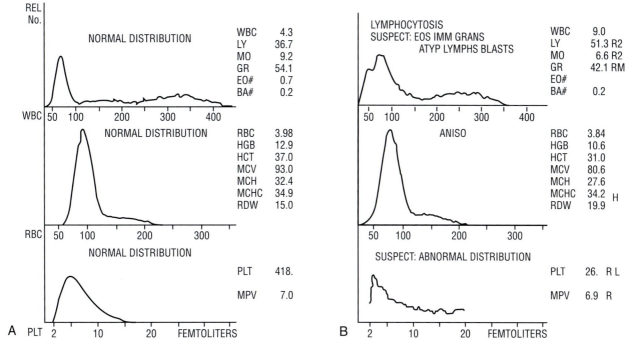

Figure 13.3 Impedance Histograms for White Blood Cells, Red Blood Cells, and Platelets. Printouts from a Coulter STKR analyzer show the complete blood count and interpretive histograms. **(A)**, Note the three distinct white blood cell *(WBC)* populations, Gaussian or normal distribution of red blood cells *(RBCs)*, and right-skewed or log-normal distribution of platelets *(PLT)*. **(B)**, Note the left shift in the WBC histogram with possible interference at the lower threshold region. The R2 flag indicates interference and loss of valley owing to overlap or insufficient separation between the lymphocyte *(LY)* and mononuclear *(MO)* populations at the 90-fL region. RM flag indicates interference at more than one region. Eosinophil *(EO)* data have been suppressed. Also note the abnormal platelet volume distribution with a low platelet count. Manual 200-cell differential counts on the same specimens: **(A)**, 52.5% neutrophils (47% segmented neutrophils, 5.5% bands), 41.5% lymphocytes, 4.0% monocytes, 1% basophils , 0.5% metamyelocytes, 0.5% reactive lymphocytes; **(B)**, 51% neutrophils (23% segmented neutrophils, 28% bands), 12% lymphocytes, 9.5% monocytes, 1% metamyelocytes, 1.5% myelocytes, 25% reactive lymphocytes, and 17 nucleated RBCs/100 WBCs. *HCT,* Hematocrit; *HGB,* hemoglobin; *GR,* granulocytes; *MCH,* mean cellular hemoglobin; *MCV,* mean cell volume; *MCHC,* mean cell hemoglobin concentration; *MPV,* mean platelet volume; *PLT,* platelet; *RDW,* red cell distribution width.

different volumes. Therefore it was not able to effectively distinguish different cells with the same volume, such as RBCs from large platelets and platelet clumps or NRBCs from lymphocytes. To more accurately discriminate between different cells with the same volume, other technologies were developed to measure additional properties of blood cells.

Radiofrequency Conductivity

Low-voltage DC impedance, as described previously, may be used in conjunction with RF conductivity to increase discrimination among cells. In addition to DC current, a high-frequency, electromagnetic RF current simultaneously flows across an aperture between the internal and external electrodes in the aperture bath (Figure 13.4).[8,9] As a cell passes through the aperture, the RF current penetrates the cell membrane and the RF current passing through the cell produces a pulse that is measured by a detector as cell conductivity. The amplitude of the pulse depends on the cell density or internal complexity. Conductivity is reduced by a high nucleus-to-cytoplasm ratio, nuclear density, and cytoplasmic granulation. When both DC and RF pulse signals are measured, the total volume of the cell is proportional to the

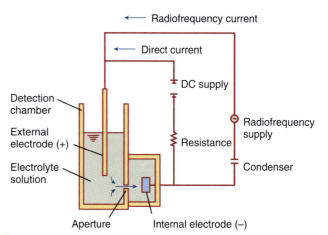

Figure 13.4 Radiofrequency/Direct Current (RF/DC) Detection Method. The simultaneous use of DC and RF in one measurement system on the Sysmex SE-9500 is depicted. (From TOA Medical Electronics Company. [1997]. *Sysmex SE-9500 Operator's Manual [CN 461-2464-2].* Kobe, Japan: TOA Medical Electronics Co.)

DC impedance and the cell interior density is proportional to the change in the RF signal.[8,9] DC and RF voltage changes can be detected simultaneously and separated by two different pulse processing circuits.[10]

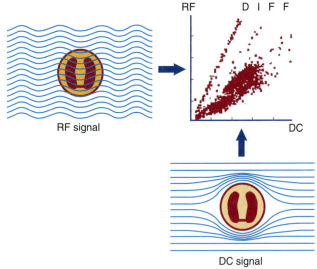

Figure 13.5 Two-Dimensional Scattergram of Direct Current *(DC)* Versus Radiofrequency *(RF)* Signals. Low-voltage DC impedance (measurement of cell volume) on the *x*-axis is plotted against RF conductivity (measurement of cell interior density and nuclear volume and complexity) on the *y*-axis to form a two-dimensional scattergram. (From TOA Medical Electronics Company. [1997]. *Sysmex SE-9500 Operator's Manual [CN 461-2464-2]*, Kobe, Japan: TOA Medical Electronics Co.)

Plotting DC on the *x*-axis and RF on the *y*-axis creates a *two-dimensional distribution scattergram* identifying three populations of WBCs: lymphocytes, monocytes, and granulocytes (Figure 13.5).[9] Such plots display the cell populations as clusters, with the number of dots in each cluster representing the concentration of that cell type. Computer cluster analysis can determine absolute counts for specific cell populations. The use of multiple methods by a given analyzer for the determination of at least two cell properties allows the separation of WBCs into a *five-part differential* (neutrophils, lymphocytes, monocytes, eosinophils, and basophils).[9]

Optical Light Scatter

Optical light scatter may be used as the primary methodology or in combination with other methods. In optical scatter systems (also called flow cytometers), a hydrodynamically focused specimen stream is directed through a flow cell past a focused light source (Figure 28.3).[11] The light source is most often laser light (*light amplification by stimulated emission of radiation*) but can be a tungsten-halogen source. Laser light is *monochromatic light* because it is emitted at a single wavelength, and it differs from brightfield light in its intensity, coherence (traveling in phase), and low divergence or spread. These characteristics allow for the detection of cell interference in the laser beam and enable differentiation and counting of cell types.[11,12]

As the cells pass through the sensing zone and interrupt the beam, light is scattered in all directions. Light scatter results from the interaction between the processes of absorption, diffraction (bending around corners or the surface of a cell), refraction (bending because of a change in speed), and reflection (backward scatter of rays caused by an obstruction).[13] The detection of scattered light and its conversion into electrical

signals is accomplished by photodetectors (photodiodes and photomultiplier tubes) at specific angles. Lenses fitted with a *blocker bar* are used to collect the scattered light in the forward direction along the light source path. The blocker bar prevents nonscattered source light from entering the detector. A series of filters and mirrors separate the varying wavelengths and present them to the photodetectors.[11,12]

Early optical scatter analyzers used only one forward, low-angle scatter measurement (primarily relying on the diffraction of light) to count and volumetrically size cells, relating the number of scatter signals to the number of cells and the size of the scatter to cell volume.[14] These one-dimensional scatter analyzers had limitations similar to those of impedance methods in that they could not reliably differentiate cells with the same volume (e.g., platelets from small RBCs, or RBCs from large platelets).[14]

Orthogonal light (90°) scatter, or *side scatter,* was introduced to further characterize blood cells.[11,12] Orthogonal light scatter results from refraction and reflection of light from larger structures inside the cell and correlates with the degree of internal complexity. This allows differentiation of five types of WBCs based on their volume and internal structure (nuclear shape, density, and cytoplasmic granules).[12] Challenges in differentiating cells without nuclei (platelets and mature RBCs) were overcome by using a reagent to volumetrically sphere RBCs and platelets (to minimize scatter irregularities) and measuring two forward light-scattering signals simultaneously, low-angle (2° to 3°) and high-angle (5° to 15°). Based on the Mie theory of light scattering of homogenous spheres, the low-angle scatter correlates with cell volume, whereas the high-angle scatter correlates with the refractive index of the cell (cell contents).[14–16] This technology is used to distinguish platelets from RBCs based on volume and refractive index (platelets have greater cytoplasmic density because of their granules),[14] and also to measure the cell hemoglobin content in RBCs.[15,16] Additional light scatter angles were added to various analyzers to further characterize cell populations and minimize cell misidentification.[10,17,18] The angles of light scatter measured by various blood cell analyzers are manufacturer and method specific.

Scatter signals at different angles can be plotted against each other to generate two- or three-dimensional dataplots, scattergrams, scatterplots, and cytograms (names of the plots vary by manufacturer) in which cells with similar properties cluster together. Computer cluster analysis of the plots is used to identify and count the various types of blood cells. Different optical scatter signals also can be plotted against signals from impedance, RF, fluorescence, or cytochemical staining.[10,17–19]

Cytochemical and Fluorescent Staining

Cytochemical staining can be used to identify and count blood cells in combination with optical scatter. For example, specific stains react with the peroxidase (PEROX) in granules of neutrophils, eosinophils, and monocytes and the light absorbance of the cells is measured and plotted against their scatter properties. This technology distinguishes neutrophils, eosinophils, and monocytes (peroxidase positive) from lymphocytes, basophils, and platelets (peroxidase negative).[19] In another example, new methylene blue or oxazine 750 stain the ribonucleic acid (RNA) in reticulocytes to distinguish them from mature RBCs and count them in combination with optical scatter.[10,19]

Fluorescent dyes bind to deoxyribonucleic acid (DNA) and RNA in WBCs, NRBCs, platelets, and reticulocytes, and they can be identified and counted in combination with optical scatter.[17,18] Fluorescent dyes absorb laser light at one wavelength and emit fluorescent light at a higher wavelength that is specific to a particular fluorescent dye (Chapter 28 and Figure 28.4). In reticulocytes and platelets, the more immature the cell, the greater is the concentration of cellular RNA and the greater is the intensity of fluorescence staining. This allows for the separation of immature cells from the mature cells and determination of their immature fractions.

Spectrophotometry for Hemoglobin Determination

The reference method of measuring hemoglobin is the cyanmethemoglobin (hemiglobincyanide) method.[20] The RBCs are lysed to release the hemoglobin, and potassium ferricyanide oxidizes the hemoglobin (Fe^{2+}) to methemoglobin (Fe^{3+}). Potassium cyanide converts methemoglobin to cyanmethemoglobin, and the absorbance at 540 nm is measured and is proportional to the hemoglobin concentration (Chapter 12). The major limitation of this method is the toxicity of the cyanide in the reagent, requiring protection of laboratory personnel from toxic exposure and special waste disposal procedures to avoid contamination of the environment. Modern analyzers have developed alternative reagents without cyanide based on the principle of the cyanmethemoglobin method to avoid the handling and disposal of toxic chemicals. Sodium laurel sulfate (SLS) is a commonly used cyanide-free reagent.

Automated blood cell analyzers have an optical component (hemoglobinometer) in which the absorbance or transmittance of the hemoglobin reaction product is measured at a specific wavelength, and the computer converts the signal to hemoglobin concentration in g/dL. A blank reading is also done to minimize interference from specimen turbidity that can falsely elevate the hemoglobin values (e.g., high WBC counts, and severe lipemia and bilirubinemia).

PRINCIPAL ANALYZERS

Overview

Automated blood cell analyzers used in the United States are produced by multiple manufacturers, including but not limited to Beckman-Coulter, Sysmex, Abbott, and Siemens Healthineers. The following descriptions are limited to the most recent US Food and Drug Administration (FDA)-cleared/approved multiparameter analyzers produced by these four manufacturers at the time of this writing. Technology continues to improve, and the newest models produced by a manufacturer may not be mentioned. Emphasis is not placed on specimen volume or handling, speed, level of automation, or comparison of analyzers. Instead, a detailed description of primary methods used by these analyzers is given to show the application of and clarify further the principles presented earlier and to enable the laboratory professional to interpret basic patient data, including analyzer-generated histograms and plots. Table 13.1 summarizes methods used for the CBC, WBC differential, NRBC, and reticulocyte and platelet analysis on the four major blood cell analyzers. Although these analyzers are capable of preparing and staining peripheral blood films and performing body fluid analysis, these functions will not be covered in this chapter. In addition, some analyzers may have a digital imaging module for visual cell morphology recognition and identification for the differential count.[17] A description of these functions is covered in Chapters 14 and E4.

Blood cell analyzers have some common basic components, including hydraulics, pneumatics, and electrical systems. The hydraulics system includes an aspirating unit, dispensers, diluters, mixing chambers, aperture baths or flow cells or both, and a hemoglobinometer. The pneumatics system generates the vacuums and pressures required for operating the valves and moving the specimen through the hydraulics system. The electrical system controls operational sequences of the total system and includes electronic analyzers and computing circuitry for processing the data generated. A data display unit receives information from the analyzer and prints results, histograms, and various plots.

Specimen handling varies among analyzers based on the degree of automation, and systems range from discrete analyzers to walkaway systems with *front-end load* capability. Computer functions also vary, with the larger analyzers having extensive microprocessor and data management capabilities. Computer software capabilities include (1) automatic startup and shutdown, with internal diagnostic self-checks and some maintenance; (2) quality control, with automatic review of quality control data, calculations, graphs, moving averages, and storage of quality control files (Chapter 3); (3) patient data storage and retrieval, with delta checks (Chapter 3), critical value flagging, and automatic verification of patient results based on user-defined algorithms; (4) host query with the laboratory or hospital information system to allow random access discrete testing capability; (5) analysis of body fluids (Chapter E4); and (6) analysis of animal specimens.

Automated blood cell analyzers are programmed to generate *flags* to notify the user about distribution abnormalities, suspect abnormal cells that cannot be definitively identified by the analyzer, results outside the reference intervals, and possible erroneous results. The flags can be defined by the analyzer manufacturer and the individual laboratory based on their patient population. Flags often require a manual review of the peripheral blood film by a laboratory professional and/or pathologist and possible corrective actions before the results can be reported. The International Society for Laboratory Hematology (ISLH) published consensus rules with criteria for action after review of automated CBC and WBC differential analysis.[21]

Beckman Coulter

The UniCel DxH 900 system from Beckman Coulter (formerly Coulter) provides the RBC, WBC, and platelet analyses listed in Box 13.1 and Figure 13.6. The analyzer uses spectrophotometry to determine the hemoglobin concentration, and three different technologies for blood cell analysis: (1) impedance, (2) RF conductivity, and (3) multiangle laser light scatter.[10]

TABLE 13.1   Methods for the Complete Blood Count, Reticulocyte, Nucleated Red Blood Cells, and White Blood Cell Differential Counts on Four Major Blood Cell Analyzers

Parameter	Beckman Coulter UniCel DxH 900	Sysmex XN-3100	Abbott CELL-DYN Sapphire	Siemens ADVIA 2120i
WBC*	Impedance	Fluorescence flow cytometry using forward scatter, side scatter, and side fluorescent light detection	Multiangle polarized scatter separation (MAPSS) at four angles with three-color fluorescent light detection	Optical scatter in the basophil channel (primary, WBC-B), and optical scatter in the peroxidase channel (secondary, WBC-P)
RBC	Impedance	DC resistance (impedance)	Impedance (primary); light scatter (secondary)	Low- and high-angle light scatter
HGB	Equivalent to the cyanmethemoglobin reference method; product measured at 525 nm with blank	Sodium lauryl sulfate-hemoglobin measured at 555 nm	Hemoglobin-imidazole complex measured at 544 nM with a blank	Cyanmethemoglobin method measured at 546 nm; or noncyanide method with monoaquomonohydroxyferri-porphyrin product measured at 565 nm
HCT	$(RBC \times MCV)/10$	Cumulative RBC pulse height detection	$(RBC \times MCV)/10$	$(RBC \times MCV)/10$
MCV	Mean of RBC volume (impedance) distribution histogram	$(HCT/RBC) \times 10$	Mean of RBC volume distribution histogram	Mean of RBC volume distribution histogram
MCH	$(HGB/RBC) \times 10$	$(HGB/RBC) \times 10$	$(HGB/RBC) \times 10$	$(HGB/RBC) \times 10$
MCHC	$(HGB/HCT) \times 100$	$(HGB/HCT) \times 100$	$(HGB/HCT) \times 100$	$(HGB/HCT) \times 100$
RDW	Derived from RBC volume histogram as RDW-CV (%) or RDW-SD (fL)	Derived from RBC volume histogram as RDW-CV (%) or RDW-SD (fL)	Derived from RBC volume histogram as RDW-CV (%)	Derived from RBC volume histogram as RDW-CV (%)
PLT	Impedance	DC resistance (impedance); if unreliable, reflex to fluorescence flow cytometry using forward scatter and side fluorescent light detection; uses platelet-specific fluorescent dye	Two-angle light scatter and fluorescent light detection (primary); impedance count for verification; optional CD61 monoclonal antibody count	Low- and high-angle light scatter
MPV	Derived from PLT volume histogram	Derived from PLT volume histogram	Derived from PLT volume histogram	Derived from PLT volume histogram
IPF	Not reported	Ratio of high-fluorescent platelets to the total platelet count; reported as a percentage and an absolute count	Not reported	Not reported
WBC differential	VCS: volume (DC impedance), conductivity (radiofrequency), and five-angle light scatter measurement	Fluorescence flow cytometry using forward scatter, side scatter, and side fluorescent light detection	Multiangle polarized scatter separation (MAPSS) and three-color fluorescent light detection	Absorbance of cytochemical (peroxidase) staining, and light scatter; for basophils, differential lysis, low- and high-angle laser light scatter
NRBC*	VCS: volume (DC impedance), conductivity (radiofrequency), and five-angle light scatter measurement	Fluorescence flow cytometry using forward scatter and side fluorescent light detection	Fluorescent staining; forward scatter and fluorescent light detection	Optical scatter in the peroxidase channel and basophil channel
Reticulocyte count	New methylene blue staining; VCS volume (DC impedance), conductivity (radiofrequency), and five-angle light scatter measurement	Fluorescence flow cytometry using forward scatter and side fluorescent light detection	Fluorescent staining; low-angle scatter and fluorescent light detection	Low- and high-angle scatter and absorbance with oxazine 750
IRF	Ratio of the count of the midrange and high scatter reticulocytes to total reticulocyte count; reported as a decimal	Ratio of the count of the medium and high fluorescent reticulocytes to total reticulocyte count; reported as a percentage	Ratio of the count of higher fluorescent reticulocytes to total reticulocyte count; reported as a decimal	Ratio of the count of the medium- and high-absorbing reticulocytes to the total reticulocyte count; not reported
Reticulocyte hemoglobin content	Not reported	Derived from light scatter signals; reported as the reticulocyte hemoglobin equivalent (RET-He) in picograms	Not reported	Derived from low- and high-angle laser light scatter; reported as the reticulocyte hemoglobin content (CHr) in picograms

*Analyzers exclude NRBCs from the WBC count when they are present.

CBC, Complete blood count; *CHr*, reticulocyte hemoglobin content; *CV*, coefficient of variation; *DC*, direct current; *HCT*, hematocrit; *HGB*, hemoglobin; *IPF*, immature platelet fraction; *IRF*, immature reticulocyte fraction; *MAPSS*, multiangle polarized scatter separation; *MCH*, mean cell hemoglobin; *MCHC*, mean cell hemoglobin concentration; *MCV*, mean cell volume; *MPV*, mean platelet volume; *NRBC*, nucleated red blood cell count; *PLT*, platelet count; *RBC*, red blood cell (or count); *RDW*, RBC distribution width; *RET-He*, reticulocyte hemoglobin equivalent; *RF*, radiofrequency; *SD*, standard deviation; *VCS, volume*, conductivity, scatter; *WBC*, white blood cell (or count).

Data from references 10 and 17-19.

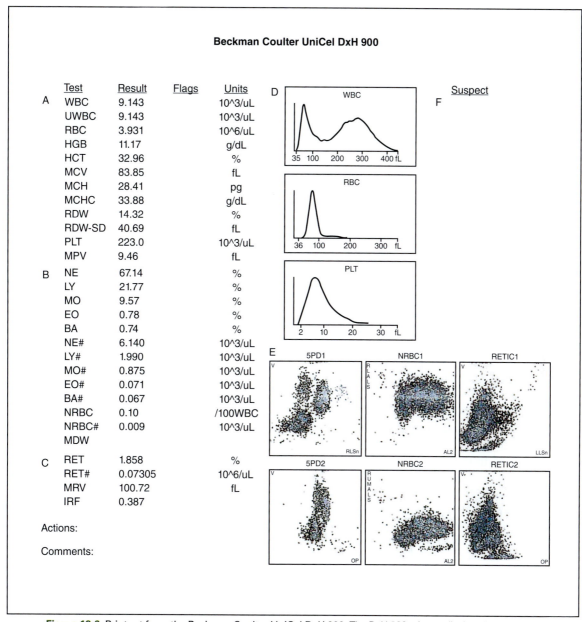

Beckman Coulter UniCel DxH 900

	Test	Result	Flags	Units
A	WBC	9.143		10^3/uL
	UWBC	9.143		10^3/uL
	RBC	3.931		10^6/uL
	HGB	11.17		g/dL
	HCT	32.96		%
	MCV	83.85		fL
	MCH	28.41		pg
	MCHC	33.88		g/dL
	RDW	14.32		%
	RDW-SD	40.69		fL
	PLT	223.0		10^3/uL
	MPV	9.46		fL
B	NE	67.14		%
	LY	21.77		%
	MO	9.57		%
	EO	0.78		%
	BA	0.74		%
	NE#	6.140		10^3/uL
	LY#	1.990		10^3/uL
	MO#	0.875		10^3/uL
	EO#	0.071		10^3/uL
	BA#	0.067		10^3/uL
	NRBC	0.10		/100WBC
	NRBC#	0.009		10^3/uL
	MDW			
C	RET	1.858		%
	RET#	0.07305		10^6/uL
	MRV	100.72		fL
	IRF	0.387		

Actions:

Comments:

Figure 13.6 Printout from the Beckman Coulter UniCel DxH 900. The DxH 900 printout displays the complete blood count (CBC), white blood cell *(WBC)* differential, and reticulocyte data for the same patient also presented in Figures 13.9, 13.12, and 13.15 using three other automated blood cell analyzers. **(A)**, CBC data. **(B)**, WBC differential data with nucleated red blood cells *(NRBCs)*. **(C)**, Reticulocyte data, including the mean reticulocyte volume *(MRV)* and the immature reticulocyte fraction *(IRF)*. **(D)**, Impedance histograms for white WBC, red blood cells *(RBC)*, and platelets *(PLT)*. **(E)**, Two-dimensional dataplots for WBCs *(5PD1* and *5PD2)*, NRBCs *(NRBC1* and *NRBC2)*, and reticulocytes *(RETIC1* and *RETIC2)*. **(F)**, *Suspect* area in which any specimen or system flags will display. *BA*, Basophils; *EO*, eosinophils; *HCT*, hematocrit; *HGB*, hemoglobin concentration; *IRF*, immature reticulocyte fraction; *LY*, lymphocytes; *MCH*, mean cell hemoglobin; *MCHC*, mean cell hemoglobin concentration; *MCV*, mean cell volume; *MDW*, monocyte distribution width; *MO*, monocytes; *MPV*, mean platelet volume; *MRV*, mean reticulocyte volume; *NE*, neutrophils; *NRBC*, nucleated red blood cell count; *PLT*, platelet count; *RBC*, red blood cell count; *RDW*, red cell distribution width coefficient of variation; *RDW-SD*, red cell distribution width standard deviation; *RET*, reticulocyte count; *UWBC*, uncorrected WBC count; *WBC*, white blood cell count.

Hemoglobin Determination

Spectrophotometric analysis is used for the direct measurement of the hemoglobin concentration using a method equivalent to the cyanmethemoglobin reference method.[10] After lysis of the RBCs in a WBC bath, the WBCs are counted and the solution moves to a hemoglobin cuvette, in which the transmittance of the solution is measured at 525 nm with a blank. Correction for turbidity resulting from high WBC count interference is made if the WBC count exceeds a specific threshold.[10]

Impedance for WBC Count and RBC and Platelet Analysis

Impedance technology is used to directly measure the WBC, RBC, and PLT counts, as well as the MCV, red cell distribution width (RDW), and mean platelet volume (MPV).[10]

The aspirated whole blood specimen is divided into two aliquots, and each is mixed with an isotonic diluent. The first dilution is delivered to the RBC aperture bath, and the second is delivered to the WBC aperture bath. In the RBC bath, RBCs and platelets are counted and discriminated by their volume using electrical impedance as the cells are pulled through each of three sensing apertures. In the WBC bath, a reagent to lyse RBCs and release hemoglobin is added before WBCs are counted simultaneously by impedance in each of three sensing apertures. (After counting cycles are completed, the WBC dilution is passed to the hemoglobinometer for the spectrophotometric determination of hemoglobin concentration.) Electrical pulses generated in the counting cycles are sent to the analyzer for pulse editing, coincidence correction, scaling, and digital conversion. The results of the three apertures in each bath are compared and, if they meet established statistical criteria, are then averaged and reported. In a process called *voting*, if the result from only one aperture does not meet the criteria, the other two are averaged and reported (called a *partial voteout*). If more than one result does not meet the criteria, the count is not reported (called a *total voteout*). Two of the three counts obtained in each bath must match within specified limits for the counts to be accepted and reported by the analyzer.[10] This multiple counting procedure prevents data errors resulting from aperture obstructions or statistical outliers.

Pulse heights for the WBC, RBC, and PLT parameters are measured, categorized, and stored to generate 256-channel volume distribution histograms (Figure 13.6D).[10] The MCV and the MPV are derived from their respective volume distribution data. The hematocrit, MCH, and MCHC are calculated from the measured values. The RDW is calculated directly from the histogram as the coefficient of variation (CV) of the RBC volume distribution or as the standard deviation of the histogram (RDW-SD) in femtoliters.[10] Algorithm analysis corrects the WBC count from NRBC interference (if NRBCs are present), and the MCV and RDW are corrected for WBC interference when the WBC count exceeds a specific threshold.[10]

VCS for WBC Differential, NRBC, and Reticulocyte Analyses

For the WBC differential, NRBC, and reticulocyte analyses, a combination of technologies are used simultaneously on each cell: (1) volumetric sizing by impedance, (2) RF conductivity, and (3) optical laser light scatter (called *volume, conductivity, scatter [VCS]* technology).[10] After RBCs are lysed and WBCs are treated with a stabilizing reagent to maintain them in a near-native state, a hydrodynamically focused specimen stream is directed through a flow cell past the sensing zone. Low-frequency DC impedance measures cell volume, whereas a high-frequency electromagnetic (RF) probe measures conductivity, an indicator of cell internal contents. The conductivity signal is corrected for cellular volume, which yields a unique measurement called *opacity*.[10] Each cell is also scanned with monochromatic laser light, which reveals information about the cell surface, such as structure, shape, and reflectivity. The VCS module uses a rotated light scatter detection method derived

from five light scatter measurements: (1) axial light loss (ALL/AL2) at 0° (which reflects the amount of light deleted as a result of absorption and scatter as a cell passes through the flow cell); (2) low-angle light scatter (LALS) at 5.1°; (3) lower median-angle light scatter (LMALS) at 10° to 20°; (4) upper median-angle light scatter (UMALS) at 20° to 42°; and (5) median-angle light scatter (MALS), which is the sum of UMALS + LMALS (Figure 13.7).[10] Using all the data collected, the computer algorithms determine the optimal separation between the cell populations so each cell type can be identified and counted. Results for the WBC differential are reported as a relative count (%) and an absolute count (number of cells per microliter).

This combination of technologies can generate two- or three-dimensional dataplots for the WBC five-part differential. The dataplot of rotated light scatter (RLSn) on the *x*-axis versus volume (V) on the *y*-axis (5PD1 dataplot) allows visualization of lymphocytes, monocytes, neutrophils, and eosinophils (Figures 13.6E and 13.8).[10] Immature granulocytes, if present, are also counted for a six-part differential. Basophils are located behind the lymphocytes on this dataplot but can be visualized by plotting opacity (OP) on the *x*-axis versus volume (V) on the *y*-axis (5PD2 dataplot). A monocyte distribution width (MDW) is also available.

For NRBCs, the dataplot of axial light loss (AL2) on the *x*-axis and rotated low-angle light scatter (RLALS) on the *y*-axis (NRBC1 dataplot) separates the NRBCs from WBCs, platelets, and cell debris so they can be counted (Figure 13.6E).[10] NRBCs,

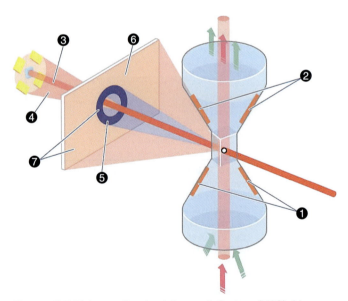

Figure 13.7 Volume, Conductivity, and Scatter (VCS) Measurements in the Beckman Coulter UniCel DxH 900. The cell enters the flow cell in a hydrodynamically focused specimen stream. As the cell passes the sensing zone, direct current impedance and radiofrequency conductivity are measured *(1,2)* in addition to five light scatter measurements: axial light loss, ALL at 0° *(3);* low-angle light scatter, LALS at 5.1° *(4);* lower median angle light scatter, LMALS at 10° to 20° *(5);* upper median-angle light scatter, UMALS at 20° to 42° *(6);* and medium-angle light scatter, MALS *(7),* which is the sum of UMALS + LMALS. (From Beckman Coulter, Inc. [2019]. UniCel DxH 900 Series with System Manager Software Coulter Cellular Analysis System. *Instructions for Use.* PN C06947AC. Brea, CA: Beckman Coulter, Inc. Figure 2.6, p. 2-10.)

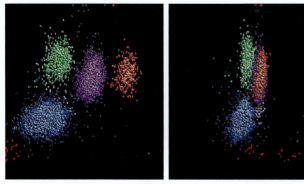

Figure 13.8 Two-Dimensional Dataplots for the Five-Part Differential on the Beckman Coulter UniCel DxH 900. Five main white blood cell populations are shown: lymphocytes *(blue)*, monocytes *(green)*, neutrophils *(purple)*, eosinophils *(orange)*, and basophils *(white)*. **(A)**, 5PD1 dataplot with rotated light scatter (RLSn) on the *x*-axis and volume (V) on the *y*-axis. **(B)**, 5PD2 dataplot with opacity (OP) on the *x*-axis and volume (V) on the *y*-axis and. (From Beckman Coulter, Inc. [2019]. UniCel DxH 900 Series with System Manager Software Coulter Cellular Analysis System. *Instructions for Use.* PN C06947AC. Brea, CA: Beckman Coulter, Inc. Figure 2.7, p. 2-11.)

when present, localize to the left of the large WBC population. An additional dataplot of axial light loss (AL2) on the *x*-axis versus rotated upper medium-angle light scatter (RUMALS) on the *y*-axis (NRBC2 dataplot) also allows visualization of the NRBC population.[10]

Reticulocytes are counted using a new methylene blue stain and VCS technology. Plotting linear light scatter (LLSn) on the x-axis versus volume (V) on the y-axis (RETIC1 dataplot) allows visualization of the reticulocyte population (Figure 13.6E).[10] The stained reticulocytes locate to the right of the mature RBC population with greater linear light scatter compared to mature RBCs. An additional dataplot of opacity (OP) on the *x*-axis versus volume (V) on the *y*-axis (RETIC2 dataplot) also visualizes the reticulocyte population.[10] Relative and absolute reticulocyte counts are reported, along with the mean reticulocyte volume (MRV) and immature reticulocyte fraction (IRF).[10] The IRF is calculated as the ratio of the reticulocytes with midrange and high light scatter to the total reticulocyte count and is reported as a fraction.[10]

Figure 13.6 represents a printout from the Beckman Coulter UniCel DxH 900 of the CBC, WBC differential, NRBC, and reticulocyte data for a patient.

Sysmex

The XN-3100 system from Sysmex Corporation, formerly TOA Medical Electronics Company, Ltd., provides the RBC, WBC, and platelet analyses listed in Box 13.1 and Figure 13.9. The analyzer uses spectrophotometry to determine the hemoglobin concentration and two different technologies for blood cell analysis: (1) DC detection and (2) fluorescence flow cytometry with multiangle scatter and fluorescence detection.[17]

Hemoglobin Determination

Spectrophotometric analysis is used for direct measurement of the hemoglobin concentration. In the hemoglobin flow cell, the RBCs are lysed and hemoglobin is oxidized and binds SLS, forming a stable SLS-hemoglobin complex, the transmittance of which is measured at 555 nm.[17]

DC Detection System for RBC Analyses and Platelet Distribution

The DC detection system is used to count and volumetrically size RBCs and platelets by the direct current resistance (impedance) method. The system features a sheathed specimen stream with hydrodynamic focusing to direct cells through the center of the aperture in single file, and a catcher tube that simultaneously pulls the specimen stream out of the flow cell.[17] This reduces coincident passage, particle volume distortion, and recirculation of blood cells around the aperture.

Particles (pulses) are counted between two discriminators (thresholds). The lower platelet discriminator is automatically adjusted in the 2- to 6-fL volume range and the upper to the 12- to 30-fL range, based on the individual specimen particle volume distribution.[17] Likewise, the RBC lower and upper discriminators are set in the 25- to 75-fL and 200- to 250-fL volume ranges, respectively.[17] These adjustable discriminators allow for the accurate counting of cell populations on a specimen-by-specimen basis and is particularly useful in separating platelets from small RBCs. The cells are displayed on a histogram (Figure 13.9E), which is checked for distribution abnormalities, and coincident passage error is accounted for in the final computer-generated results. The hematocrit also is directly measured from the RBC/platelet channel, based on the principle that the pulse heights generated by the RBCs is proportional to cell volume.[17] The hematocrit is the RBC cumulative pulse height and is considered a true relative percentage volume of erythrocytes.[17]

The MCV, MCH, MCHC, RDW-SD, RDW-CV, and MPV are calculated. RDW-SD is the RBC arithmetic distribution width measured at 20% of the height of the RBC curve, reported in femtoliters, while the RDW-CV represents 68.2% of the total RBC distribution area, reported as a percentage.[17] MPV is the average platelet volume, derived from the platelet distribution data.

Fluorescence Flow Cytometry for WBC Count, WBC Differential, NRBCs, and Reticulocyte Analyses

Fluorescence flow cytometry is used for the WBC count, WBC differential, NRBC and reticulocyte counts, and a reflex platelet count. For the WBC and NRBC counts and WBC differential, the RBCs are lysed and the WBC cell membranes are perforated to allow a fluorescent polymethine dye to penetrate the cells and bind to the intracellular nucleic acids (mostly RNA), while leaving the cells and their internal structures largely intact. A hydrodynamically focused specimen stream keeps the cells in single file as they

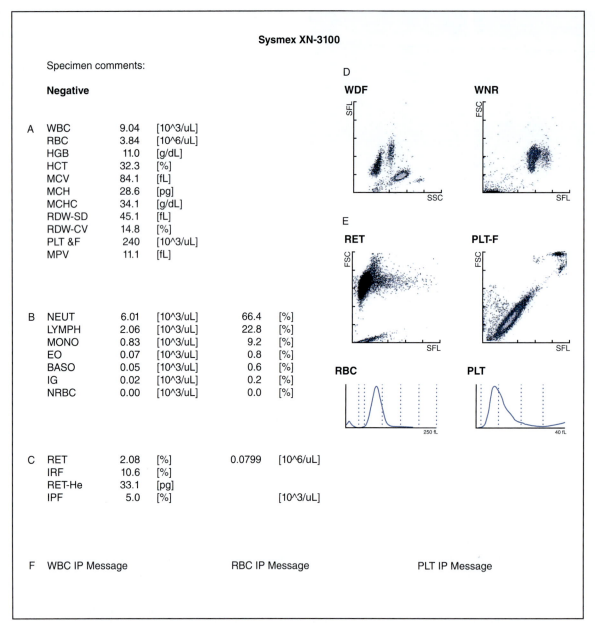

Sysmex XN-3100

Specimen comments:

Negative

A			
	WBC	9.04	[10^3/uL]
	RBC	3.84	[10^6/uL]
	HGB	11.0	[g/dL]
	HCT	32.3	[%]
	MCV	84.1	[fL]
	MCH	28.6	[pg]
	MCHC	34.1	[g/dL]
	RDW-SD	45.1	[fL]
	RDW-CV	14.8	[%]
	PLT &F	240	[10^3/uL]
	MPV	11.1	[fL]

B					
	NEUT	6.01	[10^3/uL]	66.4	[%]
	LYMPH	2.06	[10^3/uL]	22.8	[%]
	MONO	0.83	[10^3/uL]	9.2	[%]
	EO	0.07	[10^3/uL]	0.8	[%]
	BASO	0.05	[10^3/uL]	0.6	[%]
	IG	0.02	[10^3/uL]	0.2	[%]
	NRBC	0.00	[10^3/uL]	0.0	[%]

C					
	RET	2.08	[%]	0.0799	[10^6/uL]
	IRF	10.6	[%]		
	RET-He	33.1	[pg]		
	IPF	5.0	[%]		[10^3/uL]

D — WDF (SFL vs SSC) — WNR (FSC vs SFL)

E — RET (FSC vs SFL) — PLT-F (FSC vs SFL)

RBC (250 fL) — PLT (40 fL)

F   WBC IP Message   RBC IP Message   PLT IP Message

Figure 13.9 Printout from Sysmex XN-3100. The XN-3100 printout displays the complete blood count (CBC), white blood cell *(WBC)* differential, and reticulocyte data for the same patient in Figures 13.6, 13.12, and 13.15 using three other automated blood cell analyzers. **(A)**, CBC data; note the "&F" to indicate the fluorescent platelet count result. **(B)**, Six-part WBC differential including the immature granulocyte *(IG)* count, and a nucleated red blood cell *(NRBC)* count. **(C)**, Reticulocyte count *(RET)*, immature reticulocyte fraction *(IRF)*, reticulocyte hemoglobin equivalent *(RET-He)*, and immature platelet fraction *(IPF)*. **(D)**, Two scattergrams, *WDF* (lymphocytes, monocytes, neutrophils + basophils, eosinophils, and immature granulocytes, if present) and *WNR* (white blood cell count, basophils, and NRBCs). **(E)**, RET and platelet *(PLT-F)* scattergrams, and red blood cell *(RBC)* and PLT impedance histograms. **(F)**, Specimen-related flags are listed at the bottom of the printout, if any are generated. *BASO,* Basophils; *EO,* eosinophils; *HCT,* hematocrit; *HGB,* hemoglobin concentration; *IPF,* immature platelet fraction; *IRF,* immature reticulocyte fraction; *LYMPH,* lymphocytes; *MCH,* mean cell hemoglobin; *MCHC,* mean cell hemoglobin concentration; *MCV,* mean cell volume; *MONO,* monocytes; *MPV,* mean platelet volume; *NEUT,* neutrophils; *NRBC,* nucleated red blood cell count; *PLT,* platelet count; *RBC,* red blood cell count; *RDW-CV,* red cell distribution width coefficient of variation; *RDW-SD,* red cell distribution width standard deviation; *RET,* reticulocyte count; *RET-He,* reticulocyte hemoglobin equivalent; *WBC,* white blood cell count.

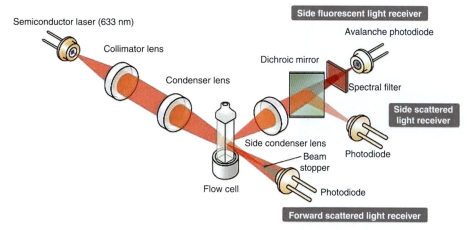

Figure 13.10 Optical Measurements in the Sysmex XN-Series. The cell suspension is stained with a fluorescent dye and enters the flow cell in a hydrodynamically focused specimen stream. As cells enter the sensing zone in the flow cell, they pass by a semiconductor laser beam, and forward scatter, side scatter, and side fluorescent light are detected. Forward scatter determines cell volume or size, side scatter measures cell contents, and side fluorescent light measures the amount of cellular nucleic acids. A dichroic mirror directs the side scatter to the side-scatter photodiode detector. The beam stopper prevents the semiconductor laser beam from reaching the forward-scatter photodiode detector. (Courtesy Sysmex Corporation.)

pass through the flow cell and sensing zone.[17,22] When a 633-nm semiconductor laser light hits the cell, three detectors measure: (1) forward scatter (FSC), which reflects cell volume; (2) side scatter (SSC), which depends on internal cell structures; and (3) side fluorescent light (SFL) in which the intensity of the fluorescence is proportional to the amount of nucleic acids in the cell (Figure 13.10).[17] The scatter signals are depicted on two-dimensional scattergrams (WDF, WNR, and WPC) in which cells with similar characteristics are separated and located to specific areas of the scattergram using algorithms.[17] The system provides a five-part differential in relative and absolute counts and also flags abnormal WBC populations.[22]

In the WDF channel, plotting SSC on the x-axis and SFL on the y-axis enables separation and counting of lymphocytes, monocytes, eosinophils, and neutrophils + basophils (Figures 13.9D and 13.11).[17,22] An immature granulocyte population is also reported when present. In the WNR channel, plotting SFL on the x-axis and FSC on the y-axis enables the determination of the total WBC count, basophils, and NRBCs (Figure 13.9D).[17,22] WBCs with high fluorescence intensity are separated from the NRBCs with low fluorescence intensity. NRBCs are excluded from the WBC count when they are present in the specimen. The WPC channel does not report WBC counts but is used to detect immature and abnormal cells for specimens flagged in the other channels.[17,22] It uses the concept of differential lysis in that the lysing reagent does not perforate the membrane of blasts and immature cells to the extent of mature cells because of differences in the lipid composition of their membrane.[22]

Therefore immature cells contain less fluorescent dye and generate lower fluorescent signals and less SSC on a scattergram that plots SSC on the x-axis and SFL on the y-axis (scatterplot not shown).[17,22]

For the reticulocyte analysis, cells are treated with a fluorescent polymethine dye and a lysis reagent to slightly perforate the membranes, which allows the dye to penetrate the cells and stain the RNA.[17,22] In the RET channel, plotting SFL on the x-axis and FSC on the y-axis enables separation of the mature RBCs from the reticulocyte population, which locates to the right on the scattergram due to their fluorescence staining (Figure 13.9E).[17] This allows for measurement of the reticulocyte count as a percentage of the total RBC population as well as the absolute reticulocyte count. The reticulocytes are further separated into low-fluorescence, medium-fluorescence, and high-fluorescence regions, with the less mature reticulocytes showing higher fluorescence.[22] The IRF is the sum of the medium- and high-fluorescence regions and indicates the ratio of immature reticulocytes to total reticulocytes in a specimen, reported as a percentage. The reticulocyte hemoglobin equivalent (RET-He) or the hemoglobin content of the reticulocytes is also measured using light scatter signals and is reported in picograms.[17,22]

The analyzer also provides for a reflex fluorescent platelet count (PLT-F) if the DC resistance platelet count is flagged as unreliable, particularly with severely low platelet counts. Cells are treated with a platelet-specific fluorescent oxazine dye that minimizes interference from other cells and particles of similar volume, and a lysis reagent to slightly perforate the platelet membranes to allow the dye to penetrate the cells and stain the

WDF scattergram

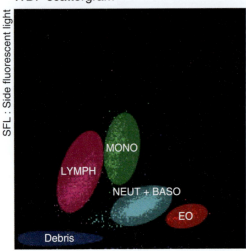

Figure 13.11 Two-Dimensional WDF Scattergram for the Five-Part Differential on the Sysmex XN-3100. The scattergram is a plot of the side scatter (SSC) on the x-axis and side fluorescent light (SFL) on the y-axis. Five main white blood cell populations are shown: lymphocytes (LYMPH, pink), monocytes (MONO, green), neutrophils + basophils (NEUT, BASO, aqua), and eosinophils (EO, red). (Courtesy Sysmex Corporation.)

RNA.[17,22] In the PLT-F channel, plotting SFL on the x-axis and FSC on the y-axis enables separation of the platelets from other cells and cell debris (Figure 13.9E).[17] The analyzer also calculates an immature platelet fraction (IPF) as the ratio of platelets with high fluorescent light intensity (most immature) to the total platelet count, and it is reported as a percentage and an absolute count.[17]

Figure 13.9 represents a printout from the Sysmex XN-3100 of the CBC, WBC differential, NRBC, and reticulocyte data for the same patient specimen for which data are given in Figure 13.6.

Abbott

Abbott's CELL-DYN Sapphire provides the RBC, WBC, and platelet analyses listed in Box 13.1 and Figure 13.12. The analyzer uses spectrophotometry to determine the hemoglobin concentration and two different technologies for blood cell analysis: (1) impedance and (2) multiangle laser light scatter with fluorescence detection.

Hemoglobin Determination

Spectrophotometric analysis is used for direct measurement of hemoglobin concentration using a noncyanide reagent that forms a hemoglobin-imidazole complex and is measured at 544 nm with a blank.[18]

Impedance for RBC and Platelet Analysis

The primary RBC count is performed using impedance technology.[18] The cells are subjected to isovolumetric sphering and

are volumetrically sized as they pass through an aperture with hydrodynamic focusing.[7] The pulse signals are displayed on a volume distribution histogram. An optical light scatter RBC analysis is used as a quality check. A secondary platelet count is also performed using impedance, whereas the primary platelet count uses optical technology.[18] The MCV and MPV are derived from RBC and platelet volume distribution histograms, respectively.[18]

Proprietary technology is used to minimize the effect of recirculating cells around the aperture. Pulses are collected and sorted in 256 channels according to their amplitudes: particles between 1 and 35 fL are included in the initial platelet data, and particles greater than 35 fL are counted as RBCs.[18] Floating thresholds are used to determine the best separation of the platelet population and to eliminate interference, such as noise, debris, or small RBCs, from the count. Coincident passage loss is corrected for in the final RBC and platelet counts. Pulse editing is applied before MCV and MPV derivation to compensate for aberrant pulses produced by nonaxial passage of cells through the aperture.

The hematocrit, MCH, and MCHC are calculated from the directly measured or derived parameters. The RDW, as a CV, is derived from the RBC histogram.[18]

MAPSS for WBC Count, WBC Differential, NRBC, Platelet, and Reticulocyte Analysis

The WBC count and differential, and the NRBC, platelet, and reticulocyte counts are derived from the optical channel using multiangle polarized scatter separation (MAPSS) technology at four angles with three-color fluorescent detection.[18] A hydrodynamically focused specimen stream is directed through a flow cell past a 488-nm laser light source. Scattered light is measured at four angles: (1) 0° forward light scatter (axial light loss [ALL]) for determination of cell volume; (2) 7° intermediate angle scatter (IAS) scatter for determination of cellular complexity (the greater the complexity, the greater the scatter); (3) 90° polarized side scatter (PSS) for determination of nuclear lobularity/segmentation; and (4) 90° depolarized side scatter (DSS) for determination of cellular granularity, specifically to distinguish neutrophils from eosinophils.[18,23] Figure 13.13 illustrates the MAPSS technology. Two detectors measure FSC at 0° and 7°. Three additional detectors measure the 90° scatter signals and/or fluorescence at specific wavelengths as follows: (1) 90° D scatter and 530-nm green fluorescence (FL1), (2) 90° scatter and 570-nm orange fluorescence (FL2), and (3) 630-nm red fluorescence (FL3).[18]

The light scatter signals are converted into electrical signals and presented graphically as scatterplots. Plotting complexity (7° scatter) on the x-axis versus lobularity (90° scatter) on the y-axis yields separation of mononuclear and polymorphonuclear subpopulations (scatterplot not shown). Plotting the polymorphonuclear subpopulation with lobularity (90° scatter) on the x-axis and granularity (90° depolarized) on the y-axis allows

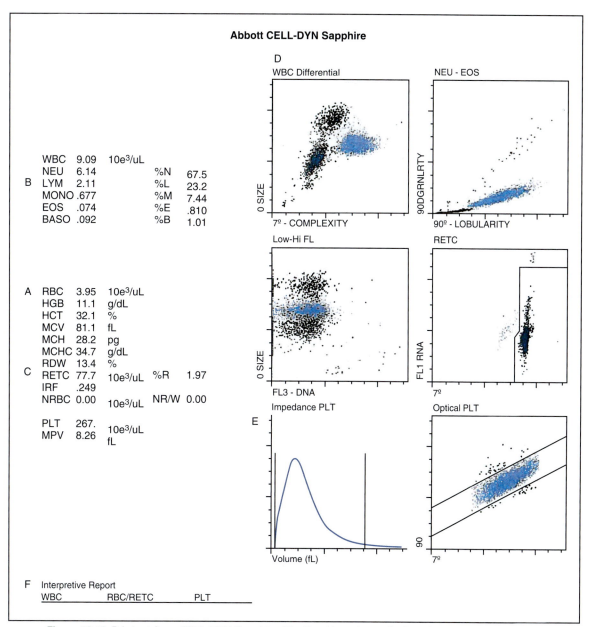

Abbott CELL-DYN Sapphire

B	WBC	9.09	10e³/uL		
	NEU	6.14		%N	67.5
	LYM	2.11		%L	23.2
	MONO	.677		%M	7.44
	EOS	.074		%E	.810
	BASO	.092		%B	1.01

A	RBC	3.95	10e³/uL		
	HGB	11.1	g/dL		
	HCT	32.1	%		
	MCV	81.1	fL		
	MCH	28.2	pg		
	MCHC	34.7	g/dL		
	RDW	13.4	%		
C	RETC	77.7	10e³/uL	%R	1.97
	IRF	.249			
	NRBC	0.00	10e³/uL	NR/W	0.00
	PLT	267.	10e³/uL		
	MPV	8.26	fL		

F Interpretive Report
WBC　　　RBC/RETC　　　PLT

Figure 13.12 Printout from CELL-DYN Sapphire. The Sapphire printout displays the complete blood count (CBC), white blood cell *(WBC)* differential, and reticulocyte data for the same patient in Figures 13.6, 13.9, and 13.15 using three other automated blood cell analyzers. **(A)**, CBC data. **(B)**, WBC differential count data. Note that the WBC count is listed with the differential instead of the CBC data. **(C)**, Reticulocyte count *(RETC)*, immature reticulocyte fraction *(IRF)*, nucleated red blood cell *(NRBC)* count, platelet count *(PLT)*, and mean platelet volume *(MPV)*. **(D)**, Scatterplot for the *WBC differential* with 7° scatter (complexity) on the x-axis and 0° scatter (size or volume) on the y-axis; and scatterplot to distinguish neutrophils from eosinophils *(NEU–EOS)* with 90° scatter (lobularity) on the x-axis and 90° depolarized (90D) scatter (granularity) on the y-axis; scatterplot for NRBCs *(Low-Hi FL)* with DNA fluorescence (FL3-DNA) on the x-axis and 0° scatter (size or volume) on the y-axis; and a scatterplot for reticulocytes *(RETC)* with 7° scatter (complexity) on the x-axis and RNA fluorescence (FL1RNA) on the y-axis. **(E)**, Impedance platelet histogram and optical platelet scatterplot with 7° scatter (complexity) on the x-axis and 90° scatter on the y-axis. **(F)**, Interpretative report comments are listed at the bottom of the printout if any are generated for the specimen. *BASO,* Basophils; *EOS,* eosinophils; *HCT,* hematocrit; *HGB,* hemoglobin concentration; *IRF,* immature reticulocyte fraction; *LYM,* lymphocytes; *MCH,* mean cell hemoglobin; *MCHC,* mean cell hemoglobin concentration; *MCV,* mean cell volume; *MONO,* monocytes; *MPV,* mean platelet volume; *NEU,* neutrophils; *NRBC,* nucleated red blood cell count; *PLT,* platelet count; *RBC,* red blood cell count; *RDW,* red cell distribution width coefficient of variation; *RETC,* reticulocyte count; *WBC,* white blood cell count.

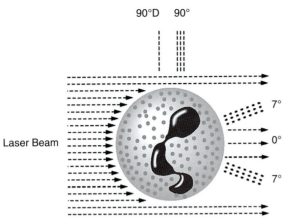

Figure 13.13 Multiangle Polarized Scatter Separation (MAPSS) Technology in Abbott Cell-Dyn Sapphire. Light scatter signals are measured at four different angles to classify white blood cell populations: 0° forward light scatter measures cell volume or size; 7° intermediate angle scatter measures cell complexity; 90° polarized side scatter measures nuclear lobularity; and 90° depolarized side scatter measures granularity. (CELL-DYN is a trademark of Abbott or its related companies. Reproduced with permission of Abbott, © 2023. All rights reserved.)

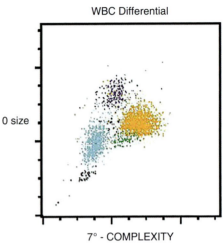

Figure 13.14 Two-Dimensional Scatterplot for the Five-Part Differential on the CELL-DYN Sapphire. Multiangle polarized scatter separation (MAPSS) technology is used to display the five major white blood cell (WBC) populations by plotting 7° scatter (complexity) on the *x*-axis and 0° scatter (size or volume) on the *y*-axis. Shown in the scatterplot are the lymphocytes (*aqua*), monocytes (*purple*), neutrophils (*orange*), eosinophils (*green*), and basophils (*black*). (CELL-DYN is a trademark of Abbott or its related companies. Reproduced with permission of Abbott, © 2023. All rights reserved.)

separation of eosinophils from neutrophils because of the unique nature of eosinophil granules, which scatter more 90° depolarized light (Figure 13.12D). Plotting complexity (7° scatter) on the *x*-axis versus size (0° scatter) on the *y*-axis displays five WBC populations: neutrophils, lymphocytes, monocytes, eosinophils, and basophils (Figures 13.12D and 13.14).[18,23] An immature granulocyte population also can be determined for a six-part differential. Absolute and relative counts of each WBC type are reported.

NRBCs are separated from WBCs and counted using light scatter and DNA fluorescence detectors. They are visualized by plotting the 630-nm red fluorescence (FL3 DNA) on the *x*-axis and size (0° scatter) on the *y*-axis as a population to the right of the scatterplot (Figure 13.12D). NRBCs are reported as the absolute number of cells per microliter and as the number per 100 WBCs (NR/W).[18]

The primary platelet count is determined using MAPSS technology (optical platelet count).[18] Platelets are separated from RBCs and identified and counted using two-angle light scatter and fluorescent detectors that provide information on cell volume and internal contents. Platelets are visualized by plotting 7° light scatter on the *x*-axis and 90° light scatter on the *y*-axis (Figure 13.12E). The MPV is derived from the impedance platelet distribution histogram.[18] An optical analysis of the RBC population is done at the same time and is used as a quality control check for the impedance RBC count, and an impedance platelet count is done as a quality check of the optical count.[18]

Further analysis of platelets can be performed using a CD61 monoclonal antibody to generate a more accurate immunoplatelet count when the platelet count is low or when there is suspected interference from nonplatelet cell debris.[18] CD61 is the GPIIIa antigen specific for the platelet membrane (Chapter 11). The reagent contains a CD61 monoclonal antibody tagged with fluorescein isothiocyanate fluorescent dye. The antibody binds specifically with the CD61 antigen on the platelet membrane, and the platelets are counted by applying an algorithm using detectors for the 7° and 90° light scatter and the 530-nm green fluorescence (FL1).[18] The immunoplatelet count, if done, replaces the optical count on the CBC report.

Reticulocytes are identified and counted using 7° light scatter and RNA fluorescence (FL1) detectors.[18] They are separated from mature RBCs and visualized by plotting complexity (7° scatter) on the *x*-axis versus the intensity of RNA staining with 530-nm green fluorescence (FL1 RNA) on the *y*-axis (Figure 13.12D). They are reported as the absolute number of cells per microliter and as a percent of the total number of RBCs determined by impedance. Because the intensity of fluorescence corresponds to reticulocyte immaturity, an IRF is determined as the fraction of reticulocytes that exceed a specific level of FL1 fluorescence.[18]

As on the previously described analyzers, user-defined distributional flags may be set, and analyzer-specific suspect flags may alert the operator to the presence of abnormal cells.

The next-generation Abbott analyzer, Alinity hq, uses only optical and fluorescent flow cytometry technologies for blood cell analysis. Along with a fluorescence detector (FL1), it uses advanced MAPSS to measure seven angles of light scatter: the four standard MAPSS detectors (ALL, IAS, PSS, and DSS) plus three narrow-angle light scatter detectors IAS1

(2.4° to 4.5°), IAS2 (4.7° to 5.7°), and IAS3 (5.9° to 7.6°).[7,23] The additional light scatter signals enables the assessment of mean cell hemoglobin content of RBCs and reticulocytes, RBC fragment flagging, and percent reticulated platelets.[7] The Alinity hq is not yet available in the United States at the time of this writing.

Figure 13.12 represents a printout from the CELL-DYN Sapphire of the CBC, WBC differential, NRBC, and reticulocyte data for the same patient specimen for which data are given in Figures 13.6 and 13.9.

Siemens Healthineers

The ADVIA 2120/2020i from Siemens Healthineers (formerly Siemens Healthcare Diagnostics) provides the RBC, WBC, and platelet analyses listed in Box 13.1 and Figure 13.15. The analyzer uses spectrophotometry to determine hemoglobin concentration and two types of technologies for blood cell analysis: (1) light scatter and (2) cytochemistry. Four independent measurement channels are used in determining the CBC, differential, and reticulocyte analyses: hemoglobin channel, RBC/platelet channel, and peroxidase and basophil-lobularity (BASO) channels.[19]

Hemoglobin Determination

Spectrophotometric analysis is used for direct measurement of hemoglobin concentration in a hemoglobin channel using a modified cyanohemoglobin method measuring light transmittance at 546 nm. A noncyanide reagent is also available that forms monoaquomonohydroxyferri-porphyrin as the reaction product which is measured at 565 nm.[19]

Light Scatter for RBC and Platelet Analyses

Laser light scatter technology is used for RBC and platelet counting and analyses. The RBCs and platelets are isovolumetrically sphered in the diluting reagent to eliminate optical orientation error in the flow cell. The specimen stream is hydrodynamically focused so that the cells enter the flow cell in single file past a laser optical assembly (laser diode light source). As each cell passes the laser beam, light scatter is measured simultaneously at two different angles: low angle (2° to 3°), correlating with cell volume, and high angle (5° to 15°), correlating with internal complexity (refractive index or hemoglobin content) (Figure 13.16).[19] This differential scatter technique, in combination with isovolumetric sphering, eliminates the adverse effect of variation in cellular hemoglobin content on the determination of RBC volume (as seen by differences in cellular deformability affecting the pulse height generated on impedance analyzers).[19]

The RBC scatter signals are plotted on a RBC cytogram (nonlinear RBC map) with high-angle light scatter (hemoglobin concentration) on the x-axis and low-angle light scatter (volume) on the y-axis. To allow easier visual assessment of the RBC population, the RBC map is converted to a linear volume/hemoglobin concentration (V/HC) cytogram with the same coordinates.[19] The RBC V/HC cytogram is divided into nine sectors separated on the x-axis by low- and high-hemoglobin

content markers at 28 and 41 g/dL, respectively, and on the y-axis by low- and high-volume markers at 60 and 120 fL, respectively (Figure 13.15E). RBCs that are normocytic and normochromic will locate in the center of the cytogram. RBC populations that cluster to the left of the low hemoglobin concentration (28 g/dL) marker are hypochromic, whereas those to the right of the high (41 g/dL) marker are reported as hyperchromic. Similarly, RBC populations below the low volume (60 fL) marker are microcytic, whereas those above the high volume (120 fL) marker are macrocytic. Independent histograms of RBC volume and RBC hemoglobin content (RBC HC) are also plotted, with the same volume and hemoglobin concentration markers for visual assessment of the RBC population (Figure 13.15D).[19]

The platelet scatter signals are counted and volumetrically sized using the same two-dimensional (low-angle and high-angle) scatter but at a higher gain that amplifies the signals. This allows better discrimination of platelets from interfering particles, such as RBC fragments and small RBCs. The scatter settings can also include platelets as large as 60 fL in the count.[19] A platelet volume distribution histogram is also plotted from the scatter signals (Figure 13.15D).

Several parameters and indices are derived from the measurements described in the previous paragraphs.[19] MCV and MPV are the mean of the RBC volume histogram and the platelet volume histogram, respectively. Hematocrit, MCH, and MCHC are mathematically computed using RBC, hemoglobin, and MCV values. RDW is calculated as the CV of the RBC volume histogram, whereas a hemoglobin distribution width (HDW), an analogous index, is calculated as the SD of the RBC hemoglobin content histogram (RBC HC). The mean cellular hemoglobin content (CH) in picograms is the mean of the RBC HC histogram. The percent microcytic, macrocytic, hypochromic, and hyperchromic cells are calculated from the RBC volume and RBC HC histograms.[19] The mean cell hemoglobin concentration (CHCM), analogous to MCHC, is derived from cell-by-cell direct scatter measures of hemoglobin concentration. Interferences with the hemoglobin colorimetric method, such as lipemia or icterus, affect the calculated MCHC but do not alter the measured CHCM. CHCM generally is not reported as a patient result but is used by the analyzer as an internal check for the MCHC and is available to the operator for calculating the cellular HGB if interferences are present.[19]

Cytochemistry and Light Scatter for WBC Count, WBC Differential, NRBCs, and Reticulocyte Analysis

Cytochemistry and optical light scatter in the PEROX and BASO channels are used to determine the WBC count and a six-part WBC differential, including neutrophils, lymphocytes, monocytes, eosinophils, basophils, and large unstained cells (LUCs). LUCs include reactive or variant lymphocytes and blasts. NRBCs and reticulocytes are also counted.[19]

In the PEROX channel, RBCs are lysed, and WBCs are stained for their peroxidase activity. The following reaction is

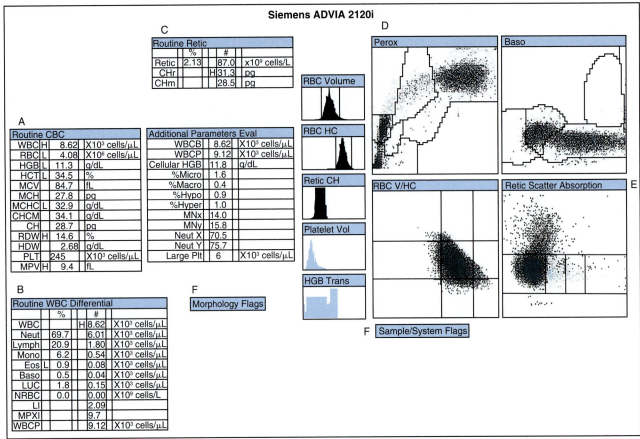

Figure 13.15 Printout from ADVIA 2120i. The printout displays the complete blood count (CBC), white blood cell *(WBC)* differential, and reticulocyte data for the same patient in Figures 13.6, 13.9, and 13.12. using three other automated blood cell analyzers. **(A)**, CBC data. **(B)**, Six-part differential, including large unstained cells *(LUC)* and nucleated red blood cells *(NRBC)*. **(C)**, Reticulocyte data including the reticulocyte count *(Retic)*, mean cell hemoglobin content of reticulocytes *(CHr)*, and mean cell hemoglobin content of the mature red blood cell population *(CHm)*. **(D)**, In the cytograms for the differential, the peroxidase *(Perox)* cytogram plots peroxidase absorbance on the *x*-axis and light scatter on the *y*-axis. In the basophil *(Baso)* cytogram, high-angle light scatter is plotted on the *x*-axis and low-angle scatter on the *y*-axis. In addition, distribution histograms of red blood cell *(RBC)* volume, hemoglobin content of mature RBCs *(RBC HC)*, hemoglobin content of mature RBCs overlaid with hemoglobin content of reticulocytes *(Retic CH)*, and platelet volume *(Vol)* are displayed. **(E)**, The *RBC* volume/hemoglobin concentration *(V/HC)* cytogram is divided into nine sectors separated on the *x*-axis by low- and high-hemoglobin content markers at 28 g/dL and 41 g/dL, respectively, and on the *y*-axis by low- and high-volume markers at 60 fL and 120 fL, respectively. The *Retic Scatter Absorption* cytogram is plotted with the absorption of cellular RNA with oxazine 750 on the *x*-axis and high-angle light scatter on the *y*-axis. **(F)**, Morphology and specimen/system flags are displayed on the bottom right of the printout, if any are generated for the specimen. *Baso*, Basophils; *Eos*, eosinophils; *CHCM*, mean cell hemoglobin concentration; *Chm*, mean cell hemoglobin content of the mature red blood cell population; *Chr*, mean cell hemoglobin content of reticulocytes; *Eos*, eosinophils; *HCT*, hematocrit; *HDW*, hemoglobin distribution width; *HGB*, hemoglobin concentration; *Lymph*, lymphocytes; *LUC*, large unstained cells; *MCH*, mean cell hemoglobin; *MCHC*, mean cell hemoglobin concentration; *MCV*, mean cell volume; *Mono*, monocytes; *MPV*, mean platelet volume; *Neut*, neutrophils; *NRBC*, nucleated red blood cell count; *PLT*, platelet count; *RBC*, red blood cell count; *RDW*, red cell distribution width; *Retic*, reticulocyte count; *WBCB*, WBC count in the Baso channel; *WBCP*, WBC count in the Perox channel.

catalyzed by cellular peroxidase, which converts the substrate to a dark precipitate in peroxidase-containing cells (neutrophils, monocytes, and eosinophils).[19]

$$H_2O_2 + \text{4-chloro-1-naphthol} \xrightarrow{\text{cellular peroxidese}} \text{dark precipitate}$$

A portion of the cell suspension is fed to a sheath-stream flow cell where a tungsten-halogen darkfield optics system is used to measure absorbance (proportional to the amount of peroxidase in each cell) and FSC (proportional to the volume of each cell).[19] Absorbance is plotted on the *x*-axis of the cytogram, and scatter is plotted on the *y*-axis (Figures 13.15D and 13.17). A total WBC count is also obtained from the optical signals in the PEROX channel (WBCP) and is used as an internal check of the primary WBC count obtained in the BASO channel (WBCB). If significant interference occurs in the WBCB count, the analyzer substitutes the WBCP value.[19]

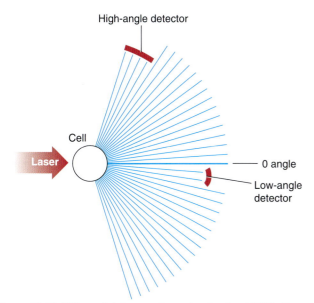

Figure 13.16 Differential Scatter Detection in the ADVIA. Forward low-angle scatter (2° to 3° correlating to cell volume) and forward high-angle scatter (5° to 15° correlating to internal complexity: refractive index or hemoglobin content) are measured for analysis of red blood cells and platelets. (From Technicon. [1993]. *Technicon H Systems Training Guide*. Tarrytown, NY: Technicon.)

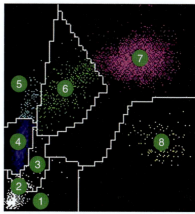

Figure 13.17 Cytogram for the Peroxidase (PEROX) Channel from the ADVIA 2120i. Blood is mixed with a reagent containing H_2O_2 and 4-chloro-1-naphthol, which reacts with the peroxidase in neutrophils, eosinophils, and monocytes, forming a dark precipitate. Detectors measure absorbance, which is proportional to the amount of peroxidase in each cell (plotted on the x-axis) and forward scatter, which is proportional to the volume of each cell (plotted on the y-axis) generating the PEROX cytogram. *1*, Noise; *2*, nucleated red blood cells; *3*, platelet clumps; *4*, lymphocytes and basophils; *5*, large unstained cells; *6*, monocytes; *7*, neutrophils; *8*, eosinophils. Basophils are counted in the basophil (BASO) channel and that value is excluded from the lymphocyte/basophil cluster to obtain the lymphocyte count. (From Siemens Healthcare Diagnostics Inc. [2010]. *ADVIA 2120/2120i Hematology Systems Operator's Guide* 067D0157-01. Tarrytown, NY: Siemens Healthcare Diagnostics Inc., p. 8-29.)

Computerized cluster analysis allows classification of the different cell populations, including abnormal clusters such as NRBCs and platelet clumps.[19] Neutrophils and eosinophils contain the most peroxidase and cluster to the right on the cytogram. Monocytes stain weakly and cluster in the midregion of the cytogram. Lymphocytes, basophils, and LUCs (including variant or reactive lymphocytes and blasts) contain no peroxidase and appear on the left of the cytogram, with LUCs appearing above the lymphocyte area. Basophils cluster with the small lymphocytes. Basophils are counted in the BASO channel and that value is excluded from the lymphocyte/basophil cluster to obtain the lymphocyte count. Absolute counts for each cell are determined and the relative (%) count is calculated. Immature granulocytes have a high volume and high peroxidase activity and appear on the right side of the neutrophil area. A mean peroxidase activity index (MPXI) reflects the staining intensity of the neutrophil population.[19] A limitation of this method is the inability to determine an accurate WBC differential and neutrophil count in patients with myeloperoxidase deficiency (Chapter 26). In such cases, the results are flagged and a manual WBC differential should be performed.[19]

In the BASO channel, cells are treated with a reagent containing a nonionic surfactant in an acidic solution. The reagent uses differential lysis in that basophils are particularly resistant to lysis in this temperature-controlled reaction, while RBCs and platelets lyse and other leukocytes (nonbasophils) are stripped of their cytoplasm.[19] Laser optics, using the same two-angle (2° to 3° and 5° to 15°) FSC system of the RBC/platelet channel, is used to analyze the treated cells. High-angle scatter (proportional to nuclear complexity) is plotted on the x-axis, and low-angle scatter (proportional to cell volume) is plotted on the y-axis. The intact basophils are identifiable by their large low-angle scatter and locate above a horizontal threshold on the BASO cytogram (Figure 13.15D).[19] The stripped nuclei of the other WBCs cluster according to their nuclear complexity and high-angle scatter. On the BASO cytogram, they locate below the basophils, with segmented cells to the right and mononuclear cells to the left along the x-axis. Blast cells cluster uniquely below the mononuclear cells. As previously noted, this channel provides the primary WBC count (WBCB).[19]

NRBCs are identified by their nuclear volume in the PEROX channel and nuclear density in the BASO channel.[19] These characteristics allow counting in the PEROX and BASO channels, and algorithms are applied to determine the absolute number and percentage of NRBCs. If NRBCs are present, the WBC count is automatically corrected.

Information from the PEROX and BASO channels is used to generate differential morphology flags indicating the possible presence of reactive lymphocytes, blasts, left shift, immature granulocytes, NRBCs, large platelets, or platelet clumps.[19]

Reticulocytes are counted in the RBC/platelet and BASO channels. The reticulocyte reagent isovolumetrically spheres the cells and stains the RNA of reticulocytes with oxazine 750, while mature RBCs do not stain.[19] As the cells in the hydrodynamically focused specimen stream pass through the flow cell, three detectors simultaneously measure low-angle scatter (2° to 3°) or volume, high-angle scatter (5° to 15°) or hemoglobin content, and absorption that is proportional to RNA content.

The retic scatter absorption cytogram is plotted with high-gain absorption of cellular RNA (cell maturation) on the x-axis versus high-angle, low-gain light scatter (cell volume) on the y-axis (Figure 13.15E).[19] This allows separation of reticulocytes (with increasing amounts of RNA with immaturity) from mature RBCs. The light scatter and the difference in absorption between the reticulocyte and mature RBC populations allows determination of the absolute number of reticulocytes per microliter and percent reticulocytes of the total RBC population. The cytogram has four subdivisions along the x-axis, going from left to right: mature RBCs, low-absorbing reticulocytes, medium-absorbing reticulocytes, and high-absorbing reticulocytes based on amount of cellular RNA. The sum of the medium-absorbing and high-absorbing cells is used to calculate the IRF.[19]

A hemoglobin content histogram (Retic CH) plots the weight of hemoglobin (in picograms) in each cell and displays the distribution of the cellular hemoglobin content of mature RBCs overlaid with the distribution of cellular hemoglobin content of reticulocytes (Figure 13.15D). Derived from this retic CH histogram are the mean cell hemoglobin content of the reticulocyte population (CHr) and the mean cell hemoglobin content of the mature RBC population (CHm).[19]

Other histograms and cytograms may be generated for quality assessment and provide unique reticulocyte indices that are not reported but may be used by the operator to further analyze the results.

Figure 13.15 represents a printout from the ADVIA 2120i of the CBC, WBC differential, NRBC, and reticulocyte data for the same patient specimen for which data are given in Figures 13.6, 13.9, and 13.12.

VALIDATION AND CALIBRATION OF AUTOMATED ANALYZERS

Implementing automation in the hematology laboratory requires critical evaluation of the analyzer's methods and limitations and the performance goals for the individual laboratory. The Clinical and Laboratory Standards Institute (CLSI) has an approved standard for evaluation of the differential count using a reference procedure[24] and guidelines for performance and evaluation of automated reticulocyte counting.[25] In addition, CLSI has an approved standard for validation, verification, and quality assurance of automated hematology analyzers.[26] This standard provides guidelines for analyzer calibration and assessment of performance criteria, including accuracy, precision, linearity, sensitivity, and specificity. The International Council for Standardization in Haematology (ICSH) also publishes guidelines for the evaluation of blood cell analyzers, including the CBC, WBC differential, and reticulocyte counting.[27] The clinical accuracy (sensitivity and specificity) of the methods should be such that the analyzer appropriately identifies patients who have disease and patients who do not have disease.[28] Quality control systems should reflect the laboratory's established performance goals and provide a high level of assurance that the analyzer is working within its specified limits.

Calibration is crucial in defining the accuracy of the data produced (Chapter 3). Calibration, or the process of electronically correcting an analyzer for analytical bias (numerical difference from the "true" value), may be accomplished by appropriate use of reference methods, reference materials, or commercially prepared calibrators.[26] Because few analyzers are precalibrated by the manufacturer, calibration must be performed at initial installation and verified at least every 6 months under the requirements of the Clinical Laboratory Improvement Act of 1988.[29] Periodic recalibration may be required after major analyzer repair requiring optical alignment or part replacement.

Whole blood calibration using fresh whole blood specimens requires the use of reference methods, materials, and procedures to determine "true" values.[30,31] The ICSH established guidelines for selecting a reference blood cell analyzer for this purpose,[27] but the cyanmethemoglobin method remains the only standard available in hematology for calibration and quality control.[20,32] Whole blood calibration, which historically has been considered the preferred method for calibration of multichannel automated blood cell analyzers, has been almost completely replaced by the use of commercial calibrators assayed using reference methods. Calibration bias is possible with the use of these calibrators because of inherent differences in stabilized and preserved cell suspensions.[33] It is essential that calibrations be carried out properly and verified by comparison with reference methods or review of quality control data after calibration and by external comparison studies such as proficiency testing.

LIMITATIONS AND INTERFERENCES

The continual improvement of automated technologies has resulted in greater sensitivity and specificity of analyzer flagging for detection of possible interferences in the data. The parallel improvement in walkaway capabilities has increased the importance of laboratory professionals' awareness and understanding of analyzer limitations, however, and of their ability to recognize factors that may interfere and cause erroneous test results. Limitations and interferences may be related to methodology or to inherent problems in the blood specimen. The more common problems are discussed below. Table 13.2 is a composite of conditions that cause interference on automated blood cell analyzers and offers action plans for obtaining correct test results.[10,17–19,34–37]

Limitations of Impedance Technology

Each analyzer has limitations related to methodology that are defined in the operation manual and in the literature. A common limitation of impedance methods alone is the analyzer's inability to reliably distinguish cells from other particles or cell fragments of the same volume. Examples include very small RBCs, RBC fragments (schistocytes), and WBC fragments (post chemotherapy) being counted as platelets and falsely increasing the platelet count. Conversely, large/giant platelets and platelet clumps may exceed the platelet threshold for counting and instead be counted as WBCs, resulting in a falsely decreased platelet count and potentially increasing the WBC count. Other examples include NRBCs and micromegakaryocytes being counted as WBCs and high WBC counts causing falsely increased RBC counts. These interferences can be minimized by combining impedance with other technologies, such as RF conductivity or light scatter that is sensitive to internal cell contents. Using multiangle light scatter, with or without cytochemical or fluorescent staining, assesses cell volume and internal cell contents to minimize these interferences. All four major analyzers count and report NRBCs and exclude them from the WBC count.

Errors in Hemoglobin Determination

In the hemoglobin determination, because of the spectrophotometric measurement, turbidity of the specimen after the RBCs are lysed can falsely increase the hemoglobin concentration. This may

TABLE 13.2   Composite of Conditions That Cause Interference on Automated Blood Cell Analyzers

Condition	Parameters Falsely Affected*	Rationale	Analyzer Indicators	Corrective Action
RBC agglutination	↓ RBC; ↑ MCV, MCHC	Agglutination of RBCs due to cold-reacting antibody; agglutinates of RBCs counted as one large cell	Flags; noncompliance with rule of three†; abnormal RBC and WBC histograms, dataplots, scattergrams, scatterplots, or cytograms	Check peripheral blood film for RBC agglutination; incubate specimen for 10–15 minutes at 37° C and repeat analysis
Severe lipemia	↑ HGB, MCH, MCHC	Causes turbidity and falsely increases spectrophotometric reading for HGB	Flags; noncompliance with rule of three†	Perform saline replacement and repeat analysis; use a plasma blank to correct for excess turbidity; CHCM (Siemens) not affected
Severe hyperbilirubinemia (serum bilirubin > 25–35 mg/dL)	↑ HGB, MCH, MCHC	Bilirubin falsely increases spectrophotometric reading for HGB	Flags; noncompliance with rule of three†	Dilute specimen with isotonic saline, repeat analysis, and correct for dilution; CHCM (Siemens) not affected
Cryoproteins, cryoglobulins	↑ WBC, HGB, MCH, MCHC; possible ↑ PLT	Precipitated cryoprotein and cryoglobulin cause turbidity and falsely increase spectrophotometric reading for HGB; precipitated proteins also may be counted as WBC or sometimes as PLTs	Flags; noncompliance with rule of three†; abnormal WBC histogram, dataplot, scattergram, scatterplot, or cytogram	Incubate specimen for 10–20 minutes at 37° C and repeat analysis
In vitro hemolysis	↓ RBC, HCT, MCV; ↑ MCH, MCHC; possibly ↑ PLT	Lysed RBCs not counted; RBC fragments can be counted as PLTs	Flags; noncompliance with rule of three†; abnormal RBC and PLT histograms	Request new specimen
Lysis-resistant RBCs	↑ WBC, HGB, MCH, MCHC	RBCs with Hb S or C may fail to lyse; will be counted as WBCs; also causes turbidity and falsely increases spectrophotometric reading for HGB	Flags; noncompliance with rule of three†; abnormal WBC histogram, dataplot, scattergram, scatterplot, or cytogram	Check peripheral blood film for Hb S or Hb C crystals; dilute specimen with isotonic saline, repeat analysis, and correct for dilution
Hyperglycemia (glucose > 600 mg/dL)	↑ MCV, HCT; ↓ MCHC	RBC cytoplasm is hypertonic due to high glucose level; when RBCs diluted with isotonic saline, osmotic movement of water into RBCs causes temporary swelling; cell volume returns to normal in approximately 5 minutes after equilibration	Noncompliance with rule of three†	Dilute specimen with isotonic saline and hold at room temperature for 10 minutes, repeat analysis, and correct for dilution
Very high WBC counts (>100 × 10⁹/L)	↑ HGB, MCH, MCHC; possible ↑ RBC, HCT, MCV, RDW	Turbidity affects spectrophotometric reading for HGB; WBCs counted with RBC count; larger WBC volume included in MCV and RDW measurements	Flags; noncompliance with rule of three†; abnormal histograms, dataplots, scattergrams, scatterplots, or cytograms	Dilute specimen with isotonic saline, repeat analysis, and correct for dilution
NRBCs, micromegakaryocytes	↑ WBC	NRBCs or micromegakaryocytes counted as WBCs	Flags; abnormal WBC dataplot, scattergram, scatterplot, or cytogram	Check peripheral blood film for abnormal cells; modern analyzers able to isolate and count NRBCs and exclude them from the WBC count; can do manual correction on uncorrected WBC count‡
Microcytes (<50 fL) or RBC fragments (schistocytes)	↑ PLT; possible ↓RBC	Volume of microcytes or RBC fragments within PLT counting threshold; possibly not counted as RBCs	Flags; abnormal PLT and RBC histograms	Check peripheral blood film for microcytes and schistocytes; estimate PLT count from blood film§; perform CD61 platelet count if available
High number of large or giant platelets	↓ PLT; ↑ WBC; possible ↑ RBC and MCV	Large or giant platelets above the PLT counting threshold, counted as WBCs, and not included in PLT count; also may be counted and sized with RBC	Flags; abnormal histograms, dataplots, scattergrams, scatterplots, or cytograms	Check peripheral blood film for large/giant platelets; estimate PLT count from blood film§; perform CD61 platelet count if available

Continued

TABLE 13.2   Composite of Conditions That Cause Interference on Automated Blood Cell Analyzers—cont'd

Condition	Parameters Falsely Affected*	Rationale	Analyzer Indicators	Corrective Action
Platelet agglutination/ clumping	↓ PLT; ↑ WBC; possible ↑ RBC and MCV	Large clumps counted as WBCs and not included in PLT count; may also be counted and sized with RBC	Flags; abnormal histograms, dataplots, scattergrams, scatterplots, or cytograms	Check peripheral blood film for platelet clumping; vortex and repeat analysis; incubate for 10–15 minutes at 37° C and repeat analysis; redraw specimen in sodium citrate anticoagulant, repeat analysis, multiply result by 1.1
Platelet satellitosis	↓ PLT	Platelets adhere to WBCs and are not included in the PLT count	Flags	Check peripheral blood film for platelet satellitosis; vortex and repeat analysis; redraw specimen in sodium citrate anticoagulant, repeat analysis, multiply result by 1.1
Fragmented WBCs	↓ WBC, ↑ PLT	WBCs may fragment during chemotherapy and fragments included in the PLT count	Flags; abnormal WBC and PLT histograms, dataplots, scattergrams, scatterplots, or cytograms	Check peripheral blood film for WBC fragments; estimate PLT count from blood film§; perform CD61 platelet count if available
WBC agglutination	↓ WBC	Agglutinated WBCs are counted as one large cell	Flags; abnormal WBC histogram, dataplot, scattergram, scatterplot, or cytogram	Check peripheral blood film for WBC clumping; vortex and repeat analysis; incubate at 37° C for 10–15 minutes and repeat analysis; redraw specimen in sodium citrate, repeat analysis, multiply result by 1.1
Inclusions in RBCs, malarial parasites	↑ RETICS	Inclusions stain with RNA dye		Check peripheral blood film for RBC inclusions
Bacteria, yeast, malarial parasites	↑ PLT; possibly ↑ WBC	Clusters of microorganisms counted as PLTs or WBCs	Flags; abnormal PLT histogram	Check peripheral blood film for microorganisms; estimate PLT count from blood film§; perform CD61 platelet count if available
Old specimen (usually > 24 hours at room temperature, > 48 hours at 2 to 8° C)	↑ MCV, MPV; ↓ PLT, WBCs	RBCs and PLTs swell as specimen ages; PLTs and WBCs degenerate with prolonged exposure to EDTA	Flags; abnormal histograms, dataplots, scattergrams, scatterplots, or cytograms	Check collection time for specimen; establish and follow specimen stability and specimen rejection criteria
Microclots, fibrin clumps	↓ Cell counts; unreliable results or no results	Cells bound in clots and cannot be reliably counted	Flags	Check specimen for clots; request new specimen

*Interferences vary by analyzer. Consult operator's manual from manufacturer for a list of limitations and interferences.
†HGB × 3 ≠ HCT ± 3.
‡Formula to correct the WBC count for NRBCs discussed in Chapter 12.
§Platelet estimate from the peripheral blood film discussed in Chapter 14.
↑, Increased; ↓, decreased;
CHCM, Mean cell hemoglobin concentration; *EDTA,* ethylenediaminetetraacetic acid; *Hb,* hemoglobin; *HCT,* hematocrit; *HGB,* hemoglobin concentration; *MCH,* mean cell hemoglobin; *MCHC,* mean cell hemoglobin concentration; *MCV,* mean cell volume; *MPV,* mean platelet volume; *NRBC,* nucleated red blood cell; *PLT,* platelet count; *RBC,* red blood cell (or count); *RDW,* red cell distribution width; *RETIC,* reticulocyte count; *WBC,* white blood cell (or count).
Data from references 10, 17-19, and 34-37.

be observed in instances of severe lipemia, severe bilirubinemia, very high WBC counts, and the presence of unlysed RBCs (e.g., cells with Hb S or Hb C) and cryoproteins/cryoglobulins. Analyzers have addressed these issues by using a blank solution and/or proprietary lysis reagents, or increasing the lysis time for lysis-resistant RBCs. The Siemens technology uses direct measurement of the CHCM (measured by low- and high-angle scatter), which allows back-calculation of the hemoglobin concentration without interference from turbidity. The saline replacement technique can be used to mitigate interference by lipemia. The specimen is centrifuged, the turbid plasma is removed and replaced with the exact amount of saline, and then the specimen is mixed and the analysis is repeated.[37] The plasma hemoglobin also can be analyzed and used as a blank in the calculation of a corrected hemoglobin value using the following formula: Corrected hemoglobin = lipemic blood hemoglobin – (1−hematorit) × lipemic plasma hemoglobin.[37]

Effects of Red Blood Cell Agglutination

RBC agglutination resulting from cold-reacting autoantibodies manifests as a classic pattern of increased MCV (often greater than

130 fL), markedly decreased RBC count, and increased MCHC (often greater than 40 g/dL). This occurs because aggregates of cells are counted as one larger cell. Careful examination of the histograms and various plots from the analyzer may yield clues to this abnormality. The peripheral blood film should be reviewed for RBC agglutinates to confirm the finding. Repeating the analysis after incubating the specimen for 10 to 15 minutes at 37° C usually reverses the autoagglutination and corrects the spurious results.

Spurious Thrombocytopenia

Falsely low platelet counts (spurious thrombocytopenia) can occur because of a high number of large or giant platelets, platelet clumping or aggregation, or platelet satellitosis (Figures 11.5, 14.1, and 14.2). Platelet clumping most often occurs with poor collection technique that results in platelet activation. Rarely platelet autoagglutination may be due to an ethylenediaminetetraacetic acid (EDTA)-dependent anti-platelet antibody that reacts at room temperature. Platelet satellitosis is also an EDTA-induced phenomenon in which the platelets surround and adhere to neutrophils (Chapter 14). The falsely lower platelet counts occur because larger platelets, platelet clumps, and platelet adherence to neutrophils exceed the platelet threshold for counting and are not counted as platelets. The peripheral blood film should be reviewed for platelet abnormalities to confirm the finding. When large or giant platelets are present, a platelet estimate may be determined from the peripheral blood film (Chapter 14), or a CD61 platelet count could be performed if available. Platelet clumping and satellitosis may be corrected by repeating the analysis after vortexing the specimen, incubating the specimen for 10 to 15 minutes at 37° C, or redrawing the specimen in sodium citrate anticoagulant and multiplying the result 1.1.[37]

Errors in Reticulocyte Counting

Falsely increased reticulocyte counts can be due to the RNA stain reacting with RBC inclusions, malarial parasites, giant platelets, and Hb S and C. Development of a stain specific for reticulocyte RNA aggregates may help to eliminate this interference.

Specimen Integrity and Stability

Specimen integrity must be taken into consideration when interpreting CBC results. A properly collected whole blood specimen in EDTA anticoagulant is required (Chapter E2). The stability of most CBC parameters to obtain acceptable results is generally 24 hours at room temperature and 48 hours at refrigerated temperature (2° to 8° C).[10,17–19,38] However, the MPV may not be reliable with prolonged storage because of cell swelling, and this is variable depending on the particular analyzer.[39] Specimen age and improper specimen handling can have profound effects on the reliability of CBC test results. These factors have even greater significance as hospitals move toward greater use of off-site testing by large reference laboratories. Specific problems with older specimens include increased WBC fragility, swelling and possible lysis of RBCs, and the deterioration of platelets. Stability studies should be performed before an analyzer is used, and

specific guidelines should be established for specimen handling and rejection.

Data Suppression and Flagging

Suppression of automated data, particularly WBC differential data, may occur when internal analyzer checks fail or cast doubt on the validity of the data. Analyzers from some manufacturers release results with specific error codes or flagging for further review. The suppression of automated differential data ensures that a manual differential count is performed, whereas the release of data with appropriate flagging mandates the need for careful review of the data and possibly a blood film examination. Each laboratory directors must establish their own criteria for reflex blood film review based on established performance goals, analyzer flagging, and inherent analyzer limitations.

It is critical that laboratory professionals have detailed knowledge of the limitations of the analyzer they are using, be able to recognize erroneous results, and take appropriate corrective action to obtain reliable results before the CBC is reported. Continued future improvements in technology will further address these limitations and eliminate or decrease the need for manual intervention to obtain accurate results.

CLINICAL UTILITY OF AUTOMATED BLOOD CELL ANALYSIS

Traditional Complete Blood Count

The CBC can be ordered with or without the differential count and reticulocyte analysis and is one of the most frequently ordered blood tests. The CBC is ordered with other blood tests for wellness screening, diagnosis of hematologic and metabolic diseases, and for monitoring therapy in nutritional anemias, and after RBC and platelet transfusions, hematopoietic stem cell transplantation, and chemotherapy regimens. The clinical utility of the traditional CBC components is described in later chapters: RBC-related components (Chapters 16 to 25); WBC-related components (Chapters 26 and 31 to 34); and platelet-related components (Chapters 37 and 38). Modern high-end automated blood cell analyzers also have modules that prepare and stain peripheral blood films based on user-defined flagging criteria, and some have modules capable of digital image analysis (Chapter 14). The importance of correlating findings of the CBC with those from the peripheral blood film examination cannot be underestimated, and that process is described in detail in Chapter 14.

The use of automated blood cell analyzers has directly affected the availability, accuracy, and clinical usefulness of the CBC, WBC differential count, and reticulocyte analysis. Some parameters that are available on modern analyzers cannot be derived by manual testing and have provided further insight into various clinical conditions. The next section will discuss these more recently developed CBC components.

Red Cell Distribution Width

The RDW is an estimate of the variation in volume of an RBC population. An increase in RDW correlates with a wider RBC histogram and anisocytosis on the peripheral blood film. Automated analyzers calculate the RDW using two formulas (Figure 13.18).[40] The RDW-CV is the CV of RBC volume, calculated as follows: RDW (%) = (SD/MCV) × 100, where SD is 1 SD of the volume of the RBC population distribution. Therefore the formula does not include the outlier cells in the RBC histogram distribution beyond 1 SD.[40] In addition, because the RDW-CV reflects the ratio of SD/MCV, it can be falsely skewed by MCV values (the denominator) that are very elevated or decreased. For example, a population of microcytes with a very low MCV can have a greater than anticipated RDW-CV compared with the observed width of the histogram. Conversely, a population of macrocytes with a very high MCV can have a lower than anticipated RDW-CV (or even one within the reference interval) compared with the observed width of the histogram.[40]

The RDW-SD is the arithmetic width of the RBC distribution histogram at the 20% frequency level and is reported in picograms. It includes some of the outlier cells beyond the ± 1 SD level and is not affected by the MCV value. Therefore it is considered a better assessment of the degree of anisocytosis in an RBC population.[40] Figure 14.14 depicts RBC histograms and corresponding RDW values in three abnormal RBC populations.

The RDW can be used with the MCV for an initial classification of an anemia, although this classification scheme is not absolute.[41,42] For example, a low MCV with a high RDW suggests iron deficiency, a low MCV with a normal RDW suggests thalassemia, and a high MCV and high RDW suggest a folate/vitamin B$_{12}$ deficiency or myelodysplasia (Table 16.4).[41,42] An increased RDW also may be the first indication of iron-deficient erythropoiesis.[43]

Reticulocyte Analysis

Automation has increased the precision and accuracy of reticulocyte counting and has expanded the analysis of immature RBCs, providing new parameters that are useful in the diagnosis and treatment of anemias. In addition to reporting the relative and absolute numbers of reticulocytes, modern blood cell analyzers also calculate the IRF and in addition, some measure the reticulocyte hemoglobin content.

The absolute reticulocyte count (Chapter 12) is an indicator of the erythropoietic activity in the bone marrow and can be used to classify types of anemia.[42,44] If a patient with anemia has an elevated absolute reticulocyte count, it indicates increased marrow erythropoiesis. Acute blood loss or a hemolytic anemia is then considered because the bone marrow is appropriately responding to the anemia by increasing erythropoiesis to compensate for the loss of RBCs from bleeding or excessive hemolysis. This process involves secretion of erythropoietin by the kidney in response to the hypoxia (Chapter 6). If a patient with anemia has a low or normal absolute reticulocyte count, it indicates decreased or ineffective erythropoiesis and an inadequate bone marrow response to the anemia. Examples of anemias in this category include aplastic anemia, iron deficiency anemia, anemia of inflammation, chronic kidney disease, and vitamin B$_{12}$ and folate deficiency (Chapter 16 and Figure 16.3).[42,44]

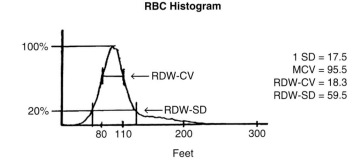

RBC Histogram

1 SD = 17.5
MCV = 95.5
RDW-CV = 18.3
RDW-SD = 59.5

1 SD = RDW-CV × MCV ÷ 100

RDW-CV = 1 SD ÷ MCV × 100

RDW-SD Particle Size Distribution

Figure 13.18 Calculation of the Red Cell Distribution Width. The red blood cell *(RBC)* histogram plots RBC volume in femtoliters on the *x*-axis and the frequency of those values on the *y*-axis. The red cell distribution width coefficient of variation *(RDW-CV)* is calculated from the width of the histogram at 1 standard deviation *(SD)* from the mean divided by mean cell volume *(MCV)* and is reported as a percentage (%). The RDW-SD is the arithmetic width of the distribution curve measured at the 20% frequency level and is reported in picograms. (Based on Munro, B. H. [2005]. *Statistical Methods for Health Care Research.* [5th ed.]. New York: Lippincott Williams and Wilkins.)

In severe anemia, *stress* or *shift* reticulocytes are released into the peripheral blood earlier than normal to compensate for the anemia. These stress reticulocytes are younger and take longer to mature in circulation; they also have a larger volume and a greater amount of cytoplasmic RNA. The IRF represents the fraction of the most immature cells in the total reticulocyte population. They are recognized by a higher staining intensity of their cellular RNA and greater optical scatter (Table 13.1). The IRF, in conjunction with the absolute reticulocyte count, can be used to assess the level of erythropoiesis. An elevated IRF is an early indicator of successful treatment after vitamin therapy in nutritional anemias, and after erythropoiesis-stimulating agent (ESA) therapy in kidney failure.[44,45] The IRF also may be useful with other tests in evaluating early bone marrow recovery after chemotherapy and detecting early erythroid regeneration after hematopoietic stem cell transplantation.[44–46]

The reticulocyte hemoglobin content (CHr, Siemens; RET-He, Sysmex) is a real-time assessment of the availability of iron for hemoglobin synthesis.[45,47] A decreased CHr/RET-He means that there is inadequate iron available for synthesis of hemoglobin in the patient's developing erythroid cells (provided there are no underlying hematopoietic disorders).[47] Therefore a decreased CHr/RET-He is an early indicator of iron deficient erythropoiesis, and is useful for early diagnosis of absolute iron deficiency (decreased or absent iron stores) in both adults and children.[45,47,48] The CHr/RET-He is also decreased in functional iron deficiency (FID). In FID, there is adequate iron in storage sites (macrophages and hepatocytes), but not enough iron is available for hemoglobin synthesis in developing erythroid cells.[45] FID occurs in ESA therapy, such as in chronic kidney disease, when iron is not released rapidly enough from storage sites to support the accelerated erythropoiesis.[45] It also occurs in anemia of inflammation, a condition in which inflammatory cytokines increase hepcidin production in the liver, causing degradation of ferroportin in the membranes of macrophages and hepatocytes. Without ferroportin, macrophages and hepatocytes are unable to export their storage iron out of the cell for hemoglobin synthesis (iron sequestration syndrome) (Chapters 9 and 17). Finally, an elevated CHr/RET-He can be an early indicator of bone marrow response after therapy with iron (oral and intravenous) in iron deficiency or after ESA therapy in chronic kidney disease.[45,47] A limitation in the use of the CHr and RET-He is the analyzer-specific methods, lack of availability on all analyzers, and lack of harmonization of the reference intervals.[44]

Platelet Analysis

Thrombocytopenia generally results from decreased production or increased destruction of platelets (Chapter 38). When there is increased destruction of platelets in the circulation (e.g., in immune thrombocytopenic purpura), thrombopoietin is secreted (mainly from the hepatocytes), which increases platelet production to compensate for the platelets lost. In the process, immature platelets are released from the bone marrow, analogous to the reticulocyte response in anemia (Chapter 11).[43] These young, immature platelets are sometimes called reticulated or stress platelets. They are larger than normal platelets (greater than 6 μm in diameter) and have an increased amount of cytoplasmic RNA (Figure 11.5).[49] Giant platelets (usually 5 to 8 μm in diameter but can reach 20 μm in diameter) occur in hereditary platelet disorders, such as Bernard Soulier syndrome (Figure 37.2) and May-Hegglin anomaly (Figure 38.2), and in myeloproliferative and myelodysplastic neoplasms (Figure 33.11).

In automated blood cell analyzers, the MPV can be measured by impedance or optical light scatter with or without staining with an RNA dye (Table 13.1). The MPV may be useful in the differential diagnosis of various platelet abnormalities. The MPV is elevated in conditions caused by increased peripheral platelet destruction (such as immune thrombocytopenic purpura) and significantly elevated in some inherited conditions (such as Bernard Soulier syndrome and May-Hegglin anomaly).[43] The MPV may be decreased in bone marrow suppression and megakaryocyte hypoplasia, and in some congenital abnormalities (e.g., Wiskott-Aldrich syndrome).[43,50,51]

Because large, immature platelets are more reactive and considered to have greater thrombotic potential, elevated MPV values are associated with higher risk of acute myocardial infarction and mortality for individuals with cardiovascular disease, and may have use in assessing a patient's risk of thrombosis.[43,51,52] However, the use of the MPV in these conditions has been hampered by the varying ability of analyzers to accurately measure MPV (especially with large and giant platelet populations that are underestimated in impedance methods), the lack of standardization of MPV reference intervals and cutoff values in various conditions (compromising comparisons in clinical studies), and the lack of well-controlled prospective studies to prove clinical utility.[43,49,51] In addition to method variations, anticoagulation and storage time also influence the MPV, which further affects the reliability and clinical utility of MPV results.[53]

An elevated MPV should always be confirmed by examining the platelet morphology on a peripheral blood film.[43]

Modern analyzers also determine the IPF, which is the proportion of very immature platelets compared to the total platelet count, based on their volume and RNA staining (Table 13.1). It is analogous to the IRF and indicates a real-time assessment of increased platelet production (megakaryopoiesis).[49] The IPF also has been studied as a risk assessment marker for adverse outcomes in cardiovascular disease.[49] Also, an increase in the IPF (along with the IRF) can be an early indication of engraftment success after hematopoietic stem cell transplant.[45,49,54] The limitations of automated IPF determinations is that the fluorescent dyes can also bind to non-RNA components of the platelet cytoplasm and falsely elevate the immature fraction.[49]

Nucleated Red Blood Cells

NRBCs are immature erythroid cells normally confined to the bone marrow (Chapter 6). However, a small number of NRBCs normally can be present in the peripheral blood of newborns but only for the first few days of life (Chapter 43; NRBC reference intervals can be found after the Index at the end of the book). NRBCs are not present in the peripheral blood of healthy adults, children, and infants after that point. When NRBCs do appear in the peripheral blood, two pathologic conditions are considered: (1) severe anemia with a compensatory bone marrow response and (2) damage or stress to the bone marrow as a result of conditions such as leukemias, myelodysplasia, or chemotherapy.[43] Circulating NRBCs may be associated with a higher risk of mortality in patients in critical care settings.[43] Automated analyzers count NRBCs based on various analyzer-dependent technologies, including impedance, conductivity, optical light scatter, and fluorescent staining (Table 13.1). Because of their serious clinical implications, NRBCs reported by an automated blood cell analyzer should be confirmed by examining a peripheral blood film before reporting the result.

ANALYZER SELECTION

Automation of the WBC differential has had a significant impact on the laboratory workflow because of the labor-intensive nature of the manual differential count. Analyzer capability has expanded in specificity and sensitivity of identifying various types of WBCs. Sophisticated histograms, dataplots, scatterplots, scattergrams, and cytograms, along with flagging, provide valuable information in the diagnosis and treatment of blood cell disorders. Manufacturers have integrated hematology workstations for the greatest automation and laboratory efficiency.

Selection of a hematology analyzer for an individual laboratory requires careful evaluation of the laboratory's needs and close scrutiny of several important analyzer issues, including specifications and system requirements, methods used, training requirements, maintenance needs, reagent usage, data management capabilities, staff response, and short-term and long-term expenditures. All analyzers claim to improve laboratory efficiency through increased automation that results in improved workflow and faster turnaround time or through the addition of new parameters that may have clinical efficacy. Automated slide maker/stainer modules can be connected directly to high-end analyzers to further improve efficiency. The slide makers/stainers can be programmed to make blood films for every specimen or to make films based on the laboratory's internal criteria for a film review. This reduces but does not eliminate the use of manual peripheral blood film review. Each laboratory must assess its own efficiency needs to determine whether a slide maker and stainer is value-added to the laboratory. The analyzer selected should suit the workload and patient population and should have a positive effect on patient outcomes. The analyzer selected for a cancer center may be different from that chosen for a community hospital. Ultimately, however, the analyzer decision may be swayed by individual preferences.

SUMMARY

- Automated cell counting provides greater accuracy and precision compared with manual cell-counting methods.
- The primary technologies used in automated blood cell analyzers include electrical (DC) impedance, radiofrequency (RF) conductivity, multiangle optical light scatter, cytochemical and fluorescent staining, and spectrophotometry for determination of hemoglobin concentration.
- The electrical impedance method measures an increase in electrical resistance between two electrodes as a cell passes through a sensing aperture. The number of pulses correlates to the cell count, and the height or amplitude of the pulses correlates with cell volume. The measurable voltage pulses are plotted on frequency distribution histograms that allow the evaluation of cell populations based on cell volume.
- RF conductivity uses high-voltage electromagnetic current that penetrates the cell. Changes in the RF signal are proportional to cell interior density. Impedance and conductivity can be plotted against each other on a two-dimensional distribution scattergram which allows the separation and counting of cell populations using cluster analysis.
- Optical scatter systems (flow cytometers) use detection of interference in a laser beam or light source to differentiate and count cell types. Forward light scatter correlates to cell volume, while low-angle, medium-angle, and 90° (orthogonal) scatter correlate to internal cell contents. Combining various angles of optical scatter, or optical scatter with DC impedance, RF conductivity, or cytochemical or fluorescent staining, allows for better discrimination between different cell types and more accurate cell counts.
- Major manufacturers of blood cell analyzers in the United States include Beckman Coulter, Sysmex, Abbott, and Siemens Healthineers. Table 13.1 summarizes the methods used for the CBC, WBC differential count, NRBC, and reticulocyte analyses for the high-end analyzer from each manufacturer.
- Reticulocyte analysis has been incorporated into all high-end automated blood cell analyzers. New methylene blue, oxazine, or fluorescent dyes stain the cellular RNA before the cells are counted using absorbance/fluorescence and light scatter. The immature reticulocyte fraction, or the fraction/percentage of very immature reticulocytes compared to the total reticulocyte count, is also determined.
- The use of various combinations of technologies and cluster analysis allows the determination of a NRBC count and the ability to exclude them from the WBC count.
- Each analyzer has limitations related to methodology that may result in flagging of specific results or suppression of automated data. Likewise, inherent specimen problems may result in flagging that indicates possible rejection of automated results.
- Automated blood cell analyzers have had a significant impact on laboratory workflow, particularly automation of the WBC differential and reticulocyte analysis.
- Newer parameters can now be measured, such as the immature reticulocyte fraction (IRF) and the reticulocyte hemoglobin content (RET-He/CHr), which have documented clinical utility.

Now that you have completed this chapter, go back and read again the case study at the beginning and respond to the questions presented. Answers can be found in Appendix C.

REVIEW QUESTIONS

Answers can be found in Appendix C.

1. Low-voltage DC resistance is used to measure:
   a. Cell volume
   b. Cell nuclear volume
   c. Cellular complexity in the nucleus
   d. Cellular complexity in the cytoplasm

2. Orthogonal or 90° light scatter is used to measure the following *except*:
   a. Cell volume
   b. Nuclear density
   c. Cellular granularity
   d. Internal complexity of the cell

3. On some blood cell analyzers, the hematocrit is a calculated value. Which of the following directly measured parameters is used in the calculation of this value?
   a. RDW
   b. MCV
   c. MCHC
   d. Hemoglobin

4. Match the cell-counting methods listed with the appropriate definition:

   ___ Impedance
   ___ RF
   ___ Optical scatter

   a. Uses diffraction, reflection, and refraction of light waves
   b. Uses high-voltage electrical waves to measure conductivity of cells
   c. Involves measurement of changes in electrical resistance between two electrodes

5. Match each analyzer listed with the technology it uses to determine WBC differential counts.

   ___ Abbott CELL-DYN Sapphire
   ___ Siemens ADVIA 2120i
   ___ Sysmex XN-3100
   ___ Beckman Coulter UniCel DxH 900

   a. Volume, conductivity, and five angles of light scatter
   b. Multiangle polarized scatter separation and three-color fluorescent light detection
   c. Peroxidase-staining absorbance and light scatter
   d. Fluorescence flow cytometry using forward and side light scatter and side fluorescent light detection

6. Using impedance technology alone, it would be difficult to distinguish:
   a. Platelets and white blood cells
   b. Giant platelets and red blood cells
   c. Small lymphocytes and neutrophils
   d. Red blood cells and white blood cells

7. The hemoglobin content of reticulocytes is derived from:
   a. Amplitude of voltage pulses of the reticulocytes
   b. Staining the hemoglobin within the reticulocytes
   c. Low- and high-angle light scatter of reticulocytes
   d. Fluorescent staining of reticulocytes

8. The *intensity* of staining of the RNA within a reticulocyte using new methylene blue, oxazine, or fluorescent dyes enables the determination of the:
   a. Reticulocyte count
   b. Immature reticulocyte fraction
   c. Nucleated red blood cell count
   d. Reticulocyte hemoglobin content

9. A patient peripheral blood film demonstrates agglutinated RBCs, and the CBC shows an elevated MCHC. What other parameters will be affected by the agglutination of the RBCs?
   a. MCV will be decreased and RBC count will be increased.
   b. MCV will be decreased and RBC count will be decreased.
   c. MCV will be increased and RBC count will be increased.
   d. MCV will be increased and RBC count will be decreased.

10. A decrease in the hemoglobin content of reticulocytes (CHr/RET-He) is an early indicator of:
    a. Iron-deficient erythropoiesis
    b. Vitamin B_{12} or folate deficiency
    c. Response to erythroid stimulating agents in kidney failure
    d. Bone marrow recovery after hematopoietic stem cell transplant

REFERENCES

1. Coulter, W. H. (1957). *High speed automatic blood cell counter and cell size analyzer* [Conference presentation, 1956, October 3]. Chicago, IL: *Proceedings of the National Electronics Conference, 1956, 12*, 1034–1042.
2. Brecher, G., Schneiderman, M., & Williams, G. Z. (1956). Evaluation of electronic red blood cell counter. *Am J Clin Path, 26*, 1439–1449.
3. Brittin, G. M., Brecher, G., & Johnson, C. A. (1969). Evaluation of the Coulter Counter Model S. *Am J Clin Path, 52*, 679–689.
4. Coulter Electronics. (1983). *Coulter Counter Model S-Plus IV with Three-Population Differential: Product Reference Manual*, PN 423560B. Hialeah, FL: Coulter Electronics.
5. Griswold, D. J., & Champagne, V. D. (1985). Evaluation of the Coulter S-Plus IV three-part differential in an acute care hospital. *Am J Clin Pathol, 84*, 49–57.
6. Coulter Corporation. (1992). *Coulter STKS Operator's Guide*, PN 423592811. Hialeah, FL: Coulter Corporation.
7. Abbott. *MAPSS* (Video). https://hematologyacademy.com/digitalresource/mapss-technology/. Accessed February 10, 2023.
8. TOA Medical Electronics Company. (1985). *Sysmex Model E-5000 Operator's Manual* (CN 461-2104-2). Kobe, Japan: TOA Medical Electronics Company.
9. TOA Medical Electronics Company. (1997). *Sysmex SE-9500 Operator's Manual* (CN 461-2464-2). Kobe, Japan: TOA Medical Electronics Company.
10. Beckman Coulter, Inc. (2019). *Instructions for Use. UniCel DxH 900 Series with System Manager Software, Coulter Cellular Analysis System*. PN C06947AC. Brea, CA: Beckman Coulter, Inc.
11. de Grooth, B. G., Terstappen, L. W. M. M., Puppels, G. J., et al. (1987). Light scattering polarization measurements, a new parameter in flow cytometry. *Cytometry, 8*, 539–544.
12. Terstappen, L. W. M. M., Mickaels, R. A., Dost, R., et al. (1990). Increased light scattering resolution facilitates multidimensional flow cytometric analysis. *Cytometry, 11*, 510–512.
13. Jovin, T. M., Morris, S. J., Striker, G., et al. (1976). Automatic sizing and separation of particles by ratios of light scattering intensities. *J Histochem Cytochem, 24*, 269–283.
14. Kunicka, J. E., Fischer, G., Murphy, J., et al. (2000). Improved platelet counting using two-dimensional laser light scatter. *Am J Clin Pathol, 114*, 283–289.
15. Tycko, D. H., Metz, M. H., Epstein, E. A., et al. (1985). Flow cytometric light scattering measurement of red blood cell volume and hemoglobin concentration. *Appl Opt, 24*, 1355–1365.
16. Mohandas, N., Kim, Y. R., Tycko, D. H., et al. (1986). Accurate and independent measurement of volume and hemoglobin concentration of individual red cells by laser light scattering. *Blood, 68*, 506–513.
17. Sysmex Corporation. (2017). *Instructions for Use. Automated Hematology Analyzer, XN series*, (XN-3000/XN-3100), CW574011. Kobe, Japan: Sysmex Corporation.
18. Abbott Laboratories. (2014). *CELL-DYN Sapphire Operator's Manual*, 9140426. Abbott Park, Illinois: Abbott Laboratories.

19. Siemens Healthcare Diagnostics Inc. (2010). *ADVIA 2120/2120i Hematology Systems Operator's Guide* 067D0157-01. Tarrytown, NY: Siemens Healthcare Diagnostics, Inc.

20. CLSI. (2000). *Reference and Selected Procedures for the Quantitative Determination of Hemoglobin in Blood.* (3rd ed., CLSI approved standard, H15-A3). Wayne, PA: Clinical and Laboratory Standards Institute.

21. Barnes, P. W., McFadden, S. L., Machin, S. J., et al. for the International Consensus Group for Hematology. (2005). The international consensus group for hematology review: suggested criteria for action following automated CBC and WBC differential analysis. *Lab Hematol, 11*, 83–90.

22. Sysmex Technologies. https://www.sysmex-europe.com/academy/clinic-laboratory/analyser-channels/wbc-differential-channel.html. Accessed February 6, 2023.

23. Lakos, G., & Wright, D. (2019). *Advances in Automated Hematology Analyzers: Optimizing Optical Technology* (white paper). Santa Clara, CA: Abbott Laboratories. https://cloud.gmo.diagnostics.abbott/hematology-analyzers-white-paper. Accessed February 10, 2023.

24. Clinical and Laboratory Standards Institute. (2007). *Reference Leukocyte (WBC) Differential Count (Proportional) and Evaluation of Instrumental Methods.* (2nd ed., approved standard, H20-A2). Wayne, PA: Clinical and Laboratory Standards Institute.

25. Clinical and Laboratory Standards Institute. (2004). *Methods for Reticulocyte Counting (Automated Blood Cell Counters, Flow Cytometry, and Supravital Dyes).* (2nd ed., CLSI approved guideline, H44-A2). Wayne, PA: Clinical and Laboratory Standards Institute.

26. Clinical and Laboratory Standards Institute. (2010). *Validation, Verification, and Quality Assurance of Automated Hematology Analyzers.* (2nd ed., CLSI approved standard, H26-A2). Wayne, PA: Clinical and Laboratory Standards Institute.

27. Briggs, C., Culp, N., Davis, B., et al. on behalf of the International Society for Laboratory Hematology. (2014). ICSH guidelines for the evaluation of blood cell analyzers including those used for differential leucocyte and reticulocyte counting. *Int J Lab Hem, 36*, 613–627.

28. Clinical and Laboratory Standards Institute. (2011). *Assessment of the Diagnostic Accuracy of Laboratory Tests using Receiver Operating Characteristic Curves.* (2nd ed., CLSI approved guideline, EP24-A2). Wayne, PA: Clinical and Laboratory Standards Institute.

29. Calibration and calibration verification. Clinical Laboratory Improvement Amendments Brochure No. 3. https://www.cms.gov/Regulations-and-Guidance/Legislation/CLIA/Downloads/6065bk.pdf. Accessed February 15, 2023.

30. Gilmer, P. R., Williams, U., Koepke, J. A., et al. (1977). Calibration methods for automated hematology instruments. *Am J Clin Pathol, 68*, 185–190.

31. Koepke, J. A. (1977). The calibration of automated instruments for accuracy in hemoglobinometry. *Am J Clin Pathol, 68*, 180–184.

32. Zwart, A., van Assendelft, O. W., Bull, B. S., et al. for the International Council for Standardization in Haematology. (1996). Recommendations for reference method for haemoglobinometry in human blood (ICSH Standard 1995) and specifications for international haemiglobincyanide standard, 4th ed. *J Clin Pathol, 49*, 271–274.

33. Savage, R. A. (1985). Calibration bias and imprecision for automated hematology analyzers: an evaluation of the significance of short-term bias resulting from calibration of an analyzer with S Cal. *Am J Clin Pathol, 84*, 186–190.

34. Cornbleet, J. (1983). Spurious results from automated hematology cell counters. *Lab Med, 14*, 509–514.

35. Zandecki, M., Genevieve, F., Gerard, J., et al. (2007). Spurious counts and spurious results on haematology analysers: a review. Part I: platelets. *Int J Lab Hematol, 29*, 4–20.

36. Zandecki, M., Genevieve, F., Gerard, J., et al. (2007). Spurious counts and spurious results on haematology analysers: a review. Part II: white blood cells, red blood cells, haemoglobin, red cell indices and reticulocytes. *Int J Lab Hematol, 29*, 21–41.

37. Gulati, G., Uppal, G., & Gong, J. (2022). Unreliable automated complete blood count results: causes, recognition, and resolution. *Ann Lab Med, 42*, 515–530.

38. Tatsumi, N., Miwa, S., & Lewis, S. M. for the International Society of Hematology and the International Council for Standardization in Haematology. (2002). Specimen collection, storage, and transmission to the laboratory for hematological tests. *Int J Hematol, 75*, 261–268.

39. Zini, G. for the International Council for Standardization in Haematology (ICSH). (2014). Stability of complete blood count parameters with storage: toward defined specifications for different diagnostic applications. *Int J Lab Hematol, 36*, 111–113.

40. Constantino, B. T. (2011). The red cell histogram and the dimorphic red cell population. *Lab Med, 42*, 300–308.

41. Bessman, J. D., Gilmer, P. R., & Gardner, F. H. (1983). Improved classification of anemia by MCV and RDW. *Am J Clin Pathol, 80*, 322–326.

42. Lin, J. C., & Benz, E. J., Jr. (2023). Approach to anemia in the adult and child. In Hoffman, R., Benz, E. J., Silberstein, L. E., et al. (Eds.), *Hematology Basic Principles and Practice.* (8th ed., pp. 463–472). St. Louis: Elsevier.

43. May, J. E., Marques, M. B., Reddy, V. V. B., et al. (2019). Three neglected numbers in the CBC: the RDW, MPV, and NRBC count. *Cleve Clin J Med, 86*, 167–172.

44. Butarello, M. (2016). Laboratory diagnosis of anemia: are the old and new red cell parameters useful in classification and treatment, how? *Int J Lab Hematol, 38* (Suppl 1), 123–132.

45. Piva, E., Brugnara, C., Spolaore, F., et al. (2015). Clinical utility of reticulocyte parameters. *Clin Lab Med, 35*, 133–363.

46. Gonçalo, A. P., Barbosa, I. L., Campilho, F., et al. (2011). Predictive value of immature reticulocyte and platelet fractions in hematopoietic recovery of allograft patients. *Transplant Proc, 43*, 241–243.

47. Ogawa, C., Tsuchiya, K., & Maeda, K. (2020). Reticulocyte hemoglobin content. *Clin Chim Acta, 504*, 138–145.

48. Ullrich, C., Wu, A., Armbsy, C., et al. (2005). Screening healthy infants for iron deficiency using reticulocyte hemoglobin content. *JAMA, 294*, 924–930.

49. Buttarello, M., Mezzapelle, G., Freguglia, F., et al. (2020). Reticulated platelets and immature platelet fraction: clinical applications and method limitations. *Int J Lab Hematol, 42*, 363–370.

50. Noris, P., Klersy, C., & Gresele, P. (2013). Platelet size for distinguishing between inherited thrombocytopenias and immune thrombocytopenia: a multicentric, real life study. *Br J Haematol, 162*, 112–119.

51. Leader, A., Pereg, D., & Lishner, M. (2012). Are platelet volume indices of clinical use? A multidisciplinary review. *Ann Med, 44*, 805–816.

52. Chu, S. G., Becker, R. C., & Berger, P. B. (2010). Mean platelet volume as a predictor of cardiovascular risk: a systematic review and meta-analysis. *J Thromb Haemost, 8*, 148–156.

53. Reardon, D. M., Hutchinson, D., Preston, F. E., et al. (1985). The routine measurement of platelet volume: a comparison of aperture-impedance and flow cytometric systems. *Clin Lab Haematol, 7*, 251–257.

54. Grabek, J., D'Elia, N., & Kelsey, G. (2021). Immature platelet fraction as a predictor of platelet count recovery following allogeneic bone marrow transplantation. *Pathology, 53*, 493–497.

14

Examination of the Peripheral Blood Film and Correlation With the Complete Blood Count

*Carolina Vilchez**

OBJECTIVES

After completion of this chapter, the reader will be able to:

1. List the specimen sources and collection processes that are acceptable for blood film preparation.
2. Describe the techniques for making peripheral blood films.
3. Describe the appearance of a well-prepared peripheral blood film, recognize a description of a slide that is consistent or inconsistent with that appearance, and troubleshoot problems with poorly prepared films.
4. Explain the principle, purpose, and basic method of Wright staining of blood films.
5. Identify and troubleshoot problems that cause poorly stained blood films.
6. Describe the proper examination of a peripheral blood film, including selection of the correct area, sequence of examination, and observations to be made at each magnification; recognize deviations from this protocol.
7. Describe how digital morphology systems automate the examination of peripheral blood films including blood cell identification and differential counting; list the advantages of using these systems.
8. Given the number of cells observed per field and the magnification of the objective, apply formulas to estimate white blood cell (WBC) and platelet counts.
9. Explain the effect that platelet satellitosis and clumping may have on automated complete blood count (CBC) results; recognize examples of results that would be consistent with these effects.
10. Follow the appropriate course of action to recognize and correct ethylenediaminetetraacetic acid-induced pseudothrombocytopenia and pseudoleukocytosis.
11. Implement a systematic approach to interpretation of CBC data that results in a summary of the numerical data and communicates the blood picture succinctly.
12. Calculate absolute WBC differential counts.

OUTLINE

Peripheral Blood Films
  Specimen Collection
  Peripheral Blood Film Preparation
  Staining of Peripheral Blood Films
  Peripheral Blood Film Examination
Summarizing Complete Blood Count Results

Organization of Complete Blood Count Results
Assessing Hematology Results Relative to Reference
  Intervals
Summarizing White Blood Cell Parameters
Summarizing Red Blood Cell Parameters
Summarizing Platelet Parameters

CASE STUDY

After studying the material in this chapter, the reader should be able to respond to the following case study. Answers can be found in Appendix C.

A healthy-looking, 56-year-old man had an automated complete blood count (CBC) performed as part of a preoperative evaluation. The results were as follows. Reference intervals can be found after the Index at the end of the book.

WBC	15.8×10^9/L	MCV	91.5 fL
RBC	4.93×10^{12}/L	MCH	30 pg
HGB	14.8 g/dL	MCHC	32.8 g/dL
HCT	45.1%	RDW	14.2%
		PLT	34×10^9/L

The peripheral blood film was examined, and the only abnormal finding was platelet clumps.

1. Comparing the patient's results with the reference intervals after the Index at the end of the book, describe the blood picture succinctly, using proper terminology for red blood cells, white blood cells, and platelets.
2. What automated CBC results should be questioned?
3. What is the best course of action to handle this problem?

*The author extends appreciation to Lynn B. Maedel and Kathryn Doig, whose work in prior editions provided the foundation for this chapter, and to Steven Marionneaux for sharing his expertise in the preparation of this chapter.

A well-made, well-stained, and carefully examined peripheral blood film can provide valuable information regarding a patient's health. More can be learned from this test than from many other routinely performed hematologic tests. White blood cell (WBC) and platelet count estimates can be achieved, relative proportions of the different types of WBCs can be obtained, and the morphology of all three cell lineages can be evaluated for abnormalities. Although routine work is now handled by sophisticated automated blood cell analyzers in most hematology laboratories, skilled and talented medical laboratory professionals are essential to the reporting of reliable test results. Accurate peripheral blood film evaluation is quite likely to be needed for some time.

The peripheral blood film evaluation is the capstone of a panel of tests called the *complete blood count* (CBC) or *hemogram*. The CBC includes enumeration of cellular elements, quantitation of hemoglobin, and statistical analyses that provide a snapshot of cell appearances. These results can be derived using the manual methods and calculations described in Chapter 12 or using the automated blood cell analyzers described in Chapter 13. Regardless of method, the numerical values should be consistent with the assessment derived by examining the cells microscopically. Careful examination of data in a systematic way ensures that all relevant results are noted and taken into consideration in the diagnosis.

This chapter begins with a discussion of the preparation and assessment of the blood film, followed by a systematic approach to review the CBC, including blood film evaluation. Such an evaluation can be applied in the hematology chapters that follow.

PERIPHERAL BLOOD FILMS

Specimen Collection

Essentially all specimens for routine testing in the hematology laboratory are collected in lavender closure tubes (Chapter E2). These tubes contain disodium or tripotassium ethylenediaminetetraacetic acid (EDTA), which anticoagulates the blood by chelating the calcium that is essential for coagulation. EDTA is the preferred anticoagulant for microscopic review of peripheral blood films because it best preserves blood cell morphology.[1] Artifactual morphologic changes in neutrophils begin to occur within 30 minutes of blood collection.[2] When EDTA-anticoagulated blood specimens are kept at room temperature, blood films should be made within 4 hours of collection to minimize storage artifacts.[3-5] When blood films are made from specimens stored at room temperature for more than 4 hours, morphology artifacts become more prominent over time.[4,5] Examples of these artifacts include neutrophil vacuolization, swelling, loss of granules, and Pelger-Huet-type nuclear changes; vacuolization of monocytes; degranulation of eosinophils and basophils; large platelets; and crenated or spherocytic RBCs.[2,4,5] Some of these artifacts may be minimized by storage of the blood at 4°C but only for a maximum of 6 hours.[4] It is important to note the collection time and storage conditions of the specimen when assessing the blood cell morphology on a peripheral blood film because morphology

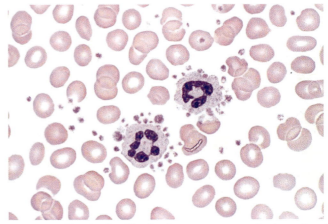

Figure 14.1 Platelet Satellitosis. An uncommon, antibody-mediated, in vitro phenomenon in which platelets adhere to neutrophils in specimens collected in ethylenediaminetetraacetate (EDTA) anticoagulant. It can potentially result in a falsely decreased platelet count (pseudothromocytopenia) in automated blood cell analyzers. (Peripheral blood, Wright-Giemsa stain, ×1000.)

artifacts can mimic features of hematologic diseases and may lead to misdiagnoses.[4,5]

The main advantages of making films from blood in the EDTA tube are that multiple slides can be made if necessary, and they do not have to be prepared immediately after the blood is drawn. In addition, EDTA generally prevents platelets from clumping on the glass slide, which makes the platelet estimate more accurate during blood film evaluation. There are purists, however, who believe that anticoagulant-free blood from a skin puncture is still the specimen of choice for evaluation of blood cell morphology.[1] Although some artifacts can be avoided in this way, specimens made from unanticoagulated, skin-puncture blood pose other problems (discussed at the end of this section).

Under certain conditions, use of a different anticoagulant or no anticoagulant may be helpful. Some patients' blood undergoes an in vitro phenomenon called *platelet satellitosis* (Figure 14.1)[6] when anticoagulated with EDTA. The platelets surround or adhere to neutrophils, which potentially causes pseudothrombocytopenia (a spuriously or falsely low platelet count) when counting is done by automated methods.[6,7] In addition, pseudothrombocytopenia and sometimes pseudoleukocytosis (a spuriously or falsely elevated WBC count) can result from platelet clumping, an in vitro phenomenon in which platelets adhere to each other (Figure 14.2).[8] The most common cause of platelet clumping in an EDTA-anticoagulated blood specimen is platelet activation resulting from improper blood collection techniques. Rarely, platelet clumping can also be caused by an anticoagulant-dependent antiplatelet antibody (usually involving EDTA), reacting at room temperature in the blood collection tube.[9] Pseudoleukocytosis occurs when platelet clumps are similar in volume to WBCs and automated blood cell analyzers cannot distinguish the two. The platelet clumps are counted as WBCs instead of platelets. In these circumstances, the examination of a blood film becomes an important quality control strategy, identifying these phenomena so that they can be corrected before the results are reported to the patient's electronic health record or health care provider.

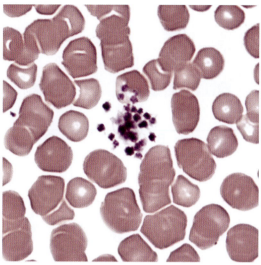

Figure 14.2 Clumped Platelets. An in vitro phenomenon in which platelets adhere to each other, forming clumps on a peripheral blood film. The most common cause is platelet activation resulting from improper blood collection techniques. Rarely, platelet clumping can also be caused by an anticoagulant-dependent antiplatelet antibody (usually involving ethylenediaminetetraacetate [EDTA]), reacting at room temperature in the blood collection tube. Platelet clumps often result in falsely decreased platelet counts (pseudothrombocytopenia) and occasionally, falsely increased white blood cell counts (pseudoleukocytosis) in automated blood cell analyzers. (Peripheral blood, Wright-Giemsa stain, ×1000.). (From Carr, J. H. [2022]. *Clinical Hematology Atlas.* [6th ed]. St. Louis: Elsevier.)

Problems such as these can be eliminated by recollecting specimens in tubes with sodium citrate anticoagulant (light blue closure), instead of EDTA, and ensuring that the proper ratio of nine parts blood to one part anticoagulant is observed (a properly filled tube). These new specimens can be analyzed in the usual way by automated blood cell analyzers; however, platelet counts and WBC counts from sodium citrate-anticoagulated specimens must be corrected for the dilution of blood with the anticoagulant. In a full-draw specimen, the blood is nine-tenths of the total tube volume (e.g., 2.7 mL of blood and 0.3 mL of sodium citrate). The "dilution factor" is the reciprocal of the dilution (i.e., 10/9 or 1.1). The WBC and platelet counts are multiplied by 1.1 to obtain accurate counts. All other CBC parameters should be reported from the original EDTA tube specimen and slide.

Another source of blood for films is from skin puncture (finger or heel) when the films are made immediately at the patient's side. There are, however, a few limitations to this procedure. First, some platelet clumping must be expected if films are made directly from a drop of blood from a skin puncture or if blood is collected in heparinized microhematocrit tubes. Generally, this clumping is not enough to interfere with platelet estimates if the films are made promptly before clotting begins in earnest. Second, only a few films can be made directly from blood from a skin puncture before the site stops bleeding. If slides are made quickly and correctly, however, cell distribution and morphology should be adequate. These problems with skin punctures can be eliminated with the use of EDTA micro-collection tubes (Chapter E2).

Peripheral Blood Film Preparation
Types of Blood Films

Manual wedge technique. The wedge film technique is probably the easiest to master. It is the most convenient and most common method used for making peripheral blood films. This technique requires at least two 3-inch × 1-inch (75-mm × 25-mm) clean glass slides. High-quality, beveled-edge microscopic slides with chamfered (beveled) corners for good lateral borders are recommended. A few more slides may be kept handy in case a good-quality film is not made immediately. One slide serves as the film slide, and the other is the pusher or spreader slide.

A drop of blood (about 2 to 3 mm in diameter) directly from a skin puncture or from a microhematocrit tube (non-heparinized for EDTA-anticoagulated blood or heparinized for skin puncture blood) is placed at one end of the slide. The drop also may be delivered using a safety dispenser such as the Alpha Scientific DIFF-SAFE dispenser. The dispenser is inserted through the rubber closure of the EDTA tube, which eliminates the need to open the tube.[10] The size of the drop of blood is important; too large a drop creates a long or thick film, and too small a drop often makes a short or thin blood film. The pusher slide, held securely in the dominant hand at about a 30- to 45-degree angle (Figure 14.3A), is drawn back into the drop of blood, and the blood is allowed to spread across the width of the slide (Figure 14.3B). It is then quickly and smoothly pushed forward to the end of the slide to create a wedge film (Figure 14.3C). It is important that the entire drop be picked up and spread. Moving the pusher slide forward too slowly accentuates poor WBC distribution by pushing larger cells, such as monocytes and granulocytes, to the very end and sides of the film. Maintaining an even, gentle pressure on the slide is essential. It is also crucial to keep the same angle all the way to the end of the film. When the hematocrit is higher than normal (i.e., >60%), as is found in patients with polycythemia or in newborns, the angle should be lowered (i.e., 25 degrees) so the film is not too short and thick. For extremely low hematocrits, the angle may need to be raised. If two or three films are made, the best one is selected for staining and the others are disposed of into an appropriate sharps disposal container. Some laboratories require two acceptable blood films and save one unstained in case another slide is required.

The procedure just described is for a push-type wedge preparation. It is called *push* because the spreader slide is pulled into the drop of blood, and the film is made by pushing the blood along the slide. The same procedure can be modified to produce a *pulled* film. In this procedure, the spreader slide is pushed into the drop of blood and pulled along the length of the slide to make the film. Although this method is much less commonly used, it also provides a satisfactory wedge preparation and may be easier for some individuals to perform. Other variations on the wedge technique include using the 3-inch side of the slide as the spreader slide or balancing the spreader slide on the fingers to avoid placing too much pressure on it. Learning to make consistently good blood films takes practice.

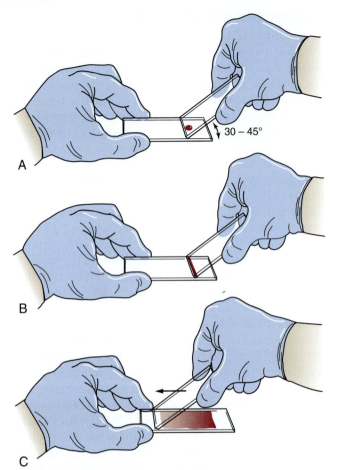

Figure 14.3 Wedge Technique of Making a Peripheral Blood Film. (A), A drop of blood is placed at one end of the slide. The pusher slide is held securely in the dominant hand at about a 30- to 45-degree angle. (B), The pusher slide is drawn back into the drop of blood, and the blood is allowed to spread across the width of the slide ensuring that the entire drop is picked up. (C), The spreader slide is then quickly and smoothly pushed forward to the end of the slide with even, gentle pressure to create a wedge film.

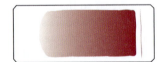

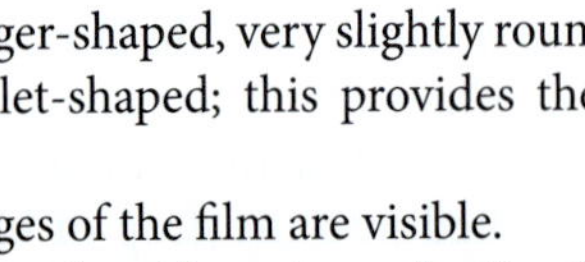

Figure 14.4 Well-Made Wedge Peripheral Blood Film.

Features of a well-made wedge peripheral blood film

1. The film is two-thirds to three-fourths the length of the slide (Figure 14.4).
2. The film is finger-shaped, very slightly rounded at the feather edge, not bullet-shaped; this provides the widest area for examination.
3. The lateral edges of the film are visible.
4. The film is smooth, without irregularities, holes, or streaks.
5. When the slide is held up to the light, the thin portion (feather edge) of the film has a "rainbow" appearance.
6. The whole drop of blood is picked up and spread.
   Figure 14.5A–H shows unacceptable films.

Semiautomated and automated slide making and staining.
Portable semiautomated devices such as the Hemaprep (J.P. Gilbert Company) are available for making wedge-type

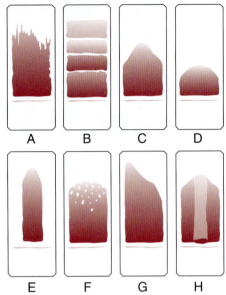

Figure 14.5 Unacceptable Peripheral Blood Films. Slide appearances associated with the most common errors are shown but note that a combination of causes may be responsible for unacceptable films. (A) Chipped or rough edge on spreader slide. (B) Hesitation in forward motion of spreader slide. (C) Spreader slide pushed too quickly. (D) Drop of blood too small. (E) Drop of blood not allowed to spread across the width of the slide. (F) Dirt or grease on the slide; may also be due to elevated lipids in the blood specimen. (G) Uneven pressure on the spreader slide. (H) Time delay; drop of blood began to dry.

peripheral blood films.[11] This device allows the operator to prepare two peripheral blood films at once, using EDTA-anticoagulated blood. The operator manually places a drop of blood on each slide and pushes a lever that mechanically activates spreader blades to spread the blood on each slide. The spreader blades are cleaned with distilled water after each use. The blood film length and thickness can be controlled by adjusting the speed of the spreader blades.[11]

The Sysmex SP-50 is an example of an automated slide-making and staining system that can be a standalone system or can be integrated with the manufacturer's automated blood cell analyzers.[12] After the analyzer has performed a CBC for a specimen, a conveyor moves the racked tube to the SP-50 module, where its barcode is read. User-definable, onboard rules built into the system determine whether a slide is required. Criteria for a manual slide review are determined by each laboratory based on its patient population. Based on the hematocrit reading, the system adjusts the volume of the drop of blood used and the angle and speed of the spreader slide in making a wedge preparation. After each blood film is prepared, the spreader slide is automatically cleaned and is ready for the next blood film to be made. The standard version of the SP-50 can make up to 30 slides per hour, and the high-speed version can make up to 75 slides per hour.[12] Patient identification information, including patient name and identification number and date for the specimen, is printed on the slide. The slide is dried, loaded into a cassette, and moved to the staining position. Based on the laboratory's desired stain protocol, stain, buffer, and rinse are added at designated times. When staining is complete, the slide is moved to a dry position and then to a collection area where it can be picked up for microscopic evaluation. Films made offline, such as bone marrow smears and cytospin preparations, may be stained using this system as well. Other blood cell analyzer manufacturers, such as Beckman Coulter, also have automated slide-making and staining modules for their analyzers.

Drying of Blood Films

Regardless of film preparation method, before staining, all blood films and bone marrow smears should be air dried as quickly as possible to avoid drying artifact (discussed in "Staining of Peripheral Blood Films"). Slides should be stained within 1 hour of blood film preparation.[3]

Staining of Peripheral Blood Films

Pure Wright stain or a Wright-Giemsa stain (Romanowsky stain)[13] is used for staining peripheral blood films and bone marrow smears. These are considered polychrome stains because they contain both eosin and methylene blue. Giemsa stains also contain methylene blue azure. The purpose of staining blood films is simply to make the cells more visible and to allow their morphology to be evaluated. Consistent day-to-day staining quality is essential.

Slides must be completely dry before staining or the thick part of the blood film may come off the slide in the staining process. Methanol in the stain fixes the cells to the slide. Actual staining of cells or cellular components does not occur until the buffer is added. Because staining reactions are pH dependent, the buffer that is added to the stain should be 0.05 M sodium phosphate (pH 6.4) or aged distilled water (distilled water placed in a glass bottle for at least 24 hours; pH 6.4 to 6.8).

Free methylene blue is a basic dye and stains acidic cellular components, such as nuclear deoxyribonucleic acid (DNA), cytoplasmic ribonucleic acid (RNA), and some granules, a blue color. These components are described as *basophilic*. Free eosin is an acidic dye and stains basic components, such as hemoglobin and some granules, a pink or orange color. Granules that stain with eosin are described as *eosinophilic*. Cellular components with a neutral pH will stain with both dyes and appear lavender in color. These components are described as *neutrophilic*. Neutrophils, basophils, and eosinophils are so named for the specific staining of their cytoplasmic granules.

Water or drying artifact has long been a nuisance to hematology laboratories. It has several appearances. It can give a moth-eaten look to the RBCs, or it may appear as a heavily demarcated central pallor or refractive (shiny) blotches on the RBCs (Figure 14.6). At other times, it manifests simply as crenated RBCs seen in the areas of the slide that dried most slowly.

Multiple factors contribute to this problem. Humidity in the air as the slide dries may add to the punched-out, moth-eaten, or crenated appearance of the RBCs. It is difficult to avoid drying artifact on films from extremely anemic patients because of the very high ratio of plasma to RBCs. Water absorbed from the air into the alcohol-based stain also can contribute.

Water or drying artifact can be minimized by drying the slide as quickly as possible and putting a stopper tightly on the stain bottle to keep out the moisture. In some laboratories, slides are fixed in pure anhydrous methanol before staining to

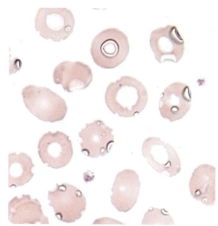

Figure 14.6 Drying Artifact on Red Blood Cells. Drying artifact appears as highly refractile areas on red blood cells on a peripheral blood film. It can occur due to slow drying of the blood film after preparation. (Peripheral blood, Wright-Giemsa stain, ×1000.) (From Carr, J. H. [2022]. *Clinical Hematology Atlas.* [6th ed]. St. Louis: Elsevier.)

help reduce water artifact. Stain manufacturers have also used 10% volume-to-volume methanol to minimize water or drying artifact.

Wright Staining Methods

Manual technique. Traditionally, Wright staining has been performed over a sink or pan with a staining rack. Slides are placed on the rack with the film side facing upward. The Wright stain may be filtered before use or poured directly from the bottle through a filter onto the slide. It is important to flood the slide completely. The stain should remain on the slide at least 1 to 3 minutes to fix the cells to the glass. Then an approximately equal amount of buffer is added to the slide. Surface tension allows very little of the buffer to run off. A metallic sheen should appear on the slide if mixing is correct (Figure 14.7). More buffer can be added if necessary. The mixture is allowed to remain on the slide for 3 minutes or more (bone marrow smears take longer to stain than peripheral blood films). Timing may be adjusted to produce the best staining characteristics. When staining is complete, the slide is rinsed with a steady but gentle stream of water with neutral pH, the back of the slide is wiped to remove any stain residue, and the slide is air dried in a vertical position.

Use of the manual Wright staining technique is desirable for staining peripheral blood films containing very high WBC counts, such as films from patients with leukemia. As with bone marrow smears, the time can be easily lengthened to enhance the staining required by the increased numbers of cells. Understaining is common when a slide from a leukemia patient is placed on an automated slide stainer. The main disadvantages of the manual technique are the increased risk of spilling the stain and the longer time required to complete the procedure. This technique is best suited for low-volume laboratories.

Automated slide stainers. Numerous automated slide stainers are commercially available. For high-volume laboratories, these instruments are essential. Once they are set up and loaded with slides, staining proceeds without operator attention. In general, it takes 5 to 10 minutes to stain a batch of slides. The processes

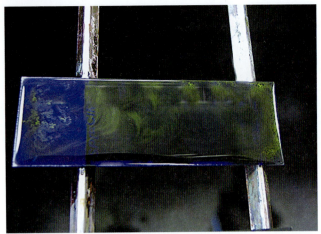

Figure 14.7 Manual Wright Staining of Slides. Note metallic sheen of stain, indicating proper mixing.

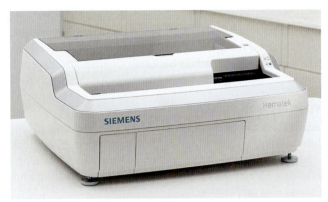

Figure 14.9 Hematek 3000 Slide Stainer. The instrument performs a Wright stain by automatically propelling the slides along a platen surface by two conveyor spirals for the fixation and staining processes. (2014 Siemens Healthineers. Photo courtesy Siemens Healthineers.)

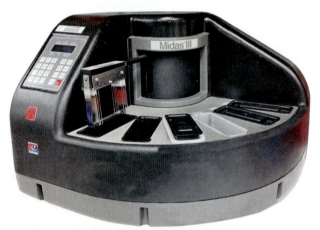

Figure 14.8 Midas III Slide Stainer. The instrument performs a Wright stain by automatically dipping the slides in stain and then in buffer, followed by a series of rinses. (Courtesy MilliporeSigma, Burlington, MA.)

of fixing, staining, and buffering are similar in practice to those of the manual method. The slides may be automatically dipped in stain and then in buffer and a series of rinses (MilliporeSigma MIDAS III) (Figure 14.8), or propelled along a platen surface by two conveyor spirals (Siemens Healthineers Hematek 3000) (Figure 14.9). In the Hematek device, stain, buffer, and rinse are pumped through holes in the platen surface, flooding the slide at the appropriate time.[14] Film quality and color consistency are usually good with any of these instruments. Some commercially prepared stain, buffer, and rinse packages do vary from lot to lot or manufacturer to manufacturer, so testing is recommended. Some disadvantages of the dip-type batch stainers are that (1) stat slides cannot be added to the batch once the staining process has begun and (2) working or aqueous solutions of stain are stable for only 3 to 6 hours and need to be prepared often. Stat slides can be added at any time to the Hematek stainer, and stain packages are stable for about 6 months.

Quick stains. Quick stains, as the name implies, are fast and easy. The whole process takes about 1 minute. Stain is purchased in a bottle as a modified Wright or Wright-Giemsa

stain. The required quantity can be filtered into a Coplin jar or a staining dish, depending on the number of slides to be stained. Aged, distilled water is used as the buffer. Stained slides are given a final rinse under a gentle stream of tap water and allowed to air dry. It is helpful to wipe off the back of the slide with alcohol to remove any excess stain. Quick stains are convenient and cost effective for low-volume laboratories such as clinics and physician office laboratories, or whenever rapid turnaround time is essential. Quality is often a concern with quick stains. With a little time and patience in adjusting the staining and buffering times, however, color quality can be acceptable.

Methanol-free stain. Cosmo Biomedical MCDh (Micro Chromatic Detection for Haematology) is a methanol-free stain that reduces staff exposure to toxic chemicals.[15] It is composed of four reagents: a mix of neutral dyes, a buffer solution, methylene blue, and a rinsing solution. MCDh is suitable for manual and automatic staining instruments and produces the typical coloration of a Wright stain.[15]

Features of a well-stained peripheral blood film. Properly staining a peripheral blood film is just as important as making a good film. Macroscopically, a well-stained blood film should be pink to purple. Microscopically, the RBCs should appear orange to salmon pink, and WBC nuclei should be purple to blue. The cytoplasm of neutrophils should be pink to tan, with violet or lavender granules. Eosinophils should have bright orange refractile granules. Faulty staining can be troublesome for reading the films, causing problems ranging from minor shifts in color to the inability to identify cells and assess morphology. Trying to interpret a poorly prepared or poorly stained blood film is extremely frustrating. If possible, a newly stained film should be examined. Hints for troubleshooting poorly stained blood films are provided in Box 14.1.

The best staining results are obtained on freshly made slides because the blood itself acts as a buffer in the staining process. Slides stained 1 week or longer after they are made turn out too blue. In addition, specimens that have increased levels of proteins (i.e., globulins) produce bluer-staining blood films, even when freshly stained.

BOX 14.1 Troubleshooting Poorly Stained Blood Films

Stain Is Too Blue	Stain Is Too Pink/Red
Appearance	**Appearance**
RBCs appear gray.	RBCs are too pale or are red.
WBCs are too dark.	WBCs are barely visible.
Eosinophil granules are gray, not orange.	
Causes	**Causes**
Stain or buffer too alkaline	Stain or buffer too acidic
Inadequate rinsing	Excessive rinsing
Prolonged staining time	Inadequate staining time
Blood film too thick	Blood film too thin
Heparinized blood specimen	

RBC, Red blood cell; *WBC,* white blood cell.
Data from Smock, K. J. (2019). Examination of the blood and bone marrow. In Greer, J. P., Rodgers, G. M., Glader, B., et al. (Eds.), *Wintrobe's Clinical Hematology.* (14th ed., pp. 1–16). Philadelphia: Lippincott Williams & Wilkins.

Peripheral Blood Film Examination

Microscopic blood film review is essential whenever automated analysis indicates that specimen abnormalities exist. The medical laboratory professional evaluates the platelet and WBC count and differential, along with WBC, RBC, and platelet morphology.

Macroscopic Examination

Examining the film before placing it on the microscope stage sometimes can give the evaluator an indication of abnormalities or test results that need rechecking. For example, a film that is bluer overall than normal may indicate that the patient has increased blood proteins, as in plasma cell myeloma, and that rouleaux may be seen on the film. A grainy appearance to the film may indicate RBC agglutination, as found in cold hemagglutinin diseases. In addition, holes all over the film could mean that the patient has increased lipid levels, and some of the automated CBC parameters should be rechecked for interferences from lipemia. Markedly increased WBC counts and platelet counts can be detected from the blue specks out at the feather edge. Valuable information might be obtained before the evaluator looks through the microscope.

Microscopic Examination

The microscope should be adjusted correctly for blood film evaluation. The light from the illuminator should be properly centered, the condenser should be almost all the way up and adjusted correctly for the magnification used, and the iris diaphragm should be opened to allow a comfortable amount of light to the eye. Many individuals prefer to use a neutral density filter over the illuminator to create a whiter light from a tungsten light source. If the microscope has been adjusted for Koehler illumination, all these conditions should have been met (Chapter E3).

10× objective examination. Blood film evaluation begins using the 10× or low-power objective lens (10× eyepiece × 10×

objective lens = 100× total magnification) (Chapter E3). Not much time needs to be spent at this magnification. However, it is a common error to omit this step altogether and go directly to the higher-power oil immersion lens. At the low-power magnification, overall film quality, color, and distribution of cells can be assessed. The feather edge and lateral edges should be checked quickly for WBC distribution. The presence of more than four times the number of cells per field at the edges or feather compared with the monolayer area of the film indicates that the film is unacceptable (i.e., a "snowplow" effect), and the film should be remade. Under the 10× objective, it is possible to check for the presence of fibrin strands; if they are present, the specimen should be rejected and another one should be collected. RBC distribution can be noted as well. Rouleaux formation or RBC agglutination is easy to recognize at this power. The film can be scanned quickly for any large, abnormal cells such as blasts, reactive lymphocytes, or even unexpected parasites. Finally, the area available for suitable examination can be assessed.

40× high-dry or 50× oil immersion objective examination. The next step is using the 40× high-dry objective (400× total magnification) or, as many laboratories now use, a 50× oil immersion objective (500× total magnification) instead. At either of these magnifications, it is easy to select the correct area of the film in which to begin the differential count and to evaluate cellular morphology. The WBC estimate also can be performed at these powers. To perform a WBC estimate, the evaluator selects an area in which the RBCs are separated from one another with minimal overlapping (where only two or three RBCs overlap). Depending on which lens is used (40× or 50×), the procedure is the same; only the multiplication factor changes. Count the WBCs in 10 fields and determine the average number of WBCs per field. The average number of WBCs per high-power field (40×) is multiplied by 2000 (if a 50× oil lens is used, multiply by 3000) to obtain an approximation of the WBC count per microliter of blood. For example, when using a 50× oil objective, if after 10 fields are scanned, it is determined that there are four to five WBCs per field, this would yield a WBC estimate of 12,000 to 15,000/μL (12 to 15 × 10⁹/L). Box 14.2 contains a summary of the procedure for the WBC count estimate. This technique can be helpful for internal quality control, although there are inherent errors in the process. Using an area of the film that is too thick (toward the origin of the film) or too thin (toward the feather edge) affects the estimates. In addition, field diameters may vary among microscope manufacturers and models, so validation of the estimation multiplication factor should be performed first (Box 14.3). Checking for a discrepancy between the estimate and the automated blood cell analyzer WBC count makes it easier to discover problems such as a film prepared using the wrong patient's blood specimen or a mislabeled film. In many laboratories, WBC estimates are performed on a routine basis; in others, these estimates are performed only as needed to confirm analyzer values.

100× oil immersion objective examination. The 100× oil immersion objective provides the highest magnification on most standard binocular microscopes (1000× total magnification). The WBC differential count generally is performed using the

BOX 14.2 Performing a White Blood Cell Estimate

1. Select an area of the blood film in which most red blood cells (RBCs) are separated from one another, with minimal overlapping of RBCs.
2. Using the 40× high-dry or 50× oil immersion objective, count the number of WBCs in 10 consecutive fields and calculate the average number of white blood cells (WBCs) per field.
3. To obtain the WBC estimate per microliter of blood, multiply the average number of WBCs per field by 2000* (if using the 40× high-dry objective) or 3000* (if using the 50× oil immersion objective).
4. Compare the WBC count from the automated blood cell analyzer with the WBC estimate from the blood film.
   Example: If an average of three WBCs were observed per field:
   Using a 40× high-dry objective, the WBC estimate is 6000/µL or 6.0 × 10^9/L.
   Using a 50× oil immersion objective, the WBC estimate is 9000/µL or 9.0 × 10^9/L.

*WBC estimation factors of 2000 (40× objective) and 3000 (50× objective) are provided as general guidelines. A WBC estimation factor should be determined and validated for each microscope in use (Box 14.3).

BOX 14.3 Validation of the White Blood Cell and Platelet Estimation Factor*

1. Perform automated white blood cell (WBC) and platelet (PLT) counts on 30 consecutive fresh patient blood specimens. Make sure the results of quality control are "in control" for WBC and PLT.
2. Prepare and stain one peripheral blood film for each specimen.
3. Using the 40× high-dry or 50× oil immersion objective for the WBC estimate and the 100× oil immersion objective for the PLT estimate, select an area of the blood film in which most red blood cells (RBCs) are separated from one another with minimal overlapping of RBCs.
4. Count the number of WBCs or PLTs in 10 consecutive fields using the magnification specified in step 3 and calculate the average number of WBCs and PLTs per field.
5. For each of the 30 specimens, divide the automated WBC count by the average number of WBCs per field (40× or 50× objective); divide the automated PLT count by the average number of PLTs per field (100× objective).
6. Add the numbers obtained in step 5 for the WBCs and divide by 30 (the number of observations in this analysis) to obtain the average ratio of the WBC count to WBCs per 40× or 50× field; add the numbers obtained in step 5 for the PLTs and divide by 30 (the number of observations in this analysis) to obtain the average ratio of the PLT count to PLTs per 100× field.
7. Round the number calculated in step 6 to the nearest whole number to obtain an estimation factor for WBCs and PLTs at the specified magnification.

*Because of the variation in the field diameter among different microscopes, an estimation factor should be determined for each microscope in use, and that number should be used to obtain the WBC and PLT estimates when using that microscope.
Modified from Terrell, J. C. (1998). Laboratory evaluation of leukocytes. In Stiene-Martin, E. A., Lotspeich-Steininger, C. A., Koepke, J. A., (Eds.), *Clinical Hematology, Principles, Procedures, Correlations*. (2nd ed., p. 337). Philadelphia: Lippincott-Raven Publishers.

100× oil immersion objective. Performing the differential normally includes counting and classifying 100 WBCs to obtain percentages of WBC types. The RBC, WBC, and platelet morphology evaluation Land the platelet estimate also are executed under the 100× oil immersion objective lens. At this magnification, the different types of WBCs can be distinguished. RBC inclusions such as Howell-Jolly bodies and WBC inclusions such as Döhle bodies can be seen easily if present. Reactive or abnormal cells are enumerated under the 100× objective as well. If present, nucleated RBCs (NRBCs) are counted and reported as NRBCs per 100 WBCs (Chapter 12).

50× oil immersion objective examination. The WBC differential and morphology examinations described for the 100× oil immersion objective also can be accomplished by experienced morphologists using a 50× oil immersion objective. The larger field of view allows more cells to be evaluated faster. Examination at this power is especially efficient for validating or verifying blood cell analyzer values when a total microscopic assessment of the film is not needed. Certain cell features that may require higher magnification can be assessed by moving the parfocal 100× objective into place and then returning to the 50× objective to continue the differential (Chapter E3). As previously mentioned, the WBC estimate also can be performed with the 50× objective, but the multiplication factor is 3000. The laboratory professional should conform to the estimation protocol of their laboratory.

Optimal assessment area. The tasks described, especially for the 100×, 40×, and 50× objectives, need to be performed in the best possible area of the peripheral blood film. That occurs between the thick area, or "heel," where the drop of blood was initially placed and spread, and the very thin feather edge. In the ideal area, microscopically, the RBCs are uniformly and singly distributed, with few touching or overlapping, and have their normal biconcave appearance (central pallor) (Figure 14.10A). An area that is too thin, in which there are holes in the film or the RBCs look flat, large, and distorted, is unacceptable (Figure 14.10B). A too-thick area also distorts the RBCs by piling them on top of one another like rouleaux (Figure 14.10C). WBCs are similarly distorted, which makes morphologic evaluation more difficult and classification potentially incorrect. When the correct area of a blood film from a patient with a normal RBC count is viewed, there are generally about 200 to 250 RBCs per 100× oil immersion field.

A common problem encountered with the oil immersion objective lens is worth mentioning. If the blood film was in focus under the 10× and 40× objectives but is impossible to bring into focus under the 100× objective, the slide is probably upside down. The 100× objective does not have sufficient depth of field to focus through the slide. The oil must be completely removed before the film is put on the stage right side up.

<4HD>*Performance of white blood cell differential.* Fewer manual differentials are performed today because of the superior accuracy of automated differentials and because of cost and time constraints (Chapter 13). When indicated, however, the manual differential always should be performed in a systematic manner. When the correct area has been selected, use of a back-and-forth serpentine, or "battlement," track pattern is preferred to minimize distribution errors (Figure 14.11)[16] and ensure that each cell is counted only once. A total of 100 WBCs are counted and classified through the use of push-down button counters (Figure 14.12A) or computer-interfaced keypads (Figure 14.12B). To increase accuracy, it is advisable to count at least

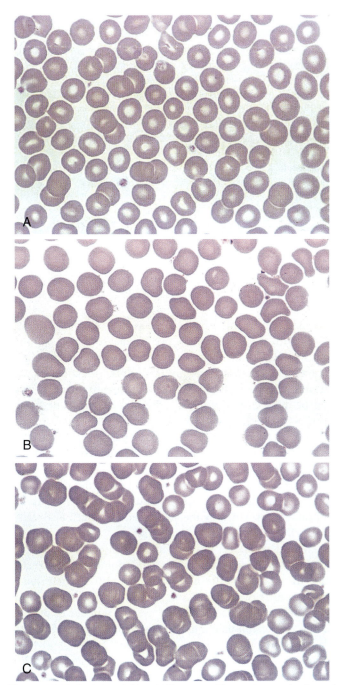

Figure 14.10 Peripheral Blood Films. (A), Photomicrograph of good area of peripheral blood film. Photomicrographs of peripheral blood film with areas **(B),** too thin and **(C),** too thick to examine. (Wright-Giemsa stain, ×1000.)

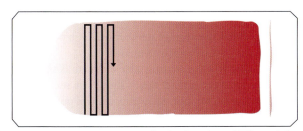

Figure 14.11 Battlement Pattern for Performing a Differential Count.

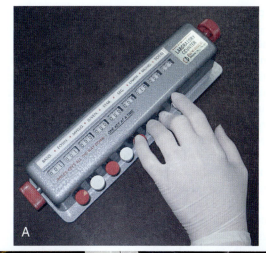

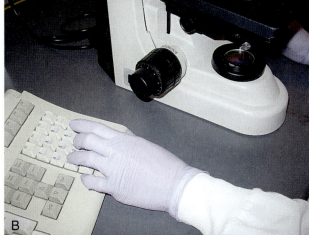

Figure 14.12 Differential Tally Counters. (A) Laboratory differential tally counter. **(B)** Computer-interfaced keypad counter.

200 cells when the WBC count is higher than 40×10^9/L. If the WBC count is 100×10^9/L or greater, it would be more precise and accurate to count 300 or 400 cells. Results are reported as percentages, for example, 54% segmented neutrophils, 6% bands, 28% lymphocytes, 9% monocytes, 3% eosinophils. The evaluator always should check to ensure that the sum of the percentages is 100.

Performing 100-cell differential counts on specimens with low WBC counts (less than 1.0×10^9/L) can become tedious and time consuming, even when the 50× oil immersion objective is used. In this situation, the differential count from the automated blood cell analyzer should be reported (if it is not flagged) because it is more accurate and precise.[17] However, if the blood cell analyzer cannot report a WBC differential or if the result is flagged, there are several options. WBCs can be concentrated by centrifugation of the specimen, and buffy coat smears can be made and examined. This practice is helpful for assessing the morphology of the cells; however, it is not recommended for performing the differential because of possible errors in cell distribution from centrifugation.[17] A truncated differential count can be done in which only 50 cells are counted on the peripheral blood film, with the result multiplied by 2 to obtain a percentage. However, because of the low number of cells counted, the accuracy of this practice is questionable, and it should be avoided if possible.[17] Another option is to simply examine the peripheral blood film or buffy coat for the presence of immature and abnormal cells, without performing a quantitative differential count.[17] In all cases, it is essential to examine the side margins of the blood film or buffy coat smear so that the larger cells such as monocytes, reactive lymphocytes, and immature cells are not missed.

In addition to counting the cells, the evaluator assesses their appearance. If present, WBC abnormalities such as toxic granulation, Döhle bodies, reactive lymphocytes, and Auer rods are evaluated and reported (Chapters 26 and 31). The International Council for Standardization in Haematology (ICSH) released guidelines and recommendations for the nomenclature and grading of RBC, WBC, and platelet abnormalities.[18] Traditionally, reactive lymphocytes were reported as a separate percentage of the 100 cells, as a percentage of the total number of lymphocytes, or semiquantitatively ("occasional" to "many"). The ICSH recommendation is to add a comment on the presence of reactive lymphocytes and to count them as a separate population of cells in the differential count if they are present in large numbers.[18] The ICSH also recommends that toxic granulation and Döhle bodies are graded as "slight" to "marked," or 1+ to 3+, and that Auer rods are reported as "present" when seen.[18] These recommendations are to be used strictly as guidelines to simplify blood film morphology reports and to help ensure better accuracy, consistency, and clinical relevance. Regardless of reporting format, each laboratory should establish criteria for reporting microscopic cell morphology.

The differential alone provides only partial information, reported in relative percentages, but absolute cell counts (number of cells per liter or microliter) can be calculated for each cell type using the total WBC count (discussed in "Summarizing White Blood Cell Parameters"). Automated blood cell analyzers report the WBC differential in both relative percentage and absolute count (Chapter 13).

Red blood cell morphology. Evaluation of RBC morphology is an important part of the blood film examination and includes an assessment of cell diameter (microcytosis, macrocytosis), variability in diameter (anisocytosis), cell color (hypochromia), cell shape (poikilocytosis and specific abnormalities in shape), and cellular inclusions (Chapter 16). Some laboratories use specific terminology for reporting the degree of abnormal morphology, such as "slight," "moderate," or "marked," or use a scale from 1+ to 3+. More recently, other laboratories employ a simpler report, using the term *present* for morphologic abnormalities that are clinically significant. Still other laboratories provide a summary statement regarding the overall RBC morphology that is consistent with the RBC indices and histogram. The latter methods are becoming more popular with increased computer interfacing in laboratories.

Review of RBC morphology can also be accomplished by digital morphology analyzers (discussed in "Automated Microscopic Examination") that provide a general assessment of RBC diameter, color, shape, and inclusions. For example, CellaVision DM analyzers can precharacterize 21 different morphologic types of RBCs.[19] The results are reported using

---

BOX 14.4 Performing a Platelet Estimate

1. Select an area of the blood film in which most red blood cells (RBCs) are separated from one another with minimal overlapping of RBCs.
2. Using the 100× oil immersion objective, count the number of platelets in 10 consecutive fields and calculate the average number of platelets per field.
3. To obtain the platelet estimate per microliter of blood, multiply the average number of platelets per field by 20,000.*
4. Compare the platelet count from the automated blood cell analyzer with the platelet estimate from the blood film.

   Example: If an average of 20 platelets were observed per 100× oil immersion field, the platelet estimate is 400,000/µL or 400 × 10⁹/L.

   In instances of significant anemia or erythrocytosis, use the following formula for the platelet estimate:

$$\frac{\text{Average number of platelets / field} \times \text{total RBC count}}{200\ \text{RBCs / field}}$$

* A platelet estimation factor of 20,000 is provided as a general guideline. A platelet estimation factor should be determined and validated for each microscope in use (Box 14.3).

---

standard semiquantitative grading as well as percent of total RBCs, with the latter a more precise measurement as thousands of RBCs are included in the analysis. According to recent ICSH recommendations for the identification, quantitation, and reporting of schistocytes, a quantitative result (%) may be more clinically significant in the diagnosis of thrombotic microangiopathy (TMA) (Chapter 38). If schistocytes above a 1% threshold are found in the peripheral blood of an adult or full-term neonate patient, there is strong suspicion of TMA.[20]

Regardless of the reporting method used, the microscopic RBC morphology assessment should be congruent with the information provided by the automated blood cell analyzer. If not, further investigation is needed.

Platelet estimate. As previously mentioned, the platelet estimate is performed under the 100× oil immersion objective lens. In an area of the film where the RBCs barely touch, with minimal overlapping, the number of platelets in 10 oil immersion fields is counted. The average number of platelets per oil immersion field multiplied by 20,000 approximates the platelet count per microliter. For example, 12 to 16 platelets per oil immersion field equals about 280,000 platelets/µL (280 × 10⁹/L) and is considered adequate. Box 14.4 contains a summary of the procedure for the platelet estimate. In situations in which the patient is anemic or has erythrocytosis, however, the relative proportion of platelets to RBCs is altered. In these instances, a more involved formula for platelet estimates may be used:

$$\frac{\text{Average number of platelets/field} \times \text{total RBC count}}{200\ \text{RBCs/field}}$$

Note that 200 is the average number of RBCs per oil immersion field in the optimal assessment area.

Regardless of whether a reportable estimate is made, verification of the analyzer platelet count should be included in the overall examination for internal quality control purposes. Blood film examination also includes an assessment of the morphology of the platelets, including diameter as well as granularity and overall appearance.

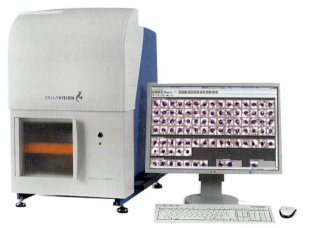

Figure 14.13 CellaVision DM9600. CellaVision analyzers automate the review of peripheral blood films by preclassifying white blood cells into 17 cell types and precharacterizing red blood cells based on 21 morphologic features. The analyzers can also characterize cell morphology on cytocentrifuged slides of cerebrospinal, peritoneal, pleural, and synovial fluids. The operator can override the analyzer's preclassification and identify cells that the analyzer could not classify. Analyzers vary in size and capacity. (Courtesy CellaVision AB, Lund, Sweden.)

Immersion oils with different viscosities do not mix well. If slides are taken to another microscope for review, oil should be wiped off first.

Automated Microscopic Examination

Digital morphology analyzers such as the CellaVision DM9600 (Figure 14.13) have automated microscopic blood cell identification.[19] This analyzer automatically identifies optimal examination areas on a slide, then locates and captures focused images of the cells. To preclassify cell images, numerous morphological characteristics are extracted from each cell and fed into a computerized visual recognition system. The digital images are presented to the operator, who reviews the cells on the screen, adjusts any classifications, enters comments about morphology, and verifies the results. Images and results are stored in a local or central database enabling remote review of cell images and results for cases needing a second review.[19] This functionality is also used by distributed laboratory networks to manage staffing when expertise in blood film review is limited. In these networks, slides are prepared and processed on small blood cell analyzers in remote laboratories, while the images and results are reviewed and reported by staff with expertise in morphology in the central laboratory.[19]

Some advantages of digital morphology analyzers include improved consistency of cell identifications and the ease of long-term storage of images for later review and comparison. The ability to compare cell images displayed side by side on the screen and quick access to an onboard library of reference cell images can help build confidence in cell identification and quality of results.[19]

Digital morphology analyzers continue to be developed. In 2020, two new compact analyzers, the CellaVision DC-1 and Scopio Labs X100, were cleared by the Food and Drug Administration (FDA).[21,22] The use of digital morphology analysis is expected to increase in smaller laboratories now with the

approval of the compact analyzers specifically designed for use in low-volume settings.[22]

SUMMARIZING COMPLETE BLOOD COUNT RESULTS

This chapter has focused so far on slide preparation and performance of a differential cell count. However, the differential is the capstone of a panel of tests collectively called the complete blood count (CBC) that includes many of the routine tests described in Chapter 12. Now that the testing for the component parts has been described, interpretation of the results for the total panel can be discussed.

The CBC has evolved over time to the typical test panel reported today, including assessment of WBCs, RBCs, and platelets. The CBC provides information about the hematopoietic system, but because abnormalities of blood cells can be caused by diseases of other organ systems, the CBC also plays a role in screening those organs for disease. The CBC provides such valuable information about a patient's health status that it is among the most commonly ordered laboratory tests performed by medical laboratory professionals.

The process of interpreting the CBC results has two phases. In phase 1, the numbers and descriptions generated by the testing are summarized using appropriate terminology. This summary provides a synopsis of the numbers that is easy to communicate to the health care provider or another laboratory professional. It is much more informative to be able to say, "The patient has a microcytic anemia," rather than, "The hemoglobin was low and the mean cell volume was also low." Phase 2 of interpretation involves recognizing a pattern of results consistent with various diseases and narrowing the diagnosis for the given patient or perhaps pinpointing it so that appropriate follow-up testing or treatment can be recommended.

The following discussion focuses on phase 1 of CBC interpretation—how to collect the pertinent information and summarize it. Phase 2 of the interpretation is the essence of the remaining chapters of this book on various hematologic conditions or other metabolic conditions that have an impact on the hematologic system.

Organization of Complete Blood Count Results

Today most laboratory professionals perform CBCs using sophisticated automated blood cell analyzers as described in Chapter 13, but the component tests can be performed using the manual methods described in Chapter 12. The blood film assessment described in this chapter is also part of a CBC. As previously mentioned, the CBC panel is essentially divided into WBC, RBC, and platelet parameters.

For phase 2 interpretation, it is sometimes important to look at all three groups of the CBC results; at other times, only one or two may be of interest. If a patient has an infection, the WBC parameters may be the only ones of interest. If the patient has anemia, all three sets, WBCs, RBCs, and platelets, may require assessment. Generally, all the parameters interpreted together provide the best information, so a complete summary of the results should be generated.

Assessing Hematology Results Relative to Reference Intervals

Proper performance of the phase 1 summary of test results requires comparison of the patient values with the reference intervals. The table of reference intervals for the CBC after the Index at the end of the book shows that there are different reference intervals for men and women, particularly for the RBC parameters. There also are different intervals for children of different ages, with the WBC changes the most notable. It is important to select the appropriate set of reference intervals in hematology for the sex and age of the patient. In addition, reference intervals for RBC parameters should be established for transgender individuals, depending on their therapy and stage of transition (Chapter 43).

CBC results can be reported in standard international (SI) units or in common units. For example, the following two sets of results in SI units and common units are equivalent:

	SI Units	Common Units
WBC count	7.2×10^9/L	7.2×10^3/µL
RBC count	4.20×10^{12}/L	4.20×10^6/µL
Hemoglobin (HGB)	128 g/L	12.8 g/dL
Hematocrit (HCT)	0.41 L/L	41%
Platelet (PLT) count	237×10^9/L	237×10^3/µL

Because either system may be used on laboratory reports, the medical laboratory professional should be able to easily interconvert CBC results between the systems. SI units are used for cell counts in this chapter.

Several strategies can help in determining the significance of the results. First, if the results are very far from the reference interval, it is more likely that they are truly outside the interval and represent a pathologic process. Second, if two or more diagnostically related parameters are slightly or moderately outside the interval in the same direction (both high or both low), this suggests that the results are clinically significant and associated with some pathologic process. Because some healthy individuals can have results slightly outside the reference interval, the best comparison for their results is not the reference interval but their own results from a prior time when they were known to be healthy.

Summarizing White Blood Cell Parameters

The WBC-related parameters of a routine CBC include the following:
1. Total WBC count (WBCs × 10^9/L)
2. WBC differential count values expressed as percentages, called *relative counts*
3. WBC differential count values expressed as the actual number of each type of cell (e.g., neutrophils × 10^9/L), called *absolute counts*
4. WBC morphology

Step 1

Start by ensuring that there is an accurate WBC count. Compare the WBC histogram and/or scatterplots with the respective cell counts to make sure they correlate with one another. Today's automated blood cell analyzers can eliminate nucleated RBCs that falsely increase the WBC count. However, manual WBC results must be corrected mathematically to eliminate the contribution of the NRBCs (Chapter 12).

Step 2

Look at the total WBC count. When the count is elevated, it is called *leukocytosis*. When the count is low, it is called *leukopenia*. As described later, increases and decreases of WBCs are associated with infections and conditions such as leukemias. Because there is more than one type of WBC, increases and decreases in the total count usually are due to changes in one of the subtypes, for example, neutrophils or lymphocytes. Determining which one is the next step.

Step 3

Examine the relative differential counts for a preliminary assessment of which cell types are affected. The relative differential count is reported in percentages. The proportion of each cell type can be described by its relative number (i.e., percent) and compared with its reference interval. Then it is described using appropriate terminology, such as a relative neutrophilia, which is an increase in neutrophils, or a relative lymphopenia, which is a decrease in lymphocytes. The terms used for increases and decreases of each cell type are provided in Table 14.1.

If the total WBC count or any of the relative values are outside the reference interval, further analysis of the WBC differential is needed. If the proportion of one of the cell types increases, then the proportion of others must decrease because the proportions are relative to one another. The second cell type may not have changed in actual number at all, however. The way to assess this accurately is with absolute differential counts.

Step 4

If not reported by the blood cell analyzer, absolute counts (cells/µL or cells/L) for each WBC type can be calculated by multiplying each relative cell count (i.e., percentage) by the total WBC count.

Examine the set of WBC results from a CBC shown in Table 14.2. On first inspection, one may look at the WBC count and recognize that a leukocytosis is present, but it is important to determine what cell type is causing the increased count. In this case, the relative counts (%) of each cell type are all within

TABLE 14.1 Terminology for Increases and Decreases in White Blood Cells

Cell Type	Increases	Decreases
Neutrophil	Neutrophilia	Neutropenia
Eosinophil	Eosinophilia	N/A
Basophil	Basophilia	N/A
Lymphocyte	Lymphocytosis	Lymphopenia (lymphocytopenia)
Monocyte	Monocytosis	Monocytopenia

N/A, Not applicable because the reference interval begins at or near zero.

TABLE 14.2 Comparison of Relative and Absolute White Blood Cell Counts

Complete Blood Count Parameter	Patient Value	Reference Interval (Examples)	Interpretation Relative to Reference Interval	Description/Summary
White blood cell count	13.2	$3.6–10.6 \times 10^9$/L	Elevated	Leukocytosis
Relative Differential				
Neutrophils	68	50%–70%	WRI	
Lymphocytes	23	18%–42%	WRI	
Monocytes	5	2%–11%	WRI	
Eosinophils	3	1%–3%	WRI	
Basophils	1	0%–2%	WRI	
Absolute Differential				
Absolute neutrophils	9.0	$1.7–7.5 \times 10^9$/L	Elevated	Absolute neutrophilia
Absolute lymphocytes	3.0	$1.0–3.2 \times 10^9$/L	WRI	
Absolute monocytes	0.70	$0.1–1.3 \times 10^9$/L	WRI	

WRI, Within reference interval.

reference intervals. There is no indication as to which cell type could be causing the increase in total numbers of WBCs.

When each relative number (e.g., neutrophils at 68% or 0.68) is multiplied by the total WBC count (13.2×10^9/L), the absolute number indicates that the neutrophils are elevated (9.0×10^9/L) compared with the reference interval provided. The absolute neutrophil count (ANC) is a very useful parameter for assessing neutropenia and neutrophilia. The absolute lymphocyte count (3.0×10^9/L) is still within the reference interval. Given this information, these results can be described as showing a leukocytosis with only an absolute neutrophilia, and the overall increase in the WBC count is due to an increase only in neutrophils. This description provides a concise summary of the WBC counts without the need to refer to every type of cell. Box 14.5 extends this concept to a convention used to describe the neutrophilic cells, and Box 14.6 addresses the clinical utility of reporting percent bands as a separate category.

When the absolute numbers of each of the individual cell types are totaled, the sum equals the WBC count (slight differences may occur because of rounding). Absolute counts are obtained directly from automated blood cell analyzers, which count actual numbers (i.e., produce absolute counts) and calculate relative values. As will be evident in later chapters, the findings in this example point toward a bacterial infection. Had there been an absolute lymphocytosis, a viral infection would be a consideration.

Step 5

Each cell type should be examined for immature cells. Immature WBCs are not normally seen in the peripheral blood, and they may indicate infections or malignancies such as leukemia. For neutrophilic cells, there is a unique term that refers to the presence of increased numbers of bands or cells younger than bands in the peripheral blood: *left shift* or *shift to the left* (Box 14.7). Some automated blood cell analyzers report an immature granulocyte count (Chapter 13).

When immature lymphocytic or monocytic cells are present, they can be reported in the differential as prolymphocytes, lymphoblasts, promonocytes, or monoblasts (Chapter 10).

Immature eosinophils or basophils are not typically staged and are included in the applicable category (e.g., eosinophilic metamyelocytes are counted as eosinophils), with comments in the interpretive section that those immature cells are present (Chapter 13).

Step 6

Any abnormalities of appearance are reported in the morphology section of the report. For WBCs, abnormal morphologic features that would be noted include changes in overall cellular appearance such as cytoplasmic toxic granulation and nuclear abnormalities such as hypersegmentation. The clinical significance of these types of changes is discussed in Chapter 26.

To summarize the WBC parameters, begin with an accurate total WBC count, followed by the relative differential, or preferably the absolute counts, noting whether any immature or abnormal cells are present in the blood. Finally, note the presence of any abnormal morphology or inclusions.

Summarizing Red Blood Cell Parameters

RBC parameters of the CBC are as follows:
1. RBC count (RBCs $\times 10^{12}$/L)
2. HGB (g/dL)
3. HCT (% or L/L)
4. Mean cell volume (MCV) (fL)
5. Mean cell hemoglobin (MCH) (pg)
6. Mean cell hemoglobin concentration (MCHC) (g/dL)
7. RBC distribution width (RDW) (%)
8. Reticulocyte count (relative and absolute) and indicators of reticulocyte maturity
9. Morphology

Step 1

Examine the hemoglobin for anemia or polycythemia by comparing the patient result with the age- and sex-specific reference intervals. Anemia is the more common condition. Hemoglobin concentration is a more reliable indicator of anemia than the hematocrit because it directly assesses the ability of the blood to

BOX 14.5 Summarizing Neutrophilia When Immature Cells Are Present

A subtle convention in assessing the differential counts involves the presence of immature cells of the neutrophilic series (e.g., bands). They typically are grouped together with the mature neutrophils in judging whether neutrophilia is present. For example, look at the following differential values and the reference intervals.

	Patient Value	Reference Interval (Examples)
White blood cells	10.6	3.6–10.6 × 109/L
Neutrophils	65	50%–70%
Bands	18	0%–10%
Lymphocytes	13	18%–42%
Monocytes	3	2%–11%
Eosinophils	1	1%–3%
Basophils	0	0%–2%

Although the mature neutrophils are within the reference interval, the bands exceed their reference interval. The total of the two, 83 (65% + 18%), exceeds the upper limit of neutrophilic cells, even when the two intervals are combined, 80 (70% + 10%), so these results would be described as a neutrophilia, even though the neutrophil value itself is within the reference interval. See steps 4 and 5 in "Summarizing White Blood Cell Parameters" for how to communicate the increase in bands.

BOX 14.6 Clinical Utility of Band Counts

An elevated band count was thought to be useful in the diagnosis of patients with infection. However, its clinical utility has been called into question, and most clinical laboratories no longer perform routine band counts. The Clinical and Laboratory Standards Institute (CLSI) recommends that bands and neutrophils be counted together and reported in one category (neutrophils) rather than in separate categories because it is difficult to consistently differentiate bands from segmented neutrophils based on their morphology.

From Cornbleet, P. J. (2002). Clinical utility of the band count. *Clin Lab Med, 22,* 101–136; and CLSI. (2007). *Reference Leukocyte (WBC) Differential Count (Proportional) and Evaluation of Instrumental Methods.* (2nd ed., approved standard, H20-A2). Wayne, PA: Clinical and Laboratory Standards Institute.

BOX 14.7 Origin of the Phrase *Left Shift*

The origin of the phrase left shift is a 1920s publication by Josef Arneth in which neutrophil maturity was correlated with segment count. A graphical representation was made and the fewer the segments, the farther left was the median—hence left shift. This was called the Arneth count or Arneth-Schilling count and was abandoned around the time Arneth died in 1955, but the term left shift lived on to describe increased numbers of immature neutrophilic cells as an indicator of infection.

TABLE 14.3 Interpretation of Mean Cell Volume Values Using the Wintrobe Terminology

Mean Cell Volume Value	Wintrobe Description
Within reference interval (80–100 fL)	Normocytic
Lower than reference interval (<80 fL)	Microcytic
Higher than reference interval (>100 fL)	Macrocytic

patient RBC abnormalities. Remember that the rule of three holds true only when overall RBC morphology is normal.

Step 2

When the hemoglobin and hematocrit values have been inspected and the rule of three applied, the next RBC parameter that should be evaluated is the MCV (Chapter 12). This value provides the average RBC volume. The MCV should be correlated with the RBC histogram from the automated blood cell analyzer and morphologic appearance of the cells using the classification first introduced by Wintrobe a century ago (Table 14.3).

The MCV is expected to be within the established reference interval (approximately 80 to 100 fL), and the RBC histogram and morphology are expected to be normal (normocytic). For a patient with anemia, classifying the anemia morphologically by the MCV narrows the range of possible causes to microcytic, normocytic, or macrocytic anemias (Chapter 16).

Step 3

Examine the MCHC to evaluate how well the cells are filled with hemoglobin. Remember that MCHC is a concentration and takes into consideration the volume of the RBCs when considering decreased or normal color. If the MCHC is within the reference interval, the cells are considered normal or *normochromic* and display typical central pallor of one-third the volume of the cell. If the MCHC is less than the reference interval, the cells are called *hypochromic,* which literally means "too little color." This correlates with a larger central pallor (hypochromia) when the cells are examined on a Wright-stained blood film.

It is possible for the MCHC to be elevated in two situations, but this does not correlate with hyperchromia. A slight elevation may be seen when cells are spherocytic (MCHC > 36 g/dL). They retain roughly normal volume but have decreased surface area. Therefore the hemoglobin is slightly more concentrated than usual, and the cells look darker with no central pallor. A more dramatic increase in MCHC (values as high as 60 g/dL) can be caused by analytical errors, often associated with patient specimen problems that falsely elevate the hemoglobin measurement. Common problems of this type include interference from lipemia, icterus, or grossly elevated WBC counts. Each of these interferes with the spectrophotometric measurement of hemoglobin, thus falsely elevating the hemoglobin and affecting the calculation of the MCHC (Chapters 12 and 13). It is worth noting that the MCHC is often best used as an internal quality control parameter.

Step 4

The RDW is determined from the histogram of RBC volumes. Briefly, when the volumes of the RBCs are about the same,

carry oxygen. In addition, the hematocrit can be influenced by the volume of the RBCs.

If the RBC morphology is normochromic and normocytic, three times the hemoglobin approximates the hematocrit; this is called the *rule of three* (Chapter 12). If the rule of three fails, it may be an indication of an analytical error due to a falsely increased or decreased hemoglobin or hematocrit. If all test results are accurate, further assessment should uncover some

Therefore the RDW provides information about the presence and degree of anisocytosis (variation in RBC volume). Only increased RDW values, and not decreased values, have clinical significance. If an RDW reference interval is 11.5% to 14.5% and a patient has an RDW of 20.6%, the patient has a more heterogeneous RBC population with more variation in cell volume (anisocytosis). If the RDW is elevated, a notation about anisocytosis is expected in the morphologic evaluation of the blood film. Using the MCV along with the RDW provides the most helpful information (Chapter 16).

Step 5

Examine the relative and absolute reticulocyte counts, if ordered. The reticulocyte count is used to assess the erythropoietic activity in the bone marrow (Chapter 12). If the patient is anemic, an elevated count indicates a bone marrow response to compensate for the anemia, as seen in the hemolytic anemias (Chapter 20). If the patient is anemic and the reticulocyte count is low, the patient has a poor bone marrow response, and bone marrow failure should be investigated (Chapter 19). Calculating the reticulocyte production index can assist in this assessment (Chapter 12). Indicators of reticulocyte maturity (such as the immature reticulocyte fraction [IRF]) that are provided on some automated blood cell analyzers are very sensitive measures of erythropoietic activity in the bone marrow (Chapter 13).

Step 6

Examine the morphology for pertinent abnormalities. Whenever anemia is indicated by the RBC parameters reported by the analyzer, and potential abnormal RBC morphology is suggested by the indices and the rule of three, a Wright-stained peripheral blood film must be reviewed. Abnormalities include abnormal volume, abnormal shape, inclusions, immature RBCs, abnormal color, and abnormal arrangement (Chapter 16). The blood film also serves as quality control because the morphologic characteristics seen through the microscope (e.g., microcytosis, anisocytosis) should be congruent with the results provided by the analyzer. When they do not agree, further investigation is necessary.

If everything in the morphology is normal, by convention, no notation regarding morphology is included. Therefore, any notation in the morphology section requires scrutiny. All RBC-related abnormal morphologic findings should be noted, including specific poikilocytosis (abnormal shape) and the presence of RBC inclusions such as Howell-Jolly bodies. One of the major challenges is in determining when the amount or degree of an abnormality is worth noting at all (i.e., when it should be reported). Laboratories strive for standardization of reporting. All laboratories must have standardized morphology criteria and competent staff whose evaluations are consistent with one another and with the standardized criteria used in that facility. Generally a semiquantitative method is used that employs terms such as *slight, moderate,* and *marked* or the numbers 1+, 2+, and 3+. Numerical ranges representing the reporting unit are defined; for example, three to six spherocytes per oil immersion field might be reported as 2+ spherocytes.

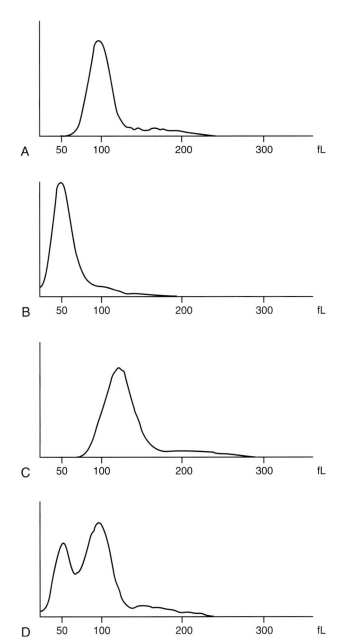

Figure 14.14 Red Blood Cell Histograms. **(A)**, Normocytic red blood cell population with MCV of 96.8 fL and RDW-CV of 14.1%. **(B)**, Microcytosis with MCV of 54.6 fL and RDW-CV of 13.2%. **(C)**, Macrocytosis and anisocytosis with MCV of 119.2 fL and RDW-CV of 23.9%. **(D)**, Dimorphic red blood cells with MCV of 80.2 fL and RDW-CV of 37.2%. Note the microcytic and the normocytic red blood cell populations. Reference intervals: *MCV*, 80 to 100 fL; *RDW-CV*, 11.5% to 14.5%. MCV, Mean cell volume; RDW-CV, red blood cell distribution width, coefficient of variation.

the histogram is narrow (Figure 14.14A). If the volumes are variable (more small cells, more large cells, or both), the histogram becomes wider. The width of the histogram, the RDW, is reflected statistically as a coefficient of variation (CV) or a standard deviation (SD). Most blood cell analyzer manufacturers provide a CV and an SD, and the operator can select which to report. Figure 14.14 depicts RBC histograms demonstrating normal, microcytosis, macrocytosis, anisocytosis, and dimorphic RBC populations.

Although this practice has been followed for many years, this semiquantitative method may not best serve the needs of providers, and many laboratories are moving toward simplifying their reports to state *present* for morphologic abnormalities. In fact, the ICSH recommends the use of qualitative grading for RBC morphology except for schistocytes because, as mentioned previously, these cells have greater clinical significance even at lower counts.[20]

The presence of immature RBCs suggests that the bone marrow is attempting to respond to an anemia. Polychromasia on the peripheral blood film indicates bone marrow response. This is manifested by the bluer color of reticulocytes that have entered the bloodstream earlier than usual in the body's attempt to improve oxygen-carrying capacity. If the anemia is severe, NRBCs also may be present. As noted earlier, it is also important to recognize NRBCs because they may falsely elevate the manual WBC count and may be an indication of an underlying disease process. A better way to assess replacement erythropoiesis is with the relative and absolute reticulocyte count, calculation of the reticulocyte production index, if appropriate, and review of the immature reticulocyte fraction available on automated blood cell analyzers (Chapters 12 and 13).

Step 7

Examine the RBC count and MCH. On a practical level, the RBC count is not the parameter used to assess anemia because there are some types of anemia, such as the thalassemias (Chapter 25), in which the RBC count is normal or even elevated. Thus the assessment of anemia would be missed by relying only on the RBC count. However, this inconsistency (low hemoglobin and high RBC count) is often helpful diagnostically.

The MCH follows the MCV; that is, smaller cells necessarily hold less hemoglobin, whereas larger cells can hold more. For this reason, it is less often used than the MCV and MCHC. In the instances in which the MCH does *not* follow the MCV, the MCHC detects the discrepancy between volume and hemoglobin content of the cell. The MCH is not crucial to the assessment of anemia when the other parameters are provided. In summary, when evaluating the RBC parameters of the CBC, examine the hemoglobin first, then the MCV, RDW, and MCHC. Finally, take note of any abnormal morphology.

Summarizing Platelet Parameters

The platelet parameters of the CBC are as follows:
1. Platelet count (platelets $\times 10^9$/L)
2. Mean platelet volume (MPV) (fL)
3. Morphology

Step 1

The platelet count should be examined for increases (thrombocytosis) or decreases (thrombocytopenia) outside the established reference interval. A patient who has unexplained bruising or bleeding may have a decreased platelet count. The platelet count should be assessed along with the WBC count and hemoglobin to determine whether all three are decreased

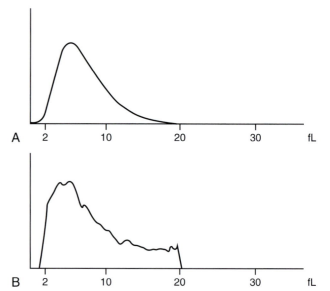

Figure 14.15 Platelet Histograms. (A), Normal with MPV of 8.0 fL. (B), Platelet population with abnormal histogram and MPV of 9.1 fL. Although the MPV is within the reference interval, the histogram shows an increase in the number of platelets with a volume between 10 and 20 fL (curve above baseline) representing giant platelets. Reference interval for the MPV for this analyzer is 6.8 to 10.2 fL. *MPV*, Mean platelet volume.

(pancytopenia) or increased (pancytosis). Pancytopenia is clinically significant because it can indicate a possible developing acute leukemia (Chapter 31) or aplastic anemia (Chapter 19). Pancytosis frequently is associated with a diagnosis of polycythemia vera (Chapter 32).

Step 2

Compare the analyzer-generated MPV with the MPV reference interval and with the platelet diameter observed on the peripheral blood film. An elevated MPV should correspond with increased platelet diameter, just as an elevated MCV reflects macrocytosis. In platelet consumption disorders such as immune thrombocytopenic purpura, an elevated MPV, accompanied by immature reticulated platelets (6 μm or larger in diameter) (Figure 11.5), reflects bone marrow release of early "stress" platelets, evidence for bone marrow compensation (Chapter 11).[23] Some automated blood cell analyzers report an immature platelet fraction (IPF) reflecting the percentage of immature platelets compared with the total number of platelets.[23] The immature platelets are counted using nucleic acid dyes, analogous to counting the IRF (Chapter 13). A platelet distribution width (PDW) is similar to the RDW. The PDW can be compared to the analyzer generated platelet count and the MPV.[24] Figure 14.15 demonstrates platelet histograms with a normal platelet population (Figure 14.15A) and one with giant platelets (Figure 14.15B).

Step 3

Examine platelet morphology and platelet arrangement. Although the MPV can recognize abnormally large platelets,

---

BOX 14.8 Applying a Systematic Approach to Complete Blood Count Summarization

A specimen from an adult male patient yields the following CBC results (refer to the reference intervals after the Index at the end of the book):

WBC	3.0×10^9/L
RBC	2.10×10^{12}/L
HGB	8.5 g/dL
HCT	26.3%
MCV	125 fL
MCH	40.5 pg
MCHC	32.3 g/dL
RDW	20.6%
PLT	105×10^9/L
MPV	8.2 fL
RETIC	0.2%

Differential:

NEUT	50%	$(1.5 \times 10^9$/L)
LYMPH	40%	$(1.2 \times 10^9$/L)
MONO	10%	$(0.3 \times 10^9$/L)

Morphology: hypersegmentation of neutrophils, anisocytosis, macrocytes, oval macrocytes, occasional teardrop cells, Howell-Jolly bodies, and basophilic stippling

The step-by-step assessment of the WBCs indicates that the WBC count is accurate and can be interpreted as leukopenia. Although the relative differential values all are within the reference intervals, calculation of absolute counts indicates an absolute neutropenia. No unexpected immature WBCs are noted, but the morphology indicates hypersegmentation of neutrophils. For the RBCs, the hemoglobin concentration (8.5 g/dL) indicates that the patient is anemic. Inspection of the MCV indicates macrocytosis because the MCV is increased to more than 100 fL, the upper limit of the reference interval. Examination of the MCHC shows it to be within the reference interval, so for these results, the RBC morphology would be described as macrocytic, normochromic. The elevated RDW indicates substantial anisocytosis. The morphologic description supports the interpretation of the RDW, with mention of anisocytosis as a result of macrocytosis and poikilocytosis characterized by oval macrocytes and occasional teardrop cells. Howell-Jolly bodies and basophilic stippling are significant RBC inclusions. The RETIC count is below the reference interval, indicating a reticulocytopenia and an inadequate response of the bone marrow to the anemia. The PLT count indicates thrombocytopenia. The MPV indicates the platelets are of normal diameter. The combined decrease in the WBC, RBC, and PLT counts indicates pancytopenia.

CBC, Complete blood count; *HCT,* hematocrit; *HGB,* hemoglobin concentration; *LYMPH,* lymphocyte count; *MCH,* mean cell hemoglobin; *MCHC,* mean cell hemoglobin concentration; *MCV,* mean cell volume; *MONO,* monocyte count; *MPV,* mean platelet volume; *NEUT,* neutrophil count; *PLT,* platelet count; *RBC,* red blood cell count; *RDW,* red cell distribution width; *RETIC,* reticulocyte count; *WBC,* white blood cell count.

BOX 14.9 Systematic Approach to Complete Blood Count Interpretation

White Blood Cells

Step 1: Ensure that the WBC count is accurate. Review WBC histogram and/or scatterplot and correlate with counts. The presence of nucleated RBCs may require correction of the WBC count.

Step 2: Compare the patient's WBC count with the laboratory's established reference interval.

Steps 3 and 4: Examine the differential information (relative and absolute) on variations in the distribution of WBCs.

Step 5: Make note of immature cells of any cell type reported in the differential that should not appear in peripheral blood in healthy states.

Step 6: Make note of any morphologic abnormalities and correlate blood film findings with the numerical values.

Red Blood Cells

Step 1: Examine the HGB concentration first to assess anemia.

Step 2: Examine the MCV to assess cell volume.

Step 3: Examine the MCHC to assess cell HGB concentration in RBC.

Step 4: Examine the RDW to assess anisocytosis. (Correlate both MCV and RDW with RBC histogram.)

Step 5: Examine the relative and absolute reticulocyte count and any indicators of reticulocyte maturity, if ordered.

Step 6: Examine the morphologic description and correlate with the numerical values. Look for evidence of a reticulocyte response.

Step 7: Review the remaining RBC parameters.

Platelets

Step 1: Examine the total platelet count.

Step 2: Examine the MPV to assess platelet volume.

Step 3: Examine platelet morphology and correlate with the numerical values.

HGB, Hemoglobin; *MCHC,* mean cell hemoglobin concentration; *MCV,* mean cell volume; *MPV,* mean platelet volume; *RBC,* red blood cell; *RDW,* RBC distribution width; *WBC,* white blood cell.

---

the morphologic evaluation also notes this. Some laboratories distinguish between large platelets (two times the normal diameter) and giant platelets (more than twice as large as normal) or compare platelet diameter with RBC diameter.

Additional morphologic descriptors include terms for reporting granularity, which is most important if missing, and in this case, the platelets are described as "hypogranular" or "agranular." Sometimes the abnormalities are too variable to classify, and the platelets are described simply as "bizarre" or dysplastic. In some cases, platelets can be clumped or adherent to WBCs (satellitosis), and these arrangements should be noted. As described previously, corrective actions can be taken to derive accurate platelet and WBC counts when these arrangements are observed on the blood film. Summarizing platelet parameters includes reporting total number, platelet diameter by either the MPV from the analyzer or morphologic evaluation, and platelet appearance.

Box 14.8 gives an example of how the entire CBC can be summarized using the steps described. When results of the CBC are properly summarized and no information has been overlooked, there is confidence that the phase 2 interpretation of the results will be reliable. Adopting a methodical approach to examining each parameter ensures that the myriad information available from the CBC can be used effectively and efficiently in patient care. Box 14.9 summarizes the systematic approach to CBC interpretation.

SUMMARY

- Much valuable information can be obtained from a well-made and well-stained peripheral blood film.
- The specimen of choice for examination of peripheral blood films is whole blood collected in ethylenediaminetetraacetic acid (EDTA) (lavender closure tube). EDTA anticoagulates blood by chelating plasma calcium and is the best anticoagulant to preserve blood cell morphology.
- Only rarely does EDTA create problems in analyzing blood of certain individuals. EDTA-induced platelet clumping or satellitosis causes automated analyzers to report falsely decreased platelet counts (pseudothrombocytopenia) and sometimes falsely increased white blood cell (WBC) counts (pseudoleukocytosis). This problem must be recognized through blood film examinations and the proper course of action followed to produce accurate results.
- The wedge film is most often used for examining a peripheral blood film, and manual, semiautomated, and automated methods are available.
- Wright or Wright-Giemsa are polychrome stains containing eosin and methylene blue. Staining reactions depend on the pH of the cellular components. Methylene blue is a basic dye that stains acidic components blue (basophilic). Eosin is an acidic dye that stains basic cell components red or pink (eosinophilic). Cellular components that have a neutral pH stain lavender (neutrophilic). Neutrophils, eosinophils, and basophils were named for the staining properties of their granules.

- Wright staining is done manually or by automated techniques depending on the laboratory and the number of slides to be processed.
- Peripheral blood films and bone marrow smears always should be evaluated in a systematic manner, beginning with the 10× objective lens and finishing with the 100× oil immersion objective lens. WBC differential and morphologic evaluation, red blood cell (RBC) and platelet morphologic evaluation, and WBC and platelet number estimate all are included.
- Digital morphology analyzers help find, capture, and identify peripheral blood cells to automate the differential count. They preclassify WBCs into various cell types and precharacterize RBCs based on morphologic features. The operator can override the analyzer's preclassification and identify cells that the analyzer could not classify. Some advantages include a quicker and more efficient evaluation of cells, large storage of morphology results, and remote consultation between colleagues.
- Use of a systematic approach to complete blood count (CBC) interpretation ensures that all valuable information is assessed and nothing is overlooked. The systematic approach to CBC interpretation is summarized in Box 14.9.

Now that you have completed this chapter, go back and read again the case study at the beginning and respond to the questions presented. Answers can be found in Appendix C.

REVIEW QUESTIONS

Answers can be found in Appendix C.

1. A laboratory science student consistently makes wedge-technique blood films that are too long and thin. What change in technique would improve the films?
   a. Increasing the downward pressure on the pusher slide
   b. Decreasing the acute angle of the pusher slide
   c. Placing the drop of blood closer to the center of the slide
   d. Increasing the acute angle of the pusher slide

2. When a blood film is viewed through the microscope, the RBCs appear redder than normal, the neutrophils are barely visible, and the eosinophils are bright orange. What is the most likely cause?
   a. The slide was overstained.
   b. The stain was too alkaline.
   c. The buffer was too acidic.
   d. The slide was not rinsed adequately.

3. A stained blood film is held up to the light and observed to be bluer than normal. What microscopic abnormality might be expected on this film?
   a. Rouleaux
   b. Spherocytosis
   c. Reactive lymphocytosis
   d. Toxic granulation

4. A laboratory professional using the 40× objective lens sees the following numbers of WBCs in 10 fields: 8, 4, 7, 5, 4, 7, 8, 6, 4, 6. Which of the following WBC counts most closely correlates with the estimate?
   a. $1.5 \times 10^9/L$
   b. $5.9 \times 10^9/L$
   c. $11.8 \times 10^9/L$
   d. $24 \times 10^9/L$

5. A blood film for a very anemic patient with an RBC count of $1.25 \times 10^{12}/L$ shows an average of seven platelets per oil immersion field. Which of the following values most closely correlates with the estimate per microliter?
   a. 14,000
   b. 44,000
   c. 140,000
   d. 280,000

6. A blood film for a patient with a normal RBC count has an average of 10 platelets per oil immersion field. Which of the following values best correlates with the estimate per microliter?
   a. 20,000
   b. 100,000
   c. 200,000
   d. 400,000

7. What is the absolute count ($\times 10^9$/L) for the lymphocytes if the total WBC count is 9.5×10^9/L and there are 37% lymphocytes?
   a. 3.5
   b. 6.5
   c. 13
   d. 37

8. Which of the following blood film findings indicates EDTA-induced pseudothrombocytopenia?
   a. The platelets are pushed to the feathered end.
   b. The platelets are adhering to WBCs.
   c. No platelets at all are on the film.
   d. The slide has a bluish discoloration when examined macroscopically.

9. Which of the following is the best area to review or perform a differential on a stained blood film?
   a. RBCs are all overlapped in groups of three or more.
   b. RBCs are mostly separated, with a few overlapping.
   c. RBCs look flattened, with none touching.
   d. RBCs are separated and holes appear among the cells.

10. Use the reference intervals provided after the Index at the end of the book. Given the following data, summarize the following blood picture:
    WBC: 86.3×10^9/L
    HGB: 9.7 g/dL
    HCT: 24.2%
    MCV: 87.8 fL
    MCHC: 33.5%
    PLT: 106×10^9/L
    a. Leukocytosis, normocytic-normochromic anemia, thrombocytopenia
    b. Microcytic-hypochromic anemia, thrombocytopenia
    c. Neutrophilia, macrocytic anemia, thrombocytosis
    d. Leukocytosis, thrombocytopenia

REFERENCES

1. Smock, K. J. (2019). Examination of the blood and bone marrow. In Greer, J. P., Rodgers, G. M., Glader, B., et al. (Eds.), *Wintrobe's Clinical Hematology*. (14th ed., pp. 1–16). Philadelphia: Lippincott Williams & Wilkins.

2. Tatsumi, N., Miwa, S., & Lewis, S. M. (2002). International Society of Hematology, and the International Council for Standardization in Haematology. Specimen collection, storage, and transmission to the laboratory for hematological tests. *Int J Hematol, 75*(3), 261–268.

3. CLSI. (2007). *Reference Leukocyte (WBC) Differential Count (Proportional) and Evaluation of Instrumental Methods*. (2nd ed., CLSI approved standard H20-A2). Wayne, PA: Clinical and Laboratory Standards Institute.

4. Vives-Corrons, J.-L., Briggs, C., Simon-Lopez, R., et al. (2014). Effect of EDTA-anticoagulated whole blood storage on cell morphology examination. A need for standardization. *Int J Lab Hematol, 36*(2), 222–226.

5. Naoum, F. A., de Oliveira Martin, F. H, Valejo, M. R., et al. (2020). Assessment of time-dependent white blood cells degeneration induced by blood storage on automated parameters and morphology examination. *Int J Lab Hematol, 42*(4), e185–e188.

6. Shahab, N., & Evans, M. L. (1998). Platelet satellitism. *N Engl J Med, 338*, 591.

7. Bartels, P. C., Schoorl, M., & Lombarts, A. J. (1997). Screening for EDTA-dependent deviations in platelet counts and abnormalities in platelet distribution histograms in pseudothrombocytopenia. *Scand J Clin Lab Invest, 57*, 629–636.

8. Lombarts, A., & deKieviet, W. (1988). Recognition and prevention of pseudothrombocytopenia and concomitant pseudoleukocytosis. *Am J Clin Pathol, 89*, 634–639.

9. Lippi, G., & Plebani, M. (2012). EDTA-dependent pseudothrombocytopenia: further insights and recommendations for prevention of a clinically threatening artifact. *Clin Chem Lab Med, 50*, 1281–1285.

10. Alpha Scientific Corp. *Diff-safe blood dispenser*. http://www.alpha-scientific.com/Diff-safe.html. Accessed November 16, 2022.

11. Hemaprep. *Automated Blood Smearing Instrument*. www.hemaprep.com/product-details/. Accessed November 16, 2022.

12. Sysmex. *SP-50*. http://www.sysmex.se/products/products-detail/sp-50.html. Accessed November 16, 2022.

13. Power, K. T. (1982). The Romanowsky stains: a review. *Am J Med Technol, 48*, 519–523.

14. Siemens Healthineers. *Hematek 3000 System*. https://www.siemens-healthineers.com/en-us/hematology/systems/hematek-3000. Accessed November 16, 2022.

15. CellaVision. *MCDh Staining*. https://www.cellavision.com/products/reagents/mcdh-staining. Accessed November 16, 2022.

16. MacGregor, R. G., Scott, R. W., & Loh, G. L. (1940). The differential leukocyte count. *J Pathol Bacteriol, 51*, 337–368.

17. Finn, W. G. (2004). *Cap Today* Q & A. http://www.captodayonline.com/Archives/q_and_a/qa_01_04.html. Accessed December 1, 2022.

18. Palmer, L., Briggs, C., McFadden, S., et al. (2015). ICSH recommendation for the standardization of nomenclature and grading of peripheral blood cell morphological features. *Int J Lab Hematol, 37*, 287–303.

19. CellaVision. *Introducing CellaVision DM9600*. http://www.cellavision.com/en/our-products/products/cellavision-dm9600. Accessed September 12, 2022.

20. Zini, G., d'Onofrio, G., Erber, W. N., et al., on behalf of the International Council for Standardization in Haematology. (2021). 2021 update of the 2012 ICSH Recommendations for identification, diagnostic value, and quantitation of schistocytes: impact and revisions. *Int J Lab Hematol, 43*, 1264–1271.

21. Katz, B. Z., Feldman, M. D., Tessema, M., et al. (2021). Evaluation of Scopio Labs X100 Full Field PBS: the first high-resolution full field viewing of peripheral blood specimens combined with artificial intelligence-based morphological analysis. *Int J Lab Hematol, 43*, 1408–1416.

22. van der Vorm, L. N., Hendriks, H. A., & Smits, S. M. (2021). Performance of the CellaVision DC-1 digital cell imaging analyser for differential counting and morphological classification of blood cells. *J Clin Pathol*. https://doi.org/10.1136/jclinpath-2021-207863.

23. Benlachgar, N., Doghmi, K., Masrar, A., et al. (2020). Immature platelets: a review of the available evidence. *Thromb Res, 195*, 43–50.

24. Reddy, V. V. B., & Morlote, D. (2021). Examination of blood and marrow cells. In Kaushansky, K., Lichtman, M. A., Prchal, J. T. et al. (Eds.), *Williams Hematology*. (10th ed., pp. 11–30). New York: McGraw-Hill.

15

Bone Marrow Examination

Kamran M. Mirza*

OBJECTIVES

After completion of this chapter, the reader will be able to:

1. Diagram bone marrow architecture and locate hematopoietic tissue.
2. List indications for bone marrow examinations.
3. Specify sites for bone marrow aspiration and biopsy.
4. List supplies for performing and assisting in bone marrow specimen collection.
5. Describe bone marrow specimen preparation after collection.
6. List the information gained from bone marrow aspirates and biopsy specimens.
7. Describe the procedures in a bone marrow aspirate smear and core biopsy specimen examination.
8. Recognize the normal hematopoietic and stromal cells of the bone marrow and their anticipated distribution.
9. Given photomicrographs and other applicable data, perform a bone marrow differential count and compute the myeloid-to-erythroid ratio.
10. Characterize features of hematopoietic and metastatic tumor cells.
11. Describe the special requirements for collection and handling of bone marrow specimens for specialized confirmatory bone marrow studies.
12. Given applicable data, prepare a systematic written bone marrow examination report.

OUTLINE

Bone Marrow Anatomy and Architecture
Indications For Bone Marrow Examination
Bone Marrow Specimen Collection Sites
Bone Marrow Aspiration and Biopsy
    Preparation
    Core Biopsy Procedure
    Aspiration Procedure
    Patient Care
Preparation of the Bone Marrow Specimen
    Direct Marrow Aspirate Smears
    Anticoagulated Aspirate Smears
    Marrow Aspirate Particle Smears

    Marrow Aspirate Concentrate (Buffy Coat) Smears
    Core Biopsy Imprints (Touch Preparations)
    Histologic Sections (Cell Block) of the Core Biopsy
    Stains for Marrow Aspirate Smears and Core Biopsy Sections
Examining Bone Marrow Aspirate or Imprint
    Low-Power (100×) Examination
    High-Power (500×) Examination
    Prussian Blue Iron Stain Examination
Examining the Bone Marrow Core Biopsy Specimen
Definitive Bone Marrow Studies
Bone Marrow Examination Reports

CASE STUDY

After studying the material in this chapter, the reader should be able to respond to the following case study. Answers can be found in Appendix C.

A patient presented with complaints of several weeks of weakness, fatigue, and malaise. Complete blood count results revealed the following. Reference intervals can be found after the Index at the end of the book.

HGB	7.5 g/dL	NEUT	21×10^9/L (70%)
HCT	21%	NEUT (Immature)	6×10^9/L (20%)
RBC	2.5×10^{12}/L	BASO	1.5×10^9/L (5%)
WBC	30×10^9/L	EO	0.3×10^9/L (1%)
PLT	540×10^9/L	LYMPH	1.2×10^9/L (4%)

Bone marrow examination revealed a hypercellular marrow with 90% myeloid precursors and 10% erythroid precursors. There were 15 megakaryocytes per low-power field (lpf).

1. What bone marrow finding provides information on blood cell production?
2. What is the myeloid-to-erythroid ratio in this patient, and what does it indicate?
3. What is the megakaryocyte distribution in bone marrow aspirates of healthy individuals?

---

*The author extends appreciation to George A. Fritsma, whose work in prior editions provided the foundation for this chapter.

BONE MARROW ANATOMY AND ARCHITECTURE

In adults, bone marrow accounts for 3.4% to 5.9% of body weight, contributes 1600 to 3700 g or a volume of 30 to 50 mL/kg, and produces roughly 6 billion blood cells per kilogram per day in a process called *hematopoiesis* (Chapter 5).[1] At birth, nearly all bones contain red hematopoietic marrow (Chapter 5). In the fifth to seventh year of life, adipocytes (fat cells) begin to replace red marrow in the long bones of the hands, feet, legs, and arms, producing yellow marrow, and by late adolescence, hematopoietic marrow is limited to the lower skull, vertebrae, shoulder, pelvis, ribs, and sternum (Figure 5.2). Although the percentage of bony space devoted to hematopoiesis is considerably reduced, the overall volume remains approximately constant as the individual matures.[2] Yellow marrow retains the ability to revert to active hematopoiesis by increasing red marrow volume in conditions such as chronic blood loss or hemolytic anemia when there is increased demand.

The arrangement of red marrow and its relationship to the central venous sinus are illustrated in Figures 5.3 and 5.4. Hematopoietic tissue is enmeshed in spongy trabeculae (bony tissue) surrounding a network of sinuses that originate at the endosteum (vascular layer just within the bone) and terminate in collecting venules.[2] Adipocytes occupy approximately 50% of the hematopoietic marrow space in adults aged 30 to 70 years, and fatty metamorphosis increases approximately 10% per decade after age 70.[3]

INDICATIONS FOR BONE MARROW EXAMINATION

Because the procedure is invasive, the decision to collect and examine a bone marrow specimen requires clinical judgment and the application of inclusion criteria. With improvements in flow cytometry immunophenotyping and increasing availability of 10-color laser instrumentation, immunohistochemistry, cytogenetic studies, and molecular diagnostics such as circulating tumor cell analysis, fluorescence in situ hybridization, polymerase chain reaction, and next-generation sequencing, peripheral blood may often provide information historically available only from bone marrow, reducing the demand for marrow specimens. On the other hand, these advanced techniques also augment bone marrow-based diagnosis and thus potentially raise the demand for bone marrow examinations in assessment of conditions not previously diagnosed through bone marrow examination.

Table 15.1 summarizes indications for a bone marrow examination.[4] Bone marrow examination may be used to diagnose and stage hematologic and nonhematologic neoplasia, to determine the cause of cytopenias, and to confirm or exclude metabolic or infectious conditions suspected on the basis of clinical symptoms and peripheral blood findings.[5]

TABLE 15.1 Indications for Bone Marrow Examination	
Indication	**Examples**
Neoplasia diagnosis	Acute leukemia (myeloid, lymphoid, mixed phenotype)
	Myeloproliferative neoplasms such as chronic myeloid leukemia, primary myelofibrosis
	Myelodysplastic neoplasms
	Lymphoproliferative disorders such as chronic lymphocytic leukemia
	Immunoglobulin disorders such as plasma cell myeloma, macroglobulinemia
	Metastatic tumors (diagnosis and/or staging)
	Unexplained organomegaly or mass lesions
	Unexplained lesion on radiologic imaging
Neoplasia diagnosis and staging	Hodgkin and non-Hodgkin lymphoma
Marrow failure: cytopenias	Unexplained, hypoplastic or aplastic anemia
	Pure red cell aplasia
	Idiosyncratic drug-induced marrow suppression
	Myelodysplastic neoplasms
	Marrow necrosis secondary to tumor
	Marrow necrosis secondary to severe infection such as parvovirus B19 infection
	Immune versus amegakaryocytic thrombocytopenia
	Sickle cell crisis
	Differentiation of megaloblastic, iron deficiency, sideroblastic, hemolytic, and blood loss anemia
	Estimation of storage iron to assess for iron deficiency
	Infiltrative processes or fibrosis
Metabolic disorders	Gaucher disease
	Mast cell disease
Infections	Granulomatous disease
	Miliary tuberculosis
	Fungal infections
	Hemophagocytic syndromes
Monitoring of treatment	After chemotherapy or radiation therapy to assess minimal residual disease
	After hematopoietic stem cell transplantation to assess engraftment

Each bone marrow procedure is ordered after thorough consideration of clinical and laboratory information. For instance, bone marrow examination is most likely unnecessary in anemia when the cause is apparent from red blood cell (RBC) indices, serum iron and ferritin levels, or vitamin B_{12} and folate levels. Multilineage abnormalities, circulating blasts in adults, and unexpected pancytopenia usually prompt marrow examination. Bone marrow puncture is prohibited in patients with coagulopathies such as hemophilia or vitamin K deficiency, although thrombocytopenia (low platelet count) is not an absolute contraindication. Special precautions such as bridging therapy may be necessary to prevent uncontrolled bleeding when a bone marrow procedure is performed on a patient receiving anticoagulant therapy, such as warfarin or heparin.

BONE MARROW SPECIMEN COLLECTION SITES

Bone marrow specimen collection is a collaborative effort between a medical laboratory professional, a nurse/advanced practice provider (APP), and a specialty physician, often a pathologist or hematologist.[6] Before bone marrow collection, a medical laboratory professional or phlebotomist typically collects peripheral blood for a complete blood count (CBC) with blood film examination. During bone marrow collection, the medical laboratory professional assists the physician by managing the specimens and producing initial preparations for examination.

Red marrow is gelatinous and amenable to sampling. Most bone marrow specimens consist of an *aspirate* (obtained by bone marrow aspiration) and a *core biopsy* specimen (obtained by trephine biopsy). Once preparation and staining are complete, both specimens are examined with light microscopy using varying magnification. Because the aspirate contains intact cells that have been dispersed by smearing, it is used to identify the types and proportions of hematologic cells (differential count) and to look for *morphologic variance*. The core biopsy specimen is formalin fixed and paraffin embedded after proper decalcification, and 4- to 5-micron-thick sections of the core are reviewed to study *bone marrow architecture:* the spatial relationship of hematologic cells to fat, connective tissue, and bony stroma. The core biopsy specimen is also used to estimate *cellularity*.

The core biopsy specimen is particularly important for evaluating diseases that characteristically produce focal lesions, rather than diffuse involvement of the marrow. Classic Hodgkin lymphoma, non-Hodgkin lymphoma, plasma cell myeloma, metastatic tumors, amyloid, and granulomas may produce predominantly focal lesions. Granulomas, or granulomatous lesions, are cell accumulations that contain *Langerhans cells*—large, activated granular macrophages that look like epithelial cells. Granulomas signal chronic inflammation. The biopsy specimen also allows for morphologic evaluation of bony spicules, which may reveal changes associated with hyperparathyroidism or Paget disease.[7]

Bone marrow collection sites include the following:
- *Posterior superior iliac crest* of the pelvis (Figure 15.1). In both adults and children, this site provides adequate red marrow and is isolated from anatomic structures that could

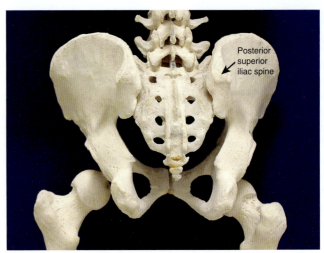

Posterior superior iliac spine

Figure 15.1 Bone Marrow Specimen Collection Site. The posterior superior iliac crest is the preferred site for obtaining the bone marrow aspirate and core biopsy specimen because it provides ample marrow and is isolated from structures that could be damaged by accidental puncture. (Courtesy Indiana Pathology Images, Indianapolis, IN.)

be damaged by accidental puncture. It is the preferred site for both aspiration and core biopsy.[6]
- *Anterior superior iliac crest* of the pelvis. This site has the same advantages as the posterior superior iliac crest, but the cortical bone is thicker. This site may be preferred for a patient who can lie only in the supine position.
- *Sternum,* below the angle of Lewis at the second intercostal space. In adults, the sternum provides ample material for aspiration but is only 1 cm thick and cannot be used for core biopsy. It is possible to accidentally pierce through the sternum and enter the pericardium, damaging the heart or great vessels.
- *Anterior medial surface of the tibia* in infants younger than 1 year of age.[6] This site may be used only for aspiration.
- *Spinous process of the vertebrae, ribs,* or other red marrow-containing bones. These locations are available but are rarely used unless one is the site of a suspicious lesion discovered on a radiograph.

Serious adverse outcomes occur in less than 0.05% of marrow collections.[6,8] Infections and reactions to anesthetics may occur, but the most common side effect is hemorrhage associated with platelet function disorders or thrombocytopenia.

BONE MARROW ASPIRATION AND BIOPSY

Preparation

A blood count and peripheral blood film examination should be obtained if these have not been collected in the previous 2 days.[9] Peripheral blood collection is often accomplished immediately before bone marrow specimen collection and seldom collected after bone marrow collection to avoid stress-related white blood cell count elevation.

Most institutions purchase or assemble disposable sterile bone marrow specimen collection trays that provide the following:
- Surgical gloves

- Shaving equipment
- Antiseptic solution and alcohol pads
- Drape material
- Local anesthetic injection, usually 1% lidocaine, not to exceed 20 mL per patient
- No. 11 scalpel blade for skin incision
- Disposable Jamshidi biopsy needle (Figure 15.2) or Westerman-Jensen needle (Figure 15.3). Both provide an obturator, core biopsy tool, and stylet. A SnareCoil biopsy needle is also an option. The SnareCoil has a coil mechanism at the needle tip that allows for capture of the bone marrow specimen without needle redirection (Figure 15.4).
- Disposable 14- to 18-gauge aspiration needle with obturator. Alternatively, the University of Illinois aspiration needle may be used for sternal puncture. The University of Illinois needle provides a flange that prevents penetration of the sternum to the pericardium.
- Microscope slides or coverslips washed in 70% ethanol
- Petri dishes or shallow circular watch glasses
- Vials or test tubes with closures
- Wintrobe hematocrit tubes
- Anticoagulant liquid tripotassium ethylenediaminetetraacetic acid (EDTA)
- Zenker fixative: potassium dichromate, mercuric chloride, sodium sulfate, and glacial acetic acid; B5 fixative: aqueous mercuric chloride and sodium acetate; or 10% neutral formalin. Controlled disposal is required for Zenker fixative and B5 fixatives that contain toxic mercury.
- Gauze dressings

The aspiration and biopsy procedure is depicted in Figure 15.5. After informed consent and a time-out procedure, in which the identity of the patient is confirmed using standard institutional procedures, the patient is asked to lie supine, prone, or in the right or left lateral decubitus position (lying on the right or left side). With attention to standard precautions, the skin is shaved if necessary, disinfected, and draped.

The physician palpates the biopsy site (Figure 15.5A), then infiltrates the skin, dermis, and subcutaneous tissue with a local anesthetic solution (Figure 15.5B) through a 25-gauge needle, producing a 0.5- to 1.0-cm papule (bubble). The 25-gauge needle is replaced with a 21-gauge needle, which is inserted through the papule to the periosteum (bone surface). With the point of the needle on the periosteum, the physician injects approximately 2 mL of anesthetic over a dime-sized area while rotating the needle and then withdraws the anesthesia needle. Next, the physician makes a 3-mm skin incision over the puncture site with a No. 11 scalpel blade to prevent skin coring during insertion of the needle.

Core Biopsy Procedure

The biopsy specimen is typically collected first because aspiration may destroy marrow architecture; however, some providers

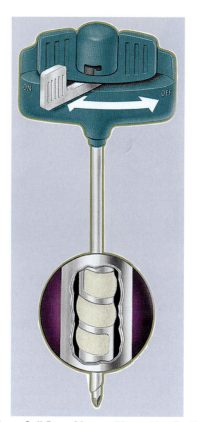

Figure 15.4 SnareCoil Bone Marrow Biopsy Needle. The coil mechanism resides within the biopsy needle as illustrated in the magnified image. The coil is turned to draw the marrow specimen into the needle. (Courtesy Tyco Healthcare/Kendall, Mansfield, MA.)

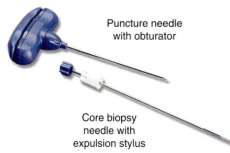

Puncture needle with obturator

Core biopsy needle with expulsion stylus

Figure 15.2 Disposable Sterile Jamshidi Bone Marrow Biopsy and Aspiration Needle. The outer puncture cannula is advanced to the medullary cavity of the bone with the obturator in place to prevent bone coring. The physician removes the obturator and slides the core biopsy needle through the cannula and into the medulla with the expulsion stylus removed. The core biopsy needle is removed from the puncture needle with the specimen in place. The specimen is expelled using the stylus. (Courtesy Care Fusion, McGaw Park, IL.)

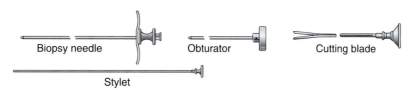

Biopsy needle   Obturator   Cutting blade

Stylet

Figure 15.3 Bone Marrow Biopsy Westerman-Jensen Needle.

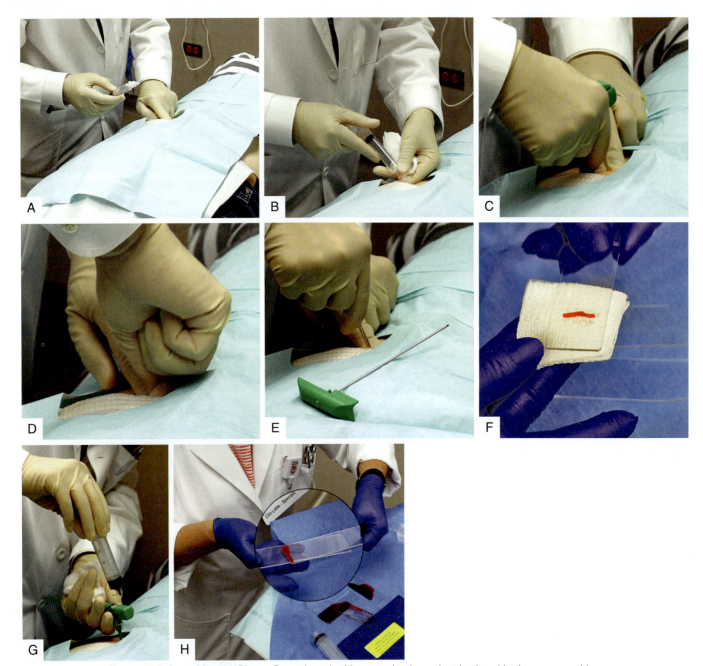

Figure 15.5 Bone Marrow Biopsy Procedure. In this example, the patient is placed in the prone position, the posterior superior iliac crest is palpated (**A**), and then local anesthetic is injected (**B**). The Jamshidi needle is inserted, and a rotating motion is used (**C** and **D**) to core through the bone. The core biopsy specimen is removed, and touch preparations of the specimen are made on glass slides (**E** and **F**). Marrow aspiration (liquid) specimens are acquired (**G** and **H**) through the same insertion point but in a separate location from the biopsy site, using an aspiration needle.

prefer to take this specimen after the aspiration; there remains no gold standard. When the Jamshidi biopsy needle is used, after the incision is made, the physician inserts the outer cannula with the obturator in place through the skin and cortex of the bone. The obturator prevents coring of skin or bone. Reciprocating rotation promotes the forward advancement of the cannula (Figure 15.5C and D). A weakening of resistance indicates penetration through the cortex to the inner medullary cavity of the bone. The physician removes the obturator, inserts the biopsy needle through the cannula, and slowly advances the

needle 2 to 3 cm with continuous reciprocating rotation along the long axis (Figure 15.5E). The physician changes the needle angle slightly to separate the core cylinder specimen from its marrow cavity attachments. The biopsy needle and cannula are withdrawn from the bone, taking the core cylinder with them. The core cylinder is 1 to 1.5 cm long and 1 to 2 mm in diameter and weighs about 150 mg. The biopsy needle is placed over an ethanol-cleaned slide, and the stylus is pushed through to dislodge the core cylinder onto the slide (Figure 15.5F). Using sterile forceps, the medical laboratory professional prepares imprints *(touch preparations)* of the core biopsy onto multiple glass slides. The core cylinder is then transferred to the chosen fixative (Zenker, B5, or formalin).

When the Westerman-Jensen needle is used, the physician punctures through the bone cortex with the needle and the obturator in place. The obturator is then removed, the cutting blades are inserted through the cannula, and the blades are advanced into the medullary cavity of the bone (Figure 15.6). The cutting blades are pressed into the medullary bone, with the outer cannula held firmly in a stationary position. The physician slowly withdraws the blades so that the cannula entraps the tissue and then withdraws the entire unit. The core cylinder is removed by inserting the probe through the cutting tip and extruding the specimen through the hub of the needle to the selected slide and fixative-containing receptacles.

Aspiration Procedure

Using the same insertion point but in a separate location from the biopsy site, the physician inserts a 14- to 18-gauge aspiration needle such as the University of Illinois needle, with obturator, through the skin and cortex of the bone. The obturator is removed, and a 10- to 20-mL syringe is attached. The physician withdraws the plunger to create negative pressure and aspirates 1.0 to 1.5 mL of marrow into the syringe (Figure 15.5G). Collecting more than 1.5 mL dilutes the hematopoietic marrow with sinusoidal (peripheral) blood. The physician detaches the syringe and passes it *immediately* to the medical laboratory professional, who expels the material onto a series of clean and sterile microscopic slides or coverslips. A series of aspirate smear slides can be made (Figure 15.5H). The physician may attach a second syringe to aspirate an additional specimen for cytogenetic analysis, molecular diagnostics, or immunophenotyping using flow cytometry. The needle is then withdrawn, and pressure is applied to the wound.

If no marrow is obtained, the physician returns the obturator to the needle, advances the needle, attaches a fresh syringe,

and tries again. The syringe and needle are retracted slightly, and the process is repeated. If this attempt is unsuccessful, the physician removes the needle and syringe, applies pressure, and begins the procedure at a new site. If the marrow is fibrotic, acellular, or packed with leukemic cells, the first and second aspiration may be unsuccessful, known as a *dry tap*. In this case, a core biopsy (described earlier) is necessary to confirm whether this is indeed a dry tap, in which case the core biopsy specimen will demonstrate a fibrotic, packed marrow (or an empty marrow in cases where the cellularity is very low) versus improper sampling. Table 15.2 summarizes the advantages and disadvantages of the marrow aspirate smear and the marrow core biopsy.

Patient Care

After bone marrow biopsy or aspiration, the physician applies a pressure dressing and advises the patient to remain in the same position for 60 minutes to prevent bleeding.

PREPARATION OF THE BONE MARROW SPECIMEN

Direct Marrow Aspirate Smears

During the bone marrow biopsy procedure, the medical laboratory professional receives the aspirate syringe from the physician at the bedside and *immediately* transfers drops of the freshly collected marrow specimen onto six (or more) ethanol-washed microscope slides (Figure 15.5H). Marrow clots rapidly, so good organization is essential. Using spreader slides, the medical laboratory professional spreads the drop into a wedge-shaped smear one-half to three-quarters the length of the slide, similar to a peripheral blood film (Chapter 14). Bony spicules 0.5 to 1.0 mm in diameter and larger fat globules follow behind the spreader and become deposited on the slide. In the direct smear preparation, the medical laboratory professional avoids crushing the spicules. Smears should be allowed to air dry.[9]

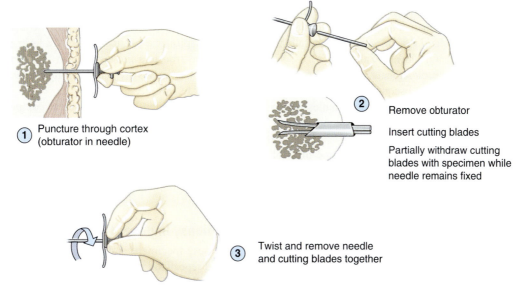

  ① Puncture through cortex (obturator in needle)

  ② Remove obturator

Insert cutting blades

Partially withdraw cutting blades with specimen while needle remains fixed

  ③ Twist and remove needle and cutting blades together

Figure 15.6 Bone Marrow Biopsy Technique Using the Westerman-Jensen Needle.

TABLE 15.2 **Advantages and Disadvantages of the Marrow Aspirate Smear and Marrow Core Biopsy**

	Marrow Aspirate Smear	Marrow Core Biopsy
Advantages	Fast Eliminates need for decalcification of specimen Can perform quantitative differential count Provides material for ancillary studies (immunophenotyping by flow cytometry, molecular diagnosis, cytogenetics)	Ability to analyze both cells and stroma Represents all cells Explains dry taps
Disadvantages	May not represent all cells Dry tap in cases of fibrosis or hypocellularity Does not represent architecture Inability to analyze the stroma	Slow processing Decalcification precludes certain ancillary studies Inability to perform quantitative differential count

---

In the syringe, the specimen consists of peripheral blood with suspended, light-colored bony spicules and fat globules. The medical laboratory professional evaluates the syringe blood for spicules. More spicules are associated with a specimen with more cells to identify and categorize. If the specimen has few fat globules or spicules, the medical laboratory professional may alert the physician to collect an additional specimen.

Anticoagulated Aspirate Smears

Anticoagulated specimens are a more leisurely alternative to direct aspirate smears. The medical laboratory professional expresses the aspirate from the syringe into a vial containing EDTA and subsequently pipettes the anticoagulated aspirate to clean glass slides, spreading the aspirate, using the same approach as in direct smear preparation. All anticoagulants distort cell morphology, but EDTA generates the least distortion.

Marrow Aspirate Particle Smears

To prepare aspirate particle smears, the medical laboratory professional expels a portion of the aspirate to a Petri dish or watch glass covered with a few milliliters of EDTA solution and spreads the aspirate over the surface with a sterile applicator. Individual bony spicules are transferred using applicators, forceps, or micropipettes (preferred) to several ethanol-washed glass slides. For each slide, the medical laboratory professional places another glass slide directly over the specimen at a right angle and presses gently to crush the spicules. The slides are separated laterally to create two rectangular smears and allowed to air dry.[9]

Some medical laboratory professionals prefer to transfer the aspirate directly to the slide, subsequently tilting the slide to drain off peripheral blood while retaining spicules. Once drained, the spicules are then crushed with a second slide as described earlier.

The medical laboratory professional may add one drop of 22% albumin to the EDTA solution, particularly if the specimen is suspected to contain prolymphocytes or lymphoblasts, which tend to rupture. The albumin reduces the occurrence of "smudge" or "basket" cells, often seen in lymphoid marrow lesions.

The aspirate particle smear may also be performed using ethanol-washed coverslips in place of slides. The coverslip method demands adroit manipulation but may yield better morphologic information because the smaller coverslips generate less cell rupture during separation. Use of glass slides offers the opportunity for automated staining, whereas coverslip preparations must first be affixed smear side up to slides and then stained manually (Chapter 14).

Marrow Aspirate Concentrate (Buffy Coat) Smears

Concentrate (buffy coat) smears are useful when there are sparse nucleated cells in the direct marrow aspirate smear or when the number of nucleated cells is anticipated to be small, as in aplastic anemia. The medical laboratory professional transfers approximately 1.5 mL of EDTA-anticoagulated marrow aspirate specimen to a narrow-bore glass or plastic tube such as a Wintrobe hematocrit tube. The tube is centrifuged at 2500g for 10 minutes and examined for four layers.

The top layer is yellowish fat and normally occupies 1% to 3% of the column. The second layer, plasma, varies in volume, depending on the amount of peripheral blood in the specimen. The third layer consists of nucleated cells and is called the *myeloid-erythroid* (ME) layer. The ME layer is normally 5% to 8% of the total column. The bottom layer is RBCs and its volume, similar to the plasma layer, depends on the amount of peripheral blood present. The medical laboratory professional records the ratio of the fat and ME layers using millimeter gradations on the tube.

Once the column is examined, the medical laboratory professional aspirates a portion of the ME layer with a portion of plasma and transfers the suspension to a Petri dish or watch glass. Marrow smears are subsequently prepared using the particle smear technique.

The concentrated buffy coat smear compensates for hypocellular marrow and allows for examination of large numbers of nucleated cells without interference from fat or RBCs. On the other hand, cell distribution is distorted by the procedure. Therefore the medical laboratory professional does not estimate numbers of different cell types or maturation stages on a buffy coat smear.

Core Biopsy Imprints (Touch Preparations)

Core biopsy specimens and clotted marrow may be held in forceps and repeatedly touched to a washed glass slide or coverslip so that cells attach and rapidly dry. When touching the specimen to the glass slide, the medical laboratory professional lifts directly upward to prevent cell distortion. Imprints are valuable when the specimen has clotted or there is a dry tap (no specimen collected with the aspiration technique). The cell morphology may closely replicate aspirate morphology, although few spicules are transferred.

Histologic Sections (Cell Block) of the Core Biopsy

After the medical laboratory professional has prepared aspirate smears and has distributed aliquots of marrow for cytogenetic, molecular, and immunophenotypic studies, the remaining core biopsy specimen, spicules, or clotted specimen is submitted to histology for preparation. The specimen is suspended in 10% formalin, Zenker glacial acetic acid, or B5 fixative for approximately 2 hours.

The fixed specimen is subsequently centrifuged, and the pellet is decalcified and wrapped in an embedding bag or lens paper and placed in a paraffin-embedding cassette. A histotechnologist sections the embedded specimen, applies hematoxylin and eosin (H&E) stain, and examines the section.

Stains for Marrow Aspirate Smears and Core Biopsy Sections

Marrow aspirate smears are stained with *Wright* or *Wright-Giemsa stains* using the same protocols as for peripheral blood film staining (Chapter 14). Some laboratory professionals prefer to increase staining time to compensate for the relative thickness of marrow smears compared with peripheral blood films. The marrow core biopsy sections are stained with H&E stain, as indicated in the preceding section.

Marrow aspirate smears and core biopsy specimens may also be stained using an acidic potassium ferrocyanide *(Prussian blue)* solution to detect and estimate marrow storage iron or iron metabolism abnormalities (Chapter 17). Further, a number of *cytochemical* stains may be used for cell identification or differentiation (Table 15.3).

EXAMINING BONE MARROW ASPIRATE OR IMPRINT

Microscopic examination of a bone marrow specimen is critical for the diagnosis of hematologic disorders. The important components of the examination, to be described in this chapter, are listed in Table 15.4. Final interpretation of the marrow should be integrated with results from the clinical history, CBC and blood film evaluation, other relevant laboratory data, immunophenotyping by flow cytometry, and molecular and cytogenetic data (Chapters 28–30).

Examination of the marrow aspirate or imprint cytology begins with a low-power review of the general organization, character, and cellular quality of the whole specimen, including the presence (or absence) of bone spicules. With reference to the patient's age and clinical indication for the marrow examination, the estimation of cellularity is made as a ratio of the nucleated cells and the presence of the adipocytes. Normal, large megakaryocytes are usually easily observed at low power, and care should be taken in noting the presence of any cohesive clusters of nonhematopoietic cells. As a rule, hematopoietic cells are always present as discohesive cells that do not form structures. The examination then follows an algorithm of intermediate- and high-power assessment that entails a detailed review of all three cell lines with the goal of assessing progressive trilineage hematopoiesis. Box 15.1 describes the uses of low- and high-power objective lenses in examining bone marrow aspirate direct smears or imprints.

Low-Power (100×) Examination

Once the marrow direct aspirate smear or imprint is prepared and stained, the medical laboratory professional or pathologist

TABLE 15.3 Cytochemical Stains Used to Identify Bone Marrow Cells and Maturation Stages

Cytochemical Stain	Application
Myeloperoxidase (MPO)	Detects myeloid cells by staining cytoplasmic granular contents
Sudan black B (SBB)	Detects myeloid cells by staining cytoplasmic granular contents
Periodic acid-Schiff (PAS)	Detects lymphocytic cells and certain abnormal erythroid cells by staining of cytoplasmic glycogen
Esterases	Distinguish myeloid from monocytic maturation stages (several esterase substrates)
Tartrate-resistant acid phosphatase (TRAP)	Detects tartrate-resistant acid phosphatase granules in hairy cell leukemia

TABLE 15.4 Components of a Bone Marrow Examination

Component	Description
Cellularity	Hypocellular, normocellular, or hypercellular classification based on ratio of hematopoietic cells to adipocytes
Megakaryocytes	Estimate using low power, 10× objective lens (100× magnification), compare with reference interval, and comment on morphology
Maturation	Narrative characterizing maturation of the myeloid and erythroid (normoblastic, rubricytic) series
Additional hematologic cells	Narrative describing numbers and morphology of eosinophils, basophils, mast cells, lymphocytes, plasma cells, monocytes, and histiocytes, if appropriate, with reference intervals
Stromal cells	Narrative describing numbers and morphology of osteoblasts, osteoclasts, bony trabeculae, fibroblasts, adipocytes, and endothelial cells; appearance of sinuses; presence of amyloid, granulomas, fibrosis, necrosis
Differential count	Numbers of all cells and cell stages observed after performing a differential count on 500 to 1000 cells and comparing results with reference intervals
Myeloid-to-erythroid ratio	Computed from nucleated hematologic cells, excluding lymphocytes, plasma cells, monocytes, and histiocytes
Iron stores	Categorization of findings as increased, normal, or decreased iron stores

BOX 15.1   Bone Marrow Aspirate Microscopic Smear Examination: Low Power and High Power

Low Power: 10× Objective Lens (100× Total Magnification)
- Assess peripheral blood dilution
- Find bony spicules and areas of clear cell morphology
- Observe fat-to-marrow ratio, estimate cellularity
- Search for tumor cells in clusters
- Examine and estimate megakaryocytes

High Power: 50× and 100× Objective Lenses (500× and 1000× Total Magnification)
- Observe granulocytic and erythroid maturation
- Distinguish abnormal distribution of cells or cell maturation stages
- Perform differential count on 500 to 1000 cells
- Compute myeloid-to-erythroid ratio

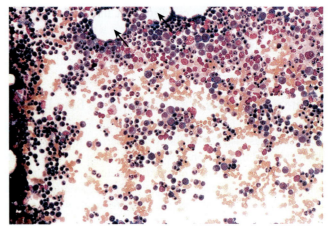

Figure 15.7 Bone Marrow Aspirate Specimen. Note the intact, contiguous cells and adipocytes *(arrows)*. This illustrates a good site for morphologic evaluation and cell counting. (Wright-Giemsa stain, ×100.)

begins the microscopic examination using the low-power (10×) dry lens, which, when linked with 10× oculars, provides a total 100× magnification. Most bone marrow examinations are performed using a teaching format that employs projection or multiheaded microscopes to allow observation by all trainees (students, residents, and fellows), laboratory staff, and physicians. The microscopist locates the bony spicules, aggregations of bone, and hematopoietic cells, all of which appear dark blue at low power (Figure 15.7). In imprints, spicules are sparse or absent; the search is for hematopoietic cells. Within these areas, the microscopist selects intact and nearly contiguous nucleated cells for examination, avoiding areas of distorted morphology or areas diluted with sinusoidal blood.

Near the spicules, cellularity is estimated by observing the proportion of *hematopoietic* cells to *adipocytes* (clear fat areas).[10] For anterior or posterior iliac crest marrow, 50% cellularity is normal for patients aged 30 to 70 years. In childhood, cellularity is 80%, and after age 70, cellularity becomes reduced. For patients older than age 70, a rule of thumb is to subtract patient age from 100% and add ±10%. Thus at age 75, the anticipated cellularity is 15% to 35%. By comparing with the age-related normal cellularity values, the microscopist classifies the observed area as *hypocellular, normocellular,* or *hypercellular.* If a core biopsy specimen was collected, it provides a more accurate estimate of cellularity than an aspirate smear because in aspirates, there is always some dilution of hematopoietic tissue with peripheral blood. In the absence of leukemia, lymphocytes should total less than 30% of nucleated cells; if more are present, the marrow specimen has been substantially diluted and should not be used to estimate cellularity.[11]

Hematopoietic cells are normally discohesive (loose intercellular connections), a feature that is helpful to visualize normal cells using the 10× objective lens. At this magnification, for screening purposes, the microscopist searches for abnormal, often molded, cell clusters (syncytia) of *metastatic tumor cells* or other abnormal infiltrating cells such as *lymphoma cells or plasma cells.* Tumor cell nuclei often stain darkly (hyperchromatic), and prominent vacuoles may be seen in the cytoplasm. Tumor cell clusters are often found near the edges of the smear because of their buoyancy.

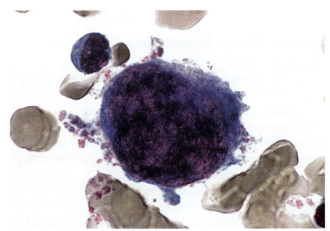

Figure 15.8 Bone Marrow Aspirate Smear Showing a Megakaryocyte. Note the platelets budding from the megakaryocyte at the plasma membrane. (Wright-Giemsa stain, ×1000.)

Although myeloid (granulocytic) cells and erythroid cells are best examined using 500× magnification, they may be more easily distinguished from each other using the 10× objective lens. The erythroid maturation stages stain more intensely, and both their nuclear and cytoplasmic margins are more sharply defined (almost perfectly round in shape), features more easily distinguished at lower magnification.

The microscopist evaluates *megakaryocytes* using low power (Figure 15.8). Megakaryocytes are the largest cells in the bone marrow, 30 to 50 μm in diameter, with multilobed nuclei (Chapter 11). Although in special circumstances, microscopists may differentiate three megakaryocyte maturation stages, *megakaryoblast, promegakaryocyte,* and *megakaryocyte* (MK-I to MK-III), a total megakaryocyte estimate is generally satisfactory. In a well-prepared aspirate or biopsy specimen, the microscopist observes 2 to 10 megakaryocytes per low-power field. Deviations yield important information and are reported as decreased or increased megakaryocytes. Bone marrow megakaryocyte estimates are essential to the evaluation of peripheral blood *thrombocytopenia* and *thrombocytosis;* for instance, in immune thrombocytopenia, an increased number of marrow megakaryocytes is not uncommon.

Abnormal megakaryocytes may be small, lack granularity, or have poorly lobulated or hyperlobulated nuclei, or widely separated nuclear lobes. Indications of abnormality may be visible using low power; however, conclusive descriptions require 500× or even 1000× total magnification.

High-Power (500×) Examination

Having located a suitable area on the slide for examination of the cells, the microscopist places a drop of immersion oil on the specimen and switches to the 50× oil immersion objective lens, providing 500× total magnification. All of the *nucleated cells* are reviewed for morphology and normal maturation. Besides megakaryocytes, cells of the granulocytic (Figures 15.9–15.12) and erythroid (rubricytic, normoblastic) (Figure 15.13) series should be present, along with eosinophils, basophils, lymphocytes, plasma cells, monocytes, and histiocytes. Chapters 5, 6, and 10 provide detailed cell and cell maturation stage descriptions. Table 15.5 lists the reference intervals for blood cells and their various maturation stages in bone marrow aspirates and imprints.

The microscopist searches for maturation gaps, misdistribution of maturation stages, and abnormal morphology. Although the specimen is customarily reviewed using the 50× oil immersion objective lens, the 100× oil immersion objective lens is often employed to detect small but significant morphologic abnormalities in the nuclei and cytoplasm of suspect cells.

The *World Health Organization (WHO) Classification of Haematolymphoid Tumours, 5th edition* (2022)[12] requires a 500-cell differential count of nucleated marrow cells. Many laboratory directors may mandate a different number, ranging from a differential count of 500 to 1000 nucleated cells. These seemingly large totals are rapidly reached in a well-prepared bone marrow smear at 500× magnification and compensate statistically for the anticipated uneven distribution of spicules and hematopoietic cells. The microscopist counts cells and maturation stages

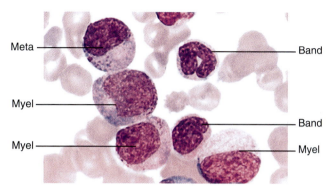

Figure 15.11 Bone Marrow Aspirate Smear. Myeloid stages include myelocytes *(Myel)*, a metamyelocyte *(Meta)*, and neutrophilic bands *(Band)*. (Wright-Giemsa stain, ×1000.)

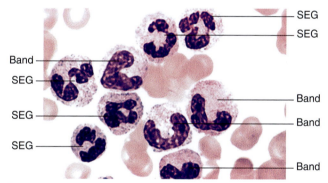

Figure 15.12 Bone Marrow Aspirate Smear. Note the neutrophilic bands *(Band)* and segmented neutrophils *(SEG)*. (Wright-Giemsa stain, ×1000.)

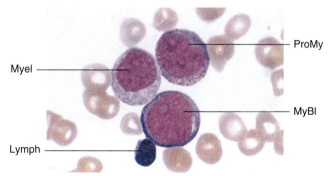

Figure 15.9 Bone Marrow Aspirate Smear. Myeloid stages include a myeloblast *(MyBl)*, promyelocyte *(ProMy)*, and myelocyte *(Myel)*. The lymphocyte *(Lymph)* diameter illustrates its size relative to the myeloid stages. The source of the lymphocyte is sinus blood. (Wright-Giemsa stain, ×1000.)

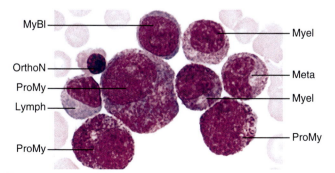

Figure 15.10 Bone Marrow Aspirate Smear. Myeloid stages include a myeloblast *(MyBl)*, promyelocytes *(ProMy)*, myelocytes *(Myel)*, and a metamyelocyte *(Meta)*. One orthochromic normoblast *(OrthoN)* and one lymphocyte *(Lymph)* are present. (Wright-Giemsa stain, ×1000.)

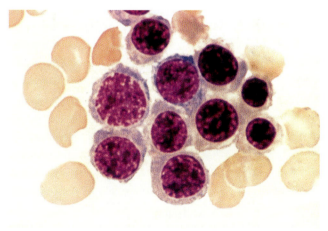

Figure 15.13 Bone Marrow Aspirate Smear. Note the island of erythroid precursors with polychromatophilic and orthochromic normoblasts. (Wright-Giemsa stain, ×1000.)

surrounding several spicules to maximize the opportunity for detecting disease-related cells. Some laboratory directors omit the differential in favor of a thorough examination of the smear.

Many microscopists choose not to differentiate the four nucleated erythroid maturation stages, and others may combine three of the four, *basophilic, polychromatophilic,* and *orthochromic normoblasts,* in a single total, counting only *pronormoblasts* (the earliest stage) separately. In normal marrow, most erythroid precursors are either polychromatophilic or orthochromic normoblasts, and differentiation yields little additional information. On the other hand, differentiation may be helpful in megaloblastic and iron deficiency anemia, and in myelodysplastic neoplasms.

The microscopist may infrequently find *osteoblasts* and *osteoclasts* in the marrow aspirate specimen. Osteoblasts (Figure 15.14) are responsible for bone formation and remodeling, and they derive from *endosteal* (inner lining) cells. Osteoblasts may resemble plasma cells, with eccentric round to oval nuclei and abundant blue, mottled cytoplasm, but they lack the prominent Golgi apparatus characteristic of plasma cells (the plasma cell "hof"). Additionally, they technically demonstrate tiny particles of eosinophilic "bone dust" within their cytoplasm. Osteoblasts are usually found in clusters resembling myeloma cell clusters. Their presence in marrow aspirates and core biopsy specimens is incidental; they do not signal disease, but they may create confusion.

Osteoclasts are nearly the diameter of megakaryocytes, but their multiple, evenly spaced nuclei distinguish them from multilobed megakaryocyte nuclei (Figure 15.15). Osteoclasts appear to derive from myeloid progenitor cells and are responsible for bone resorption, acting in concert with osteoblasts. Osteoclasts are recognized more often in core biopsy specimens than in aspirates.

Adipocytes, endothelial cells that line blood vessels, and fibroblast-like *reticular cells* complete the bone marrow composition (Chapter 5). *Stromal cells* and their extracellular matrix provide the suitable microenvironment for maturation and proliferation of hematopoietic cells but are seldom examined for diagnosis of hematologic or systemic disease. Finally, *Langerhans cells,* giant cells with "palisade" nuclei, are found in granulomas and when present, signal chronic inflammation.

Once the differential is completed, the *myeloid-to-erythroid (M:E) ratio* is computed from the total myeloid to the total nucleated erythroid cell stages. Excluded from the M:E ratio are lymphocytes, plasma cells, monocytes, histiocytes, nonnucleated erythrocytes, and nonhematopoietic stromal cells. The reference interval for the M:E ratio in adults can be found after the Index at the end of the book.

TABLE 15.5	Distribution of Cells and Cell Maturation Stages in Aspirates or Imprints		
Cell or Cell Maturation Stage	**Sample Reference Intervals***	**Cell or Cell Maturation Stage**	**Sample Reference Intervals***
Myeloblasts	0%–3%	Pronormoblasts/rubriblasts	0%–1%
Promyelocytes	1%–5%	Basophilic normoblasts/prorubricytes	1%–4%
Myelocytes	6%–17%	Polychromatophilic normoblasts/rubricytes	10%–20%
Metamyelocytes	3%–20%	Orthochromic normoblasts/metarubricytes	6%–10%
Neutrophilic bands	9%–32%	Lymphocytes	5%–18%
Segmented neutrophils	7%–30%	Plasma cells	0%–1%
Eosinophils and eosinophilic precursors	0%–3%	Monocytes	0%–1%
Basophils and mast cells	0%–1%	Histiocytes	0%–1%
Megakaryocytes	2–10 visible per low-power field	Myeloid-to-erythroid ratio	1.5:1–3.3:1

*Each laboratory must establish its own reference intervals based on its methodology and demographics of the population it serves.

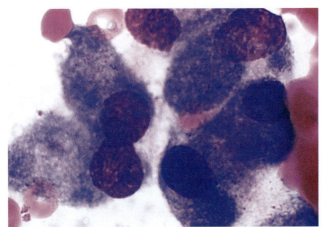

Figure 15.14 Bone Marrow Aspirate Smear Showing Osteoblasts. Note the cluster of osteoblasts that superficially resemble plasma cells. Osteoblasts have round to oval eccentric nuclei and mottled blue cytoplasm that is devoid of secretory granules. They may have a clear area within the cytoplasm but lack the well-defined central Golgi complex of the plasma cell. (Wright-Giemsa stain, ×1000.)

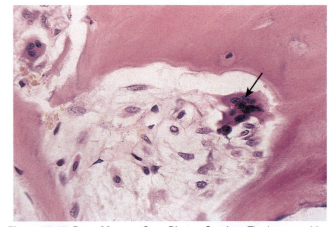

Figure 15.15 Bone Marrow Core Biopsy Section. The large, multinucleated cell near the endosteal surface is an osteoclast *(arrow)*, a cell that reabsorbs bone. The spindle-shaped cells are fibroblasts. (Hematoxylin and eosin stain, ×500.)

Prussian Blue Iron Stain Examination

A Prussian blue (acidic potassium ferrocyanide) *iron stain* is commonly used on the bone marrow aspirate smear. Figure 15.16 illustrates normal iron, absence of iron, and increased iron stores in aspirate smears. Quantitative estimates of iron stores are subject to interobserver variation and are often not reproducible. Ring sideroblasts (Figure 17.7) are defined by the presence of five or more siderotic (iron) granules encircling one-third or more of the nucleus in an iron-stained smear. At least 100 erythroblasts should be evaluated for the percentage of ring sideroblasts, if present.[9] Ring sideroblasts may be associated

with both reactive and neoplastic conditions. The iron stain may be used for core biopsy specimens, but decalcifying agents used to soften the biopsy specimen during processing may leach iron, which gives a false impression of decreased or absent iron stores. For this reason, the aspirate is preferred for the iron stain if sufficient spicules are present.

EXAMINING THE BONE MARROW CORE BIOPSY SPECIMEN

The standard stain for the core biopsy specimen is the *hematoxylin and eosin* (H&E) stain. Other stains and their purposes are listed in Table 15.6. Bone marrow core biopsy specimen and imprint (touch preparation) examinations are essential when the aspiration procedure yields a dry tap, which may be the result of hypoplastic or aplastic anemia, fibrosis, or tight packing of the marrow cavity with leukemic cells. The key advantage of the core biopsy specimen is preservation of bone marrow architecture so that cells, tumor clusters (Figure 15.17), and maturation stages may be examined relative to stromal elements. The disadvantage is that individual hematopoietic cell morphology is obscured, which is the reason why core biopsies are evaluated alongside aspirate smears.

The microscopist first examines the core biopsy specimen preparation at low power using the 10× objective lens (100× total magnification) to assess *cellularity*. Because the sample is larger, the core biopsy specimen provides a more accurate estimate of cellularity than the aspirate. The microscopist compares cellular areas with the clear-appearing adipocytes, using a method identical to that employed in examination of aspirate smears to assess cellularity. All fields are examined because cells distribute unevenly. Examples of hypocellular and hypercellular core biopsy sections are provided for comparison with normocellular marrow in Figure 15.18.

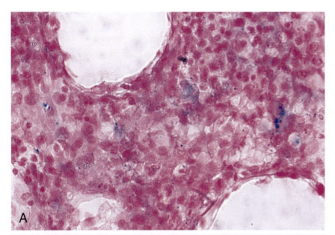
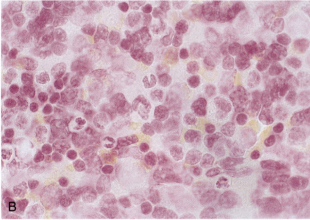
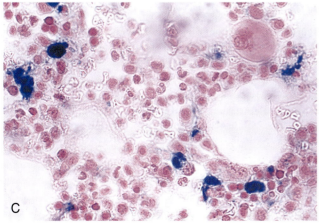

Figure 15.16 Bone Marrow Aspirate Smears Showing Iron Stores. **(A)**, Normal iron stores. **(B)**, Absence of iron stores. **(C)**, Increased iron stores. (A, B, C, Prussian blue stain, ×500.)

TABLE 15.6	**Stains Used in Examination of Bone Marrow Core Biopsy Specimens**
Stain	**Application**
Hematoxylin and eosin (H&E)	Evaluate cellularity and hematopoietic cell distribution; locate abnormal cell clusters
Prussian blue (acidic potassium ferrocyanide) iron stain	Evaluate iron stores for deficiency or excess iron; decalcification may remove iron from fixed specimens; thus EDTA chelation or aspirate smear is preferred for iron store estimation
Reticulin and trichrome stains	Examine for marrow fibrosis
Acid-fast stains	Examine for acid-fast bacilli, fungi, or bacteria in granulomatous disease
Gram stain	Examine for fungi or bacteria in granulomatous disease
Immunohistochemical stains	Establish the identity of malignant cells with stain-tagged monoclonal antibodies specific for tumor surface markers
Wright or Wright-Giemsa stain	Observe hematopoietic cell structure; cell identification is less accurate in a biopsy specimen than in an aspirate smear

EDTA, Ethylenediaminetetraacetic acid.

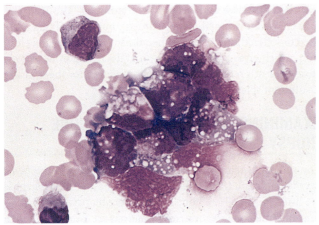

Figure 15.17 Bone Marrow Aspirate Smear Showing a Cluster or Syncytia of Tumor Cells. Nuclei are irregular and hyperchromatic, and cytoplasm is vacuolated. Cytoplasmic margins are poorly delineated. (Wright-Giemsa stain, ×500.)

Similar to what is seen on the aspirate smear, *megakaryocytes* are easily recognized by their outsized diameter and even distribution throughout the biopsy. They exhibit the characteristic lobulated nucleus, although nuclei of the more mature megakaryocytes are smaller and more darkly stained in H&E preparations than on a Wright-stained aspirate specimen. Their cytoplasm varies from light pink in maturing cells to dark pink in mature cells (Figure 15.19). Because of the greater sample volume, microscopists assess megakaryocyte numbers more accurately by examining a core biopsy section rather than an aspirate smear. Normally, there are 2 to 10 megakaryocytes per low-power field, the same as in an aspirate smear or imprint. Because the core biopsy represents a 4- to 6-micron section of a paraffin block of tissue, this is a cut section and, in contrast to the aspirate smear, *does not* represent the entire cytologic appearance of the cells. This fact is especially important when considering larger cells such as megakaryocytes because many megakaryocytes present on a core biopsy specimen will only be partially represented because they can be cut through.

Using high power (50× oil immersion objective lens), the microscopist next observes *cell distribution* relative to bone marrow stroma. For instance, in people older than age 70, normal lymphocytes may form small aggregates in nonparatrabecular regions, whereas *malignant lymphoma cell clusters* are often paratrabecular (associated with the bony region). In addition, normal lymphocytes remain as discrete cells, whereas lymphoma cells are typically pleomorphic and syncytial.

If no aspirate or imprint smears could be prepared, the core biopsy specimen may be stained using Wright, Giemsa, Wright-Giemsa, or H&E stains to make limited observations of cellular morphology. In core biopsy sections, myeloblasts and promyelocytes have oval or round nuclei with variably abundant cytoplasm (Figure 15.20). Neutrophilic myelocytes and metamyelocytes have light pink cytoplasm. Mature segmented neutrophils (segs) and neutrophilic bands (bands) are recognized by their smaller diameter and darkly stained C-shaped nuclei (bands) or nuclear segments (segs). The cytoplasm

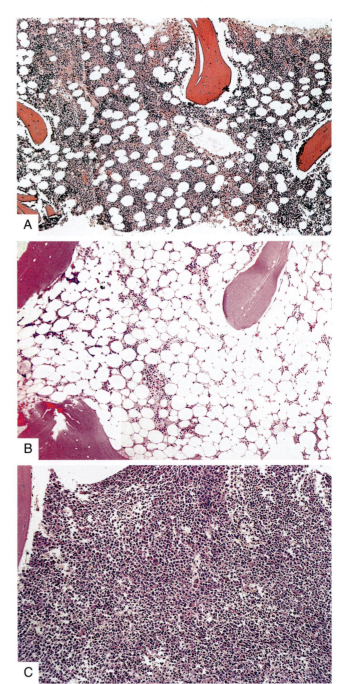

Figure 15.18 Core Biopsy Sections Showing Degrees of Cellularity. **(A)**, Normal cellularity, approximately 50% fat and 50% hematopoietic cells. (Hematoxylin and eosin stain, ×50.) **(B)**, Hypocellularity with only fat and connective tissue cells from a patient with aplastic anemia. (Hematoxylin and eosin stain, ×100.) **(C)**, Hypercellularity from a patient with chronic myeloid leukemia with virtually 100% cellularity and no fat visible. (Hematoxylin and eosin stain, 100×.) (B, Courtesy Dennis P. O'Malley, MD, director, Immunohistochemistry Laboratory, Indiana University School of Medicine, Indianapolis, IN.)

of bands and segs may be light pink or may seem unstained (Figure 15.21).

The cytoplasm of *eosinophils* stains red or orange, which makes them the most brightly stained cells of the marrow (Figure 15.21). Basophils cannot be recognized on marrow biopsy specimens fixed with Zenker glacial acetic acid solution.

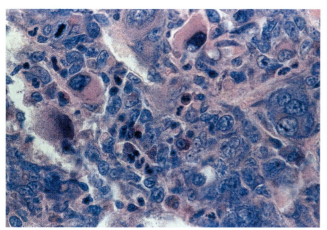

Figure 15.19 Core Biopsy Section Showing Megakaryocytes. Note the many large lobulated megakaryocytes and increased blasts. (Wright-Giemsa stain, ×400.)

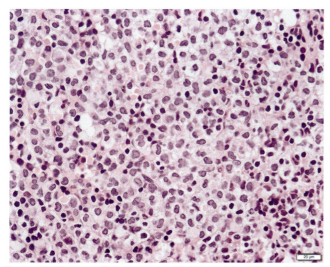

Figure 15.20 Core Biopsy Section Infiltrated by Blasts. Note the irregular nuclei and open chromatin of the blasts. (Hematoxylin and eosin stain, ×600.)

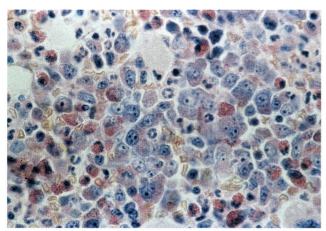

Figure 15.21 Core Biopsy Section. Note the myelocytes, metamyelocytes, bands, segmented neutrophils, and bright red-orange eosinophils. (Wright-Giemsa stain, ×400.)

The following features help differentiate the most immature granulocytic cells from the most immature erythroid cells in biopsy specimens. *Early erythroid progenitor cells* typically have two or three comma-shaped nucleoli, with one nucleolus touching the nuclear envelope. These erythroid precursors tend to cluster with more mature normoblasts and often surround histiocytes. *Polychromatophilic* and *orthochromic normoblasts,* the two most common erythroid maturation stages, have centrally placed, round nuclei that stain intensely (Figure 15.22). Their cytoplasm is not appreciably stained, but the plasma membrane margin is clearly discerned, which gives the cells of these stages a "fried-egg" appearance. Because erythroid cells have a tendency to cluster in small groups, they are more easily recognized using the 10× objective lens, although their individual morphology cannot be seen.

Lymphocytes are among the most difficult cells to recognize in the core biopsy specimen, unless they occur in clusters. Mature lymphocytes exhibit speckled nuclear chromatin in a small, round nucleus, along with a scant amount of blue cytoplasm and slightly irregular outlines (Figure 15.23).

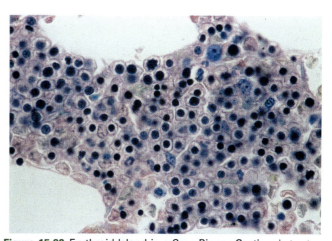

Figure 15.22 Erythroid Island in a Core Biopsy Section. Late-stage normoblasts often have a fried-egg appearance. (Wright-Giemsa stain, ×400.)

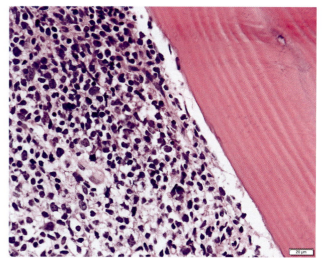

Figure 15.23 Core Biopsy With Lymphocytes. An infiltration of small mature lymphocytes is on the left (edge of bone on the right). A few are immature, with larger nuclei containing a single prominent nucleolus. (Hematoxylin and eosin stain, ×600.)

Plasma cells can be difficult to distinguish from myelocytes in H&E-stained sections but are recognized using Wright-Giemsa stain as cells with eccentric dark nuclei and blue cytoplasm and a prominent pale central Golgi apparatus (Figure 15.24). The nucleus may have a "clock-face" (irregularly condensed) appearance to the chromatin. Characteristically, plasma cells are located in clusters of a few cells in a perivascular distribution.

DEFINITIVE BONE MARROW STUDIES

Although in many cases, the aspirate smear and biopsy specimen are diagnostic, additional studies may be needed. Such studies and their applications are listed in Table 15.7. These studies require additional bone marrow specimen volume and specialized specimen collection and processing. Each study is well described in the chapter referenced in Table 15.7.

BONE MARROW EXAMINATION REPORTS

The components of a bone marrow report should be generated systematically during the microscopic review of the bone marrow specimens. In addition to the bone marrow examination components given in Table 15.4, information in the patient medical history (patient identity and age, narration of symptoms, physical findings, findings in kindred, treatment) and from the CBC and peripheral blood film examination (collected less than 2 days before the bone marrow procedure) is included. A diagnostic narrative, which is a summary of the recorded bone marrow findings and additional laboratory, chemical, microbiologic, and immunoassay tests, completes the bone marrow examination report. An example of a bone marrow examination report is provided in Figure 15.25.

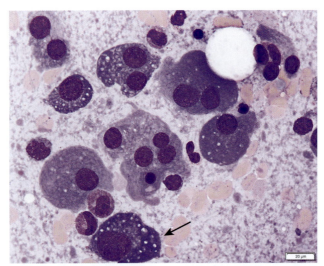

Figure 15.24 Markedly Abnormal Plasma Cells in an Aspirate Smear From a Patient With Plasma Cell Myeloma. The plasma cell highlighted by the *arrow* reveals an eccentric nucleus with a perinuclear hof (pallor). Note that most other cells have lost these normal features and demonstrate voluminous vacuolated cytoplasm and multinucleation, with some prominent nucleoli. (Wright-Giemsa stain, ×1000.)

TABLE 15.7 Definitive Studies Performed on Selected Bone Marrow Specimens			
Bone Marrow Study	**Application**	**Specimen**	**Chapter**
Iron stain	Identification of iron deficiency, iron overload	Fresh marrow aspirate	17
Cytochemical studies	Lineage identification in immature cells	Fresh marrow aspirate	31
Cytogenetic studies	Detection of numerical and structural chromosome abnormalities (such as deletions, translocations, duplications, and aneuploidy); remission studies	1 mL marrow in heparin	30
Molecular diagnostic studies	Polymerase chain reaction for diagnostic gene mutations; minimal residual disease studies; massively parallel or next-generation sequencing for identifying genetic mutations	1 mL marrow in EDTA; fresh marrow aspirate	29
Fluorescence in situ hybridization	Staining for diagnostic mutations; minimal residual disease studies	Fresh marrow aspirate	30
Flow cytometry	Immunophenotyping, usually of malignant hematopoietic cells, clonality; minimal residual disease studies	1 mL marrow in heparin, EDTA, or ACD	28

ACD, Acid-citrate dextrose; *EDTA,* ethylenediaminetetraacetic acid.

Bone Marrow Pathology Report

PATIENT INFORMATION:
LAST NAME, FIRST NAME
GENDER
AGE: DOB:
Patient ID/MRN:
Account #:

PHYSICIAN INFORMATION:
LAST NAME, FIRST NAME
NAME OF HOSPITAL/MEDICAL CENTER
ADDRESS OF MEDICAL CENTER
CITY, STATE
Tel: XXX-XXX-XXXX

FINAL DIAGNOSIS:

BIOPSY SITE; BIOPSY:
- ACUTE MYELOID LEUKEMIA WITH t(8;21)(q22;q22.1); *RUNX1::RUNX1T1,* SEE COMMENT

COMMENT:
Peripheral blood film: Leukopenia, few blasts, myelocytes, neutrophils. Relative lymphocytosis. RBCs normochromic, macrocytes, mild anisocytosis. Rare teardrop cells. Normal platelet morphology.
Bone marrow aspirate: Few spicules, blasts 65% with large nuclei with fine chromatin and needle shaped Auer rods. Moderate basophilic cytoplasm with salmon-colored graules. Few mature myeloid precursors. Erythroid precursors markedly decreased, with rare binucleate rubricytes. Few eosinophil precursors noted. Dysmorphic megakaryocytes with increased nuclear lobulation.
Bone marrow imprint: Significantly increased blasts. Few mature myeloid precursors, erythroid precursors markedly decreased.
Bone marrow biopsy: Hypercellular for age; estimated at 80% cellular. Most cells are blasts, few mature myeloid precursors. Erythroid and megakaryocytic precursors markedly reduced.
Iron stain: Stainable iron in macrophages. Sideroblasts and rare ring sideroblasts.
Flow cytometry: Analysis of the bone marrow aspirate smear demonstrates an abnormal myeloid blast population. Blasts express CD34, CD15, HLA-DR, CD33, CD19 and CD56. No phenotypic abnormalities in the lymphocytes.

Differential Counts

Date	PB	Marrow	Marrow Range (percent)		PB	Marrow	Marrow Range (percent)
Blast, unclassified	4	65	0-2	Normal lymphocytes	50	2	3-24
Myeloblasts			3-5	Reactive lymphocytes			
Promyelocytes			1-8	Lymphoblasts			
Myelocytes		14	5-21	Prolymphocytes			
Metamyelocytes			6-22	Monocytes	3		0-3
Band neutrophils			6-22	Plasma cells			0-2
Segmented neutrophils	40	4	9-27	Rubriblasts			0-4
Eosinophils	3	7		Prorubricytes			1-6
Basophils				Rubricytes			5-25
Other				Metarubricytes			1-21
Other				Erythroid		8	10-30

WBC	PLT	MPV	HGB	HCT	MCHC		
2,300	89,000	8	8.1	23	110		

Cytogenetics

ABNORMAL MALE KARYOTYPE: 45,XY,t(8;21)(q22;q22),-Y[20]

Association: This cytogenetics report renders the disease to be classified as "AML with defining genetic abnormalities" per the WHO classification 2022. There is also loss of the Y chromosome which is an incidental finding and of no clinical consequence in older male patients.

Prognosis: Good prognosis to chemotherapy and a high complete remission rate.

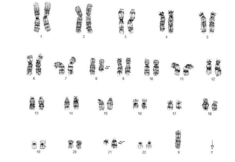

Figure 15.25 Example of a Bone Marrow Examination Report. Patient demographics, diagnosis, diagnostic comment and microscopic description, differential counts of marrow and blood with reference intervals, and cytogenetics report with karyogram can be included. *HCT,* Hematocrit; *HGB,* hemoglobin; *MCHC,* mean cell hemoglobin concentration; *MPV,* mean platelet volume; *PB,* peripheral blood; *PLT,* platelet; *RBCs,* red blood cells; *WBC,* white blood cells; *WHO,* World Health Organization.

SUMMARY

- Hematopoietic tissue in adults is located in the flat bones and the ends of the long bones. Hematopoiesis occurs within the spongy trabeculae of the bone adjacent to vascular sinuses.
- Bone marrow collection is a safe but invasive procedure performed by a pathologist or hematologist in collaboration with a medical laboratory professional to obtain specimens used to diagnose hematologic and systemic disease and/or to monitor treatment.
- The necessity for a bone marrow examination should be evaluated in light of all clinical and laboratory information. In anemias for which the cause is apparent from the red blood cell indices, a bone marrow examination may not be required. Examples of indications for bone marrow examination are numerous and include but are not limited to unexplained cytopenias, circulating blasts, and staging of lymphomas and carcinomas.
- A peripheral blood specimen should be collected for a complete blood count (CBC) and blood film examination less than 2 days before the bone marrow is collected, and the results of the CBC are reported with the bone marrow examination results.
- The preferred site for bone marrow aspiration and biopsy is the posterior iliac crest, although the anterior iliac crest can be used if the patient can lie only in the supine position. Other sites used for marrow aspirations only are the sternum (in adults) and the anterior medial surface of the tibia (in infants less than 1 year of age).

- The medical laboratory professional receives the bone marrow specimen and prepares direct aspirate smears, marrow aspirate particle smears, anticoagulated bone marrow smears, imprints, fixed biopsy sections, and specimens for confirmatory studies.
- The medical laboratory professional and pathologist collaborate with residents, fellows, attending physicians, and medical laboratory science students to review bone marrow aspirate smears, biopsy sections, and confirmatory procedure results.
- Confirmatory procedures include cytochemistry, cytogenetics, immunophenotyping by flow cytometry, and molecular diagnostics such as fluorescence in situ hybridization and next-generation sequencing.
- The medical laboratory professional and pathologist determine cellularity and megakaryocyte distribution, then perform a differential count of nucleated bone marrow cells and compute the myeloid-to-erythrocyte (M:E) ratio, comparing the results with reference intervals.
- The pathologist characterizes features of hematopoietic disease, metastatic tumor cells, and abnormalities of the bone marrow stroma, and prepares a systematic written bone marrow examination report, including a diagnostic narrative.

Now that you have completed this chapter, go back and read again the case study at the beginning and respond to the questions presented. Answers can be found in Appendix C.

REVIEW QUESTIONS

Answers can be found in Appendix C.

1. Where is most hematopoietic tissue found in adults?
   a. Liver
   b. Lungs
   c. Spleen
   d. Flat bones
2. What is the preferred bone marrow collection site?
   a. Sternum
   b. Posterior iliac crest
   c. Thoracic vertebrae
   d. Anterior head of the femur
3. The aspirate should be examined under low power to assess all of the following *EXCEPT:*
   a. Cellularity
   b. Megakaryocyte numbers
   c. Morphology of abnormal cells
   d. Presence of tumor cell clusters
4. What is the normal myeloid-to-erythroid (M:E) ratio range in adults?
   a. 1.5:1 to 3.3:1
   b. 5.1:1 to 6.2:1
   c. 8.6:1 to 10.2:1
   d. 10:1 to 12:1

5. Which are the most common erythroid stages found in the bone marrow of healthy adults?
   a. Pronormoblasts
   b. Pronormoblasts and basophilic normoblasts
   c. Basophilic and polychromatophilic normoblasts
   d. Polychromatophilic and orthochromic normoblasts
6. What cells, occasionally seen in bone marrow biopsy specimens, are responsible for the formation of bone?
   a. Macrophages
   b. Plasma cells
   c. Osteoblasts
   d. Osteoclasts
7. What is the largest hematopoietic cell found in a normal bone marrow aspirate?
   a. Osteoblast
   b. Myeloblast
   c. Pronormoblast
   d. Megakaryocyte

8. Which of the following is *NOT* an indication for a bone marrow examination?
   a. Pancytopenia (reduced numbers of red blood cells, white blood cells, and platelets in the peripheral blood)
   b. Anemia with red blood cell indices corresponding to low serum iron and low ferritin levels
   c. Detection of blasts in the peripheral blood
   d. Need for staging of Hodgkin lymphoma

9. In a bone marrow biopsy specimen, the red blood cell precursors were estimated to account for 40% of the cells in the marrow, and the other 60% were granulocyte precursors. What is the myeloid-to-erythroid (M:E) ratio?
   a. 4:6
   b. 1.5:1
   c. 1:1.5
   d. 3:1

10. On a bone marrow core biopsy sample, several large cells with multiple nuclei were noted. They were located close to the endosteum, and their nuclei were evenly spaced throughout the cell. What are these cells?
    a. Megakaryocytes
    b. Osteoclasts
    c. Adipocytes
    d. Fibroblasts

11. The advantage of a core biopsy bone marrow specimen over an aspirate is that the core biopsy specimen:
    a. Can be acquired by a less invasive collection technique
    b. Permits assessment of the architecture and cellular arrangement
    c. Retains the staining qualities of basophils owing to the use of Zenker fixative
    d. Is better for the assessment of bone marrow iron stores with Prussian blue stain

12. Which of the following features suggests involvement of the marrow by lymphoma?
    a. Paratrabecular lymphoid aggregation
    b. Lymphoid aggregates with germinal centers
    c. Nonparatrabecular lymphoid clusters
    d. Discrete, small lymphocytes with speckled nuclear chromatin

13. Using Wright-Giemsa stain, the morphologic description of an eccentric dark nuclei with deeply basophilic (blue) cytoplasm and a prominent pale central Golgi apparatus best describes a(n):
    a. Eosinophil
    b. Basophil
    c. Lymphocyte
    d. Plasma cell

REFERENCES

1. Dave, U. P., & Koury, M. J. (2021). Structure of the marrow and the hematopoietic microenvironment. In Kaushansky, K., Lichtman, M., Prchal, J. T., et al. (Eds.), *Williams Hematology.* (10th ed., pp. 47–78). New York: McGraw Hill.
2. Foucar, K., Chabot-Richards, D., Czuchlewski, D., et al. (2017). *Diagnostic Pathology: Blood and Bone Marrow.* (2nd ed.). St. Louis: Elsevier.
3. Scadden, D., & Silberstein, L. (2023). Hematopoietic microenvironment. In Hoffman, R., Benz, E. J., Silberstein, L. E., et al. (Eds.), *Hematology Basic Principles and Practice.* (8th ed., pp. 157–164). St. Louis: Elsevier.
4. Reddy, V., Marques, M. B., & Fritsma, G. A. (2013). *Quick Guide to Hematology Testing.* (2nd ed.). Washington, DC: AACC Press.
5. Smock., K. J. (2019). Examination of the blood and bone marrow. In Greer, J. P., Rodgers, G. M., Glader, B., et al. (Eds.), *Wintrobe's Clinical Hematology.* (14th ed., pp. 1–16). Philadelphia: Wolters Kluwer Health/Lippincott Williams & Wilkins.
6. Reddy, V. V. B., & Morlote, D. (2021). Examination of blood and marrow cells. In Kaushansky, K., Lichtman, M., Prchal, J. T., et al. (Eds.), *Williams Hematology.* (10th ed., pp. 11–30). New York: McGraw Hill.
7. Krause, J. R. (1981). *Bone Marrow Biopsy.* New York: Churchill Livingstone.
8. Bain, B. J. (2003). Bone marrow biopsy morbidity and mortality. *Br J Haematol, 121,* 949–951.
9. Lee, S. H., Erber, W., Porwit, A., et al., International Council for Standardization in Hematology. (2008). ICSH guidelines for the standardization of bone marrow specimens and reports. *Int J Lab Hematol, 30,* 349–364.
10. Hartsock, R. J., Smith, E. B., & Pett, C. S. (1965). Normal variations with aging of the amount of hemopoietic tissue in bone marrow from the anterior iliac crest. *Am J Clin Pathol, 43,* 326–331.
11. Loken, M. R., Chu, S-C., & Fritschle, W. (2009). Normalization of bone marrow aspirates for hemodilution in flow cytometric analyses. *Cytometry B Clin Cytom, 76,* 27–36.
12. WHO Classification of Tumours Editorial Board (2022). *Haematolymphoid tumours.* Lyon (France): International Agency for Research on Cancer; forthcoming. (WHO classification of tumours series, 5th ed.; vol. 11). https://publications.iarc.fr.

16

Anemias: Red Blood Cell Morphology and Approach to Diagnosis

Naveen Manchanda*

OBJECTIVES

After completion of this chapter, the reader will be able to:

1. Define *anemia* and recognize laboratory results consistent with anemia.
2. Describe clinical findings in anemia.
3. Discuss the importance of the history and physical examination in diagnosis of anemia.
4. Explain how the body adapts to anemia and the symptoms experienced by the patient.
5. Distinguish among effective, ineffective, and insufficient erythropoiesis when given examples.
6. List laboratory procedures that are initially performed for diagnosis of anemia.
7. Discuss the importance of the reticulocyte count in the evaluation of anemia.
8. Explain the importance of examining the peripheral blood film when investigating the cause of an anemia and distinguish important findings.
9. Describe variations in red blood cell morphology such as inclusions and changes in shape, volume, or color.
10. Use an algorithm incorporating the absolute reticulocyte count to specify three groups of anemias involving decreased or ineffective red blood cell production and give one example of each.
11. Use an algorithm incorporating the mean cell volume to narrow the differential diagnosis of anemia.

OUTLINE

Definition of Anemia
Importance of Patient History and Clinical Findings
Physiologic Adaptations in Patients With Anemia
Mechanisms of Anemia
    Ineffective and Insufficient Erythropoiesis
    Blood Loss and Hemolysis
Laboratory Diagnosis of Anemia
    Complete Blood Count With Red Blood Cell Indices
    Reticulocyte Count

Peripheral Blood Film Examination
Bone Marrow Examination
Other Laboratory Tests
Approach to Evaluating Anemias
    Morphologic Classification of Anemia Based on Mean Cell Volume
    Pathophysiologic Classification of Anemias and Reticulocyte Count

CASE STUDY

After studying the material in this chapter, the reader should be able to respond to the following case study. Answers can be found in Appendix C.

A 45-year-old woman phoned her provider and complained of fatigue, shortness of breath on exertion, and general malaise. She requested "B$_{12}$ shots" to make her feel better. The provider asked the patient to schedule an appointment to determine the cause of the symptoms before offering treatment. A point-of-care HGB determination performed in the office was 9.0 g/dL. Reference intervals can be found after the Index at the end of the book. The provider then requested additional laboratory tests, including a complete blood count (CBC) with a reticulocyte count and a peripheral blood film examination.

1. Why did the provider want the patient to come to the office before prescribing therapy?
2. How do the mean cell volume and reticulocyte count help determine the classification of the anemia?
3. Why is the examination of the peripheral blood film important in the investigation of an anemia?

*The author extends appreciation to Ann Bell and Rakesh Mehta, whose work in prior editions provided the foundation for this chapter.

Red blood cells (RBCs) perform the vital physiologic function of oxygen delivery to tissues. Hemoglobin within the RBCs has the remarkable capacity to bind oxygen in the lungs and release it appropriately in the tissues.[1] The term *anemia* is derived from the Greek word *anaimia,* meaning "without blood."[2] A decrease in the RBC count with or without a decrease in hemoglobin concentration results in decreased oxygen delivery to the tissues leading to tissue hypoxia. Anemia is a common condition, affecting an estimated 1.93 billion people worldwide.[3] Anemia should not be thought of as a disease but rather, as a manifestation of an underlying condition or deficiency.[4,5] Therefore causes of anemia should be thoroughly investigated. This chapter provides an overview of the mechanisms, diagnosis, and classification of anemia. Each anemia is discussed in detail in the following chapters.

DEFINITION OF ANEMIA

A functional definition of *anemia* is a decrease in the oxygen-carrying capacity of the blood. Anemia can arise if there is insufficient or impaired function of hemoglobin. The former is the more frequent cause.

Anemia is defined operationally as a reduction in the hemoglobin content of blood that can be caused by a decrease in the RBC count, hemoglobin, and hematocrit below the reference interval for healthy individuals of similar age, sex, and race under similar environmental conditions.[4-8] The reference intervals are derived from large pools of "healthy" individuals; however, the definition of *healthy* is different for each of these groups. Thus, these pools of healthy individuals may lack the heterogeneity required to be universally applied to any one of these populations of individuals.[6] This fact has led to the development of different reference intervals for individuals of different sex, age, and race.

Examples of hematologic reference intervals for the adult and pediatric populations are included after the Index at the end of the book. They are listed according to age and sex, but race and environmental and laboratory factors can also influence the values. Each laboratory must determine its own reference intervals based on its particular instrumentation, the methods used, and the demographic characteristics and environment of its patient population. For the purpose of discussion in this chapter, a patient is considered anemic if the hemoglobin value falls below normal as listed after the Index at the end of the book.

IMPORTANCE OF PATIENT HISTORY AND CLINICAL FINDINGS

The history and physical examination are important components in making a clinical diagnosis of anemia. A decrease in oxygen delivery to the tissues decreases the energy available to individuals to perform day-to-day activities. This gives rise to the classic symptoms associated with anemia, fatigue and shortness of breath. To elucidate the reason for a patient's anemia, one starts by obtaining a detailed history, which requires carefully questioning the patient, particularly with regard to diet, drug ingestion, exposure to chemicals, occupation, hobbies,

travel, bleeding history, race or ethnic group, family history of disease, neurologic symptoms, previous medications, previous episodes of jaundice, and various underlying disease processes that result in anemia.[4,7-9] Therefore a thorough discussion is required to elicit any potential cause of the anemia. For example, iron deficiency can lead to an interesting symptom called *pica.*[10] Patients with pica have cravings for unusual substances such as ice (pagophagia), cornstarch, or clay. Alternatively, individuals with anemia may be asymptomatic, as can be seen in mild or slowly progressive anemias where the body is able to adapt to the slowly developing anemia. However, severe anemia (e.g., hemoglobin values <7 g/dL) is always associated with symptoms.

Certain features should be evaluated closely during the physical examination to provide clues to hematologic disorders such as skin (for petechiae), eyes (for pallor or jaundice), and mouth (for mucosal bleeding). The examination should also evaluate sternal tenderness, lymphadenopathy, cardiac murmurs or arrhythmias, splenomegaly, and hepatomegaly.[4,11] Jaundice is important for the assessment of anemia because it may be due to increased RBC destruction, which suggests a hemolytic component to the anemia. Measuring vital signs is also a crucial component of the physical evaluation. Patients experiencing a rapid fall in hemoglobin typically have tachycardia (fast heart rate), whereas if the anemia is long-standing (chronic), the heart rate may be normal because of the body's ability to compensate for the anemia (discussed later).

Moderate anemias (hemoglobin of 7 to 10 g/dL) may cause pallor of conjunctivae and nail beds but may not produce clinical symptoms if the onset of anemia is slow.[4] However, depending on the patient's age and cardiovascular state, symptoms such as dyspnea, vertigo, headache, muscle weakness, and lethargy can occur.[4,8] Severe anemias (hemoglobin of less than 7 g/dL) usually produce tachycardia, hypotension, and other symptoms of volume loss, in addition to the symptoms listed earlier. Thus the severity of the anemia is gauged by the degree of reduction in hemoglobin, cardiopulmonary adaptation, and the rapidity of progression of the anemia.[4]

PHYSIOLOGIC ADAPTATIONS IN PATIENTS WITH ANEMIA

Patients who develop anemia from acute blood loss, such as with severe hemorrhage, respond with profound changes in physiologic processes to ensure adequate perfusion of vital organs and maintenance of homeostasis. In cases of severe acute blood loss, such as in trauma, blood volume decreases and hypotension develops, resulting in decreased blood supply to the brain and heart. As an immediate adaptation, there is sympathetic overdrive that results in peripheral vasoconstriction, increasing heart rate, respiratory rate, and cardiac output.[4,7,8] Blood is preferentially shunted to organs that are key to survival, including the brain, muscle, and heart.[4,7,8] This results in oxygen being preferentially supplied to vital organs, even in the presence of reduced oxygen-carrying capacity. Within hours of the initial episode of blood loss, tissue hypoxia triggers intracellular acidosis, resulting in an increase in RBC 2,3-bisphosphoglycerate

(2,3-BPG) that shifts the hemoglobin-oxygen dissociation curve to the right (decreased oxygen affinity of hemoglobin) and results in increased oxygen delivery to tissues (Chapter 8).[8,12]

With rapid blood loss, the hemoglobin and hematocrit may be initially unchanged because there is balanced loss of plasma and cells. However, a *dilutional anemia* develops as the drop in blood volume is compensated for by movement of fluid from the extravascular to the intravascular compartment or by administration of resuscitation fluid.

An increase of 2,3-BPG is also a significant mechanism in chronic anemias that enables patients with low levels of hemoglobin to remain relatively asymptomatic. Thus with slowly developing and low-grade anemia, the body develops physiologic adaptations to increase the oxygen-carrying capacity of a reduced amount of hemoglobin, which improves oxygen delivery to tissues. With persistent and severe anemia, however, patients have more symptoms such as shortness of breath and fatigue; in severe cases of anemia, the strain on the heart can ultimately lead to cardiac failure.

Reduced oxygen delivery to tissues caused by reduced hemoglobin concentration elicits an increase in *erythropoietin* (EPO), a hormone secreted by the kidneys. EPO stimulates the erythroid precursors in the bone marrow, which leads to the release of more RBCs into the circulation (Chapter 6).[7,8] Box 16.1 summarizes the body's physiologic adaptations to anemia.

MECHANISMS OF ANEMIA

The life span of an RBC in circulation is about 120 days. In a healthy individual with no anemia, each day, the bone marrow replenishes approximately 1% of RBCs that are removed from circulation because of senescence (Chapter 6). Replenishment occurs through erythropoiesis in which hematopoietic stem cells differentiate into erythroid precursor cells and the bone marrow releases reticulocytes (immature enucleated RBCs) that mature into RBCs in the peripheral circulation.

Adequate RBC production requires several nutrients such as iron, vitamin B_{12}, and folate. Globin (polypeptide chain) synthesis must also function normally. In conditions with excessive bleeding or hemolysis, the bone marrow is stimulated to increase RBC production to compensate for the lost cells. This is accomplished by releasing newly formed RBC precursors,

reticulocytes that develop into mature RBCs. Therefore maintenance of a stable hemoglobin concentration requires the production of functionally normal RBCs in sufficient numbers containing adequate hemoglobin to replace the amount lost.[4]

Ineffective and Insufficient Erythropoiesis

Erythropoiesis is the term used for bone marrow erythroid proliferative activity. Normal erythropoiesis occurs in bone marrow and is under the control of EPO and other growth factors and cytokines (Chapters 5 and 6).[7,8] When erythropoiesis is effective, bone marrow is able to produce functional RBCs that replace the daily loss of RBCs.

Ineffective erythropoiesis refers to the production of erythroid precursor cells that are defective. These often undergo apoptosis (programmed cell death) in the bone marrow before they have a chance to mature to the reticulocyte stage and be released into the peripheral circulation. Several conditions, such as megaloblastic anemia (impaired deoxyribonucleic acid [DNA] synthesis as a result of vitamin B_{12} or folate deficiency), thalassemia (deficient globin chain synthesis), and sideroblastic anemia (deficient protoporphyrin synthesis), involve ineffective erythropoiesis as a mechanism of anemia. The resulting anemia triggers an increase in EPO production leading to increased erythropoietic activity, but peripheral hemoglobin remains low.[4,11]

Insufficient erythropoiesis refers to a decrease in the number of erythroid precursors in the bone marrow, resulting in decreased RBC production and anemia. Many factors can lead to the decreased RBC production, including a deficiency of iron (inadequate intake, malabsorption, excessive loss from chronic bleeding), a deficiency of EPO (renal disease), or loss of the erythroid precursors as a result of an autoimmune reaction (aplastic anemia, acquired pure red cell aplasia) or infection (parvovirus B19). Erythropoiesis can also be suppressed by infiltration of the bone marrow space with leukemia cells or with nonhematopoietic cells (metastatic tumors, granulomas, or fibrosis), the latter called *myelophthisic anemia,* with characteristic teardrop RBCs.[4,7,12]

Blood Loss and Hemolysis

As described earlier, anemia can also develop as a result of acute blood loss (such as a traumatic injury) or chronic blood loss (such as an intermittently bleeding colonic polyp), or due to an increase in hemolysis resulting in a shortened RBC life span. With acute blood loss and excessive hemolysis, the bone marrow takes a few days to increase production of RBCs.[4,7,8] This response may be inadequate to compensate for a sudden excessive RBC loss as in traumatic hemorrhage or in conditions with a high rate of hemolysis and shortened RBC survival. The physiological adaptations to acute blood loss can occur rapidly as noted above. Numerous causes of hemolysis exist, including intrinsic defects in the RBC membrane, enzyme systems, or hemoglobin or extrinsic causes such as antibody-mediated processes, mechanical fragmentation, or infection-related destruction.[4,7,8] Chronic blood loss induces iron deficiency as a cause of anemia.

In pregnancy, a physiological dilutional anemia may develop due to a greater increase in plasma volume compared to RBC

BOX 16.1 **Adaptations to Anemia**

Response to Acute (Sudden) Loss of Blood

The following adaptations occur in minutes to hours:

- Peripheral vasoconstriction and increase in heart rate, respiratory rate, and cardiac output, which increases the flow of oxygenated blood
- Redistribution of blood flow from skin to essential organs (brain, heart, muscles)

Response to Slowly Developing Anemia

The following adaptations occur over days to weeks:

- Increase in erythrocyte 2,3-bisphosphoglycerate, which decreases hemoglobin's affinity for oxygen and allows more oxygen release to tissues
- Increase in erythropoietin production by kidneys, which increases erythropoiesis and promotes release of more red blood cells into circulation

mass. A 50% increase in plasma volume can be seen by 34 weeks of gestation and is proportional to the birth weight of the baby. Because the expansion in plasma volume is greater than the increased cell mass, there is a fall in hemoglobin by hemodilution. Note that the MCV is normal in these situations (Chapter 43).[13]

LABORATORY DIAGNOSIS OF ANEMIA

Complete Blood Count With Red Blood Cell Indices

To detect the presence of anemia, the medical laboratory professional performs a complete blood count (CBC) using an automated blood cell analyzer to determine the RBC count, hemoglobin, hematocrit (HCT), RBC indices, white blood cell (WBC) count, and platelet count (Chapter 13). The RBC indices include the mean cell volume (MCV), mean cell hemoglobin (MCH), and mean cell hemoglobin concentration (MCHC) (Chapter 12).[14] The most important of these indices, in evaluating anemias, is the MCV, a measure of the average RBC volume in femtoliters (fL). Reference intervals for these determinations are listed after the Index at the end of the book and in Table 16.1. Automated blood cell analyzers also provide the red blood cell distribution width (RDW), an index of variation of cell volume in an RBC population (discussed later). A reticulocyte count should be performed for every patient with anemia. As with RBCs, automated analyzers provide accurate measurements of reticulocyte counts.

RDW is the coefficient of variation of RBC volume expressed as a percentage.[14] It indicates the variation in RBC volume within the population measured, and an increased RDW correlates with anisocytosis (variation in RBC diameter) on the peripheral blood film. Automated analyzers calculate the RDW by dividing the standard deviation of the RBC volume by the MCV and then multiplying by 100 to convert to a percentage. Clinical usefulness of the RDW is discussed later.

Reticulocyte Count

The *reticulocyte count* is an important tool to assess the ability of the bone marrow to increase RBC production in response to anemia. Reticulocytes are young RBCs that lack a nucleus but still contain residual ribonucleic acid (RNA) to complete the production of hemoglobin. Normally, they circulate peripherally for 1 day while completing their development into a mature RBC. The adult and pediatric reference intervals for the reticulocyte count can be found after the Index at the end of the book. An *absolute reticulocyte count* is the actual number of reticulocytes in 1 L or 1 μL of blood and is determined by multiplying the percent reticulocytes by the RBC count (Table 16.1 and Chapter 12). The reference interval for the absolute reticulocyte count can be found after the Index at the end of the book and is based on an adult RBC count within the reference interval (after the Index at the end of the book).[4,7] A patient with a severe anemia may seem to be producing increased numbers of reticulocytes if only the percentage is considered. For example, an adult patient with 1.5×10^{12}/L RBCs and 3% reticulocytes has an absolute reticulocyte count of 45×10^9/L. The percentage of reticulocytes exceeds the reference interval, but the absolute reticulocyte count is within the reference interval. For the degree of anemia, however, both results are inappropriately low. In other words, production of reticulocytes within the reference interval is inadequate to compensate for an RBC count that is approximately one-third of normal.

Two successive corrections are made to the reticulocyte count to obtain a better representation of RBC production. First, to obtain a *corrected reticulocyte count*, one corrects for the degree of anemia by multiplying the reticulocyte percentage by the patient's hematocrit and dividing the result by 45 (the average normal hematocrit). If the reticulocytes are released prematurely from the bone marrow and remain in the circulation 2 to 3 days (instead of 1 day), the corrected reticulocyte count must be divided by maturation time to determine the *reticulocyte production index* (RPI) (Table 16.1). The RPI is a better indication of the rate of RBC production than the corrected reticulocyte count.[4] The reticulocyte count and derivation of RPI is discussed in Chapter 12.

In addition, state-of-the-art automated blood cell analyzers determine the fraction of immature reticulocytes among the total circulating reticulocytes, called the *immature reticulocyte fraction* (IRF). The IRF is helpful in assessing early bone marrow response after treatment for anemia and is discussed in Chapter 13.

Analysis of the reticulocyte count plays a crucial role in determining whether an anemia is due to a RBC production defect (ineffective or insufficient erythropoiesis) or to premature hemolysis and shortened survival defect. If there is shortened RBC survival, as in the *hemolytic anemias*, the bone marrow tries to compensate by increasing RBC production to release more reticulocytes into the peripheral circulation. Although an increased reticulocyte count is a hallmark of the hemolytic anemias, it can also be observed after acute blood loss (Chapter 20), which may take a few days to develop and will be enhanced

TABLE 16.1	Formulas for Reticulocyte Counts and Red Blood Cell Indices*
Test	**Formula**
Absolute reticulocyte count ($\times 10^9$/L)	= reticulocytes (%) × RBC count ($\times 10^{12}$/L)/100
Corrected reticulocyte count (%)	= reticulocytes (%) × patient's HCT (%)/45
Reticulocyte production index (RPI)	= corrected reticulocyte count/maturation time
Mean cell volume (MCV) (fL)	= HCT (%) × 10/RBC count ($\times 10^{12}$/L)
Mean cell hemoglobin (MCH) (pg)	= HGB (g/dL) × 10/RBC count ($\times 10^{12}$/L)
Mean cell hemoglobin concentration (MCHC) (g/dL)	= HGB (g/dL) × 100/HCT (%)

HGB, Hemoglobin; *HCT,* hematocrit; *RBC,* red blood cell.
*Reference intervals can be found after the Index at the end of the book. In anemia patients, the RPI should be >3.

by adequate stores of iron.[4,7,8] Chronic blood loss, on the other hand, does *not* lead to an appropriate increase in the reticulocyte count but rather, leads to iron deficiency and a subsequent low reticulocyte count. Thus an inappropriately low reticulocyte count results from decreased production of normal RBCs as a result of either insufficient or ineffective erythropoiesis.

Peripheral Blood Film Examination

An important component in the evaluation of an anemia is examination of the peripheral blood film, with particular attention to RBC diameter, shape, color, and presence of inclusions. The peripheral blood film also serves to verify the results produced by automated analyzers. Normal RBCs on a Wright-stained blood film are nearly uniform, ranging from 7 to 8 μm in diameter. Small or microcytic cells are less than 6 μm in diameter, and large or macrocytic RBCs are greater than 8 μm in diameter. Certain shape abnormalities of diagnostic value (such as sickle cells, spherocytes, schistocytes, and oval macrocytes) and RBC inclusions (such as malarial parasites, basophilic stippling, and Howell-Jolly bodies) can be detected only by studying the RBCs on a peripheral blood film (Tables 16.2 and 16.3). Examples of abnormal shapes and inclusions are provided in Figure 16.1.

Finally, a review of the WBCs and platelets may help show that a more generalized bone marrow problem is leading to the anemia. For example, hypersegmented neutrophils can be seen in vitamin B_{12} or folate deficiency, whereas blast cells and decreased platelets may be an indication of acute leukemia. Chapter 14 contains a complete discussion of the peripheral blood film evaluation. Information from the blood film examination always complements the data from the automated blood cell analyzer.

Bone Marrow Examination

The cause of many anemias can be determined from the history, physical examination, and results of laboratory tests on peripheral blood. When the cause cannot be determined, however, or the differential diagnosis remains broad, bone marrow aspiration and biopsy may help in establishing the cause of anemia.[4,8] Bone marrow examination is indicated for a patient with an unexplained anemia associated with or without other cytopenias, fever of unknown origin, or suspected hematologic malignancy. Bone marrow examination evaluates hematopoiesis and can determine whether there is an infiltration of abnormal cells into the bone marrow. Important findings in bone marrow that can point to the underlying cause of the anemia include abnormal cellularity (e.g., hypocellularity in aplastic anemia); evidence of ineffective erythropoiesis and megaloblastic changes (e.g., folate/vitamin B_{12} deficiency or myelodysplastic syndromes); lack of iron on iron stains of bone marrow (the gold standard for diagnosis of iron deficiency); and the presence of granulomata, fibrosis, infectious agents, and tumor cells that may be inhibiting normal erythropoiesis. Chapter 15 discusses bone marrow procedures and bone marrow examination in detail.

Other tests that can assist in the diagnosis of anemia can be performed on a bone marrow specimen as well. These tests include immunophenotyping of membrane antigens by flow cytometry (Chapter 28), cytogenetic studies (Chapter 30), and molecular analysis to detect specific genetic mutations and chromosome abnormalities in leukemia cells (Chapter 29).

Other Laboratory Tests

After the hematologic laboratory studies are completed, the anemia may be classified based on reticulocyte count, MCV, and peripheral blood film findings. Iron studies (including serum iron, total iron-binding capacity, transferrin saturation, and serum ferritin) are valuable if an inappropriately low reticulocyte count and a microcytic anemia are present. Serum vitamin B_{12} and serum folate assays are helpful in investigating a macrocytic anemia with a low reticulocyte count, whereas a direct antiglobulin test (DAT) can differentiate autoimmune hemolytic anemias from other hemolytic anemias. Because of the numerous potential etiologies of anemia, the specific cause needs to be determined to initiate appropriate therapy.[11]

Other laboratory tests that can assist in establishing the cause of anemia include routine urinalysis (to detect hemoglobinuria or an increase in urobilinogen), with a microscopic examination (to detect hematuria or hemosiderin) and analysis of stool (to detect occult blood or intestinal parasites). Also, certain chemistry studies are very useful, such as serum haptoglobin, lactate dehydrogenase, and unconjugated bilirubin (to detect excessive hemolysis) and renal and hepatic function tests. With more patients undergoing gastric bypass surgery for obesity, certain rare deficiencies such as insufficient copper are becoming more common as a cause of anemia.[15]

APPROACH TO EVALUATING ANEMIAS

The approach to the patient with anemia begins with taking a complete history and performing a physical examination.[4,7] For example, new-onset fatigue and shortness of breath suggest an acute drop in the hemoglobin, whereas minimal or lack of symptoms suggests a long-standing condition where adaptive mechanisms have compensated for the drop in hemoglobin. A strict vegetarian may not be getting enough vitamin B_{12} in the diet, whereas an individual with alcoholism may not be getting enough folate. A large spleen may be an indication of hereditary spherocytosis, whereas a stool positive for occult blood may indicate iron deficiency. Thus a complete history and physical examination can yield information to narrow the possible cause or causes of anemia and lead to a more rational and cost-effective diagnostic testing.

The first step in the laboratory diagnosis of anemia is detecting its presence by the accurate measurement of the hemoglobin concentration, hematocrit, MCV, and RBC count and comparison of these values with the reference interval for healthy individuals of the same age, sex, race, and environment. Knowledge of previous hematologic values is valuable as a reduction of 10% or more in these values may be the first clue that an abnormal condition may be present.[4,6,16]

There are numerous causes of anemia, so a rational algorithm to initially evaluate this condition using the previously mentioned tests is required. A reticulocyte count and a peripheral blood film examination are of paramount importance in evaluating anemia.

TABLE 16.2   Description of Red Blood Cell Abnormalities and Commonly Associated Disease States

RBC Abnormality	Cell Description	Commonly Associated Disease States
Anisocytosis	Abnormal variation in RBC volume or diameter	Hemolytic, megaloblastic, iron deficiency anemias
Macrocyte	Large RBC (>8 μm in diameter), MCV >100 fL	Megaloblastic anemia Myelodysplastic syndromes Chronic liver disease Bone marrow failure Reticulocytosis
Oval macrocyte	Large, oval RBC	Megaloblastic anemia
Microcyte	Small RBC (<6 μm in diameter), MCV <80 fL	Iron deficiency anemia Anemia of inflammation Sideroblastic anemia Thalassemia/Hb E disease and trait
Poikilocytosis	Abnormal variation in RBC shape	Severe anemia; certain shapes helpful diagnostically
Spherocyte	Small, round, dense RBC with no central pallor	Hereditary spherocytosis Immune hemolytic anemia Extensive burns (along with schistocytes)
Elliptocyte, ovalocyte	Elliptical (cigar-shaped), oval (egg-shaped) RBC	Hereditary elliptocytosis or ovalocytosis Iron deficiency anemia Thalassemia major Myelophthisic anemias
Stomatocyte	RBC with slitlike area of central pallor	Hereditary stomatocytosis Rh deficiency syndrome Acquired stomatocytosis (liver disease, alcoholism) Artifact
Sickle cell	Thin, dense, elongated RBC pointed at each end; may be curved	Sickle cell anemia Sickle cell-β-thalassemia
Hb C crystal	Hexagonal crystal of dense hemoglobin formed within the RBC membrane	Hb C disease
Hb SC crystal	Fingerlike or quartzlike crystal of dense hemoglobin protruding from the RBC membrane	Hb SC disease
Target cell (codocyte)	RBC with hemoglobin concentrated in the center and around the periphery resembling a target	Liver disease Hemoglobinopathies Thalassemia
Schistocyte (schizocyte)	Fragmented RBC caused by rupture in the peripheral circulation	Microangiopathic hemolytic anemia* (along with microspherocytes) Macroangiopathic hemolytic anemia† Extensive burns (along with microspherocytes)
Helmet cell (keratocyte)	RBC fragment in shape of a helmet	Same as schistocyte
Folded cell	RBC with membrane folded over	Hb C disease Hb SC disease
Acanthocyte (spur cell)	Small, dense RBC with few irregularly spaced projections of varying length	Severe liver disease (spur cell anemia) Neuroacanthocytosis (abetalipoproteinemia, McLeod syndrome)
Burr cell (echinocyte)	RBC with blunt or pointed, short projections that are usually evenly spaced over the surface of cell; present in all fields of blood film but in variable numbers per field‡	Uremia Pyruvate kinase deficiency
Teardrop cell (dacryocyte)	RBC with a single pointed extension resembling a teardrop or pear	Primary myelofibrosis Myelophthisic anemia Thalassemia Megaloblastic anemia

*Such as thrombotic thrombocytopenic purpura, hemolytic uremic syndrome, disseminated intravascular coagulation.
†Such as traumatic cardiac hemolysis.
‡Cells with similar morphology that are unevenly distributed in a blood film (not present in all fields) likely are due to a drying artifact in blood film preparation; these artifacts are sometimes called *crenated RBCs*.
Hb, Hemoglobin; *MCV*, mean cell volume; *RBC*, red blood cell.

TABLE 16.3 Erythrocyte Inclusions: Description, Composition, and Some Commonly Associated Disease States*

Inclusion	Appearance in Supravital Stain†	Appearance in Wright Stain	Composition of Inclusion	Associated Diseases/ Conditions
Diffuse basophilia	Dark blue granules and filaments in cytoplasm (seen in reticulocytes)	Bluish tinge throughout cytoplasm; also called *polychromasia* (seen in polychromatic erythrocytes)	RNA	Hemolytic anemia After treatment for iron, vitamin B_{12}, or folate deficiency
Basophilic stippling	Dark blue-purple, fine or coarse punctate granules distributed throughout cytoplasm	Dark blue-purple, fine or coarse punctate granules distributed throughout cytoplasm	Precipitated RNA	Lead poisoning Thalassemias Hemoglobinopathies Megaloblastic anemia Myelodysplastic syndromes
Howell-Jolly body	Dark blue-purple, dense, round granule; usually one per cell; occasionally multiple	Dark blue-purple, dense, round granule; usually one per cell; occasionally multiple	DNA (nuclear fragment)	Hyposplenism Postsplenectomy Megaloblastic anemia Hemolytic anemia Thalassemia Myelodysplastic syndromes
Heinz body	Round, dark blue-purple granule attached to inner RBC membrane	Not visible	Denatured hemoglobin	Glucose-6-phosphate dehydrogenase deficiency Unstable hemoglobins Oxidant drugs/chemicals
Pappenheimer bodies‡	Irregular clusters of small, light to dark blue granules, often near periphery of cell	Irregular clusters of small, light to dark blue granules, often near periphery of cell	Iron	Sideroblastic anemia Hemoglobinopathies Thalassemias Megaloblastic anemia Myelodysplastic syndromes Hyposplenism Postsplenectomy
Cabot ring	Rings or figure eights	Blue rings or figure eights	Mitotic spindle remnant	Megaloblastic anemia Myelodysplastic syndromes
Hb H	Fine, evenly dispersed, dark blue granules; imparts "golf ball" appearance to RBCs	Not visible	Precipitated β-globin chains of hemoglobin	Hb H disease

*Inclusions of hemoglobin crystals (Hb S, Hb C, Hb SC) are covered in Table 16.2.
†Such as new methylene blue.
‡Stain dark blue and are called *siderotic* granules when observed in Prussian blue stain.
DNA, Deoxyribonucleic acid; *Hb*, hemoglobin; *RBC*, red blood cell; *RNA*, ribonucleic acid.

The remainder of this chapter discusses the importance of individual RBC measurements, the MCV, reticulocyte count, and RDW and how they assist in classifying anemias to arrive at a specific diagnosis. Two widely used classification schemes for anemias relate to the morphology of RBCs and the pathophysiologic condition responsible for the patient's anemia.

Morphologic Classification of Anemia Based on Mean Cell Volume

The MCV is an extremely important tool and is key in the *morphologic classification* of anemia. *Microcytic anemias* are characterized by an MCV of less than 80 fL with small RBCs (less than 6 μm in diameter). Microcytosis is often associated with hypochromia (increased central pallor in RBCs) and an MCHC less than 32 g/dL. Microcytic anemias are caused by conditions that result in reduced hemoglobin synthesis. Heme synthesis is diminished in iron deficiency, iron sequestration (chronic inflammatory states), and defective protoporphyrin synthesis (sideroblastic anemia, lead poisoning). Globin chain

synthesis is insufficient or defective in thalassemia and in Hb E disease.

Iron deficiency is the most common cause of microcytic anemia; the low iron level is insufficient for maintaining normal erythropoiesis. Although iron deficiency anemia is characterized by abnormal iron studies, the early stages of iron deficiency do not result in microcytosis or anemia and are manifested only by reduced iron stores. The causes of iron deficiency vary in infants, children, adolescents, and adults, and it is imperative to find the cause before beginning treatment (Chapter 17).

Macrocytic anemias are characterized by an MCV greater than 100 fL with large RBCs (greater than 8 μm in diameter). Macrocytic anemias arise from conditions that result in megaloblastic or nonmegaloblastic RBC development in the bone marrow. Megaloblastic anemias are caused by conditions that impair synthesis of DNA, such as vitamin B_{12} and folate deficiency or myelodysplasia. Nuclear maturation lags behind cytoplasmic development as a result of the impaired DNA synthesis. This asynchrony between nuclear and cytoplasmic development

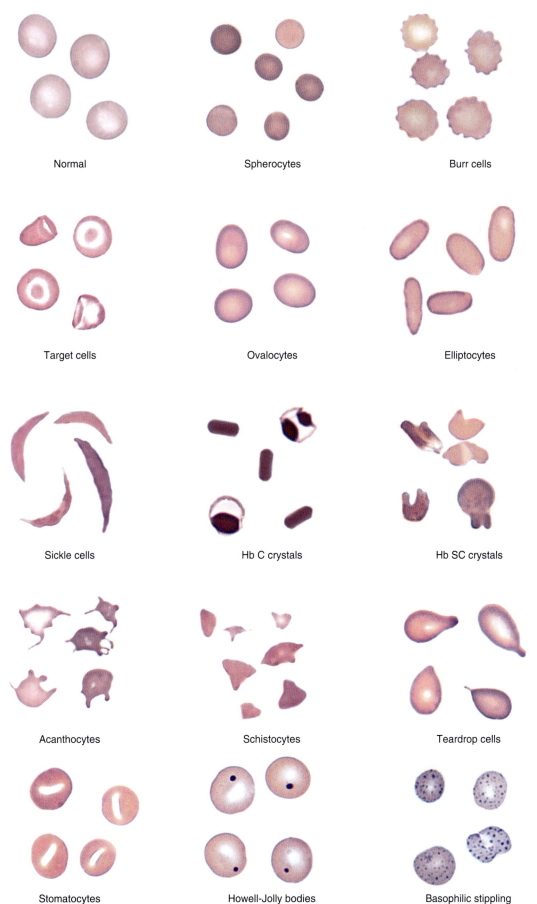

Figure 16.1 Red Blood Cells: Varied Shapes and Inclusions. Hb, Hemoglobin. (Modified from Carr, J. H. [2022]. Clinical Hematology Atlas. [6th ed.]. St. Louis: Elsevier.)

results in larger cells. All cells of the body are ultimately affected by the defective production of DNA (Chapter 18). Pernicious anemia is one cause of vitamin B_{12} deficiency, whereas pregnancy with increased requirements is a leading cause of folate deficiency. Megaloblastic anemia is characterized by oval macrocytes and hypersegmented neutrophils in the peripheral blood and by megaloblasts or large nucleated erythroid precursors in the bone marrow. The MCV in megaloblastic anemia can be markedly increased (up to 150 fL), but modest increases (100 to 115 fL) are most common.

Nonmegaloblastic forms of macrocytic anemias are also characterized by large RBCs, but in contrast to megaloblastic anemias, they are typically related to membrane changes caused by disruption of the cholesterol-to-phospholipid ratio. These macrocytic cells are mostly round, and the erythroid precursors in the bone marrow do not display megaloblastic changes. Macrocytic anemias are often seen in patients with chronic liver disease, alcohol abuse, and bone marrow failure. It is rare for the MCV to be greater than 115 fL in nonmegaloblastic anemias.

Normocytic anemias are characterized by an MCV in the range of 80 to 100 fL. The RBC morphology on the peripheral blood film must be examined to rule out a dimorphic population of microcytes and macrocytes that can yield a normal MCV. The presence of a dimorphic population can also be verified by observing a bimodal distribution on the RBC histogram produced by an automated blood cell analyzer (Chapters 13 and 14). Some normocytic anemias develop as a result of the premature destruction and shortened survival of RBCs (hemolytic anemias), and they are characterized by an elevated reticulocyte count. The hemolytic anemias can be further divided into those that result from intrinsic causes (membrane defects, hemoglobinopathies, and enzyme deficiencies) and those that result from extrinsic causes (immune and nonimmune RBC injury). A DAT helps differentiate immune-mediated RBC destruction from other causes of hemolysis. In hemolytic anemias, reviewing the peripheral blood film provides vital information for determining the cause of the hemolysis (Tables 16.2 and 16.3 and Figure 16.1). Hemolytic anemias are discussed in Chapters 20 to 24.

Other normocytic anemias develop as a result of a decreased production of RBCs and are characterized by a decreased reticulocyte count (Chapter 19). A normal MCV is also seen in dilutional anemia of pregnancy (Chapter 43). Figure 16.2 presents an algorithm for initial morphologic classification of anemia based on the MCV.

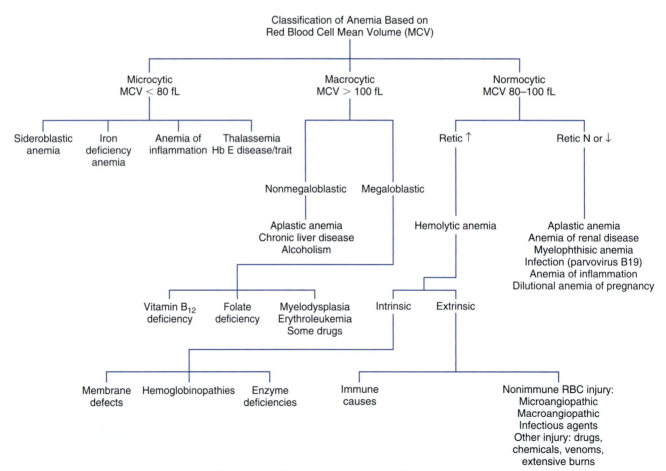

Figure 16.2 **Algorithm for Morphologic Classification of Anemia Based on Mean Cell Volume.** Anemia of chronic liver disease is multifactorial and can be macrocytic or normocytic; anemia of inflammation can be normocytic or microcytic; aplastic anemia can be macrocytic or normocytic. ↑, Increased; ↓, decreased; *Hb*, hemoglobin; *MCV*, mean cell volume; *N*, normal; *RBC*, red blood cell; *retic*, absolute reticulocyte count.

Morphologic Classification of Anemias and the Reticulocyte Count

The absolute reticulocyte count is useful in initially classifying anemias into the categories of decreased or ineffective RBC production (decreased reticulocyte count) and excessive RBC loss (increased reticulocyte count). Using the *morphologic classification* in the first category, when the reticulocyte count is decreased, the MCV can further classify the anemia into three subgroups: normocytic anemias, microcytic anemias, and macrocytic anemias. The excessive RBC loss category includes acute hemorrhage and the hemolytic anemias with shortened RBC survival. Figure 16.3 is an algorithm that illustrates how anemias can be classified based on the absolute reticulocyte count and MCV.[4,7]

Morphologic Classification and Red Blood Cell Distribution Width

The RDW can help determine the cause of an anemia when used in conjunction with the MCV. Each of the three MCV categories mentioned previously (normocytic, microcytic, macrocytic) can also be subclassified by the RDW as homogeneous (normal RDW) or heterogeneous (increased or high RDW).[7,17] For example, a decreased MCV with an increased RDW is suggestive of iron deficiency (Table 16.4). This classification is not absolute, however, because there can be an overlap of RDW values among some of the conditions in each MCV category.

Pathophysiologic Classification of Anemias and Reticulocyte Count

In a *pathophysiologic classification* of anemia, related conditions are grouped by the mechanism causing the anemia. In this classification scheme, the anemias caused by decreased RBC production have inappropriately low reticulocyte counts (e.g., disorders of DNA synthesis and aplastic anemia) and are distinguished from other anemias caused by increased RBC destruction (intrinsic and extrinsic abnormalities of RBCs) or acute blood loss, which have increased reticulocyte counts. Some anemias have more than one pathophysiologic mechanism. Box 16.2 presents a pathophysiologic classification of anemia based on the causes of the abnormality and gives one or more examples of an anemia in each classification.

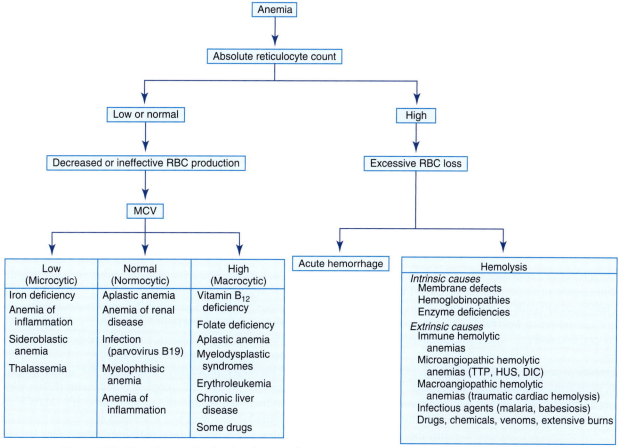

Figure 16.3 Algorithm for Evaluating Causes of Anemia Based on Absolute Reticulocyte Count and Mean Cell Volume. The list of anemias contains examples; there are numerous other causes not listed. Anemia of chronic liver disease is multifactorial and can be normocytic. *DIC,* Disseminated intravascular coagulation; *HUS,* hemolytic uremic syndrome; *MCV,* mean cell volume; *RBC,* red blood cell; *TTP,* thrombotic thrombocytopenic purpura.

TABLE 16.4 Morphologic Classification of Anemia Based on Red Blood Cell Mean Volume and Red Blood Cell Distribution Width*

	MEAN CELL VOLUME		
	Decreased	**Normal**	**Increased**
RDW Normal	α- or β-Thalassemia trait Anemia of inflammation Hb E disease/trait	Anemia of inflammation Anemia of renal disease Acute hemorrhage Hereditary spherocytosis Dilutional anemia of pregnancy	Aplastic anemia Chronic liver disease Alcoholism Chemotherapy
RDW Increased	Iron deficiency Sickle cell-β-thalassemia	Early iron, folate, or vitamin B_{12} deficiency Mixed deficiency of iron + vitamin B_{12} or folate Sickle cell anemia Hb SC disease Myelodysplastic syndromes	Folate or vitamin B_{12} deficiency Myelodysplastic syndromes Cold agglutinin disease Chronic liver disease Chemotherapy

*This classification scheme is not absolute because there can be overlap of RDW values among some of the conditions in each mean cell volume category.
Hb, Hemoglobin; *RDW,* red blood cell distribution width.
Modified from Bessman, J. D., Gilmer, P. R., & Gardner, F. H. (1983). Improved classification of anemias by MCV and RDW. *Am J Clin Pathol, 80,* 324; and Lin, J. C. (2018). Approach to anemia in the adult and child. In: Hoffman, R., Benz, E. J., Silberstein, L. E., et al. (Eds.), *Hematology: Basic Principles and Practice.* (7th ed., p. 463). Philadelphia: Elsevier.

BOX 16.2 Pathophysiologic Classification of Anemias*

Anemia Caused by Decreased Production of RBCs
Bone marrow failure: acquired and congenital aplastic anemia, pure red cell aplasia, anemia associated with marrow infiltration (myelophthisic)

Impairment of erythroid development:
- Disorders of DNA synthesis: megaloblastic anemia
- Disorders of hemoglobin synthesis: iron deficiency anemia, thalassemia, sideroblastic anemia, anemia of inflammation
- Decreased production of erythropoietin: anemia of renal disease

Anemia Caused by Increased RBC Destruction or Loss
Intrinsic RBC abnormality:
- Membrane defects: hereditary spherocytosis, hereditary elliptocytosis or pyropoikilocytosis, paroxysmal nocturnal hemoglobinuria

- Enzyme deficiencies: glucose-6-phosphate dehydrogenase deficiency, pyruvate kinase deficiency
- Globin abnormalities: sickle cell anemia, other hemoglobinopathies

Extrinsic RBC abnormality:
- Immune causes: warm-type autoimmune hemolytic anemia, cold agglutinin disease, paroxysmal cold hemoglobinuria, hemolytic transfusion reaction, hemolytic disease of the fetus and newborn
- Nonimmune RBC injuries: microangiopathic hemolytic anemia (thrombotic thrombocytopenic purpura, hemolytic uremic syndrome, HELLP syndrome, disseminated intravascular coagulation), macroangiopathic hemolytic anemia (traumatic cardiac hemolysis), infectious agents (malaria, babesiosis, bartonellosis, clostridial sepsis), other injury (chemicals, drugs, venoms, extensive burns)

Blood loss: acute blood loss anemia

* The list of anemias is not all inclusive; numerous other conditions are not listed.
Modified from Prchal, J. T. (2021). Clinical manifestations and classification of erythrocyte disorders. In: Kaushansky, K., Prchal, J. T., Burns, L.J., et al. (Eds.), *Williams Hematology.* (10th ed., pp. 553–562). New York: McGraw-Hill.
DNA, Deoxyribonucleic acid; *HELLP,* hemolysis, elevated liver enzymes, and low platelets syndrome; *RBC,* red blood cell.

SUMMARY

- *Anemia* is defined operationally as a reduction in the hemoglobin content of blood that can be caused by a decrease in the red blood cell (RBC) count, hemoglobin, and hematocrit below the reference interval for healthy individuals of the same age, sex, and race under similar environmental conditions.
- Diagnosis of anemia is based on history, physical examination, symptoms, and laboratory test results.
- Many anemias have common manifestations. Careful questioning of the patient may reveal contributing factors such as diet, medications, occupational hazards, and bleeding history.
- A thorough physical examination is valuable in determining the cause of anemia. Some of the areas that should be evaluated are skin, nail beds, eyes, mucosa, lymph nodes, heart, spleen, and liver.

- Moderate anemias (hemoglobin between 7 and 10 g/dL) may cause pallor of conjunctivae and nail beds but not manifest other clinical symptoms if the onset is slow. Severe anemias (hemoglobin of less than 7 g/dL) usually produce pallor, dyspnea, vertigo, headache, muscle weakness, lethargy, hypotension, and tachycardia.
- Laboratory procedures helpful in the initial diagnosis of anemia include the complete blood count (CBC) with RBC indices, red blood cell distribution width (RDW), and the reticulocyte count, and examination of the peripheral blood film. Examination of a peripheral blood film is especially important in the diagnosis of hemolytic anemias.
- Bone marrow examination is usually not required for diagnosis of anemia but is indicated in cases of unexplained anemia, fever of unknown origin, or suspected hematologic

neoplasm. Other tests are indicated based on the RBC indices, history, and physical examination, such as serum iron, total iron-binding capacity, and serum ferritin (for microcytic anemias) and serum folate and vitamin B_{12} (for macrocytic anemias).

- The reticulocyte count and mean cell volume (MCV) play crucial roles in investigation of the cause of an anemia.
- Morphologic classification of anemias is based on the MCV and includes normocytic, microcytic, and macrocytic anemias. The MCV, when combined with the reticulocyte count and the RDW, also can aid in classification of anemia.

- Major subgroups of the pathophysiologic classification include anemias caused by decreased RBC production and anemias caused by increased RBC destruction or acute blood loss. Anemias may have more than one pathophysiologic cause.
- The cause of anemia should be determined before treatment is initiated.

Now that you have completed this chapter, go back and read again the case study at the beginning and respond to the questions presented. Answers can be found in Appendix C.

REVIEW QUESTIONS

Answers can be found in Appendix C.

1. Which of the following patients would be considered anemic with a hemoglobin value of 14.5 g/dL? (Refer to reference intervals after the Index at the end of the book.)
   a. An adult man
   b. An adult woman
   c. A newborn boy
   d. A 10-year-old girl

2. Patients with anemia most commonly present with which one of the following set of symptoms?
   a. Abdominal pain and pressure (from splenomegaly)
   b. Shortness of breath and fatigue
   c. Chills and fever
   d. Jaundice and enlarged lymph nodes

3. Which of the following are important to consider in the patient's history when investigating the cause of an anemia?
   a. Diet and medications
   b. Occupation, hobbies, and travel
   c. Bleeding episodes in the patient
   d. All of the above

4. Which one of the following is reduced as an adaptation to long-standing anemia?
   a. Heart rate
   b. Respiratory rate
   c. Oxygen affinity of hemoglobin
   d. Volume of blood ejected from the heart with each contraction

5. An autoimmune reaction destroys the hematopoietic stem cells in the bone marrow of a young adult patient, and the amount of active bone marrow, including erythroid precursors, is diminished. Erythroid precursors that are present are normal in appearance, but there are too few to meet the demand for circulating RBCs, and anemia develops. The reticulocyte count is low. The mechanism of the anemia would be described as:
   a. Effective erythropoiesis
   b. Ineffective erythropoiesis
   c. Insufficient erythropoiesis

6. What are the INITIAL laboratory tests that are performed for the diagnosis of anemia?
   a. CBC, iron studies, and reticulocyte count
   b. CBC, reticulocyte count, and peripheral blood film examination
   c. Reticulocyte count and serum iron, vitamin B_{12}, and folate assays
   d. Bone marrow study and peripheral blood film examination

7. An increase in which of the following suggests a shortened RBC life span and hemolytic anemia?
   a. Hemoglobin
   b. Hematocrit
   c. Reticulocyte count
   d. RBC distribution width

8. Schistocytes, ovalocytes, and acanthocytes are examples of abnormal changes in RBC:
   a. Volume
   b. Shape
   c. Inclusions
   d. Hemoglobin

9. Referring to Figure 16.3, which of the following conditions would be included in the differential diagnosis of an anemic adult patient with an absolute reticulocyte count of 20 $\times 10^9$/L and an MCV of 65 fL?
   a. Aplastic anemia
   b. Sickle cell anemia
   c. Iron deficiency
   d. Folate deficiency

10. Referring to Table 16.4, which of the following conditions would be included in the differential diagnosis of an anemic adult patient with an MCV of 125 fL and an RDW of 20% (reference interval 11.5% to 14.5%)?
   a. Aplastic anemia
   b. Sickle cell anemia
   c. Iron deficiency
   d. Vitamin B_{12} deficiency

REFERENCES

1. Schecther, A. N. (2008). Hemoglobin research and the origins of molecular medicine. *Blood, 112,* 3927–3938.

2. *The American Heritage dictionary of the English language.* (4th ed.). (2001). Boston: Houghton Mifflin.

3. Kassebaum, N. J. (2016). The global burden of anemia. *Hematol Oncol Clin N Am, 30,* 247–308.

4. Means, R. T., Jr., & Glader, B. (2018). Anemia: general considerations. In: Greer, J. P., Arber, D. A., Glader, B., et al. (Eds.), *Wintrobe's Clinical Hematology.* (14th ed., pp. 588–614). Philadelphia: Wolters Kluwer.

5. Tefferi, A. (2003). Anemia in adults: a contemporary approach to diagnosis. *Mayo Clin Proc, 78,* 1274–1280.

6. Beutler, E., & Waalen, J. (2006). The definition of anemia: what is the lower limit of normal of the blood hemoglobin concentration? *Blood, 107,* 1747–1750.

7. Lin, J. C. (2023). Approach to anemia in the adult and child. In: Hoffman, R., Benz, E. J., Silberstein, L. E., et al. (Eds.), *Hematology: Basic Principles and Practice.* (8th ed., pp. 463-472). Philadelphia: Elsevier.

8. Bunn, H. F. (2016). Approach to anemias. In: Goldman, L., & Schafer, A. I. (Eds.), *Goldman-Cecil Medicine.* (25th ed., pp. 1059–1068). Philadelphia: Elsevier, Saunders.

9. Irwin, J. J., & Kirchner, J. T. (2001). Anemia in children. *Am Fam Physician, 64,* 1379–1386.

10. Kettaneh, A., Eclache, V., Fain, O., et al. (2005). Pica and food craving in patients with iron-deficiency anemia: a case-control study in France. *Am J Med, 118,* 185–188.

11. Adamson, J. W., & Longo, D. L. (2018). Anemia and polycythemia. In: Loscalzo, J., Fauci, A. S., Kasper, D.L., et al. (Eds.), *Harrison's Principles of Internal Medicine.* (21st ed., pp. 431-438). New York: McGraw-Hill.

12. Prchal, J. T. (2021). Clinical manifestations and classification of erythrocyte disorders. In: Kaushansky, K., Prchal, J. T., Burns, L.J., et al. (Eds.), *Williams Hematology.* (10th ed., pp. 553–562). New York: McGraw-Hill.

13. Rodger, M., Sheppard, D., Gándara, E., et al. (2015). Hematological problems in obstetrics. *Best Practice And Res in Clin Ob and Gyn, 29,* 671-684.

14. Smock, K. J. (2019). Examination of the blood and bone marrow. In: Greer, J. P., Arber, D. A., Glader, B., et al. (Eds.), *Wintrobe's Clinical Hematology.* (14th ed., pp. 1–16). Philadelphia: Wolters Kluwer.

15. Halfdanarson, T. R., Kumarm, N., Li, C. Y., et al. (2008). Hematological manifestations of copper deficiency: a retrospective review. *Eur J Haematol, 80,* 523–531.

16. Brill, J. R., & Baumgardner, D. J. (2000). Normocytic anemia. *Am Fam Physician, 62,* 2255–2263.

17. Bessman, J. D., Gilmer, P. R., & Gardner, F. H. (1983). Improved classification of anemia by MCV and RDW. *Am J Clin Pathol, 80,* 322–326.

17

Disorders of Iron Kinetics and Heme Metabolism

Tara Cothran Moon and Kathryn Doig

OBJECTIVES

After completion of this chapter, the reader will be able to:

1. Recognize complete blood count (CBC) results consistent with iron deficiency anemia (IDA), anemia of inflammation (AI), and sideroblastic anemias (SAs).
2. Given the results of classical iron studies as well as free erythrocyte protoporphyrin (FEP), soluble transferrin receptor (sTfR), hemoglobin content of reticulocytes, sTfR/log ferritin , and Thomas plots, distinguish findings consistent with IDA, latent iron deficiency, AI, SAs, and iron overload conditions.
3. Recognize individuals at risk for IDA by virtue of age, sex, diet, physiologic circumstances such as pregnancy and menstruation, or pathologic conditions such as chronic gastrointestinal bleeding.
4. Given a description of a Wright-stained bone marrow preparation and the appearance of bone marrow stained with Prussian blue stain, recognize results consistent with IDA, AI, or SAs.
5. Recognize clinical conditions that can predispose a patient to develop AI.
6. Define porphyria and SAs.
7. Describe in general terms the type of mutations that result in hereditary SAs and the expected peripheral blood picture and pathognomonic bone marrow finding.
8. Recognize factors contributing to development of acquired SAs and acquired porphyrias.
9. Discuss the clinical significance of increased levels of FEP.
10. Describe the pathogenesis of IDA, AI, SA secondary to lead poisoning, and hemochromatosis, generically.
11. Discuss the differences in disease etiology, laboratory diagnosis, and treatment between iron overload resulting from hereditary forms of hemochromatosis and transfusion-related hemosiderosis.
12. Describe the etiology of the erythropoietic porphyrias, expected CBC picture, diagnostic metabolites, and clinical presentation.

OUTLINE

General Concepts in Iron-Related Disorders
Iron-Restricted Anemias
  Iron Deficiency Anemia
  Anemia of Inflammation
Porphyrias
Sideroblastic Anemias
  Hereditary Sideroblastic Anemias
  Acquired Sideroblastic Anemias

Iron Overload
  Etiology
  Phenotype and Epidemiology
  Laboratory Diagnosis
  Treatment
Differential Diagnosis

CASE STUDY

After studying the material in this chapter, the reader should be able to respond to the following case study. Answers can be found in Appendix C.

An 85-year-old, slender, frail woman was hospitalized for diagnosis and treatment of anemia that was suspected during a routine examination by her health care provider. The provider noted that she appeared pale and inquired about fatigue and tiredness. Although the patient generally felt well, she admitted to feeling slightly tired when climbing stairs. A point-of-care HGB performed in the provider's office showed a dangerously low value of 3.5 g/dL, so the patient was hospitalized for further evaluation. Her hospital CBC results were as follows. Reference intervals can be found after the Index at the end of the book.

WBC	8.5×10^9/L	MCV	Calculate: _____ fL	
RBC	1.66×10^{12}/L	MCH	Calculate: _____ pg	
HGB	3.0 g/dL	MCHC	Calculate: _____ g/dL	
HCT	11%	RDW	20%	
		PLT	165×10^9/L	

WBC differential   Unremarkable
RBC morphology   Marked anisocytosis, marked poikilocytosis, marked hypochromia, marked microcytosis

Continued

GENERAL CONCEPTS IN IRON-RELATED DISORDERS

Anemia may result whenever red blood cell (RBC) production is impaired, RBC life span is shortened, or there is frank loss of RBCs from the body. The anemias associated with iron and heme typically are categorized as anemias of impaired production resulting from the lack of raw materials for hemoglobin assembly. When iron is the limiting factor, the anemias are called *iron restricted*. Two important iron-restricted anemias discussed here are iron deficiency anemia (IDA) and anemia of inflammation (AI). Inadequate production of protoporphyrin also leads to diminished production of heme and thus hemoglobin. Blockages of protoporphyrin production at various stages in the heme synthetic pathway lead to accumulations of various porphyrins. The resulting porphyrias that are accompanied by anemia are briefly discussed in this chapter. Failure to incorporate iron into protoporphyrin, chiefly due to impaired mitochondrial iron kinetics, results in anemias with excess iron accumulation in developing RBCs. These sideroblastic anemias (SAs) are rare but are discussed briefly for completeness. Iron kinetics can be perturbed, resulting in excess accumulations of iron, usually without anemia. These conditions, called *hemochromatoses*, are included here as well. There is another group of anemias with impaired iron kinetics called *iron-loading anemias*. Often, these anemias involve chronic erythroid hyperplasia, as is seen in hemoglobinopathies and thalassemias. These are diseases caused by heritable mutations affecting globin chain structure or their production. These conditions are discussed separately in Chapters 24 and 25.

An understanding of normal iron metabolism and the tests of body iron status are critical to the understanding and diagnosis of the conditions discussed in this chapter, so the reader is referred to Chapter 9, where iron kinetics and diagnostic tests are described in detail.

IRON-RESTRICTED ANEMIAS

Iron Deficiency Anemia

Etiology

Iron deficiency is a state in which there is deficient total body iron to uphold normal physiologic functions, sometimes defined by serum ferritin <15 mg/L in people >5 years old.[1] Iron deficiency develops when the intake of iron is inadequate to meet a standard level of demand, when the need for iron expands without compensated intake, when there is impaired absorption, or when there is chronic loss of hemoglobin from the body.

Inadequate intake. IDA can develop when the erythron is slowly starved for iron. Each day, approximately 1 mg of iron is lost from the body, mainly in the mitochondria of desquamated skin and sloughed intestinal epithelium.[2] Because the body tenaciously conserves all other iron from senescent cells, including RBCs, daily replacement of 1 mg of iron from the diet maintains iron balance and supplies the body's need for RBC production as long as there is no other source of loss. When the iron in the diet is consistently inadequate, over time, the body's stores of iron become depleted. Ultimately, RBC production slows to manage the iron needs for other body cells.[3,4] With approximately 1% of cells dying naturally each day, the anemia becomes apparent when the production rate is insufficient to replace lost cells.

Increased need relative to iron supply. IDA can also develop when the level of iron intake is inadequate to meet the needs of an expanding erythron. This is the case in periods of rapid growth, such as infancy (especially in prematurity), childhood, and adolescence. For example, although both infants and adult men need about 1 mg/day of iron, that corresponds to a much higher amount per kilogram of body weight for the infant. Pregnancy and nursing place similar demands on the mother's body to provide iron for the developing fetus or nursing infant in addition to her own iron needs. In each of these instances, what had previously been an adequate intake of iron for the individual becomes inadequate as the need for iron increases.

Treatment with erythropoietin is another instance when there is rapid expansion of the erythron. The demand for iron is often so great that even individuals with adequate stores of iron will experience iron-restricted erythropoiesis because it cannot be mobilized fast enough. This is called *functional iron deficiency* because iron stores are adequate, but the iron is not available to support normal erythropoiesis.

Impaired absorption. Even when the diet is adequate in iron, the inability to absorb that iron through the enterocyte into the blood will, over time, result in a deficiency of iron in the body. The impairments may be pathologic, as with malabsorption caused by celiac disease. Others may be inherited mutations to genes for iron regulatory proteins, resulting in iron-refractory iron deficiency anemia (IRIDA). One example is mutations to the gene for the matriptase-2 protein (Chapter 9) that lead to a persistent production of hepcidin, causing ferroportin in the enterocyte to be inactivated, thus preventing iron absorption in the intestine.[5] In addition, diseases that decrease stomach acidity impair iron absorption by decreasing the conversion of dietary Fe^{+3} to the absorbable Fe^{+2} form. Some loss of acidity accompanies normal aging, but gastrectomy or bariatric surgeries can impair iron absorption dramatically. Medications such as stomach acid reducers can inhibit iron absorption by decreasing gastric acidity, whereas other drugs may even bind the iron in the intestine, preventing its absorption.

Chronic blood loss. A fourth way that iron deficiency develops is with repeated blood donations, chronic hemorrhage, or hemolysis that results in the loss of small amounts of heme iron from the body over a prolonged period. Anemia develops when the iron loss exceeds iron intake over time and the storage iron is exhausted. Excessive heme iron can be lost through repeated blood donations. Chronic gastrointestinal bleeding from ulcers, tumors, parasitosis, diverticulitis, ulcerative colitis, hemorrhoids, or gastritis caused by alcohol or aspirin ingestion can also result in heme iron loss. Bleeding from mucous membranes, such as nosebleeds, can lead to heme iron loss, especially for people with arteriovenous malformations. In women, prolonged menorrhagia (heavy menstrual bleeding) or conditions such as uterine fibroid tumors or uterine malignancies can lead to heme iron loss. Heme iron can also be lost excessively through the urinary tract with kidney stones, tumors, or chronic infections. Individuals with chronic intravascular hemolytic processes, such as paroxysmal nocturnal hemoglobinuria, can develop iron deficiency as a result of the loss of iron in hemoglobin passed into the urine.

Pathogenesis

IDA develops slowly, progressing through stages that physiologically blend into one another but are useful delineations for understanding disease progression.[6] As shown in Figure 17.1, iron is distributed among three compartments: the storage compartment, principally as ferritin in the bone marrow macrophages and hepatocytes; the transport compartment of serum transferrin; and the functional compartment of hemoglobin, myoglobin, and cytochromes. Hemoglobin iron and intracellular ferritin and hemosiderin constitute nearly 90% of the total distribution of iron (Table 9.1).

For a time, as an increase in demand or increased loss of iron exceeds iron intake, essentially normal iron status continues. The body strives to maintain iron balance by accelerating absorption of iron from the intestine through a decrease in the production of hepcidin in the liver. This state of declining body iron with increased absorption is not apparent in routine laboratory test results or patient symptoms. The individual appears healthy. As the negative iron balance continues, however, a stage of iron depletion develops.

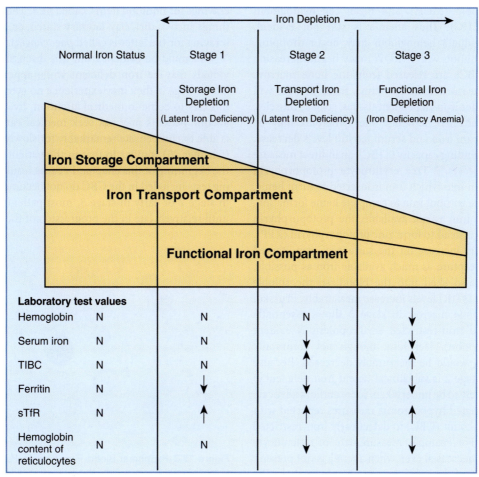

Figure 17.1 Development of Iron Deficiency Anemia. ↑, Increased; ↓, decreased; *N*, normal; *sTfR*, soluble transferrin receptor; *TIBC,* total iron-binding capacity. (From Suominen, P., Punnonen, K., Rajamaki, A., et al. [1998]. Serum transferrin receptor and transferrin receptor-ferritin index identify healthy subjects with subclinical iron deficits. *Blood, 92,* p. 2935, Figure 1.)

Stage 1. Stage 1 of iron deficiency is characterized by a progressive loss of storage iron. RBC production and development are normal throughout this phase. However, without new iron added to storage, continuing RBC production draws down the reserve. Serum ferritin levels drop over time, which indicates the decline in stored iron, and this also could be detected in an iron stain of the bone marrow. Without evidence of anemia or changes in RBC morphology, though, these tests would not be performed because individuals appear healthy (latent iron deficiency). Yet stage 1 iron deficiency is common. The prevalence of stage 1 iron deficiency in the United States has been estimated in toddlers (12 to 23 months) as 15.1%, in nonpregnant women (15 to 49 years) as 10.4%, and in pregnant women (12 to 49 years) as 16.3%.[7]

Stage 2. Stage 2 of iron deficiency is defined by the exhaustion of the storage pool of iron (Figure 17.1). For a time, RBC production continues as normal, relying on the iron available in the transport compartment and the iron being recycled from dying cells. Quickly, the hemoglobin content of reticulocytes begins to decrease, which reflects the onset of iron-restricted erythropoiesis, but because the bulk of the circulating RBCs were produced during the period of adequate iron availability, the overall hemoglobin concentration is still within the reference interval, as are the mean cell volume (MCV), mean cell hemoglobin (MCH), and mean cell hemoglobin concentration (MCHC). Thus anemia is still not evident. Although an individual's hemoglobin may begin dropping, and the RBC distribution width (RDW) may begin increasing as some smaller RBCs are released from the bone marrow, without multiple measurements over time, these changes will not be detected. Other iron-dependent tissues, such as muscles, may begin to be affected, although the symptoms may be nonspecific. The serum iron and serum ferritin levels decrease, whereas total iron-binding capacity (TIBC), an indirect measure of transferrin, increases.[8,9] Free erythrocyte protoporphyrin (FEP), the porphyrin into which iron is inserted to form heme, begins to accumulate without iron to complete heme formation. Additionally, when iron is not available, the protoporphyrin combines with zinc instead to form zinc protoporphyrin (ZPP). Transferrin receptors increase on the surface of iron-starved cells as they try to capture as much available iron as possible. The receptors are also shed into the blood, so the soluble transferrin receptor (sTfR) levels increase measurably. Prussian blue stain of the bone marrow in stage 2 shows essentially no stored iron, and iron-restricted erythropoiesis is evident (subsequent description). Hepcidin, though not commonly measured clinically, would be measurably decreased. Because iron deficiency in stage 2 is subclinical (latent iron deficiency) and testing is not likely to be undertaken, some authors advocate for the use of automated hypochromia measures reported with the complete blood count (CBC) to detect early iron-restricted erythropoiesis.[10,11] For example, measurement of reticulocyte hemoglobin can be decreased even when anemia is not present.

Stage 3. Stage 3 of iron deficiency is frank anemia. The hemoglobin concentration and hematocrit are low relative to the reference intervals. Depletion of storage iron and diminished levels of transport iron (Figure 17.1) prevent normal development of RBC precursors. Abnormal heme synthesis results in deficient hemoglobin synthesis and a delay in the signal for cell division to conclude. This causes one or more additional cell divisions during cell development and therefore a decreased size of the RBCs (microcytes).[12]

The RBCs are microcytic and hypochromic (Figure 17.2), as their ability to produce hemoglobin is restricted. As expected, serum ferritin levels are exceedingly low. Results of other iron studies (discussed later) are also abnormal, and the FEP and sTfR levels continue to increase. The hemoglobin content of reticulocytes will continue to drop, and automated hypochromia parameters will be increased. If measured, erythropoietin would be elevated but not as high as might be expected for the degree of anemia.[3,13] Hepcidin would be decreased.

In this phase the patient experiences the nonspecific symptoms of anemia, typically fatigue, weakness, and shortness of breath, especially with exertion. Pallor is evident in light-skinned individuals but also can be noted in the conjunctivae, mucous membranes, or palmar creases of dark-skinned individuals. More severe signs are not seen as often in the United States[14] but include a sore tongue (*glossitis*) due to iron deficiency in the rapidly proliferating epithelial cells of the alimentary tract and inflamed cracks at the corners of the mouth (*angular cheilosis*). *Koilonychia* (spooning of the fingernails) may be seen if the deficiency is long-standing. Patients also may experience cravings for nonfood items, called *pica*. The cravings may be for things such as dirt, clay, laundry starch, or, most commonly, ice (craving for the latter is called *pagophagia*).[14]

As should be evident from this discussion, numerous individuals may be iron deficient while appearing healthy. Until late in stage 2, they may experience no symptoms at all and are unlikely to come to medical attention. Even in stage 3, frankly anemic patients may not seek medical care because the body is able to compensate remarkably for slowly developing anemia (Chapter 16), similar to that in the patient in the case study at the beginning of this chapter. Because results of routine screening tests included in the CBC do not become abnormal until late in stage 2 or early in stage 3, most patients are not diagnosed until relatively late in the progression of the iron depletion.

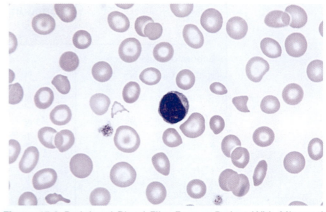

Figure 17.2 Peripheral Blood Film From a Patient With Microcytic Hypochromic Anemia. Note the variation in red blood cell (RBC) diameters compared with the lymphocyte's nuclear diameter. Variation in RBC diameters is termed *anisocytosis* and corresponds to an elevated RBC distribution width (RDW), a measure of variation in RBC volume. Hypochromia, microcytosis, and an elevated RDW may indicate iron deficiency anemia. Several target cells are seen. (Wright-Giemsa stain, ×1000.)

Epidemiology and Risk Factors

From the previous discussion, it is apparent that certain groups of individuals are more at risk to develop IDA. Menstruating women are at especially high risk. Their monthly loss of blood increases their routine need for iron, which often is not met with the standard US diet.[14] For adolescent girls, this is compounded by increased iron needs associated with growth. If women of childbearing age do not receive proper iron supplementation, pregnancy and nursing can lead to a loss of nearly 1200 mg of iron,[15] which further depletes iron stores. Succeeding pregnancies can exacerbate the problem, leading to iron-deficient fetuses.

Growing children also are at high risk. Growth requires iron for the cytochromes of all new cells, myoglobin for new muscle cells, and hemoglobin in the additional RBCs needed to supply oxygen for a larger body. The increasing need for iron as the child grows can be coupled with dietary inadequacies, especially in circumstances of poverty or neglect. Cow's milk is not a good source of iron, and infants need to be placed on iron-supplemented formula by about age 6 months, when their fetal stores of iron become depleted.[14] This assumes that the infants were able to establish adequate iron stores by drawing iron from their mothers in utero. Even though breast milk is a better source of iron than cow's milk,[16] it is not a consistent source.[17] Therefore iron supplementation is also recommended for breastfed infants after 6 months of age.[14]

Iron deficiency is relatively rare in men and postmenopausal women because the body conserves iron so tenaciously, and these individuals lose only about 1 mg/day. Gastrointestinal disease, such as ulcers, tumors, or hemorrhoids, should be suspected in iron-deficient patients in either of these groups if the diet is known to be adequate in iron. Regular aspirin ingestion and alcohol consumption can lead to gastritis and chronic bleeding. Elderly adults, particularly those living alone, may not eat a balanced diet, so pure dietary deficiency is seen among these individuals. In some elderly individuals, the loss of gastric acidity with age can impair iron absorption. Iron deficiency is associated with infection by hookworms, *Necator americanus* and *Ancylostoma duodenale*. The worm attaches to the intestinal wall and literally sucks blood from the gastric vessels. Iron deficiency is also associated with infection with other parasites, such as *Trichuris trichiura, Schistosoma mansoni,* and *Schistosoma haematobium,* in which the heme iron is lost from the body as a result of intestinal or urinary bleeding.

Soldiers subjected to prolonged maneuvers and long-distance runners also can develop iron deficiency. Iron deficiency may be seen in some athletes due to gastrointestinal bleeding, reduced iron intake, or hemoglobinuria.[18,19] Exercise-induced hemoglobinuria, also called *march hemoglobinuria,* develops when RBCs are hemolyzed by foot-pounding trauma and iron is lost as hemoglobin in the urine.[20,21] The amount lost in the urine can be so little that it is not apparent on visual inspection of the urine. Nevertheless, in rare cases, the cumulative iron loss can lead to anemia if the foot-pounding trauma is recurrent and especially severe. However, there is some evidence that well-trained professional athletes may be less subject to this effect.[22]

Laboratory Diagnosis

The early stages of iron deficiency can be detected with tests such as ferritin, but these tests are not likely to be ordered because there is virtually no physiologic evidence suggesting a declining iron state. Furthermore, these tests are not always part of comprehensive screening panels and as a result, the progressing iron deficiency can go undetected. Nevertheless, early iron deficiency might be suspected in an individual in a high-risk group and appropriate testing can be ordered. It is not until late in the progression that standard CBC parameters such as the hemoglobin and MCV fall to less than reference intervals and thus may prompt additional diagnostic testing. The tests for iron deficiency can be grouped into three general categories: screening, diagnostic, and specialized. The principles are discussed in more detail in Chapter 9.

Screening for iron deficiency anemia. When iron-restricted erythropoiesis is under way, the CBC results begin to show evidence of anisocytosis, microcytosis, and hypochromia in proportion to the severity of iron deficiency (Figure 17.2). CBC alterations and anemia become apparent after changes in iron studies. The classic picture of IDA in stage 3 includes a decreased hemoglobin concentration. An RDW greater than 15% is expected and may precede the decrease in hemoglobin.[23] For patients in high-risk groups, the elevated RDW can be an early and sensitive indicator of iron deficiency that is provided in a routine CBC.[24] As the hemoglobin concentration continues to fall, microcytosis and hypochromia become more prominent, with progressively declining values for the MCV, MCH, and MCHC. Automated measures of microcytosis and hypochromia may detect these changes before they are noticeable on the peripheral blood film.[11] The RBC count ultimately becomes decreased but lags behind the drop in indices and hematocrit due to the increased cell divisions in iron-restricted erythropoiesis. Polychromasia may be apparent early, although it is not a prominent finding. Poikilocytosis, including occasional target cells and elliptocytes, may be present, although no particular shape is characteristic or predominant. Thrombocytosis may be present due to increased commitment of progenitors toward the megakaryocyte lineage,[25,26] particularly if the iron deficiency results from chronic bleeding, but this is not a diagnostic parameter. White blood cells are typically normal in number and appearance. Iron deficiency should be suspected when the CBC findings show a microcytic hypochromic anemia with an elevated RDW but no consistent shape changes to the RBCs.

Diagnostic testing for iron deficiency. Biochemical iron studies remain the backbone for diagnosis of iron deficiency, though some argue that modern automated blood cell analyzers can supplant the biochemical studies.[27] The biochemical analyses include assays of serum iron, TIBC, transferrin saturation, and serum ferritin; Chapter 9 covers the principle of each assay and technical considerations affecting test performance and interpretation. Serum iron is a measure of the amount of iron bound to transferrin (transport protein) in the serum. TIBC is an indirect measure of transferrin and the available binding sites for iron. The percent of transferrin binding sites occupied by iron can be calculated from the total iron and the TIBC:

$$\text{Transferrin saturation}(\%) = \frac{\text{serum iron}\,(\mu g/dL) \times 100}{\text{TIBC}\,(\mu g/dL)}$$

Ferritin provides an intracellular storage repository for metabolically active iron. Yet ferritin is secreted into blood, and serum levels reflect the levels of iron stored within cells. Serum ferritin is an easily accessible surrogate for stainable bone marrow iron. Iron studies are used collectively to assess the iron status of an individual. Table 17.1 shows that, as expected, serum ferritin and serum iron values are decreased in IDA, a state called *sideropenia*. Transferrin levels increase when the hepatocytes detect low iron levels, and research shows that this is a transcriptional and posttranscriptional response to an effort to compensate for low iron levels.[8,9,28,29] The result is a decline in the iron saturation of transferrin that is more dramatic than might be expected simply from the decrease in serum iron level. The biochemical markers of iron deficiency are rarely assayed in nonanemic patients, though some results (such as serum ferritin) are abnormal during the latent period.

Instrument manufacturers have developed parameters that can be reported with a CBC to enhance detection of latent iron deficiency and that are even more sensitive to IDA. These include sensitive and quantitative detection of hypochromia and microcytosis.[11,27,30–32] Because these are early indicators of impending anemia, they can provide an early alert during the latent period. On some instruments, these newer assays remain for research use only pending approval from the US Food and Drug Administration.

Reticulocyte parameters also support the diagnosis of IDA. A low absolute reticulocyte count confirms a diminished rate of effective erythropoiesis because this is a nonregenerative anemia.[3] Automated counting of reticulocytes allows measurement of indices similar to RBC indices and can include reticulocyte volume, reticulocyte hemoglobin content, and hemoglobin concentration. (Chapter 13).[27] The hemoglobin content of reticulocytes is analogous to the MCH, but for reticulocytes only. The MCH is the average weight of hemoglobin per cell across the entire RBC population. Some of the RBCs are nearly 120 days old, whereas others are just 1 to 2 days old. If iron deficiency is developing, the MCH does not change until a substantial proportion of the cells are iron deficient, and the diagnosis is effectively delayed for weeks or months after iron-restricted erythropoiesis begins. Measuring the hemoglobin content of reticulocytes enables detection of iron-restricted erythropoiesis within days as the first iron-deficient cells leave the bone marrow and is a sensitive indicator of iron deficiency. Even in stage 2 of iron deficiency, before anemia is apparent the hemoglobin content of reticulocytes will be low.[27] One disadvantage is that a CBC is unlikely to be ordered for nonanemic patients who demonstrate no symptoms. An order for reticulocyte parameters is even less likely. It is also important to remember that individuals with thalassemia have reduced RBC/reticulocyte hemoglobin content due to decreased globin chain synthesis, and therefore this measure cannot be used reliably to diagnose IDA in this group.

Specialized tests of iron status. Other tests, although not commonly used for the diagnosis of IDA, show abnormalities that become important in the differential diagnosis of similar conditions. Test results for the accumulated porphyrin precursors to heme are elevated (Table 17.1). FEP accumulates when iron is unavailable. In the absence of iron, FEP may be preferentially chelated with zinc to form zinc protoporphyrin (ZPP).[33] FEP and zinc chelate can be assayed fluorometrically, although they are not particularly valuable in the diagnosis of IDA. The sTfR levels can be assayed using immunoassay. The concentration in serum is directly proportional to erythropoietic rate and inversely proportional to tissue iron availability. Thus levels increase as the disease progresses, and individual cells seek to take in as much iron as possible.[34]

A bone marrow assessment is not indicated for suspected uncomplicated IDA. A therapeutic trial of iron (discussed in "Response to Treatment") provides a less invasive and less expensive diagnostic assessment. However, marrow examination for iron is routinely performed when a bone marrow specimen is collected for other reasons. With routine stains, the iron-deficient bone marrow appears hyperplastic early in the progression of the disease, with a decreased myeloid-to-erythroid ratio as a result of increased erythropoiesis.[14] As the disease progresses, hyperplasia subsides, and the profound deficiency of iron leads to slowed RBC production.[4] Polychromatic normoblasts (i.e., rubricytes) show the most dramatic morphologic changes (Figure 17.3). Nuclear-cytoplasmic asynchrony is evident, with cytoplasmic maturation

TABLE 17.1	Results of Iron Studies in Microcytic Anemias				
	Iron Deficiency Anemia	**β-Thalassemia Minor**	**Anemia of Inflammation**	**Sideroblastic Anemia**	**Lead Poisoning**
Serum ferritin	↓	↑/N	↑/N	↑	N
Serum iron	↓/N	↑/N	↓	↑	Variable
TIBC	↑	N	↓	↓/N	N
Transferrin saturation	↓	↑/N	↓/N	↑	↑
FEP/ZPP	↑	N	↑	↑	↑ (marked)
sTfR	↑	N	N	N	N
Hemoglobin content of reticulocytes	↓	↓	↓	↓/N	↓/N
BM iron (Prussian blue reaction)	No stainable iron	↑/N	↑/N	↑	N
Sideroblasts in BM	None	N	None/very few	↑ (ring)	N (ring)
Other special tests		↑ Hb A₂	Specific tests for inflammatory disorders or malignancy		↑ ALA in urine ↑ Blood lead levels

↑, Increased; *↓*, decreased; *ALA*, aminolevulinic acid; *BM*, bone marrow; *FEP/ZPP*, free erythrocyte protoporphyrin/zinc protoporphyrin; *Hb*, hemoglobin; *N*, normal; *sTfR*, soluble transferrin receptor, *TIBC*, total iron-binding capacity.

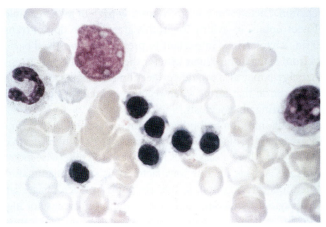

Figure 17.3 Bone Marrow Aspirate Smear From a Patient With Iron Deficiency Anemia. The later-stage nucleated red blood cells show the characteristic "shaggy" cytoplasm, which is also very blue because of delayed maturation relative to the nucleus (i.e., nuclear-cytoplasmic asynchrony). (Wright-Giemsa stain, ×1000.) (Courtesy Ann Bell, University of Tennessee, Memphis.)

lagging behind nuclear maturation. Without the pink provided by hemoglobin, the cytoplasm remains bluish after the nucleus has begun to condense. The cell membranes appear irregular and are usually described as "shaggy."

Treatment and Its Effects

Treatment. The first therapy for IDA is to treat any underlying contributing cause, such as hookworms, tumors, or ulcers. As in the treatment of simple nutritional deficiencies or increased need, dietary supplementation is necessary to replenish the body's iron stores. Oral supplements of ferrous sulfate are the standard prescription.[14] The supplements should be taken on an empty stomach to maximize absorption. Many patients experience side effects such as nausea and constipation, however, which leads to poor patient compliance. Vigilance on the part of the health care providers is important to ensure that patients complete the course of iron replacement, which usually lasts 6 months or longer.[35] Use of oral bovine lactoferrin to provide iron supplementation has been studied in some populations, and the intestinal side effects are reduced compared with ferrous sulfate while being equally effective in correcting iron deficiency.[36–38]

In some patients, such as older adults, there may be a higher incidence of intolerance of oral supplements and/or reduced absorption, and intravenous iron might be required. In rare cases in which intestinal absorption of iron is impaired (e.g., in conditions such as gastric achlorhydria, celiac disease, or matriptase-2 gene mutations causing IRIDA), intravenous administration of iron dextrans can be used. The side effects of high-molecular-weight iron dextran are notable,[14] but improved toxicity profiles for more recent iron formulations have increased safety.[39] Because of the risks associated with RBC transfusions, they are rarely warranted for the correction of uncomplicated IDA unless the patient's hemoglobin level has become dangerously low, such as the patient in this chapter's case study.

Response to treatment. When optimal treatment with iron is initiated, the effects are quickly evident. The hemoglobin content of reticulocytes will correct within 2 days.[27] Reticulocyte counts

(relative and absolute) begin to increase within 5 to 10 days.[35] The anticipated rise in hemoglobin appears in 2 to 3 weeks, and levels should return to normal for the individual by about 2 months after the initiation of adequate treatment.[40] The peripheral blood film and indices still reflect the microcytic RBC population for several months, with a biphasic population including the younger normocytic cells. The normocytic population eventually predominates. Iron therapy must continue for another 3 to 4 months to replenish the storage pool and prevent a relapse.

It is common and reasonable for health care providers to assume that iron deficiency is due to dietary deficiency because that is the case in most instances of iron deficiency. Thus supplementation should correct it. If the patient has been adherent to the therapeutic regimen, the failure to respond to iron treatment points to the need for further investigation. The patient may be experiencing continued undetected (i.e. occult) loss of blood or inadequate absorption, justifying additional diagnostics. The rare but likely underdiagnosed hereditary causes of iron deficiency should be considered. Alternatively, causes of microcytic hypochromic anemia unrelated to iron deficiency, such as thalassemia, should be investigated.

Anemia of Inflammation

Anemia is commonly associated with systemic diseases, including chronic inflammatory conditions such as rheumatoid arthritis, chronic infections such as tuberculosis or human immunodeficiency virus (HIV) infection, and malignancies. Cartwright[41] was the first to suggest that although the underlying diseases seem quite disparate, the associated anemia may be from a single cause, proposing the concept of anemia of chronic disease. This anemia, also called *anemia of inflammation* (AI) or anemia of chronic inflammation, ranks only behind IDA in incidence worldwide and is common among hospitalized patients.[42,43]

Etiology

AI occurs as part of a chronic inflammatory disorder, but the same process appears to begin acutely during virtually any infection or inflammation, including trauma or after surgery. This disorder does not include conditions that cause hemolysis or have marrow involvement. Additionally, chronic blood loss is not among the conditions leading to AI because it results in quantitative iron deficiency. The central feature of AI is sideropenia in the face of abundant iron stores. Several pathophysiologic mechanisms have been identified as contributors to AI. The cause is now understood to be largely impaired ferrokinetics and thus iron-restricted erythropoiesis. However, impaired erythropoiesis and shortened RBC life span are also contributors.

Impaired ferrokinetics. As explained in detail in Chapter 9, hepcidin is a hormone produced by hepatocytes to regulate body iron levels, particularly absorption of iron in the intestine and release of iron from macrophages and hepatocytes. Ferroportin is the iron exporting protein in the membrane of these cells. Hepcidin binds to ferroportin and causes its internalization and degradation, thus reducing the amount of iron absorbed through the intestine and recycled by macrophages and hepatocytes.[44,45] Conversely, when systemic body iron levels decrease, hepcidin production by hepatocytes decreases,[46] and enterocytes export more iron into the blood. Macrophage and hepatocyte release of iron also increases. When systemic iron levels are high, hepcidin increases, enterocytes export less iron into the blood, and macrophages and hepatocytes retain iron.

Hepcidin is an acute phase reactant.[47] During inflammation, hepatocytes increase the synthesis of hepcidin in response to interleukin-6 produced by activated *Kupffer cells* (liver macrophages) (Figure 17.4).[43,48] This increase occurs regardless of systemic iron levels in the body. As a result, during inflammation, there is a decrease in iron absorption from the intestine and iron release from macrophages and hepatocytes (Figure 17.5). Although there is plenty of iron in the body, it is unavailable to developing RBCs because it is sequestered in the macrophages and hepatocytes.

The elevation of hepcidin during inflammation may be a nonspecific defense against invading bacteria.[49] If the body can sequester iron, it reduces the iron available to bacteria and thus contributes to their demise. Although a rise in hepcidin is not harmful during disorders of short duration, chronically high levels of hepcidin sequester iron for long periods, which leads to diminished production of RBCs.

A second iron-related acute phase reactant seems to contribute to AI, although probably to a much smaller extent than hepcidin. Lactoferrin is an iron-binding protein in the granules of neutrophils. Its avidity for iron is greater than that of transferrin. Lactoferrin is important to prevent phagocytized bacteria from using intracellular iron for their metabolic processes.[50] Lactoferrin may also provide protection for the phagocyte from oxidized iron that forms when reactive oxygen species are produced during phagocytosis.[51]

During infection and inflammation, neutrophil lactoferrin is released into the blood and extracellular spaces with the death of neutrophils. There it scavenges iron that would otherwise induce oxidative damage. In this way, lactoferrin is antiinflammatory. When it is carrying iron, lactoferrin binds to macrophages and hepatocytes that take up and salvage the iron. Because of high hepcidin, however, the macrophages and hepatocytes cannot export iron and it remains sequestered away from erythroblasts. Erythroblasts cannot acquire iron salvaged by lactoferrin directly because they do not have lactoferrin receptors.

The result of these effects during chronic inflammation is a functional iron deficiency; iron is present in abundance in storage but unavailable to developing erythroblasts. This maldistribution of iron can be seen histologically with iron stains of bone marrow that show iron in macrophages but not in erythroblasts (Figure 15.16C). The effect on the developing erythroblasts is

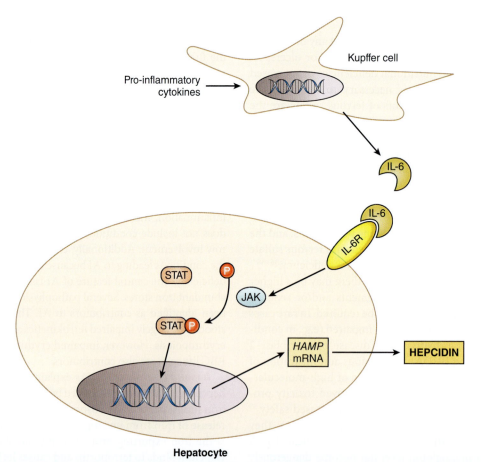

Figure 17.4 **Stimulation of Hepcidin Production During Inflammation.** Proinflammatory cytokines activate the macrophages of the liver, Kupffer cells. The Kupffer cells produce interleukin-6 *(IL-6)*. IL-6 binds to the IL-6 receptor *(IL-6R)* on hepatocytes. That binding initiates signal transduction through Janus kinase attaching a phosphate *(P)* to signal transducer and activator of transcription (JAK-STAT pathway). The hepcidin gene *(HAMP)* is upregulated, leading to production of hepcidin.

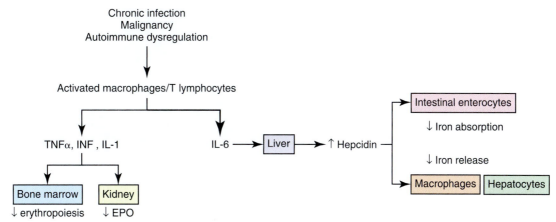

Figure 17.5 Mechanisms of Anemia in Chronic Inflammatory Conditions. Chronic infections (bacterial, viral, parasitic, or fungal), malignancy, and autoimmune dysregulation result in the release of inflammatory cytokines from activated macrophages and T lymphocytes. Interleukin-6 *(IL-6)* promotes liver production of hepcidin, an acute phase reactant that impairs iron absorption in intestinal enterocytes and iron release from macrophages and hepatocytes. Inflammatory cytokines, such as tumor necrosis factor-α *(TNF-α)*, interleukin-1 *(IL-1)*, and interferon-γ *(INF-γ)*, also inhibit erythropoiesis and decrease erythropoietin *(EPO)* production by the kidney. Although these latter mechanisms contribute to the anemia of inflammation, the hepcidin-induced inhibition of intestinal iron absorption and iron release from storage sites in macrophages and hepatocytes is the more significant cause of the anemia. (Adapted from Weiss, G., & Goodnough, L. T. [2005]. Anemia of chronic disease. *N Engl J Med, 352,* p. 1013, Figure 1.)

essentially no different from a mild iron deficiency because they are effectively deprived of the iron. So, similar to IDA, this is iron-restricted erythropoiesis.

Impaired erythropoiesis. Production of inflammatory cytokines (such as tumor necrosis factor-α and interleukin-1 from activated macrophages and interferon-γ from activated T cells) also impairs proliferation of erythroid progenitor cells, diminishes their response to erythropoietin, and decreases production of erythropoietin by the kidney (Figure 17.5).[43,52]

Shortened red blood cell life span. A third factor contributing to AI is a shortened RBC life span. The cause appears to be related to macrophage activation, vascular factors, and increased erythrophagocytosis due to antibody and complement on the surface of the RBCs.[52-55] Although inflammatory suppression and shortened RBC life span contribute to AI, the impaired ferrokinetics is the most significant cause of the anemia.

Laboratory Diagnosis

The peripheral blood picture in AI is that of a mild anemia, with hemoglobin concentration usually 8 to 10 g/dL and without reticulocytosis. The cells are usually normocytic and normochromic. Although microcytosis and hypochromia can be seen, they typically represent coexistent iron deficiency.[52] The inflammatory condition leading to the anemia also may cause other abnormalities, such as leukocytosis, a "left shift," the presence of leukemic cells, or thrombocytosis. Iron studies (Table 17.1) show low serum iron and TIBC values. Because hepatocyte production of transferrin is regulated by intracellular iron levels, the low TIBC (an indirect measure of transferrin) reflects the abundant iron stores in hepatocytes. The transferrin saturation may be normal or low. The serum ferritin level, as an acute phase reactant, is usually increased beyond the value that would be expected for the same patient in the absence of the inflammatory condition. It may not be outside the reference interval,

but it is nevertheless increased and may help rule out IDA. The failure to incorporate iron into heme results in elevation of FEP, although this test typically is not used diagnostically. The hemoglobin content of reticulocytes will be decreased, demonstrating the iron-restricted erythropoiesis, but the sTfR levels will be normal, reflecting normal intracellular iron. The bone marrow shows hypoproliferation of the RBCs, consistent with the lack of reticulocytes in the peripheral blood. Prussian blue stain of the bone marrow confirms abundant stores of iron in macrophages, although not in RBC precursors, but bone marrow examination is not usually required in the diagnostic evaluation.

Patients with IDA who have an inflammatory condition present a special diagnostic dilemma. The iron deficiency may be missed because of the increase in serum ferritin levels associated with the inflammation. Serum ferritin levels below 30 ng/mL are typically consistent with IDA. Serum ferritin values above 100 ng/mL are typically consistent with AI. Serum ferritin values in the 30 to 100 ng/mL range are most equivocal and may represent coexistent IDA and AI.[43,52,56] For patients with results in this range, IDA and AI may be distinguished, or their coexistence can be verified, by measuring sTfR levels in the serum.[57] These receptors are sloughed from cells into the blood. As noted earlier, levels increase during IDA but remain essentially normal during AI. Still, the diagnostic picture may not be clear.

Additional modifications to the use of the sTfR assay have been developed to better distinguish IDA, latent iron deficiency, and AI when ferritin results are equivocal (i.e., 30 to 100 ng/mL) (Chapter 9). One of these modifications is calculation of the sTfR/log ferritin. In AI, the numerator is essentially normal while the denominator rises, and thus a ratio <1 results.[56,58] With coexistent IDA and AI, the sTfR level rises disproportionately more than the log ferritin. A ratio >2 can be expected. The hemoglobin content of reticulocytes will be reduced in both IDA and AI. However, when graphed against the sTfR/log ferritin in a Thomas plot (Figure 9.10), the two conditions may be distinguished, sometimes better than with the sTfR/log ferritin alone (Chapter 9).[59,60] Research continues to improve the means to help resolve this diagnostic dilemma.

Treatment

Therapeutic administration of erythropoietin can correct AI,[61] but iron must be administered concurrently because stored body iron remains sequestered and unavailable (i.e., functional iron deficiency).[62] The anemia is typically not severe, however, and this costly treatment is warranted only in select patients. At present, the best course of treatment is effective control or alleviation of the underlying condition. However, various anti-hepcidin therapies are being investigated.[3,63,64]

PORPHYRIAS

Just as anemia can result from inadequate supplies of iron for production of hemoglobin, diseases that interfere with the production of protoporphyrin also can produce anemia. (Protoporphyrin synthesis is discussed in Chapter 8.) The resulting conditions include the porphyrias and SAs (which are discussed next in "Sideroblastic Anemias"). The porphyrias include both hereditary and acquired diseases in which enzymes of the heme synthetic pathway are missing or impaired. However, the term *porphyria* is most often used to refer to the hereditary conditions. Among the inherited disorders, single deficiencies of most enzymes in the synthetic pathway for heme have been identified (Figure 8.5).

When an enzyme in heme synthesis is missing, the products from earlier stages in the pathway accumulate in cells that actively produce heme, such as erythrocytes and hepatocytes. The excess porphyrins leak from the cells as they age or die and may be excreted in urine or feces, which allows diagnosis. The accumulated products also deposit in body tissues. Some of the products are fluorescent. Their accumulation in skin can lead to photosensitivity, with severe burns on exposure to sunlight. Accumulation during childhood leads to fluorescence of developing teeth and bones. Only three of the porphyrias have hematologic manifestations; the others have a greater effect on hepatocytes. Even in the porphyrias with hematologic effects, the hematologic impact is relatively minimal, and photosensitivity is a greater clinical problem. The fluorescence of accumulated compounds can be used diagnostically, for example, to measure FEP (Chapter 9). In a bone marrow preparation or peripheral blood, the erythroblasts or erythrocytes will be bright red using a fluorescent microscope (Figure 17.6). Table 17.2 summarizes the deficient enzymes, affected genes, inheritance, and clinical and laboratory features that can be used in the diagnosis of the hematologically significant porphyrias.

SIDEROBLASTIC ANEMIAS

Erythroblasts containing stainable iron (i.e., sideroblasts) are expected in the bone marrow. SAs are characterized by the presence in the bone marrow of ring sideroblasts. These are erythroblasts that, when stained with Prussian blue, demonstrate a ring of blue iron deposits around the nucleus (Figure 17.7). Electron

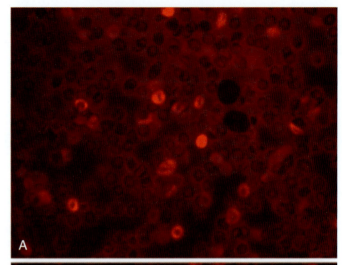
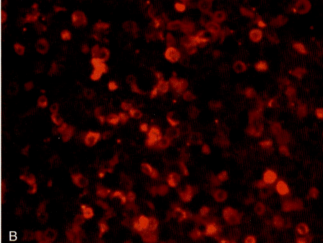

Figure 17.6 Autofluorescence of Erythroblasts and Erythrocytes in Erythropoietic Porphyria. **(A),** Erythroblasts. **(B),** Erythrocytes. (From Blagojevic, D., Schenk, T., Haas, O., et al. [2010]. Acquired erythropoietic protoporphyria. *Ann Hematol, 89*, p. 744, Figure 1.)

microscopy has demonstrated the deposits to be iron-laden mitochondria.[65] The accumulation of mitochondrial iron in SAs is due to impairments of mitochondrial iron kinetics. However, the reason that the iron-laden mitochondria encircle the nucleus is unclear. Nevertheless, *ring sideroblasts* are the hallmark of SAs. Both hereditary and acquired conditions are known (Box 17.1).

Hereditary Sideroblastic Anemias

Among the hereditary forms of SAs, X-linked and autosomal varieties are known. Hereditary SAs studied to date all have mutations in genes for proteins involved in mitochondrial processes such as heme synthesis and energy production. All hereditary SAs are quite rare, with the most common having on the order of 100 identified families.[66] Accordingly, only the most common are mentioned here. Among them is X-linked sideroblastic anemia (XLSA), which involves missense mutations to the gene for the erythroid form of aminolevulinic acid synthase 2 (ALAS2). ALAS2 catalyzes the first step in porphyrin synthesis, which uses pyridoxine (vitamin B_6) as a cofactor. Some patients with XLSA experience at least modest improvement of anemia with pharmacologic doses of pyridoxine.[67] XLSA is a microcytic

TABLE 17.2   Erythropoietic Porphyrias

		Congenital Erythropoietic Porphyria (CEP)	Erythropoietic Protoporphyria (EPP)	X-linked Erythropoietic Protoporphyria (XLEPP)
Enzyme affected		Uroporphyrinogen III synthase deficiency	Ferrochelatase deficiency	ALA synthase 2 (gain of function)
Affected gene		*UROS*	*FECH*	*ALAS2*
Inheritance		Autosomal recessive	Autosomal recessive	X-linked dominant
Clinical features		Photosensitivity, hemolytic anemia	Photosensitivity; anemia is mild if present	Photosensitivity; mild microcytic hypochromic anemia with reticulocyte response is possible
Laboratory Features				
Red blood cells	Protoporphyrin	N	↑↑↑	↑
	Uroporphyrin	↑↑↑	N	N
	Coproporphyrin	↑↑	N	N
Urine	Porphobilinogen	N	N	N
	Uroporphyrin	↑↑↑	N	N
	Coproporphyrin	↑↑	N	N
Feces	Protoporphyrin	N	↑↑	N or ↑
	Coproporphyrin	↑	N	N
Confirmatory tests		↓↓↓ Uroporphyrinogen III synthase activity Genetic testing	↓↓ Ferrochelatase activity Genetic testing	↑↑ ALA-synthase activity ↑↑ FEP/ZPP Genetic testing

↑, Minimally increased levels; *↑↑,* moderately increased levels; *↑↑↑,* markedly increased levels; *↓↓,* moderately decreased levels; *↓↓↓,* markedly decreased levels; *ALA,* aminolevulinic acid; *FEP/ZPP,* free erythrocyte protoporphyrin/zinc protoporphyrin; *N,* normal.
Modified from Desnick, R. J. & Balwani, M. (2022). The porphyrias. In Loscalzo, J., Fauci, A., Kasper, D. L., et al. (Eds.), *Harrison's Principles of Internal Medicine.* (21st ed., p. 2422). New York: McGraw Hill Education.

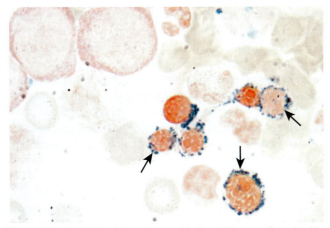

Figure 17.7 Ring Sideroblasts *(arrows)* in Bone Marrow. (Prussian blue stain, ×1000.)

BOX 17.1   Disorders Included in the Sideroblastic Anemias

Hereditary Sideroblastic Anemia
X-linked (paternal), e.g., X-linked sideroblastic anemia
Mitochondrial (maternal), e.g., Pearson marrow-pancreas syndrome
Autosomal, e.g. erythropoietic protoporphyria

Acquired Sideroblastic Anemia
Primary (clonal) sideroblastic anemia
    Myelodysplasia
    Myeloproliferative diseases
Secondary (nonclonal) sideroblastic anemias caused by drugs and bone marrow toxins
    Antitubercular drugs
    Chloramphenicol
    Alcohol
    Lead
    Chemotherapeutic agents

hypochromic anemia with ring sideroblasts in the bone marrow. As an X-linked condition, men are most often affected; however, heterozygous women may demonstrate a dimorphic population of normal RBCs with microcytic hypochromic ones.[66] Late term loss of male fetuses may occur when the mutation leads to severe anemia, evidence of the critical role of ALAS2 in hematopoiesis.[66]

Pearson marrow-pancreas syndrome (PMPS) is a form of SA that results from mitochondrial DNA deletions that code for proteins involved in energy production. Because mitochondrial DNA is inherited from the mother, the inheritance of PMPS is maternal. It is evident in childhood and, as the name suggests, may involve pancreatic exocrine insufficiency. Some children may have only erythroid effects, which may lead to misidentification as Diamond-Blackfan syndrome, but other cytopenias

are also common.[68] The RBC morphology is most often macrocytic. Individuals may be transfusion dependent.

Another relatively more frequent hereditary SA is erythropoietic protoporphyria (EPP) (Table 17.2). As described previously, the porphyrias are a group of conditions in which porphyrin production is impaired due to deficiencies or impairments of synthetic enzymes in the porphyrin production pathway. Some of the enzymes are cytoplasmic, while others are mitochondrial. In EPP, the deficiency of ferrochelatase, the enzyme that inserts iron into protoporphyrin, produces an impairment to mitochondrial iron kinetics and hence SA. As it results in a microcytic hypochromic anemia with ring sideroblasts in the bone marrow, it can be categorized as a hereditary SA or a porphyria (Figure 17.8). The hematological effects are not always prominent, and ring sideroblasts may not be numerous. X-linked erythropoietic porphyria (Table 17.2) is rarer but shares the same clinical and laboratory features as EPP.

Acquired Sideroblastic Anemias

Acquired SAs occur in both clonal (i.e., malignant or cancerous) and nonclonal forms. Mutations leading to clonal proliferations result in primary SA associated with the myeloproliferative diseases and myelodysplastic neoplasms. These are described in detail in Chapters 32 and 33. Suffice it to say here that the ring sideroblasts are a diagnostic feature in some of these conditions.

Nonclonal or secondary acquired SAs may result from exposure to various bone marrow toxins including alcohol, heavy metals such as lead, drugs such as antituberculosis treatments,[69] and chemotherapeutic agents. These exposures cause SA more frequently than the acquired clonal causes or hereditary forms of SA, so they are more frequently encountered in laboratory practice. Lead poisoning is a serious public health concern deserving of detailed discussion.

Lead Poisoning

Adults may be exposed to leaded compounds at work if proper safety precautions are not in place. Adults and children living in older homes can be exposed to lead from paints produced before the 1970s. They are at risk if dust is created during renovations or paint is permitted to peel. Toddlers and crawling infants are at special risk from getting dust on their hands and placing them in their mouths. Lead leaching from water service pipes, especially if drinking water is not properly treated, can also be a source of the toxin. Several cities in the United States have experienced this in recent years.[70–72]

Although anyone can experience lead poisoning, it is of special concern in children. The metal affects the developing central nervous system and the hematologic system, leading to impaired mental development and learning disabilities and

anemia, respectively.[72,73] In children and adults with lead poisoning, a peripheral neuropathy[74] can be seen, with abdominal cramping and vomiting or seizures.

Lead interferes with porphyrin synthesis at several steps and thus can be categorized as both an acquired porphyria and an acquired SA. The steps that are most significantly affected are as follows (Figure 8.5):

1. The conversion of aminolevulinic acid (ALA) to porphobilinogen (PBG) by ALA dehydratase (also called *PBG synthase*); the result is the accumulation of ALA.
2. The incorporation of iron into protoporphyrin IX by ferrochelatase (also called *heme synthase*); the result is accumulation of iron and protoporphyrin in the mitochondria.[75]

Anemia, when present in lead poisoning, is most often normocytic and normochromic; however, with chronic exposure to lead, a microcytic hypochromic blood picture may be seen. Coexisting iron deficiency may be a contributor. The degree of anemia in adults may not be dramatic but in children, it may be more profound. The reticulocyte count in acute poisoning may be quite elevated, which suggests that the anemia has a hemolytic component. The presence of a hemolytic component is supported by studies showing impairment of the pentose-phosphate shunt by lead,[76] which makes the cells sensitive to oxidant stress, as in glucose-6-phosphate dehydrogenase deficiency (Chapter 21). Although the bone marrow may show erythroid hyperplasia, consistent with the elevated reticulocyte count, in some patients it may be hypoplastic.[77] Basophilic stippling is a classic finding associated with lead toxicity. Lead inhibits pyrimidine 5′-nucleotidase, an enzyme involved in the breakdown of ribosomal ribonucleic acid (RNA) in reticulocytes.[78] This causes undegraded ribosomes to aggregate, forming basophilic stippling. The size of the aggregates in lead poisoning is typically large, so the stippling is heavier than that seen in many anemias and thus represents truly punctate basophilia. Because basophilic stippling is also seen in other anemias, this is not a pathognomonic finding but an expected finding, and whenever punctate basophilic stippling is seen, lead poisoning should be considered. While a bone marrow biopsy is typically not needed to establish a diagnosis of lead poisoning, the characteristic ring sideroblasts can be expected to be observed.[79] Accumulated ALA is measurable in the urine, though not typically measured diagnostically. Protoporphyrin is measurable in an extract of RBCs as FEP or ZPP. Chapter 9 describes the principles of these assays. ZPP is not recommended for screening purposes, however, due to poor sensitivity when the lead level is low and delay of elevations relative to acute lead exposure.[80]

Removal of the drug or toxin is usually successful for the treatment of acquired secondary SAs. In the case of lead poisoning, calcium disodium edetate ($CaNa_2EDTA$) and/or dimercaprol are often used to chelate the lead present in the body so that it can be excreted in the urine.[77] The other impacts of lead poisoning, such as neurological impairments in children, are often more sustained.

IRON OVERLOAD

Chapter 9 describes the body's tenacity in conserving iron. For some individuals, this tenacity becomes the basis for disease related to excess iron accumulations in nearly all cells. Iron overload may be

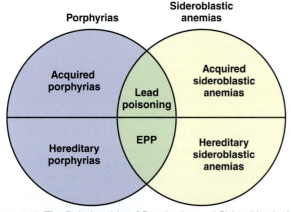

Figure 17.8 The Relationship of Porphyrias and Sideroblastic Anemias, Both Acquired and Hereditary. There is overlap between the porphyrias and the sideroblastic anemias as shown here. Some conditions such as lead poisoning and erythropoietic porphyria can be categorized as either a porphyria due to blockages in porphyrin synthesis or a sideroblastic anemia due to the presence of ring sideroblasts in the bone marrow. *EPP,* Erythropoietic porphyria.

primary, as in hereditary hemochromatosis (HH), or secondary to chronic anemias and their treatments. In both cases, the toxic effects of excess iron lead to a phenotype with serious health problems as lipids, proteins, nucleic acids, and heme iron become oxidized.

Etiology

Excess accumulation of iron results from acquired or hereditary conditions in which the body's rate of iron acquisition exceeds the rate of loss, which is usually about 1 mg/day. The body's first reaction is to store excess iron in the form of ferritin within cells. Eventually, the storage system is overwhelmed. Parenchymal cells in organs such as the liver, heart, and pancreas are damaged by uncontrolled entry of iron-producing oxidizing agents via the Fenton reaction (Chapter 9).

Acquired Iron Overload

Accumulation of excess iron may be an acquired condition. It occurs when there is a need for repeated transfusions, as in the treatment of anemias such as aplastic anemia (Chapter 19) and sickle cell anemia (Chapter 24). With repeated transfusions, the 200 to 250 mg of iron present in one unit of transfused RBCs quickly exceeds the usual 1 mg/day of iron typically added to the body's stores by a healthy diet. This is sometimes called *transfusion-related hemosiderosis.*

Some chronic anemias, usually hereditary hemolytic anemias (e.g., β-thalassemia major), are innately iron loading, even without transfusion therapy. Hemolytic anemias cause the bone marrow to develop a compensatory erythroid hyperplasia. As described in Chapter 9, erythroblasts are able to downregulate hepcidin production by secreting erythroferrone. If there are more erythroblasts than usual, as in compensatory erythroid hyperplasia, then erythroferrone is increased; hepcidin is decreased; ferroportin is active in enterocytes, macrophages, and hepatocytes; and more than the usual amount of iron is absorbed and recycled. With chronic hemolytic anemias, this leads to excessive accumulation of iron. Although this is seen most often with hereditary hemolytic anemias, the iron loading is secondary to the hereditary condition that causes the hemolysis. If the hemolysis is controlled, the iron loading subsides. Thus this is acquired iron overload in a hereditary anemia.

Hereditary Iron Overload

Iron overload may develop as a result of mutations in genes for proteins controlling iron kinetics (Table 9.2). Feedback regulation of iron is impaired, and the body continues to absorb iron, even when stores are full. This is a true hereditary iron overload called *hereditary hemochromatosis* (HH). An autosomal recessive disease was recognized for many years before modern methods allowed a molecular investigation of its cause. In the mid-1990s, a mutation was identified affecting the gene for the HH protein HFE[81] and shortly after that, additional mutations of the same gene were identified.[82,83] Nearly 100 mutations to this one gene have been identified to date.[84] Homozygosity of the most common *HFE* mutation is on the order of 0.5% among individuals of northern European descent, making it the most common hereditary condition in this group.[85]

With reliable and specific molecular tests, individuals with the phenotypic disease (i.e., excess iron accumulation in tissues and associated symptoms) who did not have *HFE* mutations were soon discovered. Trying to explain their diseases contributed to discovery of the other proteins that are now known to be involved in iron kinetics. What has emerged is a picture of HH as a group of diseases with an iron overload phenotype produced by mutations in somatic genes for iron regulatory proteins. Table 17.3 describes the features of several forms of HH, including the most common one with mutations to the *HFE* gene.

TABLE 17.3 Mutations Producing Hemochromatosis Phenotypes

Feature	Hemochromatosis, Type 1 (*HFE*-Associated Hereditary Hemochromatosis)	Hemochromatosis, Type 2A Juvenile (*HFE2*-Related Juvenile Hemochromatosis)	Hemochromatosis, Type 2B Juvenile (*HAMP*-Related Juvenile Hemochromatosis)	Hemochromatosis, Type 3 (*TFR2*-Related Hereditary Hemochromatosis)	Hemachromatosis, Type 4 (Ferroportin-Related Iron Overload)	Hemachromatosis, Type 5
Affected gene	*HFE*	*HFE2 (HJV)*	*HAMP*	*TFR2*	*SLC40A1*	*FTH1*
Mutated protein	Hereditary hemochromatosis protein	Hemojuvelin	Hepcidin	Transferrin receptor protein 2	Solute carrier family 40 member 1 (ferroportin-1)	Ferritin heavy chain
Normal function of affected protein	Participates in signaling complex for hepcidin regulation	Hepatocyte coreceptor in signaling complex for hepcidin regulation	Downregulates ferroportin-mediated iron transport in macrophages, hepatocytes, and enterocytes	Hepatic iron sensor to regulate hepcidin expression	Transports iron out of enterocytes, hepatocytes, and macrophages	Iron storage
Age of onset of symptoms (y)	30–40	Teens–20	Teens–20	20–40, mild	30–40	*
Inheritance pattern of most common alleles	Autosomal recessive	Autosomal recessive	Autosomal recessive	Autosomal recessive	Autosomal dominant	Autosomal dominant

*Found in three members of a Japanese family.

Names of hemochromatosis types from Online Mendelian Inheritance of Man: https://www.omim.org/entry/235200.
Approved gene symbols from the Human Genome Organization (HUGO) Gene Nomenclature Committee (HGNC): https://www.genenames.org.
Approved protein names from UniProt KB, 2002–2023 UniProt consortium: https://www.uniprot.org.

Phenotype and Epidemiology

Because all cells except mature RBCs require iron and have the cellular machinery for iron acquisition, most cells have the potential for iron damage. The tissues most obviously affected by iron overload are the skin, where accumulation of hemosiderin gives the skin a golden color; the liver, where cirrhosis-induced jaundice and subsequent cancer may develop; and the pancreas, where damage results in diabetes mellitus. Thus HH has been characterized as "bronzed diabetes." However, the heart muscle also is especially vulnerable to excessive iron accumulation, leading to congestive heart failure. Hepatocellular carcinoma occurs more often in patients with HH. Mutations of the *p53* tumor suppressor gene seem to contribute to the pathogenesis of the carcinoma,[86,87] and there is some evidence that the free radicals produced by iron cause the mutations in the *p53* gene.[88] Early diagnosis and treatment (discussed in "Laboratory Diagnosis" and "Treatment") can prevent the development of organ damage due to iron overload. Thus having a mutation does not equate to having disease.

In classic untreated HH (i.e., HH with *HFE* mutations), individuals usually harbor 20 to 30 g of iron by the time the disease becomes clinically evident at the age of 40 to 60 years.[89] This is almost 10 times the amount of stored iron in healthy individuals and represents just 1 to 2 mg/day of excess iron absorbed over many years.[90] In the juvenile forms of the disease associated with mutations to the genes for hepcidin or hemojuvelin, the process of iron accumulation is accelerated, so these effects may appear as early as the teenage years.

In the slower-developing diseases, phenotypic expression of the tissue damage in HH is more common in men, although the gene frequency of the somatic mutations is not higher in men. This difference is due to the blood loss associated with menstruation and childbirth, which forestalls the effects of excess iron in affected women. As a result, they usually develop clinical symptoms later in life than affected men. In each sex, homozygous individuals develop clinical disease faster than heterozygotes.

The amount of iron available in the diet for absorption affects the rate at which disease can develop. Substances that can promote iron absorption even in normal individuals, such as ascorbic acid and alcohol, also affect absorption in individuals with hemochromatosis.

The tissue effects and phenotype development are the same for individuals at risk for acquired iron overload as they are for individuals with HH. Additionally, in transfusion-related hemosiderosis, the frequency of transfusions over time affects the rate of development of clinical disease. With iron-loading anemias, iron acquisition is greatest when hemolysis is not controlled.

Laboratory Diagnosis

When individuals are diagnosed with an iron-loading anemia, such as β-thalassemia, or have an anemia requiring repeated transfusions over time, iron overload is anticipated and is a routine concern. Therefore iron overload in these situations is not a diagnostic challenge, and monitoring and treatment to prevent overload are routine, as described later in this section and in "Treatment." In HH, however, the laboratory may provide the first suggestion of the presence of the condition.

Routine Testing

Some undiagnosed individuals with HH present to their health care provider with nonspecific symptoms such as weakness, joint pain, or abdominal pain. This prompts routine laboratory testing such as CBC and metabolic panel. In other individuals with undiagnosed HH and without symptoms, HH may be discovered incidentally with abnormal results of these laboratory tests conducted as part of a routine physical examination. With or without symptoms, elevated results on common tests of liver function (e.g., elevated alanine transaminase levels) may be among the first laboratory findings that lead a care provider to order further diagnostic testing. Because inflammation is minimal, however, diminished levels of the liver's synthetic products, such as albumin, may be more suggestive of liver involvement. Hemoglobin and hematocrit may be elevated. MCV may be elevated unrelated to liver involvement. These findings suggest that the erythron will take advantage of iron when available.[84] Elevations of serum glucose are common at the time of diagnosis but only in symptomatic individuals.

Directed Testing for Diagnosis

When HH is suspected based on routine laboratory tests or symptoms, directed testing related to iron is performed. Transferrin saturation (TS) >45% or ferritin greater than 300 ng/mL for men and 200 ng/mL for women increases the suspicion for HH.[91] As macrophage ferroportin is always active, serum iron, ferritin, and TS can be elevated before tissue iron overload develops.[84]

While TS and serum ferritin can be used as screening tests in individuals with suspected HH,[92] population screening is not recommended despite how common the condition is in certain populations. This is due to the variable penetrance of the mutation[91] and the low diagnostic specificity (Chapter 3) in screening situations.[84] Diagnosis of HH ultimately relies on genetic testing to identify a patient's specific mutation, thus providing prognostic information and treatment guidance.

Directed Testing for Treatment, Monitoring, and Genetic Counseling

Directed testing in the context of known HH serves three purposes. It can be used to identify organ damage if present and thus direct treatment. It also can be used to monitor the effectiveness of the treatment. Finally, it can be used to pinpoint the mutation for family genetic counseling.

Liver function testing mentioned earlier is important in detecting early organ damage. Pancreatic function can be monitored with serum glucose. Appropriate treatment can be applied based on these results.

Determination of the actual extent of tissue damage is beyond the scope of the clinical laboratory. Liver biopsy with assessment of iron staining and degree of scarring in liver specimens is the gold standard and essential to determining the degree of organ damage. Less invasive methods are in development.[93]

Once iron overload status is determined and treatment or lifestyle practices are initiated, laboratory testing is important in lifelong monitoring. The serum ferritin level provides an assessment of the degree of iron overload and can be monitored after treatment is initiated to reduce iron stores. Hemoglobin concentration and hematocrit are inexpensive tests that can also be used to monitor treatment, as described later.

Genetic testing for known mutations provides confirmation of the diagnosis for most patients with HH. However, it is especially valuable for testing nonaffected family members who can be counseled on lifestyle changes to prevent the disease phenotype from developing or for whom early treatment interventions can prevent organ damage.

Treatment

The treatment of secondary tissue damage, such as liver cirrhosis and heart failure, follows standard protocols. Treatment of the underlying condition leading to excess iron accumulation is also needed, but HH and transfusion-related hemosiderosis require different treatment approaches. In forms of HH, withdrawal of blood by phlebotomy provides a simple, inexpensive, and effective means of removing iron from the body. The regimen calls for weekly phlebotomy early in treatment to remove about 500 mL of blood per treatment. Maintenance phlebotomies are required about every 3 months for life.[84] Ferritin and/or hemoglobin levels may be monitored.[84] A slightly low hemoglobin (i.e., mild anemia) is sought in the initiation phase and then maintained throughout life. Such monitoring is an easy and inexpensive substitute for iron studies because, as explained in the discussion of IDA, iron stores must be exhausted before anemia develops. The blood removed can be used as donor blood for transfusion under specific circumstances.[94]

Individuals who rely on transfusions to maintain hemoglobin levels and prevent anemia cannot be treated with phlebotomy. Instead, iron-chelating drugs are used to bind excess iron in the body for excretion. Deferoxamine is the classic treatment, although it is not without side effects.[95] The drug typically is administered subcutaneously with an infusion pump over 8 to 12 hours to maximize exposure time for iron binding. When absorbed into the bloodstream with its bound iron, it is readily excreted in the urine. Recently, oral iron chelators have been developed.[96–99] Although they also have side effects, the convenience of oral administration with the potential for improved patient outcomes may lead to a greater reliance on this form of treatment.

DIFFERENTIAL DIAGNOSIS

Differential diagnosis of the iron-related anemias depends on recognition of microcytosis from a low MCV (Figures 16.2 and 16.3).

The pathophysiological approach in this chapter has focused on microcytic anemias resulting from lack of iron or heme for production of hemoglobin. Globin is the third component required for hemoglobin formation, and diminished globin production can result in microcytic anemia also. Therefore the differential diagnosis of the microcytic anemias includes the anemias discussed in this chapter as well as the thalassemias (Chapter 25), which result from impairments in globin synthesis.

Initial evaluation of a microcytic anemia should include the laboratory information from the CBC including indices, reticulocyte count, and iron studies. The degree of anemia can be most significant in thalassemia and iron deficiency; AI usually does not have a hemoglobin value less than 10 g/dL. For all the microcytic anemias, low values are also expected for the MCH and MCHC; however, these indices are not markedly low with AI. Though not diagnostic, the RDW is often wider in IDA than the other conditions (Table 16.4); however, it can narrow later as the condition progresses.

When ferritin is low, the diagnosis of iron deficiency is most clear. Other iron studies meeting the IDA criteria presented in Table 17.1 will confirm the diagnosis as well as a reticulocyte count that correlates with decreased RBC production. CBC changes are proportional to the severity of iron deficiency and lag behind changes in iron studies. On the other hand, an elevated ferritin in the presence of microcytosis may be seen with AI, SAs, or thalassemia. Most likely, the special tests listed in Table 17.1 will be needed to distinguish among them. Care providers may have information about patient or family history that can direct the testing to the most likely of those causes. As mentioned previously, equivocal ferritin levels may need to be clarified by assaying the sTfR level, which rises in iron deficiency.

The time course of the development of anemia is also useful in distinguishing congenital/hereditary conditions from acquired conditions, if the time course is known. In thalassemia, IRIDA, or hereditary SAs, RBCs tend to be small from birth, and anemia is fairly consistent over time. However, iron deficiency and lead poisoning can impact infants, making it a challenge to distinguish them from the hereditary conditions. In older individuals with previously normal hematologic values, one of the acquired iron-related anemias should be considered when microcytic anemia develops. In iron deficiency, the indices fall with progression of the disease and degree of anemia.

As noted earlier, direct care providers typically have access to information that is often not available to medical laboratory staff, for example, the time course of anemia development. Family history may be important to investigate thalassemia or other genetic defects of iron kinetics. Patient history, signs, and symptoms may be important to determine the specific cause of iron deficiency (e.g., source of bleeding) or the presence of a chronic disease or inflammation. As noted earlier, iron studies are critical to distinguish these disorders. Table 17.1 lists laboratory tests that may be necessary and the pattern of results.

SUMMARY

- Impaired iron kinetics or heme metabolism can result in microcytic hypochromic anemias.
- Three conditions affecting iron kinetics can result in microcytic hypochromic anemias: iron deficiency anemia (IDA), anemia of inflammation (AI), and sideroblastic anemias (SAs), especially lead poisoning. The red blood cells (RBCs) in thalassemias also may be microcytic and hypochromic, and this condition must be differentiated from the anemias of disordered iron metabolism.
- Iron deficiency results from inadequate iron intake, increased need, decreased absorption, or excessive loss. All four of these situations create a relative deficit of body iron that over time results in a microcytic hypochromic anemia.
- Infants, children, and women of childbearing age are at greatest risk for IDA. If IDA is present in men and postmenopausal women, the possibility of gastrointestinal bleeding should be investigated because it is the primary, although not the only, cause of iron loss.
- Iron deficiency develops slowly and progresses over three stages. Stage 1 is characterized by the loss of storage iron (decreased ferritin), but hemoglobin and serum iron remain normal. In stage 2 the storage pool of iron has been exhausted and erythropoiesis is impaired. By stage 3, anemia is evident (classically microcytic and hypochromic), and all iron studies are abnormal.
- IDA is suspected when the complete blood count shows microcytic hypochromic RBCs and elevated RBC distribution width but no consistent morphologic abnormality. The diagnosis is confirmed with iron studies showing low levels of serum iron and serum ferritin, elevated total iron-binding capacity (TIBC), and decreased transferrin saturation.
- Inadequate dietary iron is treated by oral supplementation, and with good patient adherence, the anemia should be corrected within 3 months. Gastrointestinal distress resulting from iron supplements can make patient adherence a significant concern. Other causes of iron deficiency must be treated by eliminating the underlying cause or with intravenous iron administration.
- AI is associated with chronic infections, chronic inflammatory conditions, and malignancies. It may be a microcytic hypochromic anemia, but most often it is a mild normocytic normochromic anemia.
- In AI, increased levels of hepcidin, an acute phase reactant, decrease iron absorption in the intestines and sequester iron in macrophages and hepatocytes. Bone marrow macrophages show abundant stainable iron, whereas developing erythroblasts show inadequate iron (iron-restricted erythropoiesis). Inflammatory cellular products also impair the production and action of erythropoietin. RBC life span is shortened.
- Iron studies in AI show decreased serum iron level, decreased TIBC, decreased or normal transferrin saturation, and normal or increased ferritin level.
- Porphyrias are diseases in which porphyrin production is impaired. They can be acquired, such as lead poisoning, or inherited with mutations affecting enzymes in the heme synthetic pathway.
- Three hereditary porphyrias have hematologic manifestations including anemia and fluorescent erythroblasts caused by accumulated porphyrins.
- SAs develop when the synthesis of protoporphyrin or the incorporation of iron into protoporphyrin is blocked. The result is accumulation of iron in the mitochondria of developing erythroblasts. When stained with Prussian blue, the iron appears in deposits around the nucleus of the developing erythroblasts in the bone marrow. These cells are called *ring sideroblasts.*
- Hereditary SAs are quite rare. They include X-linked recessive sideroblastic anemia, Pearson marrow-pancreas syndrome with maternal inheritance, and erythropoietic porphyria with autosomal recessive inheritance.
- Acquired SAs develop due to marrow toxicities from alcohol, drugs, or heavy metals such as lead.
- Protoporphyrin synthesis and iron incorporation into protoporphyrin can be blocked when any of the enzymes of the heme synthetic pathway are deficient or impaired. Deficiencies of these enzymes may be hereditary, as in porphyrias, or acquired, as in heavy metal poisoning. The most common of the latter conditions is lead poisoning is the most common acquired condition.
- Iron studies in SAs show elevated levels of serum iron and serum ferritin, decreased or normal TIBC, and increased transferrin saturation. Test values for the accumulating products of the heme synthetic pathway, such as zinc protoporphyrin or free erythrocyte protoporphyrin, are also elevated.
- Lead interferes with several steps in heme synthesis, preventing iron incorporation into heme and resulting in a normocytic, normochromic anemia, although with long-term exposure it can be microcytic and hypochromic. Lead also impairs the pentose-phosphate shunt, which adds a hemolytic component to the anemia.
- Children are especially vulnerable to the effects of lead on the central nervous system, which may result in irreversible brain damage. Treatment consists of removing the source of lead from the patient's environment and, if necessary, chelating drug therapy to facilitate excretion of lead in the urine. Central nervous system effects are typically not reversed with treatment.
- Because the body has no mechanism for iron excretion, iron overload can occur when transfusions are used to sustain patients with chronic anemias such as β-thalassemia major (called *transfusion-related hemosiderosis*).
- Iron-loading anemias are anemias with erythroid hyperplasia that increases levels of erythroferrone leading to decreased hepcidin, increased ferroportin activity, and increased iron absorption.
- A defective hereditary hemochromatosis (HH) protein gene can lead to HH by decreased hepcidin production. Affected men develop symptoms earlier in life than women; homozygotes develop more severe disease than heterozygotes.
- Mutations of other genes affecting iron regulation can produce a phenotype similar to that of HH. When the hepcidin or hemojuvelin gene is mutated, the disease develops early in life, affecting even teenagers.

- Free iron becomes available in cells when ferritin and hemosiderin become saturated. Free iron causes tissue damage by creating free radicals that lead to cell membrane damage and perhaps mutations. The liver, pancreas, skin, and heart muscle are especially vulnerable to damage by excess iron deposition.
- Elevated transferrin saturation or serum ferritin can be an indicator of hemochromatosis that can be diagnosed fully using genetic testing to identify mutated genes.

- HH and similar diseases are treated by lifelong periodic phlebotomy to induce a mild IDA and keep body iron levels low. Transfusion-related hemosiderosis must be treated with iron-chelating drugs.

Now that you have completed this chapter, go back and read again the case study at the beginning and respond to the questions presented. Answers can be found in Appendix C.

REVIEW QUESTIONS

Answers can be found in Appendix C.

1. Below are the results of a complete blood count (CBC) and iron studies for a 28-year-old woman.
   CBC: all results within reference intervals except the RDW, which was 15%.
   Serum iron: decreased
   Total iron binding capacity (TIBC): increased
   % transferrin saturation: decreased
   Serum ferritin: decreased
   What can you conclude?
   a. The results of the iron studies reveal findings consistent with a thalassemia that was apparently previously undiagnosed.
   b. The patient is in stage 2 of iron deficiency, before frank anemia develops.
   c. The results of the iron studies are inconsistent with the CBC results, and a laboratory error should be suspected.
   d. There is no evidence of a hematologic explanation for the patient's symptoms.

2. A bone marrow biopsy was performed as part of the cancer staging protocol for a patient with Hodgkin lymphoma. Although no evidence of spread of the tumor was apparent in the bone marrow, other abnormal findings were noted, including a slightly elevated myeloid-to-erythroid ratio. White blood cell (WBC) count and red blood cell (RBC) morphology appeared normal, however. The Prussian blue stain showed abundant stainable iron in the marrow macrophages. The patient's CBC revealed a hemoglobin of 10.8 g/dL, but RBC indices were within reference intervals. RBC morphology was unremarkable. These findings are consistent with:
   a. Anemia of inflammation
   b. Sideroblastic anemia
   c. Thalassemia
   d. Iron deficiency anemia

3. Predict the iron study results for the patient with Hodgkin lymphoma described in question 2.

4. A 35-year-old woman presented to her health care provider complaining of headaches, dizziness, and nausea. The headaches had been increasing in severity over the past 6 months. This was coincident with her move into an older house, built about 1900. She had been renovating the house, including stripping paint from the woodwork. Her complete blood count (CBC) results showed a mild microcytic hypochromic anemia, with polychromasia and basophilic stippling noted. Which of the following tests would be most useful in confirming the cause of her anemia?
   a. Serum lead level
   b. Serum iron level and total iron-binding capacity (TIBC)
   c. Absolute reticulocyte count
   d. Prussian blue staining of the bone marrow to detect iron stores in macrophages

5. In men and postmenopausal women whose diets are adequate, iron deficiency anemia (IDA) most often results from:
   a. Increased need associated with aging
   b. Impaired absorption in the gastric mucosa
   c. Chronic gastrointestinal bleeding
   d. Diminished resistance to hookworm infections

6. Which one of the following individuals is at greatest risk for the development of iron deficiency anemia (IDA)?
   a. A 15-year-old boy who eats mainly junk food
   b. A 37-year-old woman who has never been pregnant and has amenorrhea
   c. A 63-year-old man with reactivation of tuberculosis from his childhood
   d. A 40-year-old man who lost blood during surgery to repair a fractured leg

7. Which of the following individuals is at the greatest risk for the development of anemia of inflammation?
   a. A 15-year-old girl with asthma
   b. A 40-year-old woman with type 2 diabetes mellitus
   c. A 65-year-old man with hypertension
   d. A 30-year-old man with severe rheumatoid arthritis

8. In what situation will increased levels of free erythrocyte protoporphyrin be present?
   a. Loss-of-function mutation to one of the enzymes in the heme synthesis pathway
   b. A mutation that prevents heme attachment to globin so that protoporphyrin remains free
   c. Any condition that prevents iron incorporation into protoporphyrin IX
   d. When red blood cells lyse, freeing their contents into the plasma

	Serum Iron Level	TIBC	% Transferrin Saturation	Serum Ferritin Level
a.	Decreased	Increased	Decreased	Decreased
b.	Increased	Normal	Increased	Normal
c.	Increased	Increased	Normal	Increased
d.	Decreased	Decreased	Normal	Normal

9. In the pathogenesis of the anemia of inflammation (AI), hepcidin levels:
   a. Decrease during inflammation and reduce iron absorption from enterocytes
   b. Increase during inflammation and reduce iron absorption from enterocytes
   c. Increase during inflammation and increase iron absorption from enterocytes
   d. Decrease during inflammation and increase iron absorption from enterocytes

10. Choose an answer below to complete the following sentence: Sideroblastic anemias (SAs) result from:
    a. Sequestration of iron in hepatocytes
    b. Inability to incorporate heme into apohemoglobin
    c. Sequestration of iron in myeloblasts
    d. Impairments to the use of iron within mitochondria

11. In general, most instances of hereditary hemochromatosis (HH) result from mutations that impair:
    a. The manner in which developing red blood cells (RBCs) acquire and manage iron
    b. The hepcidin-ferroportin iron regulatory system
    c. The transferrin receptor-transferrin (TfR-Tf) endocytic iron acquisition process for body cells other than RBCs
    d. The function of divalent metal transporter (DMT) in enterocytes and macrophages

12. In erythropoietic porphyrias, mild anemia may be accompanied by what distinctive clinical finding?
    a. Gallstones
    b. Impaired night vision
    c. Unintentional nighttime leg movements
    d. Heightened propensity for sunburn

13. A provider is concerned that a patient is developing iron deficiency from chronic intestinal bleeding caused by aspirin use for rheumatoid arthritis. The iron studies on the patient indicate the following results:

Laboratory Assay	Adult Reference Intervals	Patient Values
Serum ferritin level	12–400 ng/mL	32 ng/mL
Serum iron level	50–160 µg/dL	45 µg/dL
TIBC	250–400 µg/dL	405 µg/dL
Transferrin saturation	20%–55%	11%

How would these results be interpreted?
    a. Latent iron deficiency
    b. Functional iron deficiency
    c. Iron deficiency
    d. Equivocal for iron deficiency

14. For a patient with screening iron study values that are equivocal for iron deficiency, which of the following tests would be most helpful in determining whether iron deficiency is present or not?
    a. Zinc protoporphyrin
    b. Peripheral blood iron stain
    c. Soluble transferrin receptor
    d. Mean cell hemoglobin

Also review Chapter 9, questions 4, 10, 11, and 12, which are pertinent to the diagnostic value of various tests of iron status.

REFERENCES

1. World Health Organization. (2011). Serum ferritin concentrations for the assessment of iron status and iron deficiency in populations. Vitamin and Mineral Nutrition Information System. Geneva: World Health Organization; Publication No. WHO/NMH/NHD/MNM/11.2 https://www.who.int/vmnis/indicators/serum_ferritin.pdf. Accessed April 1, 2022.
2. Hallberg, L. (1981). Bioavailability of dietary iron in man. *Annu Rev Nutr, 1,* 123–147.
3. Kim, A., & Nemeth, E. (2015). New insights into iron regulation and erythropoiesis. *Curr Opin Hematol, 22*(3), 199–205.
4. Nai, A., Lidonnici, M. R., Rausa, M., et al. (2015). The second transferrin receptor regulates red blood cell production in mice. *Blood, 125*(7), 1170–1179.
5. Silvestri, L., Guillem, F., Pagani, A., et al. (2009). Molecular mechanisms of the defective hepcidin inhibition in TMPRSS6 mutations associated with iron-refractory iron deficiency anemia. *Blood, 113*(22), 5605–5608.
6. Suominen, P., Punnonen, K., Rajamaki, A., et al. (1998). Serum transferrin receptor and transferrin receptor-ferritin index identify healthy subjects with subclinical iron deficits. *Blood, 92,* 2934–2939.
7. Gupta, P. M., Hammer, H. C., Suchdev, P. S., et al. (2017). Iron status of toddlers, non-pregnant females, and pregnant females in the United States. *Am J Clin Nutr, 106*(Suppl 6), 1640S–1646S.
8. Rolfs, A., Kvietikova, I., Gassmann, M., et al. (1997). Oxygen-regulated transferrin expression is mediated by hypoxia-inducible factor-1. *J Biol Chem, 272*(32), 20055–20062.
9. Frise, M. C., & Robbins, P. A. (2015). Iron, oxygen, and the pulmonary circulation. *J Appl Physiol, 119*(12), 1421–1431.
10. Buttarello, M., Pajola, R., Novello, E., et al. (2016). Evaluation of the hypochromic erythrocyte and reticulocyte hemoglobin content provided by the Sysmex XE-5000 analyzer in diagnosis of iron deficiency erythropoiesis. *Clin Chem Lab Med, 54*(12), 1939–1945.
11. Urrechaga, E., Borque, L., & Escanero, J. F. (2016). Clinical value of hypochromia markers in the detection of latent iron deficiency in nonanemic premenopausal women. *J Clin Lab Anal, 30,* 623–627.
12. Stohlman Jr., F., Howard, D., & Beland, A. (1963). Humoral regulation of erythropoiesis. XII. Effect of erythropoietin and iron on cell size in iron deficiency anemia. *Proc Soc Exp Biol Med, 113,* 986–998.
13. de Klerk, G., Rosengarten, P. C. J., Vet, R. J. M., et al. (1981). Serum erythropoietin (ESF) titers in anemia. *Blood, 58*(6), 1164–1170.
14. Goodnough, L. & Nemeth, E. (2019). Iron deficiency and related disorders. In Greer, J. P., Arber, D. A., Glader, B. E., et al. (Eds), *Wintrobe's Clinical Hematology.* (14th ed, pp 1804–1883). Philadelphia: Wolters Kluwer.
15. McMahon, L. P. (2010). Iron deficiency in pregnancy. *Obstet Med, 3*(1), 17–24.

16. Saarinen, U. M., Siimes, M. A., & Dallman, P. R. (1977). Iron absorption in infants: high bioavailability of breast milk iron as indicated by the extrinsic tag method of iron absorption and by the concentration of serum ferritin. *J Pediatr, 91,* 36–39.

17. Siimes, M. A., Vuori, E., & Kuitunen, P. (1979). Breast milk iron: a declining concentration during the course of lactation. *Acta Paediatr Scand, 68,* 29–31.

18. Burden, R.J., Pollock, N., Whyte, G.P., et al. (2015). Effect of intravenous iron on aerobic capacity and iron metabolism in elite athletes. *Med Sci Sports Exerc, 47*(7), 1399–1407.

19. Coates, A., Mountjoy, M., & Burr, J. (2017). Incidence of iron deficiency and iron deficient anemia in elite runners and triathletes. *Clin J Sport Med, 27* (5), 493–498.

20. Wouthuyzen-Bakker, M., & van Assen, S. (2015). Exercise-induced anaemia: a forgotten cause of iron deficiency aneamia in young adults. *Br J Gen Pract, 65*(634), 268–269.

21. Janakiraman, K., Shenoy, S., & Sandhu, J. S. (2011). Intravascular haemolysis during prolonged running on asphalt and natural grass in long and middle distance runners. *J Sports Sci, 29*(12), 1287–1292.

22. Lippi, G., Schena, F., Salvagno, G. L., et al. (2012). Foot-strike haemolysis after a 60-km ultramarathon. *Blood Transfus, 10*(3), 377–383.

23. Thompson, W. G., Meola, T., Lipkin, M., Jr., et al. (1988). Red cell distribution width, mean corpuscular volume, and transferrin saturation in the diagnosis of iron deficiency. *Arch Intern Med, 148,* 2128–2130.

24. McClure, S., Custer, E., & Bessman, J. D. (1985). Improved detection of early iron deficiency in nonanemic subjects. *JAMA, 253,* 1021–1023.

25. Song, A. B., Kuter, D. J., Al-Samkari, H. (2020). Characterization of the rate, predictors, and thrombotic complications of thrombocytosis in iron deficiency anemia. *Am J Hematol, 95*(10), 1180–1186.

26. Xavier-Ferrucio, J., Scanlon, V., Li, X., et al. (2019). Low iron promotes megakaryocytic commitment of megakaryocytic-erythroid progenitors in humans and mice. *Blood, 134*(18), 1547–1557.

27. Brugnara, C., Schiller, B., & Moran, J. (2006). Reticulocyte hemoglobin equivalent (Ret He) and assessment of iron deficient states. *Clin Lab Haem, 29,* 303–306.

28. Cox, L. A., & Adrian, G. S. (1993). Postranscriptional regulation of chimeric human transferrin genes by iron. *Biochemistry, 32,* 4738–4745.

29. Bouri, S., & Martin, J. (2018). Investigation of iron deficiency anaemia. *Clin Med (Lond), 18*(3), 242–244.

30. Roccaforte, V., Daves, M., Lippi, G., et al. (2020). Preliminary assessment of the new Sysmex XN parameter Iron-Def for identifying iron deficiency. *Blood Transfus, 18*(5), 406–412.

31. Urrechaga, E., Borque, L., & Escanero, J.F. (2013). Biomarkers of hypochromia: the contemporary assessment of iron status and erythropoiesis. *Biomed Res Int, 2013,* 603786.

32. Hoffmann, J. J. M. L., Urrechaga, E., & Aguirre, U. (2015). Discriminant indices for distinguishing thalassemia and iron deficiency in patients with microcytic anemia: a meta-analysis. *Clin Chem Lab Med, 53*(12), 1883–1894.

33. Lamola, A. A., Joselow, M., & Yamane, T. (1975). Zinc protoporphyrin (ZPP): a simple, sensitive fluorometric screening test for lead poisoning. *Clin Chem, 21,* 93–97.

34. Huebers, H. A., Beguin, Y., Pootrakul, P., et al. (1990). Intact transferrin receptors in human plasma and their relation to erythropoiesis. *Blood, 75,* 102–107.

35. O'Sullivan, D. J., Higgins, P. G., & Wilkinson, J. F. (1955). Oral iron compounds: a therapeutic comparison. *Lancet, 2,* 482–485.

36. Abu Hashim, H., Foda, O., & Ghayaty, E. (2017). Lactoferrin or ferrous salts for iron deficiency anemia in pregnancy: a meta-analysis of randomized trials. *Eur J Obstet Gynecol Reprod Biol, 219,* 45–52.

37. Lepanto, M. S., Rosa, L., Cutone, A., et al. (2018). Efficacy of lactoferrin oral administration in the treatment of anemia and anemia of inflammation in pregnant and non-pregnant women: an interventional study. *Front Immunol, 9,* 2123.

38. El Amrousy, D., El-Afify, D., Elsawy, A., et al. (2022). Lactoferrin for iron-deficiency anemia in children with inflammatory bowel disease: a clinical trial. *Pediatr Res,* https://doi.org/10.1038/s41390-022-02136-2.

39. Abdulrehman, J., Tang, G. H., Auerbach, M., et al. (2019). The safety and efficacy of ferumoxytol in the treatment of iron deficiency: a systematic review and meta-analysis. *Transfusion, 59*(12), 3646–3656.

40. Swan, H. T., & Jowett, G. H. (1959). Treatment of iron deficiency with ferrous fumarate: assessment by a statistically accurate method. *BMJ, 2,* 782–787.

41. Cartwright, G. E. (1966). The anemia of chronic disorders. *Semin Hematol, 3,* 351–375.

42. Sears, D. A. (1992). Anemia of chronic disease. *Med Clin North Am, 76,* 567–579.

43. Poggiali, E., De Amicis, M. M., & Motta, I. (2014). Anemia of chronic disease: a unique defect of iron recycling for many different chronic diseases. *Euro J Int Med, 25,* 12–17.

44. Nemeth, E., Tuttle, M. S., Powelson, J., et al. (2004). Hepcidin regulates iron efflux by binding to ferroportin and inducing its internalization. *Science, 306,* 2090–2093.

45. Rivera, S., Liu, L., Nemeth, E., et al. (2005). Hepcidin excess induces the sequestration of iron and exacerbates tumor-associated anemia. *Blood, 105,* 1797–1802.

46. Nicolas, G., Bennoun, M., Devaux, I., et al. (2001). Lack of hepcidin gene expression and severe tissue iron overload in upstream stimulatory factor 2 (USF2) knockout mice. *Proc Natl Acad Sci U S A, 98,* 8780–8785.

47. Nicolas, G., Chauvet, C., Viatte, L., et al. (2002). The gene encoding the iron regulatory peptide hepcidin is regulated by anemia, hypoxia, and inflammation. *J Clin Invest, 110,* 1037–1044.

48. Wang, C. Y., & Babitt, J. L. (2016). Regulation in the anemia of inflammation. *Curr Opin Hematol, 23*(3), 189–197.

49. Ganz, T., & Nemeth, E. (2015). Iron homeostasis in host defense and inflammation. *Nat Rev Immunol, 15,* 500–510.

50. Masson, P. L., Heremans, J. F., & Schonne, E. (1969). Lactoferrin: an iron binding protein in neutrophilic leukocytes. *J Exp Med, 130,* 643–658.

51. Cutone, A., Rosa, L., Lepanto M. S., et al. (2017). Lactoferrin efficiently counteracts the inflammation-induced changes of the iron homeostasis system in macrophages. *Front Immunol, 8,* 705.

52. Akilesh, H. M., Buechler, M. B., Duggan, J. M., et al. (2019). Chronic TLR7 and TLR9 signaling drives anemia via differentiation of specialized hemophagocytes. *Science, 363*(6423), https://doi.org/10.1126/science.aao5213.

53. Moldawer, L. L., Marano, M. A., Wei, H., et al. (1989). Cachectin/tumor necrosis factor-alpha alters red blood cell kinetics and induces anemia in vivo. *FASEB J, 3*(5), 1637–1643.

54. Libregts, S. F., Gutiérrez, L., de Bruin, A. M., et al. (2011). Chronic IFN-γ production in mice induces anemia by reducing erythrocyte life span and inhibiting erythropoiesis through an IRF-1/PU.1 axis. *Blood, 118*(9), 2578–2588.

55. Mitlyng, B. L., Singh, J. A., Furne, J. K., et al. (2006). Use of breath carbon monoxide measurements to assess erythrocyte survival in subjects with chronic diseases. *Am J Hematol,81*(6), 432–438.

56. Weiss G., & Goodnough L, T. (2005). Anemia of chronic disease. *N Engl J Med.,352*(10), 1011–1023.

57. Mast, A. E., Blinder, M. A., Gronowski, A. M., et al. (1998). Clinical utility of the soluble transferrin receptor and comparison with serum ferritin in several populations. *Clin Chem, 44*, 45–51.

58. Castel, R., Tax, M. G., Droogendijk, J., et al. (2012). The transferrin/log(ferritin) ratio: a new tool for the diagnosis of iron deficiency anemia. *Clin Chem Lab Med, 50*, 1343–1349.

59. Thomas, C., & Thomas, L. (2002). Biochemical markers and hematologic indices in the diagnosis of functional iron deficiency. *Clin Chem, 48*, 1066–1076.

60. Leers, M. P. G., Keuren, J. F. W., & Oosterhuis, W. P. (2010). The value of the Thomas-plot in the diagnostic work up of anemic patients referred by general practitioners. *Int J Lab Hemat, 32*, 572–581.

61. Pincus, T., Olsen, N. J., Russell, I. J., et al. (1990). Multicenter study of recombinant human erythropoietin in correction of anemia in rheumatoid arthritis. *Am J Med, 89*, 161–168.

62. Arndt, U., Kaltwasser, J. P., Gottschalk, R., et al. (2005). Correction of iron-deficient erythropoiesis in the treatment of anemia of chronic disease with recombinant human erythropoietin. *Ann Hematol, 84*, 159–166.

63. Petzer, V., Theurl, I., & Weiss, G. (2018). Established and emerging concepts to treat imbalances of iron homeostasis in inflammatory diseases. *Pharmaceuticals, 11*(4):135. https://doi.org/10.3390/ph11040135

64. Malyszko, J., Malyszko, J.S., & Matuszkiewicz-Rowinska, J. (2019). Hepcidin as a therapeutic target for anemia and inflammation associated with chronic kidney disease. *Expert Opin Ther Targets, 23*(5), 407–421.

65. Bessis, M. C., & Jensen, W. N. (1965). Sideroblastic anaemia, mitochondria and erythroblastic iron. *Brit. J Haematol, 11*, 49–51.

66. Ducamp, S., & Fleming, M. D. (2019). The molecular genetics of sideroblastic anemia. *Blood, 133*(1), 59–69.

67. Horrigan, D. L., & Harris, J. W. (1964). Pyridoxine responsive anemia: analysis of 62 cases. *Adv Intern Med, 12*, 103–174.

68. Gagne, K. E., Ghazvinian, R., Yuan, D., et al. (2014). Pearson marrow pancreas syndrome in patients suspected to have Diamond-Blackfan anemia. *Blood, 124*(3), 437–440.

69. Verwilghen, R., Reybrouck, G., Callens, L., et al. (1965). Antituberculosis drugs and sideroblastic anaemia. *Br J Haematol, 11*, 92–98.

70. Sanburn J. (2016). The toxic tap. *Time, 187*(3), 32–39.

71. Fedinick, K. P. Millions served by water systems detecting lead. National Resources Defense Council. https://www.nrdc.org/resources/millions-served-water-systems-detecting-lead. Accessed May 28, 2022.

72. Hanna-Attisha, M., Lanphear, B., & Landrigan, P. (2018). Lead poisoning in the 21st century: the silent epidemic continues. *Am J Public Health, 108*(11), 1430.

73. Benson, P. (1965). Lead poisoning in children. *Dev Med Child Neurol, 7*(5), 569–571.

74. Campbell, A. M., & Williams, E. R. (1968). Chronic lead intoxication mimicking motor neurone disease. *BMJ, 4*(5630), 582.

75. Granick, S., Sassa, S., Granick, J. L., et al. (1972). Assays for porphyrins, delta-aminolevulinic acid dehydratase, and porphyrinogen synthetase in microliter samples of blood: application to metabolic defects involving the heme pathway. *Proc Natl Acad Sci U S A, 69*, 2381–2385.

76. Lachant, N. A., Tomoda, A., & Tanaka, K. R. (1984). Inhibition of the pentose phosphate shunt by lead: a potential mechanism for hemolysis in lead poisoning. *Blood, 63*, 518–524.

77. Sample, J.A. Childhood lead poisoning: Management. *UpToDate.* https://www.uptodate.com/contents/childhood-lead-poisoning-management. Accessed July 6, 2022.

78. Valentine, W. N., Paglia, D. E., Fink, K., et al. (1976). Lead poisoning. Association with hemolytic anemia, basophilic stippling, erythrocyte pyrimidine 5'-nucleotidase deficiency, and intraerythrocytic accumulation of pyrimidines. *J Clin Invest, 58*, 926–932.

79. Knollmann-Ritschel, B. E. C., & Markowitz, M. (2017). Lead poisoning. *Acad Pathol, 4*, 1–3.

80. Martin, C. J., Wentz III, C. L., & Ducatman, A. M. (2004). The interpretation of zinc protoporphyrin changes in lead intoxication: a case report and review of the literature. *Occ Med, 54*, 587–591.

81. Feder, J. N., Gnirke, A., Thomas, W., et al. (1996). A novel MHC class I-like gene is mutated in patients with hereditary haemochromatosis. *Nat Genet, 13*, 399–408.

82. Waheed, A., Parkkila, S., Zhou, X. Y., et al. (1997). Hereditary hemochromatosis: effect of C282Y and H63D mutations on association with β2-microglobulin, intracellular processing, and cell surface expression of the HFE protein in COS-7 cells. *Proc Natl Acad Sci U S A, 94*, 12384–12389.

83. Brissot, P., Bardou-Jacquet, E., Troadec, M. B., et al. (2010). Molecular diagnosis of genetic iron-overload disorders. *Expert Rev Mol Diagn, 10*, 755–763.

84. Edwards, C. Q., & Barton, J. C. (2019). Hemochromatosis. In Greer, J. P., Rodgers, G. M., Glader, B. E., et al. (Eds.), *Wintrobe's Clinical Hematology.* (14th ed., pp. 665–690). Philadelphia: Wolters Kluwer.

85. Beutler, E. (2003). The *HFE* Cys282Tyr mutation as a necessary but not sufficient cause of clinical hereditary hemochromatosis. *Blood, 101*, 3347–3350.

86. Vautier, G., Bomford, A. B., Portmann, B. C., et al. (1999). p53 mutations in British patients with hepatocellular carcinoma: clustering in genetic hemochromatosis. *Gastroenterology, 117*, 154–160.

87. Hussain, S. P., Schwank, J., Staib, F., et al. (2007). TP53 mutations and hepatocellular carcinoma: insights into the etiology and pathogenesis of liver cancer. *Oncogene, 26*(15), 166–176.

88. Hussain, S. P., Raja, K., Amstad, P. A., et al. (2000). Increased p53 mutation load in nontumorous human liver of Wilson disease and hemochromatosis: oxyradical overload diseases. *Proc Natl Acad Sci U S A, 97*, 12770–12775.

89. Niederau, C., Strohmeyer, G., & Stremmel, W. (1996). Long term survival in patients with hereditary hemochromatosis. *Gastroenterology, 110*, 1107–1119.

90. Bothwell, T. H., & MacPhail, A. P. (1998). Hereditary hemochromatosis: etiologic, pathologic, and clinical aspects. *Semin Hematol, 35*, 55–71.

91. Kane, S. F., Roberts, C., & Paulus, R. (2021). Hereditary hemochromatosis: rapid evidence review. *Am Fam Physician, 104*(3), 263–270.

92. Nadakkavukaran, I. M., Gan, E. K., & Olynyk, J. K. (2012). Screening for hereditary haemochromatosis. *Pathology, 44*, 148–152.

93. Qi, X., Liu, X., Zhang, Y., et al. (2016). Serum liver fibrosis markers in the prognosis of liver cirrhosis: a prospective observational study. *Med Sci Monit, 22*, 2720–2730.

94. Donor eligibility requirements specific to whole blood, red blood cells and plasma collected by apheresis. Subsection (2) Therapeutic phlebotomy. Code of Federal Regulation. Title 21/Chapter 1/Subchapter F/Part 630/ Subpart B/§630.15. https://www.ecfr.gov/current/title-21/chapter-I/subchapter-F/part-630/subpart-B/section-630.15. Accessed July 6, 2022.

95. Jeng, M., & Neufeld E. (2019). Thalassemia syndromes: quantitative disorders of globin chain synthesis. In Greer, J. P., Rodgers, G. M., Glader, B., et al. (Eds.), *Wintrobe's Clinical Hematology*. (14th ed., pp. 866–914). Philadelphia: Wolters Kluwer.

96. Cappellini, M. D., & Pattoneri, P. (2009). Oral iron chelators. *Annu Rev Med, 60,* 25–38.

97. Imran, F., & Phatak, P. (2009). Pharmacoeconomic benefits of deferasirox in the management of iron overload syndromes. Expert Rev Pharmacoecon *Outcomes Res, 9,* 297–304.

98. Elalfy, M. S., Adly, A. M., Wali, Y., et al. (2015). Efficacy and safety of a novel combination of two oral chelators deferasirox/deferiprone over deferoxamine/deferiprone in severely iron overloaded young beta thalassemia major patients. *Eur J Haematol, 95*(5), 411–420.

99. Hruby, M., Martínez, I. I. S., Stephan, H., et al. (2021). Chelators for treatment of iron and copper overload: shift from low-molecular-weight compounds to polymers. *Polymers, 13*(22), 3696.

18

Anemias Caused by Defects of DNA Metabolism

Tara Cothran Moon*

OBJECTIVES

After completion of this chapter, the reader will be able to:

1. Discuss the relationships among macrocytic anemia, megaloblastic anemia, and pernicious anemia, and classify anemias appropriately within these categories.
2. Discuss the physiologic roles of folate and vitamin B_{12} in deoxyribonucleic acid (DNA) production and the general metabolic pathways in which they act.
3. Describe the absorption and distribution of vitamin B_{12}, including carrier proteins and the biologic activity of various vitamin-carrier complexes.
4. Describe the biochemical basis for development of anemia with deficiencies of vitamin B_{12} and folate, and explain the cause of the accompanying megaloblastosis.
5. Recognize individuals at risk for megaloblastic anemia by virtue of age; dietary habits; or physiologic circumstance, such as pregnancy, drug regimens, or pathologic conditions.
6. Recognize complete blood count, reticulocyte count, red and white blood cell morphologies, and bone marrow findings consistent with megaloblastic anemia.
7. Correlate patient laboratory and clinical data with additional findings (e.g., serum vitamin B_{12}, serum methylmalonic acid, serum folate, plasma or serum homocysteine, and antibodies to intrinsic factor) and determine the likely cause of a patient's deficiency.
8. Recognize results of bilirubin and lactate dehydrogenase tests that are consistent with megaloblastic anemia and explain why the test values are elevated in this condition.

OUTLINE

Etiology
    Physiologic Roles of Vitamin B_{12} and Folate
    Defect in Megaloblastic Anemia Caused by Deficiency in Folate and Vitamin B_{12}
    Other Causes of Megaloblastosis
Systemic Manifestations of Folate and Vitamin B_{12} Deficiency

Causes of Vitamin Deficiencies
    Folate Deficiency
    Vitamin B_{12} Deficiency
Laboratory Diagnosis
    Screening Tests
    Specific Diagnostic Tests
Macrocytic Nonmegaloblastic Anemias
Treatment

CASE STUDY

After studying the material in this chapter, the reader should be able to respond to the following case study. Answers can be found in Appendix C.

During a holiday visit, the children noticed that their 76-year-old father seemed more forgetful than usual and had difficulty walking. Concerned about the possibility of a mild stroke, the children encouraged their father to set up an appointment with a provider. The provider diagnosed peripheral neuropathy affecting the patient's ability to walk. In addition, the physician noted that the patient was pale and slightly jaundiced and ordered a complete blood count (CBC). The CBC yielded the following results. Reference intervals can be found after the Index at the end of the book.

WBC	3.2×10^9/L	MCH	38 pg
RBC	2.22×10^{12}/L	MCHC	32 g/dL
HGB	8.5 g/dL	RDW	18.0%
HCT	27%	PLT	115×10^9/L
MCV	122 fL	RETIC	1.8%

WBC differential was unremarkable with the exception of hypersegmentation of neutrophils.

RBC morphology showed moderate anisocytosis, moderate poikilocytosis, macrocytes, oval macrocytes, few teardrop cells.

Because of these findings, additional tests were ordered, with the following results:

Serum vitamin B_{12} was decreased.

Serum folate was within reference interval.

Serum methylmalonic acid was increased.

1. Which of the CBC findings led the provider to order the vitamin assays?
2. Is the patient's reticulocyte response adequate to compensate for the anemia?
3. Based on the available test results, what can you conclude about the cause of the patient's anemia?
4. What additional testing would be helpful to diagnose the specific cause of this patient's anemia?

The author extends appreciation to Linda H. Goossen, whose work in prior editions provided the foundation for this chapter.

Impaired deoxyribonucleic acid (DNA) metabolism causes systemic effects by impairing production of all rapidly dividing cells of the body. These are chiefly the cells of the skin, the epithelium of the gastrointestinal tract, and the hematopoietic tissues. Because all these must be replenished throughout life, any impairment of cell production is evident in these tissues first. Patients may experience symptoms in any of these systems, but the blood provides a ready tissue for analysis. The hematologic effects, especially megaloblastic anemia, have come to be recognized as the hallmark of diseases affecting DNA metabolism.

ETIOLOGY

The root cause of megaloblastic anemia is impaired DNA synthesis. The anemia is named for the very large cells of the bone marrow that develop a distinctive morphology (discussed in "Laboratory Diagnosis") because of a reduction in the number of cell divisions. Megaloblastic anemia is one example of a macrocytic anemia. Box 18.1 shows the classification of macrocytic anemias. Understanding the cause of megaloblastic anemia requires a review of DNA synthesis with particular attention to the roles of vitamin B_{12} (cobalamin) and folic acid (folate).

Physiologic Roles of Vitamin B_{12} and Folate

Vitamin B_{12} (cobalamin) is an essential nutrient consisting of a tetrapyrrole (corrin) ring containing cobalt that is attached to 5,6-dimethylbenzimidazolyl ribonucleotide. It has various analogues including hydroxycobalamin and cyanocobalamin (forms often found in food and supplements) and coenzyme forms, methylcobalamin and 5′-deoxyadenosylcobalamin (Figure 18.1). Vitamin B_{12} is a coenzyme in two biochemical reactions in humans. One is isomerization of methylmalonyl coenzyme A (CoA) to succinyl CoA, which requires vitamin B_{12} (in the deoxyadenosylcobalamin form) as a cofactor and is catalyzed by the enzyme methylmalonyl CoA mutase (Figure 18.2). In the absence of vitamin B_{12}, the impaired activity of methylmalonyl CoA mutase leads to a high level of serum methylmalonic acid (MMA), which is useful for the diagnosis of vitamin B_{12} deficiency (discussed in "Laboratory Diagnosis"). The second reaction is the transfer of a methyl group from 5-methyltetrahydrofolate (5-methyl THF) to homocysteine, thereby generating methionine. This reaction is catalyzed by the enzyme methionine synthase and uses vitamin B_{12} (in the methylcobalamin form) as a coenzyme (discussed later in this section). Methylcobalamin is synthesized through reduction and methylation of vitamin B_{12}. This reaction represents the link between folate and vitamin B_{12} coenzymes and appears to account for the requirement for both vitamins in normal erythropoiesis.[1,2]

Folate is the general term used for any form of the vitamin folic acid. Folic acid is the synthetic form in supplements and fortified food. Folates consist of a pteridine ring attached to paraaminobenzoate with one or more glutamate residues (Figure 18.3). The function of folate is to transfer carbon units in the form of methyl groups from donors to receptors. In this capacity, folate plays an important role in the metabolism of amino acids and nucleotides. Deficiency of the vitamin leads to impaired cell replication and other metabolic alterations.

BOX 18.1   Classification of Macrocytic Anemias by Cause

Megaloblastic Anemia
Folate deficiency
   Inadequate intake
   Increased need
   Impaired absorption (e.g., inflammatory bowel disease)
   Impaired use due to drugs
   Excessive loss with renal dialysis
Vitamin B_{12} deficiency
   Inadequate intake
   Increased need
   Impaired absorption
      Failure to split from food
      Failure to split from haptocorrin
      Gastrectomy and gastritis
      Medications (e.g., proton pump inhibitors, metformin, nitrous oxide)
      Lack of intrinsic factor
         Pernicious anemia
         Helicobacter pylori infection
         Gastrectomy
         Hereditary intrinsic factor deficiency
      General malabsorption (e.g., inflammatory bowel disease)
      Inherited errors in absorption or transport
         Imerslund-Gräsbeck syndrome
         Transcobalamin deficiency
      Competition for the vitamin
         Diphyllobothrium latum (fish tapeworm) infection
      Blind loop syndrome
Other causes of megaloblastosis
   Myelodysplastic neoplasm
   Congenital dyserythropoietic anemia
   Certain drugs (chemotherapeutics, antiretroviral, etc., e.g., azathioprine, zidovudine)

Macrocytic, Nonmegaloblastic Anemias
Normal newborn status
Reticulocytosis
Liver disease
Chronic alcoholism
Bone marrow failure

Folate circulates in the blood predominantly as 5-methyl THF.[3] 5-Methyl THF is metabolically inactive until it is demethylated to tetrahydrofolate (THF), whereupon folate-dependent reactions may take place.

Folate has an important role in DNA synthesis. As seen in Figure 18.4, within the cytoplasm of the cell, a methyl group is transferred from 5-methyl THF to homocysteine, which converts it to methionine and generates THF. This reaction is catalyzed by the enzyme methionine synthase and requires vitamin B_{12} in the form of methylcobalamin as a cofactor. THF is then converted to 5,10-methylenetetrahydrofolate (5,10-methylene THF); the methyl group for this reaction comes from serine as it is converted to glycine. The methyl group of 5,10-methylene THF is then transferred to deoxyuridine monophosphate (dUMP), which converts it to deoxythymidine monophosphate (dTMP). This reaction is catalyzed by thymidylate synthase and results in the conversion of 5,10-methylene THF to

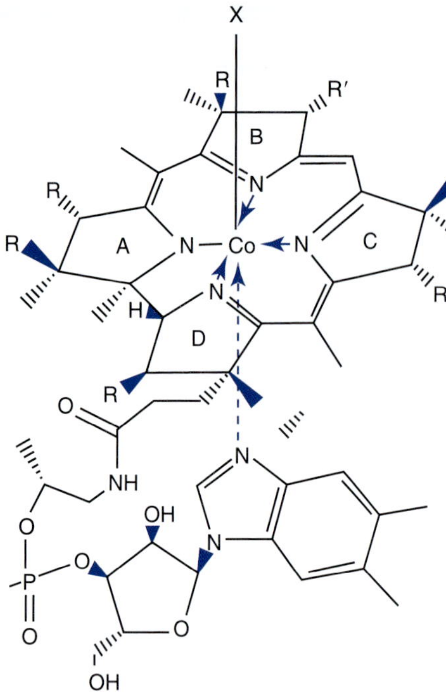

Figure 18.1 Structure of Vitamin B$_{12}$ (Cobalamin) and Its Analogs. The basic structure of cobalamin includes a tetrapyrrole (corrin) ring with a central cobalt atom linked to 5,6-dimethylbenzimidazolyl ribonucleotide. Hydroxycobalamin and cyanocobalamin are forms often found in food and supplements and methylcobalamin and 5′-deoxyadenosylcobalamin are coenzyme forms. (From Scott, J. M., & Browne, P. [2006]. Megaloblastic anemia. In Caballero, B., Allen, L., & Prentice, A. [Eds.], *Encyclopedia of Human Nutrition.* [2nd ed., p. 113]. Oxford: Academic Press.)

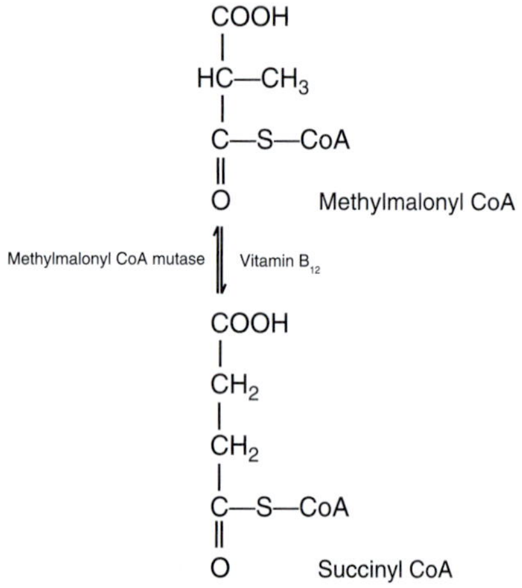

X = {
OH: hydroxycobalamin
CH$_3$: methylcobalamin
Ado: 5′-deoxyadenosylcobalamin
CN: cyanocobalamin
}

Figure 18.2 Role of Vitamin B$_{12}$ in the Metabolism of Methylmalonyl Coenzyme A (CoA). Vitamin B$_{12}$, in the 5′-deoxyadenosylcobalamin form, is a coenzyme in the isomerization of methylmalonyl CoA to succinyl CoA. The reaction is catalyzed by the enzyme methylmalonyl CoA mutase.

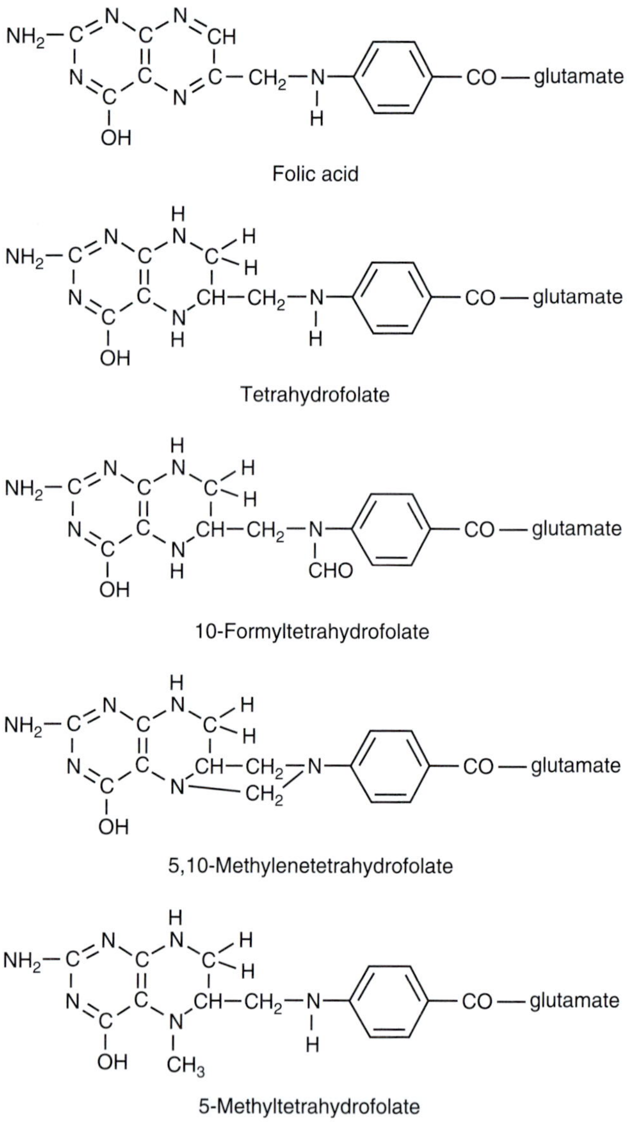

dihydrofolate (DHF). dTMP is a precursor to deoxythymidine triphosphate (dTTP) which, similar to the other nucleotide triphosphates, is a building block of the DNA molecule.

Figure 18.3 Structure of Synthetic Folic Acid and the Naturally Occurring Forms of the Vitamin. (From Scott, J. M., & Browne, P. [2006]. Megaloblastic anemia. In Caballero, B., Allen, L., & Prentice, A. [Eds.], *Encyclopedia of Human Nutrition.* [2nd ed., p. 114]. Oxford: Academic Press.)

THF is regenerated by the conversion of DHF to THF by the enzyme dihydrofolate reductase. Because some of the folate is catabolized during the cycle, the regeneration of THF also requires additional 5-methyl THF from the plasma. Once in the cell, folate is rapidly polyglutamated by the addition of one to six glutamic acid residues. This conjugation is required for retention of THF in the cell and also promotes attachment of folate to enzymes.[4]

Defect in Megaloblastic Anemia Caused by Deficiency in Folate and Vitamin B$_{12}$

When either folate or vitamin B$_{12}$ is deficient, thymidine nucleotide production for DNA synthesis is impaired. Folate deficiency has the more direct effect, ultimately preventing the methylation of dUMP. The effect of vitamin B$_{12}$ deficiency is more indirect, preventing the production of THF from 5-methyl

THF. When vitamin B_{12} is deficient, progressively more and more of the folate becomes metabolically trapped as 5-methyl THF. This constitutes what has been called the *folate trap* as 5-methyl THF accumulates and is unable to supply the folate cycle with THF. Some 5-methyl THF also leaks out of the cell if it is not readily polyglutamated. This results in a decrease in intracellular folate.[5] In addition, when either folate or vitamin B_{12} is deficient, homocysteine accumulates because methionine synthase is unable to convert it to methionine without vitamin B_{12} as a cofactor (see Figure 18.4).

In this state of diminished thymidine availability, uridine is incorporated into DNA.[6] The DNA repair process can remove the uridine, but without available thymidine to replace it, the repair process is unsuccessful. Although the DNA can unwind and replication can begin, at any point where a thymidine nucleotide is needed, there is essentially an empty space in the replicated DNA sequence, which results in many single-strand breaks. When excisions at opposing DNA strand sites coincide, double-strand breaks occur. Repeated DNA strand breaks lead to fragmentation of the DNA strand.[4] The resulting DNA is nonfunctional, and the DNA replication process is incomplete. Cell division is halted, resulting in either cell lysis or apoptosis[7] of many erythroid progenitors and precursors within the bone marrow. Cells that survive continue the abnormal maturation with a fewer number of red blood cells (RBCs) released into the circulation. This abnormal blood cell

development is called *ineffective hematopoiesis*. The dependency of DNA production on folate has been used in cancer chemotherapy (Box 18.2).

In addition to the increased apoptosis of erythroid progenitor and precursor cells in the bone marrow discussed

---

BOX 18.2   Disruption of the Folate Cycle in Cancer Chemotherapy

Folate has a complex relationship with cancer. Folate deficiency leads to DNA strand breaks, which leave the DNA vulnerable to mutation. In this way, folate deficiency is a risk factor for the initiation of cancer. The central role of folate in cell division also makes it a target for chemotherapeutic drugs used to treat cancer. Folate analogues can be used to compete for folate in DNA production and result in impaired cell division. Cells in the cell cycle, such as cancer cells and other normally rapidly dividing cells including epithelium and blood cell precursors, are most susceptible to the drug interference. Methotrexate, used in treatment of leukemia and arthritis, is an example of a folate antimetabolite drug. Methotrexate has a higher affinity for dihydrofolate reductase than tetrahydrofolate. Thus methotrexate enters the folate cycle in preference to tetrahydrofolate, and the folate cycle is blocked by the drug. Methotrexate treatment typically is followed by what is known as *leucovorin rescue*. Leucovorin is a folic acid derivative that can be administered to counteract the effects of methotrexate or other folate antagonists.

Based on Kim, S. E. (2020). Enzymes involved in folate metabolism and its implication for cancer treatment. *Nutr Res Pract, 14*(2):95–101.

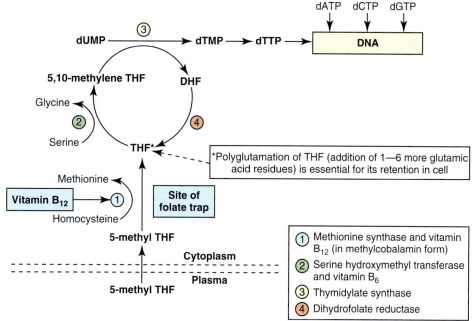

Figure 18.4 Role of Folate and Vitamin B_{12} in DNA Synthesis. Folate enters the cell as 5-methyltetrahydrofolate *(5-methyl THF)*. In the cell, a methyl group is transferred from 5-methyl THF to homocysteine, converting it to methionine and generating tetrahydrofolate *(THF)*. This reaction is catalyzed by methionine synthase and requires vitamin B_{12} as a cofactor. THF is then converted to 5,10-methylene THF by the donation of a methyl group from serine. The methyl group of 5,10-methylene THF is then transferred to deoxyuridine monophosphate *(dUMP)*, which converts it to deoxythymidine monophosphate *(dTMP)* and converts 5,10-methylene THF to dihydrofolate *(DHF)*. This reaction is catalyzed by thymidylate synthase. dTMP is a precursor of deoxythymidine triphosphate *(dTTP)*, which is used to synthesize DNA. THF is regenerated by the conversion of DHF to THF by the enzyme dihydrofolate reductase. A deficiency of vitamin B_{12} prevents the conversion of THF from 5-methyl THF; as a result, folate becomes metabolically trapped as 5-methyl THF. This constitutes the folate trap.

earlier, the remaining erythroid precursors are larger than normally seen during the final stages of erythropoiesis, and their nuclei are immature appearing compared with the cytoplasm. In contrast to the normally dense chromatin of comparable normoblasts, the nuclei of megaloblastic erythroid precursors have an open, finely stippled, reticular pattern.[5] The nuclear changes seen in the megaloblastic erythroid precursors are related to cell cycle delay, prolonged resting phase, and arrest in nuclear maturation. Electron microscopy reveals that reduced synthesis of histones is also responsible for morphologic changes in the chromatin of megaloblastic erythroid precursors.[8] Ribonucleic acid (RNA) function is not affected by vitamin B_{12} or folate deficiency because RNA contains uracil instead of thymidine nucleotides, so cytoplasmic development progresses normally. The slower maturation rate of the nucleus compared with the cytoplasm is called *nuclear-cytoplasmic asynchrony*. Together, the accumulation of cells with nuclei at earlier stages of development and cells with increased diameter and immaturity result in the appearance of erythroid precursors in the bone marrow that are pathognomonic of megaloblastic anemia.[7] Because ineffective hematopoiesis affects all three blood cell lineages, *pancytopenia* is also evident, with certain distinctive cellular changes (discussed in "Laboratory Diagnosis").

Other Causes of Megaloblastosis

Vitamin B_{12} and folate deficiency are not the only causes of megaloblastic erythroid precursors. Dysplastic erythroid precursors in myelodysplastic neoplasms (MDSs) can also have megaloblastoid features (Chapter 33). In MDSs, however, the macrocytic erythrocytes and their precursors characteristically show delayed cytoplasmic and nuclear maturation, including cytoplasmic vacuole formation, nuclear budding, multinucleation, and nuclear fragmentation, and thus may be distinguished from the megaloblastic erythroid precursors seen in the vitamin deficiencies. In addition, nuclear-cytoplasmic asynchrony and megaloblastic erythroid precursors may be seen in congenital dyserythropoietic anemia (CDA) types I and III (Chapter 19). The CDAs are rare conditions that usually manifest in childhood and may be distinguished from acquired causes of megaloblastosis by clinical history and morphologic differences. In CDA I, internuclear chromatin bridging of erythroid precursors or binucleated forms are observed, and in CDA III, giant multinucleated erythroblasts are present. In addition, treatment with any drug that affects cellular DNA biosynthesis can result in megaloblastic change. For example, these may be chemotherapeutic or antiretroviral agents.[9] Although the intended target of the drug may be malignant or abnormal cells, normal hematopoietic cells are also affected.

Although the conditions described in this section are characterized by megaloblastic morphology, they are due to acquired or inherited mutations in progenitor cells or interference with DNA synthesis and are refractory to therapy with vitamin B_{12} or folic acid.

SYSTEMIC MANIFESTATIONS OF FOLATE AND VITAMIN B_{12} DEFICIENCY

When DNA synthesis and subsequent cell division are impaired by lack of folate or vitamin B_{12}, megaloblastic anemia and its systemic manifestations develop. With either vitamin deficiency, patients may experience general symptoms related to anemia (fatigue, weakness, and shortness of breath) and symptoms related to the alimentary tract. Loss (or atrophy) of epithelium on the tongue results in a smooth surface and soreness (glossitis). Loss of epithelium along the gastrointestinal tract can result in gastritis, nausea, or constipation.

Although the blood pictures seen with the two vitamin deficiencies are indistinguishable, the clinical presentations vary. After dietary deficiency or malabsorption begins, it takes a few years to develop a vitamin B_{12} deficiency but only a few months to develop a folate deficiency, reflecting the storage capacity of each vitamin in the body. In vitamin B_{12} deficiency, neurologic symptoms may be pronounced and may even occur in the absence of anemia.[5] These include memory loss, numbness and tingling in toes and fingers, loss of balance, and further impairment of walking by loss of vibratory sense, especially in the lower limbs.[10] Neuropsychiatric symptoms may also be present, including personality changes and psychosis. These symptoms seem to be the result of demyelination of the spinal cord and peripheral nerves, as vitamin B_{12} is needed for the development and initial myelination of the central nervous system,[11] but the relationship of this demyelination to vitamin B_{12} deficiency is not entirely clear. Imaging studies of patients with vitamin B_{12} deficiency confirm the degenerative changes and abnormalities of the spinal cord.[12] The roles of increases in tumor necrosis factor-α, a neurotoxic agent, and decreases in epidermal growth factor, a neurotrophic agent, in the development of neurologic symptoms in vitamin B_{12}-deficient patients are being researched.[11,12]

At one time, folate deficiency was believed to be more benign clinically than vitamin B_{12} deficiency. Later research suggested that low levels of folate and the resulting high homocysteine levels were risk factors for cardiovascular disease.[13] More recent research has provided mixed results, with studies both refuting this association[14,15] and substantiating the association between high circulating homocysteine levels and the risk of cardiovascular disease.[16,17] Several studies suggest that high folate levels provide a cardioprotective effect in diabetic patients and certain ethnic populations.[14,18,19] The evidence at this time is unclear regarding whether persistent suboptimal folate status may have a significant long-term health impact. In addition, there is evidence of depression, peripheral neuropathy, and psychosis related to folate deficiency.[20,21] Folate levels appear to influence the effectiveness of treatments for depression.[22] Folate deficiency during pregnancy can result in impaired formation of the fetal nervous system, resulting in neural tube defects such as spina bifida,[23] despite the fact that the fetus accumulates folate at the expense of the mother. Pregnancy requires a considerable increase in folate to fulfill the requirements related to rapid fetal growth, uterine expansion, placental maturation, and expanded blood volume.[3]

Ensuring adequate folate levels in women of childbearing age is particularly important because many women are likely to be unaware of their pregnancy during the first crucial weeks of fetal development. Fortification of the US food supply with folic acid in grain and cereal products was mandated by the Food and Drug Administration in 1998 to reduce the risk of neural tube defects in the unborn.

CAUSES OF VITAMIN DEFICIENCIES

In general, vitamin deficiencies may arise because the vitamin is in relatively short supply, because use of the vitamin is impaired, or because of excessive loss. Folate deficiency can be caused by all of these mechanisms.

Folate Deficiency
Inadequate Intake
Folate is synthesized by microorganisms and higher plants. Folate is ubiquitous in foods, but a generally poor diet can result in deficiency and is the most common cause of deficiency. Good sources of folate include leafy green vegetables, dried beans, liver, beef, fortified breakfast cereals, and some fruits, especially oranges.[3,24] Folates are heat labile, and overcooking of foods can diminish their nutritional value.[3] Folate deficiency is especially common in individuals with excessive alcohol use and decreased dietary intake of fresh foods high in folate.

Increased Need
Increased need for folate occurs during pregnancy and lactation, when the mother must supply her own needs plus those of the fetus or infant. Infants and children also have increased need for folate during growth.[3] Hemolytic anemias (e.g., sickle cell anemia) can also deplete stores of folate due to increased cell turnover, and normal daily intake may not be adequate to support the increased need.

Impaired Absorption
Food folates must be hydrolyzed in the gut before absorption in the small intestine; however, only 50% of what is ingested is available for absorption.[3] A rare autosomal recessive deficiency of a folate transporter protein (proton-coupled folate transporter) severely decreases intestinal absorption of folate.[5,25] Once across the intestinal cell, most folate is transported in the plasma as 5-methyl THF unbound to any specific carrier.[10] Its entry into cells, however, is by both carrier systems and receptors.[26]

Folate absorption may also be impaired by intestinal disease, especially sprue and celiac disease. Sprue is characterized by weakness, weight loss, and steatorrhea (fat in the feces), which is evidence that the intestine is not absorbing food properly. It is seen in the tropics (tropical sprue), where its cause is generally considered to be overgrowth of enteric pathogens.[27] Celiac disease (nontropical sprue) has been traced to intolerance of gluten in some grains[27] (gluten-induced enteropathy) and can be controlled by eliminating wheat, barley, and rye products from the diet. Surgical resection of the small intestine and inflammatory bowel disease can also decrease folate absorption.

BOX 18.3   Some Drugs That May Impair Use of Folate

Impair Folate Metabolism
Methotrexate: antiarthritic, chemotherapeutic
5-Fluorouracil: chemotherapeutic
Hydroxyurea: antimetabolite
Pyrimethamine: antimalarial
Pentamidine: antimicrobial
Trimethoprim: antimicrobial

Impair Folate Absorption
Metformin: oral antidiabetic
Cholestyramine: cholesterol lowering
Oral contraceptives: hormones
Penicillins: antibiotics
Phenytoin: anticonvulsant

Impaired Use of Folate
Numerous drugs decrease absorption of folic acid or impair folate metabolism (Box 18.3).[28] Antineoplastic, antibacterial, and antiseizure agents are particularly known for this,[28] and the result is macrocytosis with frank megaloblastic anemia. Because folate deficiency results in inhibition of cell replication, several anticancer drugs, including methotrexate, are folate inhibitors.[3] In most instances, supplementation with folic acid or reduced folic acid (in the form of folinic acid) is sufficient to override the impairment and allow the patient to continue therapy.[28]

Excessive Loss of Folate
Physiologic loss of folate occurs through the kidney. The amount is small and not a cause of deficiency. Patients undergoing renal dialysis lose folate in the dialysate, however; supplemental folic acid is routinely provided to these individuals to prevent megaloblastic anemia.[10]

Vitamin B₁₂ Deficiency
Inadequate Intake
Although true dietary deficiency of vitamin B_{12} is rare, this condition is possible for strict vegetarians (vegans) who do not eat meat, eggs, or dairy products. Although it is an essential vitamin for animals, plants cannot synthesize vitamin B_{12}, and thus it is not available from vegetable sources. The best dietary sources are animal products such as liver, dairy products, fish, shellfish, and eggs.[29] In contrast to the heat-labile folate, vitamin B_{12} is not destroyed by cooking.

Increased Need
Increased need for vitamin B_{12} occurs during pregnancy, lactation, and growth. Because of the vigorous cell replication, what would otherwise be a diet adequate in vitamin B_{12} can become inadequate during these periods.

Impaired Absorption
Vitamin B_{12} in food is released from food proteins primarily in the acid environment of the stomach, aided by pepsin, and is subsequently bound by a specific salivary protein, haptocorrin,

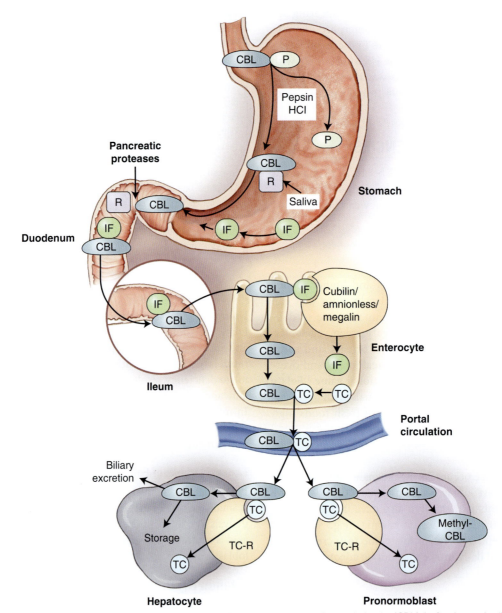

Figure 18.5 Normal Absorption of Vitamin B$_{12}$. Dietary vitamin B$_{12}$ (cobalamin *[CBL]*) is food protein *(P)* bound. In the stomach, pepsin and hydrochloric acid *(HCl)* secreted by parietal cells release CBL from P. CBL then binds haptocorrin (R protein *[R]*), released from salivary glands, and remains bound until intestinal pancreatic proteases, including trypsin, catalyze its release. Parietal cells secrete intrinsic factor *(IF)*, which binds CBL in the duodenum. Cubilin-amnionless (cubam) and megalin receptors in ileal enterocytes bind CBL-IF and, once inside the enterocyte, release CBL from IF. Enterocytes produce transcobalamin *(TC)*, which binds CBL and transports it through the portal circulation. Bone marrow pronormoblast membrane TC receptors *(TC-R)* bind CBL-TC, and release CBL from IF inside the cell, where it is converted to methylcobalamin *(methyl-CBL)*. Methyl-CBL is a coenzyme that supports homocysteine-methionine conversion. Hepatocyte TC receptors bind CBL-TC and release the CBL, which is moved to storage organelles or excreted through the biliary system.

also known as *R protein* or *transcobalamin I* (Figure 18.5). In the small intestine, vitamin B$_{12}$ is released from haptocorrin by the action of pancreatic proteases including trypsin. It is then bound by intrinsic factor, which is produced by gastric parietal cells. Vitamin B$_{12}$ binding to intrinsic factor is required for absorption by ileal enterocytes that possess receptors for the complex. These receptors are the cubilin-amnionless complex, collectively known as *cubam,* which binds the vitamin B$_{12}$-intrinsic factor complex, and megalin, a membrane transport protein.[5,26,29–32] Once in the enterocyte, the vitamin B$_{12}$

is then freed from intrinsic factor and bound to transcobalamin (previously called *transcobalamin II*) and released into the circulation. In the plasma, only 10% to 30% of the vitamin B$_{12}$ is bound to transcobalamin; the remaining 75% is bound to transcobalamin I and III, referred to as the *haptocorrins*.[29,33] The vitamin B$_{12}$-transcobalamin complex, termed *holotranscobalamin* (holoTC), is the metabolically active form of vitamin B$_{12}$. Holotranscobalamin binds to specific receptors on the surfaces of many different cells and enters the cells by endocytosis,[26] with subsequent release of vitamin B$_{12}$ from the carrier.[34] The body maintains a substantial reserve of absorbed vitamin B_{12} in hepatocytes[4] and renal cells.[26]

The absorption of vitamin B_{12} can be impaired by (1) failure to separate vitamin B_{12} from food proteins in the stomach, (2) failure to separate vitamin B_{12} from haptocorrin in the intestine, (3) lack of intrinsic factor, (4) malabsorption, (5) inherited errors of vitamin B_{12} absorption and transport, and (6) competition for available vitamin B_{12}.

Failure to separate vitamin B_{12} from food proteins. A condition known as *food-cobalamin malabsorption* is characterized by hypochlorhydria and the resulting inability of the body to release vitamin B_{12} from food or intestinal transport proteins for subsequent binding to intrinsic factor. Food-cobalamin malabsorption is caused primarily by the reduced gastric acidity in atrophic gastritis or atrophy of the stomach lining that often occurs with increasing age.[35] It also occurs with gastric bypass surgery and long-term use of histamine type 2 receptor blockers and proton pump inhibitors, which reduce gastric acidity for the treatment of ulcers and gastroesophageal reflux disease.[35]

Failure to separate vitamin B_{12} from haptocorrin. Lack of gastric acidity or lack of trypsin as a result of chronic pancreatic disease can prevent vitamin B_{12} absorption because the vitamin remains bound to haptocorrin in the intestine and unavailable to intrinsic factor.[10]

Lack of intrinsic factor. Lack of intrinsic factor is a significant cause of impaired vitamin B_{12} absorption. It is most commonly a result of autoimmune disease, as in pernicious anemia, but can also result from hereditary intrinsic factor deficiency or loss of parietal cells in *Helicobacter pylori* infection or after total or partial gastrectomy.

Pernicious anemia. Pernicious anemia is an autoimmune disorder characterized by impaired absorption of vitamin B_{12} because of an intrinsic factor deficiency.[34] This condition is called *pernicious anemia* because the disease was fatal before its cause was discovered. The incidence per year is roughly 25 new cases per 100,000 people older than 40 years of age.[5] Pernicious anemia most often manifests in the sixth decade or later but can also be found in children. Patients with pernicious anemia have an increased risk of developing gastric tumors.[4]

In pernicious anemia, autoimmune lymphocyte-mediated destruction of gastric parietal cells severely reduces the amount of intrinsic factor secreted in the stomach. Pathologic CD4 T cells inappropriately recognize and initiate an autoimmune response against the H^+/K^+-adenosine triphosphatase embedded in the membrane of parietal cells.[36] Chronic inflammatory infiltration follows, which extends into the wall of the stomach.[37] Over a period of years and even decades, there is progressive development of atrophic gastritis, resulting in the loss of the parietal cells with their secretory products, H^+ and intrinsic factor. The loss of H^+ production in the stomach constitutes *achlorhydria*. Low gastric acidity was previously an important diagnostic criterion for pernicious anemia. Serum gastrin levels can be markedly elevated as a result of the gastric achlorhydria.[4] The absence of intrinsic factor can also be detected using the Schilling test. However, because the test requires a 24-hour urine collection and the use of radioactive cobalt in vitamin

B_{12} to trace absorption, safer diagnostic tests are currently used (discussed in "Laboratory Diagnosis").

Another feature of the autoimmune response in pernicious anemia is the production of antibodies to intrinsic factor and gastric parietal cells that are detectable in serum.[38,39] The most common antibody to intrinsic factor blocks the site on intrinsic factor where vitamin B_{12} binds, which inhibits the formation of the intrinsic factor-vitamin B_{12} complex and prevents the absorption of the vitamin.[37] These blocking antibodies are present in serum or gastric fluid in 70% to 90% of patients with pernicious anemia, and their presence is highly specific for the disease.[5] Parietal cell antibodies are detectable in the serum of 50% to 90% of patients with pernicious anemia.[5,37,39]

Other causes of lack of intrinsic factor. A lack of intrinsic factor may also be related to *H. pylori* infection. Left untreated, colonization of the gastric mucosa with *H. pylori* progresses until the parietal cells are entirely destroyed, a process involving both local and systemic immune mechanisms.[40,41] In addition, partial or total gastrectomy, which results in removal of intrinsic factor-producing parietal cells, invariably leads to vitamin B_{12} deficiency.

Impaired absorption of vitamin B_{12} can also be caused by hereditary intrinsic factor deficiency. This is a rare autosomal recessive disorder characterized by the absence or impaired function of intrinsic factor. In contrast to the acquired forms of pernicious anemia, histology and gastric acidity are normal.[31]

Malabsorption. General malabsorption of vitamin B_{12} can be caused by the same conditions interfering with folate absorption, such as celiac disease, tropical sprue, and inflammatory bowel disease.

Inherited errors of vitamin B_{12} absorption and transport. Imerslund-Gräsbeck syndrome is a rare autosomal recessive condition caused by mutations in the genes for either cubilin or amnionless. This defect results in decreased endocytosis of the intrinsic factor-vitamin B_{12} complex by ileal enterocytes. Transcobalamin deficiency is another rare autosomal recessive condition resulting in a deficiency of physiologically available vitamin B_{12}.[26,31,42]

Competition for vitamin B_{12}. Competition for available vitamin B_{12} in the intestine may come from intestinal organisms. The fish tapeworm *Diphyllobothrium latum* is able to split vitamin B_{12} from intrinsic factor, rendering the vitamin unavailable for host absorption.[43] Also, *blind loops*, portions of the intestines that are stenotic as a result of surgery or inflammation, can become overgrown with intestinal bacteria that compete effectively with the host for available vitamin B_{12}.[10] In both cases, the host is unable to absorb sufficient vitamin B_{12}, and megaloblastic anemia results.

LABORATORY DIAGNOSIS

The tests used in the diagnosis of megaloblastic anemia include screening tests and specific diagnostic tests to identify the specific vitamin deficiency and perhaps its cause.

Screening Tests

Five tests used to screen for megaloblastic anemia are complete blood count (CBC), reticulocyte count, white blood cell (WBC) manual differential, serum bilirubin, and lactate dehydrogenase.

Complete Blood Count and Reticulocyte Count

Slight macrocytosis often is the earliest sign of megaloblastic anemia. Patients with uncomplicated megaloblastic anemia are expected to have decreased hemoglobin and hematocrit values, pancytopenia, and reticulocytopenia. Megaloblastic anemia develops slowly, and the degree of anemia is often severe when first detected. Hemoglobin values of less than 7 or 8 g/dL are not unusual.[4] When the hematocrit is less than 20%, erythroblasts with megaloblastic nuclei, including an occasional promegaloblast, may appear in the peripheral blood. The mean cell volume (MCV) is usually 100 to 150 fL and commonly is greater than 120 fL, although coexisting iron deficiency, thalassemia trait, or inflammation can prevent macrocytosis. The mean cell hemoglobin (MCH) is elevated by the increased volume of the cells, but the mean cell hemoglobin concentration (MCHC) is usually within the reference interval because hemoglobin production is unaffected. The RBC distribution width (RDW) is also elevated.

The characteristic morphologic findings of megaloblastic anemia in the peripheral blood include oval macrocytes (enlarged oval RBCs) (Figure 18.6) and hypersegmented neutrophils with six or more lobes (Figure 18.7).[44] Impaired cell production results in a low absolute reticulocyte count, especially in light of the severity of the anemia, and polychromasia is not observed on the peripheral blood film. Additional morphologic changes may include the presence of teardrop cells (dacryocytes), RBC fragments, and microspherocytes. These smaller cells further increase RDW. The presence of schistocytes sometimes leads to a paradoxically lower MCV than is seen in less severe cases. These erythrocyte changes reflect the severity of dyserythropoiesis and should not be taken as evidence of microangiopathic hemolysis. Nucleated RBCs, Howell-Jolly bodies, basophilic stippling, and Cabot rings may also be observed.

White Blood Cell Manual Differential Count

Hypersegmentation of neutrophils is essentially pathognomonic for megaloblastic anemia. It appears early in the course of the disease[39] and may persist for up to 2 weeks after treatment is initiated.[5] Hypersegmented neutrophils noted in the WBC differential report are a significant finding and require a reporting rule that can be applied consistently because even healthy individuals may have an occasional one. One such rule is to report hypersegmentation when there are at least 5 five-lobed neutrophils per 100 WBCs or at least 1 six-lobed neutrophil is noted.[10] Some laboratories perform a lobe count on 100 neutrophils and then calculate the mean. In megaloblastic anemia, the mean lobe count should be greater than 3.4.[10] The cause of the hypersegmentation is not understood, despite considerable investigation.[45] More recent advances in the understanding of growth factors and their impact on transcription factors may yet solve this mystery. Nevertheless, a search for neutrophil hypersegmentation on a peripheral blood film constitutes an inexpensive yet sensitive screening test for megaloblastic anemia.

Bilirubin and Lactate Dehydrogenase Levels

Although generally considered a nutritional anemia, megaloblastic anemia is in one sense a hemolytic anemia. Because many erythroid progenitors and precursors die during division in bone marrow, many RBCs never enter the circulation (ineffective hematopoiesis), so a decrease in reticulocytes occurs in the peripheral blood. The usual signs of hemolysis are evident in the serum, including an elevation in levels of total and indirect bilirubin and lactate dehydrogenase (predominantly RBC derived) (Chapter 20).

The constellation of findings, including macrocytic anemia, moderate to marked pancytopenia, reticulocytopenia, oval macrocytes, and hypersegmented neutrophils plus increased levels of total and indirect bilirubin and lactate dehydrogenase, justifies further testing to confirm a diagnosis of megaloblastic anemia and determine its cause. Occasionally the classic findings may be obscured by coexisting conditions such as iron

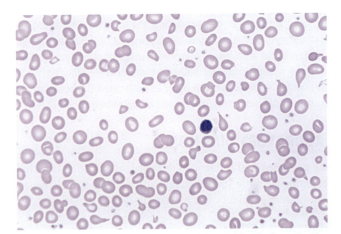

Figure 18.6 Blood Cell Morphology in Megaloblastic Anemia. Note the oval macrocytes, teardrop cells (dacryocytes), other red blood cell abnormalities, and a small lymphocyte for size comparison. (Peripheral blood, Wright-Giemsa stain, ×500.)

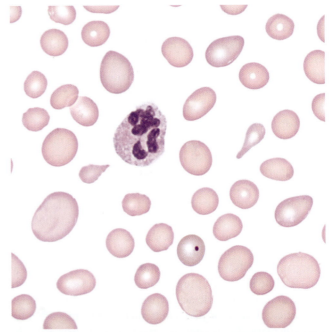

Figure 18.7 Blood Cell Morphology in Megaloblastic Anemia. Note the hypersegmented neutrophil, oval macrocytes, and a Howell-Jolly body. (Peripheral blood, Wright-Giemsa stain, ×1000.) (From Carr, J. H. [2022]. *Clinical Hematology Atlas.* [6th ed.]. St. Louis: Elsevier.)

deficiency or thalassemia, which makes the diagnosis more challenging. Most hematologic aberrations do not appear until vitamin deficiency is fairly well advanced (Box 18.4).[46]

Specific Diagnostic Tests

Bone Marrow Examination

Modern tests for vitamin deficiencies and autoimmune antibodies have made bone marrow examination an infrequently used diagnostic test for megaloblastic anemia. Nevertheless, it remains the reference confirmatory test to identify the megaloblastic appearance of the developing erythroid precursors.

Megaloblastic, in contrast to *macrocytic,* anemia refers to specific morphologic changes in the developing erythroid precursors. The cells are characterized by a nuclear-cytoplasmic asynchrony in which the cytoplasm matures as expected with increasing pinkness as hemoglobin accumulates. The nucleus lags behind, however, appearing younger than expected for the degree of maturity of the cytoplasm (Figure 18.8). This asynchrony is most striking at the stage of the polychromatic normoblast. The cytoplasm appears pinkish-blue as expected for that stage, but the nuclear chromatin remains more open than expected, similar to that in the nucleus of a basophilic

---

BOX 18.4   Sequence of Development of Megaloblastic Anemias

1. Decrease in vitamin levels
2. Hypersegmentation of neutrophils in peripheral blood
3. Oval macrocytes in peripheral blood
4. Megaloblastosis in bone marrow
5. Anemia

---

normoblast. Overall, the bone marrow is hypercellular, with a reduced myeloid-to-erythroid ratio of about 1:1 by virtue of the increased erythropoietic activity. Hematopoiesis is ineffective, however, and although cell production in the bone marrow is increased, the apoptosis of hematopoietic cells in the marrow results in peripheral pancytopenia.

The WBCs are also affected in megaloblastic anemia and appear larger than normal. This is most evident in metamyelocytes and bands because in the usual development of neutrophils, the cells should be getting smaller at these stages. The effect creates "giant" metamyelocytes and bands (Figure 18.9).

Megakaryocytes do not show consistent changes in megaloblastic anemia. They may be either increased or decreased in number and may show diminished lobulation. The latter finding is not consistently seen, however, and even when present, it is difficult to assess.

Assays for Folate, Vitamin B$_{12}$, Methylmalonic Acid, and Homocysteine

Although bone marrow aspiration is confirmatory for megaloblastosis, the invasiveness of the procedure and its expense mean that other testing is performed more often than a bone marrow examination. Furthermore, the confirmation of megaloblastic morphology in the marrow does not identify its cause. Tests for serum levels of folate and vitamin B$_{12}$ are readily available using immunoassay; serum vitamin B$_{12}$ may also be assayed by competitive binding chemiluminescence.[47] However, there are a number of interferences with these assays that can cause false increased and decreased results[5,47] (Box 18.5); reflexive testing to MMA and homocysteine (discussed next) can increase diagnostic accuracy. RBC folate levels were previously used because they did not fluctuate with diet as serum folate levels do,[48] yet they have suboptimal sensitivity and specificity. Thus the serum folate level is recommended as the initial test for evaluation of folate deficiency in the United States.[5]

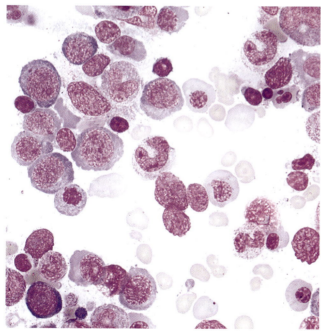

Figure 18.8 Erythroid Precursors in Megaloblastic Anemia. Note nuclear-cytoplasmic asynchrony. (Bone marrow, Wright-Giemsa stain, ×500.) (From Carr, J. H. [2022]. *Clinical Hematology Atlas.* [6th ed.]. St. Louis: Elsevier.)

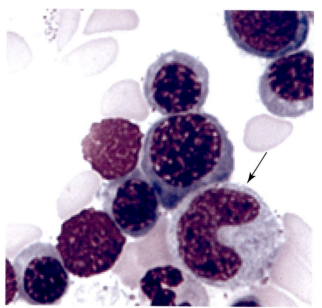

Figure 18.9 Giant Band *(arrow)* **(Early) in Megaloblastic Anemia.** (Bone marrow, Wright-Giemsa stain, original magnification ×1000.)

Data from Antony, A. C. (2023). Megaloblastic anemias. In Hoffman, R., Benz, E. J., Silberstein, L. E., et al. (Eds.), *Hematology: Basic Principles and Practice.* (8th ed., pp. 524–554). Philadelphia: Elsevier; and Oberley, M. J., & Yang, D. T. (2013). Laboratory testing for cobalamin deficiency in megaloblastic anemia. *Am J Hematol, 88,* 522–526.

Some laboratories conduct a reflexive assay for MMA if vitamin B$_{12}$ levels are low. As indicated previously, in addition to playing a role in folate metabolism, vitamin B$_{12}$ is a cofactor in the conversion of methylmalonyl CoA to succinyl CoA by the enzyme methylmalonyl CoA mutase (see Figure 18.2). If vitamin B$_{12}$ is deficient, methylmalonyl CoA accumulates. Some of it hydrolyzes to MMA, and the increase can be detected in serum and urine. Because MMA is also elevated in patients with impaired renal function, the test is not specific, and thus increased levels cannot be definitively related to vitamin B$_{12}$ deficiency.[3] MMA is assayed by gas chromatography-tandem mass spectrometry.

Homocysteine levels are affected by deficiencies in either folate or vitamin B$_{12}$. 5-Methyl THF donates a methyl group to homocysteine in the generation of methionine. This reaction uses vitamin B$_{12}$ as a coenzyme (see Figure 18.4). Thus a deficiency in either folate or vitamin B$_{12}$ results in elevated levels of homocysteine. Total homocysteine can be measured in either plasma or serum. Homocysteine may be assayed by gas chromatography-mass spectrometry, high-performance liquid chromatography, or fluorescence polarization immunoassay. Homocysteine levels are also elevated in patients with renal failure and dehydration. Figure 18.10 presents an algorithm of the analysis of these analytes in the diagnosis of vitamin B$_{12}$ and folate deficiency.

Gastric Analysis and Serum Gastrin

Gastric analysis may be used to confirm achlorhydria, an expected finding in pernicious anemia. Achlorhydria occurs in other conditions, however, including natural aging. When other causes of vitamin B$_{12}$ deficiency have been eliminated, a finding of achlorhydria is supportive, although not diagnostic, of pernicious anemia. The H$^+$ concentration is determined by pH measurement.

As a result of the gastric achlorhydria, serum gastrin levels can be markedly elevated.[4] Serum gastrin is measured by immunoassay, including chemiluminescent immunometric assays.

Antibody Assays

Antibodies to intrinsic factor and parietal cells can be detected in the sera of most patients with pernicious anemia. Various immunoassays can detect intrinsic factor-blocking antibodies; parietal cell antibodies can be detected by indirect fluorescent antibody techniques or enzyme-linked immunosorbent assays. Antiintrinsic factor antibodies are highly specific and confirmatory for pernicious anemia, but their absence does not rule out the condition. The test for parietal cell antibodies is nonspecific and not clinically useful for the diagnosis of pernicious anemia.[5]

Figure 18.11 presents an algorithm for the diagnosis of pernicious anemia using tests for serum vitamin B$_{12}$, MMA, intrinsic factor blocking antibody, and serum gastrin levels.

Holotranscobalamin Assay

Holotranscobalamin is the metabolically active form of vitamin B$_{12}$. Older methods for measuring holotranscobalamin were manual and not suitable for use in clinical laboratories. Newer, more rapid immunoassays using monoclonal antibodies specific for holotranscobalamin have been developed that are both sensitive and specific.[49,50] Recent studies support the use of holotranscobalamin to detect vitamin B$_{12}$ deficiency and recommend its use in screening for metabolic vitamin B$_{12}$ deficiency.[51–53]

Stool Analysis for Parasites

When vitamin B$_{12}$ is found to be deficient, a stool analysis for eggs or proglottids of the fish tapeworm *D. latum* may be part of the diagnostic workup.

Table 18.1 contains a summary of laboratory tests used to diagnose vitamin B$_{12}$ and folate deficiency.

MACROCYTIC NONMEGALOBLASTIC ANEMIAS

The macrocytic nonmegaloblastic anemias are macrocytic anemias in which DNA synthesis is unimpaired. The macrocytosis tends to be mild; the MCV usually ranges from 100 to 110 fL and rarely exceeds 120 fL. Patients with

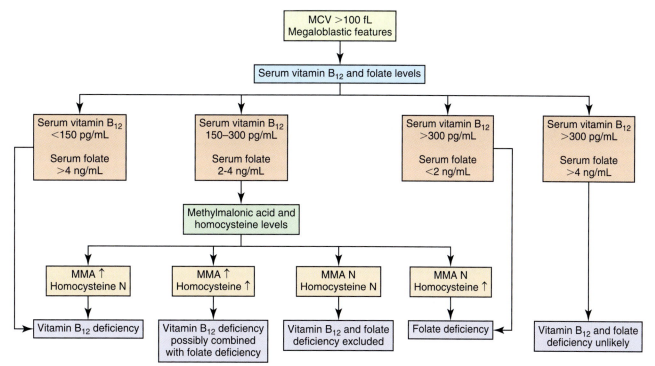

Figure 18.10 Algorithm for Diagnosis of Vitamin B$_{12}$ and Folate Deficiency. The algorithm uses serum assays for folate, vitamin B$_{12}$, methylmalonic acid, and homocysteine to differentiate the conditions. *↑*, Increased; *MCV*, mean cell volume; *MMA*, methylmalonic acid; *N*, within reference interval. (From references 5 and 40.)

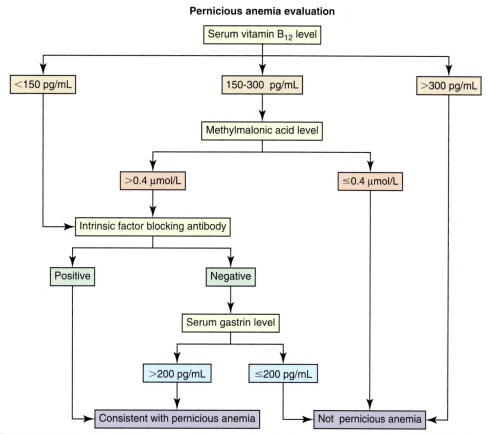

Figure 18.11 Algorithm for Diagnosis of Pernicious Anemia. (Adapted from Klee, G. G. [2000]. Cobalamin and folate evaluation: measurement of methylmalonic acid and homocysteine vs vitamin B$_{12}$ and folate. *Clin Chem, 46*, 1281.)

TABLE 18.1	**Laboratory Tests Used to Diagnose Vitamin B$_{12}$ and Folate Deficiency**		
		Folate Deficiency	**Vitamin B$_{12}$ Deficiency**
Screening Tests	Complete blood count	↓ HGB, HCT, RBCs, WBCs, PLTs ↑ MCV, MCH	Same as folate deficiency
	Manual differential count	Hypersegmented neutrophils, oval macrocytes, anisocytosis, poikilocytosis, RBC inclusions	Same as folate deficiency
	Absolute reticulocyte count	↓	↓
	Serum total and indirect bilirubin	↑	↑
	Serum lactate dehydrogenase	↑	↑
Specific Diagnostic Tests	Bone marrow examination*	Erythroid hyperplasia (ineffective) Presence of megaloblasts	Same as folate deficiency
	Serum vitamin B$_{12}$	N	↓
	Serum folate	↓	N or ↑[†]
	RBC folate	↓	N or ↓[†]
	Serum methylmalonic acid	N	↑
	Serum/plasma homocysteine	↑	↑
	Antibodies to intrinsic factor and gastric parietal cells	Absent	Present in pernicious anemia
	Serum gastrin	N	Can be markedly elevated in pernicious anemia
	Gastric analysis*	N	Achlorhydria in pernicious anemia
	Holotranscobalamin assay[‡]	N	↓
	Stool analysis for parasites	Negative	*Diphyllobothrium latum* may be the cause of deficiency

*Bone marrow examination and gastric analysis are not usually required for diagnosis.
[†]Without vitamin B$_{12}$, the cell is unable to produce intracellular polyglutamated tetrahydrofolate; therefore 5-methyltetrahydrofolate leaks out of the cell, which results in a decreased level of intracellular folate.
[‡]Holotranscobalamin level is also decreased in transcobalamin deficiency.
↑, Increased; *↓*, decreased; *HCT*, hematocrit; *HGB*, hemoglobin; *MCH*, mean cell hemoglobin; *MCV*, mean cell volume; *N*, within reference interval; *PLT*, platelet; *RBC*, red blood cell; *WBC*, white blood cell.

nonmegaloblastic, macrocytic anemia lack hypersegmented neutrophils and oval macrocytes in the peripheral blood and megaloblasts in the bone marrow. Macrocytosis may be physiologically normal, as in the newborn (Chapter 43), or the result of a pathologic condition, as in liver disease, chronic alcoholism, or bone marrow failure. Reticulocytosis is a common cause of macrocytosis. Figure 18.12 presents an algorithm for the preliminary investigation of macrocytic anemias.

TREATMENT

Treatment should be directed at the specific vitamin deficiency established by the diagnostic tests and should include addressing the cause of the deficiency (e.g., better nutrition, treatment for *D. latum*), if possible. Vitamin B$_{12}$ may be administered intramuscularly to treat pernicious anemia to bypass the need for intrinsic factor. High-dose oral vitamin B$_{12}$ treatment is increasingly popular in the treatment of pernicious anemia.[35,54,55] Regardless of the treatment modality, individuals

with pernicious anemia or malabsorption must have lifelong vitamin replacement therapy. Folic acid can be administered orally. The inappropriate treatment of vitamin B$_{12}$ deficiency with folic acid improves the anemia but does not correct or stop the progress of the neurologic damage, which may advance to an irreversible state.[3] Thus proper diagnosis before treatment is important. Iron is often supplemented concurrently to support the rapid cell production that accompanies effective treatment.

When proper treatment is initiated, the body's response is prompt and brisk and can be used to confirm the accuracy of the diagnosis. Bone marrow morphology will begin to revert to a normoblastic appearance within a few hours of treatment. A substantial reticulocyte response is apparent at about 1 week, with hemoglobin increasing toward normal levels in about 3 weeks.[11] Hypersegmented neutrophils disappear from the peripheral blood within 2 weeks of initiation of treatment.[5] Thus with proper treatment, hematologic parameters may return to normal within 3 to 6 weeks, and correction of the megaloblastic anemia may occur in 6 to 8 weeks.[56]

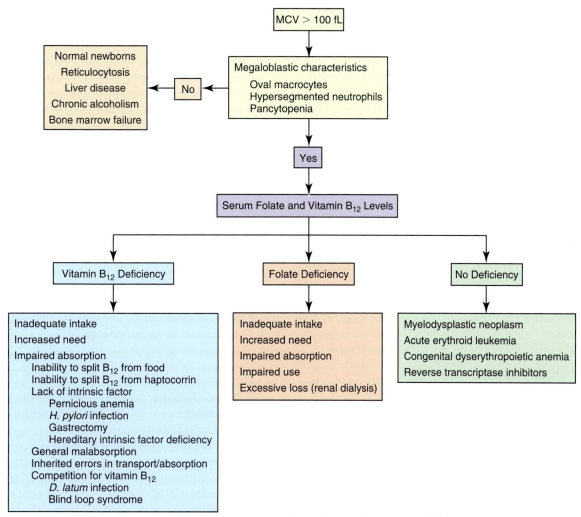

Figure 18.12 Algorithm for Preliminary Investigation of Macrocytic Anemias. *MCV,* Mean cell volume.

SUMMARY

- Impaired DNA synthesis affects all rapidly dividing cells of the body, including cells in the skin, gastrointestinal tract, and bone marrow. The effect on hematologic cells results in megaloblastic anemia.

- Vitamin B_{12} and folate are needed for the production of thymidine nucleotides for DNA synthesis. Deficiencies of either vitamin impair DNA replication, halt cell division, and increase apoptosis, which results in two major effects: ineffective hematopoiesis and megaloblastic morphology of erythroid precursors.

- Vitamin B_{12} deficiency is associated with peripheral neuropathies and neuropsychiatric abnormalities as a result of demyelinization of nerves in the peripheral and central nervous systems. Peripheral neuropathy and depression also may accompany folate deficiency. Folate deficiency in early pregnancy can lead to neural tube defects in the fetus.

- Lack of vitamin B_{12} leads to the accumulation of methylmalonic acid and homocysteine. Folate deficiency, in particular, leads to elevation of homocysteine levels and possible risk of cardiovascular disease.

- Folate deficiency may result from inadequate intake, increased need with growth or pregnancy, impaired absorption in small intestine, impaired metabolism due to drugs such as those used to treat seizures or cancer, or excessive loss via renal dialysis.

- Vitamin B_{12} deficiency arises from inadequate intake (which is uncommon because vitamin B_{12} is ubiquitous in animal products); increased need as seen in pregnancy, lactation, and growth; or inadequate absorption.

- Absorption of vitamin B_{12} depends on production of intrinsic factor by parietal cells of the stomach. Vitamin B_{12} binds to transcobalamin forming holotranscobalamin, the metabolically active form of the vitamin.

- The absorption of vitamin B_{12} can be impaired by (1) failure to separate vitamin B_{12} from food proteins in the stomach, (2) failure to separate vitamin B_{12} from haptocorrin in the intestine, (3) lack of intrinsic factor, (4) malabsorption, (5) inherited errors of vitamin B_{12} absorption and transport, and (6) competition for available vitamin B_{12}.

- Lack of intrinsic factor may result from loss of gastric parietal cells with pernicious anemia, *Helicobacter pylori* infection, gastrectomy, or inherited intrinsic factor deficiency.
- Pernicious anemia is vitamin B_{12} deficiency resulting from an autoimmune disease that causes destruction of gastric parietal cells. H^+ and intrinsic factor secretion is lost. Antibodies to parietal cells, intrinsic factor, or both are detectable in the serum.
- Classic complete blood count findings in megaloblastic anemia include decreased hemoglobin and hematocrit, pancytopenia, reticulocytopenia, elevated mean cell volume (usually greater than 120 fL), elevated RBC distribution width and mean cell hemoglobin, mean cell hemoglobin concentration within the reference interval, and oval macrocytes and hypersegmented neutrophils observed on the peripheral blood film. Additional abnormal laboratory test findings may include elevated levels of total and indirect serum bilirubin and lactate dehydrogenase as a result of the hemolysis and apoptosis of megaloblastic erythroid precursors within the bone marrow.

- The bone marrow in megaloblastic anemia is hyperplastic with increased erythropoiesis; however, it is ineffective because of increased apoptosis of developing cells. Erythroid precursors show nuclear-cytoplasmic asynchrony, with the nuclear maturation lagging behind the cytoplasmic maturation. Giant metamyelocytes and bands are evident.
- The cause of megaloblastic anemia is determined using specific immunoassays for serum folate and vitamin B_{12}. Immunoassays for holotranscobalamin and antibodies to intrinsic factor can aid in the diagnosis of pernicious anemia. Additional tests for gastrointestinal disease or parasites may be needed.
- Treatment of megaloblastic anemia is directed at correcting the cause of the deficiency and supplementing the missing vitamin.
- For pernicious anemia, lifelong supplementation with vitamin B_{12} is necessary.

Now that you have completed this chapter, go back and read again the case study at the beginning and respond to the questions presented. Answers can be found in Appendix C.

REVIEW QUESTIONS

Answers can be found in Appendix C.

1. Which of the following findings is consistent with a diagnosis of megaloblastic anemia?
   a. Hyposegmentation of neutrophils
   b. Decreased serum lactate dehydrogenase level
   c. Increase in percent reticulocytes
   d. Increased MCV
2. A patient has a clinical picture of megaloblastic anemia. The serum folate level is decreased, and the serum vitamin B_{12} level is 600 pg/mL (reference interval is 200–900 pg/mL). What is the expected value for the methylmalonic acid assay?
   a. Increased
   b. Decreased
   c. Within the reference interval
3. Which one of the following statements characterizes the relationships among macrocytic anemia, megaloblastic anemia, and pernicious anemia?
   a. Macrocytic anemias are megaloblastic.
   b. Macrocytic anemia is pernicious anemia.
   c. Megaloblastic anemia is macrocytic.
   d. Megaloblastic anemia is pernicious anemia.
4. Which of the following CBC findings is most suggestive of a megaloblastic anemia?
   a. MCV of 103 fL
   b. Hypersegmentation of neutrophils
   c. RDW of 16%
   d. HGB of 9.1 g/dL

5. In the following description of a bone marrow smear, find the statement that is INCONSISTENT with the expected picture in megaloblastic anemia.
   "The marrow appears hypercellular with a myeloid-to-erythroid ratio of 1:1 due to prominent erythroid hyperplasia. Megakaryocytes appear normal in number and appearance. WBC elements appear larger than normal, with especially large metamyelocytes, although they otherwise appear morphologically normal. Erythroid precursors also appear large. There is nuclear-cytoplasmic asynchrony, with the nucleus appearing more mature than expected for the color of the cytoplasm."
   a. Erythroid nuclei that are more mature than cytoplasm
   b. Larger than normal WBC elements
   c. Larger than normal erythroid precursors
   d. Normal appearance of megakaryocytes
6. Which one of the following findings would be INCONSISTENT with elevated titers of intrinsic factor blocking antibodies?
   a. Hypersegmentation of neutrophils
   b. Low levels of methylmalonic acid
   c. Macrocytic RBCs
   d. Low levels of vitamin B_{12}
7. Which of the following is the most metabolically active form of absorbed vitamin B_{12}?
   a. Transcobalamin
   b. Intrinsic factor-vitamin B_{12} complex
   c. Holotranscobalamin
   d. Haptocorrin-vitamin B_{12} complex
8. Folate and vitamin B_{12} work together in the production of:
   a. Amino acids
   b. RNA
   c. Phospholipids
   d. DNA

9. The macrocytosis associated with megaloblastic anemia results from:

a. Reduced numbers of cell divisions with normal cytoplasmic development

b. Activation of a gene that is typically active only in megakaryocytes

c. Reduced concentration of hemoglobin in the cells so that larger cells are needed to provide the same oxygen-carrying capacity

d. Increased production of reticulocytes in an attempt to compensate for the anemia

10. Which one of the following groups has the highest risk for pernicious anemia?

a. Malnourished infants

b. Children during growth periods

c. Adults older than 60 years of age

d. Pregnant women

REFERENCES

1. Scott, J. M. (1999). Folate and vitamin B_{12}. *Proc Nutr Soc, 58,* 441–448.

2. Wickramasinghe, S. N. (1999). The wide spectrum and unresolved issues of megaloblastic anemia. *Semin Hematol, 36,* 3–18.

3. Miller, J. W. (2013). Folic acid. In Caballero, B. (Ed.), *Encyclopedia of Human Nutrition.* (3rd ed., pp. 262–269). Amsterdam: Elsevier/Academic Press.

4. Carmel, R. (2019). Megaloblastic anemias: disorders of impaired DNA synthesis. In Greer, J. P., Arber, D. A., Glader, B. E., et al. (Eds.), *Wintrobe's Clinical Hematology.* (14th ed., pp. 927–959). Philadelphia: Wolters Kluwer.

5. Antony, A. C. (2023). Megaloblastic anemias. In Hoffman, R., Benz, E. J., Silberstein, L. E., et al. (Eds.), *Hematology: Basic Principles and Practice.* (8th ed., pp. 524–554). Philadelphia: Elsevier.

6. Wickramasinghe, S. N., & Fida, S. (1994). Bone marrow cells from vitamin B_{12}- and folate-deficient patients misincorporate uracil into DNA. *Blood, 83,* 1656–1661.

7. Koury, M. J., Horne, D. W., Brown, Z. A., et al. (1997). Apoptosis of late stage erythroblasts in megaloblastic anemia: association with DNA damage and macrocyte production. *Blood, 89,* 4617–4623.

8. Das, K. C., Das, M., Mohanty, D., et al. (2006). Megaloblastosis: from morphos to molecules. *Med Princ Pract, 14,* 2–14.

9. Aslinia, F., Mazza, J., & Yale, S. (2006). Megaloblastic anemia and other causes of macrocytosis. *Clin Med Res, 4*(3), 236–241.

10. Carmel, R., & Rosenblatt, D. S. (2003). Disorders of cobalamin and folate metabolism. In Handin, R. I., Lux, S. E., & Stossel, T. P. (Eds.), *Blood: Principles and Practice of Hematology.* (2nd ed., pp. 1361–1398). Philadelphia: Lippincott Williams & Wilkins.

11. Stabler, S. P. (2013). Vitamin B_{12} deficiency. *N Engl J Med, 368,* 149–160.

12. Pittock, S. J., Payne, T. A., & Harper, C. M. (2002). Reversible myelopathy in a 34-year-old man with vitamin B_{12} deficiency. *Mayo Clin Proc, 77,* 291–294.

13. Morrison, H. I., Schaubel, D., Desmeules, M., et al. (1996). Serum folate and risk of fatal coronary heart disease. *JAMA, 275,* 1893–1896.

14. Voutilainen, S., Virtanen, J. K., Rissanen, T. H., et al. (2004). Serum folate and homocysteine and the incidence of acute coronary events: the Kuopio Ischaemic Heart Disease Risk Factor Study. *Am J Clin Nutr, 80,* 317–323.

15. de Bree, A., Verschuren, W. M., Blom, H. J., et al. (2003). Coronary heart disease mortality, plasma homocysteine, and B-vitamins: a prospective study. *Atherosclerosis, 166,* 369–377.

16. Ganguly, P., & Alam, S. F. (2015). Role of homocysteine in the development of cardiovascular disease. *Nutr J, 10,* 14–16.

17. Humphrey, L. L., Rongwei, F., Rogers, K., et al. (2008). Homocysteine level and coronary heart disease incidence: a systematic review and meta-analysis. *Mayo Clin Proc, 83,* 1203–1212.

18. Soinio, M., Marniemi, J., Laakso, M., et al. (2004). Elevated plasma homocysteine level is an independent predictor of coronary heart disease events in patients with type 2 diabetes mellitus. *Ann Intern Med, 140,* 94–100.

19. Lindeman, R. D., Romero, L. J, Yau, C. L., et al. (2003). Serum homocysteine concentrations and their relation to serum folate and vitamin B_{12} concentrations and coronary artery disease prevalence in an urban, bi-ethnic community. *Ethn Dis, 13,* 178–185.

20. Bottiglieri, T., Laundry, M., Crellin, R., et al. (2000). Homocysteine, folate, methylation, and monoamine metabolism in depression. *J Neurol Neurosurg Psychiatry, 69,* 228–232.

21. Kronenberg, G., Colla, M., & Endres, M. (2009). Folic acid, neurodegenerative and neuropsychiatric disease. *Curr Mol Med, 9,* 315–323.

22. Alpert, J. E., Mischoulon, D., Nierenberg, A. A., et al. (2000). Nutrition and depression: focus on folate. *Nutrition, 16,* 544–546.

23. Blom, H. J., Shaw, G. M., den Heijer, M., et al. (2006). Neural tube defects and folate: case far from closed. *Nat Rev Neurosci, 7,* 724–731.

24. Gallagher, M. L. (2004). Vitamins. In Mahan, L. K., & Escott-Stump, S. (Eds.), *Krause's Food, Nutrition, and Diet Therapy.* (11th ed., pp. 74–119). Philadelphia: Saunders.

25. Qui, A., Jansen, M., Sakaris, A., et al. (2006). Identification of an intestinal folate transporter and the molecular basis for hereditary folate malabsorption. *Cell, 127,* 917–928.

26. Moestrup, S. K. (2006). New insights into carrier binding and epithelial uptake of the erythropoietic nutrients cobalamin and folate. *Curr Opin Hematol, 13,* 119–123.

27. Nath, S. K. (2005). Tropical sprue. *Curr Gastroenterol Rep, 7,* 343–349.

28. Hesdorffer, C. S., & Longo, D. L. (2015). Drug-induced megaloblastic anemia. *N Engl J Med, 373,* 1649–1658.

29. Green, R. (2013). Vitamin B_{12} physiology, dietary sources, and requirements. In Caballero, B. (Ed.), *Encyclopedia of Human Nutrition.* (3rd ed., pp. 351–356). Amsterdam: Elsevier/Academic Press.

30. He, Q., Madsen, M., Kilkenney, A., et al. (2005). Amnionless function is required for cubilin brush-border expression and intrinsic factor-cobalamin (vitamin B_{12}) absorption in vivo. *Blood, 106,* 1447–1453.

31. Watkins, D., Morel, C. F., & Rosenblatt, D. S. (2017). Inborn errors of folate and cobalamin transport and metabolism. In Sarafoglou, K., Hoffman, G. F., & Roth, K. S. (Eds.), *Pediatric Endocrinology and Inborn Errors of Metabolism.* (2nd ed., pp. 287–308). New York: McGraw-Hill.

32. Fyfe, J. C., Madsen, M., Hojrup, P., et al. (2004). The functional cobalamin (vitamin B_{12})-intrinsic factor receptor is a novel complex of cubilin and amnionless. *Blood, 103,* 1573–1579.

33. Afman, L. A., Van Der Put, N. M. J., Thomas, C. M. G., et al. (2001). Reduced vitamin B_{12} binding by transcobalamin II increases the risk of neural tube defects. *QJM, 94,* 159–166.

34. Kozyraki, R., & Cases, O. (2013). Vitamin B_{12} absorption: mammalian physiology and acquired and inherited disorders. *Biochimie, 95,* 1002–1007.

35. Dali-Youcef, N., & Andres, E. (2009). An update on cobalamin deficiency in adults. *QJM, 102,* 17–28.

36. Karlsson, F. A., Burman, P., Loof, L., et al. (1988). Major parietal cell antigen in autoimmune gastritis with pernicious anemia in the acid-producing H+, K+-adenosine triphosphatase of the stomach. *J Clin Invest, 81,* 475–479.

37. Toh, B. H., Van Driel, I. R., & Gleeson, P. A. (1997). Pernicious anemia. *N Engl J Med, 337,* 1441–1448.

38. Fernandez-Banares, F., Monzon, H., & Forme, M. (2009). A short review of malabsorption and anemia. *World J Gastroenterol, 15,* 4644–4652.

39. Wickramasinghe, S. N. (2006). Diagnosis of megaloblastic anemia. *Blood Rev, 20,* 299–318.

40. Kaferle, J., & Strzoda, C. E. (2009). Evaluation of macrocytosis. *Am Fam Physician, 79*(3), 203–208.

41. Kaptan, K., Beyan, C., Ural, A. U., et al. (2000). *Helicobacter pylori*—is it a novel causative agent in vitamin B_{12} deficiency? *Arch Intern Med, 160,* 1349–1353.

42. Morel, C. F., Watkins, D., Scott, P., et al. (2005). Prenatal diagnosis for methylmalonic acidemia and inborn errors of vitamin B_{12} metabolism and transport. *Mol Genet Metab, 86,* 160–171.

43. Nyberg, W., Gräsbeck, R., Saarni, M., et al. (1961). Serum vitamin B_{12} levels and incidence of tape worm anemia in a population heavily infected with *Diphyllobothrium latum. Am J Clin Nutr, 9,* 606–612.

44. Zittoun, J., & Zittoun, R. (1999). Modern clinical testing strategies in cobalamin and folate deficiency. *Semin Hematol, 36,* 35–46.

45. Wickramasinghe, S. N. (1999). The wide spectrum and unresolved issues in megaloblastic anemia. *Semin Hematol, 36,* 3–18.

46. Carmel, R. (1999). Introduction: beyond megaloblastic anemia. *Semin Hematol, 36,* 1–2.

47. Oberley, M. J., & Yang, D. T. (2013). Laboratory testing for cobalamin deficiency in megaloblastic anemia. *Am J Hematol, 88,* 522–526.

48. Piyathilake, C. J., Robinson, C. B., & Cornwell, P. (2007). A practical approach to red blood cell folate analysis. *Anal Chem Insights, 2,* 107–110.

49. Brady, J., Wilson, L., McGregor, L., et al. (2008). Active B_{12}: a rapid, automated assay for holotranscobalamin on the Abbott AxSYM analyzer. *Clin Chem, 54*(3), 567–573.

50. Ulleland, M., Eilertsen, I., Quadros, E. V., et al. (2002). Direct assay for cobalamin bound to transcobalamin (holo-transcobalamin) in serum. *Clin Chem, 48*(3), 526–532.

51. Heil, S. G., de Jonge, R., de Rotte, M. C. F. J., et al. (2012). Screening for metabolic vitamin B_{12} deficiency by holotranscobalamin in patients suspected of vitamin B_{12} deficiency: a multicenter study. *Ann Clin Biochem, 49,* 184–189.

52. Valente, E., Scott, J. M., Ueland, P-M., et al. (2011). Diagnostic accuracy of holotranscobalamin, methylmalonic acid, serum cobalamin, and other indicators of tissue vitamin B_{12} status in the elderly. *Clin Chem, 37*(6), 856–863.

53. Nexo, E., & Hoffmann-Lucke, E. (2011). Holotranscobalamin, a marker of vitamin B_{12} status: analytical aspects and clinical utility. *Am J Clin Nutr, 94*(1), 1S–7S.

54. Carmel, R. (2008). How I treat cobalamin (vitamin B_{12}) deficiency. *Blood, 112*(6), 2214–2221.

55. Butler, C. C., Vidal-Alaball, J., & Cannings-John, R., et al. (2006). Oral vitamin B_{12} versus intramuscular vitamin B_{12} for vitamin B_{12} deficiency: a systematic review of randomized controlled trials. *Fam Pract, 23,* 279–285.

56. Stabler, S. P. (2013). Vitamin B_{12} deficiency. *N Engl J Med, 368,* 149–160.

19

Bone Marrow Failure

Clara Lo, Bertil Glader, and Kathleen M. Sakamoto*

OBJECTIVES

After completion of this chapter, the reader will be able to:

1. Describe the clinical consequences of bone marrow failure.
2. Describe the etiology of acquired aplastic anemia and inherited/congenital bone marrow failure syndromes.
3. Discuss the pathophysiologic mechanisms of acquired aplastic anemia and inherited/congenital bone marrow failure syndromes.
4. Describe the characteristic peripheral blood and bone marrow features in aplastic anemia.
5. Classify aplastic anemia as moderate, severe, or very severe, based on laboratory tests.
6. Discuss treatment modalities for acquired aplastic anemia and inherited bone marrow failure syndromes and the patients for whom each is most appropriate.
7. Differentiate among causes of pancytopenia based on patient history and clinical and laboratory findings, and suggest further tests to confirm a diagnosis.
8. Compare and contrast the pathophysiology, clinical picture, and laboratory findings in Fanconi anemia, dyskeratosis congenita, Shwachman-Bodian-Diamond syndrome, transient erythroblastopenia of childhood, Diamond-Blackfan anemia, and congenital dyserythropoietic anemia.
9. Describe the mechanisms causing cytopenia in myelophthisic anemia and anemia of chronic kidney disease.

OUTLINE

Pathophysiology of Bone Marrow Failure
Aplastic Anemia
　　Acquired Aplastic Anemia
　　Inherited/Congenital Bone Marrow Failure Syndromes
　　Differential Diagnosis

Other Forms of Bone Marrow Failure
　　Pure Red Cell Aplasia
　　Congenital Dyserythropoietic Anemia
　　Myelophthisic Anemia
　　Anemia of Chronic Kidney Disease

CASE STUDY

After studying the material in this chapter, the reader should be able to respond to the following case study. Answers can be found in Appendix C.

A 16-year-old girl presented to her pediatrician with jaundice. The pediatrician checked liver enzyme and bilirubin levels, which were elevated. Hepatitis A, B, and C serologic tests all were negative. The patient was referred to a gastroenterologist, who diagnosed autoimmune hepatitis. With immunomodulatory treatment, her hepatitis improved. However, over the next several months, she noticed increasing fatigue and bruising. The patient also developed heavier menses, with menstrual cycles lasting up to 2 weeks. Physical examination revealed pallor and scattered ecchymoses with petechiae on her chest and shoulders, with no other abnormalities. Complete blood count results were as follows. Reference intervals can be found after the Index at the end of the book.

WBC count	2.0×10^9/L	RETIC	0.6%
HGB	7.9 g/dL	RETIC	16×10^9/L
MCV	104 fL	NEUT	0.5×10^9/L
PLT count	15×10^9/L	LYMPH	0.4×10^9/L

Serum vitamin B_{12} and folate levels were within reference intervals. Bone marrow aspirate revealed mild dyserythropoiesis but normal myelopoiesis and megakaryopoiesis. Iron stain revealed normal stores. A bone marrow biopsy specimen was moderately hypocellular (15%), with a reduction in all three cell lines. There was no increase in reticulin or blasts. Cytogenetic testing revealed a normal karyotype, and results of flow cytometry for paroxysmal nocturnal hemoglobinuria (PNH) cells were negative.

1. What term is used to describe a decrease in all cell lines in the peripheral blood?
2. Which anemia of bone marrow failure should be considered?
3. How would an increase in either reticulin or blasts alter the preliminary diagnosis?
4. How would the severity of this patient's condition be classified?
5. What treatment modality would be considered for this patient?

*The authors extend appreciation to Elaine M. Keohane, whose work in prior editions provided the foundation for this chapter.

PATHOPHYSIOLOGY OF BONE MARROW FAILURE

Bone marrow failure is the reduction or cessation of blood cell production affecting one or more cell lines. *Pancytopenia,* or decreased numbers of circulating red blood cells (RBCs), white blood cells (WBCs), and platelets, is seen in most cases of bone marrow failure, particularly in severe or advanced stages.

The pathophysiology of bone marrow failure includes (1) destruction of hematopoietic stem cells as a result of injury by drugs, chemicals, radiation, viruses, or autoimmune mechanisms; (2) premature senescence and apoptosis of hematopoietic stem cells as a result of genetic mutations; (3) ineffective hematopoiesis caused by stem cell mutations or vitamin B_{12} or folate deficiency; (4) disruption of the bone marrow microenvironment that supports hematopoiesis; (5) decreased production of hematopoietic growth factors or related hormones; and (6) loss of normal hematopoietic tissue as a result of infiltration of the marrow space with abnormal cells.

Clinical consequences of bone marrow failure vary depending on the extent and duration of the cytopenias. Severe pancytopenia can be rapidly fatal if untreated. Some patients may initially be asymptomatic, and their cytopenia may be detected during a routine blood examination. Thrombocytopenia can result in bleeding and increased bruising. Decreased RBCs and hemoglobin can result in fatigue, pallor, and cardiovascular complications. Sustained neutropenia increases the risk of life-threatening bacterial or fungal infections.

This chapter focuses on *aplastic anemia,* a bone marrow failure syndrome resulting from damaged or defective stem cells (mechanisms 1 and 2 listed earlier). Bone marrow failure resulting from other mechanisms may manifest similarly to aplastic anemia; differentiation is discussed later in "Differential Diagnosis." Because there are many mechanisms involved in the various bone marrow failure syndromes, accurate diagnosis is essential to ensure appropriate treatment.

APLASTIC ANEMIA

Aplastic anemia is a rare but potentially fatal bone marrow failure syndrome. In 1888, Ehrlich provided the first case report of aplastic anemia involving a patient with severe anemia, neutropenia, and a hypocellular marrow on postmortem examination.[1] The name *aplastic anemia* was given to the disease by Vaquez and Aubertin in 1904.[2] The characteristic features of aplastic anemia include pancytopenia, reticulocytopenia, bone marrow hypocellularity, and depletion of hematopoietic stem cells (Box 19.1). Approximately 80% to 85% of aplastic anemia

cases are acquired, whereas 15% to 20% are inherited/congenital. Box 19.2 provides an etiologic classification.[3–5]

Acquired Aplastic Anemia

Acquired aplastic anemia is classified into two major categories: idiopathic and secondary. Idiopathic acquired aplastic anemia has no known cause. Secondary acquired aplastic anemia is associated with an identified cause. Approximately 70% of all aplastic anemia cases are idiopathic, whereas 10% to 15% are secondary.[4] Idiopathic and secondary acquired aplastic anemia have similar clinical and laboratory findings. Patients may initially present with macrocytic or normocytic anemia and reticulocytopenia. Pancytopenia may develop slowly or progress at a rapid rate, with complete cessation of hematopoiesis.

Incidence

In North America and Europe, the annual incidence is approximately 1 in 500,000.[6] In Asia and East Asia, the incidence is two to three times higher than in North America or Europe, which may be due to environmental and/or genetic differences.[7] Aplastic anemia can occur at any age, with peak incidence at 15 to 25 years and the second highest frequency at older than 60 years.[6,8] There is no sex predisposition.

Etiology

As the name indicates, the cause of *idiopathic aplastic anemia* (70% of aplastic anemia cases) is unknown. *Secondary aplastic*

BOX 19.1   Characteristic Features of Aplastic Anemia

Pancytopenia
Reticulocytopenia
Bone marrow hypocellularity
Depletion of hematopoietic stem cells

BOX 19.2   Etiologic Classification of Bone Marrow Failure

Acquired Aplastic Anemia (80%–85% of Cases)
Idiopathic (70% of cases)
Secondary (10%–15% of cases)
    Dose dependent/predictable
        Cytotoxic drugs
        Benzene
        Radiation
    Idiosyncratic
        Drugs (Box 19.3)
        Chemicals
            Insecticides
            Cutting/lubricating oils
    Viruses
        Epstein-Barr virus
        Hepatitis virus (non-A, non-B, non-C, non-G)
        Human immunodeficiency virus
    Miscellaneous conditions
        Paroxysmal nocturnal hemoglobinuria
        Autoimmune diseases
        Pregnancy

Inherited/Congenital Bone Marrow Failure Syndromes (15%–20% of Cases)
Fanconi anemia
Dyskeratosis congenita
Shwachman-Bodian-Diamond syndrome

anemia (10% to 15% of aplastic anemia cases) is associated with exposure to certain drugs, chemicals, radiation, or infections, and a few miscellaneous conditions (see Box 19.2).

In secondary anemia, 10% of the cases are due to cytotoxic drugs, radiation, and benzenes that suppress the bone marrow in a predictable, dose-dependent manner.[3,8] Depending on the dose and exposure duration, the bone marrow generally recovers after withdrawal of the agent. Alternatively, approximately 70% of cases of secondary aplastic anemia are due to idiosyncratic reactions to drugs or chemicals (see Box 19.2). In idiosyncratic reactions, the bone marrow failure is unpredictable and unrelated to dose.[9] Documentation of a responsible factor or agent in these cases is difficult because evidence is primarily circumstantial, and symptoms may occur months or years after exposure. Some drugs associated with idiosyncratic secondary aplastic anemia are listed in Box 19.3.[8,10]

Generally, idiosyncratic secondary aplastic anemia is rare and likely is due to a combination of genetic and environmental factors in susceptible individuals. There are no readily available tests that predict individual susceptibility to these idiosyncratic reactions. However, genetic variations in immune response pathways or metabolic enzymes may play a role.[9] There is an approximately twofold higher incidence of human leukocyte antigen-DR2 (HLA-DR2) and its major serologic split, HLA-DR15, in patients with aplastic anemia compared with the general population, but the relationship of this finding to disease pathophysiology has not been elucidated.[11,12] There are also reports that genetic polymorphisms in enzymes that metabolize benzene increase susceptibility to toxicity, even at low exposure levels.[9,13] These include polymorphisms in glutathione *S*-transferase (GST) enzymes (GSTT1 and GSTM1), myeloperoxidase, nicotinamide adenine dinucleotide phosphate (reduced form, NADPH), quinine oxidoreductase 1, and cytochrome oxidase P450 2E1.[13] GST is important for metabolism and neutralization of chemical toxins, and deficiencies of this enzyme may increase the risk of aplastic anemia. Further study is required to assess how these genetic variations and other yet undiscovered factors contribute to aplastic anemia.

Acquired aplastic anemia occurs occasionally as a complication of infection with Epstein-Barr virus, human immunodeficiency virus (HIV), hepatitis virus, and human parvovirus B19 (see Box 19.2).[9] In 2% to 10% of patients with acquired aplastic anemia, there is a history of acute nontypable hepatitis (e.g., non-A, non-B) occurring 1 to 3 months before the onset of pancytopenia; this is thought to represent autoimmune hepatitis.[14] The acquired aplastic anemia in these cases may be mediated by such mechanisms as interferon-γ (IFN-γ) and cytokine release.

Aplastic anemia associated with pregnancy is rare, with less than 100 cases reported in the literature.[14,15] Approximately 10% of individuals with acquired aplastic anemia have a concomitant autoimmune disease,[16] and approximately 10% develop hemolytic or thrombotic manifestations of *paroxysmal nocturnal hemoglobinuria* (PNH) (see Box 19.2).[17] The overlap between acquired aplastic anemia and PNH is discussed in "Laboratory Findings."

BOX 19.3 Selected Drugs Reported to Have a Rare Association With Idiosyncratic Secondary Aplastic Anemia

Antiarthritics
Gold compounds
Penicillamine

Antibiotics
Chloramphenicol
Sulfonamides

Anticonvulsants
Carbamazepine
Hydantoins
Phenacemide

Antidepressants
Dothiepin
Phenothiazine

Antidiabetic Agents
Carbutamide
Chlorpropamide
Tolbutamide

Antiinflammatories (Nonsteroidal)
Diclofenac
Fenbufen
Fenoprofen
Ibuprofen
Indomethacin
Naproxen
Phenylbutazone
Piroxicam
Sulindac

Antiprotozoals
Chloroquine
Quinacrine

Antithyroidals
Methimazole
Methylthiouracil

Carbonic Anhydrase Inhibitors
Acetazolamide
Mesalazine
Methazolamide

Pathophysiology

The primary pathology in acquired aplastic anemia is a quantitative and qualitative deficiency of hematopoietic stem cells. Stem cells of patients with acquired aplastic anemia have diminished colony formation in methylcellulose cultures.[18] The hematopoietic stem and early progenitor cell compartment is identified by expression of CD34 surface antigens. The CD34+ cell population in the bone marrow of patients with acquired aplastic anemia can be 10% or lower than that seen in healthy individuals.[18] In addition, these CD34+ cells have increased expression of Fas receptors that mediate apoptosis and increased expression of apoptosis-related genes.[19–21]

Bone marrow stromal cells are functionally normal in acquired aplastic anemia. They produce normal or even increased quantities of growth factors and are able to support the growth of CD34+ cells from healthy donors in culture and in vivo after transplantation.[9,22] Patients with aplastic anemia also have elevated serum levels of erythropoietin, thrombopoietin, granulocyte colony-stimulating factor (G-CSF), and granulocyte-macrophage colony-stimulating factor (GM-CSF).[23] In addition, serum levels of FLT3 ligand, a growth factor that stimulates proliferation of stem and progenitor cells, is up to 200 times higher in patients with severe aplastic anemia compared with healthy controls.[23,24] However, despite their elevated levels, growth factors are generally unsuccessful in correcting the cytopenias found in acquired aplastic anemia.

The severe depletion of hematopoietic stem and progenitor cells from the bone marrow may be due to direct damage to stem cells, immune damage to stem cells, or other unknown mechanisms. Direct damage to stem and progenitor cells results from DNA injury after exposure to cytotoxic drugs, chemicals, radiation, or viruses.[8,9]

Immune damage to stem cells results from exposure to drugs, chemicals, viruses, or other agents that cause autoimmune cytotoxic T lymphocytic destruction of stem and progenitor cells.[9,25,26] An autoimmune pathophysiology was first suggested in the 1970s when aplastic anemia patients undergoing pretransplant immunosuppressive conditioning had an improvement in cell counts.[27] Further evidence supporting an autoimmune pathophysiology includes (1) elevated blood and bone marrow cytotoxic (CD8+) T lymphocytes with an oligoclonal expansion of specific T cell clones[28]; (2) increased T cell production of IFN-γ and tumor necrosis factor-α (TNF-α), cytokines that inhibit hematopoiesis and induce apoptosis[29–31]; (3) upregulation of T-bet, a transcription factor that binds to the promoter of the IFN-γ gene[32]; (4) increased TNF-α receptors on CD34+ cells[33]; and (5) improvement in cytopenias after immunosuppressive therapy (IST).[8,34] Approximately two-thirds of patients with acquired aplastic anemia respond to IST; the outcome is better in children than adults.[35,36]

Possible autoimmune mechanisms include mutation of stem cell antigens and disruption of immune regulation. Young and colleagues[34,37] showed that environmental exposures might alter self-proteins, induce expression of abnormal or novel antigens, or induce an immune response that cross-reacts with self-antigens. Solomou and colleagues[38] demonstrated that CD4+CD25+FOXP3+ regulatory T cells are decreased in aplastic anemia. These regulatory T cells normally suppress autoreactive T cells, and a deficit of these cells may facilitate an autoimmune reaction. Furthermore, a number of individuals with aplastic anemia have single nucleotide polymorphisms in IFN-γ/+874 TT, TNF-α/-308 AA, transforming growth factor-β1/-509 TT, and interleukin-6/-174 GG.[39] These polymorphisms result in cytokine overproduction and may impart a genetic susceptibility to aplastic anemia as well as contribute to its severity.[39]

The specific antigens responsible for triggering and sustaining the autoimmune attack on stem cells are unknown.[26] Candidate antigens have been identified from aplastic anemia patient sera, including kinectin,[40] diazepam-binding inhibitor-related protein 1,[41] and moesin.[42] These proteins are expressed in hematopoietic progenitor cells, but their role in the pathogenesis of aplastic anemia is not known.

Approximately one-third of patients with acquired aplastic anemia have shortened *telomeres* in their peripheral blood granulocytes compared with age-matched controls.[43,44] Telomeres protect the ends of chromosomes from damage and erosion, and cells with abnormally short telomeres undergo proliferation arrest and premature apoptosis. *Telomerase* is an enzyme complex that repairs and maintains telomeres. Approximately 10% of patients with acquired aplastic anemia and shortened telomeres have a mutation in the telomerase complex gene for either the ribonucleic acid (RNA) template *(TERC)* or the reverse transcriptase *(TERT)*.[44–46] Shortened telomeres in the other 90% of patients may be due to stress hematopoiesis or other yet unidentified mutations.[44] In stress hematopoiesis, there is an increase in progenitor cell turnover, and the telomeres become shorter with each cell division.

Approximately 4% of patients with acquired aplastic anemia and shortened telomeres have mutations in the Shwachman-Bodian-Diamond syndrome *(SBDS)* gene.[47] The *SBDS* gene product is involved in ribosome biogenesis, and its relationship to telomere maintenance is unknown. *TERT/TERC* and *SBDS* mutations also occur in the inherited bone marrow failure syndromes dyskeratosis congenita (DC) and SBDS, respectively, and some patients diagnosed with acquired aplastic anemia who have these mutations may actually have DC or SBDS.[4,9] Correct differentiation between acquired aplastic anemia and inherited bone marrow failure syndromes has important implications for appropriate treatment and prognosis. Immunosuppressive therapy is not nearly as effective in inherited bone marrow failure compared with acquired aplastic anemia. Shortened telomeres occur more often in patients whose pancytopenia does not respond to immunosuppressive therapy.[48] Defective telomere maintenance may be another pathophysiologic mechanism of stem cell injury, imparting susceptibility to aplastic anemia after an environmental insult.[44,45]

Clinical Findings

Symptoms vary in acquired aplastic anemia, ranging from asymptomatic to severe. Patients usually present with symptoms of insidious-onset anemia, with pallor, fatigue, and weakness. Severe and prolonged anemia can result in serious cardiovascular complications including tachycardia, hypotension, cardiac failure, and death. Symptoms of thrombocytopenia are also varied and include petechiae, bruising, epistaxis, mucosal bleeding, menorrhagia, retinal hemorrhages, intestinal bleeding, and intracranial hemorrhage. Fever and bacterial or fungal infections are unusual at initial presentation but may occur after prolonged periods of neutropenia. Splenomegaly and hepatomegaly are typically absent.

Laboratory Findings

Pancytopenia is typical, although initially, only one or two cell lines may be decreased. The absolute neutrophil count is decreased, and the absolute lymphocyte count may be normal or decreased. The hemoglobin is usually less than 10 g/dL, the mean cell volume is increased or normal, and the percent and absolute reticulocyte counts are decreased. Table 19.1 lists the diagnostic criteria for aplastic anemia by degree of severity (moderate, severe, and very severe).[49,50] Neutrophils, monocytes, and platelets are decreased in the peripheral blood, and the RBCs are macrocytic or normocytic (Figure 19.1). Toxic granulation may be observed in the neutrophils, but the RBCs and platelets are usually normal in appearance. Leukemic blasts and other immature blood cells are characteristically absent. The serum iron level and percent transferrin saturation may be increased, which reflects decreased iron use for erythropoiesis. Liver function test results may be abnormal in cases of hepatitis-associated aplastic anemia.

Approximately two-thirds of patients have small numbers (less than 25%) of PNH clones in the peripheral blood,[51] but only 10% of patients develop enough PNH cells to have the clinical and biochemical manifestations of PNH disease.[17] PNH is characterized by an acquired stem cell mutation resulting in lack of the glycosylphosphatidylinositol (GPI)-linked proteins CD55 and CD59. The absence of CD55 and CD59 on the surface of the RBCs renders them more susceptible to complement-mediated cell lysis. It is important to test for PNH in acquired aplastic anemia because of the potential risk of hemolytic or thrombotic complications (Chapter 21). Historically, the diagnosis of PNH depended on the Ham acid hemolysis test: patients' RBCs were placed in acidified serum, and a positive result demonstrated lysis of RBCs. However, this test was poorly sensitive because complement-mediated hemolysis was detected only in the presence of large numbers of circulating PNH cells. The Ham test has been replaced by flow cytometric analysis for proteins linked to the GPI anchor: CD55 and CD59 on RBCs and CD24 and CD14 on granulocytes and monocytes.[51,52] In addition, flow cytometry for the GPI anchor (using a fluorescein-labeled proaerolysin variant) is a high-sensitivity assay for detecting PNH cells among granulocytes (Chapter 21).[53]

Bone marrow aspirate and biopsy specimens have prominent fat cells with areas of patchy marrow cellularity. Biopsy specimens are required for accurate quantitative assessment of marrow cellularity, and severe hypocellularity is a characteristic feature of aplastic anemia (Figure 19.2). Erythroid, granulocytic, and megakaryocytic cells are decreased or absent. Dyserythropoiesis may be present, but there is typically no

dysplasia of the granulocyte or platelet cell lines. Blasts and other abnormal cell infiltrates are characteristically absent. Reticulin staining is usually normal.

In patients receiving immunosuppressive therapy, the risk of developing an abnormal karyotype is 14% at 5 years and 20% at 10 years.[54] Monosomy 7 and trisomy 8 are the most common cytogenetic abnormalities.[52,54] Cytogenetic analysis using conventional culture techniques often underestimates the incidence of karyotype abnormalities because of bone marrow hypocellularity and scarcity of cells in metaphase.[55] Alternatively, interphase fluorescence in situ hybridization (FISH) using DNA probes for specific chromosome abnormalities should be used. Compared with conventional cytogenetic analysis, FISH has greater sensitivity in the detection of chromosome abnormalities and can be performed using nondividing cells.[55] In a study performed by Kearns and colleagues,[55] FISH detected monosomy 7 or trisomy 8 in 26% of aplastic anemia patients who had a normal karyotype by conventional cytogenetic testing.

Patients with an inherited bone marrow failure syndrome may be misdiagnosed with acquired aplastic anemia if symptoms manifest in late adolescence or adulthood or if the patients lack the typical clinical and physical characteristics of an inherited marrow failure syndrome (e.g., abnormal thumbs, short stature).[4,8,9] Consideration of inherited bone marrow failure syndromes in the differential diagnosis of acquired aplastic anemia is essential because these conditions require a different therapeutic approach. The inherited bone marrow failure syndromes

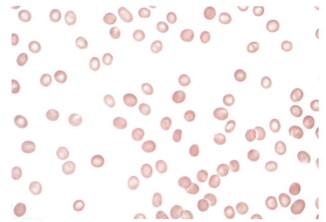

Figure 19.1 Peripheral Blood Film of a Patient With Aplastic Anemia. Note occasional macrocytes and absence of white blood cells and platelets. (Wright-Giemsa stain ×1000.)

TABLE 19.1	**Diagnostic Criteria for Aplastic Anemia**		
	MAA	**SAA**	**VSAA**
Bone marrow	Hypocellular bone marrow plus at least two of the following:	Bone marrow cellularity <25%* plus at least two of the following:	Same as SAA
Absolute neutrophil count (×10⁹/L)	0.5–1.5	0.2–0.5	<0.2
Platelet count (×10⁹/L)	20–50	<20	Same as SAA
Other	HGB ≤10 g/dL plus reticulocytes <30 × 10⁹/L	Reticulocytes <20 × 10⁹/L or <1% corrected for HCT	Same as SAA

*Or 25% to 50% cellularity with <30% residual hematopoietic cells.
HCT, Hematocrit; *HGB*, hemoglobin; *MAA*, moderate aplastic anemia; *SAA*, severe aplastic anemia; *VSAA*, very severe aplastic anemia.

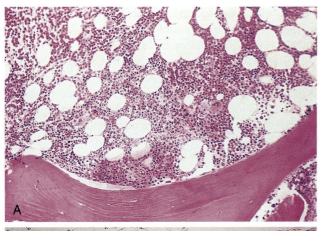

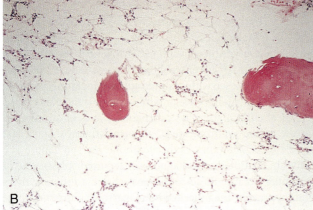

Figure 19.2 Biopsy of Normal and Hypoplastic Bone Marrow. (A), Normal bone marrow tissue section. (B), Hypoplastic bone marrow tissue section from a patient with aplastic anemia. (A, B, Hematoxylin and eosin stain, ×100.) (Courtesy Ann Bell, University of Tennessee, Memphis.)

are discussed in "Inherited/Congenital Bone Marrow Failure Syndromes."

Treatment and Prognosis

Severe acquired aplastic anemia requires immediate attention to prevent serious complications. If a causative agent is identified, its use should be discontinued. Blood product replacement should be given judiciously to avoid alloimmunization.[10] Platelets should not be transfused at counts greater than 10,000/μL, unless the patient is bleeding.[10]

One of the most important early decisions is determining whether the patient is a candidate for *bone marrow transplantation* (BMT). This clearly is the treatment of choice for patients with severe aplastic anemia who are younger than 40 years of age and have an HLA-matched related donor (MRD).[8,9,56] However, only 20% to 30% of patients meet these criteria. Historically, IST, consisting of antithymocyte globulin and cyclosporine, has been used for patients older than 40 years of age and for patients without a matched related stem cell donor.[10,17] Antithymocyte globulin decreases the number of activated T cells and cyclosporine inhibits T cell function, thereby suppressing the autoimmune reaction against the stem cells.

More recently, BMT from a high-resolution HLA-matched unrelated donor (MUD) has become an option.[10,57] With advances in modern transplantation protocols, overall survival rates with an MUD are almost as good as with an MRD.[5,8,9,58] Early identification of an MUD through international registries have prompted some centers to pursue upfront MUD BMT, particularly in centers with comparable survival outcomes to MRD BMT. Because of the increased success with MUD BMT, it has been proposed that this approach be used as initial therapy instead of IST.[56,59] Moreover, because of reported successes with haploidentical BMT for severe aplastic anemia,[60] it has been suggested that this source of stem cell donor also should be used up front rather than IST.[56] The reason for the high priority of BMT is because it is curative, while IST can be associated with late complications (aplastic anemia relapse, evolution of MDS, PNH). Individuals with PNH cells (CD55-CD59-) are almost twice as likely to respond to IST than individuals who lack these cells.[51] In addition, the presence of both PNH cells and HLA-DR2 increases the likelihood of response by 3.5-fold.[61] G-CSF, other hematopoietic growth factors, and steroids do not increase overall survival or improve the response rate; therefore they are not recommended for routine use.[10,62,63]

There have been promising results in severe aplastic anemia with the addition of a thrombopoietin mimetic, eltrombopag, to standard IST for severe aplastic anemia.[64,65] The mechanism of action of eltrombopag in aplastic anemia is unclear but may be due to stimulatory effects on stem and progenitor cells. The efficacy of eltrombopag added to standard IST for pediatric severe aplastic anemia is more controversial and may not be as good as seen in adults.[66,67]

Other supportive therapy includes antibiotic and antifungal prophylaxis in cases of prolonged neutropenia. Patients with mild to moderate aplastic anemia may not require treatment but must be monitored periodically for pancytopenia and abnormal cells.

The overall outcome for patients with acquired aplastic anemia has dramatically improved in the past two decades. Children have higher survival rates compared with adults with both BMT and IST as first-line treatment.[57] With BMT, the 10-year survival for patients aged 1 to 20 is 86% and for patients older than 40 years is 56; with IST, 10-year survival for those same age groups is 84% and 58%, respectively.[57] Additional outcomes in IST-treated patients include a 10-year risk of developing hemolytic or thrombotic PNH and a 10% to 20% risk of developing myelodysplastic syndrome (MDS) or leukemia.[17,52] Development of monosomy 7 predicts poor outcome, with a greater likelihood of unresponsiveness to IST and progression to MDS or leukemia.[54]

Inherited/Congenital Bone Marrow Failure Syndromes

Compared with acquired aplastic anemia, patients with inherited/congenital bone marrow failure syndromes present at an earlier age and may have characteristic physical stigmata.[68] The three most common inherited/congenital bone marrow failure disorders associated with pancytopenia are Fanconi anemia (FA), dyskeratosis congenita, and SBDS (see Box 19.2).[4,68–70]

Fanconi Anemia

Fanconi anemia (FA) is a chromosome instability disorder characterized by aplastic anemia, physical abnormalities, and cancer susceptibility. In 1927, Dr. Guido Fanconi first described this syndrome in three brothers with skin pigmentation, short stature, and hypogonadism.[71] FA has a prevalence of 1 to 5 cases per 1 million.[70] The carrier rate is 1 in 300 in the United States and Europe, with a threefold higher prevalence in Ashkenazi Jewish people (whose ancestors lived in Central and Eastern Europe) and South African Afrikaners.[72] FA is the most common of the inherited bone marrow failure syndromes.

Clinical findings. Patients with FA have variable features and symptoms. Physical malformations may be present at birth, though hematologic abnormalities may not appear until older childhood or adulthood. Furthermore, only two-thirds of patients have physical malformations.[4,68,70,73–75] These anomalies vary considerably, though there is a higher frequency of skeletal abnormalities (thumb malformations, radial hypoplasia, microcephaly, hip dislocation, and scoliosis); skin pigmentation (hyperpigmentation, hypopigmentation, café-au-lait lesions); short stature; and abnormalities of the eyes, kidneys, and genitals. Low birth weight and developmental delay are also common.

The symptoms associated with pancytopenia usually become apparent at 5 to 10 years of age, though some patients may not present until adulthood.[4,72] Individuals with FA also have an increased cancer risk. This includes an increased incidence of leukemia in childhood and solid tumors (e.g., oral, esophageal, anogenital, cervical) in adulthood.[75,76] In approximately 5% of cases a malignancy is diagnosed before FA is recognized.[76]

Genetics and pathophysiology. Patients with FA typically have biallelic mutations or deletions in one of at least 23 genes: *FANCA, FANCB, FANCC, FANCD1 (BRCA2), FANCD2, FANCE, FANCF, FANCG (XRCC9), FANCI, FANCJ (BRIP1/ BACH1), FANCL, FANCM, FANCN (PALB2), FANCO (RAD51C), FANCP (SLX4), FANCQ (ERCC4 or XPF), FANCR (RAD51), FANCS (BRCA1), FANCT (UBE2T), FANCU (XRCC2), FANCV (MAD2L2, REV7), FANCW (RFWD3),* and *FANCY (FAP100).*[69,70,77] The mode of inheritance is autosomal recessive except for *FANCB*, which is X-linked. Mutations in the *FANCA* gene occur with the highest frequency (60%); this is followed by *FANCC* (14%) and *FANCG* (10%), whereas mutations in the other *FANC* genes are much less common.[69,78] The relationship between mutations in the FA genes and disease pathology is not clear. Cells are highly susceptible to chromosome breakage after exposure to DNA cross-linking agents. FA cells may also have accelerated telomere shortening and apoptosis, a late S-phase cell cycle delay, hypersensitivity to oxidants, and cytokine dysregulation.[69,78]

The range of FA protein function is not completely known, but these proteins participate in a highly elaborate DNA damage response pathway. The FA pathway consists of a nuclear core complex, a protein ID complex, and effector proteins.[73,79] The FA proteins A, B, C, E, F, G, L, and M form the nuclear core complex; proteins D2 and I form the ID complex; and the effector proteins are D1, J, N, O, P, Q, R, S, T, U, V, and W.[73,77,79] The core complex facilitates the monoubiquitylation and activation of the ID complex. The ID complex then localizes with effector DNA repair proteins at foci of DNA damage to effect DNA repair.

Laboratory findings. Laboratory results are similar to those in acquired aplastic anemia, with pancytopenia, reticulocytopenia,

and a hypocellular bone marrow. Macrocytic RBCs are often the first detected abnormality, and thrombocytopenia usually precedes the development of the other cytopenias.[70,75] Fetal hemoglobin (Hb F) may be strikingly elevated.

Chromosomal breakage analysis is the diagnostic test for FA.[69,78] Patients' peripheral blood lymphocytes are cultured with the DNA cross-linking agents diepoxybutane or mitomycin C. Compared with normal lymphocytes, FA cells have a greater number of characteristic chromosome breaks and ring chromosomes, indicating increased fragility. Caution must be taken in interpreting peripheral blood results because they may be negative in the 10% to 15% of FA patients who have somatic mosaicism as a result of a reversion of one abnormal allele to the normal type.[70] Chromosome breakage studies can be performed on cultured skin fibroblasts from a skin biopsy specimen in these cases.[70,80] Diagnosis is confirmed by genetic testing for FA gene mutations.

Treatment and prognosis. More than 70% of FA patients develop bone marrow failure by 50 years of age.[81] Furthermore, one-third of patients develop MDS and/or acute myeloid leukemia (AML) by a median age of 14 years, and 25% develop solid tumors by a median age of 26 years.[76] Squamous cell carcinomas of the head and neck, anogenital region, and skin are the most common solid tumors, followed by tumors of the liver, brain, and kidney. Patients with FA have an increased risk of developing vulvar cancer (4300-fold), esophageal cancer (2300-fold), AML (800-fold), and head/neck cancer (700-fold) compared with the general population.[82] Approximately 3% of patients develop more than one type of malignancy.[83] Left untreated, death by 20 years of age secondary to bone marrow failure or malignancy is common. Patients with mutations in the *FANCC* gene experience bone marrow failure at a particularly young age and have the poorest survival rates.[70,83] Increased telomere shortening in FA cells is associated with more severe pancytopenia and a higher risk of malignancy. However, the precise role of telomere shortening in the evolution of bone marrow failure and cancer is currently unclear.

Supportive treatment for cytopenias includes transfusions and administration of cytokines (G-CSF and GM-CSF).[70,84,85] The only curative treatment for hematologic abnormalities is hematopoietic stem cell transplant, preferably from an MRD. However, with high-resolution (molecular) HLA testing, an MUD can be used, with almost the same success rate.[86] It is important to screen donor siblings for FA with DNA breakage studies and gene mutation analysis before transplant. Patients should also have decreased intensity pretransplant conditioning because of their underlying chromosomal instability.[70] Gene therapy for the hematologic problems of FA is being considered, and clinical trials for *FANCA* are now in progress.[87] It should be noted that successful treatment of hematologic failure in FA does not change the risk for development of a solid tumor malignancy.

Dyskeratosis Congenita

Telomere biology disorders (TBDs) are a heterogeneous group of diseases due to germline mutations that affect genomic stability, resulting in premature aging.[88] Some of the conditions include bone marrow failure, pulmonary fibrosis, liver cirrhosis, premature gray hair, and an increased cancer risk. *Dyskeratosis congenita* (DC) was the original TBD first observed in the early 20th century. DC is a rare inherited bone marrow failure syndrome with an incidence of approximately 4 cases per 1 million per year.[68,70,89,90]

Clinical findings. DC is characterized by mucocutaneous abnormalities, bone marrow failure, and pancytopenia. The typical clinical presentation involves a triad of abnormal skin pigmentation, dystrophic nails, and oral leukoplakia. Skin and nail findings usually appear before 10 years of age.[4,69,70] By 30 years of age, 80% to 90% of patients have bone marrow abnormalities. Patients can also manifest a wide range of multisystem abnormalities, including pulmonary fibrosis, liver disease, developmental delay, short stature, microcephaly, prematurely gray hair or hair loss, immunodeficiency, dental caries, and periodontal disease.[70,91] Patients have a 40% risk of cancer by age 50, most commonly AML, MDS, and epithelial malignancies.[89,92]

Genetics and pathophysiology. DC chromosomes have very short telomeres, and inherited defects in the telomerase complex are implicated in the pathophysiology.[92] The telomerase complex synthesizes telomere repeats to elongate chromosome ends, maintaining the telomere length needed for cell survival.

Patients with DC typically have mutations in one of at least 16 genes. The mode of inheritance is X-linked recessive, autosomal dominant, or autosomal recessive.[47,70] The best-characterized form results from one or more mutations on the long arm of the X-chromosome on the *DKC1* gene coding for dyskerin. Dyskerin is a ribonucleoprotein involved in RNA processing, and it associates with TERC (telomerase RNA component) in the telomerase complex. Autosomal dominant forms are mainly caused by mutations in the genes that encode NAF1, RPA1, TERC, TINF2 (component of the shelterin complex that regulates telomere length) or ZCCHC8.[47,91] In the autosomal recessive form, mutations in *CTC1, NHP2, NOP10, POT1, STN1* and *WRAP53* have been identified. A few genes are associated with autosomal dominant or autosomal recessive forms including *ACD, PARN, RTEL1,* and *TERT.* The proteins encoded by these genes are also involved in telomere maintenance. Although the exact pathophysiologic mechanisms are still unknown, the shortened telomeres in DC cause premature death in the rapidly dividing cells in the bone marrow and epithelium and likely lead to the genomic instability and predisposition to cancer.

Laboratory findings. Pancytopenia and macrocytic RBCs are typical peripheral blood findings. Fetal hemoglobin level also may be increased. A flow cytometry FISH (flow-FISH) test for detection of very short telomeres in WBC subsets is used as a screening test for suspected DC.[93] Patients with FA, SBDS, and acquired aplastic anemia also may have cells with shortened telomeres, though they are not found in multiple WBC subsets.[93] In contrast, DC cells often have shortened telomeres in several WBC subsets, including naïve T cells and B cells.[93] About 75% of patients have an identified mutation in one of the 11 telomerase complex genes and can be diagnosed by genetic testing.[70,91]

Treatment and prognosis. Median survival for patients with DC/TBD is 52.8 years.[92] Approximately 60% to 70% of deaths are due to bone marrow failure complications. Approximately 10% to 15% of deaths result from severe pulmonary disease, and 10% of deaths result from malignancies. Treatment with bone marrow transplantation has not been optimal because of the high incidence of fatal pulmonary fibrosis and vascular complications. Although androgen therapy produces a transient response in 50% to 70% of patients, it does not halt the progression of the bone marrow failure.

Shwachman-Bodian-Diamond Syndrome

Shwachman-Bodian-Diamond syndrome (SBDS) is a multisystem disorder characterized by pancreatic insufficiency, cytopenia, skeletal abnormalities, and a predisposition for hematologic malignancies. The incidence has been estimated to be approximately 8.5 cases per 1 million live births.[47]

Clinical findings. Patients with SBDS have peripheral blood cytopenia and decreased pancreatic enzyme secretion. The pancreatic insufficiency causes gastrointestinal malabsorption, which typically presents in early infancy. Patients have neutropenia and immune dysfunction and are at increased risk of severe infections and sepsis.[94] Nearly all SBDS patients have delayed bone maturation, and approximately 50% have failure to thrive and short stature.[95]

Genetics and pathophysiology. SBDS is most commonly an autosomal recessive disorder, and 90% of patients have biallelic mutations in the *SBDS* gene.[95] The *SBDS* gene is involved in ribosome biogenesis and mitotic spindle stability.[91,96] Other autosomal recessive pathogenic variants include *DNAJC21* and *EFL1.* Autosomal dominant pathogenic variants include *SRP54.* There are quantitative and qualitative deficiencies in CD34+ cells, dysfunctional bone marrow stromal cells, increased apoptosis and mitotic spindle destabilization in hematopoietic cells, and short telomeres in peripheral blood granulocytes.[96,97]

Laboratory findings. Nearly all patients with SBDS have neutropenia (less than 1.5×10^9 neutrophils/L).[98] Half of patients also develop anemia or thrombocytopenia, and a quarter develop pancytopenia. The RBCs are usually normocytic but can be macrocytic, and approximately two-thirds of patients have elevated Hb F. Bone marrow is usually hypocellular but can be normal or even hypercellular. Because of pancreatic insufficiency, 72-hour fecal fat testing shows increased fat excretion, and decreased serum trypsinogen and isoamylase levels compared with age-related reference intervals.[97] Compared with cystic fibrosis, which can have a similar malabsorption presentation, patients with SBDS have normal sweat chloride tests. Testing for the gene mutations is commercially available and should be done in suspected patients suspected to have SBDS and their parents.

Treatment and prognosis. In some cases, no treatment of hematologic features is needed. However, if needed, treatment consists of G-CSF for neutropenia, transfusion support for anemia and thrombocytopenia, and enzyme replacement for pancreatic insufficiency. The risk of AML and MDS is approximately 19% at 20 years and 36% at 30 years.[94,99] Allogeneic bone marrow transplantation is recommended in cases of severe pancytopenia, AML, or MDS. Despite supportive care and attempted curative therapy, however, 5-year overall survival is 60% to 72%, with many deaths occurring from severe infections and malignancy.[97,100]

Poor outcomes after transplant occur because of graft failure, transplant-related toxicities, and recurrent leukemia.

Differential Diagnosis

A distinction must be made between acquired aplastic anemia, inherited/congenital bone marrow failure syndromes, and other causes of pancytopenia, including PNH, MDS, megaloblastic anemia, and leukemia. A correct diagnosis is important because diagnostic conclusions dictate therapeutic management and prognosis. The distinguishing features of these conditions are listed in Tables 19.2 and 19.3.[101]

Alternative diagnoses include lymphoma, myelofibrosis, and mycobacterial infections, which also may manifest with pancytopenia. However, these diagnoses often can be distinguished with a careful history, physical examination, and laboratory testing. Review of a peripheral blood film by an experienced morphologist is important. If needed, bone marrow evaluation and molecular testing for chromosome abnormalities and gene mutations can further distinguish these diagnoses. Anorexia nervosa also may manifest with pancytopenia. In these cases, the bone marrow is hypocellular and has fewer fat cells. The cytopenias revert with correction of the underlying disease.

OTHER FORMS OF BONE MARROW FAILURE

Other forms of bone marrow failure include pure red cell aplasia (PRCA), congenital dyserythropoietic anemia (CDA),

myelophthisic anemia, and anemia of chronic kidney disease (CKD).

Pure Red Cell Aplasia

Pure red cell aplasia (PRCA) is a rare disorder of erythropoiesis characterized by a selective and severe decrease in erythroid precursors in an otherwise normal bone marrow. Patients have severe anemia (usually normocytic), reticulocytopenia, and normal WBC and platelet counts. PRCA may be acquired or congenital. It is important to distinguish between acquired and congenital forms because they require different therapeutic approaches.

Acquired Pure Red Cell Aplasia

Acquired PRCA may occur in children or adults and can be acute or chronic. Primary PRCA may be idiopathic or autoimmune related. Secondary PRCA may occur in association with an underlying thymoma, hematologic malignancy, solid tumor, infection, chronic hemolytic anemia, collagen vascular disease, or exposure to drugs or chemicals.[102–104] Therapy is first directed at treatment of the underlying condition, but IST may be considered if the PRCA is not responsive. Cyclosporine is associated with a higher response rate (65% to 87%) than corticosteroids (30% to 62%) and is better suited for long-term maintenance if needed.[103,105]

The acquired form of PRCA in young children is also known as *transient erythroblastopenia of childhood* (TEC). A history of

---

TABLE 19.2 Differentiation of Aplastic Anemia From Other Causes of Pancytopenia

Condition	Peripheral Blood	Bone Marrow	Laboratory Test Results	Clinical Findings
Failure of Bone Marrow to Produce Blood Cells				
Aplastic anemia	No immature WBCs or RBCs; ↓ reticulocytes; MCV ↑ or normal	Hypocellular; blasts and abnormal cells absent; reticulin normal; RBC dyspoiesis may be present; WBC and platelet dyspoiesis absent	Acquired: PNH cells* may be present; chromosome abnormalities may be present Inherited/congenital: Table 19.3	Splenomegaly absent
Increased Destruction of Blood Cells				
PNH	Reticulocytes ↑; MCV ↑ or normal; nucleated RBCs present or absent	Erythroid hyperplasia; may be hypocellular	PNH cells* present; hemoglobinuria +/–; chromosome abnormalities may be present	Splenomegaly absent; thrombosis may be present
Ineffective Hematopoiesis				
Myelodysplastic neoplasm	Variable pancytopenia; reticulocytes ↓; MCV ↑ or normal; blasts and abnormal WBCs, RBCs, and platelets may be present	Hypercellular; 20% of cases hypocellular; dyspoiesis in one or more cell lines present; blasts and immature cells present; reticulin ↑	Chromosome abnormalities usually present	Splenomegaly uncommon
Megaloblastic anemias	MCV ↑; oval macrocytes; hypersegmented neutrophils	Hypercellular with megaloblastic features	Serum vitamin B$_{12}$ or folate or both ↓	Splenomegaly absent
Bone Marrow Infiltration				
Acute leukemia	Blasts present	Hypercellular; blasts ↑; reticulin ↑	Chromosome abnormalities usually present	Splenomegaly may be present
Hairy cell leukemia	Hairy cells present; monocytes ↓	Hairy cells† and fibrosis present; reticulin ↑	Hairy cells present; TRAP +	Splenomegaly present (60%–70% of cases)

*PNH erythrocytes are detected by flow cytometry by their lack of expression of CD59; PNH granulocytes and monocytes lack CD24 and CD14 (Chapter 21).

†Hairy cells are detected by flow cytometry by their expression of CD19, CD20, CD22, CD11c, CD25, CD103, and FMC7.

↑, Increased; ↓, decreased; +, positive result; +/–, positive or negative result; *MCV*, mean cell volume; *PNH*, paroxysmal nocturnal hemoglobinuria; *RBC*, red blood cell; *TRAP*, tartrate-resistant acid phosphatase; *WBC*, white blood cell.

TABLE 19.3 Key Characteristics of Inherited/Congenital Bone Marrow Failure Anemias

Condition	Genetics*	Peripheral Blood	Bone Marrow	Laboratory Test Results	Clinical Findings
Caused by Bone Marrow Hypoplasia					
FA	AR (most), XLR; mutations identified in at least 23 genes	Pancytopenia; reticulocytes ↓; MCV ↑	Hypocellular with ↓ in all cell lines	Chromosome breakage with DEB/MMC; majority have mutations or deletions in FA genes; *FANCA* mutations occur with highest frequency (60%); Hb F may be ↑	Physical malformations may be present; risk of cancers, leukemia, MDS
DC	AR, XLR, AD; mutations identified in at least 16 genes	Pancytopenia; reticulocytes ↓; MCV ↑	Hypocellular with ↓ in all cell lines	75% have mutations or deletions in DC genes; *DKC1* mutations occur with highest frequency (30%); very short telomeres in WBC subsets by flow-FISH; Hb F may be ↑	Physical malformations may be present; pulmonary disease; risk of cancers, leukemia, MDS
SBDS	AR; mutations identified in at least 4 genes	Neutropenia; pancytopenia (25% of cases); reticulocytes ↓; MCV ↑ or normal	Hypocellular, normocellular, or hypercellular	90% have mutations in *SBDS* gene; serum trypsinogen and isoamylase ↓ for age; Hb F may be ↑	Pancreatic insufficiency; physical malformations may be present; risk of infections, leukemia, MDS
DBA	AD (most); XLR; mutations identified in at least 20 genes	Anemia; reticulocytes ↓; MCV ↑	Erythroid hypoplasia	70% have mutations or deletions in DBA genes; *RPS19* mutations occur with highest frequency (25%); erythrocyte adenosine deaminase ↑; Hb F may be ↑	Physical malformations may be present; risk of cancers, leukemia, MDS
Caused by Ineffective Hematopoiesis					
CDA I	AR; mutations identified in at least 2 genes	Anemia; reticulocytes ↓; MCV ↑; poik, baso stipp, Cabot rings	Hypercellular; erythroid precursors megaloblastoid with internuclear chromatin bridges and <5% binucleated forms	Mutations in *CDAN1* or *CDIN1* genes; spongy, "Swiss cheese" heterochromatin in erythroblasts by electron microscopy	Physical malformations may be present; iron overload; splenomegaly; hepatomegaly
CDA II	AR; mutations identified in at least 1 gene	Anemia; reticulocytes ↓; MCV normal; poik, baso stipp	Hypercellular; erythroid precursors normoblastic with 10%–35% binucleated forms	Mutations in *SEC23B* gene; positive Ham test (no longer done)	Physical malformations may be present; iron overload; jaundice; gallstones; splenomegaly
CDA III	AD; mutations identified in at least 1 gene	Mild anemia; reticulocytes ↓; MCV ↑; poik, baso stipp	Hypercellular; erythroid precursors megaloblastoid with giant multinucleated forms with up to 12 nuclei	Mutations in *KIF23* gene	Treatment usually not needed

*Gene mutations identified as of 2023; genetic discovery is ongoing.
↑, Increased; ↓, decreased; *AD*, autosomal dominant; *AR*, autosomal recessive; *baso stipp*, basophilic stippling; *CDA*, congenital dyserythropoietic anemia; *DBA*, Diamond-Blackfan anemia; *DC*, dyskeratosis congenita; *DEB*, diepoxybutane; *FA*, Fanconi anemia; *flow-FISH*, flow cytometry with fluorescence in situ hybridization; *Hb F*, fetal hemoglobin; *MCV*, mean cell volume; *MDS*, myelodysplastic neoplasm; *MMC*, mitomycin C; *poik*, poikilocytosis; *SBDS*, Shwachman-Bodian-Diamond syndrome; *XLR*, X-linked recessive; *WBC*, white blood cell.

viral infection is found in half of patients, which is thought to trigger an immune mechanism that targets RBC production.[106] The anemia is typically normocytic, and Hb F and erythrocyte adenosine deaminase levels usually are normal. RBC transfusion support is the mainstay of therapy if the child is symptomatic from anemia. Normalization of erythropoiesis occurs within weeks in the vast majority patients.

Congenital Pure Red Cell Aplasia: Diamond-Blackfan Anemia

Diamond-Blackfan anemia (DBA) is a congenital erythroid hypoplastic disorder of early infancy with an estimated incidence of 7 to 10 cases per 1 million live births.[70] Mutations have been identified in at least 20 genes: those that encode structural ribosome proteins, *RPS7, RPS10, RPS15, RPS17, RPS19, RPS24, RPS26, RPS27, RPS27a, RPS28,* and *RPS29* in the 40S subunit, and *RPL5, RPL9, RPL11, RPL15, RPL18, RPL26, RPL27, RPL31, RPL35,* and *RPL35A* in the 60S subunit, as well as the gene encoding *GATA1,* a transcription factor important for hematopoiesis, and *EPO* and *ADA2*.[70,91,107,108] Mutations in the *RPS19* gene occur with the highest frequency (25%), followed by *RPL11* and *RPS26* (approximately 7% each); the other known mutations are uncommon.[108,109] An additional 15% to 20% of cases can be accounted for by haplodeletions of these same ribosome genes, but many mutations remain unidentified. Nearly 50% of DBA mutations are linked to an autosomal dominant inheritance pattern, less than 1% have been linked to an X-linked recessive pattern (*GATA1*), and sporadic mutations have also been reported. Mutations in ribosomal proteins disrupt ribosome biogenesis in DBA, but the pathophysiologic mechanisms leading to the clinical manifestations are currently unknown.

More than 90% of patients show signs of the disorder during the first year of life, with a median age of 8 weeks; however, some patients with DBA are asymptomatic until adulthood.[110] Approximately half of patients have characteristic physical anomalies, including craniofacial dysmorphisms, short stature, and neck and thumb malformations.[70,110]

The characteristic peripheral blood finding is a severe macrocytic anemia with reticulocytopenia.[70] The WBC count is normal or slightly decreased, and the platelet count is normal or slightly increased. Bone marrow examination distinguishes DBA from the hypocellular marrow in aplastic anemia because there is normal cellularity of myeloid cells and megakaryocytes and hypoplasia of erythroid cells. The karyotype in DBA is usually normal, and genetic testing can identify a DBA-related mutation in about 70% of patients.[108] In most cases, Hb F and erythrocyte adenosine deaminase are increased; these findings distinguish DBA from TEC, in which these levels are normal.[107,111] Other features distinguishing DBA from TEC are detailed in Table 19.4.

Therapy includes RBC transfusions and corticosteroids. Although 50% to 75% of patients respond to corticosteroid therapy, side effects can be severe with long-term use, including immunosuppression and growth delay.[110] Overall survival is 75% at 40 years. Bone marrow transplantation improves outcomes, with greater than 90% overall survival in patients younger than 10 years old transplanted with an MRD and 80% in patients with an MUD.[107,108]

Congenital Dyserythropoietic Anemia

The *congenital dyserythropoietic anemias* (CDAs) are a heterogeneous group of rare disorders characterized by refractory anemia, reticulocytopenia, hypercellular bone marrow with markedly ineffective erythropoiesis, and distinctive dysplastic changes in bone marrow erythroblasts.[112] Megaloblastoid development occurs in some types, but it is not related to vitamin B_{12} or folate deficiency. Granulopoiesis and thrombopoiesis are normal. The anemia varies from mild to moderate, even among affected siblings. Secondary hemosiderosis arises from chronic intramedullary and extramedullary hemolysis as well as increased iron absorption associated with ineffective erythropoiesis. Iron overload develops even in the absence of blood transfusions. Jaundice, cholelithiasis, and splenomegaly are also common findings. CDAs do not progress to aplastic anemia or hematologic malignancies.[113]

Symptoms of CDA usually occur in childhood or adolescence but may first appear in adulthood. CDA is classified into three major types: CDA I, CDA II, and CDA III. There are rare variants that do not fall into these categories, and they have been assigned to four other groups: CDA IV through CDA VII.[112,113] Whether CDA types IV through VII are separate entities is a matter of some controversy. This merely may be a reflection of the insensitive tests to classify CDA disorders. Further gene mutation studies should clarify this issue.

CDA I is inherited in an autosomal recessive pattern and is characterized by a mild to severe chronic anemia. More than 150 cases have been reported.[114] CDA I is caused by mutations in the *CDAN1* or *CDIN1* gene. *CDAN1* (chromosome 15) encodes codanin-1, a cell-cycle regulated nuclear protein.[115,116] The exact role of *CDAN1* and *CDIN1* mutations in the pathophysiology of CDA I is unknown. Malformations of fingers or toes, brown skin pigmentation, and neurologic defects are found more often in CDA I than in the other CDA subtypes. Hemoglobin usually ranges from 6.5 to 11.5 g/dL, with a mean of 9.5 g/dL.[113] RBCs are macrocytic and may exhibit marked poikilocytosis, basophilic stippling, and Cabot rings. The erythroblasts are megaloblastoid and characteristically have internuclear chromatin bridges or nuclear stranding (Figure 19.3). There are less than 5% binucleated erythroblasts. The characteristic feature of the CDA I erythroblast is a spongy heterochromatin with a Swiss cheese appearance. Treatment includes IFN-α and iron chelation.[114]

CDA II is the most common subtype and is inherited in an autosomal recessive pattern. More than 300 cases have been

TABLE 19.4 Distinguishing Characteristics of Diamond-Blackfan Anemia and Transient Erythroblastopenia of Childhood

Test Result	DBA*	TEC*
Erythrocyte ADA ↑ at diagnosis	85%	5%
MCV ↑ at diagnosis	80%	5%
MCV ↑ in remission	80%	0%
Hb F ↑ at diagnosis	50%–85%	1%–2%
Hb F ↑ in remission	50%–85%	0%

*Percent of patients displaying the test results.

↑, Increased; *ADA*, adenosine deaminase; *DBA*, Diamond-Blackfan Anemia; *Hb F*, fetal hemoglobin; *MCV*, mean cell volume; TEC, transient erythroblastopenia of childhood.
Modified from D'Andrea, A. D., Dahl, N., Guinan, E. C., et al. (2002). Marrow failure. *Hematology Am Soc Hematol Educ Program, 58*–72.

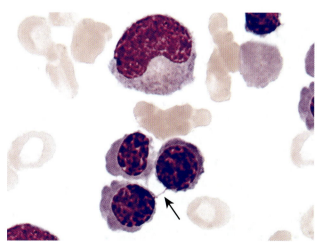

Figure 19.3 Erythroid Precursors With Nuclear Bridging *(arrow)* **Indicating Dyserythropoiesis.** (Bone marrow, Wright-Giemsa stain, ×1000.) (Modified from Carr, J. H. [2022]. *Clinical Hematology Atlas.* [6th ed.]. St. Louis: Elsevier.)

reported.[112] It results from mutations in the *SEC23B* gene on chromosome 20.[117] *SEC23B* encodes a component of the coat protein complex (COPII) that forms vesicles for transport of secretory proteins from the endoplasmic reticulum to the Golgi apparatus.[118] Its exact role in the pathophysiology of CDA II is unknown. The anemia in CDA II is mild to moderate, with hemoglobin values ranging from 9 to 12 g/dL and a mean hemoglobin of 11 g/dL.[113] On peripheral blood film, RBCs are normocytic, with anisocytosis, poikilocytosis, and basophilic stippling. The bone marrow has normoblastic erythropoiesis, with 10% to 35% binucleated forms and rare multinucleated forms. Occasional pseudo-Gaucher cells are also evident. Circulating RBCs hemolyze with the Ham acidified serum test but not with the sucrose hemolysis test.[70] For this reason, CDA II is also known as *HEMPAS* (*he*reditary *e*rythroblastic *m*ultinuclearity with *p*ositive *a*cidified *s*erum). The Ham test is no longer used for CDA II confirmation, given the difficulty of appropriate quality control and the relative lack of testing availability in most laboratories. RBCs also show abnormal migration of band 3 using sodium dodecyl sulfate-polyacrylamide gel electrophoresis. Treatment includes splenectomy and iron chelation.[114]

CDA III is the least common of the CDA subtypes, with about 60 cases reported in the literature, the majority being from one Swedish family.[119,120] This familial autosomal dominant form is associated with mutations in the *KIF23* gene, which codes for a protein involved in cytokinesis.[119] The nonfamilial or sporadic form is extremely rare, with fewer than 20 cases reported.[112] The anemia is mild, and the hemoglobin is usually in the range of 8 to 14 g/dL, with a mean of 12 g/dL.[113] RBCs are macrocytic, and poikilocytosis and basophilic stippling are evident. The bone marrow has megaloblastic changes, and giant erythroblasts with up to 12 nuclei are a characteristic feature. Patients rarely require RBC transfusions, and iron overload does not occur.

Myelophthisic Anemia

Myelophthisic anemia is due to the infiltration of abnormal cells into the bone marrow and subsequent destruction and replacement of normal hematopoietic cells. Metastatic solid tumor cells (particularly from lung, breast, and prostate), fibroblasts, and inflammatory cells (such as those found in miliary tuberculosis and fungal infections) have been implicated.[121] Cytopenia results from the release of substances such as cytokines and growth factors that suppress hematopoiesis and destroy stem, progenitor, and stromal cells. With disruption of normal bone marrow architecture by the infiltrating cells, the marrow releases immature hematopoietic cells. Furthermore, because of the unfavorable bone marrow environment, stem and progenitor cells migrate to the spleen and liver and establish extramedullary hematopoietic sites. Because blood cell production in the liver and spleen is inefficient, these extramedullary sites also release immature cells into the circulation.[122]

The severity of anemia is mild to moderate, with normocytic erythrocytes and reticulocytopenia. Peripheral blood findings include teardrop erythrocytes and nucleated RBCs as well as immature myeloid cells (*leukoerythroblastic blood picture*) and megakaryocyte fragments (Figure 19.4).[122] The infiltrating abnormal cells are detected in a bone marrow aspirate or biopsy specimen.

Anemia of Chronic Kidney Disease

Anemia is a common complication of *chronic kidney disease* (CKD), with a positive correlation between anemia and renal disease severity.[123] The Centers for Disease Control and Prevention reported that in 2017 approximately 30 million adults in the United States had CKD.[124] The primary cause of anemia in CKD is inadequate renal production of erythropoietin.[123,125] Without erythropoietin, the bone marrow lacks adequate stimulation to produce RBCs. Another contributor to the anemia of CKD is chronic inflammation. Inflammatory cytokines increase production of hepcidin by the liver, which decreases the iron available for erythropoiesis (Chapter 17). Uremia also inhibits erythropoiesis and increases RBC fragility.[126] Furthermore, hemodialysis and frequent blood draws result in chronic blood loss. Anemia of CKD is normocytic and normochromic with reticulocytopenia. Burr cells are a common peripheral blood film finding in cases complicated by uremia.

Anemia in CKD can lead to cardiovascular complications, cognitive impairment, and suboptimal quality of life. The 2012 Kidney Disease: Improving Global Outcomes (KDIGO) Clinical Practice Guideline for Anemia recommends periodic hemoglobin testing in patients with CKD and investigation of the anemia if the hemoglobin is less than 13.0 g/dL in adult men and less than 12 g/dL in adult women.[125] In adult CKD patients with anemia, a trial of oral iron (nondialysis patients) or intravenous iron (dialysis patients) is recommended when the transferrin saturation is ≤30% and serum ferritin level is ≤500 ng/mL.[125] The Guideline also recommends consideration of therapy with an erythropoiesis-stimulating agent (ESA) if the hemoglobin falls below 10 g/dL.[125] Using ESA therapy to maintain the hemoglobin at more than 11.5 g/dL is not recommended because of the increased risk of cardiovascular complications.

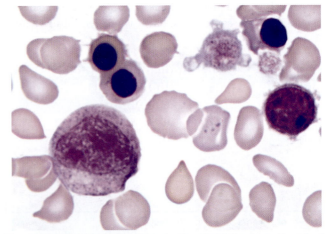

Figure 19.4 Myelophthisic Anemia Showing a Leukoerythroblastic Blood Picture. Note a myelocyte, three orthochromic normoblasts, a giant platelet with abnormal morphology, a micromegakaryocyte, and teardrop red blood cells. (Peripheral blood, Wright-Giemsa stain, ×1000.)

Successful therapy requires adequate iron stores, so plasma ferritin level and percent transferrin saturation are also periodically monitored.

Patients may become hyporesponsive to ESA therapy because of functional iron deficiency (FID). In FID, the bone marrow is unable to release iron rapidly enough to accommodate the accelerated erythropoiesis. The transferrin saturation remains less than 20%, but the serum ferritin level is normal or increased, indicating adequate iron stores.[127] Patients with FID may require intravenous iron therapy to reach or maintain target hemoglobin levels, even with high ESA doses.[127] Researchers have proposed the following diagnostic criteria for FID in CKD: decreased reticulocyte hemoglobin content and increased soluble transferrin receptor (Chapter 8) and greater than 10% hypochromic RBCs in the peripheral blood.[128] Other causes of ESA hyporesponsiveness include chronic inflammatory disease, infection, malignancy, aplastic anemia, antibody-mediated PRCA, and some hemoglobin disorders.

SUMMARY

- Bone marrow failure is the reduction or cessation of blood cell production affecting one or more cell lines. Pancytopenia (decreased red blood cells, white blood cells, and platelets) is a common finding. Sequelae of pancytopenia include weakness and fatigue, infections, and bleeding.
- Aplastic anemia may be acquired or inherited/congenital. Acquired aplastic anemia may be idiopathic or due to drugs, chemical exposures, radiation, or viruses. Acquired aplastic anemia may also occur with conditions such as paroxysmal nocturnal hemoglobinuria, autoimmune diseases, and pregnancy.
- Bone marrow failure in acquired aplastic anemia occurs from destruction of hematopoietic stem cells by direct toxic effects of a drug, autoimmune T cell targeting of stem cells, or other unknown mechanisms. The autoimmune reactions are rare adverse events after exposure to drugs, chemicals, or viruses. They are *idiosyncratic* in that they are unpredictable, and severity is unrelated to the dose or duration of exposure.
- Aplastic anemia is classified as moderate, severe, or very severe, based on bone marrow hypocellularity, absolute neutrophil count, platelet count, hemoglobin level, and reticulocyte count. The severity classification helps guide treatment decisions.
- Preferred treatment for severe acquired aplastic anemia is bone marrow transplant for younger patients with an HLA-matched related donor. For patients without a matched related donor and for older adults, immunosuppressive therapy (IST) with antithymocyte globulin and cyclosporine is typically recommended, though in centers with good matched unrelated donor transplant outcomes, upfront unrelated donor transplantation may be pursued.
- Fanconi anemia (FA), dyskeratosis congenita (DC), and Shwachman-Bodian-Diamond syndrome (SBDS) are inherited bone marrow failure syndromes with progressive bone marrow failure, and patients may present with characteristic physical malformations. FA is inherited in an autosomal recessive or X-linked pattern, and mutations in at least 23 genes have been identified. A positive chromosome breakage study with diepoxybutane is diagnostic. DC can be X-linked, autosomal dominant, or autosomal recessive, and mutations in at least 16 genes have been identified. SBDS is most commonly autosomal recessive and is primarily associated with mutations in the *SBDS* gene.
- Telomerase complex defects play a role in the pathophysiology of inherited bone marrow failure syndromes and some acquired aplastic anemias. The defects result in the inability of telomerase to elongate telomeres at the ends of chromosomes, which leads to premature hematopoietic stem cell senescence and apoptosis.
- Other forms of bone marrow failure that may be acquired or congenital include pure red cell aplasia (PRCA), congenital dyserythropoietic anemia (CDA), myelophthisic anemia, and anemia of chronic kidney disease (CKD).
- PRCA is a disorder of erythrocyte production. Acquired transient erythroblastopenia of childhood and Diamond-Blackfan anemia (DBA) are disparate subtypes with distinct causes, clinical features, and courses. Mutations in at least 20 genes have been identified in DBA.
- Patients with congenital dyserythropoietic anemia (CDA) exhibit refractory anemia, reticulocytopenia, secondary hemosiderosis, and distinct abnormalities of erythroid precursors. Three major subtypes are recognized: CDA I, CDA II, and CDA III.
- Myelophthisic anemia results from the replacement of normal bone marrow cells with abnormal cells, such as metastatic tumor cells, fibroblasts, and inflammatory cells.
- The main cause of anemia of CKD is inadequate production of erythropoietin by the kidneys.

Now that you have completed this chapter, go back and read again the case study at the beginning and respond to the questions presented. Answers can be found in Appendix C.

REVIEW QUESTIONS

Answers can be found in Appendix C.

1. The clinical consequences of pancytopenia include:
   a. Pallor and thrombosis
   b. Kidney failure and fever
   c. Fatigue, infection, and bleeding
   d. Weakness, hemolysis, and infection

2. Idiopathic acquired aplastic anemia is due to a(n):
   a. Drug reaction
   b. Benzene exposure
   c. Inherited mutation in stem cells
   d. Unknown cause

3. The pathophysiologic mechanism in acquired idiosyncratic aplastic anemia is:
   a. Replacement of bone marrow cells by abnormal cells
   b. Destruction of stem cells by autoimmune T cells
   c. Defective production of hematopoietic growth factors
   d. Inability of bone marrow stroma to support stem cells

4. Based on the criteria in Table 19.1, what is the aplastic anemia classification of a 15-year-old girl with a bone marrow cellularity of 10%, hemoglobin of 7 g/dL, absolute neutrophil count of 0.1×10^9/L, and platelet count of 10×10^9/L?
   a. Nonsevere
   b. Moderate
   c. Severe
   d. Very severe

5. The most consistent peripheral blood findings in severe aplastic anemia are:
   a. Hairy cells, monocytopenia, and neutropenia
   b. Macrocytosis, thrombocytopenia, and neutropenia
   c. Blasts, immature granulocytes, and thrombocytopenia
   d. Polychromasia, nucleated RBCs, and hypersegmented neutrophils

6. The treatment that has shown the best success rate in young patients with severe aplastic anemia is:
   a. Immunosuppressive therapy
   b. Long-term RBC and platelet transfusions
   c. Administration of hematopoietic growth factors and androgens
   d. Bone marrow transplant with an HLA-identical sibling

7. The test that is most useful in differentiating Fanconi anemia from other causes of pancytopenia is:
   a. Bone marrow biopsy
   b. Ham acidified serum test
   c. Diepoxybutane-induced chromosome breakage
   d. Flow cytometric analysis of CD55 and CD59 cells

8. In dyskeratosis congenita, mutations in genes that code for the telomerase complex may induce bone marrow failure by causing which one of the following?
   a. Resistance of stem cells to normal apoptosis
   b. Autoimmune reaction against telomeres in stem cells
   c. Decreased production of hematopoietic growth factors
   d. Premature death of hematopoietic stem cells

9. Diamond-Blackfan anemia differs from Fanconi anemia in that in the former:
   a. Reticulocyte count is increased
   b. Fetal hemoglobin is decreased
   c. Only erythropoiesis is affected
   d. Congenital malformations are absent

10. Which anemia should be suspected in a patient with refractory anemia, reticulocytopenia, hemosiderosis, and binucleated erythrocyte precursors in the bone marrow?
    a. Fanconi anemia
    b. Dyskeratosis congenita
    c. Acquired aplastic anemia
    d. Congenital dyserythropoietic anemia

11. The primary pathophysiologic mechanism of anemia associated with chronic kidney disease is:
    a. Inadequate production of erythropoietin
    b. Excessive hemolysis
    c. Hematopoietic stem cell mutation
    d. Toxic destruction of stem cells

12. Which one of the following findings is NOT consistent with myelophthisic anemia?
    a. Reticulocytosis
    b. Teardrop RBCs
    c. Extramedullary hematopoiesis
    d. Leukoerythroblastic blood picture

REFERENCES

1. Ehrlich, P. (1888). Uber einen Fall von Anamie mit Bemerkungen uber regenerative Veranderungen des Knochenmarks. *Charite Annal, 13*, 300–309.
2. Vaquez, M. H., & Aubertin, C. (1904). L'anemie pernicieuse d'apres les conceptions actuelles. *Bull Soc Med Hop Paris, 21*, 288–297.
3. Muir, K. R., Chilvers, C. E. D., Coulson, L., et al. (2003). The role of occupational and environmental exposures in the aetiology of acquired severe aplastic anaemia: a case control investigation. *Br J Haematol, 123*(5), 906–914.
4. Dokal, I., & Vulliamy, T. (2008). Inherited aplastic anaemias/bone marrow failure syndromes. *Blood Rev, 22*(3), 141–153.
5. Dufour, C., Veys, P., Carraro, E., et al. (2015). Similar outcome of upfront-unrelated and matched sibling stem cell transplantation in idiopathic paediatric aplastic anaemia. A study on behalf of the UK Paediatric BMT Working Party, Paediatric Diseases Working Party and Severe Aplastic Anaemia Working Party of EBMT. *Br J Haematol, 171*(4), 585–594.
6. Heimpel, H. (1987). Incidence of aplastic anemia: the relevance of diagnostic criteria. *Blood, 70*, 1718–1721.
7. Kojima, S. (2002). Aplastic anemia in the orient. *Int J Hematol, 76*(Suppl. 2), 173–174.
8. Young, N. S. (2018). Aplastic anemia. *N Engl J Med, 379*(17), 1643–1656.
9. Young, N. S., & Maciejewski, J. P. (2023). Aplastic anemia. In Hoffman, R., Benz, E. J, Silberstein, L. E, et al. (Eds.), *Hematology: Basic Principles and Practice.* (8th ed., pp. 369–415). Philadelphia: Elsevier.
10. Scheinberg, P., & Young, N. S. (2012). How I treat acquired aplastic anemia. *Blood, 120*(6), 1185–1196.
11. Nimer, S. D., Ireland, P., Meshkinpour, A., et al. (1994). An increased HLA DR2 frequency is seen in aplastic anemia patients. *Blood, 84*(3), 923–927.
12. Saunthararajah, Y., Nakamura, R., Nam J., et al. (2002). HLA-DR15 (DR2) is overrepresented in myelodysplastic syndrome and aplastic anemia and predicts a response to immunosuppression in myelodysplastic syndrome. *Blood, 100*(5), 1570–1574.
13. Dougherty, D., Garte, S., Barchowsky, A., et al. (2008). NQO1, MPO, CYP2E1, GSTT1 and GSTM1 polymorphisms and biological effects of benzene exposure--a literature review. *Toxicol Lett, 182*(1–3), 7–17.

14. Gonzalez-Casas, R., Garcia-Buey, L., Jones, E. A., et al. (2009). Systematic review: hepatitis-associated aplastic anaemia–a syndrome associated with abnormal immunological function. *Aliment Pharmacol Ther, 30*(5), 436–443.

15. Choudhry, V. P., Gupta, S., Gupta, M., et al. (2002). Pregnancy associated aplastic anemia-a series of 10 cases with review of literature. *Hematology, 7*(4), 233–238.

16. Stalder, M. P., Rovo, A., Halter, J., et al. (2009). Aplastic anemia and concomitant autoimmune diseases. *Ann Hematol, 88*(7), 659–665.

17. Frickhofen, N., Heimpel, H., Kaltwasser, J. P., et al. (2003). Antithymocyte globulin with or without cyclosporin A: 11-year follow-up of a randomized trial comparing treatments of aplastic anemia. *Blood, 101*(4), 1236–1242.

18. Maciejewski, J. P., Selleri, C., Sato, T., et al. (1996). A severe and consistent deficit in marrow and circulating primitive hematopoietic cells (long-term culture-initiating cells) in acquired aplastic anemia. *Blood, 88*(6), 1983–1991.

19. Philpott, N. J. Scopes, J., Marsh, J. C., et al. (1995). Increased apoptosis in aplastic anemia bone marrow progenitor cells: possible pathophysiologic significance. *Exp Hematol, 23*(14), 1642–1648.

20. Maciejewski, J. P., Selleri, C., Sato, T., et al. (1995). Increased expression of Fas antigen on bone marrow CD34+ cells of patients with aplastic anaemia. *Br J Haematol, 91*(1), 245–252.

21. Zeng, W., Chen, G., Kajigaya, S., et al. (2004). Gene expression profiling in CD34 cells to identify differences between aplastic anemia patients and healthy volunteers. *Blood, 103*(1), 325–332.

22. Novitzky, N., & Jacobs, P. (1995). Immunosuppressive therapy in bone marrow aplasia: the stroma functions normally to support hematopoiesis. *Exp Hematol, 23*(14), 1472–1477.

23. Koijima, S. (1998). Hematopoietic growth factors and marrow stroma in aplastic anemia. *Int J Hematol, 68*(1), 19–28.

24. Wodnar-Filipowicz, A., Lyman, S. D., Gratwohl, A., et al. (1996). Flt3 ligand level reflects hematopoietic progenitor cell function in aplastic anemia and chemotherapy-induced bone marrow aplasia. *Blood, 88*(12), 4493–4499.

25. Young, N. S. (1997). Autoimmunity and its treatment in aplastic anemia. *Ann Intern Med, 126*(2), 166–168.

26. Schoettler, M. L., & Nathan, D. G. (2018). The pathophysiology of acquired aplastic anemia: current concepts revisited. *Hematol Oncol Clin North Am, 32*(4), 581–594.

27. Mathe, G., Amiel, J. L., Schwarzenberg, L., et al. (1970). Bone marrow graft in man after conditioning by antilymphocytic serum. *Br Med J, 2*(5702), 131–136.

28. Risitano, A. M., Maciejewski, J. P., Green, S., et al. (2004). In-vivo dominant immune responses in aplastic anaemia: molecular tracking of putatively pathogenetic T-cell clones by TCR beta-CDR3 sequencing. *Lancet, 364*(9431), 355–364.

29. Hara, T., Ando, K., Tsurumi, H., et al. (2004). Excessive production of tumor necrosis factor-alpha by bone marrow T lymphocytes is essential in causing bone marrow failure in patients with aplastic anemia. *Eur J Haematol, 73*(1), 10–6.

30. Young, N. S. (2000). Hematopoietic cell destruction by immune mechanisms in acquired aplastic anemia. *Semin Hematol, 37*(1), 3–14.

31. Selleri, C., Sato, T., Anderson, S., et al. (1995). Interferon-gamma and tumor necrosis factor-alpha suppress both early and late stages of hematopoiesis and induce programmed cell death. *J Cell Physiol, 165*(3), 538–546.

32. Solomou, E. E., Keyvanfar, K., & Young, N. S. (2006). T-bet, a Th1 transcription factor, is up-regulated in T cells from patients with aplastic anemia. *Blood, 107*(10), 3983–3991.

33. Kasahara, S., Hara, T., Itoh, H., et al. (2002). Hypoplastic myelodysplastic syndromes can be distinguished from acquired aplastic anaemia by bone marrow stem cell expression of the tumour necrosis factor receptor. *Br J Haematol, 118*(1), 181–188.

34. Young, N. S., & Maciejewski, J. (1997). The pathophysiology of acquired aplastic anemia. *N Engl J Med, 336*(19), 1365–1372.

35. Young, N. S., Calado, R. T., & Scheinberg, P. (2006). Current concepts in the pathophysiology and treatment of aplastic anemia. *Blood, 108*(8), 2509–2519.

36. Rogers, Z. R., Nakano, T. A., Olson T. S., et al. (2019). Immunosuppressive therapy for pediatric aplastic anemia: a North American Pediatric Aplastic Anemia Consortium study. *Haematologica, 104*(10), 1974–1983.

37. Brown, K. E., Tisdale, J., Barrett, A. J., et al. (1997). Hepatitis-associated aplastic anemia. *N Engl J Med, 336*(15), 1059–1064.

38. Solomou, E. E., Rezvani, K., Mielke, S., et al. (2007). Deficient CD4+ CD25+ FOXP3+ T regulatory cells in acquired aplastic anemia. *Blood, 110*(5), 1603–1606.

39. Gidvani, V., Ramkissoon, S., Sloand, E. M., et al. (2007). Cytokine gene polymorphisms in acquired bone marrow failure. *Am J Hematol, 82*(8), 721–724.

40. Hirano, N., Butler, M. O, Von Bergwelt, M. S., et al. (2003). Autoantibodies frequently detected in patients with aplastic anemia. *Blood, 102*(13), 4567–4575.

41. Feng, X., Chuhjo, T., Sugimori, C., et al. (2004). Diazepam-binding inhibitor-related protein 1: a candidate autoantigen in acquired aplastic anemia patients harboring a minor population of paroxysmal nocturnal hemoglobinuria-type cells. *Blood, 104*(8), 2425–2431.

42. Takamatsu, H., Feng, X., Chuhjo, T., et al. (2007). Specific antibodies to moesin, a membrane-cytoskeleton linker protein, are frequently detected in patients with acquired aplastic anemia. *Blood, 109*(6), 2514–2520.

43. Ball, S. E., Gibson, F. M., Rizzo, S., et al. (1998). Progressive telomere shortening in aplastic anemia. *Blood, 91*(10), 3582–3592.

44. Calado, R. T., & Young, N. S. (2008). Telomere maintenance and human bone marrow failure. *Blood, 111*(9), 4446–4455.

45. Yamaguchi, H., Calado, R. T., Ly, H., et al. (2005). Mutations in TERT, the gene for telomerase reverse transcriptase, in aplastic anemia. *N Engl J Med, 352*(14), 1413–1424.

46. Xin, Z. T., Beauchamp, A. D., Calado, R. T., et al. (2007). Functional characterization of natural telomerase mutations found in patients with hematologic disorders. *Blood, 109*(2), 524–532.

47. Calado, R. T., Graf, S. A., Wilkerson, K. L., et al. (2007). Mutations in the *SBDS* gene in acquired aplastic anemia. *Blood, 110*, 1141–1146.

48. Brummendorf, T. H., Maciejewski, J. P., Mak, J., et al. (2001). Telomere length in leukocyte subpopulations of patients with aplastic anemia. *Blood, 97*, 895–900.

49. Camitta, B. M., Thomas, E. D., Nathan, D. G., et al. (1976). Severe aplastic anemia: a prospective study of the effect of early marrow transplantation on acute mortality. *Blood, 48*, 63–70.

50. Bacigalupo, A., Hows, J., Gluckman, E., et al. (1988). Bone marrow transplantation (BMT) versus immunosuppression for the treatment of severe aplastic anaemia (SAA): a report of the EMBT SAA working party. *Br J Haematol, 70*, 177–182.

51. Sugimori, C., Chuhjo, T., Feng, X., et al. (2006). Minor population of CD55⁻CD59⁻ blood cells predicts response to immunosuppressive therapy and prognosis in patients with aplastic anemia. *Blood, 107*, 1308–1314.

52. Socie, G., Rosenfeld, S., Frickhofen, N., et al. (2000). Late clonal diseases of treated aplastic anemia. *Semin Hematol, 37*, 91–101.

53. Sutherland, D. R., Kuek, N., Azcona-Olivera, J., et al. (2009). Use of FLAER-based WBC assay in the primary screening of PNH clones. *Am J Clin Pathol, 132*, 564–572.

54. Maciejewski, J. P., Risitano, A., Sloand, E., et al. (2002). Distinct clinical outcomes for cytogenetic abnormalities evolving from aplastic anemia. *Blood, 99*, 3129–3135.

55. Kearns, W. G., Sutton, J. F., Maciejewski, J. P., et al. (2004). Genomic instability in bone marrow failure syndromes. *Am J Hematol, 76*, 220–224.

56. Georges, G. E., Doney, K., & Storb, R. (2018). Severe aplastic anemia: allogeneic bone marrow transplantation as first-line treatment. *Blood Adv, 2*(15), 2020–2028.

57. Bacigalupo, A., Giammarco, S., & Sica, S. (2016). Bone marrow transplantation versus immunosuppressive therapy in patients with acquired severe aplastic anemia. *Int J Hematol, 104*(2), 168–174.

58. Samarasinghe, S., Veys, P., Vora, A., et al. (2018). Paediatric amendment to adult BSH Guidelines for aplastic anaemia. *Br J Haematol, 180*(2), 201–205.

59. Clesham, K., Dowse, R., & Samarasinghe, S. (2018). Upfront matched unrelated donor transplantation in aplastic anemia. *Hematol Oncol Clin North Am, 32*(4), 619–628.

60. DeZern, A. E., Zahrak, M. L., Symons, H. J., et al. (2020). Haploidentical BMT for severe aplastic anemia with intensive GVHD prophylaxis including posttransplant cyclophosphamide. *Blood Adv, 4*(8), 1770–1779.

61. Maciejewski, J. P., Follmann, D., Nakamura, R., et al. (2001). Increased frequency of HLA-DR2 in patients with paroxysmal nocturnal hemoglobinuria and the PNH/aplastic anemia syndrome. *Blood, 98*, 3513–3519.

62. Socie, G., Mary, J-Y., Schrezenmeier, H., et al. (2007). Granulocyte-stimulating factor and severe aplastic anemia: a survey by the European group for blood and marrow transplant (EBMT*). Blood, 109*, 2794–2796.

63. Gurion, R., Gafter-Gvili, A., Paul, M., et al. (2009). Hematopoietic growth factors in aplastic anemia patients treated with immunosuppressive therapy—systematic review and meta-analysis. *Hematologica, 94*, 712–719.

64. Townsley, D. M., Scheinberg, P., Winkler, T., et al. (2017). Eltrombopag added to standard immunosuppression for aplastic anemia. *N Engl J Med, 376*, 1540–1550.

65. Peffault de Latour, R., Kulasekararaj, A., Iacobelli, S., et al. (2022). Eltrombopag added to immunosuppression in severe aplastic anemia. *N Engl J Med, 386*(1), 11–23.

66. Groarke, E. M., Patel, B. A., Gutierrez-Rodrigues, F., et al. (2021). Eltrombopag added to immunosuppression for children with treatment-naive severe aplastic anaemia. *Br J Haematol, 192*(3), 605–614.

67. Filippidou, M., Avgerinou, G., Tsipou, H., et al. (2020). Longitudinal evaluation of eltrombopag in paediatric acquired severe aplastic anaemia. *Br J Haematol, 190*(3), e157–e159.

68. Furutani E., & Shimamura, A. (2019). Inherited aplastic anemia sydromes germline. In Greer J. P., Arber, D. A., Appelbaum, F. R., (Eds.), *Wintrobe's Clinical Hematology.* (14th edition, pp. 959–978). Philadelphia: Wolters Kluwer.

69. Dokal, I., Tummala, H., & Vulliamy, T. (2022). Inherited bone marrow failure in the pediatric patient. *Blood, 140*(6), 556–570.

70. Dror, Y. (2023). Inherited bone marrow failure syndromes. In Hoffman, R., Benz, E. J., Silberstein, L. E., et al. (Eds.), *Hematology: Basic Principles and Practice.* (8th ed., pp. 350–395). Philadelphia: Elsevier.

71. Fanconi, G. (1927). Familiaere infantile perniziosaartige Anaemie (pernizioeses Blutbild und Konstitution). *Jahrbuch Kinderheil, 117*, 257–280.

72. Taniguchi, T., Tischkowitz, M., Ameziane, N., et al. (2003). Disruption of the Fanconi anemia-BRCA pathway in cisplatin-sensitive ovarian tumors. *Nat Med, 9*(5), 568–574.

73. Green, A. M., & Kupfer, G. M. (2009). Fanconi anemia. *Hematol Oncol Clin North Am, 23*, 193–214.

74. Alter, B. P., & Olson, S. B. (2010). Wilms tumor, AML, and medulloblastoma in a child with cancer prone syndrome of total premature chromatid separation and Fanconi anemia. *Pediatr Blood Cancer, 54*(3), 488; author reply 489.

75. Olson, T. S. (2022). Clinical manifestations and diagnosis of Fanconi anemia, P. Newburger, Editor. *UpToDate*: Waltham, MA. https://www.uptodate.com

76. Alter, B. P. (2003). Cancer in Fanconi anemia, *1927-Cancer, 97*(2), 425–440.

77. Gueiderikh, A., Rosselli, F., & Neto, J. B. C. (2017). A never-ending story: the steadily growing family of the FA and FA-like genes. *Genet Mol Biol, 40*(2), 398–407.

78. Shimamura, A., & Alter, B. P. (2010). Pathophysiology and management of inherited bone marrow failure syndromes. *Blood Rev, 24*(3), 101–122.

79. Levitus, M., Joenje, H., & de Winter, J. P. (2006). The Fanconi anemia pathway of genomic maintenance. *Cell Oncol, 28*(1-2), 3–29.

80. Pinto, F. O., Leblanc, T., Chamousset, D., et al. (2009). Diagnosis of Fanconi anemia in patients with bone marrow failure. *Haematologica, 94*(4), 487–495.

81. Alter, B. P., Giri, N., Savage, S. A., et al. (2018). Cancer in the National Cancer Institute inherited bone marrow failure syndrome cohort after fifteen years of follow-up. *Haematologica, 103*(1), 30–39.

82. Rosenberg, P. S., Greene, M. H., & Alter, B. P. (2003). Cancer incidence in persons with Fanconi anemia. *Blood, 101*(3), 822–826.

83. Kutler, D. I., Singh, B., Satagopan, J., et al. (2003). A 20-year perspective on the International Fanconi Anemia Registry (IFAR). *Blood, 101*(4), 1249–1256.

84. Fanconi Anemia Research Fund (2020). Fanconi anemia clinical care guidelines. https://www.fanconi.org/explore/clinical-care-guidelines. Accessed December 6, 2022.

85. Olson, T. S. (2022). Management and prognosis of Fanconi anemia. P. Newburger, Editor. *UpToDate*: Waltham MA. https://www.uptodate.com

86. MacMillan, M. L., DeFor, T. E., Young, J. A., et al. (2015). Alternative donor hematopoietic cell transplantation for Fanconi anemia. *Blood, 125*(24), 3798–3804.

87. Czechowicz, A., Sevilla, J., Agarwal, R., et al. (2021). Gene therapy for Fanconi anemia (Group A): interim results of RP-L102 Clinical Trials. *Blood, 138*(Suppl. 1), 3968.

88. Kam, M. L. W., Nguyen, T. T. T., & Ngeow, J. Y. Y. (2021). Telomere biology disorders. *NPJ Genom Med, 6*(1), 36.

89. Alter, B. P., Giri, N., Savage, S. A., et al. (2009). Cancer in dyskeratosis congenita. *Blood, 113*(26), 6549–6557.

90. Olson, T. S., & Myers, K. C. (2022). Dyskeratosis congenita and other telomere biology disorders. P. Newburger, Editor. *UpToDate*. Waltham, MA. https://www.uptodate.com

91. Wegman-Ostrosky, T., & Savage, S. A. (2017). The genomics of inherited bone marrow failure: from mechanism to the clinic. *Br J Haematol, 177*(4), 526–542.

92. Niewisch, M. R., Giri, N., McReynolds, L. J., et al. (2022). Disease progression and clinical outcomes in telomere biology disorders. *Blood, 139*(12), 1807–1819.

93. Alter, B. P., Baerlocher, G. M., Savage, S. A., et al. (2007). Very short telomere length by flow fluorescence in situ hybridization identifies patients with dyskeratosis congenita. *Blood, 110*(5), 1439–1447.

94. Donadieu, J., Leblanc, T., Meunier, B. B., et al. (2005). Analysis of risk factors for myelodysplasias, leukemias and death from infection among patients with congenital neutropenia. Experience of the French Severe Chronic Neutropenia Study Group. *Haematologica, 90*(1), 45–53.

95. Myers, K. C., Rose, S. R., Rutter, M. M., et al. (2013). Endocrine evaluation of children with and without Shwachman-Bodian-Diamond syndrome gene mutations and Shwachman-Diamond syndrome. *J Pediatr, 162*(6), 1235–1240.

96. Austin, K. M., Gupta, M. L., Jr., Coats, S. A., et al. (2008). Mitotic spindle destabilization and genomic instability in Shwachman-Diamond syndrome. *J Clin Invest, 118*(4), 1511–1518.

97. Burroughs, L., Woolfrey, A., & Shimamura, A. (2009). Shwachman-Diamond syndrome: a review of the clinical presentation, molecular pathogenesis, diagnosis, and treatment. *Hematol Oncol Clin North Am, 23*(2), 233–248.

98. Dror, Y., & Freedman, M. H. (2002). Shwachman-diamond syndrome. *Br J Haematol, 118*(3), 701–713.

99. Furutani, E., Liu, S., Galvin, A., et al. (2022). Hematologic complications with age in Shwachman-Diamond syndrome. *Blood Adv, 6*(1), 297–306.

100. Myers, K., Hebert, K., Antin, J., et al. (2020). Hematopoietic stem cell transplantation for Shwachman-Diamond syndrome. *Biol Blood Marrow Transplant, 26*(8), 1446–1451.

101. Young, N. S., Scheinberg, P., & Calado, R. T. (2008). Aplastic anemia. *Curr Opin Hematol, 15*(3), 162–168.

102. LeBlanc, F. R., Maciejewski, J. P., & Loughran, T. P. (2023). Acquired disorders of red cell, white cell, and platelet production. In Hoffman, R., Benz, E. J., Silberstein, L. E., et al. (Eds.), *Hematology: Basic Principles and Practice.* (8th ed., pp. 431–450). Philadelphia: Elsevier.

103. Sawada, K., Hirokawa, M., & Fujishima, N. (2009). Diagnosis and management of acquired pure red cell aplasia. *Hematol Oncol Clin North Am, 23*(2), 249–259.

104. Means, R. T. (2016). Pure red cell aplasia. *Blood, 128*(21), 2504–2509.

105. Balasubramanian, S. K., Sadaps, M., Thota, S., et al. (2018). Rational management approach to pure red cell aplasia. *Haematologica, 103*(2), 221–230.

106. Shaw, J., & Meeder, R. (2007). Transient erythroblastopenia of childhood in siblings: case report and review of the literature. *J Pediatr Hematol Oncol, 29*(9), 659–660.

107. Lipton, J. M., & Ellis, S. R. (2009). Diamond-Blackfan anemia: diagnosis, treatment, and molecular pathogenesis. *Hematol Oncol Clin North Am, 23*(2), 261–282.

108. Da Costa, L., Leblanc, T., & Mohandas, N. (2020). Diamond-Blackfan anemia. *Blood, 136*(11), 1262–1273.

109. Boria, I., Garelli, E., Gazda, H. T., et al. (2010). The ribosomal basis of Diamond-Blackfan anemia: mutation and database update. *Hum Mutat, 31*(12), 1269–1279.

110. Lipton, J. M., Atsidaftos, E., Zyskind, I., et al. (2006). Improving clinical care and elucidating the pathophysiology of Diamond Blackfan anemia: an update from the Diamond Blackfan Anemia Registry. *Pediatr Blood Cancer, 46*(5), 558–564.

111. Glader, B. E., Backer, K., & Diamond, L. K. (1983). Elevated erythrocyte adenosine deaminase activity in congenital hypoplastic anemia. *N Engl J Med, 309*(24), 1486–1490.

112. Iolascon, A., Andolfo, I., & Russo, R. (2020). Congenital dyserythropoietic anemias. *Blood, 136*(11), 1274–1283.

113. Renella, R., & Wood, W. G. (2009). The congenital dyserythropoietic anemias. *Hematol Oncol Clin North Am, 23*(2), 283–306.

114. Heimpel, H. (2004). Congenital dyserythropoietic anemias: epidemiology, clinical significance, and progress in understanding their pathogenesis. *Ann Hematol, 83*(10), 613–621.

115. Dgany, O., Avidan, N., Delaunay, J., et al. (2002). Congenital dyserythropoietic anemia type I is caused by mutations in codanin-1. *Am J Hum Genet, 71*(6), 1467–1474.

116. Noy-Lotan, S., Dgany, O., Lahmi, R., et al. (2009). Codanin-1, the protein encoded by the gene mutated in congenital dyserythropoietic anemia type I (CDAN1), is cell cycle-regulated. *Haematologica, 94*(5), 629–637.

117. Schwarz, K., Iolascon, A., Verissimo, F., et al. (2009). Mutations affecting the secretory COPII coat component SEC23B cause congenital dyserythropoietic anemia type II. *Nat Genet, 41*(8), 936–940.

118. Kirchhausen, T. (2007). Making COPII coats. *Cell, 129*(7), 1251-1252.

119. Liljeholm, M., Irvine, A. F., Vikberg, A. L., et al. (2013). Congenital dyserythropoietic anemia type III (CDA III) is caused by a mutation in kinesin family member, *KIF23. Blood, 121*, 4791–4799.

120. Iolascon, A., Heimpel, H., Wahlin, A., et al. (2013). Congenital dyserythropoietic anemias: molecular insights and diagnostic approach. *Blood, 122*(13), 2162–2166.

121. Makoni, S. N., & Laber, D. A. (2004). Clinical spectrum of myelophthisis in cancer patients. *Am J Hematol, 76*(1), 92–93.

122. Reddy, V. V. B., & Morlote, D. (2021). Anemia associated with marrow infiltration. In Kaushansky, K., Prchal, J. T., Burns L.J., et al. (Eds.), *Williams Hematology.* (10th ed., pp. 717–720). New York: McGraw-Hill.

123. Laureano, M., & Hillis, C. (2023). Hematologic manifestations of end-organ failure. In Hoffman, R., Benz, E. J., Silberstein, L. E., et al. (Eds.), *Hematology: Basic Principles and Practice.* (8th ed., pp. 2305–2311). Philadelphia: Elsevier.

124. Centers for Disease Control and Prevention. (2023). Chronic kidney disease fact sheet, 2023. https://www.cdc.gov/kidneydisease/pdf/CKD-Factsheet-H.pdf. Accessed August 21, 2023.

125. Kidney Disease: Improving Global Outcomes (KDIGO) Anemia Work Group. (2012). KDIGO Clinical Practice Guideline for Anemia in Chronic Kidney Disease. *Kidney Inter, (*Suppl. 2), 279–335.

126. Macdougall, I. C. (2001). Role of uremic toxins in exacerbating anemia in renal failure. *Kidney Int, 59*(Suppl. 78), S67–S72.

127. Wish, J. B. (2006). Assessing iron status: beyond serum ferritin and transferrin saturation. *Clin J Am Soc Nephrol, (*Suppl. 1), S4–S8.

128. Bovy, C., Gothot, A., Delanaye, P., et al. (2007). Mature erythrocyte parameters as new markers of functional iron deficiency in haemodialysis: sensitivity and specificity. *Nephrol Dial Transplant, 22*, 1156–1162.

20

Introduction to Increased Destruction of Erythrocytes

Kathryn Doig and Susan A. McQuiston

OBJECTIVES

After completion of this chapter, the reader will be able to:

1. Define *hemolysis* and recognize its hallmark clinical findings.
2. Differentiate a hemolytic disorder from a hemolytic anemia by definition and using laboratory and clinical findings.
3. Discuss methods of classifying hemolytic anemias and apply a classification to an unfamiliar anemia.
4. Describe the processes of fragmentation (intravascular) and macrophage-mediated (extravascular) hemolysis, including sites of hemolysis, catabolic products, and relative time frame for the appearance of those products after hemolysis.
5. Describe protoporphyrin catabolism (bilirubin production), including metabolites and their sites of production and excretion.
6. Describe mechanisms that salvage hemoglobin and heme during fragmentation hemolysis.
7. Describe changes to bilirubin metabolism and iron salvage systems that occur when the rate of fragmentation or macrophage-mediated hemolysis increases.
8. Identify, explain the diagnostic value, and interpret the results of laboratory tests that indicate increased hemolysis and erythropoiesis.
9. Differentiate between hemolytic anemias and other causes of increased erythropoiesis given laboratory or clinical information.
10. Differentiate between hemolytic anemias and other causes of bilirubinemia given laboratory or clinical information.
11. Interchange conjugation terminology for bilirubin fractions with Van den Bergh reaction terminology.
12. Explain the principle of the Van den Bergh reaction to quantitate and fractionate bilirubin in body fluids.

OUTLINE

Classification of Hemolytic Disorders
    Acute Versus Chronic Hemolysis
    Inherited Versus Acquired Hemolysis
    Intrinsic Versus Extrinsic Hemolysis
    Site and Mechanism of Hemolysis
Physiologic Hemolysis
    Physiologic Macrophage-Mediated Hemolysis and Bilirubin Metabolism
    Physiologic Fragmentation Hemolysis and Plasma Hemoglobin Salvage
Pathologic Hemolysis
    Pathologic Macrophage-Mediated (Extravascular) Hemolysis
    Pathologic Fragmentation (Intravascular) Hemolysis

Clinical Features
    Anemia
    Jaundice
    Hemoglobinuria
    Miscellaneous Clinical Signs and Symptoms
Laboratory Findings
    Tests of Accelerated Red Blood Cell Destruction
    Tests of Increased Erythropoiesis
    Laboratory Tests to Identify Specific Hemolytic Processes
Differential Diagnosis

CASE STUDY

After studying the material in this chapter, the reader should be able to respond to the following case study. Answers can be found in Appendix C.

A 34-year-old patient was admitted to the hospital for a vaginal hysterectomy. Except for excessive menstrual bleeding, the patient was in otherwise good health, and all preoperative laboratory test results were within their respective reference intervals. There was no excessive blood loss during or after surgery, and recovery was uneventful except for some expected pain, for which the patient received ibuprofen. Three days after surgery, the patient began to experience abdominal pain and pass "root beer"-colored urine. A complete blood count at that time revealed a hemoglobin level of 5.8 g/dL. Reference intervals can be found after the Index at the end of the book.

1. What process is indicated by the root beer-colored urine?
2. What laboratory tests can be used to differentiate the cause of the hemolysis?
3. Based on the patient's clinical presentation, predict the results expected for each test listed for question 2.

This chapter presents an overview of the hemolytic process and provides a foundation that is applicable in the following chapters on red blood cell (RBC) disorders. The term *hemolysis* or *hemolytic disorder* refers to increased rate of destruction (lysis) of RBCs, shortening their life span. The reduced number of cells results in reduced tissue oxygenation and increased erythropoietin production by the kidney. When the patient is otherwise healthy, the bone marrow responds by accelerating erythrocyte production, which leads to reticulocytosis. A hemolytic disorder is present without anemia if the bone marrow is able to compensate by accelerating RBC production sufficiently to replace RBCs lost through hemolysis. Healthy bone marrow can increase its production of RBCs by four to eight times normal.[1,2] Therefore significant RBC destruction must occur before an anemia develops during hemolysis. A *hemolytic anemia* results when the rate of RBC destruction exceeds the increased rate of RBC production.

CLASSIFICATION OF HEMOLYTIC DISORDERS

Many anemias have a hemolytic component, including anemia associated with vitamin B_{12} or folate deficiency, inflammation, renal disease, and iron deficiency. In these conditions, hemolysis alone does not cause anemia, and so they are not typically classified as hemolytic disorders. Rather, these anemias develop as a result of the inability of bone marrow to increase production of RBCs. Because hemolysis is not the primary underlying cause, these disorders are considered anemias with a secondary hemolytic component.

When hemolysis is the primary feature, it can be classified as follows:

- Acute versus chronic
- Inherited versus acquired
- Intrinsic versus extrinsic
- Intravascular versus extravascular
- Fragmentation versus macrophage mediated

Every hemolytic condition can be classified according to each of these descriptors. Table 20.1 shows this and provides a noncomprehensive list of hemolytic anemias categorized in this way. This chapter focuses on the mechanism of hemolysis, that is, the distinction between fragmentation and macrophage-mediated hemolytic conditions. Other classifying schemes are summarized here briefly for application in the chapters that follow. Intrinsic defects leading to increased erythrocyte destruction are presented in Chapter 21, while extrinsic defects are presented in Chapters 22 and 23, and hemoglobinopathies and thalassemias are discussed in Chapters 24 and 25.

Acute Versus Chronic Hemolysis

Acute versus *chronic hemolysis* delineates the clinical presentation. Acute hemolysis has a rapid onset and either disappears

TABLE 20.1   Classification of Selected Hemolytic Anemias by Primary Cause and Type of Hemolysis

	Predominantly Fragmentation (Intravascular) Hemolysis	Predominantly Macrophage-Mediated (Extravascular) Hemolysis	
Extrinsic Defects	**Agents From Outside the RBC**		**Acquired Conditions**
	Immune hemolysis: cold antibody Microangiopathic hemolysis Infectious agents, as in malaria Thermal injury Chemicals/drugs Venoms Prosthetic heart valve	Immune hemolysis: warm antibody Drugs	
	Membrane Abnormalities		
	Spur cell anemia of severe liver disease Paroxysmal nocturnal hemoglobinuria Hereditary pyropoikilocytosis	Hereditary membrane defects such as hereditary spherocytosis	**Hereditary Conditions**
Intrinsic Defects	**Abnormalities of the RBC Interior**		
	Enzyme defects such as G6PD deficiency Hemoglobinopathies such as sickle cell disease, thalassemia		

G6PD, Glucose-6-phosphate dehydrogenase; *RBC,* red blood cell.
Green text indicates acute or episodic hemolysis.
Red text indicates chronic hemolysis.
Some conditions may exhibit mixed presentations under certain circumstances. It is evident that most hereditary conditions lead to chronic hemolysis, whereas acquired conditions are more often acute. Furthermore, the intrinsic RBC defects typically are due to hereditary conditions, whereas extrinsic factors typically lead to acquired hemolytic disorders.

or subsides between episodes. The number and periodicity of episodes can differ: episodes can be isolated, episodic, or paroxysmal. A hemolytic transfusion reaction is an example of an isolated acute incident. Sickle cell anemia is an example of an episodic hemolytic condition in which hemolysis occurs when the individual experiences deoxygenation of the RBCs. There will be multiple but unpredictable instances of deoxygenation throughout the individual's life, creating episodes of acute hemolysis. Paroxysms are events that occur in a more rhythmic or predictable frequency. *Paroxysmal nocturnal hemoglobinuria* is hemolysis that occurs when the blood pH drops during sleep. Thus the acute episodes occur with the rhythm of the sleep-wake cycle. In each of the examples of acute hemolysis, the hemolysis ends or subsides after the instance of hemolysis.

In chronic hemolysis, some level of lysis occurs in an ongoing manner and does not end. The amount of hemolysis can vary, but each individual has a baseline level. If the baseline degree of hemolysis is mild, it may not result in anemia if the bone marrow is able to compensate by increased erythropoiesis. Hereditary elliptocytosis, an abnormality of RBC membrane proteins, is one example in which the degree of hemolysis is typically low and bone marrow compensation prevents anemia.

Other chronic conditions result in persistent hemolysis that is so severe that the bone marrow cannot generate cells fast enough to compensate for the anemia. Thalassemia major is an example of such a condition. Although RBC production is brisk, each cell possesses an inadequate complement of one type of globin chain. Cells lyse in thalassemia because excess normal globin chains precipitate inside erythroid cells. The rate of hemolysis exceeds the ability of the bone marrow to compensate, so thalassemia is a persistent anemia. Hemolysis is continual, so it is chronic.

Some chronic hemolytic conditions may be punctuated over time with acute hemolytic *crises* that exceed the baseline level and do cause anemia. Glucose-6-phosphate dehydrogenase deficiency is such a condition. RBC life span is always shortened, so it is a chronic hemolytic condition, but bone marrow compensation typically prevents anemia. When the cells are challenged with oxidizing agents such as antimalarial drugs, a dramatic acute hemolytic event occurs, resulting in anemia. When the drug is withdrawn, hemolysis returns to baseline and bone marrow compensation is sufficient to overcome anemia.

Inherited Versus Acquired Hemolysis

Inherited hemolytic conditions, such as thalassemia, are passed to offspring by mutant genes from the parents. *Acquired* hemolytic disorders develop in individuals who were previously hematologically normal but acquire an agent or condition that lyses RBCs. Infectious diseases such as malaria are an example.

Intrinsic Versus Extrinsic Hemolysis

Hemolytic disorders are also classified as involving *intrinsic* or *extrinsic* RBC defects. Intrinsic hemolysis arises from conditions that affect the innate integrity of the RBC, while extrinsic hemolysis is caused by the action of agents external to the RBC. This is the classification scheme used for subsequent chapters in this book. Examples of *intrinsic* hemolytic disorders are

abnormalities of the RBC membrane, enzymatic pathways, or the hemoglobin molecule. With intrinsic defects, if RBCs of the affected patient were to be transfused into a healthy individual, they would still have a shortened life span because the defect is in the RBC. If normal RBCs are transfused into a patient who has an intrinsic defect, the transfused cells have a normal life span because the transfused cells are normal.

Extrinsic hemolytic conditions arise from agents outside the RBC, typically substances in plasma or conditions affecting the anatomy of the circulatory system. A plasma antibody against RBC antigens and a prosthetic heart valve are examples of noninfectious extrinsic agents that can damage RBCs. Infectious agents are also considered extrinsic, even though the malaria protozoa and other intracellular infectious agents are within the RBC. They are classified as extrinsic hemolytic agents because the RBC was normal until it was invaded by an outside agent. In extrinsic hemolysis, cross-transfusion studies have shown that the patient's RBCs have a normal life span in the bloodstream of a healthy individual, but normal cells are lysed more rapidly in the patient's circulation. These studies confirm that something outside the RBCs is causing the hemolysis. (Of course, in the case of intracellular parasites, a cross-transfusion study is not applicable.) Most intrinsic defects are inherited, whereas most extrinsic defects are acquired (see Table 20.1). A few exceptions exist, such as paroxysmal nocturnal hemoglobinuria, an acquired disorder involving an intrinsic defect (Chapter 21).

As mentioned earlier, intrinsic disorders are subclassified as membrane defects, enzyme defects, and hemoglobinopathies. Extrinsic hemolysis may be subclassified as immune, infectious, microangiopathic, toxic (chemicals, drugs, and venoms), or physical/mechanical (heat) (see Table 20.1).

Site and Mechanism of Hemolysis

Another classification scheme is based on the site of hemolysis and is closely related to the general mechanism of lysis. *Intravascular* hemolysis occurs due to rupture of the RBC membrane while the RBC is in the circulation, hence the designation intravascular. This results in *fragmentation* of the RBC and release of the contents into the plasma. RBCs can also lyse by fragmentation in the sinuses of the spleen, bone marrow, and liver, with the hemolysis appearing to occur just within that organ. However, the sinuses of these organs are effectively distended blood vessels, so the term *intravascular* can apply, even though it is within an organ and not distributed throughout the vasculature. Suffice it to say, if the contents of the RBCs are present in the plasma, it is intravascular hemolysis.

Macrophage-mediated hemolysis, also known as *erythrophagocytosis*, occurs when RBCs are engulfed by macrophages and lysed inside the phagocytic organelles by their digestive processes. The term *extravascular*, meaning outside the vessels, applies because the RBC is no longer in the bloodstream when the lysis occurs, hence extravascular. When the cell is ruptured, the RBC contents remain contained within the macrophage. Extravascular hemolysis occurs most often within the macrophages that reside in the spleen and liver.

Commonly, the terms *fragmentation* and *intravascular* are used interchangeably, as are *macrophage mediated* and *extravascular.* The mechanistic classifying scheme is useful because screening laboratory test results differ due to differences in the process of hemolysis, regardless of where the hemolysis occurs. Once hemolysis is detected by screening, the exact cause of the hemolysis must still be determined by targeted testing for appropriate treatment to be implemented.

PHYSIOLOGIC HEMOLYSIS

Without a nucleus to direct the replenishment of enzymes and other molecules, RBCs are doomed to die of old age at about 120 days. A loss of about 1% of RBCs daily is expected physiologically, and the body has mechanisms to process the contents of the cells and recycle iron to other cells. Physiologic RBC death occurs either by the action of macrophages that recognize aged (senescent) cells and remove them from the circulation or by rupture due to rigidity that accompanies aging.

Physiologic Macrophage-Mediated Hemolysis and Bilirubin Metabolism

Detection of hemolysis depends partly on detection of RBC breakdown products. A prominent product is bilirubin. The process of normal bilirubin production is described to clarify the relationship between hemolysis and increased bilirubin levels.

RBCs live approximately 120 days. During this time, they undergo various metabolic and chemical changes that result in membrane alterations and a loss of deformability. Under normal circumstances, macrophages of the mononuclear phagocyte system (or reticuloendothelial system) recognize these changes and phagocytize the aged erythrocytes (Chapter 6), producing a macrophage-mediated hemolytic process that removes approximately 1% of the RBCs per day. The organs involved include the spleen, bone marrow, liver, lymph nodes, and circulating monocytes, but it is primarily the macrophages in spleen and liver that process senescent RBCs. There is also minimal RBC loss due to intravascular lysis from shear stress on senescent RBCs (see "Physiologic Fragmentation Hemolysis and Plasma Hemoglobin Salvage" later).

The majority of RBC degradation occurs inside macrophages as enzymes of the macrophage phagolysosome rupture phagocytized erythrocytes and the contents are salvaged or metabolized (Figure 20.1). Hemoglobin is hydrolyzed into heme and globin; the latter is further degraded into amino acids that return to the amino acid pool within the cell or are exported to the plasma. Iron is released from heme, returned to plasma via ferroportin, bound to its protein carrier molecule (transferrin), and recycled to needy cells, thus salvaging virtually all RBC iron (Chapter 9). The protoporphyrin component is catabolized, and the products are processed in the liver, are moved to the intestines where they facilitate dietary fat absorption, and then are excreted mostly in the stool. Bilirubin and urobilinogen are the excretory products derived from the protoporphyrin component of heme.

Figure 20.2 illustrates heme catabolism. Once free heme is inside the macrophage, heme oxygenase breaks the protoporphyrin ring to yield a linear molecule, biliverdin. The lungs

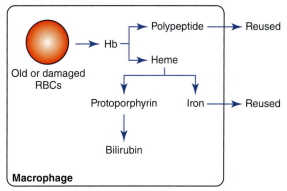

Figure 20.1 Normal Catabolism of Hemoglobin. Macrophages lyse ingested red blood cells *(RBCs)* and separate hemoglobin *(Hb)* into globin chains and heme components. Amino acids from the globin chains are reused. Heme is degraded to iron and protoporphyrin. Iron is returned to the blood to be reused. Protoporphyrin is degraded to unconjugated bilirubin.

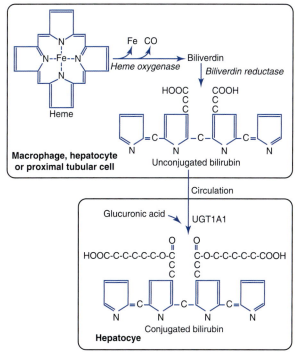

Figure 20.2 Catabolism of Heme to Bilirubin. In cells containing heme oxygenase, iron is removed from heme, and the protoporphyrin ring is opened up to form an intermediate, biliverdin. Biliverdin is converted to unconjugated bilirubin by biliverdin reductase. The unconjugated bilirubin is secreted into the blood and binds to albumin for transport to the liver. When unconjugated bilirubin enters the hepatocyte, UGT1A1 (uridine diphosphate glucuronosyltransferase family 1 member A1, formerly glucuronyl transferase) adds two molecules of glucuronic acid to form bisglucuronosyl bilirubin, also called conjugated bilirubin.

excrete a by product of that reaction, carbon monoxide. The green biliverdin is reduced to bilirubin, a nonpolar yellow molecule that is secreted into the blood (Box 20.1). This form of bilirubin is called unconjugated for reasons that will be evident shortly. Because it is hydrophobic, this form of bilirubin must bind to albumin to be transported in blood to the liver.

An understanding of blood circulation in the liver is needed to appreciate the subtleties of hepatic bilirubin metabolism.

Van den Bergh, A. A., & Muller, P. (1916). Über eine direkte und eine indirekte diazoreaktion aus bilirubin, *Biochem Z*, *77*, 90; and Hutchinson, D. W., Johnson, B., & Knell, A. J. (1972). The reaction between bilirubin and aromatic diazo compounds. *Biochem J*, *127*, 907–908.

Blood enters the liver lobule at the periphery via a hepatic artery and from a portal vein bringing blood from the intestines (Figure 5.7). Blood from each vessel enters the endothelial cell-lined sinusoids that run between rows of hepatocytes. The loose structure of the sinusoids leads to the characterization of the blood as percolating through the lobule and around the hepatocytes toward the central vein. Here, the blood drains into progressively larger veins that leave the liver to enter the inferior vena cava.

Bilirubin formed in macrophages and secreted in blood enters the liver sinusoid via the hepatic artery. In the liver sinusoid, bilirubin dissociates from albumin so that it can be carried into the hepatocyte by organic anion transporter (OAT) proteins, chiefly OATP1B3.[3,4] Once inside the hepatocyte, bilirubin is bound to glutathione S-transferase, known as ligandin, for transport to the endoplasmic reticulum.[5] There, unconjugated bilirubin is joined (i.e., conjugated) with one to two molecules of a sugar acid, glucuronic acid, by uridine diphosphate (UDP) glucuronosyltransferase family 1 member A1 (UGT1A1), previously known as glucuronyl transferase. The molecules formed include monoglucuronosyl bilirubin, with just a single glucuronic acid added, and bisglucuronosyl bilirubin, previously known as bilirubin diglucuronide, which has two glucuronic acid molecules added. The addition of the glucuronic acid molecules is an example of chemical conjugation, so the molecule is called conjugated bilirubin (Box 20.2). Thus the bilirubin originally released from macrophages that lacks glucuronic acids is termed *unconjugated bilirubin* (Box 20.2). Addition of glucuronic acids makes conjugated bilirubin polar and water soluble, while unconjugated bilirubin is not water soluble but is lipid soluble. In the structure of the liver lobule (Figure 5.7), small ducts called *canaliculi* run from the central vein outward along the lateral sides between hepatocytes. They receive the bile excreted by hepatocytes and channel it toward the exterior of the lobule where the canaliculi join into larger bile ducts that ultimately collect the bile into the common bile. Conjugated bilirubin is actively excreted by hepatocytes into the canaliculi by a unidirectional and adenosine triphosphate (ATP)-dependent membrane protein, multidrug resistant protein 2 (MRP2).[4,6] Once in the bile canaliculi, conjugated bilirubin continues down to the common bile duct and eventually into the intestines (Figure 20.3). There, it assists with the emulsification of fats for absorption from the diet.

Under normal conditions, hepatocytes at the exterior of the lobule receive the highest concentration of unconjugated bilirubin in the blood entering the sinus from the hepatic artery. Once they have absorbed and conjugated the bilirubin, they are not always able to export all of it into the bile duct. Therefore they export conjugated bilirubin into sinusoidal blood via a second MRP (MRP3), which is localized to the sinusoidal side of hepatocytes.[4] It can then be absorbed downstream by more centrilobular hepatocytes via other OAT proteins, OATP1B1 and OATP1B3, in the sinusoidal membrane.[4,5] OATP1B1 has a very high affinity for conjugated bilirubin.[4] The absorbed conjugated bilirubin can then be exported without further modification directly into the canaliculi by the downstream absorbing hepatocyte.

Once conjugated bilirubin enters the intestines, it is oxidized by gut bacteria into various water-soluble compounds, collectively called *urobilinogens*. Most urobilinogen is oxidized further to urobilin, stercobilin, and similar compounds that give the brown color to stool. This is the usual and ultimate route for excretion of most RBC-derived protoporphyrin.

Some conjugated bilirubin and urobilinogen molecules are passively absorbed from the intestines into the blood of the portal circulation (see Figure 20.3). The portal circulation (blood vessels that surround the intestines to absorb nutrients) collects these soluble bile products and carries them directly to the liver in this enterohepatic circulation. These bilirubin derivatives enter the lobule via the portal veins and flow into the sinusoidal blood. Most of the intestinally absorbed and hepatocyte-secreted conjugated bilirubin in the sinusoidal blood is absorbed into hepatocytes by OATP1B1 and recycled directly into the bile.[7]

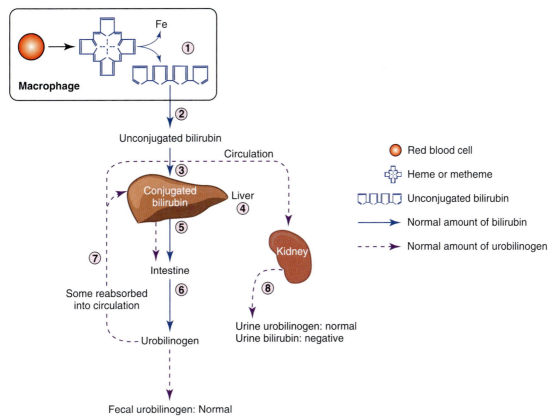

Figure 20.3 Physiologic Macrophage-Mediated Hemolysis. In a macrophage, hemoglobin is degraded to heme, the iron is released, and the protoporphyrin ring is converted to unconjugated bilirubin *(1)*. Macrophages release unconjugated bilirubin into the blood, where it binds to albumin for transport to the liver *(2)*. Unconjugated bilirubin enters the hepatocyte *(3)*. The hepatocyte converts unconjugated bilirubin to conjugated bilirubin *(4)*. Conjugated bilirubin leaves the liver in the bile and enters the small intestine *(5)*. Bacteria in the large intestine convert conjugated bilirubin to urobilinogen, most of which is excreted in the stool *(6)*. Some of the water-soluble urobilinogen is reabsorbed in the portal circulation, and most is recycled through the liver for excretion *(7)*. A small component of the reabsorbed urobilinogen is filtered and excreted in the urine *(8)*. (Modified from Brunzel, N. A. [2013]. *Fundamentals of Urine and Body Fluid Analysis.* [3rd ed., p. 141, Figure 7-8]. St. Louis: Elsevier.)

Urobilinogen is similarly recycled into the bile. A miniscule amount of conjugated bilirubin remains in the blood entering the central vein, along with a larger amount of urobilinogen. These compounds are filtered at the renal glomerulus and excreted in the urine in low concentrations. So although conjugated bilirubin is virtually undetectable in urine because of efficient recycling in the liver, a measurable amount of urobilinogen can be expected normally. This is the second but much smaller route of excretion for protoporphyrins. The yellow color of urine is not caused by the urobilinogen, however, which is colorless. It is a result of urobilin, a stool derivative of urobilinogen that is also water soluble and absorbed via the portal circulation.

Physiologic Fragmentation Hemolysis and Plasma Hemoglobin Salvage

Fragmentation hemolysis is the result of trauma to the RBC membrane that causes a rupture sufficient for the cell contents to spill directly into plasma. Approximately 10% to 20% of physiologic RBC destruction is via fragmentation,[8] usually secondary to turbulence and anatomic restrictions in the vasculature. Aged RBCs are most susceptible to these forces. The

cellular contents spilled into the plasma that are of laboratory interest include hemoglobin and lactate dehydrogenase (LDH). Physiological fragmentation hemolysis is the source of the RBC fraction of normal LDH.

Because hemoglobin is filtered through the glomerulus, some iron could be lost daily with even physiologic amounts of fragmentation hemolysis. In addition, free hemoglobin, and especially free heme, can scavenge nitric oxide and cause iron-induced oxidative damage to cells (Chapter 9). Three main mechanisms salvage hemoglobin iron and prevent oxidation. They are collectively called the *haptoglobin-hemopexin-methemalbumin system* (see Figure 20.4). A fourth mechanism involving heme carrier protein-1 (HCP-1) may also be significant.

Haptoglobin

When free in plasma, hemoglobin exists mostly as α/β globin dimers[9,10] that rapidly complex to a liver-produced plasma protein called *haptoglobin* (see Figure 20.4). Haptoglobin binds a hemoglobin dimer in a conformation that is very similar to the binding of the complementary globin dimer in the native hemoglobin structure, so the conformation of the complex has

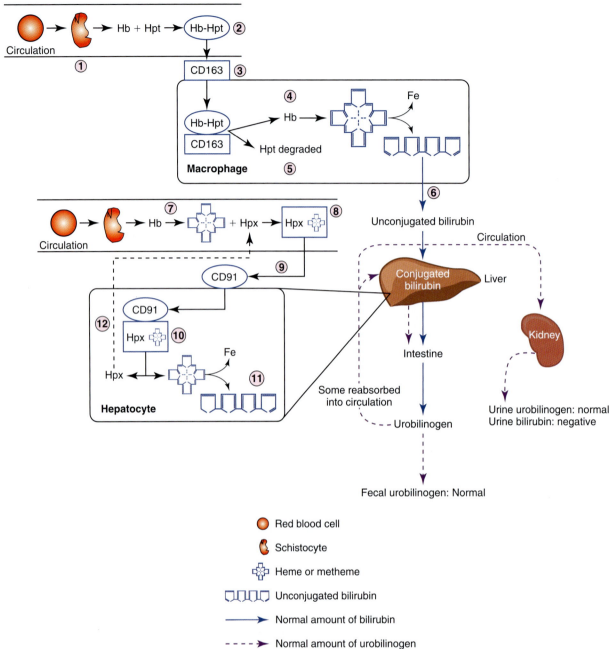

Figure 20.4 Physiologic Fragmentation Hemolysis. Normally, a small number of red blood cells lyse within the circulation, forming schistocytes and releasing hemoglobin *(Hb)* into the blood, mostly as α/β dimers *(1)*. The plasma protein haptoglobin *(Hpt)* binds a hemoglobin dimer in a complex *(2)*. The hemoglobin-haptoglobin complex binds to CD163 on the surface of macrophages in various organs *(3)*. The complex is internalized into the macrophage, where the hemoglobin dimer is released. The hemoglobin dimer is degraded to heme, the iron is released, and the protoporphyrin ring is converted to unconjugated bilirubin *(4)*. The haptoglobin is degraded *(5)*. The unconjugated bilirubin released into the blood is bound to albumin and processed through the liver as in Figure 20.3 (steps 2 to 8) *(6)*. When free hemoglobin is released into the blood with fragmentation, the iron is rapidly oxidized, forming methemoglobin, and the heme (metheme) molecule dissociates from the globin *(7)*. The plasma protein hemopexin *(Hpx)* binds free metheme into a complex *(8)*. The hemopexin-metheme complex binds to CD91 on the surface of hepatocytes *(9)*. The complex is internalized into the hepatocyte *(10)*. The iron is released from the metheme, and the protoporphyrin ring is converted to unconjugated bilirubin, ready for conjugation and further processing, as in Figure 20.3 (steps 4 to 8) *(11)*. Hemopexin may be recycled to the blood or degraded *(12)*. (Modified from Brunzel, N. A. [2013]. *Fundamentals of Urine and Body Fluid Analysis*. [3rd ed., p. 141, Figure 7-8]. St. Louis: Elsevier.)

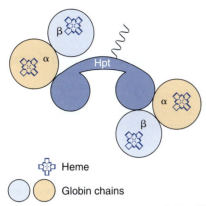

Heme

Globin chains

Figure 20.5 Haptoglobin Binding of Hemoglobin Dimers. When hemoglobin is released in plasma, it rapidly dissociates to α/β dimers. Haptoglobin *(Hpt)* is able to bind two dimers, limiting the oxidizing action of the hemes. Haptoglobin possesses a looped configuration that is able to bind to CD 163 on macrophages. This allows the complex to be endocytosed by the macrophage, thus salvaging the hemoglobin and its iron.

been termed a *pseudotetramer* (Figure 20.5).[11,12] In this complex, the hemes are sequestered, as they are in intact hemoglobin, so that cells are protected from their oxidizing properties.[11] As the plasma is carried to various tissues, the hemoglobin-haptoglobin complex (Hb-Hpt) is taken up by macrophages, principally those in the liver, spleen, bone marrow, and lung.[13] In these tissues, macrophages express CD163, the haptoglobin scavenger receptor, on their membranes. Once the Hb-Hpt complex binds to CD163, the entire complex is internalized with the receptor into a lysosome within the macrophage.[13,14] Inside the lysosome, iron is salvaged, globin is catabolized, and protoporphyrin is converted to unconjugated bilirubin, just as though an intact RBC had been ingested by the macrophage. Haptoglobin is also degraded within the lysosome. The rapid binding of the Hb-Hpt complex to the CD163 receptor prevents loss of hemoglobin iron in the urine. The degraded haptoglobin is replenished by the liver at a constant rate sufficient to salvage a day's worth of plasma hemoglobin released with physiological levels of RBC fragmentation.

Hemopexin

A second mechanism of iron salvage and oxidation prevention involves *hemopexin* (Figure 20.4). The iron in free plasma hemoglobin rapidly becomes oxidized, forming methemoglobin. The heme molecule (actually *metheme* or *hemin*) readily dissociates from the globin.[10] Free metheme has high redox activity. It is lipophilic and readily diffuses across cell membranes and into extracellular spaces oxidizing proteins, lipids, and nucleic acids. In so doing, it sensitizes cells to proinflammatory stimuli.[15] Metheme toxicity is a major factor in the lethality of systemic conditions such as sepsis or hemolytic transfusion reactions. Heme toxicity is mitigated by binding with high affinity to another liver-produced plasma protein, hemopexin.[16,17]

Hemopexin-metheme binds to lipoprotein receptor-related protein (LRP1),[18] the CD91 receptor, chiefly on hepatocytes. The complex is internalized by endocytosis (Chapter 4) into the hepatocyte.[19] Thus the heme is saved from urinary loss, and its oxidizing potential is eliminated. The fate of the internalized heme remains controversial.[19,20] The fate of the hemopexin is

similarly debated.[15,21] However, a drop in plasma hemopexin during periods of increased fragmentation hemolysis supports lysosomal degradation as its end point.

Albumin

A third mechanism of iron salvage is the metheme-albumin system. Albumin acts as a carrier for many molecules, including metheme. This is a temporary holding state for metheme, merely by virtue of the high concentration of albumin in plasma. However, metheme is rapidly transferred to hemopexin in the plasma, when available, which has a higher binding affinity for metheme than albumin.[22] The hemopexin-metheme complex then travels to the liver for processing as described previously.

Heme Carrier Protein-1

A fourth mechanism that reduces plasma heme is uptake by hepatocytes via HCP-1, also known as solute carrier family 46 member 1 (SLC46A1).[23] HCP-1 is known to import heme from the intestinal lumen into enterocytes (Chapter 9). It has also been identified on the hepatocyte membrane and shown to impact hepatocyte iron regulation.[24] Research continues to elucidate the full role of hepatocyte HCP-1 in heme salvage.

The prevailing view has been that these salvage systems work somewhat sequentially. Haptoglobin binds until it is saturated and depleted. Then hemopexin binds metheme until it is saturated. Finally, albumin binds metheme. More recent theories suggest that these systems work simultaneously, particularly during accelerated hemolysis, and that hemopexin acts to prevent heme toxicity at all times.[15,25] This may be true with HCP-1 also.

Renal Iron Salvage

The iron-related salvage systems described so far in this section are important in preventing renal iron loss, but they are highly specific and salvage only a few iron-containing compounds. Other iron-containing compounds, especially proteins, enter the glomerular filtrate daily under physiologic conditions. These include transferrin, ferritin, and lactoferrin, to name a few. In recent years, the kidney nephron has come to be considered a major contributor to body iron kinetics, as it reabsorbs these filterable iron-containing proteins.[26] Without reabsorption, physiologic daily iron loss would be sufficient to cause iron deficiency.[26]

Reabsorption of iron-containing proteins from the glomerular filtrate requires receptors on the apical side (i.e., tubule side) of the various nephron cells. Transferrin receptors appear on the apical surface of proximal tubular cells,[26,27] thus providing transferrin-specific uptake. However, the proximal tubular cells also possess the megalin-cubilin-amnionless receptor endocytosis complex.[26,28] These receptors are not specific for any heme/iron-containing proteins. Rather, they are responsible for non-specific but very efficient reabsorption of a variety of proteins from the urinary filtrate. Megalin and cubilin have each been shown to bind hemoglobin and myoglobin.[28] Additionally, megalin can bind lactoferrin, and cubilin can bind transferrin.[28]

While the proximal tubule is the major site of protein reabsorption, cells in each segment of the nephron have been shown to reabsorb iron-containing proteins using various receptors.[26,29] Additionally, divalent metal transporter-1 (DMT-1) has been identified on the luminal side of proximal tubular cells, able to transport non transferrin-bound iron.[30] These examples demonstrate that in some cases, the renal receptors, such as transferrin receptor-1 (TfR1) and DMT-1, are the same as those involved in body and cellular iron kinetics by other cells and organs (Chapter 9).

There may be multiple fates for iron reabsorbed into nephron cells in various forms. Reabsorbed iron may be used by nephron cells for their own iron needs. However, ferroportin has been identified on the *basolateral membrane* of cells all along the nephron. This suggests that renal cells are able to transfer salvaged iron back into the blood for use by other cells.[26,31] Once again, these systems evolved to manage the amount and forms of iron present in normal urinary filtrate.

PATHOLOGIC HEMOLYSIS

The physiologic hemolytic processes described in "Physiologic Hemolysis" lead to a loss of about 1% of RBCs daily. Any process that exceeds that rate is pathologic, and evidence of the accelerated hemolysis can be detected using laboratory tests.

The results will be different if the pathologic process is macrophage mediated or fragmented.

Pathologic Macrophage-Mediated (Extravascular) Hemolysis

Many hemolytic anemias are a result of increased macrophage-mediated hemolysis (Figure 20.6), during which more than the usual number of RBCs are removed from the circulation daily. Under normal circumstances, senescent RBCs display surface markers that identify them to macrophages as aged cells requiring removal (Chapter 6). Pathologic processes also lead to expression of the same markers, so cells are recognized and removed. If the number of affected cells increases beyond the quantity normally removed each day as a result of senescence, and if the bone marrow cannot compensate, anemia develops. As an example, in thalassemia, globin monomers aggregate and bind to the interior of the RBC membrane. That binding then leads to changes to the exterior of the membrane. Those changes are detected by macrophages, and the cells are removed from circulation prematurely. A similar process occurs when intracellular parasites are present or when complement or immunoglobulins

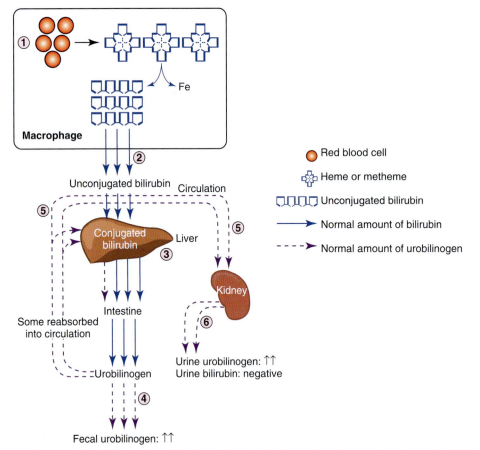

Figure 20.6 Pathologic Macrophage-Mediated Hemolysis. More than the usual number of red blood cells are ingested each day by macrophages *(1)*. An increased amount of unconjugated bilirubin is produced, released into the blood, and binds to albumin *(2)*. When increased unconjugated bilirubin is presented to the liver, an increased amount of conjugated bilirubin is made and excreted into the intestine *(3)*. When an increased amount of conjugated bilirubin is present in the intestine, an increased amount of urobilinogen is formed and excreted in the stool *(4)*. Increased urobilinogen in the intestine results in increased urobilinogen reabsorbed into the blood *(5)*. Increased urobilinogen in the blood results in increased urobilinogen filtered and excreted in the urine *(6)*. (Modified from Brunzel, N. A. [2013]. *Fundamentals of Urine and Body Fluid Analysis.* [3rd ed., p. 141, Figure 7-8]. St. Louis: Elsevier.)

TABLE 20.2 **Comparison of Laboratory Findings Indicating Accelerated Red Blood Cell Destruction in Fragmentation Versus Macrophage-Mediated Hemolysis**

Test Specimen	Result	Fragmentation Hemolysis	Macrophage-Mediated Hemolysis
Serum	Total bilirubin	↑	↑
	Indirect (unconjugated) bilirubin	↑	↑
	Direct (conjugated) bilirubin	WRI	WRI
	Lactate dehydrogenase activity (RBC fraction)	↑	sl ↑
	Haptoglobin	↓	sl ↓
	Free hemoglobin	↑	sl ↑
	Hemopexin	↓	sl ↓
Urine	Urobilinogen	↑	↑
	Free hemoglobin	Positive	Negative
	Methemoglobin	Positive	Negative
	Prussian blue staining of urine sediment	Positive	Negative
Anticoagulated whole blood	Hemoglobin, hematocrit, RBC count	↓	↓
	Schistocytes	Often present	
	Spherocytes		Often present
	Glycated hemoglobin	↓	↓
Special tests	Endogenous carbon monoxide	↑	↑
	Erythrocyte life span	↓	↓

↑, Typically increased; *sl ↑*, typically only slightly increased, minor component; *↓*, typically decreased; *sl ↓*, *typically only slightly decreased, minor component*; *RBC,* red blood cell; *WRI,* within reference interval.

are on the surface of the RBC. As defective RBCs display markers similar to those of aged RBCs, macrophage-mediated hemolysis of defective cells occurs most often in the spleen and liver, where macrophages possess receptors for those markers.

Sometimes the macrophage ingests a portion of the membrane, leaving the remainder to reseal. Little, if any, cytoplasmic volume is lost, but with less membrane, the cell becomes a spherocyte, the characteristic shape change associated with macrophage-mediated hemolysis. Although the spherocyte may enter the circulation, its survival is shortened because of its rigidity and inability to traverse the splenic sieve during subsequent passages through the red pulp. It may become trapped against the basement membrane of the splenic sinus and be fully ingested by a macrophage, or it may lyse mechanically because of its rigidity and in so doing, contribute a fragmentation component to what is otherwise a macrophage-mediated process.

In macrophage-mediated hemolytic anemias, the total plasma bilirubin level rises as RBCs are lysed prematurely. The rise of the total bilirubin is due to the increase of the unconjugated fraction (see Figure 20.6). As long as the liver is healthy, it processes the increased load of unconjugated bilirubin, producing more than the usual amount of conjugated bilirubin that enters the intestine. Increased urobilinogen forms in the intestines and is subsequently absorbed by the portal circulation and excreted by the kidney. Increased conjugated bilirubin is also absorbed into the portal (enterohepatic) circulation but is reprocessed through the hepatocytes and into the bile. Increased urobilinogen is detectable in the urine because it is (1) absorbed more than direct bilirubin into the portal circulation and (2) not reprocessed through the liver as completely as direct bilirubin. Although there is an increase in unconjugated bilirubin in the plasma, none of it appears in urine because it is bound to

albumin and cannot pass readily through the glomerulus. These findings are summarized in Table 20.2.

Hemopexin may play an especially important role in macrophage-mediated hemolysis. If macrophages ingest more than one or two erythrocytes, the released heme can be toxic to them.[25,32] They possess a membrane heme exporter, feline leukemia virus subgroup C receptor, that permits them to rid themselves of excess heme.[25] Hemopexin then is important to accept the exported free heme during macrophage-mediated hemolysis to prevent heme toxicity to other cells.[25]

Pathologic Fragmentation (Intravascular) Hemolysis

Although fragmentation hemolysis is a minor component of physiologic RBC destruction, it can be a major feature of pathologic processes. Dramatic examples of fragmentation hemolysis are the traumatic, physical lysis of RBCs caused by prosthetic heart valves or the exit of mature intracellular RBC parasites, such as malaria protozoa, bursting out of cells. In these instances, the fragmentation destruction of RBCs can cause profound anemias and organ failure (Box 20.3), as well as interference for some laboratory assays (Box 20.4).

Excessive fragmentation hemolysis is characterized by the appearance in the plasma of the contents of RBCs, chiefly hemoglobin, and thus the development of (met)hemoglobinemia. As a result, the iron salvage proteins form complexes with their respective ligands (Figure 20.7A and B): Hb-Hpt, metheme-hemopexin, and metheme-albumin. The complexes are then cleared within minutes from plasma by binding to their respective receptors on specific cells, as described previously.[17,18,21] The levels of free haptoglobin will drop because more than the usual amount of the Hb-Hpt complex will form and be taken up by macrophages (see Table 20.2). The endocytosed haptoglobin is not recycled to the plasma and there is no compensatory increase in production, so the plasma is depleted of haptoglobin during excessive fragmentation hemolysis. The levels of free hemopexin can also decrease as the heme-hemopexin complex is taken up by the hepatocyte and degraded.

If the amount of liberated hemoglobin and heme exceeds the capacity of the plasma salvage proteins, (met)hemoglobin can also appear in the glomerular filtrate in roughly the same time frame that it appears in the plasma (see Table 20.2). Increased amounts of iron-containing proteins are then presented to the proximal tubular cells for absorption (Figure 20.7C). In the case of the nonspecific megalin-cubilin-amnionless receptors, the kinetics will favor the iron-containing proteins when they are in high concentration during a hemolytic episode. However, the absorptive capacity of the nephron is limited and excess (met)hemoglobin and metheme can appear in the urine, giving it a brown color, termed *(met)hemoglobinuria*. If the conditions are suitable for the formation of casts, (met)hemoglobin-containing casts will be formed.

Proximal tubular cells are able to catabolize heme via heme-oxygenase-1,[33] thus freeing and salvaging the iron for export to the plasma by ferroportin in the basolaminal membrane (Figure 20.7D).[31] Proximal tubular cells also possess UGT1A1 to conjugate bilirubin.[34] Its disposition is uncertain at this time. MRP2 on the apical membrane may allow secretion of the conjugated bilirubin into the filtrate/urine.[35,36] However, the presence of OAT proteins in the basolaminal membrane may allow reabsorption into the plasma for ultimate liver excretion.[36] Still, the antiinflammatory role of carbon monoxide and bilirubin point to an intracellular purpose, particularly during inflammatory processes when heme-oxygenase-1 is upregulated.[37] Future research may clarify this.

Proximal tubular cell iron in excess of what can be transported into the circulation is stored as ferritin, and some is converted to hemosiderin (see Figure 20.7D). If the tubular cell is sloughed into the filtrate and appears in the urine sediment, the hemosiderin can be detected using Prussian blue stain (Chapter 9) (Figure 20.8). This provides evidence that excess iron in some form, such as hemoglobin, has been salvaged from the filtrate.

CLINICAL FEATURES

Clinical findings typical of hemolysis may be prominent if the hemolytic process is the primary cause of anemia. For patients in whom hemolysis is secondary, however, clinical features related to the primary condition may be more noticeable.

Anemia

If hemolysis is sufficient to result in anemia, patients experience the general symptoms of fatigue, dyspnea, and dizziness to a degree that is consistent with the severity and rate of development of the anemia. The associated signs of pallor and tachycardia can be expected.

Jaundice

Increase in plasma bilirubin gives a yellow tinge, not only to the plasma but also to body tissues. *Jaundice* refers to the yellow color of the skin and sclera, whereas *icterus* describes yellow plasma and tissues. Jaundice is readily evident in the sclera of the eyes of all patients as well as the skin of fair-skinned patients. In newborns experiencing hemolytic anemia, an underdeveloped blood-brain barrier permits entry of bilirubin to the brain. The lipid solubility of unconjugated bilirubin leads to deposition in the brain (Chapter 23), causing a type of brain damage called *kernicterus*, which refers to the yellow coloring (icterus) of the brain tissue.

Jaundice can result from conditions other than hemolysis, including hepatitis or gallstones. When jaundice is the result of hemolysis, it is called *hemolytic jaundice*. It is also called *prehepatic jaundice*, referring to the plasma predominance of unconjugated bilirubin before it is processed by the liver.

Hemoglobinuria

Brown urine, associated with (met)hemoglobinuria, points to a fragmentation hemolytic process. It must be differentiated from bleeding along the urinary tract or stale urine samples in which the RBCs have lysed (see "Differential Diagnosis").

Miscellaneous Clinical Signs and Symptoms

Some signs and symptoms will be different, depending on whether the hemolysis is chronic or acute.

Chronic Hemolysis

Splenomegaly can develop, particularly with chronic macrophage-mediated hemolytic processes. Gallstones (cholelithiasis) can occur whenever hemolysis is chronic. The constantly increased amount of bilirubin in the bile leads to the formation of the stones.[38] When hemolysis is chronic in children, the persistent compensatory bone marrow hyperplasia can lead to bone deformities because the bones are still forming and the enlarged marrow space enlarges the whole bone (Figure 25.3).

Acute Hemolysis

For patients in whom an acquired acute hemolytic process develops, the associated malaise, aches, vomiting, and possible fever may cause it to be confused with an acute infectious process. Profound prostration and shock may develop, particularly with acute fragmentation hemolysis. Flank pain, oliguria, or anuria develop, which lead to acute renal failure, one of the life-threatening effects of heme toxicity (see Box 20.3).

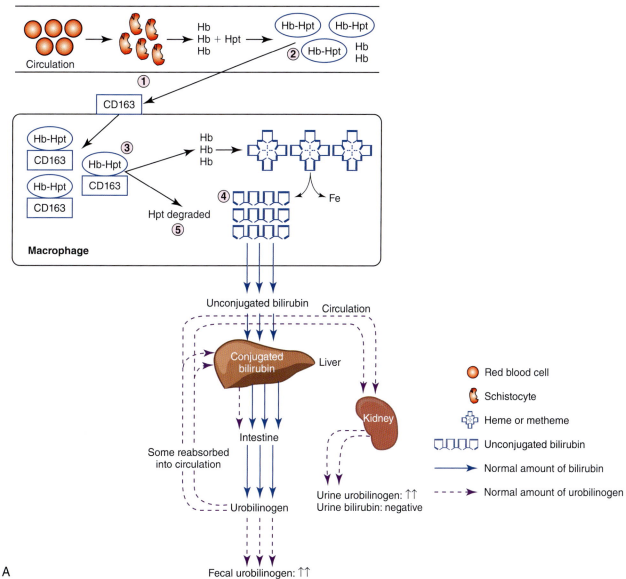

A

Figure 20.7 (A), Pathologic Fragmentation Hemolysis: The Role of Macrophages. When an increased number of red blood cells lyse by fragmentation, more than the usual amount of hemoglobin *(Hb)* is released into the blood, mostly as α/β dimers *(1)*. Haptoglobin *(Hpt)* binds the increased hemoglobin dimers, forming more than usual numbers of complexes *(2)*. The hemoglobin-haptoglobin complexes are taken up by macrophages bearing the CD163 receptor in various organs *(3)*. An increased amount of hemoglobin dimers is released from the complexes *(4)*. The hemoglobin is degraded to heme, the iron is released, and the protoporphyrin ring is converted to unconjugated bilirubin. The increased amount of unconjugated bilirubin is then transported to the liver and processed as with excess macrophage-mediated hemolysis, as in Figure 20.6 (steps 2 to 6). Degradation of haptoglobin is accelerated compared with normal *(5)*.

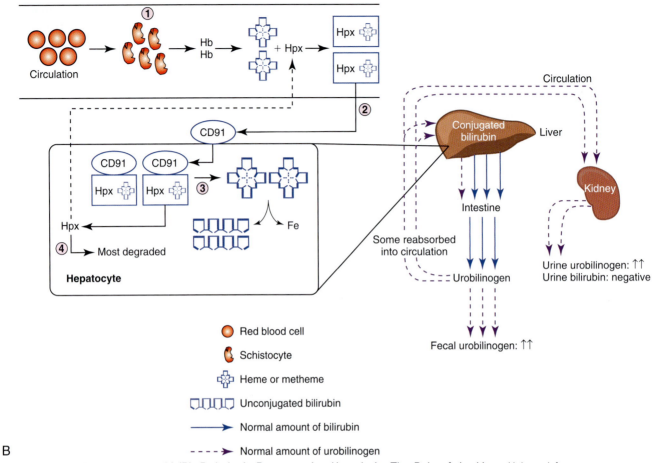

Red blood cell

Schistocyte

Heme or metheme

Unconjugated bilirubin

Normal amount of bilirubin

Normal amount of urobilinogen

B

Figure 20.7, cont'd (B), Pathologic Fragmentation Hemolysis: The Role of the Liver. Unbound free hemoglobin *(Hb)* is rapidly oxidized, forming methemoglobin, and the metheme molecule dissociates from the globin *(1)*. Hemopexin *(Hpx)* binds to metheme, and the complex is captured by the CD91 receptor on hepatocytes *(2)*. The complex is internalized by the hepatocyte, the iron is released from the metheme, and the protoporphyrin ring is converted to unconjugated bilirubin and ultimately, to conjugated bilirubin to be processed, as in Figure 20.6 (steps 3 to 6) *(3)*. Although a small of amount of hemopexin may be recycled to the blood, most is degraded *(4)*.

Continued

LABORATORY FINDINGS

In patients with the clinical features of hemolytic anemia, laboratory tests typically show evidence of increased erythrocyte destruction and the compensatory increase in the rate of erythropoiesis. Table 20.2 provides a reference throughout this section. Other tests that are specific to a particular diagnosis also may be indicated.

Tests of Accelerated Red Blood Cell Destruction
Bilirubin and Urobilinogen

In either fragmentation or macrophage-mediated hemolysis, the increased rate of hemoglobin catabolism results in increased amounts of plasma unconjugated bilirubin and carbon monoxide. The elevation of bilirubin may be evident visually in icteric serum or plasma. Serum bilirubin assays should reveal an increase indirect fraction resulting in an increase in total bilirubin. If liver function is normal, conjugated bilirubin is formed and excreted in the bile and converted to urobilinogen in the stool. The serum level of direct (conjugated) bilirubin remains within the reference interval. No bilirubin is detected in the urine because unconjugated bilirubin is bound to albumin for plasma transport and the complex is not filtered by the glomerulus. The urinary urobilinogen level may be increased, however, because there is increased urobilinogen in the stool, and more than usual amounts are absorbed by the portal circulation. In some patients, serum indirect (unconjugated) bilirubin values can be misleadingly low because the amount of bilirubin in the blood depends on the rate of RBC catabolism as well as hepatic function. If the rate of hemolysis is low and liver function is normal, the total serum bilirubin level can be within the reference interval. Quantitative measurements of fecal urobilinogen, however, would demonstrate an increase.

Plasma Hemoglobin, Urine Hemoglobin, and Urine Hemosiderin

Visual examination of plasma and urine may suggest fragmentation hemolysis. The presence of methemoglobin,

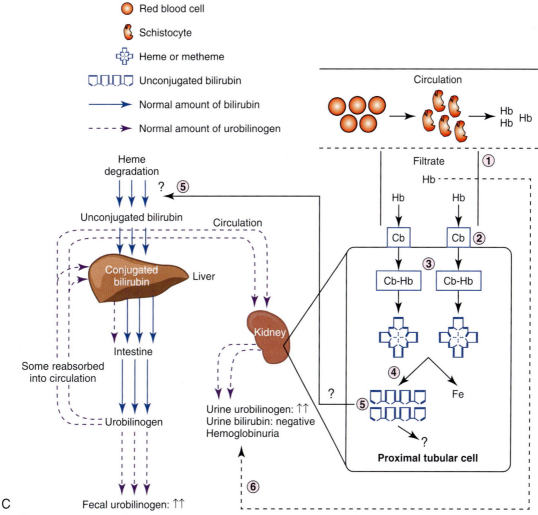

Figure 20.7, cont'd (C), Pathologic Fragmentation Hemolysis: The Role of the Kidney. When excess red blood cells lyse by fragmentation and salvage systems are saturated, free (met)hemoglobin enters the urinary filtrate *(1)*. Cubilin *(Cb)* on the luminal side of the proximal tubular cells binds proteins for reabsorption, including hemoglobin *(Hb) (2)*. Cubilin carries hemoglobin into the proximal tubular cells *(3)*. The hemoglobin is degraded to heme, the iron is released, and the protoporphyrin ring is converted to unconjugated bilirubin as in a macrophage and conjugated as in a hepatocyte *(4)*. The fate of the bilirubin is uncertain, as it may be secreted to the filtrate or reabsorbed into the blood *(5)*. When the amount of hemoglobin exceeds the capacity of the proximal tubular cells to absorb it from the filtrate, hemoglobinuria occurs *(6)*.

methemalbumin, and metheme imparts a coffee-brown color to plasma, which is strongly suggestive of fragmentation hemolysis. When these compounds are present in urine, the color is more often described as root beer- or beer-colored. In a properly collected blood specimen, physiologic fragmentation hemolysis produces a plasma hemoglobin level of less than 1 mg/dL.[39] Plasma does not become visibly red/brown until the plasma hemoglobin level is at 50 mg/dL.[39] Typical values during hemolytic processes may be as low as 15 mg/dL, so an increase in plasma hemoglobin may not always be visible.[40] As a quick

check, a urinalysis test strip for blood can be used on plasma to detect hemolysis that may not be visible.

Hemoglobin/heme from fragmentation hemolysis can be detected in urine when the capacity of the plasma salvage systems is exceeded, the reabsorptive capacity of the kidney is surpassed, and the hemoglobin/heme is filtered into the urine. The urinalysis test strip for blood can be positive, even when the hemoglobin is not present in a high enough concentration to change the color of the urine significantly. Because the product entering the urine is free hemoglobin/heme, the sediment

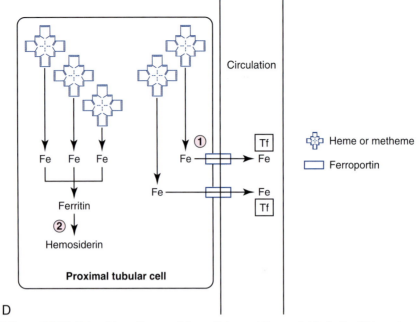

D

Figure 20.7, cont'd (D), Fate of Iron Removed From Salvaged Hemoglobin in the Kidney. Iron *(Fe)* salvaged from absorbed hemoglobin can be transported into the circulation by ferroportin on the basolaminal side of the tubular cell. In the blood, it will be bound to transferrin *(Tf)* for transport *(1)*. Iron in excess of what can be transported into the circulation is stored as ferritin, and some is converted to hemosiderin. If the tubular cell is sloughed into the filtrate and appears in the urine sediment, the hemosiderin can be detected using the Prussian blue stain *(2)*. (A–C, Modified from Brunzel, N. A. [2013]. *Fundamentals of Urine and Body Fluid Analysis.* [3rd ed., p. 141, Figure 7-8]. St. Louis: Elsevier.)

will be negative for RBCs. However, renal tubular cells sloughed into the filtrate during the period after hemoglobinuria can demonstrate deposits of hemosiderin (iron) when stained with Prussian blue stain (i.e., hemosiderinuria), resulting from absorbed hemoglobin (Figure 20.8).

Other conditions may result in a red/brown-colored urine specimen that has a positive blood strip. Bleeding along the urinary tract will likely demonstrate intact RBCs in the sediment. However, the cells may lyse depending on the pH of the specimen or if the specimen is not handled properly and is permitted to go stale. Myoglobinuria will also produce a positive blood strip without intact RBCs in the sediment.

Complete Blood Count

For a patient with a hemolytic process, a complete blood count (CBC) may provide clues to the cause. Whether the hemolysis has been sufficient to cause anemia will be reflected by the hemoglobin (HGB), hematocrit (HCT), and number of RBCs. Spherocytes can be expected to be seen with macrophage-mediated hemolysis (Table 20.2), whereas fragmented cells, or schistocytes, are noted with fragmentation hemolysis.

Haptoglobin and Hemopexin

Haptoglobin can be quantified by methods such as immunoturbidimetry. A substantial decline in the serum haptoglobin level indicates fragmentation hemolysis. In what is mostly a macrophage-mediated hemolysis, there can still be a minor component of fragmentation lysis involving spherical cells that are fragile, so a more modest decline in haptoglobin level can be seen. In short, whenever the level of hemoglobin in the plasma increases, the haptoglobin level declines. In one study, a low haptoglobin level indicated an 87% probability of hemolytic disease.[41] Haptoglobin measurement is, however, prone to both false-positive and false-negative results. Low values suggest hemolysis but may be due instead to impaired synthesis of haptoglobin caused by liver disease. Alternatively, a patient with hemolysis may have a relatively normal haptoglobin level if there is also a complicating infection or inflammation because haptoglobin is an acute phase reactant. For diagnosis of hemolysis, quantification of hemopexin may also demonstrate a low value, yet it is not often measured, relying instead on the more dramatic haptoglobin decline to detect fragmentation hemolysis. However, some researchers recommend assay of hemopexin

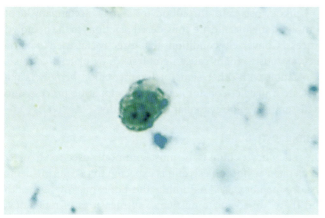

Figure 20.8 Renal Tubular Epithelial Cell Containing Hemosiderin (Urine, Prussian Blue stain, x260). (From Riley, R. S., & McPherson, R. A. [2022]. Basic examination of urine. In McPherson, R. A., & Pincus, M. R. (Eds.) *Henry's Clinical Diagnosis and Management by Laboratory Methods.* [24th ed., p. 482, Figure 29.2]. Philadelphia: Elsevier.)

and plasma heme to create a more complete picture of a patient's hemolytic process.[25] Hemopexin assays may ultimately be more valuable for detection of hemopexin depletion in conditions such as sepsis.[15]

Carbon Monoxide

Tests to determine the rate of endogenous carbon monoxide production have been developed because carbon monoxide is produced in the first step of heme breakdown by heme oxygenase. Values of 2 to 10 times the normal rate have been detected in some patients with hemolytic anemia,[42] but testing for carbon monoxide production is not typically required for clinical diagnosis.

Red Blood Cell Survival

General evidence of reduced RBC survival can be gleaned by measuring glycated hemoglobin (usually by the HbA_{1c} test).[43] Glycated hemoglobin increases over the life of a cell as it is exposed to plasma glucose. The glycated hemoglobin level usually is decreased in chronic hemolytic disease because the cells have less exposure to plasma glucose before early lysis. The magnitude of the decrease is related to the magnitude of the hemolytic process over the previous 4- to 8-week period. However, there is significant variability in RBC life span among hematologically normal individuals,[43] so use of glycated hemoglobin for detection of hemolysis is problematic without baseline values for individuals. Glycated hemoglobin levels are now widely used as an indicator of diabetes mellitus because the increased rate of glycation with elevated plasma glucose levels leads to an increase in the glycated hemoglobin value. Coexistence of hemolysis with diabetes leads to falsely lowered glycated hemoglobin values, however, and is a recognized problem in the interpretation of glycated hemoglobin values for glucose control.

A more exact RBC survival assay uses random labeling of blood with chromium-51 radioisotope. This is the reference method for RBC survival studies published by the International Committee for Standardization in Hematology.[44] A sample of

blood is collected, mixed with the isotope, and returned to the patient. The labeled cells are all ages, reflecting normal peripheral blood. This method differs from cohort labeling, in which RBCs are labeled with radioactive iron or heavy nitrogen as they are produced in the bone marrow, and thus the labeled cells are generally the same age. In both methods, the disappearance of the label from the blood is measured over time. As measured using the random chromium labeling technique, the normal half-time of chromium is 25 to 32 days.[44] A half-time of 20 to 25 days suggests mild hemolysis; 15 to 20 days, moderate hemolysis; and less than 15 days, severe hemolysis.[44] Both cohort and random techniques have significant limitations,[45] including being time consuming, being expensive, and requiring the use of radioactive isotopes. Therefore these methods are not often used clinically but are used for research, particularly in the search for improved methods of determining RBC survival. More recently, methods that use biotin as the label have been used, with the advantages of avoiding radioisotopes and requiring smaller sample volumes allowing use in children.[46]

Lactate Dehydrogenase

Serum LDH activity is often increased in patients with fragmentation hemolysis because of the release of the enzyme from ruptured RBCs, but other conditions, such as myocardial infarction or liver disease, also can cause increases. Although enzyme isoform fractionation could be used to identify LDH of RBC origin, this test is generally not needed. Rather, when other results point to fragmentation hemolysis, one should expect an increase in the level of serum LDH and other RBC enzymes and should not be misled into assuming that there is other organ damage (Table 20.2).

Tests of Increased Erythropoiesis

If bone marrow is healthy, the hypoxia associated with hemolytic anemia leads to increased erythropoiesis. Recognition of this increase may be a first clue to the presence of a hemolytic process, particularly if the liver is able to clear the unconjugated bilirubin and prevent jaundice. Laboratory findings indicating increased erythropoiesis include an increase in circulating reticulocytes and, in severe cases, nucleated RBCs, as well as associated changes in the CBC and bone marrow, described more fully in the next section (Table 20.3). These findings are persistently present in chronic hemolytic disease and are evident within 3 to 6 days after an acute hemolytic episode. Increased erythropoiesis is not unique to hemolytic anemias, however, and so it is not diagnostic. Similar results are expected after hemorrhage and with successful specific therapy for anemia caused by iron, folate, or vitamin B_{12} deficiency. An assessment of erythropoiesis can determine the effectiveness of the bone marrow response, however, and should be factored into the differential diagnosis (see "Differential Diagnosis").

Complete Blood Count and Red Blood Cell Morphology

Peripheral blood film evaluation is crucial to assessment of hemolysis. An increase in polychromatic RBCs (reticulocytes) and nucleated RBCs represents bone marrow compensation for hemolysis or blood loss. Schistocytes are expected with

TABLE 20.3 Hematologic Findings Indicating Accelerated Red Blood Cell Production

Specimen	Findings
Anticoagulated peripheral blood	Increased absolute reticulocyte count, immature reticulocyte fraction, reticulocyte production index Rising mean cell volume (compared with baseline) Polychromasia, nucleated RBCs
Bone marrow	Erythroid hyperplasia

RBC, Red blood cell.

TABLE 20.4 Morphologic Abnormalities Associated With Hemolytic Anemia

RBC Morphology	Hemolytic Disorders
Spherocytes	Hereditary spherocytosis, IgG-mediated immune hemolytic anemia, thermal injury to RBCs
Elliptocytes (ovalocytes)	Hereditary elliptocytosis
Acanthocytes	Abetalipoproteinemia, severe liver disease (spur cell anemia)
Burr cells	Pyruvate kinase deficiency, uremia
Schistocytes	Microangiopathic hemolytic anemia, traumatic cardiac hemolytic anemia, IgM-mediated immune hemolytic anemia
RBC agglutination	Cold agglutinins, immunohemolytic disease

Ig, Immunoglobulin; *RBC*, red blood cell.

excessive fragmentation hemolysis, whereas spherocytes may be seen with macrophage-mediated processes (Table 20.2). Additional morphologic changes to RBCs may point toward the cause of the hemolysis (Table 20.4).

An increase in the mean cell volume (MCV) is usually seen with extreme compensatory reticulocytosis resulting from the larger, prematurely released "shift" reticulocytes. The increase must be assessed by comparison with the value seen early in hemolysis before the shift reticulocytes have emerged. The MCV may not increase to greater than the reference interval, but rather, may be more than the baseline value for that patient. Exceptions occur if the hemolytic condition itself involves smaller cells that counter the increased volume of the reticulocytes. In hereditary spherocytosis, microspherocytes are the cause of the anemia and the MCV may be within the reference interval even when larger shift reticulocytes are generated, hence the importance of a baseline value for comparison. In other circumstances, numerous schistocytes may outnumber the reticulocytes so that the MCV remains low or normal.

The RBC distribution width (RDW) can be expected to rise with reticulocytosis. Though the MCV may not increase to more than the reference interval, the addition of larger reticulocytes can be expected to extend the range of cell volumes. Thus the previously mentioned situations where there are small cells with the larger reticulocytes may be reflected by a rise in the RDW. Alternatively, morphologic examination of the peripheral blood film can also reveal this anisocytosis.

Leukocytosis and thrombocytosis may accompany acute hemolytic anemia and are considered reactions to the hemolytic process. Conversely, conditions that directly cause leukocytosis, such as sepsis, might cause hemolysis. Low platelet counts in association with other signs of fragmentation hemolysis may indicate a platelet-consuming microangiopathic process, such as disseminated intravascular coagulopathy.

Reticulocyte Count

The reticulocyte count is the most commonly used test to detect accelerated erythropoiesis and is expected to rise during hemolysis or hemorrhage. Assuming the bone marrow is healthy and there are adequate nutrients, all measures of reticulocyte production should rise: absolute reticulocyte count, relative reticulocyte count, reticulocyte production index, and immature reticulocyte fraction. The association of reticulocytosis with hemolysis is so strong that if an anemic patient has an elevated reticulocyte count and hemorrhage is ruled out, a cause of hemolysis should be investigated. The reticulocyte increase usually correlates well with the severity of the hemolysis. Exceptions occur during aplastic crises of some hemolytic anemias and in some immunohemolytic anemias with hypoplastic marrow, which suggests that the autoantibodies were directed against the bone marrow erythroid precursors and circulating erythrocytes.[39] Chapters 12 and 16 describe the interpretation of reticulocyte indices in patients with anemia.

Bone Marrow Examination

Bone marrow examination is usually not necessary to diagnose hemolytic anemia. If conducted, however, bone marrow examination will reveal erythroid hyperplasia that results in peripheral blood reticulocytosis. As the erythroid component (the denominator) of the myeloid-to-erythroid ratio increases, the overall ratio decreases. (The myeloid-to-erythroid ratio is defined in Chapter 15.) As always, the cellularity of bone marrow should be determined on a core biopsy specimen, rather than an aspirated specimen, for a more accurate assessment.

Laboratory Tests to Identify Specific Hemolytic Processes

As noted earlier, the appearance of spherocytes or schistocytes on a peripheral blood film can point to a hemolytic cause for anemia. Other abnormalities found on the film, such as elliptocytes, acanthocytes, burr cells, sickle cells, target cells, agglutination, or parasites, may help reveal the specific disorder causing the hemolysis (see Table 20.4).

Other tests for diagnosis of specific types of hemolytic anemia are discussed in subsequent chapters. They include the direct antiglobulin test, osmotic fragility test, eosin-5′-ma-le-i-mide binding test, Heinz body test, RBC enzyme studies, and immunophenotyping.

DIFFERENTIAL DIAGNOSIS

When a patient experiences anemia, hemolysis should be considered as a general mechanism to be differentiated from hemorrhage, dilution, or diminished RBC production (Chapter 16). The diagnosis of hemolysis relies on evidence of accelerated RBC death along with evidence of an erythropoietic response. However, other anemias, with bilirubinemia and reticulocytosis, must be distinguished from hemolysis. Once hemolysis is confirmed, fragmentation versus macrophage-mediated mechanism is determined based on laboratory findings. The time course of the process may also contribute to the diagnosis.

A rapid decrease in hemoglobin concentration (e.g., 1 g/dL per week) from levels previously within the reference interval can signal hemolysis when hemorrhage and hemodilution have been ruled out. While a hemolytic process may not result in anemia if the bone marrow can compensate adequately, evidence of accelerated RBC death will still be detectable. With acute fragmentation hemolysis, the evidence of RBC destruction will be methemoglobinemia, methemoglobinuria, decreased serum haptoglobin, elevated serum LDH, and schistocytes in the peripheral blood film. The absence of these findings supports a macrophage-mediated etiology. With acute macrophage-mediated hemolysis, the only immediate finding of RBC destruction may be spherocytes on the peripheral blood film for a patient with a dropping hemoglobin value.

For a process lasting several days, evidence of accelerated RBC death will include indirect bilirubinemia and elevated urinary urobilinogen. These findings will be seen with both fragmentation and macrophage-mediated hemolysis. Regardless of the mechanism of RBC destruction, reticulocytosis is expected to follow a hemolytic event by several days if the bone marrow is healthy and has adequate resources, such as iron, for cell production.

Figure 20.9 is a graphic representation of the general time line of the events in acute fragmentation and macrophage-mediated hemolysis. In chronic hemolysis, persistence of hemoglobinemia, hemoglobinuria, decreased serum haptoglobin level, indirect bilirubinemia, elevated urinary urobilinogen, and reticulocytosis can be expected, depending on the mechanism of the hemolysis.

Hemolytic anemias must be differentiated from other anemias associated with bilirubinemia, reticulocytosis, or both. Anemia with reticulocytosis but without bilirubinemia is expected during recovery from hemorrhage not treated with transfusion or with effective treatment of deficiencies such as iron deficiency. Anemia that results from hemorrhage into a body cavity is characterized by reticulocytosis during recovery and bilirubinemia as a result of catabolism of the hemoglobin in the hemorrhaged cells. RBC morphology will remain normal throughout the event, however. Anemias associated with ineffective erythropoiesis, such as megaloblastic anemia, are essentially hemolytic, with the cell death occurring in the bone marrow. Bilirubinemia and elevated serum LDH levels are to be expected, but the reticulocyte count is low. Because most of the RBCs never reach the periphery, such anemias are typically

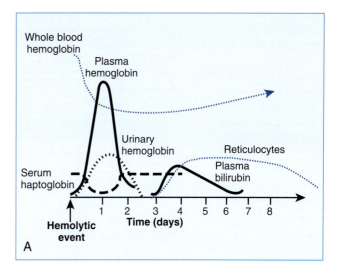

A

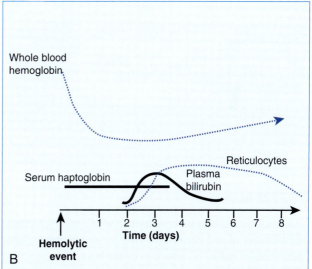

B

Figure 20.9 Hemolysis Time Lines. **(A),** Example of fragmentation (intravascular) hemolysis time line. During fragmentation hemolysis, hemoglobin is detectable in plasma and urine for a period very soon after the hemolysis occurs. Haptoglobin levels will drop as the plasma hemoglobin rises. When hemolysis ends, the hemoglobin will disappear from plasma and urine as the haptoglobin returns to normal. However, the protoporphyrin of salvaged hemoglobin will be processed to bilirubin that will rise after the hemolytic event. Assuming the hemolysis has resulted in anemia, reticulocyte indices will also rise several days after the hemolytic event. **(B),** Example of macrophage-mediated (extravascular) hemolysis time line. With macrophage-mediated hemolysis, the contents of the red blood cells do not enter the blood, so evidence of hemolysis is delayed until bilirubin and reticulocytes rise.

classified as anemias of diminished production rather than as hemolytic anemias. As summarized in Table 20.5, the differential diagnosis in each of these instances may rely on negative results of tests for increased cell destruction or accelerated production.

TABLE 20.5   Differential Diagnosis of Hemolytic Anemias Versus Other Causes of Indirect Bilirubinemia and Reticulocytosis

	Hemoglobin Level	Indirect Bilirubinemia	Reticulocytosis	Spherocytes or Schistocytes	Haptoglobin	Hemoglobinemia/ Hemoglobinuria
Hemolytic anemia—acute, fragmentation	Rapidly dropping	Delayed	Delayed	Schistocytes	Decreased	Present
Hemolytic anemia—acute, macrophage mediated	Rapidly dropping	Delayed	Delayed	Spherocytes	Normal	Not present
Hemolytic anemia—chronic, fragmentation	Persistently low	Persistent	Persistent	Schistocytes	Decreased	May be present persistently
Hemolytic anemia—chronic, macrophage mediated	Persistently low	Persistent	Persistent	Spherocytes	Normal	Not present
Acute hemorrhage	Rapidly dropping	Absent	Delayed	Absent	Normal	Not present
Hemodilution	Rapidly dropping	Absent	Absent	Absent	Normal— decreased by dilution	Not present
Recovery from hemorrhage	Rising	Absent	Present	Absent	Normal	Not present
Treated anemia (iron, vitamin B_{12}, or folate deficiency)	Rising	Absent or declining	Present	Absent	Normal	Not present
Hemorrhage into a body cavity	Rapidly dropping	Delayed	Delayed	Absent	Normal	Not present
Ineffective erythropoiesis (e.g., megaloblastic anemia)	Dropping	Persistent	Absent	Absent	Normal to decreased, depending on cause and severity	Possibly present, depending on cause and severity

SUMMARY

- A hemolytic disorder is a condition in which there is increased destruction of red blood cells (RBCs) and a compensatory acceleration in RBC production by the bone marrow.
- A hemolytic anemia develops when the bone marrow is unable to compensate for the shortened survival of the RBCs.
- Hemolytic anemias can be classified as acute or chronic, acquired or inherited, intrinsic or extrinsic, intravascular or extravascular, and fragmentation or macrophage mediated.
- Most RBC death in healthy individuals occurs via macrophages of the spleen and liver. A small amount occurs by fragmentation due to mechanical trauma.
- Hemoglobin from RBCs is converted to heme and globin within macrophages. Heme is further degraded to iron, carbon monoxide, and unconjugated bilirubin. The bilirubin is secreted into the blood, where it binds to albumin and is transported to the liver. In the liver, bilirubin is conjugated with glucuronic acid and excreted as bile into the intestines, and it is converted to urobilinogen by intestinal bacteria. Some urobilinogen is reabsorbed into the portal circulation and reexcreted through the liver. A small amount of urobilinogen remains in the blood, and it is excreted by the kidney into the urine.
- In macrophage-mediated (extravascular) hemolytic anemia, there is an increase in unconjugated bilirubin in the plasma and an increase in urobilinogen in the stool and urine. Spherocytes may be seen on the peripheral blood film.
- Signs of fragmentation (intravascular) hemolysis include (met)hemoglobinemia, (met)hemoglobinuria, elevated stool and urinary urobilinogen, and hemosiderinuria. Serum haptoglobin is markedly decreased or absent. Schistocytes may be seen on the peripheral blood film.
- Hemoglobin and heme that are present in the plasma with fragmentation hemolysis are salvaged by plasma proteins to prevent iron loss in the urine. The major salvage proteins are haptoglobin, which binds hemoglobin and carries it into macrophages, and hemopexin, which binds heme for salvage by hepatocytes. Other iron-containing proteins and molecules that enter the urinary filtrate are reabsorbed along the nephron to prevent iron deficiency.
- Jaundice can result from increased serum unconjugated bilirubin during any hemolytic anemia.

- Major clinical features of chronic inherited hemolytic anemia are varying degrees of anemia, jaundice, splenomegaly, and the development of cholelithiasis. In children, bone abnormalities may develop as a result of accelerated erythropoiesis.
- Laboratory studies providing evidence of hemolytic anemia include tests for increased RBC destruction and compensatory increase in the rate of erythropoiesis. An elevated serum indirect bilirubin level with a normal serum direct bilirubin level suggests accelerated RBC destruction. A moderate to marked decrease in serum haptoglobin level suggests a fragmentation cause of hemolysis. The reticulocyte count is the most commonly used laboratory test to identify accelerated erythropoiesis including an elevation of the immature reticulocyte fraction. On the peripheral blood smear, spherocytes are present in macrophage-mediated hemolysis, while schistocytes are the hallmark of fragmentation hemolysis. Tests specific to a particular diagnosis also may be needed.
- Hemolytic anemias must be differentiated from other anemias with reticulocytosis including post acute hemorrhage; recovery from iron, vitamin B_{12}, or folate deficiency; and bilirubinemia, such as internal bleeding.

Now that you have completed this chapter, go back and read again the case study at the beginning and respond to the questions presented. Answers can be found in Appendix C.

REVIEW QUESTIONS

Answers can be found in Appendix C.

1. The term *hemolytic disorder* in general refers to a disorder in which there is:
   a. Increased destruction of RBCs in the blood, bone marrow, or spleen
   b. Excessive loss of RBCs from the body
   c. Inadequate RBC production by the bone marrow
   d. Increased plasma volume with unchanged RBC mass
2. RBC destruction that occurs when macrophages ingest and destroy RBCs is termed:
   a. Extracellular
   b. Macrophage mediated
   c. Intraorgan
   d. Extrahematopoietic
3. A sign of hemolysis that is typically associated with both fragmentation and macrophage-mediated hemolysis is:
   a. Hemoglobinuria
   b. Hemosiderinuria
   c. Hemoglobinemia
   d. Elevated urinary urobilinogen level
4. An elderly patient is evaluated for worsening anemia, with a decrease of approximately 0.5 mg/dL of hemoglobin each week. The patient is pale, and the skin and eyes are slightly yellow. The patient complains of extreme fatigue and is unable to complete the tasks of daily living without napping in midmorning and midafternoon. The patient also tires with exertion, finding it difficult to climb even five stairs. Which of the features of this description points to a hemolytic cause for the anemia?
   a. Pallor
   b. Yellow skin and eyes
   c. Need for naps
   d. Tiredness on exertion
5. Which of the following tests provides a good indication of accelerated erythropoiesis?
   a. Urine urobilinogen level
   b. Hemosiderin level
   c. Reticulocyte count
   d. Glycated hemoglobin level
6. A 5-year-old patient was seen by a provider several days before the current visit and was diagnosed with pneumonia. The patient was prescribed a standard course of antibiotics. The patient returned to the provider again when the patient's urine began to darken after the first visit and now is alarmingly dark. The patient has no history of anemia, and there is no family history of any hematologic disorder. The CBC shows a mild anemia, polychromasia, and a few schistocytes. This anemia could be categorized as:
   a. Acquired, fragmentation
   b. Acquired, macrophage mediated
   c. Hereditary, fragmentation
   d. Hereditary, macrophage mediated
7. A patient has a personal and family history of a mild hemolytic anemia. The patient has consistently elevated levels of total and indirect serum bilirubin and urinary urobilinogen. The serum haptoglobin level is consistently decreased, whereas the reticulocyte count is elevated. The latter can be seen as polychromasia on the patient's peripheral blood film. Spherocytes are also noted. Which one of the findings reported for this patient is INCONSISTENT with a classical diagnosis of fragmentation hemolysis?
   a. Elevated total and indirect serum bilirubin
   b. Elevated urinary urobilinogen
   c. Decreased haptoglobin
   d. Spherocytes on the peripheral blood film
8. Under physiologic conditions, the major fraction of bilirubin in the plasma is:
   a. Unconjugated bilirubin secreted by the liver
   b. Conjugated bilirubin reabsorbed from the intestines
   c. Macrophage-secreted indirect bilirubin
   d. Direct bilirubin conjugated by hepatocytes

9. A patient has anemia that has been worsening over the last several months. The hemoglobin level has been declining slowly, with a drop of 1.5 g/dL of hemoglobin over about 6 weeks. Polychromasia and anisocytosis are seen on the peripheral blood film, consistent with the elevated reticulocyte count and red blood cell distribution width (RDW). Serum levels of total bilirubin and indirect fractions are within reference intervals. The urinary urobilinogen level also is normal. When these findings are evaluated, it is concluded that the anemia does not have a hemolytic component. Based on the data given here, why was hemolysis ruled out as the cause of the anemia?
   a. The decline in hemoglobin is too gradual to be associated with hemolysis.
   b. The elevation of the reticulocyte count suggests a malignant cause.
   c. Evidence of increased protoporphyrin catabolism is lacking.
   d. Elevated RDW points to an anemia of decreased production.

10. Which of the following sets of test results is typically expected with chronic fragmentation hemolysis?

	Serum Haptoglobin	Urine Hemoglobin	Urine Sediment Prussian Blue Stain
a.	Increased	Positive	Positive
b.	Decreased	Negative	Negative
c.	Decreased	Positive	Positive
d.	Increased	Positive	Negative

REFERENCES

1. Crosby, W. H., & Akeroyd, J. H. (1952). The limit of hemoglobin synthesis in hereditary hemolytic anemia. *Am J Med, 13,* 273–283.
2. Hillman, R. S., & Henderson, P. A. (1969). Control of marrow production by the level of iron supply. *J Clin Invest, 48*(3), 454–460.
3. Cui, Y., Konig, J., Leier, I., et al. (2001). Hepatic uptake of bilirubin and its conjugates by the human organic anion transporter SLC21A6. *J Biol Chem, 276,* 9626–9630.
4. Keppler, D. (2014). The roles of MRP2, MRP3, OATP1B1, and OATP1B3 in conjugated hyperbilirubinemia. *Drug Metab Dispos, 42,* 561–565.
5. Sticova, E., & Jirsa, M. (2013). New insights in bilirubin metabolism and their clinical implications. *World J Gastroent, 19*(38), 6398–6407.
6. Keppler, D., & Kartenbeck, J. (1996). The canalicular conjugate export pump encoded by the cmrp/cmoat gene. *Prog Liver Dis, 14,* 55–67.
7. van de Steeg, E., Wagenaar, E., van der Kruijssen, C. M., et al. (2010). Organic anion transporting polypeptide 1a/1b-knockout mice provide insights into hepatic handling of bilirubin, bile acids, and drugs. *J Clin Invest, 120,* 2942–2952.
8. Quigley, J. G., Means, R. T., & Glader, B. (2019). The birth, life, and death of red blood cells: erythropoiesis, the mature red blood cell, and cell destruction. In Greer, J. P., Rodgers, G. M., Glader, B., et al. (Eds.), *Wintrobe's Clinical Hematology.* (14th ed., pp. 90–131). Philadelphia: Lippincott Williams & Wilkins.
9. Schaer, D. J., Buehler, P. W., Alayash, A. I., et al. (2013). Hemolysis and free hemoglobin revisited: exploring hemoglobin and hemin scavengers as a novel class of therapeutic proteins. *Blood, 121,* 1276–1284.
10. Benesch, R. E., & Kwong, S. (1995). Coupled reactions in hemoglobin. Heme-globin and dimer-dimer association. *J Biol Chem, 270*(23), 13785–13786.
11. Andersen, C. B. F., Torvund-Jensen, M., Nielsen, M. J., et al. (2012). Structure of the haptoglobin-haemoglobin complex. *Nature, 489*(7416), 456–460.

12. Ratanasopa, K., Chakane, S., Ilyas, M., et al. (2013). Trapping of human hemoglobin by haptoglobin: molecular mechanisms and clinical applications. *Antiox Redox Signal, 18,* 2364–2374.
13. Etzerodt, A., & Moestrup, S. (2013). CD163 and inflammation: biological, diagnostic and therapeutic aspects. *Antioxid Redox Signal, 18,* 2352–2363.
14. Kristiansen, M., Graversen, J. H., Jacobsen, C., et al. (2001). Identification of the haemoglobin scavenger receptor. *Nature, 409,* 198–201.
15. Smith A: Protection against heme toxicity: hemopexin rules, OK?. In Ferreira GC, editor: *Handbook of Porphyrin Science: With Applications to Chemistry, Physics, Materials Science, Engineering, Biology and Medicine, 30.* 2014, pp 311–388.
16. Tolosano, E., & Altruda, F. (2002). Hemopexin: structure, function, and regulation. *DNA Cell Biol, 21,* 297–306.
17. Delanghe, J. R., & Langlois, M. R. (2001). Hemopexin: a review of biological aspects and the role in laboratory medicine. *Clin Chim Acta, 312,* 13–23.
18. Hvidberg, V., Maniecki, M. B., Jacobsen, C., et al. (2005). Identification of the receptor scavenging hemopexin-heme complexes. *Blood, 106,* 2572–2579.
19. Tolosano, E., Fagoonee, S., Morello, N., et al. (2010). Heme scavenging and the other facets of hemopexin. *Antioxid Redox Signal, 12,* 305–320.
20. Chiabrando, D., Vinchi, F., Fiorito, V., et al. (2014). Heme in pathophysiology: a matter of scavenging, metabolism and trafficking across cell membranes. *Front Pharmacol, 5,* 61. https://doi.org/10.3389/fphar.2014.00061.
21. Smith, A., & Morgan, W. T. (1979). Haem transport to the liver by haemopexin. *Biochem J, 182,* 47–54.
22. Morgan, W. T., Liem, H. H., Sutor, R. P., et al. (1976). Transfer of heme from heme-albumin to hemopexin. *Biochem Biophys Acta, 444,* 435–445.

23. Potter, D., Chroneos, Z. C., Baynes, J. W., et al. (1993). In vivo fate of hemopexin and heme-hemopexin complexes in the rat. *Arch Biochem Biophys*, *300*(1), 98–104.

24. Li, H., Wang, D., Wu, H., et al. (2022). SLC46A1 contributes to hepatic iron metabolism by importing heme in hepatocytes. *Metabolism*, *110*, 154306. https://doi.org/10.1016/j.metabol.2020.154306.

25. Smith, A., & McCulloh, R. J. (2016). Hemopexin and haptoglobin: allies against heme toxicity from hemoglobin not contenders. *Frontiers in Physiol*, *6*(Article 187), 1–20.

26. Thevenod, F., & Wolff, N. A. (2016). Iron transport in the kidney: implications for physiology and cadmium nephrotoxicity. *Metallomics*, *8*, 17–42.

27. Zhang, D., Meyron-Holtz, E., & Rouault, T. A. (2007). Renal iron metabolism: transferrin iron delivery and the role of iron regulatory proteins. *J Am Soc Nephrol*, *18*, 401–406.

28. Christiansen, E. I., Verroust, P. J., & Nielsen, R. (2009). Receptor-mediated endocytosis in renal proximal tubule. *Pfulgers Arch-Eur J Physiol*, *458*, 1039–1048.

29. Schmidt-Ott, K. M., Mori, K., Kalandadze, A., et al. (2006). Neutrophil gelatinase-associated lipocalin-mediated iron traffic in kidney epithelia. *Curr Opin Nephrol Hypertens*, *15*, 442–449.

30. van Swelm, R. P. L., Wetzels, J. F. M., & Swinkels, D. W. (2020). The multifaceted role of iron in renal health and disease. *Nat Rev Nephrol*, *16*(2), 77–98.

31. Wolff, N., Liu, W., Fenton, R. A., et al. (2011). Ferroportin 1 is expressed basolaterally in rat kidney proximal tubule cells and iron excess increases its membrane trafficking. *J Cell Mol Med*, *15*, 209–219.

32. Kondo, H., Saito, K., Grasso, J. P., et al. (1988). Iron metabolism in the erythrophagocytosing Kupffer cell. *Hepatology*, *8*(1), 32–38.

33. Ferenbach, D. A., Kluth, D. C., & Hughes, J. (2010). Hemeoxygenase-1 and renal ischaemia-reperfusion injury. *Exp Nephrol*, *115*, e33–e37.

34. Gaganis, P., Miners, J. O., Brennan, J. S., et al. (2007). Human renal cortical and medullary UDP-glucuronosyltransferases (UGTs): immunohistochemical localization of UGT2B7 and UGT1A enzymes and kinetic characterization of S-naproxen glucuronidation. *J Pharmacol Exp Ther*, *323*(2), 422–430.

35. Schaub, T. P., Kartenbeck, J., Konig, J., et al. (1999). Expression of the MRP2 gene-encoded conjugate export pump in human kidney proximal tubules and in renal cell carcinoma. *J Am Soc Nephrol*, *10*, 1159–1169.

36. Brandoni, A., Hazelhoff, M. H., Bulacio, R. P., et al. (2012). Expression and function of renal and hepatic organic anion transporters in extrahepatic cholestasis. *World J Gastroent*, *18*(44), 6387–6397.

37. Li Volti , G., Rodella, L. F., Giacomo, C. D., et al. (2006). Role of carbon monoxide and biliverdin in renal ischemia/reperfusion injury. *Nephron Exp Nephrol*, *104*, e135–e139. https://doi.org/10.1159/000094964.

38. Trotman, B. W. (1991). Pigment gallstone disease. *Gastroent Clin North Am*, *20*, 111–126.

39. Means, R. T. Jr., & Glader, B. (2019). Anemia: general considerations. In Greer, J. P., Rodgers, G. M., Glader, B., et al. (Eds.), *Wintrobe's Clinical Hematology*. (14th ed., pp. 588–615). Philadelphia: Lippincott Williams & Wilkins.

40. Crosby, W. H., & Dameshek, W. (1951). The significance of hemoglobinemia and associated hemosiderinuria, with particular reference to various types of hemolytic anemia. *J Lab Clin Med*, *38*, 829–841.

41. Marchand, A., Galen, R. S., & Van Lente, F. (1980). The predictive value of serum haptoglobin in hemolytic disease. *JAMA*, *243*, 1909–1911.

42. Coburn, R. F. (1970). Endogenous carbon monoxide production in man. *N Engl J Med*, *282*, 207–209.

43. Cohen, R. M., Franco, R. S., Khera, P. K., et al. (2008). Red cell life span heterogeneity in hematologically normal people is sufficient to alter HbA1c. *Blood*, *112*, 4284–4291.

44. International Committee for Standardization in Haematology. (1980). Recommended method for radioisotope red cell survival studies. *Br J Haematol*, *45*, 659–666.

45. Korell, J., Coulter, C. V., & Duffull, S. B. (2011). Evaluation of red blood cell labeling methods based on a statistical model for red blood cell survival. *J Theor Biol*, *291*, 88–98.

46. Mock, D. M., Matthews, N. I., Zhu, S., et al. (2011). Red blood cell (RBC) survival determined in humans using RBCs labeled at multiple biotin densities. *Transfusion*, *51*(5), 1047–1057.

21

Intrinsic Defects Leading to Increased Erythrocyte Destruction

*S. Renee Hodgkins**

OBJECTIVES

After completion of this chapter, the reader will be able to:

1. Describe the intrinsic cell properties that affect red blood cell (RBC) deformability.
2. Explain how defects in vertical and horizontal membrane protein interactions can result in a hemolytic anemia.
3. Compare and contrast hereditary spherocytosis, hereditary elliptocytosis, and hereditary ovalocytosis, including the inheritance pattern, mutated membrane proteins, mechanism of hemolysis, typical RBC morphology, and clinical and laboratory findings.
4. Compare and contrast the RBC morphology and laboratory findings of hereditary spherocytosis and immune-associated hemolytic anemias.
5. Explain the principle, interpretation, and limitations of the osmotic fragility, eosin-5′-maleimide binding, and ecktocytometry tests in the diagnosis of the RBC membrane disorders.
6. Describe the causes, pathophysiology, RBC morphology, and clinical and laboratory findings of hemolytic anemias characterized by stomatocytosis.
7. Describe the causes and pathophysiology of hereditary and acquired conditions characterized by acanthocytosis.
8. Describe the cause, pathophysiology, clinical manifestations, laboratory findings, and treatment for paroxysmal nocturnal hemoglobinuria.
9. Compare and contrast the inheritance pattern, pathophysiology, clinical symptoms, and typical laboratory findings of glucose-6-phosphate dehydrogenase deficiency and pyruvate kinase deficiency.
10. Given the history, symptoms, laboratory findings, and a representative microscopic field from a peripheral blood film for a patient with a suspected intrinsic hemolytic anemia, discuss possible causes of the anemia and indicate the data that support these conclusions.

OUTLINE

Red Blood Cell Membrane Abnormalities
   Red Blood Cell Membrane Structure and Function
   Hereditary Red Blood Cell Membrane Abnormalities
   Acquired Red Blood Cell Membrane Abnormalities

Red Blood Cell Enzymopathies
   Glucose-6-Phosphate Dehydrogenase Deficiency
   Pyruvate Kinase Deficiency
   Other Enzymopathies

CASE STUDY

After studying the material in this chapter, the reader should be able to respond to the following case study. Answers can be found in Appendix C.

A 45-year-old man sought medical attention for the onset of chest pain. Physical examination revealed slight jaundice and splenomegaly. The medical history included gallstones, and there was a family history of anemia. A complete blood count yielded the following results. Reference intervals can be found after the Index at the end of the book.

WBC	13.4×10^9/L	MCV	77.1 fL	
RBC	4.20×10^{12}/L	MCHC	36.7 g/dL	
HGB	11.9 g/dL	RDW	22.9%	
HCT	32.4%	PLT	290×10^9/L	

The peripheral blood film revealed anisocytosis, polychromasia, and spherocytes (Figure 21.1).

1. From the clinical information and laboratory data given, what is the most likely cause of the anemia?
2. What additional laboratory tests would be of value in establishing the diagnosis, and what abnormalities in the results of these tests would be expected to confirm your impression?
3. What is the pathophysiology of this type of anemia?

---

*The author extends appreciation to Elaine M. Keohane, whose work in prior editions provided the foundation for this chapter.

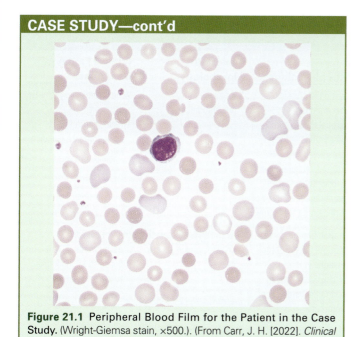

Figure 21.1 Peripheral Blood Film for the Patient in the Case Study. (Wright-Giemsa stain, ×500.). (From Carr, J. H. [2022]. *Clinical Hematology Atlas*. [6th ed.]. Philadelphia: Elsevier.)

Intrinsic hemolytic anemias comprise a large group of disorders in which defects in the red blood cells (RBCs) result in premature hemolysis and anemia. Intrinsic disorders can be divided into abnormalities of the RBC membrane, metabolic enzymes, or hemoglobin. Most of these defects are hereditary. This chapter covers defects in the RBC membrane and enzymes causing hemolytic anemia. Chapter 24 covers qualitative hemoglobin disorders (hemoglobinopathies), and Chapter 25 covers quantitative hemoglobin disorders (thalassemias).

RED BLOOD CELL MEMBRANE ABNORMALITIES

Red Blood Cell Membrane Structure and Function

The RBC maintains a biconcave discoid shape that is essential for normal function and survival for 120 days in the peripheral circulation. The key to maintaining this shape is the plasma membrane, a lipid bilayer embedded with proteins and connected to an underlying protein cytoskeleton (Figure 7.2). The insoluble lipid portion serves as a barrier to separate the vastly different ion and metabolite concentrations of the interior of the RBC from its external environment, the blood plasma. The concentration of the constituents in the cytoplasm is tightly regulated by proteins embedded in the membrane that serve as pumps and channels for movement of ions and other material between the RBC's interior and the blood plasma. Various membrane proteins also act as receptors, RBC antigens, enzymes, and support for the surface carbohydrates. The lipid bilayer remains intact because two transmembrane protein complexes embedded in the membrane anchor it to a two-dimensional protein lattice (cytoskeleton) immediately beneath its surface (Chapter 7).[1] Together the transmembrane proteins and underlying cytoskeleton provide structural integrity, cohesion, and mechanical stability to the cell.

In their life span, RBCs must repeatedly maneuver through very narrow capillaries and squeeze through the splenic sieve (narrow slits or fenestrations in the endothelial cell lining of the splenic sinuses) as they move from the splenic cords to the sinuses (Chapter 5). To accomplish this without premature lysis, the RBCs must have *deformability*, or the ability to repeatedly bend, stretch, distort, and then return to the normal discoid, biconcave shape.[2] The cellular properties that enable RBC deformability include the RBC's biconcave, discoid geometry; the elasticity (pliancy) of its membrane; and its cytoplasmic viscosity (Chapter 7).[2–4]

The biconcave, discoid geometry of the RBC is dependent on vertical and horizontal interactions between the transmembrane and cytoskeletal proteins (listed in Tables 7.5 and 7.6).[3] Two transmembrane protein complexes, the ankyrin complex and actin (protein 4.1) junctional complex, provide *vertical* structural integrity to the cell by anchoring the lipid bilayer to the underlying spectrin cytoskeleton.[3,5,6] In the ankyrin complex, ankyrin and protein 4.2 link transmembrane proteins (band 3, RhAG, and other associated proteins) to β-spectrin in the cytoskeleton.[6–8] In the actin junctional complex, protein 4.1 and actin link transmembrane proteins (band 3, GLUT1, and other associated proteins) to β-spectrin in the cytoskeleton, with protein 4.2, adducin, dematin, tropomyosin, and tropomodulin as accessory proteins (Figure 7.4).[6,9] These interactions are called *vertical* because they are perpendicular to the plane of the cytoskeleton. Vertical interactions prevent the loss of membrane, which would result in decreased surface area-to-volume ratio of the RBC.[3,5] Two major cytoskeletal proteins, α-spectrin and α-spectrin, interact laterally with each other to form antiparallel heterodimers, which link with other spectrin heterodimers to form tetramers. The ends of spectrin tetramers are joined in the actin junctional complex with the accessory proteins mentioned earlier, thus linking the spectrin tetramers in a two-dimensional lattice.[3,10,11] These proteins provide *horizontal* mechanical stability, which prevents the membrane from fragmenting in response to mechanical stress.[3,5]

Factors that affect the *elasticity* of the cell are not as clear. The viscoelastic nature of the RBC is at least in part a mechanism of the composition of the membrane.[2] Interactions between the spectrin dimers and their junctional complexes are flexible and allow for movement as the RBCs stretch and bend.[3,11] Additionally, the ability of spectrin repeats to unfold and refold is likely to be one of the determinants of membrane elasticity.[11,12]

The cytoplasmic viscosity depends on the concentration of hemoglobin, as well as the maintenance of the proper cell volume by the normal functioning of various channels and pumps that allow the passage of ions, water, and macromolecules in and out of the cell.[3] Increased concentration of hemoglobin in the RBC is a natural consequence of erythrocyte aging. When an imbalance in cation concentration occurs because of malfunction of the channels and pumps, the RBC can become overhydrated or dehydrated, which ultimately changes the cytoplasmic viscosity and decreases deformability.[2]

A defect in the RBCs that changes the membrane geometry, its elasticity, or the viscosity of the cytoplasm affects RBC deformability and can result in premature hemolysis and anemia.[3] The RBC membrane is discussed in more detail in Chapter 7;

TABLE 21.1	Characteristics of Major Hemolytic Anemias Caused by Hereditary Membrane Defects				
Condition	**Inheritance Pattern**	**Deficient Protein (Mutated Gene)**	**Pathophysiology**	**Typical RBC Morphology**	**Clinical Findings/ Comments**
Hereditary spherocytosis	75% autosomal dominant 25% nondominant	Ankyrin *(ANK1)* Band 3 *(SLC4A1)* α-Spectrin *(SPTA1)* β-Spectrin *(SPTB)* Protein 4.2 *(EPB42)*	Mutation in protein that disrupts vertical membrane interactions between transmembrane proteins and underlying cytoskeleton; loss of membrane and ↓ ratio of surface area to volume	Spherocytes, polychromasia	Varies from asymptomatic to severe Typical features: splenomegaly, jaundice, anemia
Hereditary elliptocytosis	Autosomal dominant	α-Spectrin *(SPTA1)* β-Spectrin *(SPTB)* Protein 4.1 *(EPB41)*	Mutation in protein that disrupts the horizontal linkages in the cytoskeleton; loss of mechanical stability of membrane	Few to 100% elliptocytes; schistocytes in severe cases	90% of cases asymptomatic; 10% of cases show moderate to severe anemia
Hereditary pyropoikilocytosis (rare subtype of hereditary elliptocytosis)	Autosomal recessive	α-Spectrin *(SPTA1)* β-Spectrin *(SPTB)* Homozygous or compound heterozygous	Mutation in spectrin that disrupts horizontal linkages in cytoskeleton; severe RBC fragmentation	Elliptocytes, schistocytes, microspherocytes	Severe anemia
Southeast Asian ovalocytosis	Autosomal dominant	Band 3 *(SLC4A1)*; only one known mutation	Mutation in band 3 that causes excessive membrane rigidity; only exists in heterozygous state	30% oval cells with one or two transverse ridges	Asymptomatic or mild hemolysis; prevalent in some areas of Southeast Asia
Overhydrated hereditary stomatocytosis (hereditary hydrocytosis)	Autosomal dominant	Rh-associated glycoprotein *(RHAG)* Others unknown	Mutation in protein that causes ↑ membrane permeability to sodium and potassium; high intracellular sodium causes influx of water, ↑ cell volume (↑ MCV), and ↓ cytoplasmic viscosity (↓ MCHC)	Stomatocytes (5%–50%), macrocytes	Moderate to severe hemolytic anemia; splenectomy is contraindicated because of thrombotic risk
Dehydrated hereditary stomatocytosis (hereditary xerocytosis)	Autosomal dominant	Piezo-type mechanosensitive ion channel component 1 *(PIEZO1)* Potassium calcium-activated channel subfamily N member 4 *(KCNN4)*	Mutation in protein that causes ↑ membrane permeability to potassium; low intracellular potassium causes loss of water from cell, ↓ cell volume (↓ MCV), and ↑ cytoplasmic viscosity (↑ MCHC)	Target cells, burr cells, stomatocytes (<10%), RBCs with "puddled" hemoglobin at periphery, desiccated cells with spicules	Mild to moderate anemia, splenomegaly; may lead to fetal loss, hydrops fetalis; may be accompanied by pseudohyperkalemia

↑, Increased; ↓, decreased; *MCHC*, mean cell hemoglobin concentration; *MCV*, mean cell volume; *RBC*, red blood cell.

the reader is encouraged to review that chapter when studying defects in the membrane.

Hereditary Red Blood Cell Membrane Abnormalities

Most defects in the RBC membrane that can cause hemolytic anemia are hereditary; however, acquired defects also exist. The major hereditary membrane defects are described in Table 21.1.

Hereditary membrane defects can be classified based on morphology or by the altered RBC function. For example, hereditary RBC membrane defects have historically been classified by morphologic features or shape of the RBC (e.g., spherocytes or elliptocytes). However, these defects also can be classified as those that affect membrane structure (altering geometry and elasticity) and those that affect membrane transport (altering

BOX 21.1 **Classification of Major Hereditary Membrane Defects Causing Hemolytic Anemia**

Mutations That Alter Membrane Structure
Hereditary spherocytosis
Hereditary elliptocytosis/pyropoikilocytosis
Hereditary ovalocytosis (Southeast Asian ovalocytosis)

Mutations That Alter Membrane Transport Proteins
Overhydrated hereditary stomatocytosis (hereditary hydrocytosis)
Dehydrated hereditary stomatocytosis (hereditary xerocytosis)

cytoplasmic viscosity) (Box 21.1).[11] The major disorders affecting membrane structure are hereditary spherocytosis (HS), a vertical membrane interaction defect characterized by spherocytes, and hereditary elliptocytosis (HE), a horizontal membrane interaction defect characterized by elliptical RBCs. Hereditary pyropoikilocytosis (HPP), a variant of hereditary elliptocytosis, is characterized by marked poikilocytosis and heat sensitivity. A less common membrane structure defect, hereditary ovalocytosis (Southeast Asian ovalocytosis [SAO]), is characterized by the presence of oval-shaped RBCs. Hereditary disorders that alter membrane transport proteins include overhydrated hereditary stomatocytosis (OHS; also called *hereditary hydrocytosis*) and dehydrated hereditary stomatocytosis (DHS; also called *hereditary xerocytosis [HX]*). Both of these disorders have an impact on the cation permeability of the RBC, which results in shape changes.

Diagnosis of the red cell membrane disorders requires a combination of family history, morphologic analysis of the RBC (indices, peripheral blood film), specialized tests, (osmotic fragility, flow cytometry, ektacytometry, electrophoresis) and molecular studies.

Hereditary Spherocytosis

Hereditary spherocytosis (HS) is a heterogeneous group of hemolytic anemias caused by defects in proteins that disrupt the vertical interactions between transmembrane proteins and the underlying protein cytoskeleton. HS has worldwide distribution and affects 1 in 2000 to 3000 individuals of northern European ancestry.[6,11,13] In 75% of families, it is inherited as an autosomal dominant trait and is expressed in heterozygotes who have one affected parent.[6] Homozygotes are rare; such patients present with severe hemolytic anemia but have asymptomatic parents.[13] In approximately 25% of cases, the inheritance is nondominant, with some autosomal recessive cases.[11,13]

Pathophysiology. HS results from gene mutations in which the defective proteins disrupt the vertical linkages between the lipid bilayer and the cytoskeletal network (Figure 7.5).[5] Various mutations in five known genes can result in the HS phenotype (see Table 21.1). Mutations can occur in genes for (1) cytoskeletal proteins, including *ANK1,* which codes for ankyrin (40% to 65% of cases in the United States and Europe; 5% to 10% of cases in Japan); *SPTA1,* which codes for α-spectrin (<5% of cases); *SPTB,* which codes for β-spectrin (15% to 30%

of cases); and *EPB42,* which codes for protein 4.2 (<5% of cases in the United States and Europe; 45% to 50% of cases in Japan); and (2) a transmembrane protein, band 3, which is coded by *SLC4A1* (20% to 35% of cases).[6,11] Less than 10% of cases involve de novo mutations, with most affecting the ankyrin gene.[13] A mutation database for HS lists 130 different mutations (*ANK1,* 52; *SCL4A1,* 49; *SPTA1,* 2; *SPTB,* 19; and *EPB42,* 8).[14] Because of the vertical interactions of the transmembrane proteins and cytoskeletal protein lattice, a primary mutation in one gene may have a secondary effect on another protein in the membrane. For example, primary mutations in *ANK1* result in both ankyrin and spectrin deficiencies in the RBC membrane.[13,15,16] In approximately 10% of patients, no mutation is identified.[11]

The defects in vertical membrane protein interactions cause RBCs to lose unsupported lipid membrane over time because of local disconnections of the lipid bilayer and underlying cytoskeleton. Essentially, small portions of the membrane form vesicles; the vesicles are released with little loss of cell volume.[13] The RBCs acquire a decreased ratio of surface area to volume, and the cells become spherical. These cells do not have the deformability of normal biconcave discoid RBCs, and their survival in the spleen is decreased.[4,13,15] As the spherocytes attempt to move through the narrow, elliptical fenestrations of the endothelial cells lining the splenic sinusoids (2 to 3 μm in diameter), they acquire further membrane loss or become trapped and are rapidly removed by the macrophages of the red pulp of the spleen.[4,11,13] In addition, as the RBCs are sequestered in the spleen, the membrane can acquire yet more damage, lose more lipid membrane, and become more spherical as a result of splenic conditioning.[4,13,15] The conditioning may be enhanced by the acidic conditions in the spleen and the prolonged contact of the RBCs with macrophages.[13,15] Low glucose and adenosine triphosphate (ATP) levels and phagocyte-produced free radicals, which cause oxidative damage, may also play a role (Figure 21.2).[13,15]

In HS, RBC membranes also have abnormal permeability to cations, particularly sodium and potassium, which is likely a result of disruption of the integrity of the protein cytoskeleton.[4,17] The cells become dehydrated, but the exact mechanism is not clear. Excess activity of the Na^+-K^+ ATPase may cause a reduction in intracellular cations, causing more water to diffuse out of the cell.[4,13] This results in an increase in viscosity and cellular dehydration.[13] The abnormality is not related to defects in cation transport proteins, and dehydration occurs regardless of the type of primary mutation causing the HS.[17]

Clinical and laboratory findings. Age of onset is variable, with first symptoms appearing in infancy, childhood, adulthood, or even at an advanced age.[16] There is also wide variation in symptoms. Symptomatic HS has three key clinical manifestations: anemia, jaundice, and splenomegaly.

Silent carriers are clinically asymptomatic with normal laboratory findings and usually are identified only if they are the parents of a child with recessively inherited HS.[4,13,16] Approximately 20% to 30% of patients have mild HS and are asymptomatic because an increase in erythropoiesis compensates for the RBC loss.[4,6] They usually have normal hemoglobin levels but may show subtle signs of HS, with a slight increase in serum bilirubin

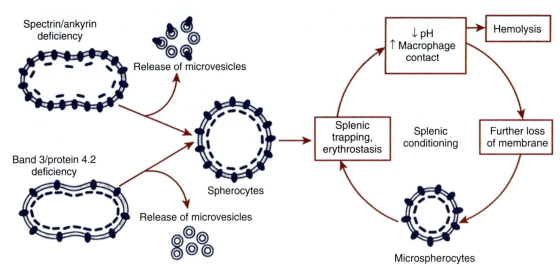

Figure 21.2 Pathophysiology of Hereditary Spherocytosis. The primary defect in hereditary spherocytosis is a loss of membrane resulting in a deficiency of membrane surface area. Decreased surface area may be produced by different mechanisms: (1) Defects of spectrin, ankyrin, or protein 4.2 lead to reduced density of the membrane skeleton, destabilizing the overlying lipid bilayer and releasing band 3–containing microvesicles. (2) Defects of band 3 lead to band 3 deficiency and loss of its lipid-stabilizing effect. This results in the loss of band 3-free microvesicles. Both pathways result in membrane loss, decreased ratio of surface area to volume, and formation of spherocytes with decreased deformability. These deformed erythrocytes become trapped in the hostile environment of the spleen (low pH, low glucose and high oxidant levels, and contact with macrophages). Splenic conditioning results either in hemolysis or further membrane damage forming microspherocytes, thus amplifying the cycle of red cell membrane injury. (From Gallagher, P. G. [2023]. Red blood cell membrane disorders. In Hoffman, R., Benz, E. J., Silberstein, L. E., et al. (Eds.), *Hematology: Basic Principles and Practice.* [8th ed., p. 653, Figure 46.2]. Philadelphia: Elsevier.)

in the range of 1.0 to 2.0 mg/dL, an increased reticulocyte count of up to 6%, and a few spherocytes on the peripheral blood film.[4,6,16] Mild HS may first become evident during pregnancy, during illnesses that cause splenomegaly (e.g., infectious mononucleosis), or in aging, when the rate of erythropoiesis starts to decline.[13,16] Approximately 60% of patients have moderate HS with incompletely compensated hemolytic anemia, hemoglobin levels greater than 8 g/dL, serum bilirubin more than 2 mg/dL, reticulocyte counts in the range of 6% to 10% (typically >8%), and spherocytes on the peripheral blood film.[4,6,11,16] Jaundice is seen at some time in about half these patients, usually during viral infections. About 5% to 10% of patients have moderate to severe HS, with hemoglobin levels usually in the range of 6 to 8 g/dL, serum bilirubin between 2 and 3 mg/dL, and reticulocyte counts greater than 10%.[4,6,16] About 3% to 5% of patients have severe HS, with hemoglobin levels less than 6 g/dL, serum bilirubin greater than 3 mg/dL, and reticulocyte counts greater than 10%.[4,6,15] Patients with severe HS are usually homozygous for HS mutations and require regular transfusions.[13] Splenomegaly is found in about half of young children and in 75% to 95% of older children and adults with HS.[4,11,15]

The hallmark of HS is spherocytes on the peripheral blood film. When present in patients with childhood hemolytic anemia and a family history of similar abnormalities, the uniform spherocytes are highly suggestive of HS. Some of these are microspherocytes, appearing as small, round, dense RBCs that are filled with hemoglobin and lack a central pallor (Figure 21.3). Normal-appearing RBCs, along with polychromasia and varying degrees of anisocytosis and poikilocytosis, are present. In addition to spherocytes, occasionally other RBC morphologic variants may be observed in some types of mutations: acanthocytes in some β-spectrin mutations,[18] pincered or mushroom-shaped cells in some cases of band 3 deficiency in patients without splenectomy,[19] and ovalostomatocytes in homozygous *EPB4.2* mutations.[20] Note that spherocytes are not specific for HS and can be seen in other hereditary and acquired conditions.

Because of the spherocytosis, patients with moderate to severe HS have an increase in the mean cell hemoglobin concentration (MCHC) greater than 36 mg/dL.[4,16,21] The mean cell volume (MCV) is variable, ranging from within the reference interval to slightly below.[6,13] MCHC is a calculated measurement of the cell hemoglobin concentration. It can be used to aid in the diagnosis of HS; however, there is variability between analyzers and mild HS cases may have a normal MCHC.[21] Several blood cell analyzers have newer technology that allows for direct measurement of a cell hemoglobin concentration mean (CHCM) of intact cells and/or parameters that estimate the hyperdense cell percentage (% Hyper) through various methods.[21] A cutoff of greater than 4% hyperchromic (hyperdense) cells has been proposed to screen patients for HS when family history and RBC indices are consistent with HS.[6,21,22] Biochemical evidence of extravascular hemolysis may be present in moderate to severe forms of HS, and the extent depends on the severity of the hemolysis. This includes a decrease in serum haptoglobin level and an increase in levels of serum indirect bilirubin and lactate dehydrogenase (Chapter 20). Bone marrow shows

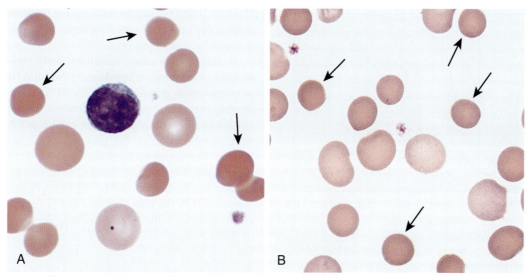

Figure 21.3 Spherocytes *(arrows)*, (A and B). (Peripheral blood, Wright-Giemsa stain, ×1000.)

erythroid hyperplasia as a result of the increased demand for RBCs to replace the circulating spherocytes that are prematurely destroyed, but bone marrow analysis is not required for diagnosis.

Additional tests. In patients with a family history of HS, splenomegaly, an increased MCHC and reticulocyte count, and spherocytes on the peripheral blood film, no further special testing is needed for the diagnosis of HS.[16] In cases in which HS is suspected but the family history and mode of inheritance are not clear or there are atypical clinical or laboratory findings, further special testing is needed to confirm a diagnosis.[16] No one method will detect all cases of HS, so a combination of methods is needed for definitive diagnosis. Testing methods include osmotic fragility, eosin-5′-maleimide (EMA) binding test, gel electrophoresis, ektacytometry, and molecular techniques. Additional techniques such as acidified glycerol lysis, autohemolysis, and cryohemolysis are less commonly performed in the United States.

Osmotic fragility is a test that demonstrates increased RBC fragility in blood specimens in which the RBCs have decreased ratios of surface area to volume. Blood is added to a series of tubes with increasingly hypotonic sodium chloride (NaCl) solutions. In each tube, water enters and leaves the RBCs until equilibrium is achieved. In 0.85% NaCl, the amount of water entering the cell is equivalent to the water leaving the cell because the intracellular and extracellular osmolarity is the same. In a hypotonic solution, more water will enter the cell to dilute the intracellular contents until equilibrium is reached between the cytoplasm and the hypotonic extracellular solution. As this phenomenon occurs, the cells swell. As the RBCs are subjected to increasingly hypotonic solutions, even more water will enter the RBCs until the internal volume is too great and lysis occurs. Because spherocytes already have a decreased ratio of surface area to volume, they lyse in less hypotonic solutions than normal-shaped, biconcave RBCs and thus have increased osmotic fragility.

In the procedure a standard volume of fresh, heparinized blood is mixed with NaCl solutions ranging from 0.85% (isotonic saline) to 0.0% (distilled water) in 0.05% to 0.1%

increments.[23] After a 30-minute incubation at room temperature, the tubes are centrifuged and the absorbance of the supernatant is measured spectrophotometrically at 540 nm.[23] The percent hemolysis is calculated for each tube as follows[23]:

$$\% \text{ Hemolysis} = \frac{A_{x\%} - A_{0.85\%}}{A_{0.0\%} - A_{0.85\%}} \times 100$$

where $A_{x\%}$ is the absorbance in the tube being measured, $A_{0.85\%}$ is the absorbance in the 0.85% NaCl tube (representing no hemolysis), and $A_{0.0\%}$ is the absorbance in the 0.0% NaCl tube (representing complete hemolysis). The hemolysis percentage for each NaCl concentration is plotted, and an osmotic fragility curve is drawn (Figure 21.4). Normal biconcave RBCs show initial hemolysis at 0.45% NaCl, and complete hemolysis generally occurs between 0.35% and 0.30% NaCl. If the curve is shifted to the left, the patient's RBCs have increased osmotic fragility with initial hemolysis at a NaCl concentration greater than 0.5%. Conversely, if the curve is shifted to the right, the RBCs have decreased osmotic fragility. Decreased osmotic fragility is found in conditions in which RBCs have increased surface area-to-volume ratios (e.g., a population of target cells in thalassemia).

Incubating the blood at 37° C for 24 hours before performing the test (called the *incubated osmotic fragility test*) allows HS cells to become more spherical and is often needed to detect mild cases. Patients who have increased osmotic fragility only when their blood is incubated tend to have mild disease and a low number of spherocytes in the total RBC population.

The osmotic fragility test is time consuming and requires a fresh heparinized blood specimen collected without trauma (to avoid hemolysis) and accurately made NaCl solutions. Specimens are stable for 2 hours at room temperature or 6 hours if the specimen is refrigerated.[23] Although the osmotic fragility test is the traditional screening method for HS, a major drawback of the test is its lack of sensitivity.[16] In a 2011 study of 150 patients with HS by Bianchi and colleagues, the

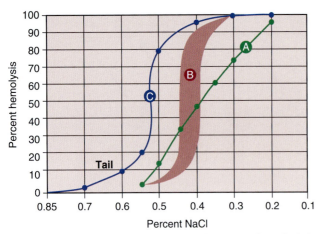

Figure 21.4 Erythrocyte Osmotic Fragility Curve. *(A)*, Curve in thalassemia showing two cell populations: one with increased fragility *(lower left of curve)* and one with decreased fragility *(upper right of curve)*. *(B)*, Normal curve. *(C)*, Curve indicating increased fragility, as in hereditary spherocytosis. The tail represents erythrocytes with increased osmotic fragility after conditioning in the spleen.

sensitivity for the unincubated test was 68%, with only a modest increase in sensitivity to 81% with the incubated test.[24] In nonsplenectomized HS patients with compensated anemia, those sensitivity figures dropped to only 53% and 64%, respectively.[24] Thus a normal osmotic fragility does not exclude a diagnosis of HS, especially in mild cases.[21] The osmotic fragility test is also nonspecific. A result indicating increased fragility does not differentiate between HS and spherocytosis caused by other conditions, such as thermal RBC injury (burns), immune hemolytic anemias, and other acquired disorders.[13,16,21] These disadvantages have led some not to recommend this test for routine use.[16] A flow cytometry–based osmotic fragility test has been developed using K2 ethylenediaminetetraacetic acid (EDTA) blood and exposing the isotonic saline–suspended RBCs to deionized water to induce hemolysis that shows a higher sensitivity (85.7%) and specificity (97.2%) for HS but may not be of value for other membrane or cation permeability defects.[21,22]

The *EMA binding* test has been proposed as a more sensitive alternative for confirmation of HS.[16] EMA is a fluorescent dye that binds to transmembrane proteins band 3, Rh, RhAg, and CD47 in the RBC membrane.[25] When measured in a flow cytometer, specimens from patients with HS show a lower mean fluorescence intensity (MFI) compared with normal controls and from patients with spherocytes caused by immune-mediated hemolysis.[25] The result is reported in percentage decrease in MFI when the patient specimen is compared with normal controls.[6,21] The sensitivity and specificity of the EMA-binding assay varies from 93% to 97% and 94% to 99%, respectively.[6,21,24,26] Positive test results can also occur with congenital dyserythropoietic anemia type II, SAO, and HPP, but these are rare conditions.[6,21,24,27] The EMA binding test offers advantages in that it is suitable for low-volume pediatric specimens, it can be performed within 3 hours, specimens are acceptable for analysis up to 7 days after collection, and gating can be used to eliminate the interference from transfused or fragmented RBCs.[6]

However, there is disagreement among laboratories on the percentage MFI decrease cutoff value for HS, and standardization is needed across laboratories.[6,21,27]

In atypical HS cases, additional tests may be required to identify the defective proteins.[16] Sodium dodecyl sulfate-polyacrylamide gel electrophoresis (SDS-PAGE) can be used to identify membrane protein deficiencies by electrophoretic separation of the various proteins in solubilized RBC membranes with quantification of the proteins by densitometry (Figure 7.3).[13,16] Membrane proteins also can be quantified by radioimmunoassay.[13] Variation in membrane surface area and cell water content can be determined by osmotic gradient *ektacytometry* (osmoscan).[28] The ektacytometer is a laser-diffraction viscometer that records the laser diffraction pattern of a suspension of RBCs exposed to constant shear stress in solutions of varying osmolality from hypotonic to hypertonic. An RBC osmotic deformability index is calculated and plotted against the osmolality of the suspending solution to generate an osmotic gradient deformability profile.[2,28] This method is available only in specialized laboratories; however, because of the advantages of distinguishing multiple RBC membrane disorders, this test may be included in future HS and other membrane defect guidelines.[1,6,13,16,28]

Several other tests have been used for diagnosis of HS (acidified glycerol lysis, autohemolysis, and hypertonic cryohemolysis), but they are cumbersome to perform; lack sensitivity and specificity, or both; and are not widely used in the United States.[4,13] The acidified glycerol lysis test measures the amount of hemolysis after patient RBCs are incubated with a buffered glycerol solution at an acid pH.[24,29] In the autohemolysis test, the patient's RBCs and serum are incubated for 48 hours, with and without glucose. The test has a sensitivity similar to that of the incubated osmotic fragility test.[4,13] The hypertonic cryohemolysis test is based on the fact that cells from HS patients are particularly sensitive to cooling at 0° C in hypertonic solutions.[30] However, increased hemolysis can also occur in SAO, some types of hereditary elliptocytosis, and congenital dyserythropoietic anemia type II.[16,30]

Molecular techniques for detection of genetic mutations are not usually required for diagnosis of HS.[13,16] Molecular studies are often performed after the identification of a deficient protein by SDS-PAGE. Because of the wide genetic diversity and shared mutations across RBC membrane defects, molecular testing often does not provide any additional information in patients whose family history confirms HS but could confirm diagnosis in a patient with no family history (recessive inheritance or de novo mutation).[22] Molecular testing also may be useful in patients who have been recently transfused because traditional methods are invalidated by the presence of donor RBCs in the patient's circulation.[31]

Complications. Although most patients with HS have a well-compensated hemolytic anemia and are rarely symptomatic, complications may occur that require medical intervention. Patients may experience various crises, classified as hemolytic, aplastic, and megaloblastic.[13] Hemolytic crises are rare and usually associated with viral syndromes. In aplastic crises there is a dramatic decrease in hemoglobin level and reticulocyte count. The crisis usually occurs in conjunction with parvovirus B19 infection, which suppresses erythropoiesis, and patients can become rapidly and severely anemic, often requiring transfusion.[16] This complication is more common in children, but it can occur in adults.[13,16] Patients with moderate and severe HS can also develop folic acid deficiency resulting from increased folate usage to support the chronic erythroid hyperplasia in the bone marrow.[13] This phenomenon is termed *megaloblastic crisis* and is particularly acute during pregnancy and during recovery from an aplastic crisis. Providing folic acid supplementation to patients with moderate and severe HS avoids this complication.[16] About half of patients, even those with mild disease, also experience cholelithiasis (bilirubin stones in the gallbladder or bile ducts) as a result of the chronic hemolysis.[13] Chronic ulceration or dermatitis of the legs is a rare complication.[13]

Treatment. Mild HS usually requires no treatment.[16] Patients with severe HS usually require regular transfusions.[13,15,16] Splenectomy is recommended for moderate to severe cases, results in longer RBC survival in the peripheral blood, and helps prevent gallstones by decreasing the amount of hemolysis and thus the amount of bilirubin produced.[13,16] The major drawbacks of splenectomy are the lifelong risk of overwhelming sepsis and death from encapsulated bacteria and an increased risk of cardiovascular disease with age.[13,16] Because infants and young children are especially susceptible to post-splenectomy sepsis, splenectomy is usually postponed until after the age of 6 years.[16] In a nationwide sample of 1657 children (aged 5 to 12 years) with HS who underwent splenectomy, there were no cases of postoperative sepsis and no fatalities from any cause during hospitalization for the surgery.[32] Partial splenectomy has been performed in young children with severe HS, but further evaluation of the risks and benefits of this procedure is needed.[13,16]

After splenectomy, spherocytes are still apparent on the blood film, and all the changes in RBC morphology typically seen after splenectomy are also observed, including Howell-Jolly bodies, target cells, and Pappenheimer bodies (Figure 21.5). Reticulocyte counts decrease to the high-reference interval, and the anemia is usually corrected. Leukocytosis and thrombocytosis are present. Bilirubin levels decrease but may remain in the high-reference interval. Occasionally a patient does not improve because of an accessory spleen missed during surgery or the accidental autotransplantation of splenic tissue during splenectomy. In these cases, hemolysis may resume years later.[13]

Differential diagnosis. HS must be distinguished from immune-related hemolytic anemia with spherocytes. Family history and evaluation of family members, including parents, siblings, and children of the patient, help differentiate the hereditary disease from the acquired disorder. Immune disorders with spherocytes are usually characterized by a positive result on the direct antiglobulin test (DAT) (Chapter 23), whereas the results are negative in HS. Increased osmotic fragility is not diagnostic of HS, because the spherocytosis found in acquired hemolytic anemia also results in increased osmotic fragility. The EMA binding test, however, shows decreased fluorescence in HS. The typical clinical and laboratory findings in HS are summarized in Table 21.2.

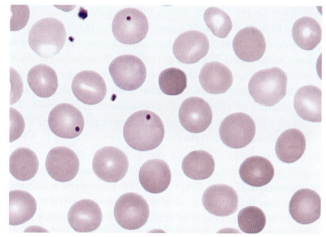

Figure 21.5 Red Blood Cell Morphology in Hereditary Spherocytosis after Splenectomy. Note the Howell-Jolly bodies and spherocytes. (Peripheral blood, Wright-Giemsa stain, ×1000.)

TABLE 21.2 Typical Clinical and Laboratory Findings in Hereditary Spherocytosis

Clinical manifestations	Splenomegaly
	Anemia*
	Jaundice (can be intermittent)
Mode of inheritance	75% autosomal dominant
	25% nondominant
Complete blood count results	↓ Hemoglobin*
	↑ Mean cell hemoglobin concentration
	↑ Reticulocyte count
	↑ Hyperchromic (hyperdense) RBCs†
Peripheral blood film findings‡	Spherocytes
	Polychromasia
Direct antiglobulin test result	Negative
Indicators of hemolysis	↓ Serum haptoglobin
	↑ Serum lactate dehydrogenase
	↑ Serum indirect bilirubin
Selected additional tests for atypical cases	Not required for diagnosis of HS with the typical features listed above
	↓ Fluorescence in eosin-5′-maleimide binding test by flow cytometry
	↑ Osmotic fragility and incubated osmotic fragility tests§
	SDS-PAGE analysis of membrane proteins

*Varies with severity of HS and ability of the bone marrow to compensate for the hemolysis.
†As measured on some automated blood cell analyzers.
‡With some rare mutations, acanthocytes, pincered cells, stomatocytes, or ovalocytes may be seen in addition to spherocytes.
§A result within the reference interval does not rule out HS; similar results can be observed in conditions other than HS.
↑, Increased; ↓, decreased; *HS,* hereditary spherocytosis *RBC,* red blood cell; *SDS-PAGE,* sodium dodecyl sulfate-polyacrylamide gel electrophoresis.

Hereditary Elliptocytosis

Hereditary elliptocytosis (HE) is a heterogeneous group of hemolytic anemias caused by defects in proteins that disrupt the horizontal or lateral interactions in the protein cytoskeleton. It reportedly exists in all of its forms in 1 in 2000 to 1 in 4000 individuals in the United States, but because the majority of cases are asymptomatic, the actual prevalence is not known.[13,33] The disease is more common in Africa and Mediterranean regions, where there is a high prevalence of malaria. The prevalence in West Africa of certain spectrin mutations associated with HE is between 0.6% and 1.6%.[13] The molecular basis for the association of elliptocytosis and malaria is unknown. The inheritance pattern in HE is mainly autosomal dominant.[11,13]

Pathophysiology. HE results from gene mutations in which the defective proteins disrupt the horizontal linkages in the protein cytoskeleton and weaken the mechanical stability of the membrane (Figure 7.5).[4,5] The HE phenotype can result from various mutations in at least three genes: *SPTA1,* which codes for α-spectrin (65% of cases); *SPTB,* which codes for β-spectrin (30% of cases); and *EPB41,* which codes for protein 4.1 (5% of cases) (see Table 21.1).[11,33] A mutation database for HE is available and lists 46 different mutations. primarily in the *SPTA1* and *SPTB* genes.[14] The spectrin mutations disrupt spectrin dimer interactions and the *EPB41* mutations result in weakened interactions between the spectrin and actin junctional complexes.[6,11] RBCs are biconcave and discoid at first but become elliptical over time after repeated exposure to the shear stresses in the peripheral circulation.[13] The extent of the disruption of the spectrin dimer interactions seems to be associated with the severity of the clinical manifestations.[11] In severe cases the protein cytoskeleton is weakened to such a point that cell fragmentation occurs. As a result, there is membrane loss and a decrease in the ratio of surface area to volume that reduces the deformability of the RBCs. The damaged RBCs become trapped or acquire further damage in the spleen, which results in extravascular hemolysis and anemia. In general, patients who are heterozygous for a mutation are asymptomatic, and their RBCs have a normal life span; those who are homozygous for a mutation or compound heterozygous for two mutations can have moderate to severe anemia that can be life threatening.[6,11]

Elliptocytosis also can be seen in patients with the Leach phenotype who lack Gerbich antigens and glycoprotein C (GPC).[4] The phenotype is due to a mutation in the genes for GPC and results in the absence of the glycoprotein in the RBC membrane.[34] The Gerbich antigens are normally expressed on the extracellular domains of GPC and thus are absent in this condition. Heterozygotes have normal RBC morphology, and homozygotes have mild elliptocytosis but no anemia.[4] The reason for the elliptocyte morphology may be a defect in the interaction between GPC and protein 4.1 in the actin junctional complex.[4]

The RBCs in HE patients all show some degree of decreased thermal stability. Cases in which the RBCs show marked RBC fragmentation on heating were previously classified as HPP. HPP is now considered a severe form of HE that exists in either the homozygous or compound heterozygous state.[11,13]

Clinical and laboratory findings. The vast majority of patients with HE are asymptomatic, and only about 10% have moderate to severe anemia.[11] Some may have a mild compensated hemolytic anemia, as evidenced by a slight increase in the reticulocyte count and a decrease in haptoglobin level or develop transient hemolysis in response to other conditions

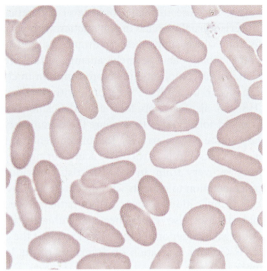

Figure 21.6 Red Blood Cell Morphology in Hereditary Elliptocytosis. (Peripheral blood, Wright-Giemsa stain, ×1000.). (From Carr, J. H. [2022]. *Clinical Hematology Atlas.* [6th ed.]. Philadelphia: Elsevier.)

such as viral infections, pregnancy, hypersplenism, or vitamin B_{12} deficiency.[13] Often an asymptomatic patient is diagnosed after a peripheral blood film is examined for another condition. However, some of these asymptomatic parents have normal RBC morphology and laboratory tests.[13] Rarely, heterozygous parents with undiagnosed, asymptomatic HE may have offspring who are homozygous or compound heterozygous for their mutations and present with moderate to severe anemia, increased osmotic fragility, and biochemical evidence of excessive hemolysis.

The characteristic finding in HE is elliptical or cigar-shaped RBCs on the peripheral blood film in numbers that can vary from a few to 100%[4] (Figure 21.6). The number of elliptocytes does not correlate with disease severity.[4] Investigation of elliptocytosis begins by taking a thorough patient and family history, performing a physical examination, and examining the peripheral blood films of the parents.[4] Other laboratory tests may be needed to rule out other conditions in which elliptocytes may be present, such as iron deficiency anemia, thalassemia, megaloblastic anemia, myelodysplastic syndrome, and primary myelofibrosis.[4] In these cases the elliptocytes usually comprise less than one-third of the RBCs.[35] An acquired defect in the gene for protein 4.1 may be found in myelodysplastic syndrome.[36]

The peripheral blood film in patients with the HPP phenotype shows extreme poikilocytosis with fragmentation, microspherocytosis, and elliptocytosis similar to that in patients with thermal burns (Figure 21.7, A). The MCV is very low (50 to 65 fL) because of the RBC fragments.[4,35] RBCs in the HPP phenotype show marked thermal sensitivity. After incubation of a blood specimen at 41° to 45° C, the RBCs fragment (Figure 21.7, B).[13] Normal RBCs do not fragment until reaching a temperature of 49° C. Thermal sensitivity is not specific for HPP, however; it also occurs in cases of HE with spectrin mutations.[4,13] RBCs with the HPP phenotype show a lower fluorescence than RBCs in HS when incubated with EMA and analyzed by flow cytometry.[37] Mutation screening using molecular tests or

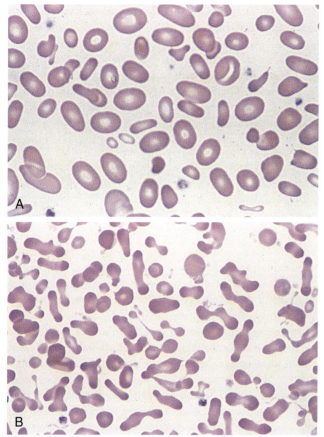

Figure 21.7 Morphology of Red Blood Cells in Hereditary Pyropoikilocytosis. **(A)**, Morphology without incubation. **(B)**, Morphology after 1 hour incubation at 45° C. (A, B, Peripheral blood, Wright-Giemsa stain, ×500.)

quantification of membrane proteins by SDS-PAGE also may be performed.

As in HS, patients with moderate or severe hemolytic anemia as a result of HE can develop cholelithiasis because of bilirubin gallstones. Hemolytic, aplastic, and megaloblastic crises can also occur.

Treatment. Asymptomatic HE patients require no treatment. HE patients who are significantly anemic and show signs of hemolysis respond well to splenectomy.[4] Transfusions are occasionally needed for life-threatening anemia.

Hereditary Ovalocytosis (Southeast Asian Ovalocytosis)

Hereditary ovalocytosis or Southeast Asian ovalocytosis (SAO) is a condition caused by a mutation in the gene for band 3 that results in increased rigidity of the membrane and resistance to invasion by malaria.[3,4] It is common in the malaria belt of Southeast Asia, where its prevalence can reach 30%.[13,38] The inheritance pattern is autosomal dominant, and all patients identified are heterozygous.[3,4]

Pathophysiology. SAO is the result of one mutation, a deletion of 27 base pairs in the gene, *SLC4A1,* and 9 amino acids in its encoded protein, band 3.[38,39] Deletion occurs at the interface between the transmembrane and cytoplasmic domains.[4,38,40] The mutation causes an increase in membrane rigidity that may be due to tighter binding of band 3 to

ankyrin, decreased lateral mobility of band 3 in the membrane, or steric hindrance of the spectrin tetramers as a result of improper folding of the cytoplasmic or first transmembrane domain of band 3.[4,13,37,38] Although band 3 is not decreased, this improper folding resulting from the deletion may cause a decreased fluorescence with EMA as the lysine residue is not available for binding.[37] RBC membranes in SAO also have decreased elasticity as measured by ektacytometry and micropipette aspiration.[2,3,37,38]

Clinical and laboratory findings. In patients with SAO, hemolysis is mild or absent. On a peripheral blood film, typical cells of SAO are oval RBCs with one to two transverse bars or ridges and usually comprise about 30% of the RBCs.[3,13] No treatment is required for this condition.

Overhydrated Hereditary Stomatocytosis (Hereditary Hydrocytosis)

RBC volume is regulated by various membrane proteins that serve as passive transporters, active transporters, and ion channels. When RBCs lose the ability to regulate volume, the cells are prematurely hemolyzed. Cell volume is determined by the intracellular concentration of cations, particularly sodium.[11] If the total cation content is increased, water enters the cell and increases the cell volume, forming a stomatocyte. If the total cation content is decreased, water leaves the cell, which decreases the cell volume and produces a dehydrated RBC, also called a *xerocyte.*

Hereditary stomatocytosis comprises a group of heterogeneous conditions in which the RBC membrane leaks monovalent cations. The two major categories are OHS (hereditary hydrocytosis) and DHS (HX). Both of these are hereditary disorders that alter membrane transport proteins and affect the intracellular cation concentration of RBCs. Molecular characterization of these conditions is ongoing and should provide a better means of classification and clearer understanding of their pathophysiology.

OHS is a very rare hemolytic anemia that results from a defect in membrane cation permeability that causes the RBCs to be overhydrated.[3,6] It is inherited in an autosomal dominant pattern.[11,13]

Pathophysiology. In OHS the RBC membrane is excessively permeable to sodium and potassium at 37° C.[41] There is an influx of sodium into the cell that exceeds the loss of potassium, which results in a net increase in the intracellular cation concentration. As a result, more water enters the cell, and the cell swells and becomes stomatocytic. Because of the water influx, the cytoplasm has decreased density and viscosity. The increase in cell volume without an increase in membrane surface area causes premature hemolysis in the spleen.[3] Most patients also have a secondary deficiency of stomatin, a transmembrane protein, but its gene is not mutated.[6,41,42] Stomatin may participate in regulation of the glycolytic pathway through the glucose transporter, Glut1.[42] Decreased amounts of stomatin may allow the cell to compensate for the increased use of ATP in attempt to compensate for the cation imbalance. Mutations in the *RHAG* gene that codes for Rh-associated glycoprotein (RhAG), along with a deficiency of the RhAG in the membrane

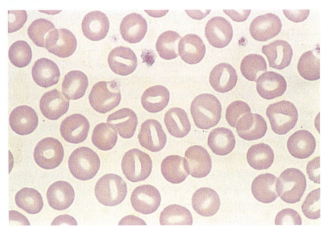

Figure 21.8 Red Blood Cell Morphology in Hereditary Stomatocytosis. (Peripheral blood, Wright-Giemsa stain, ×1000.)

have been found in some patients with OHS.[11,41,42] RhAG is a transmembrane protein involved in cation transport.[42]

Clinical and laboratory findings. OHS can cause moderate to severe hemolytic anemia. Diagnostic features include 5% to 50% stomatocytes on the peripheral blood film (Figure 21.8), macrocytes (MCV of 110 to 150 fL), decreased MCHC (24 to 30 g/dL), reticulocytosis, reduced RBC potassium concentration, elevated RBC sodium concentration, and increased net cation content in the RBCs.[3,6] Because of the increased cell volume, the RBCs have a decreased ratio of surface area to volume and increased osmotic fragility.[11] Splenectomy is not recommended in OHS because it is associated with an increased risk of thromboembolic complications.[3]

Dehydrated Hereditary Stomatocytosis (Hereditary Xerocytosis)

Dehydrated hereditary stomatocytosis (DHS) or hereditary xerocytosis (HX) is an autosomal dominant hemolytic anemia as a result of a defect in membrane cation permeability that causes the RBCs to be dehydrated.[3,4] It is the most common form of stomatocytosis.[4]

Pathophysiology. In DHS/HX the RBC membrane is excessively permeable to potassium. The potassium leaks out of the cell, but this is not balanced by an increase in sodium. Because of the reduced intracellular cation concentration, water is lost from the cell.[3,4] Most cases are due to mutations in the *PIEZO1* gene that codes for the Piezo-type mechanosensitive ion channel component 1 protein in the RBC membrane.[43–45] The PIEZO1 protein combines with other proteins to form a pore in the membrane to mediate cation transport, and it is important for RBC volume regulation.[43,45] The mutations result in an increase in ion channel activity and an increase in cation transport.[45] Mutations in the *KCNN4* gene also have been reported.[45] *KCNN4* encodes the potassium calcium-activated channel subfamily N member 4 (also called *Gardos channel*) and, when mutated, affects the transport function of the channel.[45]

Clinical and laboratory findings. Patients with DHS/HX generally have mild to moderate anemia, reticulocytosis, jaundice, and mild to moderate splenomegaly.[4,11] Fetal loss, hydrops fetalis, and neonatal hepatitis also can be

features of DHS/HX.[4] The RBCs are dehydrated with decreased MCV, increased cell viscosity and MCHC, and decreased osmotic fragility.[4,11,45] The RBC morphology includes stomatocytes (usually <10%), target cells, burr cells, desiccated cells with spicules, and RBCs in which the hemoglobin appears to be puddled in discrete areas on the cell periphery.[4,11] Most patients with DHS/HX do not require treatment. Splenectomy does not improve the anemia and is contraindicated because it increases the risk of thromboembolic complications.[3,4]

Other Hereditary Membrane Defects With Stomatocytes

Familial pseudohyperkalemia is a rare autosomal dominant disorder in which excessive potassium leaks out of the RBCs at room temperature in vitro but not at body temperature in vivo.[6] Complete blood count parameters are near the reference intervals, although some patients have a mild anemia.[6,29] Occasional stomatocytes may be observed on the peripheral blood film.[6] Mutations in the *ABCB6* gene (encoding a mitochondrial porphyrin transporter) have been identified.[45]

Cryohydrocytosis is another rare disorder that manifests as a mild to moderate hemolytic anemia with stomatocytosis caused by cold-induced leakage of sodium and potassium from the RBCs.[6,45] The RBCs have marked increase in cation permeability, cell swelling, and hemolysis when stored at 4° C for 24 to 48 hours.[29] Mutations in *SLC4A1* encoding band 3 have been identified in some patients, which cause it to leak cations out of the RBCs, whereas other patients have a deficiency in membrane stomatin or, rarely, mutations in *GLUT1 (SCL2A1)* encoding a glucose transporter.[4,6,29,45]

Rh deficiency syndrome comprises a group of rare hereditary conditions in which expression of Rh membrane proteins is absent (Rh-null) or decreased (Rh-mod).[4,13] Cases of the syndrome can be genetically divided into the amorph type (caused by mutations in Rh proteins) and the regulatory type (caused by mutations in a protein that regulates Rh gene expression).[4,13] Patients with Rh deficiency syndrome present with mild to moderate hemolytic anemia. Stomatocytes and occasional spherocytes may be observed on the peripheral blood film. Symptomatic patients may be treated by splenectomy, which improves the anemia.

Other Hereditary Membrane Defects with Acanthocytes

Acanthocytes (spur cells) are small, dense RBCs with a few irregular projections that vary in width, length, and surface distribution (Figure 21.9). These are distinct from burr cells (echinocytes), which typically have small, uniform projections evenly distributed on the surface of the RBC (Chapter 16). The differentiation is easier to make on scanning electron micrographs and on wet preparations (in which RBCs are diluted in their own plasma and examined under phase microscopy) than on dried blood films.[35] A small number of burr cells (<3% of RBCs) can be present on the peripheral blood films of healthy individuals, whereas increased numbers of burr cells are observed in uremia and pyruvate kinase (PK) deficiency.[13,35] Acanthocytes, however, are not present on peripheral blood films of healthy individuals but can be found in hereditary neuroacanthocytosis

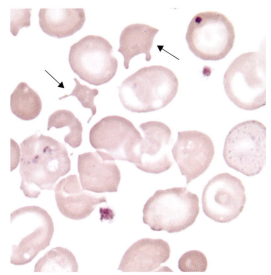

Figure 21.9 Two Acanthocytes *(arrows).* Note that cells are dense with irregularly spaced projections of varying length. (Peripheral blood, Wright-Giemsa stain, ×1000.)

(including abetalipoproteinemia [ABL]), and acquired conditions such as spur cell anemia in severe liver disease (discussed later), myelodysplasia, malnutrition, and hypothyroidism.[13]

Neuroacanthocytosis is a term used to describe a group of rare inherited disorders characterized by neurologic impairment and acanthocytes on the peripheral blood film. Three disorders are provided as examples in this group: ABL, McLeod syndrome (MLS), and chorea acanthocytosis.[4,46]

ABL is a rare autosomal recessive disorder characterized by fat malabsorption, progressive ataxia, neuropathy, retinitis pigmentosa, and acanthocytosis.[46] ABL can first manifest with steatorrhea and failure to thrive in young children (because of fat malabsorption) or as ataxia and neuropathy in young adults (because of decreased absorption of fat-soluble vitamin E).[46] ABL is caused by mutations in the microsomal triglyceride transfer protein *(MTP)* gene; *MTP* is needed to transfer and assemble lipids onto apolipoprotein B.[46] The mutations result in an absence in the plasma of chylomicrons, very-low-density lipoproteins (which transport triglycerides), and low-density lipoproteins (which transport cholesterol).[13,46] Consequently, triglycerides and cholesterol are decreased but sphingomyelin is increased in plasma.[13] Because RBC membrane lipids are in equilibrium with plasma lipids, the RBC membrane acquires increased sphingomyelin, which decreases the fluidity of the RBC membrane and results in the shape change. The shape defect is not present in developing erythroid precursors and reticulocytes but progresses as RBCs age in the circulation.[13] Other unknown mechanisms may also contribute to the formation of acanthocytes in ABL. Usually, 50% to 90% of the RBCs are acanthocytes.[4,13] Affected individuals have a mild hemolytic anemia, normal RBC indices, and normal to slightly elevated reticulocyte counts.[13] Early treatment with high doses of vitamins A and E can reduce the neuropathy and retinopathy.[13] Patients with other related disorders, such as hypobetalipoproteinemia caused by mutations in the *APOB* gene, also may have acanthocytosis and neurologic disease.[4,46]

MLS is an X-linked disorder caused by mutations in the *KX* gene.[47] *KX* codes for the Kx protein, a membrane precursor of Kell blood group antigens.[46] Men who lack Kx on their RBCs have reduced expression of Kell antigens, reduced RBC deformability, and shortened RBC survival.[46] Patients with MLS have variable acanthocytosis (up to 85%), mild anemia, and late-onset (aged 40 to 60 years), slowly progressive chorea (movement disorders), peripheral neuropathy, myopathy, and neuropsychiatric manifestations.[46,47] Some female heterozygote carriers may have acanthocytes, but neurologic symptoms are rare. Clinical manifestations in females depend on the proportion of RBCs with the normal X chromosome inactivated versus those with the mutant X chromosome inactivated.[13,47]

Chorea acanthocytosis (ChAc) is a rare autosomal recessive disorder characterized by chorea, hyperkinesia, cognitive impairments, and neuropsychiatric symptoms.[46] The mean age of onset of the neurologic symptoms is 35 years.[46] In patients with ChAc, 5% to 50% of RBCs on the peripheral blood film are acanthocytes.[46] ChAc is caused by mutations in *VPS13A*, a gene that codes for chorein, a protein with uncertain cellular functions.[47] Chorein may be involved in trafficking proteins to the cell membrane; consequently, a deficiency of chorein may lead to abnormal membrane protein structure and acanthocyte formation.[46]

Acquired Red Blood Cell Membrane Abnormalities
Acquired Stomatocytosis

Stomatocytosis may occur as a drying artifact on Wright-stained peripheral blood films. A medical laboratory professional should examine many areas on several films before categorizing the result as stomatocytosis, because in true stomatocytosis such cells should be found in all areas of the blood film. In healthy individuals, 3% to 5% of RBCs may be stomatocytes.[4] In wet preparations under phase microscopy, stomatocytes tend to be bowl shaped or uniconcave, rather than the normal biconcave shape. This technique can eliminate some of the artefactual stomatocytosis, but target cells also may appear bowl shaped in solution. Acute alcoholism and a wide variety of other conditions (e.g., malignancies and cardiovascular disease) as well as certain medications have been associated with acquired stomatocytosis.[4,13]

Spur Cell Anemia

A small percentage of patients with severe liver disease develop a hemolytic anemia with acanthocytosis called *spur cell anemia.* In severe liver disease there is excess free cholesterol because of the presence of abnormal plasma lipoproteins. The free cholesterol preferentially accumulates in the outer leaflet of the RBC membrane.[4,13] The spleen remodels the membrane into the acanthocyte shape, giving the RBC long, rigid projections.[13] Because of this remodeling, they become entrapped and hemolyzed in the spleen, which results in a rapidly progressive anemia of moderate severity, splenomegaly, and jaundice.[4,13] Spur cell anemia in end-stage liver disease has a poor prognosis. The anemia may resolve, however, if the patient is able to undergo liver transplantation.[4]

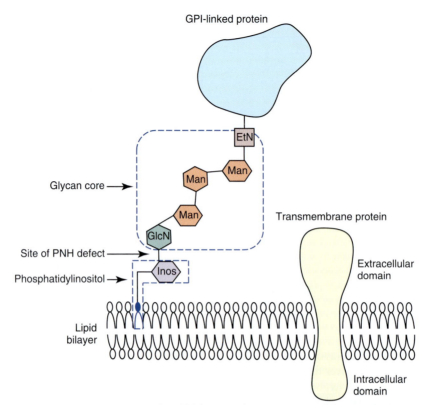

Figure 21.10 Glycosylphosphatidylinositol *(GPI)* Anchor for Attachment of Surface Proteins to the Cell Membrane. **(Left)** The structure of a GPI-anchored protein. The GPI anchor consists of phosphatidylinositol in the outer leaflet of the lipid bilayer, which is connected to a glycan core consisting of glucosamine *(GlcN),* three mannose *(Man)* residues, and ethanolamine phosphate *(EtN).* A protein is linked to the anchor at its C-terminus by an amide bond. The result is a surface protein with a fluid and mobile attachment to the cell surface. The GPI anchor and GPI-linked protein is extracellular. In paroxysmal nocturnal hemoglobinuria *(PNH),* a mutation occurs in the PIGA gene encoding phosphatidylinositol glycan anchor biosynthesis class A (PIG-A), one of seven subunits of a glycosyl transferase enzyme needed to add *N*-acetylglucosamine to the inositol *(Inos)* component of the phosphatidylinositol molecule *(arrow* shows location of the PNH defect). The mutated PIG-A enzyme subunit inhibits or prevents the first step in the biosynthesis of the GPI anchor. **(Right)** In contrast, a transmembrane protein has an extracellular domain, a short transmembrane domain, and an intracellular domain. (From Parker, C. J., & Ware, R. E. [2015]. Paroxysmal nocturnal hemoglobinuria. In Orkin, S. H., Fisher, D. E., Ginsburg, D., et al. (Eds.), *Nathan and Oski's Hematology and Oncology of Infancy and Childhood.* [8th ed., Figure 14.1]. Philadelphia: Elsevier.)

Paroxysmal Nocturnal Hemoglobinuria

Paroxysmal nocturnal hemoglobinuria (PNH) is a rare chronic intravascular hemolytic anemia caused by an acquired clonal hematopoietic stem cell mutation that results in circulating blood cells that lack glycosylphosphatidylinositol (GPI)-anchored proteins on their surfaces, such as CD55 and CD59 (Chapter 7).[48] Absence of CD55 and CD59 on the surface of the RBCs renders them susceptible to spontaneous lysis by complement. Because the mutation occurs in a hematopoietic stem cell, the defect is also found in platelets, granulocytes, monocytes, and lymphocytes.[49] PNH prevalence is difficult to assess based on criteria for inclusion. Newer estimates still indicate that PNH is rare with an annual incidence of less than 1 per 200,000.[48]

Pathophysiology of the hemolytic anemia. The GPI anchor consists of a phosphatidylinositol molecule and a glycan core (Chapter 7, Figure 7.2, B). The phosphatidylinositol is incorporated in the outer leaflet of the lipid bilayer membrane. The glycan core consists of glucosamine, three mannose residues, and ethanolamine phosphate. At least 24 genes code

for enzymes and proteins involved in the biosynthesis of the GPI anchor.[50] GPI-anchored proteins attach to the ethanolamine in the glycan core by an amide bond at their C-termini (Figure 21.10).

In PNH a hematopoietic stem cell acquires a mutation in the *PIGA* gene that codes for phosphatidylinositol glycan anchor biosynthesis class A (PIG-A), also known as phosphatidylinositol *N*-acetylglucosaminyltransferase subunit A.[51] It is one of seven subunits of a glycosyl transferase enzyme needed to add *N*-acetylglucosamine to phosphatidylinositol.[48–50] This is the first step in the biosynthesis of the GPI anchor in the endoplasmic reticulum membrane. The *PIGA* gene is located on the X chromosome, and more than 180 different mutations have been identified.[49] Without a fully functional glycosyl transferase enzyme, the hematopoietic stem cell is unable to effectively synthesize the glycan core on phosphatidylinositol in the membrane; therefore the cell is deficient in membrane GPI anchors. Without GPI anchors, all the progeny of the mutated stem cell are unable to express any of the approximately 20 currently known GPI-anchored proteins found on normal blood cells.[48] The GPI-anchored proteins are complement regulators, enzymes, adhesion molecules, blood group antigens, or receptors.[49,50] Relevant to the presence of hemolysis in PNH, two GPI-anchored proteins are absent or deficient on the RBC membrane: decay accelerating factor (DAF, or CD55) and membrane inhibitor of reactive lysis (MIRL, or CD59).[50] CD55 and CD59 are complement-inhibiting proteins. CD55 inhibits the complement alternate pathway C3 and C5 convertases, and CD59 prevents the formation of the membrane attack complex.[48] When CD55 and CD59 are absent from the RBC surface, the cell is unable to prevent the activation of complement, and spontaneous and chronic intravascular hemolysis occurs. Out of all the genes needed for GPI anchor synthesis, *PIGA* is the only one located on the X chromosome. Therefore only one acquired mutation in the *PIGA* gene is needed for the PNH phenotype in a stem cell (males have only one X chromosome, and in females one of the X chromosomes is inactivated).[48]

The *PIGA* mutant clone coexists with normal hematopoietic stem cells and progenitors, which results in a population of RBCs that is GPI-deficient and a population that is normal.[48] Some patients have a greater expansion of the mutant clone, a higher percentage of circulating GPI-deficient RBCs, and a more severe chronic hemolytic anemia.[48] On the other hand, other patients have minimal expansion of the mutant clone and have a lower percentage of circulating GPI-deficient RBCs. These patients may be asymptomatic and may not require any treatment. It is unclear why there is a greater expansion of the GPI-deficient clone and chronic hemolysis in some patients and not others.

Patients with PNH also display *phenotypic mosaicism*.[48,50] The mosaicism results when a single patient is able to harbor normal clones, as well as mutant clones with different *PIGA* mutations. Those different mutations result in variable expression of CD55 and CD59 on the RBCs within an individual patient, giving rise to three RBC phenotypes: type I, type II, and type III.[48,49] Type I RBCs are phenotypically normal, express normal amounts of CD55 and CD59, and undergo little or no complement-mediated hemolysis. Type II RBCs are the result of a *PIGA* mutation that causes only a partial deficiency of CD55 and CD59, and these cells are relatively resistant to complement-mediated hemolysis. Type III RBCs are the result of a *PIGA* mutation that causes a complete deficiency of the GPI anchor, and therefore no CD55 and CD59 proteins are anchored to the RBC surface. Type III RBCs are highly sensitive to spontaneous lysis by complement. The most common RBC phenotype in PNH is a combination of type I and type III cells, whereas the second most common has all three types.[48] When the severity of the hemolysis in PNH is being assessed, both the relative amount and the type of circulating RBCs are considered.

In addition to hemolysis, patients with PNH may have bone marrow dysfunction that contributes to the severity of the anemia. Many patients have a history of bone marrow failure caused by acquired aplastic anemia or myelodysplastic syndrome that precedes or coincides with the onset of PNH, resulting in a hypoplastic PNH presentation.[50–52]

TABLE 21.3 Clinical Manifestations in Paroxysmal Nocturnal Hemoglobinuria

Clinical Findings	Cause
Symptoms of anemia Fatigue Shortness of breath	Intravascular hemolysis; bone marrow failure
Thrombosis Budd-Chiari syndrome (hepatic vein thrombosis) Deep vein thrombosis Portal hypertension Pulmonary embolism Stroke	Intravascular hemolysis; platelet activation caused by depletion of nitric oxide by free hemoglobin
Smooth muscle dystonia Abdominal and/or back pain Dysphagia Erectile dysfunction Esophageal spasms Fatigue	Intravascular hemolysis; depletion of nitric oxide by free hemoglobin
Dark urine	Intravascular hemolysis; hemoglobinuria
Jaundice	Increased serum indirect bilirubin
Chronic kidney disease/renal tubule damage	Intravascular hemolysis; microvascular thrombosis due to platelet activation; accumulation of iron caused by repeated hemoglobinuria

Data from references 50–53.

Clinical manifestations. The onset of PNH most often occurs in the third or fourth decade, but it can occur in childhood and advanced age.[48–50] The major clinical manifestations and complications of PNH are those associated with hemolytic anemia, thrombosis, and bone marrow failure (Table 21.3).[50–53] Anemia is mild to severe, depending on the predominant type of RBC, the degree of hemolysis, and the presence of bone marrow failure. Dark urine (hemoglobinuria) and jaundice occur as a result of intravascular hemolysis. In addition, free hemoglobin released during intravascular hemolytic episodes rapidly scavenges and removes nitric oxide (NO). The decreased NO can manifest as smooth muscle dystonia (esophageal spasms, dysphagia, erectile dysfunction, abdominal and back pain) or platelet activation and thrombosis.[49,50] The most common thrombotic manifestation is hepatic vein thrombosis (called *Budd-Chiari syndrome*), which obstructs venous outflow from the liver, causing a serious, often fatal complication.[50] Patients also may develop chronic renal disease as a result of renal tubule damage from microvascular thrombosis and accumulation of iron during episodes of hemoglobinuria.[50]

Classification. The International PNH Interest Group proposed three subcategories of PNH: classic PNH, hypoplastic PNH (PNH in the setting of another specified bone marrow disorder), and subclinical PNH (Table 21.4).[48,50,52] In classic PNH there is clinical and biochemical evidence of intravascular hemolysis, reticulocytosis, a cellular bone marrow with erythroid hyperplasia and normal morphology,

TABLE 21.4 **Major Laboratory Findings in Paroxysmal Nocturnal Hemoglobinuria**

	Classical PNH	Hypoplastic PNH*	Subclinical PNH*
Hemoglobin	↓	↓	↓
Reticulocytes	↑	↓	↓
Cytopenias	Mild to moderate	Moderate to severe	Moderate to severe
Bone marrow	Normocellular to hypercellular with erythroid hyperplasia Normal to near-normal morphology Decreased iron	Evidence of bone marrow failure: Hypocellular (<25%) May have dysplastic morphology, ↑ blasts, or other myelopathy	Evidence of bone marrow failure: Hypocellular (<25%) May have dysplastic morphology, ↑ blasts, or other myelopathy
Circulating PNH granulocytes (GPI deficient)[†] by flow cytometry	>30%–50%	<20%–30%	<1%
Evidence of intravascular hemolysis[‡]	Frequent, marked	Intermittent, mild to moderate	None
DAT	Negative	Negative	Negative

*PNH in the setting of a bone marrow failure syndrome such as aplastic anemia, refractory anemia/myelodysplastic syndrome, or other myelopathy (e.g., myelofibrosis).
[†]Measured by high-sensitivity flow cytometry with anti-CD24 and fluorescein-labeled proaerolysin variant (FLAER).
[‡]Evidence of intravascular hemolysis includes elevated plasma hemoglobin, serum lactate dehydrogenase, and serum indirect bilirubin; decreased serum haptoglobin; and hemoglobinuria and hemosiderinuria.
↑, Increased; ↓ decreased; *DAT,* direct antiglobulin test.
Data from references 48, 50–52.

and a normal karyotype. In addition, more than 30% to 50% of the circulating neutrophils are GPI deficient.[48,50,52] In hypoplastic PNH, patients have evidence of hemolysis and a concomitant bone marrow failure syndrome such as aplastic anemia, refractory anemia/myelodysplastic syndrome, or other myelopathy (e.g., myelofibrosis). The number of GPI-deficient neutrophils is variable but is usually less than 20% to 30% of the total neutrophils.[48,50] In subclinical PNH, patients have no clinical or biochemical evidence of hemolysis but have a small subpopulation of GPI-deficient neutrophils that comprise less than 1% of the total circulating neutrophils.[48,52] Subclinical PNH also occurs in the setting of a bone marrow failure syndrome.

Laboratory findings. Biochemical evidence of intravascular hemolysis includes decreased levels of serum haptoglobin, increased levels of plasma hemoglobin, serum indirect bilirubin and lactate dehydrogenase, hemoglobinuria, and hemosiderinuria (Chapter 20). Hemolysis can be exacerbated by conditions such as infections, strenuous exercise, and surgery.[50] The major laboratory findings associated with classic, hypoplastic, and subclinical PNH are summarized in Table 21.4.[48,50–52] Hemoglobinuria is present in only 25% of patients at diagnosis, but it will occur in most patients during the course of the illness.[52] Very few patients report periodic hemoglobinuria at night, a symptom for which the condition was originally named.[50] Hemosiderinuria as a result of chronic intravascular hemolysis may be detected with Prussian blue staining of the urine sediment.

In classic PNH, reticulocyte counts are mildly to moderately increased, with less elevation than would be expected in other hemolytic anemias of comparable severity. The MCV may be slightly elevated because of the reticulocytosis. The DAT is negative. If the patient does not receive transfusions, iron deficiency develops as a result of the loss of hemoglobin iron in the urine, and the RBCs become microcytic and hypochromic. Serum iron studies (serum iron, total iron-binding capacity, and

serum ferritin) are performed to detect iron deficiency (Chapter 17). Folate deficiency often occurs if there is chronic erythroid hyperplasia and a greater need for folate, which leads to secondary macrocytosis. Pancytopenia may occur if there is concomitant bone marrow failure.

Bone marrow aspirate and biopsy specimens are examined for evidence of an underlying bone marrow failure syndrome, abnormal cells, and cytogenetic abnormalities.[52] The bone marrow may be normocellular to hypercellular with erythroid hyperplasia in response to the hemolysis (classic PNH), or it may be hypocellular with concomitant bone marrow failure (hypoplastic and subclinical PNH).[50] A finding of dysplasia or certain chromosome abnormalities is helpful in diagnosis of a myelodysplastic syndrome (Chapter 33). An abnormal karyotype is found in 20% of patients with PNH.[50]

Confirmation of PNH requires demonstration of GPI-deficient cells in the peripheral blood. Flow cytometric analysis (Chapter 28) of RBCs with fluorescence-labeled anti-CD59 determines the proportion of types I, II, and III RBCs and thus can provide an assessment of the severity of the hemolysis (Figure 21.11).[48,50] Type I cells with normal expression of CD59 show the highest intensity level of fluorescence; type II cells with a partial deficiency of CD59 show moderate fluorescence; and type III cells with no CD59 are negative for fluorescence. Patients with a greater proportion of type III cells (complete deficiency of GPI-anchored proteins) are expected to have a high-grade hemolysis.[48,52] Patients with a high percentage of type II cells (partial deficiency of GPI-anchored proteins) and a low percentage of type III cells may have only modest hemolysis.[48–52] A high-sensitivity two-parameter flow cytometry method using labeled anti-CD59 and anti-CD235a (anti-glycophorin A) was able to detect type III PNH RBCs with a sensitivity of 0.002% (1 in 50,000 normal cells).[54] However, flow cytometry methods to detect PNH RBCs have two major disadvantages. They underestimate the percentage of type III cells because RBCs lacking

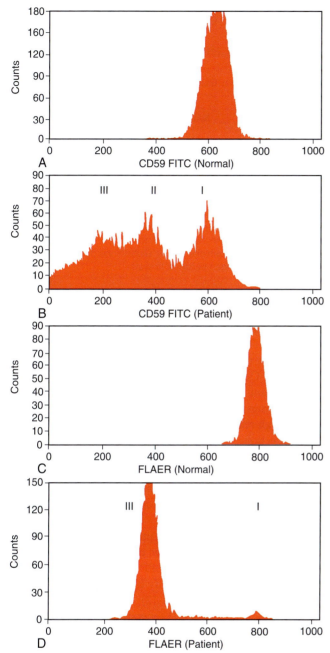

Figure 21.11 Flow Cytometric Analysis of Peripheral Blood Cells from a Patient with Paroxysmal Nocturnal Hemoglobinuria (PNH) and a Healthy (Normal) Control. **(A),** Fluorescence intensity of erythrocytes from a healthy control after staining with anti-CD59. **(B),** Fluorescence intensity of erythrocytes from an untransfused patient with PHN after staining with anti-CD59. Type II cells are "blended" between the type I (normal) and type III cells. **(C),** Fluorescence intensity of granulocytes from a healthy control stained with FLAER. **(D),** Fluorescence intensity of granulocytes from the same patient with PHN as in B after staining with FLAER. Note that the granulocytes are almost exclusively type III cells. A small population of type I granulocytes is present. *FITC,* Fluorescein isothiocyanate; *FLAER,* fluorescein-labeled proaerolysin variant. (From Araten, D. J., & Brodsky, R. A. [2023]. Paroxysmal nocturnal hemoglobinuria. In Hoffman, R., Benz, E. J., Silberstein, L. E., et al. (Eds.), *Hematology: Basic Principles and Practice.* [8th ed., p. 418, Figure 32.2]. Philadelphia: Elsevier.)

CD59 undergo rapid complement lysis in the circulation.[52] In addition, these methods cannot accurately determine the percentage of PNH RBCs after recent transfusion.

Because of the inherent problems with flow cytometry methods to detect PNH RBCs, diagnosis of PNH is accomplished by detection of the absence of GPI-anchored proteins on white blood cells (WBCs) using multiparameter flow cytometry. The absence of at least two GPI-anchored proteins in two WBC lineages (usually granulocytes and monocytes) is recommended for greater diagnostic accuracy.[50,54] Methods typically use fluorescent monoclonal antibodies to GPI-anchored proteins (e.g., CD59, CD55, CD24, CD16, CD66b, CD14), along with lineage-specific antibodies to non–GPI-anchored proteins (e.g., CD15 and CD64) to identify granulocytes and monocytes, respectively.[50,54,55] An alternative flow cytometric method uses a fluorescein-labeled proaerolysin variant (FLAER).[53–56] FLAER binds directly to the glycan core of the GPI anchor with a high signal-to-noise ratio. The absence of binding on granulocytes and/or monocytes is indicative of GPI deficiency (see Figure 21.11).[54–56] Using multiparameter flow cytometry with FLAER in combination with monoclonal antibodies to GPI-anchored antigens and lineage-specific antigens increases sensitivity and specificity for detection of GPI-deficient granulocytes and monocytes.[54,55] A high-sensitivity four-color protocol using FLAER, CD24, CD15, and CD45 for granulocytes and FLAER, CD14, CD64, and CD45 for monocytes was able to detect GPI-deficient granulocytes and monocytes with a sensitivity of 0.01% (1 in 10,000) and 0.04% (1 in 2500), respectively.[54] The results are not affected by recent transfusions because neutrophils and monocytes have a short life span in stored donor blood; therefore it can be reliably used to estimate the percentage of GPI-deficient granulocytes and monocytes in recently transfused patients.[50] The high sensitivity is also important for posttherapy monitoring of PNH clones.

The sugar water test (sucrose hemolysis test) and the Ham test (acidified serum lysis test) have insufficient sensitivity for diagnosis of PNH and have been replaced by flow cytometric techniques.

Treatment. In 2007 the US Food and Drug Administration approved eculizumab for the treatment of hemolysis in PNH.[57] Eculizumab is a humanized monoclonal antibody that binds to complement C5, prevents its cleavage to C5a and C5b, and thus inhibits the formation of the membrane attack unit.[57] Eculizumab is the treatment of choice for patients with classic PNH. It results in an improvement of the anemia and a decrease in transfusion requirements.[51,53,57,58] There is also a reduction in the lactate dehydrogenase level in the serum, reflecting a reduction in hemolysis.[57,58] In a study by Hillmen and colleagues of 195 patients taking eculizumab for a duration of 30 to 66 months, 96.4% of patients did not have an episode of thrombosis, and in 93%, markers of their chronic kidney disease stabilized or even improved.[58] Because of the inhibition of the complement system, patients taking eculizumab have an increased risk for infections with *Neisseria meningitidis* and need to be vaccinated before administration of the drug.[57] Patients continue to have a mild to moderate anemia and reticulocytosis likely because of extravascular hemolysis of RBCs sensitized with C3 (eculizumab does not inhibit complement C3).[48,59] To address this issue, research is under way to identify therapies that target the early events of complement activation, including monoclonal antibodies to C3, but a universal inhibition of C3 may increase the patient's susceptibility to infections and immune complex disease.[59]

Because of the expense and administration (intravenous) of eculizumab, novel complement inhibitors that have a longer half-life or oral administration are in high demand. Several drugs are currently in clinical trials, including C5 inhibitors, C3 inhibitors, and a complement alternative pathway inhibitor.[51,53] In 2018 the FDA approved ravulizumab, also a monoclonal antibody to C5, for the treatment of patients with PNH, which is less expensive than eculizumab with similar therapeutic outcomes.[48] A promising new therapy under investigation is a novel recombinant fusion protein (TT30) designed to prevent the formation of C3 convertase only on the membranes of GPI-deficient RBCs.[59]

Monoclonal antibodies to C5 are not curative and do not address the bone marrow failure complications of PNH. Other treatments for PNH are mainly supportive. Iron therapy is given to help alleviate the iron deficiency caused by the urinary loss of hemoglobin, and folate supplementation is given to replace the folate consumed in accelerated erythropoiesis. Administration of androgens and glucocorticoids to ameliorate anemia is not universally accepted.[48] Anticoagulants are used in the treatment of thrombotic complications. In suitable patients with severe intravascular hemolysis, hematopoietic stem cell transplantation with a human leukocyte antigen (HLA)-matched sibling donor may be an option and can be a curative therapy, but with an overall survival of only 50% to 60%.[48]

PNH is a disease with significant morbidity and mortality. Before eculizumab, thrombosis was the major cause of death, and the median survival after diagnosis was approximately 10 to 15 years.[48] Long-term studies of patients on eculizumab therapy are in progress, and early results show a decrease in the debilitating complications and an increase in survival of patients with PNH.[58]

RED BLOOD CELL ENZYMOPATHIES

For RBCs to transport oxygen over the course of their 120-day life span, they need functional enzymes to maintain glycolysis, preserve the shape and deformability of the cell membrane, keep hemoglobin iron in a reduced state, protect hemoglobin and other cellular proteins from oxidative denaturation, and degrade and salvage nucleotides. Deficiencies in RBC enzymes may impair these functions to varying degrees and decrease the life span of the cell. The most important metabolic pathways are the Embden-Meyerhof pathway (anaerobic glycolysis) and the hexose monophosphate (pentose) shunt[60] (see Figure 7.1). The most common enzymopathies are deficiencies of glucose-6-phosphate dehydrogenase (G6PD) and PK. Other RBC enzymopathies are rare.[60]

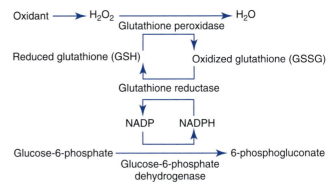

Figure 21.12 Function of Glucose-6-Phosphate Dehydrogenase (G6PD). G6PD converts glucose-6-phosphate (from the Embden-Meyerhof pathway) to 6-phosphogluconate generating the reduced form of nicotinamide adenine dinucleotide phosphate (NADPH). Glutathione reductase uses the NADPH to reduce oxidized glutathione (GSSG) to reduced glutathione (GSH). Glutathione peroxidase uses the GSH to detoxify hydrogen peroxide to water.

Glucose-6-Phosphate Dehydrogenase Deficiency

RBCs normally produce free oxygen radicals (O_2^-) and hydrogen peroxide (H_2O_2) during metabolism and oxygen transport, but they have multiple mechanisms to detoxify these oxidants (Chapter 7). Occasionally RBCs are subjected to an increased level of oxidants (oxidant stress) as a result of exposure to certain oxidizing drugs, foods, chemicals, and herbal supplements and even through reactive oxygen molecules produced in the body during infections. If allowed to accumulate in RBCs, these reactive oxygen species would oxidize and denature hemoglobin, membrane proteins, and lipids and ultimately cause premature hemolysis. Therefore the capacity of RBCs to detoxify oxidants, especially during oxidant stress, is critical to maintain their normal life span.

G6PD is one of the important intracellular enzymes needed to protect hemoglobin and other cellular proteins and lipids from oxidative denaturation. G6PD catalyzes the first step in a series of reactions that detoxify hydrogen peroxide formed from oxygen radicals (Figure 21.12). In the hexose monophosphate shunt (Chapter 7), G6PD generates reduced nicotinamide adenine dinucleotide phosphate (NADPH) by converting glucose-6-phosphate to 6-phosphogluconate. In the next step, glutathione reductase uses the NADPH to reduce oxidized glutathione (GSSG) to reduced glutathione (GSH) and NADP. In the final reaction, glutathione peroxidase uses the GSH generated in the previous step to detoxify hydrogen peroxide to water (H_2O).[60-62] GSSG is formed in the reaction and is rapidly transported out of the cell. During oxidant stress, RBCs with normal G6PD activity are able to readily detoxify hydrogen peroxide to prevent cellular damage and safeguard hemoglobin. G6PD is especially critical to the cell because it provides the only means of generating NADPH. Consequently, G6PD-deficient RBCs are particularly vulnerable to oxidative damage and subsequent hemolysis during oxidant stress.[60-62]

The *G6PD* gene is located on the X chromosome and encodes for the G6PD enzyme, which assembles into a dimer and tetramer in its functional configuration.[60] With the X-linked inheritance pattern, men can be normal hemizygotes (have the normal allele) or deficient hemizygotes (have a mutant allele). Women can be normal homozygotes (both alleles normal), deficient homozygotes (both alleles have same mutation), compound heterozygotes (each allele has a different mutation), or heterozygotes (have one normal allele and one mutant allele). The G6PD enzyme activity in female heterozygotes lies between normal and deficient because of the random inactivation of one of the X chromosomes in each cell (lyonization).[60-62] Therefore RBCs of female heterozygotes are a mosaic, with some cells having normal G6PD activity and some cells having deficient G6PD activity. Because X inactivation is random, the proportion of normal to G6PD-deficient RBCs varies among different heterozygous women.[62] Some heterozygous women experience acute hemolytic episodes after exposure to oxidants if they have a high proportion of G6PD-deficient RBCs.

G6PD deficiency is the most common RBC enzyme defect, with a prevalence of 5% of the global population, or approximately 400 million people worldwide.[63] The prevalence of G6PD deficiency varies by geographic location with African, Middle Eastern, Asian, and Mediterranean populations having the highest incidence (5% to 30% of the population) with the highest in sub-Saharan Africa (>32%).[60,63] In the United States the prevalence of G6PD deficiency in males of African ancestry is approximately 10% to 15%, whereas the carrier state is closer to 24%.[60,63] G6PD deficiency has the highest prevalence in geographic areas in which malaria is endemic because of the selective pressure of malaria.[64] Studies in Africa show that G6PD deficiency (A⁻ variant) in hemizygous males confers protection against life-threatening *Plasmodium falciparum* malaria.[65] This protective effect is not observed in heterozygous females because of their mosaicism of normal and G6PD-deficient RBCs.[65] In a 2010 case-control study in Pakistan, G6PD deficiency (Mediterranean variant) conferred protection against

Plasmodium vivax infection, also with a greater protective effect in hemizygous males.[66] This protective effect may be due to parasite susceptibility to excess free oxygen radicals produced in G6PD-deficient RBCs.[67] In addition, significant oxidative damage may occur to the RBCs early after parasite invasion so that these early-infected cells are more readily phagocytized with elimination of the parasite.[68] However, a meta-analysis of 28 malarial G6PD studies suggested a strong publication bias toward a negative correlation between G6PD deficiency and *P. falciparum*.[69] This meta-analysis failed to demonstrate a protective effect of G6PD deficiency in severe malarial infection except in studies performed in African countries. It did show, however, a negative correlation between G6PD deficiency and hyperparasitemia, suggesting that G6PD deficiency may decrease parasite load.[69]

A mutation database published in 2016 reported 217 known mutations in the *G6PD* gene, with approximately 84% of them being single missense mutations.[70] This number has increased slightly to 230 (86% single amino acid substitutions), and half of the mutations identified contribute to class I G6PD deficiency, which result in chronic nonspherocytic hemolytic anemia (CNSHA).[61] An amino acid substitution changes the structure of the enzyme and thus affects its function, stability, or both. In addition, more than 400 variant isoenzymes have been identified.[62] The normal or wild-type G6PD variant is designated G6PD-B.[60,62] Some G6PD variants have significantly reduced enzyme activity, whereas others have mild or moderately reduced activity or normal activity. The different variants of G6PD have been divided into classes by the World Health Organization, based on clinical symptoms and amount of enzyme activity (Table 21.5).[61,70] Several recent studies have shown that the severity of G6PD deficiency is determined by the catalytic activity and the protein stability of the G6PD variant.[61,71,72]

TABLE 21.5 Classification of Glucose-6-Phosphate Dehydrogenase Variants by the World Health Organization

Class	G6PD Enzyme Activity	Clinical Manifestations	Examples of Variants
I	*Severely deficient:* <1% activity or not detectable	Chronic, hereditary nonspherocytic hemolytic anemia; severity is variable; rare	G6PD-Serres G6PD-Madrid
II	*Severely deficient:* <10% activity	Severe, episodic acute hemolytic anemia associated with infections, certain drugs, and fava beans; not self-limited and may require transfusions during hemolytic episodes	G6PD-Mediterranean G6PD-Chatham
III	*Mild to moderately deficient:* 10%–60% activity	Episodic, acute hemolytic anemia associated with infections and certain drugs; self-limited	G6PD-A⁻ G6PD-Canton
IV	*Mildly deficient to normal:* 60%–150% activity	None	G6PD-B (wildtype) G6PD-A⁺*
V	*Increased:* >150% activity	None	

*May also manifest as class III
G6PD, Glucose-6-phosphate dehydrogenase.
Modified from Beutler, E., Gaetani, G., der Kaloustian, V., et al. (1989). World Health Organization (WHO) Working Group. Glucose-6-phosphate dehydrogenase deficiency. *Bull World Health Organ, 67,* 601–611; and Minucci, A., Moradkhani, K., Hwang, M. J., et al. (2012). Glucose-6-phosphate dehydrogenase (G6PD) mutations database: review of the "old" and update of the new mutations. *Blood Cells Mol Dis, 48,* 154–165.

Pathophysiology

G6PD-deficient RBCs cannot generate sufficient NADPH to reduce glutathione and thus cannot effectively detoxify the hydrogen peroxide produced on exposure to oxidative stress. Oxidative damage to cellular proteins and lipids occurs, particularly affecting hemoglobin and the cell membrane. Oxidation converts hemoglobin to methemoglobin and forms sulfhydryl groups and disulfide bridges in hemoglobin polypeptides. This leads to decreased hemoglobin solubility and precipitation as Heinz bodies.[60] Heinz bodies adhere to the inner RBC membrane, causing irreversible membrane damage (see Figure 12.12). Because of the membrane damage and loss of deformability, RBCs with Heinz bodies are rapidly removed from the circulation by intravascular and extravascular hemolysis.[62] Reticulocytes have approximately five times more G6PD activity than older RBCs, because enzyme activity decreases as the cells age. Therefore during exposure to oxidants, the older RBCs with less G6PD are preferentially hemolyzed.[64]

Clinical Manifestations

The vast majority of individuals with G6PD deficiency are asymptomatic throughout their lives. However, some patients have clinical manifestations. The clinical syndromes are acute hemolytic anemia, neonatal jaundice (hyperbilirubinemia), and CNSHA.[61,64]

Acute hemolytic anemia. Oxidative stress can precipitate a hemolytic episode, and the main triggers are certain oxidizing drugs or chemicals, infections, and ingestion of fava beans. Hemolysis secondary to drug exposure is the classic manifestation of G6PD deficiency. The actual discovery of G6PD deficiency in the 1950s was a direct consequence of investigations into the development of hemolysis in certain individuals after ingestion of the antimalarial agent primaquine.[60] Box 21.2 lists drugs that show strong evidence-based association with hemolysis in G6PD-deficient individuals or have been reported in well-documented case reports.[61,73,74] Primaquine and sulfa drugs are among the most commonly associated with hemolysis. The degree of hemolysis can vary, depending on the dosage, coexisting infection, concomitant use of other drugs, or type of mutation.[73] Exposure to naphthalene in mothballs and some herbal supplements also have been associated with hemolysis in some G6PD-deficient individuals.[60]

Individuals with class II and III G6PD deficiency are clinically and hematologically normal until the offending drug is taken. Clinical hemolysis can begin abruptly within hours or occur gradually 1 to 3 days after the drug is taken.[61,62,64] Typical symptoms include chills, fever, headache, nausea, and back pain.[60] A rapid drop in hemoglobin may occur, and the anemia can range from mild to very severe. Hemoglobinuria is a usual finding and indicates that the hemolysis is intravascular, although some extravascular hemolysis occurs. Reticulocytes increase within 4 to 6 days.[62] Generally, with class III variants such as G6PD-A⁻, the hemolytic episode is self-limiting because the newly formed reticulocytes have higher G6PD activity. With class II variants such as G6PD-Mediterranean, the RBCs are severely G6PD deficient, so the hemolytic episode may be longer, and the hemolysis is not self-limiting.[62]

Infection is another cause of hemolysis in individuals with G6PD deficiency. During the episode, the hemoglobin can drop 3 to 4 g/dL if reticulocyte production is suppressed by the infection.[60] The mechanism of hemolysis induced by acute and subacute infection is poorly understood, but the generation of hydrogen peroxide by phagocytizing leukocytes may play a role.[62] Diminished liver function may contribute further to the oxidant stress by allowing the accumulation of oxidizing metabolites. Infectious agents implicated in hemolytic episodes include bacteria, viruses, and rickettsia. Once the infection is cleared, the hemolysis resolves.[62]

Favism is a rare, severe hemolytic episode that occurs in some G6PD-deficient individuals after ingestion of fava beans. Favism can initially manifest with a sudden onset of acute intravascular hemolysis within hours of ingesting fava beans, or hemolysis can occur gradually over a period of 24 to 48 hours.[61,62] Hemoglobinuria, often described as "red wine" or "Coca-Cola" in color, is one of the first signs.[61] Specific patient factors may affect the severity of the hemolysis, including the type of mutation, the presence of underlying disorders, and the amount of fava beans ingested. Only a small percentage of G6PD-deficient individuals manifest favism, and most of these have the G6PD-Mediterranean variant.

Neonatal hyperbilirubinemia. Neonatal hyperbilirubinemia is associated with G6PD deficiency. Jaundice generally appears 2 to 3 days after birth without concomitant anemia.[64] The jaundice is mainly attributed to inefficient conjugation of indirect bilirubin by the liver rather than to excessive hemolysis.[75] These neonates must be closely monitored because the hyperbilirubinemia can be severe and cause bilirubin encephalopathy (kernicterus) and permanent brain damage.[62] Severe hyperbilirubinemia occurs more often in infants who, in addition to a mutated *G6PD* gene, are homozygous for a mutation in the promoter region of the

---

BOX 21.2 Drugs Causing Predictable Hemolysis in Glucose-6-Phosphate Dehydrogenase Deficiency

Drugs with Strong Evidence-Based Support for an Association with Drug-Induced Hemolysis

Dapsone
Methylthioninium chloride (methylene blue)
Nitrofurantoin
Phenazopyridine
Primaquine
Rasburicase
Tolonium chloride (toluidine blue)

Drugs with Well-Documented Case Reports for an Association with Drug-Induced Hemolysis

Cotrimoxazole
Quinolones
Sulfadiazine

Modified from Youngster, I., Arcavi, L., Schechmaster, R., et al. (2010). Medications and glucose-6-phosphate dehydrogenase deficiency: an evidence-based review. *Drug Saf, 33,* 713–726; and Luzzatto, L., & Seneca, E. (2014). G6PD deficiency: a classic example of pharmacogenetics with on-going clinical implications. *Br J Haematol, 164,* 469–480.

uridine diphosphate glucuronosyltransferase family 1 member A1 *(UGT1A1)* gene, which impairs their ability to conjugate and excrete indirect bilirubin.[62] In addition, the particular G6PD variant and environmental factors (e.g., drugs given to the mother or infant, the presence of infection, and gestational age) probably play an important role in the occurrence of neonatal hyperbilirubinemia, because a wide variation exists in frequency and severity in different populations with G6PD deficiency.

Chronic hereditary nonspherocytic hemolytic anemia. A small percentage of G6PD-deficient patients have CNSHA, as evidenced by persistent hyperbilirubinemia, decreased serum haptoglobin level, and increased serum lactate dehydrogenase level. Most of these patients are diagnosed at birth as having neonatal hyperbilirubinemia, and the hemolysis continues into adulthood. They usually do not have hemoglobinuria, which suggests that the ongoing hemolysis is extravascular as opposed to intravascular. RBC morphology is unremarkable. These patients also are vulnerable to acute oxidative stress from the same agents as those affecting other G6PD-deficient individuals and may have acute episodes of hemoglobinuria. The severity of CNSHA is extremely variable, likely related to the type of mutation in the *G6PD* gene.

Laboratory Findings

General tests for hemolytic anemia. The anemia occurring during a hemolytic crisis may range from moderate to extremely severe and is usually normocytic and normochromic. The morphology of G6PD-deficient RBCs is normal except during a hemolytic episode. The degree of RBC morphology change during a hemolytic episode varies, depending on the severity of the hemolysis. In some patients, the change is not striking, but in other individuals with severe variants, marked anisocytosis, poikilocytosis, spherocytosis, and schistocytosis may occur.[62] Bite cells (RBCs in which the margin appears indented and the

hemoglobin is concentrated) may be observed in rare cases of drug-induced hemolysis but should not be considered a specific feature of G6PD deficiency.[62,76] Bite cells are absent in acute and chronic hemolytic states associated with common G6PD-deficient variants, and they can also be found in other conditions.[62,76] Heinz bodies (precipitated denatured hemoglobin) can form in patients with G6PD deficiency but cannot be detected with Wright staining. They can be visualized with supravital stains, such as crystal violet, as dark purple inclusions attached to the inner RBC membrane (see Figure 12.12). The reticulocyte count is increased and may reach 30% of RBCs. Consistent with intravascular hemolysis, the serum haptoglobin level is severely decreased, the serum lactate dehydrogenase activity is elevated, and there is hemoglobinemia and hemoglobinuria. The indirect bilirubin level is also elevated. The WBC count is moderately elevated, and the platelet count varies. Importantly, the DAT is negative, indicating that an immune cause of the hemolysis is unlikely (Chapter 23). Table 21.6 contains a summary of the clinical and laboratory findings in G6PD deficiency during an acute hemolytic episode.

Tests for G6PD deficiency. The two major categories of tests for G6PD deficiency are quantitative and qualitative biochemical assays for G6PD activity (phenotypic assays) and deoxyribonucleic acid (DNA) based molecular tests for mutation detection (genotypic assays). Quantitative spectrophotometric assays are the gold standard to determine G6PD activity, make a definitive diagnosis, and assess the severity of the deficiency.[60,77] The assays are based on the direct measurement of NADPH generated by the patient's G6PD in the reaction shown in Figure 21.13. The assays require venous blood collected in heparin or EDTA anticoagulant. A hemolysate is prepared and incubated with the substrate/cofactor (glucose-6-phosphate/NADP)

TABLE 21.6 Typical Clinical and Laboratory Findings in Glucose-6-Phosphate Dehydrogenase Deficiency During Acute Hemolytic Episode

History	Recent infection, administration of drugs associated with hemolysis, or ingestion of fava beans
Clinical manifestations	Chills, fever, headache, nausea, back pain, abdominal pain Jaundice Dark urine
Complete blood count results	↓ Hemoglobin (moderate to severe) ↓ Reticulocyte count
Peripheral blood film findings	Polychromasia RBC morphology varies from normal to marked anisocytosis, poikilocytosis, spherocytosis, or schistocytosis, depending on severity
Direct antiglobulin test result	Negative
Indicators of hemolysis	↓ Serum haptoglobin (severe) ↑ Serum lactate dehydrogenase ↑ Serum indirect bilirubin ↑ Plasma hemoglobin Hemoglobinuria
Selected additional tests	↓ G6PD activity (mild to severe); may be falsely normal as a result of reticulocytosis, leukocytosis, or thrombocytosis and in individuals with mild deficiencies DNA-based mutation detection usually needed to identify heterozygous females Heinz bodies observed on supravital stain

↑, Increased; ↓, decreased; *DNA,* deoxyribonucleic acid; *G6PD,* glucose-6-phosphate dehydrogenase; *RBC,* red blood cell.

$$\text{Glucose-6-phosphate} + \text{NADP} \xrightarrow{\text{G6PD}} \text{6-Phosphogluconate} + \text{NADPH}$$

Not fluorescent   Fluorescent;
                                                                                              ↑ absorbance
                                                                                                at 340 nm

Figure 21.13 Principle of the Glucose-6-Phosphate Dehydrogenase (G6PD) Activity Assay. G6PD (in patient's hemolysate) converts glucose-6-phosphate to 6-phosphogluconate with the conversion of oxidized nicotinamide adenine dinucleotide phosphate *(NADP)* (not fluorescent) to the reduced form of nicotinamide adenine dinucleotide phosphate *(NADPH)* (fluorescent). In the quantitative assay the rate of production of NADPH is proportional to G6PD activity and is measured as an increase in absorbance at 340 nm by spectrophotometry. In the qualitative assay the appearance of a fluorescent spot under ultraviolet light when the reaction mixture is spotted on filter paper indicates normal G6PD activity.

reagent. The rate of NADPH formation is proportional to G6PD activity and is measured as an increase in absorbance at 340 nm by spectrophotometry.[60,77] The activity is typically reported as a ratio of the units of G6PD activity per gram of hemoglobin (IU/g hemoglobin [Hb]), so a standard hemoglobin assay must be done on the same specimen used for the G6PD assay. Cutoff points to determine G6PD deficiency are usually set at less than 20% of normal activity (usually <4.0 IU/g Hb), but this varies by method, laboratory, and population screened.[74]

Qualitative tests are designed as rapid screening tools to distinguish normal from G6PD-deficient patients. G6PD deficiency is defined by various methods as less than 20% to 50% of normal G6PD activity.[74,77,78] Similar to quantitative assays, these tests also incubate a lysate of heparin or EDTA-anticoagulated blood with a glucose-6-phosphate/NADP reagent to generate NADPH (see Figure 21.13). The end point in qualitative tests, however, is visually observed, and the results are reported as "G6PD-deficient" or "normal." Qualitative tests with deficient or intermediate results are reflexed to the quantitative assay for verification of the G6PD deficiency.

The fluorescent spot test is based on the principle that the NADPH generated in the reaction is fluorescent, while the NADP in the reagent is not fluorescent. Blood and glucose-6-phosphate/NADP reagent are incubated and spotted on filter paper in timed intervals. Specimens with normal G6PD activity appear as moderate to strong fluorescent spots under long-wave ultraviolet (UV) light; specimens with decreased or no activity do not fluoresce or display weak fluorescence compared with a normal control.

Dye-reduction qualitative assays use the same G6PD enzymatic reaction but have a second step in which the NADPH reduces a dye, giving a visually observed color change. An example is BinaxNOW (Alere/Abbott), which is a handheld device that uses the enzyme chromographic test (ECT) method.[79] Hemolysate is applied to one section of a lateral flow test strip in the device. The specimen migrates to the reaction pad of the strip containing the glucose-6-phosphate/NADP substrate/cofactor and a nitroblue tetrazolium dye.[79] If the specimen has normal G6PD activity, the NADPH generated reduces the dye to a formazan product that is visually observed as a brown-black color on the reaction pad.[79] This method has a sensitivity of 98% in detecting deficient specimens with G6PD activity less than 4.0 U/g Hb.[79] In another formazan-based test, the NADPH reduces a tetrazolium monosodium salt (WST-8) substrate, forming a formazan orange-colored product.[78] The dye-reduction methods have an advantage because they do not need a UV light for visualization. A disadvantage of the BinaxNOW method, however, is its higher cost compared with other assays. Rapid, point-of-care screening methods that do not require a venipuncture specimen are in development.

Biochemical qualitative screening tests are reliable to identify hemizygous males and homozygous or compound heterozygous mutant females with severe deficiency (<20% of normal activity) but lack the sensitivity to detect mild and moderate deficiencies found in some class III G6PD deficiency and in heterozygous females. They also have subjective end points that may affect test reproducibility and accuracy.

Phenotypic assays for G6PD activity have several additional limitations. As covered earlier in the chapter, reticulocytes have higher G6PD activity compared with mature RBCs. Reticulocytosis typically occurs as a response to an acute hemolytic episode and will falsely increase the patient's G6PD activity over baseline values.[60,77] G6PD deficiency should be suspected when a patient with reticulocytosis has an unexpectedly normal G6PD activity result; that is because a patient with a normal G6PD enzyme and reticulocytosis is expected to have high G6PD activity. To avoid falsely elevated or falsely normal results, biochemical assays for G6PD activity should not be performed during acute hemolysis. The testing should be performed after the reticulocyte and total RBC counts have returned to baseline, which may take 2 weeks to 2 months after the hemolytic episode.[74,77] Another limitation of phenotypic assays is that testing cannot be done after recent transfusion because the mixture of donor and patient RBCs does not reflect the patient's true G6PD activity. WBCs and platelets also contain G6PD activity, but they generally do not interfere with the assay. However, in cases of severe anemia, or in severe leukocytosis or thrombocytosis, the buffy coat should be removed from the specimen before preparing the hemolysate to avoid falsely elevating the G6PD activity.[77]

DNA-based mutation detection (genotyping) is available in larger hospital and reference laboratories. Typically the DNA is extracted from WBCs isolated from whole blood. Because the vast majority of G6PD mutations involve single nucleotide substitutions, molecular testing is straightforward. Although there are approximately 230 known mutations, rapid polymerase chain reaction–based methods can be used that target specific mutations with high prevalence in a particular geographic area, racial group, or ethnic group.[61,70,77] If targeted mutation testing is negative, whole-gene DNA sequencing is required.[77]

DNA-based testing is best suited for prenatal testing, family studies, and identification of heterozygous females who typically have indeterminate or normal biochemical (phenotypic) tests because of their mosaicism of normal and G6PD-deficient cells.[60,77] DNA-based methods can be done on patients who were recently transfused because donor WBCs have a short half-life in stored blood and will not interfere with the test. In addition, DNA-based tests are not affected by reticulocytosis and can be done during an acute hemolytic episode.

The disadvantage of DNA-based methods is the requirement for technical expertise and specialized equipment. In addition, knowing the genotype of heterozygous females does not predict the clinical phenotype in terms of the proportion of normal and G6PD-deficient cells.[74]

An additional application of tests for G6PD deficiency is screening asymptomatic patients before prescribing the drugs listed in Box 21.2. Screening is recommended for patients with a family history of G6PD deficiency or for those who are members of ethnic/racial groups with a high prevalence of G6PD variants.

Treatment

Treatment for G6PD-deficient patients with acute hemolysis begins with discontinuing drugs associated with hemolysis. Most hemolytic episodes, especially in individuals with G6PD-A$^-$, are self-limited. In patients with more severe types, such as G6PD-Mediterranean, RBC transfusions may be required. Screening is important in populations that have a high incidence of G6PD deficiency. The prevention of acute hemolytic anemia is difficult because multiple causes exist; however, some cases of acute hemolytic anemia are easily preventable, such as avoidance of fava bean consumption and drugs known to induce hemolysis. Neonates in high-risk populations should be screened for hyperbilirubinemia associated with G6PD deficiency and treated immediately to prevent kernicterus and permanent brain damage.

Favism is a relatively dangerous manifestation and potentially fatal in individuals who do not have access to appropriate medical facilities and a transfusion service. Prevention of drug-induced disease is possible by choosing alternative drugs when possible. In cases in which the offending drugs must be used, especially in individuals with G6PD-A$^-$, the dosage can be lowered to decrease the hemolysis to a manageable level. Infection-induced hemolysis is more difficult to prevent but can be detected early in the course of the episode and treated if necessary. Most episodes resolve without treatment but may be severe enough to warrant RBC transfusion. In patients with hemoglobin levels greater than 9 g/dL with persistent hemoglobinuria, close monitoring is important. Neonates with moderate hyperbilirubinemia and jaundice secondary to G6PD deficiency can be treated with phototherapy, but those with severe hyperbilirubinemia may require exchange transfusion.[60]

Pyruvate Kinase Deficiency

Pyruvate kinase (PK) is a rate-limiting key enzyme of the glycolytic pathway of RBCs. It catalyzes the conversion of phosphoenolpyruvate to pyruvate, forming ATP (see Figure 7.1). PK deficiency is an autosomal recessive disorder, with an estimated prevalence of 1 per 125,000 to as high as 1 per 20,000 in the Western population.[80] It is the most common form of hereditary nonspherocytic hemolytic anemia and is found worldwide.[60,62] PK deficiency is due to a mutation in the *PKLR* gene that codes for PK in RBCs and hepatocytes. A mutation database published in 2016 reported 256 mutations with 72% being single nucleotide substitutions (missense), about 9% deletions, and 3% insertions, while 13% affect the promoter region and introns.[81]

Symptomatic hemolytic anemia occurs in homozygotes or compound heterozygotes. Certain mutations are more common in the United States, parts of Europe, and Asia.[60,81] There is a high prevalence of PK-deficient homozygotes with the same point mutations in two isolated, consanguineous communities in the United States: an Amish kindred in Pennsylvania (1436G > A) and children born into polygamist families in a small town in the Midwest (1529G > A).[82,83]

Pathophysiology

The mechanisms causing hemolysis and premature destruction of PK-deficient cells are not completely known. Metabolic consequences of PK deficiency is a depletion of cellular ATP and an increase in 2,3-bisphosphoglycerate (2,3-BPG).[84,85] The increase in 2,3-BPG shifts the hemoglobin-oxygen dissociation curve to the right and decreases the oxygen affinity of hemoglobin[84,86] (Chapter 8). This promotes greater release of oxygen to the tissues and enables affected individuals to tolerate lower levels of hemoglobin.[60,84,85] ATP depletion also affects the ability of the cell to maintain its shape and membrane integrity.

Clinical Manifestations

Individuals with PK deficiency have a wide range of clinical presentations, varying from severe neonatal anemia and hyperbilirubinemia requiring exchange or multiple transfusions to a fully compensated hemolytic process in apparently healthy adults.[85] Most patients, however, have manifestations of chronic hemolysis, including anemia, jaundice, splenomegaly, and increased incidence of gallstones (because of the production of excessive bilirubin).[60] Rarely, folate deficiency (as a result of accelerated erythropoiesis), bone marrow aplasia (usually caused by parvovirus B19 infection), and skin ulcers can occur.[76,85] Pregnancy carries the risk of fetal loss and exacerbation of the anemia in the mother.[82,86] There is an increased risk of iron overload and organ damage that occurs with age, even in the absence of transfusions.[82,85,86] The mechanism of dysregulation of iron homeostasis is not clear but may be related to a decrease in or lack of response to hepcidin, the major iron-regulating protein.[82]

Laboratory Findings

The hemoglobin level is variable, depending on the extent of the hemolysis. Reticulocytosis is usually present, but not in proportion to the severity of the anemia, because the reticulocytes are preferentially destroyed in the spleen.[60,85] After splenectomy, the number of circulating reticulocytes can increase fivefold.[85] In addition to showing anisocytosis, poikilocytosis, and polychromasia, the peripheral blood film reveals a variable number of burr cells, or echinocytes (in the range of 3% to 30%), which increase in number after splenectomy.[85] The post-splenectomy peripheral blood film may also show Howell-Jolly bodies, Pappenheimer bodies, and target cells. The WBC and platelet counts are normal or slightly increased. Patients usually have the characteristic laboratory findings of chronic hemolysis, including increased serum indirect bilirubin and lactate dehydrogenase levels, decreased serum haptoglobin level, and increased urinary urobilinogen. The osmotic fragility is usually normal, and the DAT is negative.

The enzyme pyruvate kinase catalyzes the following reaction:

1. ADP + Phosphoenolpyruvic acid $\xrightarrow[\text{kinase}]{\text{Pyruvate}}$ ATP + Pyruvic acid

The pyruvic acid formed then takes part in the following reaction:

2. Pyruvic acid + NADH $\xrightarrow[\text{dehydrogenase}]{\text{Lactate}}$ Lactic acid + NAD
   Fluorescent → Not fluorescent; ↓absorbance at 340 mn

Figure 21.14 Principle of the Pyruvate Kinase (PK) Activity Assay. The reagent contains adenosine diphosphate (ADP), phosphoenolpyruvic acid, lactate dehydrogenase, and the reduced form of nicotinamide adenine dinucleotide (NADH). In the first step, PK (in patient's hemolysate) converts phosphoenolpyruvic acid to pyruvic acid, and a phosphate is transferred to ADP, forming adenosine triphosphate (ATP). In the second step, lactate dehydrogenase converts pyruvic acid to lactic acid with the conversion of NADH (fluorescent) to the oxidized form of nicotinamide adenine dinucleotide (NAD) (not fluorescent). In the quantitative assay, the rate of production of NAD is proportional to PK activity and is measured as a decrease in absorbance at 340 nm by spectrophotometry. In the qualitative assay the disappearance of fluorescence under ultraviolet light when the reaction mixture is spotted on filter paper indicates normal PK activity.

Tests for PK deficiency include quantitative and qualitative biochemical assays for PK activity (phenotypic assays) and DNA-based molecular tests for mutation detection (genotypic assays). In the quantitative PK assay, a hemolysate is prepared from patient's anticoagulated blood after careful removal of the WBCs. WBCs have a very high PK level, and contamination of the hemolysate with WBCs falsely increases the result (i.e., in a PK deficiency, the result could be falsely normal).[85] The reagents include phosphoenolpyruvate, adenosine diphosphate (ADP), lactate dehydrogenase, and the reduced form of NADH. In the first step of the reaction, the patient's PK converts phosphoenolpyruvate to pyruvic acid, and a phosphate is transferred to ADP, forming ATP. In the second step, lactate dehydrogenase converts the pyruvic acid to lactic acid, and the NADH is converted to its oxidized form, NAD (Figure 21.14). The rate of NAD formation is proportional to PK activity and is measured as a decrease in absorbance at 340 nm by spectrophotometry. The activity is typically reported as a ratio of the units of PK activity per gram of hemoglobin (IU/g Hb). More complex techniques may be necessary when some variant forms of PK are suspected.[85]

Qualitative tests for PK deficiency are used for screening and are based on the same principle as that described earlier; the hemolysate and reagents are incubated and spotted onto filter paper. The loss of fluorescence is visually evaluated to determine the oxidation of NADH to NAD.[87]

Mutation detection (genotypic testing) can be accomplished by sequencing the exons, flanking regions, and promoter region of the *PKLR* gene.[81,85] Molecular testing is superior in sensitivity and specificity, is applicable for use in prenatal testing, confirms patients with borderline enzyme deficiencies, and enables correlation of certain mutations with disease severity.[60,82,85]

Treatment

No specific therapy is available for PK deficiency except supportive treatment and RBC transfusion as necessary. Splenectomy is beneficial in severe cases, and after this procedure the hemoglobin level usually increases enough to reduce or eliminate the need for transfusion.[76] Splenectomy, however, results in a lifelong increased risk of sepsis by encapsulated bacteria. Additional therapeutic options include PK activators (AG-348/Mitapivat in phase 3 clinical trial) and gene therapy (phase 1 clinical trial).[86] Mitapivat has shown increased hemoglobin levels in half of the participants during its clinical trial and is a promising therapeutic option. Hematopoietic stem cell transplant may be curative for children with severe hemolytic disease who have an unaffected HLA-identical sibling for a donor; however, PK activators (once clinically available) may prove to be a better option because of the high morbidity and mortality of HSCT.[82,86]

Other Enzymopathies

Pyrimidine 5′-nucleotidase type 1 (P5′NT-1) deficiency is the third most common RBC enzyme deficiency that causes hereditary nonspherocytic hemolytic anemia (after G6PD and PK deficiencies) with only 100 cases reported worldwide.[60,88,89] P5′NT-1 is an enzyme needed for the degradation and elimination of ribosomal ribonucleic acid (RNA) in reticulocytes. P5′NT-1 removes the phosphate from pyrimidine 5′ ribonucleoside monophosphate to form ribonucleoside and inorganic phosphate. These degradation products are then able to diffuse out of the cell.[60] P5′NT-1 deficiency is inherited in an autosomal recessive manner.[60,88] The *NT5C3A* gene codes for P5′NT-1, and different mutations in this gene have been reported with each new case making detection of the deficiency increasingly challenging, particularly by LC-MS.[88,89] A recent proteomics study revealed that P5′NT-1–deficient patients also had a decrease in transketolase, an enzyme in the pentose phosphate pathway, which may offer more information on detection of P5′NT-1 deficiency.[89]

Patients who are homozygotes or compound heterozygotes for *NT5C3A* mutations develop chronic hemolytic anemia. The P5′NT-1–deficient RBCs accumulate pyrimidine ribonucleoside monophosphates, which precipitate and appear as very coarse *basophilic stippling* in the cell.[60,88] These RBCs ultimately undergo premature hemolysis. Most patients have a mild to moderate anemia with reticulocytosis, jaundice, and splenomegaly.[88] Diagnostic tests include measurement of P5′NT-1 activity, the concentration of intracellular pyrimidine nucleotides in RBCs and DNA-based testing for mutations, which has proven difficult considering the number of mutations.[88,89] Measurement of transketolase levels by western blot may serve as a reliable screening method for P5′NT-1 deficiency.[89] Therapy consists of supportive RBC transfusions as needed.

Other RBC enzymopathies are rarely encountered. In addition to PK deficiency, deficiencies of other enzymes of the RBC Embden-Meyerhof pathway that cause hereditary nonspherocytic hemolytic anemia have been described, including hexokinase, glucose-6-phosphate isomerase, 6-phosphofructokinase, fructose-bisphosphate aldolase, triosephosphate isomerase, and phosphoglycerate kinase.[62] All these deficiencies are autosomal recessive conditions, except for phosphoglycerate kinase deficiency, which is X-linked.

SUMMARY

- The red blood cell (RBC) membrane must have deformability for RBCs to maneuver through the microcirculation and the splenic pores over its life span of 120 days. Cellular properties that enable deformability are the biconcave, discoid shape of the cell; viscoelasticity of the membrane; and cytoplasmic viscosity.

- Two transmembrane protein complexes, the ankyrin complex and actin (protein 4.1) junctional complex, provide vertical structural integrity to the cell by anchoring the lipid bilayer to the underlying spectrin skeleton. α-Spectrin, β-spectrin, and their accessory proteins form a two-dimensional lattice to provide horizontal mechanical stability to the membrane.

- Hereditary spherocytosis (HS) is caused by mutations that disrupt the vertical membrane protein interactions, which results in loss of membrane, decrease in the ratio of surface area to volume, and formation of spherocytes that undergo extravascular hemolysis in the spleen. Patients with HS have anemia, splenomegaly, jaundice, an increased mean cell hemoglobin concentration (MCHC), spherocytes and polychromasia on the peripheral blood film, a negative direct antiglobulin test (DAT), and biochemical evidence of hemolysis. RBCs in HS show decreased fluorescence in the eosin-5′-maleimide binding test by flow cytometry, and osmotic fragility is usually increased.

- Hereditary elliptocytosis (HE) and hereditary pyropoikilocytosis (HPP) are caused by mutations that disrupt the horizontal interactions in the protein cytoskeleton, which results in loss of mechanical stability of the membrane. Elliptocytes are present on the peripheral blood film. Only 10% of patients with HE have moderate or severe anemia. HPP is a severe, thermal-sensitive form of HE in which extreme poikilocytosis along with schistocytes, microspherocytes, and elliptocytes are seen on the peripheral blood film.

- Hereditary ovalocytosis, also called Southeast Asian ovalocytosis (SAO), is caused by a mutation in band 3 that increases membrane rigidity. The prevalence is high in Southeast Asia, and hemolysis is mild or absent; typical cells are oval with one to two transverse bars or ridges.

- Hereditary stomatocytosis is a group of disorders characterized by an RBC membrane that leaks cations. In overhydrated hereditary stomatocytosis (OHS) or hereditary hydrocytosis, RBCs have increased mean cell volume (MCV), decreased cytoplasmic viscosity and MCHC, and stomatocytes on the peripheral blood film. In dehydrated hereditary stomatocytosis (DHS) or hereditary xerocytosis (HX), RBCs have decreased MCV and increased cytoplasmic viscosity and MCHC, and the peripheral blood film shows burr cells, target cells, few stomatocytes, and cells with puddled hemoglobin at the periphery. Stomatocytosis may also occur in Rh deficiency syndrome and in a variety of acquired conditions.

- Neuroacanthocytosis comprises a group of inherited disorders characterized by neurologic impairment and the presence of acanthocytes on the peripheral blood film. Major disorders in this group include abetalipoproteinemia (ABL), McLeod syndrome (MLS), and chorea acanthocytosis (ChAc). Acquired acanthocytosis can occur in severe liver disease (spur cell anemia).

- Paroxysmal nocturnal hemoglobinuria (PNH) is due to an acquired hematopoietic stem cell mutation that results in the lack of glycosylphosphatidylinositol (GPI)-anchored proteins on blood cell surfaces. CD55 and CD59, complement-regulating proteins, are partially or completely deficient on RBCs, which makes the RBCs susceptible to spontaneous complement lysis. Flow cytometry is a sensitive method to detect the absence of the GPI anchor and GPI-anchored proteins on cell surfaces. The rate of hemolysis in classic PNH improves after treatment with eculizumab, a complement C5 inhibitor.

- Glucose-6-phosphate dehydrogenase (G6PD) deficiency is the most common RBC enzymopathy, but the vast majority of patients are asymptomatic. Patients with class II and III G6PD variants may develop acute hemolytic anemia after infections or after ingestion of certain drugs or fava beans. A small percentage of patients have class I G6PD variant and chronic hereditary nonspherocytic hemolytic anemia (CNSHA).

- Most patients with pyruvate kinase (PK) deficiency have symptoms of hemolysis. Burr cells are commonly observed on the peripheral blood film. PK deficiency is the most common cause of CNSHA.

Now that you have completed this chapter, go back and read again the case study at the beginning and respond to the questions presented. Answers can be found in Appendix C.

REVIEW QUESTIONS

Answers can be found in Appendix C.

1. In HS, a characteristic abnormality in the CBC results is:
   a. Decreased MCH
   b. Decreased platelet and WBC counts
   c. Increased MCHC
   d. Increased MCV

2. The altered shape of the spherocyte in HS is due to:
   a. Abnormal precipitation of the hemoglobin molecule
   b. A mutated RBC membrane protein affecting vertical protein interactions
   c. A mutated RBC membrane protein affecting horizontal protein interactions
   d. Defective RNA catabolism and clearance

3. Which one of the following sets of results is consistent with HS?
   a. Decreased osmotic fragility, negative DAT result
   b. Decreased osmotic fragility, positive DAT result
   c. Increased osmotic fragility, negative DAT result
   d. Increased osmotic fragility, positive DAT result

4. The RBCs in HE are abnormally shaped and have unstable cell membranes as a result of:
   a. Defects in horizontal membrane protein interactions
   b. Deficiency in cation pumps in the RBC membrane
   c. Lack of Rh antigens in the RBC membrane
   d. Mutations in the ankyrin complex

5. The peripheral blood film for patients with mild HE is characterized by:
   a. Acanthocytes
   b. Elliptocytes
   c. Spherocytes
   d. Stomatocytes

6. Expected laboratory test results for patients with HPP include all of the following *except:*
   a. Increased MCV and normal RDW
   b. Low fluorescence when incubated with eosin-5′-maleimide
   c. Marked poikilocytosis with elliptocytes, RBC fragments, and microspherocytes
   d. RBCs that show marked thermal sensitivity at 41 C to 45° C

7. Acanthocytes are found in association with:
   a. Abetalipoproteinemia
   b. G6PD deficiency
   c. Rh deficiency syndrome
   d. Vitamin B_{12} deficiency

8. The most common manifestation of G6PD deficiency is:
   a. Acute hemolytic anemia caused by drug exposure or infections
   b. Chronic hemolytic anemia caused by cell shape change
   c. Chronic hemolytic anemia caused by intravascular RBC lysis
   d. Mild compensated hemolysis caused by ATP deficiency

9. A patient experiences an episode of acute intravascular hemolysis after taking primaquine for the first time. The provider suspects that the patient may have G6PD deficiency and orders an RBC G6PD assay 3 days after the hemolytic episode began. How will this affect the test result?
   a. Absence of enzyme activity
   b. False decrease in enzyme activity as a result of hemoglobinemia
   c. False increase in enzyme activity because of reticulocytosis
   d. No effect on enzyme activity

10. The most common defect or deficiency in the anaerobic glycolytic pathway that causes CNSHA is:
    a. Glucose-6-phosphate dehydrogenase deficiency
    b. Lactate dehydrogenase deficiency
    c. Methemoglobin reductase deficiency
    d. Pyruvate kinase deficiency

11. Which of the following laboratory tests would be best to confirm PNH?
    a. Acidified serum test (Ham test)
    b. Flow cytometry for detection of eosin-5′-maleimide binding on erythrocytes
    c. Flow cytometry for FLAER binding, CD24 on granulocytes, and CD14 on monocytes
    d. Osmotic fragility test

12. A 22-year-old man with a moderate decrease in hemoglobin level and a decrease in RBC, WBC, platelet, and reticulocyte counts has a history of infrequent and mild episodes of hemolysis with hemoglobinuria. His bone marrow showed 15% cellularity with no abnormal cells, and flow cytometry revealed that 15% of his circulating granulocytes were GPI deficient. He most likely has:
    a. A hereditary RBC membrane defect
    b. G6PD deficiency
    c. Hypoplastic PNH
    d. Pyruvate kinase deficiency

REFERENCES

1. Mohandas, N. (2018). Inherited hemolytic anemia: a possessive beginner's guide. *Hematology Am Soc Hematol Educ Program, 1,* 377–381.

2. Mohandas, N., & Chasis, J. A. (1993). Red blood cell deformability, membrane material properties and shape: regulation by transmembrane, skeletal and cytosolic proteins and lipids. *Semin Hematol, 30,* 171–192.

3. Mohandas, N., & Gallagher, P. G. (2008). Red cell membrane: past, present, future. *Blood, 112,* 3939–3948.

4. Coetzer, T. L. (2021). Erythrocyte membrane disorders. In Kaushansky, K., Prchal, J. T., Burns, L. J., et al. (Eds.), *Williams Hematology.* (10th ed., pp. 721–748). New York: McGraw-Hill.

5. Palek, J., & Jarolim, P. (1993). Clinical expression and laboratory detection of red blood cell membrane protein mutations. *Semin Hematol, 30,* 249–283.

6. Da Costa, L., Galimand, J., Fenneteau, O., et al. (2013). Hereditary spherocytosis, elliptocytosis, and other red cell membrane disorders. *Blood Rev, 27,* 167–178.

7. Bennett, V. (1983). Proteins involved in membrane-cytoskeleton association in human erythrocytes: spectrin, ankyrin, and band 3. *Methods Enzymol, 96,* 313–324.

8. Nicolas, V., Le Van Kim, C., Gane, P., et al. (2003). Rh-RhAG/ankyrin-R, a new interaction site between the membrane bilayer and the red cell skeleton, is impaired by Rh(null)–associated mutation. *J Biol Chem, 278,* 25526–25533.

9. Salomao, M., Zhang, X., Yang, Y., et al. (2008). Protein 4.1R-dependent multiprotein complex: new insights into the structural organization of the red blood cell membrane. *Proc Natl Acad Sci USA, 105,* 8026–8031.

10. An, X., Debnath, G., Guo, X., et al. (2005). Identification and functional characterization of protein 4.1R and actin-binding sites in erythrocyte beta-spectrin: regulation of the interactions

by phosphatidylinositol-4,5-bisphosphate. *Biochemistry, 44,* 10681–10688.

11. Narla, J., & Mohandas, N. (2017). Red cell membrane disorders. *Int J Lab Hem, 39*(Suppl. 1), 47–52.

12. An, X., Guo, X., Zhang, X., et al. (2006). Conformational stabilities of the structural repeats of erythroid spectrin and their functional implications. *J Biol Chem, 281,* 10527–10532.

13. Gallagher, P. G. (2023). Red blood cell membrane disorders. In Hoffman, R., Benz, E. J., Silberstein, L. E., et al. (Eds.), *Hematology: Basic Principles and Practice.* (8th ed., pp. 650–671). Philadelphia: Elsevier.

14. National Human Genome Research Institute. (2021). Red Cell Membrane Disorder Mutations Database. http://research.nhgri.nih.gov/RBCmembrane/. Accessed June 23, 2022.

15. Perrotta, S., Gallagher, P. G., & Mohandas, N. (2008). Hereditary spherocytosis. *Lancet, 372,* 1411–1426.

16. Bolton-Maggs, P. H. B., Langer, J. C., Iolascon, A., et al. (2011). Guidelines for the diagnosis and management of hereditary spherocytosis—2011 update. *Br J Haematol, 156,* 37–49.

17. De Franceschi, L., Olivieri, O., Miraglia del Giudice, E., et al. (1997). Membrane cation and anion transport activities in erythrocytes of hereditary spherocytosis: effects of different membrane protein defects. *Am J Hematol, 55,* 121–128.

18. Hassoun, H., Vassiliadis, J. N., Murray, J., et al. (1997). Characterization of the underlying molecular defect in hereditary spherocytosis associated with spectrin deficiency. *Blood, 90,* 398–406.

19. Dhermy, D., Galand, C., Bournier, O., et al. (1997). Heterogenous band 3 deficiency in hereditary spherocytosis related to different band 3 gene defects. *Br J Haematol, 98,* 32–40.

20. Bouhassira, E. E., Schwartz, R. S., Yawata, Y., et al. (1992). An alanine-to-threonine substitution in protein 4.2 cDNA is associated with a Japanese form of hereditary hemolytic anemia (protein 4.2NIPPON). *Blood, 79,* 1846–1854.

21. Farias, M. G. (2017). Advances in laboratory diagnosis of hereditary spherocytosis. *Clin Chem Lab Med, 55*(7), 944–948.

22. King, M.-J., Garçon, L., Hoyer, J. D., et al., and the International Council for Standardization in Haematology. (2015). ICSH guidelines for the laboratory diagnosis of nonimmune hereditary red cell membrane disorders. *Int J Lab Hematol, 37*(3), 304–325.

23. Hansen, D. M. (1998). Hereditary anemias of increased destruction. In Steine-Martin, E. A., Lotspeich-Steininger, C. A., & Koepke, J. A. (Eds.), *Clinical Hematology: Principles, Procedures, Correlations.* (2nd ed., pp. 255–256). Philadelphia: Lippincott.

24. Bianchi, P., Fermo, E., Vercellati, C., et al. (2012). Diagnostic power of laboratory tests for hereditary spherocytosis: a comparison study in 150 patients groups according to molecular and clinical characteristics. *Haematologica, 97,* 516–523.

25. King, M.-J., Smythe, J., & Mushens, R. (2004). Eosin-5-maleimide binding to band 3 and Rh-related proteins forms the basis of a screening test for hereditary spherocytosis. *Br J Haematol, 124,* 106–113.

26. Kar, R., Mishra, P., & Pati, H. P. (2008). Evaluation of eosin-5-maleimide flow cytometric test in diagnosis of hereditary spherocytosis. *Int J Lab Hematol, 32,* 8–16.

27. Mackiewicz, G., Bailly, F., Favre, B., et al. (2012). Flow cytometry test for hereditary spherocytosis. *Haematologica, 97,* e47.

28. Da Costa, L., Suner, L., Galimand, J., et al. (2016). Diagnostic tool for red blood cell membrane disorders: assessment of a new generation ektacytometer. *Blood Cells Mol Dis, 56*(1), 9–22.

29. King, M. J., & Zanella, A. (2013). Hereditary red cell membrane disorders and laboratory diagnostic testing. *Int J Lab Hem, 35,* 237–243.

30. Streichman, S., & Gescheidt, Y. (1998). Cryohemolysis for the detection of hereditary spherocytosis: correlation studies with osmotic fragility and autohemolysis. *Am J Hematol, 58,* 206–212.

31. Agarwal, A. M., Nussenzveig, R. H., Reading, N. S., et al. (2016). Clinical utility of next-generation sequencing in the diagnosis of hereditary haemolytic anaemias. *Br J Haematol, 174*(5), 806–814.

32. Abdullah, F., Zhang, Y., Camp, M., et al. (2009). Splenectomy in hereditary spherocytosis: review of 1,657 patients and application of the pediatric quality indicators. *Pediatr Blood Cancer, 52,* 834–837.

33. Gallagher, P. G. (2004). Hereditary elliptocytosis: spectrin and protein 4.1R. *Semin Hematol, 41,* 142–164.

34. Winardi, R., Reid, M., Conboy, J., et al. (1993). Molecular analysis of glycophorin C deficiency in human erythrocytes. *Blood, 81,* 2799–2803.

35. Gallagher, P. G. (2013). Abnormalities of the erythrocyte membrane. *Pediatr Clin N Am, 60,* 1349–1362.

36. Ideguchi, H., Yamada, Y., Kondo, S., et al. (1993). Abnormal erythrocyte band 4.1 protein in myelodysplastic syndrome with elliptocytosis. *Br J Haematol, 85,* 387–392.

37. Zaidi, A. U., Buck, S., Gadgeel, M., et al. (2020). Clinical diagnosis of red cell membrane disorders: comparison of osmotic gradient ektacytometry and eosin maleimide (EMA) fluorescence test for red cell band 3 (AE1, SLC4A1) content for clinical diagnosis. *Front Physiol, 11,* 636.

38. Mohandas, N., Winardi, R., Knowles, D., et al. (1992). Molecular basis for membrane rigidity of hereditary ovalocytosis. A novel mechanism involving the cytoplasmic domain of band 3. *J Clin Invest, 89,* 686–692.

39. Liu, S.-C., Zhai, S., Palek, J., et al. (1990). Molecular defect of the band 3 protein in Southeast Asian ovalocytosis. *N Engl J Med, 323,* 1530–1538.

40. Schofield, A. E., Tanner, M. J. A., Pinder, J. C., et al. (1992). Basis of unique red cell membrane properties in hereditary ovalocytosis. *J Mol Biol, 223,* 949–958.

41. Bruce, L. J. (2009). Hereditary stomatocytosis and cation leaky red cells—recent developments. *Blood Cells Mol Dis, 42,* 216–222.

42. Bruce, L. J., Guizouam, H., Burton, N. M., et al. (2009). The monovalent cation leak in overhydrated stomatocytic red blood cells results from amino acid substitutions in the Rh-associated glycoprotein. *Blood, 113,* 1350–1357.

43. Zarychanski, R., Schulz, V. P., Houston, B. L., et al. (2012). Mutations in the mechanotransduction protein PIEZO1 are associated with hereditary xerocytosis. *Blood, 120,* 1908–1915.

44. Bae, C., Gnanasambandam, R., Nicolai, C., et al. (2013). Xerocytosis is caused by mutations that alter the kinetics of the mechanosensitive channel PIEZO1. *Proc Natl Acad Sci USA, 110,* e1162–e1168.

45. Gallagher, P. G. (2017). Disorders of erythrocyte hydration. *Blood, 130,* 2699–2708.

46. Rampoldi, L., Danek, A., & Monaco, A. P. (2002). Clinical features and molecular bases of neuroacanthocytosis. *J Mol Med, 80,* 475–491.

47. Walker, R. H., Jung, H. H., Dobson-Stone, C., et al. (2007). Neurologic phenotypes associated with acanthocytosis. *Neurology, 68,* 92–98.

48. Parker, C. J. (2021). Paroxysmal nocturnal hemoglobinuria. In Kaushansky, K., Prchal, J. T., Burns, L. J., et al. (Eds.), *Williams Hematology.* (10th ed., pp. 625–638). New York: McGraw-Hill.

49. Besslar, M., & Hiken, J. (2008). The pathophysiology of disease in patients with paroxysmal nocturnal hemoglobinuria. *Hematol Am Soc Hematol Educ Progr,* 104–110.

50. Araten, D. J., & Brodsky, R. A. (2023). Paroxysmal nocturnal hemoglobinuria. In Hoffman, R., Benz, E. J., Silberstein, L. E., et al. (Eds.), *Hematology: Basic Principles and Practice*. (8th ed., pp. 416–430). Philadelphia: Elsevier.

51. Hill, A., DeZern, A. E., Kinoshita, T., et al. (2017). Paroxysmal nocturnal haemoglobinuria. *Nat Rev Dis Primers, 3*, 17028.

52. Parker, C., Omine, M., Richards, S., et al. (2005). Diagnosis and management of paroxysmal nocturnal hemoglobinuria. *Blood, 106*, 3699–3709.

53. Griffin, M., & Munir, T. (2017). Management of thrombosis in paroxysmal nocturnal hemoglobinuria: a clinician's guide. *Ther Adv Hematol, 8*(3), 119–126.

54. Sutherland, R. D., Keeney, M., & Illingworth, A. (2012). Practical guidelines for the high-sensitivity detection and monitoring of paroxysmal nocturnal hemoglobinuria clones by flow cytometry. *Cytometry Part B, 82B*, 195–208.

55. Preis, M., & Lowrey, C. H. (2014). Laboratory tests for paroxysmal nocturnal hemoglobinuria. *Am J Hematol, 89*, 339–341.

56. Sutherland, D. R., Kuek, N., Azcona-Olivera, J., et al. (2009). Use of FLAER-based WBC assay in the primary screening of PNH clones. *Am J Clin Pathol, 132*, 564–572.

57. Dmytrijuk, A., Robie-Suh, K., Cohen, M. H., et al. (2008). FDA report: eculizumab (Soliris) for the treatment of patients with paroxysmal nocturnal hemoglobinuria. *Oncologist, 13*, 993–1000.

58. Hillmen, P., Muus, P., Röth, A., et al. (2013). Long-term safety and efficacy of sustained eculizumab treatment in patients with paroxysmal nocturnal hemoglobinuria. *Br J Haematol, 162*, 62–73.

59. Risitano, A. M., Notaro, R., Pascariello, C., et al. (2012). The complement receptor 2/factor H fusion protein TT30 protects paroxysmal nocturnal hemoglobinuria erythrocytes from complement-mediated hemolysis and C3 fragment opsonization. *Blood, 119*, 6307–6316.

60. Gregg, X. T., & Prchal, J. T. (2023). Red blood cell enzymopathies. In Hoffman, R., Benz, E. J., Silberstein, L. E., et al. (Eds.), *Hematology: Basic Principles and Practice*. (8th ed., pp. 638–649). Philadelphia: Elsevier.

61. Luzzatto, L., Ally, M., & Notaro, R. (2020). Glucose-6-phosphate dehydrogenase deficiency. *Blood, 136*(11), 1225–1240.

62. Bartels, M., van Beers, E., & van Wijk, R. (2021). Erythrocyte enzyme disorders. In Kaushansky, K., Prchal, J. T., Burns, L. J., et al. (Eds.), *Williams Hematology*. (10th ed., pp. 749–784). New York: McGraw-Hill.

63. National Organization for Rare Disorders. (2017). Glucose-6-phosphate dehydrogenase deficiency. https://rarediseases.org/rare-diseases/glucose-6-phosphate-dehydrogenase-deficiency. Accessed June 24, 2022.

64. Luzzatto, L. (2006). Glucose 6-phosphate dehydrogenase deficiency: from genotype to phenotype. *Hematologica, 91*, 1303–1306.

65. Guindo, A., Fairhurst, R. M., Doumbo, O. K., et al. (2007). X-linked G6PD deficiency protects hemizygous males but not heterozygous females against severe malaria. *PLoS, 4*(3), e66.

66. Leslie, T., Briceno, M., Mayan, I., et al. (2010). The impact of phenotypic and genotypic G6PD deficiency on risk of *Plasmodium vivax* infection: a case-control study amongst Afghan refugees in Pakistan. *PLoS, 7*(5), e1000283.

67. Clark, I. A., & Hunt, N. H. (1983). Evidence for reactive oxygen intermediates causing hemolysis and parasite death in malaria. *Infect Immun, 39*, 1–6.

68. Cappadoro, M., Giribaldi, G., O'Brien, E., et al. (1998). Early phagocytosis of glucose-6-phosphate dehydrogenase (G6PD)-deficient erythrocytes parasitized by *Plasmodium falciparum* may explain malaria protection in G6PD deficiency. *Blood, 92*, 2527–2534.

69. Mbanefo, E. C., Ahmed, A. M., Titouna, A., et al. (2017). Association of glucose-6-phosphate dehydrogenase deficiency and malaria: a systematic review and meta-analysis. *Sci Rep, 7*, 45963.

70. Gómez-Manzo, S., Marcial-Quino, J., Vanoye-Carlo, A., et al. (2016). Glucose-6-phosphate dehydrogenase: update and analysis of new mutations around the world. *Int J Mol Sci, 17*(12), 2069.

71. Boonyuen, U., Chamchoy, K., Swangsri, T., et al. (2017). A trade off between catalytic activity and protein stability determines the clinical manifestations of glucose-6-phosphate dehydrogenase (G6PD) deficiency. *Int J Biol Macromol, 104*, 145–156.

72. Cunningham, A. D., Colavin, A., Huang, K. C., et al. (2017). Coupling between protein stability and catalytic activity determines pathogenicity of G6PD variants. *Cell Rep, 18*(11), 2592–2599.

73. Youngster, I., Arcavi, L., Schechmaster, R., et al. (2010). Medications and glucose-6-phosphate dehydrogenase deficiency: an evidence-based review. *Drug Saf, 33*, 713–726.

74. Luzzatto, L., & Seneca, E. (2014). G6PD deficiency: a classic example of pharmacogenetics with on-going clinical implications. *Br J Haematol, 164*, 469–480.

75. Kaplan, M., Muraca, M., Vreman, H. J., et al. (2005). Neonatal bilirubin production-conjugation imbalance: effect of glucose-6-phosphate dehydrogenase deficiency and borderline prematurity. *Arch Dis Child Fetal Neonatal Ed, 90*, F123–F127.

76. Prchal, J. T., & Gregg, X. T. (2005). Red cell enzymes. *Hematol Am Soc Hematol Educ Progr, 19*–23.

77. Minucci, A., Giardina, B., Zuppi, C., et al. (2009). Glucose-6-phosphate dehydrogenase laboratory assay: how, when, and why? *IUBMB Life, 61*, 27–34.

78. Tantular, I. S., & Kawamoto, F. (2003). An improved simple screening method for detection of glucose-6-phosphate dehydrogenase deficiency. *Trop Med Int Health, 8*, 569–574.

79. Tinley, K. E., Loughlin, A. M., Jepson, A., et al. (2010). Evaluation of a rapid qualitative enzyme chromatographic test for glucose-6-phosphate dehydrogenase deficiency. *Am J Trop Med Hyg, 82*, 210–214.

80. Secrest, M. H., Storm, M., Carrington, C., et al. (2020). Prevalence of pyruvate kinase deficiency: a systematic literature review. *Eur J Haematol, 105*(2), 173–184.

81. Canu, G., De Bonis, M., Minucci, A., et al. (2016). Red blood cell PK deficiency: an update of PK-LR gene mutation database. *Blood Cells Mol Dis, 57*, 100–109.

82. Rider, N. L., Strauss, K. A., Brown, K., et al. (2011). Erythrocyte pyruvate kinase deficiency in an old-order Amish cohort: longitudinal risk and disease management. *Am J Hematol, 86*, 827–834.

83. Christensen, R. D., Yaish, H. M., Johnson, C. B., et al. (2011). Six children with pyruvate kinase deficiency in one small town: molecular characterization of the PK-LR gene. *J Pediatr, 159*, 695–697.

84. van Wijk, R., & van Solinge, W. W. (2005). The energy-less red blood cell is lost: erythrocyte enzyme abnormalities of glycolysis. *Blood, 106*, 4034–4042.

85. Zanella, A., Fermo, E., Bianchi, P., et al. (2005). Red cell pyruvate kinase deficiency: molecular and clinical aspects. *Br J Haematol, 130*, 11–25.

86. Grace, R. F., & Barcellini, W. (2020). Management of pyruvate kinase deficiency in children and adults. *Blood, 136*(11), 1241–1249.

87. Tsang, S. S., & Feng, C. S. (1993). A modified screening procedure to detect pyruvate kinase deficiency. *Am J Clin Pathol, 99*, 128–131.

88. Zanella, A., Bianchi, P., Fermo, E., et al. (2006). Hereditary pyrimidine 5'-nucleotidase deficiency: from genetics to clinical manifestations. *Br J Haematol, 133*, 113–123.

89. Barasa, B., van Oirschot, B., Bianchi, P., et al. (2016). Proteomics reveals reduced expression of transketolase in pyrimidine 5'-nucleotidase deficient patients. *Proteomics Clin Appl, 10*(8), 859–869.

22

Extrinsic Defects Leading to Increased Erythrocyte Destruction—Nonimmune Causes

Catherine N. Otto[*]

OBJECTIVES

After completion of this chapter, the reader will be able to:

1. Describe the general pathophysiology and clinical laboratory findings in microangiopathic hemolytic anemia, including the characteristic red blood cell morphology.
2. Compare and contrast the pathophysiology, clinical symptoms, and typical laboratory findings in thrombotic thrombocytopenic purpura, hemolytic uremic syndrome, HELLP (*h*emolysis, *e*levated *l*iver enzymes, and *l*ow *p*latelet count) syndrome, and disseminated intravascular coagulation.
3. Explain the pathophysiology and typical laboratory features of traumatic cardiac hemolytic anemia and exercise-induced hemoglobinuria.
4. Explain the pathophysiologic mechanisms in *Plasmodium falciparum* infection that lead to anemia and neurologic manifestations.
5. Describe the pathophysiology, laboratory findings, and peripheral blood morphology in hemolytic anemia due to babesiosis, clostridial sepsis, bartonellosis, drugs, chemicals, venoms, and extensive burns.
6. Given the history, symptoms, laboratory findings, and a representative microscopic field from a peripheral blood film of a patient with suspected extrinsic nonimmune hemolytic anemia, discuss possible causes of the anemia and indicate the data that support the conclusions.

OUTLINE

Microangiopathic Hemolytic Anemia
    Thrombotic Thrombocytopenic Purpura
    Hemolytic Uremic Syndrome
    HELLP Syndrome
    Disseminated Intravascular Coagulation
Macroangiopathic Hemolytic Anemia
    Traumatic Cardiac Hemolytic Anemia
    Exercise-Induced Hemoglobinuria
Hemolytic Anemia Caused by Infectious Agents

    Malaria
    Babesiosis
    Clostridial Sepsis
    Bartonellosis
Hemolytic Anemia Caused by Other Red Blood Cell Injury
    Drugs and Chemicals
    Venoms
    Extensive Burns (Thermal Injuries)

CASE STUDY

After studying the material in this chapter, the reader should be able to respond to the following case study. Answers can be found in Appendix C.

A 24-year-old patient was brought to the emergency department with a 2-day history of fever, chills, excessive sweating, nausea, and general malaise. Because the patient had recently returned from a 3-week family trip to Ghana in Western Africa, the treating provider ordered a CBC and examination of thin and thick peripheral blood films. The following were the patient's laboratory results. Reference intervals can be found after the Index at the end of the book.

WBC	11.0×10^9/L	MCV	92 fL
HGB	8.7 g/dL	PLT	176 $\times 10^9$/L
HCT	22%		

Inclusions were noted on the thin and thick peripheral blood films (Figures 22.1 and 22.2).

Based on the results of the CBC and peripheral blood films, the patient was treated with oral quinine sulfate and doxycycline.

1. Identify the inclusions present on the thin and thick peripheral blood films.
2. What is the likely diagnosis for this patient?
3. What clues in the history support this diagnosis?
4. What are the pathophysiologic mechanisms for the anemia in this disease?

Continued

[*]The author extends appreciation to Elaine M. Keohane, whose work in prior editions provided the foundation for this chapter.

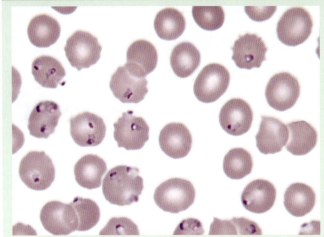

Figure 22.1 Thin Peripheral Blood Film for the Patient in the Case Study. (Wright-Giemsa stain, ×1000.)

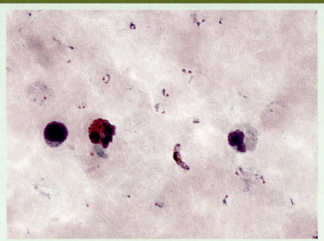

Figure 22.2 Thick Peripheral Blood Film for the Patient in the Case Study. (Wright-Giemsa stain, ×1000.) (Courtesy Linda Marler, Indiana Pathology Images, Indianapolis, IN.)

Extrinsic hemolytic anemias comprise a diverse group of disorders in which red blood cells (RBCs) are structurally and functionally normal, but a condition outside of the RBCs causes premature hemolysis. The extrinsic hemolytic anemias can be divided into conditions with nonimmune and immune causes. A common feature in the nonimmune extrinsic hemolytic anemias is the presence of a condition that causes physical or mechanical injury to the RBCs. This injury can be caused by abnormalities in the microvasculature (microangiopathic) or the heart and large blood vessels (macroangiopathic), infectious agents, chemicals, drugs, venoms, or extensive burns. The nonimmune disorders causing hemolytic anemia are discussed in this chapter and are summarized in Box 22.1. In immune hemolytic anemia, hemolysis is mediated by antibodies, complement, or both, and these conditions are covered in Chapter 23.

Examination of a peripheral blood film is important in suspected extrinsic hemolytic anemias because observation of abnormal RBC morphology, such as schistocytes, spherocytes, or the presence of intracellular organisms, provides an important clue to the diagnosis.

MICROANGIOPATHIC HEMOLYTIC ANEMIA

Microangiopathic hemolytic anemias (MAHAs) are a group of potentially life-threatening disorders characterized by RBC fragmentation and thrombocytopenia. The RBC fragmentation occurs intravascularly by mechanical shearing of RBC membranes as the cells rapidly pass through turbulent areas of small blood vessels that are partially blocked by microthrombi or damaged endothelium.[1,2] Upon shearing, RBC membranes quickly reseal with minimal escape of hemoglobin, but the resulting fragments (called *schistocytes*) are distorted and become rigid.[1] The spleen clears the rigid RBC fragments from the circulation through the extravascular hemolytic process (Chapter 20).[1]

Laboratory evidence of hemolytic anemias includes a decreased hemoglobin level, increased reticulocyte count, increased serum indirect (unconjugated) bilirubin, increased serum lactate dehydrogenase (LDH) activity, decreased serum haptoglobin level, and increased urine urobilinogen. In some cases, the fragmentation is so

severe that intravascular hemolysis occurs, with varying amounts of hemoglobinemia, hemoglobinuria, and markedly decreased levels of serum haptoglobin.[1] The presence of schistocytes on the peripheral blood film is a characteristic feature of microangiopathic hemolytic anemia. RBC shearing may also produce helmet cells and occasionally, microspherocytes. Polychromasia and nucleated RBCs may also be present on the peripheral blood film, depending on the severity of the anemia.

Thrombocytopenia is also a feature of microangiopathic hemolytic anemia due to the consumption of platelets in thrombi that form in the microvasculature.[3] Thus these disorders are sometimes called *thrombotic microangiopathies.*[4,5]

The major microangiopathic hemolytic anemias include thrombotic thrombocytopenic purpura (TTP), hemolytic uremic syndrome (HUS), HELLP (*h*emolysis, *e*levated *l*iver enzymes, *l*ow *p*latelet count) syndrome, and disseminated intravascular coagulation (DIC).[1,4,5] TTP and HUS can be difficult to differentiate because they have overlapping clinical and laboratory findings (Box 22.2). Definitive diagnosis, however, is critical because they have different etiologies and require different treatments.[3] This chapter provides an overview of these conditions. TTP, HUS, and HELLP syndrome are covered in more detail in Chapter 38. DIC is covered in more detail in Chapter 39.

Thrombotic Thrombocytopenic Purpura

TTP is a rare, life-threatening disorder characterized by the abrupt appearance of microangiopathic hemolytic anemia, severe thrombocytopenia, and markedly elevated serum LDH activity.[2,6] Neurologic dysfunction, fever, and renal failure may also occur, but they are not consistently present.[2,6] TTP is most commonly found in adults in their fourth decade, but it can manifest at any age.[5,6] There is a higher incidence in females than in males.[5]

TTP is caused by a deficiency of the von Willebrand factor (VWF)-cleaving protease ADAMTS13 (*a d*isintegrin *a*nd *m*etalloprotease with a *t*hrombo*s*pondin type 1 motif, member *13*).[6-9] ADAMTS13 regulates the size of circulating VWF by cleaving ultralong VWF (ULVWF) multimers into shorter segments that have less hemostatic potential.[6,10] VWF multimers circulate in a folded conformation so that their cleavage sites for ADAMTS13 (in the A2 domain) and binding sites for platelets (GP Ibα receptor in the A1 domain) are hidden.[5,6,10] These sites normally become accessible only when the ULVWF multimer is "unrolled or stretched out," which occurs (1) during its release from endothelial cells, (2) during passage through small blood

vessels with very high shear forces, or (3) after binding to collagen in the subendothelium after vascular injury (Chapters 36 and 38).[5,6,10] Once unrolled, ADAMTS13 binds to the cleavage sites on the ULVWF multimers and cuts them into smaller multimers.[6,10] Thus ADAMTS13 serves an important antithrombotic function by preventing VWF from excessively binding and activating platelets.[6]

When ADAMTS13 is deficient, however, the hyperreactive ULVWF multimers adhere to the endothelial cells of the microvasculature, where they readily unroll as a result of hydrodynamic shear forces.[5-7,10] Platelets are then able to bind to A1 domains of ULVWF multimers, and platelet aggregation is triggered.[5,6] Platelet-VWF microthrombi accumulate in and block small blood vessels, leading to severe thrombocytopenia; ischemia in the brain, kidney, and other organs; and hemolytic anemia due to RBC rupture as they pass through blood vessels partially blocked by microthrombi.[2,3,7] Intravascular hemolysis along with extensive tissue ischemia result in a striking increase in serum LDH activity that is characteristic of TTP.[5]

TTP can be idiopathic, secondary, or inherited. Idiopathic TTP has no known precipitating event.[5,6] In idiopathic TTP, autoantibodies to ADAMTS13 inhibit its activity, causing a severe deficiency.[5,8,9] These autoantibodies are usually of the immunoglobulin G (IgG) class but can be IgM or IgA.

Secondary TTP can be triggered by infections, pregnancy, surgery, trauma, inflammation, and disseminated malignancy, possibly by depressing the synthesis of ADAMTS13.[3,5] Other conditions may induce an inhibitory reaction to ADAMTS13, including hematopoietic stem cell transplantation; autoimmune disorders; human immunodeficiency virus (HIV); and certain drugs, such as quinine and trimethoprim.[3-6,11] Secondary TTP is heterogeneous, and the mechanisms that trigger TTP pathophysiology are not completely clear.[3]

Inherited TTP, also called Upshaw-Schulman syndrome, is a severe ADAMTS13 deficiency caused by mutations in the *ADAMTS13* gene.[5,6,12] More than 75 different mutations have been identified, and symptomatic individuals are either homozygous for one of the mutations or compound heterozygous for two different mutations.[5,12,13] Inherited TTP may manifest in infancy or childhood, with recurrent episodes throughout life; however, some patients may not be symptomatic until adulthood after their system is stressed by pregnancy or a severe infection.

Typical initial laboratory findings in all types of TTP include a hemoglobin level of 8 to 10 g/dL, a platelet count of 10 to 30 $\times 10^9$/L, and schistocytes on the peripheral blood film (Figure 22.3).[6] After the bone marrow begins to respond to the anemia, polychromasia and nucleated RBCs may also be present on the peripheral blood film. The white blood cell (WBC) count is often increased, and immature granulocytes may appear. The bone marrow shows erythroid hyperplasia and a normal number of megakaryocytes. Hemoglobinuria occurs when there is extensive intravascular hemolysis. Various amounts of protein, RBCs, and urinary casts may also be present in the urine, depending on the extent of the renal damage. Results of hemostasis tests are usually within the reference interval, which differentiates TTP

BOX 22.2 Laboratory Findings in Thrombocytopenic Purpura and Hemolytic Uremic Syndrome

Hematologic
Decreased hemoglobin
Decreased platelets
Increased reticulocyte count

Peripheral Blood Film
Schistocytes
Polychromasia
Nucleated red blood cells (severe cases)

Biochemical
Markedly increased lactate dehydrogenase activity*
Increased serum total and indirect bilirubin
Decreased serum haptoglobin level
Hemoglobinemia
Hemoglobinuria
Proteinuria, hematuria, casts†

*From systemic ischemia and hemolysis; more commonly found in thrombotic thrombocytopenic purpura.
†From acute renal failure; more commonly found in hemolytic uremic syndrome.

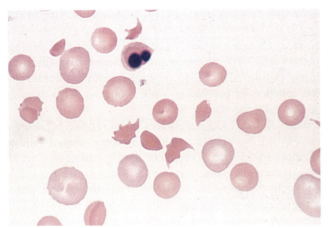

Figure 22.3 Peripheral Blood Film From a Patient With Thrombotic Thrombocytopenic Purpura. Note the schistocytes and a nucleated red blood cell. (Wright-Giemsa stain, ×1000.)

from DIC. An elevation of serum indirect bilirubin level does not occur for several days after an acute onset of hemolysis, but serum LDH activity will be markedly elevated, and the serum haptoglobin level will be reduced.

In idiopathic and inherited TTP, ADAMTS13 activity is usually severely reduced to less than 5% to 10% of normal.[4,6,7] In secondary TTP, the ADAMTS13 deficiency is not as severe. ADAMTS13 autoantibodies can be detected in idiopathic TTP but are absent in inherited TTP.[6]

Approximately 80% to 90% of patients with idiopathic TTP respond favorably to plasma exchange therapy due to the removal of the offending ADAMTS13 autoantibody and infusion of replacement ADAMTS13 enzyme from donor plasma.[6,11] Therefore it is important that this type of TTP be recognized and quickly treated with plasma exchange therapy to avoid a fatal outcome. Corticosteroids are also administered to suppress the autoimmune response.[5,6] Approximately one-third of patients who respond to plasma exchange experience recurrent episodes of TTP.[4] Rituximab (anti-CD20) is effective in suppressing an autoantibody response in some patients with relapsing TTP.[6] Patients with secondary TTP generally do not respond well to plasma exchange, and the prognosis in these cases is poor except when the TTP is related to autoimmune disease, pregnancy, or ticlopidine use.[11,13] Plasma exchange is not required in inherited TTP, which is treated by infusion of fresh frozen plasma to supply the deficient ADAMTS13 enzyme.[3,4,6]

Hemolytic Uremic Syndrome

HUS is characterized by microangiopathic hemolytic anemia, thrombocytopenia, and acute renal failure from damage to endothelial cells in the glomerular microvasculature.[3,5] There are two general types: typical and atypical HUS. Typical HUS (Shiga toxin-associated HUS [Stx-HUS]) is caused by bacteria that produce Shiga toxin and is preceded by an episode of acute gastroenteritis, often with bloody diarrhea.[5] Atypical HUS (aHUS) is caused by unregulated activation of the alternative complement pathway.[3,5] Patients with HUS have the typical laboratory findings of microangiopathic hemolytic anemia. However, the platelet count is only mildly to moderately

decreased, and evidence of renal failure is usually present, including an elevated level of serum creatinine, proteinuria, hematuria, and the presence of hyaline, granular, and RBC casts in the urine (see Box 22.2).

Stx-HUS type comprises 90% of cases of HUS.[5,14] The most common cause is infection with Shiga-like toxin-1-producing *Escherichia coli* (STEC), such as serotype O157:H7, but strains of toxin-producing *Shigella* have also been implicated.[4,5] Stx-HUS occurs most often in young children but can be found in patients of all ages. Patients initially have acute gastroenteritis, often with bloody diarrhea, and after approximately 5 to 13 days, develop oliguria and other symptoms of renal damage.[5] About one-fourth of patients also develop neurologic manifestations.[5,14]

E. coli and *Shigella* serotypes implicated in HUS release Shiga toxins (Stx-1 and Stx-2, also called *verotoxins*) that are absorbed from the intestines into the plasma. The toxins have an affinity for the Gb3 glycolipid receptors (CD77) on endothelial cells, particularly receptors in the glomerulus and brain.[4,5,15] The toxin is transported into the endothelial cells, where it inhibits protein synthesis and causes endothelial cell injury and eventual apoptosis.[5,15] Shiga toxin, together with many cytokines secreted as a result of the infection, also induces changes in endothelial cells that are prothrombotic, including expression of tissue factor, adhesion molecules, and secretion of increased amounts of ULVWF multimers.[4,5,15] Endothelial cell damage can cause stenosis (narrowing) of small blood vessels, which can be exacerbated by the activation of platelets and formation of platelet-fibrin thrombi.[3,5,15] The resultant blockages in the microvasculature of the glomeruli result in acute renal failure.[3,15] Endothelial damage and microthrombi can also occur in the microvasculature of the brain and other organs.[3,5] There is no specific treatment for Stx-HUS; patients are provided supportive care as needed, including hydration, dialysis, and transfusions.[14,15] Symptoms usually resolve spontaneously in 1 to 3 weeks, and the prognosis is favorable for most patients.[14]

aHUS comprises about 10% of cases of HUS and can first manifest in infancy, childhood, or adulthood.[5,16] The characteristic feature is uncontrolled activation of the alternative complement system, which causes endothelial cell injury, activation of platelets and coagulation factors, and formation of platelet-fibrin thrombi that obstruct the microvasculature in the glomerulus and other organs.[3,5] Approximately 50% to 70% of patients with aHUS have inherited mutations in genes that code for components of the alternative complement pathway or its regulatory proteins.[5,16] Inactivating mutations have been identified in genes for complement regulatory proteins, including complement factor H, complement factor I, membrane cofactor protein, and thrombomodulin.[3,5,16] Activating mutations have been identified in the genes for complement factors B and C3.[3,5,16] An acquired form of aHUS is associated with autoantibodies to complement factor H and accounts for approximately 5% to 10% of cases.[5] In the remaining cases, no mutation or autoantibodies have been identified.[5] aHUS may be triggered by hematopoietic stem cell therapy, pregnancy, infection, inflammation, surgery, or trauma.[3] Plasma exchange and plasma infusion have limited efficacy in aHUS.[5,16] In recent studies, therapy with eculizumab (antibody to C5) has improved platelet counts and renal function in patients with aHUS and may become the therapy of choice.[16]

Differential diagnosis of aHUS and TTP is difficult due to the similarities in their clinical presentation and initial laboratory findings (Chapter 38). Both are life-threatening disorders that require rapid action to prevent a fatal outcome; plasma exchange is most beneficial for TTP, and eculizumab is more likely to benefit patients with aHUS.[5,16] Assays for ADAMTS13 activity, ADAMTS13 inhibitors, and anti-ADAMTS13 antibodies are available and typically performed in a reflex algorithm. Current assays lack optimization and standardization; they are commonly performed only in reference laboratories. DNA analysis for complement system gene mutations is available in specialized laboratories, but the results are not timely enough to be used in initial therapy decisions.[16] More sensitive, specific, and rapid tests are needed for definitive diagnosis of these two conditions.

HELLP Syndrome

HELLP syndrome, a serious complication in pregnancy, is named for its characteristic presentation of *h*emolysis, *e*levated *l*iver enzymes, and *l*ow *p*latelet count. It occurs in approximately 0.5% to 0.9% of all pregnancies but develops in approximately 4% to 12% of pregnancies with preeclampsia and 30% to 50% of pregnancies with eclampsia, most often in the third trimester.[17,18] In preeclampsia, abnormalities in the development of placental vasculature result in poor perfusion and hypoxia. As a result, antiangiogenic proteins such as soluble vascular endothelial growth factor receptor-1 (sVEGFR-1) are released from the placenta, which bind to and inactivate placental and endothelial growth factors.[18] Continued vascular insufficiency of the placenta results in maternal endothelial cell dysfunction, which leads to platelet activation and fibrin deposition in the microvasculature, particularly in the liver.[18]

Anemia, biochemical evidence of hemolysis, and schistocytes on the peripheral blood film are found as in other microangiopathies. A low platelet count and increased serum LDH and aspartate aminotransferase (AST) activity are major diagnostic criteria for HELLP syndrome and are used to assess the severity of the disease (Chapter 38).[17,18] The platelet count, in conjunction with LDH and AST levels, serves as a predictor of maternal morbidity and mortality, with the platelet count serving as differentiation among the three risk categories.[18,19] Patients with platelet counts less than 50×10^9/L have the greatest risk of bleeding and have a greater incidence of morbidity and mortality.[18,19] Patients with platelet counts between 50 and 100×10^9/L have a moderate risk of bleeding, and patients with a platelet count greater than 100×10^9/L do not have a risk of bleeding.[18,19] Serum LDH activity is elevated, which reflects hepatic necrosis and hemolysis. Serum AST can be markedly elevated due to severe hepatocyte injury. The prothrombin time and partial thromboplastin time are within reference intervals, which distinguishes HELLP syndrome from DIC. Therapy includes delivery of the fetus and placenta as soon as possible, along with supportive care to control electrolytes, fluid balance, and hypertension and prevent seizures.[18,19]

The mortality rate is 3% to 5% for the mother and 9% to 24% for the fetus.[18]

Disseminated Intravascular Coagulation

DIC is characterized by the widespread activation of the hemostatic system resulting in fibrin thrombi formation throughout the microvasculature. Major clinical manifestations are organ damage due to obstruction of the microvasculature and bleeding due to the consumption of platelets and coagulation factors and secondary activation of fibrinolysis. DIC is a complication of many disorders, such as metastatic cancers, acute leukemias, infections, obstetric complications, crush or brain injuries, acute hemolytic transfusion reactions, extensive burns, snake or spider envenomation, and chronic inflammation (Table 39.6).

Thrombocytopenia of varying degrees is a consistent finding. Approximately half of patients have schistocytes on the peripheral blood film; however, this finding is not required for a DIC diagnosis.[20] The prothrombin time and partial thromboplastin time are prolonged, the fibrinogen level is decreased, and the D-dimer level is increased in DIC, all of which distinguish it from the other microangiopathies. Tables 39.7 and 39.8 contain the primary and specialized tests used in the diagnosis of DIC.

MACROANGIOPATHIC HEMOLYTIC ANEMIA

Traumatic Cardiac Hemolytic Anemia

Mechanical hemolysis can occur in patients with prosthetic cardiac valves due to the turbulent blood flow through and around the implanted devices.[18,21] Hemolysis is usually mild, and anemia does not generally develop due to compensation by the bone marrow.[21] Severe hemolysis is rare and is usually due to paravalvular leaks in prosthetic cardiac valves.[21] Hemolysis can also occur in patients with cardiac valve disease before corrective surgery.[18] The anemia that occurs in severe cases is usually normocytic but can be microcytic if iron deficiency develops due to chronic urinary hemoglobin loss.

Depending on the severity of the hemolysis and the ability of the bone marrow to compensate for the reduced RBC life span, patients can be asymptomatic or present with pallor, fatigue, and even heart failure.[21] Schistocytes are a characteristic feature found on the peripheral blood film due to mechanical fragmentation of the RBCs (Figure 22.4). The reticulocyte count is increased, but the platelet count is within the reference interval. Serum LDH activity and levels of serum indirect bilirubin and plasma hemoglobin are elevated, and the serum haptoglobin level is decreased. Hemoglobinuria may be observed in severe hemolysis. Hemosiderinuria and a decreased level of serum ferritin occur with chronic hemoglobinuria due to the urinary loss of iron.

Surgical repair or replacement of the prosthesis may be required if the anemia is severe enough to require transfusions. For patients with hemoglobinuria, iron supplementation is provided to replace urinary iron loss. Folic acid may also be required because deficiencies can occur due to the increased erythropoietic activity in the bone marrow.[21]

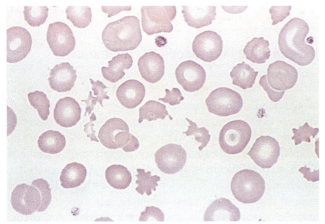

Figure 22.4 Peripheral Blood Film from a Patient with Traumatic Cardiac Hemolytic Anemia. *Note the presence of schistocytes.* (Wright-Giemsa stain, ×1000.)

Exercise-Induced Hemoglobinuria

RBC lysis, with an increase in free plasma hemoglobin and a decrease in the serum haptoglobin level, has been demonstrated in some individuals after long-distance running and, to a lesser extent, after intensive cycling and swimming[1,22–24]; however, frank hemoglobinuria after exercise is a rare occurrence.[25] Exercise-induced hemoglobinuria has been reported mainly in endurance runners but has also been observed after strenuous hand drumming.[22,26] Various causes have been proposed, including mechanical trauma from the forceful, repeated impact of the feet or hands on hard surfaces[22,23,26]; increased RBC susceptibility to oxidative stress[27]; and exercise-induced alterations in membrane cytoskeletal proteins.[28,29]

Exercise-induced hemoglobinuria does not usually cause anemia unless the hemoglobinuria is particularly severe and recurrent.[1,25] Laboratory findings include a decreased level of serum haptoglobin, an elevated level of free plasma hemoglobin, and hemoglobinuria observed after strenuous exercise. Patients also have a slight increase in mean cell volume (MCV) and reticulocyte count. Schistocytes are not present on the peripheral blood film except in rare cases.[25,26] Exercise-induced hemoglobinuria is a diagnosis of exclusion, and other possible causes of hemolysis and hemoglobinuria should be investigated and ruled out.[25] There is no treatment for the disorder other than minimizing the physical impact on the feet with padding in shoes, running on softer terrain, or, if hemolysis is severe, discontinuing the activity.

HEMOLYTIC ANEMIA CAUSED BY INFECTIOUS AGENTS

Malaria

Malaria is a potentially fatal condition caused by infection of RBCs with protozoan parasites of the genus *Plasmodium*. Most human infections are caused by *P. falciparum* and *P. vivax*, but *P. ovale*, *P. malariae*, and a fifth species, *P. knowlesi*, also infect humans.[30]

Prevalence

Approximately 3.4 billion people live in areas in which malaria is endemic and are at risk for the disease.[30] Worldwide in 2021, there were an estimated 247 million cases of malaria, with 619,000 deaths, mostly in children younger than 5 years of age.[30] The majority of deaths were in Africa (91%), followed by Southeast Asia (6%) and the Eastern Mediterranean region (2%).[30] The World Health Organization is coordinating a major global effort to control and eliminate malaria. These efforts include implementation of indoor chemical spraying, distribution of millions of insecticide-treated sleeping nets in high-risk areas, and promotion of policies for appropriate treatment in regions of endemic disease.[30]

Approximately 2000 cases of malaria are diagnosed annually in the United States, with a majority of the cases associated with travel to a malaria-endemic country.[31] *P. falciparum* and *P. vivax* cause most of the infections seen in the United States.

Pathogenesis

If an individual is bitten by an infected mosquito, the clinical outcome may be (1) no infection, (2) *asymptomatic parasitemia* (the patient has no symptoms, but parasites are present in the blood), (3) *uncomplicated malaria* (the patient has symptoms and parasitemia but no organ dysfunction), or (4) *severe malaria* (the patient has symptoms, parasitemia, and major organ dysfunction).[31,32] The clinical outcome depends on parasite factors (species, number of sporozoites injected, multiplication rate, virulence, and drug resistance), host factors (age, pregnancy status, immune status, previous exposure, genetic polymorphisms, nutrition status, coinfection with other pathogens, and duration of infection), geographic and social factors (endemicity, poverty, and availability of prompt and effective treatment), and other as yet unknown factors.[30]

In areas of high *Plasmodium* transmission, most individuals develop immunity, and major risk groups for severe malaria are children younger than 5 years of age and women in their first pregnancy.[33] Even in these risk groups, severe malaria is infrequent.[32] On the other hand, immunity is low or nonexistent in individuals living in regions with low *Plasmodium* transmission and in travelers to regions where malaria is endemic, so all age groups are at risk for severe malaria.[33] Most cases of severe malaria are due to *P. falciparum*; however, *P. vivax* and *P. knowlesi* can also cause severe disease.[30,31,33] Infection with *P. malariae* or *P. ovale*, however, is usually uncomplicated and benign. Hyperparasitemia, defined as greater than 2% to 5% of the total RBCs parasitized, is usually present in severe malaria.[33] Major complications of severe malaria include respiratory distress syndrome, metabolic acidosis, circulatory shock, renal failure, hepatic failure, hypoglycemia, severe anemia (defined as a hemoglobin level below 5 g/dL),[33] poor pregnancy outcome, and cerebral malaria.[33] Even with treatment the fatality rate of severe malaria is 10% to 20%.[33]

Causes of anemia in malaria include direct lysis of infected RBCs during schizogony, immune destruction of infected and noninfected RBCs in the spleen, and inhibition of erythropoiesis and ineffective erythropoiesis.[32] Destruction of noninfected RBCs contributes significantly to the anemia. RBCs have increased surface immunoglobulins and complement, thus enhancing their removal by the spleen.[32]

Malaria parasites metabolize hemoglobin, forming toxic hemozoin, or malaria pigment. When RBCs lyse in schizogony, the hemozoin and other toxic metabolites are released, which results in an inflammatory response, a cytokine imbalance, and macrophage-phagocytizing RBCs.[32]

Clinical and Laboratory Findings

The clinical symptoms of malaria are variable and can include fever, chills, rigors, sweating, headache, muscle pain, nausea, and diarrhea. In severe malaria, jaundice, splenomegaly, hepatomegaly, shock, prostration, bleeding, seizures, or coma may occur.[33] In patients with chronic malaria or with repeated malarial infections, the spleen may be massively enlarged.

During fevers, the WBC count is normal to slightly increased; however, neutropenia may develop during chills and rigors. In chronic malaria with anemia, the reticulocyte count is decreased due to the negative effect of inflammation on erythropoiesis. In severe malaria, one or more of the following laboratory features are found: metabolic acidosis, decreased serum glucose (less than 40 mg/dL), increased serum lactate, increased serum creatinine, decreased hemoglobin level (less than 5 g/dL), hemoglobinuria, and hyperparasitemia.[33]

Microscopic Examination

Malarial infection can be diagnosed microscopically by demonstration of the parasites in the peripheral blood.[34] Identification of malaria and its species is customarily performed in clinical microbiology. Often, malarial parasites are discovered during a review of the peripheral blood film as a component of the complete blood count (CBC) and manual differential. In the hematology laboratory, however, it is important to recognize the presence of intracellular organisms (bacteria, malaria, and other parasites) to ensure rapid diagnosis and treatment of these infections. Malarial parasite detection and species identification require specific expertise and experience. A platelet lying on top of an erythrocyte during the differential examination may be confused with a malarial parasite by an inexperienced observer (Figure 22.5).

Plasmodium species. P. vivax is widely distributed and causes 40% of human malaria cases worldwide (Figures 22.6 and 22.7).[33] It is the predominant species in Asia and South and Central America, but it also occurs in Southeast Asia, Oceania, and the Middle East.[30] It is rare in Africa and virtually absent in West Africa.[30]

P. ovale is found mainly in West Africa and India (Figure 22.8).[30]

P. malariae is found worldwide, but at low frequency (Figure 22.9). The highest prevalence is in East Africa and India.[30]

P. falciparum is the predominant species in sub-Saharan Africa, Saudi Arabia, Haiti, and the Dominican Republic (22.10; see Figure 22.1).[30] It is also found in Asia, Southeast Asia, the Philippines, Indonesia, and South America.[30] P. falciparum can produce high parasitemia (greater than 50% of RBCs infected) due to its ability to invade RBCs of all ages.

P. knowlesi is widespread in Malaysia. Cases have been reported in Myanmar, the Philippines, and Thailand (Figure 22.11).[30]

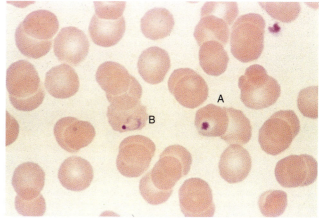

Figure 22.5 Peripheral Blood Film With a Platelet on Top of a Red Blood Cell *(A)* Compared with an Intraerythrocytic *Plasmodium vivax* Ring Form *(B)*. (Wright-Giemsa stain, ×1000.)

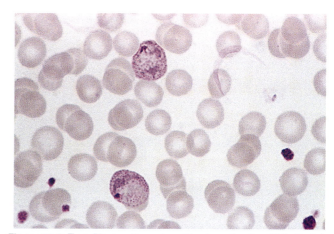

Figure 22.6 Two *Plasmodium vivax* Trophozoites in a Thin Peripheral Blood Film. Note that the infected red blood cells are enlarged and contain Schüffner stippling, and the trophozoites are large and ameboid in appearance. (Wright-Giemsa stain, ×1000.)

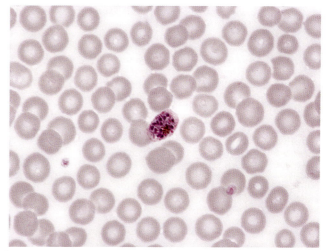

Figure 22.7 *Plasmodium vivax* Schizont in a Thin Peripheral Blood Film. Note the number of merozoites and the presence of brown hemozoin pigment. (Wright-Giemsa stain, ×1000.) (Courtesy Linda Marler, Indiana Pathology Images, Indianapolis, IN.)

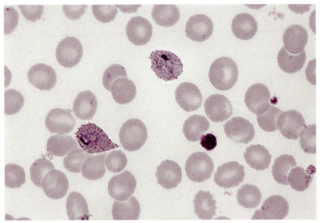

Figure 22.8 Two *Plasmodium ovale* Trophozoites in a Thin Peripheral Blood Film. Note that the infected cells are enlarged, oval, have fringed edges, and contain Schüffner stippling. (Wright-Giemsa stain, ×1000.) (Courtesy Linda Marler, Indiana Pathology Images, Indianapolis, IN.)

Babesiosis

Babesiosis is a tick-transmitted disease caused by intraerythrocytic protozoan parasites of the genus *Babesia*. There are hundreds of species of *Babesia*; a few are known to cause disease in humans. *B. microti* is the most common cause of babesiosis in the United States, where it was originally called *Nantucket fever* because the first cluster of cases was found on Nantucket Island, off Massachusetts, in 1969 and the early 1970s.[35,36] The sexual cycle of *B. microti* occurs in the tick *Ixodes scapularis*, whereas its asexual cycle primarily occurs in the white-footed mouse, the reservoir host in the United States.[37] Humans are incidental hosts and become infected after injection of sporozoites during a blood meal by infected ticks. Other *Babesia* species, such as *B. duncani* and *B. divergens*, can be found sporadically in humans.[36-38] Babesia may also be transmitted by transfusion of RBCs from asymptomatic donors.[37,38]

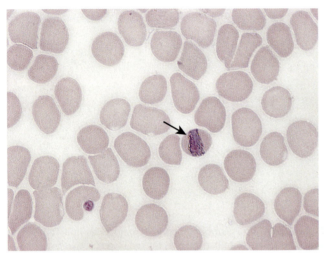

Figure 22.9 *Plasmodium malariae* Band Form *(arrow)* in a Thin Peripheral Blood Film. (Wright-Giemsa stain, ×1000.) (Courtesy Linda Marler, Indiana Pathology Images, Indianapolis, IN.)

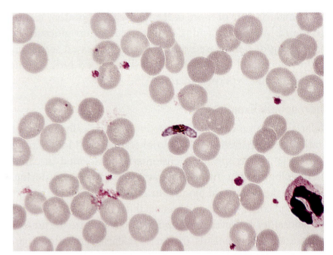

Figure 22.10 *Plasmodium falciparum* Crescent-Shaped Gametocyte in a Thin Peripheral Blood Film. (Wright-Giemsa stain, ×1000.) (Courtesy Linda Marler, Indiana Pathology Images, Indianapolis, IN.)

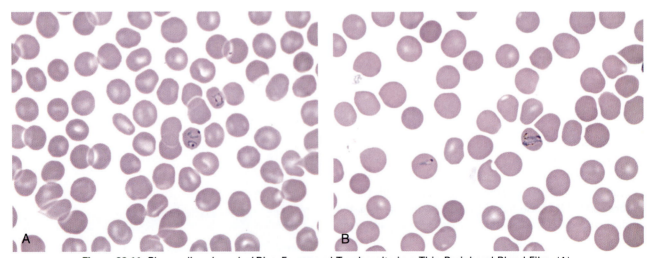

Figure 22.11 *Plasmodium knowlesi* Ring Forms and Trophozoite in a Thin Peripheral Blood Film. (A), Ring forms. (B), Ring form and trophozoite. (Wright-Giemsa stain, ×1000.) (Courtesy Wadsworth Center Laboratories, New York State Department of Health, New York, NY.)

Geographic Distribution

The areas in which *B. microti* is endemic in the United States are southern New England, New York State, New Jersey, Wisconsin, and Minnesota.[36-38] *B. duncani* occurs along the Pacific Coast (northern California to Washington); *B. divergens*-like organisms are found in Missouri, Kentucky, and Washington State; and *B. divergens* and *B. venatorum* occur in Europe.[36,38,39] Isolated cases of babesiosis have also been reported in Asia, Africa, Australia, and South America.[36,39]

Clinical Findings

The incubation period for *B. microti* infection ranges from 1 to 9 weeks.[36] Infection is asymptomatic in perhaps one-third of individuals, so the exact prevalence is unknown.[36,40] In other individuals, *B. microti* causes a mild to severe hemolytic anemia.[36,37] The patient usually experiences fever and nonrespiratory flulike symptoms, including chills, headache, sweats, nausea, arthralgias, myalgias, anorexia, and fatigue, which last from several weeks to months. Jaundice, splenomegaly, or hepatomegaly may be present. Some individuals progress to severe, life-threatening disease due to acute respiratory failure, congestive heart failure, renal shutdown, liver failure, central nervous system involvement, or DIC. Severe disease may occur at any age, but it is more common in individuals older than 50 years of age.[1,36] Immune deficiency due to asplenia, malignancy, immunosuppressive drugs, or HIV infection increases the risk of severe disease.[1,36,37]

Laboratory Findings and Diagnosis

Evidence of hemolytic anemia is usually present in symptomatic infection, including a decreased hemoglobin level, an increased reticulocyte count, a decreased serum haptoglobin level, and bilirubinemia. Leukopenia, thrombocytopenia, hemoglobinuria, and proteinuria may also be present, along with abnormal renal and liver function test results.[36]

The diagnosis of babesiosis is made by demonstration of the parasite on Wright-Giemsa-stained thin peripheral blood films in the clinical microbiology laboratory (Figures 22.12 and 22.13). Parasitemia may be low (<1% of RBCs affected) in early infections, but as many as 80% of RBCs may be infected in asplenic patients.[41] Definitive species identification requires polymerase chain reaction-based methods.[36,37]

Clostridial Sepsis

Sepsis with massive intravascular hemolysis, which is often fatal, is a rare complication of infection with *Clostridium perfringens*, an anaerobic gram-positive bacillus. *C. perfringens* grows very rapidly (7-minute doubling time) and produces an α-toxin with phospholipase C and sphingomyelinase activity that hydrolyzes RBC membrane phospholipids.[42] RBCs become spherical and extremely susceptible to osmotic lysis, which results in sudden, massive hemolysis and dark red plasma and urine.[1,42,43] The hematocrit may drop to below 10%.[1,43] Intravascular hemolysis can trigger DIC and renal failure. Spherocytes, microspherocytes, and toxic changes to neutrophils can be observed on a peripheral blood film.[1,42,43] Some conditions that increase the risk of clostridial sepsis and hemolytic anemia include malignancies (genitourinary, gastrointestinal, and hematologic), solid

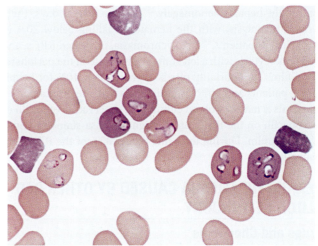

Figure 22.12 *Babesia microti* Ring Forms in a Peripheral Blood Film. Note the varying appearance of the ring forms and the presence of multiple ring forms in individual red blood cells. (Wright-Giemsa stain, ×1000.)

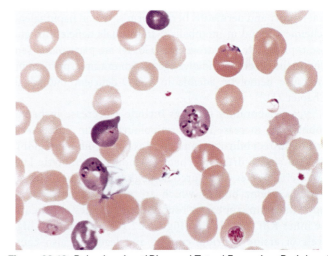

Figure 22.13 *Babesia microti* Ring and Tetrad Forms in a Peripheral Blood Film. (Wright-Giemsa stain, ×1000.)

organ transplantation, postpartum or postabortion infections, biliary surgery, acute cholecystitis, and deep wounds.[1,42,44] Rapid therapy with transfusions, antibiotics, and fluid management is critical for patient survival.[43] The prognosis is grave, and many patients die despite intensive treatment.

Bartonellosis

Human bartonellosis (Carrión disease) is transmitted by the bite of a female sandfly and is endemic in certain regions of Peru, Ecuador, and Colombia.[45,46] It is caused by *Bartonella bacilliformis*, a small, pleomorphic, intracellular coccobacillus that adheres to RBCs and causes hemolysis.[1,47] The bacteria produce a protein called *deformin* that forms pits or invaginations in the RBC membrane.[1,47] There are two clinical stages. The first stage is characterized by acute hemolytic anemia; the second stage, or chronic verruga stage, is characterized by the eruption of skin lesions and warts on the extremities, face, and trunk. The acute phase begins with fever, malaise, headache, and chills, followed by pallor, jaundice, general lymphadenopathy, and, less commonly, hepatosplenomegaly.[45–47] Over several days, there is rapid hemolysis, with the hematocrit falling below 20% in two-thirds of patients.[45,47] Polychromasia, nucleated RBCs, and mild leukocytosis with a left shift are observed on the peripheral blood film. The mortality rate is approximately 10% for hospitalized patients and 90% for individuals who are untreated.[45,46] Diagnosis is made by blood culture and observation of bacilli or coccobacilli on the RBCs on a Wright-Giemsa-stained peripheral blood film. During the acute phase, 80% of the RBCs can be involved.[1]

HEMOLYTIC ANEMIA CAUSED BY OTHER RED BLOOD CELL INJURY

Drugs and Chemicals

Hemolytic anemia of varying severity may result from drugs or chemicals that cause the oxidative denaturation of hemoglobin, leading to the formation of methemoglobin and Heinz bodies.[1] Examples of agents that can cause hemolytic anemia in individuals with normal RBCs include dapsone, a drug used to treat leprosy and dermatitis herpetiformis,[1,48] and naphthalene, a chemical found in mothballs.[49] Individuals deficient in glucose-6-phosphate dehydrogenase (G6PD) are particularly sensitive to the effects of oxidative agents. For example, primaquine can cause hemolytic anemia in G6PD-deficient individuals (Chapter 21).[33]

Typical laboratory findings include a decrease in hemoglobin level, increase in the reticulocyte count, increase in serum indirect bilirubin, and decrease in serum haptoglobin level. In severe drug- or chemical-induced hemolytic anemia, Heinz bodies (denatured hemoglobin) may be observed in RBCs. Heinz bodies, which are visualized only with a supravital stain, appear as round, blue granules attached to the inner RBC membrane (Figure 22.12). Exposure to high levels of arsine hydride, copper, and lead can also cause hemolysis.[1,50]

Venoms

Envenomation from contact with snakes, spiders, bees, or wasps can induce hemolytic anemia in some individuals. The hemolysis can occur acutely or be delayed 1 or more days after a bite or sting.[1,50] The severity of the hemolysis depends on the amount of venom injected and, in severe cases, renal failure and death can result. Some mechanisms by which venoms can induce hemolysis are direct disruption of the RBC membrane, alteration of the RBC membrane that results in complement-mediated lysis, and initiation of DIC.[50] Hemolytic anemia has been reported after bites from poisonous snakes (e.g., some cobras and pit vipers) and the brown recluse spider (*Loxosceles reclusa* and *Loxosceles laeta*), and after multiple stings (50 or more) by bees or wasps.[1,50–54]

Extensive Burns (Thermal Injuries)

Warming normal RBCs to 49°C in vitro induces RBC fragmentation and budding.[1] Patients with extensive burns manifest similar RBC injury with acute hemolytic anemia. Schistocytes, spherocytes, and microspherocytes are observed on the peripheral blood film (Figure 22.14), but the damaged RBCs are usually cleared by the spleen within 24 hours of the burn injury.[50] In addition to resulting from acute hemolysis, anemia associated with extensive burns is also caused by blood loss during surgical excision and grafting of burn wounds, nutritional deficiency, impaired metabolism, and anemia of chronic inflammation.[55] Overheating of blood in malfunctioning blood warmers before transfusion can also result in RBC fragmentation and hemolysis of the donor RBCs.[1]

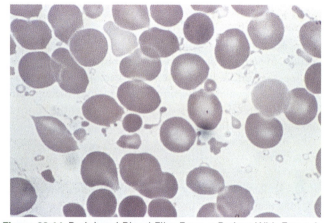

Figure 22.14 Peripheral Blood Film From a Patient With Extensive Burns. Note the presence of schistocytes, microspherocytes, and spherocytes. (Wright-Giemsa stain, ×1000.)

◼ SUMMARY

- A common feature of nonimmune extrinsic hemolytic anemias is the presence of a condition that causes physical or mechanical injury to RBCs. These conditions include microangiopathic hemolytic anemia; macroangiopathic hemolytic anemia; some infections; exposure to certain drugs, chemicals, or venoms; and extensive burns.
- Microangiopathic hemolytic anemia is characterized by the shearing of RBCs as they pass through small blood vessels partially blocked by microthrombi. Fragmented RBCs (called *schistocytes*) are formed, and premature RBC destruction results in hemolytic anemia. Ischemic injury to the brain, kidney, and other organs also occurs. Thrombocytopenia also occurs as a result of consumption in microthrombi. Major microangiopathic hemolytic anemias are thrombotic thrombocytopenic purpura (TTP), hemolytic uremic syndrome (HUS), HELLP (**h**emolysis, **e**levated **l**iver enzymes, **l**ow **p**latelet count) syndrome, and disseminated intravascular coagulation (DIC).
- TTP is a rare disorder found predominantly in adults and characterized by microangiopathic hemolytic anemia; severe thrombocytopenia; markedly increased serum lactate dehydrogenase activity; and variable symptoms of fever, neurologic

dysfunction, and renal failure. Idiopathic TTP is due to auto-immune antibodies to the von Willebrand factor-cleaving protease ADAMTS13 (*a d*isintegrin *a*nd *m*etalloprotease with a *t*hrombo*s*pondin type 1 motif, member *13*) causing a severe functional deficiency. Secondary TTP is associated with stem cell transplantation, disseminated cancer, pregnancy, and use of certain drugs. Inherited TTP is due to mutations in the *ADAMTS13* gene.

- HUS is characterized by microangiopathic hemolytic anemia, thrombocytopenia, and acute renal failure. Typical HUS (Stx-HUS) comprises 90% of cases, is found predominantly in young children, and is caused by toxin-producing strains of *Escherichia coli*. Atypical HUS (aHUS) is due to inherited mutations in genes coding for complement components and regulators or autoantibodies to complement factor H. It also occurs secondary to organ transplantation, cancer, pregnancy, human immunodeficiency virus infection, and some drugs.
- HELLP syndrome is a serious complication of pregnancy, manifesting with microangiopathic hemolytic anemia, thrombocytopenia, and elevated levels of liver enzymes.
- DIC is due to widespread intravascular activation of the hemostatic system and formation of fibrin thrombi; coagulation factors and platelets are consumed in the intravascular thrombi, and secondary fibrinolysis occurs. Schistocytes are found in approximately half of the cases.
- Macroangiopathic hemolytic anemia is caused by traumatic cardiac hemolysis (RBC fragmentation from damaged or prosthetic cardiac valves) or exercise-induced hemolysis (mechanical trauma from forceful impact on feet or hands or from strenuous exercise). The platelet count is normal in both conditions; schistocytes are seen only in traumatic cardiac hemolysis.

- Infections associated with hemolytic anemia due to invasion of RBCs include malaria and babesiosis. Hemolysis in bartonellosis is due to attachment of the bacteria to RBCs and production of a lytic protein. Hemolysis in clostridial sepsis is due to the production of α-toxin.
- Identification of parasite genus and species requires experience and expertise and is performed by laboratory professionals in clinical microbiology.
- In malaria, severe anemia is due to direct lysis of infected RBCs, immune destruction of infected and uninfected RBCs in the spleen, and inhibition of erythropoiesis.
- *Plasmodium* (five species) and *Babesia* organisms are identified by the morphology of their intraerythrocytic stages on a Wright-Giemsa-stained peripheral blood film. *Plasmodium* species are transmitted to humans by mosquitoes, whereas a tick is the vector for *Babesia*.
- Hemolytic anemia can also be caused by injury to RBCs by drugs, chemicals, venoms, and extensive burns (thermal injury). In patients with extensive burns, schistocytes, spherocytes, and microspherocytes are observed on the peripheral blood film.

Now that you have completed this chapter, go back and read again the case study at the beginning and respond to the questions presented. Answers can be found in Appendix C.

REVIEW QUESTIONS

Answers can be found in Appendix C.

1. Which one of the following is a feature found in ALL microangiopathic hemolytic anemias?
   a. Pancytopenia
   b. Thrombocytosis
   c. Intravascular RBC fragmentation
   d. Prolonged prothrombin time and partial thromboplastin time

2. Typical laboratory findings in TTP and HUS include:
   a. Schistocytosis and thrombocytopenia
   b. Anemia and reticulocytopenia
   c. Reduced levels of lactate dehydrogenase and aspartate aminotransferase
   d. Increased levels of free plasma hemoglobin and serum haptoglobin

3. The pathophysiology of idiopathic TTP involves:
   a. Shiga toxin damage to endothelial cells and obstruction of small blood vessels in glomeruli
   b. Formation of platelet-VWF thrombi due to autoantibody inhibition of ADAMTS13
   c. Overactivation of the complement system and endothelial cell damage due to loss of regulatory function
   d. Activation of the coagulation and fibrinolytic systems with fibrin clots throughout the microvasculature

4. Which of the following tests yields results that are abnormal in DIC but are usually within the reference interval or just slightly abnormal in TTP and HUS?
   a. Indirect serum bilirubin and serum haptoglobin
   b. Prothrombin time and partial thromboplastin time
   c. Lactate dehydrogenase and aspartate aminotransferase
   d. Serum creatinine and serum total protein

5. Which of the following laboratory results may be seen in BOTH traumatic cardiac hemolytic anemia and exercise-induced hemoglobinuria?
   a. Schistocytes on the peripheral blood film
   b. Thrombocytopenia
   c. Decreased serum haptoglobin
   d. Hemosiderinuria

6. Which *Plasmodium* species can infect all stages of RBCs?
   a. *P. falciparum*
   b. *P. vivax*
   c. *P. knowlesi*
   d. *P. malariae*

7. One week after returning from a vacation in Rhode Island, a 60-year-old experienced fever, chills, nausea, muscle aches, and fatigue of 2 days' duration. A complete blood count (CBC) showed a WBC count of 4.5×10^9/L, a hemoglobin level of 10.5 g/dL, a platelet count of 134×10^9/L, and a reticulocyte count of 2.7%. The medical laboratory scientist noticed tiny ameboid ring forms in some of the RBCs and some tetrad forms in others. These findings suggest:
   a. Bartonellosis
   b. Malaria
   c. Babesiosis
   d. Clostridial sepsis

8. What RBC morphology is characteristically found within the first 24 hours following extensive burn injury?
   a. Macrocytosis and polychromasia
   b. Burr cells and crenated cells
   c. Howell-Jolly bodies and bite cells
   d. Schistocytes and microspherocytes

9. Which of the following laboratory test results are abnormal in HELLP syndrome but not in DIC?
   a. Aspartate aminotransferase
   b. Prothrombin time
   c. Platelet count
   d. Hemoglobin

10. A 36-year-old patient was brought to the emergency department due to experiencing a seizure. The patient had been well until that morning, when a sudden headache and malaise developed. The patient was not taking any medications and had no history of previous surgery or pregnancy. Laboratory studies showed a WBC count of 15×10^9/L, a hemoglobin level of 7.8 g/dL, a platelet count of 18×10^9/L, and schistocytes and helmet cells on the peripheral blood film. Chemistry test results included markedly elevated serum lactate dehydrogenase activity and a slight increase in the level of total and indirect serum bilirubin. The urinalysis results were positive for protein and blood, but there were no RBCs in the urine sediment. Prothrombin time and partial thromboplastin time were within the reference interval. When the entire clinical and laboratory picture is considered, which of the following is the most likely diagnosis?
    a. HUS
    b. HELLP syndrome
    c. TTP
    d. Exercise-induced hemoglobinuria

REFERENCES

1. Mentzer, W. C., & Schrier, S. L. (2023). Extrinsic nonimmune hemolytic anemias. In Hoffman, R., Benz, E. J. Jr, Silberstein, L. E., et al. (Eds.), *Hematology: Basic Principles and Practice.* (8th ed., pp. 668–697). Philadelphia: Elsevier.

2. Moake, J. L. (2002). Thrombotic microangiopathies. *N Engl J Med, 347,* 589–600.

3. Tsai, H-M. (2013). Thrombotic thrombocytopenic purpura and the atypical hemolytic uremic syndrome. *Hematol Oncol Clin N Am, 27,* 565–584.

4. Moake, J. (2009). Thrombotic microangiopathies: multimers, metalloprotease, and beyond. *Clin Transl Sci, 2,* 366–373.

5. Gemlyn, G., & Friedman K. D. (2023). Thrombotic thrombocytopenic purpura and the hemolytic uremic syndromes. In Hoffman, R., Benz, E. J. Jr, Silberstein, L. E., et al. (Eds.), *Hematology: Basic Principles and Practice.* (8th ed., pp. 2063–2080). Philadelphia: Elsevier.

6. Kremer Hovinga, J.A., Coppo, P., Lammle, B., et al. (2017). Thrombotic thrombocytopenic purpura. *Nature Rev Dis Primers, 3,*(1), 17020. https://doi.org/10.1038/nrdp.2017.20.

7. Moake, J. L., Rudy, C. K., Troll, J. H., et al. (1982). Unusually large plasma factor VIII: von Willebrand factor multimers in chronic relapsing thrombotic thrombocytopenic purpura. *N Engl J Med, 307,* 1432–1435.

8. Furlan, M., Robles, R., Galbusera, M., et al. (1998). von Willebrand factor-cleaving protease in thrombotic thrombocytopenic purpura and the hemolytic-uremic syndrome. *N Engl J Med, 339,* 1578–1584.

9. Tsai, H-M., & Lian, E C-Y. (1998). Antibodies to von Willebrand factor-cleaving protease in acute thrombotic thrombocytopenic purpura. *N Engl J Med, 339,* 1585–1594.

10. Zhang, Q., Zhou, Y. F., Zhang, C. Z., et al. (2009). Structural specializations of A2, a force-sensing domain in the ultralarge vascular protein von Willebrand factor. *Proc Natl Acad Sci U S A, 106,* 9226–9231.

11. Kremer Hovinga, J. A., Vesely, S. K., Terrell, D. R., et al. (2010). Survival and relapse in patients with thrombotic thrombocytopenic purpura. *Blood, 115,* 1500–1511.

12. Lotta, L. A., Garagiola, I., Palla, R., et al. (2010). ADAMTS13 mutations and polymorphisms in congenital thrombotic thrombocytopenic purpura. *Hum Mutat, 31,* 11–19.

13. Mariotte, E., & Veyradier, A. (2015). Thrombotic thrombocytopenic purpura: from diagnosis to therapy. *Curr Opin Crit Care, 21,* 593–601.

14. Scheiring, J., Rosales, A., & Zimmerhackl, L. B. (2010). Clinical practice: today's understanding of the haemolytic uraemic syndrome. *Eur J Pediatr, 169,* 7–13.

15. Petruzziello, T. N., Mawji, I. A., Khan, M., et al. (2009). Verotoxin biology: molecular events in vascular endothelial injury. *Kidney Int, 75,* S17–S19.

16. Cataland, S. R., & Wu, H. F. (2014). Diagnosis and management of complement mediated thrombotic microangiopathies. *Blood Reviews, 28,* 67–74.

17. Dusse, L.M., Alpoim, P.N., Silva, J.T., et al. (2015). Revisiting HELLP syndrome. *Clin Chem Acta. 451,* 117–120.

18. Baker, K. R., & Moake, J. (2021). Fragmentation hemolytic anemia. In Kaushansky, K., Prchal, J. T., Burn, L.J. et al. (Eds.), *Williams Hematology.* (10th ed., pp. 871–878). New York: McGraw-Hill.

19. Martin, J. N. (2013). Milestones in the quest for best management of patients with HELLP syndrome (microangiopathic hemolytic anemia, hepatic dysfunction, thrombocytopenia). *Int J Gynecol Obstet, 121,* 202–207.

20. Lesesve, J. F., Martin, M., Banasiak, C., et al. (2014). Schistocytes in disseminated intravascular coagulation. *Int J Lab Hematol, 36,* 439–443.

21. Shapira, Y., Vaturi, M., & Sagie, A. (2009). Hemolysis associated with prosthetic heart valves: a review. *Cardiol Rev, 17,* 121–124.

22. Davidson, R. J. L. (1964). Exertional haemoglobinuria: a report on three cases with studies on the haemolytic mechanism. *J Clin Pathol, 17,* 536–540.

23. Telford, R. D., Sly, G. J., Hahn, A. G., et al. (2003). Footstrike is the major cause of hemolysis during running. *J Appl Physiol, 94,* 38–42.

24. Selby, G. B., & Eichner, E. R. (1986). Endurance swimming, intravascular hemolysis, anemia, and iron depletion. New perspective on athlete's anemia. *Am J Med, 81,* 791–794.

25. Shaskey, D. J., & Green, G. A. (2000). Sports haematology. *Sports Med, 29,* 27–38.

26. Tobal, D., Olascoaga, A., Moreira, G., et al. (2008). Rust urine after intense hand drumming is caused by extracorpuscular hemolysis. *Clin J Am Soc Nephrol, 3,* 1022–1027.

27. Smith, J. A., Kolbuch-Braddon, M., Gillam, I., et al. (1995). Changes in the susceptibility of red blood cells to oxidative and osmotic stress following submaximal exercise. *Eur J Appl Physiol, 70,* 427–436.

28. Beneke, R., Bihn, D., Hütler, M., et al. (2005). Haemolysis caused by alterations of alpha- and beta-spectrin after 10 to 35 min of severe exercise. *Eur J Appl Physiol, 95,* 307–312.

29. Yusof, A., Leithauser, R. M., Roth, H. J., et al. (2007). Exercise-induced hemolysis is caused by protein modification and most evident during the early phase of an ultraendurance race. *J Appl Physiol, 102,* 582–586.

30. World Health Organization. (2022). *World malaria report 2022.* Geneva: WHO Press. https://www.who.int/publications/i/item/9789240064898 Accessed December 27, 2022.

31. Centers for Disease Control and Prevention. (2022). *Malaria.* https://www.cdc.gov/malaria/about/index.html. Accessed December 21, 2022.

32. White, N. J. (2018). Anaemia and malaria. *Malar J. 17,* 371–388.

33. World Health Organization. (2022). *WHO guidelines for malaria.* Geneva: WHO Press. https://app.magicapp.org/#/guideline/6832. Accessed December 27, 2022.

34. Centers for Disease Control and Prevention. *Malaria diagnosis (U.S.) - microscopy.* https://www.cdc.gov/malaria/diagnosis_treatment/diagnostic_tools.html#tabs-1. Accessed January 22, 2023.

35. Ruebush, T. K., II, Juranek, D. D., Spielman, A., et al. (1981). Epidemiology of human babesiosis on Nantucket Island. *Am J Trop Med Hyg, 30,* 937–941.

36. Vannier, E., Diuk-Wasser, M.A., Mamoun, C. B., et al. (2015). Babesiosis. *Infect Dis Clin N Am, 29,* 357–370.

37. Centers for Disease Control and Prevention. *Babesiosis.* https://www.cdc.gov/parasites/babesiosis/. Accessed January 21, 2023.

38. Sanchez, E., Vannier, E., Wormser, G. P., et al. (2016). Diagnosis, treatment, and prevention of Lyme disease, human granulocytic anaplasmosis, and babesiosis. *JAMA, 315*(16), 1767–1777.

39. Hildebrandt, A., Zintl, A., Montero, E., et al. (2021). Human babesiosis in Europe. *Pathogens, 10,* 1165. https://doi.org/10.3390/pathogens10091165.

40. Krause, P. J., McKay, K., Gadbaw, J., et al. (2003). Increasing health burden of human babesiosis in endemic sites. *Am J Trop Med Hyg, 68,* 431–436.

41. Blevins, S. M., Greenfield, R. A., & Bronze, M. S. (2008). Blood smear analysis in babesiosis, ehrlichiosis, relapsing fever, malaria, and Chagas disease. *Cleve Clin J Med, 75,* 521–530.

42. Simon, T. G., Bradley, J., Jones, A., et al. (2014). Massive intravascular hemolysis from *Clostridium perfringens* septicemia: a review. *J Int Care Med, 29*(6), 327–333.

43. Shibazaki, S., Yasumoto, T., & Nakaizumi, T. (2018). Massive intravascular haemolysis due to *Clostridium perfringens.* *BMJ Case Rep, 2018,* bcr2017223464. https://doi.org/10.1136/bcr-2017-223464.

44. Barrett, J. P., Whiteside, J. L., & Boardman, L. A. (2002). Fatal clostridial sepsis after spontaneous abortion. *Obstet Gynecol, 99,* 899–901.

45. Maguina, C., Garcia, P. J., Gotuzzo, E., et al. (2001). Bartonellosis (Carrion's disease) in the modern world. *Clin Inf Dis. 33,* 772–779.

46. Huarcaya, E., Maguina, C., Torres, R., et al. (2004). Bartonellosis (Carrion's disease) in the pediatric population of Peru: an overview and update. *Braz J Infect Dis, 8,* 331–339.

47. Lichtman, M. A. (2021). Hemolytic anemia resulting from infections with microorganisms. In Kaushansky, K., Lichtman, M. A., Burns, L. J., et al. (Eds.), *Williams Hematology.* (10th ed., pp. 885–892). New York: McGraw-Hill.

48. Cha, Y. S., Kim, H., Kim, J., et al. (2016). Incidence and patterns of hemolytic anemia in acute dapsone overdose. *Am J Emerg Med, 34,* 366–369.

49. Kundra, T.S., Bhutatani, V., Gupta, R., et al. (2015). Naphthalene poisoning following ingestion of mothballs: a case report. *J of Clin and Diagnostic Research, 9*(8), UD01–UD002.

50. Herrmann, P. C. (2021). Erythrocyte disorders as a result of toxic agents. In Kaushansky, K., Lichtman, M. A., Burns, L. J., et al. (Eds.), *Williams Hematology.* (10th ed., pp. 879–884). New York: McGraw-Hill.

51. Athappan, G., Balaji, M. V., Navaneethan, U., et al. (2008). Acute renal failure in snake envenomation: a large prospective study. *Saudi J Kidney Dis Transpl, 19,* 404–410.

52. Chinchanikar, S., Khalaf, Z., & Mateescu, V. (2022). Brown recluse spider bite: a case report of severe hemolysis and sepsis. *Am J Clin Pathol. 158,* S114.

53. Kolecki, P. (1999). Delayed toxic reaction following massive bee envenomation. *Ann Emerg Med, 33,* 114–116.

54. Ruwanpathirana, P., & Priyankara, D. (2022). Clinical manifestations of wasp stings: a case report and a review of literature. *Trop Med Health, 50,* 82. https://doi.org/10.1186/s41182-022-00475-8.

55. Posluszny, J. A., & Gamelli, R. L. (2010). Anemia of thermal injury: combined acute blood loss anemia and anemia of critical illness. *J Burn Care Res, 31,* 229–242.

23

Extrinsic Defects Leading to Increased Erythrocyte Destruction—Immune Causes

*Ruth Perez**

OBJECTIVES

After completion of this chapter, the reader will be able to:

1. Define *immune hemolytic anemia* and describe the types of antibodies involved.
2. Compare and contrast mechanisms of immune hemolysis mediated by immunoglobulin M (IgM) and IgG.
3. Describe typical laboratory findings in immune hemolytic anemia and the importance of the direct antiglobulin test (DAT).
4. Compare and contrast four types of autoimmune hemolytic anemia in terms of immunoglobulin class involved, temperature for optimal reactivity of the autoantibody, proteins detected by the DAT on the patient's red blood cells, presence or absence of complement activation, type and site of hemolysis, and specificity of the autoantibody.
5. Relate results of the DAT to the pathophysiology and laboratory findings in autoimmune hemolytic anemia.
6. Describe two types of hemolytic transfusion reactions, the usual immunoglobulin class involved, typical site of hemolysis, and important laboratory findings.
7. Describe the cause, pathophysiology, and laboratory findings in Rh and ABO hemolytic disease of the fetus and newborn.
8. Describe three mechanisms of drug-induced immune hemolysis.
9. Compare and contrast the pathophysiology of immune hemolysis caused by drug-dependent and drug-independent antibodies, including related laboratory findings.
10. Given a patient history and results of a complete blood count, peripheral blood film examination, pertinent biochemical tests on serum and urine, DAT, and indirect antiglobulin test, determine the type of immune hemolysis.

OUTLINE

Overview of Immune Hemolytic Anemias
    Pathophysiology of Immune Hemolysis
    Laboratory Findings in Immune Hemolytic Anemia
Autoimmune Hemolytic Anemia
    Warm Autoimmune Hemolytic Anemia
    Cold Agglutinin Disease
    Paroxysmal Cold Hemoglobinuria
    Mixed-Type Autoimmune Hemolytic Anemia

Alloimmune Hemolytic Anemias
    Hemolytic Transfusion Reaction
    Hemolytic Disease of the Fetus and Newborn
Drug-Induced Immune Hemolytic Anemia
    Mechanisms of Drug-Induced Immune Hemolysis
    Antibody Characteristics
    Nonimmune Drug-Induced Hemolysis
    Treatment

CASE STUDY

After studying the material in this chapter, the reader should be able to respond to the following case study. Answers can be found in Appendix C.

A 37-year-old man sought medical attention from his general practitioner for malaise, shortness of breath, and difficulty concentrating for the past 5 days. Physical examination revealed an otherwise healthy adult with tachycardia.

There was no significant medical history, and the patient was not taking any medications. The physician ordered a complete blood count (CBC), urinalysis, comprehensive metabolic panel (CMP), and electrocardiogram (ECG). The patient's key laboratory results follow. Reference intervals can be found after the Index at the end of the book.

---

*The author extends appreciation to Elaine M. Keohane and Kim A. Przekop, whose work in prior editions provided the foundation for this chapter.

WBC	12.4×10^9/L (corrected)	RDW	17.3%
HGB	7.1 g/dL	PLT	325×10^9/L
MCV	105.4 fL	RETIC	18.1%
MCHC	36.3 g/dL	NEUT	82%

The ECG was normal. The automated blood cell analyzer printout flagged for nucleated red blood cells (RBCs) (and corrected the WBC count), 3+ anisocytosis, and reticulocytosis. The peripheral blood film had moderate spherocytes, moderate polychromasia, few macrocytes, marked anisocytosis, and 15 nucleated RBCs/100 WBCs (Figure 23.1). Occasional schistocytes and neutrophilia with a slight left shift were also observed on the blood film (not shown in Figure 23.1). The urinalysis report included 2+ protein, 2+ blood, and increased urobilinogen, with 0 to 5 RBCs seen on microscopic examination. The patient's serum was moderately icteric, and total serum bilirubin was increased. The patient was admitted for further testing. Serum haptoglobin was decreased, serum indirect (unconjugated) bilirubin and lactate dehydrogenase were elevated, and urine hemosiderin was positive.

A type and screen was ordered. The antibody screen was negative at the immediate spin and 37°C incubation phase, but showed 3+ agglutination in the antihuman globulin (AHG) phase for all panel cells and the autocontrol. The direct antiglobulin test (DAT) showed 3+ agglutination with polyspecific AHG and monospecific anti-IgG but was negative with monospecific anti-C3b/C3d (complement). An acid elution was performed on the patient's RBCs, and the eluate showed 2+ reactions with all panel cells and autocontrol at the AHG phase. The patient was diagnosed with warm autoimmune hemolytic anemia (WAIHA) and started on 1.0 mg/kg per day prednisone until the hemoglobin reached 10.0 g/dL (2 weeks of treatment). The patient was continued on prednisone for 4 months with slowly decreasing levels of the drug. He also received bisphosphonates, vitamin D, and calcium to prevent osteoporosis, an adverse effect of prednisone. At 3 weeks after

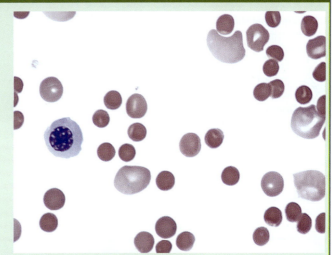

Figure 23.1 Peripheral Blood Film From the Patient in the Case Study. (Wright-Giemsa stain, ×1000.)

diagnosis, spherocytes were no longer present on the peripheral blood film, urinalysis was normal, and DAT was negative.

1. Explain why the WBC count, MCV, RDW, and reticulocyte count results were elevated.
2. Describe the immune mechanism that caused the spherocytosis, and explain why spherocytes have a shortened life span.
3. Relate the chemistry, urinalysis, and immunohematology (blood bank) results to the pathophysiology of the patient's anemia.
4. Explain why the treatment was effective, and explain if the patient's WAIHA was acute or chronic.

OVERVIEW OF IMMUNE HEMOLYTIC ANEMIAS

Immune hemolytic anemia and nonimmune hemolytic anemia are two broad categories comprising the extrinsic hemolytic anemias, disorders in which red blood cells (RBCs) are structurally and functionally normal, but a condition outside of the RBCs causes premature hemolysis. Nonimmune extrinsic hemolytic anemias are the result of physical or mechanical injury to RBCs and are discussed in Chapter 22. Immune hemolytic anemias are conditions in which RBC survival is shortened as a result of an antibody-mediated mechanism. The antibody may be an *autoantibody* (directed against a self-RBC antigen), an *alloantibody* (directed against an RBC antigen of another person), or an antibody directed against a drug (or its metabolite) taken by the patient. Some antibodies are able to activate the classical complement pathway, which results in the attachment of activated complement proteins to the RBC membrane. RBCs with bound antibody or complement are prematurely removed from the circulation extravascularly by macrophages (because of their receptors for complement and the Fc component of antibody), intravascularly by complement-mediated hemolysis, or by a combination of both mechanisms.[1] Anemia develops when the amount of hemolysis exceeds the ability of bone marrow to replace RBCs that are destroyed. The degree of anemia can vary from asymptomatic and mild to severe and life-threatening.

Immune hemolytic anemias may be classified into the following groups: autoimmune hemolytic anemia, alloimmune hemolytic anemia, and drug-induced immune hemolytic anemia (Box 23.1).[1,2] It is important to determine the cause of an immune hemolytic anemia so that the appropriate therapy can be administered to the patient.

Pathophysiology of Immune Hemolysis

In immune hemolysis, an antibody binds to an antigen on the surface of RBCs, which signals premature removal of those cells from the circulation through extravascular or intravascular hemolysis (Chapter 20). Two classes or isotypes of antibodies involved in most immune hemolytic anemias are immunoglobulin G (IgG) and IgM. IgG is a monomer in a Y-like structure with two identical heavy chains (γ H chains) and two identical light chains (either k or λ) connected by disulfide bonds.[3] At the top of the Y-like structure are two antigen-binding (Fab) domains, each formed from the N-terminus of the variable domain of one light chain and one heavy chain. IgG has one Fc domain (stem of the Y) consisting of the C-termini of the two heavy chains (Figure 23.2). IgM is a pentamer consisting of five monomeric units connected by disulfide linkages at the C-termini of their heavy chains (μ H chains).[3,4] Because the composition, structure, and size of IgG and IgM are different, their properties and mechanisms in mediating hemolysis are also different.

BOX 23.1   Classification of Immune Hemolytic Anemias

Autoimmune Hemolytic Anemia
Warm autoimmune hemolytic anemia (WAIHA)
  Idiopathic
  Secondary
    Lymphoproliferative disorders
    Nonlymphoid neoplasms
    Collagen-vascular disease
    Immunodeficiency disorders
    Viral infections
Cold agglutinin disease (CAD)
  Idiopathic
  Secondary
    Acute: infections (*Mycoplasma pneumoniae*, infectious mononucleosis,
      other viruses)
    Chronic: lymphoproliferative disorders

Paroxysmal cold hemoglobinuria (PCH)
  Idiopathic
  Secondary
    Viral infections
    Syphilis
Mixed-type autoimmune hemolytic anemia

Alloimmune Hemolytic Anemias
Hemolytic transfusion reaction (HTR)
Hemolytic disease of the fetus and newborn (HDFN)

Drug-Induced Immune Hemolytic Anemia (DIIHA)
Drug dependent
Drug independent

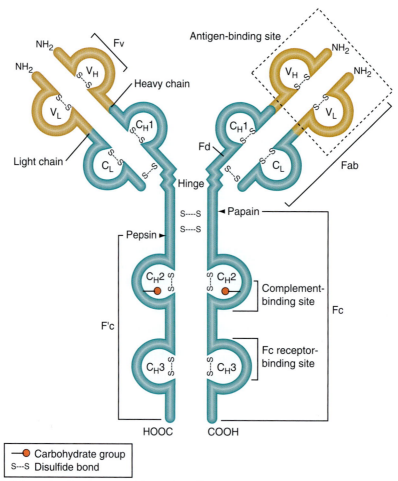

Figure 23.2 Schematic of an Immunoglobulin G (IgG) Molecule. IgG consists of two heavy chains and two light chains. Note the antigen binding sites at the amino (NH$_2$) end formed by the variable region (Fv) of one heavy chain and one light chain. Note the Fc region at the carboxyl (COOH) end of the heavy chains. The chains are held together by disulfide linkages. (From McPherson, R. A., Riley, R. S., & Massey, H. D. [2017]. Laboratory evaluation of immunoglobulin function and humoral immunity. In: McPherson, R. A. & Pincus, M. R. [Eds], *Henry's Clinical Diagnosis and Management by Laboratory Methods*. [24th ed., Figure 47.1, p. 953]. St. Louis: Elsevier.)

Classical Complement Pathway

The classical complement pathway is an important mediator of immune hemolysis. Major proteins of the classical complement pathway are designated C1 through C9, and their components or fragments are designated with lowercase suffixes. The first protein, C1, has three components: C1q, C1r, and C1s. After an antibody binds to its specific antigens on the RBC surface, C1q must bind to two adjacent antibody Fc domains to activate the pathway.[4] Theoretically, only one IgM molecule is needed for complement activation because of its larger pentameric structure with five Fc domains; however, at least two molecules of monomeric IgG in close proximity are required for C1q attachment.[4] Therefore IgM antibodies are highly effective in activating complement, whereas IgG antibodies are unable to activate the pathway unless there is a sufficient number of IgG molecules on the RBC surface.[4,5] In addition, subclasses IgG1 and IgG3 have high binding affinity for C1q, whereas subclasses IgG2 and IgG4 have minimal ability to bind complement.[4,5]

The binding of C1q to adjacent Fc domains requires calcium and magnesium ions and activates C1r, which then activates C1s. This activated C1q-C1r-C1s complex is an enzyme that cleaves C4 and then C2, which results in the binding of a small number of C4bC2a complexes to the RBC membrane. C4bC2a complex is an active *C3 convertase* enzyme that cleaves C3 in plasma; the result is the binding of many C3b molecules to C4bC2a on the RBC surface. The last phase of the classical pathway occurs when C4bC2aC3b *(C5 convertase)* converts C5 to C5b, which combines with C6, C7, C8, and multiple

C9s to form the *membrane attack complex (MAC)*. The MAC resembles a cylinder that inserts into the lipid bilayer of the membrane, forming a pore that allows water and small ions to enter the cell, causing lysis (Figure 23.3).[3] Negative regulators inhibit various complement proteins and complexes in the pathway to prevent uncontrolled activation and excessive hemolysis.[1,3,4]

Hemolysis Mediated by IgM and IgG Antibodies

Hemolysis mediated by IgM antibodies requires complement and can result in both extravascular and intravascular hemolysis.[5] When IgM molecules attach to the RBC surface in relatively low density, complement activation results in C3b binding to the membrane, but complement inhibitors prevent full activation of the pathway to the terminal MAC.[1,5] C3b-sensitized RBCs are destroyed by extravascular hemolysis, predominantly by macrophages (Kupffer cells) in the liver, which have C3b receptors. Some C3b on RBCs can be cleaved, however, which leaves the C3d fragment on the cell. RBCs sensitized with only C3d are not prematurely removed from circulation because

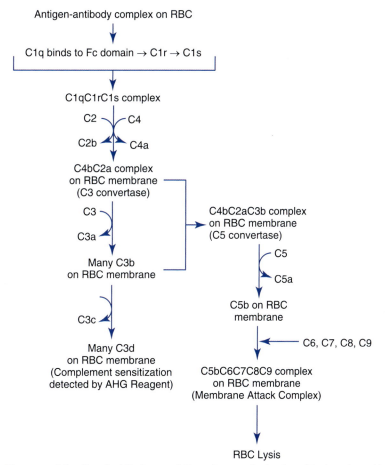

Figure 23.3 Diagram of the Classical Pathway of Complement Activation. C1q is activated by binding to adjacent Fc domains of immunoglobulin bound to RBC antigen. C1q activates C1r; C1r activates C1s, which forms the complex C1qC1rC1s. The complex activates C2 and C4 to form the C4bC2a complex (C3 convertase) on the membrane. The complex converts C3 to many C3b molecules on the membrane. If there is no further activation, C3b will degrade to C3d on the membrane, which can be detected by polyspecific AHG. C3b can also form the complex C4bC2aC3b (C5 convertase), which converts C5 to C5b on the membrane. C5b forms the membrane attack complex, C5bC6C7C8C9, which inserts into the bilipid layer, causing lysis. *AHG*, Antihuman globulin; *RBC*, red blood cell.

macrophages lack a C3d receptor.[5] In severe cases of immune hemolysis involving heavy sensitization of RBCs with IgM antibody, significantly more complement is activated, which overwhelms complement inhibitors. In these cases, complement activation proceeds from C1 to C9 and results in rapid intravascular hemolysis.[5]

Hemolysis mediated by IgG antibodies occurs with or without complement and predominantly by extravascular mechanisms.[5] RBCs sensitized with IgG are removed from circulation by macrophages in the spleen, which have receptors for the Fc component of IgG1 and IgG3.[1,5] IgG antibodies are not efficient in activating complement, and intravascular hemolysis by full activation of complement from C1 to C9 is rare (except with anti-P in paroxysmal cold hemoglobinuria).[5] However, if there is a high density of IgG1 or IgG3 bound to antigens on RBCs, some complement is activated and C3b binds to the membrane. If both IgG and C3b are on the RBC membrane, there is faster clearance from the circulation by macrophages in both the spleen and the liver.[1,5] Often, IgG-sensitized RBCs are only partially phagocytized by macrophages, which results in removal of some membrane. Spherocytes are the result of this process, and they are the characteristic cell of IgG-mediated hemolysis.[5] The spherocytes are eventually removed from circulation by entrapment in the red pulp of the spleen (splenic cords), where they are rapidly phagocytized by macrophages (Chapter 6).[5] The mechanisms of immune hemolysis are summarized in Table 23.1.

Laboratory Findings in Immune Hemolytic Anemia

Laboratory findings in immune hemolytic anemia are similar to the findings in other hemolytic anemias and include decreased hemoglobin; increased reticulocyte count; increased levels of indirect serum bilirubin and lactate dehydrogenase; and decreased serum haptoglobin level. If hemolysis is predominantly intravascular or extravascular hemolysis is severe, the haptoglobin level will be moderately to severely decreased, plasma hemoglobin will be increased, and the patient may have hemoglobinuria or even hemosiderinuria (in cases of chronic hemolysis) (Chapter 20). Mean cell volume (MCV) may be increased because of reticulocytosis and RBC agglutination (if present). Leukocytosis and

thrombocytosis may occur along with increased erythroid proliferation in bone marrow.[1] Findings on the peripheral blood film include polychromasia (as a result of reticulocytosis), spherocytes (caused by IgG-mediated membrane damage by macrophages), and occasionally RBC agglutination.[5] Nucleated RBCs, fragmented RBCs or schistocytes, and erythrophagocytosis (phagocytes engulfing RBCs) may also be observed on the peripheral blood film.[1]

To determine whether the hemolysis is due to an immune mechanism, a *direct antiglobulin test* (DAT) is performed. The DAT detects in vivo sensitization of the RBC surface by IgG, C3b, or C3d.[2] In the DAT procedure, polyspecific antihuman globulin (AHG) is added to saline-washed patient RBCs. Polyspecific AHG has specificity for the Fc portion of human IgG and complement components C3b and C3d; agglutination will occur if a critical number of any of these molecules is present on the RBC surface (Figure 23.4).[2] If the DAT result is positive with polyspecific AHG, RBCs are tested with monospecific anti-IgG and anti-C3b/C3d to identify the type of sensitization. If IgG is detected on RBCs, elution procedures are used to remove the antibody from RBCs for identification.

Specificity of the IgG antibody may be determined by assessing the reaction of the eluate with screening and panel reagent RBCs (RBCs genotyped for the major RBC antigens) using the *indirect antiglobulin test* (IAT) (Figure 23.4). Identification of any circulating alloantibodies or autoantibodies by the IAT is also important in the investigation.[2] The DAT result may be negative in patients with some immune hemolytic anemias.[2] In addition, disorders other than immune hemolytic anemia can cause a positive DAT.[2] Therefore diagnosis of immune hemolytic anemia cannot rely solely on the DAT and must take into account the patient history; symptoms; recent medications; previous transfusions; coexisting conditions, including pregnancy; and results of applicable hematologic, biochemical, and serologic tests.[2,5]

AUTOIMMUNE HEMOLYTIC ANEMIA

Autoimmune hemolytic anemia (AIHA) is a rare disorder characterized by premature RBC destruction and anemia caused

TABLE 23.1	**Major Mechanisms of Immune Hemolysis**	
	IgM Mediated	**IgG Mediated**
Extravascular hemolysis	IgM activation of classical complement pathway from C1 to C3b only; clearance of C3b-sensitized RBCs by macrophages, mainly in liver	Clearance of IgG-sensitized RBCs by macrophages, mainly in spleen Formation of spherocytes by partial phagocytosis of IgG-sensitized RBCs; spherocytes cleared by macrophages after entrapment in spleen IgG* activation of classical complement pathway from C1 to C3b only; requires high-density IgG on RBC surface; clearance of IgG- and C3b-sensitized RBCs by macrophages in spleen and liver
Intravascular hemolysis	Full IgM activation of classical complement pathway from C1 to C9 and direct RBC lysis; requires high-density IgM on RBCs to overcome complement inhibitors	Full IgG activation of classical complement pathway from C1 to C9 and direct RBC lysis; requires very-high-density IgG on RBCs for activation and to overcome complement inhibitors; uncommon

*IgG3 and IgG1 are most efficient in complement activation.
Ig, Immunoglobulin; *RBC,* red blood cell.

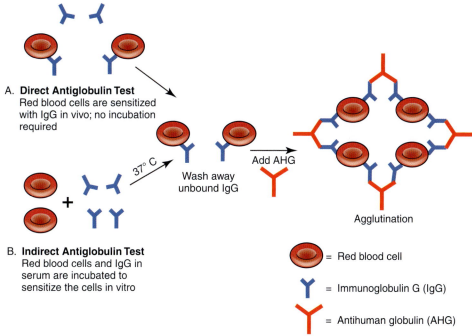

Figure 23.4 Graphic Representation of the Direct and Indirect Antihuman Globulin Reaction. **(A)**, The direct antiglobulin test detects IgG antibodies that are bound to corresponding antigens on the patient's red blood cells (RBCs) in vivo. It does not require an incubation step. **(B)**, The indirect antiglobulin test requires a 37°C incubation step to bind IgG antibodies (from patient's serum or from typing reagents) to corresponding antigens on RBCs in vitro. Polyspecific AHG is a mixture of antibodies to IgG and complement components C3d/C3b. The anti-IgG produces agglutination by binding to the Fc domain of IgG antibodies that are bound to antigens on the RBC membranes. Similarly, the anti-C3d/C3b produces agglutination by binding to the respective complement components, if present, on the RBC membranes (reaction not shown). Monospecific AHG has specificity for either IgG or C3b/C3d. Although AHG is depicted as an IgG antibody in this figure, in some reagents, it can be an IgM isotype. *AHG,* Antihuman globulin.

by autoantibodies that bind to the RBC surface, with or without complement activation. AIHA can affect both children and adults, and its annual incidence is estimated to be between 1 and 3 per 100,000 individuals.[6] In children, boys are affected more frequently, whereas in adults, women are affected more frequently.[6] Autoantibodies may arise as a result of immune system dysregulation and loss of immune tolerance, exposure to an antigen similar to an autoantigen, B lymphocyte neoplasm, or other unknown reason.[1,6] The type, amount, and duration of antigen exposure and genetic and environmental factors may also contribute to development of autoantibodies.[5] Anemia can be mild or severe, and onset can be acute or gradual. Severity of the anemia depends on autoantibody characteristics (titer, ability to react at 37°C, ability to activate complement, and specificity and affinity for the autoantigen), antigen characteristics (density on RBCs, immunogenicity), and patient factors (age, ability of bone marrow to compensate for the hemolysis, function of macrophages, complement proteins and regulators, and underlying conditions).[1,6]

Autoimmune hemolytic anemias may be divided into four major categories based on the characteristics of the autoantibody and the mechanism of hemolysis: warm autoimmune hemolytic anemia, cold agglutinin disease, paroxysmal cold hemoglobinuria, and mixed-type AIHA (Table 23.2).[2,5,6]

Warm Autoimmune Hemolytic Anemia

Etiology

Warm autoimmune hemolytic anemia (WAIHA) is the most commonly encountered autoimmune hemolytic anemia, comprising up to 70% to 80% of cases.[1,5] Autoantibodies causing WAIHA react optimally at 37°C, and the vast majority of them are IgG.[1] WAIHA may be classified as idiopathic or secondary. In patients with idiopathic WAIHA, the cause is unknown. Secondary WAIHA may occur in many conditions such as lymphoproliferative diseases (chronic lymphocytic leukemia, B-lymphocytic lymphoma, and Waldenström macroglobulinemia), nonlymphoid neoplasms (thymoma and cancers of the colon, kidney, lung, and ovary), autoimmune disorders (rheumatoid arthritis, scleroderma, polyarteritis nodosa, Sjögren syndrome, and systemic lupus erythematosus), immunodeficiency disorders, and viral infections.[1,5]

Symptoms

The onset of WAIHA is usually insidious with symptoms of anemia (fatigue, dizziness, dyspnea), but some cases can be acute and life-threatening, with fever, jaundice, splenomegaly, and hepatomegaly, especially in children with WAIHA secondary to viral infections.[1,5] Massive splenomegaly, lymphadenopathy,

TABLE 23.2	Characteristics of Autoimmune Hemolytic Anemias			
	Warm Autoimmune Hemolytic Anemia	**Cold Agglutinin Disease**	**Paroxysmal Cold Hemoglobinuria**	**Mixed-Type Autoimmune Hemolytic Anemia**
Immunoglobulin class	IgG (rarely IgM, IgA)	IgM	IgG	IgG, IgM
Optimum reactivity temperature of autoantibody	37°C	4°C; reactivity extends to greater than 30°C	4°C	4° to 37°C
Sensitization detected by direct antiglobulin test	IgG or IgG + C3d; only C3d uncommon	C3d	C3d	IgG and C3d
Complement activation	Variable	Yes	Yes	Yes
Hemolysis	Extravascular primarily	Extravascular; some intravascular	Intravascular	Extravascular and intravascular
Autoantibody specificity	Panreactive or Rh complex; rarely, specific Rh or other antigen	I (most), i (some), Pr (rare)	P	Panreactive; unclear specificity
Other laboratory findings	Polychromasia, spherocytes, occasionally decreased PLT count	RBC agglutination may be present	Polychromasia, spherocytes (common), schistocytes, NRBCs, anisocytosis, poikilocytosis, and erythrophagocytosis	Varies

Ig, Immunoglobulin; *NRBC,* nucleated red blood cell; *PLT,* platelet; *RBC,* red blood cell.

fever, petechiae, ecchymosis, or renal failure in adults suggests an underlying lymphoproliferative disorder.[1,5]

Although most autoantibodies that cause WAIHA are IgG, rare cases involving IgA autoantibodies as well as cases with fatal outcomes caused by warm-reacting IgM antibodies have been reported.[1,2] Hemolysis is predominantly extravascular in WAIHA, and cases of fulminant intravascular hemolysis are rare.[5]

Laboratory Findings

The DAT is positive in more than 95% of patients, with approximately 85% of patients having IgG alone or both IgG and C3d on their RBCs and 10% to 14% having C3d only.[1,2,5] In 1% to 4% of patients, the DAT is negative because of IgA or IgM autoantibodies that are not detected by the polyspecific AHG, IgG or C3d in an amount less than the reagent detection limit, dissociation of IgG antibodies with low avidity during the washing phase of the DAT, or various technical errors.[1,2,5] Therefore a negative DAT result does not rule out autoimmune hemolytic anemia.

Warm autoantibodies are usually panreactive; that is, they will agglutinate all screening and panel cells, donor RBCs, and the patient's own RBCs, so the specificity of the autoantibody is not apparent.[2,5] In some cases, Rh complex specificity can be demonstrated.[2,5] Rarely, a specific autoantibody to an antigen in the Rh blood group system is identified. Autoantibodies to other antigens (such as LW, Jk, K, Di, Ge, Lu, M, N, S, U, En[a], and Wr[b]) are occasionally identified.[2,5] The autoantibody can be detected in the serum in most patients (approximately 80%). Because the autoantibody is panreactive, it may mask reactions of alloantibodies with RBC panel cells. If an RBC transfusion is necessary, it is crucial to perform tests to determine whether clinically significant *allo*antibodies are also present.[5]

Anemia in WAIHA can be mild or severe, with RBC life span sometimes reduced to 5 days or less.[1] Laboratory findings for serum and urine reflect the predominantly extravascular hemolysis that occurs in IgG-mediated immune hemolysis. Polychromasia and spherocytes are typical findings on the peripheral blood film (Figure 23.1). Occasionally, WAIHA is accompanied by immune thrombocytopenic purpura and a decreased platelet count, a condition known as *Evans syndrome,* which occurs primarily in children.[6,7]

Treatment

In symptomatic but non–life-threatening WAIHA, a glucocorticosteroid such as prednisone is the initial treatment of choice.[1,2,8,9] Approximately 70% to 80% of patients show improvement with prednisone, but only about 20% to 40% achieve a long-term response.[1,8] Many adult patients need to be on a long-term maintenance dosage to remain asymptomatic.[1] A serious side effect of glucocorticosteroid treatment (initially and long term) is an increased risk of osteoporosis and bone fractures.[1] Guidelines from the American College of Rheumatology indicate that patients on glucocorticosteroids may benefit from vitamin D, calcium, and bisphosphonate therapy to prevent osteoporosis, but each patient's situation should be evaluated on an individual basis.[10]

In patients with chronic WAIHA who are refractive to prednisone therapy or require long-term, high-dose prednisone therapy, second-line therapy usually includes a choice of either splenectomy or rituximab.[1,8,9] Splenectomy achieves a favorable response only in about 50% of patients, both initially and long term.[1,8] Rituximab is a monoclonal anti-CD20 antibody that binds to the corresponding antigen found on B lymphocytes. In a recent meta-analysis of 21 studies (409 patients) of the efficacy and safety of rituximab in WAIHA, Reynaud and colleagues[11] found an overall response rate of 73% with a low incidence of adverse effects; they suggested that rituximab may be a superior choice over invasive (splenectomy) or toxic (immunosuppression) therapies. However, there are few studies on the long-term efficacy and safety of rituximab in WAIHA, and as of this publication, rituximab is not approved by the Food and Drug Administration (FDA) for this indication.[1,8] Immunosuppressive drugs, such as cyclophosphamide or azathioprine, are the third-line therapy for refractory WAIHA because the toxicity and side effects may be severe.[1,6,9] Hematopoietic stem cell transplantation (HSCT) has been used in the past for severe, refractory, life-threatening autoimmune syndromes, including hemolytic anemia and Evans syndrome but is a therapy of last resort.[9] In secondary WAIHA, successful management of the underlying condition often controls hemolysis and anemia. WAIHA with a critically low hemoglobin level requires RBC transfusion. If the autoantibody has broad specificity, all RBC units may be incompatible with the autoantibody.[1,2,5] In such cases, a check for underlying alloantibodies is performed, and extended phenotype matching for Rh, Kell, Kidd, and Ss antigens may be recommended to prevent further alloimmunization.[1] In addition, a minimum volume of RBCs is given, and the patient is carefully monitored during the transfusion.

Cold Agglutinin Disease

Etiology

Cold agglutinins are autoantibodies of the IgM class that react optimally at 4°C and are commonly found in healthy individuals. These nonpathologic cold agglutinins are polyclonal, occur in low titers (less than 1:64 at 4°C), and have no reactivity above 30°C.[1,5] Most pathologic cold agglutinins are monoclonal, occur at high titers (greater than 1:1000 at 4°C), and are capable of reacting at temperatures greater than 30°C.[2] Because pathologic cold agglutinins can react at body temperature, they may induce cold agglutinin disease (CAD). Cold agglutinins that are able to bind RBC antigens near or at 37°C (high thermal amplitude) cause more severe symptoms.[1,12,13] CAD is also recognized as a clonal lymphoproliferative B cell disorder.[6,12] It comprises approximately 15% to 20% of cases of autoimmune hemolytic anemia.[6]

In CAD, IgM autoantibodies bind to RBCs when the patient is exposed to cold temperatures, particularly in peripheral circulation and vessels of the skin, where temperatures can drop to 30°C.[13] During the brief transit of RBCs through these colder areas, IgM autoantibodies activate the classical complement pathway.[12] When RBCs return to the central circulation, the IgM antibody dissociates, but C3b components remain on the cell.[2,12] Hemolysis is predominantly extravascular by hepatic macrophages, which have receptors for C3b.[1,12] However, if the autoantibody has a high thermal amplitude or there is a deficiency in complement regulatory proteins, full complement activation and intravascular hemolysis can occur.[2,14]

Acute CAD occurs secondary to *Mycoplasma pneumoniae* infection, infectious mononucleosis, and other viral infections. These cold agglutinins are polyclonal IgM, with a normal distribution of κ and λ light chains.[2,5] Chronic CAD is a rare hemolytic anemia that typically occurs in middle-aged and elderly individuals, and the autoantibody is usually monoclonal IgM with κ light chains.[6,12,13] In a study of 86 patients with chronic CAD by Berentsen and colleagues,[12] the median age at onset was 67 years, with the median age at death reported to be 82 years. Chronic CAD can be idiopathic, but it is usually secondary to an underlying lymphoproliferative neoplasm such as B-lymphocytic lymphoma, Waldenström macroglobulinemia, or chronic lymphocytic leukemia.[12]

Symptoms

Clinical manifestations are variable in chronic CAD. Most patients have a mild anemia with a hemoglobin value ranging from 9 to 12 g/dL, but others can develop life-threatening anemia, with hemoglobin levels falling to less than 5 g/dL, especially after exposure to cold temperatures.[5,13] Patients often experience fluctuations between mild and severe symptoms, and approximately half of affected individuals require transfusions over the course of the disease.[12] Symptoms include fatigue, weakness, dyspnea, pallor (caused by the anemia), and acrocyanosis.[13] *Acrocyanosis* is a bluish discoloration of the extremities (fingers, toes, feet, earlobes, nose) as a result of RBC autoagglutination, which causes local capillary stasis and decreased oxygen delivery to the affected areas.[1,2,13] Some patients also have episodes of hemoglobinuria, especially after exposure to cold temperatures.[2,13] In contrast, patients with acute CAD may have mild to severe hemolysis that appears abruptly within 2 to 3 weeks after onset of infectious mononucleosis, other viral infection, or *M. pneumoniae* infection, but it resolves spontaneously within days to a few weeks.[13]

Laboratory Findings

The DAT result is positive with polyspecific AHG because of the presence of C3d on the RBC surface.[1] Specificity of the cold agglutinin is most often anti-I but can be anti-i or, very rarely, anti-Pr.[2,14] Virtually all adult RBCs are positive for I antigen, so anti-I will agglutinate all screening and panel cells, donor RBCs, and the patient's own RBCs at room temperature and at temperatures greater than 30°C, depending on the thermal amplitude of the autoantibody. Anti-I will show weaker or negative reactions with cord RBCs (cord cells are negative for I antigen but positive for i antigen).[2]

A cold agglutinin test determines the titer of the autoantibody at 4°C. Pathologic cold agglutinins can reach titers of 1:10,000 to 1:1,000,000 at 4°C.[1,5] Blood specimens for cold agglutinin testing must be maintained at 37°C after collection to prevent binding of the autoantibody to the patient's own RBCs, which can falsely decrease the antibody titer in the serum. Alternatively, a specimen anticoagulated with ethylenediaminetetraacetic acid (EDTA) can be warmed for 15 minutes at 37°C to dissociate autoabsorbed antibody before determining the titer.

When a high-titer cold agglutinin is present, an EDTA-anticoagulated blood specimen can show visible agglutinates in the tube at room temperature or cooler.[1] Agglutination can also be observed on the peripheral blood film (Figure 23.5). Blood specimens from patients with cold agglutinins must be warmed to 37°C for at least 15 minutes before complete blood count (CBC) analysis by automated blood cell analyzers. RBC agglutination grossly elevates the MCV, reduces the RBC count, and has unpredictable effects on other indices (Chapter 13). When the

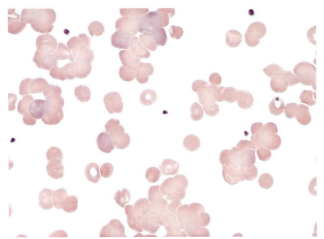

Figure 23.5 Peripheral Blood Film Showing Red Blood Cell Agglutination. (Wright-Giemsa stain, ×1000.)

specimen is warmed to 37°C, antibody dissociates from RBCs and agglutination usually disappears. If not, a new specimen is collected and maintained at 37°C for the entire time before testing. To avoid agglutination on a peripheral blood film, the slide can also be warmed to 37°C before the application of blood. Cold agglutinins can also interfere with ABO typing.[2]

Treatment

Acute CAD associated with infections is self-limiting, and cold agglutinin titers are usually less than 1:4000.[13] If hemolysis is mild, no treatment is required; however, patients with severe hemolysis require transfusion and supportive care.[13] Patients with chronic CAD and mild anemia are regularly monitored and advised to avoid cold temperatures.[1] In chronic CAD with moderate to severe symptoms, rituximab produces a partial response in about half of patients as a result of its targeting and ultimate destruction of B lymphocytes containing the CD20 antigen, but median remission is less than a year.[15] Rituximab-fludarabine and rituximab-bendamustine combination therapies have a better response rate, 76% and 71%, respectively, with the latter combination having fewer side effects and better tolerability.[16,17] Plasmapheresis is used in severe cases but provides only temporary benefit.[1] Corticosteroid therapy and immunosuppressive therapy with cyclophosphamide and chlorambucil are not effective for most patients.[13,14] Splenectomy is also not effective because C3b-sensitized RBCs in IgM-mediated autoimmune hemolysis are cleared primarily by the liver.[1,5,13]

RBC transfusion is reserved for patients with life-threatening anemia or cardiovascular or cerebrovascular symptoms.[1] If transfusion is needed, the presence of clinically significant *allo*antibodies must be ruled out.[2] In CAD cases involving an autoantibody with wide thermal amplitude, detection of coexisting warm-reactive alloantibodies can be time consuming and difficult. During transfusion, the patient is kept warm, small amounts of blood are given while the patient is observed for symptoms of a hemolytic transfusion reaction, and a blood warmer is used to minimize in vivo reactivity of the cold autoantibody.[1]

Paroxysmal Cold Hemoglobinuria

Etiology

Paroxysmal cold hemoglobinuria (PCH) is an acute form of cold-reactive hemolytic anemia. PCH can be idiopathic or secondary. Secondary PCH was associated with late-stage syphilis, but now it is most commonly seen in young children after a viral respiratory infection.[1,2,13] PCH is rare in adults. The prevalence of PCH has been reported to be as high as 32% to 40% of children with autoimmune hemolytic anemia, with a median age at presentation of 5 years.[18,19]

Anti-P autoantibody, also called the *Donath-Landsteiner antibody*, is a complement-binding IgG hemolysin with specificity for P antigen on RBCs. Anti-P autoantibody is biphasic in that at cold temperatures it binds to the P antigen on RBCs and partially activates complement (C1 to C4), but full complement activation (C3 through C9) and hemolysis occur only on warming to 37°C.[20] Anti-P autoantibody binds RBC antigen optimally at 4°C and has a thermal amplitude of less than 20°C. At warmer temperatures, anti-P autoantibody dissociates from RBCs; the titer is usually less than 1:64.[13]

Symptoms

Children typically present with acute fever, malaise, and back, leg, and/or abdominal pain 1 to 2 weeks after an upper respiratory tract infection.[13] Pallor, jaundice, and dark urine caused by hemoglobinuria are often present.[13] The abrupt onset of hemolysis causes a rapidly progressing and severe anemia, with hemoglobin levels often dropping to less than 5 g/dL.[13] Exposure to cold temperatures may precipitate hemolytic manifestations in some patients, but cold exposure is not required for the majority of patients to manifest symptoms; the reasons for this have yet to be explained.[2,19]

Laboratory Findings

Reticulocytosis is typical but can be preceded by reticulocytopenia.[13] The peripheral blood film shows polychromasia and spherocytes, but schistocytes, nucleated RBCs, anisocytosis, poikilocytosis, and erythrophagocytosis can also be observed.[13] At first, leukopenia may be present, with leukocytosis occurring later.[13] In addition, laboratory findings typical for intravascular hemolysis are found. Because anti-P autoantibody is dissociated from RBCs at body temperature, the DAT result is usually positive for C3d only.[2,18]

The classic Donath-Landsteiner screening test for anti-P is done by collecting blood specimens in two tubes (without anticoagulant), one for the patient test and the other for the patient control.[19] The patient test specimen is incubated first at 4°C for 30 minutes (to allow anti-P binding to the P antigen and partial complement activation on RBCs) and then at 37°C for 30 minutes (to allow full activation of the complement pathway to lysis). The patient control tube is kept at 37°C for both incubations (a total of 60 minutes). After centrifugation, serum is examined for hemolysis. A positive test result for anti-P is indicated by hemolysis in the patient test specimen incubated first at 4°C and then at 37°C and no hemolysis in the patient control specimen kept at 37°C. In the control tube, anti-P is not able to bind to antigen at 37°C, so complement is not activated and hemolysis does not occur.[19] Initial test results may be falsely negative as a result of low complement and/or anti-P levels in the patient specimen because of the brisk hemolysis in vivo.[19] Incubating patient serum with complement and papain-treated compatible group O RBCs increases the sensitivity of the test in detecting anti-P. Enzyme treatment provides greater exposure of the P antigen on the RBC surface for antibody binding.[19]

Treatment

PCH is severe but self-limiting and resolves in several days to a few weeks, with an excellent prognosis.[1,13,18] In most patients, anemia is severe and can be life-threatening, so transfusion is usually needed until symptoms resolve. Because anti-P autoantibody reacts only at lower temperatures and P antigen-negative blood is very rare, P-positive blood can be transfused.[2]

Mixed-Type Autoimmune Hemolytic Anemia

Mixed-type AIHA occurs very infrequently.[21] In this condition, the patient simultaneously develops an IgG autoantibody with optimum reactivity at 37°C (WAIHA) and a pathologic IgM autoantibody that reacts optimally at 0° to 10°C but has a thermal amplitude of greater than 30°C (CAD).[21] Patients with WAIHA and a nonpathogenic cold agglutinin (i.e., an agglutinin that does not react at a temperature greater than 20°C) should not be classified as having a mixed-type AIHA because the cold agglutinin is not clinically significant.[13]

Hemolysis results from a combination of extravascular and intravascular mechanisms. The disease course appears to be chronic, with intermittent episodes of severe anemia.[5,13] The DAT is positive with IgG only, C3d only, or both IgG and C3d.[2] The warm autoantibody is typically panreactive, with unclear specificity, whereas the cold-reacting antibody usually has anti-I specificity.[5] Treatment is the same as that described for WAIHA.[5]

ALLOIMMUNE HEMOLYTIC ANEMIAS

Hemolytic Transfusion Reaction

One of the most severe and potentially life-threatening complications of blood transfusion is a hemolytic transfusion reaction (HTR) caused by immune-mediated destruction of donor cells by an antibody in the recipient. The offending antibody in the recipient may be IgM or IgG, complement may be partially or fully activated or not activated at all, and hemolysis may be intravascular or extravascular, depending on the characteristics of the antibody. HTRs can have an acute or delayed onset.[2]

Acute Hemolytic Transfusion Reaction

Acute hemolytic transfusion reactions (AHTRs) occur within minutes to hours of initiation of a transfusion.[22] The most common cause of AHTR is accidental transfusion of ABO-incompatible donor RBCs into a recipient, for example, the transfusion of group A RBCs into a group O recipient. The recipient has preformed, non-RBC stimulated anti-A (IgM) that is capable of fully activating complement to C9 on binding to the A antigen on donor RBCs. There is rapid, complement-mediated intravascular hemolysis and activation of the coagulation system. ABO-incompatible RBC transfusions are usually a result of clerical error and have been estimated to occur in approximately 1 in 40,000, whereas the estimated risk of ABO HTR is 1:80,000.[2] Severity of AHTR is variable and is affected by the infusion rate and volume of blood transfused.[2,23] AHTR carries an estimated mortality rate of 2%.[22] AHTRs can occur as a result of incompatibilities involving other blood group systems, but these are rare.[22]

Symptoms of severe intravascular hemolysis found in ABO-related AHTRs begin within minutes or hours and may include chills, fever, urticaria, tachycardia, nausea and vomiting, chest and back pain, shock, anaphylaxis, pulmonary edema, congestive heart failure, and bleeding as a result of disseminated intravascular coagulation (DIC). The transfusion should be immediately terminated on first appearance of symptoms. Treatment is urgent and includes efforts to prevent or correct shock, maintain renal circulation, and control DIC.[23]

A transfusion reaction workup of the suspected HTR includes a clerical check for errors, an examination of a post-transfusion blood specimen for hemolysis, and performance of the DAT on RBCs in a posttransfusion specimen.[22] If an AHTR occurred, hemoglobinemia and hemoglobinuria are detectable and the DAT result is positive. DAT findings may be negative, however, if all the donor cells are lysed.[22] Hemoglobin and serum haptoglobin levels decrease, but serum indirect bilirubin will not begin to rise until 2 to 3 days after the episode. ABO and Rh typing, antibody screen, and cross matching are repeated on recipient and donor specimens to identify the blood group incompatibility. Coagulation tests such as D-dimer, fibrinogen, factors V and VIII, and platelet count can help reveal and assess the risk of DIC.[2]

Delayed Hemolytic Transfusion Reaction

Delayed hemolytic transfusion reaction (DHTR) may occur days to weeks after transfusion as the titer of alloantibodies increases.[2,23] Often, the patient has been alloimmunized by pregnancy or previous transfusion, but the antibody titer was lower than the level of serologic detection at the time of transfusion. The second exposure to the antigen results in an increase in titer (anamnestic response). The antibody is usually IgG, is reactive at 37°C, and may or may not be able to partially or fully activate complement. Antibodies most often implicated in DHTRs are directed against antigens in the Duffy and Kidd blood group systems.[22,23] The patient's antibody binds to transfused RBCs, which leads to extravascular hemolysis, with or without complement activation. The principal signs are an inadequate posttransfusion hemoglobin increase, positive DAT results for IgG and/or C3d, morphologic evidence of hemolysis (spherocytes, polychromasia), and an increase in serum indirect bilirubin.[22] Management of DHTR includes monitoring of kidney function, especially in acutely ill patients.[22]

Hemolytic Disease of the Fetus and Newborn

Hemolytic disease of the fetus and newborn (HDFN) occurs when an IgG alloantibody produced by the mother crosses the placenta into the fetal circulation and binds to fetal RBCs that are positive for the corresponding antigen. IgG-sensitized fetal RBCs are cleared from the circulation by macrophages in the fetal spleen (extravascular hemolysis), and an anemia gradually develops. There is erythroid hyperplasia in the fetal bone marrow and extramedullary erythropoiesis in the fetal spleen, liver, kidneys, and adrenal glands.[24] As a result, many nucleated RBCs are released into the fetal circulation. If anemia is severe in utero, it can lead to generalized edema, ascites, and a condition called *hydrops fetalis,* which is fatal if untreated.[2,24] Anti-Kell antibodies are notable because they also cause anemia by suppressing fetal erythropoiesis.[24]

Rh Hemolytic Disease of the Fetus and Newborn

In Rh HDFN, which causes the highest number of fetal fatalities, an Rh (D)-negative mother has preformed anti-D antibodies (IgG, reactive at 37°C) from exposure to the D antigen either through immunization in a previous pregnancy with a D-positive baby or from previous transfusion of blood products with D-positive RBCs. In subsequent pregnancies, the anti-D crosses the placenta and if the fetus is D positive, the anti-D binds to D antigen sites on the fetal RBCs. These anti-D-sensitized fetal RBCs are cleared from the circulation by macrophages in the fetal spleen, and anemia and hyperbilirubinemia develop. Amniocentesis is accurate at predicting severe fetal anemia, but it is an invasive procedure and carries some risk of fetal loss.[24] If severe fetal anemia and HDFN caused by anti-D are suspected, a percutaneous umbilical fetal blood specimen can be obtained and tested for the hemoglobin level to determine the severity of the anemia; in addition, a noninvasive assessment of anemia can be done by ultrasound measurement of fetal cerebral blood flow.[2,24]

Laboratory findings. ABO, Rh typing, and an antibody screen are performed on the mother when the fetus is between 10 and 16 weeks' gestation and again at 28 weeks' gestation.[24] The antibody screen during pregnancy detects antibodies other than those caused by ABO incompatibility.[2] If the antibody screen is positive for a clinically significant antibody, an RBC panel is performed to identify the specificity of the antibody. Certain antibodies may be ignored if their corresponding antigens are poorly developed at birth, such as anti-I, anti-P1, anti-Le[a], and anti-Le[b]. Mothers with initial positive antibody screens are retested with an antibody screen every month until 28 weeks, then every 2 weeks thereafter; antibody titers are reported from each specimen. Titration of the antibody does not predict the severity of HDFN; rather, it helps determine when to monitor for HDFN by additional methods, such as spectrophotometric analysis of amniotic fluid bilirubin.[2,24] After the first affected pregnancy, the antibody titer is no longer useful, and other means of monitoring the fetus are used, such as amniocentesis and ultrasonography.[24]

An unimmunized D-negative mother receives antenatal Rh immune globulin (RhIG) at 28 weeks' gestation and again within 72 hours of delivery of a D-positive infant to prevent alloimmunization to the D antigen.[2] Even one antenatal dose of 200 μg RhIG will reduce by half the risk of the mother developing anti-D antibodies and having a child with HDFN in the next

pregnancy.[25] Rh-negative women who experience spontaneous or induced abortion also receive Rh immune globulin.

At delivery, newborn testing is performed on umbilical cord blood. Neonates with Rh HDFN have a decreased hemoglobin level, increased reticulocyte count, and increased level of serum indirect bilirubin. The peripheral blood film shows polychromasia and many nucleated RBCs. ABO (only forward typing), Rh typing, and the DAT are also performed. The DAT result is positive for IgG, and anti-D can be demonstrated in an eluate of the infant's RBCs.[24]

Treatment for an affected infant. Treatment for a fetus affected by HDFN may include intrauterine transfusion, whereby pooled hemolyzed blood is removed via amniocentesis from the fetal abdomen and replaced with a small amount of fresh RBCs. This procedure can be used to correct fetal anemia and prevent hydrops fetalis.[26] Cordocentesis is also used, whereby fresh RBCs are injected into the umbilical vein. Survival rates of fetuses receiving transfusions are 85% to 90%; the risk of premature death from these procedures varies from 1% to 3%.[26] After delivery, the neonate may need exchange transfusions and phototherapy to reduce the level of serum indirect bilirubin and prevent *kernicterus* (bilirubin accumulation in the brain).[24] Prolonged postnatal anemia can be the result of a slow decrease of maternal antibody in the newborn's circulation; rare cases of prolonged anemia are documented in infants who received intrauterine transfusions.[27,28]

Hemolytic Disease of the Fetus and Newborn Caused by Other Blood Group Antibodies

ABO HDFN is more common than Rh HDFN and may occur during the first pregnancy. In contrast to Rh HDFN, ABO HDFN is asymptomatic or produces mild hyperbilirubinemia and anemia. ABO HDFN is seen in some type A or B infants born to type O mothers who produce IgG anti-A and anti-B, which are capable of crossing the placenta. The disease is milder than Rh HDFN, likely because A and B antigens are poorly developed on fetal and newborn RBCs, and other cells and tissues express A and B antigens, which reduces the amount of maternal antibody directed against fetal RBCs. The DAT result for a newborn with ABO HDFN is only weakly positive and may be negative. Spherocytes and polychromasia on the peripheral blood film are typical.[2] Table 23.3 presents a comparison of HDFN caused by ABO and Rh incompatibility.

TABLE 23.3 **Characteristics of Rh and ABO Hemolytic Disease of the Fetus and Newborn**		
	Rh	**ABO**
Blood groups	Mother: Rh (D) negative Child: Rh (D) positive	Mother: O Child: A or B
Severity of disease	Severe	Mild
Jaundice	Severe	Mild
Spherocytes on peripheral blood film	Rare	Usually present
Anemia	Severe	If present, mild
Direct antiglobulin test	Positive	Negative or weakly positive

HDFN can be caused by other IgG antibodies, particularly antibodies to the K, c, and Fy^a antigens.[2] HDFN caused by other blood group antibodies is rare.[24,29–32] Antibody screening in the first trimester can assist in identifying rare antibodies that can cause HDFN.[33] Adverse clinical outcomes in all forms of HDFN include varying degrees of anemia, jaundice, and kernicterus.

DRUG-INDUCED IMMUNE HEMOLYTIC ANEMIA

Drug-induced immune hemolytic anemia (DIIHA) is very rare, with an estimated annual incidence of about 1 per 1 million people.[34] This condition is suspected when there is a sudden decrease in hemoglobin after administration of a drug, clinical and biochemical evidence of extravascular or intravascular hemolysis, and a positive DAT result.[35] More than 125 drugs have been reported to cause DIIHA, with the most common drug categories being antimicrobial (particularly penicillins and cephalosporins), antiinflammatory, and antineoplastic drugs.[36–38] The most common drugs implicated in DIIHA in the last 10

years are piperacillin, cefotetan, and ceftriaxone.[39] Severe and even fatal cases have been reported.[34,37,40,41]

Mechanisms of Drug-Induced Immune Hemolysis

Various theories have been proposed to explain the mechanisms of DIIHA.[34,41] Three generally accepted mechanisms involve an antibody produced by the patient as a result of exposure to the drug and include drug adsorption, drug-RBC membrane protein immunogenic complex, and RBC autoantibody induction (Figure 23.6). A fourth mechanism, drug-induced nonimmunologic protein adsorption (NIPA), can result in a positive DAT result, but no drug or RBC antibody is produced by the patient. This mechanism is discussed at the end of this section.

1. *Drug adsorption:* The patient produces an IgG antibody to a drug. When the drug is taken by the patient, the drug binds strongly to the patient's RBCs. The IgG drug antibody binds to the drug attached to the RBCs, usually without complement activation. Because the offending antibody is IgG and is strongly attached to the RBCs via the drug, hemolysis is

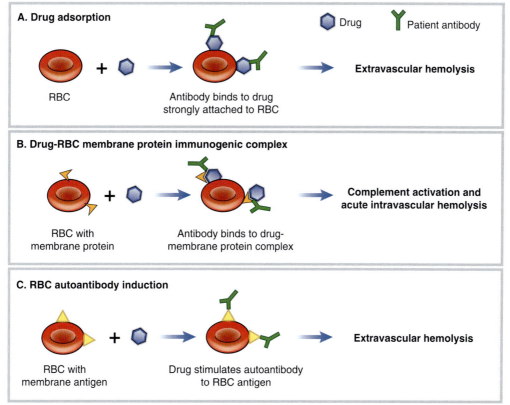

Figure 23.6 Graphic Representation of Drug-Induced Immune Hemolytic Anemia Mechanisms. (A), Drug adsorption. A drug binds (adsorbs) tightly to the RBC membrane. The patient produces an antidrug immunoglobulin G (IgG) antibody that binds to the drug. RBCs coated with adsorbed drug bound with antidrug antibodies are removed from circulation by macrophages in the spleen (extravascular hemolysis). (B), Drug-RBC membrane protein immunogenic complex. A drug loosely binds to an RBC membrane protein forming a drug-RBC protein complex. The patient produces an IgG and/or IgM (not shown) antibody that binds to the complex, causing complement activation and acute intravascular hemolysis. (C), RBC autoantibody induction. A drug induces the patient to produce IgG warm-reactive autoantibodies against RBC self-antigens. The IgG autoantibodies bind to the corresponding antigens on the RBC surface. RBCs coated with IgG autoantibodies are removed from circulation by macrophages in the spleen (extravascular hemolysis). *RBC,* Red blood cell.

extravascular by splenic macrophages, which remove the antibody- and drug-coated RBCs from the circulation.

2. *Drug-RBC membrane protein immunogenic complex:* A drug binds loosely to an RBC membrane protein to form a drug-RBC protein immunogenic complex or epitope. The patient produces an IgM and/or IgG antibody that binds to the complex on the RBCs and complement is fully activated, which causes acute intravascular hemolysis.

3. *RBC autoantibody induction:* A drug induces the patient to produce IgG warm-reactive autoantibodies against RBC self-antigens. These autoantibodies react at 37°C, and the laboratory findings are indistinguishable from those in WAIHA. Hemolysis is extravascular and is mediated by macrophages, predominantly in the spleen.

Several authors have suggested that all drug-induced immune hemolysis is explained by a single mechanism, known as the *unifying theory.* This theory proposes that a drug interacts with the RBC membrane and generates multiple immunogenic epitopes that can elicit an immune response to the drug alone, to the drug-RBC membrane protein combination, or to an RBC membrane protein alone.[2,36,42] Diagnosis of DIIHA can be made only if the antibody screen is positive and the RBC eluate contains an antibody.[1]

Antibody Characteristics

Antibodies implicated in DIIHA can be divided into two general types: drug-dependent (most common) and drug-independent antibodies.[2,36] Some drugs are able to induce a combination of both types of antibodies.[34,41,42]

Drug-Dependent Antibodies

Drug-dependent antibodies react in vitro only when the suspected drug or its metabolite is present.[2,36] There are two types of drug-dependent antibodies:

1. *Antibodies that react only with drug-treated cells*[2]: These are IgG drug antibodies that bind to the drug when it is strongly associated with the RBC surface (drug adsorption mechanism). Because they have bound IgG, RBCs are cleared from the circulation extravascularly by macrophages in the spleen, and a hemolytic anemia gradually develops. Complement is not usually activated. If the DIIHA is not recognized, the patient may continue to take the drug to a point in which life-threatening anemia develops.[2,34] Examples of drugs that elicit antibodies in this category are penicillin, ampicillin, and many cephalosporins.[2,36,38,39] Laboratory features include a positive DAT reaction with anti-IgG, whereas the reaction with anti-C3b/C3d is usually negative. In the IAT, the patient's serum and an eluate of the patient's cells react only with drug-treated RBCs and not with untreated RBCs.[2]

2. *Antibodies that react only in the presence of the drug*[2:] These IgG and/or IgM antibodies bind to the drug or its metabolite

only when it is weakly associated in a drug-RBC membrane protein complex (drug-RBC membrane protein immunogenic complex mechanism). The antibodies activate complement and trigger acute intravascular hemolysis that may progress to renal failure.[2] Hemolysis occurs abruptly after short periods of drug exposure or on readministration of the drug.[34] Examples of drugs that elicit antibodies in this category are piperacillin and some second- and third-generation cephalosporins.[2,38,39] Laboratory features include a positive DAT reaction with anti-C3b/C3d and occasionally with anti-IgG. In the IAT, the patient's serum reacts with untreated, normal RBCs only in the presence of the drug.

Drug-Independent Antibodies

Drug-independent antibodies are IgG, warm-reactive, RBC autoantibodies induced by the drug (RBC autoantibody induction mechanism). These autoantibodies have the same serologic reactivity as those causing WAIHA, and they do not require the presence of the drug for in vitro reactivity. Hemolysis is extravascular, mediated by macrophages predominantly in the spleen, usually with a gradual onset of anemia. A common example of a drug in this category is fludarabine.[2,39] Laboratory features include a positive DAT reaction with anti-IgG. In the IAT, patient's serum and an eluate of the patient's cells generally react at 37°C with all screening and panel RBCs and with the patient's own RBCs.[2]

Nonimmune Drug-Induced Hemolysis

In *drug-induced nonimmunologic protein adsorption (NIPA),* the patient does not produce an antibody to the drug or to RBCs. The mechanism is also called the *membrane modification method* because certain drugs such as high-dose clavulanate and cisplatin can alter the RBC membrane so that numerous proteins including IgG and complement adsorb onto the RBC surface.[36,41] Examples of drugs that cause NIPA and a positive DAT are cephalothin, diglycoaldehyde, cisplatin, oxaliplatin, and β-lactamase inhibitors.[2,38,39] This phenomenon is usually asymptomatic and results in a positive DAT finding but only rarely has hemolysis been reported.[38] The IAT on patient's serum and an eluate of patient's RBCs yield negative results.[2,39]

Treatment

After a DIIHA is recognized and confirmed, the first treatment is to discontinue the drug. Most patients will gradually show improvement within a few days to several weeks.[34] In cases in which a warm-reacting autoimmune antibody is present, the positive DAT result may persist for months after a hematologic recovery. If anemia is severe, the patient may require RBC transfusion or plasma exchange.[34] Regardless of mechanism, future episodes of DIIHA are prevented by avoidance of the drug.

SUMMARY

- Immune hemolytic anemias are classified into autoimmune hemolytic anemia (AIHA), alloimmune hemolytic anemia, and drug-induced immune hemolytic anemia (DIIHA).
- Hemolysis mediated by immunoglobulin M (IgM) requires complement; hemolysis may be extravascular (mainly in the liver) if complement is partially activated to C3b or intravascular if complement is fully activated to C9.
- Hemolysis mediated by IgG occurs with or without complement activation; IgG-sensitized red blood cells (RBCs) are removed from the circulation by macrophages in the spleen; partial phagocytosis produces spherocytes, which are prematurely trapped in the spleen and phagocytized; IgG- and C3b-sensitized RBCs are removed by macrophages in the spleen and liver.
- Laboratory findings in immune hemolytic anemia include decreased hemoglobin level, increased reticulocyte count, increased levels of serum indirect bilirubin and lactate dehydrogenase, and decreased serum haptoglobin level. The peripheral blood film may show polychromasia, spherocytes (IgG-mediated hemolysis), or RBC agglutination (cold agglutinins). The direct antiglobulin test (DAT) detects in vivo sensitization of RBCs by IgG and/or C3b/C3d.
- Classification of AIHA includes warm autoimmune hemolytic anemia (WAIHA), cold agglutinin disease (CAD), paroxysmal cold hemoglobinuria (PCH), and mixed-type AIHA.
- WAIHA is the most common form of AIHA and involves IgG autoantibodies with optimum reactivity at 37° C. Anemia varies from mild to severe, and characteristic morphologic features on the peripheral blood film are polychromasia and spherocytes.
- CAD is caused by an IgM autoantibody with optimum reactivity at 4° C and a thermal amplitude of greater than 30° C. RBC agglutination may be observed on a peripheral blood film, and agglutinates may cause interference with complete blood count analysis on automated blood cell analyzers.

- PCH is due to a biphasic IgG autoantibody with anti-P specificity. The antibody binds to P antigen on RBCs and partially activates complement at 4° C; complete complement activation and hemolysis occur on warming the specimen to 37° C.
- Classification of alloimmune hemolytic anemia includes hemolytic transfusion reactions and hemolytic disease of the fetus and newborn (HDFN).
- Acute hemolytic transfusion reactions occur within minutes to hours after the start of an RBC transfusion and most often involve transfusion of ABO-incompatible blood; the hemolysis is predominantly intravascular. Delayed hemolytic transfusion reactions may occur days or weeks after the transfusion and represent an anamnestic response to a donor RBC antigen; hemolysis is usually extravascular.
- HDFN occurs when an IgG alloantibody produced by the mother crosses the placenta into the fetal circulation and binds to fetal RBCs that are positive for the corresponding antigen. IgG-sensitized fetal RBCs are cleared from the circulation by macrophages in the fetal spleen, and an anemia gradually develops; the usual laboratory findings in the neonate are anemia, hyperbilirubinemia, and a positive DAT result.
- ABO HDFN is more common than Rh HDFN and produces no symptoms or mild anemia. Rh HDFN caused by anti-D results in severe anemia. Antenatal administration of Rh immune globulin to a D-negative mother when the fetus is at 28 weeks' gestation and within 72 hours after delivery of a D-positive infant prevents immunization to the D antigen.
- In DIIHA, the patient produces antibodies to (1) a drug only, (2) a complex of a drug loosely bound to an RBC membrane protein, or (3) an RBC membrane protein only. In vitro reactions of antibodies in DIIHA may be drug dependent or drug independent.

Now that you have completed this chapter, go back and read again the case study at the beginning and respond to the questions presented. Answers can be found in Appendix C.

REVIEW QUESTIONS

Answers can be found in Appendix C.

1. Immune hemolytic anemia is due to a(n):
   a. Structural defect in the RBC membrane
   b. Alloantibody or autoantibody against an RBC antigen
   c. T cell immune response against an RBC antigen
   d. Obstruction of blood flow by intravascular thrombi
2. The pathophysiology of immune hemolysis with IgM antibodies always involves:
   a. Complement
   b. Autoantibodies
   c. Abnormal hemoglobin molecules
   d. Alloantibodies

3. In hemolysis mediated by IgG antibodies, which abnormal RBC morphology is typically observed on the peripheral blood film?
   a. Spherocytes
   b. Nucleated RBCs
   c. RBC agglutination
   d. Macrocytes
4. The most important finding in the diagnostic investigation of a suspected autoimmune hemolytic anemia is:
   a. Detection of a low hemoglobin and hematocrit
   b. Observation of hemoglobinemia in a specimen
   c. Recognition of a low reticulocyte count
   d. Demonstration of IgG and/or C3d on the RBC surface

5. In autoimmune hemolytic anemia, a positive DAT is evidence that an:
   a. IgM antibody is in the patient's serum
   b. IgG antibody is in the patient's serum
   c. IgM antibody is sensitizing the patient's RBCs
   d. IgG antibody is sensitizing the patient's RBCs
6. Which of the following is NOT a mechanism of drug-induced hemolytic anemia?
   a. Drug adsorption on RBC membrane
   b. Drug-RBC membrane protein immunogenic complex
   c. RBC autoantibody induction
   d. IgM autoantibody sensitization of RBCs after exposure to cold temperatures
7. Which of the following describes a penicillin-induced DIHA?
   a. Extravascular hemolysis, positive DAT with IgG, gradual anemia
   b. Intravascular, possible renal failure, positive DAT with C3d
   c. Extravascular hemolysis, positive DAT with C3d, acute onset
   d. Intravascular hemolysis, positive DAT with IgG

8. Which one of the following statements is TRUE about DHTR?
   a. It usually is due to an ABO incompatibility.
   b. Hemoglobinemia and hemoglobinuria often occur.
   c. It is due to an anamnestic response after repeat exposure to a blood group antigen.
   d. The DAT yields a positive result for C3d only.
9. A 63-year-old man is being evaluated because of a decrease in hemoglobin of 5 g/dL after a second cycle of fludarabine for treatment of chronic lymphocytic leukemia. The patient's DAT result is strongly positive for IgG only, and antibody testing on his serum and an eluate of his RBCs yield positive results with all panel cells and the patient's own cells. This suggests which mechanism of immune hemolysis for this patient?
   a. Drug-RBC membrane protein complex
   b. Drug adsorption
   c. RBC autoantibody induction
   d. Drug-induced nonimmunologic protein adsorption
10. A group A Rh-negative mother gave birth to a group O Rh-positive baby. The baby is at risk for HDFN if:
    a. This was the mother's first pregnancy
    b. The mother has IgG ABO antibodies
    c. The mother was previously immunized to the D antigen
    d. The mother received Rh immune globulin before delivery

REFERENCES

1. Michel, M., & Jäger, U. (2023). Autoimmune hemolytic anemia. In Hoffman, R., Benz, E. J., Silberstein, L. E., et al. (Eds.), *Hematology: Basic Principles and Practice.* (8th ed., pp. 672–687). Philadelphia: Elsevier.
2. Borge, P. D. & Mansfield, P. M. (2020). The positive direct antiglobulin test and immune-mediated hemolysis. In Cohn, C. S., Delaney, M., Johnson, S. T., Katz, L. M. et al. (Eds.), *Technical Manual.* (20th ed., pp. 429–456). Bethesda, MD: American Association of Blood Banks.
3. Araten, D. J., Isenman, D. E., & Carroll, C. (2023). Complement and immunoglobulin biology leading to clinical translation. In Hoffman, R., Benz, E. J., Silberstein, L. E., et al. (Eds.), *Hematology: Basic Principles and Practice.* (8th ed., pp. 242–270). Philadelphia: Elsevier.
4. Morgan, B. P. (2013). Complement. In Paul, W. E. (Ed.), *Fundamental Immunology.* (7th ed., pp. 863–890). Philadelphia: Lippincott Williams & Wilkins.
5. Friedberg, R. C., & Johari, V. P. (2019). Autoimmune hemolytic anemia. In Greer, J. P., Arber, D. A., Glader, B., et al. (Eds.), *Wintrobe's Clinical Hematology.* (14th ed., pp. 746–765). Philadelphia: Lippincott Williams & Wilkins.
6. Michel, M. (2011). Classification and therapeutic approaches in autoimmune hemolytic anemia: an update. *Expert Rev Hematol, 4,* 607–618.
7. Dhingra, K., Jain, D., Mandal, S., et al. (2008). Evans syndrome: a study of six cases with review of literature. *Hematology, 13,* 356–360.
8. Jäger, U., Barcellini, W., Broome, C. M., et al. (2020). Diagnosis and treatment of autoimmune hemolytic anemia in adults: recommendations from the first international consensus meeting. *Blood Rev, 41,* 100648.
9. Kalfa, T. A. (2016). Warm antibody autoimmune hemolytic anemia. *Hematology Am Soc Hematol Educ Program, 2016*(1), 690–697.
10. Buckley, L., Guyatt, G., & Fink, H. A. (2017). 2017 American College of Rheumatology guideline for the prevention and treatment of glucocorticoid-induced osteoporosis. *Arthritis Care Res, 69*(8), 1095–1110.
11. Reynaud, Q., Durieu, I., Dutertre, M., et al. (2015). Efficacy and safety of rituximab in autoimmune hemolytic anemia: a meta-analysis of 21 studies. *Autoimmun Rev, 14*(4), 304–313.
12. Berentsen, S., Beiske, K., & Tjonnfjord, G. (2007). Primary chronic cold agglutinin disease: an update on pathogenesis, clinical features and therapy. *Hematology, 12,* 361–370.
13. Petz, L. (2008). Cold antibody autoimmune hemolytic anemias. *Blood Rev, 22,* 1–15.
14. Berentsen, S., Ulvestad, E., Langholm, R., et al. (2006). Primary chronic cold agglutinin disease: a population based clinical study of 86 patients. *Haematologica, 91,* 460–466.
15. Schöllkopf, C., Kjeldsen, L., Bjerrum, O. W., et al. (2006). Rituximab in chronic cold agglutinin disease: a prospective study of 20 patients. *Leuk Lymphoma, 47,* 253–260.
16. Berentsen, S., Randen, U., Vagan, A., et al. (2010). High response rate and durable remissions following fludarabine and rituximab combination therapy for chronic cold agglutinin disease. *Blood, 116,* 3180–3184.
17. Berensten, S., Randen, U., Oksman, M., et al. (2017). Bendamustine plus rituximab for chronic cold agglutinin disease: results of a Nordic prospective multicenter trial. *Blood, 130*(4), 537–541.
18. Karafin, M., Shirey, S., Ness, P., et al. (2012). A case study of a child with chronic hemolytic anemia due to a Donath-Landsteiner positive, IgM anti-I autoantibody. *Pediatr Blood Cancer, 59,* 953–955.

19. Gertz, M. (2007). Management of cold haemolytic syndrome. *Br J Haematol, 138,* 422–429.

20. Sokol, R., Hewitt, S., & Stamps, B. (1981). Autoimmune haemolysis: an 18 year study of 865 cases referred to a regional transfusion centre. *Br Med J, 282,* 2023–2027.

21. Mayer, B., Yurek, S., Kiesewetter, H., et al. (2008). Mixed-type autoimmune hemolytic anemia: differential diagnosis and critical review of reported cases. *Transfusion, 48,* 2229–2234.

22. Cohn, C. S., McCullough, J., & He, X. (2021). Blood procurement and red cell transfusion. In: Kaushansky, K., Prchal, J. T., Burns, L.J., et al. (Eds.), *Williams Hematology.* (10th ed., pp. 2483–2500). New York: McGraw-Hill.

23. Eder, A., & Chambers, L. (2007). Noninfectious complications of blood transfusion. *Arch Pathol Lab Med, 131,* 708–718.

24. Fasano, R. M., Hendrickson, J. E., & Luban, N. L. C. (2021). Alloimmune hemolytic disease of the fetus and newborn. In: Kaushansky, K., Prchal, J. T., Burns, L.J., et al. (Eds.), *Williams Hematology.* (10th ed., pp. 917–932). New York: McGraw-Hill.

25. Koelewijn, J., Haas, M., Vrijkotte, T., et al. (2008). One single dose of 200 μg of antenatal RhIG halves the risk of anti-D immunization and hemolytic disease of the fetus and newborn in the next pregnancy. *Transfusion, 48,* 1721–1729.

26. Dodd, J. M., Windrim, R. C., & van Kamp, I. L. (2012). Techniques of intrauterine fetal transfusion for women with red-cell isoimmunisation for improving health outcomes. *Cochrane Database Syst Rev, (9),* CD007096.

27. Patel, L. L., Myers, J. C., Palma, J. P., et al. (2013). Anti-Ge3 causes late-onset hemolytic disease of the newborn: the fourth case in three Hispanic families. *Transfusion, 53,* 2152–2157.

28. Dorn, I., Schlenke, P., & Hartel, C. (2010). Prolonged anemia in an intrauterine-transfused neonate with Rh-negative hemolytic disease: no evidence for anti-D-related suppression of erythropoiesis in vitro. *Transfusion, 50,* 1064–1070.

29. Michalewska, B., Wielgos, M., Zupanska, B., et al. (2008). Anti-Coa implicated in severe haemolytic disease of the foetus and newborn. *Transfus Med, 18,* 71–73.

30. Dohmen, S., Muit, J., Ligthart, P., et al. (2008). Anti-e found in a case of hemolytic disease of the fetus and newborn makes use of the IGHV3 superspecies genes. *Transfusion, 48,* 194–194.

31. van Gammeren, A. J., Overbeeke, M. A., Idema, R. N., et al. (2008). Haemolytic disease of the newborn because of rare anti-Vel. *Transfus Med, 18,* 197–198.

32. Li, B. J., Jiang, Y. J., Yuan, F., et al. (2010). Exchange transfusion of least incompatible blood for severe hemolytic disease of the newborn due to anti-Rh17. *Transfus Med, 20,* 66–69.

33. Koelewijn, J. M., Vrijkotte, T. G., van der Schoot, C. E., et al. (2008). Effect of screening for red cell antibodies, other than anti-D, to detect hemolytic disease of the fetus and newborn: a population study in the Netherlands. *Transfusion, 48,* 941–952.

34. Garratty, G. (2010). Immune hemolytic anemia associated with drug therapy. *Blood Rev, 24,* 143–150.

35. Johnson, S., Fueger, J., & Gottschall, J. (2007). One center's experience: the serology and drugs associated with drug-induced hemolytic anemia—a new paradigm. *Transfusion, 47,* 697–702.

36. Garratty, G. (2009). Drug-induced immune hemolytic anemia. *Hematology Am Soc Hematol Educ Program, 2009(1),* 73–79.

37. Garratty, G., & Arndt, P. (2007). An update on drug-induced immune hemolytic anemia. *Immunohematology, 23,* 105–119.

38. Renard, D., & Rosselet, A. (2017). Drug-induced hemolytic anemia: pharmacological aspects. *Transfus Clin Biol, 24(3),* 110–114.

39. Garratty, G., & Arndt, P. A. (2014). Drugs that have been shown to cause drug-induced immune hemolytic anemia or positive direct antiglobulin tests: some interesting findings since 2007. *Immunohematology, 30(2),* 66–79.

40. Gupta, S., Piefer, C., Fueger, J., et al. (2010). Trimethoprim-induced immune hemolytic anemia in a pediatric oncology patient presenting as an acute hemolytic transfusion reaction. *Pediatr Blood Cancer, 55,* 1201–1203.

41. Arndt, P., Garratty, G., Isaak, E., et al. (2009). Positive direct and indirect antiglobulin tests associated with oxaliplatin can be due to drug antibody and/or drug-induced nonimmunologic protein adsorption. *Transfusion, 49,* 711–718.

42. Salama, A. (2009). Drug-induced immune hemolytic anemia. *Expert Opin Drug Saf, 8,* 73–79.

24

Hemoglobinopathies (Structural Defects in Hemoglobin)

Tim R. Randolph

OBJECTIVES

After completion of this chapter, the reader will be able to:

1. Explain the difference between structural hemoglobin disorders and thalassemias, and describe the types of mutations found in the structural disorders.
2. Describe globin gene structure and the development of normal human hemoglobins throughout prenatal and postnatal life.
3. Differentiate between homozygous and heterozygous states and the terms *disease* and *trait* as they relate to the hemoglobinopathies.
4. Given the hemoglobin genotypes of parents involving common β chain variants, determine the possible genotypes of their children using a Punnett square.
5. Describe the general geographic distribution of common hemoglobin variants and the relationship of that distribution with the prevalence of malaria.
6. For disorders involving hemoglobin (Hb) S and Hb C, describe the genetic mutation, effect of the mutation on the hemoglobin molecule, inheritance pattern, pathophysiology, symptoms, clinical findings, peripheral blood findings, laboratory diagnosis, and genetic counseling and treatment considerations.
7. Describe the genetic mutation, clinical findings, and laboratory diagnosis for disorders involving Hb C-Harlem, Hb E, Hb O-Arab, Hb D, and Hb G.
8. Describe the clinical and laboratory findings for the compound heterozygous disorders of Hb S with Hb C, β-thalassemia, Hb D, Hb O-Arab, Hb Korle Bu, and Hb C-Harlem.
9. Describe the electrophoretic mobility of Hb A, Hb F, Hb S, and Hb C at an alkaline pH, and explain how other methods (including the Hb S solubility test, citrate agar electrophoresis at acid pH, and high-performance liquid chromatography) are used to distinguish Hb S and Hb C from other hemoglobins with the same alkaline electrophoresis mobility.
10. Describe the genetic mutations, inheritance patterns, pathophysiology, and clinical and laboratory findings in hemoglobin variants that result in methemoglobinemia.
11. Describe the inheritance patterns, causes, and clinical and laboratory findings of unstable hemoglobin variants.
12. Discuss the pathophysiology of hemoglobin variants with increased and decreased oxygen affinities, and explain how they differ from unstable hemoglobins.
13. Given a case history and clinical and laboratory findings, interpret test results to identify the hemoglobin variants present in the patient.

OUTLINE

Structure of Globin Genes
Hemoglobin Development
Genetic Mutations
Zygosity
Pathophysiology
Nomenclature
Hemoglobin S
  Sickle Cell Anemia
  Sickle Cell Trait
Hemoglobin C
  Prevalence, Etiology, and Pathophysiology
  Clinical Features
  Laboratory Diagnosis
  Treatment and Prognosis
Hemoglobin C-Harlem (Hemoglobin C-Georgetown)

Hemoglobin E
  Prevalence, Etiology, and Pathophysiology
  Clinical Features
  Laboratory Diagnosis
  Treatment and Prognosis
Hemoglobin O-Arab
Hemoglobin D and Hemoglobin G
Compound Heterozygosity With Hemoglobin S and Another β-Globin Gene Mutation
  Hemoglobin SC
  Hemoglobin S-β-Thalassemia
  Hemoglobin SD and Hemoglobin SG-Philadelphia
  Hemoglobin SO-Arab and Hb SD-Punjab
  Hemoglobin S-Korle Bu

Concomitant Cis Mutations With Hemoglobin S
  Hemoglobin C-Harlem
  Hemoglobin S-Antilles and Hemoglobin S-Oman
Hemoglobin M
Unstable Hemoglobin Variants
  Clinical Features
  Laboratory Diagnosis
  Treatment and Prognosis

Hemoglobins With Increased and Decreased Oxygen Affinity
  Hemoglobins With Increased Oxygen Affinity
  Hemoglobins With Decreased Oxygen Affinity
Global Burden of Hemoglobinopathies

CASE STUDY

After studying the material in this chapter, the reader should be able to respond to the following case study. Answers can be found in Appendix C.

An 18-year-old woman of African ancestry was seen in the emergency department for fever and abdominal pain. The following results were obtained on a complete blood count (CBC). Reference intervals can be found after the Index at the end of the book.

WBC	11.9×10^9/L	NEUT	75%
RBC	3.67×10^{12}/L	LYMPH	18%
HGB	10.9 g/dL	MONO	3%
HCT	32.5%	EOS	3%
RDW	19.5%	BASO	1%
PLT	410×10^9/L	RETIC	3.1%

A typical field in the patient's peripheral blood film is shown in Figure 24.1. Alkaline hemoglobin electrophoresis showed 50.9% Hb S and 49.1% Hb C.

1. Select confirmatory tests that should be performed and describe the expected results.
2. Describe the characteristic red blood cell (RBC) morphology on the peripheral blood film.
3. Based on the electrophoresis and RBC morphology results, what diagnosis is suggested?
4. If this patient were to marry a person of genotype Hb AS, what would be the expected frequency of genotypes for each of four children?

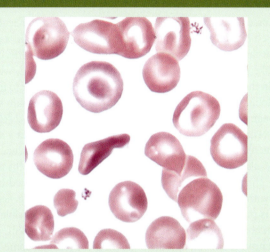

Figure 24.1 Peripheral Blood Film for the Patient in the Case Study. (Wright-Giemsa stain, ×1000.) (Courtesy Ann Bell, University of Tennessee, Memphis.)

Hemoglobinopathy refers to a disease state (opathy) involving the hemoglobin (Hb) molecule. Hemoglobinopathies are the most common genetic diseases, affecting approximately 5.2% of the world's population. Hemoglobinopathies are considered a health burden in 71% of 229 countries. These affected countries represent 89% of births globally. More than 330,000 children are born each year with some form of inherited hemoglobin disorder, with 83% having sickle cell disorder and 17% having thalassemia. The mortality rate for children younger than 5 years of age with a hemoglobinopathy is 3.4%.[1] Approximately 80% of hemoglobinopathy cases occur in middle- to low-income countries.[2] All hemoglobinopathies result from a genetic mutation in one or more genes that affect hemoglobin synthesis. The genes that are mutated can code for either proteins that make up the hemoglobin molecule (globin or polypeptide chains) or proteins involved in synthesizing or regulating synthesis of the globin chains. Regardless of the mutation encountered, all hemoglobinopathies affect hemoglobin synthesis in one of two ways: qualitatively or quantitatively. In qualitative hemoglobinopathies, hemoglobin synthesis occurs at a normal or near-normal rate, but the hemoglobin molecule has an altered amino acid sequence within the globin chains. This change in amino acid sequence can alter the structure of the hemoglobin molecule (structural defect) and its function (qualitative defect). In contrast, thalassemias result in a reduced rate of hemoglobin synthesis (quantitative), but do not affect the amino acid sequence of the affected globin chains. A reduction in the amount of hemoglobin synthesized produces an anemia and stimulates the production of other hemoglobin molecules not affected by the mutation in an attempt to compensate for the anemia. Based on this distinction, hematologists divide hemoglobinopathies into two categories: structural defects (qualitative) and thalassemias (quantitative). To add confusion to the classification scheme, many hematologists also refer to only the structural defects as hemoglobinopathies. This chapter describes the structural or qualitative defects that are referred to as hemoglobinopathies; the quantitative defects (thalassemias) are described in Chapter 25.

STRUCTURE OF GLOBIN GENES

As discussed in Chapter 8, there are six functional human globin genes located on two different chromosomes. Two of the globin genes, α and ζ, are located on chromosome 16 and are referred to as *α-like genes*. The remaining four globin genes, β, γ, δ, and ε, are located on chromosome 11 and are referred to as *β-like genes*. In the human genome there is one copy of each globin gene per chromatid, for a total of two genes per diploid nucleus, except for α and γ. There are two copies of the α and γ genes per chromatid, for a total of four genes per diploid nucleus. Each globin gene codes for the corresponding globin chain: the α-globin genes (*HBA1* and *HBA2*) are used as the template to synthesize the α-globin chains, the β-globin gene *(HBB)* codes for the β-globin chain, the γ-globin genes *(HBG1* and *HBG2)* code for the γ-globin chains, the δ-globin gene *(HBD)* codes for the δ-globin chain, the ε-globin gene *(HBE)* codes for the ε-globin chain, and the ζ-globin gene *(HBZ)* codes for the ζ-globin chain.

HEMOGLOBIN DEVELOPMENT

As discussed in Chapter 8, each human hemoglobin molecule is composed of four globin chains: a pair of α-like chains and a pair of β-like chains. During the first 3 months of embryonic life, only one α-like gene (ζ) and one β-like gene (ε) are activated, which results in the production of ζ- and ε-globin chains that pair to form hemoglobin Gower-1 ($\zeta_2\varepsilon_2$). Shortly thereafter, α and γ chain synthesis begins, which leads to the production of Hb Gower-2 ($\alpha_2\varepsilon_2$) and Hb Portland ($\zeta_2\gamma_2$). Later in fetal development, ζ and ε synthesis ceases; this leaves α and γ chains, which pair to produce Hb F ($\alpha_2\gamma_2$), also known as *fetal hemoglobin.* At about 6 months after birth, γ chain synthesis gradually decreases and is replaced by β chain synthesis so that Hb A ($\alpha_2\beta_2$), also known as *adult hemoglobin,* is produced. Three genetic loci are largely responsible for γ-globin chain repression: BCL11A (chromosome 2), HBSIL and MYB (chromosome 6), and the β-globin locus (chromosome 11). BCL11A appears to be a key element of a regulatory complex that interacts with chromatin at the HBB (hemoglobin beta) locus to repress γ-chain production. Several proposed factors may be part of the regulatory complex with BCL11A including COUP-TFII, MYB, NuRD, SOX6, KLF1, TR2/TR4, HDAC1/2, GATA1, and FOG1.[3] Another transcriptional repressor protein, NonO (non-POU domain-containing octamer-binding protein) interacts with SOX6 to bind the proximal promoter of the γ-globin gene to repress γ chain production.[4] Mutations in the gene that codes for any of these three factors result in elevated Hb F levels. The remaining δ-globin gene becomes activated around birth, producing δ chains at low levels that pair with α chains to produce the second adult hemoglobin, Hb A_2 ($\alpha_2\delta_2$). Healthy adults produce Hb A (95%), Hb A_2 (less than 3.5%), and Hb F (less than 1% to 2%).

GENETIC MUTATIONS

More than 1400 structural hemoglobin variants (hemoglobinopathies) and >500 thalassemias are known to exist throughout the world, and more are being discovered regularly (Table 24.1).[5] Each of these hemoglobin variants results from one or more genetic mutations that alter the amino acid sequence of a hemoglobin polypeptide chain. Some of these changes alter the molecular structure of the hemoglobin molecule, ultimately affecting hemoglobin function. The types of genetic mutations that occur in the hemoglobinopathies include point mutations, deletions, insertions, and fusions involving one or more of the adult globin genes, namely, α, β, γ, and δ.[5]

Point mutation is the most common type of genetic mutation occurring in the hemoglobinopathies. Point mutation is the

TABLE 24.1   Genetic Abnormalities of Hemoglobin Variants*

Total structural variants	1421
Total thalassemias	537
Amino acid substitution	1505
Deletions	242
Insertions	87
Duplications	13
Fusions	11
Total of all mutation types	1858

*Table provides a relative distribution of mutation types, including both structural variants and hemoglobinopathies. The total number of structural variants does not equal the total number of mutation types, primarily because multiple mutations can occur in the same entry. Mutations include those identified as of 2022; genetic discovery is ongoing. Data from Patrinos, G. P., Giardine, B., Riemer, W., et al. (2004). Improvements in the HbVar database of human hemoglobin variants and thalassemia mutations for population and sequence variation studies, *Nucl Acids Res, 32*(database issue), D537-541; and http://globin.cse.psu.edu/hbvar/menu.html. Accessed November 15, 2022.

replacement of one original nucleotide in the normal gene with a different nucleotide. Because one nucleotide is replaced by one nucleotide, the codon triplet remains intact, and the reading frame is unaltered. This results in the substitution of one amino acid in the globin chain product at the position corresponding to the codon containing the point mutation. As can be seen in Table 24.1, point mutations that cause an amino acid substitution are the dominant type of genetic defect among the hemoglobinopathies. It also is possible to have two-point mutations occurring in the same globin gene, which results in two amino acid substitutions within the same globin chain.[5]

Deletions involve the removal of one or more nucleotides, whereas insertions result in the addition of one or more nucleotides. Usually, deletions and insertions are not divisible by three and thus disrupt the reading frame, which leads to the nullification of synthesis of the corresponding globin chain. This is the case for the quantitative thalassemias (Chapter 25). In hemoglobinopathies, the reading frame usually remains intact, however; the result is the addition or deletion of one or more amino acids in the globin chain product, which sometimes affects the structure and function of the hemoglobin molecule.[5]

Chain extensions occur when the stop codon is mutated so that translation continues beyond the typical last codon. Amino acids continue to be added until another stop codon is reached by chance. This process produces globin chains that are longer than normal. Significant globin chain extensions usually result in degradation of the globin chain and a quantitative defect. If the extension of the globin chain is insufficient to produce significant degradation, however, the defect is qualitative and is classified as a hemoglobinopathy. Hemoglobin molecules with extended globin chains fold inappropriately, which affects hemoglobin structure and function.

Gene fusions occur when two normal genes break between nucleotides, switch positions, and anneal to the opposite gene. For example, if a β-globin gene and a δ-globin gene break in similar locations, switch positions, and reanneal, the resultant genes would be βδ and δβ fusion genes, in which the head of the fusion gene is from one original gene and the tail is from the other. If the reading frames are not disrupted and the globin chain lengths are similar, the genes are transcribed and translated into hybrid globin chains. The fusion chains fold differently, however, and affect the corresponding hemoglobin function. Eleven fusion globin chains have been identified (see Table 24.1).[5]

ZYGOSITY

Zygosity refers to the association between the number of gene mutations and the level of severity of the resultant genetic defect. Generally, there is a level of severity associated with each normal gene that is mutated and used to synthesize the globin chain product. For the normal adult globin genes, there are four copies of the α and γ genes and two copies of the β and δ genes. In theory, this could result in four levels of severity for α and γ gene mutations and two levels of severity for the β and δ gene mutations. Expressed another way, if all things were equal, it would require twice as many mutations within the α and γ genes to produce the same physiologic effect as mutations within the β and δ genes. Because the γ and δ genes are transcribed and translated at such low levels in adults, mutations of either gene have little impact on overall hemoglobin function. In addition, because the dominant hemoglobin in adults, Hb A, is composed of α and β chains, β gene mutations affect overall hemoglobin function to a greater extent than the same number of α gene mutations. This partially explains the greater number of identified β chain variants compared with α chain variants because a single β gene mutation is more likely to create a clinical condition than a single α gene mutation.

The inheritance pattern of β chain variants is referred to as *heterozygous* when only one β gene is mutated and *homozygous* when both β genes are mutated. The terms *disease* and *trait* are also commonly used to refer to the homozygous (disease) and heterozygous (trait) states.

PATHOPHYSIOLOGY

The impact of point mutations on hemoglobin function depends on the chemical nature of the substituted amino acid, where it is located in the globin chain, and the number of genes mutated (zygosity). Any change in charge and/or size of the substituted amino acid may alter the folding of the affected globin chain. A change in charge affects the interaction of the substituted amino acid with adjacent amino acids. In addition, the size of the substituted amino acid makes the globin chain either more (large amino acids) or less (small amino acids) bulky. Therefore the charge and the size of the substituted amino acid determine its impact on hemoglobin structure by potentially altering the tertiary structure of the globin chain and the quaternary structure of the hemoglobin molecule. Changes in hemoglobin structure may affect function. Location of the substitution within the globin chain also has an impact on the degree of structural alteration and hemoglobin function, based on its positioning within the molecule and the interactions with the surrounding amino acids. In the case of the sickle cell mutation, one amino acid substitution results in hemoglobin polymerization, leading to the formation of long hemoglobin crystals that stretch the red

blood cell (RBC) membrane and produce the characteristic crescent moon or sickle cell shape.

Zygosity also affects the pathophysiology of the disease. In β-hemoglobinopathies, zygosity predicts two severities of disease. In homozygous β-hemoglobinopathies, in which both β genes are mutated, the variant hemoglobin becomes the dominant hemoglobin type, and normal hemoglobin (Hb A) is absent. Examples are sickle cell disease (SCD), caused by Hb SS and Hb C disease (Hb CC). In heterozygous β-hemoglobinopathies, one β gene is mutated and the other is normal, which suggests a 50/50 distribution. In an attempt to minimize the impact of the abnormal hemoglobin, however, the variant hemoglobin is usually present in lesser amounts than Hb A. Patients with homozygous SCD (Hb SS) inherit a severe form of the disease that occurs less often but requires lifelong medical intervention which must begin early in life, whereas heterozygotes (Hb AS) are much more common but rarely experience overt symptoms.

Fishleder and Hoffman[6] divided the structural hemoglobins into four groups: abnormal hemoglobins that result in hemolytic anemia, such as Hb S and the unstable hemoglobins; abnormal hemoglobins that result in methemoglobinemia, such as Hb M; hemoglobins with either increased or decreased oxygen affinity; and abnormal hemoglobins with no clinical or functional effect. Imbalanced chain production also may be associated in rare instances with a structurally abnormal chain, such as Hb Lepore, because of reduced production of the abnormal chain. A functional classification of selected hemoglobin variants is summarized in Box 24.1.

Many of the variants are clinically insignificant because they do not produce any physiologic effect. As discussed previously, most clinical abnormalities are associated with the β chain, followed by the α chain. Involvement of the γ and δ chains does occur, but because of the small amount of hemoglobin involved, it is rarely detected and is usually of no clinical consequence. Box 24.2 lists clinically significant abnormal hemoglobins. The most commonly occurring abnormal hemoglobin and the most severe is Hb S.

NOMENCLATURE

As hemoglobins were discovered and reported in the literature, they were designated by letters of the alphabet. Normal adult hemoglobin and fetal hemoglobin were called *Hb A* and *Hb F*. By the time the middle of the alphabet was reached, however, it became apparent that the alphabet would be exhausted before all mutations were named. Currently some abnormal hemoglobins are assigned a common designation and a scientific designation. The common name is selected by the discoverer and usually represents the geographic area where the hemoglobin was identified. A single capital letter is used to indicate a special characteristic of the hemoglobin variant, such as hemoglobins demonstrating identical electrophoretic mobility but containing different amino acid substitutions, as in Hb G-Philadelphia and Hb G-Copenhagen, or Hb C and Hb C-Harlem. The variant description also can involve scientific designations that indicate the variant chain, the sequential and the helical number of the abnormal amino acid, and the

BOX 24.1   Functional Classification of Selected Hemoglobin Variants

I. Homozygous: Hemoglobin Polymorphisms: Most Common Variants

Hb S: $\alpha_2\beta_2^{6Val}$ (severe hemolytic anemia; sickling)

Hb C: $\alpha_2\beta_2^{6Lys}$ (mild hemolytic anemia)

Hb D-Punjab: $\alpha_2\beta_2^{121Gln}$ (no anemia)

Hb E: $\alpha_2\beta_2^{26Lys}$ (mild microcytic anemia)

II. Heterozygous: Hemoglobin Variants Causing Functional Aberrations or Hemolytic Anemia in the Heterozygous State

A. Hemoglobins Associated With Methemoglobinemia and Cyanosis

Hb M-Boston: $\alpha_2^{58Tyr}\beta_2$

Hb M-Iwate: $\alpha_2^{87Tyr}\beta_2$

Hb Auckland: $\alpha_2^{87Asn}\beta_2$

Hb Chile: $\alpha_2\beta_2^{28Met}$

Hb M-Saskatoon: $\alpha_2\beta_2^{63Tyr}$

Hb M-Milwaukee-1: $\alpha_2\beta_2^{67Glu}$

Hb M-Milwaukee-2: $\alpha_2\beta_2^{92Tyr}$

Hb F-M-Osaka: $\alpha_2\gamma_2^{63Tyr}$

Hb F-M-Fort Ripley: $\alpha_2\gamma_2^{92Tyr}$

B. Hemoglobins Associated With Altered Oxygen Affinity

1. Increased Affinity and Erythrocytosis

Hb Chesapeake: $\alpha_2^{92Leu}\beta_2$

Hb J-Capetown: $\alpha_2^{92Gln}\beta_2$

Hb Malmo: $\alpha_2\beta_2^{97Gln}$

Hb Yakima: $\alpha_2\beta_2^{99His}$

Hb Kempsey: $\alpha_2\beta_2^{99Asn}$

Hb Ypsi (Ypsilanti): $\alpha_2\beta_2^{99Tyr}$

Hb Hiroshima: $\alpha_2\beta_2^{146Asp}$

Hb Rainier: $\alpha_2\beta_2^{145Cys}$

Hb Bethesda: $\alpha_2\beta_2^{145His}$

2. Decreased Affinity (May Have Mild Anemia or Cyanosis)

Hb Kansas: $\alpha_2\beta_2^{102Thr}$

Hb Titusville: $\alpha_2^{94Asn}\beta_2$

Hb Providence: $\alpha_2\beta_2^{82Asn}$

Hb Agenogi: $\alpha_2\beta_2^{90Lys}$

Hb Beth Israel: $\alpha_2\beta_2^{102Ser}$

Hb Yoshizuka: $\alpha_2\beta_2^{108Asp}$

C. Unstable Hemoglobins

1. Hemoglobin May Precipitate as Heinz Bodies After Splenectomy

Severe hemolysis: no improvement after splenectomy

Hb Bibba: $\alpha_2^{136Pro}\beta_2$

Hb Hammersmith: $\alpha_2\beta_2^{42Ser}$

Hb Bristol-Alesha: $\alpha_2\beta_2^{67Asp\ or\ 67Met}$

Hb Olmsted: $\alpha_2\beta_2^{141Arg}$

Severe hemolysis: improvement after splenectomy

Hb Torino: $\alpha_2^{43Val}\beta_2$

Hb Ann Arbor: $\alpha_2^{80Arg}\beta_2$

Hb Genova: $\alpha_2\beta_2^{28Pro}$

Hb Shepherds Bush: $\alpha_2\beta_2^{74Asp}$

Hb Köln: $\alpha_2\beta_2^{98Met}$

Hb Wien: $\alpha_2\beta_2^{130Asp}$

Mild hemolysis: intermittent exacerbations

Hb Hasharon: $\alpha_2^{47His}\beta_2$

Hb Leiden: $\alpha_2\beta_2^{6\ or\ 7}$ (Glu deleted)

Hb Freiburg: $\alpha_2\beta_2^{23}$ (Val deleted)

Hb Seattle: $\alpha_2\beta_2^{70Asp}$

Hb Louisville: $\alpha_2\beta_2^{42Leu}$

Hb Zurich: $\alpha_2\beta_2^{63Arg}$

Hb Gun Hill: $\alpha_2\beta_2^{91-95}$ (5 amino acids deleted)

No disease

Hb Etobicoke: $\alpha_2^{84Arg}\beta_2$

Hb Sogn: $\alpha_2\beta_2^{14Arg}$

Hb Tacoma: $\alpha_2\beta_2^{30Ser}$

2. Tetramers of Normal Chains; Appear in α-Thalassemias

Hb Bart: γ_4

Hb H: β_4

Arg, Arginine; *Asn,* asparagine; *Asp,* aspartic acid; *Cys,* cysteine; *Gln,* glutamine; *Glu,* glutamic acid; *Hb,* hemoglobin; *His,* histidine; *Leu,* leucine; *Lys,* lysine; *Met,* methionine; *Pro,* proline; *Ser,* serine; *Thr,* threonine; *Tyr,* tyrosine; *Val,* valine.

Modified from Elghetany, M. T., Schexneider, K. I., & Banki, K. (2017). Erythrocytic disorders. In McPherson, R. A., & Pincus, M. R. (Eds.), *Henry's Clinical Diagnosis and Management by Laboratory Methods.* (23rd ed., p. 580). St. Louis: Elsevier. Originally modified from Winslow, R. M., & Anderson, W. F. (1983). The hemoglobinopathies. In Stanbury, J. B., Wyngaarden, J. B., Fredrickson, D. S., et al. (Eds.), *The Metabolic Basis of Inherited Disease.* (5th ed., pp. 2281–2317). New York: McGraw-Hill.

Updated from Patrinos, G. P., Giardine, B., Riemer, C., et al. (2004). Improvements in the HbVar database of human hemoglobin variants and thalassemia mutations for population and sequence variation studies, *Nucl Acids Res, 32* (database issue), D537–541. http://globin.cse.psu.edu/hbvar/menu.html. Accessed November 15, 2022.

---

nature of the substitution. The designation [β_6 (A$_3$) Glu→Val] for the Hb S mutation indicates the substitution of valine for glutamic acid in the A helix in the β chain at position 6.

HEMOGLOBIN S

Sickle Cell Anemia

History

Although the origin of sickle cell anemia (SCA) is difficult to determine, whole genome studies estimate the Hb S mutation to have occurred approximately 7300 years ago in the Green Sahara area of Africa.[7] Symptom tracing links the disease to one Ghanaian family back to 1670.[8] SCA was first reported in a West Indian student with severe anemia by a Chicago cardiologist, Herrick, in 1910. In 1917 Emmel recorded that sickling occurred in nonanemic patients and in patients who were severely anemic. In 1927 Hahn and Gillespie described the pathologic basis of the disorder and its relationship to the hemoglobin molecule. These investigators showed that sickling occurred when a solution of RBCs was deficient in oxygen and that the shape of the RBCs was reversible when that solution was oxygenated again.[9] In 1946 Beet reported that malarial parasites were present less often in blood films from patients with SCD than in individuals without SCD.[10] It was determined that the sickle cell trait (SCT) confers a resistance against infection with *Plasmodium falciparum* occurring early in childhood between the time that passively acquired

BOX 24.2 Clinically Important Hemoglobin Variants

I. Sickle syndromes
  A. Sickle cell trait (AS)
  B. Sickle cell disease
    1. SS
    2. SC
    3. SD-Punjab (Los Angeles)
    4. SO-Arab
    5. S-β-thalassemia
    6. S-hereditary persistence of fetal hemoglobin
    7. SE
II. Unstable hemoglobins (>185 variants)
III. Hemoglobins with abnormal oxygen affinity
  A. High affinity—familial erythrocytosis (>208 variants)
  B. Low affinity—familial cyanosis (>174 variants)
IV. M hemoglobins—familial cyanosis (9 variants): Hb M-Boston, Hb M-Iwate, Hb Auckland, Hb Chile, Hb M-Saskatoon, Hb M-Milwaukee-1, Hb M-Milwaukee-2 (Hyde Park), Hb F-M-Osaka, Hb F-M-Fort Ripley
V. Structural variants that result in a thalassemic phenotype
  A. β-thalassemia phenotype
    1. Hb Lepore (δβ fusion)
    2. Hb E
    3. Hb-Indianapolis, Hb-Showa-Yakushiji, Hb-Geneva
  B. α-thalassemia phenotype chain termination mutants (e.g., Hb Constant Spring)

Hb, Hemoglobin.
Modified from Hankins, J. S., & Wang, W. C. (2019). Sickle cell anemia and other sickling syndromes; and Verhovsek, M., & Steinberg, M. H. Hemoglobins with altered hemoglobin affinity, unstable hemoglobins, M-hemoglobins, and dyshemoglobinemias. In Greer, J. P., Arber, D. A., Glader, B., et al. (Eds.), *Wintrobe's Clinical Hematology.* (14th ed.) Philadelphia: Lippincott Williams & Wilkins.
Updated from Patrinos, G. P., Giardine, B., Riemer, C., et al. (2004). Improvements in the HbVar database of human hemoglobin variants and thalassemia mutations for population and sequence variation studies, *Nucl Acids Res, 32* (database issue), D537–541. http://globin.cse.psu.edu/hbvar/menu.html. Accessed November 15, 2022.

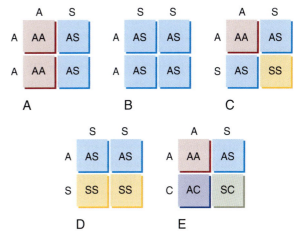

Figure 24.2 (A–E), Punnett Square Examples Illustrating the Standard Method for Predicting the Inheritance of Abnormal Hemoglobins. Each parent contributes one gene.

immunity dissipates and active immunity develops.[11] In 1949 Pauling showed that when Hb S is subjected to electrophoresis, it migrates differently than Hb A. This difference was found to be caused by an amino acid substitution in the globin chain. Pauling and coworkers[4] defined the genetics of the disorder and clearly distinguished heterozygous sickle trait (Hb AS) from the homozygous state (Hb SS).

The term *sickle cell disease* is used to describe a group of symptomatic hemoglobinopathies that have in common sickle cell formation and the associated crises. Patients with SCD are either homozygous for Hb S (SS) or are compound heterozygotes expressing Hb S in combination with another hemoglobin β chain mutation such as Hb C or β-thalassemia. SCD mutations are the most common form of hemoglobinopathy, with Hb SS and the variants Hb SC and Hb S-β-thalassemia (Hb S-β-thal) occurring most often.

Inheritance Pattern

As stated earlier, the α-like globin genes that have two copies per chromosome resulting in four loci are α (chromosome 16) and γ (chromosome 11). The β-like globin genes that have one copy per chromosome resulting in two loci are β and γ (chromosome 11). β-Hemoglobin variants are inherited as autosomal codominant, with one gene inherited from each parent.

Patients with SCD (Hb SS, Hb SC, or Hb S-β-thal) have inherited a sickle (S) gene from one parent and an S, C, or β-thalassemia gene from the other. Among patients with SCD, individuals who are homozygotes (Hb SS) usually have more severe disease than individuals who are compound heterozygotes for Hb S (Hb SC or Hb S-β-thal). Heterozygotes (Hb AS) are generally asymptomatic but may have mild symptoms and may develop adverse events when subjected to extreme exertion, as in military boot camp and high-level athletics.[12] Using Hb S and Hb C as examples, Figure 24.2 illustrates the inheritance of abnormal hemoglobins involving mutations in the β gene.

Prevalence

Globally, more than 300,000 children are born each year with SCA (Hb SS), with approximately 500 of these children dying each day from the disease. The highest frequency of the sickle cell gene is found in sub-Saharan Africa, where each year, approximately 250,000 babies are born with SCD (Hb SS), representing 0.74% of all live births occurring in this area.[2,13] Other reports estimate 1126 babies are born with SCA per 100,000 live births, or 1.1%.[14] In contrast, approximately 112/100,000 live births are born with SCA globally, with 2600 babies born annually with SCD in North America and 1300 in Europe.[13,14] Globally, the sickle cell gene occurs at the highest frequency in five geographic areas: sub-Saharan Africa, Arab-India, the Americas, Eurasia, and Southeast Asia. In 2010 these five geographic areas accounted for 64.4%, 22.7%, 7.4%, 5.4%, and 0.1% of all neonates born globally with SCT and 75.5%, 16.9%, 4.6%, 3.0%, and 0% of all neonates born globally with SCD. Three countries accounted for approximately 50% of neonates with SS and AS genotypes: Nigeria, India, and DR Congo.[15] Mortality among children with SCA in these regions ranges from 50% in urban areas to 90% in rural areas.[14] In the United States, 1 in 300 to 400 infants born to individuals of African ancestry (2000 annually) are diagnosed with SCD. Between 60% and 65% inherit two Hb S alleles (Hb SS), 25% to 30% inherit one Hb S and one Hb C allele (Hb SC), and 9% inherit a Hb S mutation with a β^0-thalasemia mutation.[16] The overall economic burden of SCD in the United States is approximately $2.98 billion per year, with health care costs for patients with SCD being 6 to 11 times higher than for patients without SCD.[14] In the United States, SCD is found mostly in individuals of African descent; however, it also has been found in individuals from the Middle East, India, and the Mediterranean region (Figure 24.3). SCD can also be found in individuals from the Caribbean and Central and South America. The sickle cell mutation is becoming more prominent in southern India, particularly in certain tribes.[17] Estimates indicate that 25,000 babies are born annually with SCA in India.[2]

Etiology and Pathophysiology

Mutation. Hb S is defined by the structural formula $\alpha_2\beta_2^{6Glu \rightarrow Val}$, which indicates that on the β chain at position 6, glutamic acid is replaced by valine. The mutation occurs in nucleotide 17, where thymine replaces adenine, resulting in a change in codon 6 and the substitution of valine (GTG) for glutamic acid (GAG) at amino acid position 6.[12] Glutamic acid has a net charge of (-1), whereas valine has a net charge of (0). This amino acid substitution produces a change in charge of $(+1)$, which affects the electrophoretic mobility of the hemoglobin molecule.

Polymerization and sickling. This amino acid substitution also affects the way the hemoglobin molecules interact with one another within the erythrocyte cytosol. Nonpolar (hydrophobic) valine is placed in the position that polar glutamic acid once held. Because glutamic acid is polar, it allows the hemoglobin tetramer to bind water and contribute to hemoglobin solubility

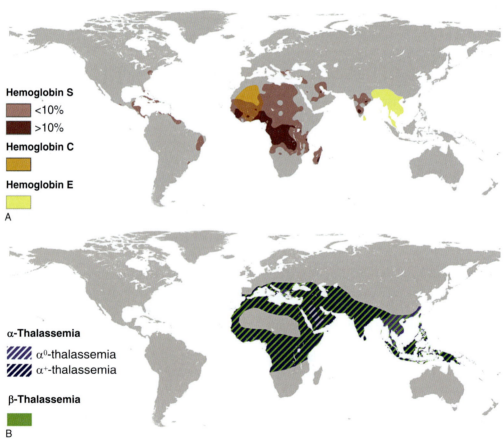

Figure 24.3 Maps of the Distribution of Inherited Disorders of Hemoglobin. **(A),** Structural hemoglobin variants. **(B),** Thalassemias. (In Piel, F. B. [2016]. The present and future global burden of the inherited disorders of hemoglobin. *Hematol Oncol Clin North Am, 30*(2), p. 328, Figure 1. Adapted from Piel, F. B., Patil, A. P., Howes, R. E., et al. [2013]. Global epidemiology of sickle haemoglobin in neonates: a contemporary geostatistical model-based map and population estimates. *Lancet, 381*, pp. 142–151; Piel, F. B., Howes, R. E., Patil, A. P., et al. [2013]. The distribution of haemoglobin C and its prevalence in newborns in Africa. *Sci Rep, 3*, p. 1671; Weatherall, D. J., & Clegg, J. B. [2001]. The *Thalassaemia Syndromes.* [4th ed.]. Hoboken, NJ: Blackwell Science; and Weatherall, D. J. [2001]. Phenotype-genotype relationships in monogenic disease: lessons from the thalassaemias. *Nat Rev Genet, 2*, pp. 245–255.)

in the cytosol. In the mutated chain the hydrophobic valine does not bind water; instead, it seeks a hydrophobic niche with which to bind. When Hb S is fully oxygenated, the quaternary structure of the molecule does not produce a hydrophobic pocket for valine. However, the natural allosteric change that occurs upon deoxygenation creates a hydrophobic pocket, which allows the valines from adjacent Hb S molecules to bind. This hemoglobin pairing creates an orientation that facilitates other hemoglobin molecules to form electrostatic bonds between amino acids and becomes the seed for polymer formation. Other hemoglobin pairs polymerize, forming a hemoglobin core composed of four hemoglobin molecules that elongate in a helical formation. An outer layer of 10 hemoglobin molecules forms around the 4-hemoglobin-molecule core, creating the long, slender Hb S polymer.[18–21] Hb S molecules within the RBCs become less soluble, forming *tactoids,* or liquid crystals of Hb S polymers that grow in length beyond the diameter of the RBC, causing sickling. In homozygotes, the sickling process begins when oxygen saturation decreases to less than 85%. In heterozygotes, sickling does not occur unless the oxygen saturation of hemoglobin is reduced to less than 40%. The blood becomes more viscous when polymers and sickle cells form.[22] Increased blood viscosity and sickle cell formation slow blood flow. In addition to a decrease in oxygen tension, there is a reduction in pH and an increase in 2,3-bisphosphoglycerate. Reduced blood flow prolongs the exposure of Hb S-containing RBCs to a hypoxic environment, and the lower tissue pH decreases oxygen affinity, which further promotes sickling. The end result is occlusion of capillaries and arterioles by sickled RBCs and infarction of surrounding tissue.

Sickle cells occur in two forms: reversible sickle cells and irreversible sickle cells.[23] Reversible sickle cells are Hb S-containing RBCs that change shape in response to oxygen tension. Reversible sickle cells circulate as normal biconcave discs when fully oxygenated but undergo hemoglobin polymerization, show increased viscosity, and change shape on deoxygenation. The vasoocclusive complications of SCD are thought to be due to reversible sickle cells that are able to travel into the microvasculature in the biconcave disk conformation because of their normal rheologic properties when oxygenated and then become distorted and viscous as they become deoxygenated, converting to the sickle cell configuration in the vessel.

In contrast, irreversible sickle cells do not change their shape regardless of the change in oxygen tension or degree of hemoglobin polymerization. These cells are seen on the peripheral blood film as elongated sickle cells with a point at each end. Irreversible sickle cells are likely recognized as abnormal by the spleen and removed from circulation, which prevents them from entering the microcirculation and causing vasoocclusion.

Intracellular hydration. Not only the oxygen tension but also the level of intracellular hydration affects the sickling process. When RBCs containing Hb S are exposed to a low oxygen tension, hemoglobin polymerization occurs. Polymerized deoxyhemoglobin S activates a membrane channel called P_{sickle} that is otherwise inactive in normal RBCs. These membrane channels open when the blood partial pressure of oxygen decreases to less than 50 mm Hg. The result of open P_{sickle} channels is an influx of Ca^{2+}, which ultimately causes an efflux of K^+ and Cl^-. The efflux of these ions leads to water efflux and intracellular dehydration, effectively increasing the intracellular concentration of Hb S and intensifying polymerization. Another contributor to K^+ and Cl^- efflux and the resultant dehydration is the K^+/Cl^- cotransporter system (KCC1). Ironically, this system is activated by dehydration and positively charged hemoglobins such as Hb S and Hb C. One potential explanation for the altered function of the membrane channels is oxidative damage triggered by Hb S polymerization. Injury to the RBC membrane induces adherence to endothelial surfaces, which causes RBC aggregation, produces ischemia, and exacerbates Hb S polymerization.[11]

Another important factor in the pathophysiology of SCD involves the redistribution of phospholipids in the RBC membrane, which contributes to hemolysis, vasoocclusive crisis (VOC), stroke, and acute chest syndrome (ACS). In the lipid bilayer membranes of normal RBCs, choline phospholipids, such as sphingomyelin and phosphatidylcholine, are located on the outer plasma layer, whereas aminophospholipids, such as phosphatidylserine (PS) and phosphatidylethanolamine, are primarily on the inner cytoplasmic layer. This asymmetric distribution of membrane phospholipids is accomplished by enzymes called *translocases* or *flippases* (Chapter 7). Inhibition of flippases and activation of an enzyme called *scramblase* cause a more random distribution of membrane phospholipids, which increases the number of choline phospholipids on the interior half of the membrane and the number of aminophospholipids on the exterior membrane surface. The sickle cells of homozygotes (Hb SS) express 2.1% PS on RBC exterior surfaces compared with 0.2% for normal Hb AA controls. Hb S polymerization may produce microparticles (discussed later) and iron complexes that adhere to the RBC membrane and generate reactive oxygen species which, along with increased intracellular calcium and protein kinase C activation, may contribute to flippase inhibition and scramblase activation. PS on the exterior surface of RBCs binds thrombospondin on vascular endothelial cells, enhancing adherence between RBCs and the vessel wall and contributing to VOC, activation of coagulation, and decreased RBC survival. In addition, RBCs with PS on the external membrane surface are vulnerable to hydrolysis by secretory phospholipase A_2 (sPLA$_2$), which generates lysophospholipids and fatty acids such as lysophosphatidic acid. This results in vascular damage that contributes to ACS.[24,25]

Dysfunctional endothelial nitric oxide synthase. A major aspect of the systemic inflammation observed in SCD is caused by dysfunctional endothelial nitric oxide synthase (eNOS). The primary function of eNOS is to generate nitric oxide (NO) to regulate blood vessel dilation to maintain blood pressure and blood flow to tissues. Increases in NO cause excessive vasodilation resulting in a sudden drop in blood pressure and associated dizziness, loss of consciousness, decreased cardiac output, and tissue cyanosis. Decreased levels of NO result in vasoconstriction and the associated symptoms of blurred vision, increase in body temperature, chronic stress, low energy, and slow recovery times. In SCD, NO can vasodilate to relax blocked blood vessels during VOCs or maintain vessel dilation to prevent VOCs. At least 10 physiologic conditions exist in the context of SCD that cause dysfunction to eNOS: endothelial arginine depletion, asymmetric dimethylarginine, complement activation, endothelial glycocalyx degradation, free fatty acids, inflammatory mediators, microparticles, oxidized low density lipoproteins, reactive oxygen species, and Toll-like receptor 4 signaling ligands.[26]

Microparticles, previously known as "cellular dust," are submicron (100 to 1000 nm in diameter), unilamellar vesicles derived from parent cells that contribute to the pathophysiology of SCD. Microparticles are generated when RBCs, platelets, endothelial cells, and monocytes undergo stimulation, activation, or apoptosis. In SCD, microparticles play a role in inflammation, coagulation, apoptosis, and angiogenesis. Inflammation and VOC can induce the release of microparticles, which in turn can further modulate the inflammatory response. It is well established that inflammation can activate white blood cells (WBCs) and promote sickling, modulate the endothelium to increase RBC adhesion, and activate coagulation through tissue factor activation, all of which promote vascular obstruction. Chronic hypercoagulability observed in patients with SCD may be initiated by tissue factor aberrantly expressed by circulating blood cells or by microparticles derived from them. It is possible that the detection, quantification, and identification of microparticle subtypes could be used diagnostically or prognostically to predict clinical outcomes.[26]

Clinical Features

Clinical manifestations of SCD can vary from no symptoms to a potentially lethal state. Symptoms also vary between ethnic groups with patients of Indian ancestry expressing a much milder disease than patients of African ancestry.[17] People with SCD can develop a variety of symptoms as listed in Box 24.3. More than 1200 hemoglobin variants are known; however, only eight genotypes cause severe disease: Hb SS, Hb S-β^0-thal, severe Hb S-β^+-thal, Hb SD-Punjab, Hb SO-Arab, Hb SC-Harlem, Hb CS-Antilles, and Hb S-Quebec-CHORI. These eight clinically significant forms are listed in order of severity and can have high morbidity and mortality rates. Three additional genotypes produce moderate disease: Hb SC, moderate Hb S-β^+-thal, and Hb AS-Oman. Three produce mild disease: mild Hb S-β^{silent}-thal, Hb SE, and Hb SA-Jamaica Plain. Two produce very mild disease: Hb S-HPFH and Hb S with a variety of mild variants.[13] Symptom variability in patients with SCD and across the genotypes listed earlier are largely caused by the intracellular ratio of Hb S to Hb F as well as factors that affect vessel tone and cellular activation. Individuals affected with SCD are characteristically symptom-free until the second half of the first year of life because of the protective effect of Hb F.[27] In the first 6 months of life, mutant β chains gradually replace normal γ chains, which causes Hb S levels to increase and Hb F levels to decrease. RBCs containing Hb S become susceptible to hemolysis, and a progressive hemolytic anemia and splenomegaly may become evident.

Many individuals with SCD experience episodes of recurring pain termed *crises*. Sickle cell crises were described by Diggs as "any new syndrome that develops rapidly in patients with

---

> **BOX 24.3** **Clinical Features of Sickle Cell Disease**
>
> I. Vasoocclusion
>   A. Causes
>   Acidosis
>   Hypoxia
>   Dehydration
>   Infection
>   Fever
>   Extreme cold
>   B. Clinical manifestations
>   1. Bones
>   Pain
>   Hand-foot dactilitis
>   Infection (osteomyelitis)
>   2. Lungs
>   Pneumonia
>   Acute chest syndrome
>   3. Liver
>   Hepatomegaly
>   Jaundice
>   4. Spleen
>   Sequestration splenomegaly
>   Autosplenectomy
>   5. Penis
>   Priapism
>   6. Eyes
>   Retinal hemorrhage
>   7. Central nervous system
>   8. Urinary tract
>   Renal papillary necrosis
>   9. Leg ulcers
> II. Bacterial infections
>   A. Sepsis
>   B. Pneumonia
>   C. Osteomyelitis
> III. Hematologic defects
>   A. Chronic hemolytic anemia
>   B. Megaloblastic episodes
>   C. Aplastic episodes
> IV. Cardiac defects
>   A. Enlarged heart
>   B. Heart murmurs
> V. Other clinical features
>   A. Stunted growth
>   B. High-risk pregnancy

SCD owing to the inherited abnormality."[28] Various crises may occur: vasoocclusive or "painful," splenic sequestration, chronic hemolytic, megaloblastic, and aplastic. These crises and other sequelae of SCD are described next.

Vasoocclusive crisis. The hallmark of SCD is VOC, which accounts for most hospital and emergency department visits. This acute, painful aspect of SCD occurs with great predictability and severity in many individuals and can be triggered by acidosis, hypoxia, dehydration, infection and fever, and exposure to extreme cold. Painful episodes manifest most often in bones, lungs, liver, spleen, penis, eyes, central nervous system (CNS), and urinary tract.

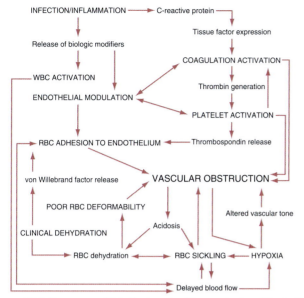

Figure 24.4 Numerous Risk Factors for Vasoocclusion, Illustrating Physiological Interrelationships. *RBC*, Red blood cell; *WBC*, white blood cell. (From Embury, S. H., Hebbel, R. P., Mohandas, N., et al. [1994]. *Sickle Cell Disease: Basic Principles and Clinical Practice.* [p. 322, Figure 5]. Philadelphia: Lippincott Williams & Wilkins.)

The pathogenesis of vasoocclusion in SCD is not fully understood, but Hb S polymerization and sickling of RBCs play a major role, with other factors also affecting this process. Most VOC events occur in capillaries and postcapillary venules. The list of possible risk factors includes polymerization, decreased deformability, sickle cell-endothelial cell adherence, endothelial cell activation, WBC and platelet activation, hemostatic activation, and altered vascular tone.[29] Interrelationships among these risk factors are shown in Figure 24.4. Vasoocclusion can be triggered by any of these factors under various circumstances. During inflammation, increased WBCs interacting with endothelium, platelet activation causing elevation of thrombospondin level, or clinical dehydration resulting in an increase in von Willebrand factor can trigger RBC adherence to endothelium, precipitating vascular obstruction. Another mechanism of obstruction can be dense cells, which are less deformable and are at greatest risk for intracellular polymerization because of their higher Hb S concentration. Vasoocclusive episodes gradually consume the patient, organ by organ, through the destructive and debilitative effects of cumulative infarcts. Approximately 8% to 10% of patients with SCD develop cutaneous manifestations in the form of ulcers or sores on the lower leg.[13]

The abnormal interaction between sickle cells and vascular endothelium seems to have a great impact on the vasoocclusive event. Endothelial adherence correlates significantly with the severity of painful episodes. In addition, sickle cell adherence to vascular endothelium results in intimal hyperplasia that can slow blood flow. Cells of patients with Hb SC disease produce less sickling with fewer adherent RBCs.[9]

The frequency of painful episodes varies from none to six per year.[9] On average, each episode persists for 4 to 5 days, although protracted episodes may last for weeks.

Rapid treatment is necessary to reduce patient suffering, morbidity, and downstream end-organ damage, and must include analgesia, supplemental oxygen, and hydration. Administration of opioids within 30 minutes of a VOC is recommended to maximize patient recovery. Providing oxygen to achieve an oxygen saturation above 95% will prevent additional sickling and reverse sickling in some RBCs. Intravenous (IV) fluids are necessary to expand blood volume to increase perfusion and improve blood flow by reducing occlusions.[30]

Splenic sequestration and infarcts. Splenic sequestration is characterized by a sudden trapping of blood in the spleen, which leads to a rapid decline in hemoglobin, often to less than 6 g/dL. This phenomenon occurs most often in infants and young children whose spleens are chronically enlarged. Children experiencing splenic sequestration episodes may have earlier onset of splenomegaly and a lower level of Hb F at 6 months of age.[9] Crises are often associated with respiratory tract infections.

Repeated splenic infarcts produce scarring resulting in diminished splenic tissue and abnormal function. Gradual loss of splenic function is referred to as *autosplenectomy* and is evidenced by the presence of Howell-Jolly and Pappenheimer bodies in RBCs on the peripheral blood film. Loss of splenic function contributes to an increased risk of bacterial infections.

Acute chest syndrome. ACS is an acute illness characterized by a new pulmonary infiltrate on chest radiograph plus any two of the following: pleuritic chest pain, hypoxemia, tachypenia, or fever. Patients may also experience other respiratory symptoms, including cough or dyspnea that occurs when the pulmonary vasculature becomes occluded. ACS is the second most common cause of hospitalization and third most common cause of death among adults with SCD.[16,31] Pulmonary infection, fat embolism, and pulmonary infarction are the most common inciting factors, resulting in a decreased alveolar oxygen tension that induces Hb S polymerization and sickle cell formation. In children, ACS generally is precipitated by infection characterized by fever, cough, and tachypnea (rapid breathing). ACS often develops within 24 to 72 hours after hospitalization for a VOC.[16] ACS is also linked with $sPLA_2$ (mentioned earlier in "Intracellular Hydration"). An increase in $sPLA_2$ is a predictor of ACS in patients with SCD and correlates with the degree of lung damage. $sPLA_2$ increases 24 to 48 hours before symptoms of ACS begin. An $sPLA_2$ level of 100 ng/mL is a predictor of impending ACS, and a subsequent transfusion has been shown to be preventive.[32] In addition to ACS symptoms (fever, hypoxia, tachypnea, and chest pain), chest radiographs and laboratory test results are helpful in making the diagnosis. The complete blood count (CBC) will often indicate a rapid decline in hemoglobin and platelet count. Creatinine and liver function tests are used to monitor organ function and predict organ failure primarily from fat emboli. Arterial blood gas testing is used to monitor lung function, and a type and screen is ordered because blood transfusions are often necessary. Blood and sputum cultures are ordered to investigate the cause of ACS and to treat underlying infections. Treatment and continuous monitoring must be initiated promptly to reduce morbidity and mortality. Oxygen is administered to maintain saturation at ≥95%, IV fluids are administered to prevent dehydration, and pain relief is essential. Incentive spirometry and chest physiotherapy are helpful to maintain adequate ventilation. Respiratory infection is presumed, so antibiotics are prescribed to all patients and tailored to treat confirmed infections. The more severe cases of ACS benefit from blood or exchange transfusions, and many patients have rapid and dramatic improvements. ACS can progress to multiorgan failure syndrome, affecting the kidneys, liver, or nervous system in addition to the lungs.[33,34]

Fat embolism syndrome and bone marrow necrosis. Fat embolism syndrome (FES) secondary to bone marrow necrosis (BMN) is a rare but often fatal sequela of SCD. Often associated with long bone fractures, FES has also been observed in nontraumatic conditions. It occurs more often in Hb SC (50%) and at similar frequency in Hb S-β⁺-thal (18%) and Hb SS (15%), with non-SS of unknown genotype accounting for the remaining 17% of cases. The cause is unknown but hypothesized to be BMN from a hypoxic event. Necrotic bone marrow material and fat particles are released into the circulation and deposit in the lung, where they fragment. Small fat droplets reenter circulation via pulmonary capillaries and terminate in various organs, causing damage. In addition, patients often experience neurologic (brain) and renal damage. Patients generally present with back, bone, and abdominal pain, and fever and fatigue associated with BMN, and may rapidly progress to respiratory failure and CNS depression from FES. Altered mental status and respiratory distress are the most consistent findings and signal rapid deterioration within hours that is often fatal if not detected and treated swiftly.[35]

The CBC results include a rapid drop in hemoglobin (>20%) and platelet count (>50%) from admission values, with many nucleated RBCs and a left shift in the differential. The reticulocyte count is low because of the BMN. Chemical analysis shows elevated lactate dehydrogenase, ferritin, creatinine, alkaline phosphatase, and bilirubin, indicating end-organ damage. A bone marrow evaluation is diagnostic, showing myeloid necrosis, focal hypoplasia, loss of fat, and eosinophilic material in the background. However, patients often die before bone marrow analysis. Rapid treatment with either multiple transfusions or RBC exchange must be administered quickly and often results in complete recovery. In contrast, delayed diagnosis and treatment often result in death or permanent neurologic damage. Mortality rates in patients receiving RBC exchange is 29% compared with simple transfusion (61%) and no transfusion (91%).[35,36]

Pulmonary hypertension. Pulmonary hypertension (PHT), defined as an elevated mean pulmonary arterial pressure, is a serious and potentially fatal sequela of SCD. PHT has a prevalence of about 33% in patients with SCD, with 10% of patients presenting with a more severe type. The mortality rate for patients with SCD who develop PHT is between 37% and 40% during the 3- to 6-year period following PHT diagnosis, compared with 17% mortality in SCD patients without PHT. Vascular endothelial damage, smooth muscle hypertrophy, and thromboembolisms likely contribute to PHT.[34] An association has been documented between the development of PHT and the NO pathway. NO is produced from the action of eNOS on arginine, which causes vasodilation. Patients with SCD have a decrease in NO, and this leads to vasoconstriction and hypertension. In addition,

low NO levels in the blood fail to inhibit endothelin-1, a potent vasoconstrictor, which results in additional vasoconstriction and hypertension. The connection between NO and SCD involves the hemolytic crisis. RBC hemolysis releases high levels of arginase, which degrades arginine; the result is less NO production from eNOS. In addition, the free hemoglobin released from hemolyzed RBCs scavenges NO, which further reduces the levels and exacerbates the vasoconstriction and hypertension.[26] Free heme causes the formation of reactive oxygen species or oxygen radicals leading to endothelial dysfunction and impaired vasodilation.[7] Blood arginine and NO levels decline a few days before the onset of ACS, a finding suggesting that the NO pathway is a connection between SCD, PHT, and asthma.[31,37] Treatment with large doses of arginine reduces pulmonary artery pressure, but the effect is not sustainable and does not reduce mortality. Increased tricuspid regurgitation velocity and blood N-terminal pro B-type natriuretic peptide (NT-proBNP) levels greater than 160 ng/L were found to be good predictors of PHT and are associated with a higher mortality rate.[29]

Acute abdominal pain (girdle syndrome). Girdle syndrome refers to acute abdominal pain caused by obstruction of mesenteric vessels, which often leads to ischemic colitis. Patients are treated by restricting food and drink (NPO), administering IV fluids for hydration, providing analgesics, and prescribing broad-spectrum antibiotics. A surgical consultation should also be obtained.[30]

Bacterial infections. Bacterial infections pose a major problem for patients with SCD, who have increased susceptibility to life-threatening infections from *Staphylococcus aureus, Streptococcus pneumoniae, Neisseria meningitidis,* and *Haemophilus influenzae.* Acute infections are common causes of hospitalization and have been the most common causes of death, especially in the first 3 years of life. Bacterial infections of the blood (septicemia) are exacerbated by the autosplenectomy effect as the spleen gradually loses its ability to function as a secondary lymphoid tissue to effectively clear organisms from the blood. Penicillin prophylaxis with the standard vaccine regimen plus *S. pneumoniae* and *H. influenzae* vaccinations have dramatically reduced childhood mortality. Nonetheless, fever can signal sepsis, so immediate empirical administration of broad-spectrum antibiotics is recommended.[34]

Acute anemia. Acute anemia is defined by a sudden decrease in hemoglobin by 2 g/dL or greater. Between 7% and 30% of patients with SCD experience one or more episodes of acute anemia. Acute anemia is usually caused by either chronic hemolysis or an aplastic crisis. Chronic hemolytic anemia is characterized by shortened RBC survival (between 16 and 20 days), with an elevated reticulocyte count and jaundice. Continuous screening and removal of sickle cells by the spleen perpetuate the chronic hemolytic anemia and autosplenectomy effect. Patients present with left upper quadrant pain and splenomegaly. Hypovolemia and shock may develop requiring rapid administration of a blood transfusion.[34] Because other conditions (such as hepatitis and gallstones) may cause jaundice, chronic hemolysis is difficult to diagnose in patients with SCD. RBC hemolysis releases free hemoglobin, which disrupts the arginine-NO pathway, resulting in the sequestration and lowering of NO. Decreased NO levels lead to endothelial cell activation, vasoconstriction, adherence of RBCs to the endothelium, and pulmonary hypertension, as previously discussed.[26] Other major sequelae of hemolysis are renal hyperfiltration and dysfunction, which can be detected early by an increased glomerular filtration rate of 140 mL/min per 1.73 m[3] or greater, found in 71% of patients with SCD.[38] Progression of renal dysfunction can be identified by detecting microalbuminuria (>4 to 5 mg/mmol), followed by proteinuria and terminating in elevated blood urea nitrogen and creatinine levels. Angiotensin-converting enzyme inhibitors (ACEIs) have been found to lower proteinuria in patients with SCD.[29]

Aplastic episodes. Aplastic episodes (bone marrow failure) are common life-threatening hematologic complications and are usually associated with infection, particularly parvovirus B19 infection. The prevalence of parvovirus infections is increased in areas of low socioeconomic status and in areas of overpopulation.[39] Aplastic episodes present clinical problems similar to those seen with other hemolytic disorders. Patients with SCD usually can compensate for the decrease in RBC survival by increasing bone marrow output. When the bone marrow is suppressed temporarily by bacterial or viral infections, however, the hematocrit decreases substantially with no reticulocyte compensation. Most aplastic episodes are short-lived, however, and require no therapy. Spontaneous recovery is characterized by the presence of nucleated RBCs and an increase in the number of reticulocytes in the peripheral blood. If anemia is severe and the bone marrow remains aplastic, transfusions are necessary. If patients are not transfused in a timely fashion, death can occur.

Megaloblastic episodes. Megaloblastic episodes result from the sudden arrest of erythropoiesis caused by folate depletion. Folic acid deficiency as a cause of exaggerated anemia in SCD is extremely rare in the United States. It is common practice to prescribe prophylactic folic acid for patients with SCD, however.[9]

Cardiac abnormalities. Cardiac complications are among the most common causes of morbidity and mortality. Approximately 32% of patients with SCD die of cardiac complications, with 70% of these patients dying of sudden cardiac events. Cardiomyopathy is associated with myocardial fibrosis, myocardial hypertrophy, diastolic dysfunction, arrhythmias, heart failure, and occasionally, myocardial infarction. In patients with severe anemia, cardiomegaly can develop as the heart works harder to maintain adequate blood flow and tissue oxygenation. Increased cardiac workload along with increased bone marrow erythropoiesis increases calorie burning, contributing to a reduced growth rate. When patients enter childbearing age, pregnancy becomes risky.[40]

Bone and skin abnormalities. Chronic anemia in SCD stimulates erythropoiesis and bone marrow hyperplasia. Concurrent hypoxia can induce bone necrosis. Together, patients with SCD experience high bone turnover and weakened architecture, exacerbating VOCs and bone death. Impaired blood supply to the head of the femur and humerus results in a condition called *avascular necrosis* (AVN). Approximately 28% of children with SCD develop AVN of the femoral head,

and about 50% of all patients with SCD develop AVN by age 35 years, resulting in joint collapse and functional impairment about 77% of the time. Physical therapy and surgery to relieve intramedullary pressure within the head of the long bones are effective, but hip and/or shoulder implants become necessary in most patients experiencing AVN. IV bisphosphonate infusions were shown to effectively reduce bone pain and did not induce sickle cell complications.[41] Similarly, leg ulcers are a common complication of SCD. Ulcers develop more frequently in the lower limbs, especially the perimalleolar areas (ankle bone), where vasoocclusion is common and fat deposits are low. Ulcers tend to heal slowly, develop unstable scars, and recur at the same site, becoming a chronic problem, with associated chronic pain.[42]

Stroke. Hemorrhagic or ischemic stroke occurs in approximately 10% of children with SCD (Hb SS and Hb S/β-thal) or 25% of all patients with SCD.[30,34] Screening children with transcranial Doppler is recommended annually between the ages of 2 and 16 years. Silent microstrokes can lead to headaches, poor school performance, reduced IQ, and overt CNS dysfunction. Neurologic examination followed by magnetic resonance imaging and, if available, transcranial Doppler ultrasonography or magnetic resonance angiography is recommended to detect microstrokes. Since the introduction of transcranial Doppler ultrasound screening, the rate of hospitalization due to stroke has decreased by 45%. Immediate treatment includes exchange transfusions, with ongoing treatment with anticoagulation. The goal is to reduce Hb S levels to less than 30% with exchange blood transfusions or to less than 60% with simple blood transfusions.[30] Following a stroke, monthly chronic transfusions are recommended to maintain Hb S levels below 30%.[34]

Retinopathy. Retinopathy occurs at a rate of 45% in patients with Hb SC, 11% in patients with Hb SS, and 17% in patients with Hb S-β-thal by early adulthood and eventually in nearly every adult.[16,34] Visual acuity is lost as a result of retinopathy caused by retinal ischemia, with secondary neovascularization and hemorrhage. Retinal detachment and central retinal artery infarction can also occur. Beginning at age 10 years, children with SCD should have annual dilated ophthalmologic examinations to detect early retinal injury. When proliferative retinopathy is detected, laser photocoagulation is performed, and vitrectomy can be done to resolve severe vitreous hemorrhage.[16,34]

Incidence With Malaria

The sickle gene occurs with greatest frequency in Central Africa, the Near East, the Mediterranean region, and parts of India. Sickle gene frequency parallels the incidence of *P. falciparum* and seems to offer some protection against cerebral falciparum malaria in young patients. Malarial parasites are living organisms within the RBCs that use the oxygen within the cells, thus reducing intracellular oxygen. This reduced oxygen tension causes the cells to sickle, which results in injury to the cells. These injured cells tend to become trapped within the blood vessels of the spleen and other organs, where they are easily phagocytized by scavenger macrophages. It has been shown that oxidative stress associated with *P. falciparum* infection stimulates the expression of mannose glycans on the RBC surface. Mannose receptors (CD206) are expressed on macrophages and endothelial cells increasing the uptake and phagocytosis of Hb S containing parasitized RBCs in the spleen. In patients with SCT, selective destruction of RBCs containing parasites decreases the number of malarial organisms and increases the time for immunity to develop. In patients with SCD, this mechanism exacerbates the anemia.[43]

Laboratory Diagnosis

When Hb S is suspected based on family history or symptoms, a CBC is performed. SCD is classified morphologically as a normocytic, normochromic anemia. The characteristic diagnostic cell observed on a Wright-stained peripheral blood film is a long, curved cell with a point at each end (Figure 24.5). Because of its appearance, the cell was named a *sickle cell*.[28] The peripheral blood film shows marked poikilocytosis and anisocytosis with normal RBCs, sickle cells, target cells, and nucleated RBCs, along with a few spherocytes, basophilic stippling, Pappenheimer bodies, and Howell-Jolly bodies. The presence of sickle cells and target cells is the hallmark of SCD. There is moderate to marked polychromasia, with a reticulocyte count between 10% and 25%, corresponding with the hemolytic state and the resultant bone marrow response. A very high reticulocyte count can increase the mean cell volume (MCV). The RBC distribution width (RDW) is increased resulting from moderate anisocytosis and reticulocytosis. An aplastic crisis can be heralded by a decreased reticulocyte count. Moderate leukocytosis is usually present (sometimes 40 to 50×10^9/L) with neutrophilia and a mild shift toward immature granulocytes. The leukocyte alkaline phosphatase score is not elevated when neutrophilia is caused by sickle cell crisis alone when no underlying infection is present. Thrombocytosis is usually present. The bone marrow shows erythroid hyperplasia, reflecting an attempt to compensate for the anemia, which results in polychromasia and an increase in reticulocytes and nucleated RBCs in the peripheral blood. Levels of immunoglobulins, particularly immunoglobulin A, are elevated in all forms of SCD. Serum ferritin levels are normal in young patients but tend to be elevated later in life. Chronic hemolysis is evidenced by elevated levels of indirect and total bilirubin with the accompanying jaundice.

The diagnosis of SCD is generally a two-step process: screening for Hb S using a hemoglobin solubility and confirmation with genotype assessment using hemoglobin electrophoresis, high-performance liquid chromatography (HPLC), or capillary electrophoresis. For more complicated cases, isoelectric focusing (IEF), tandem mass spectrometry (MS/MS), or deoxyribonucleic acid (DNA) analysis may be needed. An older screening test detects Hb S polymerization by inducing sickle cell formation on a glass slide. A drop of blood is mixed with a drop of 2% sodium metabisulfite (a reducing agent) on a slide, and the mixture is sealed under a coverslip. The hemoglobin inside the RBCs is reduced to the deoxygenated form; this induces polymerization and the resultant sickle cell formation, which can be identified microscopically. This method is slow and cumbersome and is rarely used in modern laboratories.

Hemoglobin solubility test. The most common screening test for Hb S, called the hemoglobin solubility test, capitalizes on the decreased solubility of deoxygenated Hb S in solution, producing turbidity. Blood is added to a buffered salt solution containing a reducing agent, such as sodium hydrosulfite (dithionite), and a detergent-based lysing agent (saponin). Saponin dissolves membrane lipids, causing release of hemoglobin from RBCs, and dithionite reduces iron from the ferrous to the ferric oxidation state. Ferric iron is unable to bind oxygen, converting hemoglobin to the deoxygenated form. Deoxygenated Hb S polymerizes in solution, which renders it turbid, whereas solutions containing nonsickling hemoglobins remain clear (Figure 24.6). False-positive results for Hb S can occur with hyperlipidemia, in a few rare hemoglobinopathies, and when too much blood is added to the test solution. False-negative results can occur in infants younger than 6 months and in individuals with low hematocrits. Other hemoglobin types that give a positive result on the solubility test include Hb C-Harlem (Georgetown), Hb C-Ziguinchor, Hb S-Memphis, Hb S-Travis, Hb S-Antilles, Hb S-Providence, Hb S-Oman, Hb Alexander, and Hb Porte-Alegre.[9] All these hemoglobin types have two amino acid substitutions: the Hb S substitution ($\beta^{6Glu \rightarrow Val}$) and another unrelated substitution. Hb S-Antilles

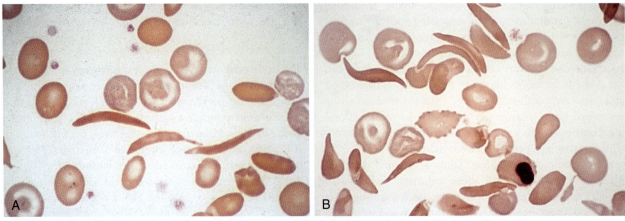

Figure 24.5 Peripheral Blood Films for a Patient With Sickle Cell Disease. (A), Note anisocytosis, polychromasia, three sickle cells, target cells, and normal platelets. **(B)**, Note anisocytosis, poikilocytosis, sickle cells, target cells, and one nucleated red blood cell. Platelets are not present in this field, but their numbers were adequate in this patient. (A, B, Wright-Giemsa stain, ×1000.) (Courtesy Ann Bell, University of Tennessee, Memphis.)

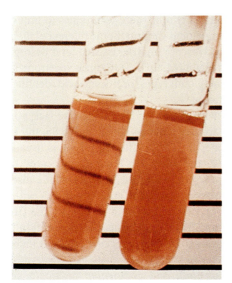

Figure 24.6 Hemoglobin Solubility Test for the Presence of Hemoglobin (Hb) S. In a negative test result *(left)*, the solution is clear, and the lines behind the tube are visible. In a positive test result *(right)*, the solution is turbid because of the polymerization of Hb S, and the lines are not visible. (Courtesy Ann Bell, University of Tennessee, Memphis.)

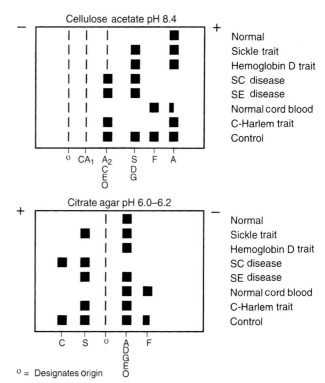

° = Designates Origin

Figure 24.7 Relative Mobilities of Normal and Variant Hemoglobins in Various Conditions Measured by Electrophoresis on Cellulose Acetate at an Alkaline pH and Citrate Agar at an Acid pH. The relative amount of hemoglobin is not proportional to the size of the band; for example, in sickle cell trait (hemoglobin [Hb] AS), the bands may appear equal, but the amount of Hb A exceeds the amount of Hb S. (From Schmidt, R. M., & Brosious, E. F. [1976]. *Basic Laboratory Methods of Hemoglobinopathy Detection.* [6th ed.]. HEW Pub. No. [CDC] 77-8266. Atlanta: Centers for Disease Control and Prevention.)

is particularly important because it can cause sickling in the heterozygous state.

Hemoglobin fractionation and quantification. Alkaline hemoglobin electrophoresis is a common first step in confirmation of hemoglobinopathies. Electrophoresis is based on the separation of hemoglobin molecules in an electric field resulting primarily from differences in total molecular charge. In alkaline electrophoresis, hemoglobin molecules assume a negative charge and migrate toward the anode (positive pole). Historically, alkaline hemoglobin electrophoresis was performed on cellulose acetate medium, but many systems use an agarose medium. Nonetheless, because some hemoglobin types have the same charge and therefore the same electrophoretic mobility patterns, hemoglobin types that exhibit an abnormal electrophoretic pattern at an alkaline pH may be subjected to electrophoresis at an acid pH for definitive separation. In an acid pH, some hemoglobin types assume a negative charge and migrate toward the anode, whereas others are positively charged and migrate toward the cathode (negative pole). For example, Hb S migrates with Hb D and Hb G on alkaline electrophoresis but separates from Hb D and Hb G on acid electrophoresis. Hb D and Hb G are further differentiated from Hb S in that they produce a negative result on the hemoglobin solubility test. Similarly, Hb C migrates with Hb E and Hb O on alkaline electrophoresis but separates on acid electrophoresis. Figure 24.7 shows electrophoretic patterns for normal and abnormal hemoglobin types. Figure 24.8 shows the electrophoretic separation of a healthy adult and a patient with SCD (Hb SS) at an alkaline pH. HPLC and capillary electrophoresis are gaining in popularity because these methods are more automated, the instruments are more user friendly, and they can be used to confirm hemoglobin variants observed with electrophoresis (Figure 24.9).

HPLC separates hemoglobin types in a cation exchange column and usually requires only one sample injection. In contrast

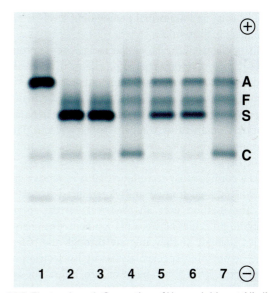

Figure 24.8 Electrophoretic Separation of Hemoglobins at Alkaline pH. Healthy adult *(1)*; A 17-year-old patient with sickle cell anemia (hemoglobin [Hb] SS) *(2, 3)*; patient with sickle cell anemia, recently transfused (note the presence of Hb A from the transfused red blood cells) *(5, 6)*; Hb A, Hb F, Hb S, and Hb C standard (Hydragel 7 Hemoglobin/Hydrasys System, Sebia Electrophoresis, Norcross, GA) *(4, 7)*. (Modified from Elghetany, M. T., Schexneider, K. I., & Banki, K. [2022]. Erythrocytic disorders. In McPherson, R. A., & Pincus, M. R. [Eds.], *Henry's Clinical Diagnosis and Management by Laboratory Methods.* [24th ed., p. 609, Figure 33.17]. St. Louis: Elsevier.)

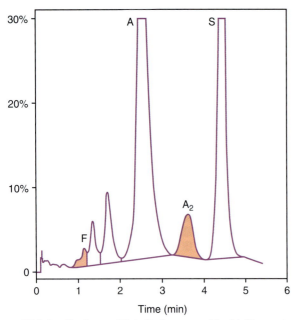

Figure 24.9 Ion-Exchange High-Performance Liquid Chromatography Separation of Hemoglobins in a Patient With Sickle Cell Trait Demonstrating Hemoglobin (Hb) F, Hb A, Hb A$_2$, and an Abnormal Hemoglobin in the Hb S Window. (Bio-Rad Variant Classic Hb Testing System, BioRad Laboratories, Philadelphia). (Modified from Elghetany, M. T., Schexneider, K. I., & Banki, K. [2022]. Erythrocytic disorders. In McPherson, R. A., & Pincus, M. R. [Eds.], *Henry's Clinical Diagnosis and Management by Laboratory Methods.* [24th ed., p. 609, Figure 33.16]. St. Louis: Elsevier.)

to electrophoresis, HPLC can identify and quantify low levels of Hb A$_2$ and Hb F, but comigration of Hb A$_2$ and Hb E occurs. Therefore HPLC is best used in the diagnosis of thalassemias rather than hemoglobinopathies because quantification of low levels of normal and abnormal hemoglobin levels is necessary to distinguish thalassemias.

Capillary electrophoresis, similar to agarose electrophoresis, separates hemoglobin types based on charge in an alkaline buffer but does so using smaller volumes and produces better separation than traditional agarose electrophoresis. Semiautomated systems allow for the testing of multiple samples in parallel with computerized analysis of results. Capillary electrophoresis is also economical because each capillary can accommodate at least 3000 runs.[44]

IEF is a confirmatory technique that is expensive and complex, requiring well-trained and experienced laboratory personnel. The method uses an electrical current to push the hemoglobin molecules across a pH gradient. The charge of the molecules changes as they migrate through the pH gradient until the hemoglobin species reaches its isoelectric point (net charge of zero). With a net charge of zero, migration stops, and the hemoglobin molecules accumulate at their isoelectric position. Molecules with isoelectric point differences of as little as 0.02 pH units can be effectively separated.[44]

Neonatal screening requires a more sophisticated approach, often using three techniques: adapted IEF, HPLC, and reverse-phase HPLC. This multisystem approach is needed to distinguish not only the multitude of hemoglobin variants but also the numerous thalassemias. More progressive laboratories use

a combination of two or more techniques to improve identification of hemoglobin variants. Some reference laboratories may use mass spectroscopy, matrix-assisted laser desorption ionization time-of-flight (MALDI-TOF) mass spectrometry, or IEF to separate hemoglobin types, or nucleic acid identification of the genetic mutation.[44]

Patients with Hb SS or Hb SC disease lack normal β-globin chains, so they have no Hb A. In Hb SS, the Hb S level is usually greater than 80%. The Hb F level is usually increased (1% to 20%), and when Hb F constitutes more than 20% of hemoglobin, it modulates the severity of the disease. This is especially true in newborns and in patients with hereditary persistence of fetal hemoglobin (HPFH).[3] The Hb A$_2$ level is usually normal. Hb A$_2$ quantification is useful in differentiating Hb SS from Hb S-β-thal because Hb A$_2$ is increased in the latter (Chapter 25).

Rapid detection and genotyping of sickle cell disease. Screening for SCD using hemoglobin solubility or the sickling test (2% sodium metabisulfite on a slide) are accessible to many clinics in underdeveloped countries. However, confirmatory methods to verify Hb S and to determine genotype are limited to only large hospitals in most of the developing nations. As a result, lateral flow immunochromatographic methods have been developed to detect Hb S, Hb C, Hb F, and Hb A that can also determine genotype. Capture antibodies specific to each hemoglobin type are solid-phase stamped in succession within the reading area of the test cassette. Labeled antihemoglobin antibodies bind to the hemoglobin molecules in the sample and wick toward the test window of the cassette. Each hemoglobin type present in the sample will be captured in the appropriate area and will form a visible band as the label accumulates at each area. A band at the control area is required for a valid test. One additional band at the Hb A position indicates a normal (Hb AA) genotype. A band at the Hb A and Hb S positions indicates SCT and only one additional band at the Hb S position indicates SCA (Hb SS). The same pattern at the Hb C position indicates Hb CC disease or a Hb AC carrier. Two additional bands at the Hb S and Hb C positions indicate Hb SC disease. Neither of the two prominent test kits on the market, Biomedomics Sickle SCAN and Sysmex HemoTypeSC, are able to detect Hb F, in newborns, in patients with concomitant HPFH, and in patients receiving hydroxyurea. However, genotyping is still possible without detection of Hb F. Sensitivity and specificity for both products are reported to be above 98%. These lateral flow methods can be used in resource-poor countries to conduct newborn screening (NBS) programs and to confirm the genotypes of existing patients.[44–47]

Treatment

Supportive care has been the mainstay of therapy for SCD and includes adequate hydration, prophylactic vitamin therapy, avoidance of low-oxygen environments, analgesia for pain, and aggressive antibiotic therapy with the first signs of infection. Hydration maintains good blood flow and reduces VOCs. Avoidance of strenuous exercise, high altitudes, and unpressurized air travel maintains high oxygen tensions and reduces the sickling phenomenon.

Infection prevention. Prophylactic oral penicillin V is recommended for children younger than 5 years to avoid infection and the associated morbidity and mortality. Pneumococcal disease has been a leading cause of morbidity and mortality in children, especially children younger than 6 years. When infections occur, prompt antibiotic treatment reduces the associated morbidity and mortality.[7,16,30] With immunization and prophylactic antibiotics, however, infections are now a preventable complication. Immunization with the 13-valent conjugate pneumococcal vaccine series is recommended to begin shortly after birth. The 23-valent pneumococcal vaccine is recommended at 2 years, with a booster at age 5 years. Standard immunizations should be given according to the schedule recommended by the US Preventive Services Task Force and the Advisory Committee for Immunization Practices (ACIP) including annual administration of influenza vaccine beginning at age 6 months. The risk of invasive bacterial infection increases in older children and adults with SCD genotypes, mainly because of reduced splenic function resulting from repeated infarcts.[7,16]

Pain care. Successful treatment of both acute and chronic pain is challenging. The ESCAPED trial reported that 54% of subjects (n = 391) had three or more hospital visits each year for acute pain episodes.[7] Treatment for acute painful episodes includes ensuring optimal hydration, rapidly treating associated infection, oxygen therapy, and effectively relieving pain. Analgesics are the foundation of pain management, with nonsteroidal antiinflammatory drugs usually given to manage mild to moderate pain and opioids given for severe pain and for VOC events. Approximately 55% of adults have chronic pain greater than 50% of their waking hours, and 29% have pain 95% of the time. Patients with SCD report using opioids at home about 78% of the days in which pain occurs, with 85% of these using long-acting opioids and 47% using short-acting opioids. Most adults report pain in three or more sites simultaneously, with the back, abdomen, and extremities being the most common locations. Pain is processed in patients with SCD using a variety of mechanisms, including nociceptive, inflammatory, neuropathic, and CNS pathways. Selective serotonin reuptake inhibitors consistently demonstrate benefit in managing chronic pain.[7] In the acute setting, parenteral opioids are used for severe pain, whereas short- and long-acting oral opioids are prescribed and closely monitored when severe pain becomes chronic. Painful crises tend to increase with age, and providers must be aware of opiate tolerance and rebound pain after opiate therapy, called central sensitization. The most appropriate response to opioid tolerance and central sensitization is a gradual dose reduction to reset the pain receptors, followed by switching to opioids that are less sensitive to this phenomenon. The patient should be examined on a regular basis, and routine testing should be done to establish baseline pain values for the patient during nonsickling periods.[7,16,30]

Children younger than 3 years often experience *hand-foot syndrome,* characterized by pain and swelling in the hands and feet. Treatment usually consists of increasing intake of fluids and analgesics for pain.

Transfusions. Transfusions can be used to prevent the complications of SCD. More specifically, chronic transfusions, given at a frequency of eight or more per year, are used to prevent stroke, symptomatic anemia, priapism, leg ulcers, pulmonary hypertension, delayed pubescence, splenomegaly, and chronic pain and to improve exercise tolerance and sense of well-being. In other circumstances, such as CNS infarction, hypoxia with infection, stroke, episodes of ACS, and preparation for surgery, transfusions are used to decrease blood viscosity and the percentage of circulating sickle cells. Before all but simple surgeries, Hb SS patients are transfused with normal Hb AA blood to achieve a hemoglobin of 10 g/dL in an effort to prevent complications in surgery. For chronically transfused children, a Hb S level of less than 30% immediately before the next transfusion is recommended.[7,16] Transfused units for all patients with SCD should be matched for C, E, and K antigens. Maintenance transfusions should be given in pregnancy if the mother experiences vasoocclusive or anemia-related problems or if there are signs of fetal distress or poor growth.[23] Blood exchange transfusion is the treatment of choice for severe VOCs and ACS. Nonetheless, transfusion therapy has the potential to cause transfusion reactions, transfusion-related infections, and iron overload. Of the three, iron overload is the most common.

Iron overload has been associated with endocrine dysfunction, hepatic fibrosis, and cardiac disease. Iron chelators have been effective in treating iron overload by chelating and removing excess iron from the body through excretion in the urine or feces. Deferoxamine, approved by the US Food and Drug Administration (FDA) in 1982, is administered by continuous pump infusion over 8 to 12 hours or by twice-daily subcutaneous injections. Oral iron chelators deferasirox (FDA approval in 2005) and deferiprone (FDA approval in 2011) are more conveniently administered in three daily doses and one daily dose, respectively. Recommendations by the National Institutes of Health (NIH) suggest that chelation therapy be initiated when the liver iron concentration exceeds 7 mg/g dry weight, cumulative transfusions of 120 mL of pure RBCs/kg of body weight, or serum ferritin levels of >1000 ng/mL. All three chelators can have adverse effects and issues with patient compliance. The use of combinations of chelators or alternating days of chelators to decrease adverse effects and improve compliance is the subject of ongoing study.[48]

Stem cell transplant. Allogeneic bone marrow or hematopoietic stem cell transplantation is the only curative therapy and has been performed in more than 1200 patients with SCD worldwide since the first transplant in 1984.[49] However, few patients qualify because of the lack of HLA-matched related donors. Between 14% and 20% of patients with SCD have HLA-identical sibling donors.[50] The risks of graft rejection, graft-versus-host disease (GVHD), and mortality must be weighed against disease severity. Pretransplant testing includes a CBC and comprehensive metabolic panel to assess hematologic status and organ function and a 24-h urine creatinine to further assess renal function. A brain magnetic resonance imaging scan is performed to detect brain infarcts and vascular abnormalities. Cardiac function (echocardiogram), pulmonary function, and dental clearance are recommended. Patients chosen for transplantation are generally children younger than age 17 with severe complications of SCD. In addition, morbidity and mortality after transplantation increase with age, which places another restriction on transplantation therapy. Pretransplant conditioning with chemotherapy such as busulfan to destroy the patient's hematopoietic cells and posttransplant immunosuppression with drugs such as cyclophosphamide to reduce the risk of GVHD are indicated. Approximately 9% of patients experience graft rejection, and 15% develop chronic GVHD.[49] Transplantation of cord blood stem cells from HLA-identical related and unrelated donors is also an option. The primary benefits of using cord blood as a source of stem cells is its lower immunogenicity as a donor source and that banking of cord blood increases the number of units available to achieve an HLA match. However, the volume of a cord blood sample often is too little for adult patients. Newer transplantation protocols involve reduced intensity conditioning and donor sample manipulations to include ex vivo CD34+ cell selection and T cell depletion.[51] Some researchers are currently focusing on the use of in utero stem cell transplantation to produce engraftment while the immune system of the fetus has the capability for HLA tolerance.

The observations that patients with homozygous HPFH are mostly asymptomatic with high quality of life and compound heterozygotes with Hb S/HPFH experience low morbidity suggest an important role of Hb F in mitigating the symptoms of SCD. Efforts to determine the mechanism of γ-chain suppression and reactivation and to identify drugs to stimulate Hb F production continue to be vigorously pursued.

Drugs to increase fetal hemoglobin. Hydroxycarbamide (hydroxyurea) therapy is the only FDA-approved drug to reactivate the production of Hb F in patients with SCD. The mechanism of γ-chain reactivation is unclear, but hydroxyurea has been shown to inhibit ribonucleotide reductase enzyme, inhibit S-phase DNA synthesis, and increase NO levels.[3] Hydroxyurea can be administered to children beginning at age 9 months with daily pediatric dose regimens. Dose escalation should occur every 2 to 3 months until the absolute neutrophil count (ANC) reaches the target level of 2.0 to 3.0×10^9/L. If the ANC drops below the target level, the dose should be reduced to the highest dose that produced the target ANC. Hydroxyurea should be withheld if the ANC falls below 1.0×10^9/L. Daily dosing for adults is higher but escalated in the same manner as in pediatric patients.[52] Daily dosing produces a better Hb F response compared with sequential weekly dosing. Because Hb F does not copolymerize with Hb S, increasing production of Hb F can avoid some complications of SCD. The severity of the disease expression and the number of irreversible sickle cells are inversely proportional to the extent to which Hb F synthesis persists. Individuals in whom Hb F levels stabilize at 12% to 20% of total hemoglobin may have little or no anemia and few, if any, vasoocclusive attacks. Levels of 4% to 5% Hb F may modulate the disease, and levels of 5% to 12% may suppress the severity of hemolysis and lessen the frequency of severe episodes.[52] However, the ratio of Hb F to F cells may be a better predictor of protection from polymerization that leads to VOC than overall Hb F concentration.[53] Hydroxyurea was shown to reduce

annual painful crises by a median of 44%, anemia, hemolysis, and inflammation, and improves quality of life and overall survival. Drug compliance is best monitored by an increasing MCV, whereas decreasing lactate dehydrogenase might be an indicator of treatment response.[29] Response to hydroxycarbamide is variable among patients with SCD, but high baseline Hb F level, neutrophil level, and reticulocyte count are the best predictors of Hb F response.[53] Because hydroxyurea is a myelosuppressive, antimetabolite chemotherapeutic drug, infertility, mutagenesis, carcinogenesis, and teratogenesis are common health concerns particularly during conception and pregnancy. However, after decades of treatment, no increased risks of these types of mutagenesis have been documented.[52]

Other drugs that have been shown to stimulate γ-chain synthesis and Hb F production either fall into the category of antineoplastic drugs (such as hydroxyurea) or are of natural origin. Sodium butyrate, azacitidine, and decitabine all have been shown to induce Hb F production but are myelosuppressive, are carcinogenic, and produce many side effects. Sodium butyrate inhibits histone deacetylase resulting in more acetylation and activation of genes. It is thought that sodium butyrate activates p38 mitogen-activated protein kinase (MAPK) stress response to increase production of Hb F. Similarly, thalidomide derivatives, lenalidomide and pomalidomide, induce Hb F production by increasing reactive oxygen species, which also activates p38 MAPK stress response. The chemotherapeutic drugs azacitidine and decitabine inhibit DNA methyltransferase activity to induce DNA hypomethylation of the promoter region of the γ-globin gene to reactivate γ-chain production. Natural ways to induce some level of Hb F production include angelicin from *Angelica arcangelica*, resveratrol from grapes, rapamycin from *Streptomyces hygroscopicus*, bergatene from *Aeglemarmelos*, and mithramycin from *Streptomyces* species.[3]

Newer drug options. L-glutamine was approved by the FDA in 2017 and has been shown to reduce acute complications of SCD in patients 5 years and older. The frequency of VOCs was reduced by 45% annually. L-glutamine is converted to free glutamine in the blood, which is taken up by RBCs and degraded, producing reduced antioxidant molecules such as nicotinamide adenine dinucleotide that neutralize oxidants to maintain RBC flexibility. In clinical trials, patients taking L-glutamine experienced fewer sickle cell crises, fewer hospital admissions and emergency visits for pain, and fewer episodes of ACS.[54] In addition to its role in reducing oxidative stress, L-glutamine enhances intestinal mucosal health, fortifies intestinal barrier functions, modifies the intestinal microbiome, and acts as an antiinflammatory agent.[55] L-glutamine can be used in combination with hydroxyurea. Another amino acid, L-arginine, reduced pain during VOCs resulting in lowered opioid doses.[7]

New treatment strategies are being investigated to protect against free hemoglobin and free heme to reduce or prevent organ damage. Haptoglobin supplementation has been found experimentally to reduce vasculotoxic injury. Haptoglobin/hemoglobin complexes are too large to penetrate endothelial cell-cell tight junctions, allowing hemoglobin to bind CD163 receptors on monocytes, macrophages, and dendritic for elimination (Chapter 20). When hemoglobin enters the subendothelial space, its NO scavenging activity causes vasculotoxic injury. Similarly, hemopexin binds free heme and directs it to hepatocytes for removal rather than to macrophages, where the heme stimulates macrophages toward the M1 proinflammatory phenotype. Combination therapy using both agents represent a natural strategy to ameliorate vasculotoxic effects and reduce or prevent organ injury.[56]

Another novel therapeutic approach is to test drugs that target adhesion of circulating blood cells to the endothelium. Crizanlizumab is a monoclonal antibody that binds P-selectin on endothelial cells and platelets to reduce the interaction between endothelial cells, platelets, RBCs, and WBCs, improving microvascular rheology. The drug was approved by the FDA in 2019 to treat patients older than 16 years with all genotypes of SCD. The recommended dose of 5 mg/kg is given as a monthly IV infusion.[57] The SUSTAIN clinical trial showed that crizanlizumab produced a reduction in annual VOC events from a median of 2.98 to 1.63 in the study population. This translates into a 45% reduction in annual VOC events.[58]

Rivipansel (GMI-1070) blocks P-selectin and E-selectin, which are highly expressed on endothelial cells and platelets of patients with SCD.[56] Rivipansel prevents WBCs from binding to the endothelium and improves blood flow by reducing cell-cell interactions and vascular occlusions. Although rivipansel failed to meet phase III trial end points, it did reduce IV opioid use and shorten hospital stay.[59]

Antisickling drugs bind to Hb S molecules and inhibit sickling by increasing oxygen affinity and maintaining Hb S in the oxyhemoglobin state. Voxelotor (also known as GBT440 or Oxbryta) was approved by the FDA in 2019 for adults and in 2021 for children 4 years and older. It functions by binding the α-globin chain of Hb S to increase oxygen binding affinity. This maintains more Hb S molecules in the oxygenated state, thus reducing polymerization and VOCs. The HOPE trial reported that oral voxelotor 1500 mg once daily resulted in rapid and durable improvements in hemoglobin concentrations (>1.0 g/dL) over 72 weeks. Hemolysis was reduced as indicated by lowered direct bilirubin levels (−26.6%) and reduced percentage of reticulocytes (−18.6%). The percentage of serious adverse events was tolerable at 28% and comparable to the placebo group at 25%.[60] 5-Hydroxymethylfurfural (5-HMF), vanillin derivatives, and trizole sulfate are currently being investigated. 5-HMF binds the N-terminal valine of the α chains that stabilizes the R state (relaxed) to increase oxygen affinity for Hb S, it inhibits P_{sickle} and Gardos channels to prevent dehydration, and it increases the ability of RBCs to generate NO to promote vasodilation and blood flow.[61] The effect of 5-HMF is improved when combined with hydroxycarbamide (hydroxyurea). Derivatives of vanillin have been found to also increase oxygen affinity of Hb S and destabilize Hb S polymer contacts. As mentioned, voxelotor binds the N-terminal valine of the α chains similar to 5-HMF, but it also influences the intradimer interface and the heme pockets to increase oxygen affinity. Triazole sulfide binds to βCys93 and βC112 and to the central water cavity to stabilize the R state and increase oxygen affinity to a greater degree than 5-HMF. The main challenge is the concentration of antisickling drug needed to bind the approximately 200 to 300 million hemoglobin molecules in each RBC. Large, nontoxic doses may be difficult to achieve and maintain, especially because most of these drugs have a short half-life.[61]

Intravenous immunoglobulin G (IVIG) is being investigated to stabilize neutrophil Mac-1 activation in VOC. Lastly, AKT2 inhibitors in combination with hydroxyurea are being tested in a mouse model to reduce neutrophil adhesion, platelet-neutrophil aggregation, endothelial E-selectin, and intercellular adhesion molecule 1 to improve survival.[56]

Gene therapy. Besides transplantation, gene therapy also offers the chance of a cure. The initial approach to gene therapy performed in mice was to transfect a wild-type β-globin gene into a lentiviral vector, expose the viral vector to patient stem cells, allow for gene integration, and transplant autologous stem cells back into the patient. Although gene integration into the patient's genome was successful, controlling the genomic position of the wild-type gene was unpredictable resulting in great variation in gene expression rates. Modifications in the gene regulatory elements and lentivirus characteristics reduced mutagenic integration and improved gene expression. This approach has been successful in a few human trials, but the insertion stimulated growth of myeloid cells with malignant potential.[51] More recently, lentiviral vectors have been used to deliver microribonucleic acid (RNA)-adapted short hairpin RNA molecules that are erythrocyte specific and designed to knock down BCL11a. BCL11a is a zinc-finger-containing transcription factor encoded on chromosome 2 that is the natural repressor of the γ-globin gene to reduce Hb F production in neonates around 6 months of age. Knocking down BCL11a reduces the repression of the γ-globin gene resulting in the production of Hb F. This approach has been shown to reactivate the γ-globin gene and is currently in early clinical development.[50]

More recently, genome-editing technologies show great promise in reversing the pathophysiology of SCD and affording the potential of a cure. The primary strategies being studied involve infusing autologous CD34+ hematopoietic stem and progenitor cells (HSPCs) that have been edited ex vivo to (1) correct the point mutation in the β-globin gene to change Hb S to Hb A production; (2) increase Hb F production by disrupting the production of γ-globin gene repressors (such as BCL11A transcription factor) to enable greater expression of the γ-globin gene; or (3) increase Hb F production by creating HPFH-like mutations in the γ-globin gene promoter to prevent it from binding the BCL11A repressor to enable greater expression of the γ-globin gene.[62,63] The primary genome-editing systems being studied include transcription activator-like effector nucleases (TALENS); zinc-finger nucleases (ZFNs); clustered regularly interspaced short palindromic repeats (CRISPR) with Cas9 nuclease; and base editing systems that work with nucleases without cleaving double-stranded DNA.[62,63] CRISPR-Cas9 has been shown to be a more versatile and effective system for genome editing and exhibits high on-target and low off-target specificity.[62,63]

CRISPRs were first reported in bacteria and in conjunction with Cas nucleases provide a mechanism for bacteria to recognize, cleave, and destroy the DNA of invading plasmids and bacteriophages.[64] CRISPR-Cas9 was engineered for genome editing in human cells, and it enables precise, targeted alterations (additions, deletions, or corrections) in the DNA sequence of a gene or its promoter/enhancers.[62–64] The CRISPR-Cas9 system includes the Cas9 nuclease complexed with an engineered single guide RNA (sgRNA) (Figure 24.10).[64] The 3′ end of the sgRNA attaches to Cas9, and the 5′ end is the recognition sequence that is homologous with the target DNA and brings the Cas9 nuclease to the exact location for target DNA cleavage.[62–64] Once introduced into a cell, the CRISPR-Cas9 complex searches for a DNA sequence that is homologous with both the sgRNA sequence and a nearby protospacer adjacent motif (PAM) sequence on the target DNA.[64] Once the sgRNA hybridizes to the target DNA, the Cas9 protein is activated to make double-stranded cuts in the DNA at that precise location.

Two different cellular DNA repair mechanisms are used to repair the break, each designed to produce a different outcome.

To correct a gene mutation, a donor template, with the wild-type (normal) sequence complementary to the coding sequence, is added to the cell. The cell then uses the donor template to repair the break using *homology directed repair* (HDR), which inserts the wild-type nucleotide(s) into the precise location in the patient's DNA.[63,64] To disrupt a gene or its promoter/enhancers, the cell repairs the break by *nonhomologous end joining* (NHEJ), forming many insertion and deletion mutations (indels) that inactivate the gene.[63,64] A more detailed explanation of CRISPR-Cas9 and other genome-editing technologies is beyond the scope of this chapter.

In 2019 the first patient with severe SCD was treated in a clinical trial involving the investigational use of CRISPR-Cas9.[50] After undergoing myeloablative conditioning, the patient received a single infusion of autologous CD34+ HSPCs in which CRISPR-Cas9 was used ex vivo to inactivate the erythroid-specific enhancer for the *BCL11A* repressor gene to allow greater expression of the γ-globin gene.[50] The patient's

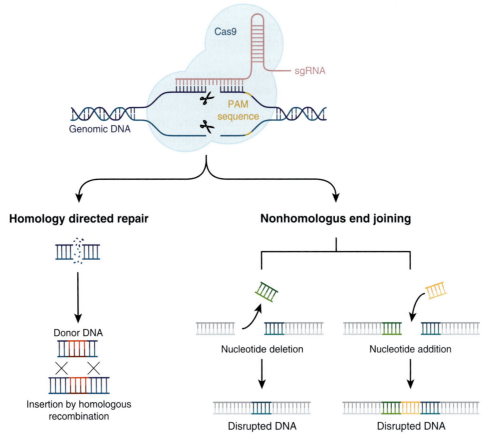

Figure 24.10 Mechanism of CRISPR-Cas9 Genome Editing. The CRISPR-Cas9 system includes the Cas9 nuclease complexed with an engineered single guide RNA *(sgRNA)*. One end of the sgRNA binds to Cas9 and the other has a recognition sequence that binds to the target DNA. The CRISPR-Cas9 complex searches for a DNA sequence that is homologous with both the guide sgRNA sequence and a nearby protospacer adjacent motif *(PAM)* sequence on the target DNA. Once the sgRNA hybridizes to the target DNA, Cas9 is activated and makes a double-stranded cut in the DNA at that precise location. To correct a gene mutation, a donor DNA template, with a wild-type (normal) sequence complementary to the coding sequence, is added. The cell then uses the donor template to repair the break using homology-directed repair, which inserts the wild-type nucleotides into the precise location on the target DNA. To disrupt a gene or its promoter/enhancers, the cell repairs the break by nonhomologous end joining, forming many insertion and deletion mutations (indels) that prevent expression of the gene. (Modified from Luthra, R., Kaur, S., & Bhandari, K. [2021]. Applications of CRISPR as a potential therapeutic. *Life Sci, 284,* 119908, Figure 1.)

hemoglobin and Hb F were 12.0 g/dL and 43.2%, respectively, 15 months after infusion (increased from a baseline of 7.2 g/dL and 9.1%). Transfusion independence was achieved with no vasoocclusive episodes; adverse events occurred but were resolved with treatment.[50] Trials using this strategy with additional patients are ongoing.[65] Other trials are being initiated for patients with severe SCD using a mutation-correction strategy. The patients will receive autologous CD34+ HSPCs in which CRISPR-Cas9 was used ex vivo to correct the Hb S mutation in the β-globin gene to change Hb S to Hb A production.[65]

Genome-editing technology involves serious risks, and long-term safety and efficacy are being carefully monitored. Off-target mutations in the edited HSPC genome can result in a loss or gain of gene function and associated serious pathologic outcomes.[62–64]

Course and Prognosis

Proper management of SCD has increased the life expectancy of patients from 14 years in 1973 to the current average life span of 54 years compared with 76 years in a matched non-SCD cohort.[66] For men and women who are compound heterozygotes for Hb SC, the average life span is more than 60 years, with a few patients living into their 70s.[27] Individuals with Hb SS can pursue a wide range of vocations and professions. They are discouraged, however, from jobs that require strenuous physical exertion or exposure to high altitudes or extreme environmental temperature variations.

Newborn screening (NBS) for hemoglobinopathies began in the 1960s as targeted population screening initiatives. In 1973, 12 public health laboratories began testing for SCD among newborns. New York was the first state to adopt a NBS program statewide in 1975. NBS programs were adopted in all 50 states within the United States in 2006. NBS has significantly reduced mortality in children with SCD by enabling prompt and comprehensive medical care. NBS programs in the United States follow a similar sequence of activities including education, screening, short-term follow-up diagnosis, management, and evaluation and long-term follow-up. Blood is collected from a heel stick usually within 24 to 72 hours of birth (or at least before hospital discharge), blotted onto paper, and sent to a designated state laboratory within 24 to 72 hours of collection to prevent degradation. The most common testing methods used in NBS programs are IEF, HPLC, and capillary electrophoresis. Less common methods include MS/MS and a variety of molecular methods.[67]

Sickle Cell Disease and Pregnancy

Managing pregnant patients with SCD is challenging and involves interventions before conception, prenatally, during delivery, and postpartum.

Preconception. Repeated microvascular occlusion in patients with SCD increases the risk of cardiomyopathy (four times greater risk), renal disease, proteinuria, pulmonary hypertension (six times greater risk), hypercoagulability, osteonecrosis, and hepatic necrosis, all of which greatly complicate pregnancy. When present, these conditions require management by a multidisciplinary approach. The father should be tested to predict the risk of the child having SCD,

and genetic counseling should be recommended as appropriate. Immunizations should be current, and the patient should be typed and screened for alloantibodies. Medications that affect pregnancy such as ACEIs or angiotensin II receptor blockers for cardiomyopathy and hydroxyurea must be discontinued before conception or switched to a safer agent.[68] Hydroxyurea is suspected to cause infertility, mutagenesis, carcinogenesis, or teratogenesis. However, decades of successful use have not produced studies to document these risks. It is common for women with SCD taking hydroxyurea to be weeks into the first trimester before learning of their pregnancy. In addition, there is evidence to suggest that hydroxyurea may benefit both mothers and fetuses during the third trimester of pregnancy.[52]

Prenatal (antenatal). Women with SCD have a sixfold increased risk of maternal death and a 2.2 times greater risk of fetal death. Fetal ultrasound should be performed during the first trimester and at 20, 32, and 36 weeks of gestation. Pregnant women should continue with folic acid at 5 mg/day or greater to prevent neural tube defects. Because pregnant patients with SCD develop blood clots five times more often, thromboembolism prophylaxis is recommended once hospitalized. Although prophylactic transfusion therapy is controversial, it may ameliorate chronic organ dysfunction, ACS, and frequent pain crises. Therapeutic transfusions are indicated if patients experience severe anemia, refractory pain crises, reticulocytopenia, septicemia, and intrapartum complications. To minimize alloimmunization, blood products should be matched for C, D, E, and Kell antigens, and leukoreduced.[68]

During delivery (intrapartum). To minimize complications, delivery is recommended between 38 and 40 weeks. To reduce sickling risk, patients should be on oxygen and kept warm and well hydrated, and local anesthesia should be used rather than general anesthesia. If a cesarean section is warranted or if the fetus has late decelerations, the patient should be transfused to maintain a hemoglobin level at 10 g/dL.[68]

Postpartum. Patients should remain hospitalized for 3 days postpartum to monitor fluid status, blood cell counts, renal function, and liver function, and for evidence of VOC, which occurs in 25% of patients. Because thromboembolism is a risk, patients should be mobilized early, and thromboprophylaxis should be restarted 12 hours after delivery and continued for 6 weeks for a cesarean section.[68] Although hydroxyurea has been contraindicated for lactating women, a recent study documented that hydroxyurea is low in breast milk and below tolerated levels.[52]

Sickle Cell Trait

The term *sickle cell trait* refers to the heterozygous state (Hb AS) and describes a benign condition that generally does not affect mortality or morbidity except under conditions of extreme exertion. In the United States, SCT occurs in approximately 1 in 13 children of African ancestry (8%) but also can be found in individuals from India, Middle East, Central and South America, Asia, and the Mediterranean region.

Individuals with SCT are generally asymptomatic and present with no significant clinical or hematologic manifestations. Under extremely hypoxic conditions, however, systemic sickling and vascular occlusion, with pooling of sickled cells in the spleen, focal necrosis in the brain, rhabdomyolysis, and even death, can occur. In circumstances such as severe respiratory infection, unpressurized flight at high altitudes, and anesthesia, in which pH and oxygen levels are sufficiently lowered, may cause sickling and the development of splenic infarcts. Failure to concentrate urine is the only consistent abnormality found in patients with SCT. This abnormality is caused by diminished perfusion of the kidney vasa recta, which impairs concentration of urine by renal tubules. Renal papillary necrosis with hematuria has been described in some patients.[9]

Although much controversy exists regarding the potential connection between strenuous exercise and severe to fatal adverse events in patients with SCT, at least 46 cases have been documented in the literature (39 military recruits and 7 athletes).[69] Deaths were due largely to cardiac or renal failure or rhabdomyolysis. These adverse events are termed exercise collapse associated with sickle cell trait (ECAST). Opponents of ECAST argue that these events occur in sickle cell-negative people, many people with SCT do not develop adverse events, sickle crisis cannot be adequately established in patients experiencing such events, and similar events have not been clearly documented in patients with SCD. However, it has been found that military recruits with SCT have a 21 times greater risk of exercise-related death than recruits with normal hemoglobin.[69] Similar data have not been established in athletes with SCT, but evidence is mounting that SCT is associated with sudden death in competitive athletes.[11] In 2010 the National Collegiate Athletic Association mandated SCT screening with the hemoglobin solubility test for all student athletes in division I sports. This mandate was implemented with division II sports in 2012 and division III sports in 2013. Athletes experiencing an adverse event present with cramping, dyspnea, muscle pain, severe weakness, fatigue, and exhaustion that evolves into a gradual deterioration over several minutes, often terminating in rhabdomyolysis. These events occur more often after strenuous physical exertion early in the athletic season, at high temperatures, at high altitudes, and after interval training. These events constitute a medical emergency that requires immediate monitoring of vital signs, administration of oxygen and IV hydration, cooling, and transport to a medical facility.[12]

The peripheral blood film in SCT has normal RBC morphology except for a few target cells. No abnormalities in the WBCs and platelets are seen. The hemoglobin solubility screening test yields positive results, and SCT is diagnosed by detecting the presence of Hb S and Hb A on hemoglobin electrophoresis or HPLC. In individuals with SCT, electrophoresis reveals approximately 40% or less Hb S and approximately 60% or more Hb A, Hb A_2 level is normal or slightly increased, and Hb F level is within the reference interval. Levels of Hb S less than 40% can be seen in patients who also have α-thalassemia or iron or folate deficiency due to decreased hemoglobin production.[23] Except in the event of ECAST, no treatment is required for this benign condition, and the patient's life span is not affected.

HEMOGLOBIN C

Hb C was the next hemoglobinopathy after Hb S to be described. In the United States it is found almost exclusively in individuals of African ancestry. Spaet and Ranney reported this disease in the homozygous state (Hb CC) in 1953.[9]

Prevalence, Etiology, and Pathophysiology

Globally, Hb C is found in 17% to 28% of people of West African ancestry, and in the United States it is found in 2% to 3% of individuals of African ancestry.[70] It is the most common non-sickling variant encountered in the United States and the third most common in the world.[4] Hb C is defined by the structural formula $\alpha_2\beta_2^{6Glu \rightarrow Lys}$, in which lysine replaces glutamic acid in position 6 of the β chain. Lysine has a +1 charge and glutamic acid has a −1 charge, so the result of this substitution is a net change in charge of +2. The amino acid substitution confers a different structural effect on the hemoglobin molecule, and the change on charge alters (slows) the electrophoresis mobility pattern compared with the Hb S substitution.

Similar to Hb S, Hb C forms polymers intracellularly. In contrast to Hb S polymers, which are long and thin, Hb C polymers form a short, thick crystal within the RBCs. The conditions under which crystals form differ in that Hb C crystals form under high oxygen tension. As a result of electrostatic interactions between the positively charged B6-lysyl side chain and the negatively charged adjacent groups, Hb C is less soluble than Hb A in RBCs and crystallizes in the oxygenated state. Band 3 within the RBC membrane serves as a nucleation center for Hb C crystal formation.[71] The shorter Hb C crystal does not alter RBC shape to the extent that Hb S does, so there is less splenic sequestration and hemolysis.

Clinical Features

Homozygous hemoglobin C disease (Hb CC) usually manifests as a mild to moderate anemia. Mild splenomegaly and hemolysis may be present. In addition, VOCs do not occur. Heterozygous hemoglobin C trait (Hb AC) is asymptomatic.

Laboratory Diagnosis

A mild to moderate, normochromic normocytic anemia occurs in homozygous Hb C disease. Occasionally, some microcytosis and mild hypochromia may be present. There is a marked increase in the number of target cells and a slight to moderate increase in the number of reticulocytes (2% to 3%). Nucleated RBCs may be present in peripheral blood.

Hexagonal crystals of Hb C form within RBCs and may be seen on the peripheral blood film (Figure 24.11). Many crystals appear extracellularly, with no evidence of a cell membrane. In some cells, hemoglobin is concentrated within the boundary of the crystal. Crystals are densely stained and vary in size and appear oblong, with pyramid-shaped or pointed ends. These crystals may be seen on wet preparations by washing RBCs and resuspending them in a solution of sodium citrate or hypertonic saline.[13,71]

Hb C yields a negative result on the hemoglobin solubility test, and definitive diagnosis is made using electrophoresis,

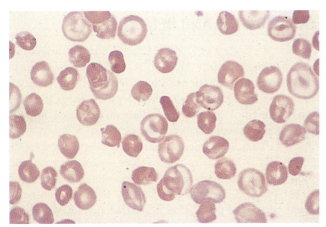

Figure 24.11 Peripheral Blood Film of a Patient With Hemoglobin (Hb) C Disease. Note one Hb C crystal and target and folded cells. (Wright-Giemsa stain, ×1000.) (Courtesy Ann Bell, University of Tennessee, Memphis.)

HPLC, or nucleic acid testing. No Hb A is present in Hb CC disease, but Hb C is present at levels of greater than 90%, with Hb F at less than 7% and Hb A_2 at approximately 2%. In Hb AC trait, about 60% Hb A is present and 30% Hb C is present. On alkaline hemoglobin electrophoresis Hb C migrates in the same position as Hb A_2, Hb E, and Hb O-Arab (see Figure 24.7). Hb C is separated from these comigrating hemoglobins on citrate agar electrophoresis at an acid pH (see Figure 24.7).

Treatment and Prognosis

No specific treatment is required. This disorder becomes problematic only if infection occurs, if splenomegaly becomes painful, or if mild chronic hemolysis leads to gallbladder disease. Genetic counseling is recommended because Hb C in combination with Hb S results in SCD and can have severe symptoms similar to Hb SS.

HEMOGLOBIN C-HARLEM (HEMOGLOBIN C-GEORGETOWN)

Hb C-Harlem (Hb C-Georgetown) has a double substitution on the β chain.[5] The substitution of valine for glutamic acid at position 6 of the β chain is identical to the Hb S substitution, and the substitution at position 73 of aspartic acid for asparagine is the same as the Hb Korle Bu mutation. The double mutation is termed *Hb C-Harlem (Hb C-Georgetown)* because the abnormal hemoglobin migrates with Hb C on alkaline hemoglobin electrophoresis. Patients heterozygous for this anomaly are asymptomatic, but patients with compound heterozygosity for Hb S and Hb C-Harlem have crises similar to those with Hb SS disease.[72]

A positive solubility test result may occur with Hb C-Harlem, and hemoglobin electrophoresis or HPLC is necessary to confirm the diagnosis. On alkaline hemoglobin electrophoresis, Hb C-Harlem migrates in the C position (see Figure 24.7). Citrate agar electrophoresis at pH 6.2, however, shows migration of Hb C-Harlem in the S position (see Figure 24.7). Because so few cases have been identified, the clinical outcome for homozygous

individuals affected with this abnormality is uncertain,[72] but heterozygotes appear normal.

HEMOGLOBIN E

Prevalence, Etiology, and Pathophysiology

Hb E was first described in 1954.[73] The variant has a prevalence of 30% in Southeast Asia and can reach rates of 50% in border areas of Cambodia, Laos, and Thailand. Hb E has also been found in Bangladesh, India, and Madagascar.[9] As a result of the influx of immigrants from these areas, Hb E prevalence has increased in the United States. It occurs infrequently in individuals of African and European ancestry. Hb E is a β chain variant in which lysine is substituted for glutamic acid in position 26 ($\alpha_2\beta_2^{26Glu\rightarrow Lys}$). As with Hb C, this substitution results in a net change in charge of +2, but because of the position of the substitution, hemoglobin polymerization does not occur. However, the amino acid substitution at codon 26 inserts a cryptic splice site at the junction of exon 1 and intron 1 that causes abnormal alterative splicing and decreased transcription of functional messenger RNA for the Hb E globin chain.[74,75] Reduced Hb E synthesis explains Hb E levels in heterozygotes of 25% to 30%.[8] Thus the Hb E mutation is both a qualitative defect (because of the amino acid substitution in the globin chain) and a quantitative defect with a β-thalassemia phenotype (because of decreased production of the mutated globin chain).[74] Hb E is often coinherited with α-thalassemia, β-thalassemia, or other hemoglobin variants, including Hb S forming Hb SE disease. This creates a wide range of clinical severities, with Hb E-β-thalassemia being the most severe.[9]

Clinical Features

The homozygous state (Hb EE) manifests as a mild anemia with microcytes and target cells. RBC survival time is shortened. The condition is not associated with clinically observable icterus, hemolysis, or splenomegaly. The main concern in identifying homozygous Hb EE is differentiating it from iron deficiency, β-thalassemia trait, and Hb E-β-thalassemia (Chapter 25).[74] Because the highest incidence of the Hb E gene is in areas of Thailand where malaria is most prevalent, it is thought that *P. falciparum* multiplies more slowly in Hb EE RBCs than in Hb AE or Hb AA RBCs and that the mutation may give some protection against malaria.[75] Hb E trait is asymptomatic. However, Hb E-β[0]-thal results in symptoms more severe than Hb EE and more closely resembles the severity β-thalassemia major, requiring regular blood transfusions.

Laboratory Diagnosis

Hb E does not produce a positive hemoglobin solubility test result and must be confirmed using electrophoresis or HPLC. In the homozygous state there is greater than 90% Hb E, mild anemia (hemoglobin 11.0 to 13.0 g/dL), a very low MCV (55 to 65 fL), few to many target cells, and a normal reticulocyte count. The heterozygous state has normal hemoglobin levels, a mean MCV of 65 fL, slight erythrocytosis, target cells (Figure 24.12), and approximately 25% to 30% Hb E. Patients with Hb E-β⁺-thal have anemia that varies in severity (hemoglobin 6.5 to 9.5

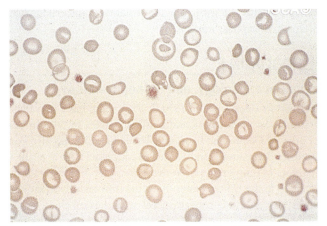

Figure 24.12 Peripheral Blood Film of a Patient With Hemoglobin E Trait. Note the microcytes and target cells. (Wright-Giemsa stain, ×1000.) (From Hematology Tech Sample H-1. [1991]. American Society of Clinical Pathologists, Chicago, IL.)

g/dL), depending on the β-thalassemia mutation, and patients with Hb E-β⁰-thal have an even more severe anemia, depending on the degree of Hb F compensation.[9] On alkaline hemoglobin electrophoresis, Hb E migrates with Hb C, Hb O, and Hb A_2 (see Figure 24.7). On citrate agar electrophoresis at an acid pH, Hb E can be separated from Hb C, but it comigrates with Hb A and Hb O (see Figure 24.7).

Treatment and Prognosis

No therapy is required with Hb E disease and trait. Some patients may experience splenomegaly and fatigue, however. Genetic counseling is recommended, and the Hb E gene mutation should be discussed in the same manner as a mild β-thalassemia allele. Patients with Hb E-β⁰-thal are given the same treatment as patients with β-thalassemia major, including chronic transfusion therapy, iron chelation therapy, splenectomy with hypersplenism, and hydroxyurea in severe cases.[9,74]

HEMOGLOBIN O-ARAB

Hb O-Arab is a β chain variant caused by the substitution of lysine for glutamic acid at amino acid position 121 ($\alpha_2\beta_2^{121Glu\rightarrow Lys}$).[5,23] It is a rare disorder found in Kenya, Israel, Egypt, and Bulgaria. In the United States, it is found in 0.4% of individuals of African ancestry.[23] No clinical symptoms are exhibited by individuals who carry this variant, except for mild splenomegaly in homozygotes. When Hb O-Arab is inherited with Hb S, however, severe clinical symptoms similar to those in Hb SS result.[5]

Homozygous individuals have mild hemolytic anemia, with many target cells on the peripheral blood film and a negative result on the hemoglobin solubility test. The presence of this hemoglobin variant must be confirmed using electrophoresis or HPLC. Because Hb O-Arab migrates with Hb A_2, Hb C, and Hb E on alkaline hemoglobin electrophoresis, citrate agar electrophoresis at an acid pH is required to differentiate it from Hb C (see Figure 24.7). Hb O-Arab is the only hemoglobin to move just slightly away from the point of application toward the cathode on citrate agar at an acid pH. No treatment is generally necessary for individuals with Hb O-Arab.

HEMOGLOBIN D AND HEMOGLOBIN G

Hb D and Hb G are a group of at least 16 β chain variants (Hb D) and 6 α chain variants (Hb G) that migrate in an alkaline pH at the same electrophoretic position as Hb S.[4,9,23] This is because their α and β subunits have one fewer negative charge at an alkaline pH than Hb A, as does Hb S. They do not sickle, however, when exposed to reduced oxygen tension.

Most variants are named for the place where they were discovered. Hb D-Punjab and Hb D-Los Angeles are identical hemoglobins in which glutamine replaces glutamic acid at position 121 in the β chain ($\alpha_2\beta_2^{121Glu\rightarrow Gln}$). Hb D-Punjab occurs in about 3% of the population in northwestern India, and Hb D-Los Angeles is seen in less than 2% of individuals of African ancestry in the United States.

Hb G-Philadelphia is an α chain variant of the G hemoglobins in which lysine replaces asparagine at position 68 ($\alpha_2^{68Asn\rightarrow Lys}\beta_2$).[5] The Hb G-Philadelphia variant is the most common G variant encountered in individuals of African ancestry and is seen with greater frequency than the Hb D variants. The Hb G variant is also found in Ghana.[4,9,23]

Hb D and Hb G do not sickle and produce a negative hemoglobin solubility test result. On alkaline electrophoresis, Hb D and Hb G have the same mobility as Hb S (see Figure 24.7). Hb D and Hb G can be separated from Hb S using citrate agar at pH 6.0 (see Figure 24.7). These variants should be suspected whenever a hemoglobin band is encountered that migrates in the S position on alkaline electrophoresis and has a negative result on the hemoglobin solubility test. In the homozygous state (Hb DD), there is greater than 95% Hb D, with normal amounts of Hb A_2 and Hb F.[33] Hb DD can be confused with the compound heterozygous state for Hb D and β⁰-thalassemia. The two disorders can be differentiated based on the MCV, levels of Hb A_2, and family studies. Hb D-β⁰-thal produces a low MCV and an elevated Hb A_2, whereas both values are usually normal in Hb DD disease.[4,9,23]

Hb D and Hb G are asymptomatic in the heterozygous state. Hb D disease (Hb DD) is marked by mild hemolytic anemia and chronic nonprogressive splenomegaly. No treatment is required.[4,9,23] When Hb D is coinherited with β⁰-thalassemia, patients have mild microcytic anemia, but when inherited with Hb S, it usually produces a mild form of SCD.[9]

COMPOUND HETEROZYGOSITY WITH HEMOGLOBIN S AND ANOTHER β-GLOBIN GENE MUTATION

Compound heterozygosity is the inheritance of two different mutant genes that share a common genetic locus, in this case the β-globin gene locus.[76] Because there are two β-globin genes, these compound heterozygotes have inherited Hb S from one parent and another β chain hemoglobinopathy or thalassemia from the other parent. Compound heterozygosity of Hb S with Hb C, Hb D, Hb O, or β-thalassemia may produce hemolytic anemia of variable severity. Inheritance of Hb S with other hemoglobins, such as Hb E, Hb G-Philadelphia, and Hb Korle Bu, causes disorders of no clinical consequence.[76]

Hemoglobin SC

Hb SC is the most common compound heterozygous syndrome that results in a structural defect in the hemoglobin molecule in which different amino acid substitutions are found on each of two β-globin chains. At position 6, glutamic acid is replaced by valine (Hb S) on one β-globin chain and by lysine (Hb C) on the other β-globin chain. In the United States and United Kingdom nearly 30% of patients with SCD are compound heterozygotes for Hb SC disease. In the United States, 1 in 941 babies are born with SCD, whereas 1 in 6173 babies are born with Hb SC disease. Hb C originated in West Africa, where Hb SC disease accounts for more than 50% of cases of SCD. Nearly 55,000 children are born with Hb SC disease worldwide.[77]

Clinical Features

Hb SC disease usually results in a milder form of SCD, but it can be severe in some cases. Growth and development are delayed compared with normal children. In contrast to Hb SS, Hb SC usually does not produce significant symptoms until the teenage years. Hb SC disease may cause all the vasoocclusive complications of SCA, but episodes are less frequent and damage is less disabling. Hemolytic anemia is moderate, and many patients exhibit moderate splenomegaly. Proliferative retinopathy is more common and more severe than in SCA. Respiratory tract infections with *S. pneumoniae* are common.[9,77]

Patients with Hb SC disease live longer than patients with Hb SS and have fewer painful episodes, but this disorder is associated with considerable morbidity and mortality, especially after age 30. In the United States the median life span for men is 60 years and for women, 68 years.[27,77]

Laboratory Diagnosis

The CBC indicates a mild normocytic normochromic anemia, with many features associated with SCA. The hemoglobin level is usually 11 to 13 g/dL, and the reticulocyte count is 3% to 5%. On the peripheral blood film there are a few sickle cells, target

cells, and intraerythrocytic crystalline structures. Crystalline aggregates of hemoglobin (SC crystals) form in some cells, where they protrude from the membrane (Figure 24.13).[76] Hb SC crystals often appear as a hybrid of Hb S and Hb C crystals. They are longer than Hb C crystals but shorter and thicker than Hb S polymers and are often branched.

The hemoglobin solubility test is positive because of the presence of Hb S. Electrophoretically, Hb C and Hb S migrate in almost equal amounts (45%) on alkaline electrophoresis, and Hb F is normal. Hb C is confirmed on citrate agar at an acid pH, where it is separated from Hb E and Hb O. Hb A_2 migrates with Hb C, and its quantification is of no consequence in Hb SC disease. Determination of Hb A_2 becomes vital, however, if a patient is suspected to have Hb C concurrent with β-thalassemia (Chapter 25).

Treatment and Prognosis

Treatment similar to that for SCD is given to individuals with Hb SC disease.[77]

Hemoglobin S-β-Thalassemia

Compound heterozygosity for Hb S and β-thalassemia is the most common cause of sickle cell syndrome in patients of Mediterranean descent and is second to Hb SC disease among all compound heterozygous sickle disorders. Hb S-β-thal usually causes a clinical syndrome resembling that of mild or moderate SCA. The severity of this compound heterozygous condition depends on the β chain production of the affected β-thalassemia gene. If there is no β-globin chain production from the β-thalassemia gene (Hb S-β⁰-thal), the clinical course is similar to Hb SS. If there is production of some level of β-globin chain (Hb S-β⁺-thal), patients tend to have a milder condition than patients with Hb SC. These patients can be distinguished from individuals with SCT because of the presence of greater amounts of Hb S than of Hb A, increased levels of Hb A_2 and Hb F, microcytosis from the thalassemia, hemolytic anemia, abnormal peripheral blood morphology, and splenomegaly (Chapter 25).[23,76]

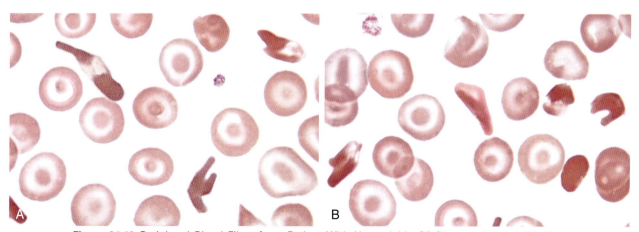

Figure 24.13 Peripheral Blood Films for a Patient With Hemoglobin SC Disease. (A) and (B), Note intraerythrocytic, blunt-ended SC crystals and target cells. (A, B, Wright-Giemsa stain, ×1000.) (Courtesy Ann Bell, University of Tennessee, Memphis.)

Hemoglobin SD and Hemoglobin SG-Philadelphia

Hb SD is a compound heterozygous sickle cell syndrome, and Hb SG-Philadelphia is a double heterozygous sickle cell syndrome.[23] Hb SG-Philadelphia is asymptomatic because Hb G is associated with an α gene mutation that still allows for sufficient Hb A to be produced. Hb SD syndrome may cause a mild to severe hemolytic anemia because both β chains are affected. Some patients with Hb SD may have severe vasoocclusive complications. Hb SD syndrome in individuals of African ancestry is usually due to the interaction of Hb S with Hb D-Los Angeles (Hb D-Punjab).

The peripheral blood film findings for Hb SD disease are comparable to those seen in less severe forms of Hb SS disease. Because Hb D and Hb G comigrate with Hb S on alkaline electrophoresis, citrate agar electrophoresis at an acid pH is necessary to separate Hb S from Hb D and Hb G. The clinical picture is valuable in differentiating Hb SD and Hb SG. The treatment for Hb SD disease is similar to treatment for patients with SCD and is administered according to the severity of the clinical condition.

Hemoglobin SO-Arab and Hb SD-Punjab

Hb SO-Arab and Hb SD-Punjab are rare compound heterozygous hemoglobinopathies that cause severe chronic hemolytic anemia with vasoocclusive episodes.[9,23] Both mutations replace glutamic acid at position 121; O-Arab substitutes lysine, and D-Punjab substitutes glutamine. Glutamic acid at position 121 is located on the outer surface of the hemoglobin tetramer, which enhances the polymerization process involving Hb S. Hb SO-Arab can be mistaken for Hb SC on alkaline electrophoresis because Hb C and Hb O-Arab migrate at the same position; however, differentiation is made on citrate agar at an acid pH because these hemoglobins do not comigrate in an acid environment. Treatment approaches are similar to what is provided to patients with SCD. Similarly, Hb D-Punjab comigrates with Hb S on alkaline electrophoresis, making this mutation look like SCA. Hb O-Arab and Hb D-Punjab are not clinically significant in either the heterozygous or the homozygous form.

Hemoglobin S-Korle Bu

Hb Korle Bu is a rare hemoglobin variant with substitution of aspartic acid for asparagine at position 73 of the β chain.[5,23] When inherited with Hb S, it interferes with lateral contact between Hb S fibers by disrupting the hydrophobic pocket for β_6 valine, which inhibits Hb S polymerization. The compound heterozygous condition Hb S-Korle Bu is asymptomatic.

CONCOMITANT CIS MUTATIONS WITH HEMOGLOBIN S

A concomitant cis mutation with Hb S involves a second mutation on the same gene along with Hb S. Three cis mutations will be described: Hb C-Harlem, Hb S-Antilles, and Hb S-Oman.

Hemoglobin C-Harlem

Hb C-Harlem has two substitutions on the β chain: the sickle mutation and the Korle Bu mutation. Patients heterozygous for only Hb C-Harlem are asymptomatic. The compound heterozygous Hb SC-Harlem state resembles Hb SS clinically. Hb C-Harlem yields a positive result on the hemoglobin solubility test and migrates to the Hb C position on alkaline electrophoresis and to the Hb S position on citrate agar electrophoresis at an acid pH.[5,23,72]

Hemoglobin S-Antilles and Hemoglobin S-Oman

Hb S-Antilles bears the Hb S mutation ($\beta^{6Glu \rightarrow Val}$), along with a substitution of isoleucine for valine at position 23.[78] Hb S-Oman also has the Hb S mutation, with a second substitution of lysine for glutamic acid at position 121.[79] In both of these hemoglobin variants, the second mutation enhances Hb S such that significant sickling can occur even in heterozygotes.[1]

Table 24.2 summarizes common clinically significant hemoglobinopathies, including general characteristics and treatment options.

HEMOGLOBIN M

Hb M is caused by a variety of mutations in the α-, β-, and γ-globin genes, all of which result in production of methemoglobin, hence the Hb M designation.[80] These genetic mutations result in a structural abnormality in the globin portion of the molecule. Most M hemoglobins involve a substitution of a tyrosine amino acid for either the proximal (F_8) or the distal (E_7) histidine amino acid in the α, β, or γ chains. These substitutions cause heme iron to autooxidize, which results in methemoglobinemia. Hb M has iron in the ferric state (Fe^{3+}) and is unable to carry oxygen, which produces cyanosis. Seven hemoglobin variants affecting the α or β chains have been classified as M hemoglobins: Hb M-Boston, Hb M-Iwate, Hb Auckland (α chain variants), Hb Chile, Hb M-Saskatoon, Hb M-Milwaukee-1, and Hb M-Milwaukee-2 (β chain variants), all named for the locations in which they were discovered. Two variants affect the γ chain, namely Hb F-M-Osaka and Hb F-M-Fort Ripley, but symptoms disappear when Hb A replaces Hb F at age 3 to 6 months.[5]

Hb M variants have altered oxygen affinity and are inherited as autosomal dominant disorders. Affected individuals have 30% to 50% methemoglobin (healthy individuals have less than 1%) and may appear cyanotic. Ingestion of oxidant drugs, such as sulfonamides, can increase methemoglobin to life-threatening levels. Methemoglobin causes the blood specimen to appear brown. Heinz bodies may be seen sometimes on wet preparations because methemoglobin causes globin chains to precipitate (Figure 12.12). Diagnosis is made by spectral absorption of the hemolysate or by hemoglobin electrophoresis. Absorption spectrum peaks are determined at various wavelengths. The unique absorption range of each Hb M variant is identified when these are compared with the spectrum of normal blood.

Before electrophoresis, all hemoglobin types are converted to methemoglobin by adding potassium cyanide to the specimen so that any migration differences observed are only the result of an amino acid substitution, not differences in iron states. On alkaline electrophoresis, Hb M migrates slightly more slowly than Hb A. The electrophoresis should be performed on agar

TABLE 24.2 Common Clinically Significant Hemoglobinopathies

Hemoglobin Disorder	Abnormal Hemoglobin	Structural Defect	Groups Primarily Affected	Hemoglobin Solubility Test Results	Hemoglobins Present	RBC Morphology	Symptoms/Organ Defects	Treatment
Sickle cell anemia (homozygous)	Hb S	$\alpha_2\beta_2^{6Glu\rightarrow Val}$	Ancestry from Africa, Middle East, India, and Mediterranean countries	Positive	0% Hb A, >80% Hb S, 1%–20% Hb F, 2%–5% Hb A$_2$	Sickle cells, target cells, nucleated RBCs, polychromasia, Howell-Jolly bodies, basophilic stippling	Vasoocclusion, bacterial infections, hemolytic anemia, aplastic episodes; affects bones, lungs, liver, spleen, penis, eyes, central nervous system, urinary tract	Transfusions, antibiotics, analgesics, bone marrow transplant, hydroxyurea
Hb C disease (homozygous)	Hb C	$\alpha_2\beta_2^{6Glu\rightarrow Lys}$	Ancestry from Africa	Negative	0% Hb A, >90% Hb C, <7% Hb F, 2% Hb A$_2$	Hb C crystals, target cells, nucleated RBCs, occasionally some microcytes	Mild splenomegaly, mild hemolysis	Usually none, antibiotics
Hb SC-Harlem* (Hb C-Georgetown)	Hb C-Harlem, Hb S	$\alpha_2\beta_2^{6Glu\rightarrow Val}$ and $\alpha_2\beta_2^{73Asp\rightarrow Asn}$ on same gene and $\alpha_2\beta_2^{6Glu\rightarrow Val}$	Rare, so uncertain; ancestry from Africa	Positive	Hb C-Harlem migrates with Hb C at alkaline pH; migrates with Hb S at acid pH	Target cells	Compound heterozygotes with Hb SC-Harlem have symptoms similar to Hb SS	Similar to Hb SS
Hb E disease (homozygous)	Hb E	$\alpha_2\beta_2^{26Glu\rightarrow Lys}$	Ancestry from Southeast Asia and Africa	Negative	0% Hb A, 95% Hb E, 2%–4% Hb A$_2$; migrates with Hb A$_2$, Hb C, and Hb O at alkaline pH	Target cells, microcytes	Mild anemia, mild splenomegaly, no symptoms	Usually none
Hb O-Arab (homozygous)	Hb O-Arab	$\alpha_2\beta_2^{121Glu\rightarrow Lys}$	Ancestry from Kenya, Israel, Egypt, Bulgaria, and Africa	Negative	0% Hb A, 95% Hb O, 2%–4% Hb A$_2$; migrates with Hb A$_2$, Hb C, and Hb E at alkaline pH	Target cells	Mild splenomegaly	Usually none
Hb D disease (rare homozygous)	Hb D-Punjab (Hb-D Los Angeles)	$\alpha_2\beta_2^{121Glu\rightarrow Gln}$	Ancestry from Middle East and India	Negative	95% Hb D, normal Hb A$_2$ and Hb F; migrates with Hb S at alkaline pH	Target cells	Mild hemolytic anemia, mild splenomegaly	Usually none
Hb G disease (rare homozygous)	Hb G, Hb G-Philadelphia	$\alpha_2\beta_2^{68Asn\rightarrow Lys}\beta_2$	Ancestry from Ghana and Africa	Negative	95% Hb G, normal Hb A$_2$ and Hb F; migrates with Hb S at alkaline pH	Target cells	Mild hemolytic anemia, mild splenomegaly	Usually none
Hb SC* disease	Hb S, Hb C	$\alpha_2\beta_2^{6Glu\rightarrow Val}$ and $\alpha_2\beta_2^{6Glu\rightarrow Lys}$	Same as Hb S	Positive	45% Hb S, 45% Hb C, 2%–4% Hb A$_2$, 1% Hb F	Sickle cells, Hb SC crystals, target cells	Same as those for Hb SS but milder	Similar to that for Hb SS but less intensive
Hb S-β-thalassemia*	Hb S + β-thalassemia mutation	$\alpha_2\beta_2^{6Glu\rightarrow Val}$ and β^0 or β^+	Same as Hb S	Positive	Hb S variable, some Hb A in β^+, increased Hb A$_2$ and Hb F	Sickle cells, target cells, microcytes	Hemolytic anemia, splenomegaly	Similar to that for Hb SS; varies depending on amount of Hb A present
Hb SD* disease	Hb S, Hb D	$\alpha_2\beta_2^{6Glu\rightarrow Val}$ and $\alpha_2\beta_2^{121Glu\rightarrow Gln}$	Same as Hb S	Positive	45% Hb S, 45% Hb D, 2%–4% Hb A$_2$, 1% Hb F; Hb S and Hb D comigrate at alkaline pH	Sickle cells, target cells	Similar to those for Hb SS but milder	Similar to that for Hb SS
Hb SG†	Hb S, Hb G	$\alpha_2\beta_2^{6Glu\rightarrow Val}$ and $\alpha_2\beta_2^{68Asn\rightarrow Lys}\beta_2$	Same as Hb S	Positive	45% Hb S, 45% Hb G, 2%–4% Hb A$_2$, 1% Hb F; Hb S and Hb G comigrate at alkaline pH	Target cells	No symptoms	Usually none
Hb SO-Arab*	Hb S, Hb O-Arab	$\alpha_2\beta_2^{6Glu\rightarrow Val}$ and $\alpha_2\beta_2^{121Glu\rightarrow Lys}$	Same as Hb S	Positive	45% Hb S, 45% Hb O, 2%–4% Hb A$_2$, 1% Hb F	Sickle cells, target cells	Similar to those for Hb SS	Similar to that for Hb SS

*Compound heterozygous.
†Double heterozygous.

Asn, Asparagine; *Asp*, aspartic acid; *Gln*, glutamine; *Glu*, glutamic acid; *Hb*, hemoglobin; *Lys*, lysine; *RBC*, red blood cell; *Val*, valine.

gel at pH 7.1 for clear separation. Further confirmation may be obtained using HPLC or DNA-based globin gene analysis. No treatment is necessary. Diagnosis is essential to prevent inappropriate treatment for other conditions, such as cyanotic heart disease.

UNSTABLE HEMOGLOBIN VARIANTS

Unstable hemoglobin variants result from genetic mutations to globin genes creating hemoglobin products that precipitate in vivo, producing Heinz bodies and causing a hemolytic anemia.[80,81] More than 185 variants of unstable hemoglobin exist.[5] The majority of these are β chain variants, and most others are α chain variants. Only a few are γ and δ chain variants. Most unstable hemoglobin variants have no clinical significance, although the majority have increased oxygen affinity. About 25% of unstable hemoglobins are responsible for hemolytic anemia, which varies from compensated mild anemia to severe hemolytic episodes.[80,81]

At one time the anemia was referred to as *congenital non-spherocytic hemolytic anemia* or *congenital Heinz body anemia*. This disorder is more properly called *unstable hemoglobin disease*. The syndrome appears at or just after birth, depending on the globin chains involved. It is inherited in an autosomal dominant pattern. All patients are heterozygous; apparently, the homozygous condition is incompatible with life. The instability of the hemoglobin molecule may be due to (1) substitution of a charged for an uncharged amino acid in the interior of the molecule, (2) substitution of a polar for a nonpolar amino acid in the hydrophobic heme pocket, (3) substitution of an amino acid in the α and β chains at the intersubunit contact points, (4) replacement of an amino acid with proline in the α helix section of a chain, or (5) deletion or elongation of the primary structure.[80,81]

Clinical Features

Unstable hemoglobin disorder is usually detected in early childhood in patients with hemolytic anemia accompanied by jaundice and splenomegaly. Fever or ingestion of an oxidant exacerbates the hemolysis. The severity of the anemia depends on the degree of instability of the hemoglobin molecule. Unstable hemoglobin precipitates in vivo and in vitro in response to factors that do not affect normal hemoglobins, such as drug ingestion and exposure to heat or cold. Hemoglobin precipitates in RBCs as Heinz bodies. Precipitated hemoglobin attaches to the inner cell membrane, causing clustering of band 3, attachment of autologous immunoglobulin, and macrophage activation. In addition, Heinz bodies can be trapped mechanically in the splenic sieve, which shortens RBC survival. Oxygen affinity of these cells is also abnormal.[80,81]

The most prevalent unstable hemoglobin is Hb Köln. Other unstable hemoglobins include Hb Hammersmith, Hb Zurich, and Hb Gun Hill.[5] Because of the large variability in the degree of instability in these hemoglobins, the extent of hemolysis varies greatly. For some of the variants, such as Hb Zurich, the presence of an oxidant is required for any significant hemolysis to occur.[80,81]

Laboratory Diagnosis

RBC morphology varies. It may be normal or show slight hypochromia and prominent basophilic stippling, which possibly is caused by excessive clumping of ribosomes. Before splenectomy, hemoglobin levels range from 7 to 12 g/dL, with a 4% to 20% reticulocyte count. After splenectomy, anemia is corrected, but reticulocytosis persists. Heinz bodies can be shown using a supravital stain (Figure 12.12). After splenectomy, Heinz bodies are larger and more numerous. Many patients excrete dark urine that contains dipyrrole.[80,81]

Many unstable hemoglobins migrate in the normal AA pattern and thus are not detected on electrophoresis. Other tests used to detect unstable hemoglobins include the isopropanol precipitation test, which is based on the principle that an isopropanol solution at 37°C weakens the bonding forces of the hemoglobin molecule. If unstable hemoglobins are present, rapid precipitation occurs in 5 minutes, and heavy flocculation occurs after 20 minutes. Normal hemoglobin does not begin to precipitate until after approximately 40 minutes. The heat denaturation test also can be used. When incubated at 50°C for 1 hour, heat-sensitive unstable hemoglobins show a flocculent precipitation, whereas normal hemoglobin shows little or no precipitation. Significant numbers of Heinz bodies appear after splenectomy, but even in individuals with intact spleens, with longer incubation and the addition of an oxidative substance such as acetylphenylhydrazine, unstable hemoglobins form more Heinz bodies than the blood from individuals with normal hemoglobins. Other techniques, such as IEF, can resolve many hemoglobin variants with only a slight alteration in their isoelectric point, and globin chain analysis can be performed by HPLC or DNA-based globin gene analysis.[80,81]

Treatment and Prognosis

Patients are treated to prevent hemolytic crises. In severe cases, the spleen must be removed to reduce sequestration and rate of removal of RBCs. Because unstable hemoglobin disease is rare, prognosis in the affected individuals is unclear. Patients are cautioned against the use of sulfonamides and other oxidant drugs. They also should be informed of the potential for febrile illnesses to trigger a hemolytic episode.[80,81]

HEMOGLOBINS WITH INCREASED AND DECREASED OXYGEN AFFINITY

More than 380 hemoglobin variants have been discovered to have abnormal oxygen affinity. Most are high-affinity variants and have been associated with familial erythrocytosis. The remaining hemoglobin variants are characterized by low oxygen affinity. Many of these are associated with mild to moderate anemia.[2]

As described in Chapter 8, normal Hb A undergoes a series of allosteric conformational changes as it converts from a fully deoxygenated to a fully oxygenated form. These conformational changes affect hemoglobin function and its affinity for oxygen. When normal hemoglobin is fully deoxygenated (tense state), it has low affinity for oxygen and other heme ligands and high affinity for allosteric effectors, such as Bohr protons and 2,3-bisphosphoglycerate. In the oxygenated (relaxed) state, hemoglobin has a high affinity for heme ligands, such as oxygen, and a low affinity for Bohr protons and 2,3-bisphosphoglycerate. The transition from the tense to the relaxed state involves a series of structural changes that have a marked effect on hemoglobin function. If an amino acid substitution lowers the stability of the tense structure, transition to the relaxed state occurs at an earlier stage in oxygen binding, and hemoglobin has increased oxygen affinity and decreased heme-heme interaction or cooperativity (Chapter 8). One example of a β chain variant is Hb Kempsey. This unstable hemoglobin variant has amino acid substitutions at sites crucial to hemoglobin function.[80,81]

Hemoglobins With Increased Oxygen Affinity

The high-affinity variants, similar to other structurally abnormal hemoglobins, show an autosomal dominant pattern of inheritance. Affected individuals have equal volumes of Hb A and the abnormal variant. Exceptions to this are compound heterozygotes for Hb Abruzzo and β-thalassemia and for Hb Crete and β-thalassemia, in which the proportion of abnormal hemoglobin is greater than 85%.[80,81]

More than 200 variant hemoglobins with high oxygen affinity have been discovered.[5] Such hemoglobins fail to release oxygen on demand, and hypoxia results. Kidneys sense the hypoxia and respond by increasing the release of erythropoietin, which leads to a compensatory erythrocytosis. These variants differ from unstable hemoglobin, which also may have abnormal oxygen affinity, in that they do not precipitate in vivo to produce hemolysis and there is no abnormal RBC morphology.[80,81]

Most individuals are asymptomatic and have no physical symptoms except a ruddy complexion. Erythrocytosis is usually detected during routine examination because the patient generally has a high RBC count, hemoglobin, and hematocrit. The WBC count, platelet count, and peripheral blood film findings are generally normal. In some cases, hemoglobin electrophoresis may establish a diagnosis. An abnormal band that separates from the A band is present on alkaline electrophoresis in some variants; however, if a band is not found, the diagnosis of increased oxygen affinity cannot be ruled out. In some cases the abnormal hemoglobin can be separated using citrate agar electrophoresis (pH 6.0). Measurement of oxygen affinity is required for definitive diagnosis.[80,81]

Patients with hemoglobins with high oxygen affinity live normal lives and require no treatment. Diagnosis should be made to avoid unnecessary treatment of the erythrocytosis as a myeloproliferative neoplasm or a secondary erythrocytosis.[80,81]

Hemoglobins With Decreased Oxygen Affinity

Hemoglobins with decreased oxygen affinity quickly release oxygen to the tissues, which results in normal to decreased hemoglobin concentration, slight anemia, and cyanosis. More than 170 variant hemoglobins with low oxygen affinity have been discovered.[5] The best known of these hemoglobins is Hb Kansas, which has an amino acid substitution of asparagine by threonine at position 102 of the β chain. These hemoglobins may be present when cyanosis and a normal arterial oxygen tension coexist, and most may be detected by starch gel electrophoresis, HPLC, or DNA-based globin gene analysis.[80,81]

GLOBAL BURDEN OF HEMOGLOBINOPATHIES

The prevalence of hemoglobinopathies has already been discussed in this chapter, and the bulk of these conditions occur in developing nations. However, as developing countries work to decrease deaths from malnutrition, infectious diseases, and other conditions, more patients with hemoglobinopathies will survive and remain consumers of the health care system. For example, in 1944 thalassemia was first identified in Cyprus. However, during the post-World War II recovery period, as the death rate decreased, the prevalence of thalassemias increased. In 1970 it was estimated that in the absence of systems to control the disease, within 40 years, 78,000 units of blood would be needed each year, requiring that 40% of the population serve as donors. If left unchecked, the cost to maintain thalassemia therapy would exceed the country's total health care budget. In contrast, efforts to develop prenatal screening and genetic counseling programs have reduced the birth rate of SCD.[2] Hemoglobinopathies are a worldwide problem, requiring planning, investment, and interventions from around the globe to optimize the impact on patients with the disease without debilitating the health care systems of developing countries where the disease is prevalent.[2]

SUMMARY

- Hemoglobinopathies are genetic disorders of globin genes that produce structurally abnormal hemoglobins with altered amino acid sequences, which can affect hemoglobin function and stability.
- Hemoglobin (Hb) S is the most common hemoglobinopathy, resulting from a substitution of valine for glutamic acid at position 6 of the β-globin chain, and primarily affects people of African descent.
- Hb S polymerizes in red blood cells (RBCs) because of abnormal interaction with adjacent tetramers when it is in the deoxygenated form, producing sickle-shaped RBCs.
- In homozygous Hb SS, polymerization of hemoglobin may result in severe episodic conditions; however, factors other

- than hemoglobin polymerization may account for vasoocclusive episodes in sickle cell patients.
- The most clinically significant hemoglobinopathies are Hb SS, Hb SC, and Hb S-β-thalassemia; Hb SS causes the most severe disease.
- Individuals with sickle cell trait (Hb AS) are clinically asymptomatic but can manifest symptoms under extreme exertion.
- Sickle cell anemia (Hb SS) is a normocytic normochromic anemia, characterized by a single band in the S position on hemoglobin electrophoresis, a single Hb S peak on high-performance liquid chromatography (HPLC), and a positive hemoglobin solubility test. The median life expectancy of patients with sickle cell disease is greater than 50 years.

- Hb C and Hb E are the next most common hemoglobinopathies after Hb S and cause mild hemolysis in the homozygous state. In the heterozygous states, these hemoglobinopathies are asymptomatic.
- Hb C is found primarily in people of African descent.
- On peripheral blood films from patients with Hb CC, hexagonal crystals may be seen with and without apparent RBC membrane surrounding them.
- Hb EE results in a microcytic anemia and is found primarily in people of Southeast Asian descent.
- Other variants, such as unstable hemoglobins and hemoglobins with altered oxygen affinity, can be identified, and many cause no clinical abnormality.

- Laboratory procedures employed for diagnosis of hemoglobinopathies are complete blood count, peripheral blood film evaluation, reticulocyte count, hemoglobin solubility test, and methods to quantify normal and variant hemoglobins, including hemoglobin electrophoresis (alkaline and acid pH), HPLC, and capillary electrophoresis.
- Advanced techniques available for hemoglobin identification include isoelectric focusing and DNA-based analysis of the globin genes.

Now that you have completed this chapter, go back and read again the case study at the beginning and respond to the questions presented. Answers can be found in Appendix C.

REVIEW QUESTIONS

Answers can be found in Appendix C.

1. A qualitative abnormality in hemoglobin may involve all of the following EXCEPT:
   a. Replacement of one or more amino acids in a globin chain
   b. Addition of one or more amino acids in a globin chain
   c. Deletion of one or more amino acids in a globin chain
   d. Decreased production of a globin chain

2. The substitution of valine for glutamic acid at position 6 of the β chain of hemoglobin results in hemoglobin that:
   a. Is unstable and precipitates as Heinz bodies
   b. Polymerizes to form tactoid crystals
   c. Crystallizes in a hexagonal shape
   d. Contains iron in the ferric (Fe^{3+}) state

3. Patients with SCD usually do not exhibit symptoms until 6 months of age because:
   a. The mother's blood has a protective effect
   b. Hemoglobin levels are higher in infants at birth
   c. Higher levels of Hb F are present
   d. The immune system is not fully developed

4. Megaloblastic episodes in SCD can be prevented by prophylactic administration of:
   a. Iron
   b. Folic acid
   c. Steroids
   d. Erythropoietin

5. Which of the following is the most definitive test for Hb S?
   a. Hemoglobin solubility test
   b. Hemoglobin electrophoresis at alkaline pH
   c. Osmotic fragility test
   d. Hemoglobin electrophoresis at acid pH

6. A patient presents with mild normochromic normocytic anemia. On the peripheral blood film, there are a few target cells, rare nucleated RBCs, and hexagonal crystals within and lying outside of the RBCs. Which abnormality in the hemoglobin molecule is most likely?
   a. Decreased production of β chains
   b. Substitution of lysine for glutamic acid at position 6 of the β chain
   c. Substitution of tyrosine for the proximal histidine in the β chain
   d. Double amino acid substitution in the β chain

7. A well-mixed specimen obtained for a CBC has a brown color. The patient is being treated with a sulfonamide for a bladder infection. Which of the following could explain the brown color?
   a. The patient has Hb M.
   b. The patient is a compound heterozygote for Hb S and thalassemia.
   c. The incorrect anticoagulant was used.
   d. Levels of Hb F are high.

8. Through routine screening, prospective parents discover that they are both heterozygous for Hb S. What percentage of their children potentially could have sickle cell anemia (Hb SS)?
   a. 0%
   b. 25%
   c. 50%
   d. 100%

9. Painful crises in patients with SCD occur as a result of:
   a. Splenic sequestration
   b. Aplasia
   c. Vasoocclusion
   d. Anemia

10. The screening test for Hb S that uses a reducing agent, such as sodium dithionite, is based on the fact that hemoglobins that sickle:
    a. Are insoluble in reduced, deoxygenated form
    b. Form methemoglobin more readily and cause a color change
    c. Are unstable and precipitate as Heinz bodies
    d. Oxidize quickly and cause turbidity

11. DNA analysis documents a patient has inherited the sickle mutation in both β-globin genes. The two terms that best describe this genotype are:
    a. Homozygous/trait
    b. Homozygous/disease
    c. Heterozygous/trait
    d. Heterozygous/disease

12. In which of the following geographic areas is Hb S most prevalent?
    a. India
    b. South Africa
    c. United States
    d. Sub-Saharan Africa

13. Which hemoglobinopathy is more common in individuals of Southeast Asian descent?
    a. Hb S
    b. Hb C
    c. Hb O
    d. Hb E

14. Which of the following Hb S compound heterozygotes exhibits the mildest symptoms?
    a. Hb S-β-thalassemia
    b. Hb SG
    c. Hb SC-Harlem
    d. Hb SC

15. Unstable hemoglobins exhibit all of the following findings EXCEPT:
    a. Globin chains that precipitate intracellularly
    b. Heinz body formation
    c. Elevated reticulocyte count
    d. Only homozygotes are symptomatic

16. A 1-year-old patient of Indian ancestry presents with anemia, and both parents claim to have an "inherited anemia" but can't remember the type. The peripheral blood shows target cells, and the hemoglobin solubility is negative. Alkaline hemoglobin electrophoresis shows a single band at the "Hb C" position and a small band at the "Hb F" position. Acid hemoglobin electrophoresis shows two bands. The most likely diagnosis is:
    a. Hb CC
    b. Hb AC
    c. Hb CO
    d. Hb SC

REFERENCES

1. Halim-Fikri, B. H., Lederer, C. W., Baig, A. A., et al. (2022). Global globin network consensus paper: classification and stratified roadmaps for improved thalassemia care and prevention in 32 countries. *J Pers Med, 12,* 552. https://doi.org/10.3390/jpm12040552.

2. Weatherall, D. J. (2011). The challenges of haemoglobinopathies in resource-poor countries. *Br J Haematol, 154,* 736–744.

3. Mukherjee, M., Rahaman, M., Ray, S. K., et al. (2021). Revisiting fetal hemoglobin inducers in beta-hemoglobinopathies: a review of natural products, conventional and combinatorial therapies. *Mol Bio Rep, 49,* 2359–2373.

4. Li, X., Chen, M., Liu, B., et al. (2021). Transcriptional silencing of fetal hemoglobin expression by NonO. *Nucleic Acids Res, 49*(17), 9711–9723.

5. Patrinos, G. P., Giardine, B., Riemer, C., et al. (2004). Improvements in the HbVar database of human hemoglobin variants and thalassemia mutations for population and sequence variation studies. *Nucl Acids Res, 32*(database issue), D537–541. http://globin.cse.psu.edu/hbvar/menu.html. Accessed August 28, 2022.

6. Fishleder, A. J., & Hoffman, G. C. (1987). A practical approach to the detection of hemoglobinopathies. Part II: the sickle cell disorders. *Lab Med, 18,* 441–443.

7. Fiocchi, J., Urits, I., Orhurhu, A., et al. (2020). A comprehensive review of the treatment and management of pain in sickle cell disease. *Curr Pain Headache Rep, 24,* 17.

8. Konotey-Ahulu, F. I. (1974). The sickle cell diseases. Clinical manifestations including the "sickle crisis." *Arch Intern Med, 133,* 611–619.

9. Natrajan, K., & Kutlar, A. (2021). Disorders of hemoglobin structure: sickle cell anemia and related abnormalities. In Kaushansky, K., Lichtman, M. A., Prchal, J. T., et al. (Eds.), *Williams Hematology.* (10th ed., pp. 825–858). New York: McGraw-Hill.

10. Serjeant, G. R. (2001). Historical review: the emerging understanding of sickle cell disease. *Br J Haematol, 112,* 3–18.

11. Park, K. W. (2004). Sickle cell disease and other hemoglobinopathies. *Int Anesth Clin, 42,* 77–93.

12. Maron, B. J., Harris, K. M., Thompson, P. D., et al. (2015). Eligibility and disqualification recommendations for competitive athletes with cardiovascular abnormalities: Task Force 14: sickle cell trait. *Circulation, 132,* e343–e345.

13. Rees, D. C., Williams, T. N., & Gladwn, M. T. (2010). Sickle-cell disease. *Lancet, 376,* 2018–2031.

14. Brown, C., Tonda, M. & Abboud, M. R. (2022). Voxelotor for the treatment of sickle cell disease in pediatric patients. *Expert Rev Hematol, 15:*(6), 485–492.

15. Piel, F. B., Patil, A. B., Howes, R. E., et al. (2013). Global epidemiology of sickle haemoglobin in neonates: a contemporary geostatistical model-based map and population estimates. *Lancet, 381,* 142–151.

16. Noronha, S. A., Sadreameli, S. C., & Strouse, J. J. (2016). Management of sickle cell disease in children. *S Med J, 109*(9), 495–502.

17. Shah, A. (2004). Hemoglobinopathies and other congenital hemolytic anemia. *Ind J Med Sci, 58,* 490–493.

18. Wishner, B. C., Ward, K. B., Lattman, E. E., et al. (1975). Crystal structure of sickle-cell deoxyhemoglobin at 5 A resolution. *J Mol Biol, 98,* 179–194.

19. Dykes, G., Crepeau, R. H., & Edelstein, S. J. (1978). Three-dimensional reconstruction of the fibers of sickle cell haemoglobin. *Nature, 272,* 506–510.

20. Dykes, G. W., Crepeau, R. H., & Edelstein, S. J. (1979). Three-dimensional reconstruction of the 14-filament fiber of hemoglobin S. *J Mol Biol, 130,* 451–472.

21. Crepeau, R. H., Edelstein, S. J., Szalay, M., et al. (1981). Sickle cell hemoglobin fiber structure altered by alpha-chain mutation. *Proc Natl Acad Sci U S A, 78,* 1406–1410.

22. Gibbs, N. M., & Larach, D. R. (2013). Anesthetic management during cardiopulmonary bypass. In Hensley, F. A., Gravlee, G. P., & Martin, D. E. (Eds.), *A Practical Approach to Cardiac Anesthesia.* (5th ed., pp. 214–237). Philadelphia: Lippincott, Williams & Wilkins.

23. Kawthalkar, S. M. (2013). Anemias due to excessive red cell destruction. In Kawthalkar, S. M. *Essentials of Hematology.* (2nd ed., pp. 171–184). New Delhi: Jaypee Brothers Medical Publishers.

24. Kuypers, F. A., (2008) Red cell membrane lipids in hemoglobinopathies. *Curr Mol Med, 8*(7), 633–638.

25. Barber, L. A., Palascak, M. B., Joiner, C. H., et al. (2009). Aminophospholipid translocation and phospholipid scramblase activities in sickle erythrocyte subpopulations. *Br J Haematol, 146,* 447–455.

26. Hebbel, R. P., & Vercellotti, G. M. (2021). Multiple inducers of endothelial NOS (eNOS) dysfunction in sickle cell disease. *Am J Hematol, 96*, 1505–1517.

27. Benkerrou, M., Alberti, C., Couque, N., et al. (2013). Impact of glucose-6-phosphate dehydrogenase deficiency on sickle cell expression in infancy and early childhood: a prospective study. *Br J Haematol, 163*, 646–654.

28. Diggs, L. W. (1965). Sickle cell crises. *J Clin Pathol, 44*, 1–19.

29. Bartolucci, P., & Galacteros, F. (2012). Clinical management of adult sickle cell disease. *Curr Opin Hematol, 19*, 149–155.

30. Monus, T., & Howell, C. M. (2019). Current and emerging treatments for sickle cell disease. *JAAPA, 32*(9), 1–5.

31. Hagar, W., & Vichinsky, E. (2008). Advances in clinical research in sickle cell disease. *Br J Haematol, 141*, 346–356.

32. Styles, L., Wagner, C. G., Labotka, R. J., et al. (2012). Redefining the value of secretory phospholipase A2 as a predictor of acute chest syndrome in sickle cell disease: results of a feasibility study (PROACTIVE). *Br J Haematol, 157*, 627–636.

33. Howard, J. (2016). Sickle cell disease: when and how to transfuse. *Hematology Am Soc Hematol Educ Program, 2016*, 625–631.

34. Kavanagh, P. L., Fasipe, T. A., & Wun, T. (2022). Sickle cell disease: a review. *JAMA, 328* (1), 57–68.

35. Tsitsikas, D. A., Bristowe, J., & Abukar, J. (2020). Fat embolism syndrome in sickle cell disease. *J Clin Med, 9*, 3601.

36. Gangaraju, R., Reddy, V. V. B., & Marquis, M. B. (2016). Fat embolism syndrome secondary to bone marrow necrosis in patients with hemoglobinopathies. *S Med J, 19*(9), 549–553.

37. Onyekwere, O. C., Campbell, A., Teshome, M., et al. (2008). Pulmonary hypertension in children and adolescence with sickle cell disease. *Pediatr Cardiol, 29*(2), 309–312.

38. Day, T. G., Drasar, E. R., Fulford, T., et al. (2011). Association between hemolysis and albuminuria in adults with sickle cell anemia. *Haematologica, 97*, 201–205.

39. Soltani, S., Zakeri, A., Tabibzadeh, A., et al. (2020). A literature review on the parvovirus B19 infection in sickle cell anemia and b-thalassemia patients. *Trop Med Health, 48*, 96.

40. Gbotosho, O. T., Taylor, M., & Malik, P. (2021). Cardiac pathophysiology in sickle cell disease. *J Thromb Thrombolysis, 52*, 248–259.

41. Grimbly, C., Escagedo, P. D., Jaremko, J. L., et al. (2022). Sickle cell bone disease and response to intravenous bisphosphonates in children. *Osteoporos Int, 33*, 2397–2408.

42. Morganti, A. & Li, D. A. (2019). Skin ulcers complicating sickle cell disease: an interlinked reparative model. *G Chir, 40*(5), 441–444.

43. Cao, H., Antonopoulos, A., Henderson, S., et al. (2021). Red blood cell mannoses as phagocytic ligands mediating both sickle cell anaemia and malaria resistance. *Nat Commun, 12*(1). https://doi.org/10.1038/s41467-021-21814-z.

44. Arishi, W. A., Alhadrami, H. A., and Zourob M. (2021). Techniques for the detection of sickle cell disease: a review. *Micromachines, 12*, 519. https://doi.org/10.3390/mi12050519.

45. Fleur, R. S., Archer, N., Hustace, T., et al. (2018). Capacity building and networking to make newborn screening for sickle cell disease a reality in Haiti. *Blood Adv, 2*(1), 54–55.

46. Nnodu, O., Isa, H., Nwegbu, M., et al. (2019). HemoTypeSC, a low-cost point-of-care testing device for sickle cell disease: promises and challenges. *Blood Cells Mol Dis, 78*, 22–28.

47. Dexter, D., & McGann, P. T. (2021). Saving lives through early diagnosis: the promise and role of point of care testing for sickle cell disease. *Br J Haematol, 196*, 63–69.

48. Bohm, N., Toussaint, B., Sarratt, S., et al. (2018). Assessment of iron overload and chelation therapy in adult in-patients with sickle cell disease. *Int Arc Clin Pharmacol, 4*, 014. http://doi.org/10.23937/2572-3987.1510014.

49. Ashorobi, D., & Bhatt R. (2022). Bone marrow transplantation in sickle cell disease. Jul 11. In: StatPearls [Internet]. Treasure Island (FL): StatPearls Publishing; 2022 Jan.

50. Frangoul, H., Altshuler, D., Cappellini, M. D., et al. (2021). CRISPR-Cas9 gene editing for sickle cell disease and b-thalassemia. *N Engl J Med, 384*, 252–260.

51. Cottle, R. N., Lee, C. M., & Bao, G. (2016). Treating hemoglobinopathies using gene-correction approaches: promises and challenges. *Hum Genet, 135*, 993–1010.

52. Power-Hays, A. & Ware, R. E. (2020). Effective use of hydroxyurea for sickle cell anemia in low-resource countries. *Curr Opin Hematol, 27*, 172–180.

53. Steinberg, M. H., Chui, D. H. K., Dover, G. J., et al. (2014). Fetal hemoglobin in sickle cell anemia: a glass half full? *Blood, 123*(4), 481–485.

54. Zaidi, A. U., Estepp, J., Shah, N., et al. (2021). A reanalysis of pain crises data from the pivotal L-glutamine in sickle cell disease trial. *Contemp Clin Trials, 110*, 106546. https://doi.org/10.1016/j.cct.2021.106546.

55. Jafri, F., Seong, G., Jang, T., et al. (2022). L-glutamine for sickle cell disease: more than reducing redox. *Ann Hematol, 101*, 1645–1654.

56. Kato, G. J. (2016). New insights into sickle cell disease: mechanisms and investigational therapies. *Curr Opin Hematol, 23*, 224–232.

57. Karki, N. R., Saunders, K., & Kutlar, A. (2022). A critical evaluation of crizanlizumab for the treatment of sickle cell disease. *Expert rev Hematol, 15*, 5–13.

58. Ataga, K. I., Kutlar, A., Kantr, J., et al. (2017). Crizanlizumab for the prevention of pain crisis in sickle cell disease. *N Eng J Med, 376*, 429–439.

59. Dampler, C. D., Telen, M. J., Wun, T., et al. (2020). Early initiation of treatment with Rivipansel for acute vaso-occlusive crisis in sickle cell disease (SCD) achieves earlier discontinuation of IV opioids and shorter hospital stay: reset clinical trial analysis. *Blood, 136*(1), 18–19.

60. Howard, J., Ataga, K., Brown, R. C., et al. (2021). Voxelotor in adolescents and adults with sickle cell disease (HOPE): long-term follow-up results of an international, randomized, double-blind, placebo-controlled, phase 3 trial. *Lancet Haematol, 8*, e323-333.

61. Oder, E., Safo, M., Abdulmalik, O., et al. (2016). New developments in anti-sickling agents: can drugs directly prevent the polymerization of sickle haemoglobin in vivo? *Br J Haematol, 175*, 24–30.

62. Park, S. H., & Bao, G. (2021). CRISPR/Cas9 gene editing for curing sickle cell disease. *Transfu Apher Sci, 60*, 103060.

63. Porteus, M. (2023). Genome editing. In Hoffman, R., Benz, E. J., Silberstein, L. E., et al. (Eds.), *Hematology: Basic Principles and Practice*. (8th ed., pp. 50–60). Philadelphia: Elsevier.

64. Luthra, R., Kaur, S., & Bhandari, K. (2021). Applications of CRISPR as a potential therapeutic. *J Life Sci 284*, 119908.

65. ClinicalTrials.gov. CRISPR-Cas9/SCD. https://clinicaltrials.gov/. Accessed January 25, 2023.

66. Lubeck, D., Agodoa, I., Bhakta, N., et al. (2019). Estimated life expectancy and income of patients with sickle cell disease compared with those without sickle cell disease. *JAMA Netw, 2*(11), e1915374.

67. El-Haj, N. & Hoppe, C. C. (2018). Newborn screening for SCD in the USA and Canada. *Int J Neonat Screen, 4*, 36.

68. Oteng-Ntim, E., Pavord, S., Howard, R., et al. (2021). Management of sickle cell disease in pregnancy: A British Society of Haematology Guideline. *Br J Haematol, 194,* 980–995.

69. Kark, J. A. & Ward, F. T. (1994). Exercise and hemoglobin S. *Semin Hematol, 31*(3), 181–225.

70. Hankins, J. S., & Wang, W. C. (2019). Sickle cell anemia and other sickling syndromes. In Greer, J. P., Arber, D. A., Glader, B., et al. (Eds.), *Wintrobe's Clinical Hematology.* (4th ed., pp. 823–865). Philadelphia: Wolters Kluwer Health/Lippincott Williams & Wilkins.

71. Hirsch, R. E., Lin, M. J., Vidugirus, G. J., et al. (1996). Conformational changes in oxyhemoglobin C (Glu beta 8 → Lys) detected by spectroscopic probing. *J Biol Chem, 271,* 372–375.

72. Steinberg, M. H. (2009). Other sickle hemoglobinopathies. In Steinberg, M. H., Forget, B. G., Higgs, D. R., et al. (Eds.), *Disorders of Hemoglobin: Genetics, Pathophysiology and Clinical Management.* (2nd ed., pp. 564–588). Cambridge: Cambridge University Press.

73. Fairbanks, V. F., Gilchrist, G. S., Brimhall, B., et al. (1979). Hemoglobin E trait reexamined: a cause of microcytosis and erythrocytosis. *Blood, 53,* 109–115.

74. Vichinsky, E. (2007). Hemoglobin E syndromes. *Hematology Am Soc Hematol Educ Program,* 2007, 79–83.

75. Jiwoo, H., Martinson, R., Iwamoto, S., et al. (2019). Hemoglobin E, malaria and natural selection. *Evol Med Public Health,* 232–241.

76. Randolph, T. R. (2008). Pathophysiology of compound heterozygotes involving hemoglobinopathies and thalassemias. *Clin Lab Sci, 21*(4), 240–248.

77. Pecker, L. H., Schaefer, B. A., & Luchtman-Jones L. (2017). Knowledge insufficient: the management of haemoglobin SC disease. *Br J Haematol, 176,* 515–526.

78. Monplaisir, N., Merault, G., Poyart, C., et al. (1986). Hemoglobin S Antilles: a variant with lower solubility than hemoglobin S and producing sickle cell disease in heterozygotes. *Proc Natl Acad Sci U S A, 83,* 9363–9367.

79. Nagel, R. L., Daar, S., Romero, J. R., et al. (1998). HbS-Oman heterozygote: a new dominant sickle cell syndrome. *Blood, 92,* 4375–4782.

80. Verhovsek, M., & Steinberg, M. (2019). Hemoglobins with altered oxygen affinity, unstable hemoglobins, M-hemoglobins, and dyshemoglobinemias. In Greer, J. P., Arber, D. A., Glader, B., et al. (Eds.), *Wintrobe's Clinical Hematology.* (4th ed., pp. 915–926). Philadelphia: Wolters Kluwer Health/Lippincott Williams & Wilkins.

81. Zur, B. (2016). Hemoglobin variants – pathomechanism, symptoms and diagnosis. *Laboratoriums Medizin, 39*(s1), 000010151520150106.

25

Thalassemias

*S. Renee Hodgkins**

OBJECTIVES

After completion of this chapter, the reader will be able to:

1. Describe the hemoglobin defect found in thalassemia.
2. Describe the worldwide geographic distribution of thalassemia and its relationship with the prevalence of malaria.
3. Name the chromosomes that contain the α-globin gene and the β-globin gene clusters and the globin chains produced by each.
4. Describe types of genetic mutations that result in α- and β-thalassemia.
5. Explain the pathophysiologic effects caused by the imbalance of globin chain synthesis in α- and β-thalassemia.
6. Describe four major clinical syndromes of β-thalassemia and the clinical expression of each heterozygous and homozygous form.
7. Recognize the pattern of laboratory findings in heterozygous and homozygous β-thalassemia, including hereditary persistence of fetal hemoglobin.
8. Correlate clinical syndromes of α-thalassemia with the number of α genes present.
9. Recognize the laboratory findings associated with various α-thalassemia syndromes.
10. Describe the treatment of transfusion-dependent thalassemia and nontransfusion-dependent thalassemia, the risks involved, and the reason it is necessary to monitor iron levels.
11. Describe clinical syndromes and pathophysiology of thalassemia associated with common structural hemoglobin variants.
12. Discuss the role of the complete blood count, peripheral blood film review, supravital stain, hemoglobin fraction quantification (using hemoglobin electrophoresis, high-performance liquid chromatography, and/or capillary zone electrophoresis), and molecular genetic testing in the diagnosis of thalassemia syndromes.
13. Discuss the current therapeutic approaches to thalassemia.
14. Differentiate β-thalassemia minor from iron deficiency anemia.
15. Given a case history and clinical and laboratory findings, interpret test results to identify the type of thalassemia present.

OUTLINE

Definitions and History
Epidemiology
Genetics of Globin Synthesis
Categories of Thalassemia
Genetic Defects Causing Thalassemia
Pathophysiology
   Mechanisms in β-Thalassemia
   Mechanisms in α-Thalassemia
β-Globin Gene Cluster Thalassemia
   Clinical Syndromes of β-Thalassemia
   Other Thalassemias Caused by Defects in the β-Globin Gene Cluster
   Screening for β-Thalassemia Minor

α-Thalassemia
   Clinical Syndromes of α-Thalassemia
Thalassemia Associated with Structural Hemoglobin Variants
   Hemoglobin S-Thalassemia
   Hemoglobin C-Thalassemia
   Hemoglobin E-Thalassemia
Diagnosis of Thalassemia
   History and Physical Examination
   Laboratory Methods
   Differential Diagnosis of Thalassemia Minor and Iron Deficiency Anemia

*The author extends appreciation to Martha Payne, Rakesh P. Mehta, and Elaine M. Keohane, whose work in prior editions provided the foundation for this chapter.

CASE STUDY

After studying the material in this chapter, the reader should be able to respond to the following case study. Answers can be found in Appendix C.

A 24-year-old male medical student in the United States was found to have a HGB level of 10.2 g/dL in a hematology laboratory class. During discussion of the family history with this student, a hematologist at the university discovered that his mother had always been anemic, had periodically been given iron therapy, and had a history of several acute episodes of gallbladder disease (attacks). Both of the student's parents had been born in Sicily. A cousin on his mother's side had two children who died of thalassemia major at ages 4 and 5 years and a third young daughter with thalassemia major who was being treated with regular blood transfusions. The student's laboratory test results were as follows. Reference intervals can be found after the Index at the end of the book.

RBC	5.74×10^{12}/L	MCV	61.0 fL
HGB	10.2 g/dL	MCH	17.8 pg
HCT	35%	MCHC	29.1 g/dL

Peripheral blood RBCs exhibited moderate microcytosis, slight hypochromia, and slight poikilocytosis with occasional target cells, and several RBCs had basophilic stippling. Hb A_2 was 4.9% of total hemoglobin by high-performance liquid chromatography. Serum ferritin level was 320 ng/mL.

1. Why was the family history so important in this case, and what diagnosis did it suggest?
2. What laboratory values helped confirm the diagnosis?
3. From what other disorders should this anemia be differentiated? What laboratory tests would be helpful? Why is differentiation important?
4. If this individual was planning to have children, what genetic counseling should be provided?

DEFINITIONS AND HISTORY

Thalassemias are a diverse group of inherited disorders caused by genetic mutations affecting the globin chain component of the hemoglobin (Hb) tetramer. Thalassemia was first described in 1925 by Cooley and Lee[1] in four children with anemia, splenomegaly, mild hepatomegaly, and facial bone changes. These characteristics would later become the typical findings in young children with untreated β-thalassemia major, often referred to as *Cooley's anemia*. Seven years later, Whipple and Bradford[2] published a paper outlining detailed autopsy studies of children who died of this disorder. Because of the high incidence of patients of Mediterranean descent with this disorder, Whipple called the disease *Thalassic* (Greek for "great sea") anemia, which was subsequently changed to *thalassemia*.

Thalassemia results from a reduced or absent synthesis of one or more of the globin chains of hemoglobin. A wide variety of mutations in hemoglobin genes lead to clinical outcomes that are wide ranging, with certain mutations causing no anemia and others leading to death in utero, during childhood, or in early adulthood. Thalassemias are named according to the chain with reduced or absent synthesis. Mutations affecting the α- or β-globin gene are most clinically significant because Hb A ($\alpha_2\beta_2$) is the major adult hemoglobin. The decreased or absent synthesis of one of the chains not only leads to a decreased production of hemoglobin, but also results in an imbalance in the α/β chain ratio.[3] The unaffected gene continues to produce globin chains at normal levels, and the accumulation of the unpaired normal chains damages red blood cells (RBCs) or their precursors, resulting in their premature destruction. This exacerbates the anemia and makes some forms of thalassemia particularly severe.

EPIDEMIOLOGY

The morbidity and mortality due to thalassemia significantly contribute to the global health burden. Across the world, an estimated 56,000 infants are conceived or born with a clinically significant thalassemia each year, with more than half requiring regular transfusions.[4] It is estimated that 5% of the world's population are carriers of an α-thalassemia mutation and 1.5% are carriers of a β-thalassemia mutation.[3,5,6] Although thalassemia occurs in all parts of the world, its distribution is concentrated in the "thalassemia belt," which extends from the Mediterranean east through the Middle East and India to Southeast Asia and south to Northern Africa (Figure 24.3).[7] The carrier frequency of β-thalassemia depends on the region, with Sardinia, Cyprus, and Greece having the highest frequency in Europe (6% to 19%), and India, Thailand, and Indonesia having the highest frequency in Asia and Southeast Asia (0.3% to 15%).[7] The carrier frequency of α-thalassemia varies considerably. In Europe, Cyprus has the highest carrier frequency at 14%.[7] The carrier frequency reaches 50% to 60% in Eastern Saudi Arabia and parts of Asia and Africa and may be as high as 75% to 80% in certain groups in Nepal, India, Thailand, and Papua New Guinea.[7]

The geographic location of the thalassemia belt coincides with areas in which malaria is prevalent (Figure 24.3). This sparked interest in studies to examine the relationship of thalassemia and resistance to malaria. A 2012 meta-analysis of 18 studies on α-thalassemia conducted by Taylor and colleagues[8] showed a decreased risk of severe malaria in α-thalassemia, both in heterozygotes (defined as– α/αα genotype) and homozygotes (defined as– α/– α and αα/– – genotypes). Interestingly, the protective effect of α-thalassemia was demonstrated only against severe malaria and not against uncomplicated malaria and asymptomatic parasitemia.[8] The researchers were unable to determine the same effect in β-thalassemia due to an insufficient number of published studies.[8] The reasons for the protective effect of thalassemia against malaria are not clear. Some mechanisms under investigation include reduced parasite invasion and growth in thalassemia cells, reduced attachment of infected thalassemia cells to endothelial cells of blood vessels, and greater binding of antimalarial antibodies to infected cells, thus increasing phagocytosis and immune clearance of parasites.[5]

GENETICS OF GLOBIN SYNTHESIS

The normal hemoglobin molecule is a tetramer of two α-like chains (α or ζ) and two β-like chains (β, γ, δ, or ε). Combinations of these chains produce six normal hemoglobins. Three are embryonic hemoglobins, Hb Gower-1 (ζ$_2$ε$_2$), Hb Gower-2 (α$_2$ε$_2$), and Hb Portland (ζ$_2$γ$_2$). The others are fetal hemoglobin (Hb F [α$_2$γ$_2$]) and two adult hemoglobins (Hb A [α$_2$β$_2$] and Hb A$_2$ [α$_2$δ$_2$]). The α-like globin gene cluster is located on chromosome 16, whereas the β-like globin gene cluster is on chromosome 11. The α-like globin gene cluster contains three functional genes: *HBZ* (ζ-globin), *HBA1* (α$_1$-globin), and *HBA2* (α$_2$-globin).[3,9,10] The β-like globin gene cluster contains five functional genes: *HBE* (ε-globin), *HBG2* (^{G}γ-globin), *HBG1* (^{A}γ-globin), *HBD* (δ-globin), and *HBB* (β-globin).[3,9] These genes are positioned in the order that corresponds to their developmental stage of expression.[9] By 10 weeks' gestation, genes for embryonic ζ and ε chains are switched off and silenced, whereas genes for α and γ chains are upregulated (this is called the *ζ to α switch* on chromosome 16 and the *ε to γ switch* on chromosome 11).[9] The γ chains combine with α chains to form Hb F (α$_2$γ$_2$), the predominant hemoglobin of fetal life. The gene for the β chain is initially activated during the second month of gestation, but β chain production occurs at low levels throughout most of fetal life.[10] Shortly before birth, however, expression of the γ-globin gene is downregulated, whereas expression of the β-globin gene is upregulated (called the *γ to β switch*). Therefore by 6 months of age and through adult life, Hb A (α$_2$β$_2$) is the predominant hemoglobin.[3] The gene for the δ chain is activated shortly before birth, but owing to its weak promoter, it produces only a relatively small amount of δ chain, resulting in a low level of Hb A$_2$(α$_2$δ$_2$) throughout life (Chapter 8 and Figure 8.6).[3,9] Table 25.1 lists the reference intervals for normal hemoglobins in adults.

γ-Globin genes code for two globin chains (^{G}γ and ^{A}γ) that differ at position 136 by a single amino acid (glycine and alanine, respectively).[10] Both of these globin chains are found in Hb F, with no functional difference identified between them. Similarly, the α-globin gene loci are duplicated on each chromosome 16 and also code for two globin chains (α$_1$ and α$_2$). Either of these genes can contribute to the two α-globin chains in the hemoglobin tetramer, and no functional difference has been identified between the two. Interspersed between the functional genes on these chromosomes are four functionless, genelike loci, or pseudogenes, that are designated by the prefixed symbol Ψ (Greek letter psi). The purpose of these pseudogenes is unknown.[10] The organization of these genes on chromosomes 16 and 11 is shown in Figure 25.1.

An individual inherits one cluster of the five functional genes on chromosome 11 from each parent. The genotype for normal β chain synthesis is designated β/β. Because two α-globin genes (α$_1$ and α$_2$) are inherited on each chromosome 16, a normal genotype is designated αα/αα.

TABLE 25.1 **Reference Intervals for Normal Hemoglobins in Adults**	
Hb A (α$_2$β$_2$)	95%–100%
Hb A$_2$ (α$_2$δ$_2$)	0%–3.5%
Hb F (α$_2$γ$_2$)	0%–2%

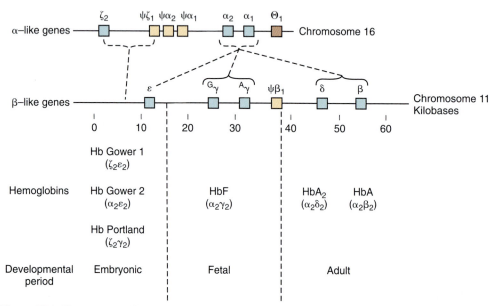

Figure 25.1 Chromosome Organization of Globin Genes and Their Expression During Development. The light blue boxes indicate functional globin genes; the tan boxes indicate pseudogenes. The scale of the depicted chromosomal segments is in kilobases of DNA. The switch from embryonic to fetal hemoglobin occurs by 10 weeks of gestation, and the switch from fetal to adult hemoglobin begins in the third trimester. *Hb*, Hemoglobin. (From Sankaran, V. G., Nathan, D. G., Orkin, S. H. [2015]. Thalassemias. In Orkin, S. H., Fisher, D. E., Ginsberg, D., et al. [Eds], *Nathan and Oski's Hematology and Oncology of Infancy and Childhood.* [8th ed., p. 716, Figure 21.2]. Philadelphia: Saunders.)

CATEGORIES OF THALASSEMIA

Thalassemias are divided into β-thalassemias, which include all the disorders of reduced globin chain production arising from the β-globin gene cluster on chromosome 11, and α-thalassemias, which involve the genes for the α_1 and α_2 chains on chromosome 16. Various deletional and nondeletional mutations can cause each of these disorders, and individuals with similar clinical manifestations are often heterogeneous at the genetic level.[3,9,10]

β-Thalassemias affect mainly β chain production but also may involve δ, $^G\gamma$, $^A\gamma$, and ε chains. In β-thalassemias, β^0 is the designation for the various mutations in the β-globin gene in which no β chains are produced. In the homozygous state (β^0/β^0), an individual does not produce Hb A ($\alpha_2\beta_2$). β^+ is the designation for the various mutations in the β-globin gene that result in a partial deficiency of β chains (ranging from 5% to 30% of normal) and a decrease in production of Hb A.[3] Some mutations in the β-globin gene lead to minimal reductions in β chain production and are associated with mild or silent clinical states. The designation β^{silent} for silent carrier has been used for those mutations. The designation $\delta\beta^0$ is used for mutations in the δ- or β-globin genes in which no δ or β chains are produced. In the homozygous state ($\delta\beta^0/\delta\beta^0$), no Hb A ($\alpha_2\beta_2$) or Hb A_2 ($\alpha_2\delta_2$) is produced. The designation $\delta\beta^{Lepore}$ indicates a fusion of the δ- and β-globin genes that produces Hb Lepore.[3,10]

The most common mutations in α-thalassemia are deletions involving the α_1- and/or α_2-globin genes.[9,11] The designation α^+ is used to indicate a deletion of *either* the α_1- or the α_2-globin gene on chromosome 16 (also called the $-\alpha$ *haplotype*). This results in decreased production of α chains from that chromosome. The designation α^0 is used to indicate a deletion of *both* the α_1- and the α_2-globin genes on chromosome 16 (also called the $--$ *haplotype*). This results in no production of α chains from that chromosome.[3,9,10] Nondeletional mutations in the α-globin gene can also result in α-thalassemia, but these are less common.[3,11] The designation α^{ND} or α^T is used for these mutations.[10] Major gene designations in thalassemia are summarized in Table 25.2.

GENETIC DEFECTS CAUSING THALASSEMIA

Types of genetic defects that cause a reduced or absent production of a particular globin chain include single nucleotide (or point) mutations, small insertions or deletions, or large deletions.[10,11] The mechanisms by which these mutations interfere with globin chain production include the following:[3,9,10]

- *Reduced or absent transcription of messenger ribonucleic acid (mRNA)* due to mutations in the promoter region or initiation codon of a globin gene or to mutations in polyadenylation sites that reduce mRNA stability
- *mRNA processing errors* due to mutations that add or remove splice sites, resulting in no globin chain or altered globin chain production
- *Translation errors* due to mutations that change the codon reading frame (frameshift mutations); substitute an incorrect amino acid codon (missense mutations); add a stop codon, causing premature chain termination (nonsense mutations); or remove a stop codon, resulting in an elongated and unstable mRNA that produces a dysfunctional globin chain
- *Deletion of one or more globin genes,* resulting in no production of the corresponding globin chains

All of these heterogeneous genetic mutations cause a reduction or lack of synthesis of one or more globin chains, resulting in the thalassemia syndromes (Figure 25.2).

TABLE 25.2 Genetic Designations in Thalassemia

Designation	Definition
Designations for Normal β-Globin and α-Globin Genes	
β	Normal β-globin gene; normal amount of β chain production; one gene located on each chromosome 11
αα	Normal α_1- and α_2-globin genes on one chromosome (haplotype αα); normal amount of α chain production; two genes located on each chromosome 16
Designations for Major Thalassemia Genes	
β^0	β-globin gene mutation that results in no β chain production
β^+	β-globin gene mutation that results in decreased β chain production varying from 5% to 30% of normal
β^{silent}	β-globin gene mutation that results in mildly decreased β chain production
$\delta\beta^0$	δβ-globin gene deletional or nondeletional mutation that results in no δ or β chain production; accompanied by some increased γ chain production
$\delta\beta^{Lepore}$	δβ-globin gene fusion that produces a small amount of fusion product, hemoglobin Lepore, and no normal δ or β chain production; accompanied by some increased γ chain production
HPFH	Hereditary persistence of fetal hemoglobin; δβ-globin gene deletional or nondeletional mutation in γ-globin gene promoter that results in no δ or β chain production; accompanied by increased γ chain production
α^0	Deletion of both α-globin genes on one chromosome (haplotype $--$) that results in no α chain production
α^+	Deletion of one α-globin gene on one chromosome (haplotype, $-\alpha$) that results in decreased α chain production
α^{ND} or α^T	Nondeletional mutation in one α-globin gene on one chromosome (haplotype $\alpha^{ND}\alpha$) that results in decreased α chain production (ND notes nondeletional; *T* denotes trait or thalassemia)
α^{CS}	Constant Spring (CS) is a known nondeletional mutation that results in an elongated alpha chain and a more severe clinical presentation.

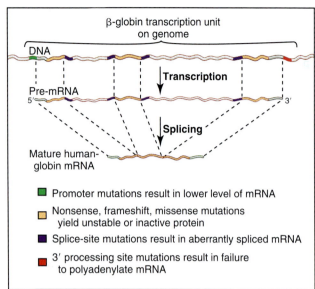

Figure 25.2 Transcription Unit of the β-Globin Gene. The nucleotide sequence of the DNA template is transcribed into a complementary pre-mRNA. The pre-mRNA is processed by removing introns and splicing together the protein coding exons (orange). The DNA sequences required for expression of a functional β-globin chain are indicated in different colors. Mutations in any of these sequences can lead to decreased or absent β-globin chain production. *DNA,* Deoxyribonucleic acid; *mRNA,* messenger ribonucleic acid. (From Corden, J. L. [2017]. Gene expression. In Pollard, T. D., Earnshaw, W. C., Lippincott-Schwartz, J., et al. [Eds.], *Cell Biology.* [3rd ed., Figure 10.2B]. Philadelphia: Elsevier.)

PATHOPHYSIOLOGY

The clinical manifestations of thalassemia stem from (1) reduced or absent production of a particular globin chain, which diminishes hemoglobin synthesis and produces microcytic hypochromic RBCs, and (2) unequal production of the α- or β-globin chains, causing an imbalance in the α/β chain ratio; this leads to markedly decreased survival of RBCs and their precursors.[3,9,10] The α/β chain imbalance is more significant and determines the clinical severity of the thalassemia.[3,12] The mechanisms and degree of shortened RBC survival are different for β-thalassemia and α-thalassemia.

Mechanisms in β-Thalassemia

Typically, individuals with severe β-thalassemia are asymptomatic during fetal life and through approximately 6 months of age because Hb F ($\alpha_2\gamma_2$) is the predominant hemoglobin. Symptoms usually begin to appear between 6 and 24 months of age, after completion of the γ to β switch.[3,10,13–15] To compensate for the decreased expression of the β-globin gene, the γ- and/or δ-globin genes are usually upregulated; however, in β-thalassemia major, this increase is insufficient to correct the α/β chain imbalance, resulting in excess α chains.[3]

In β-thalassemia, unpaired excess α chains precipitate in developing erythroid precursors forming inclusion bodies; this causes oxidative stress and damage to cellular membranes.[13,14] Apoptosis is triggered, and the damaged and apoptotic erythroid precursors are subsequently phagocytized and destroyed in the bone marrow by activated macrophages.[13,14] In addition, iron accumulation in the erythroid precursors, discussed further on in this section, and inflammatory cytokines contribute to the apoptosis.[12–14] The premature death of erythroid precursors in the bone marrow is called *ineffective erythropoiesis.*[9,12–14] In this situation, the bone marrow attempts to produce RBCs but is not able to release sufficient viable cells into the circulation. The cells that are released into the periphery are laden with inclusion bodies and are rapidly sequestered and destroyed by macrophages in the spleen (extravascular hemolysis).[9] Therefore in β-thalassemia the anemia is multifactorial and results from a combination of ineffective RBC production and increased RBC destruction.

In β-thalassemia major, profound anemia stimulates increased RBC production through increased erythropoietin (EPO) production by the kidney and results in massive (but ineffective) erythroid hyperplasia mediated through the EPO receptor and Janus kinase 2/signal transducers and activators of transcription 5 (JAK2/STAT5) pathway signaling.[3,9,12] In untreated or inadequately treated patients, marked bone changes and deformities occur due to massive bone marrow expansion. Reduction in bone mineral density and thinning of the cortex of bone increases the risk of pathologic fractures.[3,9] In children, radiographs of long bones may exhibit a lacy or lucent appearance.[3] Skull radiographs may demonstrate a typical "hair on end" appearance due to vertical striations of bony trabeculae (Figure 25.3).[3,9,14] Typical facial changes occur, with prominence of the forehead (also known as *frontal bossing*), cheekbones, and upper jaw. *Extramedullary erythropoiesis* (RBC production outside of the bone marrow) causes hepatosplenomegaly, and foci of hematopoietic tissue can appear in other body areas. Sequestration of blood cells in an enlarged spleen can worsen the anemia and can cause neutropenia and thrombocytopenia.[9] Excessive destruction of RBCs and their precursors leads to an increase in indirect bilirubin in the plasma from the breakdown of hemoglobin. The bilirubin can diffuse into the tissues, causing jaundice (Chapter 20). Patients also have an increased risk of developing thrombosis.[3,9]

Iron accumulation in various organs is a serious complication in β-thalassemia major and is a significant cause of morbidity and mortality in adults.[3] In children, excess iron causes growth retardation and absence of sexual maturity; in adults, it causes cardiomyopathy, fibrosis and cirrhosis of the liver, and dysfunction of exocrine glands.[3,14,15] The risk of organ damage due to iron accumulation begins to increase after 10 to 11 years of age.[15] On the cellular level, excess iron also promotes more α-globin precipitation and reactive oxygen species in erythroid precursors, furthering cellular damage and apoptosis.[12] Iron overload is predominantly due to the regular RBC transfusions required in β-thalassemia major (discussed later). However, the consistently elevated EPO level also promotes the upregulation and secretion of erythroferrone (ERFE) from erythroblasts.[16,17] ERFE acts on hepatocytes and traps bone morphogenetic protein, which is responsible for activating hepcidin synthesis through the Smad1/5/8 pathway, and thus prevents the production of hepcidin.[16] The low hepcidin level allows more iron absorption by intestinal enterocytes. This mechanism normally serves to provide the additional iron needed

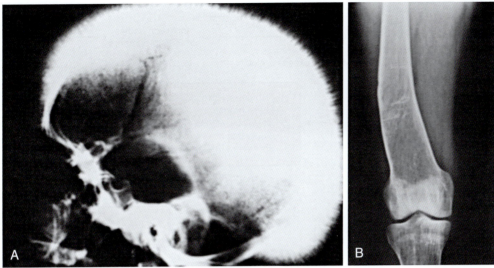

Figure 25.3 Radiologic Abnormalities in a Patient With Homozygous β-thalassemia Who Receives Blood Transfusions Infrequently (Thalassemia Intermedia). **(A)**, Skull radiograph illustrating the typical hair on end appearance. **(B)**, Severe osteoporosis, pseudofractures, thinning of the cortex, and bowing of the femur. (From Sankaran, V. G., Nathan, D. G., Orkin, S. H. [2015]. Thalassemias. In Orkin, S. H., Fisher, D. E., Ginsberg, D., et al. [Eds.], *Nathan and Oski's Hematology and Oncology of Infancy and Childhood*. [8th ed., p. 757, Figure 21.29]. Philadelphia: Saunders.)

to support EPO-stimulated erythropoiesis (Chapter 9).[3,16,17] However, in ineffective erythropoiesis, hyperabsorption of intestinal iron is not needed because iron is continually recycled back into plasma by the massive intramedullary death of erythroid precursors and hemolysis of defective α chain-laden RBCs in circulation. Thus hyperabsorption of iron further adds to the iron overload in β-thalassemia major. In nontransfusion-dependent β-thalassemia, increased ERFE levels may explain the pathologic decrease in hepcidin and the development of iron overload, even when no or very few transfusions are administered.[3,12,16,17] In support of this theory, Ganz and colleagues[18] found increased levels of serum ERFE in patients with transfusion-dependent and nontransfusion-dependent β-thalassemia, with ERFE levels declining after transfusion.

The complex pathophysiology of β-thalassemia major is summarized in Figure 25.4.

Mechanisms in α-thalassemia

In α-thalassemia, decreased production of α chains can manifest in utero because α chains are a component of both fetal (Hb F) and adult (Hb A and Hb A₂) hemoglobins. However, the accumulation of non-α chains has different consequences compared with β-thalassemia. In the fetus and newborn, a decrease in production of α chains results in an excess of γ chains. These γ chains accumulate in proportion to the number of deleted or defective α genes.[9,10] The γ chains are more stable and do not precipitate but instead form hemoglobin tetramers ($γ_4$) called *Hb Bart*.[10] After 6 months of age and through adulthood, when the γ to β switch is completed, the decrease in α chain production results in excess β chains. The excess β chains are also relatively stable and form tetramers ($β_4$), called *Hb H*.[10]

Because Hb H and Hb Bart do not precipitate to any significant degree in developing erythroid precursors in bone marrow, patients with α-thalassemia do not have severe ineffective

erythropoiesis.[9] As mature RBCs age in the circulation, however, $β_4$ tetramers in Hb H eventually precipitate and form inclusion bodies.[9] Macrophages in the spleen recognize and remove these abnormal RBCs from the circulation, and the patient manifests a moderate hemolytic anemia.

In addition to the decreased production and shortened RBC survival mechanisms, a third mechanism is involved in the anemia of α-thalassemia. Hb Bart and Hb H cannot deliver oxygen to tissues due to their very high affinity for oxygen.[10] A fetus cannot survive with only Hb Bart (found with a deletion of all four α-globin genes). The marked tissue hypoxia causes heart failure and massive edema (hydrops fetalis) and hepatomegaly, and the fetus usually dies in utero or shortly after birth.[3] This is discussed later in "α-thalassemia."

β-GLOBIN GENE CLUSTER THALASSEMIA

There is great heterogeneity in the mutations in the β-globin gene cluster that leads to the clinical syndrome of β-thalassemia.[11] More than 280 mutations have been reported in the β-globin gene itself, and more than 300 mutations are known in the entire β-globin cluster, including β-, δ-, and γ-globin genes, individually or in combination.[10,11] A small subset of mutations, however, accounts for the majority of mutant alleles within a single ethnic group or geographic area in which β-thalassemia is found.[3,15] Because multiple mutations are present in each population, most individuals with severe β-thalassemia are compound heterozygotes for two different β-thalassemia mutations.[9] A comprehensive list of hemoglobin gene mutations is maintained in the HbVar mutation database, which is available online.[11]

Clinical Syndromes of β-Thalassemia

β-Thalassemia is divided into four categories based on clinical manifestations (Table 25.3)[3,10,14]:

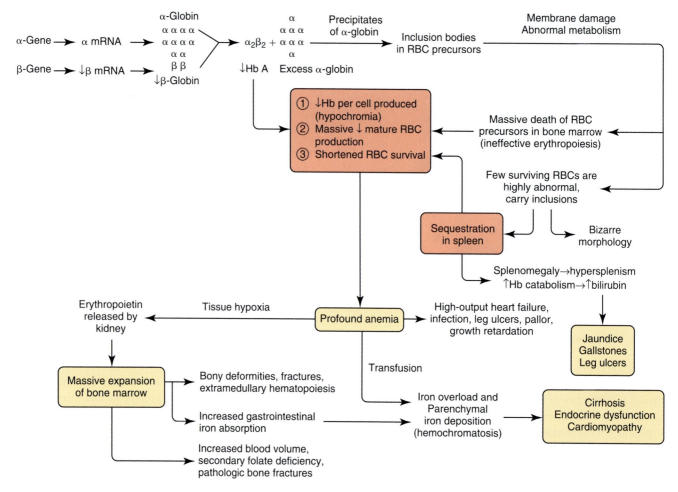

Figure 25.4 Pathophysiology of Severe Forms of β-thalassemia. The diagram outlines the pathogenesis of clinical abnormalities resulting from the primary defect in β-globin chain synthesis. *RBC,* Red blood cell. (From Sheth, S. [2023]. Thalassemia syndromes. In Hoffman, R., Benz, E. J., Silberstein, L. E., et al. [Eds], *Hematology: Basic Principles and Practice.* [8th ed., p. 560, Figure 41.6]. Philadelphia: Elsevier.)

- β-Thalassemia silent carrier (heterozygous state), with no hematologic abnormalities or clinical symptoms
- β-Thalassemia minor (heterozygous state), with mild hemolytic anemia, microcytic and hypochromic RBCs, and no clinical symptoms
- β-Thalassemia major (homozygous or compound heterozygous state), with severe hemolytic anemia, microcytic and hypochromic RBCs, severe clinical symptoms, and transfusion dependence
- β-Thalassemia intermedia, with mild to moderate hemolytic anemia, microcytic and hypochromic RBCs, moderate clinical symptoms, and no transfusion dependence

A simpler clinical classification divides symptomatic thalassemias into two broad groups based on transfusion requirements. *Transfusion-dependent thalassemia (TDT)* includes β-thalassemia major, severe Hb E-β-thalassemia, and α-thalassemia major (Hb Bart hydrops fetalis). *Non-transfusion-dependent thalassemia (NTDT)* includes β-thalassemia intermedia, mild/moderate Hb E-thalassemia, and α-thalassemia intermedia (Hb H disease).[6,19] In NTDT, occasional transfusions may be required in conditions such as infection, pregnancy, and surgery.[6,14,19] Clinical

manifestations of the various mutations depend on whether one or both of the β-globin genes are affected and the extent to which the affected gene or genes are expressed, that is, $β^0$, $β^+$, or $β^{silent}$ (see Table 25.2). β-Thalassemia is inherited in an autosomal recessive pattern. If both parents are carriers of a β-thalassemia gene mutation, they have a 25% chance of having a child with two mutated β-globin genes (homozygote or compound heterozygote) and clinical manifestations of β-thalassemia major or intermedia.

Silent Carrier State of β-Thalassemia

The designation $β^{silent}$ includes the various heterogeneous β-globin gene mutations that produce only a small decrease in production of the β chains. The silent carrier state ($β^{silent}/β$) results in nearly normal α/β chain ratios and no hematologic abnormalities.[3,9,10] It is often first recognized inadvertently, when an apparently normal parent with an unknown silent carrier state ($β^{silent}/β$) and a parent with β-thalassemia trait ($β^+/β$ or $β^0/β$) have a child with unexpected symptoms of β-thalassemia intermedia due to compound heterozygosity ($β^+/β^{silent}$ or $β^0/β^{silent}$).[10] Some individuals who are homozygous for a silent thalassemia gene mutation ($β^{silent}/β^{silent}$) have

TABLE 25.3 Clinical Syndromes of β-Thalassemia with Examples of Genotypes

Genotype	Hb A	Hb A₂	Hb F	Hb Lepore
Normal (Normal Hematologic Parameters)				
β/β	N	N	N	0
Silent Carrier State (Asymptomatic; Normal Hematologic Parameters)				
βsilent/β	N	N	N	0
Thalassemia Minor (Asymptomatic; Mild Anemia; Microcytic Hypochromic)				
β+/β	↓	↑	N to Sl ↑	0
β0/β	↓	↑	N to Sl ↑	0
δβ0/β	↓	N to ↓	5%–20%	0
δβLepore/β	↓	↓	↑	5%–15%
Thalassemia Major (Transfusion-Dependent Thalassemia; Severe Anemia; Microcytic Hypochromic)				
β+/β+	↓↓	V	↑↑	0
β+/β0	↓↓↓	V	↑↑	0
β0/β0	0	V	↑↑	0
δβLepore/δβLepore	0	0	80%	20%
Thalassemia Intermedia* (Nontransfusion-Dependent Thalassemia†; Mild to Moderate Anemia; Microcytic Hypochromic)				
βsilent/βsilent	↓	↑	↑	0
β+/βsilent or β0/βsilent	↓	↑	↑	0
δβ0/δβ0	0	0	100%	0
β0/δβ0	0	N	↑↑	0

*Other genotypes are included in this category, such as dominantly inherited β-thalassemia (heterozygous for a very severe β-globin gene mutation) and coinheritance of a triplicated α-globin gene (ααα/αα) with thalassemia minor.
†Patients with nontransfusion-dependent thalassemia do not require regular transfusions for survival but may need transfusions occasionally, such as during pregnancy, surgery, or infections.
↓, Decreased; ↑, increased; 0, absent; Hb, hemoglobin; N, normal; Sl, slight; V, variable.

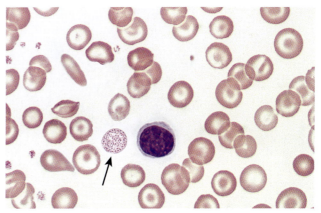

Figure 25.5 Peripheral Blood Film From a Patient With β-Thalassemia Minor. Note the microcytic hypochromic red blood cells, target cells, other poikilocytes, and basophilic stippling (arrow). (Wright-Giemsa stain, ×1000.)

slightly increased.[3] Some degree of poikilocytosis (including target cells and elliptocytes) and basophilic stippling in the RBCs may be seen on a peripheral blood film (Figure 25.5). The bone marrow shows mild to moderate erythroid hyperplasia, with minimal ineffective erythropoiesis. Hepatomegaly and splenomegaly are seen in a few patients. In the most common β-thalassemia minor syndromes (β0/β and β+/β), the Hb A level is 92% to 95%, and the Hb A₂ level is characteristically elevated and can vary from 3.5% to 7.0%.[3,10,15] The Hb F level usually ranges from 1% to 5%.[3,10] Less common types of β-thalassemia minor exist, such as δβ0/β and δβLepore/β. Other rare types have atypical features, such as Dutch β0-thalassemia minor, which shows the expected elevation in Hb A₂ level but an Hb F level in the 5% to 20% range,[21] and another mutant found in a Sardinian family in which the Hb A₂ level is within the reference interval.[22]

β-Thalassemia Major

β-Thalassemia major is characterized by a severe anemia that requires regular transfusion therapy. It is usually diagnosed between 6 months and 2 years of age (after completion of the γ to β switch) when the child's Hb A level does not increase as expected.[3,10]

In untreated β-thalassemia major, the hemoglobin level is below 7 g/dL but can fall as low as 2 to 4 g/dL.[3,10,14] The MCV ranges from 50 to 70 fL, and the MCH ranges from 12 to 20 pg.[9,14,15] The peripheral blood film shows marked microcytosis, hypochromia, anisocytosis, and poikilocytosis, including target cells, teardrop cells, and elliptocytes. Polychromasia and nucleated red blood cells (NRBCs) may be observed (Figure 25.6). RBC inclusions are commonly found, including basophilic stippling, Howell-Jolly bodies, and Pappenheimer bodies, the latter as a result of the excess nonheme iron in RBCs. The reticulocyte count is only mildly to moderately elevated and is inappropriately low in relation to the amount of erythroid hyperplasia and hemolysis present.[3] The inappropriate reticulocytosis results from apoptosis of erythroid precursors in the bone marrow (ineffective erythropoiesis).

been described.[10,20] They present with a mild β-thalassemia intermedia phenotype with an increased level of Hb F and Hb A₂.[10,20]

β-Thalassemia Minor

β-Thalassemia minor (also called β-thalassemia trait) results when one β-globin gene is affected by a mutation that decreases or abolishes its expression, whereas the other β-globin gene is normal (heterozygous state). It usually manifests as a mild asymptomatic anemia, but the hemoglobin level can range from approximately 11 to 15 g/dL in affected men and 10 to 13 g/dL in affected women.[9,15] The RBC count is within the reference interval or slightly elevated.[3,10] The RBCs are microcytic and hypochromic, with a mean cell volume (MCV) less than 75 fL and a mean cell hemoglobin (MCH) less than 26 pg.[3] The reticulocyte count is within the reference interval or

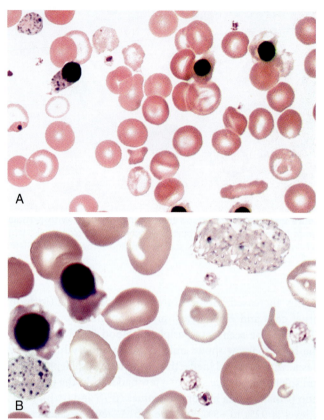

Figure 25.6 Peripheral Blood Films From a Patient With β-thalassemia Major. (**A** and **B**), Note basophilic stippling, microcytosis, hypochromia, target cells, nucleated red blood cells, and red cell fragments. (A, Wright-Giemsa stain, ×500; B, Wright-Giemsa stain, ×1000.) (Adapted from Carr, J. H. [2021]. *Clinical Hematology Atlas.* [6th ed.]. Philadelphia: Elsevier.)

Hb A is absent or decreased, depending on the specific genotype, which determines whether no β chains (β^0/β^0) are produced or a decreased amount (β^+/β^+ or β^0/β^+) of β chains is produced. In β^0/β^0, Hb F is 92% to 95%, and Hb A is absent.[14] Hb A is produced only if a β^+ mutation is present and usually ranges from 10% to 30%.[3,14,15] Hb F ranges from 70% to greater than 90%, depending on the genotype and amount of Hb A.[10,14,15] The level of Hb A_2 is variable and can be within or above the reference interval.[3,9,14] Bone marrow shows marked erythroid hyperplasia, with a myeloid-to-erythroid (M:E) ratio of 1:20 (reference interval is 1.5:1 to 3.3:1). As a result of the massive destruction of erythroid cells and release of free hemoglobin, the serum haptoglobin level is reduced or absent, and the serum lactate dehydrogenase activity is markedly elevated (Chapter 20).

Transfusion therapy is the major therapeutic option for patients with thalassemia major and typically is initiated when the hemoglobin drops to less than 7 g/dL and the patient has clinical symptoms.[3,14,23] Typically, 10 to 15 mL/kg of leukoreduced RBCs are transfused every 2 to 5 weeks.[3] RBCs that are less than 7 to 10 days old are used for transfusion to allow for maximum donor RBC

survival in the patient.[3,14] Extended typing of the patient's RBCs for major blood group antigens (or at least C, c, E, e, and Kell antigens) and transfusion of antigen-matched donor RBCs are recommended to reduce the risk of alloimmunization.[3,9,14,15]

Administration of RBC transfusions at regular intervals began in the mid-1970s. The pretransfusion hemoglobin level is usually maintained between 9 and 10.5 g/dL.[3,14,23] Such transfusion regimens are termed *hypertransfusion* and are used not only to correct the anemia, but also to suppress the marked erythropoiesis. With erythropoiesis suppressed, the marked marrow expansion does not occur; therefore the bone changes do not take place. In addition, the decrease in erythropoiesis reduces the amount of iron absorbed by intestinal enterocytes.[14,17] Children receiving this therapy do not develop hepatosplenomegaly, and their growth and development are much improved.[3]

Long-term transfusion regimens, however, lead to iron overload. Because there is no effective physiologic pathway for iron excretion in the body, iron contained in the transfused RBCs accumulates in the body. This iron is stored in organs outside the bone marrow (e.g., liver, heart, pancreas), which results in organ damage. Accumulation of iron in the liver leads to cirrhosis, and the deposition of iron in the heart leads to cardiac dysfunction and arrhythmias. In the past, with transfusion therapy alone, patients with thalassemia died in their teens, typically from cardiac failure. Now patients undergo iron chelation therapy with transfusion therapy. Iron-chelating agents bind excess iron so that it can be excreted in urine and stool. Deferoxamine, approved by the US Food and Drug Administration (FDA) in 1982, is usually administered subcutaneously with an infusion pump over 8 to 12 hours.[3,24] However, poor compliance with the regimen is seen in many patients, mainly because of the inconvenience of the infusion pump.[3,9,24] To address this concern, oral chelation agents (deferasirox, taken once daily, and deferiprone, taken 3 times daily) were approved by the FDA in 2005 and 2011, respectively.[24] All three iron-chelating agents have advantages, disadvantages, and side effects, and are not effective in all patients; studies comparing the long-term efficacy of these agents are ongoing.[23,24] Combination therapy in which agents are alternated may improve compliance and reduce the side effects.[23,24] Additional oral iron-chelating drugs are in development. Adherence to iron chelation regimens is critical to prevent iron accumulation and subsequent complications of iron overload; implementation of these regimens has extended the life expectancy of patients with β-thalassemia major into the fourth and fifth decades and beyond.[3,23]

Hematopoietic stem cell transplantation (HSCT) is the only curative therapy for thalassemia major.[3,25] Young patients (younger than 14 years of age) who have a human leukocyte antigen (HLA)-identical sibling donor and have not yet developed complications of iron overload have excellent outcomes, with overall survival rates of 90% to 96% and event-free survival rates of 83% to 93%.[25] These rates, however, drop to an overall survival rate of 80% to 82% and event-free survival rate of 74% to 76% in patients older than 14 years.[25] Because there is only a 25% chance that a sibling will have the identical HLA genotype, this option is not available to all patients. However, HSCT outcomes with well-matched unrelated donors (using high-resolution molecular typing) have been continually improving, thus providing an additional option for patients without a matched sibling donor.[23]

Hb F induction agents, such as hydroxyurea, 5-azacytidine, short-chain fatty acids, erythropoietic-stimulating agents, and thalidomide derivatives, have been evaluated for therapy in thalassemia major because of their ability to "switch on" the γ-globin gene to produce more γ chains.[26] The γ chains then combine with the excess α chains to form Hb F, thus partially correcting the α/β chain imbalance. Hydroxyurea therapy has benefited a few patients with β-thalassemia major, allowing them to become transfusion independent, but it has

not been beneficial in the majority of patients.[3,13,26] Larger and better-designed studies are needed to determine the efficacy of these agents in reducing the need for transfusions in thalassemia major.[26] Additional pharmaceuticals are being explored to enhance the production of Hb F, including thalidomide, IMR-687, and benserazide.[26,27] Each of these agents use slightly different mechanisms for increasing Hb F and balancing the α/non-α ratio.

Newer therapies are being developed for both TDT and NTDT. These therapies have targeted the globin chain imbalance, ineffective erythropoiesis, and iron load complications (Figure 25.7). Historically, HSCT was the only therapy able to address the globin chain imbalance and "cure" thalassemia; however, that required an HLA-matched sibling donor for a high success rate. Gene therapy has changed the approach to HSCT in thalassemia patients. Gene therapy (gene insertion and gene editing) is being explored through the use of

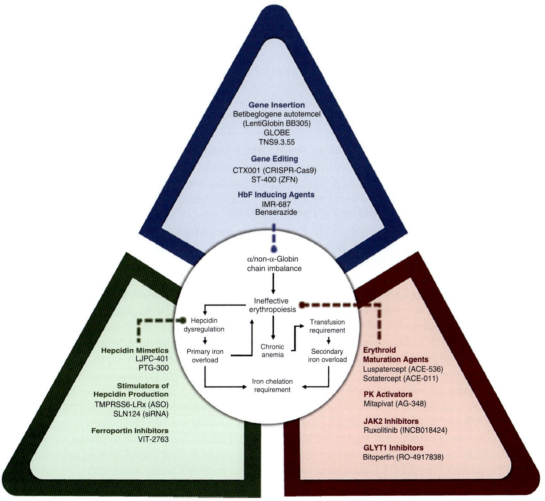

Figure 25.7 Drugs in Clinical Trial for the Treatment of Thalassemia Targeting Different Aspects of the Pathophysiology of the Disease. These treatments employ novel mechanisms such as gene editing, gene insertion, hepcidin mimetics and stimulators, and erythroid maturation activators to address the various aspects of the pathophysiology of disease: α/non-α globin chain imbalance, ineffective erythropoiesis, and iron overload. *ASO*, Antisense oligonucleotides; *CRISPR-Cas9*, clustered regularly interspaced short palindromic repeats linked to Cas9 nucleases; *GLYT1*, glycine transporter-1; *JAK2*, Janus kinase 2; *PK*, pyruvate kinase; *siRNA*, small interfering ribonucleic acid; *TMPRSS*, transmembrane serine protease; *ZFN*, zinc finger nucleases. (From Musallam, K. M., Bou-Fakhredin, R., Cappellini, M. D., & Taher, A. T. [2021]. 2021 update on clinical trials in β-thalassemia. *Am J Hematol, 96*, p. 1519, Figure 1.)

an ex vivo lentiviral vector gene transfer. These protocols use autologous CD34+ hematopoietic stem cells (HSCs) harvested from the patient and require myeloablation of the bone marrow before reinfusion of the modified HSCs. Several clinical trials have shown increased hemoglobin levels in both TDT and NTDT. In a phase 3 clinical trial, betibeglogene autotemcel, which uses a lentiviral vector to insert an amino acid substitution into Hb A (T87Q), demonstrated transfusion independence (hemoglobin >11.5 g/dL) in 88% of the participants (86% β^0/β^0 and 89% non-β^0/β^0) and was maintained on average for 20 months (HGB-207 and HGB-212 studies).[26,27] Another clinical trial for TDT (TIGET-BTHAL; ClinicalTrials.gov Identifier: NCT02453477) in phase 1/2 uses the GLOBE lentiviral vector, which encodes for the human β-globin gene, and reintroduction into the bone following ablative therapy.[26,27] Patients with severe β^+ mutations or β^0 mutations showed a reduction in transfusion requirements with several pediatric patients achieving transfusion independence. In another GLOBE clinical trial (TNS9) with four TDT patients (β^0/β^+ and β^0/β^0), at least one participant experienced significantly reduced transfusion requirements for 5 years.[26]

Several trials are also being conducted using gene editing through CRISPR/Cas9 (this methodology is explained in Chapter 24) to manipulate the genes in autologous CD34+ HSCs ex vivo to reduce the imbalance of α to non-α globin chains. In the CLIMB THAL-111 (ClinicalTrials.gov Identifier: NCT03655678) phase 1/2 trial, CTX001 modified the CD34+ HSCs at the erythroid-specific enhancer of the *BCL11A* gene, the transcription factor that controls the switch from fetal to adult hemoglobin by decreasing γ globin expression.[26,27] This switch control of Hb F production by BCL11A was discovered through research on hereditary persistence of fetal hemoglobin (HPFH).[26,28] In the CLIMB trial, the CTX001 vector (CRISPR/Cas9) increased the production of Hb F by disruption of BCL11A. By supressing BCL11A, more Hb F is produced. As seen with hydroxyurea therapy, increasing production of Hb F can reduce the clinical severity of β-thalassemia. In the CLIMB trial, participants with TDT showed increased total hemoglobin levels, increased Hb F levels, and transfusion independence for an average of almost 24 months of follow-up.[26] Another study, THALES, used a zinc-finger nuclease (ZFN) to increase the production of Hb F through BCL11A inhibition.[14,26,27] There are disadvantages to these types of therapeutics (genome editing techniques such as lentiviral vector gene insertion, CRISPR/Cas9, and ZFN) because of the requirement for myeloablative conditioning in preparation for HSCT (which uses chemotherapy and/or radiation to destroy HSCs), dependence on the ability to harvest viable CD34+ cells from the patient (required for successful treatment), and the expense of gene therapy.

Therapies targeting ineffective erythropoiesis in thalassemia by enhancing erythropoiesis also are being investigated. Luspatercept and sotatercept (activin type II receptor traps) block SMAD2/3 signaling by binding transforming growth factor-β (TGF-β) and restoring GATA-1 transcription to increase erythroid maturation and thereby circumvent the ineffective erythropoiesis seen in patients with TDT and NTDT.[27] Early data showed success in reducing transfusion, although B^0/B^0 genotypes showed lower response rates.[27] Luspatercept was approved in 2019 for use in the United States for adult patients and is currently under clinical trial for pediatric and NTDT (BEYOND trial).[26,27] Mitapivat is a pyruvate kinase activator under investigation for use in TDT (α- and β-thalassemia) to enhance erythropoiesis through adenosine triphosphate (ATP) supply.[13,26] JAK2 inhibitors (primarily ruxolitinib) have been found to be ineffective in increasing hemoglobin levels, though they have been shown to decrease splenomegaly, and trials were terminated after phase 2.[13,14,26,27]

Lastly, additional therapies to address the iron overload have been investigated for efficacy for treatment in TDT and NTDT. The iron dysregulation has been targeted through hepcidin mimetic (minihepcidins), upstream stimulators of hepcidin production, and ferroportin inhibition.[13,26,27] Figure 25.7 presents the new drug therapies for TDT and NTDT in clinical trials with their proposed mechanism of action.

β-Thalassemia Intermedia

Thalassemia intermedia is a clinical designation for syndromes in which the α/β chain imbalance and symptoms fall between those observed in β-thalassemia minor and β-thalassemia major, but without the need for regular transfusion therapy to maintain the hemoglobin level and quality of life.[3,6,9] Thalassemia intermedia is included in the NTDT group.[6,19] Patients with thalassemia intermedia typically maintain a hemoglobin level between 7 and 10 g/dL.[6]

Genotypes of thalassemia intermedia show great heterogeneity. Patients can be homozygous for mutations that cause a mild decrease in β-globin expression. Conversely, they may be compound heterozygous, with one gene causing a mild decrease in β chain production and the other causing a marked reduction in β chain production.[3,9] In rare instances, only one of the β-globin genes carries a mutation, but it is severe enough to cause a significant anemia. These cases are sometimes called *dominantly inherited* β-thalassemia.[10] Some thalassemia intermedia phenotypes result from the coinheritance of one or two abnormal β-globin genes ($\beta+$) with another hemoglobin defect, such as abnormal α-globin genes or unstable hemoglobins.[3,9] The coinheritance of α-thalassemia may permit homozygotes with more severe β-thalassemia mutations to remain transfusion independent because the α/β chain ratio is more balanced and fewer free α chains are available to precipitate and cause hemolysis.[3] Less severe clinical manifestations also occur when a β-thalassemia mutation is combined with a mutation that increases the expression of the γ-globin gene.[3] The increase in Hb F production ($\alpha_2\gamma_2$) helps to compensate for the reduction in Hb A, while helping to correct the α/β balance, as seen with the therapies mentioned in "β-thalassemia Major" that have targeted increase in Hb F and balancing of the α chains. Examples of these situations are the deletional forms of $\delta\beta^0$-thalassemia. Individuals homozygous for these mutations, or compound heterozygotes for $\delta\beta^0$-thalassemia and a β-thalassemia mutation, have thalassemia intermedia with increased γ chain and Hb F synthesis.[3,10] Conversely, coinheritance of a triplicated α-globin gene locus ($\alpha\alpha\alpha$) is also a cause of thalassemia intermedia in some individuals heterozygous for β-thalassemia due to the production of more α chains and greater imbalance of the α/β chain ratio.[3,29] The imbalanced in α chains caused by the triplication would result in increased Hb F but not the amount of Hb A_2, and present as a NTDT.[29]

Because of the genetic heterogeneity of β-thalassemia intermedia, the laboratory and clinical features vary. The degree of anemia varies between 7 and 10 g/dL, depending on the extent of the α/β chain imbalance, with an MCV between 50 and 80 fL and an MCH between 16 and 24 pg.[6] Because of the presence of splenomegaly, the platelet and neutrophil counts may be low. The clinical course varies from minimal symptoms (despite moderately severe anemia) to severe exercise intolerance and pathologic fractures.[9]

Patients with thalassemia intermedia also have iron overload, even though they do not receive regular transfusions.[3] As indicated previously, the markedly accelerated ineffective erythropoiesis suppresses hepcidin production by the liver, which results in more iron absorption by intestinal enterocytes.[17] Cardiac, liver, and endocrine complications, however, manifest 10 to 20 years later in thalassemia intermedia patients than in patients who receive regular transfusions.[3] Regular monitoring for iron overload is recommended after age 10, with periodic chelation therapy to reduce iron levels.[6] Patients also have an increased risk of thrombosis due to the effects of iron overload and α chain precipitation in RBCs, causing platelet and RBC abnormalities and endothelial cell damage.[6,19] This risk is higher after splenectomy.[6,19]

Other Thalassemias Caused by Defects in the β-globin Gene Cluster

Other thalassemias may be caused by deletion, inactivation, or fusion of a combination of genes of the β-globin gene cluster, such as HPFH, $\delta\beta^0$-thalassemia, and Hb Lepore thalassemia.[3,9,30]

Thalassemias With Increased Levels of Fetal Hemoglobin

HPFH and $\delta\beta^0$-thalassemia are closely related, heterogeneous conditions in which Hb F is expressed at increased levels beyond infancy into adulthood. These conditions have similarities but can be differentiated by the clinical presentation, hemoglobin level, MCV, and amount of Hb F produced.[10]

In HPFH, the β-globin gene cluster typically contains a deletion in the $\delta\beta$ region that leads to increased production of Hb F; however, there are also HPFH conditions that have intact β-globin gene clusters with nondeletional mutations in the promoter region of the γ-globin genes associated with HPFH.[9,10,28,30,31] Mutations in the promotor regions of the γ-globin promoter genes (deletions such as BCL11A repressor protein or enhanced activity of the transcriptional activator GATA-1) increase the transcription of γ globin and result in increased Hb F.[30,31] Because individuals with these mutations are characteristically asymptomatic, this condition is of little significance except when it interacts with other forms of thalassemia or structural

hemoglobin variants, such as Hb S. The additional γ chains produced are able to replace the missing β chains and help to restore the balance of α and non-α chains (γ or β). Significant variation is seen in heterozygotes for deletional-type HPFH, but these patients typically are asymptomatic, with a normal MCV and Hb F levels of 10% to 35%, depending on the mutation.[3,9] Homozygotes for deletional-type HPFH are also asymptomatic. They have a normal to slightly increased hemoglobin level, 100% Hb F, with slightly hypochromic and microcytic RBCs.[10] The increase in hemoglobin observed in some patients is likely a response to the slight hypoxia induced by the higher oxygen affinity of Hb F compared with Hb A.[3] Identification and quantification of Hb F levels is important when assessing thalassemia, differentiating HPFH and $\delta\beta^0$-thalassemia, and monitoring treatment that increases the Hb F levels (see "Laboratory Methods").[32]

The $\delta\beta^0$-thalassemias are also characterized by deletions in the δ- and β-globin genes and an increase in Hb F in adult life, although nondeletional types have also been described.[9] In this condition, however, the increase in production of the γ chains is not sufficient to completely restore the balance between the α and non-α chains. Individuals with heterozygous $\delta\beta^0$-thalassemia ($\delta\beta^0/\beta$) have a decreased level of Hb A, normal or decreased level of Hb A_2, and 5% to 20% Hb F.[9,10] They have a β-thalassemia minor phenotype, with a slight decrease in hemoglobin level and hypochromic microcytic RBCs. Homozygous $\delta\beta^0$-thalassemia individuals ($\delta\beta^0/\delta\beta^0$) have hypochromic microcytic RBCs, 100% Hb F, and a β-thalassemia intermedia phenotype (see Table 25.3).[9,10]

Hemoglobin Lepore Thalassemia

Hemoglobin Lepore ($\delta\beta^{Lepore}$) is a structural variant and rare type of $\delta\beta$-thalassemia caused by a fusion of the $\delta\beta$-globin genes.[11] This mutation occurs during meiosis due to nonhomologous crossover between the δ-globin locus on one chromosome and the β-globin locus on the other chromosome. The Lepore globin chain expressed by the $\delta\beta$ fusion gene contains the first 22 to 87 amino acids of the N-terminus of the δ chain and the last 31 to 97 amino acids of the C-terminus of the β chain, depending on the variant.[11] The $\delta\beta$ fusion gene produces a reduced level of the Lepore globin chain because its transcription is under the control of the δ-globin gene promoter, which is much less active than the β-globin gene promoter.[3] Conversely, in the reciprocal fusion on the other chromosome (called anti-Lepore), the β-globin gene locus is intact, so normal production of the β chain occurs.[3,10] In heterozygotes ($\delta\beta^{Lepore}/\beta$), there is a decreased level of Hb A and Hb A_2, an increase in Hb F, and approximately 5% to 15% Hb Lepore.[3,10] The clinical manifestations are similar to those of β-thalassemia minor. In homozygotes ($\delta\beta^{Lepore}/\delta\beta^{Lepore}$), there are no normal δ- or β-globin genes, no production of Hb A and Hb A_2, and approximately 80% Hb F and 20% Hb Lepore.[10] The clinical manifestations are similar to those of β-thalassemia major (see Table 25.3).[3]

Screening for β-Thalassemia Minor

Because of the high carrier frequency of β-thalassemia mutations worldwide, screening has become an important global health issue.[7] Mass screening programs in Italy and Greece combined with prenatal diagnosis have led to a significant reduction in the number of children born with β-thalassemia major.[10] Carrier parents have a 25% risk of having a child with thalassemia major or thalassemia intermedia, depending on the particular β globin gene mutations.[11] Potential β-thalassemia carriers can be initially identified by a mild decrease in hemoglobin concentration and MCV and an increase in Hb A_2, but other causes of microcytic anemias, such as iron deficiency, need to be ruled out.[10] Laboratory diagnosis of thalassemia is covered later in the chapter.

α-THALASSEMIA

In contrast to β-thalassemia, in which point mutations in the β-globin gene cluster are the most common type of mutation, in α-thalassemia, large deletions involving the $α_1$- and/or $α_2$-globin genes are the predominant genetic defect.[9-11] Nondeletional mutations also occur in α-thalassemia but are uncommon.[10,11] The extent of decreased production of the α chain depends on the specific mutation, the number of α-globin genes affected, and whether the affected α-globin gene is $α_2$ or $α_1$.[9] The $α_2$-globin gene produces approximately 75% of the α chains in normal RBCs, so mutations in the $α_2$-globin gene generally cause more severe anemia than mutations affecting the $α_1$-globin gene.[9,10,33] The notation for the normal α-globin gene complex or haplotype is αα, which signifies the two normal genes ($α_2$ and $α_1$) on one chromosome 16. A normal genotype is αα/αα.

α-Thalassemia is divided into two haplotypes: $α^0$-thalassemia and $α^+$-thalassemia. In the $α^0$-thalassemia haplotype (originally named *α-thal-1*), a deletion of both α-globin genes on chromosome 16 results in no α chain production from that chromosome. The designation – – is used for the $α^0$-thalassemia haplotype.[9,10] There are more than 20 known mutations that produce the $α^0$-thalassemia haplotype and involve deletion of both α-globin genes or the entire α-globin gene cluster (including the ζ-globin gene) on one chromosome.[11,34] The $α^0$ haplotype (– –) is found in approximately 4% of the population in Southeast Asia, is found less frequently in the Mediterranean region, and occurs infrequently in other parts of the world.[7]

In the $α^+$-thalassemia haplotype (originally named *α-thal-2*), a deletional or nondeletional mutation in one of the two α-globin genes on chromosome 16 results in decreased α chain production from that chromosome.[9] The designation – α is used for the deletional mutations, and the designation $α^Tα$ (or $α^{ND}α$) is used for the nondeletional mutations. The deletional $α^+$ haplotype (– α) is by far the most common of the α-thalassemia haplotypes. It is widely distributed throughout the thalassemia belt and central Africa (Figure 24.3), with a carrier frequency reaching 50% to 80% in some regions of Saudi Arabia, India, Southeast Asia, and Africa.[7,33] The deletional $α^+$ haplotype (– α) is also found in about 30% of individuals of African ancestry.[33] The nondeletional α+ haplotype ($α^Tα$) is relatively uncommon.[10,33] More than 70 different mutations are known, the majority of which are point mutations that affect the predominant $α_2$ gene.[6,11] The $α^Tα$ haplotype produces unstable α chains

or fewer α chains than the – α haplotype and generally results in a more severe anemia.[10,14,33]

One of the most common nondeletional α-globin gene mutations is Constant Spring ($α_2^{142Stop→Gln}$), also called $α^{CS}$ (haplotype $α^{CS}α$).[10,11] It is the result of a point mutation in the $α_2$-globin gene that changes the stop codon at 142 to a glutamine codon.[10,11,33] As a result, additional bases are added to the end of the mRNA during transcription until the next stop codon is reached. The elongated mRNA is very unstable and produces only a small amount of the $α^{CS}$ chain.[3,34,35] The $α^{CS}$ chains (with an additional 31 amino acids added to the C-terminal end) combine with β chains to form Hb Constant Spring, but incorporation of a longer α chain makes the tetramer unstable.[3,35] Because of the instability of both the mRNA and the hemoglobin tetramer, the circulating level of Hb Constant Spring is very low (<1%).[3,10,35] Consequently, Hb Constant Spring is difficult to detect by alkaline hemoglobin electrophoresis and, when present, is visualized as a faint, slow-moving band near the point of origin.[10]

Clinical Syndromes of α-Thalassemia

α-Thalassemia has four clinical syndromes, which are determined by the number of genes affected and the amount of α chains produced (Table 25.4):[3,9,10]

- Silent carrier state (– α/αα)
- α-Thalassemia minor/trait homozygous $α^+$ (– α/– α) or heterozygous $α^0$ (– –/αα)
- Hb H disease/α-thalassemia intermedia (– –/– α)
- Hb Bart hydrops fetalis syndrome/α-thalassemia major (– –/– –)

Silent Carrier State

Deletion of one α-globin gene, leaving three functional α-globin genes (– α/αα), is the major cause of the silent carrier state. The α/β chain ratio is nearly normal, and no hematologic abnormalities are present.[9,10] Because one α-globin gene is absent, there is a slight decrease in α chain production. When not enough α chains are present, the non-α chains γ (primarily produced during fetal life) and β (adult globin) can form tetramers (four of each chain) to create Hb Bart ($γ_4$) or Hb H ($β_4$). In this case, the decrease in alpha chain production results in a slight excess of γ chains only at birth that form Hb Bart ($γ_4$) in the range of 1% to 2%.[9,10] A nondeletional $α^+$ mutation (ND or T for trait) in one α-globin gene ($α^{ND}α/αα$ or $α^Tα/αα$) also results in the silent carrier state. An example of a nondeletional mutation, Constant Spring (CS), $α^{CS}α/αα$, results in Hb Constant Spring as less than 1% of the total hemoglobin.[10] There is no reliable way to diagnose silent carrier state other than genetic analysis.

α-Thalassemia Minor (α-Thalassemia Trait)

Deletion of two α-globin genes is the major cause of α-thalassemia minor. It exists in two forms: homozygous $α^+$ (– α/– α) or heterozygous $α^0$ (– –/αα), where + represents a partial deletion and 0 represents complete deletion of α on one chromosome.[9,10] This syndrome is asymptomatic and characterized by a mild microcytic anemia with an MCV of less than 80 fL and an MCH of less than 27 pg.[6,14] At birth, the proportion of Hb Bart ($γ_4$) is

TABLE 25.4 Clinical Syndromes of α-Thalassemia

Genotype	Hb A	Hb Bart (in Newborn)	Hb H (in Adult)	Hb Constant Spring
Normal (Normal Hematologic Parameters)				
αα/αα	N	0	0	0
Silent Carrier State (Asymptomatic; Normal Hematologic Parameters)				
−α/αα	N	1%–2%	0	0
$\alpha^{CS}\alpha/\alpha\alpha$	N	1%–3%	0	<1%
α-Thalassemia Minor (Asymptomatic; Mild Anemia; Microcytic Hypochromic)				
−−/αα	Sl↓	5%–15%	0	0
−α/−α	Sl↓	5%–15%	0	0
$\alpha^{CS}\alpha/\alpha^{CS}\alpha$*	Sl↓	5%–15%	0	<6%
Hb H Disease, α-Thalassemia Intermedia (Nontransfusion-Dependent Thalassemia†, Mild to Moderate Anemia; Microcytic Hypochromic)				
−−/−α	↓	10%–40%	1%–40%	0
$−−/\alpha^{CS}\alpha$‡	↓	↑↑	↑↑	<1%
Hb Bart Hydrops Fetalis Syndrome, α-Thalassemia Major (Transfusion-Dependent Thalassemia; Severe Anemia; Usually Death in Utero or Shortly after Birth)				
−−/−−	0	80%–90% (remainder Hb Portland)	NA	0

*$\alpha^{CS}\alpha/\alpha^{CS}\alpha$ genotype results in mild to moderate hemolytic anemia with jaundice and hepatosplenomegaly.
†Patients with nontransfusion-dependent thalassemia do not require regular transfusions for survival but may need transfusions occasionally, such as during pregnancy, surgery, or infections.
‡$−−/\alpha^{CS}\alpha$ genotype and other nondeletional genotypes ($−−/\alpha^{ND}\alpha$) result in Hb H disease that is moderate to severe and may require more frequent transfusions than the deletional $−−/−\alpha$ genotype.
↑↑, Increased more than $−−/−\alpha$; 0, absent; ↓, decreased; CS, Constant Spring; Hb, hemoglobin; N, normal; NA, not applicable.

in the range of 5% to 15%.[10] In adults, the production of α and β chains is reduced only slightly, so Hb H (β_4) is not usually present.[9] Homozygosity for nondeletional mutations in both α_2-globin genes ($\alpha^{ND}\alpha/\alpha^{ND}\alpha$) may have a more severe clinical presentation and produce a mild to moderate hemolytic anemia, often with jaundice and hepatosplenomegaly.[10,35,36] In the homozygous mutation, $\alpha^{CS}\alpha/\alpha^{CS}\alpha$, Hb Constant Spring is 5% to 6% of the total hemoglobin, and the hemoglobin concentration is 9 to 11 g/dL.[9,10,35]

Hemoglobin H Disease (α-Thalassemia Intermedia)

Deletion of three α-globin genes is the major cause of Hb H disease, in which only one α-globin gene remains to produce α chains ($−−/−\alpha$).[9,10] This genetic abnormality is particularly common in individuals of Southeast Asian, Mediterranean, and Middle Eastern descent because of the prevalence of the α^0 gene haplotype (−−). It is characterized by the accumulation of excess unpaired β chains that form tetramers of Hb H (β_4) in adults. In the newborn, Hb Bart (γ_4) comprises 10% to 40% of the hemoglobin, with the remainder being Hb F ($\alpha_2\gamma_2$) and Hb A ($\alpha_2\beta_2$). After the γ to β switch, Hb H replaces most of the Hb Bart, so Hb H is in the range of 1% to 40%, with a reduced amount of Hb A_2 ($\alpha_2\delta_2$), traces of Hb Bart, and the remainder Hb A.[9,10,33,34] The nondeletional α^+ haplotype, when combined with the α^0 haplotype ($−−/\alpha^{ND}\alpha$), generally produces a more severe Hb H disease with a higher level of Hb H than the α^0 interaction with the deletional α^+ haplotype ($−−/−\alpha$) such as Hb H-Hb Constant Spring ($−−/\alpha^{CS}\alpha$).[9,10,33,35,36]

Hb H disease is characterized by a mild to moderate, chronic hemolytic anemia with hemoglobin concentrations averaging 7 to 10 g/dL and reticulocyte counts of 3% to 10%, although a wide variability in clinical and laboratory findings exists.[6,9] Patients with deletional Hb H disease generally have higher hemoglobin levels compared with patients with nondeletional types.[6,9,10] Bone marrow exhibits erythroid hyperplasia, and the spleen is usually enlarged. Hb H disease is classified as an NTDT; that is, patients do not require regular transfusions. However, infection, pregnancy, or exposure to oxidative drugs may cause a hemolytic crisis, requiring transfusions on a temporary basis.[6,10,19]

Hemolytic crises often lead to detection of the disease because individuals with Hb H disease may otherwise be asymptomatic. RBCs are microcytic and hypochromic, with marked poikilocytosis, including target cells and bizarre shapes (Fig. 25.8). Hb H is vulnerable to oxidation and gradually precipitates in the circulating RBCs to form inclusion bodies of denatured hemoglobin.[9] Hb H inclusions alter the shape and viscoelastic properties of the RBCs, contributing to decreased RBC survival. The inclusions are typically removed as the RBC passes through the spleen; however, after splenectomy, most RBCs have many inclusions. Hb H inclusions are visualized with supravital staining (discussed later in "Laboratory Methods").

Two distinct conditions are associated with Hb H disease and congenital physical and intellectual abnormalities: ATR-16 syndrome and α-thalassemia X-linked intellectual disability (ATRX) syndrome. Patients with ATR-16 syndrome inherit or acquire a large deletion in the short arm of chromosome 16, which removes the ζ- and α-globin genes and all the flanking genes to the terminus of the chromosome.[34] Patients have physical deformities, intellectual disabilities, and Hb H disease.[33,34,36]

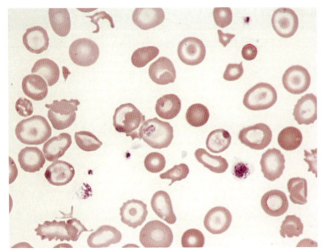

Figure 25.8 Peripheral blood film showing poikilocytosis (target cells, schistocytes, acanthocytes), microcytosis, hypochromasia, anisocytosis, and Howell-Jolly bodies from a postsplenectomy 67-year-old man of Turkish Cypriot descent with Hb H disease (- - ^{MED}/αNDα). (Wright-Giemsa stain, ×1000). (From Spencer-Chapman, M., Luqmani, A., Layton, D. M., et al. [2018] Unusual inclusions in hemoglobin H disease post-splenectomy. *Am J Hematol*, 93, p. 963.)

ATRX syndrome is due to mutations of the *ATRX* gene located on the X chromosome.[37,38] The ATRX protein is a component of a large complex that regulates expression of various genes, including the α-globin genes.[34,38] The regulation is accomplished by deoxyribonucleic acid (DNA) remodeling and/or methylation, thus affecting transcription, replication, and repair of the target genes.[33,34,38] Therefore when the *ATRX* gene is mutated, patients have decreased α chain production.[33,34,36,38] Affected males with ATRX syndrome have pronounced intellectual disability, physical deformities, developmental delay, and Hb H disease. An acquired Hb H disease with mutations in the *ATRX* gene has been found in myelodysplastic syndrome.[34,38,39]

Hemoglobin Bart Hydrops Fetalis Syndrome (α-Thalassemia Major)

Homozygous α⁰-thalassemia (– –/– –) results in the absence of all α chain production. It usually results in death in utero or shortly after birth, although a small number survive with aggressive transfusion therapy, including intrauterine transfusions.[3,9,34] It is included in the TDT category because if the neonate survives, lifelong transfusions are required.[19]

Without intrauterine transfusion, the fetus becomes severely anemic, which leads to cardiac failure and edema in fetal subcutaneous tissues (hydrops fetalis). Hb Bart (γ₄) is the predominant hemoglobin, along with a small amount of Hb Portland (ζ₂γ₂) and traces of Hb H (β₄).[3,9] Hb Bart has a very high oxygen affinity; it does not deliver oxygen to the tissues.[9,10,34] The fetus can survive until the third trimester because of Hb Portland, but this hemoglobin cannot support the later stages of fetal growth and the affected fetus becomes severely anoxic (severely deficient in oxygen).[3,9] The fetus is delivered prematurely and is usually stillborn or dies shortly after birth. In addition to anemia, edema,

and ascites, the fetus has gross hepatosplenomegaly and cardiomegaly.[3,9] At delivery, there is a severe microcytic hypochromic anemia (hemoglobin concentration of 3 to 8 g/dL), with high reticulocyte counts and numerous NRBCs in the peripheral blood.[34] The bone marrow cavity is expanded and marked erythroid hyperplasia is present, along with foci of extramedullary erythropoiesis.

Hydropic pregnancies are hazardous to the mother, resulting in toxemia and severe postpartum hemorrhage.[9,14,34] Hydropic changes are detected in midgestation by ultrasound testing.[40] If both parents carry one α⁰-thalassemia haplotype (– –/αα), prenatal diagnosis of homozygosity can be made by molecular genetic testing of fetal cells from chorionic villus sampling or amniotic fluid.[34] Absence of the α-globin genes establishes the diagnosis. Early termination of the pregnancy prevents the serious maternal complications.[9] Patients with a family history of α-thalassemia are encouraged to seek prenatal genetic counseling and antenatal screening.

THALASSEMIA ASSOCIATED WITH STRUCTURAL HEMOGLOBIN VARIANTS

Hemoglobin S-Thalassemia

Sickle cell anemia (Hb SS)-α-thalassemia is a genetic abnormality that is due to the coinheritance of two abnormal β-globin genes for Hb S and an α-thalassemia haplotype. Hb SS-α⁺-thalassemia is fairly common because the genes for Hb S and the α⁺-thalassemia haplotype, – α, are common in populations of African ancestry. Individuals with Hb SS-α⁺-thalassemia have a milder anemia, with higher hemoglobin levels and lower reticulocyte counts than individuals with sickle cell anemia alone.[41] In one study, Hb SS individuals with the genotypes αα/αα, – α/αα, and – α/– α had average hemoglobin concentrations of 8.4, 9.0, and 9.5 g/dL, respectively, and reticulocyte counts of 10.8%, 8.8%, and 6.9%, respectively.[41]

Hb S-β-thalassemia is a compound heterozygous condition that results from the inheritance of a β-thalassemia gene from one parent and an Hb S gene from the other. This syndrome has been reported in the populations of Africa, the Mediterranean area, the Middle East, and India.[10] The clinical expression of Hb S-β-thalassemia depends on the type of β-thalassemia mutation inherited.[9,10] Individuals with Hb S-β⁺-thalassemia produce variable amounts of normal β chains. Patients have mostly Hb S with slightly elevated Hb A₂ and variable amounts of Hb F and Hb A, depending on the specific abnormal β⁺ gene inherited. These patients can be distinguished from patients with sickle cell anemia by the presence of microcytosis, splenomegaly, an elevated Hb A₂ level, and an Hb A level that is less than the Hb S level.

The interaction of β^silent-thalassemia (in which β chains are produced at mildly reduced levels) and Hb S results in a condition that may be slightly more severe than sickle cell trait. Typically, there is mild hemolytic anemia with splenomegaly. These patients can be distinguished from patients with sickle cell trait by the presence of microcytosis and splenomegaly. Hemoglobin electrophoresis or HPLC confirms this condition when the quantity of Hb S exceeds that of Hb A. In sickle cell trait, Hb A is the predominant hemoglobin.

The combination of β^0-thalassemia and Hb S produces a phenotype similar to sickle cell anemia, with a similar incidence of stroke and a similar life expectancy.[10,42] Both conditions lack Hb A and produce severe, painful crises as the predominant symptom. Typically, the microcytosis and elevated Hb A_2 level in Hb S-β^0-thalassemia distinguish it from sickle cell anemia.

Hemoglobin C-Thalassemia

Hb C-β-thalassemia produces moderately severe hemolysis, splenomegaly, hypochromia, microcytosis, and numerous target cells. The hemoglobin electrophoresis pattern varies, depending on the type of β-thalassemia gene defect, with higher Hb C concentrations in patients when there is minimal or no β chain production.[10]

Hemoglobin E-Thalassemia

Hb E-β-thalassemia is a significant concern in Southeast Asia and Eastern India owing to the high prevalence of both genetic mutations.[10] Hb E is due to a point mutation that inserts a splice site in the β-globin gene and results in decreased production of Hb E.[3] In the homozygous state (Hb EE), the clinical symptoms are similar to a mild β-thalassemia (Chapter 24). When the mutations are coinherited in the compound heterozygous state, there is a marked reduction of β chain production. The clinical symptoms are similar to β-thalassemia intermedia or β-thalassemia major, depending on the particular β-globin gene mutation.[10] Severe Hb E-β-thalassemia manifests a hemoglobin concentration ranging from 4 to 5 g/dL and is classified and managed as a TDT.[6] Mild and moderate Hb E-β-thalassemias (hemoglobin concentration of 9 to 12 g/dL and 6 to 7 g/dL, respectively) are classified and managed as NTDTs.[6]

Table 25.5 summarizes some compound heterozygous states of β-thalassemia combined with a structural β-globin defect.

DIAGNOSIS OF THALASSEMIA

History and Physical Examination

Individual and family histories are paramount in the diagnosis of thalassemia. The ethnic background of the individual should be investigated because of the increased prevalence of specific gene mutations in certain populations. In the clinical examination, findings that suggest thalassemia include pallor due to anemia; jaundice due to hemolysis; splenomegaly due to sequestration of the abnormal RBCs, excessive extravascular hemolysis, and some extramedullary erythropoiesis; and skeletal deformities due to massive expansion of the bone marrow cavities. These findings are particularly prominent in untreated or partially treated β-thalassemia major.[10] Carrier states will not have outward signs of thalassemia or anemia but may have decreased MCV (<80 fL) and mean cell hemoglobin concentration (MCHC) (<27 pg) and elevated or borderline levels of Hb A2.[42] Coexpression of gene mutations in β-, α-, and δ-globin chains and iron deficiency can lead to borderline levels of Hb A_2 (3.3% to 3.9%).[42]

Laboratory Methods

Table 25.6 contains a summary of tests for the diagnosis of thalassemia.

Complete Blood Count With Peripheral Blood Film Review

Although most thalassemias result in a microcytic and hypochromic anemia, laboratory results can vary from borderline abnormal to markedly abnormal; this depends on the type and number of globin gene mutations. The hemoglobin and hematocrit are decreased, but the RBC count can be disproportionately high relative to the degree of anemia, which can generate a very low MCV and MCH. The MCHC is also decreased. The RBC distribution width (RDW) is elevated (reflecting anisocytosis) in untreated β-thalassemia major, but it is often normal in β-thalassemia minor. On a peripheral blood film, the RBCs are typically microcytic and hypochromic except in silent carrier phenotypes, in which RBCs appear normal. In β-thalassemia minor, α-thalassemia minor, and Hb H disease, the cells are microcytic, with target cells and slight to moderate poikilocytosis. In homozygous and compound heterozygous β-thalassemia, extreme poikilocytosis may be present, including target cells and elliptocytes, in addition to polychromasia, basophilic stippling, Howell-Jolly bodies, Pappenheimer bodies, and NRBCs.

TABLE 25.5	β-Thalassemia Associated with Structural β-Globin Variants (Compound Heterozygotes)						
Genotype	Hb A	Hb A_2	Hb F	Other Hb	RBC Morphology	Clinical Manifestations*	Treatment
Hb S-β^+-thalassemia	↓↓	↑	N to ↑	Hb S > Hb A	Microcytes, sickle cells, target cells	Ranges from mild to severe anemia with recurrent vaso-occlusive crises	Ranges from no treatment to transfusion support and pain control
Hb S-β^0-thalassemia	0	↑	N to ↑	Hb S			
Hb C-β^+-thalassemia	↓↓	†	↑	Hb C > Hb A	Microcytes, Hb C crystals, target cells	Ranges from moderate to severe anemia	Usually no treatment needed
Hb C-β^0-thalassemia	0	†	↑	Hb C			
Hb E-β^+-thalassemia	↓↓	†	↑↑	Hb E > Hb A	Microcytes, target cells	Ranges from mild to severe anemia with transfusion dependency	Ranges from no treatment to transfusion support
Hb E-β^0-thalassemia	0	†	↑↑	Hb E			

*Clinical manifestations depend on the amount of Hb A produced; compound heterozygotes with the β^0 gene have more severe symptoms.
†Not all methods can quantitate Hb A_2 in the presence of the abnormal hemoglobin. High-performance liquid chromatography can separate Hb A_2 from Hb C; capillary zone electrophoresis can separate Hb A_2 from Hb E.
↓, Decreased; ↑, increased; 0, absent; *Hb*, hemoglobin; *N*, normal; *RBC*, red blood cell.

TABLE 25.6 Laboratory Diagnosis of Thalassemia

Screening Tests	Complete blood count Peripheral blood film review Iron studies (to rule out IDA)	HGB, HCT, MCV, MCH, MCHC: ↓ RETIC: sl to mod ↑ Varying degrees of microcytosis, hypochromia, target cells, anisocytosis, poikilocytosis, RBC inclusions, NRBCs Serum ferritin and serum iron: N to ↑↑
Presumptive Diagnosis	Supravital stain Hemoglobin fraction quantification by electrophoresis, HPLC, and/or CZE	α-thal: Hb H inclusions β-thal: Hb A ↓ or 0; Hb A₂ ↑ (carriers); Hb F usually ↑; Hb Lepore and other mutants may be present α-thal: Hb A ↓ or 0 (hydrops fetalis); Hb A₂ ↓; Hb Bart, Hb H, Hb Constant Spring, and other mutants may be present
Definitive Diagnosis	Molecular genetic tests* β-thal: >290 mutations in *HBB* α-thal: >110 mutations in *HBA1* and/or *HBA2*	β-thal: initial DNA sequence analysis or PCR-based screen for four to six most common mutations if specific ethnic group known; if negative, deletion/duplication analysis, such as MLPA or gene-targeted microarray analysis α-thal: initial targeted deletional analysis for five most common deletions; if negative, DNA sequence analysis; if negative, deletion/duplication analysis as above

*Required for prenatal diagnosis, preconception risk assessment/carrier detection in couples, or diagnosis of rare or complex mutations.
↓, Decreased; ↑, increased; ↑↑, markedly increased; 0, absent; *CZE,* capillary zone electrophoresis; *Hb,* hemoglobin; *HCT,* hematocrit; *HGB,* hemoglobin concentration; *IDA,* iron deficiency anemia; *MCH,* mean cell hemoglobin; *MCHC,* mean cell hemoglobin concentration; *MCV,* mean cell volume; *MLPA,* multiplex ligation-dependent probe amplification; *mod,* moderate; *NRBC,* nucleated red blood cells; *PCR,* polymerase chain reaction; *RETIC,* reticulocyte count; *RBC,* red blood cell; *sl,* slight; *thal,* thalassemia.
Data from references 3, 11, 15, and 34.

Reticulocyte Count

The reticulocyte count is elevated, which indicates that the bone marrow is responding to a hemolytic process. In Hb H disease, the typical reticulocyte count is 5% to 10%.[10] In homozygous β-thalassemia it is typically 2% to 8%, disproportionately low relative to the degree of anemia.[3,10] This relatively low reticulocyte count reflects the inadequate production of reticulocytes due to ineffective erythropoiesis.

Supravital Staining

In Hb H disease, α-thalassemia minor, and silent carrier α-thalassemia, brilliant cresyl blue or new methylene blue stain may be used to induce precipitation of the intrinsically unstable Hb H.[43] Hb H inclusions (denatured β₄ tetramers) typically appear as small, multiple, irregularly shaped greenish-blue bodies that are uniformly distributed throughout the RBC. They produce a pitted pattern on the RBC surface, similar to the pattern of a golf ball or raspberry (Figure 25.9). In Hb H disease, almost all RBCs contain Hb H inclusions.[36] In α-thalassemia minor, only a few cells may contain these inclusions, and in silent carrier α-thalassemia, only a rare cell does. These inclusions appear different from Heinz bodies, which are larger and fewer in number and most often appear attached to the inner membrane of the RBC. This staining technique is very sensitive in detecting Hb H in α-thalassemia syndromes.[43]

Assessment of Hemolysis

Because thalassemias have a hemolytic component to their pathophysiology, tests for hemolysis are part of the overall assessment. Typically, there are increases in unconjugated (indirect) bilirubin and lactate dehydrogenase and a decrease in haptoglobin (Chapter 20).

Assessment of Normal and Variant Hemoglobins

The major clinical laboratory methods used to identify and quantify normal and variant hemoglobins include hemoglobin

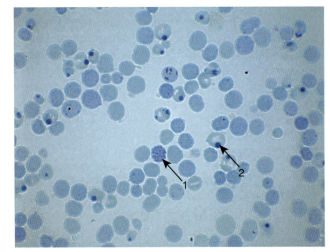

Figure 25.9 Supravital stain of red blood cells (RBCs) from an Hb H preparation slide from the same patient in Figure 25.8. Note the fine, evenly dispersed granular inclusions and the "golf ball" appearance on several of the RBCs in this field *(1)*. Heinz bodies are also present *(2)*. (Magnification not specified.) (From Spencer-Chapman, M., Luqmani, A., Layton, D. M., et al. [2018] Unusual inclusions in hemoglobin H disease post-splenectomy *Am J Hematol, 93,* p. 963.)

electrophoresis, cation-exchange HPLC, and capillary zone electrophoresis (CZE).[44] Each of these methods has advantages and limitations, and no one method is able to identify and quantify all hemoglobin variants. Therefore a combination of at least two of the above-mentioned methods is used for confirmation of a hemoglobin variant.[45]

Hemoglobin electrophoresis at an alkaline pH has been the traditional tool for thalassemia and hemoglobinopathy diagnosis. In this method, the patient's RBC lysate is spotted on a solid support (e.g., agarose) and subjected to an electrical current in an alkaline buffer. Normal and variant hemoglobins will migrate and separate on the support according to their charge. The support is stained, and each hemoglobin band is quantified by scanning densitometry and reported as a percentage of the total hemoglobin.[45] This technique is able to distinguish the common hemoglobins (e.g., Hb A, Hb F, Hb S, and Hb C) and the fast-moving hemoglobins (Hb H and Hb Bart).[44-46] Electrophoresis, however, has the following limitations: it is labor intensive, has low resolution, and cannot accurately quantify Hb A_2 and Hb F. In addition, Hb S and Hb C must be confirmed by another method because Hb D and Hb G comigrate with Hb S, and Hb E and Hb O^{Arab} comigrate with Hb C.[45] Methods used for confirmation usually include electrophoresis at an acid pH, HPLC, and CZE, or in the case of Hb S the hemoglobin solubility test (Figures 24.6–24.9). Figure 25.10 shows the relative hemoglobin mobilities in alkaline electrophoresis for various thalassemias and hemoglobinopathies.

In HPLC, the patient's RBC lysate in buffer is injected into a cation-exchange column. Both normal and variant hemoglobins will bind to the column. An elution buffer is injected and forms a gradient of varying ionic strength.[45] The various hemoglobin types will be differentially eluted from the column, each having a specific column retention time. As each hemoglobin fraction passes near the end of the column, a detector measures the absorbance of the fraction at 415 nm, which is recorded as a peak on a chromatogram.[45] The area under the peak is used to quantify the hemoglobin fraction, which is reported as a percentage of total hemoglobin. With the availability of fully automated instruments, HPLC has replaced hemoglobin electrophoresis in many laboratories as the routine screening method for analysis of hemoglobins.[44] The method is ideal for β-thalassemia screening because it can accurately and quickly quantify Hb A, Hb A_2, and Hb F with 100% sensitivity and 90% specificity if no hemoglobin variants are present (Figure 25.11).[46]

The precise and accurate quantification of Hb A_2 is particularly important in screening individuals for β-thalassemia minor (trait). HPLC can also presumptively identify and quantify hemoglobin variants even in low concentration.[44,45] However, HPLC requires specialized instrumentation and extensive experience and training to accurately interpret the complex chromatograms.[44,45,47] Additional limitations of HPLC include the following: Hb A_2 and Hb E have the same retention time and therefore cannot be accurately quantified by this method; Hb A_2 can be overestimated in the presence of Hb S due to overlapping peaks and underestimated in the presence of Hb D^{Punjab}; and HPLC is not able to identify all variants.[44-48] A manual microcolumn method is also available for the measurement of Hb

A_2.[45] Mutations in the δ-globin gene may interfere with diagnosis of β-thalassemia carrier states, as the Hb A_2 can be lower than 2% and may have an Hb A_2 variant spike on HPLC/CZE.[49]

In CZE, the patient's RBC lysate is introduced into a thin, silica glass capillary tube in an alkaline buffer. When a current is applied, various hemoglobin fractions migrate to the cathode at different velocities due to electroendosmotic flow.[45] As each hemoglobin fraction passes near the end of the capillary, a detector measures the absorbance of the fraction at 415 nm, which is recorded as a peak on a electrophoretogram. The instrument calculates the percentage of each hemoglobin fraction using an integration of the area under the peak and the migration time.[45] Fully automated systems are available that provide rapid and accurate identification and quantification. The peaks are placed into zones in the electrophoretogram for easier identification, and the method can presumptively identify hemoglobin variants, including those in low concentration (see Figure 25.11).[45] An advantage of CZE over HPLC is that it can separate and quantify Hb A_2 in the presence of Hb E.[44,48] However, because there is overlap in the peaks for Hb A_2 and Hb C, it cannot quantify Hb A_2 in the presence of Hb C.[44] As with HPLC, it also cannot detect all variants.[44,45] Complementing HPLC with CZE or electrophoresis has minimized the limitations of these methods.[47] Other technologies, such as isoelectric focusing and mass spectrometry, are used in newborn screening programs for detection of common hemoglobin variants.[44,45]

Molecular Genetic Testing

Molecular genetic testing is required to detect specific mutations in globin genes and definitively identify the type of thalassemia. Molecular genetic testing is not usually required in adults with typical findings on the complete blood count (CBC), electrophoresis, and/or HPLC, but it is required for prenatal diagnosis, preconception risk assessment/carrier detection in couples, and diagnosis of rare or complex mutations.[15,34,44,48]

In β-thalassemia, point mutations in the *HBB* gene are the most common abnormality.[11,48] Therefore, DNA sequence analysis is a practical initial approach and can identify almost 100% of mutations; however, it is not optimal for detection of deletions.[15,48] Targeted mutation analysis employing polymerase chain reaction (PCR)-based methods can also be used for detection and quantification of the four to six most common mutations in genetically homogeneous populations if an individual's ethnicity is known.[3,48] If sequencing is not successful,

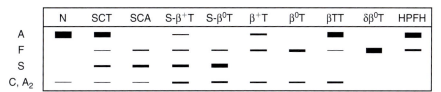

Figure 25.10 Relative Electrophoretic Mobilities at Alkaline pH of Various Hemoglobins Important in the Diagnosis of Thalassemia Syndromes and Hemoglobinopathies. *β⁰T*, β0-thalassemia major, β0/β0 (no Hb A, increased Hb F, slight increase in Hb A_2); *β⁺T*, β+ -thalassemia major, β+/β+ (decreased Hb A, increased Hb F, slight increase in Hb A_2); *βTT*, β-thalassemia minor (slight decrease in Hb A, increased Hb A_2, some Hb F); *δβ⁰T*, δβ0-thalassemia, homozygous, δβ0/δβ0 (100% Hb F); *HPFH*, hereditary persistence of fetal hemoglobin, heterozygous (mostly Hb A, some Hb F, no Hb A_2); *N*, normal; *SCA*, sickle cell anemia (no Hb A, mostly Hb S, increased Hb F, normal Hb A_2); *SCT*, sickle cell trait (Hb A > Hb S, normal Hb A_2 and Hb F); *S-β⁰T*, sickle cell-β0-thalassemia (no Hb A, increased Hb A_2 and F, mostly Hb S); *S-β⁺T*, sickle cell-β+-thalassemia (Hb A < Hb S, increased Hb A2 and Hb F).

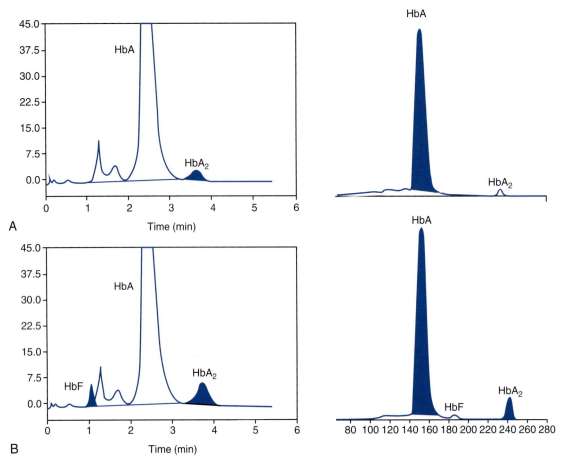

Figure 25.11 Separation and Quantification of Hemoglobin Fractions by High-Performance Liquid Chromatography (Bio-Rad, *left*) and Capillary Electrophoresis (Sebia, *right*). (A), Healthy adult with Hb F <1% and Hb A_2 <3.5%. (B), Adult with β-thalassemia minor with increased Hb F and Hb A_2. (Modified from Giordano, P. C. [2013]. Strategies for basic laboratory diagnostics of the hemoglobinopathies in multiethnic societies: interpretation of results and pitfalls. *Int J Lab Hematol*, 35, p. 472, Figure 3.)

testing can reflex to deletion/duplication analysis, such as multiplex ligation-dependent probe amplification or gene-targeted microarray analysis (Chapter 29).[15,48]

For *HBA1* or *HBA2* mutations in which 95% are deletions, PCR-based targeted mutation analysis, such as gap-PCR, can be initially performed for the five most common deletional mutations.[34,48] This strategy detects approximately 85% of all deletions.[34] If this analysis is not successful, DNA sequencing of the *HBA1* and *HBA2* genes or deletion/duplication analysis can be performed.[34,48]

When the parents' mutation is known, analysis for the specific mutation in fetal cells can be done on specimens from amniocentesis (at 15 to 18 weeks' gestation), by chorionic villus sampling (at 10 to 12 weeks' gestation), or with preimplantation genetic diagnosis using a cell from a 3-day-old embryo after in vitro fertilization.[15,34] Noninvasive methods for detection of the paternal mutation in fetal DNA isolated from maternal circulation are also available.[15,34]

Other Procedures

The classic 2-minute *alkali denaturation* test is accurate and precise to quantify Hb F in the 0.2% to 50% range.[32,50] Most human hemoglobins are denatured on exposure to a strong alkali, but Hb F is not. The Hb F can be separated and its concentration

compared with that of other hemoglobins.[50] However, automated HPLC is now most often used to quantify Hb F.[32,46]

In the Kleihauer-Betke acid elution slide test (traditionally used to assess fetal maternal hemorrhage), peripheral blood films are prepared with ethanol fixation and immersed in a citrate phosphate buffer (pH 3.3). Adult hemoglobins are eluted from the RBCs, but Hb F resists acid elution and remains in the cell. When the cells are subsequently stained, RBCs containing Hb F will take up the stain, whereas RBCs containing only adult hemoglobin will appear as "ghosts." In the context of thalassemia, this test can determine if the Hb F distribution in RBCs is pancellular (found in all RBCs as expected in deletional HPFH cases) or heterocellular (found in some but not all RBCs in β-globin gene cluster thalassemias and nondeletional HPFH cases).[32,46,50]

In underdeveloped countries with limited technology, a single-tube osmotic fragility test (OFT) has been used to screen populations for thalassemia carriers.[3,9,51] This is based on the fact that carriers have hypochromic RBCs, resulting in decreased osmotic fragility.[46,51] An aliquot of anticoagulated blood is incubated in 0.36% or 0.375% saline for 5 minutes.[44,51] Because the solution is hypotonic, normal RBCs will lyse, and the solution will clear. However, patients with thalassemia have hypochromic RBCs that will not lyse in 0.36% or 0.375% saline, and the solution will remain turbid. This test is not specific for thalassemia and will be positive for any condition causing hypochromia, including iron deficiency anemia (IDA). Tatu and Sweatman[51] evaluated hemolysis area (HA) as a screening test for thalassemia trait. HA uses a portable spectrophotometer to quantify OFT-based results (low HA means lower rate of hemolysis), whereas OFT is typically read visually and can have interobserver errors. HA had a lower sensitivity but higher specificity and positive predictive value (91.5%, 90.8%, and 79.6%, respectively) compared with 0.45% OFT (97.6%, 72.9%, and 33.6%) and was similar to 0.36% OFT (80.9%, 96.6%, and 90.5%).[51] Because of the portability and ease of use, the OFT and HA could be used as screening methods in areas of high prevalence.[51]

Ultimately, the recommendation for detection of thalassemia carriers would be evaluation of CBC (MCV <79 fL, MCHC <27 pg) and hemoglobin identification through HPLC or CZE, with quantification of Hb F and Hb A_2.[52] OFT and HA could be helpful in support of a diagnosis where the results are unclear.[52]

Differential Diagnosis of Thalassemia Minor and Iron Deficiency Anemia

RBCs in thalassemia minor are microcytic and hypochromic, and this disease must be differentiated from IDA and other microcytic hypochromic anemias to avoid unnecessary tests or treatments. An incorrect presumption that a patient has iron deficiency may lead to inappropriate iron therapy or to unnecessary diagnostic procedures such as colonoscopy to detect gastrointestinal bleeding.

The clinical history is crucial. A family history of thalassemia raises the suspicion for this diagnosis. A history of previously normal hemoglobin levels and RBC indices, significant bleeding, or pica (cravings for nonfood items such as clay or dirt) leads to the diagnosis of iron deficiency (Chapter 17). The most common pica symptom in the United States is pagophagia, the craving to chew on ice.

IDA and β-thalassemia minor are best differentiated using the serum ferritin level, serum iron level, total iron-binding capacity, transferrin saturation, and Hb A_2 level, along with a CBC and examination of a peripheral blood film (Table 17.1).[45,52-54] Additional testing may include soluble transferrin receptor and less commonly, zinc protoporphyrin levels.

Before the Hb A_2 level is evaluated for β-thalassemia minor, iron deficiency should be ruled out first, as patients with thalassemia can have IDA as a comorbidity. Low iron levels in patients with β-thalassemia minor reduce the Hb A_2 level; therefore iron stores should be replenished before laboratory analysis for Hb A_2 is undertaken to avoid detection of falsely decreased (or normal rather than elevated) levels of Hb A_2 due to the lack of iron.[45] This is particularly important in carrier states, as it can lead to incorrect interpretation that thalassemia is not present.

A mild erythrocytosis (high RBC count) and marked microcytosis (low MCV) are found more commonly in β-thalassemia

minor. In IDA, the RBC count and MCV may be normal or decreased, depending on whether the deficiency is developing or longstanding (early depletion of iron stores vs. chronic iron depletion) (Chapter 9). The RDW can be normal or increased in both β-thalassemia minor and IDA, with a significant overlap of values; therefore the RDW alone cannot distinguish these conditions.[52-55] Basophilic stippling can be observed on the peripheral blood film in β-thalassemia minor, which can distinguish it from IDA. Target cells can be found in both conditions; thus their presence does not help discriminate between the two disorders.

Because of the challenges of differentiating IDA and thalassemia minor, discrimination indices (a set of values or calculations used to evaluate for the presence of a disease) with a high sensitivity and specificity have been actively sought. More than 40 discrimination indices have been proposed to distinguish β-thalassemia minor from IDA, using an individual parameter such as the RBC count, hemoglobin concentration, MCV, MCH, or RDW, or simple calculations based on various parameters such as the Mentzer index (MCV/RBC), Green and King index ($MCV^2 \times RDW/100 \times Hb$), or microcytic RBC %/hypochromic RBC % ratio (M/H ratio).[53-55] A 2015 meta-analysis published by Hoffmann and colleagues[55] on the 12 most common discrimination indices in the literature found that results were variable among individual studies and populations, and their sensitivity in discriminating β-thalassemia minor and IDA ranged from 62% to 92% with similar results found in other studies.[53,54] Low sensitivity leads to a high number of false-negative results and inability to adequately discriminate between thalassemia and IDA. The various discrimination indices available for screening for β-thalassemia minor should be properly validated and used with caution. and may have limited value.[3,9,52-54]

Newer instrumentation values such as mean reticulocyte hemoglobin (CHr, MCHCr, and Ret-He), mean reticulocyte volume (MCVr), and immature reticulocyte fraction (IRF) have led to additional studies and development of new discrimination indices for differentiating between IDA and β-thalassemia trait.[56] One study evaluated an index that combined CHr with RBC parameters ([RBC × MCHC × 50/ MCV]/CHr) to discriminate between thalassemia and IDA (sensitivity 96%, specificity 97%, and accuracy 96.4%).[56] In addition to discrimination indices, another interesting approach by Jahangiri and colleagues[57] compared the application of a Bayesian decision tree and machine learning (data mining techniques) with classification and regression trees to evaluate IDA and β-thalassemia trait with a sensitivity of 96% and a specificity of 93% in the test data sets using more of an algorithmic approach. Techniques and calculations to easily and accurately differentiate thalassemia minor/trait and IDA continue to be explored and evaluated. Discrimination indices and decision trees to distinguish IDA from β-thalassemia trait could be particularly useful in areas where there is limited access to advanced technology (e.g., molecular testing, HPLC) and thalassemia prevalence is high.

SUMMARY

- Thalassemias are a group of heterogeneous disorders in which one or more globin chains are reduced or absent.
- Thalassemias result in a hypochromic microcytic anemia due to decreased production of hemoglobin. The imbalance of globin chain synthesis causes an excess of the normally produced globin chain that damages the red blood cells (RBCs) or their precursors and results in premature hemolysis and ineffective erythropoiesis.
- β-Thalassemia is caused by mutations that affect the β-globin gene complex. It is clinically manifested as a silent carrier state, β-thalassemia minor, β-thalassemia intermedia, and β-thalassemia major. Symptomatic thalassemia can also be classified as transfusion-dependent thalassemia or nontransfusion-dependent thalassemia, which guides treatment decisions.
- New therapies target the thalassemia pathophysiology: α/non-α-globin imbalance (gene editing by CRISPR-Cas9, Hb F-inducing agents, gene insertion by lentiviral vector), ineffective erythropoiesis (agents that enhance erythroid maturation and JAK2 inhibitors), and iron overload (chelation, hepcidin mimetics or stimulators, ferroportin inhibitors).
- In the silent carrier state (β^{silent}/β), the blood picture is completely normal. β-Thalassemia minor or trait is a heterozygous state, with one β-globin gene mutation and a slight reduction in β chain production and Hb A. It results in a mild, asymptomatic, microcytic hypochromic anemia, usually characterized by an elevated Hb A_2 level, which aids in diagnosis.
- β-Thalassemia major is a homozygous or compound heterozygous state with two β-globin gene mutations, resulting in a reduction or absence of β chain production and thus a reduction in or absence of Hb A. It is a severe anemia characterized by α/β chain imbalance and precipitation of excess α chains in erythroid precursors, causing ineffective erythropoiesis. Patients are dependent on transfusions for life. Severe iron overload develops due to repeated transfusions and increased iron absorption by intestinal enterocytes, requiring ongoing iron chelation therapy.
- β-Thalassemia intermedia manifests abnormalities with a severity between those of β-thalassemia major and β-thalassemia minor. Patients are not dependent on transfusions but can develop iron overload due to increased iron absorption, requiring periodic iron chelation therapy.
- α-Thalassemia is most commonly caused by a deletion of one, two, three, or all four of the α-globin genes, resulting in reduced or absent production of α chains. In the fetus, unpaired γ chains form γ_4 tetramers, called *Hb Bart*. In infancy through adulthood, unpaired β chains form β_4 tetramers, called *Hb H*. Both Hb Bart and Hb H have a high oxygen affinity and are unable to effectively transport oxygen to the tissues.
- α-Thalassemia is divided clinically into a silent carrier state, α-thalassemia minor, Hb H disease, and Hb Bart hydrops fetalis syndrome.
- Silent carrier α-thalassemia is a result of the deletion (or, rarely, a nondeletional mutation) of one of four α-globin genes ($-\alpha/\alpha\alpha$) or ($\alpha^{ND}\alpha/\alpha\alpha$); it is associated with a normal RBC profile and is asymptomatic. α-Thalassemia minor is a result of the deletion of two α-globin genes ($-\alpha/-\alpha$ or $--/\alpha\alpha$) and is clinically similar to β-thalassemia minor except that Hb A_2 is not increased.
- Hb H disease is a result of the deletion of three of the four α-globin genes ($--/-\alpha$); Hb H inclusions (β_4 tetramers) precipitate in older circulating RBCs, causing a hemolytic anemia. The RBCs are microcytic and hypochromic, and the disease is clinically similar to β-thalassemia intermedia.
- In Hb Bart hydrops fetalis syndrome, all four of the α-globin genes are deleted ($--/--$). There is severe anemia, and fetal death usually occurs in utero or shortly after birth. The predominant hemoglobin in the fetus is Hb Bart (γ_4).
- The preliminary diagnosis of thalassemia is made from the complete blood count results and RBC morphology, iron studies, supravital staining, and hemoglobin fraction quantification by hemoglobin electrophoresis, high-performance liquid chromatography, and/or capillary zone electrophoresis. Molecular genetic testing is required for definitive diagnosis in prenatal testing, preconception risk assessment/carrier detection in couples, and identification of rare or complex mutations.
- Thalassemia trait must be differentiated from other microcytic hypochromic anemias, especially iron deficiency anemia. Iron studies are important for this differentiation.

Now that you have completed this chapter, go back and read again the case study at the beginning and respond to the questions presented. Answers can be found in Appendix C.

REVIEW QUESTIONS

Answers can be found in Appendix C.

1. Thalassemia is caused by:
   a. Structurally abnormal hemoglobins
   b. Absent or reduced synthesis of a globin chain of hemoglobin
   c. Excessive absorption of iron
   d. Reduced or absent protoporphyrin synthesis

2. Thalassemia is more prevalent in individuals from areas along the tropics because it confers:
   a. Resistance to heat in heterozygotes with a thalassemia mutation
   b. Selective advantage against tuberculosis
   c. Resistance to severe malaria in heterozygotes with a thalassemia mutation
   d. Selected advantage against tick-borne illnesses

3. The hemolytic anemia and ineffective erythropoiesis associated with β-thalassemia is due to:
   a. A structurally abnormal hemoglobin
   b. Oxidation of hemoglobin to Heinz bodies
   c. Uncoupling of the RBC membrane from the cytoskeleton
   d. Precipitation of excess α chains in RBCs and their precursors

4. β-Thalassemia minor (heterozygous) usually exhibits:
   a. Increased Hb H
   b. 10% to 35% Hb F
   c. No Hb A
   d. Increased Hb A_2

5. RBC morphologic features in β-thalassemia major usually include:
   a. Microcytes, hypochromia, target cells, RBC inclusions, NRBCs
   b. Macrocytes, acanthocytes, target cells, polychromasia, NRBCs
   c. Microcytes, hypochromia, target cells, sickle cells, elliptocytes
   d. Macrocytes, hypochromia, target cells, RBC inclusions, NRBCs

6. β-thalassemia major of the genotype $β^0/β^0$ can be differentiated from the $β^+/β^+$ genotype by the amount of:
   a. Hb A
   b. Hb A_2
   c. Hb F
   d. Hb H

7. Homozygotes for deletional-type HPFH are characterized by:
   a. 10% to 35% Hb F with normal RBC morphology
   b. 100% Hb F with slightly hypochromic microcytic RBCs
   c. 1% Hb F with normal RBC morphology
   d. 5% to 15% Hb F with slightly hypochromic microcytic RBCs

8. What abnormal hemoglobin is present in adults with α-thalassemia, genotype $(– –/α –)$?
   a. A_2
   b. F
   c. H
   d. Bart

9. Hb Bart is composed of:
   a. Two α and two β chains
   b. Two ε and two γ chains
   c. Four β chains
   d. Four γ chains

10. When one α gene is deleted $(α –/αα)$, a patient has:
    a. Normal hemoglobin levels
    b. Mild anemia (hemoglobin range 9 to 11 g/dL)
    c. Moderate anemia (hemoglobin range 7 to 9 g/dL)
    d. Marked anemia requiring regular transfusions

11. In which part of the world is the α gene mutation causing Hb Bart hydrops fetalis $(– –/– –)$ most common?
    a. Northern Africa
    b. Mediterranean
    c. Middle East
    d. Southeast Asia

12. A patient with a hemoglobin concentration of 8.0 g/dL and an MCV of 62 fL had microcytes, target cells, and a few sickle cells on his peripheral blood film. High-performance liquid chromatography showed 25% Hb A, 65% Hb S, 6% Hb A_2, and 4% Hb F. These results are most compatible with:
    a. Sickle cell trait
    b. Sickle cell anemia
    c. Hb S-$β^0$-thalassemia
    d. Hb S-$β^+$-thalassemia

13. Hb H inclusions in a supravital stain preparation appear as:
    a. A few large, blue, round bodies in the RBCs with aggregated reticulum
    b. Uniformly stained blue cytoplasm in the RBC
    c. Small, evenly distributed, greenish-blue granules that pit the surface of RBCs
    d. Uniform round bodies that adhere to the inner RBC membrane

14. Which of the following laboratory findings is INCONSISTENT with β-thalassemia minor?
    a. A slightly elevated RBC count and marked microcytosis
    b. Target cells and basophilic stippling on the peripheral blood film
    c. Hemoglobin level of 10 to 13 g/dL
    d. Elevated MCHC and spherocytic RBCs

15. A 9-month-old infant of Asian heritage is seen for severe fatigue and pallor. Her hemoglobin concentration is 6.5 g/dL with an MCV of 59 fL; microcytosis, hypochromia, poikilocytosis, basophilic stippling, Howell Jolly bodies, Pappenheimer bodies, and nucleated RBCs are noted on the peripheral blood film. High-performance liquid chromatography showed 0% Hb A, 96% Hb F, and 4% Hb A_2. These findings should lead the provider to suspect:
    a. β-thalassemia major, $β^0/β^0$
    b. β-thalassemia major, $β^+/β^+$
    c. Severe iron deficiency anemia
    d. Homozygous α-thalassemia $(– –/– –)$

REFERENCES

1. Cooley, T. B., & Lee, P. (1925). A series of cases of splenomegaly in children with anemia and peculiar bone changes. *Trans Am Pediatr Soc, 37,* 29–33.
2. Whipple, G. H., & Bradford, W. L. (1932). Racial or familial anemia of children associated with fundamental disturbances of bone and pigment metabolism (Cooley-von Jaksch). *Am J Dis Child, 44,* 336–365.
3. Sheth, S. (2023). Thalassemia syndromes. In Hoffman, R., Benz, E. J., Silberstein, L. E., et al. (Eds.), *Hematology: Basic Principles and Practice.* (8th ed., pp. 555–584). Philadelphia: Elsevier.
4. Modell, B., & Darlison, M. (2008). Global epidemiology of haemoglobin disorders and derived service indicators. *Bull World Health Org, 86,* 480–487.
5. Goheen, M. M., Campino, S., & Cerami, C. (2017). The role of the red blood cell in host defense against falciparum malaria: an expanding repertoire of evolutionary alterations. *Br J Haematol, 179,* 543–556.

6. Taher, A., Musallam, K., & Cappellini, M. (Eds.) (2017). *Guidelines for the Management of Non-Transfusion-Dependent Thalassaemia (NTDT).* 2nd ed. Nicosia, Cyprus: Thalassaemia International Federation. https://thalassaemia. org.cy/publications/tif-publications/guidelines-for-the-clinical-management-of-non-transfusion-dependent-thalassaemias-updated-version/ Accessed January 25, 2023.

7. Weatherall, D. J., & Clegg, J. B. (2001). Inherited haemoglobin disorders: an increasing global health problem. *Bull World Health Organ, 79,* 704–712.

8. Taylor, S. M., Parobek, C. M., & Fairhurst, R. M. (2012). Haemoglobinopathies and the clinical epidemiology of malaria: a systematic review and meta-analysis. *Lancet Infect Dis, 12* (6), 457–468.

9. Jeng, M., & Neufeld, E. (2018). Thalassemia syndromes: quantitative disorders of globin chain synthesis. In Greer, J. P., Arber, D. A., Glader, B., et al. (Eds.), *Wintrobe's Clinical Hematology.* (14th ed., pp. 865–914). Philadelphia: Wolters Kluwer Health.

10. Sheth, S., & Thein, S. L. (2021). Thalassemias: a disorder of globin synthesis. In Kaushansky, K., Prchal, J. T., Burns, L. J., et al. (Eds.), *Williams Hematology.* (10th ed., pp. 725–758). New York: McGraw-Hill Education.

11. Giardine, B., Borg, J., Viennas, E., et al (2014). Updates of the HbVar database of human hemoglobin variants and thalassemia mutations. *Nucleic Acids Res, 42*(Database issue), D1063–D1069. https://doi.org/10.1093/nar/gkt911.

12. Camaschella, C., & Nai, A. (2016). Ineffective erythropoiesis and regulation of iron status in iron loading anaemias. *Br J Haematol, 172,* 512–523.

13. Longo, F., Piolatto, A., Ferrero, G. B., et al. (2021). Ineffective erythropoiesis in β-thalassaemia: key steps and therapeutic options by drugs. *Int J Mol Sci, 22,* 7229.

14. Cappellini, M. D., Farmakis, D., Porter, J., et al. (Eds) (2021). *2021 Guidelines for the Management of Transfusion Dependent Thalassaemia (TDT).* 4th ed. Version 2.0. Nicosia, Cyprus: Thalassaemia International Federation.https://www.thalassemia. org/wp-content/uploads/2021/06/TIF-2021-Guidelines-for-Mgmt-of-TDT.pdf Accessed January 25, 2023.

15. Origa, R. Beta-thalassemia. 2000 Sep 28 [Updated 2021 Feb 04]. In: Adam, M. P., Mirzaa, G. M., Pagon, R. A., et al., editors. *GeneReviews® [Internet].* Seattle (WA): University of Washington, Seattle; 1993-2022. https://www.ncbi.nlm.nih.gov/books/ NBK1426/. Accessed July 26, 2022.

16. Srole, D. N., & Ganz, T. (2021). Erythroferrone structure, function, and physiology: iron homeostasis and beyond. *J Cell Physiol, 236*(7), 4888–4901.

17. Kim, A., & Nemeth, E. (2015). New insights into iron regulation and erythropoiesis. *Curr Opin Hematol, 22,* 199–205.

18. Ganz, T., Jung, G., Naeim, A., et al. (2017). Immunoassay for human serum erythroferrone. *Blood, 130,* 1243–1246.

19. Musallam, K. M., Rivella, S., Vichinsky, E., et al. (2013). Non-transfusion-dependent thalassemias. *Haematologica, 98,* 833–844.

20. Asadov, C., Alimirzoeva, Z., Mammadova, T., et al. (2018). β-Thalassemia intermedia: a comprehensive overview and novel approaches. *Int J Hematol 108*(1), 5–21.

21. Gilman, J. G., Huisman, T. H., & Abels, J. (1984). Dutch beta 0-thalassaemia: a 10 kilobase DNA deletion associated with significant gamma-chain production. *Br J Haematol, 56,* 339–348.

22. Oggiano, L., Pirastu, M., Moi, P., et al. (1987). Molecular characterization of a normal Hb A2 beta-thalassaemia determinant in a Sardinian family. *Br J Haematol, 67,* 225–229.

23. Cappellini, M. D., Porter, J. B., Viprakasit, V., et al. (2018). A paradigm shift on beta-thalassaemia treatment: how will we manage this old disease with new therapies? *Blood Rev, 32*(4), 300–311.

24. Marsella, M., & Borgna-Pignatti, C. (2014). Transfusional iron overload and iron chelation therapy in thalassemia major and sickle cell disease. *Hematol Oncol Clin North Am, 28,* 703–727.

25. Baronciani, D., Angelucci, E., Potschger, U., et al. (2016). Hemopoietic stem cell transplantation in thalassemia: a report from the European Society for Blood and Bone Marrow Transplantation Hemoglobinopathy Registry, 2000–2010. *Bone Marrow Transplant, 51,* 536–541.

26. Musallam, K. M., Bou-Fakhredin, R., Cappellini, M. D., et al. (2021). 2021 update on clinical trials in β-thalassemia. *Am J Hematol, 96*(11), 1518–1531.

27. Motta, I., Bou-Fakhredin, R., Taher, A. T., et al. (2020). Beta thalassemia: new therapeutic options beyond transfusion and iron chelation. *Drugs, 80*(11), 1053–1063.

28. Wienert, B., Martyn, G. E., Funnell, A. P. W., et al (2018). Wake-up sleepy gene: reactivating fetal globin for β-hemoglobinopathies. *Trends Genet, 34*(12), 927–940.

29. Payán-Pernía, S., Bernal Noguera, S., Rojas Rodríguez, E., et al. (2020). Mild thalassemia intermedia due to interaction of δβ-thalassemia with triplicated α-globin genes. *Hemoglobin, 44*(4), 294–296.

30. Hariharan, P., Kishnani, P., Sawant, P., et al. (2020). Genotypic-phenotypic heterogeneity of δβ-thalassemia and hereditary persistence of fetal hemoglobin (HPFH) in India. *Ann Hematol, 99*(7), 1475–1483.

31. Doerfler, P. A., Feng, R., Li, Y., et al. (2021). Activation of γ-globin gene expression by GATA1 and NF-Y in hereditary persistence of fetal hemoglobin. *Nat Genet, 53*(8),1177–1186.

32. Stephens, A. D., Angastiniotis, M., Baysal, E., et al. (2012). ICSH recommendations for measurement of haemaglobin F. *Int J Lab Hematol, 34,* 14–20.

33. Chui, D. H. K., Fucharoen, S., Chan, V. (2003). Hemoglobin H disease: not necessarily a benign disorder. *Blood, 101,* 791–800.

34. Tamary H., & Dgany, O. Alpha-thalassemia. 2005 Nov 1 [Updated 2020 Oct 1]. In: Adam, M. P., Mirzaa, G. M., Pagon, R. A., et al., editors. *GeneReviews® [Internet].* Seattle (WA): University of Washington, Seattle; 1993–2022. Available from: https://www. ncbi.nlm.nih.gov/books/NBK1435/ Accessed August 5, 2022.

35. Singsanan, S., Fucharoen, G., Savongsy, O., et al. (2007). Molecular characterization and origins of Hb Constant Spring and Hb Pakse in Southeast Asian populations. *Ann Hematol, 86,* 665–669.

36. Fucharoen, S., & Viprakasit, V. (2009). Hb H disease: clinical course and disease modifiers. *Am Soc Hematol Educ Program,* 26–34.

37. Wilkie, A. O., Zeitlin, H. C., Lindenbaum, R. H., et al. (1990). Clinical features and molecular analysis of the alpha thalassemia/mental retardation syndromes. II. Cases without detectable abnormality of the alpha globin complex. *Am J Hum Genet, 46,* 1127–1140.

38. Higgs, D. R. (2004). Gene regulation in hematopoiesis: new lessons from thalassemia. *Hematology Am Soc Hematol Educ Program,* 1–13.

39. Wykretowicz, J., Song, Y., McKnight, B., et al. (2019). A diagnosis of discernment: identifying a novel ATRX mutation in myelodysplastic syndrome with acquired α-thalassemia. *Cancer Genet, 231–232,* 36–40.

40. Sun, X., Shen, J., & Wang, L. (2021). Insights into the role of placenta thickness as a predictive marker of perinatal outcome. *J Int Med Res, 49*(2), 300060521990969.

41. Steinberg, M. H., Rosenstock, W., Coleman, M. B., et al. (1984). Effects of thalassemia and microcytosis on the hematologic and vasoocclusive severity of sickle cell anemia. *Blood, 63,* 1353–1360.

42. Colaco, S., Colah, R., & Nadkarni, A. (2022). Significance of borderline Hb A2 levels in β thalassemia carrier screening. *Sci Rep, 12*(1), 5414.

43. Pan, L. L., Eng, H. L., Kuo, C. Y., et al. (2005). Usefulness of brilliant cresyl blue staining as an auxiliary method of screening for alpha-thalassemia. *J Lab Clin Med, 145,* 94–97.

44. Gallivan, M. V. E., & Giordano, P. C. (2012). Analysis of hemoglobinopathies, hemoglobin variants and thalassemias. In Kottke-Marchant, K., & Davis, B. H. (Eds.), *Laboratory Hematology Practice.* West Sussex, UK: Wiley-Blackwell.

45. Stephens, A. D., Angastiniotis, M., Baysal, E., et al. (2012). ICSH recommendations for the measurement of haemoglobin A2. *Int J Lab Hematol, 34,* 1–13.

46. Giordano, P. C. (2013). Strategies for basic laboratory diagnostics of the hemoglobinopathies in multi-ethnic societies: interpretation of results and pitfalls. *Int J Lab Hematol, 35,* 465–479.

47. Chopra, P., Bhardwaj, S., Negi, P., et al. (2020). Comparison of two high-pressure liquid chromatography instruments Bio-Rad Variant-II and Tosoh HLC-723G11 in the evaluation of hemoglobinopathies. *Indian J Hematol Blood Transfus, 36*(4), 725–732.

48. Sabath, D. E. (2017). Molecular diagnosis of thalassemias and hemoglobinopathies: an ACLPS critical review. *Am J Clin Pathol, 148,* 6–15.

49. Mahmud, N., Maffei, M., Mogni, M., et al. (2021). Hemoglobin A2 and heterogeneous diagnostic relevance observed in eight new variants of the delta globin gene. *Genes, 12*(11), 1821.

50. Wild, B. J., & Bain, B. J. (2004). Detection and quantitation of normal and variant haemoglobins: an analytic review. *Ann Clin Biochem, 41,* 355–369.

51. Tatu, T., & Sweatman, D. (2018). Hemolysis area: a new parameter of erythrocyte osmotic fragility for screening of thalassemia trait. *J Lab Physicians, 10*(2), 214–220.

52. Traeger-Synodinos, J., Harteveld, C. L., Old, J. M., et al. (2015). EMQN haemoglobinopathies best practice meeting. EMQN best practice guidelines for molecular and haematology methods for carrier identification and prenatal diagnosis of the haemoglobinopathies. *Eur J Hum Genet, 23*(4), 426–437.

53. Ntaois, G., Chatzinikolaou, A., Saouli, Z., et al. (2007). Discrimination indices as screening tests for β-thalassemia trait. *Ann Hematol, 86,* 487–491.

54. Nalbantoglu, B., Guzel, S., Buyukyalcin, V., et al. (2012). Indices used in differentiation of thalassemia trait from iron deficiency anemia in pediatric population. Are they reliable? *Pediatr Hematol Oncol, 29,* 472–478.

55. Hoffmann, J. J. M. L., Urrechaga, E., & Aguirre, U. (2015). Discriminant indices for distinguishing thalassemia and iron deficiency in patients with microcytic anemia: a meta-analysis. *Clin Chem Lab Med, 53,* 1883–1894.

56. Vicinanza, P., Vicinanza, M., Cosimato, V., et al (2018). Mean reticulocyte hemoglobin content index plays a key role to identify children who are carriers of β-thalassemia. *Translational medicine @ UniSa, 17,* 31–36.

57. Jahangiri, M., Rahim, F., Saki, N., et al. (2021). Application of Bayesian decision tree in hematology research: differential diagnosis of β-thalassemia trait from iron deficiency anemia. *Comput Math Methods Med,* 1–10.

26

Nonmalignant Leukocyte Disorders

Steven Marionneaux*

After the completion of this chapter, the reader will be able to:

1. Compare the genetic defects, pathologic mechanisms, and clinical and laboratory findings in the primary immunodeficiencies discussed in the chapter.
2. Explain how the presence of Pelger-Huët cells during blood film review could be misinterpreted as a neutrophilic left shift.
3. Describe peripheral blood film abnormalities in Alder-Reilly anomaly and May-Hegglin anomaly and their similarity to other conditions.
4. Associate various lysosomal storage diseases with their underlying pathologic conditions and clinical and laboratory manifestations.
5. Define neutrophilia, neutropenia, lymphocytosis, lymphocytopenia, monocytosis, monocytopenia, eosinophilia, and basophilia.
6. List acquired conditions associated with quantitative changes in leukocyte subtypes.
7. Compare in vivo and in vitro alterations in leukocyte morphology with normal cells.
8. Outline the pathogenesis and clinical and laboratory features of infectious mononucleosis.
9. Given the patient history, clinical and laboratory findings, and representative cells from a peripheral blood film or bone marrow smear, interpret results to determine the type of nonmalignant leukocyte disorder, and recommend additional tests to confirm a diagnosis.

Primary Immunodeficiency Disorders/Inborn Errors of Immunity
  Severe Combined Immune Deficiency
  Wiskott-Aldrich Syndrome
  22q11.2 Deletion Syndrome
  Bruton Tyrosine Kinase Deficiency
  Chédiak-Higashi Syndrome
  Congenital Defects of Phagocyte Number and/or Function
Lysosomal Storage Disorders
  Mucopolysaccharidoses
  Sphingolipidoses
Morphologic Abnormalities of Leukocytes Without Associated Immune Deficiency
  Pelger-Huët Anomaly
  Pseudo– or Acquired Pelger-Huët Anomaly

  Neutrophil Hypersegmentation
  Alder-Reilly Anomaly
  May-Hegglin Anomaly
Quantitative Abnormalities of Leukocytes
  Quantitative Abnormalities of Neutrophils
  Quantitative Abnormalities of Eosinophils
  Quantitative Abnormalities of Basophils
  Quantitative Abnormalities of Monocytes
  Quantitative Abnormalities of Lymphocytes
Secondary Morphologic Changes in Leukocytes
  Storage Artifacts in Leukocytes
  Secondary Changes in Neutrophils and Monocytes
  Eosinophils and Basophils
  Lymphocytes
Infectious Mononucleosis

*The author extends appreciation to Scott Dunbar for his assistance with some of the figures in this chapter.

CASE STUDY

After studying the material in this chapter, the reader should be able to respond to the following case study. Answers can be found in Appendix C.

A 25-year-old woman was seen by her primary care physician with a complaint of fatigue. Physical examination revealed pale conjunctiva. The remainder of the examination was unremarkable. The patient indicated she was experiencing heavier than normal bleeding during menses. Complete blood count results were as follows. Reference intervals can be found after the Index at the end of the book.

WBC	8.1 × 10⁹/L	MCHC	29 g/dL
HGB	8.6 g/dL	PLT	172 × 10⁹/L
MCV	65 fL		

WBC 8.1 × 10^9/L MCHC 29 g/dL
HGB 8.6 g/dL PLT 172 × 10^9/L
MCV 65 fL

Because of the low mean cell volume, a blood film review was performed. Apparent immature granulocytes were present (Figure 26.1) and a manual differential was performed:

Segmented neutrophils	9	Lymphocytes	30
Bands	21	Monocytes	7
Metamyelocytes	16	Eosinophils	2
Myelocytes	14	Basophils	1

1. Do you agree with the classification of the immature granulocytes shown? If not, provide an explanation in morphologic terms.
2. The patient was subsequently diagnosed with iron deficiency anemia. Based on the cell images shown, what other hematologic diagnosis is suspected?

3. Provide an approach to correcting the results of the WBC differential that does not require repeating the test.
4. What are clinical implications of reporting the manual differential results above if a left shift does not actually exist?

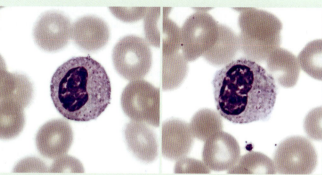

Figure 26.1 Examples of Cells Classified as Immature Granulocytes in the Differential for the Patient in the Case. (Peripheral blood, Wright-Giemsa stain, Cellavision DC-1, ×1000.) (Courtesy Cellavision AB, Lund, Sweden.)

This chapter focuses on leukocyte disorders not associated with clonal or neoplastic changes in hematopoietic precursor cells. The cause of these disorders can be genetic or acquired, and result in quantitative, functional, and/or morphologic changes in one or more lineages: neutrophils, lymphocytes, monocytes, eosinophils, and/or basophils. Some of these disorders are associated with significant clinical manifestations.

PRIMARY IMMUNODEFICIENCY DISORDERS/ INBORN ERRORS OF IMMUNITY

As of June 2022, nearly 500 (inherited) inborn errors of immunity (IEI) or primary immunodeficiency disorders have been identified, each originating from a single germline genetic abnormality affecting the innate or adaptive immune system.[1] Most individual IEIs are rare; however, as a group, the prevalence of diagnosed IEIs the United States is approximately 1 in 1200 individuals.[2]

The mechanisms of disease, clinical manifestations, and disease severity among the IEIs can vary based on the nature of the gene defect and its pattern of inheritance. In each IEI, a missense mutation, deletion, or frame shift mutation leads to a reduced quantity and/or quality of the encoded protein, altering normal functioning within the innate or adaptive immune system. This can have a wide range of effects from life-threatening manifestations that arise in infants to manageable disorders diagnosed in adults.

This section illustrates the heterogenous clinical presentations associated with IEI by reviewing a select number of diseases within the classification schema from the International Union of Immunological Societies Expert Committee[1] and will mainly include diseases associated with peripheral blood morphologic abnormalities.

Severe Combined Immune Deficiency

Severe combined immune deficiency (SCID) includes a group of IEIs associated with defects in both cellular and humoral immunity.[1] Nearly all patients with SCID experience a marked decrease in circulating T cells, poorly functioning B cells, hypogammaglobulinemia, and profound clinical symptoms that manifest in infancy. Left untreated, most patients with SCID die within the first 2 years of life from overwhelming bacterial, viral, and/or fungal infections. Potentially curative options in SCID are allogeneic hematopoietic stem cell transplantation (HSCT) and gene therapy, in which the goal is reconstitution of the failed immune system. The outcomes in patients treated with HSCT have improved over the past decade. Most patients with SCID who undergo HSCT can expect to survive well into adulthood.[3] In the United States, gene therapy is not yet approved for SCID. However, gene therapy is an option for patients treated in clinical trials in which there has been promising success. However, even with gene therapy, there remains a significant risk of leukemic transformation in SCID patients.[1]

Common Gamma Chain Deficiency/X-Linked Severe Combined Immune Deficiency

Common gamma chain deficiency/X-linked SCID is classified as T–B+ SCID[1] and is the most common SCID. This disease initiates from a mutation in *IL2RG* located at Xq13.1. *IL2RG* normally encodes the gamma chain protein within receptor complexes that bind interleukin-2 (IL-2), IL-4, IL-7, IL-9, IL-15, and IL-21. These interleukins provide growth, differentiation, and survival signals for T and natural killer (NK) lymphocytes. In common gamma chain deficiency, a mutation in *IL2RG* leads to truncated gamma chain proteins and faulty signal transduction that impairs T and NK cell development. Infants with the disease have no thymus, tonsils, or lymph nodes and often experience severe life-threatening infections within the first few months of life as protective maternal immunoglobulins are depleted. Prompt diagnosis of common gamma chain deficiency is key in implementing preventive measures in anticipation of these infections. The white blood cell (WBC) count in affected infants is decreased as a result of severely decreased T and NK lymphocytes. B cells are generally adequate in number but are dysfunctional without T cell signaling. In common gamma chain deficiency, there is failure to thrive and death usually occurs before 2 years without HSCT.

Adenosine Deaminase Deficiency (ADA-SCID)

Adenosine deaminase deficiency (ADA-SCID) is classified as T–B– SCID[1] and represents 10% to 20% of SCID cases. It is an autosomal recessive disorder caused by a mutation in the *ADA* gene located at chromosome 20q13.12. Adenosine deaminase is a key component in the metabolic breakdown of adenosine triphosphate (ATP) and RNA in all cells. In ADA-SCID, there is intracellular and extracellular accumulation of toxic levels of adenosine and deoxyadenosine in lymphocytes, causing profound decreases in T, B, and NK cells. Patients with ADA-SCID experience severe recurring, life-threatening bacterial, viral, and fungal infections beginning early in life. Additional manifestations include skeletal abnormalities, neurologic deficits, and skin rashes.[1]

Wiskott-Aldrich Syndrome

Wiskott-Aldrich syndrome (WAS) is classified as a combined immunodeficiency with associated or syndromic features.[1] WAS is a rare X-linked disease caused by one of more than 450 mutations in the *WAS* gene,[4] which results in decreased Wiskott-Aldrich syndrome protein (WASP) expression. Disease severity and clinical manifestations in WAS can vary based on the type of mutation present and its impact on WASP expression. WASP controls RNA polymerase II–dependent transcription and has a critical role in actin cytoskeleton remodeling of hematopoietic cells. Low WASP levels have an impact on the stability of the immunologic synapse, the site where T-cells and antigen-presenting cells interact. Abnormal reorganization of the cytoskeleton results in defective T cell function and impaired interaction with lymphocytes, leading to decreased B cells. NK cells are normal or increased in number but have diminished cytotoxic activity. Regulatory T cells involved in autoimmunity are dysfunctional.[5] WASP deficiency also diminishes neutrophil chemotaxis, phagocytosis and other steps involved in the killing of microorganisms, which increases susceptibility to infections. There is a risk of bleeding because of thrombocytopenia, small abnormal platelets, and shortened platelet survival, which is the result of increased immune-related and nonimmune-related destruction and ineffective megakaryocytopoiesis.

WAS diagnosis is typically confirmed through *WAS* gene sequencing in patients with suspected disease. HSCT can be curative in patients with human leukocyte antigen (HLA)-matched donors.[6,7] Gene therapy is a promising approach most appropriate for patients with WAS who lack a matched donor.[8]

There is, however, a significant risk for the development of acute leukemia.

22q11.2 Deletion Syndrome

22q11.2 deletion syndrome (22DS)/DiGeorge syndrome/velocardiofacial syndrome is classified as a combined immunodeficiency with associated syndromic features.[1] The genetic aberration in 22DS is a heterozygous microdeletion of 1.5 to 3 million base pairs on chromosome 22 at q11.2 resulting in a loss of over 100 genes and their encoded protein products.[9,10] The deletion breakpoint and genes lost in the deletion can differ among patients, contributing to the variable clinical phenotype. Haploinsufficiency caused by the loss of T-box transcription factor 1 gene (*TBX1*), DiGeorge Syndrome Critical Region 8 (*DGCR8*), and several microRNAs result in congenital malformations and other clinical manifestations in 22DS.[10] Variable degrees of thymic hypoplasia proportionally affect the severity of immune dysfunction, autoimmunity, and T lymphopenia.

Abnormal development of the embryonic pharyngeal system during gestation produces characteristic cardiac anomalies, thymus and parathyroid hypoplasia, and craniofacial deformations in 22DS patients. A wide array of additional clinical findings includes intrauterine growth restriction, major infections, failure to thrive, short stature, skeletal defects, neuropsychiatric diseases, developmental delays, gastrointestinal diseases, ophthalmologic disorders, hypocalcemia, immune thrombocytopenia, and autoimmune hemolytic anemia. Genetic testing confirms the 22DS diagnosis in patients with the characteristic presentation. The survival of affected infants is often less than 1 year without thymic tissue transplantation or HLA-matched HSCT with memory T cells. Graft-versus-host disease is a common complication after HSCT. In a survey of 17 athymic patients with 22DS who underwent HSCT between 1995 and 2006, 41% were alive at a median followup of 5.8 years.[11]

Bruton Tyrosine Kinase Deficiency

Classified as an antibody deficiency, Bruton tyrosine kinase (BTK) deficiency/X-linked agammaglobulinemia is caused by a mutation in the gene encoding BTK (Xq21.3-Xq22), a signal transduction protein that promotes B-cell lineage development.[1] A mutation in *BTK* leads to marked reduction in B cells, absent tonsils and adenoids, inability to produce plasma cells, and therefore severe decreases in all immunoglobulin isotypes and grossly defective antibody responses. The lack of a humoral immune response leaves the patient susceptible to infections from encapsulated bacteria, bloodborne enteroviruses, and certain fungal and parasitic infections.

The disease manifests clinically after maternal antibodies clear from the BTK-deficient infant's circulation, between 3 and 18 months. Recurrent otitis, conjunctivitis, diarrhea, and sinus and skin infections are common. The disease is often first suspected when the child experiences a severe life-threatening bacterial infection. Molecular genetic testing is needed to confirm the diagnosis. The management of BTK deficiency consists primarily of immunoglobulin replacement therapy. Most patients diagnosed today will live well into adulthood because of earlier recognition, advancements in immunoglobulin therapies, and improvements

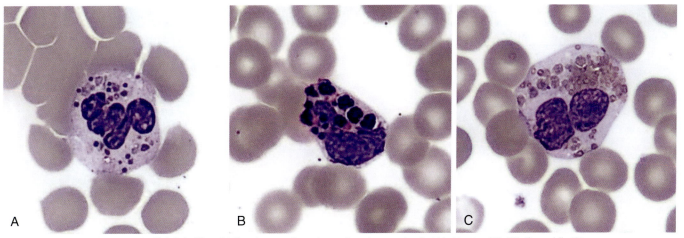

Figure 26.2 Chédiak-Higashi Syndrome. Fused cytoplasmic granules in (A), Neutrophil. (B), Basophil. (C), Eosinophil. (Peripheral blood, Wright-Giemsa stain, Cellavision DC-1, ×1000.) (Courtesy Cellavision AB, Lund, Sweden.)

in antimicrobials. Recent studies of gene therapy to restore normal BTK function in mice have shown promising findings.[12]

Chédiak-Higashi Syndrome

Chédiak-Higashi syndrome (CHS) is a rare autosomal recessive disease of immune dysregulation classified as a familial hemophagocytic lymphohistiocytosis syndrome with hypopigmentation.[1,13] CHS is caused by a mutation in the lysosomal trafficking regulator (*LYST*) gene on chromosome 1q42.3. The mutation leads to the formation of giant fused cytoplasmic granules/inclusions in leukocytes, platelets, fibroblasts, melanocytes, and other granulated cells in nerve tissue, kidney, and gastric mucosa. On peripheral blood films, the inclusions can be seen in granulocytes (Figure 26.2), monocytes, large granular lymphocytes (NK and cytotoxic T cells), and platelets. Patients with CHS often have cytopenias, particularly neutropenia. Clinical manifestations present in infancy as partial albinism, severe recurrent life-threatening bacterial infections, mild bleeding, easy bruising, and progressive neurologic impairment. In suspected patients, genetic testing for mutations in *LYST* is done to confirm the diagnosis. Patients with CHS are at high risk of developing an aggressive, life-threatening syndrome of excessive immune activation known as hemophagocytic lymphohistiocytosis. Most children with CHS will succumb to the disease before 7 years unless treated with HSCT.[14] HSCT using matched donors has proven successful; however, it does not prevent neurologic deterioration.[15]

Pseudo–Chédiak-Higashi (PCH) granules/inclusions resemble the fused lysosomal granules in CHS. PCH granules are seen most often in acute myeloid leukemia (AML). One study reported PCH granules in the leukemic cells of 5 of 20 children with AML.[16] PCH granules are also associated with chronic myeloid leukemia, myelodysplastic neoplasms (MDSs), and rarely, in acute lymphoblastic leukemia.[17]

Congenital Defects of Phagocyte Number and/or Function

The congenital defects of phagocytes include a heterogeneous group of qualitative and quantitative disorders affecting phagocytic cells of the innate immune system, primarily neutrophils, monocytes, and/or macrophages. As of 2022, there were 42 distinct disease entities, each originating from a unique genetic abnormality.[1] These diseases are organized into four subgroups, (1) congenital neutropenias, (2) defects of motility, (3) defects of respiratory burst, and (4) other nonlymphoid defects. A common thread in all phagocyte diseases is an increased susceptibility to bacterial and fungal infections. Dermatologic symptoms, delayed wound healing, growth failure, and inflammation of the oral mucosa are also common. A wide array of additional clinical symptoms are associated with the individual diseases. This section highlights several phagocyte disorders that arise from different underlying mechanisms.

Congenital Neutropenia

Congenital neutropenia (absolute neutrophil count [ANC] less than $1.5 \times 10^9/L$) is associated with a variety of nonmalignant conditions covered in this chapter in which the decrease in neutrophils results from decreased production, increased destruction, or apoptosis. The congenital neutropenias (CNs) are a group of inherited diseases in which the primary defect is in the production of neutrophils.[1] Common to all CNs is early clinical onset, frequently in infancy, and an increased risk of primarily bacterial and fungal infections arising from neutropenia rather than some other immune deficiency. In some CNs, there are nonhematologic manifestations such as neurologic/cognitive defects, dysmorphic features, and organ dysfunction.

Severe congenital neutropenia. Severe congenital neutropenia (SCN) is a subset of CN characterized by an ANC less than $0.5 \times 10^9/L$ (often less than $0.2 \times 10^9/L$) and recurring, severe, often life-threatening bacterial and fungal infections with or without nonhematologic manifestations and an increased risk of malignancy, frequently MDS or AML. Mutations in the neutrophil elastase gene *ELANE* (causing SCN1) are responsible for 50% to 60% of all SCN cases.[18] Ten subtypes of SCN are listed in Table 26.1.[1,19,20]

Bone marrow examination in patients with SCN shows a maturation arrest in the neutrophil series at the myelocyte/promyelocyte stage and dysmorphic changes in neutrophilic cells.

TABLE 26.1   Severe Congenital Neutropenias

Subtype	Gene	Inheritance	Location	Disease	Associated Features*
SCN1	ELANE	AD	19p13.3	Elastase deficiency	Mild anemia, thrombocytopenia, monocytosis, eosinophilia, osteopenia
SCN2	GFI1	AD	1p22.1	GFI1 deficiency	Monocytosis, lymphopenia, IG
SCN3	HAX1	AR	1q21.3	Kostmann disease	Neurologic defects
SCN4	G6PC3	AR	17q21.31	G6PC3 deficiency	BM dysplasia, anemia, thrombocytopenia, HSM; cardiac, urogenital, skeletal, endocrine, and vascular abnormalities, deafness
SCN5	VPS45	AR	1q21.2	VPS45 deficiency	BM fibrosis, EMH, anemia, anisopoikilocytosis, thrombocytopenia, NRBC, enlarged kidneys, HSM, delayed development, blindness, no response to G-CSF in some
SCN6	JAGN1	AR	3p25.3	JAGN1 deficiency	Short stature, facial dysmorphia, hypothyroidism, urogenital anomalies
SCN7	CSFCR	AR	1p34.3	GCSF receptor deficiency	No response to G-CSF
SCN8	SRP54	AD	14q13.2	SRP54 deficiency	Groups A and B patients: short stature, pancreas dysfunction, poor response to G-CSF. Group B also has developmental delay, autism
SCN9	CLPB	AD	11q13.4	3-Methylglutaconic deficiency	Neurocognitive defects, cataracts, cardiac defects, facial dysmorphia, hypothroidism
SCNX	WAS	XL	Xp11.23	X-linked neutropenia	Low normal platelets, monocytopenia

*SCN1–SCN9 and SCNX are all associated with severe neutropenia and recurring acute, severe, life-threatening infections.
AD, Autosomal dominant; *AR*, autosomal recessive; *BM*, bone marrow; *EMH*, extramedullary hematopoiesis; *HSM*, hepatosplenomegaly; *IG*, immature granulocytes in blood; *NRBC*, nucleated red blood cells in peripheral blood; *SCN*, severe congenital neutropenia; *XL*, sex-linked.

The mainstay of treatment in SCN is long-term granulocyte colony-stimulating factor (G-CSF), which is effective in most patients at increasing the absolute neutrophil count and decreasing the rate of infections and mortality. While the risk of malignancy in SCN is thought to be a complication of the disease, long-term G-CSF therapy increases this risk.[21] After 15 years on G-CSF, the cumulative risk of AML/MDS is 22%.[22] Patients who do not respond to G-CSF or require higher doses to maintain adequate neutrophil counts and infection prophylaxis are often considered for HSCT.

Cyclic neutropenia. Cyclic neutropenia is a CN caused by *ELANE* mutations but is a less severe disease compared to SCN1, which also stems from *ELANE* mutations. Patients with cyclic neutropenia experience characteristic episodes of severe neutropenia (less than 0.2×10^9/L) together with absolute monocytosis in approximately 21-day cycles, each lasting 3 to 5 or more days. During the ANC nadir, patients often experience mouth ulcers, sore throat, gingivitis, rash, fatigue, fever, and/ or cervical lymphadenopathy. The risk of life-threatening infections in cyclic neutropenia is much lower than in SCN1 and there is no increased risk of malignant transformation.

Shwachman-Diamond syndrome. Shwachman-Diamond syndrome (SDS) is classified as a CN with associated neutrophil functional defects.[1] SDS is a rare disease but a common bone marrow failure syndrome. SDS is caused by a mutation in *SBDS* which encodes SBDS, a key component in ribosome maturation, cell proliferation, and maintenance of the bone marrow microenvironment. Biallelic mutations in *SBDS* occur in most patients, resulting in a truncated nonfunctional SBDS protein and both neutropenia and impaired neutrophil chemotaxis. Patients are usually diagnosed in infancy with pancreatic insufficiency and associated malabsorption and steatorrhea. There are also skeletal abnormalities, severe infections, and failure to thrive. Additional manifestations of SDS often include developmental delays and bone marrow failure with dysplasia, cytopenias, and increased risk of AML or MDS, particularly in patients who develop multiple hematopoietic cell clones with *TP53* mutations.[23] The diagnosis of SDS in suspected patients is achieved though molecular genetic testing, typically DNA sequencing. G-CSF is used in patients with neutropenia and severe infections. Allogeneic HSCT can potentially cure SDS patients with bone marrow failure and MDS or AML; however, there is no effect on the nonhematologic manifestations. Outcome data in SDS patients treated with HSCT are limited.

Defects of Motility

As leukocytes (primarily neutrophils and monocytes) leave circulation to move to a site of infection, they adhere to the vascular endothelium and tissue matrix and roll along the vessel wall. Adhesion molecules such as selectins and integrins expressed on endothelial cells and leukocytes mediate this process, interacting with ligands on the surface of leukocytes to slow the speed of neutrophils in circulation. Ligand binding induces high-affinity attachment of integrins with endothelial cell receptors, facilitating leukocyte transmigration between gaps in endothelial cells (diapedesis) (Chapter 10).

Leukocyte adhesion disorders. Leukocyte adhesion disorders (LADs) are rare autosomal recessive primary immunodeficiency disorders characterized by the inability of neutrophils and monocytes to move from peripheral circulation to sites of infection. Patients with LAD have recurring infections and impaired wound healing and, depending on the LAD subtype, they may also have developmental abnormalities and/or increased risk of bleeding. Absolute neutrophilia is present in LAD, especially evident during infections. LAD subtype is determined through genetic testing, typically DNA sequencing. Allogeneic HSCT has been shown to be a potentially curative therapy in severe LAD-I and LAD-III. A 2021 review of transplant data in 84 patients from 33 sites found a 3-year overall survival estimate of 83%.[24] There are three subtypes of LAD.

Leukocyte adhesion disorder type I. LAD-1 is the most common type, caused by a mutation in *ITGB2*, which encodes the CD18 subunit of β2 integrins. The mutation leads to decreased production or a truncated form of β2 integrin and diminished neutrophil adhesion to endothelial cells, recognition of bacteria, and outside-in signaling. In LAD-I, neutrophils accumulate in peripheral circulation but cannot reach sites of infection in tissues because of the adhesion problem. T-cell function is also impaired in LAD-I. As of March 2023, 177 different mutations had been described[25] that can have differing effects on the quantity and quality of the encoded β2 integrin. Shortly after birth, LAD-I infants experience severe recurring infections, most often of the skin, oral mucosa, gastrointestinal tract, respiratory tract, and perirectal area.

In addition, LAD-I infants usually have lymphadenopathy, splenomegaly, neutrophilia, and lack of pus formation. The clinical severity of LAD-I is heterogeneous and largely related to the specific *ITGB2* mutation and its impact on β2 integrins.[25]

Leukocyte adhesion disorder type II. LAD-II is caused by 1 of 16 mutations in SLC35C1, which codes for a fucose transporter in the Golgi system.[25] The mutation leads to a lack of or a dysfunctional transporter and diminished fucosylation of cell surface glycoproteins that serve as ligands for L-selectins on leukocytes. The adhesion and rolling of leukocytes along endothelial cells of the vessel wall toward the site of infection depends on the binding of L-selectins on leukocytes with E or P selectins on endothelial cells, with their matching ligands on opposite cells. Therefore in LAD-II, a lack of fucosylated glycoprotein ligands for L-selectin decreases the adhesion of leukocytes to the vascular endothelium and impairs their transmigration to sites of infection. Fortunately, β2 integrins are also activated through alternate pathways not affected by the *SLC35C1* mutation. This provides partial functioning leukocyte adhesion and transmigration that is less impaired than that in LAD-I. Consequently, infections in LAD-II patients tend to be fewer and less severe than in LAD-I. On the other hand, the lack of fucosylation in LAD-II affects glycoproteins other than selectins, leading to severe cognitive impairment, skeletal abnormalities, growth retardation, and distinctive facial features.

Leukocyte adhesion disorder type III. LAD-III is caused by 1 of 31 mutations in *FERMT3*.[25] *FERMT3* encodes kindlin-3 (fermitin family homolog 3), which is required for normal inside-out signaling of hematopoietic cells and activation of β1, β2, and β3 integrins. In LAD-III, integrin expression is normal;

however, the integrins fail to respond to external signals, which limits neutrophil adhesion, NK cell activity, and platelet function. Patients with LAD-III experience severe recurrent infections, osteoporosis, and bleeding. Without treatment with HSCT, the prognosis of infants with LAD-III is poor.

Defects of Respiratory Burst: Chronic Granulomatous Disease

Chronic granulomatous disease (CGD) is a rare condition caused by the decreased ability of neutrophils, monocytes, macrophages, and eosinophils to kill phagocytized bacteria and yeast. This is due to a failure in the respiratory burst and failed production of powerful antimicrobial superoxide anions and other reactive oxygen species, including hydrogen peroxide, hypochlorous acid, and others. The failed respiratory burst in CGD is caused by a mutation in one of six genes that encode protein components in the reduced form of nicotinamide adenine dinucleotide phosphate (NADPH) oxidase, which is required in the respiratory burst. Approximately two-thirds of CGD cases are inherited as X-linked recessive and one-third are autosomal recessive. X-linked recessive patients generally have a more severe disease course with shortened survival compared with autosomal recessive patients. In normal individuals, phagocytosis of foreign organism leads to phosphorylation and binding of cytosolic p47phox and p67phox. Primary granules containing antibacterial neutrophil elastase and cathepsin G and secondary granules containing the cytochrome complex gp91phox and p22phox migrate to the phagolysosome. NADPH oxidase forms when p47phox and p67phox, along with p40phox and RAC2, combine with the cytochrome complex. The principal antimicrobial agent, superoxide, is generated in the phagolysosome during the respiratory burst, when an electron from NADPH is added to oxygen. In addition, NADPH has regulatory functions in the generation of other antimicrobial agents. Most cases of CGD are due to mutations in the genes coding for gp91phox or p47phox. The six genes implicated in CGD and their encoded protein products are listed in Table 26.2.[26]

Patients with CGD experience life-threatening catalase-positive bacterial and fungal infections, as well as inflammatory complications such as colitis and granuloma formation in the gastrointestinal tract, urinary tract, and other organs. Neutrophil

TABLE 26.2 Genes Involved in Chronic Granulomatous Disease

Gene	Location	Inheritance	Protein Product
CYBB	Xp21.1	XLR	gp91phox
CYBA	16q24	AR	p22phox
NCF1	7q11.23	AR	p47phox
NCF2	1q25	AR	p67phox
NCF4	22q13.1	AR	p40phox
CYBC1(EROS)	17q25.3	AR	Essential for reactive oxygen species (EROS)

AR, Autosomal recessive; *XLR,* sex-linked recessive.

function tests such as dihydrorhodamine 123 or nitroblue tetrazolium test can be used to screen suspected patients. Positive screening tests are followed with DNA sequencing to confirm the diagnosis. The optimal management of mild to moderately severe CGD involves long-term antimicrobial prophylaxis plus quick recognition and aggressive treatment of acute infections and inflammatory complications. Over the past two decades, studies using HSCT in CGD have shown significant improvements in outcomes and reductions in morbidity and mortality. A 2018 review of data from nine studies reported an overall event-free survival of more than 80% and overall survival of approximately 90% at 3 years after HSCT.[27]

Enzymatic White Blood Cell Defects: Myeloperoxidase Deficiency

Myeloperoxidase (MPO) deficiency is the most common inherited disorder of phagocytes. MPO is an enzyme found in high concentration in primary azurophilic granules of neutrophils and in lower concentration in the lysosomal granules of monocytes. In neutrophils, MPO catalyzes the conversion of H_2O_2 to HOCL and other microbicidal reactive oxygen intermediates. MPO plays an important role in the killing of phagocytized bacteria and yeast and participates in the formation of neutrophil extracellular traps (NETs), another mechanism for eliminating microorganisms.[28] The *MPO* gene is located on chromosome 17q23. Pathogenic mutations lead to decreased MPO production, limiting its participation in microbicidal activities. Nevertheless, most MPO-deficient individuals are asymptomatic. This is because neutrophils employ additional pathways for generating microbicidal agents. Although less potent, these pathways provide adequate protection against pathogens in the majority of individuals with MPO deficiency. However, there have been reports of increased susceptibility to fungal infections in MPO deficiency when comorbid diseases are present.[29,30]

Automated hematology analyzers that use MPO in the WBC differential method are limited in the analysis of MPO-deficient patients (Chapter 13).

LYSOSOMAL STORAGE DISORDERS

The inborn errors of metabolism consist of 1450 disorders divided into 24 categories and 124 groups.[31] These are mostly single gene defects affecting enzymes that metabolize substrates into various components. In most cases, the enzyme deficiency leads to a buildup of toxic substances that are the source of clinical manifestations. The inborn errors of metabolism include the lysosomal storage disorders (LSDs) a group of over 70 inherited diseases. In the LSDs, single gene mutations negatively affect the production, transport and secretion of lysosomal enzymes.[32] Failed degradation of macromolecules and gradual buildup ("storage") of undigested substrates within lysosomes result in cell dysfunction, cell death, and a variety of clinical symptoms. All cells containing lysosomes are potentially affected. LSDs are classified according to the undigested macromolecule(s) that accumulates in the cell. Subtypes of LSDs include sphingolipidoses, pseudobasophilia, mucolipidoses, mucopolysaccharidoses (MPSs), lipoprotein storage disorders, and lysosomal transport defects. The more common LSDs are presented in this chapter.

Mucopolysaccharidoses

The MPSs are a rare group of inherited disorders of mucopolysaccharide or glycosaminoglycan degradation. The combined incidence in the United States for all subtypes is 1 per 100,000 live births.[33] MPS types I, II, and III have the highest incidence. As of 2021, only four cases of MPS type IX had been reported.[33] The MPSs are caused by reduced activity in enzymes necessary for the degradation of one or more substrates: dermatan sulfate, heparan sulfate, keratan sulfate, chondroitin sulfate, and hyaluronan. The partially degraded material builds up in lysosomes, causing serious clinical consequences and shortened survival. Table 26.3 provides genetic, biological, and clinical information about MPS subtypes, along with the deficient enzymes and accumulated substrates.[32,34,35]

The peripheral blood films of patients with MPS may show metachromatic Reilly bodies (acquired Alder-Reilly anomaly [ARA]) in neutrophils, monocytes, and lymphocytes. Bone marrow macrophages (histiocytes) also can demonstrate cytoplasmic metachromatic material. Diagnosis relies on assays that measure the specific enzymes deficient in each subtype. Genetic testing to identify pathologic mutations can be performed for diagnostic confirmation. MPS treatment includes supportive care, enzyme replacement therapy, and/or HSCT. Gene therapy is a promising treatment approach and clinical studies are ongoing in patients with MPS types I, II, IIIA, and IV.[36]

Sphingolipidoses

The sphingolipidoses are a group of LSDs with functional deficiencies in enzymes needed for lysosomal breakdown of sphingolipids, causing harmful accumulation of various phospholipids in tissues. The pathways involved in sphingolipid catabolism, specific enzyme deficiencies, and corresponding storage diseases are outlined in Figure 26.3. Gaucher disease and Niemann-Pick disease are examples of sphingolipidoses and are described in more detail in the following sections.

Gaucher Disease

Gaucher disease (GD) is the most common LSD. It is an autosomal recessive disorder triggered by a defect or deficiency in the catabolic enzyme β-glucocerebrosidase, which is necessary for glycolipid metabolism. As a result, unmetabolized substrate sphingolipid glucocerebroside accumulates in the lysosomes of macrophages throughout the body, including osteoclasts in bone and microglia in the brain.[37] GD stems from a mutation in *GBA* located at 1q21-q22. More than 400 pathogenic mutations have been reported and, although some correlations have been found between specific mutations and patient outcomes, most clinical phenotypes cannot be predicted by genotype.[38]

There are three types of GD, and type I is by far the most common. Neurologic symptoms are key factors in differentiating subtypes. The phenotype is quite heterogeneous. Some patients are asymptomatic, whereas others experience a multitude of clinical problems. Clinical information associated with the three types of GD is provided in Table 26.4.

TABLE 26.3 Mucopolysaccharidoses

Name	Also Known As	Enzyme Deficiency	AS	Gene and Location	Clinical Features
MPS I	Hurler syndrome,* Hurler-Scheie syndrome,† and Scheie syndrome†	Alpha-L-iduronidase	DS + HS	IDUA 4p16.3	*Severe phenotype (Hurler):* coarse facial features, skeletal abnormalities, severe intellectual disability, hepatosplenomegaly, corneal clouding, umbilical hernia, frequent upper respiratory tract infections
MPS II	Hunter syndrome	Iduronate 2-sulfatase	DS + HS	IDS Xq28	*Severe phenotype:* coarse facial features, hepatosplenomegaly, short stature, skeletal deformities, cardiovascular disorders, deafness, neurocognitive issues
MPS III A	Sanfilippo syndrome	N-Sulfoglucosamine sulfohydrolase	HS	SGSH 17q25.3	Hirsutism, coarse facial features, behavioral problems, aggressive behavior, speech delay, hepatomegaly
MPS III B	Sanfilippo syndrome	Alpha-N-acetylglucosaminidase	HS	NAGLU 17q21.2	Cardiomegaly, coarse facial features, progressive dementia, convulsions,
MPS III C	Sanfilippo syndrome	Heparan-alpha-glucosaminide N-acetyltransferase	HS	HGSNAT 8p11.21	Delayed psychomotor development, behavioral problems, sleep disorder, hearing loss, coarse facial features, recurring infections, diarrhea, epilepsy, and retinitis pigmentosa
MPS IV A	Morquio syndrome	N-Acetylgalactosamine-6-sulfatase	KS + CS	GALNS 16q24.3	Musculoskeletal abnormalities, short stature, pulmonary and cardiac dysfunction, hearing loss, corneal clouding
MPS IV B	Morquio syndrome	Beta-galactosidase	KS	GLB1 3p22.3	Musculoskeletal abnormalities, short stature, pulmonary and cardiac dysfunction, hearing loss, corneal clouding
MPS VI	Maroteaux-Lamy syndrome	Arylsulfatase B	DS + CS	ARSB 5q14.1	*Severe form:* coarse facial features, severe skeletal abnormalities, joint stiffness, respiratory disease, cardiac disease, sleep apnea, pulmonary hypertension, corneal clouding, hepatosplenomegaly, macrocephaly, hearing loss
MPS VII	Sly disease	Beta-glucuronidase	HS + DS + CS	GUSB 7q11.21	Varies widely *Infantile:* hydrops fetalis *Severe:* like MPS I (Hurler) *Intermediate:* skeletal abnormalities, coarse facial features, variable cognitive impairment *Mild:* skeletal abnormalities
MPS IX	Natowicz syndrome	Hyaluronidase-1	HYAL	HYAL1 3p21.31	Facial dysmorphism; hepatosplenomegaly; cardiac, respiratory, and skeletal involvement; and neurologic, hematologic, and ocular symptoms

*Most severe.
†Attenuated phenotype.
AS, Accumulated substrate; *CS,* chondroitin sulfate; *DS,* dermatan sulfate; *HYAL,* hyaluronan; *HS,* heparin sulfate; *KS,* keratan sulfate; *MPS,* mucopolysaccharidoses.

In GD, macrophages containing excess glucocerebroside accumulate in the spleen, liver, and bone marrow and are primarily responsible for the disease manifestations. Gaucher cells are lysosome-engorged macrophages with eccentric nuclei and abundant fibrillar blue-gray cytoplasm with a striated or wrinkled appearance (sometimes described as onion skin-like) (Figure 26.4). Gaucher cells stain positive with trichrome, aldehyde fuchsin, periodic acid-Schiff (PAS) and acid phosphatase.[39] In untreated patients, Gaucher cells infiltrate the hematopoietic space in bone resulting in anemia and thrombocytopenia.

A commercially available test for β-glucosidase (glucocerebrosidase) is available to confirm the GD diagnosis. Genetic testing performed in suspected patients to screen for the most common mutations, including *N370S, 84GG, IVS2 +1G>A,* and *L444P.*[39] All three types of GD have been associated with an increased risk for developing hematopoietic neoplasms, most frequently plasma cell (multiple) myeloma.[40,41]

Treatment of GD includes enzyme replacement therapy and substrate reduction therapy.[42] HSCT offers the potential for cure; however, it is not often used because treatment-related mortality is high.[43] Gene therapy, genome editing, and chaperone therapy are additional modalities being pursued.

Pseudo-Gaucher cells. Pseudo-Gaucher cells are seen in bone marrow specimens from patients with thalassemia, myeloid neoplasms,[44,45] acute lymphoblastic leukemia,[46] non-Hodgkin lymphoma,[46] and plasma cell neoplasms.[47] In these diseases, pseudo-Gaucher cells are thought to result from increased cell turnover overwhelming the glucocerebrosidase enzyme, causing accumulation of glucosylceramide in macrophages. Therefore pseudo-Gaucher cells result from a relative rather than true decrease in enzyme. Pseudo- and true

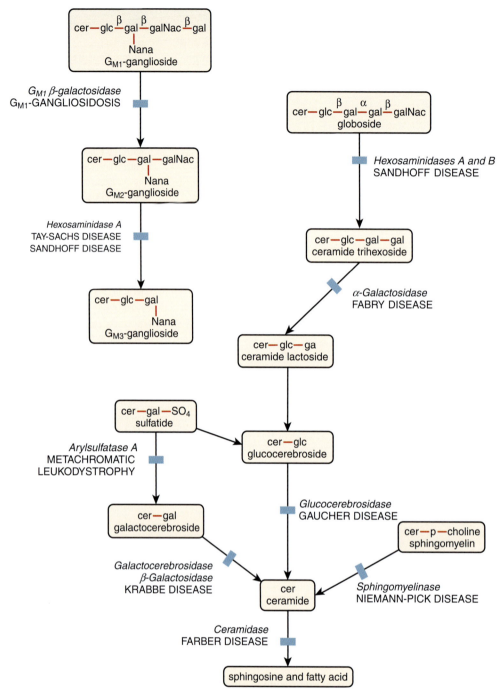

Figure 26.3 Pathways and Diseases of Sphingolipid Metabolism. (From Orkin, S. H., Fisher, D. E., & Look, A. T., et al. [2009]. *Nathan and Oski's Hematology of Infancy and Childhood*. [7th ed.]. Philadelphia: Saunders.)

TABLE 26.4	**Clinical Subtypes of Gaucher Disease***		
	Type I: Nonneuronopathic	**Type II: Acute Neuronopathic**	**Type III: Subacute Neuronopathic**
Age at presentation	Childhood/adulthood	Infancy	Childhood/adulthood
Hepatosplenomegaly	+ → +++	+	+ → +++
Skeletal abnormality	− → +++	−	++ → +++
CNS disease	−	+++	+ → +++
Life span	6–80+ years	<2 years	2–60 years
Ethnicity	Ashkenazi Jews	Panethnic	Panethnic, Swedes

*Severity of disease features are indicated as − to +++.
CNS, Central nervous system.

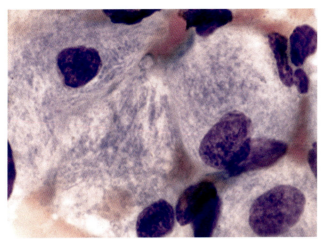

Figure 26.4 Characteristic Macrophages in Patient with Gaucher Disease. Note cytoplasmic striations in the cytoplasm. (Bone marrow, hematoxylin and eosin stain, ×1000.)

Gaucher cells are usually indistinguishable using routine stains. However, electron microscopy shows that pseudo-Gaucher cells contain needle-like inclusions, not the tubular inclusions found in Gaucher cells.

Niemann-Pick Disease

Niemann-Pick (NP) disease has three subtypes. Types A and B, also known as acid sphingomyelinase deficiency (ASMD), are characterized by an accumulation of fat in cellular lysosomes of vital organs, impairing their function and leading to a range of clinical manifestations. NP types A and B are caused by recessive mutations in the *SMPD1* gene on chromosome 11p15.4. The mutations result in a deficiency of lysosomal hydrolase enzyme acid sphingomyelinase (ASM) and a subsequent buildup of the substrate sphingomyelin in the liver, spleen, and lungs. More than 200 pathogenic mutations in *SMPD1* have been identified.[48]

Foam cells and *sea-blue histiocytes* are found in bone marrow specimens from patients with all three types of NP. Foam cells are macrophages with cytoplasm packed with lipid-filled lysosomes that appear as small vacuoles (foam) after staining (Figure 26.5). Sea-blue histiocytes are also lipid-filled macrophages, containing ceroid, a product of cytoplasmic oxidation and polymerization of unsaturated lipids that appear blue on Romanowsky-type staining. In addition to NP disease, bone marrow sea-blue histiocytes are seen in chronic myeloid leukemia (CML), MDS, lymphoma, and other diseases.

NP type A (acute neuronopathic form). NPA manifests in infancy in which there is a failure to thrive, lymphadenopathy, hepatosplenomegaly, vision problems, and rapid neurodegenerative decline that ends in death, usually by 4 years. In NPA, there is less than 5% normal sphingomyelinase activity.

NP type B (nonneuronopathic form). NPB has approximately 10% to 20% normal enzyme activity. NPB presents in the first decade to adulthood with a variable clinical course. Although there is no neurocognitive impairment, patients experience massive hepatosplenomegaly, heart disease, and pulmonary insufficiency.

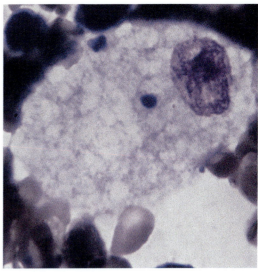

Figure 26.5 Niemann-Pick Cell. Note eccentric nucleus and bubble-like pattern of storage deposits in the cytoplasm. (Bone marrow, hematoxylin and eosin stain, ×1000.) (From Carr, J. H. [2022]. *Clinical Hematology Atlas.* [6th ed.]. St. Louis: Elsevier.)

To confirm the diagnosis of NPA and NPB, guidelines recommend enzymatic quantitation of sphingomyelinase activity in peripheral blood lymphocytes or cultured skin fibroblasts as first-line testing. Gene sequencing to identify *SMPD1* mutations can be done in patients who demonstrate sphingomyelinase deficiency in initial testing.[49] Genetic testing screens for three genes responsible for more than 90% of cases in the Ashkenazi Jewish population and one gene in approximately 90% of type B patients from North Africa.[39,50] Treatment of NPA and NPB primarily consists of enzyme replacement therapy (ERT), although it is ineffective at slowing the progression of neurologic disease in patients with NPA. Most patients with type A succumb to the disease within the first 3 years of life. The prognosis in type B can vary, with some patients living into adulthood; however, quality of life in these patients is often significantly affected by disease-related issues. In 2022, the US Food and Drug Administration (FDA) approved the ERT olipudase alfa as the first disease-modifying treatment for NPA and NPB.[51] Its impact on survival has yet to be determined.

NP type C. NPC is a rare autosomal recessive LSD caused by a mutation in the *NPC1* or *NP2* gene (95% and 5% of cases, respectively). The mutation leads to impaired cellular trafficking and homeostasis of cholesterol and subsequent buildup of unesterified cholesterol in lysosomes. The clinical presentation in NPC is heterogeneous regarding age of onset, type and severity of neurologic and psychiatric symptoms, and visceral involvement. Early diagnosis of NPC is key because substrate reduction therapy can slow the progression of neurologic damage; however, because of its heterogeneous presentation, diagnosis of NPC is often challenging. A suspicion index tool for NPC has proven to be highly sensitive and specific at making a presumptive diagnosis.[52]

Current guidelines recommend serum biomarker testing of oxysterols, lyso-SM-509, and/or lysosphingomyelin as first-line screening for NPC.[53] Mutation analysis of the *NPC1* and *NP2*

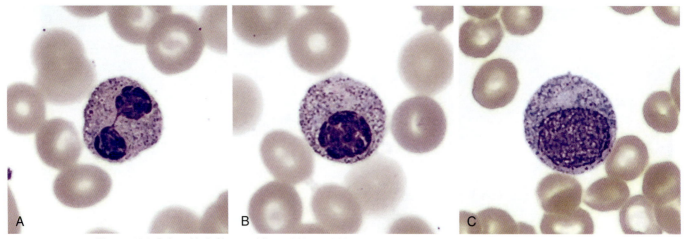

Figure 26.6 Pelger-Huët Neutrophils and Normal Myelocyte. **(A)**, Pince-nez or bilobed Pelger-Huët neutrophil. **(B)**, Unilobed Pelger-Huët neutrophil. **(C)**, Normal myelocyte. Note the hypercondensed, chunky chromatin pattern in the Pelger-Huët neutrophils and other differentiating morphologic characteristics between the unilobed Pelger-Huët neutrophil and myelocyte. (Peripheral blood, Wright-Giemsa stain, ×1000.) (Courtesy Cellavision AB, Lund, Sweden.)

genes follows positive screening tests to confirm the suspected diagnosis. As of February 2023, there were no approved treatments for NPC. Current therapies focus on symptom relief. NPC has a poor prognosis, with a median age of death of 13 years.[54]

MORPHOLOGIC ABNORMALITIES OF LEUKOCYTES WITHOUT ASSOCIATED IMMUNE DEFICIENCY

Pelger-Huët Anomaly

Pelger-Huët anomaly (PHA), or true/congenital PHA, is a benign autosomal dominant disorder characterized by neutrophils with decreased nuclear segmentation and a distinctive, coarse chromatin pattern. PHA is typically seen in neutrophils, although similar nuclear abnormalities are sometimes observed in other leukocytes. The prevalence of PHA is approximately 1 in 4785 in the United States.[55] The disorder stems from a mutation in the lamin B receptor *(LBR)* gene. The encoded lamin B receptor is an inner nuclear membrane protein involved in leukocyte nuclear segmentation and chromatin organization during normal cell maturation. Nearly all cases of PHA are heterozygous, with approximately 50% expression of the lamin B receptor.[56] Most neutrophils in the heterozygote exhibit coarse chromatin and bilobed nuclei connected by a thin filament, the classic "pince-nez" appearance most often associated with PHA (Figure 26.6, A). However, PHA nuclei also may be round, ovoid, and/or peanut shaped (Figure 26.6, B); however, these variants seem to be unfamiliar to some morphologists, who may confuse them with immature neutrophils (Figure 26.6, C). PHA neutrophils, regardless of nuclear shape, all exhibit the same characteristic coarse, chunky chromatin and are regarded as fully mature neutrophils. PHA neutrophils, appear to function normally, and heterozygotes are clinically well. In the rare homozygote, trace amounts of the lamin B receptor are produced, resulting in failed lobulation of the nuclei of neutrophils

and other WBCs. In homozygous PHA, cognitive impairment, heart defects, and skeletal abnormalities have been reported.[57]

Pseudo- or Acquired Pelger-Huët Anomaly

In pseudo-Pelger-Huët anomaly (PPHA), neutrophils with the distinctive nuclei can be seen in MDS, AML, and myeloproliferative neoplasms (MPNs). The underlying cause has been linked to the loss of nuclear lamin-B1 *(LMNB1)* gene on chromosome 5q, which can be disrupted in myeloid neoplasms.[58] PPHA neutrophils in MDS are indicative of granulocyte lineage dysplasia, a morphologic feature of the disease with diagnostic implications. PPHA is also associated with autoimmune diseases, severe bacterial infections, HIV, tuberculosis, mycoplasma pneumonia, and COVID-19 infection, in which disease severity has been shown to correlate with the number of PPHA neutrophils.[59,60] Drugs associated with PPHA morphology include immunosuppressants, chemotherapies, valproate, sulfisoxazole, fluconazole, ganciclovir, hematopoietic growth factors, ibuprofen, and others.[61]

Differences Between Pelger-Huet Neutrophils and Immature Granulocytes

The cytologic characteristics of Pelger-Huët (PH) type neutrophils can trigger morphologic flags on automated hematology analyzers[62] and subsequent microscopic examination of the blood film. Otherwise, PH neutrophils are an incidental finding during microscopic review for a different purpose. Either way, PH neutrophils must be recognized and not falsely reported as immature neutrophils. Because PH nuclei can be round, oval, or peanut shaped, the cells may be mistaken for myelocytes, metamyelocytes, or band neutrophils. The misclassification of PH neutrophils can lead to unnecessary tests, misdiagnosis, and inappropriate treatment. PH neutrophils are mature neutrophils, and guidelines state that these cells should be classified as *segmented neutrophils* with an attached interpretive comment.[36,63]

There are morphologic differences between PH neutrophils and immature neutrophils that can aid in their differentiation

(Figure 26.6). PH neutrophils are smaller and the nucleus-to-cytoplasm (N:C) ratio is lower than in immature neutrophils. PH neutrophils have darker, coarser, and more densely clumped chromatin than normal mature neutrophils, metamyelocytes, and myelocytes. Metamyelocytes and myelocytes generally show some degree of cytoplasmic basophilia, whereas PH neutrophils typically exhibit mature nonbasophilic cytoplasm with normal granulation, except that pseudo-PHA neutrophils in MDS may appear hypogranular.

Differentiating Between Pseudo- and True Pelger-Huët Neutrophils

Differentiating between PHA and PPHA can be difficult. It is important to consider the number of neutrophils exhibiting PH morphology. In PHA, the number of affected neutrophils is typically higher than in PPHA (greater than 68% versus less than 35%, respectively).[64,65] In PHA, all WBC lineages can be affected in terms of nuclear shape and chromatin structure, although it is not a common observation. In PPHA, the phenomenon is restricted to neutrophils. Furthermore, if PHA is suspected, careful examination of peripheral blood films of family members will often reveal PH morphology. Clinical correlation may also help in differentiating true from pseudo-PHA. Molecular testing can make the distinction if needed.

Neutrophil Hypersegmentation

Normal neutrophils contain three to five nuclear lobes separated by filaments. Hypersegmented neutrophils have more than five lobes and are most often associated with megaloblastic anemia (Chapter 18), in which these neutrophils are usually larger than normal (Figure 26.7). Hypersegmented neutrophils also can be seen in MDS, where they represent a form of dysplasia. In rare cases, hypersegmented neutrophils are an indication of hereditary neutrophil hypersegmentation. In this disorder, individuals are asymptomatic and have no signs of megaloblastic anemia.

Alder-Reilly Anomaly

Alder-Reilly anomaly (ARA) is a rare inherited disorder characterized by granulocytes (and sometimes monocytes and lymphocytes) filled with large, dark-staining metachromatic cytoplasmic granules (Figure 26.8). A more common acquired form is most often associated with mucopolysaccharidoses, discussed earlier in this chapter. The metachromatic granules are known as Reilly bodies, composed of partially digested mucopolysaccharides. Leukocyte function is not affected in ARA. Reilly bodies in neutrophils may be confused with toxic granulation; however, Reilly bodies also can be present in monocytes and lymphocytes, whereas toxic granulation is seen only in neutrophils. Also, neutrophilia with left shift, Döhle bodies, or both often accompany toxic granulation. These findings are not associated with ARA.

May-Hegglin Anomaly

May-Hegglin anomaly (MHA) is a rare autosomal-dominant disorder characterized by variable thrombocytopenia, giant platelets, and large Döhle body-like inclusions in

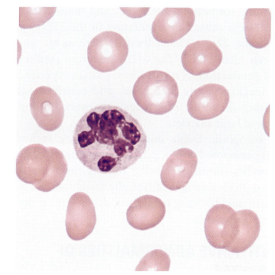

Figure 26.7 Hypersegmented Neutrophil. (Peripheral blood, Wright-Giemsa stain, ×1000.) (From Carr, J. H. [2022]. *Clinical Hematology Atlas*. [6th ed.]. St. Louis: Elsevier.)

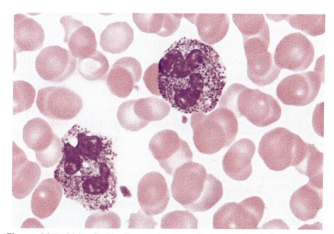

Figure 26.8 Alder-Reilly Anomaly. Note dark granules in both neutrophils. Similar granules also can be seen in eosinophils and basophils. (Peripheral blood, Wright-Giemsa stain, ×1000.) (Courtesy Dennis R. O'Malley, US Labs, Irvine, CA.)

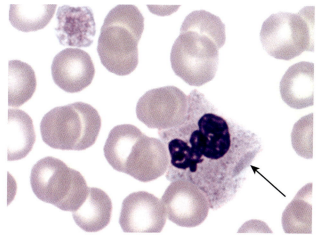

Figure 26.9 Neutrophil and Giant Platelet from a Patient with May-Hegglin Anomaly. Note the large, elongated, bluish inclusion *(arrow)* in the neutrophil cytoplasm. (Peripheral blood, Wright-Giemsa stain, ×1000.)

neutrophils, eosinophils, basophils, and monocytes (Figure 26.9). MHA is caused by a mutation in the *MYH9* gene on chromosome 22q12-13. At least 33 pathogenic mutations have been identified.[66] The MHA mutation results in disordered production of myosin heavy chain type IIA, which affects megakaryocyte maturation and platelet fragmentation during shedding from megakaryocytes, leading to the presence of large platelets.

The basophilic Döhle body-like leukocyte inclusions in MHA are composed of precipitated myosin heavy chains. True Döhle bodies consist of lamellar rows of rough endoplasmic reticulum. PHA patients are typically asymptomatic; however, some have mild bleeding tendencies, depending on the degree of thrombocytopenia.

QUANTITATIVE ABNORMALITIES OF LEUKOCYTES

Quantitative Abnormalities of Neutrophils

Neutrophils (bands plus segmented forms) normally represent around 50% to 70% of circulating WBCs in adults and an ANC of approximately 2 to 7×10^9/L. The ANC reference interval in children is about 1.5 to 8.5×10^9/L. Some clinicians prefer to also include metamyelocytes and myelocytes (if present) in the ANC calculation; however, this is not a common practice. The relative (%) concentrations of cells in the WBC differential should not be used to define neutrophilia, neutropenia, or other increases and decreases in different cell lineages.

Neutrophilia

Neutrophilia is an absolute increase in neutrophils greater than 7.0×10^9/L in adults or 8.5×10^9/L in children. Neutrophilia can result from a catecholamine-induced shift in neutrophils from the marginal pool (cells normally adhering to vessel walls) to the circulating pool. More often, neutrophilia occurs when there is an increase in bone marrow production or transfer of neutrophils from the bone marrow storage pool to the circulating pool (Chapter 10). An increase in circulating neutrophils often includes immature neutrophils such as metamyelocytes and myelocytes, defined as "left shift." Box 26.1 lists conditions associated with neutrophilia.

Leukemoid Reaction

The term leukemoid reaction (LR) is defined as an "extreme" reactive neutrophilic leukocytosis that often includes a left shift. The lower threshold to define an LR varies from 25 to 50×10^9/L. LRs are most associated with infections, including bacterial, viral, mycobacterial, treponemal, and occasionally COVID-19.[67] Toxic vacuoles in neutrophils when present in LRs suggest an infectious etiology.[68] LRs are also associated with nonmyeloid cancers, medications (steroids, lithium, minocycline, myeloid growth factors), intoxications, hemorrhage, hemolysis, and splenectomy. The mortality rate in hospitalized patients with a LR is approximately 45%.[68] Suspected cases of LR should be differentiated from CML, which has overlapping features. Characteristics helpful in differentiating between LR and CML are listed in Table 26.5.

Leukoerythroblastic Reaction

Leukoerythroblastic reaction (LER), also known as leukoerythroblastic picture or leukoerythroblastosis, refers to the presence of immature neutrophils and nucleated red blood cells in a peripheral blood film (Figure 19.4). Teardrop RBCs, when present in LER, suggest the presence of extramedullary hematopoiesis and myelofibrosis, most notably primary myelofibrosis. LER is most often associated with cancers involving space-occupying metastasis, lymphoma, leukemia, and primary myelofibrosis. LER is sometimes observed in hemolytic disorders, infections, hemorrhage, and other conditions.[69]

Neutropenia

Neutropenia is a decrease in the ANC to less than 1.5×10^9/L. The risk of infection increases as the ANC falls below 1.5×10^9/L. Severe neutropenia (less than 0.5×10^9/L) increases the risk of opportunistic infections, particularly in patients undergoing myelosuppressive treatments for cancer, and is often the threshold at which prophylactic antimicrobial therapy is initiated. Agranulocytosis refers to a neutrophil count of less than 0.1×10^9/L. The underlying mechanisms of neutropenia include

---

BOX 26.1   Causes of Neutrophilia

Emotional stress
Strenuous exercise
Trauma/injury
Pregnancy: labor and delivery
Eclampsia
Surgery
Infections: bacterial, some viral, including COVID-19
Burns
Myocardial infarction
Pancreatitis
Vasculitis
Colitis
Autoimmune disease
Acute hemorrhage
Chronic blood loss
Hemolysis
Smoking
Chronic blood loss
Metabolic ketoacidosis
Uremia
Leukocyte adhesion deficiency
Familial cold urticaria
Hereditary neutrophilia
Myeloproliferative neoplasm including chronic myeloid leukemia
Steroids (oral, injection)
Lithium
Colony-stimulating factors (G-CSF, GM-CSF)
Cortisol
Epinephrine

Adapted from Dale, D. C., & Welte, K. (2016). Neutropenia and neutrophilia. In Kaushansky, K., Lichtman, M. A., Prchal, J. T., et al. (Eds.), *Williams Hematology*. (9th ed., pp. 991–1004). New York: McGraw-Hill; and Reichard, K. (2010). Non-neoplastic granulocytic and monocytic disorders, excluding neutropenia. In Foucar, K., Reichard, K., & Czuchlewski, D. (Eds.), *Bone Marrow Pathology*. (3rd ed., Vol 1, pp. 180–205). Chicago: American Society for Clinical Pathology Press.

TABLE 26.5 Distinguishing Characteristics of Leukemoid Reaction and Chronic Myeloid Leukemia

	Leukemoid Reaction	Chronic Myeloid Leukemia
Eosinophils and basophils	Normal count and morphology	Often elevated; may show abnormal/immature morphologic features
Neophil morphology	Toxic granulation and Döhle bodies (more common if infectious cause)	May see pseudo–Pelger-Huët forms, hypogranular neutrophils, or both
Platelet count	Normal	May be increased earlier in chronic phase; decreased in accelerated and blast phases
Platelet morphology	Normal	May be abnormal, with large/giant, hypogranular, and/or bizarre forms
Hemoglobin	Normal	Often anemic
LAP score	Elevated	Decreased
Genetics	Normal	Positive for t(9;22); *BCR::ABL1*

LAP, Leukocyte alkaline phosphatase.

(1) increased rate of removal or destruction of peripheral blood neutrophils; (2) fewer neutrophils are released from bone marrow to peripheral blood because of decreased production of neutrophils or ineffective hematopoiesis, in which neutrophils are present in the bone marrow but are not released into circulation because they are defective; (3) decrease in the ratio of circulating versus marginal pool of neutrophils; or (4) a combination of these.

Acquired neutropenia. Neutropenia is most often an acquired condition. There are numerous causes of acquired neutropenia that are listed in Box 26.2.

Drug-induced neutropenia. Medications are the source of most cases of acquired neutropenia. Neutropenia has been associated with almost all classes of drugs and is due to myeloid suppression or immunologic response. Many agents used to treat cancer are known to induce neutropenia, including traditional myelosuppressive chemotherapeutics, targeted therapies, and immunotherapies. The mortality rate from neutropenia associated with cancer therapy is estimated at 12.5%.[70] Nonchemotherapy drug-induced severe neutropenia (ANC less than 0.5×10^9/L) most often manifests as an idiosyncratic reaction and has a mortality rate of approximately 5%.[71] The annual rate of occurrence of nonchemotherapy drug-induced neutropenia (ANC less than 1.5×10^9/L) is 2.3 to 15.4 cases per million in the United States, with a mortality rate of 10% to 16%.[72]

Neonatal alloimmune neutropenia. In neonatal alloimmune neutropenia (NAN), maternal immunoglobulin G (IgG) crosses the placenta and binds to paternal human neutrophil antigens (HNA) found on fetal leukocytes. These antibody-coated neutrophils are removed from circulation through the reticuloendothelial system, generally resulting in an ANC of less than 0.5×10^9/L, often within 1 week of birth. Of the nine

BOX 26.2 Causes of Acquired Neutropenia

Drugs

Anticancer: chemotherapy,* immunologics

Analgesics/antiinflammatories: acetaminophen, aspirin,* diclofenac, ibuprofen, indomethacin, linezolid, naproxen, sulfasalazine*

Antibiotics: β-lactams, cephalosporins, chloramphenicol, clindamycin, gentamicin, penicillin,* sulfonamides, trimethoprim-sulfamethoxazole,* tetracycline, vancomycin*

Antivirals: acyclovir, ganciclovir,* abacavir, zidovudine

Antifungals: terbinafine, amphotericin B

Anticonvulsants: carbamazepine, phenytoin, valproate

Antihistamines: brompheniramine, chlorphenamine, cimetidine, famotidine, ranitidine

Antimalarials: chloroquine, dapsone,* quinine

Antithyroids: propylthiouracil,* methimazole,* carbimazole*

Cardiovascular: amiodarone, captopril, clopidogrel, flecainide, furosemide, methyldopa, procainamide,* propranolol, quinidine, spironolactone, thiazide diuretics, ticlopidine*

Antianxiety/hypnotics: benzodiazepines, meprobamate

Psychotropics: amitriptyline, amoxapine, clozapine,* doxepin, olanzapine, phenothiazines, risperidone

Hypoglycemics: chlorpropamide, tolbutamide

Phenothiazines: chlorpromazine, phenothiazines

Other

Levamisole (adulterated cocaine)

Immunologic

Radiation

Toxins

Overwhelming infections

Splenomegaly

Hemodialysis

Aplastic anemia

Copper deficiency

Alcoholism

Tumor metastasis to bone marrow/space-occupying lesion

Hematologic malignancy
    Myelodysplastic neoplasms
    Large granular lymphocyte syndrome
    Leukemia
    Plasma cell neoplasm

* More common cause.

Adapted from Andrès, E., & Maloisel, F. (2008). Idiosyncratic drug-induced agranulocytosis or acute neutropenia. *Curr Opin Hematol, 15*(1), 15–21; Andrès, E., & Mourot-Cottet, R. (2017). Nonchemotherapy drug-induced neutropenia—an update. *Exp Opin Drug Saf, 16*(11), 1235–1242; Gibson, C., & Berliner, N. (2014). How we evaluate and treat neutropenia in adults. *Blood, 124*(8), 1251–1258; and Pick, A. M., & Nystrom, K. K. (2014). Nonchemotherapy drug-induced neutropenia and agranulocytosis: could medications be the culprit? *J Pharm Pract, 27*(5), 447–452.

HNAs located on Fcγ-receptor IIIb (FcγRIIIb, CD16b), HNA-1 and HNA-3 were most often implicated as the cause of NAN in a 2021 study of 10,000 neonates,[73] although HNA-2 has historically been reported to be a common cause.[74] The 2021 incidence of NAN in the United States was 0.9%.[73] Infections that develop during NAN are most often not life-threatening. Recovery and normalization of the ANC generally occurs within 6 months, after maternal IgG is cleared from circulation.

Autoimmune neutropenia. Autoimmune neutropenia (AIN) is defined as an ANC below the age-specific reference interval and the presence of IgG autoantibodies against one or more HNA.

Primary AIN. Primary AIN occurs in approximately 1 per 100,000 children under 10 years.[75] Primary AIN typically manifests around 7 to 9 months as a mild infection that is usually manageable with conservative approaches.[76] Routine antibiotic prophylaxis is not routinely used in diagnosed patients.[77] Primary AIN tends to be self-limiting, with most patients spontaneously recovering by 4 to 5 years.

Secondary AIN. Secondary AIN is more common in adults and is associated with connective tissue disorders, Felty syndrome, hematopoietic neoplasms, solid tumors, primary immunodeficiencies, bacterial and viral infections, transplant, and as idiosyncratic reactions to a number of medications. Immunologic mechanisms involved in drug-induced neutropenia include formation of immune complexes, haptens, drug-induced formation of neutrophil autoantibodies, and T-lymphocyte toxicity.

Quantitative Abnormalities of Eosinophils

Several factors influence the number of eosinophils in circulation: bone marrow proliferation rate and release into the bloodstream, movement from circulation into extravascular tissues, and cell survival and destruction after eosinophils leave the circulation. The proliferation and differentiation of eosinophils precursors is regulated by granulocyte-macrophage colony-stimulating factor (GM-CSF) and IL-3 and IL-5. The release of eosinophils into circulation is controlled mostly by IL-5 and also IL-3.

Eosinophilia

Eosinophilia is defined as an absolute eosinophil count greater than 0.4×10^9/L. Eosinophilia is associated with various infectious diseases, most notably helminth parasites, ectoparasites, protozoa, fungi, and viruses. Eosinophilia is also found in allergic reactions, including asthma, rhinitis, atopic dermatitis, and drug hypersensitivity; autoimmune disorders; congenital immunodeficiency; radiation exposure; hematopoietic neoplasms; solid tumors; and primary eosinophilic disorders.[78]

Quantitative Abnormalities of Basophils

Basophilia is defined as an absolute basophil count greater than 0.10×10^9/L. Basophilia is associated with MPNs, most notably CML. Basophil counts in CML are generally higher than in other conditions. In CML, the basophil count is used in the differential diagnosis, diagnosis of the accelerated phase, assessment of treatment response, and assessment of prognosis.[79-81] Basophilia is a feature of AML with t(6;9)(p23;q34.1), therapy-related acute leukemia, therapy-related MDS with multilineage dysplasia, and acute basophilic leukemia (Chapter 31).[79] In addition to myeloid neoplasms, basophilia is associated with atopic disorders, chronic iron deficiency, classic Hodgkin lymphoma, smallpox, and chickenpox.

There have been several published reports of unreliable basophil counts affecting popular automated hematology analyzers.[82-86] Falsely increased automated basophil counts are a chronic problem familiar to many laboratory scientists as a source of unnecessary blood film reviews and longer turnaround times.[82,86-88] The consistent findings of pseudobasophilia in certain conditions has been used as a suspect flag for abnormal lymphocytes and dengue fever.[87,89] In CML, basophils are often undercounted by hematology analyzers, diminishing its value as a marker of accelerated disease.[90-92] Decreased confidence in the automated basophil count has prompted a call to remove this cell class from the automated WBC differential.[83]

Quantitative Abnormalities of Monocytes
Monocytosis

Monocytosis is defined as an absolute monocyte count greater than 1.0×10^9/L.[83] Monocytosis is seen in a variety of conditions because of the monocyte's role in acute and chronic inflammation and infections, immunologic conditions, hypersensitivity reactions, and tissue repair. Monocytosis is often the first sign of recovery after myelosuppression. It is also seen in cyclic neutropenia, in which monocytosis occurs during periods of neutropenia in a 21-day cycle. Conditions associated with monocytosis are listed in Box 26.3.

BOX 26.3 Conditions Associated with Monocytosis

Infection
 Tuberculosis
 Brucellosis
 Leishmaniasis
 Fungal
 Subacute bacterial endocarditis
 Malaria
Recovery from acute infection
Recovery from myelosuppression
Immunologic/autoimmune
 Systemic lupus erythematosus
 Rheumatoid arthritis
 Autoimmune neutropenia
 Inflammatory bowel disease
 Myositis
 Sarcoidosis
Cyclic neutropenia
Postsplenectomy
Drugs
 Colony-stimulating factors
 Olanzapine
Malignancy
 Hodgkin lymphoma
 Myelodysplastic/myeloproliferative neoplasms
 Myelodysplastic neoplasms
 Acute myeloid leukemia involving the monocyte lineage

Adapted from Lynch, D. T., & Foucar, K. F. (2016). Ask the hematopathologists: diagnostic approach to monocytosis. *Hematologist, 13*(4), 4; Robinson, R. L., Burk, M. S., & Raman, S. (2003). Fever, delirium, autonomic instability, and monocytosis associated with olanzapine. *J Postgrad Med, 49*(1), 96; and Tsolia, M., Drakonaki, S., Messaritaki, A., et al. (2002). Clinical features, complications and treatment outcome of childhood brucellosis in central Greece. *J Infect, 44*(4), 257–262.

Monocytopenia

Monocytopenia is defined as an absolute monocyte count of less than 0.2×10^9/L and is most often observed in combination with cytopenias of other lineages because of aplastic anemia or myelosuppressive therapies. Monocytopenia has also been associated with patients receiving steroid therapy, those on hemodialysis, and in patients with sepsis. Viral infections, especially those caused by the Epstein-Barr virus (EBV), are also associated with monocytopenia. Profound monocytopenia is characteristic of hairy cell leukemia and in certain myeloid neoplasms with germline *GATA2* mutations.[79]

Quantitative Abnormalities of Lymphocytes

Lymphocytosis

In adults, lymphocytosis is defined as a count greater than 5.0×10^9/L. In children between 2 weeks and 9 years, lymphocytosis is defined as greater than 10.0×10^9/L. In newborns, lymphocytosis is defined as greater than 5.0×10^9/L. Lymphocytosis is usually accompanied by reactive or malignant changes in morphology. It is highly unusual for lymphocytes with normal morphology to increase in number beyond the reference interval. Box 26.4 lists disorders associated with reactive lymphocytosis.

Lymphopenia

Lymphopenia in children is defined as an absolute lymphocyte count less than 2.0×10^9/L, whereas in adults, it is less than 1.0×10^9/L. Nonmalignant causes of lymphopenia may be inherited or acquired and are listed in Box 26.4.

SECONDARY MORPHOLOGIC CHANGES IN LEUKOCYTES

Storage Artifacts in Leukocytes

The potential presence of in vitro storage artifacts/defects in all types of leukocytes and other blood cells should always be considered when examining blood films. Time-dependent degenerative morphologic changes in blood cells stored in EDTA (storage artifacts) can be observed as early as 2 hours after specimen collection. The Clinical Laboratory Standards Institute (CLSI) has stated that blood films should be prepared within 4 hours of collection.[93] Some morphologic characteristics of cells in blood stored over 4 hours mimic true abnormalities (storage artifact). If reported, the provider may interpret them as clinically significant findings. Two common storage artifacts, autophagic vacuoles and pyknotic/apoptotic neutrophils, are discussed in this chapter. The reader is referred elsewhere for information on other forms of storage artifacts in leukocytes, RBCs, and platelets.

Secondary Changes in Neutrophils and Monocytes

Physiologic responses to infection, inflammation, stress, or administration of recombinant colony-stimulating factors (G-CSF or GM-CSF) usually include neutrophilia. An increase in neutrophils will often but not always include immature neutrophils, known as a left shift. The severity of infection, inflammation, or dose of G-CSF influences the rise in the ANC and number/type of neutrophilic cells released into circulation.

Reactive changes in neutrophil morphology can accompany neutrophilia, especially in cases of infection and inflammation, including toxic granulation, Döhle bodies, and toxic vacuolation, summarized in Table 26.6. These reactive changes occur when various cytokines are expressed during infection, inflammation, and tissue injury from trauma and burns. The cytokine

---

BOX 26.4 Causes of Nonmalignant Lymphocytosis and Lymphopenia

Lymphocytosis	Lymphopenia
Reactive Morphology	**Congenital Immunodeficiencies**
Infections	Severe combined immunodeficiency disease
Infectious mononucleosis	Common variable immune deficiency
Cytomegalovirus infection	Ataxia-telangiectasia
Hepatitis	Wiskott-Aldrich syndrome
Acute HIV infection	
Adenovirus	
Chickenpox	**Infections**
Herpes	Acquired immunodeficiency syndrome
Influenza	Severe acute respiratory syndrome
Paramyxovirus (mumps)	COVID-19*
Rubella (measles)	West Nile virus
Roseola	Hepatitis
β-Hemolytic streptococci	Influenza
Brucellosis	Herpes
Paratyphoid fever	Measles
Toxoplasmosis	Tuberculosis
Typhoid fever	Typhoid fever
Listeria	Pneumonia
Mycoplasma	Rickettsiosis
Syphilis	Ehrlichiosis
	Sepsis
Other Causes	Malaria
Idiosyncratic drug reactions	
Postvaccination	**Other Causes**
Sudden onset of stress from myocardial infarction	Immunosuppressive agents
	Stevens-Johnson syndrome
Allergic reaction	Chemotherapy
Hyperthyroidism	Radiation
Malnutrition	Aplastic anemia
	Platelet or stem cell apheresis
Nonreactive Morphology	Major surgery
Bordetella pertussis (whooping cough)	Autoimmune disease
	Hodgkin lymphoma
Polyclonal B-lymphocytosis	Advanced cancers
	Primary myelofibrosis
	Protein-losing enteropathy
	Renal failure
	Ethanol abuse
	Zinc deficiency

* *Note.* Although patients with COVID-19 typically have lymphopenia, lymphocytes can show reactive morphology.
Adapted from Vasu, S., & Caligiuri, M. A. (2016). Lymphocytosis and lymphocytopenia. In Kaushansky, K., Lichtman, M. A., Prchal, J. T., et al. (Eds.), *Williams Hematology.* (9th ed., pp. 1199–1210). New York: McGraw-Hill; and Foucar, K. (2010). Non-neoplastic disorders of lymphoid cells. In Foucar, K., Reichard, K., & Czuchlewski, D. (Eds.), *Bone Marrow Pathology.* (3rd ed., Vol 2, pp. 448–473). Chicago: American Society for Clinical Pathology Press.

G-CSF, administered to stimulate neutrophil production, can also induce toxic changes.

Toxic Granulation

Toxic granules (TGs) are dark, pronounced, and readily visible in the cytoplasm of segmented and band neutrophils. TGs contain enzymes normally found in primary (azurophilic) and secondary (specific) granules. TGs contain increased acid mucosubstance, which is thought to enhance neutrophil bactericidal activity.[94] There is a positive correlation between the level of C-reactive protein (an acute phase protein) and the number of neutrophils with TGs, suggesting an association with inflammation.[95] TGs also can be observed in infections, in pregnancy, and in patients who have received G-CSF. Grading the level of TGs during a morphologic review can be challenging because TGs are often irregularly distributed at different levels of intensity among the neutrophils (Figure 26.10). Toxic granulation can mimic AR bodies. However, AR bodies are typically present in other types of WBCs, which can help differentiate it from toxic granulation.

Döhle Bodies

Döhle bodies are pale, blue-gray, single or multiple cytoplasmic inclusions consisting of aggregates of denatured ribosomal ribonucleic acid (RNA) or remnants of rough endoplasmic reticulum. Döhle bodies are usually found in band and segmented neutrophils and can sometimes appear together with toxic granulation. They can vary in size and shape between 1 and 5 μm in diameter and are often indistinct, usually located near the cell membrane (Figure 26.11). Döhle bodies are associated with severe and/or systemic infections, burns, trauma, pregnancy, cancer, and G-CSF administration. Döhle bodies are similar in appearance to the inclusions found in MHA. However, in MHA, the Döhle body-like inclusions also can be observed in eosinophils, basophils, and monocytes.

Neutrophil Vacuolation

Toxic vacuoles. Neutrophils with cytoplasmic vacuoles are encountered less often than TGs and Döhle bodies. Neutrophil vacuoles found in cells with toxic granulation and/or Döhle bodies are called *toxic vacuoles* (Figure 26.12, A) and are a general indication of phagocytic activity. Toxic vacuoles are more closely associated with infections than are toxic granulation and/or Döhle bodies without vacuoles.[96] Toxic vacuoles can be variable in size (up to 6 μm in diameter), irregularly distributed within the cell, and may (rarely) contain microorganisms (discussed later). Toxic vacuoles sometimes coalesce and distort cellular morphology.

Autophagic vacuolation. Autophagic vacuolation is a cellular degradation process involved in most aspects of neutrophil biology and pathophysiology. The process of autophagy includes the formation of small vacuoles, approximately 2 μm in diameter (Figure 12.12, B), often with wider distribution in the cytoplasm than toxic vacuoles. These vacuoles are not associated with toxic granulation and Döhle bodies. Autophagy occurs during cell death. Autophagic vacuoles in neutrophils and other leukocytes

TABLE 26.6	Reactive (Toxic) Morphology in Neutrophils	
Reactive Change	**Appearance**	**Associated with**
Toxic granulation	Dark, blue-black cytoplasmic granules	Inflammation, infection, pregnancy, G-CSF administration
Döhle bodies	Intracytoplasmic, pale blue round or elongated bodies between 1 and 5 μm in diameter, usually adjacent to cellular membranes; can be indistinct	Inflammation, infection, pregnancy, G-CSF administration
Cytoplasmic vacuoles	Small to large circular clear areas in cytoplasm; rarely may contain organism	Bacterial infection, autophagy secondary to drug ingestion, acute alcoholism, or storage artifact

G-CSF, Granulocyte colony-stimulating factor.

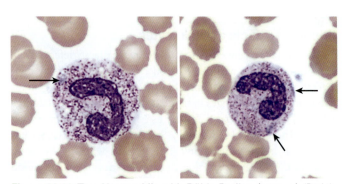

Figure 26.11 Two Neutrophils with Döhle Bodies *(arrows).* (Peripheral blood, Wright-Giemsa stain, Cellavision DC-1, ×1000.) (Courtesy Cellavision AB, Lund, Sweden.)

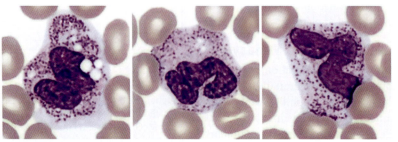

Figure 26.10 Toxic Granulation in Neutrophils. Note the uneven distribution of toxic granules among a patient's neutrophils. Other patients may show a more homogeneous presentation. (Peripheral blood, Wright-Giemsa stain, Cellavision DC-1, ×1000.) (Courtesy Cellavision AB, Lund, Sweden.)

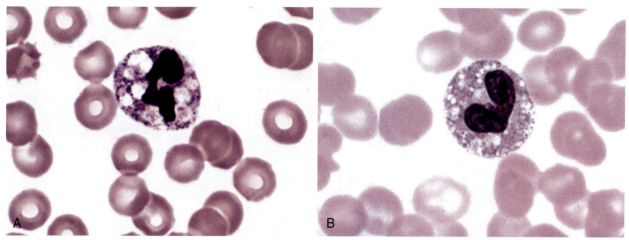

Figure 26.12 Cytoplasmic Vacuoles. **(A)**, Phagocytic vacuoles. Note their larger size. **(B)**, Autophagic vacuoles. Note their smaller size. (Peripheral blood, Wright-Giemsa stain, ×1000.)

are often associated with a delay in preparing the blood film after specimen collection. Autophagy is also seen in hypoxia; starvation; chemical exposure, including alcohol poisoning; toxic levels of radiation; and a newly described syndrome called VEXAS (vacuoles, E1 enzyme, X-linked, autoinflammatory, somatic).[97,98] In VEXAS, vacuoles are also present in other hematopoietic cells.

Pyknosis and Apoptosis in Neutrophils

Pyknotic nuclei. Pyknotic nuclei often indicate imminent cell death. In a pyknotic nucleus, water has been lost and the chromatin becomes dense and dark; however, chromatin or filaments are still visible between the nuclear lobes of segmented neutrophils.

Apoptotic nuclei. Apoptotic nuclei are found in dead neutrophils. They are rounded, dense nuclear fragments without visible filaments or chromatin pattern (Figure 26.13). Apoptotic neutrophils are sometimes confused with nucleated RBCs. A key difference is the presence of granules in apoptotic neutrophils. Nucleated RBCs are agranular. Like autophagic vacuoles, pyknotic neutrophils often suggest an excessive delay occurred between specimen collection and blood film preparation.

Intracellular Organisms in Neutrophils and Monocytes

Bacteria and fungal organisms. Neutrophils and (less often) monocytes with engulfed fungal elements (Figure 26.14, A and B) or bacteria (Figure 26.14, C and D) are a rare finding in patients with disseminated infections and generally associated with a poor outcome. In these patients, neutrophils may also exhibit TGs and Döhle bodies. The identification of intracellular bacteria in blood films is not necessarily an ominous finding because they have been noted in asymptomatic patients with indwelling catheters[99] and in patients undergoing surgical and dental procedures.

Cases of such tickborne illnesses, as human granulocytic anaplasmosis (HGA) and human monocytic ehrlichiosis (HME), have been increasing in the United States. The etiologic bacteria are *Anaplasma phagocytophilum* in HGA and *Ehrlichia chaffeensis* (less commonly *Ehrlichia ewingii*) in HME, both

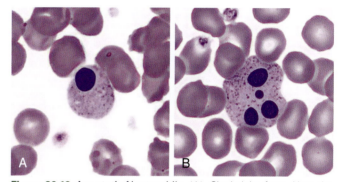

Figure 26.13 Apoptotic Neutrophils. **(A)**, Single-lobe form. Note the presence of residual neutrophil granules can help differentiate this cell from a nucleated red blood cell. **(B)**, Multilobe form. (Peripheral blood, Wright-Giemsa stain, Cellavision DM-9600, ×1000.) (Courtesy Cellavision AB, Lund, Sweden.)

transmitted to humans and other vertebrate hosts through a tick bite. The primary animal reservoirs are the white-footed mouse in HGA and white-tailed deer in HME. These small, obligate, intracellular bacteria appear in clusters (morulae) within neutrophils (HGA) (Figure 26.14, D) and monocytes (HME). HGA and HME present clinically as mild to severe acute illnesses during spring and summer months with overlapping clinical manifestations; however, HME is often more severe, with many cases requiring hospitalization. Patients with HGA and HME frequently have fever, chills, malaise, myalgia, headache, and less often nausea, vomiting, arthralgia, neurologic symptoms, and/or rash. Leukopenia (secondary to neutropenia or lymphopenia), left-shifted neutrophils, thrombocytopenia, and elevated hepatic enzymes are common laboratory findings. Nonhemolytic anemia develops in about half of these patients.

A patient with a history of outdoor exposure in endemic regions who presents with fever, leukopenia, and/or thrombocytopenia should be considered highly suspect for HMA or HME. Up to 80% of HMA patients will demonstrate neutrophils with intracellular morulae on peripheral blood or buffy coat film review.[100] This finding rapidly confirms the diagnosis in patients presenting with the described clinical and laboratory findings. Otherwise, polymerase chain reaction (PCR) testing

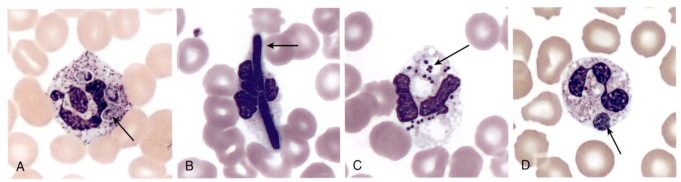

Figure 26.14 Neutrophils with Intracellular Organisms *(arrows).* (A), *Histoplasma capsulatum.* (B), *Candida* species. (C), *Enterococcus faecium.* (D), *Anaplasma phagocytophilum.* (Peripheral blood, Wright-Giemsa stain, Cellavision DC-1, ×1000.) (Courtesy Cellavision AB, Lund, Sweden.)

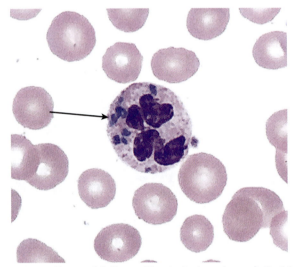

Figure 26.15 Neutrophil Green-Blue Inclusions *(arrow).* (Peripheral blood, Wright-Giemsa stain, ×1000.) (Courtesy Woo Cheal Cho, MD Anderson Cancer Center, Houston, TX.)

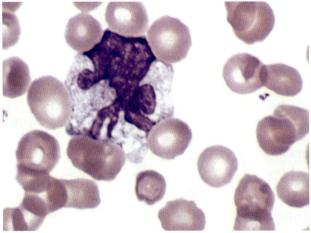

Figure 26.16 Reactive Monocyte. (Peripheral blood, Wright-Giemsa stain, ×1000.)

can be used to confirm the diagnosis. It is important that morulae not be confused with Döhle bodies. Approximately 5% of HME patients will show morulae within monocytes.[101] Early detection and treatment with doxycycline is effective at treating HMA and HME and lowers the risk of serious complications.

Green-Blue Inclusions in Neutrophils and Monocytes

Green-blue inclusions in neutrophils and monocytes (critical blue-green inclusions/crystals of death) were seldom reported before 2009; however, increased awareness and enhanced visibility, largely through digital morphology, have spurred numerous publications in recent years.[102] The inclusions are described as bluish-green or mostly green amorphous, refractile, shiny bodies of irregular shape, size, and number, contained in cytoplasm of neutrophils (Figure 26.15) and occasionally in monocytes. The inclusions are thought to contain lipofuscin released from necrotic liver parenchymal cells in critically ill patients with acute liver failure, multiorgan failure, lactic acidosis, COVID-19 infection, sepsis, and yellow fever.[103–105] In many cases, the presence of blue-green inclusions is a sign of impending death.[103,104]

Reactive Monocytes

Reactive morphology in monocytes is associated with infections, including COVID-19,[106] recovery from myelosuppression, and administration of GM-CSF (Figure 26.16). Reactive monocytes have more immature chromatin patterns, small nucleoli, increased N:C ratio, deepened cytoplasmic basophilia, increased vacuoles, and distinct granulation. Differentiating between benign reactive monocytes and immature or abnormal malignant monocytes is notoriously challenging, especially in cases with monocytes. However, it is an important distinction to make.[107]

Eosinophils and Basophils
Ruptured and Smudged Eosinophils

Eosinophils are fragile cells that sometimes rupture during slide preparation. Guidelines state that ruptured or damaged eosinophils should be counted with intact eosinophils in microscopic WBC differentials.[63] Overlooking damaged eosinophils or classifying them as smudge cells leads to falsely decreased eosinophil counts. Hypogranular eosinophils and eosinophils with mixed granulation are typically associated with myeloid neoplasms.

Hypogranular Basophils

Basophil granules are water soluble and can wash away during staining. Affected basophils may show only a residual pinkish tinge in or around the cell (Figure 26.17). This might be the only clue that these cells are not neutrophils. Hypogranular basophils (in vivo induced) also can be observed in some myeloid neoplasms.

Lymphocytes

Reactive Lymphocytes

Various terms haven been used over the years to identify lymphocytes showing reactive morphology: Turk cells, Downey cells, immunoblasts, and reactive, variant, atypical, transformed,

effector, and plasmacytoid lymphocytes. The International Committee for Standardization in Hematology (ICSH) recommends a simple and logical nomenclature for nonnormal lymphocytes that is based on two cell classes, (1) "reactive lymphocyte" applies to lymphocytes with morphologic changes associated with a benign cause, and (2) "abnormal lymphocyte" applies to lymphocytes with morphology stemming from a suspected malignant or clonal origin.[63] The goal of the ICSH guidelines are to reduce the use of an assortment of terms for the same cell and improve consistency and recognition among individuals, laboratories, and clinical centers around the world.

Reactive lymphocytes are occasionally observed in peripheral blood films of healthy individuals. However, reactive lymphocytes more than approximately 5% of total leukocytes are most often associated with absolute lymphocytosis in patients with infection or other conditions listed in Box 26.4.

Reactive changes occur when lymphocytes are stimulated by antigen. Lymphocyte activation results in the transformation of small resting lymphocytes into proliferating larger cells (Figure 26.18). These reactive lymphocytes often appear in a heterogeneous population of different shapes and sizes in a peripheral blood film. There is variation in the N:C ratio, nuclear shape, and chromatin pattern, which is often condensed; however, some cells may show more immature chromatin. Nucleoli may be visible. An increase in basophilic cytoplasm that differs in intensity within and between cells is a common finding. The reactive lymphocyte's cytoplasm may be indented by surrounding RBCs. A plasmacytoid lymphocyte is a type of reactive lymphocyte that shares some characteristics of plasma cells (Figure 26.19).

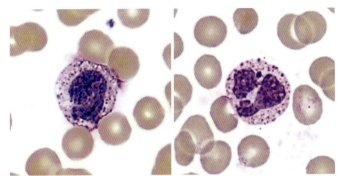

Figure 26.17 Basophils with Decreased Granulation. Basophil granules were lost during slide staining. Note the residual pinkish tinge in the cytoplasm. (Peripheral blood, Wright-Giemsa stain, Cellavision DC-1, ×1000.) (Courtesy Cellavision AB, Lund, Sweden.)

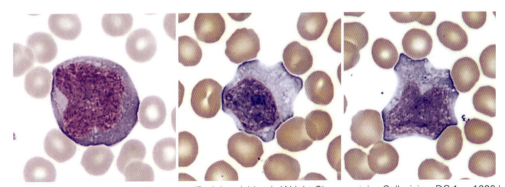

Figure 26.18 Reactive Lymphocytes. (Peripheral blood, Wright-Giemsa stain, Cellavision DC-1, ×1000.) (Courtesy Cellavision AB, Lund, Sweden.)

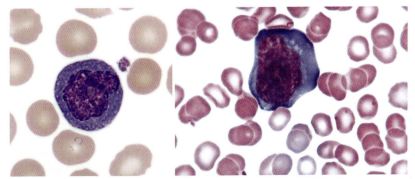

Figure 26.19 Reactive (Plasmacytoid) Lymphocytes. (Peripheral blood, Wright-Giemsa stain, Cellavision DC-1, ×1000.) (Courtesy Cellavision AB, Lund, Sweden.)

A few plasmacytoid lymphocytes are often admixed in a heterogeneous population with other morphologic forms of reactive lymphocytes in a range of nonmalignant conditions (Box 26.4). A higher number and/or more homogeneous population of plasmacytoid lymphocytes should raise the suspicion of a lymphoid neoplasm.

INFECTIOUS MONONUCLEOSIS

EBV is the etiologic agent in infectious mononucleosis (IM). IM occurs most often in 15- to 24-year-olds; however, asymptomatic EBV infections are common in younger children.[108] EBV is widely disseminated because up to 95% of adults are seropositive,[108] although (symptomatic) IM is uncommon in adults. EBV also has been implicated in lymphoid neoplasms and other cancers, posttransplant lymphoproliferative disease, chronic fatigue syndrome, multiple sclerosis, autoimmune diseases, and vitamin D deficiency.

The incubation period of IM is approximately 3 to 7 weeks. During this time, EBV preferentially infects B lymphocytes through attachment of viral envelope glycoprotein 350/220 to CD21 (C3d complement receptors) and CD35 (complement receptor type 1). The oropharynx epithelial cells are also infected, but the mechanism is unclear because these cells do not express CD21 or CD35. BMRF2 is an EBV glycoprotein that may facilitate EBV entry into epithelial cells through binding with β1, α5, and α3 integrins on epithelial cells.[109] The cellular response in IM is important in controlling the infection and is marked by proliferation and activation of NK lymphocytes, CD4+ T cells, and CD8+ memory cytotoxic T cells (EBV-CTLs) in response to B-cell infection. Reactive lymphocytes observed in IM represent CD8+ cytotoxic T cells activated during the cellular response.

Common clinical manifestations in IM include sore throat (with or without tonsillar exudate), dysphagia, fever, chills, posterior cervical lymphadenopathy, fatigue, loss of appetite, and headache. More than half of patients also have splenomegaly.[108] Initial testing includes complete blood count with differential and rapid heterophile antibody test. Most patients have an absolute lymphocytosis with 10% to 50% or more reactive (often referred to as "atypical") lymphocytes. On blood films, the population of reactive lymphocytes is mostly pleomorphic. The classic IM reactive lymphocyte is a larger cell with abundant variably basophilic cytoplasm that hugs surrounding RBCs resembling "ballerina skirting." Historically, these cells in IM were referred to as Downey type II cells.[110] The detection of significant numbers of reactive lymphocytes in symptomatic patients with lymphocytosis but negative with heterophile antibody tests can help diagnose IM at remote or resource-limited centers unable to reflex to sophisticated EBV tests.[111]

Up to 20% of IM patients experience additional symptoms, including abdominal pain, nausea, vomiting, hepatomegaly (with abnormal liver function tests), rash, petechiae, and eyelid edema. In rare cases, patients develop aplastic anemia, hemolytic anemia, thrombocytopenia, disseminated intravascular coagulation, and/or neurologic complications.

Patients with acute IM produce IgM heterophile antibodies that cross react with mammalian RBCs, forming the basis of most rapid screening tests. These simple tests are widely available and can confirm an IM diagnosis with a sensitivity and specificity of 87% and 91%, respectively.[112] However there are significant limitations, including a 40% false-negative rate in children less than 5 years old.[112] Also, approximately 25% of older-age, newly infected individuals may fail to produce a positive result.[113,114] Further, false-positive results can occur in patients with other infections, autoimmune disorders, and cancer.

Heterophile-negative patients with a high degree of clinical suspicion may require testing with a panel of EBV antigens and antibodies, including EBV viral capsid antigen (VCA), EBV nuclear antigen (EBNA), and IgG/IgM antibodies against VCA and EBNA. These tests offer greater sensitivity and specificity compared to rapid heterophile antibody tests; however, they can be expensive, with longer turnaround times. Patients who remain negative for EBV antigen and antibody tests may have cytomegalovirus mononucleosis syndrome, which has clinical features nearly identical to those of EBV IM.

■ SUMMARY

- Inborn errors of immunity are a group of inherited diseases of the innate or adaptive immune system often associated with severe clinical manifestations.
- Common gamma chain deficiency and adenosine deaminase deficiency are examples of severe combined immune deficiency (SCID), characterized by defects in cellular and humoral immunity and associated with a wide range of severe clinical manifestations and early death unless treated with hematopoietic stem cell transplantation (HSCT).
- Wiskott-Aldrich syndrome is a combined immunodeficiency disease with phagocyte dysfunction and abnormal platelets in which HSCT can be curative in human leukocyte antigen (HLA)-matched donors.
- 22q11.2 deletion syndrome (DiGeorge syndrome) is caused by a deletion of a string of base pairs on chromosome 22. The deletion breakpoint differs between patients and the clinical heterogeneity is related to which genes were lost in the deletion. Disease manifestations include severe decrease in T cells and other hematologic abnormalities, physical malformations, severe infections, neuropsychiatric issues, and other problems.
- Bruton tyrosine kinase deficiency is associated with a profound decrease in B cells and antibody production, resulting in severe bacterial, fungal, and parasitic infections. Advancements in immunoglobulin and antimicrobial therapies have greatly improved outcomes.
- Chédiak-Higashi syndrome is a rare condition affecting various granulated hematopoietic and nonhematopoietic cells throughout the body in which the formation of giant fused cytoplasmic granules disrupts normal cell functions, leading to a wide range of serious clinical symptoms and early death.

- The severe congenital neutropenias are a group of diseases in which genetic mutations lead to a maturation arrest in the neutrophil series at the myelocyte/promyelocyte stage. Absolute neutrophil counts (ANCs) of less than 0.5×10^9/L, severe, recurring, often life-threatening bacterial and fungal infections, and an increased risk of leukemic transformation are found.
- Leukocyte adhesion disorders (LADs) arise because of impaired ability of phagocytes to move from circulation to sites of infection. Clinical findings can include recurring severe infections, organomegaly, neurologic defects, skeletal defects, facial dysmorphia, bleeding, and osteoporosis.
- Shwachman-Diamond syndrome is characterized by exocrine pancreatic insufficiency, digestive problems, infections, physical anomalies, neurologic defects, bone marrow failure, and increased risk of leukemia.
- Chronic granulomatous disease stems from a failure in the neutrophil respiratory burst. Patients experience severe recurring infections and inflammatory disorders, including granuloma formation in various organs. Advances in antimicrobials, long-term antimicrobial prophylaxis, quick recognition, and aggressive treatment have led to significantly improved outcomes.
- Pelger-Huët anomaly (PHA) is a mostly benign genetic disorder resulting in hypolobulated mature leukocytes that function normally. Pelger-Huët neutrophils resemble immature neutrophils that can lead to erroneous reporting, clinical confusion, unnecessary diagnostic investigations, and inappropriate treatment. Pseudo-Pelger-Huët anomaly (PPHA) is the presence of hypolobulated neutrophils in association with myeloid neoplasms and other conditions.
- Alder-Reilly anomaly (ARA) is a rare inherited disorder characterized by metachromatic cytoplasmic granules in leukocytes, which can be confused with toxic granulation. A more common acquired form is most often associated with mucopolysaccharidoses.
- May-Hegglin anomaly (MHA) is characterized by thrombocytopenia, giant platelets, and Döhle body-like inclusions in leukocytes. Most cases are asymptomatic.
- Lysosomal storage disorders are congenital deficiencies of lysosomal enzymes and impaired digestion of macromolecules, which accumulate and impair cellular functions leading to a range of clinical symptoms.
- Gaucher disease is a lysosomal storage disorder characterized by a deficiency in β-glucocerebrosidase and accumulation of sphingolipids in cells leading to a serious clinical manifestations and increased risk for malignant transformation.
- Niemann-Pick disease is a lysosomal storage disorder caused by a deficiency in sphingomyelinase and buildup of fats in various organs in the body, resulting in neurologic defects, organomegaly, failure to thrive, and early death.
- Reactive changes in neutrophils include left shift, Döhle bodies, toxic granulation, and toxic vacuoles.
- Reactive changes in lymphocytes include increased diameter, increased basophilic cytoplasm, and morphologic heterogeneity.

Now that you have completed this chapter, go back and read again the case study at the beginning and respond to the questions presented. Answers can be found in Appendix C.

REVIEW QUESTIONS

Answers can be found in Appendix C.

1. Which one of the following inherited leukocyte disorders is caused by a mutation in the lamin B receptor?
   a. Pelger-Huët anomaly
   b. Chédiak-Higashi disease
   c. Alder-Reilly anomaly
   d. May-Hegglin anomaly

2. Which one of the following inherited leukocyte disorders involves mutations in nonmuscle myosin heavy-chain IIA?
   a. Pelger-Huët anomaly
   b. Chédiak-Higashi disease
   c. Alder-Reilly anomaly
   d. May-Hegglin anomaly

3. Which one of the following morphologic leukocyte abnormalities is a common manifestation of the mucopolysaccharidoses?
   a. Pelger-Huët anomaly
   b. Chédiak-Higashi disease
   c. Alder-Reilly anomaly
   d. May-Hegglin anomaly

4. Which one of the following lysosomal storage diseases is characterized by macrophages with striated cytoplasm and storage of glucocerebroside?
   a. Sanfilippo syndrome
   b. Gaucher disease
   c. Fabry disease
   d. Niemann-Pick disease

5. The neutrophils in chronic granulomatous disease are incapable of producing:
   a. Hydrogen peroxide
   b. Hypochlorous acid
   c. Superoxide
   d. All of the above

6. Individuals with X-linked SCID have a mutation that affects their ability to synthesize:
   a. Deaminase
   b. Oxidase
   c. IL-2 receptor
   d. IL-8 receptor

7. An absolute lymphocytosis with reactive lymphocytes suggests which of the following conditions?
   a. DiGeorge syndrome
   b. Bacterial infection
   c. Parasitic infection
   d. Viral infection

8. What leukocyte cytoplasmic inclusion is composed of ribosomal RNA?
   a. Primary granules
   b. Toxic granules
   c. Döhle bodies
   d. Howell-Jolly bodies

9. The expected complete blood cell (CBC) results for women in active labor would include:
   a. High total white blood cell (WBC) count with increased lymphocytes
   b. High total WBC count with a slight shift to the left in neutrophils
   c. Normal WBC count with increased eosinophils
   d. Low WBC count with increased monocytes

10. Which one of the following is true of an absolute increase in lymphocytes with reactive morphology?
    a. The population of lymphocytes appears morphologically homogeneous.
    b. They are usually effector B cells.
    c. The reactive lymphocytes have increased cytoplasm with variable basophilia.
    d. They are most commonly seen in bacterial infections.

REFERENCES

1. Tangye, S. G., Al-Herz, W., Bousfiha, A., et al. (2022). Human inborn errors of immunity: 2022 update on the classification from the International Union of Immunological Societies Expert Committee. *J Clin Immunol, 42*, 1473–1507.
2. Boyle, J. M., & Buckley, R. H. (2007). Population prevalence of diagnosed primary immunodeficiency diseases in the United States. *J Clin Immunol, 27*, 497–502.
3. Slatter, M. A., & Gennery, A. R. (2022). Advances in the treatment of severe combined immunodeficiency. *Clin Immunol, 242*, 109084.
4. Cooper, D. N., Ball, E. V., Stenson, A. D., et al. *The Human Gene Mutation Database.* Cardiff: Institute of Medical Genetics in Cardiff. https://www.hgmd.cf.ac.uk/ac/index.php. Accessed June 16, 2023.
5. Sudhakar, M., Rikhi, R., Loganathan, S. K., et al. (2021). Autoimmunity in Wiskott-Aldrich syndrome: updated perspectives. *Appl Clin Genet, 14*, 363–388.
6. Burroughs, L. M., Petrovic, A., Brazauskas, R., et al. (2020). Excellent outcomes following hematopoietic cell transplantation for Wiskott-Aldrich syndrome: a PIDTC report. *Blood, 135*, 2094–2105.
7. Elfeky, R. A., Furtado-Silva, J. M., Chiesa, R., et al. (2018). One hundred percent survival after transplantation of 34 patients with Wiskott-Aldrich syndrome over 20 years. *J Allergy Clin Immunol, 142*, 1654–1656.
8. Mallhi, K. K., Petrovic, A., & Ochs, H. D. (2021). Hematopoietic stem cell therapy for Wiskott-Aldrich syndrome: improved outcome and quality of life. *J Blood Med, 12*, 435–447.
9. Lindsay, E. A., Goldberg, R., Jurecic, V., et al. (1995). Velo-cardio-facial syndrome: frequency and extent of 22q11 deletions. *Am J Med Genet, 57*, 514–522.
10. Du, Q., de la Morena, M. T., & van Oers, N. S. C. (2019). The genetics and epigenetics of 22q11.2 deletion syndrome. *Front Genet, 10*, 1365.
11. Janda, A., Sedlacek, P., Honig, M., et al. (2010). Multicenter survey on the outcome of transplantation of hematopoietic cells in patients with the complete form of DiGeorge anomaly. *Blood, 116*, 2229–2236.
12. Seymour, B. J., Singh, S., Certo, H. M., et al. (2021). Effective, safe, and sustained correction of murine XLA using a UCOE-BTK promoter-based lentiviral vector. *Mol Ther Methods Clin Dev, 20*, 635–651.
13. Kaplan, J., De Domenico, I., & Ward, D. M. (2008). Chediak-Higashi syndrome. *Curr Opin Hematol, 15*, 22–29.
14. Boztug, K. (2023). Chediak Higashi syndrome. L. D. Notarangelo, Editor. *UpToDate*: Waltham, MA. https://www.uptodate.com.
15. Nagai, K., Ochi, F., Terui, K., et al. (2013). Clinical characteristics and outcomes of Chediak-Higashi syndrome: a nationwide survey of Japan. *Pediatr Blood Cancer, 60*, 1582–1586.
16. Aonuma, K., Komiyama, A., & Akabane, T. (1990). Pseudo-Chediak-Higashi anomaly in acute myeloid leukemia (M2) of childhood. *Acta Paediatr Jpn, 32*(6), 651–655.
17. Qiang, X., Tao, T., & Chen, X. (2022). Pseudo-Chediak-Higashi granules in a case of acute lymphoblastic leukemia mimicking acute myeloid leukemia. *Turk J Haematol, 39*, 213–214.
18. Xia, J., Bolyard, A. A., Rodger, E., et al. (2009). Prevalence of mutations in *ELANE, GFI1, HAX1, SBDS, WAS* and *G6PC3* in patients with severe congenital neutropenia. *Br J Haematol, 147*, 535–542.
19. OMIM. (2023). *Online Mendelian Inheritance in Man, OMIM.* https://www.omim.org/. Accessed June 16, 2023.
20. Skokowa, J., Dale, D. C., Touw, I. P., et al. (2017). Severe congenital neutropenias. *Nat Rev Dis Primers, 3*, 17032.
21. Dale, D. C., Bolyard, A. A., Shannon, J. A., et al. (2022). Outcomes for patients with severe chronic neutropenia treated with granulocyte colony-stimulating factor. *Blood Adv, 6*, 3861–3869.
22. Rosenberg, P. S., Zeidler, C., Bolyard, A. A., et al. (2010). Stable long-term risk of leukaemia in patients with severe congenital neutropenia maintained on G-CSF therapy. *Br J Haematol, 150*, 196–199.
23. Rogers, Z. R., & Myers, K. C. (2022). Shwachman-Diamond syndrome. P. Newburger, & M. B. Heyman, Editors. *UpToDate*: Waltham, MA. https://www.uptodate.com.
24. Bakhtiar, S., Salzmann-Manrique, E., Blok, H. J., et al. (2021). Allogeneic hematopoietic stem cell transplantation in leukocyte adhesion deficiency type I and III. *Blood Adv, 5*, 262–273.
25. Roos, D., van Leeuwen, K., Madkaikar, M., et al. (2023). Hematologically important mutations: leukocyte adhesion deficiency (second update). *Blood Cells Mol Dis, 99*, 102726.
26. Arnadottir, G. A., Norddahl, G. L., Gudmundsdottir, S., et al. (2018). A homozygous loss-of-function mutation leading to CYBC1 deficiency causes chronic granulomatous disease. *Nat Commun, 9*(1), 4447.
27. Connelly, J. A., Marsh, R., Parikh, S., et al. (2018). Allogeneic hematopoietic cell transplantation for chronic granulomatous disease: controversies and state of the art. *J Pediatric Infect Dis Soc, 7*, S31–S39.
28. Wei, Y., Kim, J., Ernits, H., et al. (2021). The septic neutrophil-friend or foe. *Shock, 55*, 147–155.
29. Lehrer, R. I., & Cline, M. J. (1969). Leukocyte myeloperoxidase deficiency and disseminated candidiasis: the role of myeloperoxidase in resistance to *Candida* infection. *J Clin Invest, 48*, 1478–1488.
30. Koziol-Montewka, M., Magrys, A., Paluch-Oles, J., et al. (2006). MPO and cytokines in the serum of cancer patients in the context of *Candida* colonization and infection. *Immunol Invest, 35*, 167–179.
31. Ferreira, C. R., Rahman, S., Keller, M., et al. (2021). An international classification of inherited metabolic disorders (ICIMD). *J Inherit Metab Dis, 44*, 164–177.
32. Platt, F. M., d'Azzo, A., Davidson, B. L., et al. (2018). Lysosomal storage diseases. *Nat Rev Dis Primers, 4*, 27.
33. Puckett, Y., Mallorga-Hernandez, A., & Montano, A. M. (2021). Epidemiology of mucopolysaccharidoses (MPS) in United States: challenges and opportunities. *Orphanet J Rare Dis, 16*, 241.
34. Kubaski, F., de Oliveira Poswar, F., Michelin-Tirelli, K., et al. (2020). Diagnosis of mucopolysaccharidoses. *Diagnostics, 10*, 172.

35. McBride, K. L., & Flanigan, K. M. (2021). Update in the mucopolysaccharidoses. *Semin Pediatr Neurol, 37*, 100874.

36. Penon-Portmann, M., Blair, D. R., & Harmatz, P. (2022). Current and new therapies for mucopolysaccharidoses. *Pediatr Neonatol, 64*(Suppl 1), S10–S17.

37. Beutler, E., Nguyen, N. J., Henneberger, M. W., et al. (1993). Gaucher disease: gene frequencies in the Ashkenazi Jewish population. *Am J Hum Genet, 52*, 85–88.

38. Jezela-Stanek, A., Kleinotiene, G., Chwialkowska, K., et al. (2021). Do not miss the (genetic) diagnosis of Gaucher syndrome: a narrative review on diagnostic clues and management in severe prenatal and perinatal-lethal sporadic cases. *J Clin Med, 10*, 4890.

39. Ferreira, C. R., & Gahl, W. A. (2017). Lysosomal storage diseases. *Transl Sci Rare Dis, 2*, 1–71.

40. Rosenbloom, B. E., Weinreb, N. J., Zimran, A., et al. (2005). Gaucher disease and cancer incidence: a study from the Gaucher Registry. *Blood, 105*, 4569–4572.

41. Mistry, P. K., Taddei, T., vom Dahl, S., et al. (2013). Gaucher disease and malignancy: a model for cancer pathogenesis in an inborn error of metabolism. *Crit Rev Oncog, 18*, 235–246.

42. Kong, W., Lu, C., Ding, Y., et al. (2022). Update of treatment for Gaucher disease. *Eur J Pharmacol, 926*, 175023.

43. Styczynski, J., Tridello, G., Koster, L., et al. (2020). Death after hematopoietic stem cell transplantation: changes over calendar year time, infections and associated factors. *Bone Marrow Transplant, 55*, 126–136.

44. Cho-Vega, J. H., & Loghavi, S. (2022). Pseudo-Gaucher cells in a myeloid neoplasm with *PDGFRB* rearrangement: imitating the imitator. *Blood, 140*, 664.

45. Roldan Galiacho, V., Moreno Gamiz, M., & Echebarria-Barona, A. (2021). Aggregates of pseudogaucher cells in a pediatric patient with chronic myeloid leukemia. *J Pediatr Hematol Oncol, 43*, 224–225.

46. Carrington, P. A., Stevens, R. F., & Lendon, M. (1992). Pseudo-Gaucher cells. *J Clin Pathol, 45*, 360.

47. Beaton, B., Ramaswami, U., Hughes, D. A., et al. (2018). Abundant pseudo-Gaucher cells result in delay in diagnosis of plasma cell myeloma. *Br J Haematol, 182*, 465.

48. Pinto, C., Sousa, D., Ghilas, V., et al. (2021). Acid sphingomyelinase deficiency: a clinical and immunological perspective. *Int J Mol Sci, 22*, 12870.

49. Nordli, D. R. (2022). Overview of Niemann-Pick disease. M. J. Aminoff, Editor. *UpToDate*: Waltham, MA. https://www.uptodate.com.

50. Schuchman, E. H. (2009). The pathogenesis and treatment of acid sphingomyelinase-deficient Niemann-Pick disease. *Int J Clin Pharmacol Ther, 47*(Suppl 1), S48–57.

51. FDA. (2022). *FDA Approves First Treatment for Acid Sphingomyelinase Deficiency, a Rare Genetic Disease*. https://www.fda.gov/news-events/press-announcements/fda-approves-first-treatment-acid-sphingomyelinase-deficiency-rare-genetic-disease. Accessed June 16, 2023.

52. Pineda, M., Jurickova, K., Karimzadeh, P., et al. (2019). Evaluation of different suspicion indices in identifying patients with Niemann-Pick disease Type C in clinical practice: a post hoc analysis of a retrospective chart review. *Orphanet J Rare Dis, 14*, 161–172.

53. Geberhiwot, T., Moro, A., Dardis, A., et al. (2018). Consensus clinical management guidelines for Niemann-Pick disease type C. *Orphanet J Rare Dis, 13*, 50–62.

54. Bianconi, S. E., Hammond, D. I., Farhat, N. Y., et al. (2019). Evaluation of age of death in Niemann-Pick disease, type C: utility of disease support group websites to understand natural history. *Mol Genet Metab, 126*, 466–469.

55. Colella, R., & Hollensead, S. C. (2012). Understanding and recognizing the Pelger-Huet anomaly. *Am J Clin Pathol, 137*, 358–366.

56. Hoffmann, K., Dreger, C. K., Olins, A. L., et al. (2002). Mutations in the gene encoding the lamin B receptor produce an altered nuclear morphology in granulocytes (Pelger-Huet anomaly). *Nat Genet, 31*, 410–414.

57. Oosterwijk, J. C., Mansour, S., van Noort, G., et al. (2003). Congenital abnormalities reported in Pelger-Huet homozygosity as compared to Greenberg/HEM dysplasia: highly variable expression of allelic phenotypes. *J Med Genet, 40*, 937–941.

58. Reilly, A., Creamer, J. P., Stewart, S., et al. (2022). Lamin B1 deletion in myeloid neoplasms causes nuclear anomaly and altered hematopoietic stem cell function. *Cell Stem Cell, 29*, 577–592 e578.

59. Dusse, L. M., Moreira, A. M., Vieira, L. M., et al. (2010). Acquired Pelger-Huet: what does it really mean? *Clin Chim Acta, 411*, 1587–1590.

60. Berber, I., Cagasar, O., Sarici, A., et al. (2021). Peripheral blood smear findings of COVID-19 patients provide information about the severity of the disease and the duration of hospital stay. *Mediterr J Hematol Infect Dis, 13*, e2021009.

61. Wang, E., Boswell, E., Siddiqi, I., et al. (2011). Pseudo-Pelger-Huet anomaly induced by medications: a clinicopathologic study in comparison with myelodysplastic syndrome-related pseudo-Pelger-Huet anomaly. *Am J Clin Pathol, 135*, 291–303.

62. Nieto-Borrajo, E., & Bermejo-Rodriguez, A. (2019). Acquired Pelger-Huet anomaly in a patient treated with valganciclovir. *BMJ Case Rep, 12*, e230958.

63. Palmer, L., Briggs, C., McFadden, S., et al. (2015). ICSH recommendations for the standardization of nomenclature and grading of peripheral blood cell morphological features. *Int J Lab Hematol, 37*, 287–303.

64. Skendzel, L. P., & Hoffman, G. C. (1962). The Pelger anomaly of leukocytes: forty-one cases in seven families. *Am J Clin Pathol, 37*, 294–301.

65. Shetty, V. T., Mundle, S. D., & Raza, A. (2001). Pseudo Pelger-Huet anomaly in myelodysplastic syndrome: hyposegmented apoptotic neutrophil? *Blood, 98*, 1273–1275.

66. Untanu, R. V., & Vajpayee, N. (2022). May Hegglin anomaly. In *StatPearls*. https://www.ncbi.nlm.nih.gov/pubmed/28722981. Accessed June 16, 2023.

67. Tarekegn, K., Ramos, A. C., Gross, H. G. S., et al. (2021). Leukemoid reaction in a patient with severe COVID-19 infection. *Cureus, 13*, e13598.

68. Karakonstantis, S., Koulouridi, M., Pitsillos, K., et al. (2019). A prospective study of hospitalized patients with leukemoid reaction; causes, prognosis and value of manual peripheral smear review. *Rom J Intern Med, 57*, 241–247.

69. Calvache, E. T., Calvache, A. D. T., & Faulhaber, G. A. M. (2020). Systematic review about etiologic association to the leukoerythroblastic reaction. *Int J Lab Hematol, 42*, 495–500.

70. Sereeaphinan, C., Kanchanasuwan, S., & Julamanee, J. (2021). Mortality-associated clinical risk factors in patients with febrile neutropenia: a retrospective study. *IJID Reg, 1*, 5–11.

71. Pick, A. M., & Nystrom, K. K. (2014). Nonchemotherapy drug-induced neutropenia and agranulocytosis: could medications be the culprit? *J Pharm Pract, 27*, 447–452.

72. Andres, E., & Mourot-Cottet, R. (2017). Non-chemotherapy drug-induced neutropenia – an update. *Expert Opin Drug Saf, 16*, 1235–1242.

73. Abbas, S. A., Lopes, L. B., Moritz, E., et al. (2021). Serologic and molecular studies to identify neonatal alloimmune neutropenia in a cohort of 10,000 neonates. *Br J Haematol, 192*, 778–784.

74. Tomicic, M., Starcevic, M., Zach, V., et al. (2007). Alloimmune neonatal neutropenia due to anti-HNA-2a alloimmunization

with severe and prolonged neutropenia but mild clinical course: two case reports. *Arch Med Res, 38,* 792–796.

75. Lyall, E. G., Lucas, G. F., & Eden, O. B. (1992). Autoimmune neutropenia of infancy. *J Clin Pathol, 45,* 431–434.

76. Afzal, W., Owlia, M. B., Hasni, S., et al. (2017). Autoimmune neutropenia updates: etiology, pathology, and treatment. *South Med J, 110,* 300–307.

77. Fioredda, F., Calvillo, M., Bonanomi, S., et al. (2012). Congenital and acquired neutropenias consensus guidelines on therapy and follow-up in childhood from the Neutropenia Committee of the Marrow Failure Syndrome Group of the AIEOP (Associazione Italiana Emato-Oncologia Pediatrica). *Am J Hematol, 87,* 238–243.

78. Weller, P. F., & Klion, A. D. (2023). Eosinophil biology and causes of eosinophilia. P. Newburger, Editor. *UpToDate*: Waltham, MA. http://www.uptodate.com.

79. Swerdlow, S. H., Campo, E., Harris, N. L., et al. (2017). *WHO Classification of Tumours of Haematopoietic and Lymphoid Tissues* (4 ed., Vol. 2). Lyon, France: International Agency for Research on Cancer (IARC).

80. Hochhaus, A., Baccarani, M., Silver, R. T., et al. (2020). European LeukemiaNet 2020 recommendations for treating chronic myeloid leukemia. *Leukemia, 34,* 966–984.

81. Aijaz, J., Junaid, N., Naveed, M. A., et al. (2020). Risk stratification of chronic myeloid leukemia according to different prognostic scores. *Cureus, 12,* e7342.

82. Feriel, J., Depasse, F., & Genevieve, F. (2020). How I investigate basophilia in daily practice. *Int J Lab Hematol, 42,* 237–245.

83. Hoffmann, J. (2020). Basophil counting in hematology analyzers: time to discontinue? *Clin Chem Lab Med, 59,* 813–820.

84. Tosato, F. (2021). The role of laboratory hematology between technology and professionalism: the paradigm of basophil counting. *Clin Chem Lab Med, 59,* 821–822.

85. Ducrest, S., Meier, F., Tschopp, C., et al. (2005). Flowcytometric analysis of basophil counts in human blood and inaccuracy of hematology analyzers. *Allergy, 60,* 1446–1450.

86. Mannem, C., Krishanmurthy, T., Gayathri, B. R., et al. (2017). Characterization of pseudobasophilia on Sysmex-XT 1800i automated hematology analyser. *Int J Res Med Sci, 5,* 2912.

87. Manuel, K., Ambroise, M. M., Ramdas, A., et al. (2021). Pseudobasophilia as a screening tool in dengue: a single center study. *J Lab Physicians, 13,* 156–161.

88. Hur, M., Lee, Y. K., Lee, K. M., et al. (2004). Pseudobasophilia as an erroneous white blood cell differential count with a discrepancy between automated cell counters: report of two cases. *Clin Lab Haematol, 26,* 287–290.

89. Chandrashekar, V. (2013). Basophil differentials as a marker for atypical lymphocyte morphologic characteristics. *Lab Med, 44,* 133–135.

90. Chopra, P. B. S., & Arora, A. (2021). Comparison of basophil count by Beckman Coulter UniCel DxH 800, Sysmex XN-1000, and manual microscopy in cases of suspected chronic myeloid leukemia. *Iraqi J Hematol, 10,* 91–96.

91. Shah, H. P., Tormey, C. A., & Siddon, A. J. (2022). Automated analysers underestimate atypical basophil count in myeloid neoplasms. *Int J Lab Hematol, 44,* 831–836.

92. Hoffmann, J. (2022). Basophil counting by hematology analyzers in cases of suspected chronic myeloid leukemia. *Iraqi J Hematol, 11,* 89–90.

93. CLSI. (2007). *Reference Leukocyte (WBC) Differential Count (Proportional) and Evaluation of Instrumental Methods.* (2nd ed., CLSI approved standard H20-A2). Wayne, PA: Clinical Laboratory Standards Institute.

94. Schofield, K. P., Stone, P. C., Beddall, A. C., et al. (1983). Quantitative cytochemistry of the toxic granulation blood neutrophil. *Br J Haematol, 53,* 15–22.

95. van de Vyver, A., Delport, E. F., Esterhuizen, M., et al. (2010). The correlation between C-reactive protein and toxic granulation of neutrophils in the peripheral blood. *S Afr Med J, 100,* 442–444.

96. Zieve, P. D., Haghshenass, M., Blanks, M., et al. (1966). Vacuolization of the neutrophil. An aid in the diagnosis of septicemia. *Arch Intern Med, 118,* 356–357.

97. Beck, D. B., Ferrada, M. A., Sikora, K. A., et al. (2020). Somatic mutations in UBA1 and severe adult-onset autoinflammatory disease. *N Engl J Med, 383,* 2628–2638.

98. Yu, Y., & Sun, B. (2020). Autophagy-mediated regulation of neutrophils and clinical applications. *Burns Trauma, 8,* tkz001–tkz001.

99. Torlakovic, E., Hibbs, J. R., Miller, J. S., et al. (1995). Intracellular bacteria in blood smears in patients with central venous catheters. *Arch Intern Med, 155,* 1547–1550.

100. Bakken, J. S., Krueth, J., Wilson-Nordskog, C., et al. (1996). Clinical and laboratory characteristics of human granulocytic ehrlichiosis. *JAMA, 275,* 199–205.

101. McClain, M. T. (2023). Human ehrlichiosis and anaplasmosis. S. L. Kaplan, & D. J. Sexton, Editors. *UpToDate*: Waltham, MA. http://www.uptodate.com.

102. Merino, A., Molina, A., Rodriguez-Garcia, M., et al. (2021). Detection and significance of green inclusions in peripheral blood neutrophils and monocytes. *Int J Lab Hematol, 43,* e92–e94.

103. Soos, M. P., Heideman, C., Shumway, C., et al. (2019). Blue-green neutrophilic inclusion bodies in the critically ill patient. *Clin Case Rep, 7,* 1249–1252.

104. Cantu, M. D., Towne, W. S., Emmons, F. N., et al. (2020). Clinical significance of blue-green neutrophil and monocyte cytoplasmic inclusions in SARS-CoV-2 positive critically ill patients. *Br J Haematol, 190,* e89–e92.

105. Martins, N. N. N., Jardim, L. L., Pereira, L. S., et al. (2022). Blue-green cytoplasmic inclusions in neutrophils/monocytes of patients with yellow fever. *Int J Lab Hematol, 44,* e168–e171.

106. Lusky, K. (2021). Close-up on abnormal monocyte morphology in peripheral blood smears. *CAP Today, 35,* 1–40.

107. Lynch, D. T., Hall, J., & Foucar, K. (2018). How I investigate monocytosis. *Int J Lab Hematol, 40,* 107–114.

108. Aronson, M. D., & Auwaerter, P. G. (2023). Infectious mononucleosis. M. S. Hirsch, & S. L. Kaplan, Editors. *UpToDate*: Waltham, MA. http://www.uptodate.com.

109. Bu, G. L., Xie, C., Kang, Y. F., et al. (2022). How EBV infects: the tropism and underlying molecular mechanism for viral infection. *Viruses, 14*(11), 2372.

110. Downey, H. A. L., & Stasney, J. (1935). Infectious mononucleosis: part II hematologic studies. *JAMA, 105,* 764–768.

111. Feder, H. M., Jr., & Rezuke, W. N. (2020). Infectious mononucleosis diagnosed by Downey cells: sometimes the old ways are better. *Lancet, 395,* 225.

112. Sylvester, J. E., Buchanan, B. K., & Silva, T. W. (2023). Infectious mononucleosis: rapid evidence review. *Am Fam Physician, 107,* 71–78.

113. Hoagland, R. J. (1975). Infectious mononucleosis. *Prim Care, 2,* 295–307.

114. Fugl, A., & Andersen, C. L. (2019). Epstein-Barr virus and its association with disease – a review of relevance to general practice. *BMC Fam Pract, 20,* 62–73.

27

Introduction to Hematologic Neoplasms

Constantine E. Kanakis and Kamran M. Mirza*

OBJECTIVES

After completion of this chapter, the reader will be able to:

1. Describe the difference between a leukemia and lymphoma.
2. Compare and contrast acute versus chronic leukemias.
3. Describe etiologic factors associated with hematologic neoplasms including environmental exposures, viruses, and hereditary cancer predisposition syndromes.
4. Describe the difference between the French-American-British (FAB) and World Health Organization (WHO) systems of classification of hematologic neoplasms.
5. Describe how mutations in genes for key hematopoietic cell proteins and processes can lead to malignant transformation.
6. Compare and contrast oncogenes and tumor suppressor genes in terms of their normal functions, mechanisms by which each produces malignant transformation, effect of mutations on cells, and whether they act in a dominant or recessive manner, and provide an example of each.
7. Explain how mutation or loss of DNA repair genes can result in malignant transformation.
8. Explain why localized treatments are rarely used for hematologic neoplasms.
9. Briefly describe various types of therapies used for hematologic neoplasms.

OUTLINE

General Characteristics of Hematologic Neoplasms
Incidence, Prevalence, and Etiology
Classification Schemes
Molecular Pathogenesis
    Cellular Processes Perturbed in Hematologic Neoplasms
    Epigenetic Mechanisms
    Oncogenes
    Tumor Suppressor Genes
    DNA Repair Genes

Therapy
    Chemotherapy
    Radiation Therapy
    Supportive Therapy
    Targeted Therapy
    Hematopoietic Stem Cell Transplantation

CASE STUDY

After studying the material in this chapter, the reader should be able to respond to the following case study. Answers can be found in Appendix C.

A 66-year-old, previously healthy man presented to his primary care provider with a 5-day history of progressive weakness, fever, and bruising. Physical examination was unremarkable except for generalized ecchymoses. A complete blood count (CBC) was ordered, and the key results were as follows. Reference intervals can be found after the Index at the end of the book.

WBC	3.2×10^9/L	HGB	8.9 g/dL
NEUT	0.5×10^9/L	PLT	12×10^9/L

In the differential count, 44% of the white blood cells were similar to those in Figure 27.1, and a markedly decreased number of platelets and neutrophils were observed on his peripheral blood film.

1. Describe the nucleated cells in the figure, indicate how you would report them in the differential count, and identify the inclusions at the arrows and their significance.
2. What is the most likely diagnosis?
3. What additional laboratory testing should be performed to confirm the identity of the cells and the diagnosis?
4. Correlate the findings of weakness, fever, and ecchymoses with the applicable CBC results.
5. Discuss molecular mechanisms that can cause maturation arrest in acute leukemia.
6. Does the analyzer platelet count from the CBC correlate with the findings in the representative field of the peripheral blood film in the figure? What term is used to describe this finding?

Continued

*The authors extend appreciation to Peter D. Emanuel and Elaine M. Keohane, whose work in prior editions provided the foundation for this chapter.

CASE STUDY—cont'd

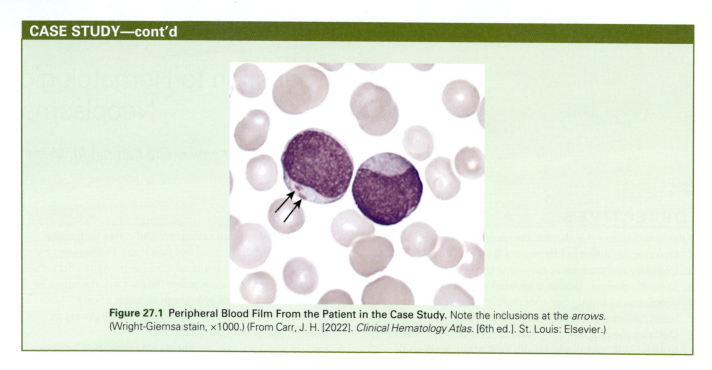

Figure 27.1 Peripheral Blood Film From the Patient in the Case Study. Note the inclusions at the *arrows.* (Wright-Giemsa stain, ×1000.) (From Carr, J. H. [2022]. *Clinical Hematology Atlas.* [6th ed.]. St. Louis: Elsevier.)

GENERAL CHARACTERISTICS OF HEMATOLOGIC NEOPLASMS

Hematologic neoplasms result from abnormal growth of cells of the hematopoietic system. In the context of this and the chapters that follow, discussion focuses on malignant neoplasms or hematologic malignancies. They are acquired genetic diseases; that is, most patients are not born with the condition but acquire it sometime later.

Hematologic neoplasms were the first human cancers in which a consistent genetic defect was identified. In 1960 Nowell and Hungerford[1] published an abstract that described a consistent shortened chromosome in seven patients with chronic myeloid leukemia (CML). This shortened chromosome was later named the Philadelphia chromosome for the city in which it was discovered. In 1973 Rowley[2] reported the t(9;22) translocation in CML, and in 1982 Taub and colleagues[3] reported the t(8;14) translocation in Burkitt lymphoma. Since then, with development of increasingly sensitive methods, a multitude of other mutations have been and continue to be identified in hematologic neoplasms with many serving as specific targets for therapy.

Hematologic neoplasms include several lineage-based categories: *leukemias, lymphomas,* and *myeloid proliferations and neoplasms.* These are broad terms that refer to large heterogeneous groups of disorders. They initiate in a hematopoietic cell as a result of acquisition of one or more mutations in key genes that regulate cell growth (proliferation), survival, differentiation, or maturation. They occur in hematopoietic cells of all lineages and at various stages of their development.

Most hematologic neoplasms are systemic (diffusely involving the peripheral blood and/or bone marrow) at initiation of the malignant process. Leukemias originate in the bone marrow, and leukemia cells readily pass into the peripheral blood, but they can also infiltrate lymphoid tissues (spleen, liver, lymph nodes) as well as other organs and tissues of the body. Lymphomas are solid tumors often composed of mature lymphoid cells that usually originate in the lymphatic system and proliferate in lymph nodes and other lymphoid organs and tissues. Lymphoma cells also can circulate in peripheral blood. With rare exceptions, most treatments for hematologic neoplasms given with curative intent cannot be localized, as with radiation or surgery, but must by nature be systemic-type treatments.

Leukemias are divided into lymphoid, myeloid, or mixed-phenotype lineages and further by presenting phenotype and cell count into acute (precursor cell) and chronic (mature cell) categories. In acute leukemias, onset is sudden, progression is rapid, and the outcome is often fatal in weeks or months if left untreated. The white blood cell (WBC) count is variable, and there is an excess accumulation of precursor hematopoietic cells or blasts of a specific lineage in bone marrow and peripheral blood because of a blockade in differentiation (maturation arrest). In chronic leukemias, the onset is insidious, and progression is slower, with a longer survival compared with acute leukemia. The WBC count is usually elevated, and there is a proliferation and accumulation of mature and maturing cells of a specific lineage. In all untreated leukemias, most normal hematopoietic cells in bone marrow are eventually replaced by leukemia cells, thus affecting normal bone marrow function. Because of the rapid expansion of blasts in the bone marrow in acute leukemia, bleeding as a result of thrombocytopenia, fever caused by neutropenia-induced infection, and fatigue as a result of decreased hemoglobin concentration are often found at presentation. Symptoms of chronic leukemias at presentation are generally nonspecific and variable; some patients may be asymptomatic and diagnosed after an incidental finding of an elevated WBC count or abnormal peripheral blood film. Table 27.1 compares acute and chronic leukemias.

TABLE 27.1	General Characteristics of Acute and Chronic Leukemia	
	Acute Leukemia	**Chronic Leukemia**
Predominant cell type	Precursor cell or blast	Mature
Onset	Sudden	Insidious
Symptoms at presentation	Fever (as a result of neutropenia-induced infection) Mucocutaneous bleeding (as a result of thrombocytopenia) Fatigue (as a result of anemia)	Variable, nonspecific; some asymptomatic
White blood cell count	Variable	Increased
Progression without treatment	Rapid; weeks to months	Slower; months to years

This chapter presents an overview of hematologic neoplasms as an introduction to the chapters that follow. In addition to the complete blood count (Chapters 12 and 13), peripheral blood film examination (Chapter 14), and bone marrow examination by aspiration and biopsy (Chapter 15), laboratory methods used to diagnose and monitor hematologic neoplasms include immunophenotyping by flow cytometric analysis (Chapter 28), molecular diagnostics (Chapter 29), and cytogenetics (Chapter 30). Specific hematologic neoplasms that are discussed include acute lymphoblastic and myeloid leukemias (Chapter 31), myeloproliferative neoplasms (Chapter 32), myelodysplastic neoplasms (Chapter 33), and mature lymphoid neoplasms (Chapter 34).

INCIDENCE, PREVALENCE, AND ETIOLOGY

The National Cancer Institute Surveillance, Epidemiology, and End Results (SEER) Program projected an estimated 60,650 new cases of leukemia, 80,470 cases of non-Hodgkin lymphoma, and 8540 cases of Hodgkin lymphoma for 2022 in the United States, representing 3.2%, 4.2%, and 0.4% of all cancers, respectively.[4–6] SEER estimated the prevalence of leukemia and lymphoma in the United States to be 472,714 in 2019, down from 1.3 million people in 2015.[4–6] Certain types of leukemia are more prevalent in a particular age group; for example, acute lymphoblastic leukemia is more common in young children, whereas chronic lymphocytic leukemia and myelodysplastic neoplasms are generally more common in older adults.

For most hematologic neoplasms, causes directly related to development of the malignancy are often unknown. There are, however, a few exceptions. Environmental toxins can induce genetic changes, leading to a malignant phenotype. Environmental exposures known to lead to hematologic neoplasms include radiation exposure, as experienced by survivors of atomic explosions, and exposure to organic solvents, such as benzene. In addition, as more cancer survivors live longer, it is clear that some alkylating agents and other types of chemotherapy used to treat various cancers can induce deoxyribonucleic acid (DNA) damage in hematopoietic cells, leading to hematologic neoplasms. This has led to the establishment of a World Health Organization (WHO) classification of *secondary myeloid neoplasm, post cytotoxic therapy* and reflects the complex interactions between a particular cytotoxic agent and the hematopoietic microenvironment; this was last updated in 2022.[7]

Some viruses have been implicated in hematologic neoplasms as a result of their ability to insert into host cell genomes,

cause genetic and epigenetic changes, and/or produce oncoproteins that interfere with normal cell processes that protect cells from malignant transformation.[8] Examples include human T-cell lymphotropic virus type 1 (HTLV-1), a retrovirus that invades CD4[+] lymphocytes and can cause adult T-cell leukemia/lymphoma,[9] and Epstein-Barr virus, a DNA virus that invades mainly B lymphocytes and has been implicated as a contributing causal factor in Burkitt and other non-Hodgkin lymphomas and in a subset of classic Hodgkin lymphoma.[10] Furthermore, immunosuppression resulting from human immunodeficiency virus type 1 (HIV-1) infection also causes an increased risk of non-Hodgkin lymphoma.[11]

In hereditary cancer predisposition syndromes, germline mutations in more than 140 different genes impart an increased risk of developing a hematologic neoplasm to varying degrees.[12] Some examples include congenital bone marrow failure syndromes (Chapter 19) such as Fanconi anemia (caused by mutation in one of the *FA* genes needed for DNA repair) and dyskeratosis congenita (caused by mutation in genes for telomere maintenance).[12] Other examples include Li-Fraumeni syndrome (usually caused by mutations in *TP53*) and ataxia telangiectasia (caused by mutations in *ATM*).[12] *TP53* (also called the *guardian of the genome*) is a tumor suppressor gene and nuclear transcription factor that promotes cell cycle arrest and apoptosis or programmed cell death (Chapter 4) when damaged cellular DNA cannot be repaired. ATM kinase is a component of the DNA damage response signaling pathway.[13,14] These proteins are part of a highly complex system of molecular checks and balances that prevents cells with damaged DNA from progressing through the cell cycle (Chapter 4). When mutated or deleted, they help sustain malignant cell phenotypes, allowing them to increase in number. Down syndrome (trisomy 21) is another condition that is associated with an increased risk of leukemia, but the genetic mechanisms involved are not fully understood.[15]

CLASSIFICATION SCHEMES

The French-American-British (FAB) classification of acute leukemias was devised in the 1970s and 1980s. FAB schemas were based largely on morphologic characteristics and relied heavily on examination of routine histologic stain preparations to distinguish lymphoid neoplasms from myeloid neoplasms (Figure 31.2). Although these types of diagnostic criteria have not been abandoned, more precise classifications such as WHO and concurrent International Consensus Classification (ICC) are now being used.[7,16,17] WHO periodically convenes an expert panel of hematopathologists, geneticists, and clinicians to determine consensus opinion on the classification scheme for hematologic neoplasms. The 2022 WHO classification considers cell lineage, dominant clinical attributes, and dominant biologic attributes. The classification uses broad categories of mature lymphoid neoplasms, myeloid neoplasms, and acute leukemia that will be discussed in detail in the chapters that follow.[7]

MOLECULAR PATHOGENESIS

Cellular Processes Perturbed in Hematologic Neoplasms

Cellular processes involved in hematopoiesis and its regulation are highly complex (Chapter 5), and mutations can cause dysregulation in stimulatory as well as inhibitory pathways. The types of mutations found in hematologic neoplasms include chromosomal rearrangements (such as translocation or inversion), gains or losses of chromosomes (aneuploidy), total or partial gene deletions, point mutations, insertions, and gene duplication/amplification (Chapters 29 and 30). Mutations may change or delete the functionality of essential genes for hematopoiesis or may disrupt regulatory mechanisms involved in their expression. The latter are called *epigenetic* mechanisms because the DNA sequence of the gene itself is not altered, but there is a heritable abnormality in how that gene is expressed (discussed in "Epigenetic Mechanisms").

Leukemogenesis (initiation and maintenance of leukemia) is a stepwise process in which a hematopoietic cell accumulates multiple, independent mutations, or "multiple hits," that affect various cellular pathways, which eventually advance the proliferation of a malignant clone. There are exceptions, however, such as in CML, in which apparently only one genetic mutation, the t(9;22) translocation with fusion of the *BCR::ABL1* genes (yielding a constitutively active tyrosine kinase), is required for initiation of the leukemia (Chapter 32).[18,19] However, this initiating mutation in CML causes genetic instability in the cell, and as the malignant clone rapidly proliferates, additional mutations accumulate causing more genetic defects, which lead to the terminal blast transformation stage.[20]

In hematologic neoplasms, mutations or deletions disrupt key genes coding for various cellular proteins (Box 27.1) and processes and may result in one or more of the following four major tenets of oncogenesis (malignant transformation of cells into cancer)[21]:

- Uncontrolled proliferation caused by mutation in genes coding for *signal transduction proteins* or *growth factor receptors*;

BOX 27.1   Examples of Cell Proteins Altered in Hematologic Neoplasms

Cell cycle regulatory proteins
Checkpoint control proteins
DNA repair proteins
Growth factor receptors
Nuclear transcription factors
Proapoptotic and antiapoptotic proteins
Signal transduction proteins

this leads to activation without stimulus and without ability to suppress the response.

- Loss of DNA repair capability and cell cycle control as a result of inactivating mutation or deletion of genes coding for *DNA repair proteins, cell cycle proteins* that regulate the cell cycle, or *checkpoint control proteins* that arrest the cell cycle when DNA is damaged; inactivation or loss of one or more of these proteins allows cells with damaged DNA to progress through the cell cycle and proliferate.
- Block in differentiation due to mutation in genes coding for *nuclear transcription factors* or aberrant changes in their *epigenetic regulation*; this leads to maturation arrest or dysplastic changes.
- Continued cell survival and inhibition of apoptosis as a result of mutation or deletion of genes coding for *proapoptotic* and other related proteins; this leads to persistence of *leukemic stem cells* that retain self-renewal properties. In the hematopoietic environment, apoptosis is essential to contain and control the massive cell expansion that occurs in the hematopoietic system during times of stress, infection, hemolysis, or hemorrhage.

Epigenetic Mechanisms

Epigenetic mechanisms control how genes are expressed and silenced (Table 27.2). They are important for normal gene expression in all types of cells and are critical for complex processes such as embryogenesis and cell differentiation. Heritable aberrant epigenetic changes can occur in hematopoietic cells, and those changes are retained in their progeny. Aberrant epigenetic mechanisms can initiate and maintain many hematologic neoplasms much like the multiple hits discussed previously. Examples include the following:

1. Hypermethylation and hypomethylation of CpG islands in gene promoters and other noncoding DNA regions by DNA methyltransferases (DNMTs) that inhibit gene transcription or cause inappropriate gene expression.

TABLE 27.2	Examples of Epigenetic Mechanisms That Control Gene Expression
DNA methylation	Hypermethylation of CpG islands in gene promoters and other noncoding DNA regions by DNA methyltransferases prevents gene transcription and expression.
Histone acetylation	Histone acetyltransferases keep DNA chromatin in an open configuration so that transcription can occur.
	Histone deacetylases keep DNA chromatin in a closed configuration so genes are unavailable for transcription, replication, and repair.
miRNAs	miRNAs (small 22 nucleotide RNA segments) inhibit gene expression by specifically binding to targeted mRNA transcripts, blocking their translation to protein, and causing their destabilization and degradation.

miRNA, MicroRNA; *mRNA*, messenger RNA.

2. Mutations in histone acetyltransferases or excessive recruitment of histone deacetylases to transcription sites that keep DNA chromatin in a closed, inactive state so that genes are unavailable for transcription, replication, and repair.

3. MicroRNAs (miRNAs, small 22-nucleotide ribonucleic acid [RNA] segments) that inhibit gene expression by specifically binding to targeted messenger RNA (mRNA) transcripts, blocking their translation to protein and causing their destabilization and degradation.[22,23]

Examples of transcriptional epigenetic repression of hematopoietic genes causing a block in differentiation are the t(8;21) translocation and fusion of the core-binding transcription factor gene, *RUNX1,* with the *RUNX1T1* gene in acute myeloid leukemia, and the t(15;17) translocation and fusion of the retinoic acid receptor gene, *RARA,* with the *PML* gene in acute promyelocytic leukemia (APL) (Chapter 31). Hypermethylation is also a common method of silencing tumor suppressor genes (discussed in "Tumor Suppressor Genes").

Oncogenes

Oncogenes originally were identified in tumor-forming retroviruses but are derived from normal human cellular homologues called proto-oncogenes. The DNA sequence of proto-oncogenes is highly conserved, and the protein products they encode are essential for normal cellular function. They are important in signaling pathways, cell proliferation, cell differentiation, and apoptosis. Mutation of a proto-oncogene can convert it to an oncogene with leukemogenic potential.[21] These are considered dominant disorders because only one mutated copy of the oncogene is required to contribute to leukemogenesis. Activation of the dominant oncogene alters the gene product or its expression and transforms the cell into a malignant phenotype, even in the presence of a residual normal allele. Most chromosome translocations in leukemias involve oncogenes. Mutations cause constitutive (continuous) and unregulated activation of the oncogene and therefore are called *gain-of-function* mutations. In hematologic neoplasms, the type of proto-oncogenes usually involved are signal transduction proteins (such as tyrosine kinases), growth factor receptors, or transcription factors.

Mutations that activate proto-oncogenes can be qualitative or quantitative. Qualitative alterations involve a structural change to the proto-oncogene and production of an *abnormal protein product.* The structural change results in dysregulation and constitutive activation of the abnormal oncogene product. A common qualitative mutation is a *translocation* that results in a chimeric fusion gene, such as the t(9;22) translocation forming the *BCR::ABL1* fusion gene in CML and in some cases of acute lymphoblastic leukemia. The abnormal *BCR::ABL1* fusion gene is transcribed and translated to a fusion protein with dysregulated tyrosine kinase activity that is inappropriately expressed (Chapter 32). Other genetic mechanisms that cause dysregulation of a tyrosine kinase include *point mutations* such as the *JAK2* p.Val617Phe (c.1849G>T) mutation in polycythemia vera (Chapter 32) and *internal tandem* duplication such as the *FLT3*-ITD mutation in acute myeloid leukemia (Chapter 31). *JAK2* encodes a nonreceptor tyrosine kinase associated with the intracellular domain of growth factor receptors, such as the erythropoietin receptor, and

normally transmits an intracellular signal for proliferation when the appropriate growth factor ligand binds to the extracellular domain of the receptor. *FLT3* codes for a receptor tyrosine kinase preferentially expressed on the membrane of hematopoietic stem and progenitor cells that promotes hematopoietic cell proliferation and differentiation when bound with its ligand (Chapters 4 and 5). The common feature of these examples is constitutive activation of the mutated kinase and its intracellular signaling for proliferation in the absence of ligand binding, with an inability to suppress or turn off the signal.

In quantitative mutations, there is an *overexpression of a normal proto-oncogene* in a hematopoietic cell. An example of this type of mechanism is found in B-lymphoid neoplasms in which a proto-oncogene becomes oncogenic by translocation next to the promoter of the immunoglobulin heavy chain (*IGH*) locus on chromosome 14. The *IGH* gene is normally actively transcribed in B cells, so when a normal proto-oncogene comes under the control of the *IGH* promoter, there is an *overexpression* of its normal proto-oncogene product. Examples include the t(14;18) translocation in follicular lymphoma with overexpression of the *BCL2* gene, normally located on chromosome 18, and t(11;14) translocation in mantle cell lymphoma with overexpression of the *CCND1* gene, normally located on chromosome 11, that codes for cyclin D1. BCL2 protein inhibits apoptosis, and cyclin D1 regulates the cell cycle (Chapters 4 and 34). Excess production of either of these proteins causes dysregulation in apoptosis or the cell cycle contributing to malignant transformation.

Another mechanism that results in overexpression of a normal proto-oncogene product is *gene amplification.* By increasing the gene copy number in each cell, there is an increased production of the protein product and oncogenic potential. This mechanism, however, is uncommon in hematologic neoplasms. Gene expression can also be increased by aberrant epigenetic mechanisms and by an increase in the number of chromosomes, such as in trisomy (presence of three copies of a chromosome and three copies of its coded genes, instead of the normal two copies).

Tumor Suppressor Genes

Tumor suppressor genes are so named because they code for proteins that protect cells from malignant transformation. These gene products differ from oncogenes in that they normally slow down cell division or promote apoptosis. Whereas proto-oncogenes become oncogenic when activated, tumor suppressor genes promote malignant transformation when they are inactivated or deleted. They do not act in a dominant fashion as in oncogenes; rather, cells are transformed into a malignant phenotype only after both alleles are deleted or inactivated (*loss-of-function* mutations), the so-called two-hit mechanism proposed by Knudson.[24] Mechanisms for loss of function of tumor suppressor genes include gene deletion, inactivating mutation, and epigenetic silencing.

Numerous tumor suppressor genes have now been identified, and many have been found to be associated with autosomal dominant familial cancer predisposition syndromes. Some well-known examples of loss or inactivation of tumor suppressor genes include *TP53* in Li-Fraumeni syndrome (mentioned in

TABLE 27.3	Comparison of Oncogenes and Tumor Suppressor Genes	
	Oncogenes	**Tumor Suppressor Genes**
Normal functions	Promote cell proliferation and differentiation, signal transduction, apoptosis	Detect damaged DNA and delay cell cycle to allow for DNA repair or apoptosis
Effect of mutations	Leukemogenic when inappropriately activated (gain-of-function mutation); causes constitutive (continuous), dysregulated, and/or overexpression of oncogene product	Leukemogenic when inactivated or deleted (loss-of-function mutation); causes inability to prevent cells with damaged DNA from progressing through the cell cycle; helps sustain malignant phenotypes
Genetics	Dominant; only one mutant allele needed for leukemogenesis	Recessive; deletion or inactivation of both alleles needed for leukemogenesis
Examples of mutations	Chromosomal rearrangement (translocation, inversion), point mutation, internal tandem duplication, gene amplification	Deletion, inactivating mutation, epigenetic silencing
Examples relevant to hematologic neoplasms	*ABL1, JAK2, BCL2*	*TP53, RB1, WT1*

"Incidence, Prevalence, and Etiology"), *RB1* involved in familial retinoblastoma, and *WT1* in Wilms tumor. More importantly, these tumor suppressor genes are deleted or inactivated in many sporadic (nonfamilial) cancers, including hematologic neoplasms, which leads to accumulation of additional mutations and a more clinically aggressive state. An example is chronic lymphocytic leukemia, which has a more aggressive course when the *TP53* gene is deleted or mutated, warranting a different approach to therapy (Chapter 34).[25]

Table 27.3 compares characteristics of oncogenes and tumor suppressor genes.

DNA Repair Genes

Mutations in *DNA repair genes* are also involved in hematologic neoplasms. Mutations in these genes cause genetic instability and increased mutation rates, leading to an increased risk of malignant transformation. An example is the Fanconi anemia gene, *FA,* which is important for maintaining genomic stability in hematopoietic tissues (mentioned in "Incidence, Prevalence, and Etiology").

Regardless of the type of chromosome or genetic abnormality, oncogene activation or the loss or inactivation of tumor suppressor or DNA repair genes has adverse molecular effects on proliferation, differentiation, maturation, survival, apoptosis, cell cycle control, and DNA repair mechanisms in hematopoietic cells and an increased risk of malignant transformation. The list of chromosomal and molecular aberrations known to occur in various hematologic neoplasms continues to grow on an almost daily basis. Indexing this list is far beyond the scope of this chapter, but specific examples will be discussed in the chapters that follow.

THERAPY

Treatment for leukemia and lymphoma may involve chemotherapy, radiation, supportive therapy, targeted therapies, and hematopoietic stem cell transplantation (HSCT) (Box 27.2). Research in leukemia-specific therapy using molecular targets and immunotherapy and cellular therapy is ongoing and rapidly advancing. New schemes for risk stratification and treatment modalities have resulted in prolonged survival and cures for conditions that were uniformly fatal with conventional

BOX 27.2	General Categories of Therapy for Hematologic Neoplasms

Chemotherapy
   Cell cycle effects: phase-specific or phase-nonspecific agents
   Biochemical mode of action: alkylating agents, plant alkaloids, antimetabolites, antitumor antibiotics, glucocorticoids
Radiation therapy
Supportive therapy
   Growth factors and cytokines
Targeted therapy
   Targeted molecular therapy
   Immunotherapy
   Cellular therapy
Hematopoietic stem cell transplantation
   Syngeneic
   Allogeneic
   Autologous

treatment. In contrast to many solid tumors, numerous hematologic neoplasms now have cure rates that are substantially higher than they were two or three decades ago. Many exciting new therapies that are less toxic are now under development or are already employed in patient settings. These therapies are bringing more optimism to the care of patients with hematologic neoplasms. Selection of the best therapy must start, however, with an accurate diagnosis. Even the most effective therapies do not work if they are applied in the wrong circumstances.

Curative treatment strategies are now a realistic goal for patients with Hodgkin lymphoma, CML, hairy cell leukemia, some forms of non-Hodgkin lymphoma, and for children with acute lymphoblastic leukemia. Cure may be attainable in other patients with acute lymphoblastic or myeloid leukemia, and long-term remissions may be achievable in adults with multiple myeloma. For patients with other hematologic neoplasms such as mantle cell lymphoma, chronic lymphocytic leukemia, or a therapy-related leukemia, cure remains elusive, and therapy must be directed more toward attaining remissions or providing supportive care.

Chemotherapy

Chemotherapy is oral or parenteral cancer treatment with compounds that possess antitumor properties. Methods of action of chemotherapy drugs vary considerably. Chemotherapy agents can be classified in two ways: by their effects on the cell cycle and by their biochemical mechanism of action. Some chemotherapy drugs can affect cells only in specific phases of the cell cycle (phase specific), whereas other drugs act during any phase of the cell cycle (phase nonspecific). A general biochemical classification of chemotherapy agents includes alkylating agents, plant alkaloids, antimetabolites, antitumor antibiotics, and glucocorticoids. Chemotherapy drugs are usually given in combination according to various published protocols or in the context of a clinical trial.

Chemotherapy is usually administered in three phases: induction, consolidation, and maintenance. The goal of induction is to rapidly decrease the tumor burden and achieve remission. There are different types of remission depending on the leukemia and the sensitivity of methods used for detection of malignant cells. For example, a *hematologic* remission in acute leukemia may include a normocellular bone marrow, recovery of peripheral blood cell counts, and no microscopic evidence of leukemia cells, whereas a *cytogenetic* remission is the absence of the cytogenetic defect determined by karyotyping methods (Chapter 30). A *molecular* remission is the absence of leukemia cell nucleic acid sequences using highly sensitive molecular methods capable of detecting one leukemia cell among 10^5 or 10^6 normal cells (Chapter 29). After hematologic remission is achieved, millions of leukemia cells may still be undetected in the body (called *minimal residual disease*), so a consolidation phase is done with different chemotherapy agents to further reduce the number of leukemia cells. A maintenance phase may be incorporated in the treatment plan, which is continued for a longer period with less intensive agents to eradicate any remaining leukemia cells to prevent a relapse.

Chemotherapy agents affect both malignant and normal cells. Their effects are most pronounced on rapidly dividing cells, such as those in gastrointestinal mucosa and bone marrow. This limits dosage and usually determines the maximum tolerated dose for a patient. Neutrophil and platelet counts are routinely monitored because they are the first cells to decrease after chemotherapy because of their shorter life spans.

Radiation Therapy

Radiation kills cells by producing unstable ions that damage DNA and may cause instant or delayed death of cells. Toxic effects of radiotherapy can occur during therapy or much later. Complications can be reduced through use of combined anterior and posterior treatment ports and application of maximal shielding techniques to prevent damage to normal tissues. The hematopoietic system, gastrointestinal tract, and skin are most often affected during radiotherapy. Spinal and pelvic irradiation can cause marrow suppression, sometimes lowering blood counts to life-threatening levels. Toxic effects are usually reversible when radiation is stopped.

Supportive Therapy

Numerous substances that are naturally produced in the human body have now been developed using recombinant technologies. Some are commercially produced and cleared by the US Food and Drug Administration (FDA) for supportive care of patients with cancer, including patients with hematologic neoplasms. Growth factors and colony-stimulating factors (CSFs), a class of cytokines, normally act in the bone marrow microenvironment to stimulate blood cell formation (Chapter 5). Erythropoietin promotes red blood cell formation, and recombinant forms are administered to cancer patients with anemia induced by chemotherapy. Similarly, granulocyte colony-stimulating factor (G-CSF) and granulocyte-macrophage colony-stimulating factor (GM-CSF) are used to rapidly expand the number of mature neutrophils to fight or prevent infection. Recombinant forms of G-CSF and GM-CSF are administered to cancer patients with chemotherapy-induced neutropenia. These agents not only have improved patients' quality of life but also have allowed more efficient and effective delivery of chemotherapy regimens by preventing delays of or dosage reductions in chemotherapy courses as a result of low blood cell counts.

Targeted Therapy

As more has been learned about specific genetic lesions that cause hematologic neoplasms, researchers have worked to develop targeted therapies that act specifically on malignant cells and leave normal cells untouched. As a result of these advances, cancer therapy is realizing the dream of targeted therapeutics and is moving away from nonspecific therapies such as chemotherapy and radiation. In 2001 the FDA cleared imatinib mesylate for treatment of chronic-phase CML as the first rationally designed molecular targeted therapy for a cancer.[26] The t(9;22) translocation in CML results in production of the *BCR::ABL1* gene fusion, creating a fusion protein with constitutive and unregulated tyrosine kinase activity. Imatinib is an orally administered, small tyrosine kinase inhibitor (TKI) molecule that binds to the ABL1 domain of the fusion protein and selectively blocks its tyrosine kinase activity.[26,27] It reduces the massive cell proliferation and induces apoptosis of CML cells and remission with very few side effects.[27] Imatinib is now the first-line treatment for chronic-phase CML and has resulted in long-term remissions of 10 years and longer (Chapter 32).[26,27] Newer and more potent TKIs have also been developed (such as dasatinib and nilotinib) to treat imatinib resistance that develops in some patients with CML; these second-generation drugs have also been cleared by the FDA for first-line treatment in CML.[26-28] Imatinib is also used in combination with chemotherapeutic agents to treat *BCR::ABL1* positive acute lymphoblastic leukemia.[28] Other TKIs are in development, and their effectiveness and safety are being evaluated in other hematologic neoplasms with dysregulated kinases, such as JAK2 inhibitors in polycythemia vera and FLT3 inhibitors in acute myeloid leukemia.[29,30]

In APL, the t(15;17) translocation, results in fusion of the retinoic acid receptor gene, *RARA,* with the *PML* gene. RARA protein is a ligand-dependent transcription factor that when bound to retinoic acid, upregulates expression of target genes required for myeloid differentiation.[31] However, RARA in the *PML::RARA* fusion does not respond to retinoic acid, resulting in silencing of transcription of genes needed for differentiation and a block in maturation beyond the promyelocytic stage.[31] Now the prognosis of patients with APL is dramatically improved with the availability of differentiation therapy using all-trans retinoic acid (ATRA) as first-line treatment along with chemotherapeutic agents (Chapter 31). ATRA binds to RARA in the fusion protein and overcomes the block, allowing transcription and expression of genes needed for myeloid differentiation and maturation.[31]

In lymphoid neoplasms, treatment includes immunotherapy using monoclonal antibodies for targeted therapeutic strategies. Monoclonal antibodies generally must be delivered intravenously or subcutaneously. An example is rituximab (anti-CD20), which binds to the CD20 antigen present on malignant cells in many B-lymphoid neoplasms and has shown efficacy in non-Hodgkin lymphoma and chronic lymphocytic leukemia.[32] The antibody targets CD20+ lymphocytes for destruction by antibody-mediated and complement-mediated cytotoxicity.[32] Additional modifications of immunotherapy are now being developed, such as the bispecific T cell engager (BiTE) monoclonal antibody, blinatumomab.[33] It can bind both CD19 and CD3, bringing CD3+ T-lymphoid cells closer to CD19+ B-lymphoid cells to promote their destruction by cytokines.[33] It has shown efficacy in relapsed or refractory non-Hodgkin lymphoma and precursor acute lymphoblastic leukemia.[33] Monoclonal antibodies can also be conjugated with toxins (called *immunoconjugates*) to kill target cells. An example is inotuzumab ozogamicin, an anti-CD22 monoclonal antibody conjugated with calicheamicin, an antibiotic with cytotoxic activity.[34] The conjugated antibody binds to CD22+ B-lymphoid cells, bringing the toxin close to the cell where it rapidly enters, binds to, and damages DNA and induces apoptosis.[34] It has been used with encouraging results in relapsed or refractory acute lymphoblastic leukemia.[34]

Cellular therapy is also being implemented, with high efficacy in patients with high-risk hematologic neoplasms. One such therapy uses CD19-specific chimeric antigen receptor T (CAR-T) cells, in which patient T cells are collected by pheresis and are genetically engineered ex vivo using lentiviral or retroviral vectors to express protein complexes that recognize only the patient's leukemia cells.[35] Engineered CAR-T cells then specifically bind to patient's leukemia cells and target them for destruction.[35] CAR-T cells have been successful in achieving remission in patients with high-risk, refractory, or relapsed acute lymphoblastic leukemia and non-Hodgkin lymphoma.[35] Gene editing technologies, such as CRISPR/Cas9 targeted nuclease, are also being used to improve the potency and safety of CAR-T cells.[35]

Epigenetic therapies are also used in hematologic neoplasms to reverse epigenetic silencing of gene transcription. For example, histone deacetylase inhibitors are being used in cutaneous T-cell lymphoma to prevent deacetylation, allowing chromatin to open so that repressed genes can be transcribed and expressed.[22,36] Likewise, hypomethylating treatment, using drugs that remove methyl groups from gene promoters allowing expression of genes, is used in high-risk myelodysplastic neoplasms.[22,37]

These and other targeted therapies will be discussed in more detail in chapters covering specific hematologic neoplasms. Development and optimization of targeted therapies is an area of intense research, and their use will continue to improve patient outcomes and survival as they more specifically target malignant cells and not patients' normal cells.

Hematopoietic Stem Cell Transplantation

As more has been learned about hematopoietic stem cells (HSCs), the therapeutic method of *bone marrow transplantation* has evolved to be more aptly termed *hematopoietic stem cell transplantation* (HSCT) because different sources in addition to bone marrow can be used to obtain HSCs. Along with bone marrow, peripheral blood and umbilical cord blood (UCB) are rich sources. Bone marrow is harvested through multiple needle aspirations, typically from the posterior iliac crests, and it is done in a sterile surgical environment, usually under general or regional anesthesia.[38] Collection of peripheral blood stem cells is less invasive in that they are harvested by pheresis after mobilization out of bone marrow by cytokines and chemokines such as G-CSF and plerixafor.[38] UCB is collected by inserting a sterile needle into the umbilical vein after the infant is delivered and the cord is clamped and cut, either before or after delivery of the placenta.[38] Regardless of the source, HSCs are considered *adult stem cells,* even when they come from umbilical cord blood, as opposed to *embryonic stem cells,* which are the subject of considerable ethical debate. HSCT remains an expensive and difficult treatment alternative.

When the decision to perform HSCT has been made and a donor has been found, an extensive hospital stay is usually required. Pretransplantation conditioning regimens use high-dose therapy to kill the patient's malignant cells and normal bone marrow cells. This regimen reduces the body's immunity to dangerously low levels and necessitates special protective isolation. Granulocyte counts approaching zero are commonly seen immediately before and after transplantation. After infusion of donor HSCs, the recipient remains in a severely immunosuppressed condition for 2 weeks or longer. Strict isolation at this point is crucial. Prophylactic antibiotics and intravenous nutrition are also essential to keep the patient alive until marrow engraftment. Recovery of granulocytes, reticulocytes, and platelets to normal levels is monitored closely in peripheral blood. Evaluation and management of red blood cell and platelet transfusions are crucial components of HSCT. After discharge, peripheral blood cell counts and bone marrow continue to be monitored to measure the progress of engraftment of donor HSCs.

HSCs for treatment of malignant disease come from donors of three general types: (1) *syngeneic,* or from an identical twin; (2) *allogeneic,* usually from an HLA-identical sibling or HLA-matched unrelated donor; or (3) *autologous,* in which the patient's own marrow or peripheral blood stem cells are used (Figure 27.2). Most HSC donors are allogeneic, but for optimal outcomes, it is important to match as many HLA antigens as possible. Within any given family, there can be only four HLA haplotypes (two maternal and two paternal), and there is one chance in four that a sibling will be HLA identical. If an HLA-identical sibling or fully HLA-matched unrelated donor is not available, HLA-partially matched, related, or unrelated donors have been used.

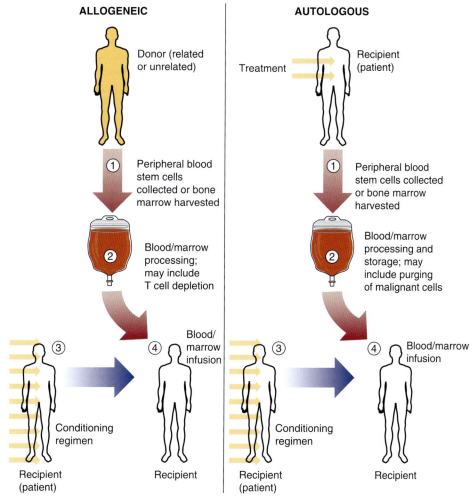

Figure 27.2 Overview of Hematopoietic Stem Cell Transplantation in Allogeneic and Autologous Donors.

Even with continued improvement in technique and supportive care, HSCT carries many risks. Death after transplantation is caused by complications of the conditioning regimens, such as infections or bleeding from bone marrow suppression, graft-versus-host disease, regrowth of malignant cells, and failure of donor HSCs to engraft.

SUMMARY

- Most neoplasms of the hematopoietic system are acquired genetic diseases. They include leukemias, lymphomas, and myeloid proliferations and neoplasms.
- Leukemias originate in bone marrow, and leukemia cells readily pass into peripheral blood, but they can also infiltrate lymphoid tissues (spleen, liver, lymph nodes) as well as other organs and tissues of the body. Lymphomas are solid tumors of lymphoid cells that usually originate in the lymphatic system and proliferate in lymph nodes and other lymphoid organs and tissues.
- Leukemias are divided into lymphoid, myeloid, and mixed-phenotype lineages, and further into acute (precursor cell) and chronic (mature cell) categories. In acute leukemias, onset is sudden, progression is rapid, and the outcome is often fatal in weeks or months if left untreated. In chronic leukemias, onset is insidious, and progression is slower, with a longer survival compared with acute leukemia.

- For most hematologic neoplasms, causes directly related to development of the malignancy are unknown, but a few exceptions exist. Some known causes include environmental toxins, certain viruses, previous chemotherapy, and familial predisposition.
- Classification schemes for hematologic neoplasms include the older French-American-British (FAB) system, based primarily on morphology and cytochemical staining, and the World Health Organization (WHO) system, which retains some elements of the FAB scheme but emphasizes molecular and cytogenetic abnormalities.
- Types of mutations found in hematologic neoplasms include chromosomal rearrangements (such as translocation or inversion), gains or losses of chromosomes (aneuploidy), total or partial gene deletions, point mutations, insertions, and gene duplication/amplification.

- Hematologic neoplasms illustrate that a single mutation, or more commonly a series of mutations, can lead to malignant transformation by disrupting the molecular machinery of hematopoietic cells.
- Most chromosomal translocations in leukemias involve oncogenes. Activation of the dominant transforming oncogene alters its gene product or its expression and transforms the cell into a malignant phenotype, even in the presence of a residual normal allele.
- In contrast to oncogenes, tumor suppressor genes contribute to the malignant process only if both alleles have been lost or otherwise inactivated.
- Activation of oncogenes or the loss or inactivation of tumor suppressor or DNA repair genes has adverse molecular effects on proliferation, survival, differentiation, and maturation of hematopoietic cells.

- Most hematologic neoplasms are systemic (diffusely involving the peripheral blood and/or bone marrow) at initiation of the malignant process. Therefore with rare exceptions, most treatments for hematologic neoplasms given with curative intent are not localized, such as radiation or surgery, but must by nature be systemic treatments.
- Current treatments for hematologic neoplasms can be generally divided into the following categories: chemotherapy, radiation therapy, supportive therapy, targeted therapy, and hematopoietic stem cell transplantation.

Now that you have completed this chapter, go back and read again the case study at the beginning and respond to the questions presented. Answers can be found in Appendix C.

REVIEW QUESTIONS

Answers can be found in Appendix C.

1. Lymphomas differ from leukemias in that they are:
   a. Solid tumors
   b. Not considered systemic diseases
   c. Never found in peripheral blood
   d. Do not originate from hematopoietic cells
2. Which one of the following viruses is known to CAUSE lymphoid neoplasms in humans?
   a. HIV-1
   b. HTLV-1
   c. Hepatitis B
   d. Parvovirus B
3. Loss of function of tumor suppressor genes increase the risk of hematologic neoplasms by:
   a. Suppressing cell division
   b. Activating tyrosine kinases, which promote proliferation
   c. Promoting excessive apoptosis of hematopoietic cells
   d. Allowing cells with damaged DNA to progress through the cell cycle
4. Oncogenes are said to act in a dominant fashion because:
   a. Leukemia is a dominating disease that is systemic
   b. The oncogene product is a gain-of-function mutation
   c. A mutation in only one allele is sufficient to promote a malignant phenotype
   d. They are inherited by autosomal dominant transmission
5. Which one of the following is NOT one of the cellular abnormalities produced by oncogenes?
   a. Constitutive activation of a growth factor receptor
   b. Constitutive activation of a signaling protein
   c. Acceleration of DNA catabolism
   d. Dysregulation of apoptosis

6. Which one of the following is an example of a tumor suppressor gene?
   a. *ABL1*
   b. *RARA*
   c. *TP53*
   d. *JAK2*
7. G-CSF is provided as supportive treatment during leukemia treatment regimens to:
   a. Suppress GVHD
   b. Overcome anorexia
   c. Prevent anemia
   d. Reduce the risk of infection
8. Imatinib is an example of what type of leukemia treatment?
   a. Supportive care
   b. Chemotherapy
   c. Bone marrow conditioning agent
   d. Targeted therapy
9. Which one of the following statements is FALSE about epigenetic mechanisms?
   a. Epigenetic mechanisms control how genes are expressed and silenced.
   b. MicroRNAs can bind to specific mRNAs and block their translation.
   c. Hypermethylation of CpG islands in gene promoters results in their overactivation.
   d. Histone deacetylases keep chromatin of target genes in a closed inactive state.
10. Which one of the following is NOT a source of hematopoietic stem cells for transplantation?
    a. Spleen
    b. Bone marrow
    c. Peripheral blood
    d. Umbilical cord blood

REFERENCES

1. Nowell, P. C., & Hungerford, D. A. (1960). A minute chromosome in human granulocytic leukemia (Abstract). *Science, 132,* 1497.

2. Rowley, J. D. (1973). A new consistent chromosomal abnormality in chronic myelogenous leukemia identified by quinacrine fluorescence and Giemsa staining. *Nature, 243,* 290–293.

3. Taub, R., Kirsch, I., Morton, C., et al. (1982). Translocation of the *c-myc* gene into the immunoglobulin heavy chain locus in human Burkitt lymphoma and murine plasmacytoma cells. *Proc Natl Acad Sci USA, 79,* 7837–7841.

4. National Cancer Institute, Surveillance, Epidemiology, and End Results Program (SEER). *Cancer Stat Facts: Leukemia.* https://seer.cancer.gov/statfacts/html/leuks.html. Accessed December 28, 2022.

5. National Cancer Institute, Surveillance, Epidemiology, and End Results Program (SEER). *Cancer Stat Facts: Non-Hodgkin Lymphoma.* https://seer.cancer.gov/statfacts/html/nhl.html. Accessed December 28, 2022.

6. National Cancer Institute, Surveillance, Epidemiology, and End Results Program (SEER). *Cancer Stat Facts: Hodgkin Lymphoma.* https://seer.cancer.gov/statfacts/html/hodg.html. Accessed December 28, 2022.

7. WHO Classification of Tumours Editorial Board. *Haematolymphoid tumours. Lyon (France): International Agency for Research on Cancer; forthcoming.* (WHO classification of tumours series, 5th ed.; vol. 11). https://publications.iarc.fr.

8. Gaglia, M. M., & Munger, K. (2018). More than just oncogenes: mechanisms of tumorigenesis by human viruses. *Curr Opin Virol, 32,* 48–59.

9. Fiore, D., Cappelli, L. V., Broccoli, A., et al. (2020). Peripheral T cell lymphomas: from the bench to the clinic. *Nat Rev Cancer, 20,* 323–342.

10. Yin, H., Qu, J., Peng, Q., et al. (2019). Molecular mechanisms of EBV-driven cell cycle progression and oncogenesis. *Med Microbiol Immunol, 208,* 573–583.

11. Baptista, M. J., Tapia, G., Muñoz-Marmol, A. M., et al. (2022). Genetic and phenotypic characterisation of HIV-associated aggressive B-cell non-Hodgkin lymphomas, which do not occur specifically in this population: diagnostic and prognostic implications. *Histopathology, 81,* 826–840.

12. Sweet-Cordero, E. A., & Biegel, J. A. (2019). The genomic landscape of pediatric cancers: implications for diagnosis and treatment. *Science, 363,* 1170–1175.

13. Zhang, C., Liu, J., Xu, D., et al. (2020). Gain-of-function mutant p53 in cancer progression and therapy. *J Mol Cell Biol, 12,* 674–687.

14. Huang, R. X., & Zhou, P. K. (2020). DNA damage response signaling pathways and targets for radiotherapy sensitization in cancer. *Signal Transduct Target Ther, 5,* 1–27.

15. Labuhn, M., Perkins, K., Matzk, S., et al. (2019). Mechanisms of progression of myeloid preleukemia to transformed myeloid leukemia in children with Down syndrome. *Cancer Cell, 36,* 123–138.

16. Campo, E., Jaffe, E. S., Cook, J. R., et al. (2022). The international consensus classification of mature lymphoid neoplasms: a report from the clinical advisory committee. *Blood, 140,* 1229–1253.

17. Arber, D. A., Orazi, A., Hasserjian, R. P., et al. (2022). International consensus classification of myeloid neoplasms and acute leukemias: integrating morphologic, clinical, and genomic data. *Blood, 140,* 1200–1228.

18. Stam, K., Heisterkamp, N., & Grosveld, G. (1985). Evidence of a new chimeric bcr/c-abl mRNA in patients with chronic myelocytic leukemia and the Philadelphia chromosome. *N Engl J Med, 313,* 1429–1433.

19. Daley, G. Q., Van Etten, R. A., & Baltimore, D. (1990). Induction of chronic myelogenous leukemia in mice by the P210 *bcr/abl* gene of the Philadelphia chromosome. *Science, 247,* 824–830.

20. Ko, T. K., Javed, A., Lee, K. L., et al. (2020). An integrative model of pathway convergence in genetically heterogeneous blast crisis chronic myeloid leukemia. *Blood, 135,* 2337–2353.

21. Lodish, H., Birk, A., Kaiser, C. A., et al. (2021). *Cancer. In Molecular Cell Biology.* (9th ed., pp.). New York: W.H. Freeman MacMillan.

22. Yang, H., & Green, M. R. (2020). Harnessing lymphoma epigenetics to improve therapies. *Blood, 136,* 2386–2391.

23. Weiss, C. N., & Ito, K. (2017). A macro view of microRNAs: the discovery of microRNAs and their role in hematopoiesis and hematologic disease. *Int Rev Cell Mol Biol, 334,* 99–175.

24. Knudson, A. G. (1985). Hereditary cancer, oncogenes, and antioncogenes. *Cancer Res, 45,* 1437–1443.

25. Zenz, T., Eichhorst, B., Busch, R., et al. (2010). TP53 mutation and survival in chronic lymphocytic leukemia. *J Clin Oncol, 28,* 4473–4479.

26. Sampaio, M. M., Santos, M. L. C., Marques, H. S., et al. (2021). Chronic myeloid leukemia-from the Philadelphia chromosome to specific target drugs: a literature review. *World J Clin Oncol, 12,* 69–94.

27. Hochhaus, A., Larson, R. A., Guilhot, F., et al. (2017). Long-term outcomes of imatinib treatment for chronic myeloid leukemia. *N Eng J Med, 376,* 917–927.

28. Haddad, F. G., & Short, N. J. (2022). Evidence-based minireview: what is the optimal tyrosine kinase inhibitor for adults with newly diagnosed Philadelphia chromosome-positive acute lymphoblastic leukemia? *Hematology Am Soc Hematol Educ Program, 2022,* 213–217.

29. Springuel, L., Renauld, J. C., & Knoops, L. (2015). JAK kinase targeting in hematologic malignancies: a sinuous pathway from identification of genetic alterations towards clinical indications. *Hematologica, 100,* 1240–1253.

30. Kennedy, V. E., & Smith, C. C. (2020). *FLT3* mutations in acute myeloid leukemia: key concepts and emerging controversies. *Front Oncol, 10,* 612880.

31. Liquori, A., Ibanez, M., Sargas, C., et al. (2020). Acute promyelocytic leukemia: a constellation of molecular events around a single *PML::RARA* fusion gene. *Cancers, 12,* 624.

32. Feugier, P. (2015). A review of rituximab, the first anti-CD20 monoclonal antibody used in the treatment of B non-Hodgkin's lymphomas. *Future Oncol, 11,* 1327–1342.

33. Goebeler, M. E., & Bargou, R. (2016). Blinatumomab: a CD19/CD3 bispecific T cell engager (BiTE) with unique anti-tumor efficacy. *Leuk Lymphoma, 57,* 1021–1032.

34. Kantarjian, H. M., DeAngelo, D. J., Stelljes, M., et al. (2016). Inotuzumab ozogamicin versus standard care for acute lymphoblastic leukemia. *N Engl J Med, 375(8),* 740–753.

35. Perales, M. A., Kebriaei, P., Kean, L. S., et al. (2018). Building a safer and faster CAR: seatbelts, airbags, and CRISPR. *Biol Blood Marrow Transplant, 24,* 27–31.

36. Duvic, M. (2015). Histone deacetylase inhibitors for cutaneous T-cell lymphoma. *Dermatol Clin, 33,* 757–764.

37. Voso, M. T., Lo-Coco, F., & Fianchi, L. (2015). Epigenetic therapy of myelodysplastic syndromes and acute myeloid leukemia. *Curr Opin Oncol, 27,* 532–539.

38. Zubair, A. C., & Rowley, S. D. (2023). Practical aspects of hematologic stem cell harvesting and mobilization. In Hoffman, R., Benz, E. J., Silberstein, L. E., et al. (Eds.), *Hematology: Basic Principles and Practice.* (8th ed., pp. 1653–1666). Philadelphia: Elsevier.

28

Flow Cytometric Analysis in Hematologic Disorders

Magdalena Czader

OBJECTIVES

After completion of this chapter, the reader will be able to:

1. Discuss technical aspects of flow cytometry including specimen triage and processing, instrumentation, data collection, and a design of an antibody panel.
2. Describe the pattern recognition approach to analysis of flow cytometric data for diagnosis and follow-up of hematologic malignancies.
3. Identify basic cell populations defined by flow cytometric parameters.
4. Recognize key immunophenotypic features of normal bone marrow, peripheral blood, and lymph node tissue and specimens from patients with acute leukemia or lymphoma.
5. Discuss applications of flow cytometry beyond the immunophenotyping of hematologic malignancies.

OUTLINE

Specimen Processing
Flow Cytometry: Principle and Instrumentation
Analysis of Flow Cytometric Data
    Concept of Gating
    Analysis of Flow Cytometric Data
Cell Populations Identified By Flow Cytometry
    Granulocytic Lineage
    Monocytic Lineage
    Erythroid Lineage
    Megakaryocytic Lineage
    Lymphoid Lineage
Flow Cytometric Analysis of Myeloid Neoplasms (Acute Myeloid Leukemias and Chronic Myeloid Neoplasms)

Acute Myeloid Leukemias With Defining Genetic Abnormalities
Acute Myeloid Leukemias Defined by Differentiation
Myeloproliferative, Myelodysplastic, and Overlap Neoplasms
Flow Cytometric Analysis of Lymphoid Neoplasms (Lymphoblastic Leukemia/Lymphoma and Mature Lymphoid Neoplasms)
    B-Lymphoblastic Leukemia/Lymphoma
    T-Lymphoblastic Leukemia/Lymphoma
    Mature Lymphoid Neoplasms
Other Applications of Flow Cytometry Beyond Immunophenotyping of Hematologic Malignancies

CASE STUDIES

After studying the material in this chapter, the reader should be able to respond to the following case studies. Answers can be found in Appendix C.

Case 1

A 58-year-old man had a 5-month history of extensive right cervical lymphadenopathy and night sweats. His complete blood count (CBC) results were within reference intervals. Physical examination showed additional bilateral axillary lymphadenopathy. A cervical lymph node was excised. Histologic examination revealed nodular architecture, with predominantly medium-sized lymphoid cells with irregular nuclear outlines. Flow cytometric data are presented in Figure 28.1.

1. What cell population predominates on the forward scatter (FS)/side scatter (SS) scattergram?
2. List antigens positive in this population.
3. Does the pattern of light chain expression support the diagnosis of lymphoma?

Case 2

A 3-year-old girl was brought to the physician due to fatigue and fevers. The CBC revealed a WBC of 3×10^9/L, HGB of 8.3 g/dL, and PLT of 32×10^9/L. Reference intervals can be found after the Index at the end of the book. Review of the peripheral blood film showed rare undifferentiated blasts with occasional cytoplasmic blebs. No granules or Auer rods were identified. Bone marrow examination showed a marked increase in blasts (79%) and decreased trilineage hematopoiesis. Flow cytometric analysis was performed. In addition to the markers shown in Figure 28.2, the population of interest was positive for CD34, CD33, CD41, and HLA-DR.

1. What abnormal features are observed on the CD45/SS scattergram?
2. What is the most likely diagnosis, considering the constellation of markers expressed by the predominant population?

CASE STUDIES—cont'd

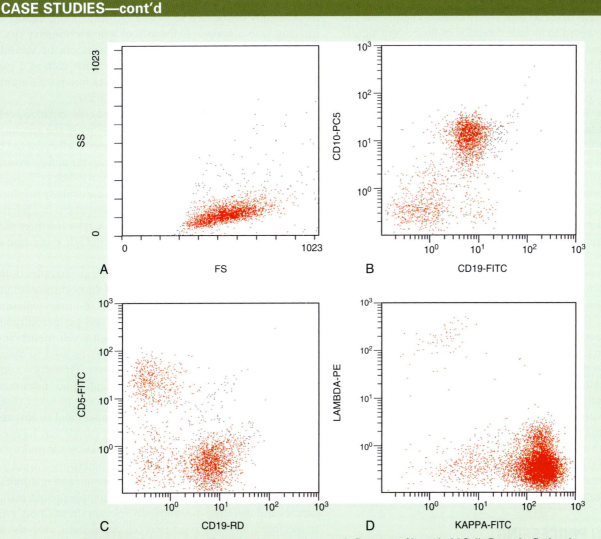

Figure 28.1 Scattergrams Showing Immunophenotypic Features of Lymphoid Cells From the Patient in Case 1. *FITC,* Fluorescein isothiocyanate; *FS,* forward scatter; *PC5,* phycoerythrin-cyanine 5; *PE,* phycoerythrin; *RD,* rhodamine; *SS,* side scatter.

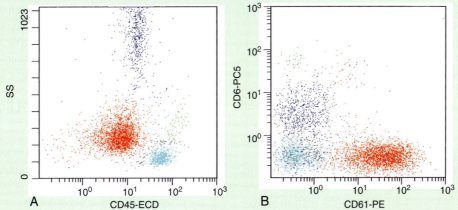

Figure 28.2 Predominant Bone Marrow Population for the Patient in Case 2. *ECD,* Phycoerythrin-Texas red; *PC5,* phycoerythrin-cyanine 5; *PE,* phycoerythrin; *SS,* side scatter.

Flow cytometry was originally designed to measure physical properties of cells based on their ability to deflect light. Over the years, it has evolved to include detection of fluorescent signals emitted by dyes bound directly to specific molecules or attached to proteins through monoclonal antibodies. The development of monoclonal antibodies has been the most significant factor contributing to today's broad application of flow cytometry. Although the term *flow cytometry* implies the measurement of a cell, this technique is also applied to study other particles including chromosomes, microorganisms, and proteins. The main advantage of flow cytometry over other techniques of cell analysis is its ability to rapidly and simultaneously analyze multiple parameters in a large number of cells, which not only enables cell populations to be characterized, but also rare-event cells to be identified and quantified in a heterogeneous cellular background. Therefore flow cytometry is not only applied to analysis of cell lineage in acute leukemia or detection of clonality in lymphoid populations but also makes it possible to discern abnormal populations in chronic myeloid neoplasms, quantitate minimal residual disease, and monitor immunodeficiency states. The World Health Organization (WHO) classification of hematolymphoid neoplasms recommends integrating flow cytometry with morphologic and molecular genetic data for a definitive diagnosis.[1] This approach emphasizes the central role of flow cytometry in a hematopathology laboratory.

This chapter is focused on the use of flow cytometry in a routine hematopathology laboratory. The chapter follows a "life" of a flow cytometric specimen that begins with specimen processing and ends with a final diagnosis. The discussion is divided into preanalytical (specimen processing), analytical (flow cytometric instrumentation and analysis), and postanalytical (immunophenotypic features of hematopoietic disorders) sections.

SPECIMEN PROCESSING

Flow cytometric analysis is particularly useful in diagnosing hematologic disorders. Bone marrow, peripheral blood, and lymphoid tissues are the most commonly analyzed specimens. In addition, immunophenotyping is often performed on body cavity fluids and solid tissues when they are suspected to harbor a hematologic malignancy.[2]

Prolonged transport or transport under inappropriate conditions may result in decreased viability and selective cell loss leading to suboptimal results. Peripheral blood and bone marrow specimens should be processed within 24 to 48 hours from the time of collection, depending on the anticoagulant used. Certain specimens, such as body cavity fluids or specimens from neoplasms with a high proliferative activity, often require immediate processing.[3]

When cells are suspended in a fluid, as in peripheral blood and bone marrow, minimal specimen preparation is required. These specimens are collected into a tube or container with an anticoagulant, most commonly heparin or ethylenediaminetetraacetic acid (EDTA), and are transported to a flow cytometry laboratory at room temperature. Bone marrow biopsy specimens and solid tissue specimens, including core needle biopsies, are submitted in culture media such as RPMI (Roswell Park Memorial

Institute Medium) to maintain viability. Tissue fragments are mechanically dissociated to yield a cell suspension, usually by mincing with a scalpel. Cellularity of a flow cytometry specimen obtained from small biopsy specimens can be variable. Therefore when only a small biopsy specimen such as a core needle biopsy can be obtained, a concurrent fine-needle aspiration is the preferred material for flow cytometry.[4]

To obtain a pure population of nucleated cells, red blood cells (RBCs) are lysed. The cellularity and viability of the specimen can be assessed before the specimen is stained. Cell count can be obtained using an automated blood cell analyzer or flow cytometry. The specimen is stained with propidium iodide or 7-amino actinomycin to test viability. The latter is particularly helpful if the laboratory receives a high number of specimens in a referral setting, when the transport is prolonged. A cytocentrifuge slide (Chapter E4) can be prepared for a morphologic inspection of a cell suspension.

As soon as these initial processing steps are completed, the specimen is stained with a combination of fluorochrome-conjugated monoclonal antibodies. The analysis of intracytoplasmic markers requires an additional fixation and permeabilization step to allow antibodies to pass through a cell membrane. A predetermined panel of antibodies may be used to detect membrane-bound and intracellular markers. Typically, a combination of 8 to 15 markers is used depending on instrumentation and individual laboratory preferences.[5] In select cases, particularly in patients with prior diagnoses and in low cellularity specimens, customized antibody panels may be used. Simultaneous analysis of multiple markers, known as *multicolor* or *multiparameter flow cytometry*, has numerous advantages. It facilitates visualization of antigen expression and maturation patterns, which are often disturbed in hematolymphoid malignancies and therefore diagnostically relevant. In addition, even in specimens with heterogeneous cell populations, analysis can be accomplished using few tubes and with a lower total number of cells, which saves reagents, time, and data storage. There is no consensus on the standardized panel of antibodies to be used in routine flow cytometric evaluation, nevertheless recommendations have been made for individual disease entities and/or specific applications.[6] The US-Canadian Consensus Project in Leukemia/Lymphoma Immunophenotyping recommends the comprehensive approach with multiple markers for myeloid and lymphoid lineage.[6] Selected markers commonly analyzed by flow cytometry are presented in Table 28.1.

FLOW CYTOMETRY: PRINCIPLE AND INSTRUMENTATION

The most significant discovery that led to the advancement of flow cytometry and its subsequent widespread application in clinical practice was the development of *monoclonal antibodies*.[7] In the original *hybridoma* experiments, lymphocytes with predetermined antibody specificity were cocultured with a myeloma cell line to form immortalized hybrid cells producing specific monoclonal antibodies. For this discovery, which not only fueled the development of flow cytometry but also had innumerable research and clinical applications, Köhler and Milstein received

TABLE 28.1	Lineage-Associated Markers Commonly Analyzed in Routine Flow Cytometry
Lineage	**Markers**
Immature	CD34
	CD117
	Terminal deoxynucleotidyl transferase
Granulocytic/monocytic	CD33
	CD13
	CD15
	CD14
Erythroid	CD71
	Glycophorin A
Megakaryocytic	CD41
	CD42
	CD61
B lymphocytes	CD19
	CD20
	CD22
	κ Light chain
	λ Light chain
T lymphocytes	CD2
	CD3
	CD4
	CD5
	CD7
	CD8

a Nobel Prize in 1984. Over the years, numerous antibodies were produced and tested for their lineage specificity. Categorization of these antibodies and associated antigens is accomplished through workshops on human leukocyte differentiation antigens that have been held regularly since 1982. These workshops provide a forum for reporting new antigens and antibodies and define a cluster of antibodies recognizing the same antigen, called *cluster of differentiation* (CD) (Tables 28.1 and 28.2). Consecutive numbers are assigned to each new reported antigen. The Tenth International Conference on Human Leukocyte Differentiation Antigens listed more than 370 clusters of differentiation.[8]

Monoclonal antibodies have numerous diagnostic applications and are increasingly used in immunotherapy. Common routine diagnostic methods using monoclonal antibodies are immunohistochemistry, immunofluorescence, and Western blot. These methods study cellular proteins in fixed tissues or in cellular extracts; however, they do not examine antigens in their native state and cannot analyze multiple antigens in composite cell populations with a complex antigen makeup. In contrast, flow cytometry can define antigen expression on viable cells. Multiple antigens can be detected simultaneously on an individual cell, and numerous cells are tested at the same time. This is accomplished by the conjugation of monoclonal antibodies to a variety of fluorochromes that can be detected directly by a flow cytometer. In a flow cytometer, particles stained with such monoclonal antibodies are suspended in a fluid and pass one by one in front of a light source. As antibodies with fluorochromes

are illuminated, they emit fluorescent signals registered by detectors. Registered fluorescence signals are analyzed using flow cytometry software.

The flow cytometer consists of fluidics, a light source (laser), a detection system, and a computer. A brief discussion of these basic components is presented in the following paragraph. To be analyzed as individual events, cells must pass separately, one by one, through the illumination and detection system of a flow cytometer. This is accomplished by injecting a cell suspension into a stream of sheath fluid. This technique, called *hydrodynamic focusing,* creates a central core of individually aligned cells surrounded by a sheath fluid (Figure 28.3). The central alignment is essential for consistent illumination of cells as they pass before a laser light source.

A laser is composed of a tube filled with gas, most commonly argon or helium-neon, and a power supply. Current is applied to the gas to raise electrons of a gas to an excited state. When electrons return to a ground state, they emit photons of light. Through an amplification system, a strong beam of light with light waves of identical direction, polarization plane, and wavelength is produced. This narrow, coherent beam of light is used to illuminate individual cells, each stained with antibodies conjugated to specific fluorochromes.

After exposure to and absorption of laser light, the electrons of fluorochromes are raised from a ground state to a higher energy state (Figure 28.4). The return to the original ground level is accompanied by a loss of energy, emitted as light of a specific wavelength. Flow cytometers are equipped with several photodetectors, each specific for light of a unique wavelength. The fluorescence from an individual cell is partitioned into different wavelengths through a series of filters (dichroic mirrors) and directed to the corresponding photodetector. Thus fluorescent signals derived from different fluorochromes attached to particular antibodies are recorded separately.

In addition to fluorescence, laser light scattered on contact with cells is recorded. The detector situated directly in line with the illuminating laser beam measures forward scatter (FS or FSC), which is proportional to particle volume or size. A photodetector located to the side measures side scatter (SS or SSC), which reflects surface complexity and internal structures such as granules and vacuoles. FS, SS, and fluorescence are displayed simultaneously and are analyzed using flow cytometry software.

ANALYSIS OF FLOW CYTOMETRIC DATA

Concept of Gating

Cell populations with similar physical properties such as similar size, cytoplasmic complexity, and expression of a specific antigen form *clusters* on data displays generated by flow cytometers. A *gate* is an electronic boundary used by an operator to enclose these cell clusters for further analysis. Thus gating is a process of selecting a population of interest as defined by one or more flow cytometric parameters.

Gating can be applied at the time of analysis of flow cytometry data or at the time of data acquisition (live gate). In routine

TABLE 28.2 Hematolymphoid Antigens Commonly Used in Clinical Flow Cytometry

Cluster of Differentiation	Function	Cellular Expression
CD1a	T cell development	Precursor T cells
CD2	T cell activation	Precursor and mature T cells, NK cells
CD3	Antigen recognition	Precursor and mature T cells
CD4	Coreceptor for HLA class II	Precursor T cells, helper T cells, monocytes
CD5	T cell signaling	Precursor and mature T cells, subset of B cells
CD7	T cell activation	Precursor and mature T cells, NK cells
CD8	Coreceptor for HLA class I	Precursor T cells, suppressor/cytotoxic T cells, subset of NK cells
CD10	B cell regulation	Precursor B cells, germinal center B cells, granulocytes
CD11b	Cell adhesion	Granulocytic and monocytic lineage, NK cells
CD13	Monocyte adhesion to endothelial cells	Granulocytic and monocytic lineage
CD14	Monocyte activation	Mature monocytes
CD15	Ligand for selectins	Granulocytic and monocytic lineage
CD16	Low-affinity IgG Fc receptor	Granulocytic and monocytic lineage, NK cells
CD18	Cell adhesion and signaling	Granulocytic and monocytic lineage
CD19	B cell activation	Precursor and mature B cells
CD20	B cell activation	Precursor and mature B cells
CD22	B cell activation and adhesion	Precursor and mature B cells
CD31	Cell adhesion	Megakaryocytes, platelets, leukocytes
CD33	Cell proliferation and survival	Granulocytic and monocytic lineage
CD34	Cell adhesion	Hematopoietic stem cells
CD36	Cell adhesion	Megakaryocytes, platelets, erythroid precursors, monocytes
CD38	Cell activation and proliferation	Hematopoietic cells, including activated lymphocytes and plasma cells
CD41	Cell adhesion	Megakaryocytes, platelets
CD42b	Receptor for von Willebrand factor	Megakaryocytes, platelets
CD45	T and B cell receptor activation	Hematopoietic cells
CD56	Cell adhesion	NK cells, subset of T cells
CD61	Cell adhesion	Megakaryocytes, platelets
CD62P	Homing	Platelets
CD63	Cell development, activation, growth, and motility	Platelets
CD64	High-affinity IgG Fc receptor	Granulocytic and monocytic lineage
CD71	Iron uptake	High density on erythroid precursors, low to intermediate density on other proliferating cells
CD79a	B cell receptor signal transduction	Precursor and mature B cells
CD117	Stem cell factor receptor	Hematopoietic stem cells, mast cells

Ig, Immunoglobulin; *NK*, natural killer.

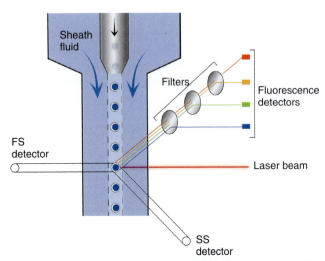

Figure 28.3 Diagram of a Flow Cytometer. As cells are injected into pressurized sheath fluid, they are positioned in the center of the stream and one by one, exposed to the laser light. Forward scatter and side scatter are collected by separate detectors. *FS*, Forward scatter; *SS*, side scatter.

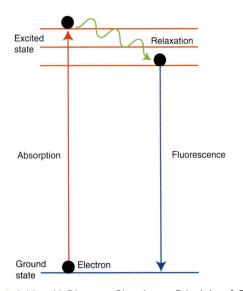

Figure 28.4 Jablonski Diagram Showing a Principle of Fluorescence. When electrons absorb energy, they are raised to the excited state. Subsequently, on their return to ground state, the absorbed energy is emitted in a form of fluorescence.

Analysis of Flow Cytometric Data

As with microscopic examination, an evaluation of flow cytometric data is based on an inspection of visual patterns. First, scattergrams displaying most commonly two parameters at a time are scanned to detect abnormal populations. Subsequent analysis focuses on antigenic properties of abnormal cells.

Analysis begins with inspection of scattergrams (dot plots) presenting cell size, cytoplasmic complexity, and expression of pan-hematopoietic antigen CD45. As in microscopic examination at low magnification, an operator detects specific cell populations based on their physical properties (Figure 28.5). The identification of particular populations can be confirmed and further resolved on the scattergram of CD45 antigen and SS (Figure 28.6). This display also provides information on relative proportions of specific cell populations in a flow cytometric specimen. Lymphocytes show the highest density of CD45, with approximately 10% of the cell membrane occupied by this antigen. Granulocytic series show intermediate CD45 density; late erythroid precursors and megakaryocytes are negative for CD45. The CD45/SS display is particularly useful for detection of blasts, which overlap with lymphocytes, monocytes, or both on the FS/SS displays.[9]

The FS/SS and CD45/SS dot plots allow for identification of a target population. Further analysis focuses on patterns of antigen expression, including qualitative data (antigen presence or absence) and fluorescence intensity as a relative measure of an antigen density.

CELL POPULATIONS IDENTIFIED BY FLOW CYTOMETRY

Surface and cytoplasmic markers expressed in hematologic malignancies resemble those of normal hematopoietic cell differentiation. Often, neoplastic cells are arrested at particular stages of development and show aberrant antigen expression. Diagnosis and classification of hematologic neoplasms is based on the knowledge of normal hematopoietic maturation pathways.

In the past, differentiation of hematopoietic cells was defined by morphologic criteria. Over time, it became clear that specific morphologic stages of development are accompanied by distinct changes in immunophenotype. Approximate morphologic-immunophenotypic correlates exist; however, because hematopoiesis is a continuous process, transitions between various developmental phases represent a continuum.

All hematopoietic progeny are derived from pluripotent stem cells. These cells are not solely recognized by morphology but are defined by their functional and antigenic features. They usually express a combination of CD34, CD117 (*c-kit*), CD38, and HLA-DR antigens.[10,11] As hematopoietic cells mature, they lose stem cell markers and acquire lineage-specific antigens. A brief discussion of the maturation sequence of major hematopoietic cell lineages is presented in the following sections.

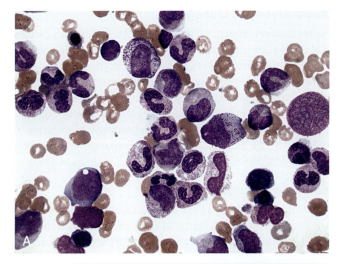

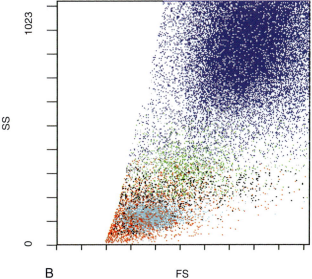

Figure 28.5 Main Cell Subpopulations of Normal Bone Marrow. **(A),** Bone marrow is composed of a heterogeneous population of cells of different sizes and variable complexity of cytoplasm. (Wright-Giemsa stain, ×1000.) **(B),** Dot plot of forward scatter (cell size) versus side scatter (internal complexity) reflects the heterogeneity of bone marrow subpopulations. Lymphocytes are smallest with a negligible amount of agranular cytoplasm and are located closest to the origins of the axes *(aqua)*. Monocytes are slightly larger with occasional granules and vacuoles *(green)*. Granulocytic series shows prominent granularity *(navy)*. *FS,* Forward scatter; *SS,* side scatter.

diagnostic flow cytometry, data are collected ungated; that is, all events detected by the flow cytometer are recorded. This allows for comprehensive analysis of all cells in a given specimen, including unexpected abnormal populations and retention of positive and negative internal controls. In this scenario, gating is most commonly used during analysis of flow cytometry data. "Live gating," or selectively acquiring a specific cell population during running of a flow cytometry experiment, was more common in the past and is no longer routinely used due to advances in computing.

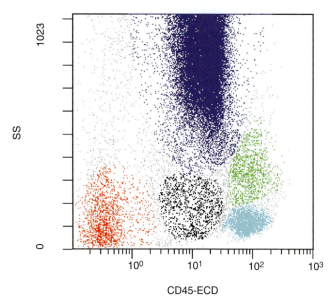

Figure 28.6 Scattergram Showing Differential Densities of Pan-Hematopoietic Marker CD45 on Bone Marrow Leukocytes. Lymphocytes *(aqua)* and monocytes *(green)* show highest densities of CD45 antigen. Intermediate expression of CD45 is seen in the granulocytic population *(navy)* and blasts *(black)*. Erythroid precursors *(red)* are CD45 negative. *ECD,* Phycoerythrin-Texas red; *SS,* side scatter.

Granulocytic Lineage

The developmental stages of granulocytic lineage as defined by the expression of specific antigens correspond closely to the morphologic sequence.[12] The first morphologically recognizable cell committed to the granulocytic lineage is a myeloblast (Chapter 10). A myeloblast is characterized by an expression of immature cell markers CD34, CD38, HLA-DR, and stem cell factor receptor CD117. Pan-myeloid markers CD13 and CD33, present on all myeloid progeny, are first expressed at this stage. As a myeloblast matures to a promyelocyte, it loses CD34 and HLA-DR and acquires CD15 antigen. Further maturation to a myelocyte stage leads to an expression of CD11b, a temporary loss of CD13, and a gradual decrease in the density of CD33. Finally, as granulocytic cells near a band stage, CD16 is acquired, and the density of CD13 increases.

Monocytic Lineage

The earliest immunophenotype stage of monocytic development is defined by a gradual increase in the density of CD13, CD33, and CD11b antigens. Subsequent acquisition of CD15 and CD14 marks the transition to a promonocyte and mature monocyte. In contrast to the granulocytic series, strong expression of CD64 and HLA-DR antigens persists throughout monocytic maturation, starting at earliest stages of monocytic development.

Erythroid Lineage

The majority of erythroid precursors do not express pan-hematopoietic marker CD45. The earliest marker of erythroid differentiation is the transferrin receptor, CD71. The density of this antigen increases starting in the pronormoblast stage and is rapidly downregulated in reticulocytes.[13] In contrast, glycophorin A (CD235a), although present on reticulocytes and erythrocytes, first appears at the basophilic normoblast stage.

Megakaryocytic Lineage

The maturation sequence of megakaryocytes is less well defined. CD41 and CD61, referred to as glycoprotein IIb/IIIa complex, appear as the first markers of megakaryocytic differentiation. These antigens are present on a small subset of CD34+ cells believed to represent early megakaryoblasts.[10] CD31 and CD36, although not entirely specific for megakaryocytic lineage, also are present on megakaryoblasts. Subsequent maturation to megakaryocytes and platelets is characterized by the appearance of additional glycoproteins, CD42, CD62P, and CD63.

Lymphoid Lineage

The B and T lymphocytes are derived from lymphoid progenitors that express CD34, terminal deoxynucleotidyl transferase (TdT), and HLA-DR. Lymphoid differentiation is characterized by a continuum of changes in the expression of surface and intracellular antigens. The earliest B cell markers include CD19, cytoplasmic CD22, and cytoplasmic CD79.[14] As B cell precursors mature, they acquire the CD10 antigen. The appearance of the mature B cell marker CD20 coincides with the decrease in the expression of CD10 (Figure 10.17). Another specific immature B cell marker is the cytoplasmic μ chain that eventually is transported to the surface and forms the B cell receptor. At this stage, the immunoglobulin chains in so-called naïve B cells have become rearranged. The normal mature B cell population shows a mix of κ and λ light chain-expressing cells. The exclusive expression of only κ or λ light chain is a marker of clonality, seen often in mature B cell neoplasms. The differentiation of mature naïve B cells, often recapitulated by B cell malignancies, is discussed in detail in Chapter 34.

Similar to B cell precursors, bone marrow-based early T cell precursors express CD34 and TdT.[15] The first markers associated with T cell lineage are CD2, CD7, and cytoplasmic CD3. CD2 and CD7 are also present in natural killer (NK) cells and, along with the CD56 molecule, are used to detect NK cell-derived neoplasms. In T cells, the expression of CD2, CD7, and cytoplasmic CD3 is followed by the appearance of CD1a and CD5, and coexpression of CD4 and CD8 antigens. Finally, the CD3 antigen appears on a cell surface, and CD4 or CD8 is lost. The sequential transition from double-negative (CD4−CD8−) through double-positive (CD4+CD8+) stages generates a population of mature helper (CD4+) and suppressor (CD8+) T cells (Figure 10.21). The latter stages of T cell differentiation occur in thymus. Normal T cells express a diverse, polyclonal complement of T cell receptors (TCRs). The latter can be analyzed by flow cytometry to facilitate detection of neoplastic-monoclonal T cells using monoclonal antibodies against TCR variable β chains, or TCR constant β chain-1.[16,17]

FLOW CYTOMETRIC ANALYSIS OF MYELOID NEOPLASMS (ACUTE MYELOID LEUKEMIAS AND CHRONIC MYELOID NEOPLASMS)

In myeloid malignancies, flow cytometry is used for initial diagnosis, follow-up, and prognostication. Specific immunophenotypes are associated with select cytogenetic abnormalities. Because most myeloid malignancies are stem cell disorders, evaluation of both blast population and maturing myeloid component is performed. Blast gate typically includes cells with a low-density expression of CD45 antigen and low SS. In normal bone marrow, a blast gate includes a relatively low number of cells showing the immature myeloid immunophenotype (see Figure 28.6). In acute myeloid and lymphoblastic leukemias, this blast gate becomes densely populated by immature cells, which reflects the increased number of blasts seen in a bone marrow specimen (Figure 28.7). The location of the immature population on the CD45/SS scattergrams depends on the subtype of acute myeloid leukemia (AML). In this chapter, the immunophenotypic features of AML and chronic myeloid neoplasms are discussed in the context of the WHO classification, which includes categories defined by recurrent cytogenetic abnormalities.[1] These leukemias often show specific immunophenotypes and are discussed separately in the following sections.

Acute Myeloid Leukemias With Defining Genetic Abnormalities

In most cases, AML with *RUNX1::RUNX1T1* fusion shows an immature myeloid immunophenotype with high-density CD34 and coexpression of CD19 and other B cell markers (Figure 28.8).[18] In addition, numerous myeloid antigens, including CD13, myeloperoxidase, and often weak CD33, are expressed. Often, there is asynchronous coexpression of CD34 and CD15. TdT is commonly present.

AML with *CBFB::MYH11* fusion is characterized by the presence of immature cells with expression of CD34, CD117, and TdT, and subpopulations of maturing cells showing monocytic (CD14, CD11b, CD4) and granulocytic (CD15) markers.[19] The aberrant coexpression of CD2 on the monocytic population is common.

Acute promyelocytic leukemia with *PML::RARA* fusion shows a specific immunophenotype. In contrast to most less-differentiated AMLs, the majority of cases of acute promyelocytic leukemia manifest with high SS, which reflects the granular cytoplasm of leukemic cells (Figure 28.9). The constellation of immunophenotypic features used to diagnose acute promyelocytic leukemia includes lack of CD34, HLA-DR, and leukocyte integrin antigens (CD11a, CD11b, CD18); presence of homogeneous strong CD33 along with myeloperoxidase and CD117; and variable CD13 and CD15.[20] The lack of CD34 and HLA-DR is a sensitive indicator of *PML::RARA* rearrangement; however, it is also seen in approximately 30% of other AMLs, including those with mutated *NPM1* and with *FLT3* internal tandem duplication.[21]

AMLs with *KMT2A* rearrangement in adults most commonly manifest with monocytic differentiation. The immunophenotypic features are nonspecific and can be seen in any acute myelomonocytic or monocytic leukemia (negative for CD34 and positive for CD33, CD13, CD14, CD4, CD11b, and CD64).

Acute Myeloid Leukemias Defined by Differentiation

In the least-differentiated AMLs, AML with minimal differentiation and AML without maturation, blasts are present in the region of low-density CD45 antigen and display low SS reflecting their relatively agranular cytoplasm. By definition, even the least differentiated AML is positive for a minimum of two myeloid-associated markers. The expression of CD13, CD33, and CD117 is common. Primitive hematopoietic antigens such as CD34, HLA-DR, and even TdT are often seen. Myeloperoxidase is absent or expressed in only a few cells. The immunophenotypic profile of AML with maturation is similar, but more mature myeloid markers such as CD15 and myeloperoxidase are often expressed.

In AMLs, aberrant antigen coexpression falls into two categories. Simultaneous expression of early and late markers of myeloid differentiation on the leukemic blasts is not uncommon (asynchronous antigen expression). Similarly, markers

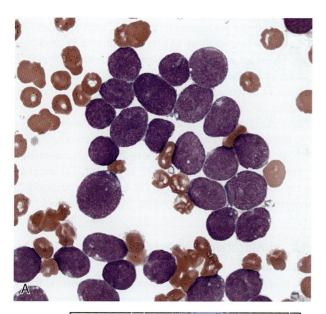

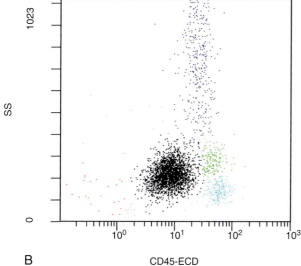

Figure 28.7 Bone Marrow Specimen Showing Acute Leukemia. Note uniform cytologic and flow cytometric characteristics. **(A),** Bone marrow aspirate from a patient with lymphoblastic leukemia/lymphoma. (Wright-Giemsa stain, ×500.) **(B),** CD45 versus side scatter plot shows a homogeneous population of blasts *(black)* with a marked decrease in normal hematopoietic elements. Compare with the heterogeneous pattern of normal bone marrow in Figure 28.5. *ECD,* Phycoerythrin-Texas red; *SS,* side scatter.

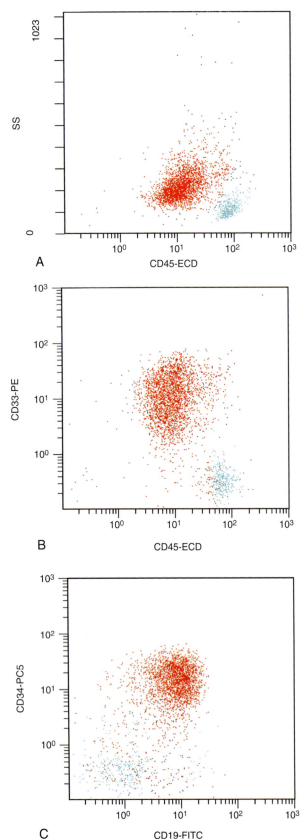

Figure 28.8 Acute Myeloid Leukemia with *RUNX1::RUNX1T1* Fusion. **(A),** CD45 versus side scatter showing increase in blasts *(red)* with residual lymphocytes *(aqua).* **(B** and **C),** Blasts are positive for CD33 and CD34 with characteristic coexpression of CD19 antigen. *ECD,* Phycoerythrin-Texas red; *FITC,* fluorescein isothiocyanate; *PC5,* phycoerythrin-cyanine 5; *PE,* phycoerythrin; *SS,* side scatter.

specific for other lineages, such as lymphoid lineage, may be seen on myeloid blasts. The most common example is CD7 antigen, which is typically considered a T/NK cell-associated marker (Figure 28.10).

Acute myelomonocytic leukemia and acute monocytic leukemia usually show higher expression of CD45, similar to that seen in normal monocytic precursors. In addition, in acute myelomonocytic leukemia, a population of primitive myeloid blasts is often seen (Figure 28.11). Acute monocytic leukemias express myeloid markers and antigens associated with monocytic lineage, such as CD14, CD4, CD11b, and CD64. Although CD14 is present on all mature monocytes, it may be absent in monocytic leukemias.[22] More immature monocytic markers, such as high-density CD64, are more consistently expressed.

In acute erythroid leukemia, leukemic cells are positive for erythroid markers such as CD71, glycophorin A, and hemoglobin. However, in more immature erythroid leukemias, glycophorin A and hemoglobin may be absent. In these cases, the diagnosis is based on the absence of myeloid markers, high expression of CD71, and scatter characteristics.

Acute megakaryoblastic leukemia usually shows low SS and low to absent CD45. Early megakaryocytic markers, CD41 and CD61, are often expressed (see Figure 28.2).[23] Occasionally, the late megakaryocytic marker CD42b is present. The expression of stem cell markers CD34 and HLA-DR on the population of leukemic megakaryoblasts varies. Myeloid markers may be positive.

Myeloproliferative, Myelodysplastic, and Overlap Neoplasms

The knowledge of antigen expression in the normal myeloid differentiation helps to define the aberrant expression patterns commonly seen in chronic myeloid neoplasms. The abnormalities detected by flow cytometry reflect morphologic features (e.g., hypogranulation of neutrophils in myelodysplastic syndrome detected by low SS) and show changes in antigen expression. Qualitative (presence or absence of a particular antigen) and quantitative abnormalities (number of antigen molecules) can be used for diagnostic purposes. The interested reader is referred to review articles discussing the details of immunophenotyping in myelodysplastic syndromes and myeloproliferative neoplasms.[24–29] A few examples are highlighted to illustrate the role of flow cytometry in diagnosing these diseases.

SS abnormalities related to hypogranular neutrophils are seen in approximately 70% of myelodysplastic neoplasms (Figure 28.12). In high-grade myelodysplastic neoplasms and myeloproliferative neoplasms undergoing transformation, blast percentage is increased. Blasts have a variety of aberrant immunophenotypic features, most commonly coexpression of CD7 and CD56 antigens. Blasts and maturing granulocytic precursors may show asynchronous expression of myeloid markers, including retention of CD34 and HLA-DR in late stages of maturation or late myeloid markers manifesting early in differentiation, such as CD15 on myeloblasts. Asynchronous coexpression of markers can also be seen in monocytic and erythroid

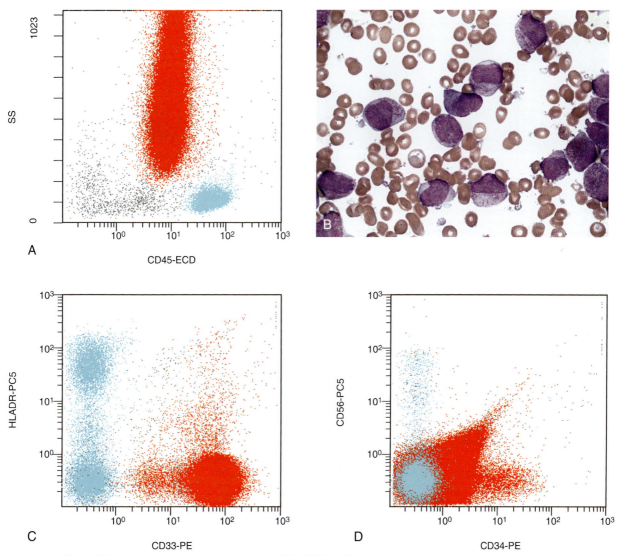

Figure 28.9 Acute Promyelocytic Leukemia With *PML::RARA* Fusion. **(A),** Typical side scatter pattern in acute promyelocytic leukemia corresponding to prominent granularity of leukemic cells *(red)*. Residual lymphocytes are shown in *aqua.* **(B),** Numerous leukemic promyelocytes with distinct granules and occasional Auer rods. (Wright-Giemsa stain, ×500.) **(C),** Leukemic cells show high-density expression of CD33 antigen and lack HLA-DR. **(D),** Similarly, CD34 antigen is absent or present in only a few leukemic cells. *ECD,* Phycoerythrin-Texas red; *PC5,* phycoerythrin-cyanine 5; *PE,* phycoerythrin; *SS,* side scatter.

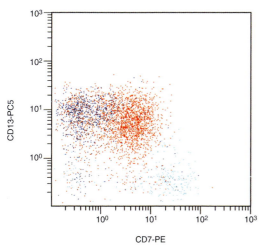

Figure 28.10 Myeloblasts of Acute Myeloid Leukemia Show Aberrant Coexpression of CD7 Antigen. *PC5,* Phycoerythrin-cyanine 5; *PE,* phycoerythrin.

lineages. Aberrant immunophenotypes are seen in 98% of cases of myelodysplastic neoplasms. More importantly, immunophenotypic abnormalities can be seen in cases with minimal or no morphologic dysplasia.[24,30] Other studies underscore the significance of immunophenotypic abnormalities in predicting the outcome after stem cell transplantation.[27] Flow cytometry can also be useful in myelodysplastic/myeloproliferative neoplasms. A prime example is chronic myelomonocytic leukemia, in which flow cytometry not only defines the blast immunophenotype but also determines the subtype of monocytes (classical vs. nonclassical vs. intermediate). The monocyte subtype is helpful in diagnosing chronic myelomonocytic leukemia, especially in cases which do not fulfill diagnostic criteria set by the WHO.[31] The utility of flow cytometry in myeloproliferative neoplasms is less well established. Specifically, the application of flow cytometry as a diagnostic tool in chronic myeloid leukemia is limited to an accelerated or blast phase, in which a lineage of a blast

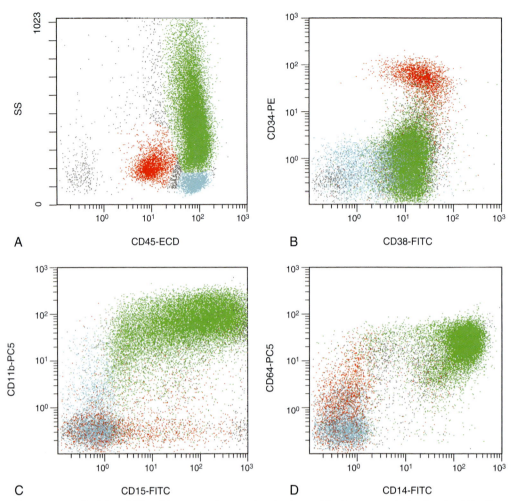

Figure 28.11 Peripheral Blood Immunophenotyping in Acute Myelomonocytic Leukemia. **(A),** CD45 versus side scatter display shows myeloid blasts *(red)* and a monocytic population *(green).* **(B–D),** Primitive leukemic blasts are positive for CD34 and negative for CD14. In contrast, the monocytic population does not express CD34 and shows positivity for mature monocyte marker CD14 and characteristic monocytic pattern of CD11b and CD15 expression. *ECD,* Phycoerythrin-Texas red; *FITC,* fluorescein isothiocyanate; *PC5,* phyco-erythrin-cyanine 5; *PE,* phycoerythrin; *SS,* side scatter.

population needs to be determined. In a chronic phase, the presence of *BCR::ABL1* rearrangement (Philadelphia chromosome) demonstrated by conventional karyotyping or molecular studies remains the defining diagnostic feature. Other myeloproliferative neoplasms are not well studied. In general, flow cytometric abnormalities are seen in most cases with abnormal karyotype.[26] No consistent set of immunophenotypic features that can be routinely used in the workup of myeloproliferative states has been described.

FLOW CYTOMETRIC ANALYSIS OF LYMPHOID NEOPLASMS (LYMPHOBLASTIC LEUKEMIA/ LYMPHOMA AND MATURE LYMPHOID NEOPLASMS)

Similar to myeloid neoplasms, a diagnosis of lymphoid malignancies relies on the expression of lineage-associated markers corresponding to specific stages of lymphoid development. No single marker can be used for lineage

assignment, and a diagnosis is typically based on the presence of several B cell or T cell antigens. The sentinel feature of mature B and T cells is the presence of surface receptor complexes. The immune system responds to a wide array of antigens; in healthy individuals, B and T cells express a great diversity of surface immunoglobulin and TCR complexes (polyclonal populations), respectively. A neoplastic lymphoid population is characterized by an expression of a monoclonal B cell receptor or TCR. In most cases, a clonality confirms the malignant nature of lymphoid proliferation. In contrast, lymphoid precursors are generally negative for surface immunoglobulin and TCRs and instead carry markers of immaturity such as CD34 or TdT. In lymphoblastic (precursor-derived) neoplasms, an expansion of a population with homogeneous marker expression, rather than clonality, is diagnostic of malignancy. This section presents the key immunophenotypic features of lymphoblastic leukemias and lymphomas. Selected examples of associations between the immunophenotype and the genotype are discussed.

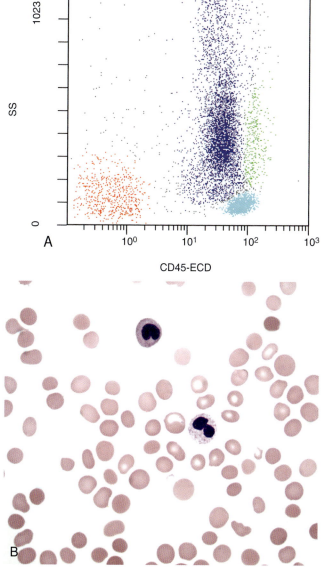

Figure 28.12 Myelodysplastic Neoplasm. **(A),** Low side scatter of hypogranular neutrophils seen in most cases of myelodysplastic neoplasm *(navy).* **(B),** Corresponding photomicrograph of markedly dysplastic, hypogranular neutrophils in myelodysplastic neoplasm. (Wright-Giemsa stain, ×500.) *ECD,* Phycoerythrin-Texas red; *SS,* side scatter.

B-Lymphoblastic Leukemia/Lymphoma

B-lymphoblastic leukemia/lymphoma (B-ALL/B-LBL) is derived from lymphoblasts and is positive for CD19, CD22, CD79a, HLA-DR, and TdT (Figure 28.13). The expression of CD34 and CD10 is often seen. Surface immunoglobulin light chains are not present. Cytoplasmic μ chain or surface immunoglobulin M (IgM) may be detected, however. Because B-LBL can arise at any stage of B cell differentiation, the presence of several specific markers usually defines early precursor, intermediate, and pre-B stages. The Fifth Edition of the WHO Classification of Haematolymphoid Tumours and International Consensus Classification introduced a number of new genetically defined B-LBL entities.[1] Often, immunophenotypes correlate with the genetic and clinical features. However, in routine practice, confirmation of cytogenetic abnormality using conventional karyotyping or molecular techniques is necessary. A few common examples of genetically defined B-LBL entities are discussed in the following sections.

B-Lymphoblastic Leukemia/Lymphoma With *KMT2A* Rearrangement

KMT2A gene rearrangements occur most often in infant B-LBL. In contrast to other B-LBLs, blasts in this leukemia are negative for CD10 antigen.[32] CD19, CD34, TdT, and occasionally myeloid markers are present. The more mature B cell marker CD20 is absent.

B-Lymphoblastic Leukemia/Lymphoma With *BCR::ABL1* Fusion

Philadelphia chromosome, t(9;22), *BCR::ABL1,* is a hallmark of chronic myeloid leukemia but also can occur in de novo pediatric and adult B-LL. These cases benefit from an addition of tyrosine kinase inhibitor to the chemotherapy regimen, and therefore it is important to identify them promptly. Most *BCR::ABL1*-positive cases have a classic intermediate or common B-LBL immunophenotype, with the expression of CD19, CD10, CD34, and TdT. The presence of myeloid markers CD13 and CD33 and the lack or decreased expression of CD38 antigen on leukemic blasts are common. The density of antigens and their homogeneous or heterogeneous expression within leukemic populations correlate closely with the presence of *BCR::ABL1.*[33]

B-Lymphoblastic Leukemia/Lymphoma With *BCR::ABL1*-like Features

BCR::ABL1-like B-LBL does not have *BCR::ABL1* rearrangement; however, it shows a gene expression pattern similar to *BCR::ABL1*-positive cases and often has rearrangements of other tyrosine kinase genes.[34] It occurs in 10% to 25% of patients diagnosed with B-LBL. Diagnosis can be challenging without gene expression profiling. Flow cytometry can be used as a screening tool to identify overexpression of CRLF2 protein (Figure 28.13D), which is seen in approximately 40% to 50% of *BCR::ABL*-like B-LL cases. Patients with this leukemia are treated using regimens including tyrosine kinase inhibitors.

T-Lymphoblastic Leukemia/Lymphoma

T-lymphoblastic leukemia/lymphoma (T-LBL) is derived from immature cells committed to T cell lineage. T-LL expresses a combination of markers reflecting the stage of T cell differentiation. CD3 is the most specific T cell marker. As with normal T cells, this antigen is seen initially in the cytoplasm before appearing on the cell surface. Other T cell antigens include CD2, CD7, CD5, CD1a, CD4, and CD8. Typically, a sequence of T cell antigens is detected, recapitulating the T cell differentiation (Figure 28.14). CD34 and CD10 may be present. As in other lymphoid neoplasms, a combination of markers determines leukemia subtype.

Mature Lymphoid Neoplasms

B and T cell lymphomas display immunophenotypes resembling their normal counterparts. The immunophenotypic features of

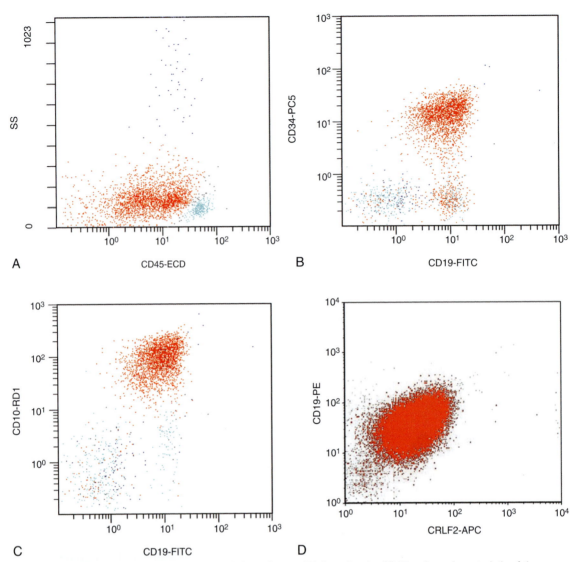

Figure 28.13 B-Lymphoblastic Leukemia/Lymphoma. **(A),** Low-density CD45 antigen characteristic of the blast population. **(B),** Uniform expression of CD34 and CD19 on leukemic blasts. **(C),** High-density CD10 on CD19+ blasts. **(D),** Leukemic blasts positive for CRLF2 antigen are seen in a proportion of cases of B lymphoblastic leukemia/lymphoma with *BCR::ABL1*-like features. *APC,* Allophycocyanin; *ECD,* phycoerythrin-Texas red; *FITC,* fluorescein isothiocyanate; *PC5,* phycoerythrin-cyanine 5; *PE,* phycoerythrin; *RD1,* rhodamine; *SS,* side scatter.

lymphomas are discussed in detail in Chapter 34 and are summarized in Table 34.2. Lymphomas are clonal neoplasms, which implies that the malignant population is derived from a single precursor cell. Therefore all neoplastic cells typically show similar genetic and immunophenotypic features. This stands in strong contrast to variable immunophenotypes of normal lymphoid populations, reflecting a process of antigen-driven selection.

Mature B Cell Neoplasms

Normal precursor B cells randomly rearrange immunoglobulin heavy and light chain genes. As a result, a mature B cell population expresses a mix of heavy and light chains (Figure 28.15A). In contrast, a monoclonal (monotypic) surface light chain expression, exclusively κ or λ, is seen in most B cell lymphomas (Figure 28.15B). In the appropriate clinical context and/

or when expressed on a significant number of cells, monotypic light chain along with the expression of pan-B cell markers is diagnostic of B cell lymphoma. Rarely, lymphomas may lose the expression of surface light chains, a feature not seen in normal mature B cells.[35] In most cases of plasma cell myeloma, neoplastic plasma cells lack surface immunoglobulin light chains and express only cytoplasmic κ or λ. Caution is warranted when interpreting small monoclonal populations of B cells. Small clones or oligoclonal B cell populations can be seen in reactive conditions such as autoimmune diseases.

Mature T Cell Neoplasms

In an appropriate clinical context, a robust population of clonal T cells indicates malignancy. In the majority of laboratories, the clonality of T cells is confirmed by a molecular analysis of TCR genes. However, flow cytometry can also be

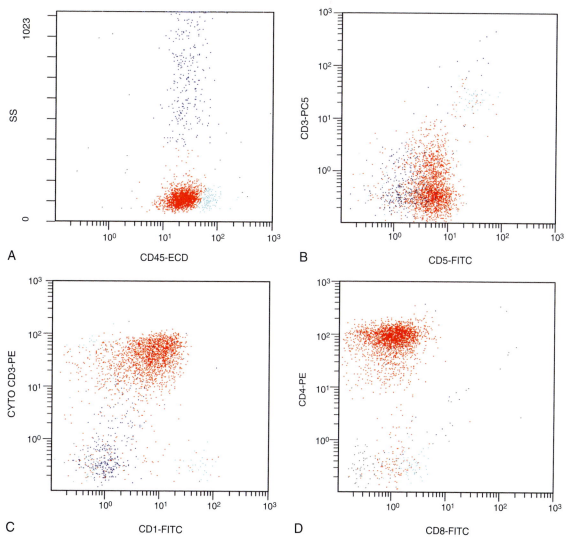

Figure 28.14 T-Lymphoblastic Leukemia/Lymphoma. **(A),** Predominant population in the blast gate. **(B** and **C),** Although CD3 antigen is absent from the surface of leukemic cells, it is present in blast cytoplasm, confirming the precursor T cell origin of the leukemia. **(C),** Note residual normal T cells *(aqua)* positive for surface CD3 and CD5 antigens. **(D),** Simultaneous expression of CD4 and CD8 antigens. *ECD,* Phycoerythrin-Texas red; *FITC,* fluorescein isothiocyanate; *PC5,* phycoerythrin-cyanine 5; *PE,* phycoerythrin; *SS,* side scatter.

used to detect clonality in most cases of T cell lymphoma.[16,17] However, until recently, the flow cytometric evaluation of T cell clonality was not widely available, and therefore a diagnosis of T cell lymphoma was often based on an aberrant T cell immunophenotype. In most cases, a loss or atypical expression of a lymphoid marker can be shown using flow cytometry. For example, mycosis fungoides is characterized by a mature T cell immunophenotype with expression of CD2, surface CD3, CD5, and CD4 and a loss of the CD7 and CD26 antigens (Figure 28.16). Over the years, it has been shown that the aberrant immunophenotype is a reliable diagnostic feature when the neoplastic population is sizeable. However, small numbers of T cells with unusual antigen makeup can appear in inflammatory conditions;[36] thus the aberrant immunophenotype alone cannot be considered pathognomonic of T cell malignancy.

OTHER APPLICATIONS OF FLOW CYTOMETRY BEYOND IMMUNOPHENOTYPING OF HEMATOLOGIC MALIGNANCIES

The immunophenotyping of hematolymphoid neoplasms is one of many applications of flow cytometry. Other common applications include diagnosis and monitoring of immunodeficiency states, diagnosis of paroxysmal nocturnal hemoglobinuria (PNH), hematopoietic stem cell enumeration, cell cycle analysis, detection of fetal hemoglobin, and monitoring of sepsis.

Select primary (inherited) and secondary (acquired) immunodeficiencies can be diagnosed using flow cytometry. Both a loss of specific antigens (e.g., CD11/CD18 in leukocyte adhesion deficiency) and functional defects (e.g., oxidative burst evaluation in chronic granulomatous disease) can be assayed by flow cytometry.

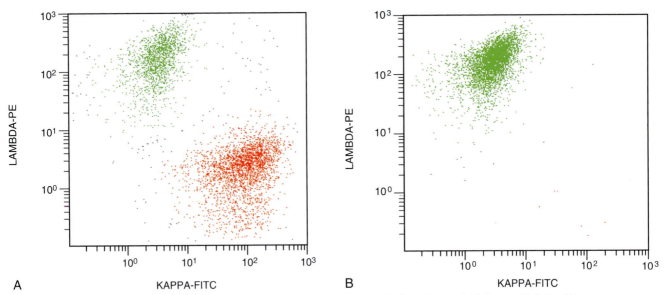

Figure 28.15 Comparison of Surface Light Chain Expression in Reactive and Malignant B Cells. **(A),** Reactive B cells show heterogeneous expression of κ and λ. **(B),** B cell lymphomas are monoclonal (monotypic), with the entire lymphoma population expressing only one type of light chain. *FITC,* Fluorescein isothiocyanate; *PE,* phycoerythrin.

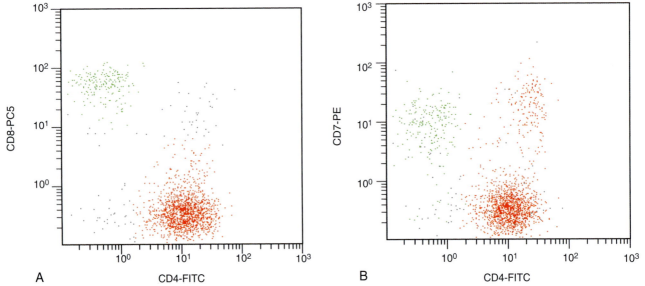

Figure 28.16 Mycosis Fungoides. **(A),** T cell population is positive for CD4 antigen *(red).* **(B),** Neoplastic T cells show loss of CD7 *(green). FITC,* Fluorescein isothiocyanate; *PC5,* phycoerythrin-cyanine 5; *PE,* phycoerythrin.

Human immunodeficiency virus (HIV) infection causes a progressive decrease in the number of CD4+ helper T cells. The absolute number of helper T cells in peripheral blood correlates with the stage of the disease and with patient prognosis. The enumeration of T cells and their subsets is easily accomplished by flow cytometry using antibodies against CD4 and CD8 antigens. The absolute numbers are derived by performing a routine white blood cell (WBC) count on the concurrent peripheral blood specimen or by running calibrating beads simultaneously with the patient specimen. The CD4:CD8 ratio in healthy individuals is typically greater than 1. A significant decrease in numbers of CD4-positive T cells in HIV-positive

patients leads to a reversed CD4:CD8 ratio. Because the CD4 lymphocyte depletion is associated with various infections, the absolute number of CD4-positive lymphocytes serves also as a guide for antibiotic prophylaxis in HIV-positive patients.

The diagnostic approach to PNH is a prime example of how an application of flow cytometry increases understanding of hematologic disorders and directly contributes to clinical decision making (Chapter 21).[37] Before the development of the flow cytometric assays, PNH diagnosis was based on detection of increased susceptibility of RBCs to lysis by the Ham or sucrose hemolysis tests, both of which showed inconsistent sensitivity. Flow cytometry significantly improved the sensitivity and specificity of PNH testing. The decreased expression of glycosylphosphatidylinositol-anchored proteins on RBCs, granulocytes, and monocytes of PNH patients can be measured by flow cytometry. The loss of these proteins is diagnostic of PNH and correlates with clinical symptoms. Typically, several markers are investigated simultaneously, including CD59, CD24, CD14, and aerolysin. The latter is not present on human cells in vivo; however, it binds to glycosylphosphatidylinositol anchors in an in vitro assay (Figure 28.17).

Another important application of flow cytometry is cell sorting. During sorting, a heterogeneous cell population is physically divided into subsets according to their physical or immunophenotypic properties. High-speed sorting is achieved by charging droplets containing individual cells of interest. As the charged droplet passes through the electrostatic field, it is isolated from the remainder of the specimen and collected into a separate container. The primary clinical application of cell sorting is in hematopoietic stem cell transplantation. More recently, cell sorting has been used to isolate rare cells for genetic analysis.

Initially, flow cytometry was primarily confined to the hematopathology and research laboratories. Over the years, its use expanded to hematopoietic stem cell transplantation, transfusion medicine, coagulation, microbiology, molecular pathology, and drug development. Examples of these applications include tissue typing, molecular testing for neoplasia-associated translocations, and evaluation of drug response such as monitoring platelet activation after antiplatelet therapy or after cellular therapies such as chimeric antigen receptor T cells after infusion.

Even though flow cytometry is a mature field, in recent years, it experienced a revival, with a focus on high-throughput testing for simultaneous analysis of multiple biologic constituents.

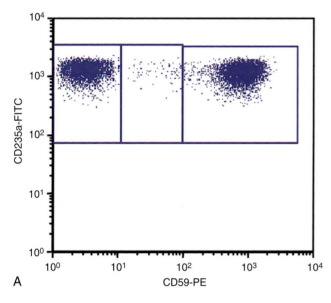

A

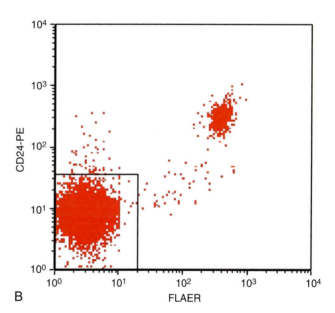

B

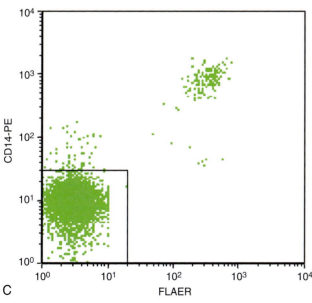

C

Figure 28.17 Diagnosis of Paroxysmal Nocturnal Hemoglobinuria (PNH) Based on the Decreased Expression of Glycosylphosphatidylinositol-Linked Molecules. Different levels of glycosylphosphatidylinositol-anchored proteins are best visualized in red blood cells (RBCs) using an antibody against CD59 antigen. **(A),** RBCs from a patient diagnosed with PNH. Three populations of RBCs are seen, with variable expression of CD59 molecule. Type I cells show normal level of CD59 expression *(rightmost box)*. A few cells show a slight decrease in CD59 level (type II cells). A prominent population of RBCs negative for CD59 antigen is also seen (type III cells) *(leftmost box)*. **(B),** Granulocytes in PNH show a complete loss of CD24 and fluorescent aerolysin *(black box)*. A small population of normal granulocytes positive for CD24 and fluorescent aerolysin is also seen. **(C),** PNH monocytes negative for CD14 and FLAER and a few normal monocytes positive for both antigens are seen. *FITC,* Fluorescein isothiocyanate; *FLAER,* fluorescent aerolysin; *PE,* phycoerythrin.

New approaches to a single cell analysis such as spectral flow cytometry and an integration of mass spectrometry with single-cell fluidics provide a superior resolution and expand the number of parameters that can be measured in any given cell. Mass cytometry allows analysis of 40 to 50 antigens through tagging the antibodies with heavy metals.[38] These methodologies are still predominantly research tools; however, they have opened new avenues to diagnostic immunophenotyping in hematopathology.[39,40]

SUMMARY

- Flow cytometry measures physical, antigenic, and functional properties of particles suspended in a fluid.
- Multiparameter flow cytometry is a technique routinely used for diagnosis and follow-up of hematologic disorders.
- The characterization of complex specimens is achieved through analysis of multiple parameters in individual cells and the simultaneous display of data for thousands of cells. The cell size, cytoplasmic complexity, and immunophenotypic features detected by monoclonal antibodies conjugated to various fluorochromes are analyzed in clinical specimens.
- A key starting point in flow cytometric analysis is a fresh, high-quality specimen.
- A flow cytometer consists of fluidics, a light source (laser), multiple detectors, and a computer.
- As with microscopic examination, an evaluation of flow cytometric data is based on the inspection of visual patterns. Initially, the entire specimen is scanned for the presence of abnormal populations. Subsequently, detailed immunophenotypic features of cell subsets are studied.
- The immunophenotyping of hematologic specimens is based on knowledge of the maturation patterns of hematopoietic cells. Compared with normal cells, malignant myeloid and lymphoid cells and cell populations in nonneoplastic hematologic disorders show significant qualitative and quantitative differences in antigen expression.
- Flow cytometric analysis of acute leukemia determines a lineage of leukemic cells. In select entities, immunophenotype corresponds to the underlying genetic lesion.
- Immunophenotyping of myelodysplastic, myeloproliferative, and myelodysplastic/myeloproliferative neoplasms contributes to morphologic and molecular genetic diagnosis.
- The clonality of mature B cell and T cell neoplasms can be detected by flow cytometry.
- Flow cytometric analysis is also used for diagnosis and monitoring of immunodeficiencies, hematopoietic stem cell enumeration, detection of fetal hemoglobin, tissue typing, molecular analysis, and drug testing.

Now that you have completed this chapter, go back and read again the case studies at the beginning and respond to the questions presented. Answers can be found in Appendix C.

REVIEW QUESTIONS

Answers can be found in Appendix C.

1. What is the most common clinical application of flow cytometry?
   a. Diagnosis of platelet disorders
   b. Detection of fetomaternal hemorrhage
   c. Diagnosis of leukemias and lymphomas
   d. Anemia diagnosis

2. Which of the following is true of CD45 antigen?
   a. It is present on every cell subpopulation in the bone marrow, peripheral blood, and lymphoid tissues.
   b. It is expressed on all hematopoietic cells with the exception of megakaryocytes and late erythroid precursors.
   c. It is not measured routinely by flow cytometry and is more commonly used by immunohistochemistry.
   d. It is commonly present on nonhematopoietic cells and therefore not useful in differential diagnoses.

3. Erythroid precursors are characterized by the expression of:
   a. CD71
   b. CD20
   c. CD61
   d. CD3

4. In Figure 28.2A, the cell population colored in aqua represents:
   a. Monocytes
   b. Nonhematopoietic cells
   c. Granulocytes
   d. Lymphocytes

5. Antigens commonly expressed by B-lymphoblastic leukemia/lymphoma include:
   a. CD3, CD4, and CD8
   b. CD19, CD34, and CD10
   c. CD42b, CD61, and CD41
   d. CD33, CD13, and HLA-DR

6. Which of the following is true of flow cytometric gating?
   a. It is defined as selection of a target population for flow cytometric analysis.
   b. It can be done only at the time of initial data acquisition.
   c. It can be done only at the time of analysis and data interpretation.
   d. It is accomplished by adjusting flow rate.

7. Collection of ungated events:
   a. Facilitates comprehensive analysis of all cells
   b. Does not help in detection of unexpected abnormal populations
   c. Allows the collection of data on a large number of rare cells
   d. Is used for leukemia diagnosis only

8. Mycosis fungoides is characterized by:
   a. Loss of certain antigens compared with the normal T cell population
   b. Polyclonal T cell receptor as determined by flow cytometry
   c. Immunophenotype indistinguishable from that of normal T cells
   d. Expression of CD3 and CD8 antigens
9. Mature granulocytes show the expression of:
   a. CD15, CD33, and CD34
   b. CD15, CD33, and CD41
   c. CD15, CD33, and CD13
   d. CD15, CD33, and CD7
10. During the initial evaluation of flow cytometric data, cell size, cytoplasmic complexity, and expression of certain antigens are used to define cell subpopulations. Which of the following parameters defines cytoplasmic complexity/granularity?
    a. SS
    b. FS
    c. CD45
    d. HLA-DR
11. The most important feature of the mature neoplastic B cell population is:
    a. A presence of specific immunophenotype with expression of CD20 antigen
    b. A clonal light chain expression (i.e., exclusively κ- or λ-positive population)
    c. An aberrant expression of CD10 antigen on CD19+ cells
    d. An aberrant expression of CD5 antigen on CD19+ cells

REFERENCES

1. WHO Classification of Tumours Editorial Board. *Haematolymphoid tumours*. Lyon (France): International Agency for Research on Cancer; forthcoming. (WHO classification of tumours series, 5th ed.; vol. 11). https://publications.iarc.fr.WHO 2023.
2. Czader, M., & Ali, S. Z. (2003). Flow cytometry as an adjunct to cytomorphologic analysis of serous effusions. *Diagn Cytopathol, 29,* 74–78.
3. Del Principe, M. I., Gatti, A, Johansson, U., et al. (2020). ESCCA/ISCCA protocol for the analysis of cerebrospinal fluid by multiparametric flow-cytometry in hematological malignancies. *Cytometry B Clin Cytom, 100,* 269–281.
4. Czader, M., Chiu, A., Perkins, S., et al. (2014). Core needle biopsy in lymphoma diagnosis: a multiinstitutional study. *Mod Pathol, 27,* 344A.
5. Rajab, A., Axler, O., Leung, J., et al. (2017). Ten-color 15-antibody flow cytometry panel for immunophenotyping of lymphocyte population. *Int J Lab Hematol, 39,* 76–85.
6. Kalina, T. (2020). Reproducibility of flow cytometry through standardization: opportunities and challenges. *Cytometry A, 97,* 137–147
7. Kohler, G., & Milstein, C. (1975). Continuous cultures of fused cells secreting antibody of predefined specificity. *Nature, 256,* 495–497.
8. Human Cell Differentiation Molecules. http://hcdm.org. Accessed December 15, 2022.
9. Borowitz, M. J., Guenther, K. L., Shults, K. E., et al. (1993). Immunophenotyping of acute leukemia by flow cytometric analysis. Use of CD45 and right-angle light scatter to gate on leukemic blasts in three-color analysis. *Am J Clin Pathol, 100,* 534–540.
10. Macedo, A., Orfao, A., Ciudad, J., et al. (1995). Phenotypic analysis of CD34 subpopulations in normal human bone marrow and its application for the detection of minimal residual disease. *Leukemia, 11,* 1896–1901.
11. Laurenti, E., & Gottgens, B. (2018). From haematopoietic stem cells to complex differentiation landscapes. *Nature, 553,* 418–426.
12. Terstappen, L. W., Safford, M., & Loken, M. R. (1990). Flow cytometric analysis of human bone marrow. III. Neutrophil maturation. *Leukemia, 4,* 657–663.
13. Loken, M. R., Shah, V. O., Dattilio, K. L., et al. (1987). Flow cytometric analysis of human bone marrow: I. Normal erythroid development. *Blood, 69,* 255–263.
14. Ciudad, J., Orfao, A., Vidriales, B., et al. (1998). Immunophenotypic analysis of CD19+ precursors in normal human adult bone marrow: implications for minimal residual disease detection. *Haematologica, 83,* 1069–1075.
15. Terstappen, L. W., Huang, S., & Picker, L. J. (1992). Flow cytometric assessment of human T-cell differentiation in thymus and bone marrow. *Blood, 79,* 666–677.
16. Beck, R. C., Stahl, S., O'Keefe, C. L., et al. (2003). Detection of mature T-cell leukemias by flow cytometry using anti–T-cell receptor Vβ antibodies. *Am J Clin Pathol, 120,* 785–794.
17. Horna, P., Shi, M., Olteanu, H., et al. (2021). Emerging role of T-cell receptor constant beta chain-1 (TRBC1) expression in the flow cytometric diagnosis of T-cell malignancies. *Int J Mol Sci, 22,* 1817–1837.
18. Andrieu, V., Radford-Weiss, I., Troussard, X., et al. (1996). Molecular detection of t(8;21)/AML1-ETO in AML M1/M2: correlation with cytogenetics, morphology and immunophenotype. *Br J Haematol, 92,* 855–865.
19. Adriaansen H. J., te Boekhorst, P. A., Hagemeijer, A.M., et. al. (1993). Acute myeloid leukemia M4 with bone marrow eosinophilia (M4Eo) and inv(16)(p13q22) exhibits a specific immunophenotype with CD2 expression. *Blood, 81,* 3043–3051.
20. Lo Coco, F., Avvisati, G., Diverio, D., et al. (1991). Rearrangements of the RAR-alpha gene in acute promyelocytic leukaemia: correlations with morphology and immunophenotype. *Br J Haematol, 78,* 494–499.
21. Gajendra, S., Gupta, R., Thakral, D., et al. (2023). CD34 negative HLA-DR negative acute myeloid leukaemia: a higher association with NPM1 and FLT3-ITD mutations. *Int J Lab Hematol, 45,* 221–228.
22. Krasinskas, A. M., Wasik, M. A., Kamoun, M. et al. (1998). The usefulness of CD64, other monocyte-associated antigens, and CD45 gating in the subclassification of acute myeloid leukemias with monocytic differentiation. *Am J Clin Pathol, 110,* 797–805.
23. Helleberg, C., Knudsen, H., Hansen, P. B., et al. (1997). CD34+ megakaryoblastic leukaemic cells are CD38-, but CD61+ and glycophorin A+: improved criteria for diagnosis of AML-M7? *Leukemia, 11,* 830–834.

24. Stetler-Stevenson, M., Arthur, D. C., Jabbour, N., et al. (2001). Diagnostic utility of flow cytometric immunophenotyping in myelodysplastic syndrome. *Blood, 98*, 979–987.

25. Porwit, A., van de Loosdrecht, A. A., Bettelheim, P., et al. (2014). Revisiting guidelines for integration of flow cytometry results in the WHO classification of myelodysplastic syndromes-proposal from the International/European LeukemiaNet Working Group for Flow Cytometry in MDS. *Leukemia, 28*, 1793–1798.

26. Kussick, S. J., & Wood, B. L. (2003). Four-color flow cytometry identifies virtually all cytogenetically abnormal bone marrow samples in the workup of non-CML myeloproliferative disorders. *Am J Clin Pathol, 120*, 854–865.

27. Wells, D. A., Benesch, M., Loken, M. R., et al. (2003). Myeloid and monocytic dyspoiesis as determined by flow cytometric scoring in myelodysplastic syndrome correlates with the IPSS and with outcome after hematopoietic stem cell transplantation. *Blood, 102*, 394–403.

28. Zhang, S., Zhou, J., Nassiri, M., et al. (2013). Diagnostic approach to myelodysplastic syndrome. In: Sayar H. (Ed.), *Myelodysplastic Syndrome*. (1st ed., pp. 25–60). Hauppauge, NY: Nova Science Publishers.

29. Kern, W., Westers, T. M., Bellos, F., et al. (2023). Multicenter prospective evaluation of diagnostic potential of flow cytometric aberrancies in myelodysplastic syndromes by the ELN iMDS flow working group. *Cytometry B Clin Cytom, 104*, 51–65.

30. Della Porta, M. G., Picone, C., Pascutto, C., et al. (2012). Multicenter validation of a reproducible flow cytometric score for the diagnosis of low-grade myelodysplastic syndromes: results of a European LeukemiaNET study. *Haematologica, 97*, 1209–1217.

31. Wagner-Ballon, O., Bettelheim, P., Lauf, J., et al. (2023). ELN iMDS flow working group validation of the monocyte assay for chronic myelomonocytic leukemia diagnosis by flow cytometry. *Cytometry B Clin Cytom, 104*, 66–76

32. Harbott, J., Mancini, M., Verellen-Dumoulin, C., et al. (1998). Hematological malignancies with a deletion of 11q23: cytogenetic and clinical aspects. European 11q23 Workshop participants. *Leukemia, 12*, 823–827.

33. Tabernero, M. D., Bortoluci, A. M., Alaejos, I., et al. (2001). Adult precursor B-ALL with BCR/ABL gene rearrangements displays a unique immunophenotype based on the pattern of CD10, CD34, CD13 and CD38 expression. *Leukemia, 15*, 406–414.

34. Den Boer, M. L., van Slegtenhorst, M., De Menezes, R. X., et al. (2009). A subtype of childhood acute lymphoblastic leukaemia with poor treatment outcome: a genome-wide classification study. *Lancet Oncol, 10*, 125–134.

35. Li, S., Eshleman, J. R., & Borowitz, M. J. (2002). Lack of surface immunoglobulin light chain expression by flow cytometric immunophenotyping can help diagnose peripheral B-cell lymphoma. *Am J Clin Pathol, 118*, 229–234.

36. Alaibac, M., Pigozzi, B., Belloni-Fortina, A. et al. (2003). CD7 expression in reactive and malignant human skin T-lymphocytes. *Anticancer Res, 23*, 2707–2710.

37. Dezern, A. E., & Borowitz, M. J. (2018). ICCS/ESCCA consensus guidelines to detect GPI-deficient cells in paroxysmal nocturnal hemoglobinuria (PNH) and related disorders part 1 - clinical utility. *Cytometry B Clin Cytom, 94*, 16–22.

38. Jager, S. J., & Davis, K. L. (2021). Mass cytometry of hematopoietic cells. *Mol Biol, 2185*, 65–76.

39. Sanders, C. K., & Mourant, J. R. (2013). Advantages of full spectrum flow cytometry. *J Biomed Opt, 18*, 037004. https://doi.org/10.1117/1.JBO.18.3.037004.

40. Behbehani, G. K. (2017). Applications of mass cytometry in clinical medicine: the promise and perils of clinical CyTOF. *Clin Lab Med, 37*, 945–964.

29

Molecular Diagnostics in Hematopathology

Cynthia L. Jackson and Shashi Mehta*

OBJECTIVES

After completion of this chapter, the reader will be able to:

1. Describe the structure of DNA, including the composition of a nucleotide, the double helix, and the antiparallel complementary strand orientation.
2. Predict the nucleotide sequence of a complementary strand of DNA or RNA, given the nucleotide sequence of a DNA template.
3. Explain the relationship between DNA structure and protein structure.
4. Discuss the process of DNA replication, including replication origin, replication fork, primer, DNA polymerase, Okazaki fragments, and leading and lagging strands.
5. Determine the appropriate patient specimen required for DNA isolation to identify an inherited or somatic mutation.
6. Discuss common methods of DNA and RNA isolation.
7. Explain the principle of the polymerase chain reaction (PCR) and reverse transcription PCR.
8. Describe the methods for detecting amplified target DNA, including capillary gel electrophoresis, and restriction fragment length polymorphism methods, and multiplex ligation-dependent probe amplification.
9. Compare and contrast qualitative real-time PCR and endpoint PCR.
10. Discuss the principle and use of quantitative real-time PCR and digital PCR for monitoring minimal residual disease.
11. Explain the principle and clinical applications of traditional Sanger DNA sequencing and contrast this method with pyrosequencing and next-generation sequencing.
12. Describe the use of comprehensive genome profiling in the detection of mutations.
13. Describe the use of microarray-based comparative genomic hybridization and single nucleotide polymorphism array karyotyping for the detection of chromosome copy number alterations.
14. Describe how optical genome mapping can be applied to replace conventional cytogenetics.

OUTLINE

Structure and Function of DNA
  The Central Dogma: DNA to RNA to Protein
  DNA at the Molecular Level
  Transcription and Translation
  DNA Replication and the Cell Cycle
Molecular Diagnostic Testing Overview
Nucleic Acid Isolation
  Isolating DNA from Clinical Specimens
  Isolating RNA from Clinical Specimens
Amplification of Nucleic Acids by Polymerase Chain Reaction
  Polymerase Chain Reaction for Amplifying DNA
  Reverse Transcription Polymerase Chain Reaction for Amplifying RNA
Detection of Amplified DNA
  Capillary Gel Electrophoresis

  Restriction Endonuclease Methods
Real-Time Polymerase Chain Reaction
  Qualitative Real-Time Polymerase Chain Reaction
  Quantitative Real-Time Polymerase Chain Reaction
  Minimal Residual Disease in Leukemia
  Digital Polymerase Chain Reaction
  Multiplex Ligation-Dependent Probe Amplification
  Mutation Enrichment Strategies
Nucleic Acid Sequencing
  DNA Sequencing by Capillary Electrophoresis
  Next-Generation Sequencing
Chromosomal Microarrays
Pathogen Detection and Infectious Disease Load
Current Developments

---

*The authors extend appreciation to Mark E. Lasbury, whose work in prior editions provided the foundation for this chapter.

CASE STUDY

After studying the material in this chapter, the reader should be able to respond to the following case study. Answers can be found in Appendix C.

A 55-year-old man presented to his hematologist for a followup visit for a 3-year history of thrombocytosis thought to be reactive in the setting of chronic retained kidney stones. He had a basal cell carcinoma removed a year ago, and he stated that his dermatologist was satisfied with the removal. He also has a history of chronic back pain from a herniated disk, which he elected to treat conservatively. He reported overall good quality of life, with the exception of occasional right toe numbness. In the current visit, his spleen was slightly palpable. The following were the results of his complete blood count (CBC). Reference intervals may be found after the Index at the end of the book.

WBC	13.6×10^9/L	HCT	51.4%
RBC	5.70×10^{12}/L	PLT	605×10^9/L
HGB	17.2 g/dL		

Based on the CBC results, a bone marrow biopsy was done, which showed a hypercellular marrow with trilineage hematopoiesis and hyperplasia of granulocytes. A reticulin stain of the bone marrow showed a grade 2/3 fibrosis. Given the clinical history and laboratory results, a myeloproliferative neoplasm, such as polycythemia vera, was considered. The hematologist ordered an erythropoietin level, which was 3.0 mU/mL (reference interval 4.0 to 19.5 mU/mL), and a real-time PCR Taqman probe assay for the *JAK2* c.1849G>T (p.Val617Phe) mutation. Figure 29.1 illustrates the assay results.

1. What type of specimen is appropriate for *JAK2* mutation testing?
2. Based on the real-time PCR curves with wild-type and mutant probes, in which reaction does the patient specimen amplify?
3. Does the patient have a *JAK2* p.Val617Phe mutation? If so, is it heterozygous or homozygous?
4. Based on the test results, what is the probable diagnosis?

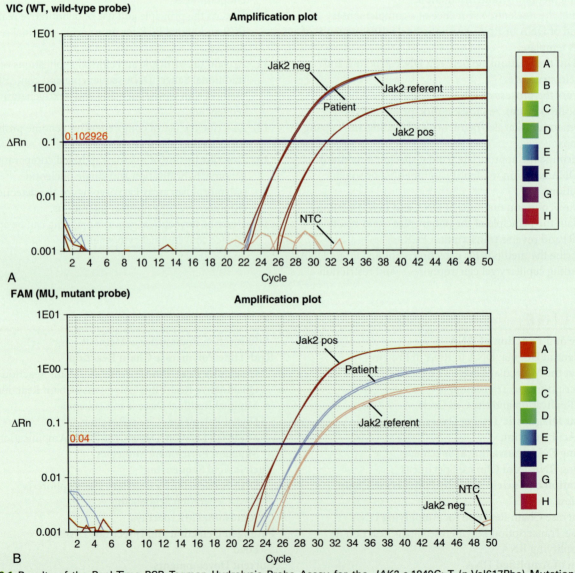

Figure 29.1 Results of the Real-Time PCR Taqman Hydrolysis Probe Assay for the *JAK2* c.1849G>T (p.Val617Phe) Mutation for the Patient in the Case Study. **(A),** Real-time amplification curves, with a probe complementary to the wild-type allele (labeled *VIC*). Curves are shown for the positive control *(Jak2 pos)*, negative control *(Jak2 neg,* wild-type), no-template control *(NTC)*, referent (sensitivity) control, and the patient. **(B),** Real-time amplification curves with a probe complementary to the mutant allele (labeled *FAM*). Curves are shown for the positive control *(Jak2 pos)*, negative control *(Jak2 neg,* wild-type), no-template control *(NTC)*, referent (sensitivity) control, and the patient.

Continued

CASE STUDY—cont'd

Specimen	Vic (WT)	Fam (MU)	Ratio (MU/WT)	Average
Negative control	2.973	0.804	0.270	
Negative control	2.986	0.756	0.253	0.262
Positive control	1.073	3.395	3.130	
Positive control	1.109	3.359	3.061	3.096
No template control	0.066	0.026	0.394	
No template control	0.069	0.027	0.391	
Sensitivity control	2.999	1.074	0.358	
Sensitivity control	2.989	1.077	0.359	0.359
Patient	3.06	2.695	0.881	0.898
Patient	3.008	2.75	0.914	

C

Figure 29.1—contd' (C), Table of the fluorescent values after 35 cycles of PCR showing the relative ratio of FAM/VIC fluorescence for each of the specimens. Specimens with a FAM/VIC ratio greater than the sensitivity or referent control are considered mutant.

Molecular biology techniques have become an essential tool in the diagnostic team's ability to predict or identify an increasing number of diseases in the clinical laboratory. Molecular techniques enable providers to diagnose a disease, monitor disease progression during treatment, make accurate prognoses, and predict the response to therapeutics. The short interval required to perform most molecular diagnostic tests and analyze their results is an additional positive aspect of this type of testing, resulting in more efficient patient management, especially in cases of infection.

Five main areas of hematologic molecular testing include detection of mutations, gene rearrangements, and chromosomal abnormalities for diagnosis and prognosis of hematologic malignancies (Box 29.1); detection and quantification of minimal residual disease to monitor treatment of hematologic malignancies; detection of mutations in inherited hematologic disorders (Box 29.2); pharmacogenetic testing to detect genetic variation affecting certain drug therapies (Box 29.3); and identification of hematologically important infectious diseases (Box 29.4).

STRUCTURE AND FUNCTION OF DNA

The Central Dogma: DNA to RNA to Protein

Most of the stored information needed to carry out cell processes resides in deoxyribonucleic acid (DNA); therefore proper cellular storage, maintenance, and replication of DNA are necessary to ensure homeostasis. Because molecular testing takes advantage of DNA structure and replication, a review of molecular biology is helpful.

The central dogma in genetics is that information stored in DNA is *replicated* to daughter DNA, *transcribed* to messenger ribonucleic acid (mRNA), and *translated* into a functional

---

BOX 29.1   Major Hematologic Malignancies in Which Molecular Methods Are Performed for Diagnosis and Monitoring Minimal Residual Disease

For Diagnosis

Acute leukemias
  Myeloid
  Lymphoblastic
Myeloproliferative neoplasms
  Chronic myeloid leukemia
  Polycythemia vera
  Essential thrombocythemia
  Primary myelofibrosis
Myelodysplastic neoplasms
Mature lymphoid neoplasms
  Chronic lymphocytic leukemia
  Lymphomas

For Monitoring Minimal Residual Disease

Acute leukemias
  Quantification of fusion mRNA transcripts resulting from translocations
  Quantification of specific B and T cell receptor rearrangements
Chronic myeloid leukemia
  Quantification of fusion messenger ribonucleic acid (mRNA) transcripts resulting from translocation

---

protein (Figure 29.2). This process is essential for carrying out cellular functions while preserving a record of the stored DNA information. In eukaryotes, the initial DNA sequence is composed of *translated* exons separated by *untranslated* introns. The introns are enzymatically excised following transcription from DNA to RNA, and the mature mRNA sequence is then

---

BOX 29.2   Inherited Hematologic Disorders Detected by Molecular Methods

Erythrocyte disorders
  Hemoglobinopathies/thalassemias
  Membrane abnormalities
  Enzyme deficiencies
  Erythropoietic porphyrias
Leukocyte disorders
  Quantitative disorders
  Functional disorders
  Storage disorders
Platelet disorders
  Quantitative disorders
  Functional disorders
Bone marrow failure syndromes
Coagulopathies
  Thrombophilia
  Bleeding disorders

BOX 29.3   Testing for Genetic Variation Affecting Therapy

Warfarin sensitivity
  Cytochrome P450 2C9 variants, CYP2C9*2, CYP2C9*3
  VKORC1 variants
Clopidogrel sensitivity
  Cytochrome P450 2C19 variants, CYP2C19*17, others
Thiopurine sensitivity
  Thiopurine S-methyltransferase, TPMT*2, TPMT*3C, TPMT*3A
Tyrosine kinase inhibitor/resistance
  ABL1 mutation analysis

BOX 29.4   Hematologically Important Pathogens Detected by Molecular Methods

Parasitic pathogens
  Plasmodium
  Filaria
  Babesia
  Leishmania
  Trypanosoma
Fungal pathogens
Bacterial pathogens
Viral pathogens
  Parvovirus B19
  Cytomegalovirus
  Epstein-Barr virus
  Human immunodeficiency virus types 1 and 2
  Human T-cell lymphotropic virus type 1
  SARS-CoV-2

Modified from Paessler, M., & Bagg, A. (2005). Use of molecular techniques in the analysis of hematologic diseases. In Hoffman, R., Benz, E. J. Jr., Shattil, S. J., et al (Eds.), *Hematology: Basic Principles and Practice*. (4th ed., pp. 2713–2726). Philadelphia: Churchill Livingstone.

translated. Translation is an enzymatic process in which mRNA three-nucleotide base sequences, called *codons*, drive the addition of encoded amino acids to the growing peptide. The mature protein then carries out its cellular function, which may be structural or may involve recognition, regulation, or enzymatic activity.

The structural units that carry DNA's message are called *genes*. The human β-globin gene *(SBB)*, part of the hemoglobin molecule, provides a good example of replication and transcription because it was one of the first sequenced and demonstrates the result of aberrant sequence maintenance. A normal (or wild-type) β-globin gene contains a sequence of bases that code for a β-globin peptide of 146 amino acids (Chapter 8). In hemoglobin S (Hb S), one inherited mutation changes a single DNA base. This is called a *point mutation*. The mutation occurs in the sequence that codes for the sixth amino acid of β-globin, and it substitutes the amino acid valine for glutamic acid in the growing peptide. Valine modifies the overall charge, producing a protein that polymerizes in a low-oxygen environment. This leads to sickled erythrocytes, circulatory ischemia and its sequelae, and chronic hemolytic anemia (Chapter 24).[1] Mutation in one of the two copies *(alleles)* of this gene inherited from the parents results in a *heterozygous* condition, or sickle cell trait. Heterozygotes are asymptomatic, with rare exceptions (i.e., during times of

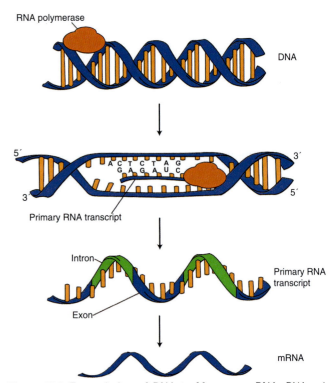

Figure 29.2 Transcription of DNA to Messenger RNA. RNA polymerase binds to a sequence of DNA called the promoter region, which causes the DNA strands to separate. Using one of the DNA strands as a template, RNA polymerase moves along and simultaneously reads (transcribes) the DNA strand, forming the primary messenger RNA *(mRNA)* transcript by joining the complementary ribonucleotides. The primary mRNA transcript consists of sequences called exons, which provide coding information, and introns, which are excised from the mature mRNA. The spliced mRNA then leaves the nucleus and enters the cytoplasm, where ribosomes translate the mRNA into protein.

extreme physical stress or low-oxygen conditions). If both alleles are mutated, there is overt *homozygous* sickle cell disease, and the symptoms are usually severe.

Every active gene is translated. Human somatic (nongamete) cells contain 20,000 to 25,000 genes in 2 meters of DNA, with approximately 3 billion DNA base pairs.[2] Significant packing takes place to reduce the volume of the nucleic acid to the size of chromosomes (Figure 30.3).

DNA at the Molecular Level

DNA is a duplex molecule composed of two complementary, hydrogen-bonded *nucleotide* strands (Figure 29.3). Deoxyribonucleotides and ribonucleotides are the building blocks of DNA and RNA, respectively. Each nucleotide is composed of a 5-carbon sugar (pentose), a nitrogenous base, and a phosphate group. The numbers one prime (1′) to five prime (5′) designate the pentose's carbons. In DNA the pentose is a ribose in which the hydroxyl group on the 2′ carbon is replaced by a hydrogen molecule, hence 2′-deoxyribose (Figure 29.4, A). In RNA the 2′ ribose retains the 2′ hydroxyl group. The hydroxyl group present on the 3′ carbon of the sugar is crucial for polymerization of the nucleotide monomers to form the nucleic acid strand.

The nitrogenous base is linked to the sugar by a glycosidic bond at the 1′ carbon. Four different bases form DNA, but the linkage to the sugar is the same for each. The phosphate group is linked to the sugar at the 5′ carbon by a phosphodiester bond (Figure 29.4, B–C). The phosphate group is also crucial for addition of nucleotides to the growing polymer. A sugar, whether ribose or deoxyribose, linked to a nitrogenous base but without a phosphate group, is called a *nucleoside*. A nucleoside cannot be incorporated into DNA, and neither can a nucleotide consisting of only one phosphate group (deoxynucleotide monophosphate [dNMP]). To be incorporated into a growing strand of DNA, the nucleotide must have three phosphate groups linked to one another, referred to as α-, β-, and γ-phosphates, with the α-phosphate linked to the sugar (Figure 29.5).

Synthesis of a DNA strand requires the enzyme DNA polymerase. This enzyme recognizes the hydroxyl group on the 3′ carbon of the deoxyribose. It then forms a phosphodiester bond between the 3′ hydroxyl group of the last nucleotide and the 5′ α-phosphate group of the next nucleotide to be added (Figure 29.5). Polymerization of subsequent nucleotides forms a DNA strand.

DNA consists of two strands that are antiparallel and complementary (Figure 29.6). One strand begins with a phosphate group attached to the 5′ carbon of the first nucleotide and ends with the hydroxyl group on the 3′ carbon of the last nucleotide. This strand is in the 5′ to 3′ direction. The other strand runs in the 3′ to 5′ direction, or antiparallel. Nucleotide sequences composing these strands provide the encoded messages of the genes. Therefore addition of nucleotides to a DNA strand is highly regulated.

One regulation mechanism arises from the complementary characteristic of the nucleotides. A nucleotide's identity depends

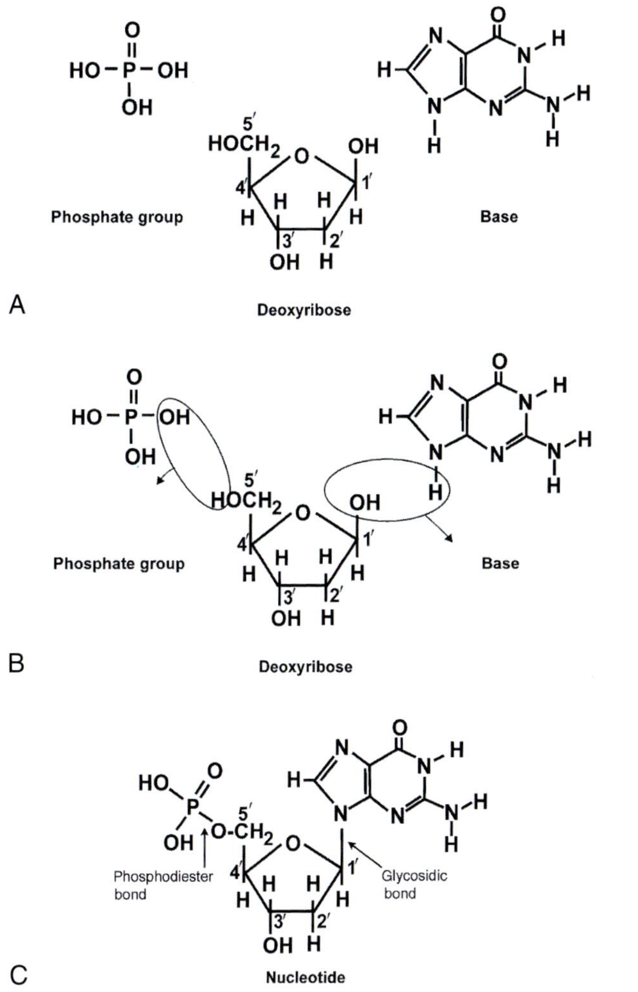

Figure 29.4 DNA Nucleotide Structure. (A), The pentose sugar, deoxyribose, a phosphate group, and a nitrogenous base compose a DNA nucleotide. The carbons of the deoxyribose molecule are numbered 1′ through 5′. The hydroxyl group on the 2′ carbon of ribose is replaced by a hydrogen molecule, making the structure a deoxyribose. **(B),** A nucleotide results from the formation of a glycosidic bond between the nitrogenous base and the hydroxyl group on the 1′ carbon of deoxyribose and a phosphodiester bond between the phosphate group and the hydroxyl group on the 5′ carbon of deoxyribose. **(C),** A nucleotide illustrating the glycosidic and phosphodiester bonds.

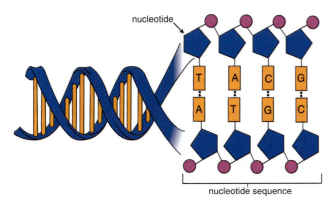

Figure 29.3 DNA Structure. DNA is a double-stranded helical macromolecule consisting of nucleotide subunits joined in sequence by deoxyribose molecules *(pentagons)* and phosphate radicals *(circles)*. The bases thymine *(T)*, adenine *(A)*, cytosine *(C)*, and guanine *(G)* are illustrated in their standard pairs: thymine to adenine, cytosine to guanine.

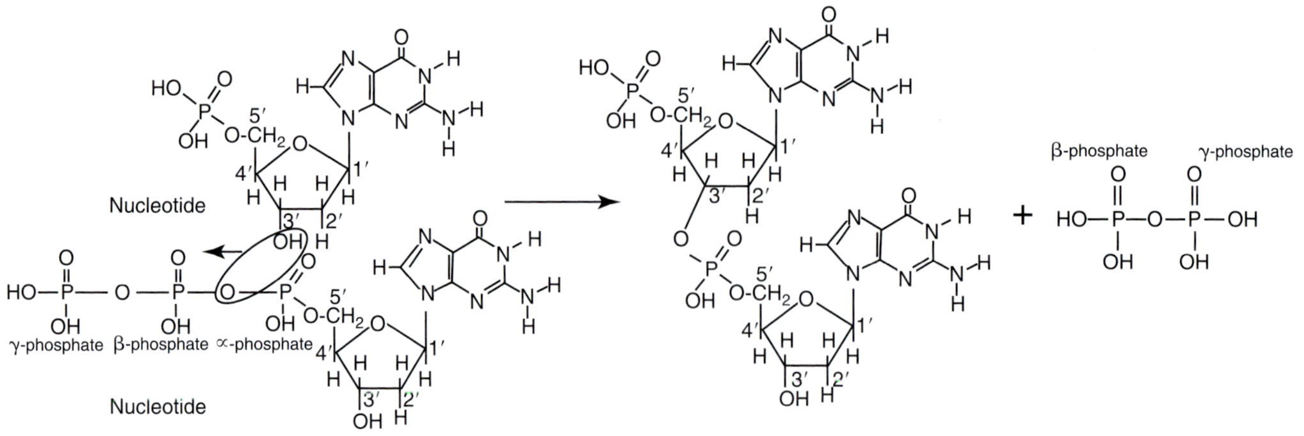

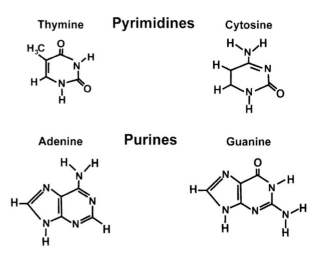

Figure 29.5 Action of DNA Polymerase. The enzyme DNA polymerase catalyzes the formation of a phosphodiester bond between the hydroxyl group on the 3′ carbon of one nucleotide with the phosphate group on the 5′ carbon of the downstream nucleotide *(circled area on left)*. The α-phosphate group is split with release of the β- and γ-phosphates.

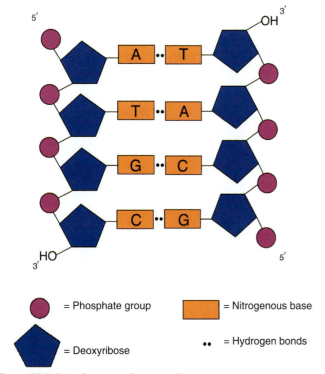

= Phosphate group = Nitrogenous base

= Deoxyribose •• = Hydrogen bonds

Figure 29.6 DNA Structure Showing Two Antiparallel and Complementary Strands. One strand begins with a 5′ phosphate group and ends with a 3′ hydroxyl group. This strand is read in the 5′ to 3′ direction. The other strand begins with a 3′ hydroxyl group and ends with a 5′ phosphate group. This strand is shown in the 3′ to 5′ orientation.

on the type of its nitrogenous base. There are two categories of nitrogenous bases in nucleic acids: purines and pyrimidines (Figure 29.7). Adenine (A) and guanine (G) are double-ringed purines, whereas thymine (T) and cytosine (C) are single-ringed pyrimidines. Adenine forms hydrogen bonds at two points with thymine (A:T), whereas guanine forms hydrogen bonds at three points with cytosine (G:C). If a strand has a 5′-CTAG-3′ sequence, the complementary nucleotides on the 3′ to 5′ strand are 3′-GATC-5′. Hydrogen bonds between A:T and G:C hold the strands together (Figure 29.8). In RNA the pyrimidine

Figure 29.7 Structure of Pyrimidines and Purines. The single-ringed pyrimidines (thymine and cytosine) and the double-ringed purines (adenine and guanine) are the code-carrying nitrogenous bases of DNA.

uracil (U) takes the place of thymine and can form hydrogen bonds with adenine. RNA is most often single stranded but can have significant secondary structure.

DNA resembles a ladder, with the repeating sugar and phosphate groups forming the sides of the ladder and the bases forming the rungs. The pairing of a double-ringed purine on one strand with a single-ringed pyrimidine on the other maintains a consistent distance between the DNA strands. This makes DNA flexible, which allows the molecule to twist into a helix. Twisting stabilizes the molecule and protects the bases from their environment.

Transcription and Translation

Transcription is the process of conversion of the DNA nucleotide code to mRNA by the enzyme RNA polymerase, which recognizes initiation sequences called *promoters*. Promoters lie upstream of coding sequences and bind RNA polymerase, which separates the DNA strands. The enzyme then slides along the 3′ to 5′ template DNA strand, "reading" the code and polymerizing (assembling) the complementary ribonucleotides in the 5′ to 3′

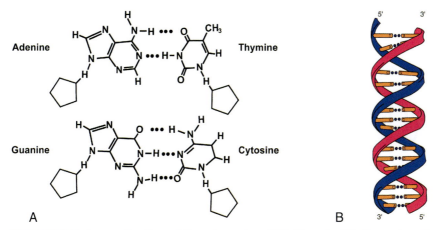

Figure 29.8 Hydrogen Bonding of Complementary DNA Strands. **(A)**, The purine adenine forms two hydrogen bonds with the pyrimidine thymine. The purine guanine forms three hydrogen bonds with the pyrimidine cytosine. **(B)**, The two strands maintain a consistent distance from each other, which allows DNA to twist into a helix.

direction. As the complementary ribonucleotides form hydrogen bonds with the bases of the exposed DNA strand, the RNA polymerase creates phosphodiester bonds to extend the single-stranded primary RNA transcript (see Figure 29.2). If the nucleotide sequence of the template DNA strand is 3'-CTAG-5', the primary RNA transcript is 5'-GAUC-3', in which uracil is substituted for thymine.

Primary mRNA transcripts are composed of introns and exons. Introns are untranslated, intervening sequences located between the coding portions of genes. Their many functions are being actively investigated, particularly their role in regulation of gene expression and alternative splicing.[3] Exons are sequences that encode the gene product. Before mRNA can serve as a translation template, introns must be excised from the primary transcript and the exons adjoined. The mature mRNA is completed by the addition of a 5' cap and a tail of many repeated adenine nucleotides (polyA tail).[4] The mature mRNA leaves the nucleus and enters the cytoplasm to be translated by ribosomes.

Ribosomes translate the mRNA code into a peptide sequence. Complexes of proteins and structural ribosomal RNAs (rRNAs) form both large and small ribosome subunits. Mature cytoplasmic mRNA is bound by the small ribosomal subunit at the translation initiation site. At this point, another series of elements is introduced, transfer RNAs (tRNAs), each bound to its specific amino acid. Because there are 20 natural amino acids, there are 20 tRNAs. Each tRNA has a specific nucleic acid sequence located at the point of interaction with the mRNA, complementary to the nucleotide sequence of the mRNA. Each tRNA interacting sequence (anticodon) complements a specific three-nucleotide sequence (codon) of the mRNA.

The mRNA codon AUG is the most common translation initiation site and codes for the amino acid methionine. The first step in translation is hydrogen bonding of the tRNA (with a bound methionine) to the initiation codon of the mRNA. The appropriate tRNA is then bonded to the adjacent codon, and a peptide bond is catalyzed between the two amino acids. The peptide bond forms between the carboxyl terminus of the methionine in the existing peptide chain and the amino

terminus of the amino acid to be added. Hydrogen bonding of tRNAs to the codons and the formation of the peptide bonds are mediated by the ribosome. With the addition of more amino acids, translation proceeds until a termination codon is reached. Three termination codons exist that do not code for any amino acid and terminate translation: UAA, UAG, and UGA. The ribosome then dissociates, and the peptide folds into its functional shape.

DNA Replication and the Cell Cycle

After cells carry out their functions, they either divide by mitosis or die by apoptosis, also called programmed cell death. The cell cycle progresses through a defined sequence of G_1 (gap 1), S (DNA synthesis), G_2 (gap 2), and M (mitosis) phases, with various checkpoints along the cycle (Chapter 4 and Figure 4.6). The checkpoints have complex mechanisms to stop the progression of the cell cycle if a problem is detected, at which point the cell will undergo apoptosis. Some cells exit the cell cycle during the G_1 phase and enter a phase called G_0 (quiescence). Cells in G_0 normally do not reenter the cell cycle and remain alive, performing their function until apoptosis occurs.

DNA replication during the S phase requires a complex orchestration of events; this discussion focuses on those events that are exploited for molecular diagnostic testing. Contained within the double-stranded DNA helix are multiple origins of replication. At each origin the enzyme helicase disrupts the hydrogen bonds, untwisting and separating the DNA strands, producing two replication forks. Here, a deoxyribonucleotide (deoxynucleotide triphosphate [dNTP]) polymerizes to form new complementary strands (Figure 29.9). DNA replication occurs bidirectionally from the two replication origin sites. Each DNA strand in the replication fork serves as a template for the formation of a daughter or complementary strand through the activity of DNA polymerase.[5] The DNA polymerase substrate is the free hydroxyl group located on the 3' carbon of a deoxyribonucleotide. DNA polymerase recognizes this group and catalyzes the joining of the complementary deoxyribonucleotide. DNA polymerase reads the DNA template in the 3' to

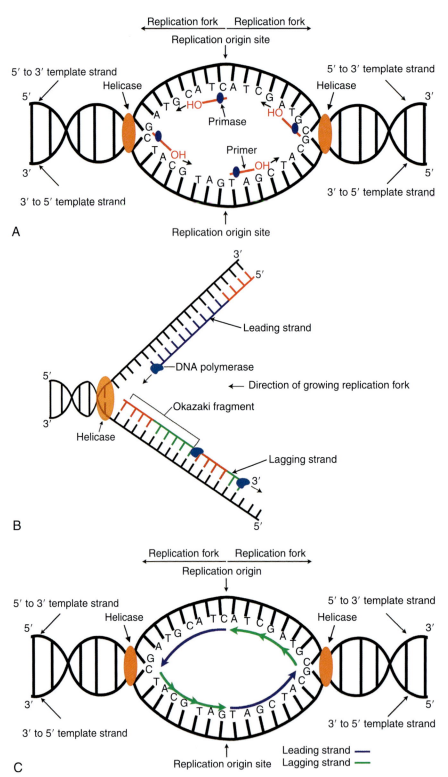

Figure 29.9 DNA Replication. **(A)**, Primases synthesize RNA primers that anneal to the single-stranded template strands. The primers must be oriented in such a way that the hydroxyl group on the 3′ end of the primers is available for deoxyribonucleotide addition by DNA polymerase. **(B)**, DNA polymerase extends the primer located on the 5′ to 3′ coding strand, producing the complementary leading strand *(blue)*. On the 3′ to 5′ template strand, DNA polymerase extends the primers, producing Okazaki fragments. The primer ribonucle-otides *(red)* are replaced with deoxynucleotides by DNA polymerase to produce the complementary lagging strand *(green)*. **(C)**, Bidirectional DNA replication, in which the 5′ to 3′ parent strand serves as the template for producing the continuous leading strands on a replication fork to the left of an origin. The 3′ to 5′ parent strand is the template for the lagging strands, which are produced in a discontinuous manner. The continuous and discontinuous strands are reversed on the replication fork to the right.

5′ direction, and the complementary strand is synthesized in the 5′ to 3′ direction.

A primer is required to provide the free 3′ hydroxyl group that is necessary for DNA polymerase activity. The enzyme primase synthesizes short RNA polymers complementary to the template that serve as primers to initiate DNA synthesis. At the replication origin, the primer hybridizes to the 3′ end of the 5′ to 3′ (top) template strand (see Figure 29.9). Then DNA polymerase recognizes the free hydroxyl group on the 3′ carbon of the last nucleotide in the primer and catalyzes the formation of phosphodiester bonds between the correct complementary nucleotide triphosphate and the primer, releasing the β- and γ-phosphate groups. DNA polymerase continues, adding deoxyribonucleotides along the replication fork, going to the left of the replication origin, producing the complementary strand called the *leading strand.*

The second template strand, called the *lagging strand,* is also read in the 3′ to 5′ direction. To form a complementary strand, a primer hybridizes to the exposed 3′ end of the replication fork. To proceed in the 5′ to 3′ direction, nucleotides are added in fragments toward the origin of replication. As the left replication fork extends to open more of the template strands for replication, additional primers are hybridized, and DNA polymerase uses the primers to initiate the formation of the complementary strand, continuing until it meets a previously hybridized primer.

DNA polymerase not only joins nucleotides but also degrades the RNA primers and fills in the correct complementary deoxyribonucleotides. Because the replication of the lagging strand produces many small fragments, it is called *discontinuous replication,* and the fragments are called *Okazaki fragments.* Finally, the enzyme ligase joins the discontinuous fragments. The replication fork to the right (downstream) is replicated in the same fashion, although the lagging strand is now formed complementary to the top (5′ to 3′) strand and the leading strand is formed from the 3′ to 5′ strand; the opposite of the situation described occurs for the left replication fork (see Figure 29.9).

The cell cycle is highly regulated. At certain critical points within the cycle, decisions are made to continue or begin cell death by apoptosis. This decision may depend on the state of the DNA replicated. Normally the cell detects errors made during replication and either corrects them or begins apoptosis. This prevents the persistence of daughter cells with genetic errors. If the sensing molecules fail, cell division may continue. Pathogenic mutations in proteins that mediate cell cycle control may result in tumor formation. In summary, DNA synthesis and accurate cell cycle control demand that the integrity of the nucleotide sequence be maintained during DNA replication.

MOLECULAR DIAGNOSTIC TESTING OVERVIEW

DNA or RNA sequences are used to diagnose and monitor solid tumors, acute leukemias, myeloproliferative neoplasms, myelodysplastic neoplasms, inherited hematologic disorders, and viral, parasitic, fungal, and bacterial infections. Molecular diagnostic testing exploits the enzymes and processes of DNA replication. Most molecular testing methods use replication—for

example, polymerase chain reaction (PCR)—to make millions of *amplicons* (copies) of a DNA sequence of interest. The creation of synthetic DNA requires the use of short sequences used as either primers or probes to locate specific DNA or RNA sequences within vast populations of nucleic acids.

Specific mutations are associated with hematologic disease but as the number and heterogeneity of disease drivers has increased, multiple testing modalities often are required.[6,7] Detection may involve allele-specific amplification methods, Sanger sequencing, next-generation sequencing (NGS), and occasionally, by restriction fragment length polymorphism analysis of amplified DNA. Messenger and ribosomal RNA also may be amplified through a process called *reverse transcription PCR* (RT-PCR). Using mRNA as the target, the existence of mutations that are being actively translated can be detected. Assessment of mRNA shows whether a mutation is expressed in a certain cell type or tissue and can be used to quantitatively determine the level of transcription of a gene. It also can be used to detect and monitor chromosome translocations that produce novel chimeric mRNA transcripts in conditions in which the breakpoints are too widely separated to be detected by PCR amplification of DNA.

Most molecular tests use DNA amplification (e.g., PCR), generating multiple amplicons of the target sequence. Amplification is meant to be specific to the sequence of interest in the specimen being tested; however, it will amplify any DNA that is present in the reaction. Consequently, it is critical to eliminate contamination of newly isolated target DNA with amplicons from previously amplified specimens. Contamination can be avoided by designating separate laboratory locations for each step, having a unidirectional work flow, and employing appropriate controls. Operators routinely use ultraviolet (UV) light and bleach to induce strand breaks in contaminating DNA on work surfaces, and a uracil-*N*-glycosylase system that destroys previously amplified DNA also can be incorporated into the PCR reactions.

In genetically based hematologic disease, sequence variants can occur that do not affect function. Individuals vary in genetic sequences coding for identical proteins. Such single nucleotide polymorphisms (SNPs) are commonly detected but might not be associated with disease. With these caveats in mind, several techniques are presented, and an example from hematopathology is given for each. Box 29.5 presents a summary of molecular methods with hematopathology applications.

NUCLEIC ACID ISOLATION

Isolating DNA from Clinical Specimens

Most molecular diagnostic tests begin with isolation of DNA or RNA from a patient specimen. To test for a mutation in patient DNA, the patient's DNA is isolated. To test for microorganism DNA, as in an infection, DNA is also isolated from the patient specimen because it will include the organism DNA. The preferred nucleic acid for clinical diagnosis is DNA because it is inherently more stable than RNA and is less labor intensive to isolate; however, NGS of RNA is increasingly employed to detect fusions.

The molecular laboratory isolates nucleic acid from a wide variety of clinical specimen types. Patient specimens for human DNA isolation may include peripheral blood, bone marrow, tissue biopsy specimens (both fresh and formalin-fixed, paraffin-embedded), needle aspirates, body fluids, saliva, and cheek swabs. Blood, saliva, or cheek swab specimens are all appropriate for identifying an inherited defect, although blood is the most common specimen type. Every nucleated cell contains a full complement of DNA. If individuals inherit a mutation, it is present in the DNA of all their nucleated cells, both gamete and nongamete (somatic) cells. Thus the DNA in the nucleus of white blood cells (WBCs) can reveal inherited mutations. In solid tumors, somatic (acquired) mutations are detected by analyzing DNA from the suspect tissue. For identification of infectious disease organisms by molecular techniques, DNA also must be isolated from the affected tissues. Peripheral blood is adequate for infections with viruses (e.g., the human immunodeficiency virus [HIV] and cytomegalovirus [CMV]) that infect blood cells, whereas CSF is required for meningeal infections.

Whole blood is collected preferentially in an ethylenediaminetetraacetic acid (EDTA) tube to prevent clotting and to inhibit enzymes that may digest DNA, although other blood collection tubes also may be acceptable. The red blood cells (RBCs) are removed by taking advantage of the differential lysis in a hypotonic buffer because of differing osmotic fragility between WBCs and RBCs. Incubation in hypotonic buffer will result in the lysis of RBCs, thus allowing the WBCs to be removed from

the hemoglobin and lysed RBCs by centrifugation. Hemoglobin is a potent inhibitor of PCR and other downstream procedures.[8]

DNA from tissue suspected of being malignant can be isolated from formalin-fixed, paraffin-embedded tissue sections mounted on glass microscope slides or whole sections cut directly into a microfuge tube. Tissue is obtained from the entire section or from a portion of the section by microdissection, either by scraping or by laser. The tissue is degraded by an enzyme called *proteinase K* to break open the cells and release the DNA. The specimen is then purified using an automated or manual extraction kit as described below.[9] In addition to paraffin-embedded specimens, fresh or frozen tissue specimens are appropriate for DNA isolation. Quickly thawing and mincing the frozen tissue prepares the specimen for DNA isolation. The minced tissue is mixed with an extraction buffer to release the DNA from the cells and is then purified.

There are a number of automated extraction systems, in addition to manual extraction kits, available for DNA extraction. Most of these systems use a solid phase extraction system that takes advantage of the binding of DNA to silica under high-salt conditions. Manual kits use columns that can be spun in a microcentrifuge, with the eluent collected in microfuge tubes. Cells that have been lysed and protease treated are applied to a column in a high-salt buffer. The column is washed to remove impurities, and the DNA is eluted in a low-ionic-strength buffer and collected in a microfuge tube.[10] Automated extractors have packaged reagents and can be programmed to extract and purify the DNA automatically. There are a variety of models to choose from, depending on the number and type of specimens. Isolated DNA can be stored at −20° C. If a delay in the molecular testing is necessary, the isolated DNA specimen can be stored at −80° C indefinitely.

Isolating RNA from Clinical Specimens

RNA isolation poses greater technical challenges than DNA isolation. Ubiquitous ribonucleases (RNases) degrade RNA. These enzymes are the body's primary defense against pathogens and are found on mammalian epidermal surfaces; therefore they contaminate all laboratory surfaces.[11] Clinical laboratories that isolate RNA must be RNase-free, which necessitates additional precautions and decontamination steps.[12]

Isolated total RNA includes mRNA, rRNA, and tRNA, all of which participate in protein synthesis. Depending on cell type, mRNA may comprise only 3% to 5% of the total cellular RNA; therefore a large-volume specimen may be needed to obtain adequate mRNA. The mRNA does not represent all the information stored in the DNA, only those genes being expressed. Consequently, mRNA provides quantitative information on the genes being expressed in a cell at the time the specimen was collected.

RNA may be purified using either liquid or solid phase procedures. The steps of RNA isolation using a liquid phase method are (1) RNA release by cell lysis combined with RNase inhibition by homogenization or incubation in a strongly denaturing solution containing chemical agents such as urea or guanidine isothiocyanate, (2) protein and DNA removal, and (3) RNA precipitation using alcohols. In step 2, extraction is performed using acidic phenol chloroform and guanidine isothiocyanate.

These steps separate the DNA and protein into the organic phase, whereas the RNA remains in the aqueous phase. RNA resists an acidic pH, whereas DNA is readily depurinated because acid cleaves the bond between the purine base and the deoxyribose sugar. Therefore acidic phenol preferentially isolates and preserves RNA, whereas the genomic DNA is partitioned along with contaminating proteins, lipids, and carbohydrates. Precipitating the RNA from the aqueous phase requires the addition of salt to neutralize the charge of the phosphodiester backbone and ethanol to make the nucleic acid insoluble.[13] Purification of RNA using column-based methods is similar to DNA except that the RNA is suspended in a high-salt buffer that preferentially binds RNA greater than 200 nucleotides to the column to remove smaller RNAs, such as tRNA and 5S RNA.

AMPLIFICATION OF NUCLEIC ACIDS BY POLYMERASE CHAIN REACTION

Polymerase Chain Reaction for Amplifying DNA

PCR is the principal technique in the clinical molecular laboratory. PCR is an enzyme-based method for amplifying a specific target sequence to allow its detection from a small amount of highly complex material.[14] As an example, sickle cell anemia results from a single β-globin gene nucleotide substitution (point mutation) in which adenine is replaced by thymine (*HBB* c.20A>T). Detecting this mutation from among 3 billion base pairs (bp) in the human genome would be like finding a needle in a haystack if only a few cells were assessed. When millions of β-globin copies are produced in PCR, however, the mutation is easily detected.[15] There are two categories of PCR reactions: endpoint PCR and real-time PCR. Amplification for both categories is basically the same. The major difference is in the method of detection of the PCR product. With endpoint PCR, the amplification products must be detected at the end of the amplification phase (when all the amplification cycles are completed) using another technique, such as capillary gel electrophoresis. In real-time PCR, the amplicons are detected during each PCR cycle using fluorescence detection. Detection methods are described later in the chapter.

As with natural DNA replication, PCR amplification requires primers that anneal (bind) to complementary nucleotide sequences on either side of the target region. In testing for the sickle cell mutation, for example, selected primers flank (i.e., bind on either side of) the β-globin gene sequence containing the mutation. The total base pair length of the primer sequences plus the target sequence can vary but in this example, it is 110 bp for the β-globin gene, a typical sequence length for many PCR assays (Figure 29.10).[15] Besides primers, the PCR master mix reagents include a heat-insensitive DNA polymerase (e.g., Taq polymerase) isolated from the thermophilic bacterium *Thermus aquaticus* and a mixture of the four deoxyribonucleotides—deoxyadenosine triphosphate (dATP), deoxythymidine triphosphate (dTTP), deoxyguanosine triphosphate (dGTP), and deoxycytidine triphosphate (dCTP)—in a magnesium-containing buffer.

The DNA is first denatured at 95° C, which separates the strands; then cooled to the primer annealing (binding) temperature of 40° C to 60° C; and then warmed to 72° C to promote specific chain extension, in which nucleotides are added to the primers by DNA polymerase. The annealing temperature is optimized for each set of primers. A thermocycler is used to accurately produce and monitor the rapid temperature changes.

Once double-stranded DNA is denatured, one primer anneals to the 3′ end of the 5′ to 3′ strand and the other primer to the 3′ end of the complementary 3′ to 5′ strand. Both primers possess a free 3′ hydroxyl group. The DNA polymerase recognizes this hydroxyl group, reads the template, and catalyzes formation of the phosphodiester bond joining the first complementary deoxyribonucleotide to the primer. The polymerase rapidly continues down the template strands at 1000 nucleotides per second, extending the complementary strand in the 5′ to 3′ direction to eventually produce complete daughter strands that continue to the 5′ end of the template.[16] This completes one PCR cycle. In the second cycle, the temperature changes are repeated, and the first-cycle products become the template for additional daughter strands. After the second cycle, daughter strands are produced that are bounded by the primer sequences at the 5′ and 3′ ends, resulting in a fragment of DNA of the desired length. After 25 to 40 subsequent cycles, double-stranded DNA of specific length and sequence, called an *amplicon,* is reproduced millions of times.[17,18]

Primer annealing accounts for PCR specificity, and primer design is crucial for achieving confidence in the test results regardless of the application. Wherever primers anneal, specifically or nonspecifically, they become starting points for extension by DNA polymerase.

Commercial kits contain primer sets that have been tested for annealing specificity, but care must be taken to use the optimal annealing temperature. Even if the primer is properly designed, it can anneal to noncomplementary regions if the annealing temperature is too low. Several online primer design programs are available from genome centers and company websites. One such program that can help determine the uniqueness, and therefore specificity, of the primers is the Basic Local Alignment Sequence Tool (BLAST).[19] These programs will also analyze pairs of primers to avoid complementarity between the primers themselves; this prevents primer hybridization to each other, which forms undesirable primer dimers.

Controls are essential for the accurate interpretation of a PCR result. The three controls required for PCR are the negative, positive, and no-DNA or no-template control (NTC). All three are included in each run. In addition, in most applications, a sensitivity control will be included that consists of a low positive specimen near the lowest concentration detected. The negative control consists of DNA known to lack the sequence of interest; the positive control contains the target sequence. Comparison of the amplification in the patient specimen to results in the negative and positive controls determines whether the target DNA sequence is present in the patient's DNA. The NTC detects master mix contamination. Amplification in the NTC indicates DNA contamination, which renders the entire test result unreliable.[20]

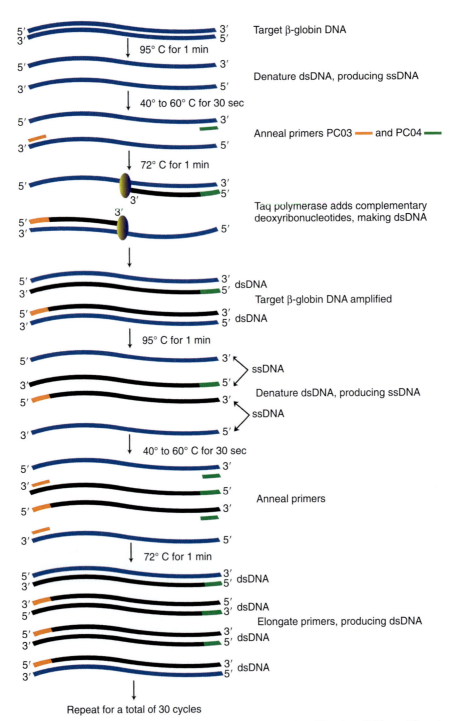

Figure 29.10 Application of PCR to Target β-Globin DNA Amplification. PCR amplifies the target DNA, making millions of copies of the target DNA after 30 cycles. Flanking forward and reverse primers (*PCO3* and *PCO4*) are used to amplify the target β-globin DNA segment. One primer (*PCO3, orange*) anneals to the 3′ end of the 3′ to 5′ DNA strand. The other primer (*PCO4, green*) anneals to the 3′ end of the 5′ to 3′ DNA strand. These primers provide the 3′-OH end for extension in the 5′ to 3′ direction during the PCR reaction and set the boundaries for the size of the amplicon. *dsDNA,* Double-stranded DNA; *ssDNA,* single-stranded DNA.

Reverse Transcription Polymerase Chain Reaction for Amplifying RNA

Some hematology molecular tests, such as those for translocations, require mRNA as the starting material. Genetically altered mRNA sequences often translate to an altered protein. The classic example is the Philadelphia chromosome (Ph′), carrying the chromosome translocation t(9;22)(q34;q11.2) (Chapter 32). This translocation is present in 95% of chronic myeloid leukemia (CML) cases, in 20% of adult acute lymphoblastic leukemia (ALL) cases, in 5% of pediatric ALL cases, and in rare instances, in acute myeloid leukemia.[21,22] Ph′ results from a reciprocal translocation of the *ABL1* gene on chromosome 9 to the breakpoint cluster region (*BCR*) of chromosome 22, producing a *BCR::ABL1* hybrid or chimeric gene (Figure 29.11, A).[23,24] Transcription of *BCR::ABL1* produces a chimeric mRNA made up of exons from both the *BCR* and *ABL1* genes. Translation generates a fusion protein with tyrosine kinase activity that alters normal cell cycle control, resulting in unrestrained cell proliferation.[25] RT-PCR of the chimeric mRNA is the standard method to detect this mutation (Figure 29.11, B). Although the mutation is present at the DNA level, the nucleotide position at which the two chromosome sections join is variable. The DNA also includes untranslated introns, which make the chimera too long to replicate. The physiologic excision and splicing of mRNA yields a much shorter target that is more easily amplified.

In RT-PCR, the *reverse* transcriptase enzyme produces complementary DNA (cDNA) from mRNA present in a total RNA specimen extracted from patient specimens such as blood or bone marrow (Figure 29.11, B). PCR subsequently amplifies the cDNA.

The first step is to transcribe the RNA into DNA using reverse transcriptase and a primer to produce an RNA-cDNA hybrid. The primer can be oligo(dT), a series of thymine nucleotides complementary to the string of adenine nucleotides on

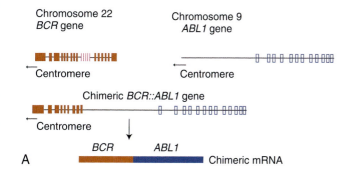

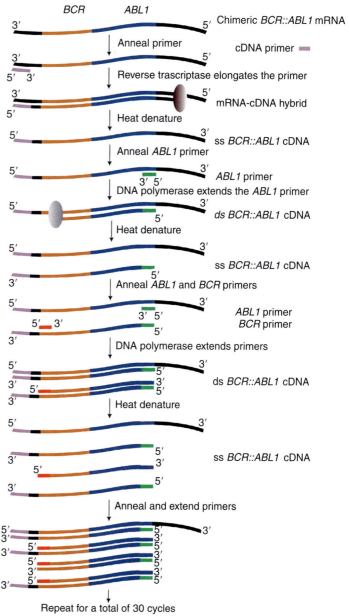

Figure 29.11 Formation and Detection of *BCR::ABL1* mRNA. (A), The *BCR* gene is present on chromosome 22 and the *ABL1* gene is located on chromosome 9. The Ph' chromosome results from the translocation of the *ABL1* gene to chromosome 22, which places the *ABL1* gene next to the *BCR* gene and produces a chimeric *BCR::ABL1* gene. The transcription of the *BCR::ABL1* gene produces a chimeric messenger RNA (mRNA) consisting of a portion of the *BCR* gene and a portion of the *ABL1* gene. **(B)**, Reverse transcription polymerase chain reaction (RT-PCR) produces complementary DNA (cDNA) from messenger RNA (mRNA). This diagram shows the RT-PCR steps used to produce amplified *BCR::ABL1* cDNA. Initially a gene-specific primer or short random primers anneal to the chimeric *BCR::ABL1* mRNA. Reverse transcriptase elongates the primer, producing an mRNA-cDNA hybrid. Heat denaturation breaks the hydrogen bonds, holding the hybrid molecule together, releasing the single-stranded (ss) *BCR::ABL1* cDNA. Next, a primer specific for the *ABL1* gene is annealed to the cDNA. DNA polymerase elongates the primer, producing the double-stranded (ds) *BCR::ABL1* cDNA. The cDNA becomes single-stranded by heat denaturation. Then the *ABL1* primer, in addition to a primer specific for the *BCR* gene, anneals to the ss cDNA. DNA polymerase elongates the primers, producing ds *BCR::ABL1* cDNA. The cycle is repeated 20 to 40 times, producing millions of copies of the ds *BCR::ABL1* cDNA.

the 3′ end of most mRNAs, called the *polyA tail;* a set of short random primers that prime the cDNA synthesis more evenly; or a specific primer for the gene of interest. The primer anneals to the complementary sequence of the mRNA. Reverse transcriptase recognizes the 3′ hydroxyl group on the last nucleotide of the primer and reads the mRNA template strand, then adds the correct complementary deoxyribonucleotide. Reverse transcriptase continues along the mRNA template strand, joining the complementary deoxyribonucleotides to the growing cDNA strand to form the mRNA-cDNA hybrid. Subsequently, heat denaturation breaks the hydrogen bonds between the mRNA-cDNA hybrid, separating the two strands. The cDNA strand then acts as a template for replication by DNA polymerase. The cDNA synthesis can be done separately from the PCR amplification step in a two-step procedure or combined with the PCR in a single reaction. For example, with the *BCR::ABL1* translocation, the single-stranded cDNA is amplified as in DNA-based PCR, using one primer specific for a target sequence in the *BCR* gene and a second primer specific for the *ABL1* gene. DNA polymerase extends the primers, forming a double-stranded cDNA of a specific region of the target chimeric gene. Only the cDNA containing the translocation and therefore both primer binding sites will be amplified, resulting in millions of copies of the *BCR::ABL1* sequence.[26,27]

DETECTION OF AMPLIFIED DNA

Although many molecular tests are now performed using real-time PCR, there are still circumstances in which amplicons are produced using endpoint PCR, and the product must be detected using downstream techniques. PCR-amplified target DNA may be detected by capillary gel electrophoresis using fluorescent dyes alone, or following restriction enzyme digestion of the amplicons, or by DNA sequencing by capillary electrophoresis (discussed later in the chapter).

Capillary Gel Electrophoresis

Nucleic acid phosphate groups confer a net negative charge to DNA fragments. Consequently, in electrophoresis, the rate at which DNA fragments (amplicons) migrate through gels is proportional to their mass only and, unlike proteins, not their relative charge. DNA fragment mass is a function of the length in base pairs or kilobase pairs (kb, $1000 \times$ bp).

In capillary gel electrophoresis, long, fused silica capillaries filled with derivatized acrylamide polymer are used for separation of single-stranded, negatively charged DNA fragments on the basis of size or number of base pairs. Specimen is applied to the capillary using electrokinetic injection, and the DNA fragments are separated using a high voltage as they migrate through the capillary from the negative electrode to the positive electrode. Smaller DNA fragments move faster through the polymer in the capillary compared to larger fragments. Detection of the separated fragments occurs by incorporating a fluorescent label into the PCR-amplified DNA. Before reaching the positive electrode, the fluorescently labeled DNA fragments cross the path of a laser beam and detector. When the laser beam hits a fluorescent DNA fragment, light is emitted at a specific wavelength. The light emission is read by the detector, and the signal produces a peak on an electropherogram (Figure 29.12).

Capillary electrophoresis offers a number of advantages over traditional gel electrophoresis. Injection, separation, and detection of the fragments are automated. Separation can be quite rapid with excellent resolution. Time of fragment elution and peak height information are stored for easy retrieval. Size ladders can be labeled with different fluorescent dyes and run in the same capillary as the specimen providing more accurate sizing.[28] This method of separation is used in a number of applications, including B and T cell clonality testing, bone marrow engraftment analysis, and screening for the internal tandem duplication mutation in the *FLT3* gene in acute myeloid leukemia (Chapter 31).[29]

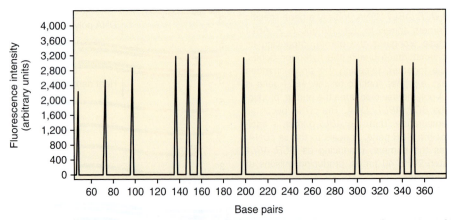

Figure 29.12 An Electropherogram of Capillary Gel Electrophoresis Showing the Separation of Fluorescently Labeled DNA Fragments by Size (Number of Base Pairs). Fragments migrate through the matrix in the capillary from the negative to the positive pole and emerge from the capillary in size order (smaller fragments first). Before reaching the positive electrode, the fluorescently labeled DNA fragments are detected by passing one at a time between a laser beam and the detector. Each fragment is represented by a peak on the electropherogram.

Restriction Endonuclease Methods

One method to determine whether an amplified target DNA fragment contains a mutation of interest uses enzymes derived from bacteria called *restriction endonucleases* (also known as restriction enzymes). Each restriction enzyme recognizes a specific nucleotide sequence and cuts both strands of the target DNA at the sequence, producing restriction fragments. The number of restriction fragments produced depends on the number of restriction sites present in the amplified target.[30,31] Enzyme action at one restriction site produces two restriction fragments, action at two restriction sites produces three restriction fragments, and so on.

A restriction enzyme detects even a single base substitution if the mutation alters the recognition sequence and prevents digestion at the site or creates a new site resulting in an additional fragment. A restriction fragment length polymorphism (RFLP) is a mutation or polymorphism-induced change in the restriction enzyme recognition site of the target DNA template that alters the length (number of base pairs) of the restriction fragments. A mutation in the tyrosine kinase domain of the *FLT3* gene is an example of an RFLP used in a PCR-based mutation detection assay.[32]

REAL-TIME POLYMERASE CHAIN REACTION

In contrast to endpoint PCR, real-time PCR measures the change in nucleic acid amplification as replication progresses using fluorescent marker dyes. There are several commercially available instruments that vary in their capacity, specimen volume, and optics.[33] A variety of choices are available in the optics for fluorescent detection. A tungsten lamp is commonly used for excitation, and different filters are used to select the excitation and emission wavelength. Light-emitting diodes or lasers for excitation also can be coupled with emission detection, depending on the instrument. Real-time PCR can be used in quantitative or qualitative assays. The time interval (expressed as the number of replication cycles) required to reach a selected fluorescence threshold is proportional to the copy number of target molecules in the original specimen.[34] The PCR cycle at which amplification crosses the threshold is denoted as the Ct for threshold value or the Cp for crossing point value. Importantly, these values are calculated from the exponential portion of the amplification curve. The Ct value is inversely related to the amount of target so that the more starting DNA or cDNA that is present in the reaction, the number of PCR cycles required to reach the threshold and exponential phase of the reaction is lower (Figure 29.13).

Real-time PCR requires the use of fluorescent detection, and there are several different options available. The simplest and the most straightforward option is to add a fluorescent dye, such as SYBR green, to the PCR reaction. These dyes bind to double-stranded DNA so that the fluorescence increases in proportion to the number of copies of the PCR product. The disadvantage of this approach is that these dyes do not differentiate between specific and nonspecific PCR amplicons, so the PCR reaction must be free of mispriming and primer dimers (primers that partially anneal to one another and are extended

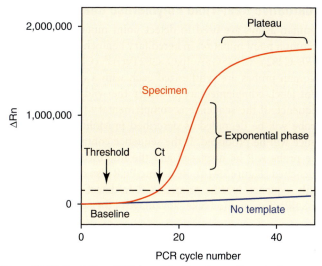

Figure 29.13 Real-Time PCR Amplification Curve. Note the important features of the curve, including the threshold *Ct* value and the exponential phase of the curve.

by the polymerase, forming very short amplicons). This method is commonly followed by a melting curve analysis to confirm the specificity of the amplification. Melting curves are often run in conjunction with real-time PCRs to confirm specificity of the product by heating the amplicon in increasing intervals from 65° C to 95° C and measuring the fluorescence. When the double-stranded DNA melts, the fluorescence will sharply decrease. Each amplicon has a specific melting point, depending on its size and base pair composition.

A more specific method of detection adds a probe in addition to the forward and reverse PCR primers, which also binds to the amplicon, providing additional specificity.

Several methods are commonly used, including hybridization probes, Taqman or hydrolysis probes, and molecular beacon and Scorpion probes. Hybridization probes use two oligonucleotide probes that bind to the amplicon adjacent (within one to five bases) to one another. One of the oligos has a 3′ donor fluorophore and the other a 5′ acceptor. The 3′ fluorophore is excited and the energy is transferred to the acceptor, which then fluoresces at a detectable wavelength. This is called fluorescence resonance energy transfer (FRET).[35] Hybridization probe technology in combination with melting curve analysis is used in some commercial thrombophilia assays.

Taqman probes consist of a single oligonucleotide that anneals between the forward and reverse primers. This probe contains a fluorophore on the 5′ end and a quencher on the 3′ end. This method takes advantage of the 5′ to 3′ exonuclease activity of DNA polymerase. As the amplicon is synthesized by DNA polymerase, the probe is degraded, which is why it is called a hydrolysis probe. This separates the fluorophore from the quencher and results in fluorescence. As the number of amplicons increases, there is more target to anneal to the probe and greater fluorescence as the probes are degraded.[36]

Molecular beacons and Scorpion probes use a hairpin structure to juxtapose the reporter and quencher. When the probe binds to the target, the hairpin unfolds and separates the fluorophore from the quencher and fluorescence is detected.[37]

Qualitative Real-Time Polymerase Chain Reaction

Taqman assays are used to detect point mutations, such as a common point mutation in hereditary hemochromatosis type1, *HFE* C282Y (c.845G>A [p.Cys282Tyr])[38] (Chapter 17). Two Taqman probes are synthesized each with a different fluorescent label, complementary to either the wild-type or mutant sequence. If the sequence is complementary to the target, the probe will be degraded as described previoiusly, and fluorescence will be produced. If the sequence contains a mismatch, the probe will be displaced and the fluorescence will remain quenched (Figure 29.14). Real-time PCR also can be combined with sequence-specific primer PCR to detect point mutations or SNPs. This method takes advantage of the fact that the 3′ end

of a primer in PCR must match the template sequence exactly to be extended by the polymerase. This is in contrast to the 5′ end of the primer, which can have additional nucleotides added. By using primers complementary to either the wild-type or mutant nucleotide, the presence or absence of a mutation can be determined by the reaction that produces the PCR product.[39] There are several modifications of this technique. One widely used technique, called SnaPshot, uses dideoxynucleotides, each labeled with a different fluorophore and primers of different size in a multiplex reaction to detect several different nucleotide changes simultaneously. The different-sized PCR products are then identified by size fractionation using capillary gel electrophoresis.[40,41] There are other variations on this

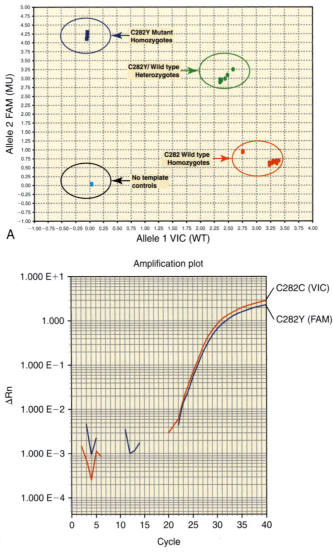

Figure 29.14 Qualitative Real-Time PCR for Hereditary Hemochromatosis, *HFE* C282Y Gene Mutation Detection (c.845G>A [p.Cys282Tyr]). The mutation replaces the amino acid cysteine (C) with tyrosine (Y) in position 282 of the HFE protein. The method uses two Taqman amplification probes, one for the wild-type (normal) and one for the mutant allele, each labeled with a different fluorescent reporter. **(A)**, Taqman allelic discrimination plot demonstrating the three genotypic populations for the *HFE* gene and no template controls. The scatter plots are derived from the total fluorescence of the amplification curve for both fluorescent probes. The genotype can be determined from the position on the scatter plot. **(B)**, Real-time PCR amplification curves of a heterozygous C282C/Y mutant patient showing fluorescence with the two Taqman probes: VIC for the wild-type and FAM for the mutant allele.

technique that are not discussed here. It is clear, however, that there are an increasing number of applications of real-time PCR in hematology, and multiple different techniques can be used to detect the same mutation. Applications of these techniques include the detection of translocations such as the *PML::RARA* translocation[42] and resistance mutations in viruses or bacteria, in addition to somatic mutations in cancer cells and germline mutations in genetic diseases.

Quantitative Real-Time Polymerase Chain Reaction

Real-time quantitative PCR can be done in two ways: relative quantitation, which normalizes to a reference gene used when measuring gene expression, or absolute quantitation, in which a standard curve of a known copy number of diluted standards is run along with the patient specimens. Once the relationship between the copy number of the standards and the Ct value is determined using the standard curve, the copy number of the patient specimen can be determined from the crossing point value. This assay is used to monitor minimal residual disease in chronic myeloid leukemia by quantifying the amount of the *BCR::ABL1* transcript (Figure 29.15) (Chapter 32) and also viral loads in infectious disease.[43,44] For *BCR::ABL1* quantification, a normalized copy number (NCN) is generated by dividing the *BCR::ABL1* copies by the control gene copy number. If an international standard is included in the assay, the NCN value can be converted to an International Standard NCN (ISNCN). This value should be reproducible across different laboratories and is the preferred value to be used to follow patients being treated with tyrosine kinase inhibitors.[45,46]

Minimal Residual Disease in Leukemia

Various therapies reduce leukemia cells to undetectable levels when assessed by visual examination of a peripheral blood film or bone marrow smear. However, residual leukemia cells may still be present in the patient after treatment that are not detected by conventional morphology assessment; this is called *minimal residual disease* (MRD).[47] More sensitive methods are required to detect MRD. Real-time quantitative PCR provides the opportunity to follow disease burden and to measure MRD in leukemia, a key indicator of treatment efficacy, clinical remission, and prognosis.[47]

Real-time quantitative PCR identifies the specific nucleic acid sequence in residual leukemia cells and helps guide the types and intensity of therapy, with the goal of *molecular remission*. Real-time reverse transcription quantitative PCR to assess the fusion transcript levels in CML is regarded as the gold standard for the detection and quantification of MRD. Subsequent to remission, periodic real-time quantitative PCR assays are used to detect early relapse and drug resistance, enabling the hematologist to initiate appropriate follow-up therapy.[48]

Real-time quantitative PCR is able to detect a few malignant cells within a population of a million cells, providing unparalleled sensitivity. Current assays to assess MRD can detect one leukemia cell among 10^5 to 10^6 normal cells. Current applications include detection of *BCR::ABL1* transcripts in CML and some acute leukemias (Figure 29.16); *JAK2* mutations in the myeloproliferative neoplasms, such as polycythemia

vera, essential thrombocythemia, and primary myelofibrosis (Chapter 32); the t(15;17) or *PML::RARA* fusion transcript in acute promyelocytic leukemia (Chapter 31); and gene rearrangements in mature lymphoid neoplasms (Chapter 34).[49]

A major issue with quantitative assays has been the lack of reproducibility between different laboratories because of the specimen type and quality, the choice of housekeeping gene for normalization, and the specific assay used. An international standard for *BCR::ABL1* quantification has been developed and made available by the World Health Organization (WHO). This standard serves as a universal standard and allows for interlaboratory comparison.[50]

Digital Polymerase Chain Reaction

Digital PCR (ddPCR) is a technique that can be used to quantify a target with very high sensitivity (Figure 29.17). For example, ddPCR can be used to detect resistance mutations to tyrosine kinase inhibitors used to treat CML (e.g., the T315I resistance mutation in the *BCR::ABL1* gene)[51] (Chapter 32) or to quantify virus copy number.[52] This technique uses various methods, for example, a droplet generator to create nanoliter droplets that partition template molecules, which are then amplified by endpoint PCR. The amplicons are detected by fluorescence and either read by a droplet reader or by some other detection mechanism. The distinguishing feature of ddPCR is that it does not require a standard curve. The absolute quantification is based on the number of positive (amplified droplets) divided by the total number of droplets generated. For translocation detection, wells containing an amplified housekeeping gene, translocation product, or both are then quantified. This method is extremely sensitive, detecting a few molecules per specimen, and can be used in both DNA and RNA applications.[53,54]

Multiplex Ligation-Dependent Probe Amplification

Multiplex ligation-dependent probe amplification (MLPA) is a method that can detect multiple copy number changes in a single reaction. It can also detect genomic deletions, duplications, and point mutations. It involves the use of two oligonucleotides that comprise the MLPA probes. Each oligonucleotide contains a primer sequence and a hybridization sequence complementary to the target. The probes hybridize to the denatured DNA target adjacent to each other and are ligated by a thermostable DNA ligase. A universal PCR primer pair which is fluorescently labeled amplifies the ligated target. For multiplex reactions, the probes are designed to produce different size fragments. To accomplish this, a stuffer fragment can be added to make the PCR products different sizes. The products are resolved using capillary gel electrophoresis. This has been applied to testing for genetic diseases such as thalassemia as well as malignancies (Figure 29.18).[55,56]

Mutation Enrichment Strategies

To detect low levels of disease or emerging resistance, it is helpful to be able to enrich for the presence of the mutation. There are currently several methods to accomplish this, all of which seek to selectively amplify the mutant sequence in the presence of an excess of wild-type sequence. Peptide-nucleic acid (PNA)

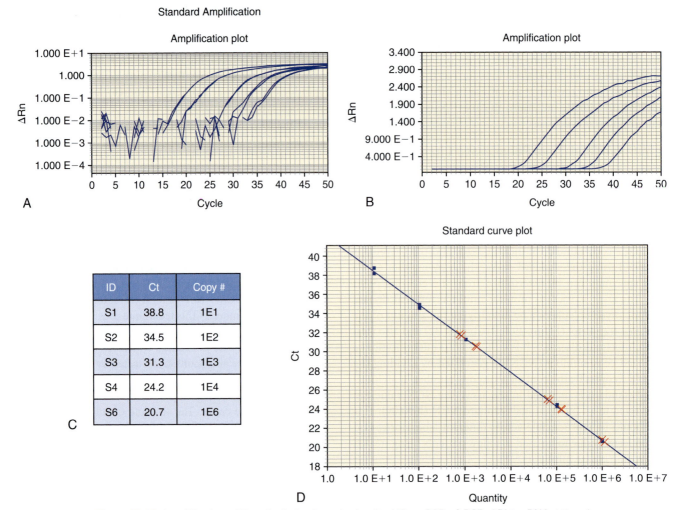

Standard Amplification

Figure 29.15 Amplification of Standards for Quantitative Real-Time PCR of *BCR::ABL1* mRNA. (A) and (B), Amplification curves for a series of standards of known copy number. (C), Table listing the Ct value and copy number of the standards containing known copy numbers of *BCR::ABL1* transcripts. (D), Graph of the Ct value versus the log of the copy number of the standards to generate a standard curve.

and locked nucleic acid (LNA) both contain normal nucleotide bases for hybridization but different backbones from the phosphodiester backbone of DNA and RNA.[57] This gives these probes the ability to hybridize more tightly when used as probes in PCR reactions. When the probes span and match the wild-type sequence, they can inhibit the amplification of the wild-type allele, thus enriching for the mutant allele.[58]

NUCLEIC ACID SEQUENCING

DNA Sequencing by Capillary Electrophoresis

The ability to read the sequence of the nucleic acid has been just as important as PCR in the development of molecular biology. A combination of these two important techniques (cycle sequencing) has made DNA sequencing an integral part of molecular diagnostics. In cycle sequencing, the order of the nucleotide bases is determined after amplification.[59] Cycle sequencing is applied in molecular testing to assess amplified sequences for insertions, deletions, or point mutations, such as *CEBPA* mutations that occur in some cases of AML (Chapter 31), or *JAK2*

exons 12 to 15 mutations that occur in some cases of *BCR::ABL1*-negative myeloproliferative neoplasms (Chapter 32).[60,61]

Cycle sequencing is based on dideoxynucleotide terminator sequencing.[62] Addition of nucleotides to a growing DNA polymer requires a 3′ hydroxyl group on the last added nucleotide and a triphosphate group on the 5′ end of the next nucleotide to be added (see Figure 29.5). If a nucleotide lacks the 3′ hydroxyl group, it can be incorporated into the newly synthesized strand of the DNA but cannot be extended, so the fragment terminates at the "defective" base. If low concentrations of the terminators—dideoxyadenosine triphosphate, dideoxycytosine triphosphate, dideoxyguanine triphosphate, and dideoxythymine triphosphate—are included in the single primer PCR master mix used for sequencing, over a number of cycles, a series of DNA fragments is produced that terminate at each successive base, with each fragment differing in length by one nucleotide. This is called a *ladder* or *nested series* of fragments.

In the dye terminator method, each of the four dideoxynucleotides in the PCR reaction is labeled with a different fluorescent dye so that each DNA fragment terminates in a labeled

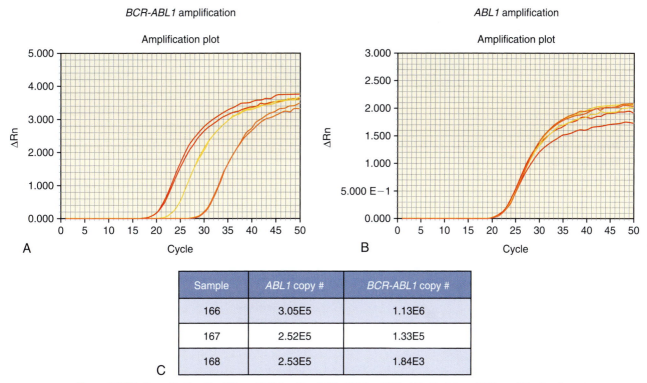

Sample	*ABL1* copy #	*BCR-ABL1* copy #
166	3.05E5	1.13E6
167	2.52E5	1.33E5
168	2.53E5	1.84E3

Figure 29.16 Quantitative Real-Time PCR for the *BCR::ABL1* mRNA. **(A)**, Real-time PCR amplification for *BCR::ABL1* transcripts. **(B)**, Real-time PCR amplification for the control gene, *ABL1*, as a measure of specimen quality. **(C)**, Table listing the copy numbers for *ABL1* and *BCR::ABL1* for three specimens derived from standard curves, such as the one illustrated in Figure 29.15.

dideoxynucleotide corresponding to the sequence of the target DNA (Figure 29.19, A). The specific fluorescent color of the DNA fragment identifies the terminal nucleotide. Alternatively, in the dye primer method, the primers are labeled with four different fluorescent dyes (corresponding to each nucleotide), and in separate tubes, each labeled primer is subjected to PCR with unlabeled dideoxynucleotides (Figure 29.19, B). As in the dye terminator method, the specific fluorescent color of the DNA fragments corresponds to the terminal nucleotide.

Fluorescently labeled fragments are subjected to capillary electrophoresis (described earlier in the chapter). DNA fragments migrate through the capillary and separate based on their size. Near the end of the capillary, fragments pass one by one through the beam of a laser in an order based on their base pair length (with the shortest fragments emerging first). A detector reads the specific fluorescent color of each fragment and displays the signal as a peak on an electropherogram; this allows the sequence to be read (Figure 29.19, C).

To read the nucleotide at each position unambiguously, the PCR reaction for cycle sequencing contains only a single primer that produces single-sided PCR. Two separate reactions are typically carried out, one using the forward primer and a second using the reverse primer. This produces complementary sequences from both strands. After the cycle sequencing reactions, the nested products are purified and denatured before loading on the capillary sequencer. Injection, separation, and detection are automated, but the operator can set the parameters, such as amount of specimen injected, length of capillaries, and type of polymer. Capillary DNA sequencing instruments

are equipped with base calling software that will read the base sequence of the DNA fragment sequenced. Software packages will also identify alterations in the sequence, such as SNPs, point mutations, and insertions or deletions based on comparison to a specific reference sequence.

Pyrosequencing is another sequencing method that is useful for the determination of point mutations and short sequence analysis. This method uses a "sequencing by synthesis" principle and the detection of pyrophosphate release upon nucleotide incorporation. Nucleotides are added sequentially to a single-stranded template and when the complementary base is added, it is incorporated, resulting in pyrophosphate release. The pyrophosphate released is then converted to adenosine triphosphate (ATP) by sulfurylase in the presence of adenosine 5′ phosphosulfate. This reaction is coupled to the luminescent conversion of luciferin to oxyluciferin by the enzyme luciferase, resulting in the release of light. Luminescent reactions resulting from the incorporation of nucleotides are represented as peaks on a pyrogram. The intensity of the light determines if there are multiple nucleotides that are identical because the peak height in the pyrogram will be proportional to the number of nucleotides.[63]

Sanger DNA sequencing has been considered the gold standard for the detection of germline point mutations and SNPs. With a point mutation, for example, sequencing of either strand will show whether the mutation (e.g., adenine to thymine) is present by comparison of the sequence to the reference sequence. Each cell has two copies (alleles) of somatic genes; therefore sequencing will produce a nested series of fragments from each allele. If the patient is a homozygote, the two nested series of

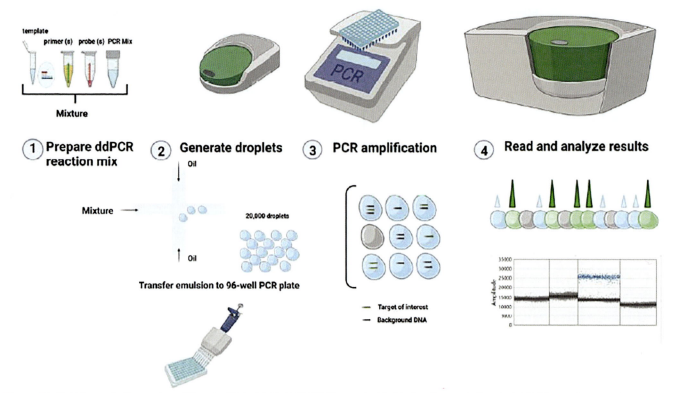

Figure 29.17 Schematic Illustration of Droplet Digital PCR (ddPCR) (**Created with** Bio.Render.com). A typical ddPCR workflow. *(1)* For the assay, a quantity of ddPCR mix, (buffer, dNTPs, primers, and probes) and the DNA sample are loaded in a multichannel cartridge with droplet generation mineral oil. *(2)* The droplet generator creates a vacuum with negative pressure crosswise the cartridge. In this way, the negative pressure subdivides the DNA sample into water-in-oil droplets at the same time. *(3)* Subsequently, these partitions will be individually amplified under specific thermal cycling conditions. *(4)* After PCR amplification is complete, the plate is placed in the droplet reader, which analyzes each droplet individually. (From Lambrescu, I., Popa, A., Manole, E., et al. (2022). Application of droplet digital PCR technology in muscular dystrophies research. *Int J Mol Sci, 23,* 4802.)

fragments will be identical, whether wild-type or mutant. If the patient is a heterozygote, both wild-type and mutant fragments will be produced in the single-sided PCR, generating two nested series of fragments. In analysis of this sequence, both signals will be present at the position of the mutation, but half the templates will contain each sequence.

Next-Generation Sequencing

Next-generation sequencing (NGS), also known as massively parallel sequencing (MPS), is a technique that is being increasingly applied in all areas of molecular diagnostics, including hematology.[64–66] Large-scale sequencing efforts, such as The Cancer Genome Atlas (TCGA) and The 1000 Genomes Project, have greatly expanded the number of clinically relevant genes and gene variants.[67,68] Important variants have been identified in oncogenes and in genes coding for tumor suppressors, receptors and other signaling molecules, and metabolic enzymes. Many of these genes have diagnostic, prognostic, or therapeutic implications in hematologic malignancies.[69–70] As the number of clinically significant variants has increased, so has the need for a unified platform for testing. Therefore NGS plays an increasingly important role in clinical practice. The technology is still evolving, but the most commonly used methods sequence short fragments multiple times lend use bioinformatics to reassemble the sequence and detect sequence variants.

Most clinical NGS tests for hematologic malignancies and genetic diseases involve the selection of a panel of clinically relevant genes for testing.[71–73] These panels can detect single nucleotide variants, small insertions and deletions (indels), and in some cases, copy number variants. There are also RNA-based panels for the detection of fusion genes resulting from translocations.

The process of NGS can be divided into several steps, including template and library preparation, sequencing and detection, and finally, data analysis and assembly (Figure 29.20). Currently available commercial systems use a variety of methods. There are two common methods of template selection: amplicon based or capture based.[64,65] Amplicon-based target selection uses multiplex PCR reactions to amplify the sequences of interest, whereas capture-based target selection first uses baits to hybridize and capture the targets of interest, followed by PCR amplification. The libraries are prepared by the addition of indexing primers to identify each specimen. One commonly used method for sequencing involves immobilization of molecules on a solid phase followed by amplification to produce clonally amplified clusters. Sequencing by synthesis reactions are carried out using cyclic reversible terminators in two or four colors and fluorescent detection by lasers after each base addition. A second commonly used method also amplifies the sequencing template but uses emulsion PCR

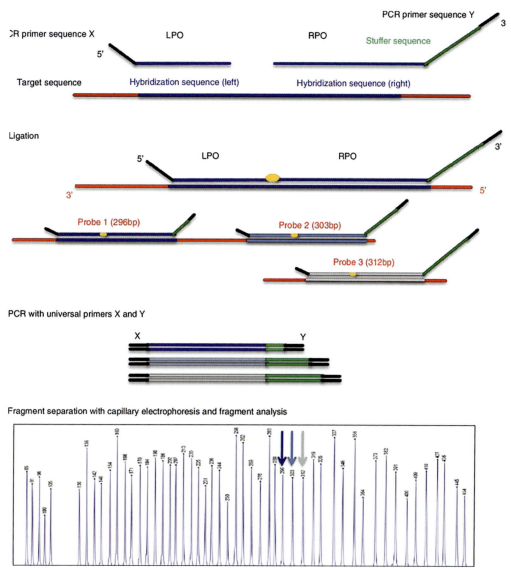

Figure 29.18 Overview of Multiplex Ligation-Dependent Probe Amplification (MLPA) Technology for Copy Number Detection. An outline of the MLPA technique: (1) MLPA probes consist of two hemiprobes: a 5′ oligonucleotide, called the left probe oligonucleotide *(LPO)*, and the 3′ oligonucleotide, called the right probe oligonucleotide *(RPO)*, which target adjacent sequences *(blue)* and a polymerase chain reaction (PCR) primer sequence *(black)*. The RPO has a nonhybridizing stuffer sequence *(green)*, which gives the probe a specific length. To begin the reaction, the MLPA probe mix is added to denatured DNA for approximately 16 hours of hybridization. (2) After successful hybridization to their target sequences in the sample DNA, the bound probe oligonucleotides are enzymatically ligated, creating a template for the subsequent PCR reaction. (3) In the PCR reaction, all MLPA probes are amplified by the same PCR primer pair (X and Y), allowing semiquantitative amplification of the probes. (4) Because of the different lengths of the stuffer sequences, the amplification products of different MLPA probes can be separated, identified, and quantified by capillary electrophoresis. This allows the use of up to 50 probes in a single MLPA reaction. Relative amounts of probe amplification products, as compared with a reference DNA sample, reflect the relative copy number of the target. (From Hömig-Hölzel, C., & Savola, S. (2012). Multiplex ligation-dependent probe amplification (MLPA) in tumor diagnostics and prognostics. *Diagn Mol Pathol, 21,* 189–206.)

to accomplish it. The sequencing technology takes advantage of the hydrogen ion released when a base is added and uses semiconductor technology to translate the release of a hydrogen ion into a nucleotide sequence by the sequential addition of bases and the measurement of the voltage produced when the correct nucleotide base is added. Both methods use proprietary software to produce a base calling FASTQ file as the primary analysis. The secondary analysis involves demultiplexing and alignment to a reference sequence to produce a binary alignment map (BAM) file, followed by production of a variant call file (VCF). There are also numerous programs

available as open source or from commercial vendors for generation of a pipeline for analysis. The tertiary analysis involves the clinical annotation of the variants identified. This can be done manually by searching publicly available databases such as the Catalog of Somatic Mutations in Cancer (COSMIC),[74] ClinVar,[75] or mycancergenome.org and searching the published literature or alternatively, using commercially available annotation software.

As with any assay, there are quality measures that are evaluated. All NGS reactions are given a quality score (Q score) and the number of reads (the number of times a target is sequenced)

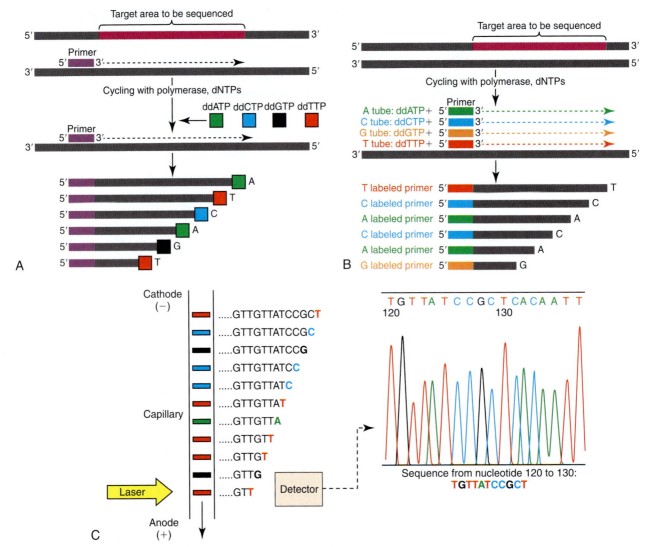

Figure 29.19 Dideoxy Chain Termination (Sanger) DNA Sequencing. Cycle sequencing of a DNA template produces a nested series of fragments that differ by one nucleotide each. The template is amplified by polymerase chain reaction (PCR), using a single primer sequence (single-sided PCR). The PCR master mix includes small amounts of dideoxynucleotides. When a dideoxynucleotide is incorporated into the growing DNA polymer, chain extension terminates. **(A)**, Dye terminator method, in which each of the four dideoxynucleotides are labeled with a different fluorescent dye. The identity of the terminal nucleotide corresponds to its specific fluorescent color. **(B)**, Dye primer method, in which the primer is labeled with four different fluorescent dyes, corresponding to each nucleotide. Again, the identity of the terminal nucleotide corresponds to the specific color of the primer. **(C)**, Capillary gel electrophoresis, in which fluorescently labeled fragments pass between a laser and detector in size order (smallest fragments first). The fluorescent color of the fragment identifies the terminal nucleotide. The signals appear as peaks on an electropherogram, with each peak representing a specific terminal nucleotide in sequence order.

is evaluated. The variant allele fraction (VAF), usually given as the percent of variant reads over the total reads, is also evaluated to confirm it is above the limit of detection. Several consensus documents have been issued with respect to NGS, including laboratory standards by the College of American Pathologists (CAP) and[76] joint standards and guidelines on validating oncology panels and bioinformatics pipelines by CAP and the Association for Molecular Pathology (AMP),[77,78] as well as joint standards and guidelines for interpreting and reporting sequence variants in cancer by CAP, AMP, and the American Society of Clinical Oncology.[79] Current clinical applications for NGS have

been mainly limited to the sequencing of panels of genes associated with a particular disease. This makes the bioinformatics analyses more manageable and limits the number of variants of unknown significance (VUS) that are identified. NGS clinical assays are in routine clinical use for many different hematologic diseases, including myeloid, lymphoid, and erythroid malignancies.[80-82] In addition to sequencing panels of genes, this technology has been used to sequence whole genomes and exomes (the coding exons), as well as RNA sequencing (RNAseq).[83,84] Comprehensive genome profiling (CGP) increasingly is being applied to all types of hematologic diseases, especially oncology.

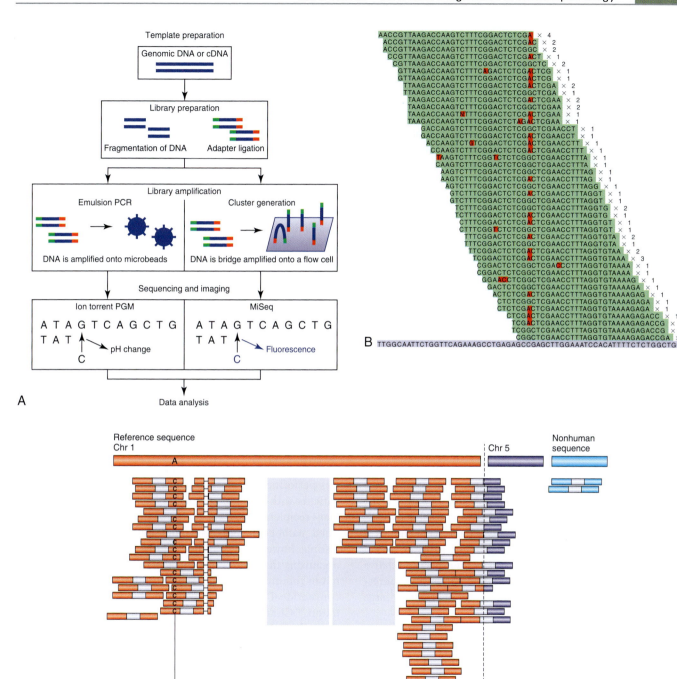

Figure 29.20 Next-Generation Sequencing. (A), Diagram of the procedure for next-generation sequencing (NGS) using the two most common technologies. (B), An illustration of a number of NGS reads for a 32-nucleotide sequence aligned with the genomic reference sequence in *blue* on the *bottom* (sequence mismatches are in *red*). The center of the alignment shows a variant present in the heterozygous state. (C), Sequenced fragments are depicted as bars, with colored tips representing the sequenced ends and the unsequenced portion of the fragment in *gray*. Reads are aligned to the reference genome (e.g., mostly chromosome 1 in this example). The colors of the sequenced ends show where they align. Different types of genomic alterations can be detected. *Left to right,* Point mutations (in this example, *A* to *C*) and small insertions and deletions (indels) (in this example, a deletion shown by a *dashed line*) are detected by identifying multiple reads that show nonreference sequence; changes in sequencing depth (relative to a normal control) are used to identify copy number changes (*shaded boxes* represent absent or decreased reads in a tumor specimen); paired ends that map to different genomic loci (in this case, chromosome 5) are evidence of rearrangements; and sequences that map to nonhuman sequences are evidence for the potential presence of genomic material from pathogens. (*A* from Grada, A., & Weinbrecht, K. [2013]. Next-generation sequencing: methodology and application. *J Invest Dermatol, 133,* 248–251; *B* from Almomani, R., van der Heijden, J., Ariyurek, Y., et al. [2011]. Experiences with array-based sequence capture: toward clinical applications. *Eur J Hum Genet, 19,* 50–55; and *C* from Meyerson, M., Gabriel, S., & Getz, G. [2010]. Advances in understanding cancer genomes through second generation sequencing. *Nat Rev Genet, 11,* 685–696.)

CGP is the use of an NGS assay testing both DNA and RNA to identify multiple categories of genetic alterations, including SNVs, CNVs, indels, and fusions. In addition, there is an increased recognition of germline predisposition identified by NGS that has been incorporated into current guidelines.[85,86] NGS technology is also being applied to the determination of epigenome modifications such as methylation that affect gene regulation and expression. NGS will continue to play an increasingly important role in molecular diagnostics.

CHROMOSOMAL MICROARRAYS

Chromosomal microarray analysis is a methodology used to measure gains and losses of genomic DNA. The advantage of a microarray compared with conventional karyotyping is that it is a higher-resolution method and will detect genetic changes that cannot be observed by karyotyping (Chapter 30). In addition, chromosomal microarrays have the advantage of also detecting aneuploidy and large chromosomal duplications and insertions.

There are two different types of chromosomal microarrays: comparative genomic hybridization (aCGH) and single nucleotide polymorphism array (SNP-A) karyotyping. Both types of arrays can identify variation in copy number. Because of the differences in methodology, however, they detect different types of variants (Figures 29.21, 30.28, and 30.29).

In array-based assays, the specimen DNA is isolated, denatured, and hybridized to a chip or an array containing thousands of probes with known sequences. For comparative genome hybridization, the patient DNA and a control DNA are labeled with different fluorescent dyes and after hybridization, the relative intensity of the two fluorescent signals is used to determine if there are any genomic gains or losses. Duplications result in a higher-intensity fluorescence relative to control and deletions result in a lower-intensity fluorescence. CGH is most useful in the detection of relatively large duplications or deletions.[87]

In SNP arrays, only the patient DNA is labeled, denatured, and hybridized to an array containing probes with known SNPs. The fluorescent intensity is compared to a reference set of controls that have been previously run and normalized. The signal intensity is used to determine the copy number. SNP arrays are also able to detect runs of homozygosity that can indicate uniparental disomy or consanguinity.[88] Because each of these methods has both advantages and disadvantages, array platforms have been developed that contain both types of sequences: SNPs and larger clones used in CGH. This provides a more uniform coverage over the entire genome. Array procedures have improved such that in addition to DNA isolated from peripheral blood, DNA isolated from formalin-fixed, paraffin-embedded specimens also can be used. In certain situations, arrays are replacing or are used as an adjunct to conventional karyotyping and fluorescence in situ hybridization (FISH) (Chapter 30). Arrays are useful to detect copy number variants but do not detect balanced translocations.[87]

PATHOGEN DETECTION AND INFECTIOUS DISEASE LOAD

Box 29.4 contains a list of hematologically important pathogens detected by molecular methods. Real-time quantitative PCR can detect and quantify a number of blood borne viruses: hepatitis B and C viruses, human papillomavirus, CMV, Epstein-Barr virus, and HIV.[89] Human bacterial pathogens, such as β-hemolytic *Streptococcus* from throat swabs, anaerobes from wound swabs, and bacteria from urine or other body fluids, can be detected within hours of collection. Antibacterial therapy can be initiated based on the rapid results of molecular susceptibility testing. Real-time quantitative PCR is the reference method for detection and quantification of methicillin-resistant *Staphylococcus aureus* (MRSA), vancomycin-resistant *Enterococcus,* and opportunistic *Clostridioides.* Molecular diagnostic techniques are effective in identifying and monitoring malarial and other bloodborne parasites. The challenge to primer and probe developers is to select sequences that are specific enough to avoid false-positive results caused by nonpathogenic strains, sensitive enough to positively identify infectious strains, and flexible enough to remain effective as pathogenic microorganisms mutate and evolve. There are currently multiple FDA-approved assays for the detection of viral, bacterial, and parasitic pathogens. A current listing of these tests can be found on the FDA's website (https://www.fda.gov/medical-devices/in-vitro-diagnostics/nucleic-acid-based-tests). Recently, NGS was performed on plasma from immunocompromised adult patients with hematologic malignancies and stem cell transplant recipients. NGS appears to be highly sensitive and identified pathogenic organisms not detected by conventional testing; however, it was not highly specific and identified organisms that were not clinically relevant, and is currently not in common practice. It is best used in patients negative by conventional testing and in conjunction with clinical presentation.[90] Clinical relevance is important when assessing infectious disease using molecular techniques. These methods allow millions of copies to be generated from a single DNA or RNA sequence from a microorganism or virus. Theoretically, the presence of a single organism can lead to a positive test result, but a single organism may not be clinically relevant. Standard curves of template number are crucial to data interpretation. Also, because DNA survives the organism, a positive result on a test for a given sequence does not guarantee that the organism was viable at the time of sampling.

CURRENT DEVELOPMENTS

Molecular diagnostics is a rapidly growing area of the clinical laboratory, and in many situations, is standard of care. The technology continues to develop. It promises to revolutionize laboratory techniques in all disciplines, and the technologies of genomics are being extended to proteomics (the molecular analysis of proteins) and metabolomics (the molecular

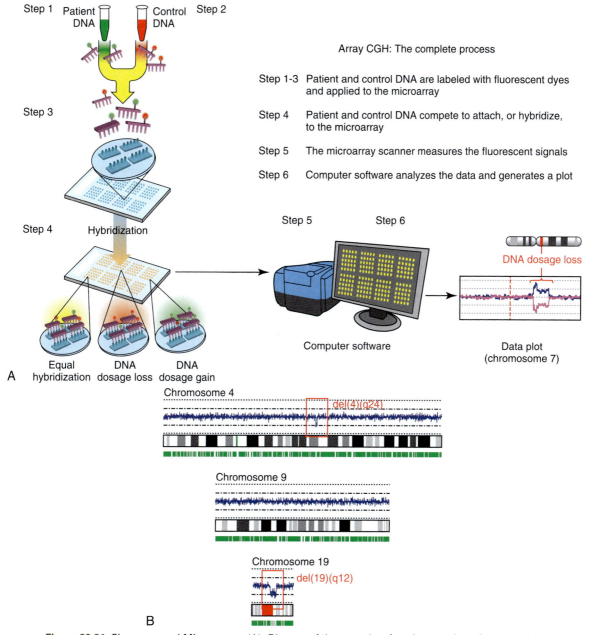

Figure 29.21 Chromosomal Microarrays. **(A)**, Diagram of the procedure for microarray-based comparative genomic hybridization (aCGH). The data plot shows patient DNA loss on chromosome 7 *(pink)*, with a control plot *(blue)*. **(B)**, An example of a single nucleotide polymorphism array (SNP-A) karyogram from a patient with a secondary acute myeloid leukemia, with microdeletions on chromosomes 4 and 19 and a normal chromosome 9. (*A* © 2008 SLACK, Inc. Modified from Shaffer, L. G., & Bejjani, B. A. [2009]. Using microarray-based molecular cytogenetic methods to identify chromosome abnormalities. *Pediatr Ann, 38,* 440–447; *B* from Gondek, L. P., Dunbar, A. J., Szpurka, H., et al. [2007]. SNP array karyotyping allows for the detection of uniparental disomy and cryptic chromosomal abnormalities in MDS/MPD-U and MPD. *PLoS ONE, 2*(11), e1225. https://doi.10.1371/journal.pone.0001225.)

analysis of metabolism). Methods continue to be automated and miniaturized, providing ever-greater sensitivity and reliability coupled with short turnaround time and technical simplification. There are automated systems for NGS library preparation and even the sequencing and data analysis. In many situations, assays are moving from single analyte assays to multiplex assays detecting panels of analytes of multiple types. The updated WHO guidelines for lymphoid and myeloid diseases incorporate genetic testing on multiple levels for diagnosis, prognosis, and therapy.[69,70]

Another technique being applied to the detection of mutation panels is matrix-assisted laser desorption/ionization-time of flight (MALDI-TOF) mass spectrometry. This methodology uses PCR coupled to a single-base extension reaction that adds labeled nucleotides so that the extension products containing different mutations have different masses. These reactions are also multiplexed to increase throughput, detecting hundreds of mutations in a single panel assay. This has been applied to pharmacogenetic testing.[91]

Circulating tumor DNA is a promising technique using a minimally invasive specimen type for the monitoring of genetic alterations in solid tumors (e.g., lymphomas), which may shed DNA into the bloodstream. This technique, known as liquid biopsy, can potentially be used instead of a tissue biopsy to monitor for residual disease or the development of resistance to targeted drug therapy. The circulating tumor DNA can be tested using a variety of downstream techniques, including real-time PCR, digital PCR, or NGS.[92,93] It is in clinical use for lung adenocarcinomas and other solid tumors. Application to hematologic malignancies has been complicated by the possibility of clonal hematopoiesis of undetermined potential (CHIP), which can complicate interpretation.

Optical genome mapping (OGM) is a technique that has been used in genome sequencing and is being applied to replace conventional cytogenetics (Figure 29.22). OGM uses imaging of high-molecular-weight DNA and very long linear single DNA molecules (median size >250 kb), which are labeled at multiple specific sites. It uses whole genome imaging analysis to identify structural variation. This is accomplished using microfluidics, high-resolution microscopy, and automated image analysis. Two pipelines are used to identify both structural variants and CNVs.[94,95]

In addition to techniques such as OGM, nanopores are also being used in the generation of long sequencing reads greater than 10,000 bases from single DNA molecules. The technique called single-molecule real-time sequencing (SMRT) uses a zero-mode wave (ZMW) guide with DNA polymerase attached to identify nucleotides as they are incorporated using fluorescent detection. DNA molecules are circularized using hairpin ligation adapters for sequencing, and multiple molecules can be sequenced simultaneously by the use of a chip with multiple ZMWs. The technology and bioinformatics continue to improve, but the major disadvantage is the high error rate, estimated to be approximately 10%, in contrast to standard NGS, where the error rate is estimated to be 0.2% to 0.5%.[96,97]

Evidence gained from bulk analyses of hematologic malignancies has identified significant cellular heterogeneity. This can encompass the development of changing subclones within the malignant cells as well as involving cellular hierarchies and surrounding cellular components. NGS sequencing of multicellular specimens is limited in its ability to identify these changes at the individual cell level. Novel single-cell technologies are being developed and applied to address this heterogeneity. For example, single cells can be isolated and sequenced using RNA-seq to determine the expression of thousands of genes simultaneously.

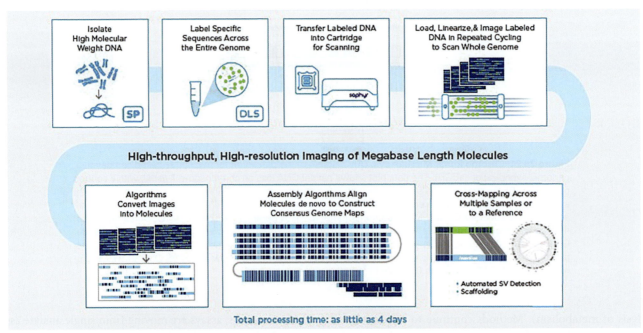

Figure 29.22 Optical Genome Mapping. This technology images ultralong linearized DNA molecules labeled at specific sequence motifs. Comparative analysis of the label patterns over long contiguous reads across the whole genome reveals structural variants (>500 bp) at sensitivities as high as 99%, with false-positive rates below 2%. All major types of large structural variants can be detected, even at allele fractions. (From 30149-Saphyr-Brochure.pdf [bionanogenomics.com].)

Multimodal profiling, defined as the simultaneous detection of multiple types of molecules, can interrogate DNA, DNA methylation status, RNA, and proteins in single cells. Bioinformatic approaches allow the clustering of cell populations and tracking changes in cells with disease progression.[98] This has important consequences in identifying factors critical in prognosis and resistance to therapy.

Small microRNAs (miR, ~290 nucleotides long) that were once thought to be insignificant are evolving as biomarkers for the progression of hematologic malignancies. The dysregulation of miRs affects normal hematopoiesis, and their atypical expression has begun to be established in T and B cell leukemias and lymphomas. These miRs target genes in the 3′ UTR (3′ untranslated region) and are hypothesized to inhibit the translation of mRNAs to proteins. These miRs can be detected by many molecular-based techniques, such as PCR, NGS, and microarray technology. Their clinical role in hematologic cancer therapy as a prognostic marker is now starting to be recognized. Multiple studies demonstrate that the ability to measure the expression of miR has expanded the repertoire of diagnostic, prognostic, and therapeutic efficacy markers in hematologic malignancies.[99]

Much of the descriptions of technologies in this chapter have been directed at identifying and characterizing disease states; however, the ultimate goal is to reverse and ultimately prevent hematologic disease. Recent advances in gene editing techniques using the CRISPR CAS9 system have made advances in the treatment of sickle cell disease by increasing expression of the γ-globin gene. More recently, this technique has been applied to the correction of the mutant HbS in SCD patients (Chapter 24 and Figure 24.10).

In the future, molecular technologies will increase the efficiency and sensitivity for detection of all types of genome alterations, including point mutations, insertion and deletion mutations, copy number variants, chromosome rearrangements, and gene expression analysis. These new or improved techniques will facilitate the discovery of new chromosome rearrangements, in addition to the diagnosis of microbial infections. This will result in refined classification and improved treatment of hematologic diseases.

SUMMARY

- DNA directs cell function, as described by the central dogma. DNA retains the genetic code and reproduces itself through replication.
- The genetic code is transcribed from DNA to mRNA. The mRNA consists of coding exons and noncoding introns that are excised after transcription. The processed mRNA then transports the code from the nucleus to the cytoplasm, where it is translated to a peptide by the cytoplasmic ribosomes.
- DNA consists of a five-carbon sugar (deoxyribose), a phosphate group, and a nitrogenous base. Bases are either purines or pyrimidines. The purines are adenine (A) and guanine (G); the pyrimidines are thymine (T) and cytosine (C).
- DNA is a double-stranded molecule held together by hydrogen bonding between the bases, A to T and G to C. Heat denatures double-stranded DNA by breaking the hydrogen bonds, producing single-stranded DNA. DNA strands are antiparallel; that is, 5′ to 3′ strands anneal to 3′ to 5′ complementary strands.
- DNA replication occurs in the 5′ to 3′ direction and requires a template, primer, four nucleotides (A, C, G, T), and DNA polymerase to add nucleotides that are complementary to the template.
- RNA is a single-stranded molecule that contains the sugar ribose instead of deoxyribose and the pyrimidine uracil in place of thymine.
- During transcription, RNA polymerase recognizes a sequence of deoxyribonucleotides, called the *promoter,* within DNA. RNA polymerase binds to the promoter, separates the DNA strands, and begins adding ribonucleotides that are complementary to the DNA template, forming a primary RNA transcript consisting of introns and exons. The exons provide the coding information. The introns are excised and the exons are spliced together, forming a mature

mRNA that enters the cytoplasm and is translated to protein by ribosomes.
- Translation depends on tRNA, small RNA molecules designed to transport and add amino acids to growing peptide chains in cytoplasmic ribosomes.
- Five areas of hematologic molecular testing include detection of mutations, gene rearrangements, and chromosomal abnormalities for diagnosis and prognosis of hematologic malignancies; detection and quantification of minimal residual disease to monitor treatment of hematologic malignancies; detection of mutations in inherited hematologic disorders; pharmacogenetic testing to detect genetic variation affecting certain drug therapies; and identification of hematologically important infectious diseases.
- Peripheral blood, bone marrow, tissue biopsy specimens (both fresh and formalin-fixed paraffin-embedded), fine-needle aspirates, body fluids, saliva, and cheek swabs are specimens used for DNA and RNA isolation.
- Specific DNA sequences are amplified by endpoint polymerase chain reaction (PCR) and real-time PCR. RNA targets can be amplified by PCR by first converting the RNA target to complementary DNA (cDNA) using reverse transcriptase.
- In endpoint PCR, amplified DNA is detected by capillary gel electrophoresis or DNA sequencing. Endpoint PCR also can be combined with restriction enzyme digestion of amplicons, followed by detection of the restriction fragments by one of the methods mentioned above. In real-time PCR, the amplicons are detected during the PCR cycles by fluorescence detection.
- Real-time PCR can be used qualitatively to determine the presence or absence of a target or can quantify the copy number of a target DNA or RNA. Digital PCR can also be used to quantify copy numbers of a target.

- Multiplex ligation-dependent probe amplification (MLPA) is an alternative method that can be used to identify multiple types of DNA alterations.
- The dideoxy chain termination (Sanger) method for DNA sequencing is based on the principle that synthesis of a DNA polymer is terminated upon incorporation of a dideoxynucleotide. The target DNA template is amplified over a number of cycles, which produces a series of DNA fragments that terminate at each successive base, with each fragment differing in length by one nucleotide. DNA fragments are detected by labeling either the dideoxynucleotide or the primer with a fluorescent dye. Other methods for DNA sequencing include pyrosequencing and next-generation sequencing (NGS).
- NGS is a parallel sequencing technique in which multiple DNA fragments are sequenced simultaneously. This technique can be used to sequence panels of genes to identify mutations and small insertions and deletions (indels), as well as fusions and copy number variants.
- Chromosomal microarrays measure gains and losses of genomic DNA. They provide much greater sensitivity in detecting small genomic changes compared to conventional karyotyping. There are two types: microarray-based comparative genomic hybridization (aCGH) and single nucleotide polymorphism array (SNP-A) karyotyping. CGH requires the use of a control DNA.
- Molecular testing permits providers to make more accurate diagnostic, therapeutic, and prognostic decisions. It also allows a more sensitive assessment of minimal residual disease and therapeutic efficacy, resulting in better patient management.

Now that you have completed this chapter, go back and read again the case study at the beginning and respond to the questions presented. Answers can be found in Appendix C.

REVIEW QUESTIONS

Answers can be found in Appendix C.

1. If the DNA nucleotide sequence is 5′-ATTAGC-3′, then the mRNA sequence transcribed from this template is:
   a. 5′-GCUAAU-3′
   b. 5′-AUUAGC-3′
   c. 5′-TAATCG-3′
   d. 5′-UAAUCG-3′

2. Cells with damaged DNA and mutated or nonfunctioning cell cycle regulatory proteins:
   a. Are arrested in G_1 and the DNA is repaired
   b. Continue to divide, which leads to tumor progression
   c. Divide normally, producing identical daughter cells
   d. Go through apoptosis

3. To start DNA replication, DNA polymerase requires an available 3′ hydroxyl group found on the:
   a. Leading strand
   b. mRNA
   c. Parent strand
   d. Primer

4. Ligase joins Okazaki fragments of the:
   a. 5′ to 3′ template strand
   b. Lagging strand
   c. Leading strand
   d. Primer fragments

5. A 40-year-old patient enters the hospital with a rare form of cancer caused by faulty cell division regulation. This cancer localized in the patient's spleen. An ambitious laboratory developed a molecular test to verify the type of cancer present. This molecular test would require patient specimens taken from which two tissues?
   a. Abnormal growths found on the skin and in the bone marrow
   b. Normal splenic tissue and cancerous tissue
   c. Cancerous tissue in spleen and bone marrow
   d. Peripheral blood and cancerous tissue in the spleen

6. One main difference between PCR and reverse transcription PCR is that:
   a. PCR requires primers.
   b. PCR uses reverse transcriptase to elongate the primers.
   c. Reverse transcription PCR uses cDNA as a template.
   d. Reverse transcription PCR requires ligase to amplify the target DNA.

7. Which one of the following statements about capillary gel electrophoresis is FALSE?
   a. Fluorescent detection occurs when the fragments pass by a laser.
   b. A buffer solution is required to maintain the electrical current.
   c. The matrix of a capillary is derivatized polyacrylamide gel.
   d. The larger DNA fragments will migrate faster through the capillary.

8. In which of the following applications would it be most appropriate to use NGS technology?
   a. Testing for a point mutation in the *FV* gene
   b. Testing for the *BCR::ABL1* translocation in CML
   c. Sequencing a B-cell lymphoma genome
   d. Determining the karyotype in AML

9. One major difference between endpoint PCR and real-time PCR is that:
   a. Endpoint PCR requires thermostable DNA polymerase, deoxynucleotides, and primers.
   b. Endpoint PCR requires a separate step to detect the amplicons formed in the reaction.
   c. Real-time PCR uses capillary gel electrophoresis to detect amplicons during PCR cycling.
   d. Real-time PCR detects and quantifies amplicons using cleavage-based signal amplification.

10. Which of the following statements about minimal residual disease is TRUE?
    a. Clinical remission of hematologic cancers is determined by molecular techniques such as PCR and flow cytometry.
    b. Real-time, quantitative PCR-determined copy number of *BCR::ABL1* transcripts will always be lower in molecular remission than in clinical remission.
    c. Qualitative PCR that uses a known copy number of a target sequence is of use in determining minimal residual disease levels.
    d. Minimal residual disease assessment can aid providers in making treatment decisions but does not yet offer insights into prognosis.

REFERENCES

1. Rees, D. C., Williams, T. N., & Gladwin, M. T. (2010). Sickle-cell disease. *Lancet, 376*(9757), 2018–2031.
2. National Human Genome Research Institute. *A Brief Guide to Genomics.* https://www.genome.gov/about-genomics/fact-sheets/A-Brief-Guide-to-Genomics. Accessed March 12, 2023.
3. Hubé, F., & Francastel, C. (2015). Mammalian introns: when the junk generates molecular diversity. *Int J Mol Sci, 16*(3), 4429–4452.
4. Lewin, B. (2018). Messenger RNA. In Krebs, J. E., Goldstein, E. S., & Kilpatrick, S. T. (Eds.), *Lewin's Genes XII.* (12th ed., pp. 543–563). Sudbury, MA: Jones & Bartlett.
5. Lodish, H., Berk, A., Kaiser, C. A., et al. (2021). Fundamental molecular genetic mechanisms. In *Molecular Cell Biology.* (9th ed., pp. 34–52). New York, NY: WH Freeman.
6. Arber, D., Orazi, A., Hasserjian, R., et al. (2022). International consensus classification of myeloid neoplasms and acute leukemia: integrating morphological, clinical and genomic data. *Blood, 140*, 1200–1228.
7. Campo, E., Jaffe E., Cook, J., et al. (2022). The International Consensus Classification of mature lymphoid neoplasms: a report from the clinical advisory committee. *Blood, 140*, 1229–1253.
8. Bartlett, J. M. S., & White, A. (2003). Extraction of DNA from whole blood. In Bartlett, J. M. S., & Stirling, D. (Eds.), *PCR Protocols.* (2nd ed., pp. 29–31). Totowa, NJ: Humana Press.
9. Shimizu, H., & Burns, J. C. (1995). Extraction nucleic acids: sample preparation from paraffin-embedded tissues. In Innis, M. A., Gelfand, D. H., & Sninsky, J. J. (Eds.), *PCR Strategies.* (pp. 32–38). San Diego: Academic Press.
10. Cao, W., Hashibe, M., Rao, J. Y., et al. (2003). Comparison of methods for DNA extraction from paraffin-embedded tissues and buccal cells. *Cancer Detect Prevent, 27*, 397–404.
11. Harder, J., & Schroder, J. M. (2002). RNase 7, a novel innate immune defense antimicrobial protein of healthy human skin. *J Biol Chem, 277*, 46779–46784.
12. Bogner, P. N., & Killeen, A. A. (2006). Extraction of nucleic acids. In Coleman, W. B., & Tsongalis, G. J. (Eds.), *Molecular Diagnostics for the Clinical Laboratorian.* (pp. 25–30). Totowa, NJ: Humana Press.
13. Killeen, A. A. (2004). Methods in molecular pathology. In *Principles of Molecular Pathology.* (pp. 89–139). Totowa, NJ: Humana Press.
14. Mullis, K. B., & Faloona, F. A. (1987). Specific synthesis of DNA in vitro via a polymerase-catalyzed chain reaction. *Methods Enzymol, 155*, 335–350.
15. Saiki, R. K., Scharf, S., Faloona, F., et al. (1985). Enzymatic amplification of β-globin genomic sequences and restriction site analysis for diagnosis of sickle cell anemia. *Science, 230*, 1350–1354.
16. Studwell, P. S., & O'Donnell, M. (1990). Processive replication is contingent on the exonuclease subunit of DNA polymerase III holoenzyme. *J Biol Chem, 265*, 1171–1178.
17. Saiki, R. K., Gelfand, D. H., Stoffel, S., et al. (1988). Primer-directed enzymatic amplification of DNA with a thermostable DNA polymerase. *Science, 239*, 487–491.
18. Cha, R. S., & Thilly, W. G. (1995). Specificity, fidelity and efficiency of PCR. In Dieffenbach, C. W., & Dveksler, G. S. (Eds.), *PCR Primer: A Laboratory Manual.* (pp. 37–52). Cold Spring Harbor, NY: Cold Spring Harbor Press.
19. Altschul, S. F., Gish, W., Miller, W., et al. (1990). Basic local alignment search tool. *J Mol Biol, 215*, 403–410.
20. Mifflin, T. E. (2003). Setting up a PCR laboratory. In Dieffenbach, C. W., & Dveksler, G. S. (Eds.), *PCR Primer: A Laboratory Manual.* (2nd ed., pp. 5–14). Cold Spring Harbor, NY: Cold Spring Harbor Laboratory Press.
21. Najfeld, V. (2023). Conventional and molecular cytogenomic basis of hematologic malignancies. In Hoffman, R., Benz, E. J., Silberstein, L. E., et al. (Eds.), *Hematology: Basic Principles and Practice.* (8th ed., pp. 813–899). Philadelphia: Elsevier.
22. Bhatt, V. R., Akhtari, M., Bociek, R. G., et al. (2014). Allogeneic stem cell transplantation for Philadelphia chromosome-positive acute myeloid leukemia. *J Natl Compr Canc Netw, 12*, 963–968.
23. Bartram, C. R., de Klein, A., Hagemeijer, A., et al. (1983). Translocation of the c-abl oncogene correlates with the presence of a Philadelphia chromosome in chronic myelocytic leukemia. *Nature, 306*, 277–280.
24. Heisterkamp, N., Stephenson, J. R., Groffen, J., et al. (1983). Localization of the c-abl oncogene adjacent to a translocation break point in chronic myelocytic leukemia. *Nature, 306*, 239–242.
25. Clark, S. S., McLaughlin, J., Crist, W. M., et al. (1987). Unique forms of the abl tyrosine kinase distinguish Ph1-positive CML from Ph1-positive ALL. *Science, 235*, 85–88.
26. Preudhomme, C., Revillion, F., Merlat, A., et al. (1999). Detection of BCR-ABL transcripts in chronic myeloid leukemia (CML) using a "real-time" quantitative RT-PCR assay. *Leukemia, 13*, 957–964.
27. Luu, M. H., & Press, R. D. (2013). BCR-ABL PCR testing in chronic myelogenous leukemia: molecular diagnosis for targeted cancer therapy and monitoring. *Expert Rev Mol Diagn, 13*, 749–762.
28. Dubrow, R. S. (1992). Capillary gel electrophoresis. In Grossman, P. D., & Colburn, J. C. (Eds.), *Capillary Gel Electrophoresis Theory and Practice.* (pp. 146–154). San Diego: Academic Press.
29. Van Dongen, J., Langerak, A. W., Bruggemann, M., et al. (2003). Design and standardization of PCR primers and protocols for the detection of immunoglobulin and T cell receptor gene rearrangements in suspect lymphoproliferations. Report of the BIOMED-2 Concerted Action BMH4-CT98-3936. *Leukemia, 12*, 2257–2317.
30. Nathans, D., & Smith, H. O. (1975). Restriction endonucleases in the analysis and restructuring of DNA molecules. *Annu Rev Biochem, 44*, 273–293.
31. Ross, D. W. (1990). Restriction enzymes. *Arch Pathol Lab Med, 114*, 906.

32. Murphy, K. M., Levis, M., Hafez, M. J., et al. (2003). Detection of FLT3 internal tandem duplication and D835 mutations by a multiplex polymerase chain reaction and capillary electrophoresis. *J Mol Diagn, 5*(2), 96–102.

33. Templeton, K. E., & Claas, E. C. J. (2003). Comparison of four real-time PCR detection systems. In Dieffenbach, C. W., & Dveksler, G. S. (Eds.), *PCR Primer: A Laboratory Manual.* (2nd ed., pp. 187–198). Cold Spring Harbor, NY: Cold Spring Harbor Laboratory Press.

34. van der Velden, V. H. J., Hochhaus, A., Cazzaniga, G., et al. (2003). Detection of minimal residual disease in hematologic malignancies by real-time quantitative PCR: principles, approaches, and laboratory aspects. *Leukemia, 17*, 1013–1034.

35. Ahmad, A. I., & Ghasemi, J. B. (2007). New FRET primers for quantitative real-time PCR. *Anal Bioanal Chem, 387*, 2737–2743.

36. Luthra, R., & Medeiros, L. J. (2006). TaqMan reverse transcriptase-polymerase chain reaction coupled with capillary electrophoresis for quantification and identification of bcr-abl transcript type. *Methods Mol Biol, 335*, 135–145.

37. Tan, W., Wang, K., & Drake, T. J. (2004). Molecular beacons. *Curr Opin Chem Biol, 8*, 547–553.

38. Olynyk, J. K., & Ramm, G. A., (2022) Hemochromatosis. *N Engl J Med, 37*, 2159–2170.

39. Rudert, W. A., Braun, E. R., & Faas, S. J. (1997). Double labeled fluorescent probes for 5′ nuclease assays: purification and performance evaluation. *BioTechniques, 22*, 1140–1145.

40. Fanis, P., Kousiappa, I., Phylactides, M., et al. (2014). Genotyping of BCL11A and HBSIL-MYB SNPs associated with fetal haemoglobin levels: a SNaPshot minisequencing approach. *BMC Genomics, 15*, 108. doi:10.1186/1471-2164-15-108.

41. Latini, F. R., Gazito, D., Amoni, C. P., et al. (2014). A new strategy to identify rare blood donors: single polymerase chain reaction multiplex SNaPshot reaction for detection of 16 blood group alleles. *Blood Transfus, 12*(Suppl. 1), s256–s263.

42. Bolufer, P., Colomer, D., Gomez, M. T., et al. (2004) Quantitative assessment of *PML::RARAα* and *BCR::ABL* by two real-time PCR instruments: multi-institutional laboratory trial. *Clin Chem, 50*, 1088–1092.

43. Jennings, L. J., Smith, F. A., Halling, K. C., et al. (2012). Design and analytic validation of *BCR::ABL1* quantitative reverse transcription polymerase chain reaction assay for monitoring minimal residual disease. *Arch Pathol Lab Med, 136*, 33–40.

44. Wittek, M., Stürmer, M., Doerr, H. W., et al. (2007). Molecular assays for monitoring HIV infection and antiretroviral therapy. *Expert Rev Mol Diagn, 7*, 237–746.

45. Gabert, J., Beillard, E., van der Velden, V. H., et al. (2003). Standardization and quality control of "real-time" quantitative reverse transcriptase polymerase chain reaction of fusion transcripts for residual disease detection in leukemia: a Europe Against Cancer program. *Leukemia, 17*, 2318–2357.

46. Press, R. D., Kamel-Reid, S., & Ang, D. (2013). *BCR::ABL1* RT-qPCR for monitoring the molecular response to tyrosine kinase inhibitors in chronic myeloid leukemia. *J Mol Diagn, 15*, 565–576.

47. Kantarjian, H., Schiffer, C., Jones, D., et al. (2008). Monitoring the response and course of chronic myeloid leukemia in the modern era of BCR-ABL tyrosine kinase inhibitors: practical advice on the use and interpretation of monitoring methods. *Blood, 111*, 1774–1780.

48. Parker, W. T., Lawrence, R. M., Ho, M., et al. (2011). Sensitive detection of *BCR::ABL1* mutations with chronic myeloid leukemia after imatinib resistance is predictive of outcome during subsequent therapy. *J Clin Oncol, 29*, 4250–4259.

49. Lobetti-Bodoni, C., Mantoan, B., Monitillo, L., et al. (2013). Clinical implications and prognostic role of minimal residual disease detection in follicular lymphoma. *Ther Adv Hematol, 4*, 189–198.

50. White, H. E., Matejtschuk, P., Rigsby, P., et al. (2010). Establishment of the first World Health Organization International Genetic Reference Panel for quantitation of BCR-ABL mRNA. *Blood, 116*, e111–e117

51. Jennings, L. J., George, D., Czech, J., et al. (2014). Detection and quantification of *BCR::ABL1* fusion transcripts by droplet digital PCR. *J Mol Diagn, 16*, 174–179.

52. Wood-Bouwens, C., Lau, B. T., Hande, C. M., et al. (2017). Single-color digital PCR provides high-performance detection of cancer mutations from circulating DNA. *J Mol Diagn, 19*(5), 697–710.

53. Huggett, J. F., Cowen, S., & Foy, C. A. (2015). Considerations for digital PCR as an accurate molecular diagnostic tool. *Clin Chem, 61*(1), 79–88.

54. Galimberti, S., & Baldacci, S. (2022). Digital droplet PCR in hematologic malignancies: a new useful molecular tool. *Diagnostics, 12*, 1305.

55. Stuppia, L., Antonucci, I., Palka, G., et al. (2012). Use of the MLPA assay in the molecular diagnosis of gene copy number alterations in human genetic diseases. *Int J Mol Sci, 13*, 3245–3276.

56. Konialis, C., Savola, S., Karapanou, S., et al. (2014) Routine application of a novel MLPA-based first-line screening test uncovers clinically relevant copy number aberrations in haematological malignancies undetectable by conventional cytogenetics. *Hematology, 19*, 217–224.

57. Porcheddu, A., & Giacomelli, G. (2005). Peptide nucleic acids (PNAs), a chemical overview. *Curr Med Chem, 12*, 2561–2599.

58. Oh, J. E., Lim, H. S., An, C. H., et al. (2010). Detection of low-level KRAS mutations using PNA-mediated asymmetric PCR clamping and melting curve analysis with unlabeled probes. *J Mol Diagn, 12*, 418–424.

59. Buckingham, L. (2019). DNA sequencing. In Buckingham, L. (Ed.), *Molecular Diagnostics: Fundamentals, Methods, and Clinical Applications.* (3rd ed., pp. 223–257). Philadelphia: FA Davis.

60. Behdad, A., Weigelin, H. C., Elenitoba-Johnson, K. S., et al. (2015). A clinical grade sequencing-based assay for CEBPA mutation testing: report of a large series of myeloid neoplasms. *J Mol Diagn, 17*, 76–84.

61. Alghasham, N., Alnouri, Y., Abalkhail, H., et al. (2016). Detection of mutations in *JAK2* exons 12-15 by Sanger sequencing. *Int J Lab Hematol, 38*, 34–41.

62. Sanger, F., Nicklen, S., & Coulson, A. R. (1977). DNA sequencing with chain-terminating inhibitors. *Proc Natl Acad Sci U S A, 74*, 5463–5467.

63. Fakhrai-Rad, H., Pourmand, N., & Ronaghi, M. (2002). Pyrosequencing: an accurate detection platform for single nucleotide polymorphisms. *Hum Mutat, 19*, 479–485.

64. Goodwin, S., McPherson, J. D., & McCombie, W. R. (2016). Coming of age: ten years of next-generation sequencing technologies. *Nat Rev Genet, 17*, 333–351.

65. Levy, S. E., & Myers, R. M. (2016). Advancements in next-generation sequencing. *Annu Rev Genomics Hum Genet, 17*, 95–115.

66. Ramkissoon, L. A., & Montgomery, N. D. (2021). Application of next-generation sequencing in hematologic malignancies. *Hum Immunol, 82*, 859–870.

67. National Cancer Institute, National Human Genome Research Institute. *The Cancer Genome Atlas.* https://cancer.gov/ccg/research/genome-sequencing/TCGA. Accessed March 14, 2023.

68. The 1000 Genomes Consortium. (2015). A global reference for human genetic variation. *Nature, 526,* 68–74.

69. Alaggio, R., Amador, C., Anagnostopoulos, J., et al. (2022). The 5th edition of the World Health Organization classification of haematolymphoid tumours: lymphoid neoplasms. *Leukemia, 36,* 1720–1748.

70. Khoury, J. D., Solary, E., Abla, O., et al. (2022). The 5th edition of the World Health Organization classification of haematolymphoid tumours: myeloid and histiocytic/dendritic neoplasms. *Leukemia, 36,* 1703–1719.

71. He, J., Abdel-Wahab, O., Nahas, M. K., et al. (2016). Integrated genomic DNA/RNA profiling of hematologic malignancies in the clinical setting. *Blood, 127,* 3004–3014.

72. Kluk, M. J., Lindsley, R. C., Aster, J. C., et al. (2016). Validation and implementation of a custom next-generation sequencing clinical assay for hematologic malignancies. *J Mol Diagn, 18,* 507–515.

73. Zhang, B. M., & Keegan, A. (2021). An overview of characteristics of clinical next-generation sequencing-based testing for hematologic malignancies. *Arch Pathol Lab Med, 145,* 1110–1116.

74. COSMIC. https://www.cancer.sanger.ac.uk/cosmic. Accessed March 15, 2023.

75. ClinVar. National Library of Medicine. https://www.ncbi.nlm.nih.gov/clinvar/. Accessed March 15, 2023.

76. Aziz, N., Zhao, Q., Bry, L., et al. (2015). College of American Pathologists' laboratory standards for next-generation sequencing clinical tests. *Arch Pathol Lab Med, 139,* 481–493.

77. Jennings, L. J., Arcila, M. E., Corless, C., et al. (2017). Guidelines for the validation of next-generation sequencing based oncology panels: a joint consensus recommendation of the Association for Molecular Pathology and College of American Pathologists. *J Mol Diagn, 19,* 341–365.

78. Roy, S., Coldren, C., Karunamurthy, A., et al. (2018). Standards and guidelines for validating next-generation sequencing bioinformatics pipelines: a joint recommendation of the Association for Molecular Pathology and the College of American Pathologists. *J Mol Diagn, 20*(1), 4–27.

79. Li, M. M., Datto, M., Duncavage, E. J., et al. (2017). Standards and guidelines for the interpretation and reporting of sequence variants in cancer. A joint consensus recommendation of the Association for Molecular Pathology, American Society of Clinical Oncology, and College of American Pathologists. *J Mol Diagn, 19,* 4–23.

80. Stamatopoulos, B., Timbs, A., & Bruce, D. (2017). Targeted deep sequencing reveals clinically relevant subclonal IGHV rearrangements in chronic lymphocytic leukemia. *Leukemia, 31,* 837–845.

81. Mata, E., Diaz-Lopez, A., Martin-Moreno, A. M., et al. (2017). Analysis of the mutational landscape of classic Hodgkin lymphoma identifies disease heterogeneity and potential therapeutic targets. *Oncotarget, 8,* 111386–111395.

82. Duncavage, E. J., Bagg, A., Hasserjian, R. P., et al. (2022). Genomic profiling for clinical decision making in myeloid neoplasms and acute leukemia. *Blood, 140,* 2228–2247.

83. Ferreira, P. G., Jares, P., Rico, D., et al. (2014). Transcriptome characterization by RNA sequencing identifies a major molecular and clinical subdivision in chronic lymphocytic leukemia. *Genome Res, 24,* 212–226.

84. Migita, N. A., Jotta, P. Y., do Nascimento, N. P., et al. (2023). Classification and genetics of pediatric B-other acute lymphoblastic leukemia by targeted RNA sequencing. *Blood Adv, 7*(13), 2957–2971.

85. Fukuhara, S., Oshikawa-Kumade, Y., Kogure, Y., et al. (2022). Feasibility and clinical utility of comprehensive genomic profiling of hematological malignancies. *Cancer Sci, 113,* 2763–2777.

86. Hiemenz, M. C., Oberley, M. J., Doan, A., et al. (2021). A multimodal genomics approach to diagnostic evaluation of pediatric hematologic malignancies. *Cancer Genet, 254,* 25–33.

87. Shao, L., Kang, S-H., Li, J., et al. (2010). Array comparative genomic hybridization detects chromosomal abnormalities in hematological cancers that are not detected by conventional cytogenetics. *J Mol Diagn, 12,* 670–679.

88. Hagenkord, J., & Chang, C. C. (2009). The reward and challenges of array-based karyotyping for clinical oncology applications. *Leukemia, 23,* 829–833.

89. Kimura, H., & Kwong, Y-L. (2019). EBV viral loads in diagnosis, monitoring and response assessment. *Front Oncol, 9,* 1–6.

90. Yu, J., & Diaz, J. D. (2021). Impact of next-generation sequencing cell-free pathogen DNA test on antimicrobial management in adults with hematological malignancies and transplant recipients with suspected infections. *Transplant Cell Ther, 27,* 500.e1–500.e6.

91. Pratt, V. M., Wang, W. Y., Boone, E. C., et al. (2022). Characterization of reference materials for TPMT and NUDT15: a GeT-RM collaborative project. *J Mol Diagn, 24,* 1079–1088.

92. Rolfo, C., Cardona, A. F., Cristofanilli, M., et al. (2020). Challenges and opportunities of cfDNA analysis implementation in clinical practice: perspective of the International Society of Liquid Biopsy (ISLB). *Crit Rev Oncol Hematol, 151,* 102978.

93. Cheng, A. P., Cheng, M. P., Loy, C. J., et al. (2022). Cell-free DNA profiling informs all major complications of hematopoietic cell transplantation. *PNAS, 119,* e2113476118.

94. Neveling, K., Mantere, T., Vermeulen, S., et al. (2022). Next-generation cytogenetics: comprehensive assessment of 52 hematological malignancy genomes by optical genome mapping. *Am J Hum Genet, 108,* 1423–1435.

95. Rack, K., De Bie, J., Ameye, G., et al. (2021). Optimizing the diagnostic workflow for acute lymphoblastic leukemia by optical genome mapping. *Am J Hematol, 97,* 548–561.

96. Clarke, J., Wu, H-C., Jayasinghe, L., et al. (2009). Continuous base identification for single-molecule nanopore DNA sequencing. *Nat Nanotechnol, 4,* 265–270.

97. Luo, S., Chen, X., Zeng, D., et al. (2022). The value of single-molecule real-time technology in the diagnosis of rare thalassemia variants and analysis of phenotype- genotype correlation. *J Hum Genet, 67,* 183–195.

98. Brierley, C. K., & Mead, A. J. (2020). Single-cell sequencing in hematology. *Curr Opin Oncol 32,* 139-145. https://doi.10.1097/cco.0000000000000613.

99. Han, Z., Rosen, S. T., & Querfeld, C. (2020). Targeting microRNAs in hematologic malignancies. *Curr Opin Oncol, 32*(5), 536–544.

30

Cytogenetics

Gail H. Vance

OBJECTIVES

After completion of this chapter, the reader will be able to:

1. Describe chromosome structure and the methods used in G-banded chromosome identification.
2. Explain the basic laboratory techniques for preparing chromosomes for analysis.
3. Differentiate between numeric and structural chromosome abnormalities.
4. Discuss the importance of karyotype in the diagnosis of hematologic malignancies.
5. Explain the basic technique of fluorescence in situ hybridization (FISH).
6. Discuss the advantage of using FISH analysis in conjunction with G-banded analysis of cells.

7. Describe the types of chromosomal abnormalities that are detectable with cytogenetic methods.
8. Given a diagram of a G-banded chromosome, name the chromosome structures identifiable by light microscopy.
9. Given the designation of a chromosome abnormality, determine whether the abnormality is numeric or structural, which chromosomes are affected, what type of abnormality it is, and what segment of the chromosome is affected.
10. Define chromosomal microarray analysis and describe the genomic nature and advantage of this test.

OUTLINE

Reasons for Chromosome Analysis
Chromosome Structure
    Cell Cycle
    Chromosome Architecture
    Metaphase Chromosomes
Chromosome Identification
    Chromosome Number
    Chromosome Size and Type
Techniques for Chromosome Preparation and Analysis
    Chromosome Preparation

Chromosome Banding
Metaphase Analysis
Fluorescence In Situ Hybridization
Cytogenetic Nomenclature
Chromosome Abnormalities
    Numeric Abnormalities
    Structural Abnormalities
Cancer Cytogenetics
    Leukemia
    Solid Tumors
Chromosomal Microarray Analysis

CASE STUDY

After studying the material in this chapter, the reader should be able to respond to the following case study. Answers can be found in Appendix C.

An 80-year-old male came to his physician with painful right neck swelling in the last 10 days. No fever, history of fatigue, or weight loss was reported. A neck CT scan showed extensive cervical adenopathy, greater on the right side. A lymph node biopsy was performed and a diagnosis of diffuse large B-cell lymphoma was rendered. For additional subclassification and prognostication, a paraffin-embedded tissue section was received in the laboratory for fluorescence in situ hybridization (FISH) testing. FISH studies using a panel of

probes for lymphoma, including the following genes: *BCL6, MYC/IGH, MYC,* and *IGH/BCL2* (Abbott Molecular, Des Plaines, IL), was requested. Results were positive for t(8;14) *(MYC::IGH),* rearrangement of *MYC,* and also positive for t(14;18) *(IGH::BCL2)* (Figures 30.1 and 30.2). The results of FISH testing classified the patient's disease as recently described diffuse large B-cell lymphoma/high-grade B-cell lymphoma with *MYC* and *BCL2* rearrangements. In cases associated with a pathologic diagnosis of diffuse large B-cell lymphoma, "double hit" lymphoma is associated with aggressive disease and a poor response to therapy.

CASE STUDY—cont'd

A bone marrow aspirate was sent for G-band analysis and FISH with the lymphoma panel. The karyotype was 46,XY[20] and FISH results were normal, indicating the tumor had not invaded the bone marrow.

1. What is G-banded chromosome analysis?

2. Are the described FISH results examples of numeric or structural abnormalities? What type? Which chromosomes are involved? Explain.

3. What is FISH and how does it complement standard chromosome analysis?

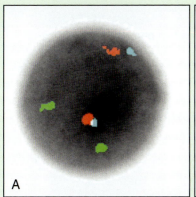
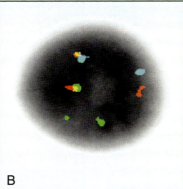
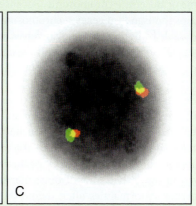
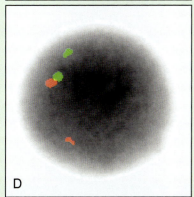

Figure 30.1 Interphase Fluorescence In Situ Hybridization (FISH) Procedure from the Patient in the Case Study using t(8;14) *MYC::IGH* Probes and *MYC* Break Apart Probes. **(A),** A normal interphase pattern, RRGGAA, for the probe set with two copies each of *MYC (red), IGH (green)*, and the chromosome 8 centromere *(aqua).* **(B),** An abnormal dual-color, dual-fusion signal pattern representing a t(8;14) *(two yellow).* **(C),** A normal *MYC* break apart probe pattern, FF *(two yellow).* **(D),** A *MYC* rearrangement pattern, RGF *(red, green, yellow).* Probes from Abbott Molecular, Des Plaines, IL. (Courtesy the Cytogenetics Laboratory, Indiana University School of Medicine, Indianapolis, IN.)

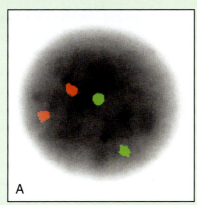
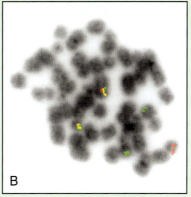

Figure 30.2 Interphase and Metaphase Fluorescence in Situ Hybridization (FISH) Procedure from the Patient in the Case Study using t(14;18) *IGH::BCL2* Probes. **(A),** A normal interphase pattern, RRGG, for the probe set with two copies each of *IGH (green)* and *BCL2 (red).* **(B),** An abnormal dual-color, dual-fusion pattern in metaphase cells. The fusion signals *(yellow)* represent the translocated chromosomes 14 and 18 (der(14) and der(18)). The *red* signal represents the unrearranged *BCL2* locus. There are two *green* signals representing the unrearranged *IGH* locus and an additional chromosome 14 with the *IGH* signal (RGGFF). Probes from Abbott Molecular, Des Plaines, IL. (Courtesy the Cytogenetics Laboratory, Indiana University School of Medicine, Indianapolis, IN.)

Human cytogenetics is the study of chromosomes, their structure, and their inheritance. There are between 20,000 and 25,000 genes in the human genome, most of which reside on the 46 chromosomes normally found in each somatic cell.[1]

Chromosome disorders are classified as structural or numeric and involve the loss, gain, or rearrangement of either a piece of a chromosome or the entire chromosome. Because each chromosome contains thousands of genes, a chromosomal abnormality that is observable by light microscopy involves, on average, 3 to 5 megabases (Mb) of DNA and represents the disruption or loss of hundreds of genes. Such disruptions often have a profound clinical effect.

Chromosomal abnormalities are observed in approximately 0.65% of all live births.[2] The gain or loss of an entire chromosome, other than a sex chromosome, is usually incompatible with life and accounts for approximately 50% of first-trimester spontaneous abortions.[3] In leukemia, cytogenetic abnormalities are observed in more than 50% of bone marrow specimens.[4] These recurring abnormalities often define the leukemia and frequently indicate clinical prognosis.

REASONS FOR CHROMOSOME ANALYSIS

Chromosome analysis is an important diagnostic procedure in clinical medicine. Not only are chromosomal anomalies major causes of reproductive loss and birth defects, but also nonrandom chromosome abnormalities are recognized in many forms of cancer.

Physicians who care for patients of all ages may order chromosome analysis or karyotyping for patients with intellectual disability, infertility, ambiguous genitalia, short stature, fetal loss, risk of genetic or chromosomal disease, and cancer (Table 30.1). In the following discussion, basic cytogenetic concepts are presented. Supplementation of this chapter with the material in Chapter 29 is recommended.

CHROMOSOME STRUCTURE

Cell Cycle

The cell cycle is divided into four stages: G_1, the growth period before synthesis of DNA; S phase, the period during which DNA synthesis (replication) takes place; G_2, the period after DNA synthesis; and M, the period of mitosis, or cell division, the shortest phase of the cell cycle (Figure 4.6). During mitosis, chromosomes are maximally condensed. While in mitosis, cells can be chemically treated to arrest cell progression through the cycle so that the chromosomes may be isolated and analyzed.

Chromosome Architecture

A chromosome is formed from a double-stranded DNA molecule that contains a series of genes. The complementary double-helix structure of DNA was established in 1953 by James Watson and Francis Crick.[5] The backbone is a sugar-phosphate polymer. The sugar is deoxyribose. Attached to the backbone and filling the center of the helix are four nitrogen-containing bases. Two of these, adenine (A) and guanine (G), are purines; the other two, cytosine (C) and thymine (T), are pyrimidines (Figure 29.6).

TABLE 30.1   Common Translocations in Hematopoietic and Lymphoid Neoplasia and Sarcoma*

Tumor Type	Karyotype	Genes
Chronic Myeloid Leukemia		
Chronic myeloid leukemia	t(9;22)(q34.1;q11.2)	BCR::ABL1
B-Cell Leukemias/Lymphomas		
B-lymphoblastic leukemia/lymphoma	t(12;21)(p13.2;q22.1)	ETV6::RUNX1
	t(1;19)(q23.3;p13.3)	PBX1::TCF3
	t(4;11)(q21.3;q23.3)	AFF1::KMT2A
Burkitt lymphoma	t(8;14)(q24.2;q32.3)	MYC::IGH
	t(2;8)(p11.2;q24.2)	IGK::MYC
	t(8;22)(q24.2;q11.2)	MYC::IGL
Mantle cell lymphoma	t(11;14)(q13.3;q32.3)	CCND1::IGH
Follicular lymphoma	t(14;18)(q32.3;q21.3)	IGH::BCL2
Diffuse large B-cell lymphoma	t(3;14)(q27.3;q32.3)	BCL6::IGH
Lymphoplasmacytic lymphoma	t(9;14)(p13.2;q32.3)	PAX5::IGH
MALT lymphoma	t(14;18)(q32.3;q21.3)	IGH::MALT1
	t(11;18)(q22.2;q21.3)	BIRC3::MALT1
	t(1;14)(p22.3;q32.3)	BCL10::IGH
T-Cell Leukemias/Lymphomas		
T-lymphoblastic leukemia	del(1)(p33p33)	STIL::TAL1
	t(7;11)(q34;p13)	TRB::LMO2
Anaplastic large cell leukemia	t(2;5)(p23.2;q35.1)	ALK::NPM1
Sarcomas and Tumors of Bone and Soft Tissue		
Alveolar rhabdomyosarcoma	t(2;13)(q36.1;q14.1)	PAX3::FOXO1A
	t(1;13)(p36.13;q14.1)	PAX7::FOXO1A
Ewing sarcoma/PNET	t(11;22)(q24.3;q12.2)	FLI1::EWSR1
	t(21;22)(q22.2;q12.2)	ERG::EWSR1
	t(7;22)(p21.2;q12.2)	ETV1::EWSR1
Clear cell sarcoma	t(12;22)(q13.1;q12.2)	ATF1::EWSR1
Myxoid liposarcoma	t(12;16)(q13.3;p11.2)	DDIT3::FUS
	t(12;22)(q13.3;q12.2)	DDIT3::EWSR1
Synovial sarcoma	t(X;18)(p11.2;q11.2)	SSX1 or SSX1::SS18
Alveolar soft part sarcoma	t(X;17)(p11.2;q25.3)	TFE3::ASPSCR1

*Modified according to the Hugo Nomenclature Database, November 2022. *MALT,* Mucosa-associated lymphoid tissue; *PNET,* primitive neuroectodermal tumor.

The chromosomal DNA of the cell resides in the cell's nucleus. This DNA and its associated proteins are referred to as *chromatin.* During the cell cycle, at mitosis, the nuclear chromatin condenses approximately 10,000-fold to form chromosomes.[6] Each chromosome results from progressive folding, compression, and compaction of the entire nuclear chromatin. This condensation is achieved through multiple levels of helical coiling and supercoiling (Figure 30.3).

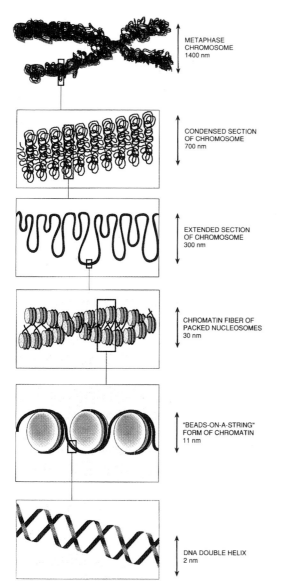

METAPHASE CHROMOSOME 1400 nm

CONDENSED SECTION OF CHROMOSOME 700 nm

EXTENDED SECTION OF CHROMOSOME 300 nm

CHROMATIN FIBER OF PACKED NUCLEOSOMES 30 nm

"BEADS-ON-A-STRING" FORM OF CHROMATIN 11 nm

DNA DOUBLE HELIX 2 nm

Figure 30.3 Chromosome Structure. The folding and twisting of the DNA double helix. (From Gelehrter, T. D., Collins, F. S., Ginsberg, D. [1998]. *Principles of Medical Genetics*. (2nd ed.). Philadelphia: Lippincott Williams & Wilkins.)

Metaphase Chromosomes

Metaphase is the stage of mitosis in which the chromosomes align on the equatorial plate. Electron micrographs of metaphase chromosomes have provided models of chromosome structure. In the "beads-on-a-string" model of chromatin folding, the DNA helix is looped around a core of histone proteins.[7] This packaging unit is known as a *nucleosome* and measures approximately 11 nm in diameter.[8] Nucleosomes are coiled into twisted forms to create an approximately 30-nm chromatin fiber. This fiber, called a *solenoid*, is condensed further and bent into a loop configuration. These loops extend at an angle from the main chromosome axis.[9]

CHROMOSOME IDENTIFICATION

Chromosome Number

In 1956 Tijo and Levan[10] identified the correct number of human chromosomes as 46. This is the *diploid* chromosome

number and is determined by counting the chromosomes in dividing somatic cells. The designation for the diploid number is 2n. Gametes (ova and sperm) have half the diploid number (23). This is called the *haploid* number of chromosomes and is designated as n. Different species have different numbers of chromosomes. The reindeer has a relatively high chromosome number for a mammal (2n = 76), whereas the Indian muntjac, or barking deer, has a very low chromosome number (2n = 7 in the male and 2n = 6 in the female).[11]

Chromosome Size and Type

In the 1960s, before the discovery of banding, chromosomes were categorized by overall size and the location of the centromere (primary constriction) and were assigned to one of seven groups, A through G. Group A includes chromosome pairs 1, 2, and 3. These are the largest chromosomes, and their centromeres are located in the middle of the chromosome; that is, they are metacentric. Group B chromosomes, pairs 4 and 5, are the next largest chromosomes; their centromeres are off center, or submetacentric. Group G consists of the smallest chromosomes, pairs 21 and 22, whose centromeres are located at one end of the chromosomes and are designated as acrocentric (Figure 30.4).

TECHNIQUES FOR CHROMOSOME PREPARATION AND ANALYSIS

Chromosome Preparation

Tissues used for chromosome analysis contain cells with an inherently high mitotic rate (bone marrow cells) or cells that can be stimulated to divide in culture (peripheral blood lymphocytes). Special harvesting procedures are established for each tissue type. Mitogens such as phytohemagglutinin or pokeweed mitogen are added to peripheral blood cultures to induce cell division. Phytohemagglutinin primarily stimulates T lymphocytes to divide,[12] whereas pokeweed preferentially stimulates B lymphocytes.[13]

Chromosomes may be obtained from replicating cells by arresting the cell in metaphase. Cells from the peripheral blood or bone marrow are cultured in media for 24 to 72 hours. In standard peripheral blood cultures, because the cells are terminally differentiated, a mitogen is added to stimulate cellular division. Neoplastic cells are spontaneously dividing and generally do not require stimulation with a mitogen. After the cell cultures have grown for the appropriate period, demecolcine (Colcemid), an analog of colchicine, is added to disrupt the mitotic spindle fiber attachment to the chromosome. Following culture and treatment with demecolcine, cells are transferred to a conical tube and exposed to a hypotonic (potassium chloride) solution that lyses red cells and causes the chromosomes to spread apart from one another. A fixative solution of 3:1 methanol and acetic acid is added to the cell suspension. The fixative serves to "harden" cells and remove proteinaceous material. Cells are dropped onto cold, wet glass slides to achieve optimal dispersal of the chromosomes. The slides are then aged, typically by exposure to heat, before banding.

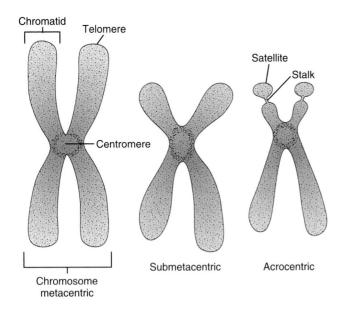

Figure 30.4 Chromosome Morphology. The three shapes of chromosomes are metacentric, submetacentric, and acrocentric. This figure also shows the position of the centromere and telomere, in addition to the two sister chromatids that comprise a metaphase chromosome.

Chromosome Banding

Analysis of each chromosome is made possible by staining with a dye. The name chromosome is derived from the Greek words *chroma,* meaning "color," and *soma,* meaning "body." Hence *chromosome* means "colored body." In 1969 Caspersson and colleagues[14] were the first investigators to stain chromosomes successfully with a fluorochrome dye. Using quinacrine mustard, which binds to adenine-thymine–rich areas of the chromosome, they were able to distinguish a banding pattern unique to each chromosome. This banding pattern, called *Q-banding,* differentiates the chromosome into bands of differing widths and relative brightness (Figure 30.5). The most brightly fluorescent bands of the 46 human chromosomes include the distal end of the Y chromosome, the centromeric regions of chromosomes 3 and 4, and the short arms of the acrocentric chromosomes (13, 14, 15, 21, and 22).

Other stains are used to identify chromosomes, but in contrast to Q-banding, these methods normally necessitate some pretreatment of the slide to be analyzed. Giemsa (G) bands are obtained by pretreating the chromosomes with the proteolytic enzyme trypsin. *GTG-banding* means "G-banding by Giemsa with the use of trypsin." Giemsa, like quinacrine mustard, stains AT-rich areas of the chromosome. The dark bands are called *G-positive*(+) bands. Guanine-cytosine–rich areas of the chromosome have little affinity for the dye and are referred to as *G-negative*(−) bands. G+ bands correspond with the brightly fluorescing bands of Q-banding (Figures 30.6 and 30.7). G-banding is the most common method used for staining chromosomes.

C-banding stains the centromere (primary constriction) of the chromosome and the surrounding condensed heterochromatin. Constitutive heterochromatin is a special type of late-replicating repetitive DNA that is located primarily at the centromere of the chromosome. In C-banding, the chromosomes are treated first with an acid and then with an alkali (barium hydroxide) before Giemsa staining. C-banding is most intense in human chromosomes 1, 9, and 16, and the Y chromosome. Polymorphisms from different individuals are also observed in the C-bands. These polymorphisms have no clinical significance (Figure 30.8).

Specific chromosomal regions that are associated with the nucleoli in interphase cells are called *nucleolar organizer regions* (NORs). NORs contain tandemly repeated RNA genes. NORs can be differentially stained in chromosomes by a silver stain in a method called *AG-NOR–banding.*

Chromosome banding is visible after chromosome condensation, which occurs during mitosis. The banding pattern observed depends on the degree of condensation. By examination of human chromosomes early in mitosis, it has been possible to estimate a total haploid genome (23 chromosomes) with approximately 2000 AT-rich (G+) bands.[15] The later the stage of mitosis, the more condensed is the chromosome and the fewer are the total G+ bands observed.

Metaphase Analysis

After banding, prepared slides with dividing cells are scanned under a light microscope with a low-power objective lens (10×). When a metaphase cell has been selected for analysis, a 63× or 100× oil immersion objective lens is used. Each metaphase cell is analyzed first for the number of chromosomes, then each chromosome pair is analyzed for its banding pattern. A normal somatic cell contains 46 chromosomes, which includes two sex chromosomes and 22 pairs of autosomes (chromosomes 1 through 22). The laboratory scientist records a summary of the analysis using chromosome nomenclature. This summary is called a *karyotype.* Any variation in number and banding pattern is recorded by the laboratory scientist. At least 20 metaphase cells are analyzed from leukocyte cultures. If abnormalities are noted, the laboratory scientist may need to analyze additional cells. Computer imaging is used to confirm and record the microscopic analysis. A picture of all the chromosomes aligned from 1 to 22, including the sex chromosomes, is called a *karyogram.*

Fluorescence In Situ Hybridization

The use of molecular methods coupled with standard karyotype analysis has improved chromosomal abnormality detection beyond that of the light microscope. DNA or RNA probes labeled with either fluorescent or enzymatic detection systems are hybridized directly to metaphase or interphase cells on a glass microscope slide. These probes usually belong to one of three classes: probes for repetitive DNA sequences, primarily generated from centromeric DNA; whole chromosome probes that include segments of an entire chromosome; and specific loci or single-copy probes.

Fluorescence in situ hybridization (FISH) is a molecular technique commonly used in cytogenetic laboratories. FISH studies are a valuable adjunct to the diagnostic workup. In FISH, the DNA or RNA probe is labeled with a fluorophore. Target DNA is treated with heat and formamide to denature the

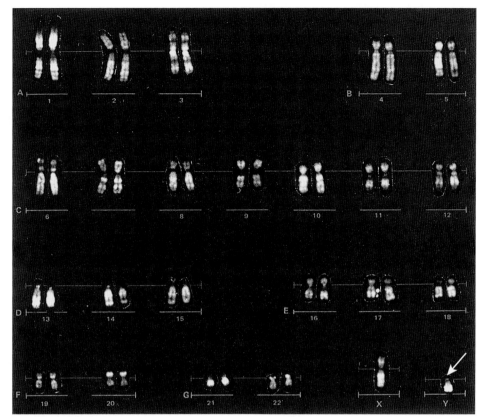

Figure 30.5 Q-Banded Preparation. Note the intense brilliance of Yq *(arrow)*. (Courtesy Cytogenetics Laboratory, Indiana University School of Medicine, Indianapolis, IN.)

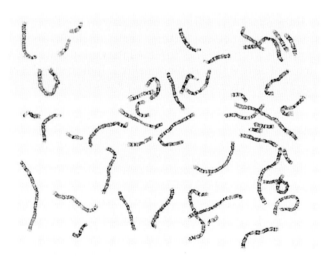

Figure 30.6 Normal Male Metaphase Chromosomes.

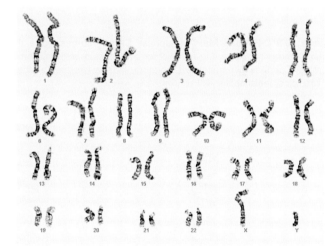

Figure 30.7 Normal Male Karyogram, GTG-Banded Preparations. (Courtesy Cytogenetics Laboratory, Indiana University School of Medicine, Indianapolis, IN.)

double-stranded DNA, which renders it single stranded. The target DNA anneals to a similarly denatured, single-stranded, fluorescently labeled DNA or RNA probe with a complementary sequence. After hybridization, the unbound probe is removed through a series of stringent washes, and the cells are counterstained for visualization (Figure 30.9).

In situ hybridization with centromere or whole chromosome painting probes can be used to identify individual chromosomes (Figure 30.10). Marker chromosomes represent chromatin material that has been structurally altered and cannot be identified by a G-band pattern. FISH using a centromere or paint probe, or both, is often helpful in identifying the chromosome(s) of origin (Figure 30.11).[16] Specific loci probes can be used to detect both structural and numeric abnormalities but are especially helpful in identifying chromosomal translocations or inversions.

The FISH procedure has many advantages and has advanced the detection of chromosomal abnormalities beyond that of

G-banded analysis. Both dividing (metaphase) and nondividing (interphase) cells can be analyzed with FISH. Performance of FISH on uncultured cells, such as bone marrow smears, provides a quick test result that can be reported within 24 hours. Also, in cultured bone marrow specimens submitted for G-band analysis, the number of dividing cells may be insufficient for cytogenetic diagnosis. In such cases, FISH performed on interphase (nondividing) cells with probes for a specific translocation or structural abnormality may provide the diagnosis. A distinct advantage of FISH is the application of fluorescent probes to nondividing cells in both cell suspension and paraffin-embedded tissues. FISH can detect tumor heterogeneity for both major and minor clonal abnormalities. The use of multicolor probes enables the localization and detection of multiple targets simultaneously.

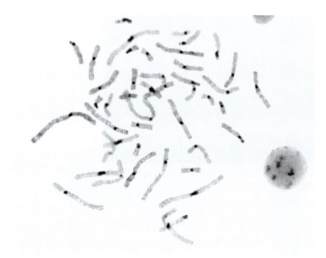

Figure 30.8 C-Banded Male Metaphase Chromosomes. Note the stain at the centromere and heterochromatic regions of the chromosomes. (Courtesy Cytogenetics Laboratory, Indiana University School of Medicine, Indianapolis, IN.)

CYTOGENETIC NOMENCLATURE

Banding techniques enabled scientists to identify each chromosome pair by a characteristic banding pattern. In 1971, a Paris conference for nomenclature of human chromosomes was convened to designate a system to describe the regions and specific bands of the chromosomes. The chromosome arms were designated *p* (petite) for the short arm and *q* for the long arm. The regions in each arm and the bands contained within each region were numbered consecutively, from the centromere outward to the telomere or end of the chromosome. To designate a specific region of the chromosome, the chromosome number is written first, followed by the designation of either the short or long arm, then the region of the arm, and finally the specific band. *Xq21* designates the long arm of the X chromosome, region 2, band 1. To designate a sub band, a decimal point is placed after the band designation, followed by the number assigned to the sub-band, as in Xq21.1 (Figure 30.12).

Cytogenetic/cytogenomic nomenclature represents a uniform code used by cytogeneticists around the world to communicate chromosome abnormalities. The International System for Human Cytogenomic Nomenclature represents current nomenclature guidelines.[17] Each nomenclature string begins with the modal number of chromosomes, followed by the sex chromosome designation. A normal male karyotype is designated 46,XY and a normal female karyotype is designated 46,XX. If abnormalities are observed in the cell, the designation is written to include abnormalities of modal chromosome number, sex chromosomes, and then the autosomes. A cell from a bone marrow specimen with trisomy of chromosome 8 (three copies of chromosome 8) in a male is written as 47,XY,+8 (no intervening spaces). The number of cells with this abnormality is indicated in brackets. If 20 cells were examined, trisomy 8 was found in 10 cells,

General FISH Protocol

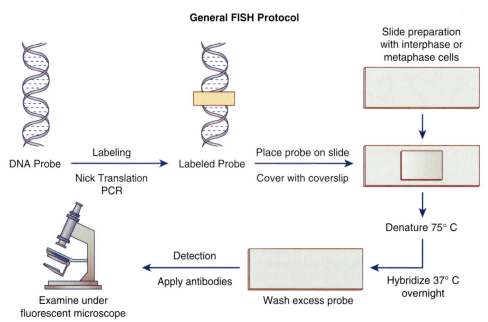

Figure 30.9 General Protocol for Fluorescence In Situ Hybridization (FISH). PCR, Polymerase chain reaction.

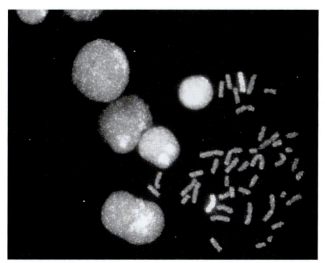

Figure 30.10 Metaphase Preparation is "Painted" with Multiple Probes for Chromosome 7, Producing a Fluorescent Signal. (Courtesy Cytogenetics Laboratory, Indiana University School of Medicine, Indianapolis, IN.)

Locus-specific probes Chromosome paint probes Centromere probes	
Detection of numerical chromosome abnormalities	**Detection of structural chromosome abnormalities**
Trisomy Monosomy Polyploidy	Deletions Duplications Inversions Translocations Ring chromosomes Marker chromosomes Dicentric chromosomes

Figure 30.11 Applications of Fluorescence In Situ Hybridization in the Clinical Laboratory.

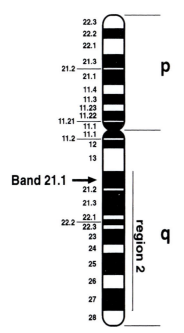

Figure 30.12 Banding Pattern of the Human X Chromosome at the 550 Average Band Level. *Arrow* indicates the location of Xq21.1.

and the remainder were normal, the findings would be written as 47,XY,+8[10]/46,XY[10].

Translocations (exchange of material between two chromosomes) are designated *t,* with the lowest chromosome number listed first. Thus a translocation between the short arm of chromosome 12 at band p13 and the long arm of chromosome 21 at band q22 is written as t(12;21)(p13;q22). A semicolon is used to separate the chromosomes and the band designations. A translocated chromosome is called a *derivative chromosome.* Using the previous example, chromosomes 12 and 21 are referred to as der(12) and der(21). Deletions are written with the abbreviation del preceding the chromosome. A deletion of the long arm of chromosome 5 at band 31 is written as del(5)(q31). No spaces are entered in these designations except between abbreviations.[17]

CHROMOSOME ABNORMALITIES

There are many types of chromosome abnormalities, such as deletions, inversions, ring formations, trisomies, and polyploidy. These defects can be grouped into two major categories: defects involving an abnormality in the *number* of chromosomes and defects involving structural *changes* in one or more chromosomes.

Numeric Abnormalities

Aneuploidy refers to any abnormal number of chromosomes that is not a multiple of the haploid number (23 chromosomes). Numeric abnormalities often are subclassified as aneuploidy or polyploidy. The common forms of aneuploidy in humans are trisomy (the presence of an extra chromosome) and monosomy (the absence of a single chromosome). Aneuploidy is the result of nondisjunction, the failure of chromosomes to separate normally during cell division. Nondisjunction can occur during either of the two types of cell division: mitosis or meiosis. During normal mitosis, a cell divides once to produce two cells that are identical to the parent cell. In mitosis, each daughter cell contains 46 chromosomes. Meiosis is a special type of cell division that generates male and female gametes (sperm and ova). In contrast to mitosis, meiosis entails two cell divisions: meiosis I and meiosis II, resulting in 23 chromosomes, which is the haploid number (n).

In polyploidy, the chromosome number is higher than 46 but is always an exact multiple of the haploid chromosome number of 23. A karyotype with 69 chromosomes is called *triploidy (3n)* (Figure 30.13). A karyotype with 92 chromosomes is called *tetraploidy (4n)*.

In cancer, numeric abnormalities in the karyotype may be classified further, based on the modal number of chromosomes in a neoplastic clone. *Hypodiploid* refers to a cell with fewer than 45 chromosomes; *near-haploid* cells have from 23 up to approximately 34 chromosomes (Figure 30.14); *hyperdiploid* cells have more than 47 chromosomes. *High hyperdiploidy* refers to a chromosome number of more than 50.[18] Finally, the term *pseudodiploid* is used to describe a cell with 46 chromosomes and structural abnormalities.[17]

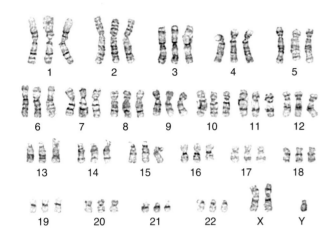

Figure 30.13 Triploid Karyotype, 69,XXY. (Courtesy Cytogenetics Laboratory, Indiana University School of Medicine, Indianapolis, IN.)

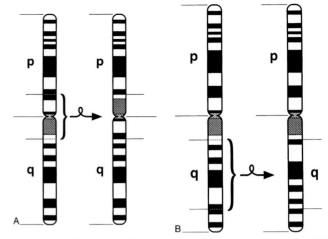

Figure 30.15 Examples of Pericentric and Paracentric Inversion. **(A)**, Pericentric inversion involves the centromere. **(B)**, Paracentric inversion occurs in either the short or long arm of the chromosome.

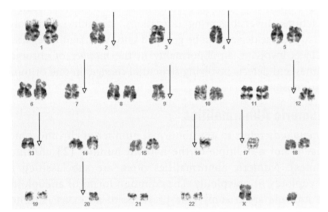

Figure 30.14 Hypodiploid Karyotype with 36 Chromosomes. *Arrows* indicate missing chromosomes. (Courtesy the Cytogenetics Laboratory, Indiana University School of Medicine, Indianapolis, IN.)

Structural Abnormalities

Structural rearrangements result from breakage of a chromosome region, with loss or subsequent rejoining in an abnormal combination. Structural rearrangements are defined as *balanced* (no loss or gain of genetic chromatin) or *unbalanced* (gain or loss of genetic material). Structural rearrangements of single chromosomes include inversions, deletions, isochromosomes, ring formations, insertions, translocations, and duplications. Inversions (inv) involve one or two breaks in a single chromosome, followed by a 180-degree rotation of the segment between the breaks, with no loss or gain of material. If the chromosomal material involves the centromere, the inversion is called *pericentric*. If the material that is inverted does not include the centromere, the inversion is called *paracentric* (Figure 30.15).

Interstitial *deletions* arise after two breaks in the same chromosome arm and loss of the segment between the breaks. Terminal deletions (loss of chromosomal material from the end of a chromosome) and interstitial deletions involve the loss of genetic material. The clinical consequence to the individual with a deletion depends on the extent and location of the deleted chromosomal material (Figure 30.16, A).

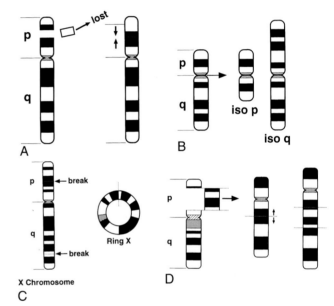

Figure 30.16 Structural Abnormalities of Chromosomes. **(A)**, Interstitial deletion. **(B)**, Isochromosome. **(C)**, Ring chromosome. **(D)**, Insertion.

Isochromosomes arise from either abnormal division of the centromeres, in which division is perpendicular to the long axis of the chromosome rather than parallel to it, or from breakage and reunion in chromatin adjacent to the centromere. Each resulting daughter cell has a chromosome in which the short arm or the long arm is duplicated (Figure 30.16, B).

Ring chromosomes can result from breakage and reunion of a single chromosome, with loss of chromosomal material outside the break points. Alternatively, one or both telomeres (chromosome ends) may join to form a ring chromosome without significant loss of chromosomal material (Figure 30.16, C).

Insertions involve movement of a segment of a chromosome from one location of the chromosome to another location of the same chromosome or to another chromosome. The segment is released as a result of two breaks, and the insertion occurs at the site of another break (Figure 30.16, D).

Duplication means partial trisomy for part of a chromosome. This can result from an unbalanced insertion or unequal crossing over in meiosis or mitosis.

Translocations occur when there is breakage in two chromosomes and each of the broken pieces reunites with another chromosome. If chromatin is neither lost nor gained, the exchange is called a *balanced reciprocal translocation*. A reciprocal translocation is balanced if all chromatin material is present. The loss or gain of chromatin material results in partial monosomy or trisomy for a segment of the chromosome, which is designated an *unbalanced rearrangement*.

Another type of translocation involving breakage and reunion near the centromeric regions of two acrocentric chromosomes is known as a *Robertsonian translocation*. Effectively, this is a fusion between two whole chromosomes, rather than an exchange of material, as in a reciprocal translocation. These translocations are among the most common balanced structural rearrangements seen in the general population, with a frequency of 0.09% to 0.1%.[19] All five human acrocentric autosomes (13, 14, 15, 21, and 22) may form a Robertsonian translocation. In this case, the resulting balanced karyotype has only 45 chromosomes, which includes the translocated chromosome (Figure 30.17).

CANCER CYTOGENETICS

Cancer cytogenetics is a field that has been built on discovery of nonrandom chromosome abnormalities in many types of cancer. In hematologic neoplasia, specific structural rearrangements are associated with distinct subtypes of leukemia that have characteristic morphologic and clinical features. Cytogenetic analysis of malignant cells may determine the diagnosis and often the prognosis of a hematologic malignancy, assist the oncologist in the selection of appropriate therapy, and aid in monitoring the effects of therapy. Bone marrow is the tissue most frequently used to study the cytogenetics of a hematologic malignancy. Unstimulated peripheral blood and bone marrow trephine biopsy specimens also may be analyzed. Cytogenetic analysis of cancers involving other organ systems may be performed using solid tissue obtained during surgery or by needle biopsy. Chromosomal defects in cancer include a wide range of numeric abnormalities and structural rearrangements, as discussed earlier (see Table 30.1).

Cancer results from multiple and sequential genetic mutations occurring in a somatic cell. At some juncture, a critical mutation occurs, and the cell becomes self-perpetuating or clonal. A clone is a cell population derived from a single progenitor.[17] A cytogenetic clone exists if two or more cells contain the same structural abnormality or supernumerary marker chromosome, or if three or more cells are missing the same chromosome. The primary aberration, or stemline, of a clone is a cytogenetic abnormality that is frequently observed as the sole abnormality associated with the cancer. The secondary aberration, or sideline, includes abnormalities additional to the primary aberration.[17] In chronic myeloid leukemia (CML), the primary aberration is the Philadelphia chromosome, resulting from a translocation between the long arms of chromosomes 9 and 22, t(9;22)(q34.1;q11.2). A sideline of this clone would include secondary abnormalities, such as trisomy for chromosome 8, written as +8,t(9;22)(q34.1;q11.2).

Leukemia

Leukemias are clonal proliferations of malignant leukocytes that arise initially in the bone marrow before disseminating to the peripheral blood, lymph nodes, and other organs. They are broadly classified by the type of blood cell giving rise to the clonal proliferation (lymphoid or myeloid) and by the clinical course of the disease (acute or chronic). The four main leukemia categories are acute lymphoblastic leukemia (ALL), acute myeloid leukemia (AML), chronic lymphocytic leukemia (CLL), and CML. The World Health Organization (WHO) Classification of Haematolymphoid Tumours has largely replaced the French-American-British (FAB) classification.[20,21] The WHO category of AML has three categories. One of these, AML with defining genetic abnormalities, further categorizes AML into 13 subtypes with cytogenetic and molecular abnormalities (Box 30.1).[20]

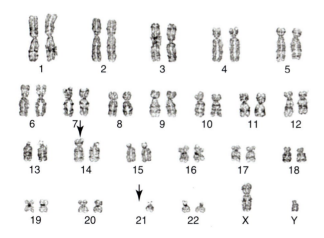

Figure 30.17 Balanced Robertsonian Translocation Between Chromosomes 14 and 21. The nomenclature for this karyogram is written 45,XY,der(14;21)(q10;q10). *Arrows* indicate sites of the translocation on chromosomes 14 and 21. (Courtesy Cytogenetics Laboratory, Indiana University School of Medicine, Indianapolis, IN.)

BOX 30.1	Acute Myeloid Leukemia with Defining Genetic Abnormalities*

Acute promyelocytic leukemia with *PML::RARA* fusion
Acute myeloid leukemia with *RUNX1::RUNX1T1* fusion
Acute myeloid leukemia with *CBFB::MYH11* fusion
Acute myeloid leukemia with *DEK::NUP214* fusion
Acute myeloid leukemia with *RBM15::MRTFA* fusion
Acute myeloid leukemia with *BCR::ABL1* fusion
Acute myeloid leukemia with *KMT2A* rearrangement
Acute myeloid leukemia with *MECOM* rearrangement
Acute myeloid leukemia with *NUP98* rearrangement
Acute myeloid leukemia with *NPM1* mutation
Acute myeloid leukemia with *CEBPA* mutation
Acute myeloid leukemia, myelodysplasia-related
Acute myeloid leukemia with other defined genetic alterations

*Updated according to the Hugo Nomenclature Database, November 2022.
WHO Classification of Tumours Editorial Board. *Haematolymphoid tumours.* Lyon (France) International Agency for Research on Cancer, forthcoming. *WHO Classification of Tumors Series.* (vol. 11; 5th ed.). https://publications.iarc.fr

Chronic Myeloid Leukemia

The first malignancy to be associated with a specific chromosome defect was CML, in which approximately 95% of patients were found to have the Philadelphia chromosome translocation, t(9;22)(q34.1;q11.2) by G-banded analysis.[22,22] The Philadelphia chromosome (derivative chromosome 22) is characterized by a balanced translocation between the long arms of chromosomes 9 and 22 (Figure 30.18). At the molecular level, the gene for *ABL1*, an oncogene on chromosome 9, joins a gene on chromosome 22 named *BCR*. The result of the fusion of these two genes is a new fusion protein of about 210 kD with growth promoting capabilities that override normal cell regulatory mechanisms (Figures 30.19 through 30.21)

(Chapter 32).[24] The fusion protein activates tyrosine kinase signaling to drive proliferation of the cell. This signaling may be blocked by imatinib mesylate or another tyrosine kinase inhibitor.[25] The patient's response to imatinib is monitored by cytogenetic analysis, FISH, and molecular testing.

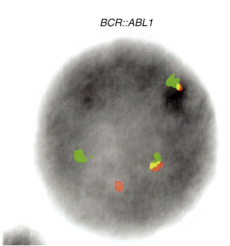

BCR::ABL1

Figure 30.20 Abnormal Bone Marrow Interphase Cell with the *BCR (green)* and *ABL1 (red)* Probes in a Fluorescence In Situ Hybridization Procedure. (Abbott Molecular, Des Plaines, IL.) One *red* signal represents the normal *ABL1* gene on chromosome 9, one *green* signal represents the normal *BCR* gene on chromosome 22, and two fusion signals *(yellow)* are from the derivative chromosomes 9 and 22, indicating a positive result for the translocation. (Courtesy Cytogenetics Laboratory, Indiana University School of Medicine, Indianapolis, IN.)

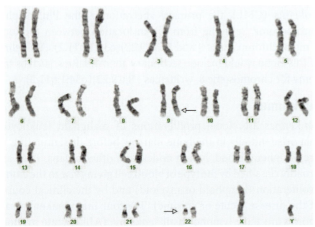

Figure 30.18 Translocation between Chromosomes 9 and 22 in Chronic Myeloid Leukemia. *Arrows* show sites of the translocation on chromosomes 9 and 22. Note the shorter chromosome 22 (Philadelphia chromosome). (Courtesy the Cytogenetics Laboratory, Indiana University School of Medicine, Indianapolis, IN.)

BCR::ABL1

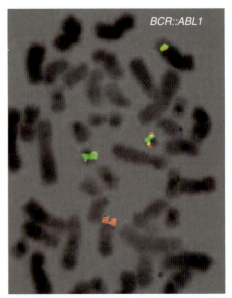

BCR::ABL1

Figure 30.21 Abnormal Bone Marrow Metaphase Cell with the *BCR* (*green*) and *ABL1* (*red*) Probes in a Fluorescence In Situ Hybridization Procedure (Abbott Molecular, Des Plains, IL). One *red* signal represents the normal *ABL1* gene on chromosomes 9 and one *green* signal represents the normal *BCR* gene on chromosome 22. The fusion signals *(yellow)* represent the translocated chromosomes 9 and 22 (der(9) and der(22)). (Courtesy the Cytogenetics Laboratory, Indiana School of Medicine, Indianapolis, IN.)

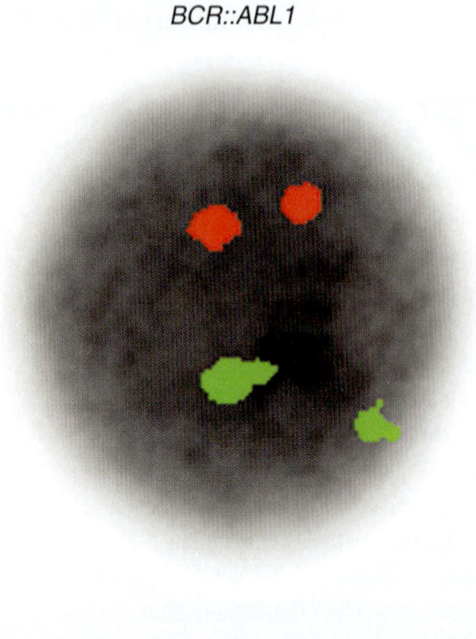

Figure 30.19 Normal Bone Marrow Interphase Cell Hybridized with the *BCR (green)* and *ABL1 (red)* Probes in a Fluorescence In Situ Hybridization Procedure. (Abbott Molecular, Des Plaines, IL.) The two *red* and two *green* signals represent the genes on the normal chromosomes 9 and 22. (Courtesy Cytogenetics Laboratory, Indiana University School of Medicine, Indianapolis, IN.)

At diagnosis, the characteristic karyotype is the presence of the Philadelphia chromosome in all cells analyzed. After treatment with imatinib for several months, the karyotype typically has a mixture of abnormal and normal cells, indicating the patient's response to therapy. A complete cytogenetic response is defined as a bone marrow karyotype with only normal cells. The therapeutic response is often monitored using peripheral blood instead of a bone marrow aspirate. In contrast to the bone marrow, the peripheral blood often does not contain spontaneously dividing cells. As a result, chromosomal analysis of a specimen of unstimulated peripheral blood may be unsuccessful because of the absence of dividing cells. In these cases, FISH with probes for the specific abnormality is performed on 200 or more interphase (nondividing) cells of the peripheral blood specimen to search for chromosomally abnormal cells. The detection of cytogenetic abnormalities in interphase (nondividing) cells is an important advantage of FISH technology.

Acute Leukemia

The Philadelphia chromosome is also observed in acute leukemia. It is seen in about 25% of adults with ALL, 2% to 5% of children with ALL, and 1% of patients with AML.[26–28] In childhood ALL, the chromosome number is critical for predicting the severity of the leukemia. Children whose leukemic cells contain more than 50 chromosomes (high hyperdiploid karyotype) have the best prognosis for complete recovery with therapy. Recurring translocations observed in ALL include t(4;11)(q21.3;q23.3), t(12;21)(p13.2;q22.1), and t(1;19)(q23.3;p13.3). Each translocation is associated with a prognostic outcome, which assists oncologists in determining the patient's therapy. The t(4;11) translocation is the one most commonly found in infants with acute lymphoblastic leukemia. Rearrangements of the *AFF1* gene on chromosome 4 and the *KMT2A* (formerly *MLL*) gene on chromosome 11 occur in this translocation.[29,30] Disruption of the *KMT2A* gene is seen in both ALL and AML (Figures 30.22 and 30.23).

AMLs were historically subdivided into several morphologic classifications, ranging from M0 to M7 according to the FAB classification (Chapter 31).[31,32] Characteristic chromosome translocations are associated with some subgroups and were incorporated into the WHO classification. Among them is a translocation between the long arms of chromosomes 8 and 21, t(8;21)(q22.3;q22.1), which is representative of AML with maturation. Acute promyelocytic leukemia is associated with a translocation between the long arms of chromosomes 15 and 17, t(15;17)(q24.1;q21.1) (Figure 30.24). A pericentric inversion of chromosome 16, inv(16)(p13.1q22.1), is seen in AML with increased eosinophils. The inversion juxtaposes the core the binding factor beta *(CBFB)* gene on 16q with the myosin heavy chain gene *(MYH11)* on 16p to form a new fusion gene and protein (Figure 30.25).[33] These recurring rearrangements have enabled researchers to localize genes important for cell growth and regulation. As with acute lymphoblastic leukemia, the specific translocation in AML often predicts the patient's prognosis and response to

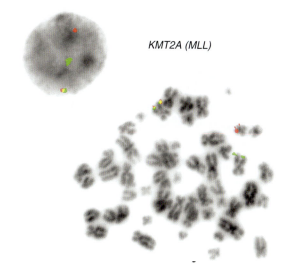

Figure 30.22 Bone Marrow Metaphase Cell Showing a Disruption of the *KMT2A* (*MLL*) Gene in a Fluorescence In Situ Hybridization Procedure with Break-Apart Probes. *Green* and *red* probes hybridize to different regions of the *KMT2A* gene. A *yellow* fusion signal represents an intact *KMT2A* gene on the normal chromosome 11. Split *red* and *green* signals indicate a disruption of the *KMT2A* gene because of a rearrangement. (Courtesy Cytogenetics Laboratory, Indiana University School of Medicine, Indianapolis, IN.)

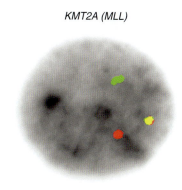

Figure 30.23 Bone Marrow Interphase Cell Showing a Disruption of the *KMT2A* (*MLL*) Gene in a Fluorescence in Situ Hybridization Procedure with Break-Apart Probes. Green and red probes hybridize to different regions of the *KMT2A* gene. A *yellow* fusion signal represents an intact *KMT2A* gene on the normal chromosome 11. Split *red* and *green* signals indicate a disruption of the *KMT2A* (*MLL*) gene because of a rearrangement. (Courtesy Cytogenetics Laboratory, Indiana University School of Medicine, Indianapolis, IN.)

therapy. Understanding the molecular consequences of the cytogenetic abnormalities, such as the *BCR::ABL1* translocation, provides the fundamental information for the development of targeted therapies.

Solid Tumors

Just as recurring structural and numeric chromosome defects have been observed in the hematologic malignancies, a wide range of nonrandom abnormalities also have been found in

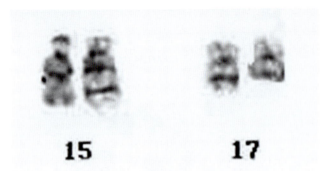

Figure 30.24 Bone Marrow Metaphase Chromosomes 15 and 17 Homologues Showing a Translocation Between the Long Arms of Chromosomes 15 and 17, t(15;17)(q24.1;q21.1). This translocation is diagnostic of acute promyelocytic leukemia. The abnormal chromosomes are on the right. (Courtesy Cytogenetics Laboratory, Indiana University School of Medicine, Indianapolis, IN.)

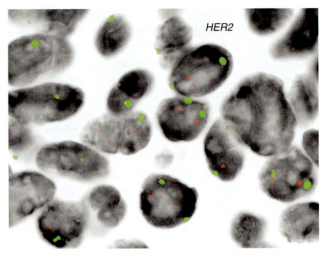

Figure 30.26 Normal Interphase Nuclei from a Paraffin-Embedded Tissue Section Hybridized with Probes for *HER2 (red)* and the Chromosome 17 Centromere *(green)* in a Fluorescence In Situ Hybridization Procedure (Abbott Molecular, Des Plaines, IL). Two *green* and two *red* signals are seen per cell.

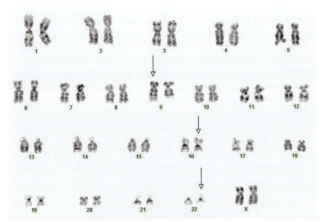

Figure 30.25 Bone Marrow Karyogram for a Patient with Acute Myeloid Leukemia (AML) Showing a Translocation, t(9;22)(q34.1;q11.2), and an Inverted Chromosome 16, inv(16)(p13.1q22.1). *Arrows* show the abnormal chromosomes. (Courtesy Cytogenetics Laboratory, Indiana University School of Medicine, Indianapolis, IN.)

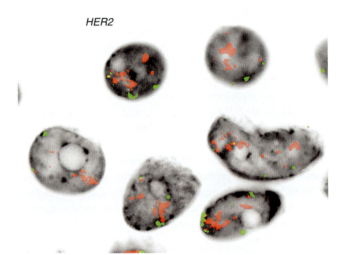

Figure 30.27 Tissue Section from a Breast Cancer Patient Demonstrating Amplification of *HER2*. The tissue was hybridized with fluorescence in situ hybridization probes for *HER2 (red)* and the chromosome 17 centromere probe *(green)* (Abbott Molecular, Des Plaines, IL). The number of *HER2* signals exceeds the number of centromere signals, which indicates selective amplification of *HER2*.

solid tumors. Most of these abnormalities confer a proliferative advantage on the malignant cell and serve as useful prognostic indicators. Amplification (increased copy number) of the gene *HER2* (also called *ERBB2*) on chromosome 17, a transmembrane growth factor receptor, is associated with an aggressive form of invasive breast cancer.[34,35] FISH with probes for the *HER2* gene and an internal control (17 centromere) can determine if there is gene amplification in the tumor (Figure 30.26).[36] If FISH testing shows amplification to be present, the patient is eligible for targeted therapy with a monoclonal antibody, trastuzumab (Figure 30.27).[37] FISH for *HER2* typically is performed on tissue sections from the paraffin-embedded tumor block.

CHROMOSOMAL MICROARRAY ANALYSIS

Chromosomal microarray (CMA) is a fluorescence-based molecular technique for submicroscopic analysis of genomic DNA. CMA testing increases the detection of clinically significant imbalances over a karyotype.[38] CMA is performed using a glass slide or chip platform. CMAs, like standard cytogenetic analysis, look at the entire genome but with higher levels of resolution (base pair or kilobase level) determined by the number and composition of targets on the array. Using a single nucleotide polymorphism (SNP)-based array, the patient's DNA is hybridized to a chip composed of more than 2 million markers that detect copy number variation (gains and losses) and SNPs. SNP probes detect position-specific markers that have different forms (polymorphic). Analysis of the SNP data from a specimen allows for detection of copy neutral loss of heterozygosity or uniparental disomy, in addition to copy

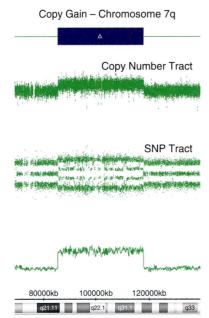

Figure 30.28 Chromosomal Microarray Diagram Demonstrating Approximately a 32.4 Mb Gain of Genetic Material Between Bands 7q21 and 7q31. (Courtesy Cytogenetics Laboratory, Indiana University School of Medicine, Indianapolis, IN.)

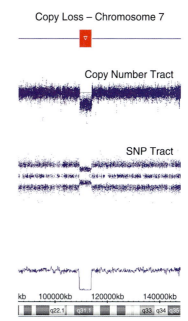

Figure 30.29 Chromosomal Microarray Diagram Demonstrating Approximately a 4.6 Mb Loss at Band 7q31.1. (Courtesy Cytogenetics Laboratory, Indiana University School of Medicine, Indianapolis, IN.)

number variants (gains and losses of genomic DNA). Copy number variants (CNV) in the patient's specimen are assessed relative to a reference control. In the constitutional setting, chromosomal microarray (CMA) analysis has achieved great success in delineating new genomic disorders and identifying genes with importance in dosage sensitivity. The yield of detection of abnormalities is increased because of the high resolution of the array (Figures 30.28 and 30.29).[38–40] This technique is used for diagnosis of constitutional (inherited) and neoplastic disease.[40]

SUMMARY

- Cytogenetics is the study of chromosome structure and inheritance.
- Chromosome disorders are secondary to structural or numeric chromosomal abnormalities involving the rearrangement or the loss or gain of either a piece of a chromosome or the entire chromosome.
- Nonrandom chromosome abnormalities are observed in constitutional (germline) genetic syndromes as well as cancer.
- A chromosome is composed of a double-helix strand of DNA. Attached to the backbone of deoxyribose are adenine (A), guanine (G), cytosine (C), and thymine (T).
- During mitosis, cells can be chemically treated to arrest cell progression in metaphase so that chromosomes can be analyzed.
- Q-banding differentiates chromosomes into bands of different widths and relative brightness, revealing a banding pattern unique to each individual chromosome.
- Other stains used to identify chromosomes may require pretreatment of the slide for analysis. These include G-banding, C-banding, and AG-NOR-banding.
- Fluorescence in situ hybridization (FISH), a molecular cytogenetic technique, uses DNA or RNA probes and fluorescence microscopy to identify individual chromosomes and targeted chromosomal loci. Metaphase and interphase cells may be analyzed by FISH.

- Tissues used for chromosome analysis typically include bone marrow cells and peripheral blood lymphocytes, amniotic fluid, nonneoplastic tissue, and tumors.
- A normal cell contains 46 chromosomes, which include 2 sex chromosomes (XX or XY).
- Defects in chromosomes can be categorized as numeric or structural. Numeric abnormalities may be subclassified as aneuploidy and polyploidy.
- Structural rearrangements include inversions, deletions, isochromosomes, ring formations, insertions, translocations, and duplications.
- Specific structural rearrangements are associated with distinct subtypes of leukemias and may assist in diagnosis, prognosis, and monitoring of therapy. Solid tumors also may be analyzed using cytogenetic analysis.
- Chromosomal microarray testing uses an array platform to detect abnormalities at a submicroscopic level of resolution. The higher resolution increases the detection of chromosomal abnormalities, typically gains and losses.

Now that you have completed this chapter, go back and read again the case study at the beginning and respond to the questions presented. Answers can be found in Appendix C.

REVIEW QUESTIONS

Answers can be found in Appendix C.

1. G-banding refers to the technique of staining chromosomes:
   a. To isolate those in the G group (i.e., chromosomes 21 and 22)
   b. In the G_0 or resting stage
   c. Using Giemsa stain
   d. To emphasize areas high in guanine residues

2. Which of the following compounds is used to halt mitosis in metaphase for chromosome analyses?
   a. Imatinib
   b. Fluorescein
   c. Trypsin
   d. Demecolcine

3. One arm of a chromosome has 30 bands. Which band would be nearest the centromere?
   a. Band 1
   b. Band 15
   c. Band 30

4. Which of the following is NOT an advantage of the use of FISH?
   a. It can be used on nondividing cells.
   b. It can be used on paraffin-embedded tissue.
   c. It can detect mutations that do not result in abnormal banding patterns.
   d. It must be performed on dividing cells.

5. Which of the following types of mutations would likely NOT be detectable with cytogenetic banding techniques?
   a. Point mutation resulting in a single amino acid substitution
   b. Transfer of genetic material from one chromosome to another
   c. Loss of genetic material from a chromosome that does not appear on any other chromosome
   d. Duplication of a chromosome resulting in 3n of that genetic material

6. Which of the following describes a chromosomal deletion?
   a. Point mutation resulting in a single amino acid substitution
   b. Transfer of genetic material from one chromosome to another
   c. Loss of genetic material from a chromosome that does not appear on any other chromosome
   d. Duplication of a chromosome resulting in 3n of that genetic material

   For questions 7 to 9: The chromosome analysis performed on a patient's leukemic cells is reported as 47,XY,+4,del(5)(q31)[20].

7. This patient's cells have which of the following abnormalities?
   a. Loss of the entire number 31 chromosome
   b. Loss of the entire number 5 chromosome
   c. Loss of a portion of the short arm of chromosome 4
   d. Loss of a portion of the long arm of chromosome 5

8. What other mutation is present in this patient's cells?
   a. Polyploidy
   b. Tetraploidy
   c. An extra chromosome 4
   d. Four copies of chromosome 5

9. This patient's leukemic cells demonstrate:
   a. Structural chromosomal defects only
   b. Numeric chromosomal defects only
   c. Both structural and numeric chromosomal defects

10. Aneuploidy describes the total chromosome number:
    a. That is a multiple of the haploid number
    b. That reflects a loss or gain of a single chromosome
    c. That is diploid but has a balanced deletion and duplication of whole chromosomes
    d. In gametes; diploid is the number in somatic cells

REFERENCES

1. International Human Genome Sequencing Consortium. (2004). Finishing the euchromatic sequence of the human genome. *Nature, 431*, 931–945.
2. Benn, P. (2010). Prenatal diagnosis of chromosomal abnormalities through amniocentesis. In Milunsky, A., & Milunsky, J. M. (Eds.), *Genetic Disorders and the Fetus.* (6th ed., pp. 194–195). Baltimore: Wiley-Blackwell.
3. Boué, J., Boué, A., & Lazar, P. (1975). Retrospective and prospective epidemiological studies of 1500 karyotyped spontaneous human abortions. *Teratology, 12*, 11–26.
4. Rowley, J. D. (2008). Chromosomal translocations: revisited yet again. *Blood, 112*, 2183–2189.
5. Watson, J. D., & Crick, F. H. C. (1983). Molecular structure of nucleic acids: a structure for deoxyribose nucleic acid. *Nature, 171*, 737–738.
6. Earnshaw, W. C. (1988). Mitotic chromosome structure. *Bioessays, 9*, 147–150.
7. Olins, A. L., & Olins, D. E. (1974). Spheroid chromatin units. *Science, 183*, 330–332.
8. Oudet, P., Gross-Bellard, M., & Chambon, P. (1975). Electron microscopic and biochemical evidence that chromatin structure is a repeating unit. *Cell, 4*, 281–300.
9. Rattner, J. B. (1988). Chromatin hierarchies and metaphase chromatin structure. In Adolph, K. W., (Ed.), *Chromosomes and Chromatin,* (vol. 3, p. 30). Boca Raton, FL: CRC Press.
10. Tijo, J. H., & Levan, A. (1956). The chromosome number of man. *Hereditas, 42*, 1–6.
11. Hsu, T. C. (1979). *Human and Mammalian Cytogenetics.* (pp. 6–7). New York, NY: Springer-Verlag.
12. Nowell, P. C. (1960). Phytohemagglutinin: an initiator of mitosis in culture of normal human leukocytes. *Cancer Res, 20*, 462–466.

13. Farnes, P., Barker, B. E., Brownhill, L. E., et al. (1964). Mitogenic activity of *Phytolacca americana* (pokeweed). *Lancet, 2,* 1100–1101.

14. Caspersson, T., Zech, L., Modest, E. J., et al. (1969). Chemical differentiation with fluorescent alkylating agents in *Vicia faba* metaphase chromosomes. *Exp Cell Res, 58,* 128–140.

15. Stein, C. K. (2017). Applications of cytogenetics in modern pathology. In McPherson, R. A., Pincus, M. R. (Eds.), *Henry's Clinical Diagnosis and Management by Laboratory Methods.* (23rd ed., p. 1337). Philadelphia, PA: Saunders.

16. Plattner, R., Heerema, N. A., Yurov, Y. B., et al. (1993). Efficient identification of marker chromosomes in 27 patients by stepwise hybridization with alpha satellite DNA probes. *Hum Genet, 91,* 131–140.

17. McGowan-Jordan, J., Hastings, R. J., & Moore S. (Eds.). (2020). *ISCN 2020: An International System for Human Cytogenomic Nomenclature.* Basel, Switzerland: S. Karger.

18. Moorman, A. V., Richards, S. M., Martineau, M., et al. (2003). Outcome heterogeneity in childhood high-hyperdiploid acute lymphoblastic leukemia. *Blood, 102,* 2756–2762.

19. Turleau, C., Chavin-Colin, F., & de Grouchy, J. (1979). Cytogenetic investigation in 413 couples with spontaneous abortions. *Eur J Obstet Gynecol Reprod Biol, 9,* 65–74.

20. World Health Organization Classification of Tumours Editorial Board. *Haematolymphoid Tumors.* Lyon (France) International Agency for Research on Cancer, forthcoming. *WHO Classification of Tumors Series.* (5th ed.; Vol. 11). https://publications.iarc.fr.

21. Bennett, J. M., Catovsky, D., Daniel, M. T., et al. (1976). Proposals for classification of the acute leukaemias. French-American-British (FAB) Co-operative Group. *Br J Haematol, 33,* 451–458.

22. Nowell, P. C., & Hungerford, D. A. (1960). A minute chromosome in human chronic granulocytic leukemia. *Science, 132,* 1497 (abstract).

23. Rowley, J. D. (1973). A new consistent chromosomal abnormality in chronic myelogenous leukemia identified by quinacrine fluorescence and Giemsa staining. *Nature, 243,* 290–293.

24. Ben-Neriah, Y., Daley, G. Q., Mes-Masson, A., et al. (1986). The chronic myelogenous leukemia-specific P210 protein is the product of the *BCR/ABL* hybrid gene. *Science, 233,* 212–214.

25. Druker, B. J., Tamura, S., Buchdunger, E., et al. (1996). Effects of a selective inhibitor of the Abl tyrosine kinase on the growth of *BCR-ABL* positive cells. *Nat Med, 2,* 561–566.

26. Moorman, A. V., Harrison, C. J., Buck, G. A. N., et al. (2007). Karyotype is an independent prognostic factor in adult acute lymphoblastic leukemia (ALL): analysis of cytogenetic data from patients treated on the Medical Research Council (MRC) UKALLXII/Eastern Cooperative Oncology Group (ECOG) 2993 trial. *Blood, 109,* 3189–3197.

27. Hunger, S. P., & Mullighan, C. G. (2015). Acute lymphoblastic leukemia in children. *N Engl J Med, 373,* 1541–1552.

28. Crist, W., Carroll, A., Shuster, J., et al. (1990). Philadelphia chromosome positive acute lymphoblastic leukemia: clinical and cytogenetic characteristics and treatment outcome. A Pediatric Oncology Group study. *Blood, 76,* 489–494.

29. Morrissey, J., Tkachuk, D. C., Milatovich, A., et al. (1993). A serine/proline-rich protein is fused to HRX in t(4;11) acute leukemias. *Blood, 81,* 1124–1131.

30. Hayne, C. C., Winer, E., Williams, T., et al. (2006). Acute lymphoblastic leukemia with a 4;11 translocation analyzed by multi-modal strategy of conventional cytogenetics, FISH, morphology, flow cytometry, molecular genetics and review of the literature. *Exp Mol Pathol, 81,* 62–71.

31. Bennett, J. M., Catovsky, D., Daniel, M. T., et al. (1985). Proposed revised criteria for the classification of acute myeloid leukemia: a report of the French-American-British Cooperative Group. *Ann Intern Med, 103,* 620–625.

32. Bennett, J. M., Catovsky, D., Daniel, M. T., et al. (1985). Criteria for the diagnosis of acute leukemia of megakaryocytic lineage (M7): a report of the French-American-British Cooperative Group. *Ann Intern Med, 103,* 460–462.

33. Claxton, D. F., Liu, P., Hsu, H. B., et al. (1994). Detection of fusion transcripts generated by the inversion 16 chromosome in acute myelogenous leukemia. *Blood, 83,* 1750–1756.

34. Slamon, D. J., Godolphin, W., Jones, L. A., et al. (1989). Studies of the *HER-2* proto-oncogene in human breast and ovarian cancer. *Science, 244,* 707–712.

35. Perez, E. A., Roche, P. C., Jenkins, R. B., et al. (2002). *HER2* testing in patients with breast cancer: poor correlation between weak positivity by immunohistochemistry and gene amplification by fluorescence in situ hybridization. *Mayo Clin Proc, 77,* 148–154.

36. Wolff, A. C., Hammond, M. E. H., Allison, K. H., et al. (2018). Human epidermal growth factor receptor 2 testing in breast cancer: American Society of Clinical Oncology/College of American Pathologists clinical practice guideline focused update. *J Clin Oncol, 36*(20), 2105–2122.

37. Slamon, D. J., Leyland-Jones, B., Shak, S., et al. (2001). Use of chemotherapy plus a monoclonal antibody against *HER2* for metastatic breast cancer that overexpresses *HER2. N Engl J Med, 344,* 783–792.

38. Miller, D. T., Adam, M. P., Aradhya, S., et al. (2010). Consensus statement: chromosomal microarray is the first-tier clinical diagnostic test for individuals with developmental disabilities or congenital anomalies. *Am J Hum Genet, 86,* 749–764.

39. South, S. T., Lee, C., Lamb, A. N., et al. (2013). ACMG standards and guidelines for constitutional cytogenomic microarray analysis, including postnatal and prenatal applications: revision 2013. *Genet Med, 15*(11), 901–909.

40. Shao, L., Akkari, Y., Cooley, L. D., et al. (2021). Chromosomal microarray analysis, including constitutional and neoplastic disease applications, 2021 revision: a technical standard of the American College of Medical Genetics and Genomics (ACMG). *Genet Med, 23,* 1818–1829.

31

Acute Leukemias

Mark A. Russell and Ameet R. Kini*

OBJECTIVES

After completion of this chapter, the reader will be able to:

1. Discuss the causes and development of acute leukemia.
2. List the laboratory tests performed and their diagnostic contribution in the investigation of a suspected acute leukemia.
3. Characterize the diagnostic criteria used for acute myeloid and acute lymphoblastic leukemias.
4. Compare and contrast acute lymphoblastic and myeloid leukemias by morphology, presenting signs and symptoms, laboratory findings, and prognosis.
5. Given the patient history, clinical and laboratory findings, including representative cells on the peripheral blood film or bone marrow smear, interpret results of diagnostic tests to determine the type of leukemia and recommend additional tests to confirm a diagnosis.
6. Discuss tumor lysis syndrome, including risk, cause, and laboratory findings.
7. Discuss the cell staining patterns for the myeloperoxidase, Sudan black B, and esterase stains.

OUTLINE

Classification Schemes for Acute Leukemias
Acute Lymphoblastic Leukemia
    Clinical Presentation and Diagnosis
    World Health Organization Classification
    Morphology
    Prognosis
    Immunophenotyping
    Genetic and Molecular Findings
Acute Myeloid Leukemia
    Clinical Presentation and Diagnosis
    World Health Organization Classification

Risk Categories of Acute Myeloid Leukemia
Acute Myeloid Leukemia with Defining Genetic
    Abnormalities
Acute Myeloid Leukemia, Defined by Differentiation
Myeloid Sarcoma
Myeloid Neoplasms, Secondary
Acute Leukemias of Ambiguous Lineage
Cytochemical Stains and Interpretations
    Myeloperoxidase
    Sudan Black B
    Esterases

CASE STUDY

After studying the material in this chapter, the reader should be able to respond to the following case study. Answers can be found in Appendix C.

A 5-year-old child was seen by her family physician because of weakness and headaches. She had been in good health except for the usual communicable diseases of childhood. Physical examination revealed a pale, listless child with multiple bruises. The WBC count was 15×10^9/L, the HGB was 8 g/dL, and the PLT was 90×10^9/L. Reference intervals can be found after the Index at the end of the book. She had "abnormal cells" in her peripheral blood (Figure 31.1). Cytogenetic studies revealed hyperdiploidy.

1. What is the most likely diagnosis?
2. What characteristics of this disease indicate a positive prognosis?
3. What prognosis is associated with the hyperdiploidy?

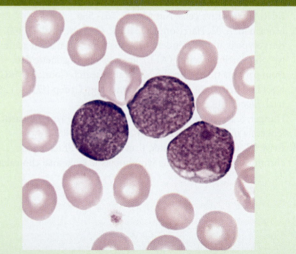

Figure 31.1 Peripheral Blood Film for the Patient in the Case Study. (Wright-Giemsa stain, ×1000.) (From Carr, J. H. [2022]. *Clinical Hematology Atlas.* [6th ed.]. St. Louis: Elsevier.)

*The authors extend appreciation to Reeba A. Omman, Bernadette F. Rodak, Woodlyne Roquiz, and Pranav Gandhi, whose work in prior editions provided the foundation for this chapter.

The broad term leukemia is derived from the ancient Greek words *leukos* (λενκός), meaning "white," and *haima* (αἷμα), meaning "blood."[1] As defined today, acute leukemia refers to the rapid clonal proliferation in the bone marrow of lymphoid or myeloid progenitor cells known as *lymphoblasts* and *myeloblasts*, respectively. When proliferation of blasts overwhelms the bone marrow, blasts are seen in the peripheral blood, and the patient's symptoms reflect suppression of normal hematopoiesis.

For most cases of acute leukemia, the causes directly related to the development of malignancy are unknown. The exceptions that exist are certain toxins that can induce genetic changes, leading to a malignant phenotype. Environmental exposures known to lead to hematopoietic malignancies include radiation and exposure to organic solvents, such as benzene. Rarely, leukemias can be seen in patients with known familial cancer predisposition syndromes. Alkylating agents and other forms of chemotherapy used to treat various forms of cancer can induce deoxyribonucleic acid (DNA) damage in hematopoietic cells, leading to therapy-related leukemias.

Regardless of the mechanism of initial genetic damage, the development of leukemia is currently thought to be a stepwise progression of mutations or "multiple hits" involving mutations in genes that give cells a proliferative advantage, in addition to mutations that hinder differentiation.[2,3] These mutations result in transformation of normal hematopoietic stem cells or precursors into leukemic stem cells (LSCs). The LSCs then initiate, proliferate, and sustain the leukemia.[4]

CLASSIFICATION SCHEMES FOR ACUTE LEUKEMIAS

The French-American-British (FAB) classification of the acute leukemias was devised in the 1970s and was based on morphologic examination along with cytochemical stains to distinguish lymphoblasts from myeloblasts (Figure 31.2). The use of cytochemical stains continues to be a useful but infrequent adjunct for differentiation of hematopoietic diseases, especially acute

leukemias. The details of the cytochemical stains are addressed at the end of this chapter.

Laboratory diagnosis of acute leukemias begins with the complete blood count, peripheral blood film examination, and bone marrow aspirate and biopsy examination, followed by immunophenotyping by flow cytometry, molecular diagnostic studies, cytogenetic analysis, and occasionally, cytochemical staining (Table 31.1). Findings of these techniques are discussed throughout the chapter in relation to specific leukemias.

Hematologists and pathologists are now moving toward more precise classification of many of the leukocyte neoplasms based on recurring chromosomal and genetic lesions found in many patients. These lesions are related to disruptions of oncogenes, tumor suppressor genes, and other regulatory elements that control proliferation, maturation, apoptosis, and other vital cell functions. In 2001 the World Health Organization (WHO) published classification schemes for nearly all the tumors of hematopoietic and lymphoid tissues,[5] and in some cases WHO blended the older morphologic schemes with the newer schemes. For instance, in the WHO classification scheme for acute myeloid leukemias (AMLs), there are some remnants of the old FAB classification, but new classifications were introduced for leukemias associated with consistently recurring chromosomal translocations. According to the WHO classification, a finding of at least 20% blasts in the bone marrow is required for diagnosis of the majority of AMLs, and testing must be performed to detect the presence or absence of genetic anomalies. Although there is no specific blast percentage required for acute lymphoblastic leukemias (ALLs), a diagnosis of ALL is usually not made if blasts are less than 20%. The most recent (2022) WHO classification was released because of further insights into the molecular biology of the entities, with updates reflected in some of the classifications.[6] In-depth discussion of each of the subclassifications is beyond the scope of this book; only the most common subtypes of ALL and AML are described.

Additionally, in 2022, the International Consensus Classification of Myeloid Neoplasms and Acute Leukemias was

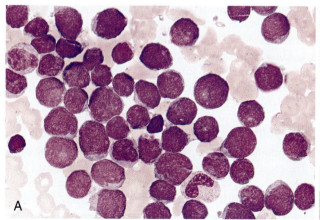
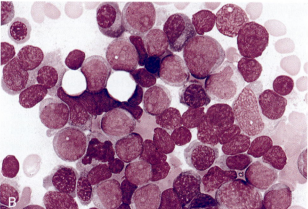

Figure 31.2 Lymphoblasts and Myeloblasts. (A), Lymphoblasts have a diameter two to three times the normal lymphocyte diameter, scant blue cytoplasm, open to moderately coarse chromatin, deeper staining than myeloblasts, and inconspicuous nucleoli. **(B),** Myeloblasts have a diameter three to five times the lymphocyte diameter, moderate gray cytoplasm, uniform fine chromatin, two or more prominent nucleoli, and possibly Auer rods. (A and B, Bone marrow, Wright-Giemsa stain, ×500.)

TABLE 31.1 Laboratory Tests for Diagnosis of Acute Leukemias

Laboratory Test	Contribution	Chapters
Complete blood count	Provides quantitative assessment of WBCs, RBCs, and PLTs in peripheral blood; screens for immature and abnormal cells	12,13
Peripheral blood film examination	Provides relative % of WBC types (differential); assesses WBC, RBC, PLT morphology; identifies abnormal and immature cells	14
Bone marrow examination	Provides relative % of WBC and RBC types, including % blasts (differential); assesses morphology/degree of maturation, cellularity, megakaryocyte number, M:E ratio, other bone marrow cells and architecture; identifies abnormal cells and abnormal distribution of cells	15
Immunophenotyping by flow cytometry	Assesses the pattern of expression of surface and cytoplasmic antigens on immature blood cell populations to quantify and determine their lineage and clonality; identifies patterns of expression associated with particular leukemias; assesses minimal residual disease after treatment	28
Molecular diagnostics	Identifies genetic abnormalities associated with particular leukemias and their prognosis; assesses clonality; assesses minimal residual disease after treatment	29
Cytogenetics	Provides an assessment of chromosome number and structure; identifies chromosome abnormalities associated with particular leukemias and their prognosis	30
Cytochemical stains	Used infrequently to assist in identifying the lineage of immature blood cell populations	End of this chapter

M:E, Myeloid to erythroid; *PLT,* platelet; *RBC,* red blood cell; *WBC,* white blood cell.

published, which built upon the prior WHO 4th edition classification released in 2017. This second classification system has some key differences from the most recent WHO classification; however, there are many similarities. The entities addressed in this chapter will be based on the WHO Classification of Haematolymphoid Tumours (5th edition).

ACUTE LYMPHOBLASTIC LEUKEMIA

ALL is primarily a disease of childhood and adolescence, accounting for 25% of childhood cancers and up to 75% of childhood leukemia.[7] The peak incidence of ALL in children is between 2 and 5 years.[8] Although ALL is rare in adults, risk increases with age; most adult patients are older than 50 years. The subtype of ALL is an important prognostic indicator for survival.[6,9] Adults have a poorer outlook: 80% to 90% experience complete remission, but the cure rate is less than 40%.[10,11]

Clinical Presentation and Diagnosis

Patients with B cell ALL (B-ALL) typically present with fatigue (caused by anemia), fever (caused by neutropenia and infection), and mucocutaneous bleeding (caused by thrombocytopenia). Lymphadenopathy, including enlargement, is often a symptom.[12] Enlargement of the spleen (splenomegaly) and of the liver (hepatomegaly) may be seen. Bone pain often results from intramedullary growth of leukemic cells.[12] Eventual infiltration of malignant cells into the meninges, testes, or ovaries occurs frequently, and lymphoblasts can be found in the cerebrospinal fluid.[13] Patients with ALL often have decreased neutrophil counts, regardless of whether their total white blood cell (WBC) count is low, normal, or elevated. The prevalence and severity of infections are inversely correlated with the absolute neutrophil count (ANC). Infections are common when the ANC is less than 500/μL, and they are especially severe when it is less than 100/μL.

In T cell ALL (T-ALL), there may be a large mass in the mediastinum, leading to compromise of regional anatomic structures. Similar to B-ALL, T-ALL may manifest with anemia, thrombocytopenia, organomegaly, and bone pain, although the degree of leukopenia is often less severe.[14]

World Health Organization Classification

B-lymphoblastic leukemia/lymphoma (B-ALL/B-LBL) is subdivided into 11 defined subtypes that are associated with recurrent cytogenetic abnormalities and an additional subsection including provisional subtypes.[6] These entities are linked with unique clinical, phenotypic, or prognostic features (Table 31.2). Cases of B-ALL that do not exhibit the specific genetic abnormalities are classified as B-lymphoblastic leukemia/lymphoma, not otherwise specified (NOS). When testing is pending, a diagnosis of B-lymphoblastic leukemia/lymphoma, not further classified, can be rendered. Approximately 50% to 70% of patients with T-lymphoblastic leukemia/lymphoma have abnormal gene rearrangements, and proposals have been made to subclassify T-ALL.[15] However, the 2022 WHO classification continues to subcategorize T-ALL into early T-precursor lymphoblastic leukemia/lymphoma, which has limited early T cell differentiation, and T-ALL, NOS.[6]

Morphology

Lymphoblasts vary in size but fall into two morphologic types. The most common type seen is a small lymphoblast (1.0 to 2.5 times the size of a normal lymphocyte) with scant blue cytoplasm and indistinct nucleoli (see Figure 31.2, A); the second type of lymphoblast is larger (two to three times the size of a lymphocyte) with prominent nucleoli and nuclear membrane irregularities (Figure 31.3).[14] These cells may be confused with the blasts of AML.

TABLE 31.2 2022 WHO Classification and Prognosis of B-Lymphoblastic Leukemias/Lymphomas

Classification	Prognosis
B-lymphoblastic leukemia/lymphoma with high hyperdiploidy	Very favorable prognosis
B-lymphoblastic leukemia/lymphoma with hypodiploidy	Poor prognosis
B-lymphoblastic leukemia/lymphoma with iAMP21	High relapse risk on standard therapy
B-lymphoblastic leukemia/lymphoma with *BCR::ABL1* fusion	Relatively poor prognosis
B-lymphoblastic leukemia/lymphoma with *BCR::ABL1*-like features	Inferior overall 5-year survival
B-lymphoblastic leukemia/lymphoma with *KMT2A* rearrangement	Poor prognosis
B-lymphoblastic leukemia/lymphoma with *ETV6::RUNX1* fusion	Very favorable prognosis
B-lymphoblastic leukemia/lymphoma with *ETV6::RUNX1*-like features	Currently undefined (too few cases)
B-lymphoblastic leukemia/lymphoma with *TCF3::PBX1* fusion	Intermediate/relatively favorable
B-lymphoblastic leukemia/lymphoma with *IGH::IL3* fusion	Currently undefined (too few cases)
B-lymphoblastic leukemia/lymphoma with *TCF3::HLF* fusion	Dismal prognosis
B-lymphoblastic leukemia/lymphoma with other defined genetic alterations	Variable prognosis based on genetic alteration
B-lymphoblastic leukemia/lymphoma, NOS	Intermediate prognosis

NOS, Not otherwise specified; *WHO,* World Health Organization.
WHO Classification of Tumours Editorial Board (Eds). (2022). *Haematolymphoid Tumours* [Internet; beta version ahead of print] 5th ed. (International Agency for Research on Cancer).

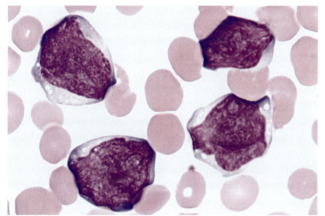

Figure 31.3 Acute Lymphoblastic Leukemia. Note large lymphoblasts with prominent nucleoli and membrane irregularities. (Peripheral blood, Wright-Giemsa stain, ×1000.) (From Carr, J. H. [2022]. *Clinical Hematology Atlas.* [6th ed.]. St. Louis: Elsevier.)

Prognosis

Prognosis in ALL has improved dramatically over the past decades as a result of improvement in algorithms for treatment.[16] The prognosis for ALL depends on age at the time of diagnosis, lymphoblast load (tumor burden), immunophenotype, and genetic abnormalities (see Table 31.2). Children, rather than infants or teens, have the best survival. Chromosomal translocations are the strongest predictor of adverse treatment outcomes for children and adults. Peripheral blood lymphoblast counts greater than 20 to 30×10^9/L, hepatosplenomegaly, and lymphadenopathy all are associated with a worse outcome. The effects of other variables previously associated with a poorer prognosis, such as sex and ethnic group, have been eliminated when patients have been given equal access to treatment in trials carried out at a single institution.[17] The more frequent use of minimal residual

TABLE 31.3 Immunophenotypic Characteristics of Acute Lymphoblastic Leukemia

ALL Subtype	Immunophenotype
Early (pro/pre-pre) B-ALL	CD34, CD19, cytoplasmic CD22, TdT
Intermediate (common) B-ALL	CD34, CD19, CD10, cytoplasmic CD22, TdT
Pre-B-ALL	CD34 +/−, CD19, cytoplasmic CD22, cytoplasmic μ, TdT (variable)
T-ALL	CD2, CD3, CD4, CD5, CD7, CD8, TdT

ALL, Acute lymphoblastic leukemia; *TdT,* terminal deoxynucleotidyl transferase.

disease testing in ALL has allowed for the reduction or intensification of chemotherapy with better patient outcomes.[16]

Immunophenotyping

Although morphology is the first tool used to distinguish ALL from AML, immunophenotyping and genetic analysis are the most reliable indicators of a cell's origin. Because both B and T cells are derived from lymphoid progenitors, both usually express CD34, terminal deoxynucleotidyl transferase (TdT), and human leukocyte antigen, DR subregion (HLA-DR). Historically, four types of ALL have been identified by immunologic methods: early B-ALL (pro-B, or pre-pre-B), intermediate (common) B-ALL, pre-B-ALL, and T-ALL (Table 31.3). B-ALL is characterized by specific B cell antigens that are expressed at different stages of B cell development. In general, B cells express CD19, CD20, CD22, CD24, C79a, CD10, cytoplasmic μ, and PAX-5 (B cell-specific activator protein). While blast phenotype alone was historically used to guide treatment decision making, using a combined phenotype and genetic-based classification is the current recommendation.[6] In the earliest stage of differentiation (pre-pre-B or pro-B), blasts express CD34, CD19, cytoplasmic CD22, and TdT. The incidence of pro-B-ALL is about 5% in children and 11% in adults. In intermediate, or common, B-ALL, CD10 is expressed. The most mature B-ALL is called pre-B-ALL, in which CD34 is typically negative, but there is characteristic expression of cytoplasmic μ heavy chain. Pre-B-ALL accounts for 15% of childhood cases and 10% of adult B-ALL.[18]

T-ALL is seen most often in teenaged males with a mediastinal mass, elevated peripheral blast counts, meningeal involvement, and infiltration of extramedullary sites.[19,20] The common T cell markers CD2, CD3, CD4, CD5, CD7, and CD8 are usually present. Most cases express TdT. A distinct subtype of T-ALL, early T-precursor ALL (ETP-ALL) often shows expression of myeloid makers and is thought to be derived from T cell precursor cells that have the capacity for myeloid differentiation.[9] Early studies showed poor response to therapy in ETP-ALL; however, more recent studies have suggested that the prognosis is the same as with other T-ALL with optimal therapy, although this may be a consequence of more aggressive treatment in ETP-ALL.[6,9]

Genetic and Molecular Findings

Cytogenetic abnormalities are seen in the majority of B-ALL and T-ALL, which produce changes that affect normal B and T cell development and underlie the pathogenesis of these neoplasms. A majority of T-ALL have been shown to have gain-of-function mutations involving the *NOTCH1* gene, which alters the Notch receptor signaling pathway responsible for normal T cell development.[21] These NOTCH1 alterations, when combined with inactivation of the *INK4/ARF* locus, are characteristically seen in T-ALL. A molecular-based classification for T-ALL has been proposed in a study of 264 T-ALL cases from pediatric and young adult patients, with 8 subgroupings based on alterations of the following genes: *TAL1, TAL2, TLX1, TLX3, HOXA, LMO1/2, LMO2-LYL1,* and *NKX2-1.*[15] In T-ALL, however, the cytogenetic alterations show less specificity and less correlation with the prognosis and treatment outcome than in B-ALL. The 2022 WHO classification of B-ALL/LBL is now largely defined by cytogenetic and/or molecular abnormalities, as listed in Table 31.2. "B-ALL/LBL, NOS" should be used only when an underlying defining genetic abnormality is not discovered after comprehensive testing.

B-lymphoblastic leukemia/lymphoma with the t(9;22)(q34;q11.2), *BCR::ABL1* fusion (Philadelphia chromosome-positive ALL) has the worst prognosis among ALLs. It is more common in adults than in children. Tyrosine kinase inhibitors, such as imatinib, have shown success in treating chronic myeloid leukemia, improving survival (Chapter 32). B-lymphoblastic leukemia/lymphoma with *KMT2A* rearrangement is more common in very young infants, and the translocation may even occur in utero.[22] This leukemia has a very poor prognosis. About 25% of childhood ALL cases show a t(12;21)(p13.2;q22.1), *ETV6::RUNX1* translocation and appear to derive from a B cell progenitor rather than the hematopoietic stem cell.[23] This translocation is rare in adults. In children, it carries an excellent prognosis, with a cure rate of over 90%. High

hyperdiploidy in B-lymphoblastic leukemia/lymphoma is common in childhood B-ALL, accounting for 25% of cases, but it is much less common in adults. This genotype is associated with a very favorable prognosis in children. Conversely, hypodiploidy (fewer than 46 chromosomes) conveys a poor prognosis in both children and adults.[6]

ACUTE MYELOID LEUKEMIA

AML is the most common type of leukemia in adults, and the incidence increases with age. AML is less common in children. The FAB classification of AML was based on morphology and cytochemistry; the WHO classification relies heavily on molecular characterization and cytogenetics (Chapters 29 and 30).[6]

Clinical Presentation and Diagnosis

The clinical presentation of AML is nonspecific but reflects decreased production of normal bone marrow elements. Most patients with AML have a total WBC count between 5 and 30 × 10⁹/L, although the WBC count may range from 1 to 200 × 10⁹/L. Myeloblasts are present in the peripheral blood in 90% of patients. Anemia, thrombocytopenia, and neutropenia give rise to the clinical findings of pallor, fatigue, fever, bruising, and bleeding. In addition, disseminated intravascular coagulation and other bleeding abnormalities can be significant.[24] Infiltration of malignant cells into the gums and other mucosal sites and skin also can be seen.

Splenomegaly is seen in half of AML patients, but lymph node enlargement is rare. Cerebrospinal fluid involvement in AML is rare and does not seem to be as ominous a sign as in ALL. Patients with AML tend to have few symptoms related to the central nervous system, even when it is infiltrated by blasts.

Common abnormalities in laboratory test results include hyperuricemia (caused by increased cellular turnover), hyperphosphatemia (due to cell lysis), and hypocalcemia (the latter two are also involved in progressive bone destruction). Hypokalemia is also common at presentation. During induction chemotherapy, especially when the WBC count is quite elevated, tumor lysis syndrome may occur. Tumor lysis syndrome is a group of metabolic complications that can occur in patients with malignancy, most notably lymphomas and leukemias, with and without treatment of the malignancy. These complications are caused by the breakdown products of dying cancer cells, which in turn cause acute uric acid nephropathy and renal failure. Tumor lysis syndrome is characterized by hyperkalemia, hyperphosphatemia, hyperuricemia and hyperuricosuria, and hypocalcemia.[25] The hyperkalemia alone can be life-threatening. Aggressive prophylactic measures to prevent or reduce the clinical manifestations of tumor lysis syndrome are critical.[26]

World Health Organization Classification

Laboratory diagnosis of AML begins with a complete blood count, peripheral blood film examination, and bone marrow aspirate and biopsy specimen examination. The total WBC count may be normal, increased, or decreased; anemia is usually present, along with significant thrombocytopenia. The bone marrow is usually hypercellular, and greater than

20% of cells typically are blasts, although if certain genetic abnormalities are present, the 20% blast threshold is not necessary for the diagnosis of AML.[6] The 2022 WHO classification for myeloid malignancies has categorized AMLs into two broad categories, those defined by genetic abnormalities and those defined by differentiation, in addition to a section for myeloid sarcoma, as shown in Box 31.1. The subtypes under the category defined by genetic abnormalities are listed in Table 31.4.[6] The subtypes defined by genetic abnormalities no longer require 20% blasts for diagnosis, except for AML with BCR::ABL1 and AML with CEBPA mutation. Fluorescence in situ hybridization, next-generation sequencing (NGS), polymerase chain reaction-based mutational analysis, and chromosomal analysis by karyotyping are commonly employed modalities to assess underlying genetic abnormalities (Chapters 28 to 30).

BOX 31.1 2022 WHO Classification of Acute Myeloid Leukemia

Acute myeloid leukemia with defining genetic abnormalities
Acute myeloid leukemia, defined by differentiation
Myeloid sarcoma

Data from WHO Classification of Tumours Editorial Board (Eds). (2022). *Haematolymphoid Tumours* [Internet; beta version ahead of print] 5th ed. (International Agency for Research on Cancer). WHO, World Health Organization.

TABLE 31.4 2022 WHO Classification and Prognosis of Acute Myeloid Leukemia with Defining Genetic Abnormalities

Classification	Prognosis
APL with PML::RARA fusion	Long-term cure rates >90%
AML with RUNX1::RUNX1T1 fusion	High rates of complete remission and disease-free survival
AML with CBFB::MYH11 fusion	Favorable prognosis
AML with DEK::NUP214 fusion	Poor prognosis
AML with RBM15::MRTFA fusion	No uniform prognosis
AML with BCR::ABL1 fusion	Poor response to standard induction chemotherapy
AML with KMT2A rearrangement	Prognosis depends on fusion partner
AML with MECOM rearrangement	Aggressive disease with short survival
AML with NUP98 rearrangement	Poor prognosis
AML with NPM1 mutation	Typically shows good response to standard chemotherapy
AML with CEBPA mutation	Variable prognosis depending on CEBPA mutation type
AML, myelodysplasia-related	Poor prognosis
AML with other defined genetic alterations	Prognosis based on specific alteration

AML, Acute myeloid leukemia; *APL*, acute promyelocytic leukemia; *WHO*, World Health Organization.
Data from WHO Classification of Tumours Editorial Board (Eds). (2022). *Haematolymphoid Tumours* [Internet; beta version ahead of print] 5th ed. (International Agency for Research on Cancer).

Risk Categories of Acute Myeloid Leukemia

The European Leukemia Network regularly publishes updates on AML in relation to diagnosis, risk stratification, and management decision making. The most recent update was released in 2023. In the context of common intensive therapy for AML patients, the majority of the stratification is based on underlying genetic aberrations, similar to the WHO 5th edition Classification (Table 31.4). Favorable risk includes AML with RUNX1::RUNX1T1 fusion, AML with CBFB::MYH11 fusion, AML with NPM1 mutation, and AML with CEBPA mutation. Intermediate risk includes AML with a specific KMT2A rearrangement, MLLT3::KMT2A, in addition to AML with FLT3-ITD mutations. Several AML subtypes are labeled as adverse risk, including but not limited to those with BCR::ABL1 fusion, DEK::NUP214 fusion, MECOM rearrangements, or mutations in myelodysplasia-related genes and/or TP53.[27]

Acute Myeloid Leukemia with Defining Genetic Abnormalities

Acute Myeloid Leukemia with RUNX1::RUNX1T1

The t(8;21)(q22;q22.1), RUNX1::RUNX1T1 translocation is found in 1% to 5% of AML cases. It is the most common core binding factor (CBF) rearrangement in patients with AML (55% to 70% of CBF AML). CBF is a heterodimeric protein complex involved in the transcriptional regulation of normal hematopoiesis. AML with this CBF translocation has large myeloblasts with basophilic and granular cytoplasm and perinuclear hofs, and single Auer rods are commonly seen. Chédiak-Higashi-like granules also may be seen. About 90% of cases show increased blasts and myeloid precursors with some maturation (Figure 31.4); however, approximately 10% of cases show AML without maturation. In the neutrophil lineage, morphologic dysplasia, such as pseudo-Pelger-Huët cells and hypogranulation, can be seen. Dysplasia is uncommon in other cell lines. Marrow eosinophilia is frequent. Immunophenotypically, the blasts may show aberrant expression of B cell antigens (CD19, CD79a, PAX-5).[6] At least one additional mutation is seen in most cases, with some having higher mutation burden (≥2). Prognosis is generally favorable but may be negatively affected if unfavorable additional abnormalities, such as KIT mutations, CD56 expression, and/or monosomy 7 occur.[6,28] A predictive scoring system, I-CBFit, has been proposed to guide therapy decision making.[29] The diagnosis of this subtype is based on the genetic abnormality in the context of increased peripheral blood and/or bone marrow blasts, which may be less than 20%.[6]

Acute Myeloid Leukemia with CBFB::MYH11

This AML subgroup accounts for approximately 5% to 8% of AML cases in younger adults and decreases in incidence with age.[6] The chromosomal aberration inv(16) is sufficient for diagnosis in the context of increase blasts that may be less than 20%.[6,30] The blasts usually show myelomonocytic differentiation. Marrow eosinophilia with morphologically abnormal eosinophils with large dark-purple granules on Romanowsky type stains is a unique feature and is frequently seen (Figure 31.5). Additional chromosomal aberrations are somewhat common (~ 45% of cases) and most cases (>90% of cases) have

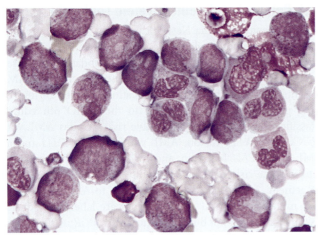

Figure 31.4 Acute Myeloid Leukemia with t(8;21). Note myeloblasts with granular cytoplasm and some maturation. (Bone marrow aspirate, Wright-Giemsa stain, ×500.)

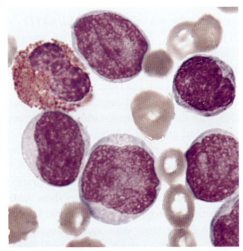

Figure 31.5 Acute Myeloid Leukemia with *CBFB::MYH11,* inv(16). There is an increase in myeloid and monocytic lineages. Eosinophilia may also be present. (Peripheral blood, Wright-Giemsa stain, ×1000.) (From Carr, J. H. [2022]. *Clinical Hematology Atlas.* [6th ed.]. St. Louis: Elsevier.)

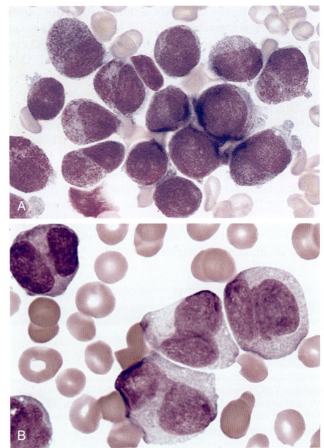

Figure 31.6 Acute Myeloid Leukemia with t(15;17) or Promyelocytic Leukemia. **(A),** Hypergranular variant (more common). **(B),** Microgranular variant showing bilobed nuclear features. (A, B, Peripheral blood, Wright-Giemsa stain, A, ×500, B, ×1000.)

somatic mutations (commonly involving *NRAS* or *KRAS* followed by *KIT*).[6,31] The incidence of extramedullary disease is higher than in most types of AML, and the central nervous system is a common site for relapse.[6,30] The remission rate is good, but only half of patients are cured.[30]

Acute Promyelocytic Leukemia with *PML::RARA*

Acute promyelocytic leukemia comprises 5% to 8% of AML cases. It occurs in all age groups but is seen most commonly in young adults. This disorder is characterized by a differentiation block at the promyelocytic stage. The abnormal promyelocytes are considered to be comparable to blasts for the purpose of diagnosis. Detection of the t(15;17) translocation is sufficient for diagnosis in the presence of the characteristic atypical promyelocytes or microgranular blasts. A blast percentage of 20% is not required.[6,28] Characteristic of the more common hypergranular APL are the abnormal hypergranular promyelocytes, some with Auer rods (Figure 31.6, A). By flow

cytometry, hypergranular promyelocytes show high side scatter and forward scatter and are typically CD34 and HLA-DR negative, although positive for CD117. When promyelocytes release primary granule contents, their procoagulant activity initiates disseminated intravascular coagulation; however, thromboembolic events may occur at presentation and during treatment.[32] In one variant of APL, the granules are so small that because of the limits of light microscopy, the cells give the appearance of having no granules (Figure 31.6, B). This microgranular variant, accounting for 30% to 40% of APL cases, may be confused with other presentations of AML, but the presence of occasional Auer rods, the "butterfly" or "coin-on-coin" nucleus, and the clinical presentation are clues. Microgranular blasts are frequently located in the traditional blast gate by flow cytometry side scatter versus CD45 plots and are more likely to express CD34 than the hypergranular promyelocytes. Microgranular APL presents with very high WBC counts with short doubling time.

The treatment of APL is significantly different from all other types of AML, and it is therefore important to arrive at an accurate diagnosis. Treatment includes all-trans-retinoic acid (ATRA) and arsenic trioxide.[33] ATRA is a vitamin A analog and induces differentiation of the malignant promyelocytes. In adults who achieve a complete remission, the prognosis is better than for any other type of AML.[28] At the time of diagnosis, the

WBC count may be used to stratify patients into low, intermediate, and high risk subsets. Treatment with ATRA and arsenic trioxide is largely curative in low-/intermediate-risk APL. There are a few variant RARA translocations that confer a less favorable prognosis because the cells do not respond to ATRA therapy.[6]

Acute Myeloid Leukemia with *KMT2A* Rearrangement

The 2022 WHO classification has updated *KMT2A* rearranged AML to include all fusion partners in addition to the previously described t(9;11)(p22;q23); *KMT2A::MLLT3*.[6] *KMT2A* rearrangements are detected at all ages, are present in more than 50% of infant AML cases, and have a decreasing incidence with age. *KMT2A::MLLT3* is the most common rearrangement in adults with *KMT2A* rearranged AML. *KMT2A* rearrangements may be seen after topoisomerase II inhibitor therapy, and such cases should be classified as a myeloid neoplasm post cytotoxic therapy; an example of such is *KMT2A::CREBBP*. Clinically, extramedullary involvement is common, often involving the gingiva or skin. The WBC count varies, ranging from leukopenia to leukocytosis up to 200 × 10⁹/L. Histologically, the blasts in AML with *KMT2A* rearrangement often show monocytic, monoblastic, or myelomonocytic features, although a wide spectrum is seen. AML with t(9;11) presents with an increase in monoblasts and immature monocytes (Figure 31.7). The blasts are large, with abundant cytoplasm and fine nuclear chromatin. The cells may have motility, with pseudopodia seen frequently. Granules and vacuoles can be observed in the blasts. The prognosis may be dependent on the fusion partner. In adults, *KMT2A::MLLT3* has an intermediate risk of relapse compared to the poorer prognosis of other fusion partners. In children, the evidence is not as clear.

Acute Myeloid Leukemia with *DEK::NUP214*, Acute Myeloid Leukemia with *MECOM* Rearrangement, Acute Myeloid Leukemia with *RBM15::MRTFA*, Acute Myeloid Leukemia with *BCR::ABL1*, Acute Myeloid Leukemia with *NUP98* Rearrangement, and Other Defined Genetic Alterations

These are rare leukemias included in the 2022 WHO classification.[6] Detailed description of these entities is beyond the scope of this chapter.

Acute Myeloid Leukemia with *NPM1* Mutation and Acute Myeloid Leukemia with *CEBPA* Mutation

AML with *NPM1* mutation and AML with *CEBPA* mutation are included in the 2022 WHO classification as defined entities. AML with *CEBPA* mutation now includes single mutations in the basic leucine zipper region of the gene in addition to biallelic mutations.[6]

AML with *NPM1* mutation and AML with *CEBPA* mutation are associated with a better prognosis.[34] The blasts of AML with *NPM1* mutation often show monocytic features and "cuplike" nuclear indentations.

Acute Myeloid Leukemia, Myelodysplasia-Related

AML, myelodysplasia-related (AML-MR) affects primarily older adults and has a poor prognosis. Diagnosis requires at least 20% blasts with specific cytogenetic or molecular

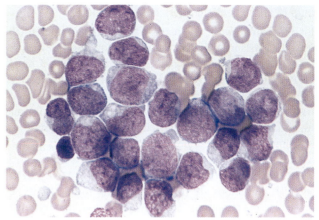

Figure 31.7 Acute Myeloid Leukemia with t(9;11). Both monoblasts and immature monocytes are increased. (Bone marrow aspirate, Wright-Giemsa stain, ×500.)

abnormalities and may arise de novo or after a known myelodysplastic neoplasm (MDS) or myelodysplastic/myeloproliferative neoplasm (MDS/MPN) (Chapters 32 and 33). Cases meeting requirements for AML with defining genetic abnormalities should be classified as such. Morphologic criteria for dysplasia have been removed.[6] The list of defining cytogenetic abnormalities includes complex karyotype (≥3 abnormalities), 5q deletion or loss, monosomy 7 or 7q deletion or loss, 11q deletion, 12p deletion or loss, monosomy 13 or 13q deletion, 17p deletion or loss, i(17q), and idic(X)(q13). The list of defining somatic mutations includes *SRSF2, SF3B1, U2AF1, ZRSR2, ASXL1, EZH2, BCOR,* and *STAG2*.

Acute Myeloid Leukemia, Defined by Differentiation

AML lacking the genetic abnormalities seen in the WHO subtypes described earlier, are grouped according to morphology, flow cytometric phenotyping (Chapter 28), and limited cytochemical reactions, similar to the FAB classification. The FAB classification was based on the cell of origin, degree of maturity, cytochemical reactions, and limited cytogenetic features (Table 31.5).[35,36] A blast percentage of at least 20% in the peripheral blood or bone marrow is required for diagnosis. This category accounts for about 25% of all AML, but as more genetic subgroups are recognized, the number in this group will diminish.[37]

Acute Myeloid Leukemia with Minimal Differentiation

The blasts in AML with minimal differentiation typically show expression of two or more myeloid markers (e.g., CD13, CD33, and/or CD117). Most cases express CD34 and approximately 30% of cases express CD7 and/or TdT. Granulocytic, monocytic, and B cell markers are often absent (Figure 31.8).[6,38] Auer rods typically are absent, and there is no clear evidence of cellular maturation, including cytoplasmic granulation. The cells yield negative results with the cytochemical stains myeloperoxidase (MPO) and Sudan black B (SBB). These cases account for less than 5% of AML, and patients are generally either infants or older adults. Although not specific, rearrangements of *BCL11B* on chromosome 14q32 are seen in approximately 30% of AML with minimal differentiation.

Acute Myeloid Leukemia without Maturation

Closely aligned with the blasts in minimally differentiated AML, the blasts in AML without maturation also show expression of two or more myeloid markers (e.g., CD13, CD33, and/or CD117). CD34 is positive in the majority of cases (Figure 31.9). CD7 and/or CD56 expression is seen in one third of cases.[6] Blasts may comprise 90% of nonerythroid cells in the bone marrow, and fewer than 10% of the leukocytes show maturation to the promyelocyte stage or beyond. At least 3% of blasts give positive results with MPO or SBB stains.[6,28] Most cases (two-thirds) have a normal karyotype. *DNMT3A, RUNX1, ASXL1, IDH2,* and *IDH1* mutations are frequent (ranging from 20% to 30% of cases). Some mutations seen in AML without maturation are now included in the list of mutations diagnostic for AML-MR, as described earlier.

Acute Myeloid Leukemia with Maturation

AML with maturation is a common variant that manifests with more than 20% blasts, at least 10% maturing cells of neutrophil lineage (Figure 31.10), and fewer than 20% precursors with monocytic lineage. Auer rods are often present.[6] The blasts show expression of MPO, are usually positive for CD34, and show expression of two or more myeloid markers (e.g., CD13, CD33, and/or CD117). A normal karyotype is seen in two-thirds of cases. *ASXL1, RUNX1, STAG2, IDH2,* and *DNMT3A* are frequently mutated (ranging from 20% to 40%), which may reclassify the case as AML-MR.[6]

Acute Basophilic Leukemia

Acute basophilic leukemia (ABL) is a rare type of AML. Blasts are 20% or greater of cellular elements and are medium to large, with cytoplasm containing coarse basophilic granules. Auer rods are not seen. The blasts show expression of two or more myeloid markers (e.g., CD13, CD33, and/or CD117), although CD117 expression is usually weak, as opposed to mast cell leukemia, which has strong CD117 expression. CD9 and/or CD203c expression may be seen. HLA-DR is negative. Immature and mature basophils are increased (20% to 80% of cellular elements). The blasts show metachromasia on toluidine blue staining. They are negative for MPO, SBB, napththol AS-D chloracetate esterase, and nonspecific esterase cytochemistry stains. A recurrent translocation, *MYB::GATA1,* has been seen in male infants with ABL, although no clear molecular pathway has been identified.[6]

Acute Myelomonocytic Leukemia

Acute myelomonocytic leukemia is characterized by the presence of myeloid (≥20%) and monocytoid cells (≥20%) in the bone marrow. Monocytic cells (monoblasts and promonocytes) constitute at least 20% of all marrow cells (Figure 31.11). The monoblasts are large, with abundant cytoplasm containing small granules and pseudopodia. The nucleus is large and immature and may contain multiple nucleoli. Promonocytes also are present and may have contorted nuclei. The peripheral blood involvement usually shows an increase in monocytes, which are typically more mature than those in the bone marrow. The cells are positive for the myeloid antigens CD13 and

TABLE 31.5 French-American-British (FAB) Classification of the Acute Myeloid Leukemias

Subtype	Description
M0	Acute myeloid leukemia, minimally differentiated
M1	Acute myeloid leukemia without maturation
M2	Acute myeloid leukemia with maturation
M3	Acute promyelocytic leukemia
M4	Acute myelomonocytic leukemia
M4eo	Acute myelomonocytic leukemia with eosinophilia
M5a	Acute monocytic leukemia, poorly differentiated
M5b	Acute monocytic leukemia, well differentiated
M6	Acute erythroleukemia
M7	Acute megakaryocytic leukemia

From Bennett, J. M., Catovsky, D., Daniel, M. T., et al. (1976). Proposals for the classification of the acute leukaemias. French-American-British (FAB) co-operative group. *Br J Haematol, 33*(4), 451–458; and Bennett, J. M., Catovsky, D., Daniel, M. T., et al. (1985). Proposed revised criteria for the classification of acute myeloid leukemia. A report of the French-American-British Cooperative Group. *Ann Intern Med, 103*(4), 620–625.

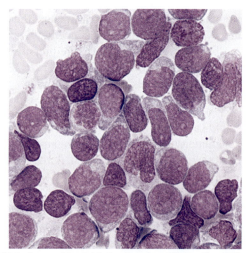

Figure 31.8 Acute Myeloid Leukemia, Minimally Differentiated (French-American-British Classification M0). Blasts lack myeloid morphologic features and yield negative results with myeloperoxidase and Sudan black B staining. Auer rods are not seen. CD34 is frequently expressed. (Bone marrow aspirate, Wright-Giemsa stain, ×500.)

CD33 and the monocytic antigens CD14, CD4, CD11b, CD11c, and CD64. The blasts are positive for MPO, and nonspecific esterase is usually positive in the monoblasts, promonocytes, and monocytes. Most cases have a normal karyotype. Frequent mutations include *TET2, RUNX1,* and *ASXL1;* some of the mutations found may reclassify acute myelomonocytic leukemia as AML-MR.[6]

Acute Monocytic Leukemia

In acute monocytic leukemia, 80% or greater of leukemic cells are of monocytic lineage. By definition, monoblasts and promonocytes are 20% or greater of bone marrow or peripheral

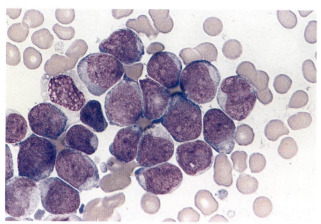

Figure 31.9 Acute Myeloid Leukemia without Maturation (French-American-British Classification M1). Blasts constitute 90% of the nonerythroid cells; there is less than 10% maturation of the granulocytic series beyond the promyelocyte stage. (Bone marrow aspirate, Wright-Giemsa stain, ×500.)

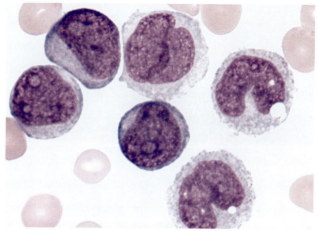

Figure 31.11 Acute Myelomonocytic Leukemia. Both myeloid and monocytic cells are present. Monocytic cells comprise at least 20% of all marrow cells, with monoblasts and promonocytes present. (Peripheral blood, Wright-Giemsa stain, ×1000.) (From Carr, J. H. [2022]. *Clinical Hematology Atlas*. [6th ed.]. St. Louis: Elsevier.)

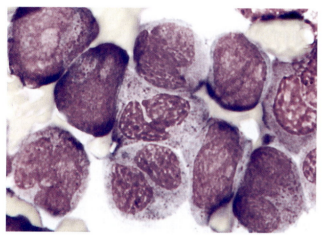

Figure 31.10 Acute Myeloid Leukemia with Maturation. Blasts constitute 20% or more of the nucleated cells of the bone marrow, and there is maturation beyond the promyelocyte stage in more than 10% of the nonerythroid cells. (Bone marrow aspirate, Wright-Giemsa stain, ×1000.)

blood cells, and maturing granulocytic cells are less than 20% of cells. The leukemic cells are positive for CD14, CD4, CD11b, CD11c, and CD64. Blasts are large, with abundant, often agranular cytoplasm and large prominent nucleoli (Figure 31.12, A). When some evidence of maturation is present, the cells are called promonocytes. Promonocytes in monocytic leukemias with differentiation are considered to be blast equivalents (Figure 31.12, B). Nonspecific esterase testing usually yields positive results. Acute monocytic leukemia is seen in all ages, with the immature form more common in younger individuals. Extramedullary involvement, including cutaneous and gingival infiltration, and bleeding disorders are common. Nonspecific cytogenetic abnormalities are seen in most cases.[6,39]

Acute Erythroid Leukemia

Also known as pure erythroid leukemia, acute erythroid leukemia (AEL) is a neoplastic proliferation of erythroid cells (≥80%

of marrow elements) that show a maturation arrest (≥30% of leukemic cells are pronormoblasts/erythroblasts).[40–42] The myeloblast component is not significant. Biallelic loss of *TP53* is characteristic of AEL. Complex rearrangements and hypodiploid chromosome number are common. Chromosomes 5 and 7 are frequently affected.[6]

The more mature red blood cell (RBC) precursors have significant dysplastic features, such as multinucleation, megaloblastoid asynchrony, and vacuolization. The nucleated RBCs in the peripheral blood may account for more than 50% of the total number of nucleated cells. Ring sideroblasts, Howell-Jolly bodies, and other inclusions may be present (Figure 31.13). Abnormal megakaryocytes may be seen. AEL has an aggressive and rapid clinical course.[6]

Acute Megakaryoblastic Leukemia

Patients with acute megakaryoblastic leukemia (AMKL) usually have cytopenias, although some may have thrombocytosis. Diagnosis requires the presence of at least 20% blasts of megakaryocyte origin. AMKL can be divided into three clinical groupings: children with Down syndrome, children without Down syndrome, and adults.

Megakaryoblast diameters vary from that of a small lymphocyte to three times their size. Chromatin is delicate, with prominent nucleoli. Immature megakaryocytes may have light blue cytoplasmic blebs (Figure 31.14, A). Megakaryoblasts are identified by immunostaining, using antibodies specific for cytoplasmic von Willebrand factor or platelet membrane antigens CD41 (glycoprotein IIb), CD42b (glycoprotein Ib) (Figure 31.14, B), or CD61 (glycoprotein IIIa).[6]

The RAM phenotype is seen in a subset of AMKL and is characterized by strong CD56 expression, variable CD34 and CD117, and negative CD7, CD11b, CD13, CD36, CD45, CD38, and HLA-DR. This phenotype is specifically associated with *CBFA2T3::GLIS2* fusion and is associated with extremely poor prognosis.[6]

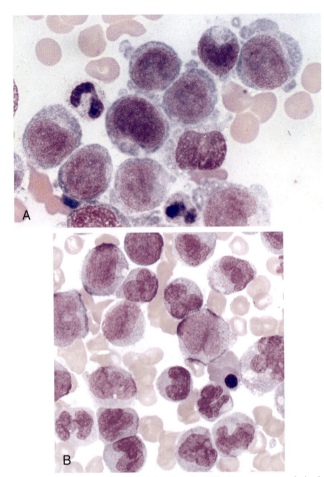

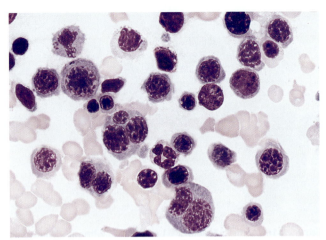

Figure 31.13 Acute Erythroid Leukemia. Erythroid precursors showing dysplastic features, including multinucleation and megaloblastic asynchrony. (Bone marrow aspirate, Wright-Giemsa stain, ×500.) (From Carr, J. H. [2022]. *Clinical Hematology Atlas*. [6th ed.]. St. Louis: Elsevier.)

Figure 31.12 Acute Monocytic Leukemia. **(A),** Acute monocytic leukemia, poorly differentiated, with more than 80% of the bone marrow cells of monocytic origin. **(B),** Acute monocytic leukemia, well differentiated, with promonocytes. Promonocytes are considered blast equivalents. (A, B, Bone marrow aspirate, Wright Giemsa stain, ×500.)

Myeloid Sarcoma

Myeloid sarcoma refers to extramedullary proliferation of blasts of one or more myeloid lineages that disrupts tissue architecture. Tissue architecture must be effaced for the neoplasm to qualify for this diagnosis. Tissues commonly affected include skin, gastrointestinal tract, and lymph nodes.[6,28]

Myeloid Neoplasms, Secondary

Secondary myeloid neoplasms include those associated with post cytotoxic therapy, germline predisposition, and Down syndrome.

A subset of myeloid neoplasms post cytotoxic therapy (MN-pCT) with 20% or more blasts are classified as AML and develop in a patient with history of DNA-damaging cytotoxic chemotherapy (e.g., alkylating agents, topoisomerase II inhibitors, antimetabolites, antitubulin agents, and PARP1 inhibitors) or large-field radiation therapy. If also meeting criteria for an AML with defining genetic abnormalities, the neoplasm should be classified as such, with a descriptor of "post cytotoxic therapy" included (e.g., AML with *CBFB::MYH11* fusion post cytotoxic therapy). MN-pCT usually arises within 10 years of the last treatment, with those secondary to topoisomerase II inhibitors

typically arising in 1 to 3 years and those secondary to alkylating agents or radiation arising 5 to 7 years after therapy. AML-pCT secondary to alkylating agents and ionizing radiation typically manifests with a pre-MDS phase and harbors *TP53* mutations and unbalanced chromosomal aberrations. These cases have particularly poor outcome compared to those secondary to topoisomerase II inhibitor therapy, which typically manifest as overt AML without prior MDS, have more balanced translocations, and have somewhat more favorable outcome (comparable to de novo AML if the respective therapy can be administered).[6]

Similarly, a subset of myeloid neoplasms associated with germline predisposition meet criteria for AML with 20% or more blasts. Broad subtypes are classified based on the presence or absence of preexisting platelet disorders or organ dysfunction. It is beyond the scope of this chapter to further elucidate the many entities within this category.

Two entities are included in the myeloid proliferations associated with Down syndrome: transient abnormal myelopoiesis (TAM) and myeloid leukemia of Down syndrome (ML-DS). Both entities show mutations in exon 2 or 3 of *GATA1*, which is only leukemogenic in the presence of trisomy 21 and is required in the diagnostic criteria of both entities. ML-DS also shows additional mutations in epigenetic regulator genes or tyrosine kinase genes. TAM occurs in 25% to 30% of newborns with Down syndrome. TAM often manifests within the first 7 days of life, with a wide range of clinical features and commonly with leukocytosis with increased blasts in the peripheral blood. Anemia is uncommon and platelet counts are variable. Bone marrow involvement is usually mild. More than 90% of patients will resolve without treatment in 2 to 3 months, whereas 20% of patients will later develop ML-DS. In comparison, ML-DS mainly involves the bone marrow and presents later in age, with a median age of onset of 1.6 years. It is usually preceded by MDS with pancytopenia. Approximately half of patients with ML-DS have a history of TAM. Bone marrow fibrosis is common in ML-DS. Blast counts may be less than 20% in this entity. ML-DS has a better prognosis than AML in children without Down syndrome.[6]

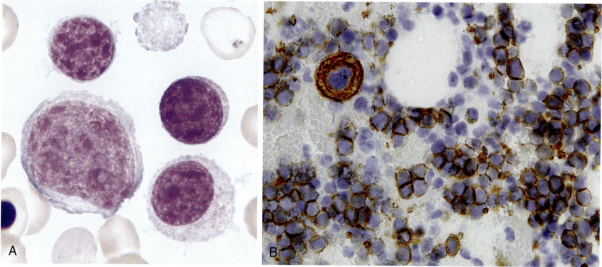

Figure 31.14 Acute Megakaryocytic Leukemia. **(A),** Megakaryoblasts showing morphologic heterogeneity with one small blast with scant cytoplasm, two with cytoplasmic blebbing, and one quite large. **(B),** Positive reaction for CD42b, a marker for megakaryocytic lineage. (A, Peripheral blood, Wright-Giemsa stain, ×1000; B, Bone marrow aspirate, Immunostain, ×1000.)

ACUTE LEUKEMIAS OF AMBIGUOUS LINEAGE

Acute leukemias of ambiguous lineage (ALALs) include leukemia in which there is no clear evidence of differentiation along a single cell line; leukemias of this type are commonly referred to as acute undifferentiated leukemias (AULs). Other cases of ALAL that demonstrate a multiplicity of antigens in which it is not possible to determine a specific lineage are called mixed phenotype acute leukemias (MPALs). MPALs may be biphenotypic, in which markers for multiple lineages are expressed in a single cell line, or bilineal, in which multiple populations are identified. The entities in this category require 20% or more blasts for diagnosis. Lineage criteria are based on immunophenotype. B lineage is assigned based on CD19 expression. Strong CD19 expression requires one or more of CD10, CD22, and/or CD79a also strongly expressed, whereas weak CD19 expression requires two or more. T lineage is based on CD3 expression, either greater than 50% of the intensity of mature T cell expression by flow cytometry or nonzeta chain positivity by immunohistochemistry. Myeloid lineage is based on MPO (>50% the intensity of mature neutrophil expression) or monocytic differentiation (positive for two or more of the following: nonspecific esterase, CD11c, CD14, CD64, and/or lysozyme). It is increasingly being recognized that specific molecular alterations are associated with ambiguous phenotype. Thus the 2022 WHO classification has significantly revised the criteria for this designation; a summary of the category is shown in Box 31.2.[6,37]

CYTOCHEMICAL STAINS AND INTERPRETATIONS

Techniques such as flow cytometry, cytogenetic analysis, and molecular testing are now commonly used in the diagnosis of acute leukemias. However, older techniques, such as cytochemical stains, still retain their importance. An advantage of

---

BOX 31.2 2022 WHO Classification of Acute Leukemias of Mixed or Ambiguous Lineage

Acute leukemia of ambiguous lineage with defining genetic abnormalities
Mixed-phenotype acute leukemia with *BCR::ABL1* fusion
Mixed-phenotype acute leukemia with *KMT2A* rearrangement
Acute leukemia of ambiguous lineage with other defined genetic alterations
Acute leukemia of ambiguous lineage, immunophenotypically defined
Mixed-phenotype acute leukemia, B/myeloid
Mixed-phenotype acute leukemia, T/myeloid
Mixed-phenotype acute leukemia, rare types
Acute leukemia of ambiguous lineage, NOS
Acute undifferentiated leukemia

NOS, Not otherwise specified.
From WHO Classification of Tumours Editorial Board (Eds). (2022). *Haematolymphoid Tumours* [Internet; beta version ahead of print] 5th ed. (International Agency for Research on Cancer).

---

cytochemical stains is that they are relatively inexpensive and can be performed by laboratories throughout the world, including in areas where resources and access to advanced techniques are limited. The cytochemical stains are summarized in Table 31.6.

Myeloperoxidase

MPO (Figures 31.15 and 31.16) is an enzyme found in the primary granules of granulocytic cells (neutrophils, eosinophils, and, to a certain extent, monocytes). Lymphocytes do not exhibit MPO activity. This stain is useful for differentiating the blasts of AML from those of ALL.

Interpretation

MPO is present in the primary granules of most granulocytic cells, beginning at the promyelocyte stage and continuing throughout maturation. Leukemic myeloblasts are usually positive for MPO.

TABLE 31.6 Acute Leukemia Cytochemical Reactions

Condition	MPO	SBB	NASDA	ANBE	ANAE
ALL	–	–	–	–/+ (focal)	–/+ (focal)
AML	+	+	+	–	–
AMML	+	+	+	+ (diffuse)	+ (diffuse)
AMoL	–	–/+	–	+ (diffuse)	+ (diffuse)
Megakaryocytic leukemia	–	–			+ (localized)

+, Positive reaction; –, negative reaction; –/+, negative or positive reaction; *ALL*, acute lymphoblastic leukemia; *AML*, acute myeloid leukemia; *AMML*, acute myelomonocytic leukemia; *AMoL*, acute monocytic leukemia; *ANAE*, α-naphthyl acetate esterase; *ANBE*, α-naphthyl butyrate esterase; *MPO*, myeloperoxidase; *NASDA*, naphthol AS-D chloroacetate esterase; *SBB*, Sudan black B.

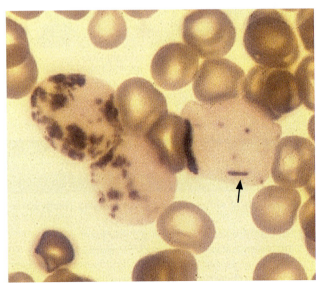

Figure 31.15 Positive Reaction with Myeloperoxidase Stain in Early Myeloid Cells. Note Auer rod at arrow. (Bone marrow aspirate, myeloperoxidase stain, ×1000.)

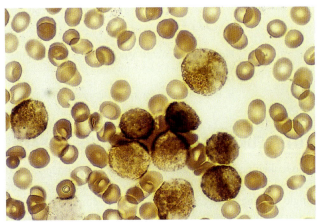

Figure 31.16 Strong Positive Reaction with Myeloperoxidase Stain in Leukemic Promyelocytes. From a patient with acute promyelocytic leukemia. (Bone marrow aspirate, myeloperoxidase stain, ×1000.)

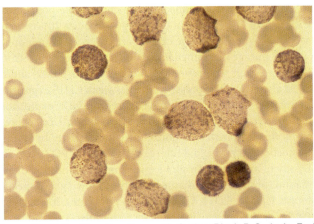

Figure 31.17 Positive Reaction with Sudan Black B Stain in Early Myeloid Cells. Positivity increases with the maturity of the myeloid cell. (Bone marrow aspirate, Sudan black B stain, ×1000.)

In many cases of the AMLs (without maturation, with maturation, and promyelocytic leukemia), it has been found that more than 80% of the blasts show MPO activity. Auer rods found in leukemic blasts and promyelocytes test strongly MPO positive.

In contrast, lymphoblasts in ALL and lymphoid cells are MPO negative. It is important that the reaction only in the blast cells be used as the determining factor for the differentiation of acute leukemias. This is true for MPO and for other cytochemical stains used in determining cell lineage described in this chapter. Maturing granulocytes are MPO positive; this is a normal finding and has little or no diagnostic significance.

Sudan Black B

SBB staining (Figure 31.17) is another useful technique for the differentiation of AML from ALL. SBB stains cellular lipids. The staining pattern is similar to that of MPO; SBB staining is possibly a little more sensitive for the early myeloid cells.

Interpretation

Granulocytes (neutrophils) show a positive reaction to SBB from the myeloblast through the maturation series. The staining becomes more intense as the cell matures as a result of the increase in the numbers of primary and secondary granules. Monocytic cells can demonstrate negative to weakly positive staining due to various changes that occur during differentiation. Lymphoid cells generally do not stain.

Esterases

Esterase reactions are used to differentiate myeloblasts and neutrophilic granulocytes from cells of monocytic origin. Nine isoenzymes of esterases are present in leukocytes. Two substrate esters commonly used are α-naphthyl acetate and α-naphthyl butyrate (both nonspecific). Naphthol AS-D chloroacetate (specific) also may be used. "Specific" refers to the fact that only granulocytic cells show staining, whereas nonspecific stains also may produce positive results in other cells.

Interpretation

Esterase stains can be used to distinguish acute leukemias that are granulocytic from leukemias that are primarily of monocytic origin. When naphthol AS-D chloroacetate is used as a substrate, the reaction is positive in the granulocytic cells and negative to weak in the monocytic cells (Figure 31.18). Chloroacetate esterase is present in the primary granules of neutrophils. Leukemic myeloblasts generally show a positive reaction. Auer rods also show positivity.

α-Naphthyl acetate, in contrast to naphthol AS-D chloroacetate, reveals strong esterase activity in monocytes that can be inhibited with the addition of sodium fluoride.[43,44] Granulocytes and lymphoid cells generally show a negative result on nonspecific esterase staining (Figure 31.19).

A diffuse positive α-naphthyl butyrate esterase reaction is seen in monocytes. α-Naphthyl butyrate is less sensitive than α-naphthyl acetate, but it is more specific. Granulocytes and lymphoid cells generally show a negative reaction (Figure 31.20), although a small positive dot may be seen in lymphocytes. In myelomonocytic leukemia, positive AS-D chloroacetate activity and positive α-naphthyl butyrate or α-naphthyl acetate activity should be seen because myeloid and monocytic cells are present. In myelomonocytic leukemia, at least 20% of the cells must show monocytic differentiation that is nonspecific esterase positive and is inhibited by sodium fluoride. In the pure monocytic leukemias, 80% or more of the blasts are nonspecific esterase positive and specific esterase negative.

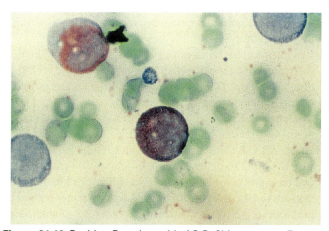

Figure 31.18 Positive Reaction with AS-D Chloroacetate Esterase Stain in Two Early Myeloid Cells. (Bone marrow aspirate, AS-C chloroacetate esterase stain, ×1000.)

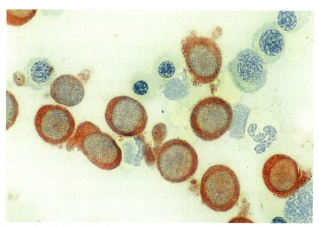

Figure 31.20 Positive Reaction with α-Naphthyl Butyrate Esterase in Cells of Monocytic Origin. Note the negative reaction of myeloid and erythroid precursors. (Bone marrow aspirate, α-naphthyl butyrate esterase stain, ×1000.)

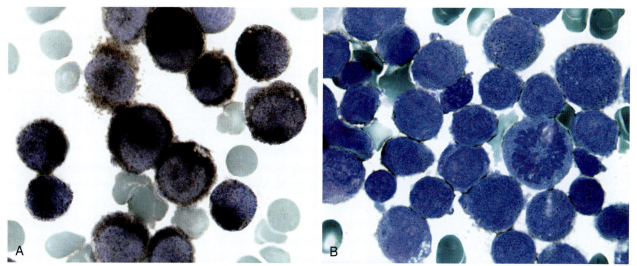

Figure 31.19 α-Naphthyl Acetate Esterase Stain in Cells of Monocytic Origin. **(A),** Positive reaction with α-naphthyl acetate esterase stain in immature monocytic cells. **(B),** Same specimen with addition of sodium fluoride to the stain, showing a negative reaction. Fluoride inhibits the esterase reaction in the immature monocytic cells. (A, B, Bone marrow aspirate, α-naphthyl acetate esterase stain, ×1000.)

SUMMARY

- The development of leukemia is a stepwise progression of mutations, or "multiple hits," involving mutations that give leukemic stem cells a proliferative advantage and also hinder differentiation.
- For most acute leukemias, causes directly related to the development of the malignancy are unknown, but a few exceptions exist. Some known causes include environmental toxins, certain viruses, previous chemotherapy, and familial predisposition.
- There are several classification schemes for leukocyte neoplasia, including the FAB system, based primarily on morphology and cytochemical staining, the WHO system, which retains some elements of the FAB scheme but emphasizes molecular and cytogenetic changes, and the International Consensus Classification system, which differs slightly from the WHO.
- Only half of patients with acute lymphoblastic leukemia (ALL) have leukocytosis, some patients have circulating lymphoblasts, but neutropenia, thrombocytopenia, and anemia are usually present.
- In children ALL is a disease in which the "good prognosis" subtypes are associated with a 95% rate of complete remission, but adults with ALL have a poor prognosis.
- Infiltration of malignant cells into the meninges can occur in ALL, with lymphoblasts found in the cerebrospinal fluid, testes, and ovaries.
- Prognosis in ALL depends primarily on age at the time of diagnosis, lymphoblast load (tumor burden), immunophenotype, and genetic abnormalities. Chromosomal translocations seem to be the strongest predictor of adverse treatment outcomes for children and adults.
- The t(12;21) *ETV6::RUNX1* translocation is found in about 25% of patients with childhood ALL and has an excellent prognosis with a cure rate of over 90%.
- There are two main subtypes of ALL, according to the WHO classification system: B-lymphoblastic leukemia/lymphoma and T-lymphoblastic leukemia/lymphoma.

- Tumor lysis syndrome is an increasingly common complication of treatment, especially in patients with a high tumor burden.
- Although morphology is the first tool in distinguishing ALL from acute myeloid leukemia (AML), immunophenotyping is often the only reliable indicator of a cell's origin.
- The incidence of AML in adults increases with age.
- The clinical presentation of a patient with AML is nonspecific and reflects the decreased production of normal bone marrow elements, an elevated WBC count, and the presence of myeloblasts. Anemia, thrombocytopenia, and neutropenia give rise to the clinical findings of pallor, fatigue, bruising and bleeding, and fever with infections.
- The classification of AML is complicated by the presence or absence of multiple cell lines defined as "myeloid" in origin, specific cells within these cell lines, and specific karyotype abnormalities.
- Leukemias with ambiguous lineage include leukemias in which there is no clear evidence of differentiation along a single cell line.
- Cytochemical techniques can still be used in conjunction with morphologic analysis, immunohistochemical methods, flow cytometry, cytogenetic analysis, and molecular techniques in establishing a diagnosis.
- Myeloperoxidase (MPO) stains primary granules and is useful in differentiating granulocytic from lymphoid cells. Sudan black B (SBB) stains lipids and results parallel those with the MPO stain. Esterases help differentiate granulocytes and their precursors from cells of monocytic origin. Butyrate esterase testing gives positive results in monocytes but not in granulocyte precursors, whereas naphthol AS-D chloroacetate esterase stains granulocyte precursors.

Now that you have completed this chapter, go back and read again the case study at the beginning and respond to the questions presented. Answers can be found in Appendix C.

REVIEW QUESTIONS

Answers can be found in Appendix C.

1. According to the WHO classification, except in leukemias with defining genetic abnormalities, the minimal percentage of blasts necessary for a diagnosis of acute leukemia is:
   a. 10%
   b. 20%
   c. 30%
   d. 50%

2. A 20-year-old patient has an elevated WBC count with 70% blasts, 4% neutrophils, 5% lymphocytes, and 21% monocytes in the peripheral blood. Eosinophils with abnormally large, dark purple-violet granules are seen in the bone marrow. AML with which of the following karyotypes would be most likely to be seen?
   a. AML with *RUNX1::RUNX1T1* fusion
   b. AML with *CBFB::MYH11* fusion
   c. APL with *PML::RARA* fusion
   d. AML with *KMT2A* rearrangement

3. Which of the following would be considered a sign of potentially favorable prognosis in children with ALL?
   a. High hyperdiploidy
   b. Presence of CD19 and CD20
   c. Absence of trisomy 8
   d. Presence of *BCR::ABL1* gene

4. Signs and symptoms of cerebral infiltration with blasts are more commonly seen in:
   a. AML with defining cytogenetic abnormalities
   b. AML post cytotoxic therapy
   c. AML, myelodysplasia-related
   d. ALL

5. An oncology patient exhibiting signs of renal failure with seizures after initial chemotherapy may potentially develop:
   a. Hyperleukocytosis
   b. Tumor lysis syndrome
   c. Acute leukemia post cytotoxic therapy
   d. Myelodysplasia

6. Disseminated intravascular coagulation is more often seen in association with leukemia characterized by which of the following mutations?
   a. t(12;21)(p13;q22), *ETV6::RUNX1*
   b. t(9;22)(q34;q11.2), *BCR::ABL1*
   c. inv(16)(p13;q22), *CBFB::MYH11*
   d. t(15;17)(q22;q12), *PML::RARA*

7. Which of the following leukemias affects primarily children, is characterized by an increase in monoblasts and monocytes, and often is associated with gingival and skin involvement?
   a. Pre-B-lymphoblastic leukemia
   b. Acute erythroid leukemia
   c. AML with *KMT2A* rearrangement
   d. APL with *PML::RARA* fusion

8. A 20-year-old patient presents with fatigue, pallor, easy bruising, and swollen gums. Bone marrow examination reveals 82% cells with delicate chromatin and prominent nucleoli that are positive for CD14, CD4, CD11b, and CD36. Which of the following acute leukemias is likely?
   a. Minimally differentiated leukemia
   b. Leukemia of ambiguous lineage
   c. Acute monocytic leukemia
   d. Acute megakaryoblastic leukemia

9. The WHO diagnostic criteria for acute erythroid leukemia includes which of the following bone marrow findings?
   a. ≥70% erythroid cells of which ≥20% are pronormoblasts
   b. ≥80% erythroid cells of which ≥30% are pronormoblasts
   c. ≥90% erythroid cells of which ≥15% are pronormoblasts
   d. ≥95% erythroid cells of which ≥35% are pronormoblasts

10. A patient with normal chromosomes has a WBC count of $3.0 \times 10^9/L$ and dysplasia in all cell lines. There are 60% blasts of varying sizes. The blasts stain positive for CD61. The most likely type of leukemia is:
    a. Acute lymphoblastic
    b. Acute megakaryoblastic
    c. Acute monocytic
    d. APL with *PML::RARA*

11. SBB stains which of the following component of cells?
    a. Glycogen
    b. Lipids
    c. Structural proteins
    d. Enzymes

12. The cytochemical stain α-naphthyl butyrate is a nonspecific esterase stain that shows diffuse positivity in cells of which lineage?
    a. Erythroid
    b. Monocytic
    c. Granulocytic
    d. Lymphoid

REFERENCES

1. Anderson, K., Anderson, L. E., & Glanze, W. D. (Eds.) (1994). *Mosby's Medical, Nursing, and Allied Health Dictionary.* (4th ed.). St. Louis: Mosby.

2. Bachas, C., Schuurhuis, G. J., Hollink, I. H. I. M., et al. (2010). High-frequency type I/II mutational shifts between diagnosis and relapse are associated with outcome in pediatric AML: implications for personalized medicine. *Blood, 116,* 2752–2758.

3. Reilly, J. T. (2005). Pathogenesis of acute myeloid leukaemia and inv(16)(p13;q22): a paradigm for understanding leukaemogenesis? *Br J Haematol, 128,* 18–34.

4. Lane, S. W., & Gilliland, D. G. (2010). Leukemia stem cells. *Semin Cancer Biol, 20,* 71–76.

5. Jaffe, E. S., Harris, N. L., Stein, H., et al. (Eds.). (2001). *Pathology and Genetics of Tumours of Haematopoietic and Lymphoid Tissues.* Lyon, France: IARC Press.

6. WHO Classification of Tumours Editorial Board. (2022). *Haematolymphoid Tumours* [Internet; beta version ahead of print] 5th ed. International Agency for Research on Cancer. https://

tumourclassification.iarc.who.int/chapters/63. Accessed October 31, 2023.

7. Stanulla, M., & Schrauder, A. (2009). Bridging the gap between the north and south of the world: the case of treatment response in childhood acute lymphoblastic leukemia. *Haematologica, 94,* 748–752.

8. Inaba, H., Greaves, M., & Mullighan, C. G. (2013). Acute lymphoblastic leukaemia. *Lancet, 381,* 1943–1955.

9. Swerdlow, S. H., Campo, E., Harris, N. L., et al. (2017). *WHO Classification of Tumours of Haematopoietic and Lymphoid Tissues.* (4th ed.) Lyon, France: IARC Press.

10. Advani, A., Jin, T., Bolwell, B., et al. (2009). A prognostic scoring system for adult patients less than 60 years of age with acute lymphoblastic leukemia in first relapse. *Leuk Lymphoma, 50,* 1126–1131.

11. Pui, C. H., & Evans, W. E. (2006). Treatment of acute lymphoblastic leukemia. *N Engl J Med, 354,* 166–178.

12. Redaelli, A., Laskin, B. L., Stephens, J. M., et al. (2005). A systematic literature review of the clinical and epidemiological burden of acute lymphoblastic leukaemia (ALL). *Eur J Cancer Care, 14,* 53–62.

13. Hutter, J. J. (2010). Childhood leukemia. *Pediatr Rev, 31*, 234–241.

14. Onciu, M. (2009). Acute lymphoblastic leukemia. *Hematol Oncol Clin North Am, 23*, 655–674.

15. Liu, Y., Easton, J., Shao, Y., et al. (2017). The genomic landscape of pediatric and young adult T-lineage acute lymphoblastic leukemia. *Nat Genet, 49*, 1211–1218.

16. Pieters, R., de Groot-Kruseman, H., Van der Velden, V., et al. (2016). Successful therapy reduction and intensification for childhood acute lymphoblastic leukemia based on minimal residual disease monitoring: study ALL10 from the Dutch Childhood Oncology Group. *J Clin Oncol, 34*, 2591–2601.

17. Pilozzi, E., Pulford, K., Jones, M., et al. (1998). Co-expression of CD79a (JCB117) and CD3 by lymphoblastic lymphoma. *J Pathol, 186*(2), 140–143.

18. Burns, M. A., Gutierrez, A., & Silverman, L. B. (2023). Pathobiology of acute lymphoblastic leukemia. In Hoffman, R., Benz, E. J., Silberstein, L. E., et al. (Eds.), *Hematology: Basic Principles and Practice.* (8th ed., pp. 1049–1065). Philadelphia: Elsevier.

19. Attarbaschi, A., Mann, G., Dworzak, M., et al. (2002). Mediastinal mass in childhood T-cell acute lymphoblastic leukemia: significance and therapy response. *Med Pediatr Oncol, 39*, 558–565.

20. Goldberg, J. M., Silverman, L. B., Levy, D. E., et al. (2003). Childhood T-cell acute lymphoblastic leukemia: the Dana-Farber Cancer Institute acute lymphoblastic leukemia consortium experience. *J Clin Oncol, 21*, 3616–3622.

21. Van Vlierberghe, P., & Ferrando, A. (2012). The molecular basis of T cell acute lymphoblastic leukemia. *J Clin Invest, 122*, 3398–3406.

22. Gale, K. B., Ford, A. M., Repp, R., et al. (1997). Backtracking leukemia to birth: identification of clonotypic gene fusion sequences in neonatal blood spots. *Proc Natl Acad Sci U. S. A., 94*, 13950–13954.

23. Castor, A., Nilsson, L., Astrand-Grundström, I., et al. (2005). Distinct patterns of hematopoietic stem cell involvement in acute lymphoblastic leukemia. *Nat Med, 11*, 630–637.

24. Uchiumi, H., Matsushima, T., Yamane, A., et al. (2007). Prevalence and clinical characteristics of acute myeloid leukemia associated with disseminated intravascular coagulation. *Int J Hematol, 86*, 137–142.

25. Montesinos, P., Lorenzo, I., Martín, G., et al. (2008). Tumor lysis syndrome in patients with acute myeloid leukemia: identification of risk factors and development of a predictive model. *Haematologica, 93*, 67–74.

26. Cairo, M. S., & Bishop, M. (2004). Tumour lysis syndrome: new therapeutic strategies and classification. *Br J Haematol, 127*, 3–11.

27. Shimony, S., Stahl, M., & Stone, R. M. (2023). Acute myeloid leukemia: 2023 update on diagnosis, risk-stratification, and management. *Am J Hematol, 98*, 502–526.

28. Heerema-McKenney, A., & Arber, D. A. (2009). Acute myeloid leukemia. *Hematol Oncol Clin North Am, 23*, 633–654.

29. Ustun, C., Morgan, E., Moodie, E. E. M., et al. (2018). Core-binding factor acute myeloid leukemia with t(8;21): risk factors and a novel scoring system (I-CBFit). *Cancer Med, 7*, 4447–4455.

30. Mrózek, K., Marcucci, G., Paschka, P., et al. (2008). Advances in molecular genetics and treatment of core-binding factor acute myeloid leukemia. *Curr Opin Oncol, 20*, 711–718.

31. Opatz, S., Bamopoulos, S. A., Metzeler, K. H., et al. (2020). The clinical mutatome of core binding factor leukemia. *Leukemia, 34*, 1553–1562.

32. Stein, E., McMahon, B., Kwaan, H., et al. (2009). The coagulopathy of acute promyelocytic leukaemia revisited. *Best Pract Res Clin Haematol, 22*, 153–163.

33. Nasr, R., Lallemand-Breitenbach, V., Zhu, J., et al. (2009). Therapy-induced PML/RARA proteolysis and acute promyelocytic leukemia cure. *Clin Cancer Res, 15*, 6321–6326.

34. Falini, B., Mecucci, C., Tiacci, E., et al. (2005). Cytoplasmic nucleophosmin in acute myelogenous leukemia with a normal karyotype. *N Engl J Med, 352*, 254–266.

35. Bennett, J. M., Catovsky, D., Daniel, M. T., et al. (1985). Proposed revised criteria for the classification of acute myeloid leukemia. A report of the French-American-British Cooperative Group. *Ann Intern Med, 103*, 620–625.

36. Bennett, J. M., Catovsky, D., Daniel, M. T., et al. (1976). Proposals for the classification of the acute leukaemias. French-American-British (FAB) co-operative group. *Br J Haematol, 33*, 451–458.

37. Vardiman, J. W., Thiele, J., Arber, D. A., et al. (2009). The 2008 revision of the World Health Organization (WHO) classification of myeloid neoplasms and acute leukemia: rationale and important changes. *Blood, 114*, 937–951.

38. Kaleem, Z., Crawford, E., Pathan, M. H., et al. (2003). Flow cytometric analysis of acute leukemias. Diagnostic utility and critical analysis of data. *Arch Pathol Lab Med, 127*, 42–48.

39. Villeneuve, P., Kim, D. T., Xu, W., et al. (2008). The morphological subcategories of acute monocytic leukemia (M5a and M5b) share similar immunophenotypic and cytogenetic features and clinical outcomes. *Leuk Res, 32*, 269–273.

40. Kowal-Vern, A., Cotelingam, J., & Schumacher, H. R. (1992). The prognostic significance of proerythroblasts in acute erythroleukemia. *Am J Clin Pathol, 98*, 34–40.

41. Lessard, M., Struski, S., Leymarie, V., et al. (2005). Cytogenetic study of 75 erythroleukemias. *Cancer Genet Cytogenet, 163*, 113–122.

42. Liu, W., Hasserjian, R. P., Hu, Y., et al. (2011). Pure erythroid leukemia: a reassessment of the entity using the 2008 World Health Organization classification. *Mod Pathol, 24*, 375–383.

43. Scott, C. S., Den Ottolander, G. J., Swirsky, D., et al. (1993). Recommended procedures for the classification of acute leukaemias. International Council for Standardization in Haematology (ICSH). *Leuk Lymphoma, 11*(1-2), 37–50.

44. Head, D. R. (1996). Revised classification of acute myeloid leukemia. *Leukemia, 10*(11), 1826–1831.

Myeloproliferative Neoplasms

Tim R. Randolph

OBJECTIVES

After completion of this chapter, the reader will be able to:

1. Define myeloproliferative neoplasms (MPNs), list the four most common diseases included in the World Health Organization classification of MPNs, and recognize their abbreviations.
2. Define chronic myeloid leukemia (CML) and describe the cell lines involved, the clinical phases and the expected clinical manifestations, key peripheral blood and bone marrow findings, and diagnostic criteria applicable to each stage.
3. Discuss the cytogenetics, molecular genetics, and molecular pathophysiology of CML and relate it to treatment approaches, monitoring minimal residual disease, and mechanisms of drug resistance.
4. Discuss the driver mutations (*JAK2, MPL, CALR*) and the proposed pathogenic mechanism in MPNs.
5. Briefly discuss disease progression, including transitions between essential thrombocythemia (ET), polycythemia vera (PV), and primary myelofibrosis (PMF).
6. Define ET, including the clinical features, pathophysiology, laboratory findings, diagnostic criteria, and two complications that may occur in patients with ET.
7. Define PV and describe the clinical features, laboratory findings, diagnostic criteria, and complications.
8. Define PMF and describe the clinical features, laboratory findings, diagnostic criteria, and complications.
9. Describe the mutations that occur in MPNs and relate them to disease progression and current therapy.
10. Briefly describe the other myeloproliferative neoplasms, other than the main four, outlined in this chapter.
11. Given the patient history and clinical and laboratory findings, including representative cells on the peripheral blood film or bone marrow smear, interpret results of diagnostic tests to determine the type of MPN, and recommend additional tests to confirm a diagnosis.

OUTLINE

BCR::ABL1-Positive Myeloproliferative Neoplasms
  Chronic Myeloid Leukemia
BCR::ABL1-Negative Myeloproliferative Neoplasms
  Background
  Essential Thrombocythemia
  Polycythemia Vera
  Primary Myelofibrosis
Other Myeloproliferative Neoplasms
  Chronic Neutrophilic Leukemia
  Chronic Eosinophilic Leukemia

  Juvenile Myelomonocytic Leukemia
  Myeloproliferative Neoplasm–Not Otherwise Specified
Myeloid/Lymphoid Neoplasms
Mastocytosis
  Incidence
  Clinical Presentation
  Diagnosis
  Pathogenetic Mechanism
  Prognosis

CASE STUDY

After studying the material in this chapter, the reader should be able to respond to the following case study. Answers can be found in Appendix C.

A 34-year-old woman presented to the provider with a 2-month history of increasing weakness, persistent nonproductive cough, fever and chills accompanied by night sweats, and a 13-lb weight loss over a 6-month period. Results of chest radiographs and purified protein derivative test (for tuberculosis) were negative. The patient was treated with ciprofloxacin and her cough improved, but she continued to grow weaker and was able to consume only small quantities of food. The patient appeared pale and cachectic. Tenderness and fullness were present in the left upper quadrant, and the spleen was palpable below the umbilicus. No hepatomegaly or peripheral adenopathy was noted. Her laboratory results were as follows. Reference intervals can be found after the Index at the end of the book.

WBC	248×10^9/L	LYMPH	10%
HGB	9.5 g/dL	EO	3%
HCT	26.3%	BASO	7%
PLT	449×10^9/L	Myelocyte	30%
RETIC	3%	Promyelocyte	1%
NEUT	44%	Myeloblast	1%
BANDS	4%	NRBC	2 per 100 WBCs

Continued

Myeloproliferative neoplasms (MPNs) are clonal hematopoietic disorders caused by genetic mutations in the hematopoietic stem cells (HSCs) that result in expansion, excessive production, and accumulation of mature erythrocytes, granulocytes, and platelets. Each MPN is characterized by the clonal expansion of one or more myeloid cell lines, but usually one cell line in particular dominates. The World Health Organization (WHO) classification of tumors of the hematopoietic system classifies MPNs into four predominant disorders, *chronic myeloid leukemia (CML)*, *essential thrombocythemia (ET)*, *polycythemia vera (PV)*, and *primary myelofibrosis (PMF)*, and four less common subtypes, *chronic neutrophilic leukemia (CNL)*, *chronic eosinophilic leukemia (CEL)*, *juvenile myelomonocytic leukemia (JMML)*, and *myeloproliferative neoplasm–not otherwise specified (MPN-NOS)*.[1] As originally described by Dameshek in 1951, MPNs have pathogenetic similarities as well as common clinical and laboratory features resulting in the classification of MPNs.[2]

The four main MPNs are subdivided into two categories: *BCR::ABL1*-positive and *BCR::ABL1*-negative MPNs. CML is the prototype *BCR::ABL1*-positive neoplasm and is characterized by neutrophilia, a significant left shift to include all stages of myeloid development, and the presence of the Philadelphia (Ph) chromosome translocation and/or the *BCR::ABL1* fusion gene. In contrast, *BCR::ABL1*-negative MPNs are genetically related based on the presence of the Janus kinase 2 (*JAK2*) mutation in most cases and the absence of the Ph chromosome or *BCR::ABL1* fusion gene in all cases. Each of these three MPNs manifest with proliferation of one primary myeloid element: thrombocytosis in ET; erythrocytosis in PV; and neutrophilia, a left shift, and eventual fibrosis in PMF. PMF is a combination of overproduction of hematopoietic cells and stimulation of fibroblast production leading to bone marrow fibrosis that results in ineffective hematopoiesis with resultant peripheral blood cytopenias.

MPNs typically manifest as stable chronic disorders that may transform first to a subacute and then to an aggressive cellular growth phase, such as acute myeloid leukemia (AML) or acute lymphoblastic leukemia (ALL). They may manifest a demonstrate cellular phase, such as bone marrow hypoplasia, or exhibit clinical symptoms and morphologic patterns characteristic of subacute disease, followed by a more aggressive cellular expression. Familial MPNs have been described in families in which two or more members are affected.[3]

BCR::ABL1-POSITIVE MYELOPROLIFERATIVE NEOPLASMS

Chronic Myeloid Leukemia

CML is an MPN that arises from a single genetic translocation in a pluripotential HSC producing a clonal overproduction of the myeloid cell line and resulting in a preponderance of immature neutrophilic cells in the granulocytic cell line. CML begins with a chronic clinical phase and, if untreated, progresses to an accelerated phase in 3 to 4 years and often terminates as an acute leukemia. Progression to acute leukemia can be of the myeloid type (AML) or the lymphoid type (ALL). The clinical features are frequent infection, anemia, bleeding, and splenomegaly secondary to massive pathologic accumulation of myeloid progenitor cells in bone marrow, peripheral blood, and extramedullary tissues. Neutrophilia with all maturational stages present, basophilia, eosinophilia, and often thrombocytosis are commonly observed in peripheral blood.

Incidence

CML occurs at rate of approximately 35,000 cases globally each year, with about 9000 cases occurring in the United States. CML occurs at all ages but is seen predominantly in adults age 46 to 53 years. It represents about 15% to 20% of all cases of leukemia and is slightly more common in men than in women.[4] Before the development of imatinib mesylate, 5-year survival was 22%, and it is now estimated to be as much as 90%. Imatinib is a tyrosine kinase inhibitor (TKI) that has changed the prognosis and treatment for CML and is described in detail later. Symptoms associated with clinical onset are usually of minimal intensity and include fatigue, decreased tolerance of exertion, anorexia, abdominal discomfort, weight loss, and symptomatic effects from splenic enlargement.

Cytogenetics of the Philadelphia Chromosome

The Ph chromosome is a unique chromosome that is present in proliferating HSCs and their progeny in CML. Mutagens producing chromosomal breakage can cause the Ph chromosome to form, but it appears more often in populations exposed to ionizing radiation.[5,6] In most patients, a cause cannot be identified. The Ph chromosome was first identified as a short chromosome 22 in 1960 by Nowell and Hungerford in Philadelphia.[7] In 1973 Rowley at the University of Chicago discovered that the Ph chromosome is a reciprocal translocation between the long arms of

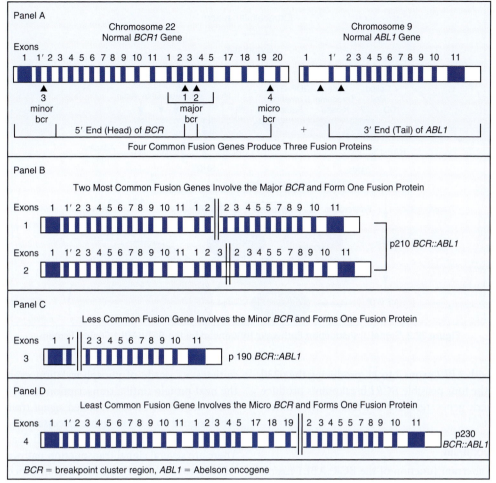

Figure 32.1 Molecular Biology of the *BCR::ABL1* Fusion Gene. **(A),** Normal *BCR1* gene on chromosome 22 and *ABL1* gene on chromosome 9. **(B),** Two *BCR* fusion gene products from the major *BCR*. **(C),** Fusion gene product from the minor *BCR*. **(D),** Fusion gene product from the micro *BCR*.

chromosomes 9 and 22 (Chapter 30).[8] This acquired somatic mutation specifically reflects the translocation of an *ABL1* proto-oncogene from band q34 of chromosome 9 to the breakpoint cluster region (BCR) of band q11 of chromosome 22, resulting in a unique chimeric gene, *BCR::ABL1*.[9] This new gene produces a 210-kD BCR::ABL1 fusion protein (p210 BCR::ABL1) that expresses enhanced tyrosine kinase activity from the ABL1 moiety compared with its natural enzymatic counterpart.

Molecular Genetics

The t(9;22) translocation that produces the *BCR::ABL1* chimeric gene has been identified in four primary molecular forms that produce three versions of the BCR::ABL1 chimeric protein: p190, p210, and p230 (Figure 32.1). The four genetic variations are based on the area of the *BCR* gene that houses the breakpoint on chromosome 22 because the breakpoint on chromosome 9 occurs in the same location. The wild-type (normal) *ABL1* gene on chromosome 9 is a relatively large gene of approximately 230 kb containing 11 exons. The breakpoint consistently occurs 5′ of the second exon such that exons 2 to 11 contributed to the *BCR::ABL1* fusion gene.[9]

There are four *BCR* genes in the human genome: *BCR1, BCR2, BCR3,* and *BCR4*. The *BCR1* gene is involved in the Ph

translocation. The wild-type (normal) *BCR1* gene is approximately 100 kb, with 20 exons. In 1984, Groffen and colleagues[10] identified the BCR on chromosome 22 as a 5-exon region involving exons 12 to 16 that was the area of breakage in the traditional t(9;22) translocation. This area was later termed the *major BCR*. Two other areas of breakage were identified on chromosome 22, one near the 5′ (head) of the *BCR1* gene, called the *minor BCR,* and one in the 3′ end (tail) of the *BCR1* gene, termed the *micro BCR*. Therefore two areas of breakage in the major BCR, one breakpoint area in the minor BCR, and one breakpoint region in the micro BCR produce four versions of the *BCR* gene that combine with exons 2 to 11 of the *ABL1* gene to form four versions of the *BCR::ABL1* chimeric gene.

Within the major BCR, two specific breakpoints account for the t(9;22) translocation involved in the development of CML. Breakage in the *BCR1* gene in the major BCR contributes exons 1 to 13 or 1 to 14, whereas the *ABL1* gene contributes exons 2 to 11. Because the two breakpoints in the major BCR differ by only one exon, the chimeric protein product is essentially the same size and is designated as the p210 protein. Breakage in the minor BCR contributes only exon one from *BCR1*, which joins with the same exons 2 to 11 of *ABL1* to produce a p190 protein. The micro BCR breakpoint contributes exons 2 to 19 from

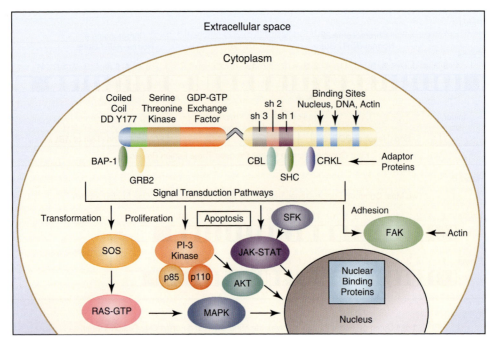

Figure 32.2 Signal Transduction Pathways Influenced by the BCR::ABL1 Fusion Protein.

BCR1, which fuse with *ABL1* exons 2 to 11, producing the p230 protein. Therefore the four possible *BCR1* breakpoints produce four different chimeric genes, resulting in a total of three different protein products.[11]

Pathogenetic Mechanism

To understand the aberrant function of the BCR::ABL1 fusion protein, it is first helpful to understand the functions of both the normal BCR and ABL1 proteins. The wild-type ABL1 protein, when in its usual location on chromosome 9, codes for p125, which exhibits normal tyrosine kinase activity. The *BCR1* gene produces p160, expresses serine and threonine kinase activity, is a guanine nucleotide exchange factor, and is thought to function in the regulation of cell growth. Protein kinases are enzymes that catalyze the transfer of phosphate groups from adenosine triphosphate (ATP), guanosine triphosphate (GTP), and other phosphate donors to receiver proteins. A tyrosine kinase transfers the phosphate group to a tyrosine amino acid on the receiver protein. For the kinase activity of the ABL1 protein to occur, the ABL1 protein must first be phosphorylated. This is often accomplished through autophosphorylation. The ABL1 protein has three primary domains called *SH1, SH2,* and *SH3* that together express and regulate the kinase activity. SH1 is the binding site for ATP; SH2 is the docking point for phosphate receiver proteins; and SH3 is the domain that controls the phosphorylation activity. When ATP binds to the ATP binding site, the phosphate is transferred to the SH2 region of the ABL protein, which initiates a conformational change that alters the tertiary structure of the protein and exposes the active site of the kinase enzyme. When a second ATP binds the ATP binding site and a receiver protein docks in the SH2 domain, the phosphate group is transferred to the receiver protein. In most physiologically normal intracellular pathways, protein phosphorylation activates the receiver protein (Figure 32.2). This phosphorylation

initiates a cascade of phosphorylation events, each activating the next protein until a transcription factor becomes activated. These activation cascades, called *signal transduction pathways,* are designed to activate genes necessary to control cell proliferation, differentiation, and natural cell death, called *apoptosis.* There are several signal transduction pathways activated by the ABL1 tyrosine kinase that function in concert to activate these genes in a precise order and at the required level of activation to control these cellular events.[11–14]

In the case of CML, the *BCR::ABL1* translocation occurs next to the SH3 domain of the *ABL1* moiety, which is designed to control the rate and timing of phosphorylation. Therefore the BCR::ABL1 tyrosine kinase loses the ability to shut off kinase activity and is said to have constitutive tyrosine kinase activity. The BCR::ABL1 enzyme continuously adds phosphate groups to tyrosine residues on cytoplasmic proteins, activating several signal transduction pathways. These pathways stimulate gene expression, keeping the myeloid cells proliferating, reducing differentiation, reducing adhesion of cells to bone marrow stroma, and virtually eliminating apoptosis. The result is increased clonal proliferation of myeloid cells secondary to a reduction in or loss of sensitivity to protein regulators. There is an increase in growth factor–independent cellular proliferation from activation of the *RAS* gene and a decrease in or resistance to apoptosis. New clones of stem cells vulnerable to additional genetic changes lead to disease progression.[11,12]

The *BCR::ABL1* fusion gene is also identified with Ph chromosome–positive ALL. The chromosome appears in 25% of adults and 3% to 5% of children with this disease. The minor chimeric *BCR::ABL1* gene that transcribes and translates to a p190 protein is present in 50% of Ph chromosome–positive ALL cases in adults and 90% of Ph chromosome–positive ALL cases in children. The micro *BCR,* when fused with the *ABL1* gene, produces a large p230 protein and is the least common version found.[15]

Peripheral Blood and Bone Marrow

Between 85% and 90% of patients with CML are diagnosed in chronic phase.[13] They present with a median white blood cell (WBC) count of 38×10^9/L, but it can be as high as 300 to 400 $\times$ 10^9/L. Anemia is usually absent, but thrombocytopenia is common with a median platelet count of 487×10^9/L with counts as high as 1000 to 2000 $\times$ 10^9/L. There are dramatic morphologic changes in the peripheral blood and bone marrow that reflect the expansion of the granulocyte pool, particularly in the later maturational stages. Figure 32.3 illustrates a common pattern in the peripheral blood of chronic phase CML at the time of diagnosis. Leukocytosis is readily apparent at scanning microscopy powers. Segmented neutrophils, bands, metamyelocytes, and myelocytes predominate, and immature and mature eosinophils and basophils are increased. A deep left shift is expected with median myelocytes at 11.5% and metamyelocytes at 3%, respectively. Basophilia may be a sensitive and specific screening tool to suggest CML over other causes of leukocytosis.[16] Table 32.1 lists the qualitative changes in the peripheral blood, bone marrow, and extramedullary tissues that are commonly observed at the time of diagnosis.

Extramedullary granulopoiesis may involve sinusoids and medullary cords in the spleen and sinusoids, portal tract zones, and solid areas of the liver. Bone marrow changes are illustrated in Figure 32.4. An intense hypercellularity is present, resulting from granulopoiesis, marked by broad zones of immature granulocytes, usually perivascular or periosteal, differentiating into more centrally placed mature granulocytes. Normoblasts appear reduced in number. Megakaryocytes are normal or increased in number and, when increased, may appear in clusters and exhibit dyspoietic cytologic changes. They often appear small with reduced nuclear size (by approximately 20%) and reduced nuclear lobulations. Reticulin fibers are increased in approximately 20% of patients. Increased megakaryocyte density is associated with an increase in myelofibrosis.

Other Laboratory Findings

In patients with the typical peripheral blood findings discussed earlier, diagnosis of CML is confirmed by demonstrating the presence of the t(9;22) translocation by cytogenetic analysis (Figure 30.18), detection of the *BCR::ABL1* fusion gene using fluorescence in situ hybridization (Figures 30.19–30.21), and/or detection of the fusion transcript by quantitative reverse transcription polymerase chain reaction (RT-PCR) (Figures 29.11, 29.15, and 29.16).

Although molecular techniques are more commonly used to diagnose CML, initial testing of the cells for leukocyte alkaline phosphatase (LAP) enzyme activity may be useful in some settings for preliminary differentiation of CML from a leukemoid reaction caused by severe infection (Chapter 26). LAP is an enzyme found in the membranes of secondary granules of neutrophils. To perform the LAP, a blood film is incubated with a naphthol-phosphate substrate and diazo dye at an alkaline pH. The LAP enzyme hydrolyzes the substrate and the liberated naphthol reacts with the dye, producing a colored precipitate on the granules. The slide is examined microscopically, and 100 segmented neutrophils and bands are counted and rated from

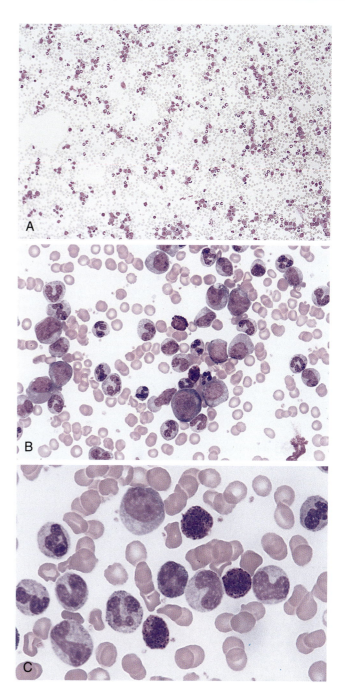

Figure 32.3 Peripheral Blood Films From a Patient in Chronic Phase Chronic Myeloid Leukemia. **(A),** Leukocytosis is evident at scanning power (Wright-Giemsa stain, ×100.) **(B),** Bimodal population of segmented neutrophils and myelocytes (Wright-Giemsa stain, ×500.) **(C),** Increased basophils and immature neutrophils (Wright-Giemsa stain, ×1000.)

0 to 4+, based on the intensity of the staining. The LAP score is calculated by multiplying each score by the number of cells and adding the products. For example, 5 cells with 4+ staining, 5 cells with 3+, 25 cells with 2+, 45 cells with 1+, and 20 cells with 0 staining are calculated as a LAP score of 130. Because scoring is subjective, the mean score of two examiners is reported, and they should agree within 10%. A sample reference interval for the LAP score is 15 to 170, but every laboratory establishes its own reference interval. The LAP score is decreased in

TABLE 32.1   Common Morphologic Changes in Chronic Myeloid Leukemia

Peripheral Blood

Erythrocytes	Normal or decreased
Reticulocytes	Normal
Nucleated red blood cells	Present
Total white blood cells	Increased
Lymphocytes	Normal or increased
Neutrophils	Increased
Basophils	Increased
Eosinophils	Increased
Myelocytes	Increased
Leukocyte alkaline phosphatase	Decreased
Platelets	Normal or increased

Bone Marrow

Cellularity	Increased
Granulopoiesis	Increased
Erythropoiesis	Decreased
Megakaryopoiesis	Increased or normal
Reticulin	Increased

Macrophages

Gaucher-like	Sea blue
Green-gray crystals	Increased

Megakaryocytes

Small	Increased

Extramedullary Tissue

Splenomegaly	Present
Sinusoidal	Present
Medullary	Present
Hepatomegaly	Present
Sinusoidal	Present
Portal tract	Present
Local infiltrates	Present

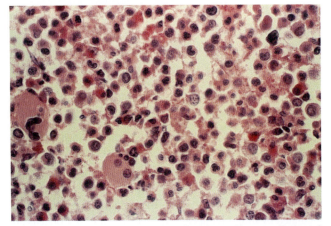

Figure 32.4 Bone Marrow Biopsy Specimen From a Patient in Chronic Phase Chronic Myeloid Leukemia. Note the hypercellularity with increased granulocytes and megakaryocytes. (Hematoxylin and eosin stain, ×400.)

untreated CML and normal or increased in leukemoid reactions. Individuals with PV or individuals in the third trimester of pregnancy can also have higher LAP scores.

Progression

Three stages of progression have been described for CML: chronic phase, high-risk chronic phase (previously known as accelerated phase), and blast phase. Before use of imatinib, most cases of CML would eventually reach blast phase and transform into acute leukemia within 3 to 4 years.[13] Disease progression is accompanied by an increase in the frequency and number of clinical symptoms, adverse changes in laboratory values, and poorer response to therapy than in the chronic phase. Additional chromosome abnormalities reflect evolution of the malignant clone and may appear associated with enhanced dyshematopoietic cell maturation patterns and increases in morphologic and functional abnormalities in blood cells. There is often an increasing degree of anemia and, in the peripheral blood, fewer mature leukocytes, more basophils, and fewer platelets, with a greater proportion of abnormal platelets, dwarf megakaryocytes, and megakaryocytic fragments. As the circulating blast count increases to 10% to 19%, anemia and thrombocytopenia either emerge or worsen.

Blast phase involves the peripheral blood, bone marrow, and extramedullary tissues. Based on definition of acute leukemia, blasts constitute more than 20% of total bone marrow cellularity, and the peripheral blood exhibits increased blasts. Blast phase leukemia usually is AML (70%) or ALL (30%), but origins from other hematopoietic clonal cells are possible.[13] Extramedullary growth may occur as lymphocytic or myeloid cell proliferations; the latter are often referred to as *myeloid sarcoma.* Myeloid sarcoma is observed at many sites or locations in the body and may precede a marrow blast crisis. The clinical symptoms of blast phase mimic those of acute leukemia, including severe anemia, leukopenia of all WBCs except blasts, and thrombocytopenia. Accumulation of genetically unstable hematopoietic progenitor cells driven by the BCR::ABL1 fusion protein is vulnerable to additional genetic mutations which, in combination with *BCR::ABL1*, stimulate disease progression. Certain disease-modulating mutations produce protein products that function to deregulate cell apoptosis and proliferation, such as epidermal growth factor receptor *(EGFR)*, tumor protein p53 *(TP53)*, and Schmidt-Ruppin A-2 proto-oncogene *(SRC)*; affect cell adhesion, such as catenin beta 1 *(CTNNB1)*; regulate hematopoiesis, such as runt-related transcription factor 1 *(RUNX1)*; result in chromatin remodeling, such as additional sex combs like 1 *(ASXL1)*; or regulate lymphoid differentiation, Ikaros zinc finger 1 *(IKZF1)*. Other genetic mutations are associated with transforming growth factor-β (TGF-β) such as SKI-like proto-oncogene *(SKIL)*, transforming growth factor beta 1 *(TGFB1)*, and transforming growth factor beta 2 *(TGFB2)*. Still other mutations occur in genes associated with tumor necrosis factor-α (TNF-α) pathways such as tumor necrosis factor alpha *(TNFA)* and nuclear factor kappa B subunit 1 *(NFKB1)*.[17,18]

Ph chromosome is sometimes found in patients with AML and ALL. It is understood that some of these cases likely represent undiagnosed CML that rapidly progressed to an acute leukemia before diagnosis. However, because rapidly dividing malignant cells are more prone to genetic mutation, the presence of Ph chromosome in acute leukemias may reflect a

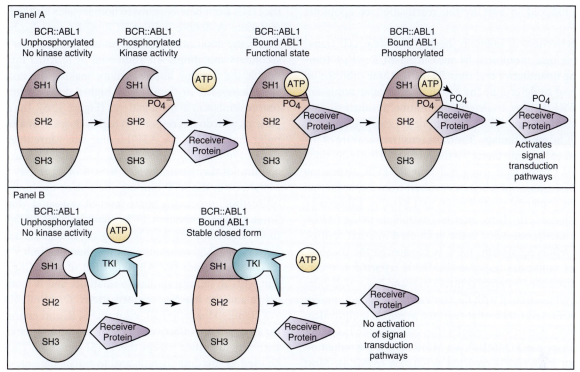

Figure 32.5 Mechanism of TKI Inhibition of BCR::ABL1 Tyrosine Kinase Activity. **(A),** Mechanism of tyrosine kinase activity of the BCR::ABL1 fusion protein. **(B),** Mechanism of tyrosine kinase inhibition by imatinib mesylate. *ATP,* Adenosine triphosphate; *TKI,* tyrosine kinase inhibitor.

late-stage mutation that contributed little to acute leukemia leukemogenesis.

Treatment

Early treatment approaches for CML were unable to produce remission, so the goal of therapy became the reduction of tumor burden. The first forms of therapy for CML included alkylating agents such as nitrogen mustard,[19] introduced in the late 1940s, and busulfan,[20] which came into use in the early 1950s. Later, busulfan in combination with 6-thioguanine was used to achieve the goal of tumor burden reduction. Other drugs such as hydroxyurea and 6-mercaptopurine were introduced later and found to improve patient survival. The discovery of interferon-α in 1983 dramatically improved outcomes of patients with CML by inducing the suppression of the Ph chromosome, reducing the rate of cellular progression to blast cells, and increasing the frequency of long-term patient survival, especially when combined with cytarabine.[21,22] Using former cytoreductive treatment approaches, most patients would experience disease progression and eventually succumb to their disease.

During this period, bone marrow transplantation with either autologous or allogeneic HSCs were the best hope of cure, especially in patients younger than age 55. Relapses occurred, but long-term, disease-free survival was possible. Optimal survival occured when the patient was treated during the chronic phase within 1 year of diagnosis and was younger than age 50. Treatment required ablative chemotherapy, followed by transplantation of mobilized normal progenitor cells that exhibited CD34+ surface markers. Allogeneic bone marrow transplants were more successful in patients up to age 55 with donors matched for HLA antigens A, B, and DR. Donor-matched lymphocyte infusions after allogeneic transplantation of marrow from a sibling donor may assist in producing complete remissions or to restore lost remission if reinfused.[14]

Current first-line therapy involves the use of synthetic proteins (TKIs) that bind the abnormal BCR::ABL1 protein, blocking the constitutive tyrosine kinase activity and reducing signal transduction activation. Imatinib mesylate was the first synthetic TKI designed to selectively bind the ATP binding site and thus inhibit the tyrosine kinase activity of the BCR::ABL1 fusion protein. When imatinib binds the ATP binding site, ATP is unable to bind to provide the phosphate group necessary for kinase activity. Imatinib binds the BCR::ABL1 protein in the inactive conformation, which precedes the autophosphorylation necessary to generate the kinase active site (Figure 32.5).[23] Imatinib has also been shown to bind the ATP binding site of other tyrosine kinases, including TEL::ABL1, stem cell factor receptor (a-KIT, b-KIT, c-KIT), and platelet-derived growth factor receptor (PDGFR), lymphocyte-specific kinase (Lck), vascular endothelial growth factor receptor-1 (VEGFR-1), VEGFR-2, VEGFR-3, colony-stimulating factor receptor-1 (CSFR-1), nicotinamide adenine dinucleotide phosphate (NAD[P]H), dehydrogenase, quinone 2 (NQ02), and c-Raf in most tissues. Therefore imatinib may be a useful treatment option in other conditions, but it raises questions about clinical efficacy and toxicity.[24]

Goals of therapy include complete hematologic, cytogenetic, and molecular remission as indicated by a normalized complete blood count (CBC) and differential, absence of Ph chromosome by karyotype analysis, and absence of measurable *BCR::ABL1* transcripts, respectively. Complete remission from imatinib therapy is induced in part by the reactivation of apoptotic pathways.[25]

The effectiveness of imatinib therapy and stem cell transplantation is best monitored by measuring *BCR::ABL1* transcripts using quantitative real-time RT-PCR. These monitoring tools are used to determine the extent of molecular remission following TKI therapy, to determine minimal residual disease following stem cell transplants, and to detect early relapse following both forms of therapy. The most sensitive measure of the effectiveness of imatinib therapy is the number of log reductions of *BCR::ABL1* transcripts using real-time RT-PCR. Reporting of *BCR::ABL1* transcript levels has evolved from log reduction to *BCR::ABL1*/internal control ratios as a percent, adjusted by the international scale. Three internal controls are in use (*ABL1, GUSB,* and *BCR*), but *ABL1* is the most used internal control. Using this reporting system, 100% is considered the baseline, and a major molecular response (MMR) is reported as a percentage (*BCR::ABL1*/internal control ratio) and has a molecular response level associated with the equivalent log reduction. For example, *BCR::ABL1* transcript reported as ≤0.1% is equivalent to a 3-log reduction in transcript level and is designated as major molecular response 3 (MMR3). An MMR4 is a 4-log reduction in transcript level and is reported as <0.01% (MMR4). Most assay systems report a maximum sensitivity of 4.5 log reduction or 0.0032% on the international scale.[14] Remission milestones indicating effective imatinib therapy are complete hematologic remission in 3 to 6 months, complete cytogenetic response in 6 months to 1 year, and a 2- to 3-log reduction in *BCR::ABL1* transcripts. Sustained remission is best predicted by the rate to achieve MMR3 and if MMR4 is achieved. Patients who sustained MMR4 for 12 months are unlikely to drop below MMR3 (*BCR::ABL1* >0.1%) within 1 year (0%) or 5 years (2.6%). For patients achieving MMR3 but not MMR4, the odds of loss of MMR3 are higher at year 1 (4.4%) and year 5 (25.4%). Loss of MMR is attributed to both a loss of compliance and drug resistance.[26] However, discontinuation of imatinib therapy in patients who achieve a more than 4-log reduction usually results in relapse.

Although imatinib has proven to be a successful form of therapy, a major limitation is the development of imatinib resistance resulting in relapse. Approximately 25% to 30% of patients with newly diagnosed CML will discontinue imatinib therapy within 5 years because of lack of remission or the development of resistance or toxicity. About 17% of these patients develop imatinib resistance at 5 years.[27] The two major categories of imatinib resistance are primary and secondary. Primary resistance is defined as the inability to reach the remission milestones. This form of resistance accounts for most treatment failures and probably results from the presence of mutations other than the *BCR::ABL1* mutation at the time of diagnosis. Secondary resistance involves the loss of a previous response and occurs at a rate of 16% at 42 months. The majority of cases of imatinib resistance result from two primary causes: acquisition of additional *BCR::ABL1* mutations and expression of point mutations in the ATP binding site (33% to 50%). Additional *BCR::ABL1* mutations can occur through the usual translocation of the remaining unaffected chromosomes 9 and 22, which converts

the HSCs from heterozygous to homozygous for the *BCR::ABL1* mutation. A double dose of *BCR::ABL1* can also be acquired from gene duplication during mitosis and accounts for 10% of secondary mutations. An additional *BCR::ABL1* mutation will double the tyrosine kinase activity, making the imatinib dosage inadequate. In these cases, higher doses of imatinib will restore remission in most patients (Figure 32.6). The majority of patients who do not respond to higher doses of imatinib express point mutations in the ATP binding site. More than 60 mutations have been identified in the ATP binding site, and these account for the remaining 50% to 90% of secondary mutations. Mutations in the ATP binding site reduce the binding affinity of imatinib, producing some level of resistance (Figure 32.7). Three second-generation TKIs—dasatinib, nilotinib, and bosutinib—overcome the ATP binding site mutations because they have a much higher binding affinity than imatinib.[27–29]

Dasatinib binds the ABL1 portion of the BCR::ABL1 protein with an affinity similar to imatinib, and it binds both the active and the inactive conformations. Dasatinib also inhibits SRC family kinases (SFK), c-kit, PDGFR, and ephrin A receptor kinase.[24] It is effective against all imatinib-resistant mutants currently identified except the T315I mutation. Dasatinib can be used as first-line therapy and to rescue patients resistant to imatinib therapy unless the T315I mutation has been identified.

Nilotinib binds to the ATP binding site of the ABL1 protein in the inactive conformation with 30 times greater potency than imatinib. Structurally, nilotinib is a derivative of imatinib and binds more specifically than imatinib to ABL1, stabilizing the ABL1 protein. Nilotinib also binds PDGFR and kit family kinases.[24] Similar to dasatinib, nilotinib can be used as first-line therapy and to rescue patients with imatinib resistance against all mutants currently identified except the T315I mutation.

Bosutinib binds both the active and the inactive conformations of ABL1 and is 10 times more potent than imatinib. It inhibits ABL1 and SRC kinases, fibroblast growth factor receptor (FGFR), and mitogen-activated protein kinase (MAPK), but does not significantly inhibit PDGFR or c-kit. Similar to dasatinib and nilotinib, it is effective against most imatinib-resistant mutants except the T315I mutation, showing a complete hematologic response in 83% and a complete cytogenetic response in 23% of imatinib- and dasatinib-resistant patients. Because the T315I mutation is not treatable by any of the first- and second-generation TKIs, other non-TKI therapies have also been developed. First-line treatment with second-generation TKIs is showing superior results, with earlier and more profound remissions and fewer relapses from TKI resistance in patients with newly diagnosed CML compared with inatinib.[15]

All three second-generation TKIs are approved by the US Food and Drug Administration (FDA) for first-line therapy and are effective at rescuing patients resistant to imatinib except for patients (about 15%) who have developed the T315I mutation. The T315I mutation places a large, bulky isoleucine residue in the center of the ATP binding site, and all four FDA-approved TKIs are resistant to this mutation. However, a third-generation TKI, ponatinib, inhibits the T315I mutation.[27–29]

Ponatinib was approved by the FDA in 2012 as a rescue therapy for patients resistant to imatinib, dasatinib, and nilotinib

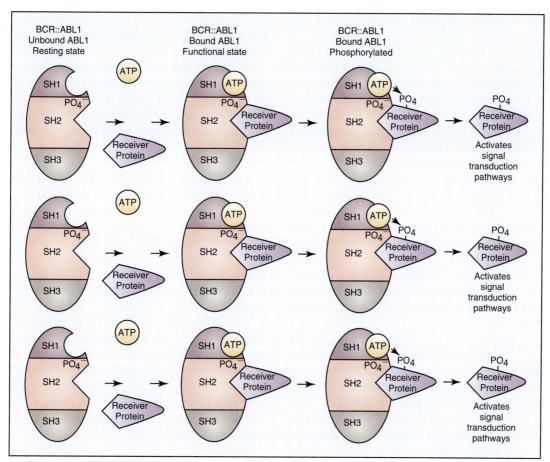

Figure 32.6 Mechanism of TKI Resistance due to an Increased Copy Number of *BCR::ABL1* Genes. The increased copies produce more BCR::ABL1 fusion proteins, which results in increased tyrosine kinase activity, requiring a higher dosage of imatinib to restore remission. *ATP*, Adenosine triphosphate; *TKI*, tyrosine kinase inhibitor.

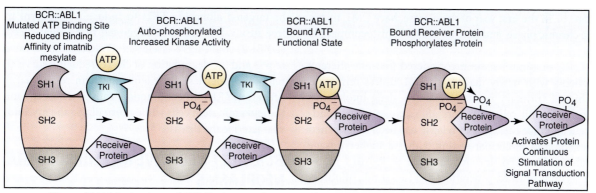

Figure 32.7 Mechanism of TKI Resistance Because of Point Mutations in the ATP Binding Site. The mutations reduce the binding affinity of imatinib, allowing ATP to bind; this restores the increased tyrosine kinase activity that drives the phenotype and pathogenesis of the disease. *ATP*, Adenosine triphosphate; *TKI*, tyrosine kinase inhibitor.

when administered as a tablet taken once a day. Ponatinib was shown to rescue about 70% of patients who developed the T315I mutation in response to first- and second-generation TKI therapy.[13] In addition to inhibiting the T315I mutation, it can also inhibit a wide range of tyrosine kinases, including PDGFR, c-kit, SFK, FGFR, VEGFR-1, VEGFR-2, VEGFR-3, Flt-3, RET, and ARG.[24,30] In 2013, ponatinib was given a revised warning notice, listing a thrombotic risk of about 13% per year.[31]

The newest third-generation TKI, asciminib, was approved by the FDA in 2021 for CML patients in chronic phase previously treated with two or more TKIs or who developed the T315I mutation. Asciminib binds the myristoyl site of the BCR::ABL1 protein, converting it to an inactive conformation. Binding outside the ATP binding site allows tyrosine kinase inhibition in the presence of the T315I mutation. Rescues from TKI relapses are occurring in patients on asciminib with restored hematologic remission (92%), complete cytogenetic remission (54%), and major molecular remission (28%).[31]

Homoharringtonine was originally discovered and used for CML therapy before the development of TKIs. It was reintroduced as a supplemental therapy to TKIs to rescue patients who developed TKI resistance. Homoharringtonine is a plant alkaloid that induces apoptosis, inhibits protein synthesis, and upregulates B cell chronic lymphocytic leukemia/lymphoma (BCL-2)-associated X protein (BAX) and caspase-mediated cleavage of poly (ADP) ribose polymerase (PARP).[24]

Omacetaxine is a semisynthetic derivative of homoharringtonine and was approved by the FDA as rescue therapy in 2012 and received full approval in 2014. It was designed for more efficient manufacturing compared with homoharringtonine. Omacetaxine is administered as subcutaneous injection twice daily for 14 days of a 28-day cycle for the induction phase, followed by 7 days of a 28-day cycle for maintenance. Omacetaxine has been shown to induce apoptosis but by downregulating myeloid cell leukemia sequence-1 (Mcl-1), which is *BAX* independent.[24]

The development of a care plan for treating patients with newly diagnosed CML is an ongoing commitment requiring not only the formulation of alternative approaches to achieve and maintain complete cellular remission but also the establishment of laboratory monitoring parameters to follow and confirm long-term success of therapy. Historically, chemotherapy has provided cellular remission but usually has not prevented clinical progression to accelerated or blast phases. During this period, bone marrow transplantation was the preferred approach for curative treatment available for patients who qualify. However, the long-term success (cure) rate remains at 50% to 70%, and most patients will not qualify. For a patient to qualify for transplantation, the patient must be younger than 50 years of age, be in the first year of the disease, have CML that is still in the chronic phase, and have an available histocompatible donor.

Since 2001, imatinib has been considered first-line therapy for all patients with newly diagnosed CML unless remission is not achieved (primary resistance), unless drug intolerance is indicated, or until relapse occurs after remission (secondary resistance). Once the cause of relapse has been determined by cytogenetic and molecular testing, either a higher dosage of imatinib can be given (for an additional *BCR::ABL1* mutation) or a second- or third-generation TKI (dasatinib, nilotinib, bosutinib) can be prescribed, unless the T315I mutation is present in the ATP binding site. In this case the patient can be given ponatinib or an A-loop inhibitor (ONO12380), or other drugs like omacetaxine, MK 0457, or BIRB-796 that inhibit the T315I mutation.[25] Dasatinib, nilotinib, and bosutinib are being used as first-line therapy in hopes that TKIs with higher binding affinities will extend remissions by reducing the rate of mutation-induced relapses. Among the second-generation TKIs, bosutinib shows the most promise because it demonstrates high potency; has the ability to overcome most P-loop mutations (except T315I); and shows fewer side effects such as neutropenia, thrombocytopenia, cardiotoxicity, and pancreatitis compared with nilotinib and dasatinib. Ponatinib and A-loop

inhibitors can be used to rescue patients treated with second-generation TKIs, particularly patients who develop the T315I mutation.[27]

Treatment-free remission is being explored in patients who developed and maintained a deep molecular remission. Several studies report maintenance of a deep molecular remission approaching 50% (38% to 65%) for 5 to 10 years following the discontinuation of first-line TKI therapy. Conversely, about half of patients relapse when TKI therapy is discontinued. Findings most predictive of relapse following discontinuation were length of total TKI therapy (should to be >74.8 months), *BCR::ABL1* levels at TKI discontinuation (should be <0.0023% [MMR4.5]), immune cell numbers (high natural killer cells and low regulatory T cells and monocyte-derived myeloid suppressor cells), and halving time of *BCR::ABL1* levels on initial therapy (should be <9.35 days). Relapse rate after 2 years of TKI discontinuation is about 14%. If relapse occurs following TKI discontinuation, patients tend to retain TKI sensitivity once treatment is resumed.[31]

Gene expression studies on peripheral blood, bone marrow samples, CD34+ cells, and single cells are beginning to demonstrate genetic and epigenetic events responsible for causing loss of remission, other than ATP binding site mutations, following TKI therapy. Gene expression studies have not identified a specific gene expression signature that predicts loss of remission, but this approach is showing promise in tailoring therapy for patients with CML.[32]

Relapse following TKI discontinuation suggests that the leukemic stem cell population is responsible for the chemoresistance. TKIs target and inhibit proliferation of developing myeloid cells resulting in the various levels (hematology, cytogenetic, molecular) of remission that most patients with CML achieve. However, the leukemic stem cell population must be targeted alongside TKIs to induce a long-term treatment-free survival. It has been suggested that a dual-specific kinase (DYRK2) could serve as a target. DYRK2 controls the activation of p53 and the degradation of cMYC reducing survival and self-renewal properties of the leukemic stem cells. Dual therapy to activate DYRK2 in conjunction with TKI therapy may inhibit the leukemic stem cells while normalizing the myeloid cells that characterize the disease.[33]

BCR::ABL1-NEGATIVE MYELOPROLIFERATIVE NEOPLASMS

Background

The *BCR::ABL1* negative MPNs are composed mainly of three specific disorders: ET, PV, and primary myelofibrosis (PMF). These conditions primarily affect older people between 53 and 64 years of age. These MPNs are clonal stem cells disorders that present with an increase in one or more myeloid cells lines (platelets, erythrocytes, myelocytes) that are morphologically and functionally normal. Overproduction of normal cells explains the long survival (decades) compared to other hematologic neoplasms (months to years). ET must present with thrombocytosis but can also exhibit leukocytosis and a left shift; PV must present with erythrocytosis but also shows leukocytosis two thirds of the time and thrombocytosis half the time; PMF initially presents with a leukocytosis and a left shift but can also exhibit thrombocytosis. As the name implies, PMF slowly develops fibrosis in the bone marrow that inhibits hematopoiesis, eventually resulting in pancytopenia. Overlap in cell production results in disease mimicry that complicates accurate diagnosis. Several clinical scoring systems have been developed to attempt standardization of diagnoses and track progression. These MPNs can convert from one to another, further complicating the diagnostic process. ET can convert to either PV or secondary MF (sMF), and PV can transform into sMF. Once myelofibrosis commences, prognosis worsens and overall survival is reduced. Any of the three disorders can progress from a myeloproliferative neoplasm in the chronic phase (MPN-CP) to a myeloproliferative neoplasm in the blast phase (MPN-BP) and can terminate in an acute leukemia.[34]

Molecular Pathophysiology

ET, PV, and PMF share three common gain-of-function driver mutations: (1) JAK2 (JAK2 V617F); (2) calreticulin (CALR); and (3) myeloproliferative leukemia virus oncogene (MPL), also called thrombopoietin (TPO) receptor (TPOR). These driver mutations result in the constitutive activation of the thrombopoietic receptor (TPOR or MPL) resulting in continuous activation of the JAK2 signaling pathway. JAK2 V617F and CALR mutations were found in 3.1% and 0.16%, respectively, of the general population suggesting that these mutations may occur years before symptom onset, in childhood and possibly as early as infancy.[35] The MPL receptor is the only hematopoietic receptor on HSCs, and it is essential to maintaining quiescence or stimulating proliferation. Controlling quiescence maintains normal proliferation rates, while uncontrolled proliferation results in increasing numbers of megakaryocytic, erythrocytic, and myelocytic cells. Because all three driver mutations act to stimulate the TPO receptor, thrombocytosis is a common feature in ET, PV, and PMF. The driver mutations occur in the HSCs, gradually resulting in accumulation of mutated HSCs, while the overproduction of mature myeloid cells occurs at the level of the committed stem cell. The degree of accumulation of mutated HSCs produces a clonal HSC burden that predicts overall survival. Clonal burden is lowest in ET, highest in PMF, and variable in PV.[34]

The normal JAK2 protein is a tyrosine kinase enzyme much like the ABL1 moiety of the BCR::ABL1 fusion gene found in CML. Normally the JAK2 protein is closely associated with cytokine receptors, mainly erythropoietin, TPO, and granulocyte colony-stimulating factor (G-CSF), and functions near the cell membrane. When a cytokine receptor binds its ligand, the JAK2 protein becomes activated through transphosphorylation when bound to the cytoplasmic region of the receptor. Once activated, the kinase activity of JAK2 phosphorylates signal transducers and activators of transcription (STAT) proteins, eventually generating transcription proteins that bind promoter regions and signal gene expression. The JAK-receptor complex also activates other signaling pathways.[36]

The normal JAK2 protein controls transphosphorylation through conformational inhibition. JAK2 has seven domains

(JH1 through JH7), but two domains (JH1 and JH2) control the kinase activity. JH1 has kinase activity and JH2 does not have kinase activity (pseudokinase). Normally, JH2 folds and interacts with the JH1 domain to inhibit kinase activity and to modulate or regulate receptor signaling.[41] Mutations in the JH2 domain remove this inhibitory function.[37]

The most common JAK2 mutation, JAK2 V617F, is detected in more than 95% of patients with PV and is found on chromosome band 9p24. Shortly after the JAK2 V617F mutation was reported, several groups corroborated the finding using other approaches and reported that the mutation is acquired, clonal, present in the HSCs, constitutively active, and capable of activating the erythropoietic signal transduction pathway in the absence of erythropoietin.[38,39] The point mutation replaces guanine with thymine at exon 14 of the gene, which changes the amino acid at position 617 from valine to phenylalanine in the pseudokinase domain. This one amino acid change prevents the inhibition conformation of the tyrosine kinase, causing it to remain in the active conformation. More specifically, the phenylalanine mutation in the kinase domain is unable to bind the corresponding amino acid in the pseudokinase domain, as can the valine in the wild-type counterpart, which prevents the protein from folding into the inactive conformation (Figure 32.8).[40–42]

Normally, erythropoietin is released from the kidney into the blood in response to hypoxia and binds to erythropoietin receptors on the surface of erythroid precursor cells. The resulting conformational change in the erythropoietin receptor causes two erythropoietin receptors to dimerize. This produces a docking point for the head of the inactive JAK2 protein at the FERM domain (Band-4.1, ezrin, radixin, and moesin).[43,44] Docking of JAK2 stimulates a phosphorylation event, causing a conformational change, and the valine releases from the pseudokinase domain, converting it to an active tyrosine kinase. JAK2 can also bind to several other receptors, including MPL (also known as TPO receptor), G-CSF receptor, prolactin receptor, growth hormone receptor (GHR), granulocyte-macrophage colony-stimulating factor (GM-CSF) receptor, cytokine receptor-like factor 2, interleukin-3 receptor (IL-3-R), IL-5-R, and interferon-γ2 receptor (IFN-γ2-R).[3,42] The diversity in ligand receptor binding of JAK2 partially explains the range of myeloid proliferation observed in the MPNs in which the JAK2 mutation is found: PV (erythroid), ET (thrombopoietic), and neutrophilic (PMF). Once activated, JAK2 phosphorylates several cytoplasmic proteins, primarily through the STAT proteins producing activated transcription factors that activate a host of genes designed to drive and control cell proliferation and differentiation, while also initiating apoptosis (Figure 32.9).

Constitutive tyrosine kinase activity of the mutated JAK2 protein causes continuous activation of several signal transduction pathways that are normally activated after erythropoietin stimulation via the erythropoietic receptor. Mutated JAK2 is active and will phosphorylate STAT proteins in the absence of erythropoietin or will overphosphorylate in its presence (Figure 32.10).[37] HSCs that bear the JAK2 mutation are resistant to erythropoietin-deprivation apoptosis by upregulation of BCL-X, an antiapoptotic protein. JAK2-bearing progenitor cells do not divide more rapidly but accumulate because they do not die

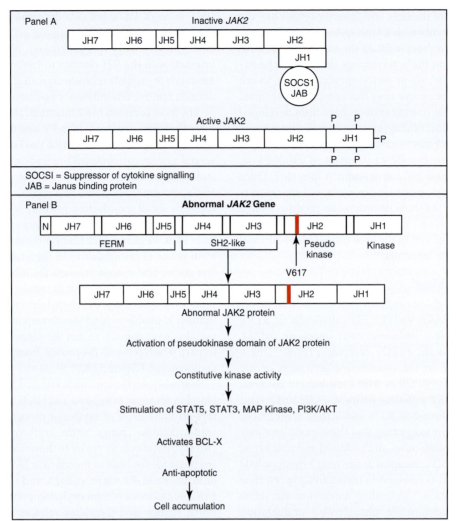

Figure 32.8 Normal Regulation of JAK2 Function and Loss of Regulation from the *JAK2* V617F Mutation. **(A)**, Normal function of the *JAK2* protein and regulation of phosphorylation by *JAK2* intrachain folding and the binding of JAK2 inhibitors SOCS1 and JAB proteins. **(B)**, The *JAK2* V617F mutation and the loss of normal JAK2 folding and inhibitor binding resulting in phosphorylation, activation, and the stimulation of STAT, MAP kinase, and PI3K/AKT signal transduction pathways. *JAK2*, Janus-activated kinase 2; *MAP*, mitogen-activated protein; *PI3K*, phosphoinositide-3 kinase; *STAT*, signal transducer and activator of transcription.

normally.[45–48] In addition to the role of mutated JAK2 in the abrogation of STAT signaling, it has also been shown to influence chromatin structure[49,50] and to decrease methyltransferase activity.[51–53]

JAK2 V617F is found in about 95% of patients with PV, with approximately 1% to 2% of the remaining 5% harboring another *JAK2* mutation in exon 12,[54] usually between amino acid residues 536 and 547, also resulting in a gain of function similar to *JAK2* V617F.[53] Exon 12 is not located in the pseudokinase domain, but it is hypothesized that the mutation can modify the structure of the JH2 domain, rendering the protein incapable of forming the inactive conformation.[55] *JAK2* exon 12 mutations have been found in 3% of patients with PV and are not associated with ET or PMF, but can be found in patients who progress to secondary myelofibrosis.[55,56]

JAK2 V617F is found in approximately 50% to 60% of ET and PMF patients, with most of the remaining patients expressing mutations in MPL (5% to 10%) or CALR (25% to 40%).[52]

A minority of patients with *BCR::ABL1*-negative MPN are negative for all three driver mutations, so-called triple-negative.[57]

Since the original discovery of a mutation in the thrombopoietic receptor gene *MPL* in 2006,[58] several gain-of-function mutations have been identified. *MPL* mutations occur in at least 3% of patients with ET and 5% of patients with PMF, with some reports as high as 5% to 10%.[54] Most *MPL* mutations occur in exon 10, where tryptophan 515 is substituted for a leucine, lysine, asparagine, or alanine.[59–61] Tryptophan 515 is located on the cytosolic side of the membrane and is key in transducing the signal that TPO has bound to the receptor. These mutations cause the MPL receptor to be hypersensitive to TPO and in some cases, to assume the active conformation in the absence of TPO. A similar mutation, *MPL* S505N, was initially described in familial PV but has since been found in sporadic MPN.[42]

Experts hypothesize that mutations in signaling molecules alone are insufficient to initiate MPNs, suggesting that other mutations are necessary before *JAK2* V617F to induce disease

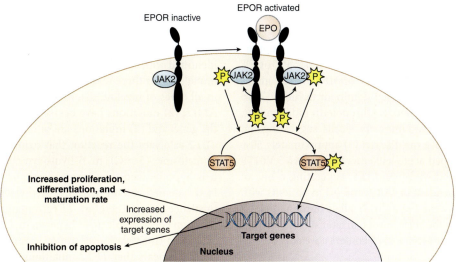

Figure 32.9 Activation of the Erythropoietin Receptor by Erythropoietin. The EPOR on erythroid precursors has an extracellular domain, a single-transmembrane domain, and a cytoplasmic tail with many associated JAK2 molecules (only one shown associated with each receptor). One EPO molecule binds the extracellular domain of two EPORs, resulting in dimerization and a conformational change that triggers activation *(P)* of the associated JAK2 kinases by transphosphorylation and autophosphorylation. Multiple tyrosine residues in the EPOR cytoplasmic domain are also phosphorylated. This results in activation of various signal transduction pathways, the predominant one involving the STAT5 or the JAK/STAT5 pathway. JAK2 phosphorylates STAT5 transcription factors, which enter the nucleus, bind to promoters, and initiate transcription and expression of numerous target genes. Other signal transduction pathways are also activated, such as the MAPK and PI3K pathways (not shown). The result is an increase in proliferation, differentiation, and maturation rate and inhibition of apoptosis in erythroid precursors. *EPO,* Erythropoietin; *EPOR,* erythropoietin receptor; *JAK2,* Janus-activated kinase 2; *MAPK,* mitogen-activated protein kinase; *PI3K,* phosphoinositide-3 kinase; *STAT5,* signal transducer and activator of transcription 5. (From Kremyanskaya, M., Najfeld, V., Mascarenhas, J., et al. [2023]. The polycythemias. In Hoffman, R., Benz, E. J., Silberstein, L. E., et al. [Eds.], *Hematology Basic Principles and Practice.* [8th ed., pp. 1129–1168]. St. Louis: Elsevier; and Bhoopalan, S. V., Huang, L. J., & Weiss, M. J. [2020]. Erythropoietin regulation of red blood cell production: from bench to bedside and back. *F1000Res, 9,* 1153.)

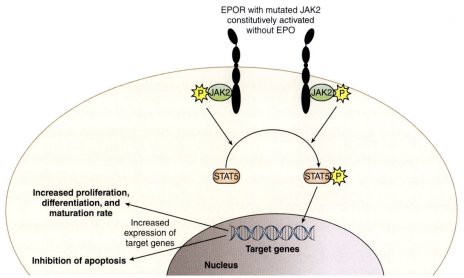

Figure 32.10 Erythropoietin Receptor With Associated Mutant *JAK2* Showing Activation in Absence of Erythropoietin. The EPOR on erythroid precursors has an extracellular domain, a single-transmembrane domain, and a cytoplasmic tail with many associated JAK2 molecules (only one shown associated with each receptor). Mutation in *JAK2* results in constitutive activation of various signal transduction pathways in the absence of erythropoietin. The predominant pathways involve the STAT5 or the JAK/STAT5 pathway. JAK2 phosphorylates STAT5 transcription factors, which enter the nucleus, bind to promoters, and initiate transcription and expression of numerous target genes. Other signal transduction pathways are also activated, such as the MAPK and phosphoinositide-3 kinase pathways (not shown). The result is an increase in proliferation, differentiation, and maturation rate and inhibition of apoptosis in erythroid precursors without erythropoietin stimulation. *EPO,* Erythropoietin; *EPOR,* erythropoietin receptor; *JAK2,* Janus-activated kinase 2; *MAPK,* mitogen-activated protein kinase; *STAT5,* signal transducer and activator of transcription 5. (From Kremyanskaya, M., Najfeld, V., Mascarenhas, J., et al. [2023]. The polycythemias. In Hoffman, R., Benz, E. J., Silberstein, L. E., et al. [Eds.], *Hematology Basic Principles and Practice.* [8th ed., pp. 1129–1168]. St. Louis: Elsevier; and Bhoopalan, S. V., Huang, L. J., & Weiss, M. J. [2020]. Erythropoietin regulation of red blood cell production: from bench to bedside and back. *F1000Res, 9,* 1153.)

and later, to drive progression. Four lines of evidence support this hypothesis: (1) familial MPN expresses a classic PV or ET phenotype in the absence of *JAK2* V617F or *MPL* W515L mutations and transmits in an autosomal dominant fashion; (2) in some ET and PV clones that were erythropoietin independent, *JAK2* V617F was identified in a minority of cells, suggesting that a pre-*JAK2* mutation drove the disease; (3) approximately 50% of patients who developed acute leukemia from a *JAK2* V617F form of MPN expressed wild-type *JAK2*, suggesting a line of clonal evolution independent of *JAK2*; and (4) in patients with PV and ET at diagnosis, the *JAK2* V617F allele burden in HSCs was low compared with the allele burden in later stages of hematopoiesis, suggesting that *JAK2* V617F confers a weak proliferative advantage to HSCs.[41]

Three reports in 2010 identified a germline haplotype block that predisposes patients to *JAK2* mutations.[62–64] This haplotype block was identified as a single nucleotide polymorphism (rs10974944) located in intron 12 of the *JAK2* gene, increasing the development of MPN by three- to fourfold.[40]

Disease Progression

Hyperproliferation predisposes HSCs to additional mutations resulting in disease progression down a variety of paths. ET can progress to PV, and either ET or PV can progress to sMF. Progression can also occur as the conversion of any of the MPNs in chronic phase (MPN-CP) to blast phase (MPN-BP) or to an overt acute leukemia. Leukemic progression is far more common in PMF. In some cases, initial progression of disease results from a loss of *JAK2* heterozygosity resulting in enhanced mutational allele frequencies caused by a second *JAK2* mutation of the other allele, uniparental disomy, or chromosomal duplication. Loss of heterozygosity enhances the cytokine-independent proliferation already present in the MPNs. However, driver mutations alone (*JAK2*, *MPL*, and *CALR*) may play a lesser role in disease progression, as triple-negative PV patients (negative for *JAK2*, *MPL*, and *CALR*) have a greater risk of leukemic transformation than PV patients with a high *JAK2* allele burden.

There is much overlap in the plethora of additional mutations identified thus far in MPNs, but they are not unique to the MPNs and contribute to disease progression. Most of these mutations appear to fall into three primary categories: mutations in epigenetic modifiers (i.e., *TET2*, *IDH 1/2*, *EZH2*, *ASXL1*, *DNMT3a*), mutations in transcription factors and signal transduction genes (i.e., *TP53*, *RUNX1*, *IK2F1*, *NRAS*, *SH2B3*[LNK], *CBL*, *NF1*, *FLT3*), and mutations in splicing factors (i.e., *SF3B1*, *U2AF1*, *SRSF2*, *ZRSR2*).[57] Not only do these mutations contribute to the progression of ET or PV to sMF and from MPN-CP to MPN-BP, but progression can demonstrate myelodysplastic cellular features also.

Epigenetic Modifiers *(TET2, IDH 1/2, EZH2, ASXL1, DNMT3a)*

Somatic mutations have been identified in genes that control DNA methylation in patients with PV and other MPNs. The most notable are *TET2* (ten eleven translocation 2), *IDH1* (isocitrate dehydrogenase 1), and *IDH2*. *TET2* is one of three members

of the *TET* family of genes (*TET1* and *TET3*) and the only one identified with sequence alterations. *TET2* appears to be highly mutagenic for three reasons: (1) mutations have been identified in all types of myeloid disorders, including MPNs, MDSs, and AMLs; (2) mutations have been found in all coding regions of the gene; and (3) mutations are often biallelic (homozygous).[65] *TET2* catalyzes the reaction that oxidizes the 5-methyl group of cytosine (5-mC) to 5-hydroxymethycytosine (5-hmC).[66] It is hypothesized that 5-hmC serves as an intermediate base in the demethylation of DNA. Methylation of histones serves to silence genes. Therefore *TET2* mutations produce a loss-of-function effect, resulting in hypermethylation and a loss of gene activation (inactivation of tumor suppressor genes).[40] In addition, it appears that *TET2* mutations precede *JAK2* mutations based on three observations: (1) *TET2* mutations are expressed in CD34[+] HSCs; (2) *TET2* mutations have been identified in all forms of myeloid disorders; and (3) all patients with both *TET2* and *JAK2* mutations produced clones with both mutations and clones that were *TET2* positive and *JAK2* negative, but none that were *JAK2* positive and *TET2* negative. Therefore *TET2* mutations may create abnormal clones that predispose to *JAK2* mutations.[65] *TET2* mutations have been identified in 9.8% to 16% of PV patients, 4.4% to 5% of ET patients, and 7.7% to 17% of PMF patients.[40]

Mutations in the genes that code for the citric acid cycle enzymes isocitrate dehydrogenase 1 (IDH1) and isocitrate dehydrogenase 2 (IDH2) have been associated with hypermethylation of DNA in patients with MPN and AML.[67] Normally, these enzymes function to convert isocitrate to α-ketoglutarate, requiring the reduction of NAD(P)[+] to NADPH as the energy source. In patients with MPNs, mutations in *IDH1/2* occur most often at the *IDH2* R140 residue, the *IDH1* R132 residue, and the *IDA2* R172 residue.[68] These mutations are thought to alter enzyme function, causing the conversion of α-ketoglutarate to 2-hydroxyglutarate.[69] It is hypothesized that because *TET2* is dependent on α-ketoglutarate, the *IDH1/2* mutations would result in less α-ketoglutarate, thus impairing the function of *TET2* and exacerbating the hypermethylation function of mutated *TET2* protein products.[67] *IDH1/2* mutations occur most often (21.6% of patients) in patients with late-stage PV and ET during blast transformation compared with an incidence of 1% to 5% in patients with early PV (1.9%), ET (0.8%), and PMF (4.2%).[58] As expected, *IDH1/2* mutations are associated with adverse overall survival, raising the potential of using *IDH1/2* mutational analysis or 2-hydroxyglutarate detection as indicators of poor prognosis.

Mutations in two additional genes involved in epigenetic modification, *EZH2* and *ASXL1*, have been implicated in MPN, MDS, and MDS/MPN and along with *TET2*, may precede *JAK2* V617F mutations. *EZH2* and *EZH1* function as two of several proteins that form the polychrome repressive complex 2 (PRC2) that regulates chromatin structure. More specifically, *EZH1* and *EZH2* provide the functional domain for the PRC2 complex to methylate histone H3 at lysine 27.[70] The array of mutations noted in *EZH2* to date function to either eliminate protein production or abrogate methyltransferase activity. Mutations in *EZH2* have been identified in 3% of PV patients,

13% of PMF patients, 12.3% of MDS/MPN patients, and 5.8% to 23% of MDS patients.[71,72] *ASXL1* mutations have been identified in most myeloid malignancies and at a frequency similar to *TET2*.[41] *ASXL1* normally functions in conjunction with *ASXL2* and *ASXL3* to deubiquinate histone H2 to balance the activity of PRC1 to monoubiquinate target genes to modify chromatin structure.[73,74] Ubiquination tags proteins for natural removal, thus regulating their function. The function of *ASXL1* in hematopoiesis is poorly understood, but the loss-of-function mutations have been identified in less than 7% of PV and ET patients and 19% to 40% in PMF patients.[75,76]

Transcription Factors and Signal Transduction Genes (TP53, RUNX1, IK2F1, NRAS, SH2B3[LNK], CBL, NF1, FLT3)

Disease progression to blast crisis occurs in less than 10% of PV and ET patients, but several genetic mutations are implicated in this transformation.[77,78] In addition to mutations that modulate epigenetic changes previously discussed (in *IDH1/2* and *TET2*), mutations in *TP53* and *RUNX1* are involved in blast transformation. *TP53* gene produces the P53 protein that is known to be a tumor suppressor. P53 controls cell cycle checkpoints and apoptosis, and loss-of-function mutations are implicated in a host of cancers, including disease progression in the classic MPNs. *TP53* mutations have not been identified in MPNs in the chronic phase but have been found in 20% of patients with MPNs who have progressed to AML.[79-81] The protein product of the *RUNX1/AML1* gene is a transcription factor that is important in hematopoiesis. *RUNX1* mutations were identified in 30% of post-MPN-AML patients, making it a candidate for the most common mutation involved in MPN transformation to AML.[41]

Mutations in Splicing Factors (SF3B1, U2AF1, SRSF2, ZRSR2)

Splicing factors convert pre-messenger ribonucleic acid (mRNA) into mature mRNA by splicing out intron segments. Small nuclear ribonucleoprotein (snRNP) complexes composed largely of U1 and U2 associate with other proteins such as SF3B1, U2AF1, SRSF2, and ZRSR2 to form the spliceosome. Mutations in any of these splicing factors can result in mRNA that is longer than normal (contains additional exons or intron segments), is shorter than normal (exon splicing), or contains alternative exons. Any of these mutations can result in protein products with alternative functions. Splicing factor mutations are found more commonly in PMF than in ET or PV.[54]

Mutations in *ASXL1, IDH1/2, EZH2,* and *SRSF2* are detected in about one-third of patients with PMF and predict a shorter overall survival and a shorter leukemia-free survival. It is also suggested that mutations in *SRSF2, U2AF1, SF3B1, IDH1/2,* and *EZH2* correlate with the development of bone marrow fibrosis. Chromosomal aberrations identified from karyotype analysis are most influential in the final progression to acute leukemia.[35]

Inflammation has also been shown to contribute to disease progression by stimulating fibrosis formation in the bone marrow. Bone marrow cells from the malignant clone, normal hematopoietic cells, and nonhematopoietic cells each produce cytokines that stimulate "myofibroblasts" to produce fibrotic

tissue. A plethora of cytokines have been reported to contribute to the formation of fibrotic tissue, but IL-8 and IL-1β best predict progression from PMF to MPN-BP, and TNF-α is instrumental in the progression of any MPN to MPN-BP. Dysplastic megakaryocytes appear to be a major contributor to fibrosis by producing cytokines that stimulate the formation of myofibroblasts. Elevated levels of reactive oxygen species promote disease progression by promoting inflammation, enhancing JAK-STAT signaling to facilitate clonal dominance, and causing genomic instability, resulting in oxidative DNA damage.[35]

Clinically, disease progression may manifest as the development of thromboembolic events, major bleeding, pruritus, night sweats, fever, weight loss, or fatigue. Laboratory biomarkers to detect disease progression include an increasing WBC count, left shift on the differential, anemia, blasts, and increasing bone marrow fibrosis.

Diagnosis

Symptoms usually motivate patients to be evaluated and often include weakness, fatigue, bruising, bleeding, and thrombosis or, in the case of PV, hyperviscosity syndrome causing tinnitus, ruddy complexion, and blurred vision. Thrombotic events are more common in ET and PV. Sometimes MPNs are discovered serendipitously from CBC results indicating one or more myeloid cytoses. Regardless, elevated counts on the CBC that appear normal morphologically suggest MPNs, which are often confirmed by bone marrow analysis. There is much overlap in the clinical and laboratory presentation of MPNs, so accurate diagnosis is difficult, especially in non-*BCR::ABL1* MPNs. Certainly, the presence of the *BCR::ABL1* mutation confirms CML, and the *JAK2* mutation suggests *BCR::ABL1*-negative MPNs. It is suggested that *JAK2* mutations may occur decades before the *JAK2*-positive clone expands to the point of bone marrow detection or producing clinical symptoms. Detection of disease before clinical manifestations or cell count elevations may allow early interventions to prolong the asymptomatic, chronic phase of the disease or even disease reversal. Bone marrow disease precedes peripheral blood changes, but early disease is often undetected by bone marrow analysis because any given bone marrow sample is likely not to include sparse pockets containing the abnormal clone. Serial bone marrow sampling is not practical or efficacious. A variety of imaging techniques (ultrasound, computed tomography, positron emission tomography, and magnetic resonance imaging) show potential to provide early detection of disease. Magnetic resonance imaging has been shown to evaluate bone marrow fat content as a surrogate marker for bone marrow cellularity in PMF and possibly in ET and PV. Molecular imaging using radioactive uptake is also being studied and shows promise in identifying inflammation or malignant proliferation.[35]

Treatment

Standard treatment for ET and PV include hydroxyurea and anagrelide to prevent vascular events. JAK2 inhibitors such as ruxolitinib are most effective in PMF to reduce splenomegaly and other symptoms. Some patients can be resistant or intolerant to these therapies. First-line therapy for PV in the early stages is therapeutic phlebotomy. However, these treatments are not considered disease-modifying interventions and are not capable of eradicating the malignant clone. Interferon-α (IFN-α), especially pegylated IFN-α, has been shown to induce hematologic and molecular responses in patients with ET and PV, occasionally reaching complete remission. IFN-α and pegylated IFN-α are not as effective in PMF but may augment the effects of ruxolitinib if used together. Stem cell transplantation is the only therapy with curative potential but is reserved for the minority of patients who qualify.

JAK2 inhibitors. Ruxolitinib was the first JAK2 inhibitor approved by the FDA in 2011 for PMF and hydroxyurea-resistant or intolerant PV. Ruxolitinib binds with high affinity to the ATP-binding site of the active form of JAK1, JAK2, JAK3, and wild-type JAK proteins as well as the *JAK2* V617F mutation. In addition, ruxolitinib was tested against 26 other tyrosine kinases and found to have a low binding affinity for all 26 proteins.[24] Patients treated with ruxolitinib have demonstrated reduced splenomegaly and improvement in constitutional symptoms. Patients treated for PMF experience improved overall survival, improved medullary fibrosis, and in some patients, a reduced allelic load. In contrast, side effects include onset of anemia and thrombocytopenia in the early phases of treatment, opportunistic infections, skin cancer, and secondary malignant tumors following long-term use.[35]

Momelotinib is not only a JAK inhibitor, but it also inhibits type 1 activin receptors. Inhibition of the type 1 activin receptor downregulates hepcidin production in the liver, resulting in improved iron absorption from the gut and release of stored iron from macrophages.[82] Myelofibrosis, whether PMF or post ET/PV myelofibrosis, causes fibrosis in the bone marrow and anemia. Primary treatment with hydroxyurea and anagrelide can also induce anemia. Although momelotinib did not outperform ruxolitinib in reducing splenomegaly or symptom reduction, it did show evidence of improving the associated anemia. The MOMENTUM clinical trial is under way to evaluate the antianemia effects of momelotinib.[57]

Pacritinib is a JAK2 and FLT3 kinase inhibitor that is non-myelosuppressive. Because myelofibrosis eventually produces pancytopenia and thrombocytopenia, suggesting a poor prognosis, a JAK2 inhibitor that does not exacerbate anemia and thrombocytopenia may have clinical benefits.[55] The PERSIST-1 clinical trial indicated improved hemoglobin and platelet levels in patients with myelofibrosis and decreased splenomegaly.[83] The PACIFICA study is evaluating the efficacy of pacritinib in patients with myelofibrosis and severe thrombocytopenia.[84]

Fedratinib is a JAK2 and FLT3 inhibitor that was approved by the FDA in 2019 for post-ET and post-PV myelofibrosis. It was shown to reduce Total Symptom Score (TSS) and splenomegaly and is currently being considered for patients with myelofibrosis who are resistant to or have suboptimal responses to other JAK2 inhibitors such as ruxolitinib. Fedratinib continues to be studied in the FREEDOM trial involving myelofibrosis patients previously exposed to ruxolitinib.[57]

Jakitinib is an inhibitor for both JAK1 and JAK2 kinases and is being studied in clinical trials in patients with intermediate- to high-risk myelofibrosis, both primary and secondary, who are resistant to or have had suboptimal responses to ruxolitinib. Jakitinib is showing promise to reduce splenomegaly and potentially TSS and transfusion dependence.[57]

Combination therapies. Ruxolitinib is also being studied in clinical trials in combination with other drugs to either increase efficacy or improve tolerability by acting on other molecular targets. For example, luspatercept is an erythroid maturation agent that can counteract the erythrocyte suppression effect common with ruxolitinib therapy. When used in combination, luspatercept produced increased hemoglobin levels and reduced the need for transfusions. Parsaclisib is a phosphoinositol-3 kinase δ inhibitor that appears to work synergistically with ruxolitinib to reduce TSS and splenomegaly in patients with partial responses to ruxolitinib alone. Navitoclax is a nonselective inhibitor of B cell lymphoma-2 (Bcl-2) to regulate apoptosis. In combination with ruxolitinib, myelofibrosis patients with resistance or suboptimal responses to ruxolitinib showed decreases in splenomegaly, TSS, bone marrow fibrosis, and cytokine dysregulation. Pelabresib is a bromodomain and extraterminal domain (BET) inhibitor. In combination with ruxolitinib, patients with resistance or suboptimal responses to ruxolitinib showed decreases in splenomegaly, TSS, and bone marrow fibrosis and improvements in anemia.57

Non-JAK inhibitors. Several non-JAK inhibitor drugs are in clinical trials to study their ability to rescue myelofibrosis patients who have become resistant to ruxolitinib and have lost their clinical response. Imetelstat is a telomerase enzyme complex inhibitor that demonstrated a reduction in splenomegaly and TSS and improved overall survival.[85] KRT232 is an MDM2 (mouse double minute 2) inhibitor, which acts to reduce MDM2 levels. MDM2 binds p53 stimulating ubiquitization to produce proteolytic degradation of p53. KRT-232 stimulation lifts the inhibition of p53 to increase p53 levels and reduce uncontrolled cell growth. *JAK2* V617F may inhibit p53, so administration of KRT-232 may stimulate TP53 expression by inhibiting MDM2 expression. In myelofibrosis patients with nonmutated TP53 who relapsed or are refractory to ruxolitinib, KRT-232 showed improvements in splenomegaly and TSS. Bomedemstat is a lysine-specific demethylase 1 (LSD1) inhibitor being studied to reduce thrombocytosis in myelofibrosis and ET. Early results show symptom reduction, reduced splenic volume, reduced bone marrow fibrosis, and mutant allele burden reduction. Rusfertide is structurally similar to hepcidin and functions to reduce iron absorption and release from stores by degrading ferroportin. It is being studied in patients with phlebotomy-dependent PV to reduce erythrocyte counts and the frequency of phlebotomies. Ropeginterferon α-2b is a monopegylated interferon that has been studied in patients with PV needing cytoreduction. Preliminary results suggest higher complete hematologic remission rates and lower *JAK2* V617F allele burden compared with hydroxyurea supplemented with pegylated IFN-α-2a and JAK2 inhibitors. Givinostat is a histone deacetylase inhibitor that prevents the synthesis of mutated *JAK2* through epigenetic suppression. It is being studied in patients with PV requiring cytoreduction. Preliminary results suggest some level of hematologic remission and reductions in splenomegaly, itching, and allelic load. Givinostat may also work synergistically with hydroxyurea to better control overall symptoms and hematocrit levels.[57]

Essential Thrombocythemia

ET is a clonal MPN with increased megakaryopoiesis and sustained thrombocytosis and a risk of thrombosis and/or hemorrhage. The platelet count is usually greater than 600×10^9/L and sometimes greater than 1000×10^9/L. However, WHO criteria require a sustained thrombocytosis with a platelet count of 400×10^9/L or greater. Over the years, ET has been known as *primary thrombocytosis, idiopathic thrombocytosis,* and *hemorrhagic thrombocythaemia.*[1]

Incidence

In the absence of a well-defined diagnostic algorithm, determining the true incidence of ET has been difficult. When the diagnostic system developed by the Polycythemia Vera Study Group (PVSG) is applied, however, the incidence is estimated to be between 0.6 and 2.5 cases per 100,000 persons per year. The SEER study reported an overall incidence rate of 1.55/100,000 person-years.[86] The majority of cases occur in individuals between the ages of 50 and 60 years, but a second peak occurs primarily in women of childbearing age, approximately 30 years of age.[87]

Pathogenetic Mechanism

As previously described, *JAK2, MPL,* and *CALR* are considered driver mutations for ET and occur at a rate of 64.1% *(JAK2)* (range, 31.3% to 72.1%), 4.3% *(MPL)* (range, 0.9% to 12.5%), and 15.5% *(CALR)* (range, 12.6% to 50%). Some patients with ET are negative for both *JAK2* and *MPL,* but 10% to 15% of these patients are positive for the *CALR* mutation. The remaining patients, about 16%, are negative for all three driver mutations and are referred to as triple-negative patients. Most triple-negative patients have been found to express new somatic mutations in *JAK2* and *MPL* or an uncommon hereditary version.[88,89] Mutations in the erythropoietin and G-CSF cytokine receptors may activate *JAK2* in *JAK2* V617F-negative patients.

In ET, one *JAK2* V617F mutation is more common, but in PV, two *JAK2* V617F mutations are more common. Therefore *JAK2* V617F burden is thought to be critical in the transformation of ET to PV and in disease progression in PV.

As previously discussed, two *MPL* mutations (*MPL* W515L and *MPL* W515K) occur in approximately 4% of patients with *JAK2* V617F-negative ET and 10% with PMF. This mutation results in cytokine-independent growth and constitutive downstream signaling pathways and favors the ET phenotype.[42]

CALR, similar to *JAK2* and *MPL,* modulates the JAK-STAT pathway. Two type 1 (quantitative) and two type 2 (qualitative) mutations have been described in *CALR*. ET patients with a *CALR* mutation show 45% type 1 mutations and 39% type 2 mutations. These mutations occurred in the last exon that codes for the C-terminal amino acids. CALR proteins normally locate to the endoplasmic reticulum, but these mutations alter the subcellular localization. The *CALR* mutation was associated with a higher platelet count, but patients experience thrombosis rates half those of ET patients with a *JAK2* mutation. ET patients with the *CALR* mutation have lower WBC and hemoglobin levels

compared with ET patients with a *JAK2* mutation, and most do not progress to PV.[88]

Several other mutations previously discussed also occur in ET, including *TET2* (4.4% to 5%), *ASXL1* (5.6%), *LNK* (3% to 6%), and *IDH1/2* (0.8%).[88] The manner in which these mutations alter normal cellular functions was previously described.

Clinical Presentation

In more than half of patients diagnosed with ET, the disorder is discovered in the laboratory from an unexpectedly elevated platelet count on a routine CBC; the remaining patients see a physician because of vascular occlusion or hemorrhage. Vascular occlusions are often the result of microvascular thromboses in the digits or thromboses in major arteries and veins that occur in a variety of organ systems, including splenic or hepatic veins, as in Budd-Chiari syndrome. Repeated splenic infarcts can result in splenic atrophy. Thrombosis can result in pulmonary emboli and neurologic complications such as headache, paresthesia of the extremities, visual impairments, and tinnitus. Arterial thrombi can cause myocardial infarction, transient ischemic attack, and cerebrovascular accident.[87] Bleeding occurs most often from mucous membranes in the gastrointestinal, skin, urinary, and upper respiratory tracts.

A minimally palpable spleen that can result in abdominal fullness is seen in about half of patients with ET. Fatigue, weight loss, and night sweats can also occur, along with Raynaud syndrome and gout.[87]

Diagnosis

ET must be differentiated from secondary or reactive thrombocytoses and from other MPNs. Thrombocytosis may be secondary to chronic active blood loss, hemolytic anemia, chronic inflammation, infection, or nonhematologic neoplasia. The identification of the *JAK2* V617F and *MPL* W515K/L mutations excludes cases of reactive thrombocytosis.

The 2022 WHO classification of tumors requires that all four major criteria be met, or the first three major criteria plus any one of the minor diagnostic criteria be met for the diagnosis of ET.[1] The WHO major diagnostic criteria are as follows: (1) platelet count >450 × 10⁹/L; (2) bone marrow biopsy showing (a) proliferation of mainly the megakaryocytic lineage, with increased numbers of enlarged, mature megakaryocytes with hyperlobulated nuclei; (b) no significant increase or left shift in neutrophil granulopoiesis; (c) very rarely, minor (grade 1) increase in reticulin fibers; (3) must not meet WHO criteria for *BCR::ABL1*-positive CML, PV, PMF, MDS, or other myeloid neoplasms; (4) must demonstrate *JAK2* V617F, *CALR,* or *MPL* mutations. Minor criteria include the presence of a clonal marker or absence of evidence of reactive thrombocytosis.

Peripheral Blood and Bone Marrow

The most consistent finding in the peripheral blood is thrombocytosis that must exceed 400×10^9/L to meet WHO criteria but often ranges from 1000 to 5000×10^9/L. Platelets often appear normal, but giant bizarre platelets, platelet aggregates, micromegakaryocytes, and megakaryocyte fragments can also be observed. Figure 32.11 shows a peripheral blood film that

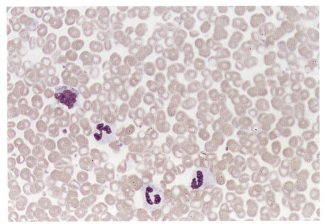

Figure 32.11 Peripheral Blood Film From a Patient in the Stable Phase of Essential Thrombocythemia. Note the increased numbers of platelets and mature neutrophils. (Wright-Giemsa stain, ×500.)

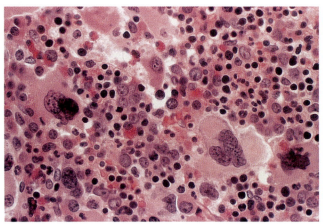

Figure 32.12 Bone Marrow Biopsy Specimen From a Patient With Essential Thrombocythemia. Note the marked number of megakaryocytes. (Hematoxylin and eosin stain, ×400.)

exhibits early phase thrombocytosis with variation in platelet diameter and shape, including giantism, agranularity, and pseudopods. Platelets commonly are present in clusters and tend to accumulate near the thin edge of the blood film. Abnormal platelet function testing can occur.

In the early stages of the disease, most patients are not anemic unless bleeding induces anemia. Erythrocytes are normocytic and normochromic unless iron deficiency is present secondary to excessive bleeding. Significant bleeding can also stimulate reticulocytosis, producing polychromasia on the peripheral blood smear. Splenic infarction can result in Howell-Jolly bodies, nucleated erythrocytes, and poikilocytosis. About one-third of patients present with a mild erythrocytosis, which must be distinguished from PV.

Leukocytosis is usually present and ranges from 22 to 40 × 10^9/L. Segmented neutrophils may be increased and occasionally metamyelocytes and myelocytes are seen. Basophils and eosinophils are usually normal but can be mildly elevated.

Early phase bone marrow has marked megakaryocytic hypercellularity, clustering of megakaryocytes, and increased megakaryocyte diameter with nuclear hyperlobulation and density (Figure 32.12). Special studies reveal increased numbers of smaller and less mature megakaryocytes. Increased granulopoiesis and erythropoiesis may contribute to bone marrow hypercellularity and, in about 25% of patients, reticulin fibers may be increased. However, significant fibrosis is usually not seen. The major peripheral blood, bone marrow, and extramedullary findings are listed in Table 32.2.

Careful analysis of the bone marrow biopsy specimen is useful in distinguishing ET from MDSs associated with the del(5q) mutation, refractory anemia with ringed sideroblasts with thrombocytosis, and the prefibrotic phase of PMF. A diagnosis of ET is questionable in patients with a platelet count of more than 400 × 10^9/L if certain features are observed on the bone marrow biopsy specimen. For example, increased erythropoiesis or granulopoiesis in the bone marrow is a questionable finding for ET and suggests an alternative diagnosis of PV or PMF, respectively, especially if bizarre or significantly atypical megakaryocytes are also identified. Dyserythropoiesis or dysgranulopoiesis suggests

TABLE 32.2 Common Morphologic Changes in Essential Thrombocythemia

Peripheral Blood	
Hemoglobin	Slightly decreased
Hematocrit	Slightly decreased
Red blood cell volume	Normal
Total white blood cells	Normal or slightly increased
Neutrophils	Normal or slightly increased
Platelets	Increased
Platelet function	Decreased
Bone Marrow	
Normoblasts	Normal or increased
Granulocytes	Normal or slightly increased
Megakaryocytes	
Clusters	Present
Large	Present
Hyperlobulated	Present
Dense nuclei	Present
Variability in size	Increased
Reticulin	Normal or slightly increased
Extramedullary Tissue	
Splenomegaly	Present
Sinusoidal	Present
Medullary	Present
Megakaryocytic proliferation	Present

a myelodysplastic disorder and should prompt an investigation for (del)5q, (inv)3, or t(3;3).[87]

Treatment and Prognosis

Patients with thrombocytosis without a history of thrombosis or cardiovascular risk factors may not require treatment; otherwise, treatment is initiated to reduce the platelet count and control thrombosis. Treatment involves prevention or early alleviation of hemorrhagic or vasoocclusive complications that occur as the platelet count increases. Plateletpheresis can be used to quickly reduce the platelet count, but cytoreductive therapy is needed for ongoing control. The production of platelets must be reduced by suppressing marrow megakaryo-cyte production with an alkylating agent such as hydroxyurea or anagrelide. Hydroxyurea is preferred in ET patients with concomitant thrombocytosis and leukocytosis because it targets both cell lines, whereas anagrelide is preferred if only the platelet count is elevated because of fewer side effects compared with hydroxyurea. Patients with ET treated with hydroxyurea may incur an increased risk for disease transformation to acute leukemia or myelofibrosis. However, malignant transformation occurs at a frequency of less than 5%.[87] Hydroxyurea therapy may achieve a desired reduction of peripheral platelets without the risk of complications experienced with myelosuppressive agents. This may relate to the youth of ET patients, in whom the risk of leukemic transformation seems relatively low. Low-dose aspirin is also recommended to prevent thrombosis and is particularly recommended for intermediate- and high-risk patients or patients with the *JAK2* V617F mutation.[87,90]

JAK2 inhibitors are being investigated in patients with ET who are refractory or intolerant to hydroxyurea or are otherwise high risk. Ruxolitinib and lestaurtinib show the most promise but with meager effects on cell counts and symptoms.

Patients with ET experience relatively long survival provided that they remain free of serious thromboembolic or hemorrhagic complications. Clinical symptoms associated with thromboembolic vasoocclusive events include the syndrome of erythromelalgia (throbbing and burning pain in the hands and feet, accompanied by mottled redness of areas), transient ischemic attacks, seizures, and cerebral or myocardial infarction. Other symptoms include headache, dizziness, visual disturbances, and dysesthesias (decreased sensations). Hemorrhagic complications include bleeding from oral and nasal mucous membranes or gastrointestinal mucosa and the appearance of cutaneous ecchymoses (Chapter 38).

The median survival for patients with ET is 20 years, including cases in which the process arises in younger patients.[87,91] According to risk stratification, low-risk patients have a long-term survival that does not reach median, intermediate-risk patients have a median survival of 24.5 years, and high-risk patient have a survival of 13.8 years. Within 10 years of diagnosis, patients with ET progress to MPN-BP at a rate of 1%. Patients progress to MF at a rate of 10% and acute leukemia at a rate of 5%. The *JAK2* mutation increases the risk of transformation into PV. The most common cause of death is thrombosis and bleeding. Patients whose cells manifest chromosome abnormalities may have a poorer prognosis.[91]

Polycythemia Vera

PV is a neoplastic clonal MPN producing erythrocytosis, often accompanied by increased granulocytes and platelets in the peripheral blood. The *JAK2* V617F and *JAK2* exon 12 mutations are strongly associated with PV, with an associated risk of hemorrhage and venous and arterial thrombosis.[1] Splenomegaly is common. The disease arises in an HSC and is clonal in nature.

Incidence

PV is the most common MPN. The annual incidence of PV varies by country, with Japan reporting 2 cases per 1 million, Australia and Europe reporting 13 cases per 1 million, and the United States averaging 8 to 10 cases per 1 million. PV rarely occurs in children and occurs most often between the ages of 40 and 60 years, with a peak incidence after the age of 60 years, particularly in men. Peak incidence for women is <40 years of age.[34] It occurs more often in men than women and is more common in people of Jewish descent.[93] A familial predisposition for PV may exist because it has been reported in several members of the same family.

Pathogenetic Mechanism

In PV, neoplastic clonal stem cells are hypersensitive to, or function independently of, erythropoietin for cell growth. Trace levels of erythropoietin in serum stimulate the growth of erythroid progenitor cells in in vitro colony-forming growth systems. There is preservation of hypersensitive and normosensitive erythroid colony-forming units, however, which indicates some level of normal hematopoiesis. Adverse clinical progression seems to correlate with the propagation of the erythropoietin-sensitive colony-forming units.

As previously discussed, the *JAK2* V617F mutation is detected in more than 95% of patients with PV (range, 46.7% to 100%) with 1% to 2% of the remaining 5% harboring another *JAK2* mutation in exon 12. The other two driver mutations, *MPL* and *CALR,* rarely occur in patients with PV.[89] However, an increasing allele burden for *JAK2* mutations correlates with disease progression in PV patients, as do mutations in epigenetic modifiers (i.e., *TET2, IDH1/2, EZH2, ASXL1, DNMT3a*), transcription factors, and signal transduction genes (i.e., *TP53, RUNX1, IK2F1, NRAS, SH2B3 [LNK], CBL, NF1, FLT3*) and mutations in splicing factors (i.e., *SF3B1, U2AF1, SRSF2, ZRSR2*). Karyotype abnormalities contribute most to leukemic transformation.[35]

Diagnosis

Based on 2022 WHO standards, the diagnosis of PV requires that all three major criteria be met, or the first two major criteria plus the one minor criterion be met. The three major criteria are (1) an elevated hemoglobin (>16.5 g/dL in men and >16.5 g/dL in women) or elevated hematocrit (>49% in men and >48% in women); (2) bone marrow showing hypercellularity for age with trilineage growth (panmyelosis) including prominent erythroid, granulocytic, and megakaryocytic proliferation with pleomorphic, mature megakaryocytes; and (3) the identification of the *JAK2* V617F mutation or the *JAK2* exon 12 mutation. The one minor criterion is low serum erythropoietin levels.[1] Additional features of PV include an arterial oxygen saturation of 92% (normal) or greater, splenomegaly, thrombocytosis of greater than 400×10^9 platelets/L, leukocytosis of greater than 12×10^9 cells/L without fever or infection, increases in LAP, serum vitamin B_{12}, or unbound vitamin B_{12} binding capacity. WHO criteria for the diagnosis of PV are summarized in Box 32.1.

It is not always easy to assign an early diagnosis of PV. Erythrocytosis secondary to hypoxia or erythropoietin-producing neoplasms are the most difficult to diagnose correctly. In individuals with these conditions, the bone marrow exhibits erythroid hyperplasia without granulocytic or megakaryocytic hyperplasia. Patients with stress or spurious erythrocytosis

BOX 32.1   WHO Diagnostic Criteria

Polycythemia Vera (PV)

Major Criteria

1. Hemoglobin >16.5 g/dL in men and >16.0 g/dL in women *or* Hematocrit >49% in men and >48% in women
2. Bone marrow showing hypercellularity for age, with trilineage growth (panmyelosis) including prominent erythroid, granulocytic, and megakaryocytic proliferation, with pleomorphic, mature megakaryocytes (difference is size)
3. Presence of *JAK2* V617F or *JAK2* exon 12 mutation

Minor Criterion

1. Subnormal serum erythropoietin level

Prefibrotic Primary Myelofibrosis (Pre-PMF)

Major Criteria

1. Megakaryocytic proliferation and atypia, without reticulin fibrosis >grade 1, accompanied by increased age-adjusted bone marrow cellularity, granulocytic proliferation, and often, decreased erythropoiesis
2. Not meeting WHO criteria for *BCR::ABL1* + CML, PV, ET, MDS, or other myeloid neoplasms
3. Presence of *JAK2, CALR,* or *MPL* mutation or, in the absence of these mutations, presence of another clonal marker or absence of minor reactive bone marrow reticulin fibrosis

Minor Criteria

1. Presence of at least one of the following, confirmed in two consecutive determinations:
   a. Anemia not attributed to a comorbid condition
   b. Leukocytosis >11 × 10^9/L
   c. Palpable splenomegaly
   d. LD increased to above upper limit of institution's reference range
   e. Leukoerythroblastosis

   Diagnosis of pre-PMF requires meeting all three major criteria and at least one minor criteria.

Overt Primary Myelofibrosis

Major Criteria

1. Megakaryocytic proliferation and atypia, accompanied by reticulin and/or collagen fibrosis grades 2 or 3

2. Not meeting WHO criteria for *BCR::ABL1* + CML, PV, ET, MDS, or other myeloid neoplasms
3. Presence of *JAK2, CALR,* or *MPL* mutation or, in the absence of these mutations, presence of another clonal marker or absence of minor reactive bone marrow myelofibrosis

Minor Criteria

1. Presence of at least one of the following, confirmed in two consecutive determinations:
   a. Anemia not attributed to a comorbid condition
   b. Leukocytosis >11 × 10^9/L
   c. Palpable splenomegaly or detected by imaging
   d. LD increased to above upper limit of institution's reference range
   e. Leukoerythroblastosis

   Diagnosis of overt PMF requires meeting all three major criteria and at least one minor criterion.

Chronic Neutrophilic Leukemia

1. Peripheral blood leukocytosis >25 × 10^9/L

   Bands and segmented neutrophils of WBC count ≥80%

   Immature granulocytes (promyelocytes, myelocytes, metamyelocytes) of WBC count <10%

   Myeloblasts rarely observed

   Monocyte count <1 × 10^9/L (<10%)

   No dysgranulopoiesis
2. Hypercellular bone marrow

   Neutrophilic granulocytes increased in percentage and number

   Myeloblasts <5% of nucleated cells

   Neutrophil maturation appears normal
3. Not meeting WHO criteria for *BCR::ABL1* + CML, PV, ET, or PMF
4. No rearrangement of *PDGFRA, PDGFRB, FGFR1,* or *PCM1::JAK2*
5. Presence of *CSF3R* T618I or other activating *CSF3R* mutation
6. Presence of *CSF3R* T618I or another *CSF3R* activating mutation *or*

   Persistent neutrophilia for at least 3 months; splenomegaly; no identifiable cause of reactive neutrophilia, including the absence of a plasma cell neoplasm; *or*

   If a plasma cell neoplasm is present, demonstration of clonality of myeloid cells by cytogenetic or molecular studies

CML, Chronic myeloid leukemia; *ET,* essential thrombocytopenia; *LD,* lactate dehydrogenase; *MDS,* myelodysplastic syndrome; *WBC,* white blood cell; *WHO,* World Health Organization.

From WHO Classification of Tumours Editorial Board. (2022). Haematolymphoid tumours [Internet, beta version ahead of print]. WHO Classification of Tumours Series. (5th ed; vol 11). https://tumourclassification.iarc.who.int/chapters/63. Accessed February 8, 2023.

exhibit increased hemoglobin and hematocrit without increased erythrocyte mass or splenomegaly.

Peripheral Blood and Bone Marrow

Common peripheral blood, bone marrow, and tissue findings in the early or proliferative phase of PV are listed in Table 32.3. Figures 32.13 and 32.14 show common morphologic patterns in peripheral blood and bone marrow morphologic and cellular changes. Not only are quantitative changes seen, but also bone marrow normoblasts may collect in large clusters; megakaryocytes are enlarged and exhibit lobulated nuclei; and bone marrow sinuses are enlarged, without fibrosis. Approximately 80% of patients manifest bone marrow panmyelosis, and 100% of bone marrow volume may exhibit hematopoietic cellularity. Although the bone marrow pattern

may mimic that of other MPNs, the peripheral blood cells appear normal, with normocytic normochromic erythrocytes; mature granulocytes; and normal-sized, granulated platelets. The other 20% of patients exhibit lesser degrees of cellularity in the bone marrow and peripheral blood. Splenomegaly, hepatomegaly, generalized vascular engorgement, and circulatory disturbances increase the risk of hemorrhage, tissue infarction, and thrombosis.

Clinical Presentation

Patients with PV often present with a history of mild symptoms occurring for several years, although some patients are diagnosed serendipitously from laboratory values of asymptomatic patients. PV initially manifests in a proliferative phase independent of normal regulatory mechanisms that is associated with increased

TABLE 32.3 Common Morphologic Changes in Polycythemia Vera

Peripheral Blood

Hemoglobin	Increased
Hematocrit	Increased
Red blood cell volume	Increased
Erythrocyte morphology	Normocytic/normochromic
Total white blood cells	Increased
Granulocytes	Increased
Platelets	Increased
Leukocyte alkaline phosphatase	Normal or increased

Bone Marrow

Normoblasts	Increased
Granulocytes	Increased
Megakaryocytes	Increased
Reticulin	Increased

Extramedullary Tissue

Splenomegaly	Present
Sinusoidal	Present
Medullary	Present
Hepatomegaly	Present
Sinusoidal	Present

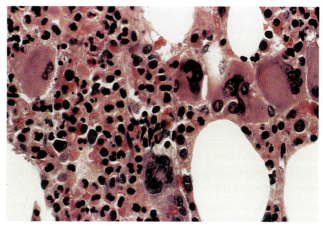

Figure 32.14 Bone Marrow Biopsy Specimen From a Patient in the Stable Phase of Polycythemia Vera. Note the panmyelosis. (Hematoxylin and eosin stain, ×400.)

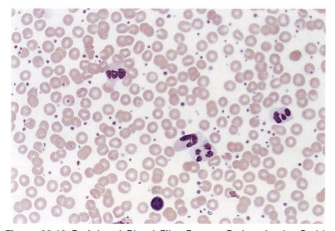

Figure 32.13 Peripheral Blood Film From a Patient in the Stable Phase of Polycythemia Vera. Note the essentially normocytic, normochromic erythrocytes. (Wright-Giemsa stain, ×500.)

red blood cell (RBC) mass. The increased RBC mass produces blood hyperviscosity, often resulting in cardiovascular disease. In the early stages of the disease, before treatment, extended periods of high hematocrit (>60%) and hyperviscosity produce hypertension in about 50% of patients with PV. Presenting symptoms are associated with hyperviscosity and hyperproliferation and include headache, weakness, pruritus, weight loss, and fatigue. Pruritus has been associated with elevated blood histamine and is often not associated with a visible rash.

About half of patients with PV have thrombocytosis, and one-third experience thrombotic or hemorrhagic episodes. PV patients older than 60 years of age or with a history of thrombosis are considered high risk for thrombotic or hemorrhagic events. Similarly, PV patients have an intermediate risk if concomitant risk factors exist, including uncontrolled

hypertension, diabetes, smoking, obesity, or hypercholesterolemia. Thrombotic risk is reduced if the calreticulin (*CALR*) mutation is identified, especially in patients with ET.[86] Other thrombosis-related events such as myocardial infarctions, retinal vein thrombosis, thrombophlebitis, and cerebral ischemia can occur at any stage of the disease and occasionally, are the first indication of the disease.

The stable phase of PV can progress to a spent phase in a few patients, usually within 10 years from diagnosis. In the spent phase, patients experience progressive splenomegaly or hypersplenism and pancytopenia. They may also exhibit the triad of bone marrow fibrosis, splenomegaly, and anemia with teardrop-shaped poikilocytes. The latter pattern is called *post-polycythemic myeloid metaplasia* and develops in about 30% of PV patients within 20 years. This phase of PV is morphologically similar to PMF and must be carefully differentiated. Peripheral WBC and RBC counts vary, and nucleated erythrocytes, immature granulocytes, and large platelets are present. Usually, splenomegaly is due to extramedullary hematopoiesis. Myelofibrosis occurs within the bone marrow and may come to occupy a significant proportion of bone marrow volume, with subsequent ineffective hematopoiesis.

Treatment and Prognosis

Treatment options for PV can be placed into three groups: therapeutic phlebotomy, myelosuppressive therapy, and targeted molecular therapy. The treatment of choice for PV in low-risk patients (<60 years old and no thrombosis history) is low-dose aspirin and therapeutic phlebotomy at a frequency necessary to maintain the hematocrit at less than 45% for men and 42% for women.[92] RBC mass testing can be used to estimate the number of phlebotomies needed to reach target hematocrit levels. In most cases, 500 to 1500 mL of blood must be removed to normalize the RBC mass, after which monthly hematocrit measurements can dictate the phlebotomy schedule.[34] Therapeutic phlebotomy decreases erythrocyte counts and expands plasma volume to reduce blood viscosity, thus restoring normal blood flow and blood pressure to ameliorate the associated symptoms of headache, weakness, fatigue, and pruritus. Blood removal also reduces available iron, which inhibits erythropoiesis and delays the return of erythrocytosis.

Pruritus is a common clinical feature of PV. Patients are instructed to avoid hot baths, to towel dry gently to reduce skin irritation, and to take an antihistamine such as diphenhydramine as needed. In extreme cases, selective serotonin reuptake inhibitors such as paroxetine and fluoxetine are being evaluated in clinical trials.

In high-risk patients with PV (>60 years old with thrombosis history), the alkylating agent hydroxyurea is recommended as first-line therapy in conjunction with phlebotomy and low-dose aspirin. Pegylated IFN-α can be substituted in young patients or women of childbearing age.[92] The risk of thrombosis and bleeding is increased in patients treated with phlebotomy alone, so the use of alkylating myelosuppressive agents may be required to control these complications.

Treatment with modern JAK inhibitors such as ruxolitinib has provided important benefits to patients with PV. Ruxolitinib binds with high affinity to the ATP-binding site of the active form of JAK1, JAK2, JAK3, and wild-type JAK proteins as well as the *JAK2* V617F mutation. In addition, ruxolitinib was tested against 26 other tyrosine kinases and found to have a low binding affinity for all 26 proteins.[29] Ruxolitinib is becoming the first choice as second-line therapy following hydroxyurea failure or intolerance. Patients show reductions in severe pruritus, reduced spleen volume, and reduction of symptoms associated with post-PV myelofibrosis.[92]

Several other drugs are in clinical trials for the treatment of PV, including epigenetic modifiers such as idasanutlin (MDM2 inhibitor); telomerase inhibitors such as imetelstat; and TKIs such as momelotinib, erlotinib, dasatinib, and imatinib. However, one of the more promising drugs to treat PV is another epigenetic modifier, givinostat, a potent inhibitor of histone deacetylases I and II. Givinostat has been shown to induce apoptosis in neoplastic cells, inhibit the synthesis of several proinflammatory cytokines, reduce proliferation of *JAK2* V617F cells, and promote growth of nonmutated hematopoietic cells. Clinical trials report complete (11%) and partial (89%) hematologic remissions, lowered hematocrit and reduced spleen size (56%), reduced *JAK2* V617F allele burden (22%), and low incidence of thrombosis in 2.3% of patients per year.[92]

About half of PV patients survive 15 months without treatment, and survival is extended to 14 years with phlebotomy as the only treatment. Age, abnormal karyotype, leukocytosis, and a history of thrombosis are factors that adversely affect survival. The median survival for PV patients stratified by risk into high-, medium-, and low-risk groups using criteria of age, WBC count, and thrombosis is 10.9, 18.9, and 27.8 years, respectively.[86] Overall median survival exceeds 10 to 20 years.[90] Within 10 years of diagnosis, about 4% of patients with PV progress to MPN-BP. PV in the spent phase transitions into acute leukemia in 5% to 10% of patients. Overall, PV progresses to acute leukemia in 15% of patients. The use of myelosuppressive therapy increases the risk, whereas only 1% to 2% of patients treated with phlebotomy alone experience leukemic transformation.

Primary Myelofibrosis

PMF, previously known as *chronic idiopathic myelofibrosis, agnogenic myelofibrosis,* and *myelofibrosis with myeloid metaplasia,* is a clonal HSC MPN characterized by a proliferation of abnormal megakaryocytes and granulocytes in the bone marrow with an accompanying polyclonal increase in fibroblasts producing progressive marrow fibrosis. The bone marrow demonstrates ineffective hematopoiesis associated with areas of marrow hypercellularity (leukoerythroblastosis), extramedullary hematopoiesis, fibrosis, and increased megakaryocytes. It is the least common but most aggressive form of MPN. PMF can form de novo or as an evolutionary consequence of PV or ET. Megakaryocytes are enlarged, with pleomorphic nuclei, coarse segmentation, and areas of hypochromia. The peripheral blood film exhibits immature granulocytes and normoblasts, dacryocytes (teardrop-shaped RBCs), and other bizarre RBC shapes. PMF is further subdivided into prefibrotic/early stage PMF and overt fibrotic stage PMF.[1]

WHO 2022 diagnostic criteria for prefibrotic myelofibrosis requires that all three major and one minor criteria, confirmed in two consecutive determinations, be met. Major criteria are as follows: (1) megakaryocytic proliferation and atypia, without reticulin grade >1, accompanied by age-adjusted bone marrow cellularity, granulocyte proliferation, and usually a decreased erythropoiesis; (2) not meeting WHO criteria for *BCR::ABL1*-positive CML, PV, ET, myelodysplastic syndromes, or other myeloid neoplasms; (3) presence of mutations in *JAK2, CALR,* or *MPL, or* presence of another clonal marker, *or* absence of minor reactive marrow reticulin fibrosis. Minor criteria for prefibrotic PMF are as follows: (1) anemia not attributed to a comorbid condition; (2) leukocytosis $\geq 11 \times 10^9/L$; (3) splenomegaly detected clinically and/or by imaging; (4) lactate dehydrogenase level above the upper limit of the international reference range; (5) leukoerythroblastic.[1]

Myelofibrosis

Fibroblasts are normally found in the bone marrow and produce collagen to provide structural support for HSCs. In PMF a reactive process causes overproduction of collagen that eventually disrupts the normal architecture of the bone marrow and replaces hematopoietic tissue resulting in pancytopenia. In approximately 30% of patients, biopsy specimens show no fibrosis. Increases in collagen are not part of the clonal proliferative process but are considered secondary to an increased release of fibroblastic growth factors such as platelet-derived growth factor (PDGF), TGF-α and TGF-β, TNF-α, IL-1α, and IL-1β. Vascular endothelial growth factor, PDGF, fibroblast growth factor, epidermal growth factor, hepatocyte growth factor, and insulin-like growth factor are contained in the α-granules of megakaryocytes and platelets, and they collectively stimulate the growth and proliferation of endothelial cells, blood vessels, and fibroblasts. The abnormal release or leakage of PDGF from the platelet results in reduced platelet concentrations of PDGF and increased levels of serum PDGF that are characteristic of PMF. PDGF does not stimulate synthesis of collagen, laminin, or fibronectin, but TGF-β stimulates increased expression of genes for fibronectin and collagen, whereas it decreases synthesis of collagenase-like enzymes. Thus the net effect is the accumulation of bone marrow stromal elements.[93] Marrow fibrosis causes expansion of marrow sinuses and vascular volume, with an increased rate of blood flow. Bone marrow fibrosis is not the sole criterion for the diagnosis of PMF because increases in marrow fibrosis may reflect a reparative response to injury from benzene or ionizing radiation, may be a consequence of immunologically mediated injury, or may represent a reactive response to other hematologic conditions.

Hematopoiesis and Extramedullary Hematopoiesis

Extramedullary hematopoiesis, clinically recognized as hepatomegaly or splenomegaly, is caused by the release of clonal stem cells into the circulation. The cells accumulate in the spleen, liver, or other organs, including adrenals, kidneys, lymph nodes, bowel, breasts, lungs, mediastinum, mesentery, skin, synovium, thymus, and lower urinary tract. There is an increase in circulating unilineage and multilineage HPCs, and the number of CD34+ cells may be 300 times normal.[96] The increase in circulating CD34+ cells separates PMF from other MPNs and predicts the degree of splenic involvement and risk of conversion to acute leukemia. Body cavity effusions containing hematopoietic cells may arise from extramedullary hematopoiesis in the cranium; the intraspinal epidural space; or the serosal surfaces of pleura, pericardium, and peritoneum.

Pathogenetic Mechanism

As with ET and PV, most patients with PMF have a somatic mutation in one of three driver genes, *JAK2* (V617F), *CALR,* or *MPL,* that affect the JAK-STAT pathway. About 60% (range, 25% to 87.5%) of PMF patients have the *JAK2* V617F mutation, 30% (range, 10% to 100%) have a mutation in *CALR*, and 5% (range, 0% to 17.1%) have an *MPL* mutation.[40,89,94] A small number of PMF patients are negative for all three driver mutations (termed triple negative) and have a worse prognosis. Mutations in genes that regulate epigenetic modification rather than the JAK-STAT pathway have also been identified in PMF, including *TET2* (7.7% to 17%), *ASXL1* (13% to 23%), DNA methyltransferase 3A *(DNMT3A),* and enhancer of Zeste homolog 2 *(EZH2).*[40,94] In addition, 6% of patients with PML expressed a *CBL* mutation that is more typically found in JMML or chronic myelomonocytic leukemia (CMML).[95] Lastly, other mutations previously discussed (*LNK* [3% to 6%], *EZH2* [13%], and *IDH1/2* [4.2%]) have also been identified in PMF.[40]

Incidence and Clinical Presentation

PMF occurs in patients older than age 60 and equally among men and women. The disease may be asymptomatic and usually progresses as a slow, chronic condition. Occasionally, it can follow a rapid, acute course marked by rapid fibrosis formation and the associated pancytopenia. Symptoms result from anemia, myeloproliferation, or splenomegaly. The most common constitutional symptoms encountered by patients with PMF include fatigue (84%), bone pain (47%), night sweats (56%), pruritus (50%), and fever (18%).[96,97] Splenomegaly is present in 90% of patients with PMF, and 50% have hepatomegaly.[98,99]

Major hemolytic episodes occur in 15% of PMF patients during the course of their disease, and 10% of patients demonstrate hemosiderinuria and decreased blood haptoglobin levels suggesting intravascular hemolysis. Some patients develop bleeding diathesis resulting from a combination of thrombocytopenia, abnormal platelet function, and hemostatic abnormalities suggestive of chronic disseminated intravascular coagulation.[100]

Peripheral Blood and Bone Marrow

Patients with PMF demonstrate a broad range of changes in laboratory test values and peripheral blood film results that reflect both quantitative and qualitative abnormalities. In the early stages, anemia, leukocytosis with a left shift, and thrombocytosis are associated with MPN. Between 34% and 54% of PMF patients present with hemoglobin less than 10 g/dL.[98,99] However, as the fibrosis evolves in the bone marrow, blood cell counts fall and pancytopenia eventually develops, along with leukoerythroblastosis, anisocytosis, and poikilocytosis. Examination of the bone marrow biopsy specimen provides most of the information for diagnosis. Changes commonly observed in peripheral blood and bone marrow examinations are summarized in Table 32.4.

Abnormalities in erythrocytes noted on peripheral blood films include the presence of dacryocytes (teardrop cells), other bizarre shapes, nucleated RBCs, and polychromatophilia in the context of a normocytic and normochromic anemia. Reticulocytosis is common, ranging from 2% to 15%.

Granulocytes can be increased, normal, or decreased in number at presentation but fall as the disease progresses. The differential indicates immature granulocytes producing a left shift, blasts (<5%), and cells with nuclear or cytoplasmic anomalies. Eosinophilia, basophilia, and pseudo-Pelger-Huët anomaly can also be identified. LAP is variable but often elevated or normal.

Platelets may be normal, increased, or decreased in number, with a mixture of normal and abnormal morphologic features (Figure 32.15). Thrombocytosis is more common early in the disease and thrombocytopenia is more common in the later stages. Micromegakaryocytes may be observed (Figure 32.16), with naked micromegakaryocytic nuclei, megakaryocyte fragments, and cytoplasmic blebbing.

Bone marrow biopsy specimens are difficult to obtain and often yield a dry tap. If an aspirate is obtained, the sample will often appear normal, making a biopsy critical to assess fibrosis. The bone marrow biopsy specimen exhibits intense fibrosis, granulocytic and megakaryocytic hypercellularity, dysmegakaryopoiesis, dysgranulopoiesis, and numerous dilated sinuses containing luminal hematopoiesis.

Treatment and Prognosis

PMF is by far the worst MPN, and patients are at risk for fatal outcomes associated with disease progression, leukemic transformation, thrombohemorrhagic complications, and infections. All patients, regardless of risk, should be evaluated for allogeneic HSC transplantation eligibility. For the large number of patients in whom HSC transplantation is not an option, treatments to alleviate symptoms should be initiated. A diverse spectrum of

TABLE 32.4 Common Morphologic Changes in Primary Myelofibrosis

Peripheral Blood

Hemoglobin	Normal or decreased
Anisocytosis	Present
Poikilocytosis	Present
Teardrop-shaped erythrocytes	Present
Nucleated red blood cells	Present
Polychromasia	Normal or increased
Total white blood cells	Normal, decreased, or increased
Immature granulocytes	Increased
Blasts	Present
Basophils	Present
Leukocyte anomaly	Present
Leukocyte alkaline phosphatase	Increased, normal, or decreased
Platelets	Increased, normal, or decreased
Abnormal platelets	Present
Megakaryocytes	Present

Bone Marrow

Cellularity	Increased
Granulopoiesis	Increased
Megakaryocytes	Increased
Erythropoiesis	Normal or increased
Myelofibrosis	Increased
Sinuses	Increased
Dysmegakaryopoiesis	Present
Dysgranulopoiesis	Present

Extramedullary Tissue

Splenomegaly	Present
Sinusoidal	Present
Medullary	Present
Hepatomegaly	Present
Sinusoidal	Present
Portal tract	Present
Local infiltrates	Present
Other tissues	Present

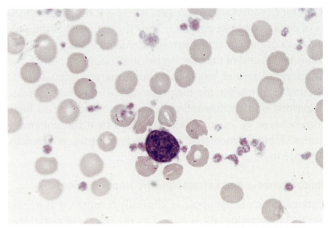

Figure 32.16 Peripheral Blood Film From a Patient With Primary Myelofibrosis. Note the increased platelets and a micromegakaryocyte. (Wright-Giemsa stain, ×1000.)

approaches have historically been palliative. Treatment has been targeted at the amelioration of anemia, hepatosplenomegaly, and constitutional symptoms.

Before commencing disease-targeted therapy, risk stratification of patients is needed to maximize benefits and minimize adverse outcomes. Although there is no consensus on the best tool to assess prognosis, the goals of care, symptom burden, medical fitness, and laboratory values must be considered when evaluating risk of therapy.

For higher-risk patients, ruxolitinib, fedratinib, or hydroxyurea is considered first-line therapy. Ruxolitinib and fedratinib are effective at reducing splenomegaly and other symptoms but have not been shown to modify the disease course or prolong survival. Ruxolitinib should not be initiated during an active infection and should be administered in lower doses in the context of thrombocytopenia, renal disease, and liver dysfunction. Fedratinib should not be administered to patients with severe liver disease and has been associated with serious and sometimes fatal encephalopathies, cardiovascular death, myocardial infarction, stroke, and liver toxicity. Hydroxyurea should be used for patients who are not candidates for ruxolitinib or fedratinib and when cytoreduction is warranted. Hydroxyurea should be used with caution when cytopenias are present. For patients who are ineligible for HSC transplantation and when the other treatments fail, surgical splenectomy, splenic irradiation, or IFNs may be considered. Momelotinib, a JAK1/2 inhibitor, pacritinib, a JAK2/FLT3 inhibitor, and lestaurtinib, a non-JAK inhibitor, have been evaluated in clinical trials and found to be less effective than ruxolitinib and fedratinib.[101–103]

For low-risk patients who are asymptomatic, observation only is warranted, with followup visits every 3 to 6 months with history taking, symptom assessment, clinical examination, CBC, and tests to assess liver and renal function. As symptoms emerge, HSC transplantation, palliative care, and targeted therapy should be initiated.

Anemia is usually managed by transfusion therapy because patients with PMF rarely respond to erythropoietin. Splenectomy should be considered only if the discomfort of splenomegaly outweighs the extramedullary hematopoiesis

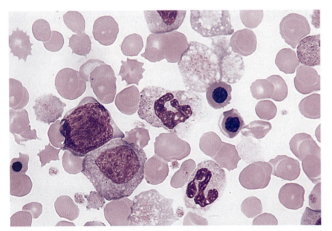

Figure 32.15 Peripheral Blood Film From a Patient With Primary Myelofibrosis. Note the nucleated red blood cells, giant platelets, and immature myeloid cells. (Wright-Giemsa stain, ×1000.)

therapies are available to alleviate symptoms or modify clinical problems in patients with PMF. Except for allogeneic HSC transplantation, none have been disease modifying, so treatment occurring in the spleen. In some patients, danazol[104] (androgen to treat endometriosis, fibrocystic breast disease, and hereditary angioedema) has been shown to improve anemia and reduce the transfusion requirement. If danazol is ineffective, either thalidomide[105,106] or lenalidomide[107] with prednisone has been shown to improve anemia in about 25% to 33% of PMF patients. Approximately 20% of patients with severe anemia respond, with an average duration of 1 to 2 years. Thalidomide and lenalidomide must be used with caution because of the occurrence of neuropathies and myelosuppression, particularly if the patient has been identified with del(5q31).[108] Pomalidomide has been found to produce anemia and symptom relief without neuropathy and myelosuppression.[109]

Leukemic transformation is the most common cause of death in patients with PMF, and there is no standard treatment available. There are three primary approaches to the treatment of leukemic transformation: (1) inductive chemotherapy with or without HSC transplantation (curative); (2) nonintensive chemotherapy (improves survival); (3) supportive/palliative care (symptom relief). Curative approaches improve median survival by a few months to 2 years. Cytarabine, azacytidine, and decitabine are common chemotherapeutic drugs used.

Average survival from the time of diagnosis is about 5 years, but patients have lived as long as 15 years. During this time, increasing numbers and pleomorphism of megakaryocytes lead to progressive marrow failure. Marrow blasts may increase. Adverse prognostic indicators include more severe anemia and thrombocytopenia, greater hepatomegaly, unexplained fever, and hemolysis. Within 10 years of diagnosis, approximately 20% of patients with PMF will progress to MPN-BP. Mortality is associated with infection, hemorrhage, postsplenectomy complications, cardiac failure, and transformation to acute leukemia.[110]

OTHER MYELOPROLIFERATIVE NEOPLASMS

Chronic Neutrophilic Leukemia

CNL is largely a clonal disorder in which a hyperproliferation of neutrophilic cells in the bone marrow produces sustained neutrophilia in the peripheral blood and hepatosplenomegaly. While most cases are clonal, some follow cytotoxic chemotherapy, with a few reports of familial/germline predisposition. The BCR::ABL1 translocation must be absent to distinguish the disease from CML.[1] The bone marrow is hypercellular because of increased neutrophilic granulocyte proliferation, but dysplasia is absent.[110,111]

Incidence

CNL is a rare disorder, with 0.1 to 1.0 new case each year per 1 million people. The median age at diagnosis is 65 years, with men affected slightly more often than women (1.6/1.0 ratio).[1,111]

Clinical Presentation

At the time of diagnosis, most patients are asymptomatic or experience minimal symptoms associated with mild splenomegaly. The initial period may last for several months to years before evolving into symptomatic disease. Some patients present with fatigue, weight loss, pruritus, easy bruising, bone pain, night sweats, and recurrent episodes of gout. As CNL progresses, hepatosplenomegaly and bleeding diatheses develop, sometimes accompanied by low-grade fever.

Mild to moderate splenomegaly is present in about 40% of cases at diagnosis and progresses to severe splenomegaly in nearly all cases. Occasionally massive splenomegaly is seen and is sometimes painful but rarely requires palliative splenectomy. Hepatomegaly is less common, and lymphadenopathy is a rare event.

Bleeding diathesis is an important clinical feature because it can contribute to the cause of death. Bleeding is often predictable, based on the degree of thrombocytopenia, but it is sometimes disproportionate, suggesting concomitant qualitative platelet malfunction. Studies have reported prolonged bleeding time and abnormal platelet aggregation response to ADP, collagen, and epinephrine. A variety of erythematous and/or hemorrhagic skin lesions are common in CNL, and the severity of the lesions mirror the disease activity and severity. Approximately half of patients report a history of thrombosis.

Patients with CNL often develop severe, life-threatening, or even fatal infections due to the qualitative defects in neutrophil function. Mycobacteria and fungi are the most common serious infectious agents. A diagnosis of CNL mat be obscured by a secondary infection, resulting in a delayed diagnosis.[110,111]

Peripheral Blood and Bone Marrow

Patients present with a WBC count of more than 25×10^9/L (WHO criteria), but it may reach levels of 100×10^9/L or even 500×10^9/L. Mature neutrophils dominate (>80%, WHO criteria), but the increase in bands, metamyelocytes, myelocytes, and promyelocytes in combination must comprise less than 10% of WBCs but are often <5%. Monocytosis, basophilia, and eosinophilia must be absent to help distinguish CNL from myelodysplastic disorders and other myeloproliferative disorders such as CML. Neutrophils appear normal, with no evidence of dysplasia, and often contain toxic granules without Döhle bodies. CNL neutrophils contain normal granular content but often exhibit functional defects including motility, deformability, chemotaxis, and the respiratory burst.

RBC count is often normal but can show a mild to moderate normocytic normochromic anemia. Platelet count is often normal but can be decreased or, rarely, increased, with normal platelet morphology. Thrombocytopenia can develop as the disease progresses, largely because of splenomegaly or progression to acute myeloid leukemia.

The bone marrow reflects the peripheral blood in that it is hypercellular, with predominantly a proliferation of neutrophils, including myelocytes, metamyelocytes, bands, and segmented neutrophils without dysplasia. The myeloid-to-erythroid ratio is greater than 10:1 and often 20:1. Erythrocyte and megakaryocyte morphology is normal, and megakaryocyte hyperplasia is common.[110,111]

Diagnosis

WHO 2022 diagnostic criteria require that CNL be differentiated from CML, myelodysplasia, a reactive neutrophilic process, and other MPNs using the following criteria: (1) peripheral blood leukocyte count of >25 × 10^9/L with >80% normal segmented and band neutrophils, a monocyte count of 1 × 10^9/L or less, and <10% monocytes with myeloblasts rarely observed and immature neutrophilic cells (promyelocytes, myelocytes, and metamyelocytes) at ≤10% of the differential; (2) a hypercellular bone marrow with mostly normal-appearing neutrophilic cells and myeloblasts <5%; (3) must not meet WHO criteria for BCR::ABL1-positive CML, PV, ET, or PMF; (4) no evidence of PDGFRA, PDGFRB, FGFR1, or PCM::JAK2 fusion; (5) presence of CSF3R T618I or another activating CSF3R mutation or persistent neutrophilia of greater than 3 months, splenomegaly, and no identifiable cause of reactive neutrophilia including absence of plasma cell neoplasm or, if a plasma cell neoplasm is present, demonstration of clonality of myeloid cells by cytogenetic or molecular studies.[1] Megakaryocytes are normal or slightly left shifted. Splenomegaly must be present and is often accompanied by hepatomegaly. Reactive neutrophilia must be excluded by eliminating infection, inflammation, and tumors as a cause of the neutrophilia. A diagnosis of CNL can still be made in the presence of a reactive process if clonality of the myeloid line can be documented by karyotyping or molecular analysis. In the rare instance where the CSF3R T618I mutation is absent, the following must be present: persistent neutrophilia for 3 months; splenomegaly; and no identifiable cause of reactive neutrophilia, including the presence of a plasma cell neoplasm or demonstration of clonality of myeloid cells by cytogenetic or molecular studies. Lastly, there can be no evidence of PV, PMF, ET, MDS, or MDS/MPN disorders.[1]

Pathogenetic Mechanism

The apparent driver mutation for CNL is in the CSF3R gene, mainly at the T618I or T640N mutations. Normally, the CSF3R protein serves as a transmembrane receptor for G-CSF to regulate neutrophil production by committing myeloid precursors to granulocytic differentiation, accelerating the production of the postmitotic neutrophilic pool, prolonging the survival of neutrophils and their precursors, and enhancing neutrophil function. Binding of G-CSF to CSF3R stimulates homodimerization of CSF3R, leading to the activation of primarily JAK/STAT pathways and to a lesser extent, phosphatidylinositol-3-kinase (PI3K)/AKT and MAPK/ERK pathways. The T618I or T640N mutation of CSF3R causes a ligand-independent activation of the G-CSF pathway, resulting in increased proliferation. Conversely, CSF3R mutations that fail to bind G-CSF have been shown to cause severe congenital neutropenia and chronic idiopathic neutropenia.

Although CSF3R is thought to be a driver mutation, other disease-modifying mutations include genes involved in epigenetic and transcriptional regulation (ASXL1 [77%], TET2 [21%]), spliceosome assembly (SRSF2 [44%], U2AF1 [15%]), and SETBP1 [41%].[110,111] Most cases demonstrate four unique point mutations that suggest a sequential conference of mutations in an HSC.[1]

Approximately 90% of patients with CNL have a normal karyotype, but chromosomal abnormalities are identified, particularly as the disease progresses, including +8, +9, +21, del(20q), del(11q), and del(12p). The Ph chromosome or a BCR::ABL1

translocation cannot be expressed in CNL; otherwise, a diagnosis of CML is required. JAK2 mutations rarely have been identified. As stated earlier, there must be no rearrangements of the PDGFRA, PDGFRB, FGRF1, or PCM1::JAK2 genes, and the CSF3R T618I mutation or other activating CSF3R mutation should be present.[110,111]

Therapy

The only curative treatment for CNL is allogeneic stem cell transplantation for patients who qualify. For all other patients, first-line therapy is hydroxyurea if the CSF3R mutation is proximal and dasatinib if the CSF3R mutation is truncating. Approximately 75% of patients show clinical improvement on hydroxyurea, but the drug is not disease modifying. Historically, IFN-γ has been used as first-line therapy, but data are insufficient to warrant use. Patients who fail hydroxyurea or dasatinib are treated with ruxolitinib, but rescue is uncommon. Therapeutic responses generally last about 12 months.[110,111]

Prognosis

CNL is a slow, smoldering condition, and patient survival ranges from 6 months to longer than 20 years. Median survival is 2 years. Prognosis worsens with a WBC count >50 × 10^9/L, a platelet count of <160 × 10^9/L, and the ASXL1 mutation. CNL progresses to an accelerated phase that exhibits progressive neutrophilia, anemia, thrombocytopenia, and splenomegaly that are unresponsive to treatment. Blasts and other immature cells can be present in the peripheral blood, and some patients develop myelodysplasia that can transform into AML.

Chronic Eosinophilic Leukemia

CEL is a clonal proliferation of eosinophils from eosinophil precursors that dominate in the bone marrow and peripheral blood. Eosinophils are found in other peripheral tissues, including heart, lungs, central nervous system, gastrointestinal tract, and skin. Hepatosplenomegaly occurs in approximately 30% to 50% of patients. Infiltrating eosinophils degranulate to release cytokines, enzymes, and other granular proteins that damage the surrounding tissue, which results in organ dysfunction.[112]

Clinical Presentation

Although some patients with eosinophilia may be asymptomatic, most have signs and symptoms of fever, fatigue, cough, angioedema, muscle pain, and pruritus. A more severe sequela of CEL involves the heart. Fibrosis can form in the heart (endomyocardial fibrosis), which can evolve into cardiomegaly. Within the heart, scar tissue may form in the mitral and tricuspid valves, affecting valve function and predisposing to thrombi formation. Other serious complications include peripheral neuropathy, central nervous system dysfunction, pulmonary symptoms from eosinophilic infiltrates, and rheumatologic problems.[112] CEL occurs most often in men in the seventh decade of life. Very few cases of peripheral eosinophilia (1.2%) meet the criteria for CEL.[1]

Peripheral Blood and Bone Marrow

Peripheral eosinophilia (>1.5 × 10^9/L) must be observed, with the majority of eosinophils appearing normal. Some evidence of eosinophil abnormality is found, however, and includes the presence of eosinophilic myelocytes and metamyelocytes, hypogranulation, and vacuolization. Neutrophilia is a common finding; other features such as mild monocytosis, basophilia, and the presence of blasts are less common. The bone marrow is hypercellular because of eosinophilic proliferation, and the M:E ratio is increased. Eosinophils can demonstrate Charcot-Leyden crystals. Myeloblast numbers are elevated but less than the 20% threshold necessary to classify the disorder as an acute leukemia. Erythrocytes and megakaryocytes are normal in number, but megakaryocytes often demonstrate dysplastic morphologic features. Erythrocytic and granulocytic cells usually appear normal but can exhibit mild dysplasia.[1]

Diagnosis

The diagnosis of CEL requires eosinophilia with a count of more than 1.5×10^9 cells/L on at least two occasions within a 4-week period, evidence of clonality, abnormal bone marrow morphology, and the elimination of reactive eosinophilia and other malignancies that have concomitant eosinophilia. Reactive conditions such as parasitic infections, allergies, Löffler syndrome (pulmonary disease), cyclical eosinophilia, angiolymphoid hyperplasia of the skin, collagen vascular disorders, and Kimura disease must be excluded in the differential diagnosis. Likewise, other malignancies that can produce a concomitant eosinophilia include T cell lymphoma, Hodgkin lymphoma, systemic mastocytosis, CMML, atypical CML, and ALL. These disorders lead to the release of a variety of interleukins that can drive a secondary eosinophil reaction. No single genetic abnormality is specific for CEL. This criterion excludes *PCM1::JAK2*, which is observed in the group of disorders called myeloid/lymphoid neoplasms with eosinophilia and rearrangement of *PDGFRA, PDGFRB,* or *FGFR1*.[1,112]

Treatment

No standard of care has been established for patients with CEL. Hydroxyurea can be used to control leukocytosis, eosinophilia, and splenomegaly, and IFN-α has been used for refractory patients, producing hematologic and cytogenetic remissions in some patients. Allogeneic HSC transplantation has produced long-term remission in a few patients.

Prognosis

Survival is variable, around 2 years, but the prognosis is considered poor. In a small case series of 10 participants with CEL, the median survival was 22 months, with 50% transforming to AML.[115] The most common causes of death include infection, bleeding, and disease-related organ failure. Features of megakaryocyte dysplasia, thrombocytopenia, an increase in karyotype abnormalities, or bone marrow fibrosis indicate an unfavorable prognosis.[112]

Juvenile Myelomonocytic Leukemia

JMML is a MPN of early childhood involving HSCs driven by RAS pathway activation, resulting in granulocytosis and monocytosis that frequently infiltrate organs. JMML is a rare condition, affecting about 1.2 children per 1 million and occurring in boys twice as often as girls. JMML has been observed between birth and 14 years of age, but the peak incidence is between 4 months and 4 years of age.[1]

Clinical Presentation

More than half of patients with JMML present with pallor and fever, while others experience respiratory infections with a cough, bleeding, rashes, and gastrointestinal symptoms. Most patients will demonstrate splenomegaly (90%), hepatomegaly (80%), lymphadenopathy (50%), and skin rash (30%), reflecting leukemic infiltrates.[1]

Peripheral Blood and Bone Marrow

The CBC usually shows a leukocytosis, often between 25×10^9/L and 30×10^9/L, composed mostly of granulocytes, some immature, and monocytes ($>1 \times 10^9$/L). Some dysplastic features are seen, particularly in the monocytic element. Anemia and thrombocytopenia are common, and blasts average about 2% in the peripheral blood. The bone marrow reflects the granulopoiesis with occasional erythroid hyperplasia but, in contrast to the peripheral blood, the monocytoid elements are not prominent. Blasts may be moderately elevated but rarely approach the 20% criterion of acute leukemia.[1]

Diagnosis

Diagnosis of JMML requires meeting all five clinical, hematologic, and laboratory criteria, plus either one molecular criterion or two nonmolecular criteria. The five initial criteria include monocytosis $>1 \times 10^9$/L, blast/promonocyte counts of <20% in blood and bone marrow, organ infiltration (usually splenomegaly), absence of Ph1 or *BCR::ABL1* fusion, and absence of *KMT2A (MLL1)* gene rearrangement. In addition, one of the following molecular criteria must be met: mutations in RAS genes or RAS regulator genes, including *PTPN11, KRAS, NRAS, NF1,* or *CBL*; or mutations in genes upstream of RAS that activate RAS, including *ALK, PDGFR-B, ROS1,* or others. If the molecular criteria cannot be met, two or more of the following must be met to replace the molecular requirement: increased Hb F for age; myeloid and erythroid precursors in the peripheral blood; thrombocytopenia with decreased megakaryocytes in the bone marrow; and documented hypersensitivity of myeloid progenitors to GM-CSF.[1]

RAS gene mutations or *RAS* regulator gene mutations are seen in more than 90% of cases. Documenting one or more of these mutations supports the diagnosis of JMML. These mutations increase the sensitivity of myeloid progenitors to GM-CSF to stimulate overproduction of granulocytes and monocytes. In about 40% of somatically acquired mutations, the initial mutational event can be traced to birth, suggesting the mutation may have occurred in utero. Additional somatic mutations in other RAS genes, other gene targets, and altered DNA methylation are associated with disease progression and poor outcomes.[1]

Prognosis

The diversity of driver mutations makes prognostic predictions challenging. While some subtypes have demonstrated spontaneous remission, there are several poor prognostic indicators. Prognosis worsens with age older than 2 years; platelet counts below 33×10^9/L; elevated Hb F; somatic variants in *PTPN11* or *NF1*; secondary somatic mutations of *SETBP1*, *ASXL1*, and *EZH2*; and DNA hypermethylation. Blast crisis occurs in about 30% of patients.[1]

Myeloproliferative Neoplasm–Not Otherwise Specified

The category MPN-NOS is designed to capture disorders that clearly express myeloproliferative features but either fail to meet the criteria of a specific MPN or have features that overlap two or more specific MPNs. Most patients with MPN-NOS fall into one of four groups: patients with an early stage of PV, ET, or PMF in which the criteria that define the disorders are not yet fully developed; patients with portal or splanchnic vein thrombosis; patients presenting with features indicative of advanced disease resulting from clonal evolution or fibrosis that masks the potential underlying condition; and patients who have clear evidence of an MPN but who have a concomitant condition such as a second neoplasm or an inflammatory condition that alters the MPN features. MPN-NOS may account for as many as 10% to 15% of MPN disorders, but meticulous application of diagnostic criteria should reduce this prevalence to <5%.[1]

Diagnosis

MPN-NOS is considered a diagnosis by exclusion. Clinical, morphologic, laboratory, and molecular features of MPN must be present, but criteria for specific MPNs must not be met. While there are no specific diagnostic criteria for MPN-NOS, the MPN driver mutations (*JAK2*, *CALR*, and *MPL*) are present, as well as the triple-negative type. Other mutations such as *PDGFRA*, *PDGFRB*, or *FGFR1*, or fusions involving *JAK2* or *ABL1* must be absent to rule out similar neoplastic conditions. Caution should be exercised so that morphologic changes caused by the patient's cytotoxic drug therapy, growth factor therapy, or poor collection of samples are not confused with the features of MPN-NOS. In patients with MPN-NOS in the early stages of development or with a concomitant disorder such as inflammation, the MPN-NOS may be reclassified to a specific category of MPN once the disease begins to express typical features or the secondary condition subsides. Likewise, in patients with an advanced MPN, the disorder may be reclassified as an acute leukemia once the blast criterion of more than 20% blasts in the bone marrow is met.[1]

Prognosis

Prognosis varies depending largely on whether the patient best fits the early stage MPN-NOS model or the advanced-stage model. Rising blast counts of >10% signal disease progression. Blast counts of between 10% and 19% indicate the accelerated phase of the disease. Allogeneic HSC transplantation represents the only strategy to achieve long-term survival.[1]

MYELOID/LYMPHOID NEOPLASMS

Although the myeloid/lymphoid neoplasms are not included in the MPN diagnostic category, these entities are discussed in this chapter. This group of myeloid or lymphoid neoplasms is characterized by a corresponding eosinophilia and a defining gene rearrangement. The 2022 WHO classification system identifies seven categories defined by a gene rearrangement in the following genes: *PDGFRA*, *PDGFRB*, *FGFR1*, *JAK2*, *FLT3*, *ETV6::ABL1*, and other tyrosine kinase fusion genes.

The myeloid/lymphoid neoplasms with eosinophilia and defining gene rearrangements were segregated into their own category for three primary reasons: (1) each disorder has an underlying neoplasm of either the myeloid or the lymphoid type; (2) these conditions usually have an associated eosinophilia; (3) the mutations listed result in a constitutive activation of a tyrosine kinase. *PDGFRA* and *PDGFRB* respond to TKIs such as imatinib and ponatinib, whereas the others take a more aggressive course with variable sensitivity to TKI therapy. Therefore allogeneic HSC transplantation remains the best chance for long-term disease-free survival in non-*PDGFRA* and non-*PDGFRB* neoplasms.[1]

The most common mutation involving *PDGFRA* is a fusion gene involving *FIP1L1::PDGFRA*, which occurs more often in men. This fusion gene and most of the other *PDGFRA* rearrangements respond well to imatinib. Most patients achieve complete hematologic remission and complete molecular remission on imatinib therapy. Imatinib resistance is rare, but when it does occur, it is usually attributed to a specific mutation (T674I) that occurs in the ATP binding site of *PDGFRA*, similar to the T315I mutation in the *BCR::ABL1* fusion gene.[1]

Although more than 30 distinct fusion genes have been identified with *PDGFRB*, the most common rearrangement is *ETV6::PDGFRB*. Similar to the fusion genes associated with *PDGFRA*, those involving *PDGFRB* are also sensitive to imatinib and consistently produce complete hematologic remission as well as cytogenetic remission (92%) and molecular remission (86%). The 10-year survival with imatinib is 90%, with an 88% 6-year, progression-free survival rate.[1,112]

There have been 14 different fusion genes associated with *FGFR1*, resulting in a myeloproliferative syndrome with variable eosinophilia or with a leukemia/lymphoma picture. *ZMYM2::FGFR1* is associated with a high incidence of T lymphoblastic lymphoma transformation. *BCR::FGFR1* and *TPR::FGFR1* are associated with MPNs, with basophilia resembling CML. The *CEP43::FGFR1* and *CNTRL::FGFR1* fusion genes are often associated with features of CMML, whereas at other times, the *CEP43G::FGFR1* mutation resembles a PV phenotype without eosinophilia. The clinical course is more aggressive and not responsive to imatinib, nilotinib, or dasatinib, with minimal response to ponatinib. Chemotherapy did not produce sustained complete remission, leaving allogeneic HSC transplantation as the only treatment with the potential for long-term remission or cure.[1]

PCM1::JAK2 fusion gene, t(8;9), is the most common fusion gene in this category. Two other, less common rearrangements have been described, involving *ETV6::JAK2*, t(9;12), and *BCR::JAK2*, t(9;9). Patients present with features of a chronic myeloid neoplasm, with either eosinophilia or bone marrow fibrosis 50% to 70% of the time. The male-to-female ratio is a staggering 27:5, with the median age of diagnosis in the fifth decade of life. The clinical course is aggressive, with rapid transformation to AML or occasionally ALL. Treatment with ruxolitinib has produced complete hematologic remission, but it is usually short-lived, with relapse occurring after 18 to 24 months. Similar to the *FGFR1* rearrangements, allogeneic stem cell transplantation offers the best hope of long-term survival and potential for cure in patients with the *PCM1::JAK2* fusion gene.[1]

There are several partner genes identified thus far that pair with *FLT3*, but the most common is *ETV6::12p131*. FLT3 fusion proteins constitutively phosphorylate growth factor/ligand-independent proliferation. The disease generally follows an aggressive clinical course. Small-molecule FLT3 inhibitors such as sorafenib, sunitinib, and midostaurin have been used, with variable responses, most of which are generally short-lived. Allogeneic HSC transplantation is the best curative strategy for eligible patients.[1]

The *ETV6::ABL1* translocation leads to the activation of a nonreceptor tyrosine kinase ABL1. As one might predict, the laboratory features of the *ETV6::ABL1* sometimes resemble CML. However, other cases more closely resemble MDS/MPN with neutrophilia, CEL, or other MDS/MPNs. The prognosis is generally poor, but remissions have been reported using TKIs such as dasatinib, nilotinib, imatinib, bosutinib, and ponatinib.[1]

The last entry in this group involves myeloid and lymphoid neoplasms with eosinophilia resulting from tyrosine kinase fusion genes other than those previously defined. Examples include *ETV6::FGFR2, ETV6::LYN, ETV6::NTRK3, RANBP2::ALK, BCR::RET,* and *FGFR1OP::RET*. Due to a low number of cases and a wide range of potential fusion genes, determining a prognosis in this category is difficult. Based on a few reported cases, these neoplasms follow a more aggressive clinical course, are refractory to treatment, and are associated with a poor prognosis.[1]

MASTOCYTOSIS

Mastocytosis is not considered a subgroup of the MPNs in the WHO classification, but it will still be discussed in this chapter. Mastocytosis is a heterogeneous group of disorders caused by a clonal neoplastic proliferation of mast cells, which accumulate in one or more organ systems, but it can manifest differently and within a range of severities. The WHO group has classified mastocytosis into three subcategories: cutaneous mastocytosis, systemic mastocytosis, and MC sarcoma.[1]

Incidence

Mastocytosis can occur at any age, with cutaneous mastocytosis seen most often in children. Infants can be born with cutaneous mastocytosis, and half of affected children develop the disease before 6 months of age. In contrast, systemic mastocytosis generally occurs after the second decade of life. Approximately 80% of patients with mastocytosis have skin involvement, regardless of the type of mastocytosis diagnosed. Cutaneous mastocytosis occurs in the skin; systemic mastocytosis usually involves the bone marrow and other organ systems such as the spleen, lymph nodes, liver, and gastrointestinal tract; and MC leukemia is characterized by MCs in the peripheral blood.[1]

Clinical Presentation

Patients present with urticarial lesions with a wheal and flare appearance that may become activated when stroked on physical examination. Skin lesions also tend to have melanin pigmentation. Four categories of symptom severity have been described in mastocytosis: constitutional systems such as fatigue and weight loss; skin manifestations; mediator-related systemic events such as abdominal pain, gastrointestinal distress, headache, and respiratory symptoms; and musculoskeletal symptoms such as bone pain, arthralgias, and myalgias. Hematologic findings include anemia, leukocytosis, eosinophilia, neutropenia, and thrombocytopenia. In patients with systemic mastocytosis with associated clonal hematologic non-MC lineage disease, the most common associated hematologic finding is CMML, but any myeloid or lymphoid malignancy can occur, although myeloid versions predominate.[1]

Diagnosis

The typical skin lesion is the first diagnostic clue to mastocytosis. Cutaneous mastocytosis occurs in three forms: macropapular cutaneous mastocytosis (also known as urticaria pigmentosa), diffuse cutaneous mastocytosis, and mastocytoma, all of which occur predominantly in children. In macropapular cutaneous mastocytosis, MCs are confined to the skin and form aggregates in the dermis, whereas in diffuse cutaneous mastocytosis, MCs are found in more than one cutaneous location. Cutaneous mastocytosis is usually found in children and has a good prognosis, often resulting in natural lesion disappearance during puberty. In contrast, systemic mastocytosis often develops in adults, and MCs are identified in various internal organs and in the bone marrow. To establish a diagnosis of systemic mastocytosis, either one major and one minor criterion or three minor criteria must be met. Major criteria involve multifocal dense infiltrates of MCs (≥15 MCs in aggregates) in bone marrow biopsy specimens and/or in sections of other extracutaneous organs. Minor criteria include the following: (1) more than 25% of MCs are atypical cells (type I or type II) on bone marrow smears or are spindle shaped in MC infiltrates detected on sections of visceral organs; (2) MCs must express a *KIT* mutation at codon 816 in the bone marrow or other extracutaneous organ; (3) MCs in bone marrow, blood, or extracutaneous organs must express CD2, CD25, or CD30; and (4) total serum tryptase must be greater than 20 ng/mL. Key diagnostic features distinguish the five types of systemic mastocytosis: bone marrow mastocytosis, indolent systemic mastocytosis, smoldering systemic mastocytosis, aggressive systemic mastocytosis (ASM), systemic mastocytosis with associated hematologic (non-MC lineage) neoplasm, and MC leukemia. Indolent systemic mastocytosis is characterized by a low MC burden. Smoldering systemic mastocytosis exhibits a prognosis that is less favorable than indolent systemic mastocytosis but more favorable than ASM or MC leukemia. Systemic mastocytosis with associated hematologic (non-MC lineage) neoplasm manifests with myelodysplastic syndrome, MPN, AML, lymphoma, or another hematopoietic neoplasm. ASM usually does not manifest with skin lesions or MCs in circulation but does have MCs in bone marrow, dysplastic hematopoietic changes, and/or hepatosplenomegaly. ASM has been subdivided into two variants: untransformed variant and variant in transformation (ASM-t), in which bone marrow MCs are 5% to 20%. MC leukemia is characterized by more than 20% atypical MCs in the bone marrow. MC leukemia is subdivided into two types: classical MC leukemia, where more than 10% MCs are found in the peripheral blood, and aleukemic MC leukemia, in which less than 10% MCs are found in the peripheral blood. It has been proposed to further subdivide MC leukemia into acute MC leukemia (with organ damage) and chronic MC leukemia (without organ damage). MC sarcoma manifests as a single unifocal MC tumor with high-grade pathologic characteristics. Extracutaneous mastocytoma also exhibits a unifocal MC tumor, but it is pathologically low grade. A provisional subentity of systemic mastocytosis, termed *bone marrow mastocytosis* with no skin lesions, a low MC burden, and a good prognosis, is being discussed. Concurrently, extracutaneous mastocytoma was removed from the classification system because of its rarity.[1]

Pathogenetic Mechanism

The most common genetic mutation in patients with mastocytosis involves codon 816 in the *KIT* gene and occurs in about 80% of adults and 35% to 40% of children with systemic mastocytosis. This mutation replaces aspartic acid with valine, which alters the tyrosine kinase receptor activity, causing constitutive kinase activity in the absence of ligand. Usually the mutation is somatic, but a few cases of familial *KIT* mutations have been reported. Additional mutations can push proliferation of hematopoietic clones, causing systemic mastocytosis with associated clonal hematologic non-MC lineage disease, including *TET2, SRSF2, ASXL1,* and *JAK2.*[1]

Prognosis

Cutaneous mastocytosis in children has a favorable prognosis and may regress spontaneously around puberty. Milder versions such as cutaneous mastocytosis and indolent cutaneous mastocytosis follow a benign course and are associated with a normal life span. Hematologic involvement usually evolves into the corresponding hematologic disease. Patients with aggressive systemic mastocytosis, MC leukemia, and MC sarcoma are often treated with cytoreductive chemotherapy but may survive only a few months after diagnosis. Signs and symptoms that predict a poorer prognosis include elevated lactate dehydrogenase and alkaline phosphatase, anemia, thrombocythemia, abnormal peripheral blood morphology, bone marrow hypercellularity, and hepatosplenomegaly.[1]

▌ SUMMARY

- Myeloproliferative neoplasms (MPNs) are clonal hematopoietic stem cell disorders that result in excessive production and overaccumulation of erythrocytes, granulocytes, and platelets in some combination in bone marrow, peripheral blood, and body tissues.
- Within the classification of MPN, the four major conditions are chronic myeloid (myelogenous) leukemia (CML), polycythemia vera (PV), essential thrombocytopenia (ET), and primary myelofibrosis (PMF).
- In CML, there are large numbers of myeloid precursors in the bone marrow, peripheral blood, and extramedullary tissues.
- The peripheral blood exhibits leukocytosis with increased myeloid series, particularly the later maturation stages, often with increases in eosinophils and basophils.
- The Philadelphia chromosome, t(9;22), either at the chromosomal or molecular (*BCR::ABL1*) level, must be present in all cases of CML.
- In CML, the bone marrow exhibits intense hypercellularity with a predominance of myeloid precursors. Megakaryocyte numbers are normal to increased.
- Patients with CML can progress from a chronic stable phase through a high-risk chronic phase and blast phase.

- Bone marrow transplantation has been successful in CML, and imatinib mesylate, a tyrosine kinase inhibitor, produces remission in most cases.
- Approximately 4% of patients with CML given imatinib as first-line therapy develop imatinib resistance.
- Dosage escalation or administration of second- or third-generation tyrosine kinase inhibitors restores remission in most patients with imatinib resistance except those with the T315I mutation.
- PV manifests with panmyelosis in the bone marrow with increases in erythrocytes, granulocytes (66%), and platelets (50%).
- Based on the World Health Organization (WHO) standards, the diagnosis of PV requires that all three major criteria or the first two major criteria and one minor criterion be met. The clinical diagnosis of PV requires hemoglobin greater than 16.5 g/dL in men and women or elevated hematocrit (>49% for men or >48% for women) (first major criterion); bone marrow hypercellularity and panmyelosis with pleomorphic, mature megakaryocytes (second major criterion); and the presence of *JAK2* V617F or the *JAK2* exon 12 mutation. The one minor criterion is low serum erythropoietin levels.

- The *JAK2* V617F mutation is found in >95% of patients with PV and contributes to the pathogenesis of the disease.
- PV is treated with phlebotomy, hydroxyurea, *JAK2* inhibitors, and low-dose aspirin.
- ET involves an increase in megakaryocytes with a sustained platelet count greater than 450×10^9/L.
- WHO diagnosis requires that all four major criteria be met or three major criteria and one minor criterion be met. Major criteria are (1) platelet count >450×10^9/L; (2) bone marrow showing megakaryocytic proliferation, no significant increase in left shift or neutrophil granulopoiesis, and very rarely, an increase in reticulin fibers; (3) must not meet WHO criteria for a diagnosis of *BCR::ABL1*-positive CML, PV, PMF, MDS, or other myeloid neoplasm; and (4) must demonstrate *JAK2* V617F, *CALR*, or *MPL* mutations. The two minor criteria are presence of a clonal marker and absence of evidence of reactive thrombocytosis.
- In the early phases of ET, peripheral blood shows increased numbers of platelets with abnormalities in size and shape. Bone marrow megakaryocytes are increased in number and in size.
- Complications of ET include thromboembolism and hemorrhage.
- Treatment can include watch and wait, plateletpheresis, hydroxyurea, or anagrelide.
- The *JAK2* V617F mutation is observed in 50% to 60% of patients with ET and PMF and contributes to the pathogenesis of the disorders.
- PMF manifests with ineffective hematopoiesis, sparse areas of marrow hypercellularity (especially with increased megakaryocytes), bone marrow fibrosis, splenomegaly, and hepatomegaly.
- The peripheral blood in PMF exhibits immature granulocytes and nucleated RBCs; teardrop-shaped cells are a common finding.
- Platelets may be normal, increased, or decreased in number with abnormal morphology. Micromegakaryocytes may be present.

- WHO diagnostic criteria for prefibrotic myelofibrosis requires all three major and one minor criterion be met on two separate demonstrations. Major criteria are (1) bone marrow cellularity demonstrating megakaryocytic proliferation with atypia, granulocyte proliferation, and usually decreased erythropoiesis; (2) do not meet WHO criteria for *BCR::ABL1*-positive CML, PV, ET, MDSs, or other myeloid neoplasms; and (3) presence of *JAK2*, *CALR*, or *MPL, or* presence of another clonal marker, *or* absence of minor reactive marrow reticulin fibrosis. Minor criteria include (1) anemia not attributed to a comorbid condition; (2) leukocytosis >11×10^9/L; (3) splenomegaly; (4) elevated lactate dehydrogenase; and (5) leukoerythroblastosis.
- Treatment for low-risk patients who are asymptomatic warrants observation only with followup visits every 3 to 6 months. As the disease progresses, hematopoietic stem cell transplantation should be considered. For higher-risk patients, JAK inhibitors such as ruxolitinib, fedratinib, or hydroxyurea are considered first-line therapy. Hydroxyurea should be used for patients who are not candidates for ruxolitinib or fedratinib and when cytoreduction is warranted.
- JAK inhibitors improve splenomegaly and constitutional symptoms in patients with PMF to a greater degree than in patients with ET or PV.
- Other MPNs include chronic neutrophilic leukemia, chronic eosinophilic leukemia, juvenile myelomonocytic leukemia, and myeloproliferative neoplasms–not otherwise specified.
- Neoplasms not classified within the myeloproliferative group but included in this chapter include myeloid/lymphoid neoplasms with eosinophilia and rearrangement of *PDGFRA*, *PDGFRB*, or *FGFR1* or with *PCM1::JAK2* and mastocytosis.

Now that you have completed this chapter, go back and read again the case study at the beginning and respond to the questions presented. Answers can be found in Appendix C.

REVIEW QUESTIONS

Answers can be found in Appendix C.

1. A peripheral blood film that shows increased neutrophils with a left shift, basophils, eosinophils, and platelets is highly suggestive of:
   a. AML
   b. CML
   c. MDS
   d. Multiple myeloma
2. Which of the following chromosome abnormalities is associated with CML?
   a. t(15;17)
   b. t(8;14)
   c. t(9;22)
   d. Monosomy 7

3. A patient has a WBC count of 30×10^9/L and the following WBC differential:
   Segmented neutrophils—38%
   Bands—17%
   Metamyelocytes—7%
   Myelocytes—20%
   Promyelocytes—10%
   Eosinophils—3%
   Basophils—5%
   Which of the following test results would be helpful in determining whether the patient has CML?
   a. Nitroblue tetrazolium reduction product increased
   b. Myeloperoxidase increased
   c. Periodic acid-Schiff staining decreased
   d. FISH positive for *BCR::ABL1* fusion

4. A patient in whom CML has previously been diagnosed has circulating blasts and promyelocytes that total 30% of leukocytes. The disease is considered to be in what phase?
   a. Chronic stable phase
   b. High-risk chronic phase
   c. Transformation to acute leukemia
   d. Temporary remission

5. The most common mutation found in patients with primary PV is:
   a. *BCR::ABL1*
   b. Philadelphia chromosome
   c. *JAK2* V617F
   d. t(15;17)

6. The peripheral blood in PV typically manifests:
   a. Erythrocytosis only
   b. Erythrocytosis and thrombocytopenia
   c. Erythrocytosis with thrombocytosis, and granulocytosis most of the time
   d. Anemia and thrombocytopenia

7. A patient has a platelet count of 700×10^9/L with abnormalities in the size, shape, and granularity of platelets; a WBC count of 12×10^9/L; and hemoglobin of 11 g/dL. The Philadelphia chromosome is not present. The most likely diagnosis is:
   a. PV
   b. ET
   c. CML
   d. Leukemoid reaction

8. Complications of ET include all of the following EXCEPT:
   a. Thrombosis
   b. Hemorrhage
   c. Seizures
   d. Infections

9. Which of the following patterns is characteristic of the peripheral blood in patients with PMF?
   a. Teardrop-shaped erythrocytes, nucleated RBCs, immature granulocytes
   b. Abnormal platelets only
   c. Hypochromic erythrocytes, immature granulocytes, and normal platelets
   d. Spherocytes, immature granulocytes, and increased numbers of platelets

10. Bone marrow fibrosis associated with PMF results in:
    a. Increased blast production
    b. Leukocytosis
    c. Pancytopenia
    d. Hepatosplenomegaly

REFERENCES

1. WHO Classification of Tumours Editorial Board. *Haematolymphoid Tumors* [Internet, beta version ahead of print]. Lyon (France): International agency for research on cancer; 2022 [cited 2023/February/10]. (WHO classification of tumours series, 5th ed; vol 11). https://tumourclassification.iarc.who.int/chapters/63. Accessed February 8, 2023.

2. Dameshek, W. (1951). Some speculations on the myeloproliferative syndromes. *Blood, 6,* 372.

3. Berg, S., Diaz, M. O., Nand, S., et al. (2019). Germline mutations predispose to familial myeloproliferative neoplasms. *Blood, 134,* 2969.

4. Lin, C., Mao, L., Shao, L., et al. (2020). Global, regional, and national burden of chronic myeloid leukemia, 1990-2017: a systemic analysis for the global burden of disease study 2017. *Front Oncol, 10:580759,* 1–12.

5. Bizzozero, O. J., Johnson, K. G., & Ciocco, A. (1966). Radiation-related leukemia in Hiroshima and Nagasaki, 1946-1964: I. Distribution, incidence, and appearance time. *N Engl J Med, 274,* 1095–1101.

6. Brown, W. M., & Doll, R. (1965). Mortality from cancer and other causes after radiotherapy for ankylosing spondylitis. *BMJ, 5474,* 1327–1332.

7. Nowell, P., & Hungerford, D. A. (1960). A minute chromosome in human granulocytic leukemia. *Science, 132,* 1497–1499.

8. Rowley, J. D. (1973). A new consistent chromosome abnormality in chronic myelogenous leukemia identified by quinacrine fluorescence and Giemsa banding. *Nature, 243,* 290–293.

9. Stam, K., Heisterkamp, N., Grosveld, G., et al. (1985). Evidence of a new chimeric bcr/c-abl mRNA in patients with chronic myelocytic leukemia and the Philadelphia chromosome. *N Engl J Med, 313,* 1429–1433.

10. Groffen, J., Stephenson, J. R., Heisterkamp, N., et al. (1984). Philadelphia chromosomal breakpoints are clustered within a limited region, bcr, on chromosome 22. *Cell, 36*(1), 93–99.

11. Faderl, S., Talpaz, M., Estrov, Z., et al. (1999). Mechanisms of disease: the biology of chronic myeloid leukemia. *N Engl J Med, 341*(3), 164–172.

12. Randolph, T. R. (2005). Chronic myelocytic leukemia part I: history, clinical presentation, and molecular biology. *Clin Lab Sci, 18*(1), 38–48.

13. Braun, T. P., Eide, C. A. & Druker, B. J. (2020). Response and resistance to BCR-ABL1-targeted therapies. *Cancer Cell, 37,* 530.

14. Bradford, S. & Apperley, J. F. (2022). Measurable residual disease in chronic myeloid leukemia. *Haematol, 107,* 2794–2809.

15. Bernt, K. M. & Hunger, S. P. (2014). Current concepts in pediatric Philadelphia chromosome-positive acute lymphoblastic leukemia. *Front Oncol, 4,* 1–22.

16. Ogasawara, A., Matsushita, H., Tanaka, Y., et al. (2019). A simple screening method for the diagnosis of chronic myeloid leukemia using the parameters of a complete blood count and differentials. *Clinica Chimica Acta, 489,* 249–253.

17. Abdulmawjooh, B., Costa, B., Roma-Rodrigues, C., et al. (2021). Genetic biomarkers in chronic myeloid leukemia: What have we learned so far? *Int J Mol Sci, 22,* 12516.

18. Ochi, Y. Genetic landscape of chronic myeloid leukemia. *Int J Hematol, 117,* 30–36.

19. Wintrobe, M. M., Huguley, C. M., McLennan, M. T., et al. (1947). Nitrogen mustard as a therapeutic agent for Hodgkin's disease, lymphosarcoma and leukemia. *Ann Intern Med, 27*, 529–539.

20. Galton, D. A. (1953). The use of myleran in chronic myeloid leukemia: results of treatment. *Lancet, 264*, 208–213.

21. Lion, T., Gaiger, A., Henn, T., et al. (1995). Use of quantitative polymerase chain reaction to monitor residual disease in chronic myelogenous leukemia during treatment with interferon. *Leukemia, 9*, 1353–1360.

22. Guilhot, F., Chastang, C., Michallet, M., et al. (1997). Interferon alpha 2b combined with cytarabine versus interferon alone in chronic myelogenous leukemia. *N Engl J Med, 337*, 223–229.

23. Atwell, S., Adams, J. M., Badger, J., et al. (2004). A novel mode of Gleevec binding is revealed by the structure of spleen tyrosine kinase. *J Biol Chem, 279*, 55827–55832.

24. Green, M. R., Newton, M. D., & Fancher, K. M. (2016). Off-target effects of BCR-ABL and JAK2 inhibitors. *Am J Clin Oncol, 39*, 76–84.

25. Druker, B. J., Talpaz, M., Resta, D. J., et al. (2001). Efficacy and safety of a specific inhibitor of the BCR-ABL tyrosine kinase in chronic myeloid leukemia. *N Engl J Med, 344*, 1031–1037.

26. Claudiani, S., Gatenby, A., Szydlo, R., et al. (2019). MR4 sustained for 12 months is associated with stable deep molecular responses in chronic myeloid leukemia. *Haematologica, 104*, 2206–2214.

27. Bhamidipati, P. K., Kantarjian, H., Cortex, J., et al. (2013). Management of imatinib-resistant patients with chronic myeloid leukemia. *Ther Adv Hem, 4*, 103–117.

28. Nardi, A., Azam, M., & Daley, G. O. (2004). Mechanisms and implications of imatinib resistance mutations in BCR-ABL. *Curr Opin Hematol, 11*, 35–43.

29. Kantarjian, H. M., Talpaz, M., Giles, F., et al. (2006). New insights into the pathophysiology of chronic myeloid leukemia and imatinib resistance. *Ann Intern Med, 145*, 913–923.

30. Narayanan, V., Pollyea, D. A., Gutman, J. A., et al. (2013). Ponatinib for the treatment of chronic myeloid leukemia and Philadelphia chromosome-positive acute lymphoblastic leukemia. *Drugs Today, 49*, 261–269

31. Harrington, P., & de Lavallade, H. (2021). Novel developments in chronic myeloid leukemia. *Curr Opin Hematol, 28*, 122–127.

32. Krishnan, V., Kim, D. H., Hughes, T. P., et al. (2022). Integrating genetic and epigenetic factors in chronic myeloid leukemia risk assessment: toward gene expression-based biomarkers. *Haematologica, 107*, 358–370.

33. Park, C. S., & Lacorazza, D. (2020). DYRK2 controls a key regulatory network in chronic myeloid leukemia stem cells. *Exp Mol Med, 52*, 1663–1672.

34. Spivak, J. L. (2021). Advances in polycythemia vera and lessons learned for acute leukemia. *Best Pract Res Clin Haematol, 34*, 1-12.

35. Baumeister, J., Chatain, N., Sofias, A. M., et al. (2021). Progression of myeloproliferative neoplasms (MPN): diagnostic and therapeutic perspectives. *Cells, 10*, 3551.

36. Torres, D. G., Paes, J., da Costa, A. G., et al. (2022). JAK2 variant signaling: genetic, hematologic and immune implications in chronic myeloproliferative neoplasms. *Biomolecules, 12*, 291.

37. Hubbard, S. R. (2018). Mechanistic insights into regulation of JAK2 tyrosine kinase. *Front Endocrinol, 8*, 361.

38. Tefferi, A., Thiele, J., & Vardiman, J. W. (2009). The World Health Organization classification system for myeloproliferative neoplasms: order out of chaos. *Cancer, 115*, 3842–3847.

39. Kralovicics, R., Guan, Y., & Prchal, J. T. (2002). Acquired uniparental disomy of chromosome 9p is a frequent stem cell defect in polycythemia vera. *Exp Hematol, 30*, 229–236.

40. Wahab-Abdel, O. (2011). Genetics of the myeloproliferative neoplasms. *Curr Opin Hematol, 18*, 117–123.

41. Vainchenker, W., Delhommeau, F., Constantinescu, S. N., et al. (2011). New mutations and pathogenesis of myeloproliferative neoplasms. *Blood, 118*, 1723–1735.

42. Constantinescu, S. N., Vainchenker, W., Levy, G., et al. (2021). Functional consequences of mutations in myeloproliferative neoplasms. *HemaSphere, 5*, e578.

43. Suresh, S., Rajvanshi, P. K., & Noguchi, C. T. (2020). The many facets of erythropoietic physiologic and metabolic response. *Front Physiol, 10*, 1534.

44. Virtanen, A. T., Haikarainen, T., Sampathkumar, P., et al. (2023). Identification of novel small molecule ligands for JAK2 pseudokinase domain. *Pharmaceuticals, 16*, 75.

45. Rumi, E., Barate, C., Benevolo, G., et al. (2019). Myeloproliferative disorders: state of the art. *Hematol Oncol, 38*, 121–128.

46. James, C., Ugo, V., Le Couedic, J. P., et al. (2005). A unique clonal JAK2 mutation leading to constitutive signaling causes polycythemia vera. *Nature, 434*, 1144–1148.

47. Baxter, E. J., Scott, L. M., Campbell, P. J., et al. (2005). Acquired mutation of the tyrosine kinase JAK2 in human myeloproliferative disorders. *Lancet, 365*, 1054–1061.

48. Levine, R. L., Wadleigh, M., Cools, J., et al. (2005). Activating mutation in the tyrosine kinase JAK2 in polycythemia vera, essential thrombocythemia, and myeloid metaplasia with myelofibrosis. *Cancer Cell, 7*, 387–397.

49. Shi, S., Calhgoun, H. C., Xai, F., et al. (2006). JAK signaling globally counteracts heterochromatic gene silencing. *Nat Genet, 38*, 1071–1076.

50. Shi, S., Larson, K., Guo, D., et al. (2008). Drosophila STAT is required for directly maintaining HP1localization and heterochromatin stability. *Nat Cell Biol, 10*, 489–496.

51. Liu, F., Zhao, X., Pema, F., et al. (2011). JAK2V617F-mediated phosphorylation of PRMT5 downregulates its methyltransferase activity and promotes myeloproliferation. *Cancer Cell, 19*, 283–294.

52. Pastore, F., Bhagwat, N., Pastore, A., et al. (2020). PRMT5 inhibition modulates E2F1 methylation and gene regulatory networks leading to therapeutic efficacy in JAK2V617F mutant MPN. *Cancer Disc, 10*, 1742–1757.

53. Li, L., Kim, J. H., Lu, W., et al. (2022). HMGA1 chromatin regulators induce transcriptional networks involved in GATA2 and proliferation during MPN progression. *Blood, 139*, 2797–2815.

54. Hautin, M., Mornet, C., Chauveau, A., et al. (2020). Splicing anomalies in myeloproliferative neoplasms: paving the way for new therapeutic venues. *Cancers, 12*, 2216.

55. Scott, L. M., Tong, W., Levine, R. L., et al. (2007). JAK2 exon 12 mutations in polycythemia vera and idiopathic erythrocytosis. *N Engl J Med, 356*, 459–468.

56. Passamonti, F., Elena, C., Schnittger, S., et al. (2011). Molecular and clinical features of the myeloproliferative neoplasm associated with JAK2 exon 12 mutations. *Blood. 117*, 2813–2816.

57. Penna, D. (2021). New horizons in myeloproliferative neoplasm treatment: a review of current and future therapeutic options. *Medicina, 57*, 1181.

58. Pikman, Y., Lee, B. H., Mercher, T., et al. (2006). MPLW515L is a novel somatic activating mutation in myelofibrosis with myeloid metaplasia. *PLoS Med, 3,* e270.

59. Beer, P. A., Campbell, P. J., Scott, L. M., et al. (2008). MPL mutations in myeloproliferative disorders; analysis of the PT-1 cohort. *Blood, 112,* 141–149.

60. Boyd, E. M., Bench, A. J., Goday-Fernandez, A., et al. (2010). Clinical utility of routing MPL exon 10 analysis in the diagnosis of essential thrombocythaemia and primary myelofibrosis. *Br J Haematol, 149,* 250–257.

61. Chaligne, R., Tonetti, C., Besancenot, R., et al. (2008). New mutations in MPL in primitive myelofibrosis: only the MPL W515L mutations promote a G1/S-phase transition. *Leukemia, 22,* 1557–1566.

62. Jones, A. V., Chase, A., Silver, R. T., et al. (2009). JAK2 haplotype is a major risk factor for the development of myeloproliferative neoplasms. *Nat Genet, 41,* 446–449.

63. Kilpivaara, O., Mukherjee, S., Schram, A. M., et al. (2009). A germline JAK2 SNP is associated predisposition to the development of JAK2(V617F)-positive myeloproliferative neoplasms. *Nat Genet, 41,* 455–459.

64. Olcaydu, D., Harutyunyan, A., Jager, R., et al. (2009). A common JAK2 haplotype confers susceptibility to myeloproliferative neoplasms. *Nat Genet, 41,* 450–454.

65. Delhommeau, F., Dupont, S., Della Valle, V., et al. (2009). Mutations in TET2 in myeloid cancers. *N Engl J Med, 360,* 2289–2301.

66. Tahiliani, M., Koh, K. P., Shen, Y., et al. (2009). Conversion of 5-methylcytosine to 5-hydroxymethylcytosine in mammalian DNA by MLL partner TET1. *Science, 324,* 930–935.

67. Figueroa, M., Abdel-Wahab, O., Lu, C., et al. (2010). Leukemic IDH1 and IDH2 mutations result in a hypermethylation phenotype, disrupt TET2 function, and impair hematopoietic differentiation. *Cancer Cell, 18,* 553–567.

68. Tefferi, A., Lasho, T. L., Abdel-Wahab, O., et al. (2010). IDH1 and IDH2 mutation studies in 1473 patients with chronic-, fibrotic-, or blast-phase essential thrombocythemia, polycythemia vera or myelofibrosis. *Leukemia, 24,* 1302–1309.

69. Dang, L., White, D. W., Gross, S., et al. (2009). Cancer-associated IDH1 mutations produce 2-hydroxyglutarate. *Nature, 462,* 739–744.

70. Cao, R. & Zhang, Y. (2004). The functions of E(Z)/EZH2-mediated methylation of lysine 27 in histone H3. *Curr Opin Genet Dev, 14,* 155–164.

71. Ernest, T., Chase, A. J., Score, J., et al. (2010). Inactivating mutations of the histone methyltransferase gene EZH2 in myeloid disorders. *Nat Genet, 42,* 722–776.

72. Nikoloski, G., Langemeijer, S. M., Kuiper, R. P., et al. (2010). Somatic mutations of the histone methyltransferase gene EZH2 in myelodysplastic syndromes. *Nat Genet, 42,* 665–667.

73. Sauvageau, M., & Sauvaheau, G. (2010). Polycomb group proteins: multi-faceted regulators of somatic stem cells and cancer. *Cell Stem Cell, 7,* 299–313.

74. Scheuermann, J. C., de Ayala Alonso, A. G., Oktaba, K., et al. (2010). Histone H2A deubiquitinas activity of the Polycomb repressor complex PR-DUB. *Nature, 465,* 243–247.

75. Carbuccia, N., Murati, A., Trouplin, A., et al. (2009). Mutations of ASXL1 gene in myeloproliferative neoplasms. *Leukemia, 23,* 2183–2186.

76. Tefferi, A. (2010). Novel mutations and their functional clinical relevance in myeloproliferative neoplasms: JAK2, MPL, TET2, ASXL1, CBL, IDH and IKZF1. *Leukemia, 24,* 1128–1138.

77. Campbell, P. J., Baxter, E. J., Beer, P. A., et al. (2006). Mutation of JAK2 in the myeloproliferative disorders: timing, clonality studies, cytogenetic associations, and role in leukemic transformation. *Blood, 108,* 3548–3555.

78. Mesa, R. A., Li, C. Y., Ketterling, R. P., et al. (2005). Leukemic transformation in myelofibrosis with myeloid metaplasia: a single-institution experience with 91 cases. *Blood, 105,* 973–977.

79. Beer, P. A., Delhommeau, F., LeCouedic, J. P., et al. (2010). Two routes to leukemic transformation after a JAK2 mutation-positive myeloproliferative neoplasm. *Blood, 115,* 2891–2900.

80. Harutyunyan, A., Klampfl, T., Cazzola, M., et al. (2011). p53 lesions in leukemic transformation. *N Engl J Med, 364,* 488–490.

81. Beer, P. A., Ortmann, C. A., Campbell, P. J., et al. (2010). Independently acquired biallelic JAK2 mutations are present in a minority of patients with essential thrombocythemia. *Blood, 116,* 1013–1014.

82. Asshoff, M., Petzer, V., Warr, M. R., et al. (2017). Momelotinib inhibits ACVR1/ALK2, decreases hepcidin production, and ameliorates anemia of chronic disease in rodents. *Blood, 129,* 1823–1830.

83. Mesa, R. A., Vannucchi, A. M., Mead, A., et al. (2017). Pacritinib versus best available therapy for the treatment of myelofibrosis irrespective of baseline cytopenias (PERSIST-1): An international, randomized, phase 3 trial. *Lancet Haematol, 4,* e255–e236.

84. Harrison, C. N., Gerds, A. T., Kiladjian, J. J., et al. (2019). Pacifica: a randomized, controlled phase 3 study of pacritinib vs. physician's choice in patients with primary myelofibrosis, post polycythemia vera myelofibrosis, or post essential thrombocythemia myelofibrosis with severe thrombocytopenia (platelet count <50,000/mL). *Blood, 134,* 4175.

85. Mascarenhas, J., Komrokji, R. S., Cavo, M., et al. (2018). Imetelstat is effective treatment for patients with intermediate-2 or high-risk myelofibrosis who have relapsed or are refractory to Janus Kinase inhibitor therapy: results of a phase 2 randomized study of two dose levels. *Blood, 132,* 685.

86. Verstovsek, S., Yu, J., Scherber, R. M., et al. (2022). Changes in the incidence and overall survival of patients with myeloproliferative neoplasms between 2002 and 2016 in the United States. *Leuk Lymphoma, 63,* 694–702.

87. Aruch, D., & Mascarenhas J. (2016). Contemporary approach to essential thrombocythemia and polycythemia vera. *Curr Opin Hematol, 23,* 150–160.

88. Passamonti, F., Mora, B., & Maffioli, M. (2016). New molecular genetics in the diagnosis and treatment of myeloproliferative neoplasms. *Curr Opin Hematol, 23,* 137–143.

89. Mejia-Ochoa, M., Toro, P. A. A., & Cardona-Arias, J. A. (2019). Systematization of analytical studies of polycythemia vera, essential thrombocythemia and primary myelofibrosis, and a meta-analysis of the frequency of JAK2, CALR and MPL mutations: 2000-2018. *BMC Cancer, 19,* 590.

90. Pardanani, A., & Tefferi, A. (2011). Targeting myeloproliferative neoplasms with JAK inhibitors. *Curr Opin Hematol, 18,* 105–110.

91. Passamonti, F., Rumi, E., Arcaini, L., et al. (2008). Prognostic factors for thrombosis, myelofibrosis, and leukemia in essential thrombocythemia: a study of 605 patients. *Haematologica, 93,* 1645–1651.

92. Benevolo, G., Vassallo, F., Urbino, I., et al. (2021). Polycythemia vera (PV): update on emerging treatment options. *Ther Clin Risk Manag, 17,* 209–221.

93. Prchal, J. T. & Lichtman, M. A. (2021). Primary myelofibrosis. In Kaushansky, K., Prchal, J. T., Burns, L. J., et al. (Eds.), *Williams Hematology*, 10e. McGraw-Hill. https://accessmedicine.mhmedical.com/content.aspx?bookid=2962&sectionid=252541674.

94. Hobbs, G. S., & Rampal, R. K. (2015). Clinical and molecular genetic characterization of myelofibrosis. *Curr Opin Hematol, 22*, 177–183.

95. Grand, F. H., Hidalgo-Curtis, C. E., Ernst, T., et al. (2009). Frequent CBL mutations associated with 11q acquired uni-parental disomy in myeloproliferative neoplasms. *Blood, 113*, 6182–6192.

96. Mesa, R. A., Schwager, S., Radia, D., et al. (2009). The Myelofibrosis Symptom Assessment Form (MFSAF): an evidence-based brief inventory to measure quality of life and symptomatic response to treatment in myelofibrosis. *Leuk Res, 33*, 1199–1203.

97. Mesa, R. A., Niblack, J., Wadleigh, M., et al. (2007). The burden of fatigue and quality of life in myeloproliferative disorders (MPDs): an international Internet-based survey of 1179 MPD patients. *Cancer, 109*, 68–76.

98. Gangat, N., Caramazza, D., Vaidya, R., et al. (2011). DIPSS-Plus: a refined dynamic international prognostic indicator system (DIPSS) for primary myelofibrosis that incorporates prognostic information from karyotype, platelet count and transfusion status. *J Clin Oncol, 29*, 392–397.

99. Cervantes, F., Dupriez, B., Pereira, A., et al. (2009). New prognostic scoring system for primary myelofibrosis based on a study of the International Working Group for Myelofibrosis Research and Treatment. *Blood, 113*, 2895–2901.

100. Venugopal, S., Najfeld, V., Keyzner, A., et al. (2023). Primary myelofibrosis and chronic neutrophilic leukemia. In Hoffman, R., Benz, E. J., Jr., Silberstein, L. E., et al. (Eds.), *Hematology: Basic Principles and Practice*. (8th ed., pp. 1193–1224). Philadelphia: Elsevier.

101. Scherber, R., & Mesa, R. A. (2011). Future therapies for the myeloproliferative neoplasms. *Curr Hematol Malig Rep, 6*, 2–27.

102. Stein, B. L., Crispino, J. D., & Moliterno, A. R. (2011). Janus kinase inhibitors: an update on the progress and promise of targeted therapy in the myeloproliferative neoplasms. *Curr Opin Oncol, 23*, 609–616.

103. Verstovsek, S., & Komrokji, R. S. (2015). A comprehensive review of pacritinib in myelofibrosis. *Future Oncol, 11*(20), 2819–2830.

104. Cervantes, S., Mesa, R., & Barosi, G. (2007). New and old treatment modalities in primary myelofibrosis. *Cancer J, 13*, 377–383.

105. Elliott, M. A., Mesa, R., & Barosi, G. (2002). Thalidomide treatment in myelofibrosis with myeloid metaplasia. *Br J Haematol, 117*, 288–296.

106. Thomas, D. A., Giles, F. J., Albitar, M., et al. (2006). Thalidomide therapy for myelofibrosis with myelometaplasia. *Cancer, 106*, 1974–1984.

107. Tefferi, A., Cortez, J., Verstovsek, S., et al. (2006). Lenalidomide therapy in myelofibrosis with myeloid metaplasia. *Blood, 108*, 1158–1164.

108. Tefferi, A., Lasho, T. L., Mesa, R. A., et al. (2007). Lenalidomide therapy in del(5)(q31)-associated myelofibrosis: cytogenetic and JAK2V617F molecular remissions. *Leukemia, 21*, 1827–1828.

109. Mesa, R. A., Pardanani, A. D., Hussein, K., et al. (2010). Phase 1/-2 study of pomalidomide in myelofibrosis. *Am J Hematol, 85*, 129–130.

110. Maxson, J. E., & Tyner, J. W. (2017). Genomics of chronic neutrophilic leukemia. *Blood, 129*, 715–722.

111. Thomopoulos, T. P., Symeonidis, A., Kourakli, A., et al. (2022). Chronic neutrophilic leukemia: a comprehensive review of clinical characteristics, genetic landscape and management. *Front Oncol, 12*, 891–961.

112. Reiter, A., & Gotlib, J. (2016). Myeloid neoplasms with eosinophilia. *Blood, 129*, 704–714.

33

Myelodysplastic Neoplasms

*Nicholas C. Brehl**

OBJECTIVES

After completion of this chapter, the reader will be able to:

1. Define myelodysplastic neoplasms (MDS).
2. Explain the etiology of MDS.
3. Recognize morphologic features of dyspoiesis in bone marrow and peripheral blood.
4. Discuss abnormal functions of granulocytes, erythrocytes, and platelets in MDS.
5. Correlate peripheral blood, bone marrow, and cytogenetic and molecular findings in MDS with classification systems.
6. Compare and contrast subclassifications of MDS using the 2022 World Health Organization classification model and International Consensus Classification model.
7. Review the epidemiology of MDS and apply it as a contributor in differential diagnosis.
8. Explain the rationale for the category of myelodysplastic/myeloproliferative neoplasms (MDS/MPN).
9. Correlate peripheral blood, bone marrow, and cytogenetic findings in MDS/MPN with disease classification.
10. Given the patient history, clinical and laboratory findings, including representative cells on the peripheral blood film or bone marrow smear, interpret results of diagnostic tests to determine the type of MDS and recommend additional tests to confirm a diagnosis.
11. Discuss prognostic indicators in MDS.
12. Discuss modes of management and treatment in MDS, including novel therapies.

OUTLINE

Etiology
Morphologic Abnormalities in Peripheral Blood and Bone Marrow
  Dyserythropoiesis
  Dysmyelopoiesis
  Dysmegakaryopoiesis
Differential Diagnosis
Abnormal Cellular Function
Classification of Myelodysplastic Neoplasms
  French-American-British Classification
  World Health Organization Classification
  International Consensus Classification
Myelodysplastic Neoplasms with Defining Genetic Abnormalities
  Myelodysplastic Neoplasm with Low Blasts and Isolated 5q Deletion
  Myelodysplastic Neoplasm with Low Blasts and *SF3B1* Mutation
  Myelodysplastic Neoplasm with Biallelic *TP53* Inactivation
Myelodysplastic Neoplasms, Morphologically Defined
  Myelodysplastic Neoplasm with Low Blasts

  Myelodysplastic Neoplasm, Hypoplastic
  Myelodysplastic Neoplasm with Increased Blasts
Childhood Myelodysplastic Neoplasms
  Childhood Myelodysplastic Neoplasm with Low Blasts
  Childhood Myelodysplastic Neoplasm with Increased Blasts
Myelodysplastic/Myeloproliferative Neoplasms
  Chronic Myelomonocytic Leukemia
  MDS/MPN with Neutrophilia
  MDS/MPN with *SF3B1* Mutation and Thrombocytosis
  MDS/MPN, Not Otherwise Specified
Cytogenetics, Molecular Alterations, and Epigenetics
  Cytogenetics
  Molecular Alterations
  Epigenetics
Prognosis
Treatment
  Future Directions

*The author extends appreciation to Bernadette. F. Rodak, whose work in prior editions provided the foundation for this chapter.

CASE STUDY

After studying the material in this chapter, the reader should be able to respond to the following case study. Answers can be found in Appendix C.

A 43-year-old man experienced fatigue and malaise. He presented with pancytopenia (WBC of 2.2×10^9/L, HGB of 6.1 g/dL, and PLT of 51×10^9/L). The MCV was 132 fL. Reference intervals can be found after the Index at the end of the book. The WBC differential, vitamin B_{12}, and folate levels were within reference intervals. The bone marrow was normocellular, with a myeloid-to-erythroid ratio of 1:1 and adequate megakaryocytes. The erythroid component was dysplastic, with megaloblastic features. No abnormal localization of immature precursors was noted. Chromosome analysis indicated direct duplication of chromosome

1q. The patient was maintained with transfusions over the next 6 years. At that time his bone marrow revealed increased erythropoiesis, decreased granulopoiesis, and megakaryopoiesis, all with dysplastic changes. There were 50% to 60% ring sideroblasts.

1. What should be included in the differential diagnosis of patients with pancytopenia and elevated MCV?
2. Given the vitamin B_{12} and folate levels were within the reference intervals, what is the patient's probable diagnosis?
3. In which World Health Organization 2022 classification does this disorder belong?

For decades, laboratory professionals have observed a group of morphologic abnormalities in peripheral blood films and bone marrow smears of elderly patients. The findings were heterogeneous and affected all cell lines, and the condition either remained stable for years or progressed rapidly to death.

Historically this pattern of abnormalities was referred to as *refractory anemia, smoldering leukemia, oligoblastic leukemia,* or *preleukemia.*[1,2] In 1982 the French-American-British (FAB) Cooperative Leukemia Study Group proposed terminology and a specific set of morphologic criteria to describe what were known as *myelodysplastic syndromes* (MDS).[3] In 1997 a group from the World Health Organization (WHO) proposed a new classification that included molecular, cytogenetic, and immunologic criteria in addition to morphologic features.[4,5] The WHO classification was revised in 2008, 2016, and 2022. Emphasis in this chapter is placed on the WHO 2022 classification model, which renamed *myelodysplastic syndromes* as *myelodysplastic neoplasms* but kept the abbreviated form as MDS.[6]

MDS are a group of acquired clonal hematologic disorders characterized by progressive cytopenias in the peripheral blood, reflecting defects in erythroid, myeloid, and/or megakaryocytic maturation.[6,7] There is an increased risk, especially among certain subtypes, for the disease to transform into acute myeloid leukemia (AML).[6,7] The median age at diagnosis is 77 years.[8] MDS rarely affects individuals younger than age 40 unless preceded by chemotherapy, radiation, or a germline mutation.[1,9,10] However, cases in young adults and children have been reported.[10,11] The incidence of MDS seems to be increasing, but this apparent increase is best attributable to improved techniques for identifying these diseases and to improved classification.[8] Familiarity with MDS is an essential part of the body of knowledge required by medical laboratory professionals.

ETIOLOGY

As a clonal hematopoietic disorder, it was previously thought that the cell of origin for MDS was a myeloid progenitor because erythroid, myeloid, and megakaryocytic cells are commonly affected. However, a myeloid progenitor did not explain the increased risk that patients with MDS had for developing a lymphoid malignancy or the presence of somatic mutations in both myeloid and lymphoid cells. Phenotypically normal hematopoietic stem cells (HSCs) were found to be the cell of origin for MDS.[7,12] These HSCs exist in low frequency in the bone marrow

and may harbor one or more somatic mutations. The mutations in the affected HSCs drive clonal expansion at the expense of normal HSCs.[12,13]

Driven by advances in next-generation sequencing, the concept of pre-MDS conditions is now well established. As humans age, somatic mutations are acquired by hematopoietic cells. Some of these mutations confer a competitive survival advantage to the mutated cell leading to clonal hematopoiesis. Over 95% of patients over age 50 harbor durable and long-lasting clonal hematopoiesis of HSCs.[14] Although many of these patients are otherwise healthy, clonal hematopoiesis confers an increased risk of progression to MDS, other hematopoietic malignancy, or nonhematopoietic disorder. Clonal cytopenia of unknown significance (CCUS) and clonal hematopoiesis of indeterminate potential (CHIP) are both clonal disorders that do not meet the criteria for classification as MDS because they lack either dysplasia and an MDS-related mutation (CCUS) or dysplasia and a peripheral cytopenia (CHIP).[15] The complex interactions among additional cytogenetic aberrations, somatic mutations, epigenetic modifications, the bone marrow microenvironment, and environmental stimuli determine whether CCUS, CHIP, and other pre-MDS conditions develop into MDS (or another malignancy), the severity of the subsequent disorder, and its risk for transformation into AML.[12,13,15–18]

The genetic mutations in the HSC that lead to MDS come from a variety of sources. De novo mutations (primary MDS) account for most of the cases. The mutations may also arise as a result of therapy (myeloid neoplasm post cytotoxic therapy), secondary to exposure to chemicals or radiation (not associated with prior disease treatment), or they may be inherited (myeloid neoplasms associated with germline predisposition or myeloid proliferations associated with Down syndrome). Inherited mutations, also known as germline mutations, predispose patients to MDS and other malignancies to variable degrees and may not manifest until the patient is elderly.[10]

Myeloid neoplasm post cytotoxic therapy (MN-pCT, previously known as therapy-related MDS) develops in patients after treatment history of exposure to DNA-damaging cytotoxic chemotherapy and/or large-field radiation therapy. Although causality is impossible to determine, the effects of some leukemogenic chemotherapies and therapeutic radiation are known to cause genetic mutations and cellular disruptions.[19,20] Median onset of MN-pCT is usually 4 to 7 years after therapy was initiated but may vary dependent upon the agents used.[19,20] In addition to inducing genetic change in hematopoietically active cells, evidence is accumulating that chemotherapy may apply a selective pressure to the bone marrow, which allows preexisting mutations to accumulate.[20,21] Patients who have received cytokines, such as G-CSF or GM-CSF, for bone marrow stimulation are also at an increased risk for developing MN-pCT.[22] MN-pCT is aggressive and may evolve quickly into AML.[19,20]

The 2022 WHO classification recognizes patients who have a predisposition to develop MDS from germline mutations (myeloid neoplasms with germline predisposition). Patients with inherited bone marrow failure syndromes such as Fanconi anemia, Diamond-Blackfan anemia, and Shwachman-Diamond syndrome are at a significantly increased risk for developing MDS, particularly in childhood or adolescence (Chapter 19).[23] Other mutations, such as those commonly identified in de novo MDS, may be inheritable and confer increased risk for development of MDS.[23]

MDS is characterized by the presence of progressive cytopenias despite a cellular bone marrow, ineffective hematopoiesis, dysplasia in one or more cell lines, and clonal hematopoeisis evidenced by the presence of cytogenetic abnormalities and/or molecular mutations.[24] The characteristic cytopenias found in MDS are caused by ineffective hematopoiesis. It is now understood that this process is characterized by activation of an inflammatory cell death pathway known as pyroptosis.[25,26] In MDS, ineffective hematopoiesis is increased in early disease, when peripheral blood cytopenias are evident. Later in MDS, when progression toward leukemia is more apparent, complex changes driven by additional genetic mutations, epigenetic changes, downstream effects of inflammatory cytokines and pyroptosis, and reciprocal interactions between the MDS cells and the microenvironment occur, which allows increased neoplastic cell survival and expansion of the abnormal clone.[18,25,26]

MORPHOLOGIC ABNORMALITIES IN PERIPHERAL BLOOD AND BONE MARROW

In MDS, each of the three major myeloid cell lines may have dyspoietic morphologic features. The following sections provide descriptions of common abnormal morphologic findings.[3,24] The WHO recommends that a threshold of at least 10% of cells within a lineage is used when determining whether dysplasia is significant for the diagnosis of MDS.[24] These descriptions are not all inclusive.

Dyserythropoiesis

In peripheral blood the most common morphologic finding in dyserythropoiesis is the presence of oval macrocytes (Figure 33.1). When these cells are seen in the presence of normal vitamin B_{12} and folate values, MDS should be included in the differential diagnosis. Hypochromic microcytes in the presence of adequate iron stores also are seen in MDS. A dimorphic red blood cell (RBC) population (Figure 33.2) is another indication of the clonality of this disease. Poikilocytosis, basophilic stippling, Howell-Jolly bodies, and siderocytes also are indications that the erythrocyte has undergone abnormal development.[27]

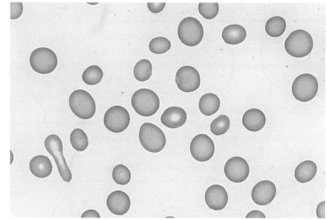

Figure 33.1 Oval Macrocytes. (Peripheral blood, Wright-Giemsa stain, ×1000.)

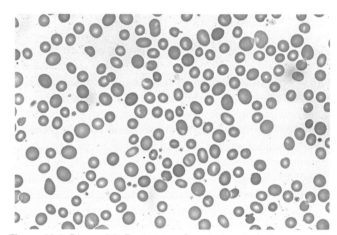

Figure 33.2 Dimorphic Erythrocyte Population. Includes macrocytic and microcytic cells. (Peripheral blood, Wright-Giemsa stain, ×500.)

Dyserythropoiesis in the bone marrow is evidenced by RBC precursors with more than one nucleus or abnormal nuclear shapes. The normally round nucleus may have lobes or buds (Figure 33.3). Nuclear fragments may be present in the cytoplasm. Internuclear bridging is occasionally present (Figure 33.4).[28] Abnormal cytoplasmic features may include basophilic stippling or heterogeneous staining (Figure 33.5). Ring sideroblasts are a common finding. Megaloblastoid development in the presence of normal vitamin B_{12} and folate values is another indication of MDS. The bone marrow may have erythrocytic hyperplasia or hypoplasia. Morphologic features of dyserythropoiesis are summarized in Box 33.1.

Dysmyelopoiesis

Dysmyelopoiesis in the peripheral blood is suspected when there is a persistence of basophilia in the cytoplasm of otherwise mature white blood cells (WBCs), indicating nuclear-cytoplasmic asynchrony (Figure 33.6). Abnormal granulation of the cytoplasm of neutrophils, in the form of larger than normal granules, hypogranulation, or the absence of granules, is a common finding. Agranular bands can be easily misclassified as monocytes (Figure 33.7). Abnormal nuclear features may include hyposegmentation and pseudo-Pelger-Huët anomaly (Chapter 26), hypersegmentation, or nuclear rings (Figure 33.8).[29]

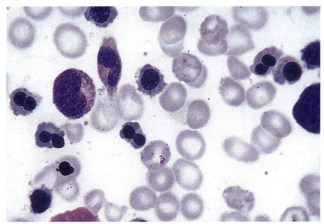

Figure 33.3 Erythroid Hyperplasia and Nuclear Budding in Erythroid Precursors. (Bone marrow, Wright-Giemsa stain, ×1000.)

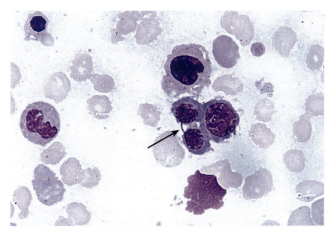

Figure 33.4 Erythroid Precursors Showing Nuclear Bridging. *(arrow)* (Bone marrow, Wright-Giemsa stain, ×1000.)

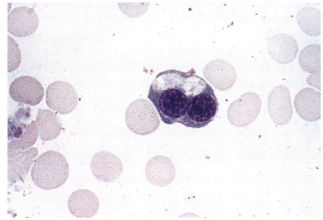

Figure 33.5 Heterogeneous Staining in a Bilobed Erythroid Precursor. (Bone marrow, Wright-Giemsa stain, ×1000.)

In the bone marrow, dysmyelopoiesis may be represented by nuclear cytoplasmic asynchrony. Cytoplasmic changes include uneven staining, such as a dense ring of basophilia around the periphery with a clear, unstained area around the nucleus, or whole sections of cytoplasm unstained, with the remainder of the cytoplasm stained normally (Figure 33.9). There may be abnormal

BOX 33.1 Morphologic Features of Dyserythropoiesis
Megaloblastoid development including oval macrocytes and nuclear-cytoplasmic asynchrony Dimorphic red blood cell (RBC) population with hypochromic microcytes RBC precursors with more than one nucleus, nuclear budding, abnormal nuclear shapes, internuclear bridging, or heterogenous cytoplasmic staining RBC inclusions including Howell-Jolly bodies, basophilic stippling, and Pappenheimer bodies Ring sideroblasts

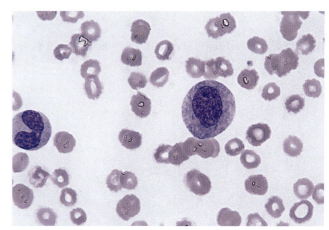

Figure 33.6 Myeloid Cells. This myelocyte *(right)* has a nucleus with clumped chromatin and a basophilic immature cytoplasm showing asynchrony. Note also the agranular myeloid cell *(left)* (Peripheral blood, Wright-Giemsa stain, ×1000.)

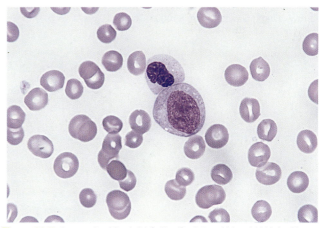

Figure 33.7 Agranular Myeloid Cells. (Peripheral blood, Wright-Giemsa stain, ×1000.)

granulation of the cytoplasm in which promyelocytes or myelocytes or both are devoid of primary granules (Figure 33.10), primary granules may be larger than normal, or secondary granules may be reduced in number or absent, and there may be an occasional Auer rod.[30,31] Agranular promyelocytes may be mistaken for blasts; this could lead to misclassification of the disease as an AML. Abnormal nuclear findings may include hypersegmentation or hyposegmentation and possibly ring-shaped nuclei. Morphologic features of dysmyelopoiesis are summarized in Box 33.2.

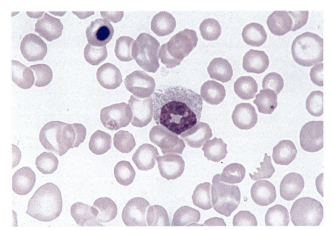

Figure 33.8 Nuclear Ring in Myeloid Cell. (Peripheral blood, Wright-Giemsa stain, ×1000.)

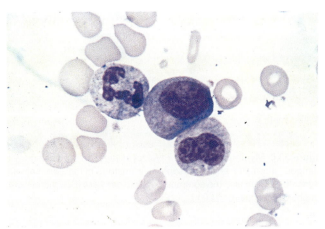

Figure 33.9 Uneven Staining of White Blood Cell Cytoplasm. (Bone marrow, Wright-Giemsa stain, ×1000.)

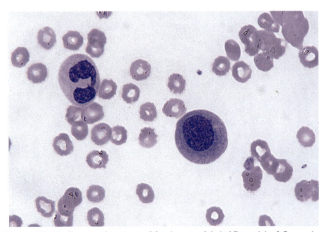

Figure 33.10 Promyelocyte or Myelocyte *(right)* Devoid of Granules and an Agranular Neutrophil *(left).* (Bone marrow, Wright-Giemsa stain, ×1000.)

The bone marrow may exhibit granulocytic hypoplasia or hyperplasia. Monocytic hyperplasia is a common finding in dysplastic marrows.

Abnormal localization of immature precursors is a characteristic finding in bone marrow biopsy specimens from patients with MDS.[32] Normally, myeloblasts and promyelocytes reside

> **BOX 33.2** **Morphologic Features of Dysmyelopoiesis**
>
> Nuclear-cytoplasmic asynchrony with persistent cytoplasmic basophilia
> Abnormal cytoplasm in myeloid cells: larger granules, hypogranulation, or absence of granules; uneven staining
> Abnormal nuclei in neutrophils: hyposegmentations and peudo-Pelger-Huët anomaly, hypersegmentation, or nuclear rings

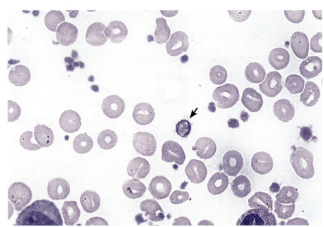

Figure 33.11 Abnormal Platelet Granulation *(arrow).* (Peripheral blood, Wright-Giemsa stain, ×1000.)

along the endosteal surface of the bone marrow. In some cases of MDS, these cells tend to cluster centrally in marrow sections.[32]

Dysmegakaryopoiesis

Platelets also exhibit dyspoietic morphology in the peripheral blood. Common changes include giant platelets and abnormal platelet granulation, either hypogranulation or agranulation (Figure 33.11). Some platelets may possess large fused granules. Circulating micromegakaryocytes may be present in peripheral blood from patients with MDS (Figure 33.12).[9]

The megakaryocytic component of the bone marrow may exhibit abnormal morphology: large mononuclear megakaryocytes, micromegakaryocytes, or micromegakaryoblasts. The nuclei in these cells may be bilobed or have multiple small, separated nuclei (Figure 33.13). Morphologic features of dysmegakaryopoiesis are summarized in Box 33.3.[9]

DIFFERENTIAL DIAGNOSIS

Dysplasia by itself is not sufficient evidence for MDS because several other conditions can cause similar morphologic features. Some examples are vitamin B_{12} or folate deficiency, which can cause pancytopenia and dysplasia, and exposure to heavy metals. Copper deficiency may cause reversible myelodysplasia.[9] Some congenital hematologic disorders, such as Fanconi anemia and congenital dyserythropoietic anemia, may also manifest with dysplasia. Parvovirus B19 and some chemotherapeutic agents may give rise to dysplasia similar to that in MDS. Paroxysmal nocturnal hemoglobinuria and aplastic anemia have similar features, as does infection with human immunodeficiency virus (HIV).[33,34] Therefore a thorough history and

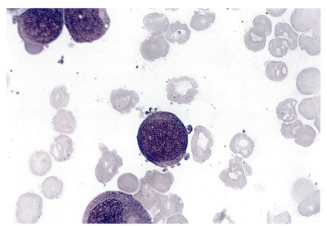

Figure 33.12 Micromegakaryocyte. (Peripheral blood, Wright-Giemsa stain, ×1000.)

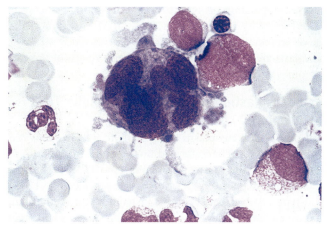

Figure 33.13 Megakaryocyte with Small, Separated Nuclei. (Bone marrow, Wright-Giemsa stain, ×1000.)

BOX 33.3 Morphologic Features of Dysmegakaryopoiesis

Giant platelets
Abnormal platelet granulation: hypogranulation, agranulation, or large fused granules
Circulating micromegakaryocytes
Bone marrow: micromegakaryocytes and micromegakaryoblasts; large mononuclear megakaryocytes; megakaryocytes with bilobed or multiple small nuclei

---

physical examination, including questions about exposure to drugs and chemicals, are essential.[9]

ABNORMAL CELLULAR FUNCTION

The cells produced by abnormal maturation not only have an abnormal appearance but also have abnormal function.[9,35] The granulocytes may have decreased adhesion,[36,37] deficient phagocytosis,[37] decreased chemotaxis,[36,37] or impaired microbicidal capacity.[38] Decreased levels of myeloperoxidase and alkaline phosphatase may be found.[39] The RBCs may exhibit shortened survival,[40] and erythroid precursors may have a

decreased response to erythropoietin that may contribute to anemia.[41] Patients may experience bleeding despite adequate platelet numbers, abnormal platelet function tests, or hyperaggregation.[9,42,43] The type and degree of dysfunction depend on the mutation present in the HSC.

CLASSIFICATION OF MYELODYSPLASTIC NEOPLASMS

French-American-British Classification

In an effort to standardize the diagnosis of MDS, the FAB created five classes of MDS, each with a specific set of morphologic criteria. The categories were organized by morphology, the amount of dysplasia, and the number of blasts in the bone marrow. Although rarely referenced today, the FAB classification provided a framework for discussion of a seemingly heterogeneous group of disorders. The WHO classification builds upon the FAB classification system while incorporating advances in medical knowledge such as clinical, molecular, cytogenetic, and immunologic characteristics of these disorders.

World Health Organization Classification

The WHO classification system maintained some of the organization initiated in the FAB system, but it also has undergone significant updates in pace with scientific research. The threshold for dysplasia, a requirement for the diagnosis of MDS, is defined as 10% dysplastic cells in any hematopoietic lineage.[44] The percentage of blasts required for diagnosis of an acute leukemia has decreased to 20% from FAB's threshold of 30%. The 2022 WHO classification system is outlined in Box 33.4 and briefly detailed in Table 33.1. The classification is extensive, and only the highlights are presented in this chapter.

International Consensus Classification

A division within the scientific field concerning authorship and the deliberative process occurred following the 2016 WHO classification, resulting in the creation of a new classification system called the International Consensus Classification (ICC) in 2022.[45] Although there are many similarities between the 2022 WHO classification system and the ICC, each system is unique and stands on its own. Unlike the 2022 WHO classification system, ICC preserved the name myelodysplastic syndromes for MDS. One of the more notable changes is the ICC's creation of the MDS/AML category for adult patients who present with 10% to 19% blasts.[45] This category, largely synonymous with WHO 2022 MDS with increased blasts 2, emphasizes the biologic continuum between MDS and AML.[45] In this chapter, emphasis is placed on the 2022 WHO classification system, but Table 33.1 provides comparisons between the 2022 WHO and ICC classification systems when appropriate.

MYELODYSPLASTIC NEOPLASMS WITH DEFINING GENETIC ABNORMALITIES

Myelodysplastic Neoplasm with Low Blasts and Isolated 5q Deletion

Myelodysplastic neoplasm with low blasts and isolated 5q deletion (MDS-5q) is a well-defined neoplasm largely unchanged

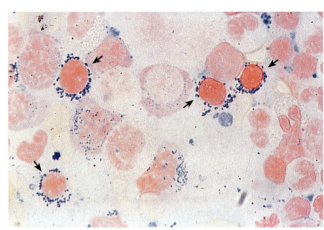

Figure 33.14 Ring Sideroblast *(arrows)*. (Bone marrow, Prussian blue stain, ×1000.)

from the 2016 WHO classification. The interstitial deletion of 5q may occur in isolation or in the presence of another cytogenetic abnormality, with the exception of monosomy 7 or 7q deletion.[44] MDS-5q predominantly affects females and occurs at a median age of 67.[46,47] These patients typically have anemia without other cytopenias and dysplastic megakaryocytes.[48] Some present with thrombocytosis and/or erythroid hypoplasia.[49–50] There are less than 2% blasts in the peripheral blood and less than 5% blasts in the bone marrow.[44] Auer rods are not seen.[48] Patients with MDS-5q are typically classified at lower risk than many other MDS with the median survival of patients ranging from 54 to 146 months.[47,49,51] A thalidomide analog, lenalidomide, is often effective in patients with MDS-5q.[47–51]

Myelodysplastic Neoplasm with Low Blasts and *SF3B1* Mutation

A mutation in the spliceosome gene *SF3B1* characterizes 90% of the cases of MDS with more than 5% ring sideroblasts in the bone marrow.[48] A ring sideroblast is an erythroid precursor containing at least five iron granules per cell, and these iron-containing mitochondria must circle at least one-third of the nucleus (Figure 33.14).[52] The 2016 and 2022 WHO classification systems group MDS with *SF3B1* mutation together with MDS without an *SF3B1* mutation that presents with 15% or more ring sideroblasts. The renaming of this category in the 2022 WHO classification emphasizes the unique biology and favorable prognosis conferred by the *SF3B1* mutation versus other driver mutations. However, patients with an unmutated *SF3B1* mutation and 15% or more ring sideroblasts are still included in this group. Patients with MDS with low blasts and *SF3B1* mutation have anemia and dyserythropoiesis.[48] The peripheral blood often demonstrates a dimorphic picture, with a mixed population of hypochromic cells and normochromic cells. This entity accounts for 17% of all MDS with a median age of presentation between 70 and 75 years old.[48] MDS with low blasts and *SF3B1* mutation has one of the most favorable outcomes in comparison to other MDS.[48,53]

Myelodysplastic Neoplasm with Biallelic *TP53* Inactivation

Myelodysplastic neoplasm with biallelic *TP53* inactivation (MDS-bi*TP53*) is characterized by the multi-hit mutation of both copies of the tumor suppressor gene *TP53* or mutation of one copy followed by deletion of the other copy.[44] Loss of wild-type *TP53* leads to genomic instability, which contributes to most patients with MDS-bi*TP53* having complex karyotypes and a poor prognosis.[44] *TP53* mutations account for 5% to 10% of de novo MDS.[48,54]

MYELODYSPLASTIC NEOPLASMS, MORPHOLOGICALLY DEFINED

Myelodysplastic Neoplasm with Low Blasts

Myelodysplastic neoplasm with low blasts (MDS-LB) is defined, by the presence of cytopenia and dysplasia in at least one cell lineage, with less than 5% blasts in the bone marrow and less than 2% blasts in the peripheral blood.[48] The presence of dysplasia in a single lineage (MDS with low blasts and single lineage dysplasia) or multiple lineages (MDS with low blasts and multilineage dysplasia) provide an option to further subclassify this group. Molecular and cytogenetic evaluations are recommended for prognostic evaluation, but MDS-LB is not defined by either.

Myelodysplastic Neoplasm, Hypoplastic

Hypoplastic MDS (h-MDS) is associated with an age-adjusted, profoundly hypocellular bone marrow with cytopenia and dysplasia.[48] The hypocellularity is frequently the result of T-cell mediated targeting of HSCs.[44,48] Cytogenetic and molecular diagnostic testing are necessary to distinguish MDS-h from aplastic anaemia and paroxysmal nocturnal hemoglobinuria, which have significant overlap in their manifestations. h-MDS accounts for 10% to 15% of MDS and is diagnosed at a lower median age than other MDS.[48,55]

TABLE 33.1 Comparison of the 2022 World Health Organization (WHO) Classification and International Consensus Classification (ICC) of MDS

WHO 2022 Classification	International Consensus Classification
MDS with Defining Genetic Abnormalities	
MDS with low blasts and isolated 5q deletion (MDS-5q) <5% BM blasts and <2% PB blasts	MDS with del(5q) (MDS-del5q) <5% BM blasts and <2% PB blasts

MDS with low blasts and *SF3B1* mutation (MDS-*SF3B1*)
  SF3B1 mutation or ≥15% ring sideroblasts
  <5% BM blasts and <2% PB blasts
	MDS with mutated *SF3B1* (MDS-*SF3B1*)*
	  Requires *SF3B1* mutation
	  <5% BM blasts and <2% PB blasts

MDS with biallelic *TP53* inactivation (MDS-bi*TP53*) <20% blasts in BM and PB	MDS with mutated *TP53* (MDS-*TP53*) <10% blasts in BM and PB
	MDS/AML with mutated *TP53* 10%–19% blasts in BM and PB
MDS, Morphologically Defined	
MDS with low blasts (MDS-LB)	

MDS-LB single lineage dysplasia†
    <5% BM blasts and <2% PB blasts
    Dysplasia in 1 cell lineage
	MDS, NOS with single lineage dysplasia†
	  <5% BM blasts and <2% PB blasts
	  Dysplasia in 1 cell lineage

MDS-LB multilineage dysplasia†
    <5% BM blasts and <2% PB blasts
    Dysplasia in 2 or 3 cell lineages
	MDS, NOS with multilineage dysplasia†
	  <5% BM blasts and <2% PB blasts
	  Dysplasia in 2 or 3 cell lineages

MDS, hypoplastic (MDS-h) <5% BM blasts and <2% PB blasts	
MDS with increased blasts (MDS-IB)	

MDS-IB1
    5%–9% BM blasts or 2%–4% PB blasts
	MDS with excess blasts (MDS-EB)
	  5%–9% BM blasts or 2%–9% PB blasts

MDS-IB2
    10%–19% BM blasts or 5%–19% PB blasts or Auer rods
	MDS/AML
	  10%–19% BM blasts or PB blasts

MDS with fibrosis 5%–19% BM blasts; 2%–19% PB blasts	
Childhood MDS	**Pediatric and/or Germline Mutation-Associated Disorders**

Childhood MDS with low blasts (cMDS-LB)
  <5% BM blasts and <2% PB blasts
  Hypocellular
  NOS
	Refractory cytopenia of childhood

Childhood MDS with increased blasts (cMDS-IB) 5%–19% BM blasts and 2%–19% PB blasts	
MDS/MPN	

Chronic myelomonocytic leukemia‡
  Myelodysplastic CMML (WBC<13 × 10⁹/L)
  Myeloproliferative CMML (WBC≥13 × 10⁹/L)
	Chronic myelomonocytic leukemia‡
	  Myelodysplastic CMML (WBC<13 × 10⁹/L)
	  Myeloproliferative CMML (WBC≥13 × 10⁹/L)

MDS/MPN with neutrophilia (MDS/MPN-N)	Atypical chronic myeloid leukemia (aCML)

MDS/MPN with *SF3B1* mutation and thrombocytosis
  Requires *SF3B1* mutation with concurrent *JAK2* p.V617F or biological similar mutation
  If *SF3B1* mutation is not detected, diagnosis can be supported with ≥15% ring sideroblasts
	MDS/MPN with *SF3B1* mutation and thrombocytosis
	  Requires *SF3B1* mutation
	  JAK2 p.V617F or similar mutation supports diagnosis but is not required
	MDS/MPN with ring sideroblasts and thrombocytosis, NOS
	  SF3B1 mutation not detected but ≥15% ring sideroblasts are found

MDS/MPN, NOS	MDS/MPN, NOS

*Classify as MDS, NOS for cases with ≥15% ring sideroblasts and unmutated *SF3B1*.
†Dysplasia is defined as ≥10% dysplastic cells in a cell lineage.
‡Monocytes ≥0.5 × 10⁹/L and ≥10% of PB WBCs; <20% blasts and promonocytes in PB and BM.
AML, Acute myeloid leukemia; *BM,* bone marrow; *CMML,* chronic myelomonocytic leukemia; *MDS,* myelodysplastic neoplasms (WHO) and myelodysplastic syndromes (ICC); *MPN,* myeloproliferative neoplasm; *NOS,* not otherwise specified; *PB,* peripheral blood; *WBC,* white blood cells.
Data from references 44 and 45.

Myelodysplastic Neoplasm with Increased Blasts

Myelodysplastic neoplasm with increased blasts (MDS-IB) is defined by having 5% to 19% blasts in the bone marrow and/or 2% to 19% blasts in the peripheral blood.[44,48] MDS-IB accounts for 28% to 39% of MDS cases.[48] MDS-IB can be further subclassified by percent of blasts and the presence of fibrosis. Overall survival and the period until transformation into AML is worse for patients with MDS-IB2.[53,56] The boundary between MDS presenting with increased blasts and AML has hinged on a 20% blast cutoff under multiple revisions of the WHO classification.[48] The 2022 WHO revision retains the cutoff but acknowledges it as arbitrary and not reflective of the biologic processes underlying the pathology. The risk of lowering the blast cutoff for AML may lead to overtreating patients; therefore the 20% blast cut remains. However, MDS with more than 10% blasts should be considered as an AML equivalent for therapeutic decisions and clinical trials when appropriate.[44,57]

CHILDHOOD MYELODYSPLASTIC NEOPLASMS

Childhood Myelodysplastic Neoplasm with Low Blasts

Myelodysplastic neoplasms in people younger than 18 years are uncommon and are biologically distinct from MDS in adults. Cases often present with somatic mutations involving pathways distinct from adult MDS and present with hypocellular bone marrows.[57] Childhood myelodysplastic neoplasm with low blasts (cMDS-LB) is a neoplasm characterized by cytopenia, dysplasia, less than 5% bone marrow blasts, and less than 2% blasts in the peripheral blood.[48] Children and adolescents may present de novo, but some have an inherited bone marrow failure syndrome or a germline predisposition. Cytogenetic and molecular diagnostic testing are helpful in differentiating cMDS-LB from bone marrow failure syndromes, germline disorders, metabolic diseases, and other overlapping conditions. This category is subdivided into cMDS-LB, hypocellular and cMDS-LB not otherwise specified. Eighty percent of the cases are cMDS-LB, hypocellular.[58]

Childhood Myelodysplastic Neoplasm with Increased Blasts

Childhood myelodysplastic neoplasm with increased blasts (cMDS-IB) is defined as having 5% to 19% blasts in the bone marrow and/or 2% to 19% blasts in the peripheral blood.[48] cMDS-IB is more likely to have RAS-pathway mutations than cMDS-LB.[48] Diagnosis of cMDS-IB requires the exclusion of Down syndrome, juvenile myelomonocytic leukemia, and AML with defining genetic abnormalities.[48]

MYELODYSPLASTIC/MYELOPROLIFERATIVE NEOPLASMS

The MDS/MPN category includes myeloid neoplasms with clinical, laboratory, and morphologic features that are characteristic of both MDS and MPN, namely the presence of cytopenias and cytoses. Included in this classification are chronic myelomonocytic leukemia (CMML); MDS/MPN with neutrophilia, MDS/ MPN with *SF3B1* mutation and thrombocytosis, and MDS/ MPN, not otherwise specified (Box 33.5). The 2022 WHO classification has reclassified juvenile myelomonocytic leukemia as a myeloproliferative neoplasm.

Chronic Myelomonocytic Leukemia

CMML is a clonal disorder characterized by a persistent monocytosis of more than 0.5×10^9/L and more than 10% in the peripheral blood; less than 20% blasts and promonocytes in the peripheral blood and bone marrow; and not meeting diagnostic criteria for any myeloproliferative neoplasm or myeloid/ lymphoid neoplasms with eosinophilia and defining gene rearrangements (*PDGFRA*, *PDGFRB*, *FGFR1*, or *JAK2*).[48] Dysplasia in at least one cell line, acquired cytogenetic or molecular abnormality, and atypical portioning of monocyte subsets may also be required or used to support the diagnosis of CMML. CMML is subtyped into myelodysplastic CMML (WBC $<13 \times 10^9$/L) and myeloproliferative CMML ($\geq 13 \times 10^9$/L).[48] Patients with myelodysplastic CMML often present with symptoms consistent with cytopenias such as fatigue, bruising, or recurrent infections, whereas patients with myeloproliferative CMML often present with weight loss, bone pain, and splenomegaly. The mutational landscape of CMML is complex, with some patients having 8 to 14 distinct mutations in coding sequences.[59] Mutations have been found in more than 90% of CMML cases with *TET2*, *SRSF2*, *ASXL1*, and *RUNX1* being the most common.[59–61] The accumulation of mutations occurs in a discernable pattern, starting with epigenetic genes followed by mutations in splicing genes and then signaling genes. Cytogenetic abnormalities such as trisomy 8 and loss of all or portions of chromosome 7 are also common.[59–61]

MDS/MPN with Neutrophilia

The 2022 WHO classification renamed atypical chronic myeloid leukemia to myelodysplastic/myeloproliferative neoplasm with neutrophilia (MDS/MPN-N) to avoid confusion with chronic myeloid leukemia (CML).[44] MDS/MPN-N is characterized by leukocytosis with morphologically dysplastic neutrophils and their precursors. Basophilia may be present, but it is not a prominent feature. Multilineage dysplasia is common. The *BCR::ABL1* fusion gene is not present, but karyotype abnormalities are seen in a third of patients, with essentially all patients demonstrating at least one gene mutation.[62] Dyspoiesis may be seen in all cell lines, but it

---

> **BOX 33.5   The 2022 World Health Organization Classification of Myelodysplastic/ Myeloproliferative Neoplasms**
>
> Chronic myelomonocytic leukemia (CMML)
>   Myelodysplastic CMML (MD-CMML)
>   Myeloproliferative CMML (MP-CMML)
> MDS/MPN with neutrophilia
> MDS/MPN with *SF3B1* mutation and thrombocytosis
> MDS/MPN, not otherwise specified

MDS/MPN, Myelodysplastic/myeloproliferative neoplasms. Adapted from Khoury, J. D., Solary, E., Abla, O., et al. (2022). The 5th edition of the World Health Organization classification of haematolymphoid tumors: myeloid and histiocytic/dendritic neoplasms. *Leukemia, 36,* 1703–1719.

is most remarkable in the neutrophils, which may exhibit pseudo-Pelger-Huët cells, hypogranularity, and bizarre segmentation.[63,64] The prognosis is poor for patients with MDS/MPN-N because they commonly progress to AML or succumb to bone marrow failure.[60,65]

MDS/MPN with *SF3B1* Mutation and Thrombocytosis

The 2022 WHO classification renamed MDS/MPN with ring sideroblasts and thrombocytosis as MDS/MPN with *SF3B1* mutation and thrombocytosis (MDS/MPN-*SF3B1*-T). MDS/MPN-*SF3B1*-T presents with 15% or more ring sideroblasts, anemia, and dysplasia in at least the erythroid lineage.[48] Platelet count is persistently elevated, $450 \times 10^9/L$ or greater. Molecular analysis typically demonstrates concurrent mutations in *SF3B1* and *JAK2* p.V617F, although other mutations involving spliceosome factors and cell signaling are admissible. MDS/MPN-*SF3B1*-T has the most favorable prognosis of any MDS/MPN, with a median overall survival of 76 to 128 months.[48]

MDS/MPN, Not Otherwise Specified

The designation MDS/MPN, NOS is used for cases that meet the criteria for MDS/MPN but do not fit into one of the aforementioned subcategories. The time of diagnosis, clinical history, and the detection of molecular aberrations are important factors in properly diagnosing this condition.

CYTOGENETICS, MOLECULAR ALTERATIONS, AND EPIGENETICS

Cytogenetics

Chromosome abnormalities are found in about 50% of cases of de novo MDS and 90% to 95% of MDS-pCT.[19,66,67] Karyotype has a major effect on prognosis in MDS patients, and detection of specific karyotypes can be cautiously applied to predict response to treatment.[67] Balanced translocations, which are common among patients with AML, are found only rarely in cases of de novo MDS.[66,67] Except for del(5q), no cytogenetic abnormality is specific to a subtype of MDS. The most common abnormalities involve chromosomes 5, 7, 8, 18, 20, and 13.[9,66] The most common single abnormalities besides del(5q) are trisomy 8 and monosomy 7, 12p–, iso 17, –21, and loss of the Y chromosome.[66]

Molecular Alterations

Advances in molecular genetics have made testing more available for routine use, and such information is strengthening prognostic scoring models. Likewise, identification of mutations may allow the development of targeted therapies.[68,69] About 90% of patients with MDS have at least one mutation, with a median of nine mutations within the coding sequence per patient.[70–72] There are at least 47 different genes that harbor these mutations and many of them are not specific to MDS.[71,72] These mutations affect five major groups of genes: RNA splicing, DNA methylation, activated cell signaling, myeloid transcription factors, and chromatin modifiers.[73] The most common mutations include *TET2, SF3B1, ASXL1, SRSF2, DNMT3A,* and *RUNX1*.[70–72] The prognostic value of these gene mutations are varied. For instance, *SF3B1* confers a favorable prognosis, whereas others,

such as *TP53,* confer a negative prognosis and predict a higher risk of transformation to AML.[74,75]

Epigenetics

The term *epigenetics* describes changes in gene expression that occur without altering the DNA sequence. Gene function is affected through selective activation or inactivation, rather than a change in the primary nucleotide sequence itself.[76,77] The three different ways in which epigenetics may facilitate oncogenesis are methylation of CpG islands, histone modification, and alteration of microRNA expression (Chapter 27).[78,79] Mutations in *TET2, ASXL1,* and other epigenetic regulators play important roles in altering CpG island methylation and histone methylation, respectively.[78,79] Changes in epigenetic regulation lead to unique gene expression profiles for MDS subtypes. Treatment with demethylating agents may slow the progression of MDS.[80–82]

PROGNOSIS

The 2022 WHO classification system described in this chapter categorizes MDS based on similarities in morphologic, molecular, cytogenetic, immunologic, and clinical characteristics, but it has limited ability to provide a prognosis. The clinical phenotypes for patients with MDS are heterogeneous. Some patients are mostly asymptomatic, whereas other patients experience severe symptoms coinciding with a rapid transformation to AML and leading to shortened survival. Several prognostic scoring models have been developed to predict outcomes for patients with MDS, including the International Prognostic Scoring System (IPSS),[83] WHO Classification-Based Prognostic Scoring System (WPSS),[84] MD Anderson Prognostic Scoring System (MDAPSS),[85] Revised International Prognostic Scoring System (IPSS-R),[56] and the Molecular International Prognostic Scoring System.[53] Each of these systems considers cytopenias, percentage of blasts, and cytogenetics in the stratification of patients.[86,87] Each scoring system has its respective strengths, limitations, and intended uses.[87,88] As a brief example, some scoring systems were not developed or validated to be used for patients with secondary MDS, postcytotoxic therapy MDS, MDS/MPN neoplasms, or for patients at different points in the disease course, stages of therapy, and posttherapy failure.[89–91] Additionally, scoring systems vary in their consideration of patient age and comorbidities, which may dramatically influence patient survival.[92] For brevity, IPSS, IPSS-R, and IPSS-M are the only models discussed.

IPSS and IPSS-R are the most widely used prognostic scoring models for MDS.[73,56,89,93] IPSS was introduced in 1997.[83] IPSS-R was introduced in 2012 to address growing concerns with IPSS.[56] Compared with IPSS, IPSS-R improves stratification of patients by identifying five risk categories instead of the original three.[94] IPSS-R includes additional cytogenetic abnormalities and is more sensitive to the percentage of blasts and the degree of cytopenias.[81] Other clinical features that affect survival but not transformation into AML include patient age, serum ferritin, patient performance status, and lactate dehydrogenase levels.[81] IPSS-R is not validated for all patient populations and thus needs to be applied with care.[89–91]

As knowledge of somatic mutations in MDS increases, our understanding of their effects on prognosis becomes more refined. Mutations in over 40 different genes have been identified in patients with MDS.[71,72,95] Some of these mutations have an independent ability to predict poor outcomes such as *TP53, EZH2, ETV6, RUNX1,* and *ASXL1*.[95–98] Conversely, mutations in *SF3B1* are significant for predicting positive outcomes.[96–98] The observed heterogeneity in MDS is driven by these somatic mutations, their interaction with other coexisting mutations, allele burden, karyotype abnormalities, cytokine concentrations, bone marrow microenvironment, clinical context, and numerous other factors.[88] In 2022, IPSS-M was published, which integrates hematologic parameters, cytogenetics, and mutations in 31 genes.[53] IPSS-M has better discrimination and improved prognostic accuracy for overall survival, leukemia-free survival, and AML transformation. IPSS-M provides a continuous score that can be interpreted in a six-category risk schema.[53] IPSS-M is applicable for secondary and postcytotoxic therapy MDS.[53]

Although many different prognostic scoring systems have been developed, it is important that users recognize limitations inherent in each one. The type of MDS or MDS/MPN, time since diagnosis, history of treatment, presence of genetic and epigenetic aberrations, age, comorbidities, and numerous other factors play important roles in deciding which prognostic system to use and how it should be applied to patient care.

TREATMENT

Treatment of patients with MDS is challenging because many are older and have coexisting illnesses, and the heterogeneity of the disease makes the use of one standard treatment impossible. When looking at all subtypes of MDS together, patients have a 31% 5-year overall survival, with most succumbing to AML or effects of bone marrow failure such as infection and bleeding.[8,92] Prognostic scoring systems are often used to direct patient therapy by categorizing patients into low-risk and high-risk groups.

Patients who are stratified into low-risk categories are treated less aggressively than patients with high-risk MDS. Patients with low-risk MDS are kept under observation and provided supportive therapy aimed at overcoming deficiencies in hematopoiesis as needed. Patient interventions may include transfusions, erythroid-stimulating agents, thrombopoietin, granulocyte colony-stimulating factor, antibiotics, and iron chelation.[68,69,86,99] Immunosuppressive therapy with drugs such as antithymocyte globulin and cyclosporine has resulted in decreased risk of leukemic transformation in subsets of patients.[99–101] Lenalidomide and azanucleosides are also prescribed for patients with low-risk MDS.[68,69,99]

Four drugs (lenalidomide, azacitidine, decitabine, and luspatercept) have been cleared by the US Food and Drug Administration (FDA) that show promise when used either alone or in combination with other therapies.[68,69,99,102] Azacitidine and decitabine belong to a group of drugs called azanucleosides. Azanucleosides deplete intracellular methyltransferases (DMNTs); are effective in low dose, with minimal side effects; and have improved the quality of life for patients with high-grade MDS.[68,103] Unfortunately, as many as 50% of patients will not respond to these agents.[68,69,99,102,104]

Lenalidomide, a thalidomide analog, was cleared by the FDA in 2005 for use in patients with low- or intermediate-risk MDS.[105,106] Lenalidomide has immunomodulatory and antiangiogenic effects.[105,106] It has shown remarkable promise, especially in patients with del(5q), resulting in transfusion independence for many patients.[106] Complete cytogenetic remission was seen in more than 50% of patients with MDS taking lenalidomide, whereas in MDS patients taking erythropoietin, cytogenetic remission is rare.[106] Lenalidomide also has been given to patients without 5q deletions, with 26% of patients becoming transfusion independent for a duration of 10 to 18 months.[68,107,108] The apparent efficacy of lenalidomide explains its widespread adoption for the treatment of patients with del(5q), despite its myelosuppressive action in 50% to 60% of patients.[68,105,106]

Luspatercept is a recombinant fusion protein that enhances late state erythroid maturation, thereby reducing transfusion dependence. Luspatercept is approved by the FDA for myelodysplastic neoplasm with ring sideroblasts and myelodysplastic neoplasm/myeloproliferative neoplasm with ring sideroblasts and thrombocytosis, though studies investigating its use in other low-risk MDS are ongoing.[68]

The standard of care for patients with high-risk MDS include treatment with hypomethylating agents such as azacitidine and decitabine.[68,69,76,77,99,103,107] As previously mentioned, these azanucleosides have a low response rate and their median response duration is about a year.[68,69,99]

The only cure for MDS is hematopoietic stem cell transplantation (HSCT). Patients with an IPSS score of intermediate 2 or higher and patients with more than 10% blasts should be considered for allogeneic HSCT.[109,110] Additionally, patients who have failed to respond to hypomethylating agents or have mutations that confer a poor prognosis are also potential candidates.[99,111] HSCT is most successful in patients younger than age 70 with no comorbidity, although emerging research suggests that patients of older age should still be considered for HSCT.[9,112] Intensive chemotherapy is rarely successful in achieving a durable remission, so it is typically considered a bridge therapy for high-risk MDS until HSCT.[68]

Future Directions

As research addressing the role of pyroptosis in MDS continues, future therapies may be aimed at controlling immune signaling. These interventions may even take place before the diagnosis of MDS, based on the mutations present in patients with CHIP or CCUS. Additional therapies for patients who fail hypomethylating agents or relapse after HSCT should be developed.[68,86,99] Recently the FDA cleared therapies for AML with mutations in either *IDH1/2* or *BCL2* that may be beneficial to patients with MDS who also harbor mutations in these genes. Because effective treatment for MDS remains limited, it has been suggested that patients be provided with information on the prognosis for their type of MDS, available therapies, and success rates, and should take part in making decisions regarding their treatment.[113,114] As more is learned about the molecular biology of MDS and points of intervention to slow its progress, it may be possible to develop customized treatment plans for individual patients.[69,115]

SUMMARY

- Myelodysplastic neoplasms (MDS) are a group of clonal disorders characterized by progressive cytopenias and dyspoiesis of the myeloid, erythroid, and megakaryocytic cell lines.
- The dyspoiesis is evidenced by abnormal morphologic appearance and abnormal function of the cell lines affected.
- The World Health Organization (WHO) classification of MDS is based on morphologic, molecular, cytogenetic, and immunologic characteristics of blood cell lines.
- Prognosis in MDS depends on several factors, including percentage of bone marrow blasts, depth of cytopenias, and karyotypic abnormalities.

- Treatment of MDS depends on the prognosis. If the prognosis is favorable, patients may receive only supportive therapy.
- Other treatments that have met with limited success include chemotherapeutic agents and epigenetic modifiers.
- Currently, the only cure for MDS is hematopoietic stem cell transplantation.
- Future treatment possibilities include the use of drugs targeting novel therapeutic pathways.

Now that you have completed this chapter, go back and read again the case study at the beginning and respond to the questions presented. Answers can be found in Appendix C.

REVIEW QUESTIONS

Answers can be found in Appendix C

1. MDS are most common in which age group?
   a. 2 to 10 years
   b. 15 to 20 years
   c. 25 to 40 years
   d. Older than 50 years
2. What is a major indication of MDS in the peripheral blood and bone marrow?
   a. Dyspoiesis
   b. Leukocytosis with left shift
   c. Normal bone marrow with abnormal peripheral blood features
   d. Thrombocytosis
3. An alert hematologist should recognize all of the following peripheral blood abnormalities as diagnostic clues in MDS EXCEPT:
   a. Oval macrocytes
   b. Target cells
   c. Agranular neutrophils
   d. Circulating micromegakaryocytes
4. For an erythroid precursor to be considered a ring sideroblast, the iron-laden mitochondria must encircle how much of the nucleus?
   a. One-quarter
   b. One-third
   c. Two-thirds
   d. Entire nucleus
5. According to the WHO classification of MDS, what percentage of blasts would constitute transformation to an acute leukemia?
   a. 5%
   b. 10%
   c. 20%
   d. 30%

6. A patient has anemia, oval macrocytes, and hypersegmented neutrophils. Which of the following tests would be most efficient in differential diagnosis of this disorder?
   a. Serum iron and ferritin levels
   b. Erythropoietin level
   c. Vitamin B_{12} and folate levels
   d. Chromosome analysis
7. A 60-year-old woman comes to the physician with fatigue and malaise. Her hemoglobin is 8 g/dL, hematocrit is 25%, RBC count is 2.00×10^{12}/L, platelet count is 550×10^9/L, and WBC count is 3.8×10^9/L. Her WBC differential is unremarkable. Bone marrow shows erythroid hypoplasia and hypolobulated megakaryocytes; granulopoiesis appears normal. Ring sideroblasts are rare. Chromosome analysis reveals the deletion of 5q only. Based on the classification of this disorder, what therapy would be most appropriate?
   a. Supportive therapy; lenalidomide if the disease progresses
   b. Aggressive chemotherapy
   c. Hematopoietic stem cell transplantation
   d. Low-dose cytosine arabinoside, accompanied by *cis*-retinoic acid
8. Which of the following is LEAST likely to contribute to the death of patients with MDS?
   a. Neutropenia
   b. Thrombocytopenia
   c. Organ failure
   d. Neuropathy
9. Into what other hematologic disease does MDS often convert?
   a. Megaloblastic anemia
   b. Aplastic anemia
   c. AML
   d. Myeloproliferative disease
10. Chronic myelomonocytic leukemia is classified in the WHO system as:
    a. A myeloproliferative neoplasm
    b. Myelodysplastic syndrome, unclassified
    c. MDS/MPN
    d. Acute leukemia

REFERENCES

1. Layton, D. M., & Mufti, G. J. (1986). Myelodysplastic syndromes: their history, evolution and relation to acute myeloid leukemia. *Blood, 53*(6), 423–436.
2. Steensma, D. P. (2012). Historical perspectives on myelodysplastic syndromes. *Leuk Res, 36*(12), 1441–1452.
3. Bennett, J. M., Catovsky, D., Daniel, M. T., et al. (1982). Proposals for the classification of the myelodysplastic syndromes. *Br J Haematol, 51*(2), 189–199.
4. Harris, N. L., Jaffe, E. S., Diebold, J., et al. (2000). The World Health Organization classification of hematological malignancies report of the Clinical Advisory Committee Meeting, Airlie House, Virginia, November 1997. *Mod Pathol, 13*(2), 193–207.
5. Vardiman, J. W., Harris, N. L., & Brunning, R. D. (2002). The World Health Organization (WHO) classification of the myeloid neoplasms. *Blood, 100*(7), 2292–2302.
6. Shastri, A., Will, B., Steidel, U., et al. (2017). Stem and progenitor cell alterations in myelodysplastic syndromes. *Blood, 129*(12), 1586–1594.
7. Sperling, A. S., Gibson, C. J., & Ebert, B. L. (2017). The genetics of myelodysplastic syndrome: from clonal haematopoiesis to secondary leukaemia. *Nat Rev Cancer, 17*(1), 5–19.
8. Zeidan, A. M., Shallis, R. M., Wang, R., et al. (2019). Epidemiology of myelodysplastic syndromes: why characterizing the beast is a prerequisite to taming it. *Blood Rev, 34*, 1–15.
9. Gibson, C. J., & Steensma, D. P. (2023). Myelodysplastic syndromes. In Hoffman, R., Benz, E. J., Silberstein, L. E., et al. (Eds.), *Hematology: Basic Principles and Practice*. (8th ed. pp. 977–1000). St. Louis: Elsevier.
10. Avagyan, S., & Shimamura, A. (2022). Lessons from pediatric MSA: approaches to germline predisposition to hematologic malignancies. *Front Oncol, 12*, 813149.
11. Niemeyer, C. M., & Baumann, I. (2008). Myelodysplastic syndrome in children and adolescents. *Semin in Hematol, 45*(1), 60–70.
12. Woll, P. S., Kjällquist, U., Chowdhury, O., et al. (2014). Myelodysplastic syndromes are propagated by rare and distinct human cancer stem cells in vivo. *Cancer Cell, 25*(6), 794–808.
13. Kennedy, J. A., & Ebert, B. L. (2017). Clinical implications of genetic mutations in myelodysplastic syndrome. *J Clin Oncol, 35*(9), 968–974.
14. Young, A. L., Challen, G. A., Birmann, B. M., et al. (2016). Clonal haematopoiesis harbouring AML-associated mutations is ubiquitous in healthy adults. *Nat Commun, 7*, 12484.
15. Valent, P. (2019). ICUS, IDUS, CHIP, and CCUS: diagnostic criteria, separation from MDS and clinical implications. *Pathobiology, 86*, 30–38.
16. Calvi, L. M., Li, A. J., & Becker, M. W. (2019). What is the role of the microenvironment in MDS? *Best Prac Res Clin Haematol, 32*, 101113.
17. Menssen, A. J., & Walter, M. J. (2020). Genetics of progression from MDS to secondary leukemia. *Blood, 136*(1), 50–60.
18. Medyouf, H. (2017). The microenvironment in human myeloid malignancies: emerging concepts and therapeutic implications. *Blood, 129*(12), 1617–1626.
19. Zahr, A. A., Kavi, A. M., Mukherjee, S., et al. (2017). Therapy-related myelodysplastic syndromes, or are they? *Blood Rev, 31*(3), 119–128.
20. Ganser, A., & Heuser, M. (2017). Therapy-related myeloid neoplasms. *Curr Opin Hematol, 24*(2), 152–158.
21. Mossner, M., Jann, J., Wittig, J., et al. (2016). Mutational hierarchies in myelodysplastic syndromes dynamically adapt and evolve upon therapy response and failure. *Blood, 128*(9), 1246–1259.
22. Hershman, D., Neugut, A. I., Jacobson, J. S., et al. (2007). Acute myeloid leukemia or myelodysplastic syndrome following use of granulocyte colony-stimulating factors during breast cancer adjuvant therapy. *J Natl Cancer Inst, 99*(3), 196–205.
23. Bannon, S. A., & DiNardo, C. D. (2016). Hereditary predispositions to myelodysplastic syndrome. *Int J Mol Sci, 17*(6), 838.
24. Khoury, J. D., & Campbell, P. (2022). Myelodysplastic neoplasms: introduction. In: Swerdlow, S. H., Campo, E., Harris, N. L., et al. (Eds.), *WHO Classification of Tumours of Haematopoietic and Lymphoid Tissues*. (4th ed., pp. 98–106). Lyon, France: IARC Press.
25. Basiorka, A. A., McGraw, K. L., Eksioglu, E. A., et al. (2016). The NLRP3 inflammasome functions as a driver of the myelodysplastic syndrome phenotype. *Blood, 128*(25), 2960–2975.
26. Sallman, D. A., & List, A. (2019). The central role of inflammatory signaling in the pathogenesis of myelodysplastic syndromes. *Blood, 133*(10), 1039–1048.
27. Rodak, B. F., & Leclair, S. J. (2002). The new WHO nomenclature: introduction and myeloid neoplasms. *Clin Lab Sci, 15*(1), 44–54.
28. Head, D. R., Kopecky, K., Bennett, J. M., et al. (1989). Pathologic implications of internuclear bridging in myelodysplastic syndrome. An Eastern Cooperative Oncology Group/Southwest Oncology Group Cooperative Study. *Cancer, 64*(11), 2199–2202.
29. Langenhuijsen, M. M. (1984). Neutrophils with ring-shaped nuclei in myeloproliferative disease. *Br J Haematol, 58*(2), 227–230.
30. Doll, D. C., & List, A. F. (1989). Myelodysplastic syndromes. *West J of Med, 151*(2), 161–167.
31. Seymour, J. F., & Estey, E. H. (1993). The prognostic significance of Auer rods in myelodysplasia. *Br J Haematol, 85*(1), 67–76.
32. Tricot, G., De Wolf-Peeters, R., Vlietinck, R., et al. (1984). Bone marrow histology in myelodysplastic syndromes II. Prognostic value of abnormal localization of immature precursors in MDS. *Br J of Haematol, 58*(2), 217–225.
33. Leguit, R. J., & van den Tweel, J. G. (2010). The pathology of bone marrow failure. *Histopathology, 57*(5), 655–670.
34. Tanaka, T. N., & Bejar, R. (2019). MDS overlap disorders and diagnostic boundaries. *Blood, 133*(10), 1086–1095.
35. Barbui, T., Cortelazzo, S., Viero, P., et al. (1993). Infection and hemorrhage in elderly acute myeloblastic leukemia and primary myelodysplasia. *Hematol Oncol, 11*(suppl 1), 15–18.
36. Mazzone, A., Ricevuti, G., Pasotti, D., et al. (1993). The CD11/CD18 granulocyte adhesion molecules in myelodysplastic syndromes. *Br J Haematol, 83*(2), 245–252.
37. Mittelman, M., Karcher, D., Kammerman, L., et al. (1993). High Ia (HLA-DR) and low CD11b (Mo1) expression may predict early conversion to leukemia in myelodysplastic syndromes. *Am J Hematol, 43*(3), 165–171.
38. Toma, A., Fenaux, P., Dreyfus, F., et al. (2012). Infections in myelodysplastic syndromes. *Haematologica, 97*(10), 1459–1470.
39. Boogaerts, M. A., Nelissen, V., Roelant, C., et al. (1983). Blood neutrophil function in primary myelodysplastic syndromes. *Br J Haematol, 55*(2), 217–227.
40. Verhoef, G. E., Zachee, P., Ferrant, A., et al. (1992). Recombinant human erythropoietin for the treatment of anemia in the

myelodysplastic syndromes: a clinical and erythrokinetic assessment. *Ann Hematol, 64*(1), 16–21.

41. Merchav, S., Nielsen, O. J., Rosenbaum, H., et al. (1990). In vitro studies of erythropoietin-dependent regulation of erythropoiesis in myelodysplastic syndromes. *Leukemia, 4*(11), 771–774.

42. Lintula, R., Rasi, V., Ikkala, E., et al. (1981). Platelet function in preleukemia. *Scand J Haematol, 26*(1), 65–71.

43. Mittelman, M., & Zeidman, A. (2000). Platelet function in the myelodysplastic syndromes. *Int J Hematol, 71*(2), 95–98.

44. Khoury, J. D., Solary, E., Abla, O., et al. (2022). The 5th edition of the World Health Organization classification of haematolymphoid tumours: myeloid and histiocytic/dendritic neoplasms. *Leukemia, 36*, 1703–1719.

45. Arber, D. A., Orazi, A., Hasserjian, R. P., et al. (2022). International consensus classification of myeloid neoplasms and acute leukemias: integrating morphologic, clinical and genomic data. *Blood, 140*(11), 1200–1228.

46. Strupp, C., Nachtkamp, K., Hildebrandt, B., et al. (2017). New proposals of the WHO working group (2016) for the diagnosis of myelodysplastic syndromes (MDS): characteristics of refined MDS types. *Leuk Res, 57*, 78–84.

47. Gurney, M., Patnaik, M. M., Hanson, C. A., et al. (2017). The 2016 revised world health organization definition of 'myelodysplastic syndrome with isolated del(5q)'; prognostic implications of single versus double cytogenetic abnormalities. *Br J Haematol, 178*(1), 57–60.

48. WHO Classification of Tumours Editorial Board. Haematolymphoid tumours. Lyon (France) International Agency for Research on Cancer, forthcoming. *WHO Classification of Tumours series* (5th ed., vol. 11). https://publications.iarc.fr.

49. Giagounidis, A. A., Germing, U., Haase, S., et al. (2004). Clinical, morphological, cytogenetic, and prognostic features of patients with myelodysplastic syndromes and del(5q) including band q31. *Leukemia, 18*(1), 113–119.

50. Giagounidis, A. A., Haase, S., Heinsch, M., et al. (2007). Lenalidomide in the context of complex karyotype or interrupted treatment: case reviews of del(5q) MDS patients with unexpected responses. *Ann Hematol, 86*(2), 133–137.

51. Fenaux, P., Giagounidis, A., Selleslag, D., et al. (2017). Clinical characteristics and outcomes according to age in lenalidomide-treated patients with RBC transfusion-dependent lower-risk MDS and del(5q). *J Hematol Oncol, 10*(1), 131.

52. Mufti, G. J., Bennett, J. M., Goasguen, J., et al. (2008). Diagnosis and classification of myelodysplastic syndrome: International Working Group on Morphology of Myelodysplastic Syndrome (IWGM-MDS) consensus proposals for the definition and enumeration of myeloblasts and ring sideroblasts. *Haematologica, 93*(11), 1712–1717.

53. Bernard, E., Tuechler, H., Greenberg, P. L., et al. (2022). Molecular international prognostic scoring system for myelodysplastic syndromes. *NEJM Evid, 1*(7), 1–14.

54. Daver, N. G., Maiti, A., Kadia, T. M., et al. (2022). TP53-mutated myelodysplastic syndrome and acute myeloid leukemia: biology, current therapy, and future directions. *Cancer Discov, 12*(11), 2516–2529.

55. Bono, E., McLornan, D., Travaglino, E., et al. (2019). Clinical, histopathological and molecular characterization of hypoplastic myelodysplastic syndrome. *Leukemia, 33*, 2495–2505.

56. Greenberg, P. L., Tuechler, H., Schanz, J., et al. (2012). Revised international scoring system for myelodysplastic syndromes. *Blood, 120*, 2454–2465.

57. Falini, B., & Martelli, M. P. (2023). Comparison of the international consensus and 5th WHO edition classifications of adult myelodysplastic syndromes and acute myeloid leukemia. *Am J Hematol, 2023, 98*(3), 1–12.

58. Baumann, I., Führer, M., Behrendt, S., et al. (2012). Morphological differentiation of severe aplastic anemia from hypocellular refractory cytopenia of childhood: reproducibility of histopathological diagnostic criteria. *Histopathology, 61*, 10–17.

59. Deininger, M. W. N., Tyner, J. W., & Solary, E. (2017). Turning the tide in myelodysplastic/myeloproliferative neoplasms. *Nat Rev Cancer, 17*(7), 425–440.

60. Mughal, T. I., Cross, N. C. P., Pardron, E., et al. (2015). An international MDS/MPN working group's perspective and recommendations on molecular pathogenesis, diagnosis and clinical characterization of myelodysplastic/myeloproliferative neoplasms. *Haematologica, 100*(9), 1117–1130.

61. Palomo, L., Meggendorfer, M., Hutter, S., et al. (2020). Molecular landscape and clonal architecture of adult myelodysplastic/myeloproliferative neoplasms. *Blood, 136*(16), 1851–1862.

62. Patnaik, M. M., Barraco, D., Lasho, T. L., et al. (2017). Targeted next generation sequencing and identification of risk factors in world health organization defined atypical chronic myeloid leukemia. *Am J Hematol, 92*, 542–548.

63. Xubo, G., Xingguo, L., Xianguo, W., et al. (2009). The role of peripheral blood, bone marrow aspirate and especially bone marrow trephine biopsy in distinguishing atypical chronic myeloid leukemia from chronic granulocytic leukemia and chronic myelomonocytic leukemia. *Eur J Haematol, 83*, 1292–1301.

64. Locatelli, F., Nöllke, P., Zecca, M., et al. (2005). Hematopoietic stem cell transplantation (HSCT) in children with juvenile myelomonocytic leukemia (JMML): results of the EWOG-MDS/EBMT trial. *Blood, 105*, 410–419.

65. Vardiman, J. W., Bennett, J. M., Bain, B. J., et al. (2008). Atypical chronic myeloid leukemia, BCR-ABL1 negative. In Swerdlow, S. H., Campo, E., Harris, N. L., et al. (Eds.), *WHO Classification of Tumours of Haematopoietic and Lymphoid Tissues*. (4th ed., pp. 80–81). Lyon, France: IARC Press.

66. Haase, D., Germing, U., Schanz, J., et al. (2007). New insights into the prognostic impact of the karyotype in MDS and correlation with subtypes: evidence from a core dataset of 2124 patients. *Blood, 110*, 4385–4395.

67. Pedersen-Bjergaard, J., Andersen, M. T., & Andersen, M. K. (2007). Genetic pathways in the pathogenesis of therapy-related myelodysplasia and acute myeloid leukemia. *Hematology Am Soc Hematol Educ Program*, 392–397.

68. Saygin, C., & Carraway, H. E. (2021). Current and emerging strategies for management of myelodysplastic syndromes. *Blood Rev, 48*, 100791.

69. Hellström-Lindbert, E., Tobiasson, M., & Greenburg, P. (2020). Myelodysplastic syndromes: moving towards personalized management. *Haematologica, 150*(7), 1765–1779.

70. Ogawa, S. (2019). Genetics of MDS. *Blood, 133*(10), 1049–1059.

71. Haferlach, T., Nagata, Y., Grossmann, V., et al. (2014). Landscape of genetic lesions in 944 patients with myelodysplastic syndromes. *Leukemia, 28*, 241–247.

72. Papaemmanuil, E., Gerstung, M., Malcovati, L., et al. (2013). Clinical and biological implications of driver mutations in myelodysplastic syndromes. *Blood, 122*, 3616–3627.

73. Haider, M., Duncavage, E. J., Afaneh, K. F., et al. (2017). New insight into the biology, risk stratification, and targeted treatment of myelodysplastic syndromes. In Dizon, D. S. (Ed.),

American Society of Clinical Oncology 2017 Educational Book: Making a Difference in Cancer Care With You (480–494). Alexandria, VA: ASCO.

74. Bejar, R., Stevenson, K., Abdel-Wahab, O., et al. (2011). Clinical effect of point mutations in myelodysplastic syndromes. *N Engl J Med, 364*, 2496–2506.

75. Malcovati, L., Karimi, M., Papaemmanuil, E., et al. (2015). *SF3B1* mutation identifies a distinct subset of myelodysplastic syndrome with ring sideroblasts. *Blood, 126*, 233–241.

76. Nakao, M. (2001). Epigenetics: interaction of DNA methylation and chromatin. *Gene, 278*, 25–31.

77. Musolino, C., Sant'Antonio, E., Penna, G., et al. (2010). Epigenetic therapy in myelodysplastic syndromes. *Eur J Haematol, 84*, 463–473.

78. Milunović, V., Rogulj, I. M., Planinc-Peraica, A., et al. (2016). The role of microRNA in myelodysplastic syndromes: beyond DNA methylation and histone modification. *Eur J Haematol, 96*, 553–563.

79. Issa, J. J. (2013). The myelodysplastic syndrome as a prototypical epigenetic disease. *Blood, 121*, 3811–3817.

80. Scott, L. J. (2016). Azacitidine: a review in myelodysplastic syndromes and acute myeloid leukemia. *Drugs, 76*, 889–900.

81. Fenaux, P., Mufti, G. J., Hellstrom-Lindberg, E., et al. (2009). Efficacy of azacitidine compared with that of conventional care regimens in the treatment of higher-risk myelodysplastic syndromes: a randomized, open-label, phase III study. *Lancet Oncol, 10*, 223–232.

82. Kantarjian, H., Oki, Y., Garcia-Manero, G., et al. (2007). Results of a randomized study of 3 schedules of low-dose decitabine in higher-risk myelodysplastic syndrome and chronic myelomonocytic leukemia. *Blood, 109*, 52–57.

83. Greenberg, P., Cox, C., & LeBeau, M. M. (1997). International scoring system for evaluating prognosis in myelodysplastic syndromes. *Blood, 89*, 2079–2088.

84. Malcovati, L., Germing, U., Kuendgen, A., et al. (2007). Time-dependent prognostic scoring system for predicting survival and leukemic evolution in myelodysplastic syndromes. *J Clin Oncol, 25*, 3503–3510.

85. Kantarjian, H., O'Brien, S., Ravandi, F., et al. (2008). Proposal for a new risk model in myelodysplastic syndrome that accounts for events not considered in the original International Prognostic Scoring System. *Cancer, 113*, 1351–1361.

86. Garcia-Manero, G. (2015). Myelodysplastic syndromes: 2015 update on diagnosis, risk-stratification and management. *Am J Hematol, 90*, 832–841.

87. Nazha, A., & Sekeres, M. A. (2016). Improving prognostic modeling in myelodysplastic syndromes. *Curr Hematol Malig Rep, 11*, 395–401.

88. Bejar, R. (2013). Prognostic models in myelodysplastic syndromes. *Hematol Am Soc Hematol Educ Program, 2013*(1), 504–510.

89. Zeidan, A. M., Sekeres, M. A., Garcia-Manero, G., et al. (2016). Comparison of risk stratification tools in predicting outcomes of patients with higher-risk myelodysplastic syndromes treated with azanucleosides. *Leukemia, 30*, 649–657.

90. Cazzola, M., Della Porta, M. G., Travaglino, E., et al. (2011). Classification and prognostic evaluation of myelodysplastic syndromes. *Semin Oncol, 38*, 627–634.

91. Nazha, A., Komrokji, R. S., Garcia-Monero, G., et al. (2016). The efficacy of current prognostic models in predicting outcome of patients with myelodysplastic syndromes at the time of hypomethylating agent failure. *Haematologica, 101*, 224–227.

92. Nachtkamp, K., Stark, R., Strupp, C., et al. (2016). Causes of death in 2877 patients with myelodysplastic syndromes. *Ann Hematol, 95*, 937–944.

93. Della Porta, M. G., Tuechler, H., Malcovati, L., et al. (2015). Validation of WHO classification-based prognostic scoring system (WPSS) for myelodysplastic syndromes and comparison with the revised international prognostic scoring system (IPSS-R). A study of the international working group for prognosis in myelodysplasia (IWG-PM). *Leukemia, 29*, 1502–1513.

94. Neukirchen, J., Lauseker, M., Blum, S., et al. (2014). Validation of the revised international prognostic scoring system (IPSS-R) in patients with myelodysplastic syndrome: a multicenter study. *Leuk Res, 38*, 57–64.

95. Montalban-Bravo, G., Takahashi, K., Wang, F., et al. (2016). Clinical relevance of driver mutations and number of driver mutations in patients with myelodysplastic syndromes and chronic myelomonocytic leukemia. *Blood, 128*, 54.

96. Nazha, A., Narkhede, M., Radivoyevitch, T., et al. (2016). Incorporation of molecular data into the revised international prognostic scoring system in treated patients with myelodysplastic syndromes. *Leukemia, 30*, 2214–2220.

97. Nazha, A., Al-Issa, K., Hamilton, B. K., et al. (2017). Adding molecular data to prognostic models can improve predictive power in treated patients with myelodysplastic syndromes. *Leukemia, 31*(12), 2848–2850.

98. Bejar, R., Papaemmanuil, E., Haferlach, T., et al. (2015). Somatic mutations in MDS patients are associated with clinical features and predict prognosis independent of the IPSS-R: analysis of combined datasets from the international working group for prognosis in MDS-molecular committee. *Blood, 126*, 907.

99. Platzbecker, U. (2019). Treatment of MDS. *Blood, 133*(10), 1096–1107.

100. Sloand, E. M., Wu, C. O., Greenberg, P., et al. (2008). Factors affecting response and survival in patients with myelodysplasia treated with immunosuppressive therapy. *J Clin Oncol, 26*, 2505–2511.

101. Ganán-Gómez, I., Wei, Y., Starczynowski, D. T., et al. (2015). Deregulation of innate immune and inflammatory signaling in myelodysplastic syndromes. *Leukemia, 29*, 1458–1469.

102. Steensma, D. P., Baer, M. R., Slack, J. L., et al. (2009). Multicenter study of decitabine administered daily for 5 days every 4 weeks to adults with myelodysplastic syndromes: the alternative dosing for outpatient treatment (ADOPT) trial. *J Clin Oncol, 27*, 3842–3848.

103. Griffiths, E. A., & Gore, S. D. (2013). Epigenetic therapies in MDS and AML. *Adv Exp Med Biol, 754*, 253–283.

104. Gore, S. D., Fenaux, P., Santini, V., et al. (2013). A multivariate analysis of the relationship between response and survival among patients with higher-risk myelodysplastic syndromes treated within azacitidine or conventional care regimens in the randomized AZA-001 trial. *Haematologica, 98*, 1067–1072.

105. Talati, C., Sallman, D., & List, A. (2017). Lenalidomide: myelodysplastic syndromes with del(5q) and beyond. *Semin Hematol, 54*, 159–166.

106. Giagounidis, A., Mufti, G. J., Germing, U., et al. (2014). Lenalidomide as a disease-modifying agent in patients with del(5q) myelodysplastic syndromes: linking mechanism of action to clinical outcomes. *Ann Hematol, 93*, 1–11.

107. Greenberg, P. L., Stone, R. M., Al-Kali, A., et al. (2017). Myelodysplastic syndromes, version 2.2017: clinical practice guidelines in oncology. *J Natl Compr Canc Netw, 15*, 60–87.

108. Raza, A., Reeves, J. A., Feldman, E. J., et al. (2008). Phase 2 study of lenalidomide in transfusion-dependent, low-risk, and intermediate-1-risk myelodysplastic syndromes with karyotypes other than deletion 5q. *Blood, 111*, 86–93.

109. Appelbaum, F. R. (2011). The role of hematopoietic cell transplantation as therapy for myelodysplasia. *Best Pract Res Clin Haematol, 24*, 541–547.

110. Gerds, A. T., & Deeg, H. J. (2012). Transplantation for myelodysplastic syndrome in the era of hypomethylating agents. *Curr Opin Hematol, 19*, 71–75.

111. Della Porta, M. G., Gallì, A., Bacigalupo, A., et al. (2016). Clinical effects of driver somatic mutations on the outcomes of patients with myelodysplastic syndromes treated with allogeneic hematopoietic stem-cell transplantation. *J Clin Oncol, 34*, 3627–3637.

112. Muffly, L., Pasquini, M. C., Martens, M., et al. (2017). Increasing use of allogeneic hematopoietic cell transplantation in patients aged 70 years and older in the United States. *Blood, 130*, 1156–1164.

113. Sekeres, M. A., Stowell, S. A., Berry, C. A., et al. (2013). Improving the diagnosis and treatment of patients with myelodysplastic syndromes through a performance improvement initiative. *Leuk Res, 37*, 422–426.

114. Besson, D., Rannou, S., Elmaaroufi, H., et al. (2012). Disclosure of myelodysplastic syndrome diagnosis: improving patients' understanding and experience. *Eur J Haematol, 90*, 151–156.

115. Scott, B. L., & Deeg, H. J. (2010). Myelodysplastic syndromes. *Annu Rev Med, 61*, 345–358.

34

Mature Lymphoid Neoplasms

Steven Marionneaux and Peter Maslak

OBJECTIVES

After completing this chapter, the reader will be able to:

1. Compare and contrast similarities and differences between leukemia and lymphoma with respect to clinical and laboratory findings.
2. Explain the approach to the diagnosis of the mature lymphoid neoplasms as outlined by the World Health Organization classification.
3. Differentiate monoclonal B-cell lymphocytosis, chronic lymphocytic leukemia (CLL)/small lymphocytic lymphoma (SLL), prolymphocytic progression of CLL/SLL, hairy cell leukemia, and large granular lymphocytic leukemia using key laboratory results and peripheral blood findings.
4. Differentiate various types of non-Hodgkin lymphoma using key laboratory test results and morphologic features of circulating malignant cells.
5. Describe the different forms of Hodgkin lymphoma.
6. Differentiate various types of plasma cell neoplasms using key laboratory test results and morphologic features of malignant cells.
7. Given the patient history, clinical and laboratory findings, including representative cells on the peripheral blood film, bone marrow smear, or lymph node biopsy, interpret results of diagnostic tests to determine the type of mature lymphoid neoplasm and recommend additional tests to confirm a diagnosis.
8. Describe how prognostic assessment and staging systems are used in the evaluation and management of leukemias and lymphomas.

OUTLINE

Genetic Abnormalities
Classification Schemas Based on Cell Differentiation
Approach to Diagnosis: Interface Between Clinical and Laboratory Medicine
　Clinical Signs and Symptoms
Diagnostic Procedures
　Clinical Laboratory Testing
　Anatomic Pathology Testing
　Imaging Studies
Diagnostic Evaluation
　Staging Systems
　Prognostic Assessment
Leukemias
　Chronic Lymphocytic Leukemia (CLL)/Small Lymphocytic Lymphoma (SLL)
　Monoclonal B-Cell Lymphocytosis (MBL)
　T-Prolymphocytic Leukemia (T-PLL)
　Hairy Cell Leukemia (HCL)
　Large Granular Lymphocytic (LGL) Leukemia
Non-Hodgkin Lymphoma
　Adult T-Cell Leukemia/Lymphoma (ATLL)

Burkitt Lymphoma (BL)
Follicular Lymphoma (FL)
Mantle Cell Lymphoma (MCL)
Diffuse Large B-Cell Lymphoma (DLBCL)
Marginal Zone Lymphoma (MZL)
Mycosis Fungoides/Sézary Syndrome (MF/SS)
Anaplastic Large Cell Lymphoma (ALCL)
Peripheral T-Cell Lymphoma, Not Otherwise Specified (PTCL-NOS)
Hodgkin Lymphoma
　Clinical and Laboratory Findings
　Treatment
Plasma Cell Neoplasms
　Monoclonal Gammopathy of Undetermined Significance (MGUS)
　Plasma Cell (Multiple) Myeloma (MM)
　Plasmacytoma
　Waldenström Macroglobulinemia and Heavy Chain Disease
　Treatment

CASE STUDY

After studying the material in this chapter, the reader should be able to respond to the following case study. Answers can be found in Appendix C.

  A 75-year-old healthy man was seen in the emergency department for pain in his right forearm after a fall on ice. Imaging studies revealed a fractured radius. A complete blood count (CBC) and chemistry panel were also performed at admission. His CBC results are as follows. Reference intervals can be found after the Index at the end of the book.

WBC	9.5×10^9/L	HCT	43%
HGB	14.5 g/dL	PLT	195×10^9/L

NEUT	30%	MONO	9%
LYMPH	60%	EO	1%

  Peripheral blood film review revealed a marked increase in smudge cells. Lymphocytes appeared mature with a dense nuclear chromatin pattern. Chemistry test results were all within reference intervals.

1. What is the significance of the CBC results?
2. Identify the most appropriate next steps to investigate these results.
3. Describe the diagnostic criteria for the suspected condition. How would it be staged, and what are the tests frequently performed to assess prognosis?

Mature lymphoid neoplasms are a diverse collection of disease entities with varying clinical presentations and natural histories. However, identification with a particular lineage is common to all. Most disease entities can be identified with a normal counterpart in the blood, bone marrow, or lymph nodes. Neoplastic transformation of these cells results in abnormal changes in growth and differentiation patterns, resulting in lymphoma.

Lymphoid cells are intimately involved in immunity and, not surprisingly, those tissues that function in the immune system are the areas most involved in cases of lymphoma. Broadly speaking, lymphoid neoplasms in which the primary site of involvement is the blood or bone marrow are classified as *leukemias* (leukemic phase), whereas those in which the focus of disease is the lymph nodes, spleen, or other extranodal sites are classified as *lymphomas*. These categories are not mutually exclusive; there are diseases such as chronic lymphocytic leukemia/small lymphocytic lymphoma (CLL/SLL) in which the neoplastic cells are prominent in the blood (CLL component) but also involve the spleen and lymph nodes (SLL component). Likewise, mantle cell lymphoma (MCL) may have a leukemic phase in which lymphoma cells are found in the peripheral blood. Although not identified as a leukemia, plasma cell neoplasms (PCNs) such as plasma cell (multiple) myeloma (MM) tend to occur in the bone marrow; however, extramedullary involvement can be an important part of the clinical presentation.

This chapter illustrates the significant role of the clinical laboratory in the diagnosis and management of mature lymphoid neoplasms. As the most current World Health Organization (WHO) classification lists approximately 100 different diseases spread among several different categories, this chapter highlights the more common or well-known disorders that may be encountered in the clinical laboratory.[1,2]

GENETIC ABNORMALITIES

The generation of immunologic diversity is an inherently complex process with many steps. Such complexity can lend itself to error, and many of the genetic abnormalities that characterize the various types of B-cell and T-cell lymphomas involve the immunoglobulin and T-cell receptor (TCR) genes, respectively. A mutation in an individual gene can result in a defective gene with an altered product, which has fundamental implications for the growth or function of the cell. Alternatively, chromosomal translocations can cause various genes to become "misplaced," exposing them to either stimuli or suppression and resulting in

an altered expression pattern. If such genes are involved in growth or maturation, these changes may have profound implications for the cell and result in clinical disease.[1-4] Common examples of translocated genes are *MYC,* which stimulates entry into the cell cycle; *BCL2,* which suppresses apoptosis; and *BCL6,* which can suppress the transcription of genes needed for cell growth. In addition, other chromosomal abnormalities (e.g., inversions, deletions, trisomy) and specific gene mutations can contribute to the development and progression of a lymphoid neoplasm. Some of the more common chromosome and gene abnormalities found in mature lymphoid neoplasms are summarized in Table 34.1.[2-4]

CLASSIFICATION SCHEMAS BASED ON CELL DIFFERENTIATION

Most mature lymphoid neoplasms represent neoplastic transformation of normal lymphoid cells (cells of origin) at various stages of development. Morphology is the first step in interpreting patterns of involvement but is imperfect because different diseases can show lymphoid cells in the peripheral blood that have a similar appearance. Immunophenotyping by flow cytometry (Chapter 28) and/or immunohistochemistry are important tools that can help define a particular disorder according to the cell differentiation schema. This model fits some diseases better than others. For example, Hodgkin lymphoma (HL) and hairy cell leukemia (HCL) are recognized as B-cell neoplasms, although the normal counterparts of the transformed cells remain elusive. CLL can arise in two circumstances: one version with unmutated heavy chains, representing a pregerminal center event; and one with hypermutated heavy chains, suggesting a later stage of development. The unmutated form has more clinically aggressive disease, with a poorer prognosis.[5]

Although useful in grouping similar disease entities, a schema based on the degree of cell maturation is not reflective of clinical behavior. Acute lymphoblastic leukemia (ALL) is more commonly found in the pediatric population and has a stem cell or precursor phenotype. ALL is generally aggressive and has a fulminant clinical presentation, yet is curable in more than 90% of patients. On the other hand, diseases involving cells at the terminal end of differentiation such as MM also can be clinically aggressive but are often more difficult to cure with current therapies. Therefore natural history and clinical behavior are not reflective of the phenotype of a particular disorder but of the underlying genetic changes that determine tumor growth and response to therapy. The typical clinical behavior of some of the more common mature lymphoid neoplasms are summarized in Box 34.1.

TABLE 34.1 Some Chromosome and Gene Abnormalities in Mature Lymphoid Neoplasms

Disease	Chromosome Abnormalities	Gene Abnormalities*
CLL	del(13)(q14)	*MIR15A/MIR16-1*
		DLEU/DLEU1
	9q34.3	*NOTCH1*
	del(11)(q23)	*ATM*
		BIRC3
	2q33.1	*SF3B1*
	del(17)(p13)	*TP53*
	Trisomy 12	
T-PLL	14q11.2	*TRA*
	14q32	*TCL1A*
	t(X;14)(q28;q11)	*MTCP1::TRA*
	8q24.21	*MYC*
HCL	7q34	*BRAF* V600E
BL	t(8;14)	*MYC::IGH*
	t(2;8)	*IGK::MYC*
	t(8;22)	*MYC::IGL*
FL	t(14;18)	*IGH::BCL2*
	1p36	*TNFRSF14*
MCL	t(11;14)	*CCND1::IGH*
	11q22.3	*ATM*
	17p13.1	*TP53*
DLBCL	3q27	*BCL6*
	t(14;18)	*IGH::BCL2*
		MYC/BCL2/BCL6 (double or triple hit)
	6p25.3	*IRF4*
MZL, MALT	t(11;18)	*BIRC3::MALT1*
	t(1;14)	*BCL10::IGH*
	t(14;18)	*IGH::MALT1*
	t(3;14)	*FOXP1::IGH*
MZL, SMZL	Trisomy 3	
	del(7)(q21)	
LPL/ Waldenström	3p22.2	*MYD88*
	2q22.1	*CXCR4*
ALCL, ALK-positive	t(2;5)	*ALK::NPM1*
	t(1;2)	*TPM3::ALK*
	t(2;3)	*ALK::TFG*
	t(2;17)	*ALK::CLTC*
	inv(2)	*ATIC::ALK*
ALCL, ALK-negative	6p25	*DUSP22*
		IRF4
PTCL-NOS	t(5;9)	*ITK::SYK* (follicular variant)
	10p14	*GATA3*
	17q21.32	*TBX21*
MM	Hyperdiploidy/hypodiploidy	UD
	t(11;14)	*CCND1::IGH*
	t(4;14)	*FGFR3/NSD2::IGH*
	t(14;16)	*IGH::CMIP*
	t(14;20)	*IGH::MAFB*
	del(17)(p13)	*TP53*
	del(13)/monosomy 13	*RB1*
		DIS3

*Gene names updated according to the HUGO Database, December 2023.

ALCL, Anaplastic large cell lymphoma; *BL,* Burkitt leukemia/lymphoma; *CLL,* chronic lymphocytic leukemia; *DLBCL,* diffuse large B-cell lymphoma; *FL,* follicular lymphoma; *HCL,* hairy cell leukemia; *LPL,* lymphoplasmacytic lymphoma; *MALT,* mucosa associated lymphoid tissue lymphoma; *MCL,* mantle cell lymphoma; *MM,* plasma cell (multiple) myeloma; *MZL,* marginal zone lymphoma; *PTCL-NOS,* peripheral T-cell lymphoma, not otherwise specified; *SMZL,* splenic marginal zone lymphoma; *T-PLL,* T-prolymphocytic leukemia; *UD,* undetermined.

Data from Liu, Y., Corcoran, M., Rasool, O., et al. (1997). Cloning of two candidate tumor suppressor genes within a 10 kb region on chromosome 13q14, frequently deleted in chronic lymphocytic leukemia. *Oncogene, 15*(20), 2463–2473; Dave, B. J., Nelson, M., & Sanger, W. G. (2011). Lymphoma cytogenetics. *Clin Lab Med, 31*(4), 725–761; Swerdlow, S. H., Campo, E., Harris, N. L., et al. (2017). *WHO Classification of Tumours of Haematopoietic and Lymphoid Tissues* (4th ed., vol. 2). International Agency for Research on Cancer (IARC); and Taylor, J., Xiao, W., & Abdel-Wahab, O. (2017). Diagnosis and classification of hematologic malignancies on the basis of genetics. *Blood, 130,* 410–423.

BOX 34.1   Clinical Behavior of Mature Lymphoid Neoplasms

Aggressive Disease
Adult T-cell leukemia/lymphoma
Prolymphocytic leukemia
Anaplastic large cell lymphoma
Mantle cell lymphoma
Sézary syndrome
Diffuse large B-cell lymphoma
Peripheral T-cell lymphoma
Plasma cell (multiple) myeloma
Burkitt leukemia/lymphoma

Generally Indolent Disease
Chronic lymphocytic leukemia/small lymphocytic lymphoma
Large granular lymphocytic leukemia
Hairy cell leukemia
Mycosis fungoides
Lymphoplasmacytic lymphoma (Waldentröm macroglobulinemia)
Marginal zone lymphoma
Follicular lymphoma
Solitary plasmacytoma
Smoldering multiple myeloma

An appreciation of the ontogeny of B, T, and natural killer (NK) lymphocytes is useful for understanding some of the biological behaviors of the diseases and forms the basis for classification of these disorders. Neoplastic counterparts of lymphoid cells that localize to the germinal center of lymphoid tissues will likewise gravitate to these areas of involvement. The WHO has developed a classification system based on a multiparameter approach to diagnosis.[2] A summary of the 2022 WHO classification for the mature lymphoid neoplasms is shown in Box 34.2.[1]

APPROACH TO DIAGNOSIS: INTERFACE BETWEEN CLINICAL AND LABORATORY MEDICINE

Clinical Signs and Symptoms

Given the broad spectrum of diseases contained in this chapter, the presenting signs and symptoms range from asymptomatic disease detected during routine laboratory testing to fulminant illness characterized by fever, weight loss, night sweats, adenopathy, and severe functional compromise. In all cases, the history and physical examination are of utmost importance and the first step in arriving at an accurate diagnosis. Manifestations of disease can be interpreted differently depending on the clinical context. For example, lymphadenopathy is a common manifestation in lymphoma but also can be seen in a number of infections and inflammatory conditions. The recognition of a symptom as abnormal then triggers a diagnostic workup that relies on the laboratory to further define the underlying pathologic condition.

Although manifesting symptoms may be nonspecific, they are often reflective of involvement of a particular organ system by the tumor. In patients with lymphadenopathy, the pattern of lymph node involvement may be characteristic in some forms of lymphoma, with painless cervical adenopathy in the young adult most likely associated with HL. Systematic B symptoms include (1) unexplained weight loss (>10% body weight in 6 months before staging, (2) unexplained persistent fever (>38.0° C), and (3) recurrent, drenching night sweats. B symptoms are associated with increased concentrations of inflammatory proteins and cytokines such as C-reactive protein and interleukin-6 (IL-6), respectively. B symptoms are present at diagnosis in approximately 2% to 31% of patients with non-Hodgkin lymphoma (NHL)[6] and in 25% and 76% of patients with early stage and advanced-stage HL, respectively.[7,8] The development of B symptoms in a patient with low-grade lymphoma or CLL who previously had been without complaints may herald the histologic transformation of the disease to a more aggressive form. In HL, patients may present with unique complaints of alcohol intolerance, pruritus, or skin rash on starting ampicillin. Gastrointestinal (GI) complaints (e.g., early satiety or nausea) may not only relate to direct involvement of the GI tract with tumor but also may have an indirect cause such as hepatosplenomegaly. Tumor infiltration of skin can occur diffusely or be localized and appear as nodules. Although more common in T-cell neoplasms, skin involvement also can be seen in several B-cell neoplasms such as marginal zone lymphoma (MZL).

Body fluid analysis of the cerebrospinal fluid (CSF) or pleural fluid to check for tumor cells is often performed in patients presenting with central nervous system (CNS) symptoms or dyspnea as a result of pleural effusion. Positive findings in body fluids indicate progressive systemic disease and often a dismal prognosis. Cytopenias can result from bone marrow involvement with lymphoma, myelosuppressive treatment, or, less often, autoimmune anemia or thrombocytopenia. Some forms of lymphoma have a leukemic phase in which lymphoma cells are found on the peripheral blood film. Alternatively, abnormalities of the peripheral blood that are distinct from tumor involvement may be important for patient management. For example, Reed Sternberg (RS) cells in HL are almost never seen in the peripheral blood, but reactive leukocytosis or the development of lymphopenia has prognostic implications in this disease.

DIAGNOSTIC PROCEDURES

Clinical Laboratory Testing

The complete blood count (CBC) is one of the first laboratory tests ordered to investigate a patient's symptoms. A quantitative abnormality in the CBC may be the first indication of an underlying pathologic condition. Lymphocytosis usually triggers examination of the peripheral blood film to further characterize the abnormality. In healthy adults an absolute increase in lymphocytes reflects either a reactive response to an underlying stimulus or the presence of a lymphoid neoplasm. Changes in lymphocyte morphology are often suggestive of the underlying cause of the lymphocytosis. A separate classification of reactive and abnormal lymphocytes in the manual white blood cell (WBC) differential or a comment indicating the presence of these cells can be helpful in the clinical evaluation of the patient. These findings may lead to further testing by other techniques

BOX 34.2   2022 WHO Classification of Mature Lymphoid Neoplasms*

MATURE B-CELL NEOPLASMS
Preneoplastic and Neoplastic Small Lymphocytic Proliferations
Monoclonal B-cell lymphocytosis
Chronic lymphocytic leukemia/small lymphocytic lymphoma

Splenic B-Cell Lymphomas and Leukemias
Hairy cell leukemia
Splenic marginal zone lymphoma
Splenic diffuse red pulp small B-cell lymphoma
Splenic B-cell lymphoma/leukemia with prominent nucleoli

Lymphoplasmacytic Lymphoma
Lymphoplasmacytic lymphoma

Marginal Zone Lymphoma
Extranodal marginal zone lymphoma of mucosa-associated lymphoid tissue
Primary cutaneous marginal zone lymphoma
Nodal marginal zone lymphoma
Pediatric marginal zone lymphoma

Follicular Lymphoma
In situ follicular B-cell neoplasm
Follicular lymphoma
Pediatric-type follicular lymphoma
Duodenal-type follicular lymphoma

Cutaneous Follicle Center Lymphoma
Primary cutaneous follicle center lymphoma

Mantle Cell Lymphoma
In situ mantle cell neoplasm
Mantle cell lymphoma
Leukemic nonnodal mantle cell lymphoma

Transformations of Indolent B-Cell Lymphomas
Transformations of indolent B-cell lymphomas

Large B-Cell Lymphomas
Diffuse large B-cell lymphoma, NOS
T-cell/histiocyte-rich large B-cell lymphoma
Diffuse large B-cell lymphoma/high grade B-cell lymphoma with *MYC* and *BCL2* rearrangements
ALK-positive large B-cell lymphoma
Large B-cell lymphoma with *IRF4* rearrangement
High-grade B-cell lymphoma with 11q aberrations
Lymphomatoid granulomatosis
EBV-positive diffuse large B-cell lymphoma
Diffuse large B-cell lymphoma associated with chronic inflammation
Fibrin-associated large B-cell lymphoma
Fluid overload-associated large B-cell lymphoma
Plasmablastic lymphoma
Primary large B-cell lymphoma of immune-privileged sites
Primary cutaneous diffuse large B-cell lymphoma, leg type
Intravascular large B-cell lymphoma
Primary mediastinal large B-cell lymphoma
Mediastinal gray zone lymphoma
High-grade B-cell lymphoma, NOS

Burkitt Lymphoma
Burkitt lymphoma

KSHV/HHV8-Associated B-Cell Lymphoid Proliferations and Lymphomas
Primary effusion lymphoma
KSHV/HHV8-positive diffuse large B-cell lymphoma
KSHV/HHV8-positive germinotrophic lymphoproliferative disorder

Lymphoid Proliferations and Lymphomas Associated with Immune Deficiency and Dysregulation
Hyperplasias arising in immune deficiency/dysregulation
Polymorphic lymphoproliferative disorders arising in immune deficiency/dysregulation
EBV-positive mucocutaneous ulcer
Lymphomas arising in immune deficiency/dysregulation
Inborn error of immunity-associated lymphoid proliferations and lymphomas

Hodgkin Lymphoma
Classic Hodgkin lymphoma
Nodular lymphocyte predominant Hodgkin lymphoma

PLASMA CELL NEOPLASMS AND OTHER DISEASES WITH PARAPROTEINS
Monoclonal Gammopathies
Cold agglutinin disease
IgM monoclonal gammopathy of undetermined significance
Non-IgM monoclonal gammopathy of undetermined significance
Monoclonal gammopathy of renal significance

Diseases with Monoclonal Immunoglobulin Deposition
Immunoglobulin-related (AL) amyloidosis
Monoclonal immunoglobulin deposition disease

Heavy Chain Diseases
Mu heavy chain disease
Gamma heavy chain disease
Alpha heavy chain disease

Plasma Cell Neoplasms
Plasmacytoma
Plasma cell myeloma
Plasma cell neoplasms with associated paraneoplastic syndrome
    POEMS syndrome
    TEMPI syndrome
    AESOP syndrome

MATURE T-CELL AND NK-CELL NEOPLASMS
Mature T-Cell and NK-Cell Leukemias
T-prolymphocytic leukemia
T-large granular lymphocytic leukemia
NK-large granular lymphocytic leukemia
Adult T-cell leukemia/lymphoma
Sézary syndrome
Aggressive NK-cell leukemia

Primary Cutaneous T-Cell Lymphomas
Primary cutaneous CD4-positive small or medium T-cell lymphoproliferative disorder
Primary cutaneous acral CD8-positive lymphoproliferative disorder
Mycosis fungoides
Primary cutaneous CD30-positive T-cell lymphoproliferative disorder: lymphomatoid papulosis
Primary cutaneous CD30-positive T-cell lymphoproliferative disorder: primary cutaneous anaplastic large cell lymphoma
Subcutaneous panniculitis-like T-cell lymphoma

BOX 34.2 **2022 WHO Classification of Mature Lymphoid Neoplasms*—cont'd**

Primary cutaneous gamma/delta T-cell lymphoma
Primary cutaneous CD8-positive aggressive epidermotropic cytotoxic T-cell lymphoma
Primary cutaneous peripheral T-cell lymphoma, NOS

Intestinal T-Cell and NK-Cell Lymphoid Proliferations and Lymphomas
Indolent T-cell lymphoma of the gastrointestinal tract
Indolent NK-cell lymphoproliferative disorder of the gastrointestinal tract
Enteropathy-associated T-cell lymphoma
Monomorphic epitheliotropic intestinal T-cell lymphoma
Intestinal T-cell lymphoma, NOS

Hepatosplenic T-Cell Lymphoma
Hepatosplenic T-cell lymphoma

Anaplastic Large Cell Lymphoma
ALK-positive anaplastic large cell lymphoma
ALK-negative anaplastic large cell lymphoma
Breast implant-associated anaplastic large-cell lymphoma

Nodal T-Follicular Helper (TFH) Cell Lymphoma
Nodal TFH cell lymphoma, angioimmunoblastic type
Nodal TFH cell lymphoma, follicular type
Nodal TFH cell lymphoma, NOS

Other Peripheral T-Cell Lymphomas
Peripheral T-cell lymphoma, NOS

EBV-Positive NK/T-Cell Lymphomas
EBV-positive nodal T- and NK-cell lymphoma
Extranodal NK/T-cell lymphoma

EBV-Positive T- and NK-Cell Lymphoid Proliferations and Lymphomas of Childhood
Severe mosquito bite allergy
Hydroa vacciniforme lymphoproliferative disorder
Systemic chronic active EBV disease
Systemic EBV-positive T-cell lymphoma of childhood

*Leukemias/lymphomas in red font are discussed in the chapter.
AESOP, *A*denopathy and *e*xtensive *s*kin patch *o*verlying a *p*lasmacytoma syndrome; *AL*, *a*myloidosis *l*ight chain; ALK, anaplastic lymphoma kinase; EBV, Epstein-Barr virus; *NK*, natural killer; *NOS*, not otherwise specified; *POEMS*, *p*olyneuropathy, *o*rganomegaly, *e*ndocrinopathy, *m*onoclonal plasma cell disorder, *s*kin changes syndrome; *TEMPI*, *t*elangiectasias, *e*levated erythropoietin level and erythrocytosis, *m*onoclonal gammopathy, *p*erinephric fluid collections, and *i*ntrapulmonary shunting syndrome; *WHO*, World Health Organization.
From Alaggio, R., Amador, C., Anagnostopoulos, I., et al. (2022). The 5th edition of the World Health Organization classification of haematolymphoid tumours: lymphoid neoplasms. *Leukemia, 36,* 1720–1748, Tables 1 and 2.

such as flow cytometry to document clonality and establish an immunophenotype, and cytogenetic studies such as fluorescence in situ hybridization (FISH) to detect genetic changes associated with disease.

Although the current generation of automated blood cell analyzers employ powerful tools to detect a wide variety of abnormalities in the peripheral blood (Chapter 13), they are not perfect. Lymphoid neoplasms can present distinct challenges for these analyzers as the physical properties of the abnormal lymphocytes (as defined by light scatter, fluorescence, or histochemical methodologies used by the analyzer) may not be sufficiently sensitive to detect the morphologic qualities of the malignant lymphoid cells. This may be particularly true if there are no quantitative abnormalities present and the automated differential is autovalidated without a review of the blood film. The absence of flags in an automated differential does not always rule out the presence of abnormal cells in the peripheral blood. Therefore clinical context is most important and communication between the provider and the laboratory staff is key. Certain circumstances, such as the presence of lymphadenopathy, may require a microscopic review of the blood film to detect abnormal lymphoid cells, even if the CBC was normal. The presence of these cells may prompt further diagnostic procedures such as a biopsy of the bone marrow or an enlarged lymph node. An example of a potential disparity between the automated and manual differential is illustrated in Figure 34.1.

Flow cytometry is the diagnostic tool that, when used as an adjunct to morphologic evaluation, often may provide useful information capable of separating reactive from clonal disorders and discriminating among the mature lymphoid disorders that manifest with peripheral blood involvement. Immunophenotyping is undertaken with standard consensus panels and the pattern of staining with a series of monoclonal antibodies associated with lineages and degree of maturation establishes an immunologic profile.[9] Various T-cell and B-cell disorders have typical immunologic profiles, and these are summarized in Table 34.2.

Often, the first information obtained from this immunologic screen is to establish the lineage of the cells of interest as lymphoid. For B cells, the next step is to determine if the population is clonal by detecting the presence of light chain restriction. The absence of light chain restriction in immature lymphoid neoplasms such as ALL does not rule out malignancy and morphologic differentiation of the blasts remains of paramount importance. Likewise, Burkitt lymphoma (BL) cells appear markedly different from normal mature lymphocytes, and flow cytometry is hardly needed to define them as abnormal. However, both disorders may lack characteristics associated with mature lymphoid morphology, and flow cytometry is needed to define the degree of maturation (pre-B versus mature B cells) and guide the provider to the proper management for that disorder.

Although it may be relatively straightforward to define a population as being of T or NK lineage, the variability in the phenotypic abnormalities in these lymphomas often makes the precise diagnosis based on immunophenotyping alone difficult. T-cell disorders are generally characterized by some "mismatch" in

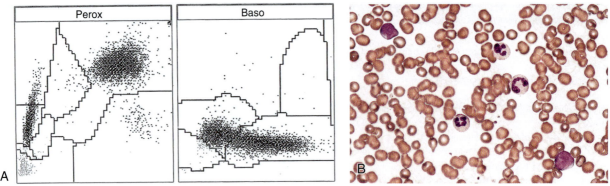

Figure 34.1 Disparity Between Automated and Manual Differentials. **(A)**, Cytogram generated by an automated blood cell analyzer for an 11-year-old boy with a history of acute lymphoblastic leukemia *(ALL)* who was treated with hematopoietic stem cell transplantation. The cytogram shows a relatively normal pattern in which suspect/morphologic flags (e.g., "blast" or "variant lymphocyte") were not generated. **(B)**, Upon manual review by the medical laboratory scientist, circulating blasts were noted, consistent with relapsed disease. This underscores the inability of modern instrumentation to always detect lymphoid abnormalities. *Baso,* Basophils; *Perox,* peroxidase. (34.1, B: Peripheral blood, Wright-Giemsa stain, ×100.)

TABLE 34.2   Common Immunophenotypes in Mature Lymphoid Neoplasms

Neoplasm	Immunophenotypes
CLL	CD19+, CD20+ (dim), CD5+, CD23+, CD200+, ROR1+, surface immunoglobulin (dim), CD10–, FMC7 dim or –, CD79b dim or –
T-PLL	CD4+ or CD4+/CD8+ (dual), TCL1+, CD2+, CD3+, CD7+, CD52+, Tdt –
HCL	CD20+ (bright), CD25+, CD103+, CD11c+, surface immunoglobulin (bright), CD19+, CD22+
LGL	T cell: CD8+, CD3+, CD57+, CD16+, CD2+, CD5+ (dim), CD7+ (dim) or – NK cell: CD56+, CD3–, CD16+, CD2+, CD4–, CD8–, CD7+ (dim) or –, CD57+ (dim) or –
ATLL	CD2+, CD5+, CD3+ or dim, CD7–, CD4+, CD25+ (bright), FOXP3+
BL	CD19+, CD20+, CD22+, CD10+, surface immunoglobulin (bright), Ki67+, Tdt–, CD79a+
FL	CD19+, CD20+ CD10+, surface immunoglobulin (bright), CD5–, CD23 variable, HLA-DR+, CD21+, CD79a+
MCL	CD19+, CD20+, CD5+, CD23–, CD200–, FMC7+, CD22+, CD79b+, CD10+/–, CD43+
DLBCL	CD19+, CD20+, CD79a+, CD22+ (bright), CD10+/–, CD45+
MZL	CD19+, CD20+, CD22+, CD79b+, surface immunoglobulin (bright), FMC7+, CD5–, CD10–, CD23–
ALCL	CD30+, ALK+/–, CD3–, CD2+, CD5+, CD4+, TIA1+
MF/SS	CD2+, CD3+, CD5+, CD7–, CD4+, CD26–
MM	CD45 dim or –, CD38+, CD138+, CD56+, monotypic cytoplasmic light chains
CHL	High forward scatter (large cells), CD30+, CD40+ (bright), CD15+, CD20–, CD64–

ALCL, Anaplastic large cell lymphoma; *ATLL,* adult T-cell leukemia/lymphoma; *BL,* Burkitt leukemia/lymphoma; *CHL,* classic Hodgkin lymphoma; *CLL,* chronic lymphocytic leukemia; *DLBCL,* diffuse large B-cell lymphoma; *FL,* follicular lymphoma; *HCL,* hairy cell leukemia; *LGL,* large granular lymphocytic leukemia; *MCL,* mantle cell lymphoma; *MF/SS,* mycosis fungoides/Sézary syndrome; *MM,* plasma cell (multiple) myeloma; *MZL,* marginal zone lymphoma; *T-PLL,* T-prolymphocytic leukemia.
Data from Swerdlow, S. H., Campo, E., Harris, N. L., et al. (2017). *WHO Classification of Tumours of Haematopoietic and Lymphoid Tissues* (4th ed., vol. 2). International Agency for Research on Cancer (IARC).

T-cell antigenic patterns not found in normal mature cells. These may take the form of an absence of a marker usually expressed in normal T cells (i.e., CD7) or in the expression of a primitive marker such as TdT, which is not ordinarily found in a mature T cell. The ability to measure TCR Vβ repertoire as a marker of T-cell clonality can be used to identify potentially clonal populations. No laboratory technique is without potential for error, and there may be clonal populations present that fall outside of the restricted pattern tested for by the commercially available kits used for this purpose. Such cases would therefore require

molecular testing (Chapter 29), which remains the gold standard to establish the presence of clonal disease. NK cells do not rearrange immunoglobulins or TCRs in ways that are detectable by the techniques described earlier; thus no standard method is available to define clonality in this lineage. Instead, some laboratories have relied on the detection of an abnormal pattern of killer Ig-like receptors (KIRs) expression in much the same way T-cell mismatch helps define an abnormal population.[10]

Biochemical analysis may be useful for three purposes: (1) evaluating organ systems for compromise because of tumor involvement, (2) serving as an indirect measure of tumor burden, and (3) assessing prognosis. An indication of organ compromise is then used to guide further diagnostic workup through imaging studies or biopsy. Biochemical testing panels are a good indicator of the patient's ability to tolerate therapies used to treat the neoplasm. For example, serum creatinine levels are used to assess renal function in patients receiving treatment known to affect the kidneys. Baseline measurements of uric acid may be indicated, particularly in disorders with high tumor cell turnover. Patients may undergo assessment for a monoclonal protein with protein electrophoresis, immunofixation, and, if indicated, quantitative immunoglobulin testing. Patients presenting with unexpected anemia may require a reticulocyte count, haptoglobin level, and a direct antiglobulin test (DAT) to rule out an associated autoimmune hemolytic anemia. Lactate dehydrogenase (LD) and β_2 microglobulin have utility as an estimate of tumor burden and have been incorporated into scoring systems that have prognostic value. Likewise, measurement of erythrocyte sedimentation rate (ESR) is indicated in HL as elevated levels have been found to be predictive of early relapse and decreased survival. Testing for hepatitis B should be undertaken before the institution of therapy. Patients who have evidence of hepatitis B surface antigen positivity require prophylactic antiviral therapy to avoid the severe complications that accompany viral reactivation. Human immunodeficiency virus (HIV) should be routinely tested before institution of therapy because it may have a significant impact on overall management.

Analyzing the peripheral blood is relatively easy, but it may not yield sufficient information to make a tissue diagnosis. Because lymphadenopathy is common in mature lymphoid neoplasms, it is logical to attempt to secure tissue from an area that is highly likely to be involved with disease. Alternatively, if malignant lymphoid cells are found in peripheral blood, bone marrow aspiration and biopsy may be needed. Although lymphadenopathy is common in CLL/SLL, a peripheral blood specimen may be sufficient to make the diagnosis, thus avoiding an invasive procedure. Even in cases presenting with peripheral adenopathy, it may be worthwhile to obtain a CBC before lymph node biopsy.

Anatomic Pathology Testing

An excisional biopsy remains the gold standard for lymphoma diagnosis; however, fine-needle aspiration (FNA) has become increasingly popular because of the relative ease in which specimens can be obtained. FNA, coupled with the advances in flow cytometry and FISH analysis, have made this a feasible approach for diagnosis of certain disorders and may be particularly useful as a screening procedure for differentiating reactive lymphadenopathy from malignant disease. Yet, FNA may not be suitable in all cases, and it is important to be aware of the limitations associated with this approach. In lymphoid neoplasms with focal involvement or in which the malignant cells make up only a minor population in the lymph node, an FNA may miss the relevant population entirely. The paucity of tissue obtained by FNA may also limit the testing that can be accomplished on suboptimal specimens. In certain cases, FNA cytology can be problematic and the tissue architecture from the biopsy is key in providing the necessary information to arrive at an accurate diagnosis.

Imaging Studies

Establishing a tissue diagnosis is followed by studies designed to delineate the extent of tumor involvement for disease staging. Accurate staging of the tumor is fundamental in developing a treatment plan. Newer imaging studies and the emergence of certain forms of molecular analysis have changed the way imaging is approached. As discussed previously, abnormalities in biochemical testing may be early evidence of tumor involvement in a particular organ system. Radiographic imaging is frequently employed to verify the presence of tumor and extent of disease. CT scans have become a standard part of the diagnostic workup for both HL and NHL. Conventional radiographic studies are routinely supplemented by a functional assessment of tumor biology using positron emission tomography (PET) with fluorodeoxyglucose (FDG) as a tracer. When combined with CT scanning, PET allows greater localization of tumor and is more sensitive in delineating areas of disease than standard imaging alone. However, the utility of PET is limited by the biologic characteristics of the lymphoid tumor in question. Some forms of lymphoma are FDG avid (have high affinity for), whereas other lymphomas have variable uptake of FDG, which makes interpretation of the scan more problematic. Among the FDG-avid tumors are HL, BL, nodal MZL, lymphoblastic lymphoma, diffuse large B-cell lymphoma (DLBCL), and follicular lymphoma (FL). Peripheral T-cell lymphoma and some of the more indolent lymphoid neoplasms such as CLL/SLL and extranodal MZL are less avid for FDG making PET/CT less clinically useful in these settings.

DIAGNOSTIC EVALUATION

Staging Systems

In addition to detecting areas of occult disease, PET scanning may be useful for defining areas to be biopsied for diagnosis. This is particularly true when there is a clinical suspicion of histologic transformation of an indolent lymphoma, such as CLL/SLL. Combined PET/CT scans may define a highly avid area for biopsy, maximizing the potential for making an accurate diagnosis. Following the completion of therapy, PET/CT scans may be useful in differentiating between areas of residual disease versus residual scar tissue. The patient with residual scar tissue could be spared from additional biopsies or therapy because there is no evidence of active disease.

Incorporation of data obtained from these studies is used to supplement the findings noted on physical examination and has resulted in the development of formalized staging systems. The Ann Arbor staging system was first applied to HL to quantify nodal and extranodal sites of involvement (see Table 34.3).[11] The staging system was further qualified by the absence or presence of B symptoms. The ultimate clinical utility of this system is to define limited versus extensive disease because treatment differs between the two.

Ann Arbor staging has also been applied to NHL but is less useful in these diseases because of biological differences.[12] Even among indolent subtypes, few patients present with truly localized disease and there is no appreciable difference in therapy for patients of any subtype who have stage III or stage IV disease.

TABLE 34.3 Staging Hodgkin Lymphoma/Primary Nodal Non-Hodgkin Lymphoma

Stage	Ann Arbor	Lugano
	Limited Disease	
I	1 node involved or single extranodal site (E)	1 node or group of nodes; single extranodal lesion without nodal involvement
II	≥2 nodes/groups or lymphatic structures on same side of diaphragm or involvement of limited contiguous extralymphatic organ or tissue (IIE)	≥2 nodes or nodal groups on same side of diaphragm; stage I or II by nodal extent with limited contiguous extranodal involvement. II bulky defined as a single or nodal abdominal mass of ≥10 cm or a mediastinal mass ≥⅓ the internal transverse diameter of the thorax
	Advanced Disease	
III	Nodes on both sides of diaphragm (III) with involvement of spleen (IIIS) or limited contiguous extralymphatic organ or tissue involvement (IIIE) or both (IIIES)	Nodes on both sides of diaphragm Nodes above the diaphragm with spleen involvement
IV	Diffuse or disseminated foci of involvement of ≥1 extralymphatic organ or tissue with or without associated lymphatic involvement	Additional noncontiguous extralymphatic involvement

Data from Carbone, P. P., Kaplan, H. S., Musshoff, K., et al. (1971). Report of the committee on Hodgkin's disease staging classification. *Cancer Res, 31*(11), 1860–1861; Rosenberg, S. A. (1977). Validity of the Ann Arbor staging classification for the non-Hodgkin's lymphomas. *Cancer Treat Rep, 61*, 1023–1027; Lister, T. A., Crowther, D., Sutcliffe, S. B., et al. (1989). Report of a committee convened to discuss the evaluation and staging of patients with Hodgkin's disease: Cotswolds meeting. *J Clin Oncol, 7*, 1630–1636; and Cheson, B. D., Fisher, R. I., Barrington, S. F., et al. (2014). Recommendations for initial evaluation, staging, and response assessment of Hodgkin and non-Hodgkin lymphoma: the Lugano classification. *J Clin Oncol, 32*, 3059–3068.

The Lugano classification, a simplification of the original Ann Arbor staging, is currently used in NHL (see Table 34.3).[13] It groups patients into limited (stages I and II) and advanced (stages III and IV) disease, recognizing that the intrinsic properties of the disease have more bearing on clinical outcome than extent of disease as described by anatomic distribution.

Prognostic Assessment

The high number of risk factors in NHL has prompted further modification of prognostic models to include the most clinically relevant features that predict patient response to therapy. The Internal Prognostic Index (IPI) was developed in accordance with these principles and has largely supplanted anatomic staging as the primary prognostic tool.[14] The analysis was based on data generated from over 2000 patients with aggressive histologic lymphoma who were treated with standard anthracycline-containing regimens. The analysis identified four significant parameters:

(1) age (≤60 versus >60 years), (2) serum LD to indicate tumor burden (within the reference interval versus above the reference interval), (3) performance status (0/1 versus 2 to 4), (4) stage (limited versus advanced), and (5) extranodal involvement (≤1 site versus >1 site). Based on a scoring system assigned to the parameters, patients are grouped into four prognostic groups, with differing overall survival (OS) rates at 5 years: (1) low risk: 73%, (2) low to intermediate risk: 51%, (3) high to intermediate risk: 43%, and (4) high risk: 26%. This model has subsequently undergone slight modification with the introduction of rituximab, a CD20 targeted monoclonal antibody, which has improved survival across all subgroups.[15]

Although it was initially established in large cell lymphoma, the IPI has applicability across other types of lymphoma. Despite this, there is recognition that the different disease entities have unique features that can play an important role in determining overall prognosis, and the IPI has been adapted to fit this. A separate model, the Follicular Lymphoma International Prognostic Index (FLIPI/FLIPI2), has been developed to account for the pattern of disease seen in FL. Other disease-specific systems incorporating biological features that are particular to those disorders have been developed for T-cell lymphoma and MCL.

Although some of the basic principles discussed previously are shared among the different entities considered under the umbrella of the mature lymphoid disorders, the clinical course and management largely depend on the underlying biology of each individual disease as reflected in histologic features, immunophenotype, and, increasingly, molecular genetics. Familiarity with these characteristics is of utmost importance to the laboratorian and the provider in arriving at the correct diagnosis and formulating an effective treatment strategy. The unique features of some of the more common or unique diseases are highlighted in the following section.

LEUKEMIAS

Chronic Lymphocytic Leukemia (CLL)/Small Lymphocytic Lymphoma (SLL)

CLL/SLL is the most common leukemia in the adult population. Even so, it constitutes about 1% of all new cancer cases in the United States in a single year.[16] CLL is a malignancy of B lymphocytes. Although some of the earlier literature discussed a T-cell variety, these disorders probably have been reclassified among the mature T-cell neoplasms, and some are discussed in this chapter.

CLL/SLL is generally a disease of the older adult. The median age at diagnosis is approximately 69 years, with a slight male preponderance. The annual incidence in the United States is approximately 4.6 cases per 100,000 persons.[16] Because of the long natural history of CLL/SLL in many patients, the prevalence is probably much higher.

Most CLL/SLL patients are asymptomatic on presentation. The disease is often detected by an abnormality in the CBC during routine health screening. Alternatively, lymphadenopathy or splenomegaly may be noted in the physical examination. The International Workshop on Chronic Lymphoid Leukemia (IWCLL) has developed specific criteria to establish the diagnosis of CLL. It requires the sustained presence of at least 5×10^9/L circulating B lymphocytes with documentation of clonality by flow cytometry.[17]

Morphology

On a blood film, the typical CLL/SLL lymphocyte is described as small and mature appearing, with a minimal amount of cytoplasm and a dense nucleus having a condensed chromatin pattern and inconspicuous nucleolus. The chromatin pattern has been labeled as "cobblestone," and the overall appearance of the nucleus has been likened to that of a "soccer ball," "pepperoni pizza," or "cracked earth" (Figure 34.2). A few larger lymphocytes, clefted forms, and/or prolymphocytes can sometimes be found among the typical CLL/SLL lymphocytes. When prolymphocytes are more than 15% in the blood and/or bone marrow, the diagnosis is further defined by the WHO as "prolymphocytic progression of CLL/SLL."[1] These patients have been shown to experience more aggressive disease and have shorter survival times.[18]

Smudge cells are commonly observed on CLL/SLL blood films and represent fragile CLL lymphocytes that are damaged during blood film preparation. Smudge cells are sometimes overlooked when the manual differential is performed on a CLL/SLL blood film; however this practice diminishes the accuracy of the differential cell counts. Therefore it is recommended that smudge cells be counted as lymphocytes in the WBC differential in cases of CLL.[19,20] Alternative approaches include reporting the results of the automated differential or using an albuminized blood film to perform the differential. There are limitations associated with these procedures that should be considered before implementation. Untreated CLL/SLL patients with 30% or more smudge cells on routine blood films have been shown to have a better prognosis than those with less than 30% smudge cells.[21]

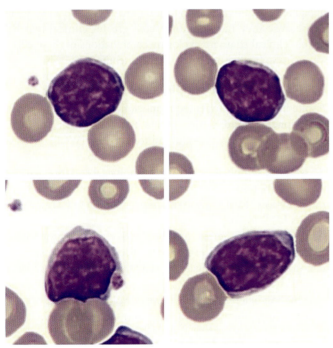

Figure 34.2 Chronic Lymphocytic Leukemia (CLL). Leukemia cells have a high nuclear-to-cytoplasmic ratio, and the nuclear chromatin has a "cracked earth," or "soccer ball" appearance. (Peripheral blood, Wright-Giemsa stain, ×1000.) (Courtesy Cellavision AB, Lund, Sweden.)

Diagnosis

CLL/SLL lymphocytes express B-cell markers CD19, CD20, and CD23 but also aberrantly coexpresses the T-cell antigen CD5, key in recognizing most cases. Although CLL/SLL cells typically demonstrate surface immunoglobulin, the level of expression may be dim and the ability to discern light chain restriction, indicating B-cell clonality, may be difficult. There is, however, some variability in the expression of cell markers, and not all cases fit into a classical CLL/SLL profile. In an effort to account for this variability yet retain the ability to differentiate CLL from other mature B-cell neoplasms, a scoring system has been developed (Box 34.3).[22] Each criterion is given 1 point and the total score is cumulative. A combined score of 4 or greater is consistent with CLL/SLL. Low scores of 1 to 2 are more associated with NHL. An intermediate score of 3 remains problematic, and such cases may require biopsy of a lymph node or molecular test(s) to establish the diagnosis.[22]

Guidelines allow for the diagnosis of CLL/SLL to be made from the peripheral blood.[23,24] However, such cases may require a cytospin slide stained for cyclin D1 or FISH for t(11;14) to rule out MCL. In the past, a bone marrow biopsy was recommended to establish the pattern of involvement as a prognostic marker, but biopsies have largely been superseded by other important biomarkers, including cytogenetic abnormalities and the mutational status of the heavy chain immunoglobulin gene (IGHV). Although peripheral blood may suffice to establish a CLL/SLL diagnosis in uncomplicated patients who are to be monitored without therapy, a more extensive workup is needed for symptomatic patients who require treatment. Such testing may include a full cytogenetic panel and a bone marrow biopsy.

Staging and Prognosis

Like NHL, the extent of disease involvement in CLL/SLL as reflected in staging systems is an important prognostic determinant and helps dictate clinical management. Both the Rai and the Binet staging systems have been used toward this end.[25,26] Both systems divide patients into risk categories that reflect the degree of organomegaly/lymphadenopathy or compromise of marrow function (Table 34.4). An important caveat is the presence of autoimmune phenomena affecting up to 25% of CLL/SLL patients at some point in the disease. For patients with unexplained anemia or thrombocytopenia, an

---

BOX 34.3 Catovsky-Matutes Scoring for Chronic Lymphocytic Leukemia Diagnosis

Score 1 point for each of following:
- Weak expression of surface immunoglobulin
- Expression of CD5
- Expression of CD23
- No expression of FMC7
- Absent or weak expression of CD79b or CD22

A combined score of 4 or greater is consistent with a diagnosis of CLL, whereas a lower score is suggestive of some other lymphoid neoplasm.

CLL, Chronic lymphocytic leukemia.
Data from Matutes, E., & Polliack, A. (2000). Morphological and immunophenotypic features of chronic lymphocytic leukemia. *Rev Clin Exp Hematol, 4,* 22–47.

TABLE 34.4 Staging for Chronic Lymphocytic Leukemia

Rai Classification (Revised)	Binet Classification
Low Risk (formerly Stage 0)	**Stage A**
Lymphocytosis >5 × 10⁹/L	Hemoglobin ≥10 g/dL and platelets ≥100 × 10⁹/L and <3 enlarged nodal areas
Intermediate Risk (formerly Stages I and II)	**Stage B**
Lymphocytes >5 × 10⁹/L and (lymphadenopathy + splenomegaly) or hepatomegaly, or both	Hemoglobin ≥ 10 g/dL and platelets ≥100 × 10⁹/L and ≥3 enlarged nodal areas
High Risk (formerly Stages III and IV)	**Stage C**
Lymphocytes >5 × 10⁹/L and hemoglobin <11 g/dL or platelets <100 × 10⁹/L	Hemoglobin <10 g/dL or platelets <100 × 10⁹/L and any number of enlarged nodal areas

Data from Rai, K. R., Sawitsky, A., Cronkite, E. P., et al. (1975). Clinical staging of chronic lymphocytic leukemia. *Blood, 46,* 219–234; and Binet, J. L., Auquier, A., Dighiero, G., et al. (1981). A new prognostic classification of chronic lymphocytic leukemia derived from a multivariate survival analysis. *Cancer, 48,* 198–206.

underlying autoimmune process needs to be ruled out to avoid inadvertently "upstaging" the patient. The therapeutic approach to autoimmune cytopenia differs from CLL/SLL therapy and the occurrence of such a complication is not alone an indication to start anti-CLL chemotherapy.

The Rai and Binet staging systems are based on clinical criteria. A wide range of biological features have now been identified as having prognostic implications in CLL/SLL.[5,27–29] The underlying karyotype is a strong predictor of survival. Del(17p) and/or *TP53* abnormalities are the worst prognostic indicators and predict resistance to standard chemoimmunotherapy approaches. The *IGHV* mutational status is a marker for two different CLL/SLL subtypes; a less mature form with unmutated *IGHV* and another with a more mature phenotype associated with *IGHV* mutation. Patients with the unmutated, pre-germinal center form have a more aggressive clinical course, often accompanied by additional unfavorable genetic changes. Patients with mutated *IGHV* have better outcomes and, if required, do better with standard chemoimmunotherapy approaches. CD49d, CD38, and ZAP70 expression are cell markers with independent prognostic value for an unfavorable prognosis. CLL/SLL lymphocytes expressing C49d may have a higher proliferative capacity and may represent a clone with a higher potential for progression over time.[30] Testing for CD38 has been incorporated into standard immunophenotyping panels for CLL/SLL, and the significant cutoff (number of cells expressing CD38) with prognostic significance has been established. ZAP70 is a tyrosine kinase, and testing for its expression has been more problematic because there is variability in inter-laboratory testing and reproducibility between laboratories has been an issue. More recently, methylation states of ZAP70 have

been reported to be more reproducible, but this testing is not available in most clinical laboratories and remains restricted to research laboratories. DNA sequencing has identified abnormalities in *NOTCH1, SF3B,* and *BIRC3* as having negative prognostic value; however, they have not yet been integrated into routine clinical practice.[31–33]

Given the number of prognostic markers for CLL/SLL that now exist, a few studies have undertaken the formulation of a prognostic score similar to the IPI used in NHL. Most systems agree that *TP53* abnormalities, *IGHV* mutational status, serum beta 2-microglobulin, Rai/Binet stage, and age are important independent prognostic factors. These factors were, however, identified in the context of standard chemoimmunotherapy approaches. It has not been established if they are still relevant with the newer BTK or BCL2 targeted agents (discussed later).

Treatment

The therapy of CLL/SLL has undergone profound changes. In the past, treatment consisted largely of oral alkylating agents such as chlorambucil or cyclophosphamide. For younger, "fit" patients, these drugs were eventually replaced by the nucleoside analogue fludarabine and later, the anti-CD20 monoclonal antibody rituximab. Combination therapy with the alkylating agent bendamustine and rituximab has found application in older patient populations. The introduction of targeted agents has caused a fundamental paradigm shift in CLL/SLL therapeutics. These newer agents include BTK inhibitors (ibrutinib, acalabrutinib), PI3k inhibitors (idelalisib), and BCL2 inhibitors (venetoclax).[34–37] Furthermore, new monoclonal antibodies such as obinutuzumab have been designed to be more efficacious and are gradually replacing rituximab in combination regimens. BTK inhibitor-based and venetoclax-based regimens have largely supplanted traditional chemoimmunotherapy as "upfront" therapy because they have demonstrated greater clinical benefit. Current clinical trials are exploring combinations of these effective agents to further improve patient outcomes.

Monoclonal B-Cell Lymphocytosis (MBL)

Despite having a documented monoclonal B-cell population in the peripheral blood, some patients have fewer than 5 × 10⁹/L circulating B lymphocytes and fail to meet the IWCLL criteria to establish a CLL/SLL diagnosis. Patients who are asymptomatic, without lymphadenopathy, organomegaly, cytopenias, or systemic symptoms, are referred to as having monoclonal B-cell lymphocytosis (MBL).[25] The risk of progression to CLL in MBL patients is 1% to 2% per year.[24]

Individuals with fewer than 5 × 10⁹/L circulating monoclonal B lymphocytes and evidence of disease elsewhere such as adenopathy or organomegaly are classified as having small lymphocytic lymphoma (SLL). SLL patients may require histologic confirmation of a lymph node biopsy or biopsy of other tissues. Clinical management of SLL is often like that used in CLL.

T-Prolymphocytic Leukemia (T-PLL)

Prolymphocytic leukemia (PLL) has historically been subclassified as B-cell PLL (B-PLL) and T-cell PLL (T-PLL); however, the 5th edition of the WHO classification system (2022) no longer recognizes B-PLL as a distinct entity.[1] In view of the heterogeneous nature of B-PLL, these cases are now classified as either (1) MCL positive for the *IGH::CCND1* fusion gene, (2) CLL/SLL with prolymphocytic progression, or (3) splenic B-cell lymphoma/leukemia with prominent nucleoli.

T-PLL is a rare disorder that constitutes only about 2% of the mature lymphoid leukemias.[2] T-PLL has a distinct clinical course that differs from other mature lymphoid neoplasms. It is generally a disease of the elderly, with a median age at diagnosis of approximately 65 years and equal distribution among the sexes.

T-PLL is largely an aggressive disorder with primary manifestations in the peripheral blood, bone marrow, and spleen. The typical clinical presentation is characterized by massive splenomegaly, with a WBC count often exceeding 100×10^9/L consisting mainly of prolymphocytes. Lymphadenopathy tends to be minimal, although there is a high incidence of tissue involvement in T-PLL with skin as a common area of infiltration.

Laboratory Findings

Prolymphocytes in T-PLL may be confused with normal lymphocytes as they are smaller in size compared with B prolymphocytes and the nucleolus is generally less distinct. The nucleus of T prolymphocytes may be round, oval, or have an irregular contour and a cerebriform appearance. T prolymphocytes commonly exhibit cytoplasmic protrusions or blebbing (Figure 34.3). Immunophenotyping and genetic studies may be useful in distinguishing T-PLL from other chronic T-cell neoplasms. Unlike the other postthymic T-cell disorders, CD7 is usually expressed, and the TCL-1 antigen can be detected by either flow cytometry or immunohistochemistry. FISH analysis may reveal inv(14) in approximately 80% of patients.[2] T-PLL can resemble CLL if one relies on the automated differential alone. Automated blood cell analyzers would detect the increased WBC count; however, the smaller sized T prolymphocytes may be classified as normal lymphocytes in the automated differential. A morphology flag may

or may not be present, depending on the degree of morphologic abnormalities exhibited by the prolymphocytes. Regardless, all cases of absolute lymphocytosis detected in the CBC mandate careful review of the peripheral blood film if one has not previously been done.

Treatment

Unfortunately, therapies for these diseases are suboptimal. T-PLL has been treated with the anti-CD52 monoclonal antibody alemtuzumab, and this remains the standard of care. Complete responses can occur in up to 90% of patients, but these are often relatively short lived.[38] Responding patients often proceed to hematopoietic stem cell transplantation (HSCT) in an effort to achieve a long-term response, but durable remissions are only achieved in about 20% to 30% of patients treated with this therapy.

Hairy Cell Leukemia (HCL)

HCL is an indolent disease of B-cell lineage predominantly diagnosed in middle-aged individuals (median age at diagnosis is 50 years). The major nidus of disease is in the spleen, blood, and bone marrow. Patients typically present with splenomegaly and cytopenias.

Laboratory Findings

Hairy cells are sometimes misclassified as monocytes in the automated differential count. However, the true monocyte count in patients with HCL is characteristically decreased. A low number of hairy cells may be present, so in cases in which HCL is suspected, careful examination of the blood film or bone marrow aspirate smear is key to making the diagnosis. The characteristic hairy cells have round to ovoid or kidney bean-shaped nuclei that lack nucleoli and relatively abundant blue-gray cytoplasm with ragged, hairlike projections that extend circumferentially around the cell (Figure 34.4). Few morphologic variants exist in which the hairy cells have less prominent or absent "hairs," but they still exhibit the distinctive kidney bean-shaped

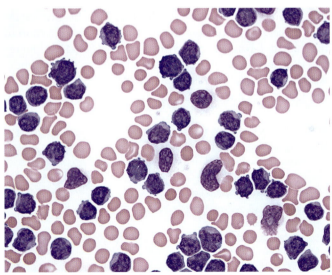

Figure 34.3 T-Prolymphocytic Leukemia (T-PLL). Small leukemia cells have high nuclear-to-cytoplasmic ratios, clumped chromatin, nucleoli, and cytoplasmic protrusions (blebbing). (Peripheral blood, Wright-Giemsa stain, X400.) (Courtesy Michael G. Bayerl, MD, Penn State Health.)

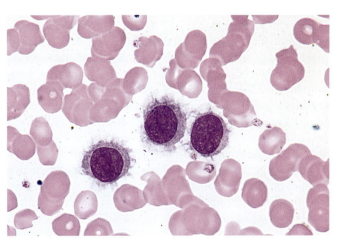

Figure 34.4 Hairy Cells. The leukemia cells are small to medium, with round-oval nuclear shape, moderately clumped chromatin, and pale blue cytoplasm with a "shaggy" cytoplasmic border. Hairy cells may also appear without cytoplasmic projections. (Peripheral blood, Wright-Giemsa stain, ×1000.)

nucleus. Bone marrow aspirate may be difficult to obtain in some cases because of marrow fibrosis, resulting in a "dry tap" (Chapter 15). In such instances, the bone marrow biopsy is of the utmost importance in establishing the diagnosis. Patterns of bone marrow involvement may be interstitial or patchy. Immunohistochemistry with an anti-CD20 antibody may help identify clusters of abnormal cells. Annexin A is specific to HCL and can be used to differentiate HCL from other B-cell neoplasms such as splenic marginal zone lymphoma (SMZL), which can have similar morphology.

Treatment

Historically, patients have been treated with splenectomy, which removes a large reservoir of disease. Splenectomy has largely been replaced by treatment with the purine analogues cladribine (2-CDA) and pentostatin, which induce durable remissions with successful restoration of blood counts.[39] However, it is not uncommon in these patients to find evidence of measurable residual disease using high-sensitivity flow cytometry or molecular testing. In 2011, genomic sequencing studies discovered the presence of the *BRAF* V600E mutation, the causal genetic event in HCL found in more than 97% of patients.[40] This led to development of the BRAF inhibitor vemurafenib, which has been found to be highly effective in treating patients refractory to the purine analogues.[41] Combination therapy with the BRAF inhibitor and rituximab result in longer remissions with less measurable residual diseases. The *Pseudomonas* exotoxin-linked recombinant anti-CD22 antibody, moxetumomab, also has been shown to be effective for relapsed refractory disease.[41]

Large Granular Lymphocytic (LGL) Leukemia
Laboratory Findings

Large granular lymphocytes (LGLs) have abundant pale blue cytoplasm with distinct medium to large azurophilic cytoplasmic granules. LGLs represent up to 15% of circulating lymphocytes or less than 0.6×10^9/L in healthy adults. LGLs should be counted with normal lymphocytes in the WBC differential, and a comment added when they are increased in number.[42] LGL leukemia is a rare disease characterized by an increase in circulating LGLs to more than 2×10^9/L.[2] LGL leukemia is a disease of older adults (median age at diagnosis is 60 years). Although many patients with LGL leukemia are asymptomatic and have LGLs noted on examination of the peripheral blood film, many present with cytopenias, usually in the form of neutropenia or anemia. The increase in circulating LGLs in these patients may trigger a morphology flag on the automated blood cell analyzer because of their size. An increase in peripheral blood LGLs also can be seen in autoimmune disease and after HSCT or chemotherapy. Therefore it is important to document the persistence of the LGL population for longer than 6 months and note the absence of any associated condition that could cause a similar blood picture.

Diagnosis

LGL leukemia is listed as two separate entities under the 2022 WHO classification system. T-large granular lymphocytic leukemia is a clonal expansion of cytotoxic T cells expressing CD3, CD8, and CD57. Clonality can be confirmed by detection of TCR gene rearrangements. The other form of LGL leukemia is of NK origin and categorized as NK-large granular lymphocytic leukemia. This disease is a clonal expansion of NK cells. These cells are typically negative for CD3 but express CD56. Restricted KIR expression may be used to demonstrate clonality of this population. Both disorders usually have an indolent course, although the NK form can be associated with transformation to a more aggressive form.

Treatment

Most therapy used to treat this disease is instituted in response to the severity of the cytopenias. Myeloid growth factors are often used to treat isolated neutropenia. Although there is no standard approach to therapy, immunosuppressive agents such as low doses of methotrexate, cyclophosphamide, or cyclosporin A have been used to suppress the clone and improve peripheral blood counts.

NON-HODGKIN LYMPHOMA

The primary sites of disease in lymphoma are extramedullary areas such as the lymph nodes and spleen. Some lymphomas have a characteristic morphology or immunophenotype, and most require biopsy of involved tissue with an assessment of the tissue architecture to establish the diagnosis.

Many types of lymphoma have a leukemic phase (Box 34.4), defined as the presence of lymphoma cells in the peripheral blood. The morphology of these lymphoid cells can vary widely depending on the type of lymphoma present. The International Counsel for Standardization in Haematology (ICSH) guidelines recommend using the term "abnormal lymphocyte" to identify and separately classify monoclonal lymphoid cells in the WBC differential.[42] Once a diagnosis has been established, "abnormal lymphocyte" can be replaced with a more specific term that identifies the neoplastic cell.

Adult T-Cell Leukemia/Lymphoma (ATLL)

ATLL is a postthymic neoplastic disorder of T cells that has the unique feature of being associated with retroviral infection by the human T-lymphotropic virus type I (HTLV-1). Although first described in Japan, the virus is endemic in the Caribbean islands, Africa, South America, the Middle East, and northern Oceania. The virus is acquired through transplacental

---

BOX 34.4   Leukemic Phase of Non-Hodgkin Lymphoma

Small lymphocytic lymphoma
Adult T-cell leukemia/lymphoma
Burkitt leukemia/lymphoma (sporadic/HIV related)
Follicular lymphoma
Mantle cell lymphoma
Marginal zone lymphoma
Lymphoplasmacytic lymphoma (Waldentröm macroglobulinemia)
Sézary syndrome/advanced mycosis fungoides
Diffuse large B-cell lymphoma (rare)
Peripheral T-cell lymphoma

transmission, breastfeeding, blood transfusion, or sex. Despite this, the estimated lifetime risk of developing ATLL among HTLV-1 carriers is approximately 5%.[43]

Clinical and Laboratory Findings

Patients typically present with widespread disease and peripheral blood involvement. Of the four clinical subtypes of ATLL, the acute form is the most well known. This disease typically has an aggressive clinical course marked by extensive extranodal involvement of the peripheral blood and skin. Complications of tumor involvement include osteolytic lesions, hypercalcemia, and profound immunosuppression resulting in infections. These complications represent the major source of morbidity and mortality in this disease.

There is often marked leukocytosis in the leukemic phase of ATLL in which the ATLL cells have a distinctive appearance. The prototypical ATLL cells are medium to large in size and have accentuated nuclei with irregular contours, coarsely clumped chromatin, and deeply basophilic cytoplasm (Figure 34.5). The term "flower cell" has been coined for this morphology. Not all ATLL cells have this distinctive appearance, and there can be a spectrum of morphologic variants. The ATLL cells can be smaller in size with a pleomorphic appearance reminiscent of other peripheral T-cell lymphomas such as Sézary syndrome. The ATLL immunophenotype is generally consistent with the T helper cell; CD3 and CD4 are expressed while CD7 and CD8 are absent. CD25 and CCR4 are also highly expressed, causing some to postulate whether this disease represents a neoplastic transformation of T helper 2 (T_H2)/T regulatory (T_{reg}) cells. An increase in the soluble form of IL-2 has prognostic significance and can be used as a tumor marker for assessing disease status.

Treatment

Despite extensive clinical trial experience, therapy of ATLL remains suboptimal; therefore participation in clinical trials is encouraged. Aggressive antilymphoma regimens have been used to treat the acute subtype, with dismal response rates. The median survival is 8 months, with only 11% of patients alive at 4 years.[44] Patients with indolent forms of ATLL tend to have a better prognosis. A combination of interferon-α and azidothymidine (AZT) has shown some efficacy against the HTLV-1 virus. The best outcomes were again noted in the chronic, more indolent subtypes. Studies with other experimental agents such as the anti-CCR4 monoclonal antibody mogamulizumab have shown some efficacy, and combination therapy with multidrug lymphoma regimens has improved outcomes. These results, however, may come at the cost of toxicity, which can limit downstream therapeutic options. HSCT has been investigated in this disease, and some long-term survivors have been reported. Some studies have used mogamulizumab before HSCT and reported inferior outcomes when these two modalities are combined because toxicity was found to increase with combination therapy.

Burkitt Lymphoma (BL)

BL is an aggressive malignancy of mature B cells characterized by a rapid tumor growth with an often-fulminant clinical presentation. BL has three subtypes: endemic, sporadic, and immunodeficiency-associated. The endemic form is found primarily in children in equatorial Africa along a geographic distribution similar to malaria. Extranodal involvement is common with the orbits and mandible as typical sites of disease. Also, in nearly all cases of endemic BL, the Epstein-Barr virus (EBV) genome is present in the neoplastic cells.

In contrast, sporadic BL is seen in the United States and Western Europe and manifests mostly as abdominal disease. Extranodal involvement is a common finding, however, and various tissues can be involved. Lymphoma cells infiltrate the bone marrow in up to 70% of cases, and evidence of CNS disease can be found in about one-third of patients. Immunodeficiency-associated BL is associated with HIV, post-transplantation, and congenital immunodeficiency. Unlike in the other subtypes, the blood and bone marrow are the primary sites of disease in immunodeficiency-associated BL.

Clinical and Laboratory Findings

A leukemic phase may develop in a subset of patients with BL in whom circulating tumor cells have a characteristic morphology. BL cells are intermediate sized, have finely clumped chromatin, and have deeply basophilic cytoplasm with distinct vacuoles. The bone marrow biopsy may show sheets of infiltrating medium-sized cells with scant cytoplasm (Figure 34.6). Both bone marrow and lymph node biopsies may have a classic "starry sky" appearance that results from the interspersed tingible body macrophages suspended in a "sea" of malignant cells.

The immunophenotypic profile is that of a mature B cell in which both surface immunoglobulin and light chain restriction are present along with the expression of CD10, but immature markers such as CD34 and TdT are absent. Specimens sent for flow cytometric analysis need to be processed quickly because the high cell turnover that characterizes BL may result in poor viability, which reduces the quality of the results. The characteristic cytogenetic and molecular findings are presented in Table 34.1.

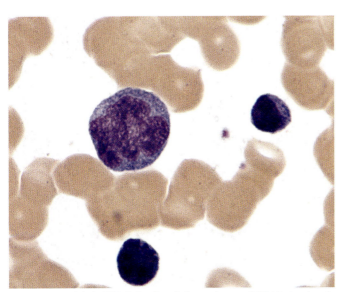

Figure 34.5 Adult T-Cell Leukemia/Lymphoma (ATLL). Leukemia cells can range in size. Some have distinctive nuclear lobulation and have been termed "flower cells." (Peripheral blood, Wright-Giemsa stain, ×1000.)

Treatment

Despite its relatively fulminant manifestation, BL is highly responsive to chemotherapy and is curable in more than 90% of patients with early stage disease and 60% to 80% of patients with more advanced stages. Intensive supportive care is key to success as the chemotherapy regimens used are of high intensity and cycled over relatively short periods of time. Given the high tumor cell turnover that occurs with BL treatment, tumor lysis syndrome should be anticipated, and supportive efforts with aggressive intravenous hydration and antihyperuricemia medications are indicated before the start of cytotoxic chemotherapy.[45]

Follicular Lymphoma (FL)

FL represents a neoplastic disorder of germinal B cells and is the second most common form of NHL. FL is generally a disease of middle-aged to older adults. Although it typically has an indolent course, FL generally tends to be incurable with current therapies. The clinical pattern is one of serial responses to treatment followed by recurring relapse until death.

Clinical and Laboratory Findings

Most patients with FL present with painless lymphadenopathy but are otherwise asymptomatic. Peripheral blood involvement with FL cells is seen in about 10% of cases. Circulating lymphoma cells are small to medium in size, with scant cytoplasm and heavily condensed chromatin, and often show distinct deep nuclear clefts at sharp angles (Figure 34.7). A few large cells with immature features also may be noted. Bone marrow biopsy reveals characteristic localization of tumor cells in a paratrabecular distribution. There also may be a variable degree of interstitial infiltration. The characteristic effacement of normal architecture seen in the lymph node is typically absent in the marrow. In tissue section, the lymphoma cells appear small and irregular, with an angular appearance (centrocytes), or larger, with round to ovoid nuclei containing 1 to 3 nucleoli located on the border within the nucleus (centroblasts). Histologically, FL is graded according to the number of larger cells. This grading is correlated with clinical outcome of the patients, with grade 3 disease having the poorest outcomes.

Treatment

As most FL patients are asymptomatic, a "watch and wait" strategy is appropriate.[44] A separate scoring system (FLIPI1/FLIPI2) has been developed to aid in making clinical decisions. For patients who require treatment, a standard treatment regimen has not been established, although therapy with an anti-CD20 monoclonal antibody either alone or in combination with multidrug chemotherapy (e.g., bendamustine + rituximab [BR]/rituximab, cyclophosphamide, doxorubicin hydrochloride, vincristine sulfate, and prednisone [R-CHOP]) is often the first regimen employed. More recently specific agents targeted to unique biological features such as surface antigen expression (CD20, CD22, or CD37), B-cell receptor signaling pathway, genes implicated in lymphomagenesis (*BCL2, p53*), or epigenetic modifications have been piloted and found to be of benefit. For relapsed disease, both autologous and allogeneic HSCT have produced long-term remission in patients responding to salvage chemotherapy. More recently, anti-CD19-directed chimeric antigen receptor (CAR)-T cell therapy (Chapter 27) has been found to be highly effective in patients who historically have been difficult to treat.[46]

Mantle Cell Lymphoma (MCL)

MCL constitutes approximately 6% of NHL cases.[47] The median age at diagnosis is 68 years and males are affected more often than females.

Clinical and Laboratory Findings

MCL is generally a clinically aggressive disorder, although an indolent type has been described. Most patients present with extensive lymphadenopathy. Extranodal disease is not uncommon, with the GI tract acting as a primary area of involvement. Patients with the indolent form of MCL tend to have the disease restricted to the blood, bone marrow, and spleen.

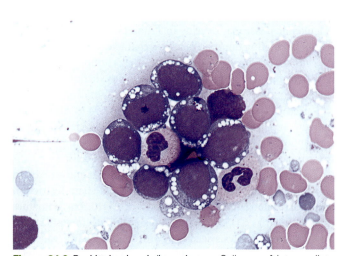

Figure 34.6 Burkitt Leukemia/Lymphoma. Cells are of intermediate size with deeply basophilic cytoplasm and distinct cytoplasmic vacuoles. (Bone marrow aspirate, tetrachrome stain, ×400.)

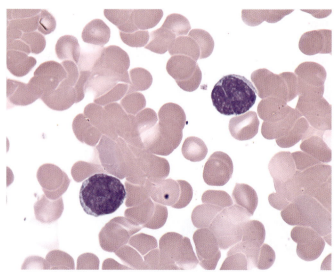

Figure 34.7 Follicular Lymphoma. Follicular lymphoma cells circulating in the peripheral blood can appear as small, cleaved lymphoid cells. (Peripheral blood, Wright-Giemsa stain, ×400.)

Bone marrow and peripheral blood involvement is common in MCL. At diagnosis, 75% of patients show lymphoma cells on the peripheral blood film and more than 50% have an absolute lymphocytosis. MCL cells in peripheral blood are cytologically similar cells to those found in tissue specimens. A spectrum of morphologic variants has been recognized, and arriving at correct diagnosis may be somewhat problematic. The different presentations of mantle cells in the peripheral blood include:

- Small to medium cells with notched, clefted, or otherwise irregularly shaped nuclei, with condensed chromatin and scant cytoplasm that may not be visible in some cells (most common presentation)
- Small, mature-appearing lymphocytes that can easily be mistaken for CLL/SLL (Figure 34.8). Similar cells with frayed cytoplasmic projections can resemble HCL or splenic MZL
- Large, immature blastlike cells that are often confused with acute leukemia or large cell lymphoma
- Large, pleomorphic atypical cells with ovoid or irregularly shaped nuclei exhibiting clefts, immature chromatin, small but distinct nucleoli, and variable amounts of cytoplasm. These cells may resemble large cell lymphoma in some patients. In other cases, the cells have large, prominent single nucleoli that mimic prolymphocytes.

Accurate diagnosis of MCL requires demonstration of either t(11,14) by FISH or overexpression of cyclin D1 by immunohistochemistry. Expression of SOX11, a transcription factor, may be useful in the 5% of cases that are cyclin D1 negative.

Treatment

In the indolent form of the MCL, a "watch and wait" strategy is appropriate. A separate prognostic index (MIPI) has been developed and may be useful in determining clinical management. Patients who develop bulky disease or B symptoms often require therapy. Age is a major discriminator for determining the therapeutic approach. Patients typically are treated with chemoimmunotherapy regimens (BR/R-CHOP), followed by consolidation with autologous HSCT and maintenance with rituximab. Those patients who are unable to undergo HSCT may receive rituximab alone as maintenance. Younger, more "fit" patients have been treated with more intensive multidrug regimens used in high-grade lymphoma, such as R-Hyper CVAD (rituximab, cyclophosphamide, vincristine, doxorubicin, and dexamethasone). The B-cell receptor signaling inhibitors, ibrutinib, acalabrutinib, and zanubrutinib, have been found to be effective agents in treated patients who have relapsed. The proteosome inhibitor bortezomib has been shown to be active in treating MCL, and this is increased when combined with other antilymphoma chemotherapy regimens. Anti-CD19-directed CAR-T cell therapy (brexucabtagene autoleucel) has been shown to have high overall response rates in patients with MCL and resulted in lasting remission in a subgroup of patients.[48]

Diffuse Large B-Cell Lymphoma (DLBCL)

DLBCL is the most common form of NHL, representing about 30% of all cases. It is generally a disease of the elderly but can occur in younger patients. DLBCL can arise de novo or as a transformation from a more indolent form of lymphoma such as SLL, FL, or MZL. Although it has an aggressive clinical course, DLBCL is curable in approximately two-thirds of patients when treated with combination chemoimmunotherapy. However, the disease is somewhat heterogeneous because various subgroups are recognized based on morphologic or genetic criteria.

Clinical and Laboratory Findings

The most common clinical manifestation is rapidly expanding painless lymphadenopathy in one or more sites. Extranodal involvement is typically found in the GI tract, testis, or bone. Clinical symptoms depend on the areas of involvement. The bone marrow is infiltrated with lymphoma cells in approximately 30% of patients. Bone marrow involvement may be diagnostically concordant to the node/extranodal site and show DLBCL; however, in some cases bone marrow involvement is morphologically discordant, with nodal disease showing DLBCL and bone marrow showing a low-grade lymphoma. Approximately one-third of patients with bone marrow involvement have lymphoma cells in the peripheral blood that appear highly pleomorphic with large, round, or irregularly shaped nuclei; prominent nucleoli; variably clumped chromatin; and variable amounts of basophilic cytoplasm (Figure 34.9). The DLBCL cells can be confused with leukemic blasts.

On microscopic examination of an affected lymph node, DLBCL cells appear large and typically efface tissue architecture with a diffuse pattern. Morphologic variants of DLBCL cells have been described. In addition, several disorders (e.g., plasma cell [multiple] myeloma and anaplastic large cell lymphoma) may include highly pleomorphic forms that can be confused with one of the DLBCL subtypes. Such cases require immunohistochemistry and molecular/genetic testing to rule out the other entities to confirm the diagnosis.

Genetic testing reveals translocations involving the *BCL6* gene in about 30% of DLBCL cases. Interestingly, translocation of the *BCL2* gene, a marker associated with t(14;18) and FL is

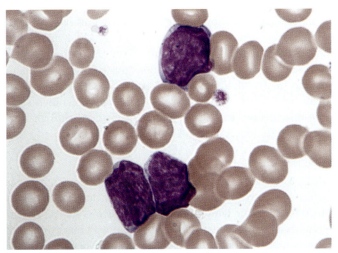

Figure 34.8 Mantle Cell Lymphoma. Mantle cells can have a variable appearance. Some cases can be confused with chronic lymphocytic leukemia/small lymphocytic lymphoma (CLL/SLL), and immunophenotyping/cytogenetic analysis is needed to differentiate between the disorders. In this case, the chromatin in the lymphoma cells has a more open chromatin pattern than is typically seen in CLL lymphocytes. (Peripheral blood, Wright-Giemsa stain, ×1000.)

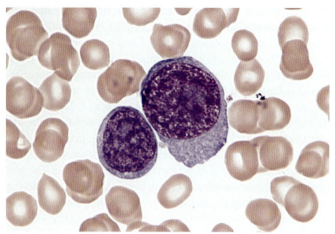

Figure 34.9 Diffuse Large B-Cell Lymphoma. Peripheral blood involvement is generally rare. The lymphoma cells may be large, with moderate amounts of cytoplasm and several nucleoli. Cells may also resemble blasts in acute leukemia. (Peripheral blood, Wright-Giemsa stain, ×1000.)

present in 20% to 30% of DLBCL cases and may complicate diagnosis. *MYC*, a gene typically associated with BL, is rearranged in about 10% of DLBCL patients. These findings demonstrate that isolated genetic differences do not define the lymphoma subtype but instead need to be considered in the context of clinical and morphologic criteria. Up to 70% of patients with *MYC* abnormalities also have concurrent *BCL2* and/or *BCL6* abnormalities. These cases have been labeled "double- (or triple-) hit" lymphoma and have an exceptionally poor prognosis.[49,50] The WHO classifies this type of DLBCL "diffuse large B-cell lymphoma/high-grade B-cell lymphoma with *MYC* and *BCL2* rearrangements."[2]

DLBCL is an example of a disease in which advances in molecular technology have had a fundamental effect on the approach to treatment. Gene expression profiling has been used to define two primary subtypes, based largely on corresponding normal stages of B-cell development: germinal center (GC) and activated B cell (ABC or nongerminal center).[51] These subtypes have prognostic implications, with the GC variety having a more favorable outcome. Gene expression profiling is not readily available in many clinical laboratories; therefore surrogate scoring systems based on immunohistochemical algorithms have been developed to identify subtypes. It is important to note, however, these algorithms do not have 100% correlation with the molecular profile, and assigning therapy based on surrogate scoring systems does not represent the current standard of care. New molecular testing may be introduced in the future that will provide similar information with better correlation and reproducibility, replacing the current immunohistochemical analyses.[15]

Treatment

Although DLBCL typically has an aggressive course, it is curable in many patients. As previously discussed, the IPI was initially developed from a cohort of patients with DLBCL and remains a useful tool for the provider. The incorporation of rituximab to standard combination chemotherapy (R-CHOP) greatly improved patient outcomes and currently represents the

standard of care for most patients. Patients with unfavorable subtypes ("double hit" or "double expressor") remain a challenge, and some of the newer targeted agents are currently being tested in ongoing clinical trials.

In the relapsed setting, CD19-directed CAR-T cell therapy (axicabtagene ciloleucel, tisagenlecleucel) has demonstrated significant activity, with high response rates and sustained remissions after 1 to 2 years of followup. Toxicities associated with CAR-T cell therapy can be severe, and specialized training and experience is required for administration.[46]

Marginal Zone Lymphoma (MZL)

MZL is an indolent B-cell lymphoma typically associated with chronic antigen stimulation in the setting of either infection or autoimmunity. Three main subtypes of MZL are extranodal marginal zone lymphoma of mucosa associated lymphoid tissue (MALT), splenic marginal zone lymphoma (SMZL), and nodal marginal zone lymphoma (NMZL).[52]

MALT Lymphoma

MALT lymphoma is the most common subtype of MZL, representing 7% to 8% of B-cell lymphomas. The median age at diagnosis is 61 years. It is typically associated with organs that seemingly lack obvious lymphoid tissue. These organs have been subjected to chronic inflammation; this in turn increases B cell proliferation, in which errors during class switching and hypermutation lead to uncontrolled growth and malignant transformation. The stomach is most often involved and is also the site most closely associated with *Helicobacter pylori* infection. The salivary gland, ocular adnexa, thyroid, skin, and small intestine also can be affected but are associated with different infectious stimuli. A distinct variant of MALT lymphoma, immunoproliferative small intestine disease, is seen in the Middle East, Africa, and the Mediterranean and is associated with severe malabsorption. As in the gastric-centered MALT, disease spread beyond the small intestine region (including peripheral blood) is uncommon, although transformation to a more aggressive histologic subtype has been described. Treatment of MALT lymphoma is centered upon relief of symptoms. With *H. pylori*-associated disease, treating the underlying infection with triple antibiotic therapy may result in remission. A similar observation has been made with antibiotic therapy for immunoproliferative small intestine disease. Radiation therapy of involved sites also has been used for local control of the disease.

Splenic Marginal Zone Lymphoma (SMZL)

SMZL accounts for less than 1% of NHL and is most common in adults over 50 years. Areas of involvement include white pulp of the spleen, splenic lymph nodes, bone marrow, and very often, peripheral blood. Patients typically present with massive splenomegaly and an absolute lymphocytosis in the peripheral blood characterized by the presence of villous lymphocytes or cells like those seen in CLL (Figure 34.10).[53] These villous lymphocytes may easily be confused with hairy cells. However, the cytoplasmic projections in the villous lymphocytes tend to have a polar distribution as opposed to the circumferential pattern seen in hairy cells. In SMZL, CD103 is negative and annexin A staining

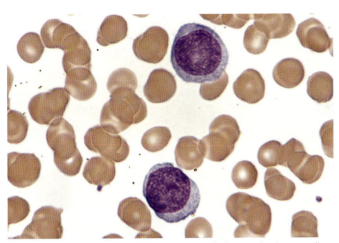

Figure 34.10 Marginal Zone Lymphoma. Cells may be intermediate in size, with round nuclei. They tend to have a more open chromatin pattern compared with normal lymphocytes. (Peripheral blood, Wright-Giemsa stain, ×1000.)

is absent with immunohistochemical staining of the biopsy. That is used to differentiate SMZL from HCL because the morphology of cells can appear similar. Extranodal sites of disease other than blood and bone marrow are rare. Approximately one-third of patients, especially those with advanced disease, have a low level of monoclonal protein. Patients may develop severe anemia and thrombocytopenia secondary to splenic sequestration.

Patients with asymptomatic SMZL are generally followed with a "watch and wait" strategy. Rituximab monotherapy is the treatment of choice for most patients when therapy is indicated. Recent experience has demonstrated efficacy with a combination of rituximab and chemotherapy.[53]

Nodal Marginal Zone Lymphoma (NMZL)

NMZL accounts for 1% of NHL and is most common in adults over 50 years of age. NMZL is primarily localized to the lymph nodes, although the bone marrow also can be involved. Within the lymph node, NMZL cells extend from the mantle-marginal zone interface, disrupting the interfollicular region. In some sense, the NMZL diagnosis represents a generic term for disorders that morphologically appear like other low-grade B-cell malignancies but lack distinguishing characteristics (i.e., cyclin D1 expression, *BCL2* abnormalities) that would identify it as one of the other well-defined disorders. An association with hepatitis C virus has been noted and NMZL patients with hepatitis C infection will often have cryoglobulinemia as well. There is no standard recommended therapy for NMZL. The current generation of targeted agents used to treat other NHL may represent a new approach as data from ongoing clinical trials becomes available.[54]

Mycosis Fungoides/Sézary Syndrome (MF/SS)

Mycosis fungoides (MF)/Sézary syndrome (SS) is the most familiar form of cutaneous T-cell lymphoma. SS and MF are closely related diseases but differ in cell of origin and clinical characteristics and are therefore considered to be separate entities. Both MF and SS are diseases of the elderly, with a slight male preponderance. MF is the more common disorder, making

up approximately 60% to 70% of cutaneous T-cell lymphoma cases. MF remains largely confined to the skin, although in the later stages of the disease, dissemination to lymph nodes, organs, and peripheral blood can be seen. MF is generally an indolent disease with a slow, progressive course. SS is an aggressive systemic disorder with peripheral blood involvement and a worse prognosis than MF.

Clinical and Laboratory Findings

Both SS and MF are generally disorders of CD4+ T cells. More recently, some have argued that they are distinct diseases arising from totally separate precursors. The malignant clone in MF has been shown to have an effector memory phenotype, whereas Sézary cells are associated with central memory T cells. The malignant T cells in MF and SS have an abnormal appearance, with scant cytoplasm, a cerebriform, folded nucleus, variably condensed chromatin, and inconspicuous nucleoli. The Sézary cells in SS can be both large (most common) and small (Figure 34.11). A single case of SS can manifest with small cells, large cells, or both types. Patients also can undergo a transformation from the small to the large cell variety.

Diagnosis of MF in the early stages can be problematic. Patients may present with psoriatic-like skin lesions requiring repeated biopsy before a definitive diagnosis can be made. Longitudinal followup of initially nondiagnostic lesions may be required before morphologic confirmation of disease. Skin biopsy specimens can have characteristic localization of atypical cells in Pautrier microabscesses in the epidermis, but this occurs in only a minority of cases.

Clinically, SS is characterized by erythroderma, generalized lymphadenopathy, and the presence of clonal T cells (Sézary cells) in skin, lymph nodes, and peripheral blood. The diagnosis is based on the presence of all three characteristics, plus at least one of the following: an increased number CD4+ T cells resulting in a CD4/CD8 ratio of 10 or greater, a loss of at least one T-cell antigen, or an absolute Sézary cell count greater than 1000 cells/μL in the peripheral blood.[2] Flow cytometry is often used to enumerate Sézary cells; alternatively, the cells may be counted microscopically using a Wright-stained peripheral blood film.[1,2] Pruritus can be severe for patients with SS and difficult to control with symptomatic therapy alone. In addition, patients have profound immunosuppression and infection remains a major source of morbidity and mortality.

Treatment

The prognosis of patients with MF and SS are different. Only 10% to 20% of SS patients are alive at 5 years compared with 68% of patients with MF. Therapy for early stage MF consists largely of agents used to treat the symptoms of the disease, including localized therapy with topical steroids, nitrogen mustard, or phototherapy. More advanced disease is mostly incurable, and patients are generally urged to participate in clinical trials or pursue allogenic HSCT, the only treatment with the potential for cure. Given the aggressive nature of advanced MF and SS, a wide variety of agents have been tested in clinical trials. Therapeutic approaches have included single-agent chemotherapy, biological response modifiers (interferons), monoclonal antibodies directed to CD52

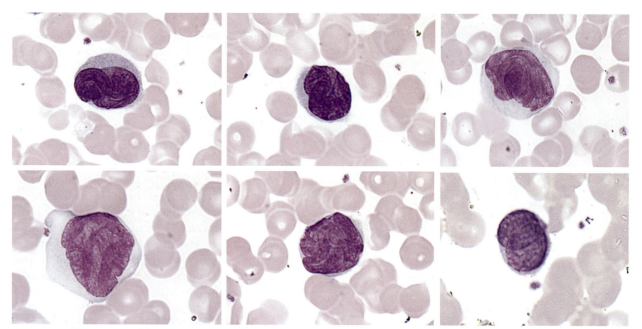

Figure 34.11 **Sézary Syndrome.** Sézary lymphoma cells can vary in appearance. Most commonly, the cells are large with cerebriform or folded nuclei. However, in some cases, the cells are smaller with nuclear irregularities/atypia. (Peripheral blood, Wright-Giemsa stain, ×1000.)

(alemtuzumab), CD4 (zanolimumab), or CCR4 (mogamulizumab), as well as histone deacetylases and retinoids. More recently, CRISPR-CAS 9—engineered allogeneic CAR-T cell therapy has entered clinical trials for relapsed refractory mature T-cell disorders such as SS/MF, and such an approach could represent a new paradigm of therapy for these diseases. Despite the wide range of investigative activity, improving outcomes of SS and advanced MF remains challenging.[55]

Anaplastic Large Cell Lymphoma (ALCL)

ALCL is a T-cell disorder that is associated with large pleomorphic cells. There is, however, heterogeneity in morphologic appearance, and some of the cells are small to medium in size. Invariably, the tumor cells express CD30. The disease can be divided into two subtypes, depending on the expression of the anaplastic lymphoma kinase (ALK) protein. ALK+ tumors generally tend to occur in a younger cohort and have a better prognosis than most other peripheral T-cell lymphomas. ALK+ ALCL constitutes approximately 10% to 30% of childhood lymphomas. The ALK– form is more common in older patients, with a median age at diagnosis of about 57 years. A subtype of ALK– ALCL has been associated with breast implants.[56,57]

Clinical and Laboratory Findings

The clinical presentation of ALK+ and ALK– ALCL are similar. Most patients present with advanced-stage disease (stages III and IV) and B symptoms. ALCL involves the lymph nodes and extranodal sites such as skin, bones, and soft tissue such as liver and lung. There is a cutaneous variant in which the disease is localized only to the skin. Bone marrow is involved in 10% to 30% of cases. Bone marrow involvement in ALCL may be subtle, and immunohistochemical stains may be required to detect disease. Rare cases of ALCL with a leukemic phase have been reported (Figure 34.12).

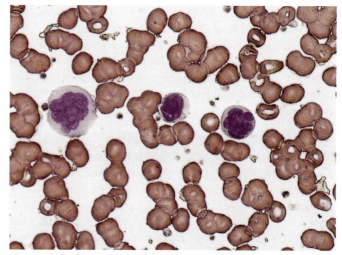

Figure 34.12 **Anaplastic Large Cell Lymphoma.** Lymphoma cells range in size and have irregular, lobulated nuclei. In some cases, the lymphoma cells resemble blasts. (Peripheral blood, Wright-Giemsa stain, ×400.)

Treatment

The primary approach to treatment of ALCL is combination chemotherapy with relatively standard regimens containing an anthracycline such as CHOP. The ALK+ variety has been reported to have a 5-year survival of approximately 70% to 90% using this approach. Given several distinct disease-related features in ALCL, several targeted therapies have been explored. These include the anti-CD30 immunoconjugate brentuximab vedotin (BV), which has been approved by the US Food and Drug Administration (FDA) for use in relapsed disease. Patients responding to treatment often proceed to either autologous or allogeneic HSCT to achieve long term survival.

Peripheral T-Cell Lymphoma, Not Otherwise Specified (PTCL-NOS)

PTCL-NOS is a heterogeneous group of disorders. Diseases classified in this WHO category lack defining features that would place them in another category.[57] They are disorders of postthymic T cells with rearrangement of the TCR.

Clinical and Laboratory Findings

Immunophenotypically, the abnormal cells are characterized by T-cell antigen mismatch, with the absence of CD7 or CD5 expression as the most common finding. More recently, gene expression profiling has underscored this heterogeneity, although deregulation of genes associated with proliferation, apoptosis, and cell adhesion (consistent with an activated T-cell state) have been noted.

The clinical course of PTCL-NOS can be variable, reflecting tumor heterogeneity. Most patients present with disseminated disease and poor performance status. An intermediate to high risk IPI score is found in 50% to 70% of PTCL-NOS patients. There is often diffuse lymph node involvement, with extranodal spread to sites such as the skin and GI tract. Bone marrow is invaded with lymphoma in 20% to 30% of patients. Eosinophilia, as well as anemia and thrombocytopenia, can be seen in a subset of patients (Figure 34.13).

Treatment

Given the fulminant nature of the PTCL-NOS, standard therapy consists of combination chemotherapy. However, approximately 30% of patients are refractory to standard regimens. For patients with CD30-positive disease, brentuximab vedotin (BV)-based chemotherapy regimens have improved outcomes. Patients who do respond tend to relapse within a relatively short period of time. HSCT has been investigated to prolong remissions in patients who respond to treatment. However, given the relatively rare nature of this disease, there is no large clinical data set to confirm the efficacy of HSCT. For relapsed disease, targeted agents that are used in ALCL are currently under investigation.

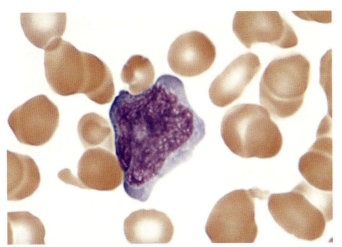

Figure 34.13 Peripheral T-Cell Lymphoma. Peripheral blood involvement is uncommon. Lymphoma cells are larger, basophilic, and have a pleomorphic appearance. (Peripheral blood, Wright-Giemsa stain, ×1000.)

HODGKIN LYMPHOMA

HL is primarily a nodal-based disease that is distinct from nodal NHL. It can also involve extranodal sites. HL is a relatively rare cancer, with an estimated US incidence of 2.6 cases per 100,000 persons per year. Historically, HL is associated with unique biological and clinical features. It was one of the first tumor types that could be cured with combination chemotherapy and therefore serves as a model for the evolution of therapeutics in modern oncology. HL patients who relapse can still be cured with current available therapies.[58] This is an uncommon outcome in oncology. Approximately 86% of HL patients are alive 5 years after diagnosis. Because this is a disease of a younger patient cohort, effective chemotherapy survival data provides useful information regarding toxicity and the long-term effects of cancer therapy.

Clinical and Laboratory Findings

There are two distinct forms of HL that differ pathologically and clinically: classic HL (CHL) and nodular lymphocyte predominant HL (NLPHL) (also known as nodular lymphocyte predominant B-cell lymphoma). The diagnosis of each type is established with lymph node biopsy.

CHL accounts for about 95% of cases and has a bimodal age distribution with peaks in the 30s and again after age 50 years. CHL is characterized by the presence of Reed-Sternberg (RS) cells, which are large binucleated/multinucleated cells with abundant cytoplasm and distinct nuclei. Morphologic variants exist among the various subtypes of HL. RS cells are of B cell origin, although they lack expression of most B cell markers. Immunophenotyping shows that RS/RS variants primarily express CD30 and often coexpress CD15 (Figure 34.14). RS/RS-like cells reside in lymph nodes (not peripheral blood) in a "sea" of reactive cells that includes lymphocytes, histiocytes, granulocytes, eosinophils, and plasma cells. There are four recognized histologic subtypes of CHL: nodular sclerosis, mixed cellularity, lymphocyte rich, and lymphocyte depleted. The histologic subtype is primarily a result of the background in which the RS or RS-like cells are found. Previously, the histologic subtype was thought to be of prognostic significance, but this more likely was a function of stage and all subtypes of CHL are treated similarly. Although RS cells are recognized to be of B cell lineage, the lineage of the tumor cells in HL long remained problematic because they are relatively scarce compared to the reactive component of the lymph node. The large number of other cell types skewed attempts at identifying the origin of these cells until more advanced diagnostic techniques became available.

NLPHL is a distinct yet uncommon form of HL, diagnosed most often in young adults. Instead of the RS cell found in CHL, the malignant cell is a lymphocytic histiocytic (L&H) variant. The L&H tumor cells are large, with scant cytoplasm and a folded single nucleus, and are labeled "popcorn" cells because of this distinct morphology. The H&L cells are negative for CD15 and CD30 expression, and about 50% of them express epithelial membrane antigen (EMA). These cells exist in a nodular background composed primarily of small lymphocytes. This disorder is also of B cell origin, although the level of transformation is different from that in CHL.

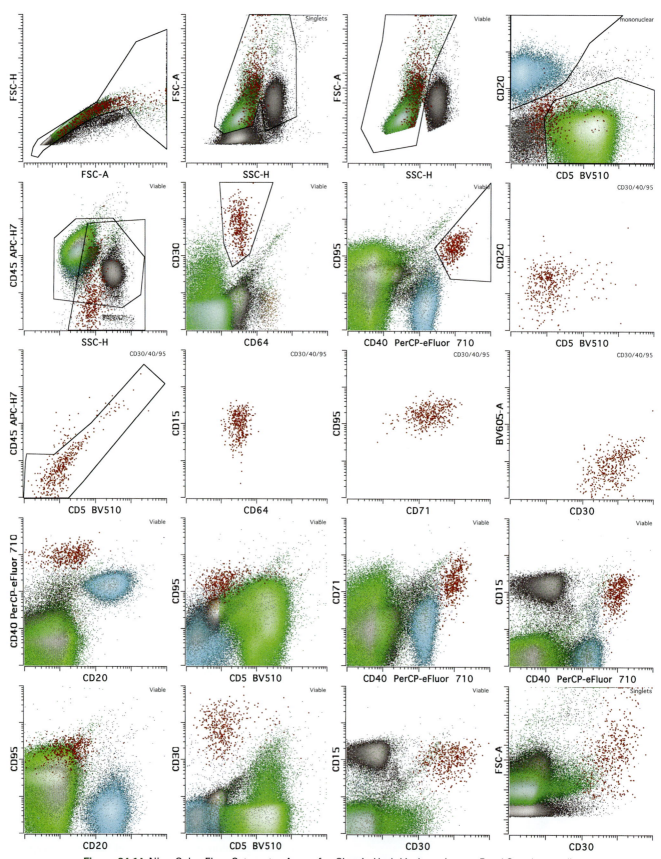

Figure 34.14 Nine-Color Flow Cytometry Assay for Classic Hodgkin Lymphoma. Reed-Sternberg cells *(red)* are large and typically have high forward and side scatter. The cells express CD30, CD40, CD95, and CD15 but lack CD64. T cells express CD5 *(green)*, whereas B cells express CD20 *(light blue)*. Flow cytometry is largely used as a confirmatory test in cases with problematic morphology. (Courtesy Qi Gao, Memorial Sloan Kettering Cancer Center, NY.)

The clinical manifestation of CHL and NLPHL can differ. Patients with CHL may present with cervical/supraclavicular and mediastinal adenopathy that spreads in a contiguous manner. Patients with NLPHL have peripheral lymphadenopathy and mediastinal adenopathy is uncommon. In addition, nodal involvement is not contiguous and extranodal involvement is rare. B symptoms occur more frequently in CHL than in NLPHL. Treatment decisions are based on the Ann Arbor stage.

Treatment

HL is one of the initial successes associated with combination chemotherapy. The original regimen, MOPP (mechlorethamine, vincristine, procarbazine, and prednisone), was found to be effective even in advanced disease. Radiotherapy was used for patients found to have localized disease and to supplement therapy in cases in which there was bulky lymphadenopathy. Although highly effective, treatment-related toxicity issues began to emerge as more patients survived for longer periods. These complications included cardiac toxicity (for those who received radiation as part of therapy to the mediastinum) and secondary malignancies. Secondary malignancies became a major concern as patients developed solid tumors in the radiation field more than 10 years after the completion of this therapy. Patients who received high cumulative doses of alkylating agents were found to be at risk for developing myelodysplastic neoplasms (MDS) or acute myeloid leukemia (AML) within a shorter time frame. Eventually, newer regimens such as ABVD (doxorubicin, bleomycin, vinblastine, dacarbazine) were introduced and found to be superior and less toxic than MOPP. These regimens have largely replaced MOPP as the standard of care. The addition of BV to ABV has increased disease-free survival for patients with advanced disease when given as initial therapy. As chemotherapy-based regimens combined with radiation to the involved areas began to be used more frequently in limited-stage disease, attempts to attenuate the total dose of chemotherapy administered and hence minimize any associated toxicity have been adopted into clinical practice.[59–62]

HL is a tumor that is highly sensitive to chemotherapy and radiotherapy. For some patients, dose attenuation designed to minimize toxicity may result in less effective disease control and result in tumor recurrence. Such patients, however, can still be cured. For chemotherapy relapses, high-dose therapy followed by rescue autologous HSCT is an effective salvage therapy, resulting in approximately 55% of patients free from relapse at 3-year followup.[63] Patients with CHL who relapse after autologous HSCT may still achieve disease control following treatment with BV.[64] Immune checkpoint blockade inhibitors targeting PD-1 (nivolumab/pembroluzumab) have demonstrated significant clinical activity given the biology of the RS cell, and have been incorporated into the treatment strategy for disease relapse following BV/autologous HSCT.[58]

PLASMA CELL NEOPLASMS

PCNs are malignant disorders of terminally differentiated B cells. Although PCNs constitute only about 1% to 2% of cancers, they are the second most common hematologic malignancy after CLL. The prototypical PCN, plasma cell (multiple) myeloma (MM), is generally a disease of the elderly, with a median age at diagnosis of 69 years. Less than 2% of MM patients are below the age of 40. PCNs are slightly more common in males than females.

The ability of the clonal plasma cells to secrete monoclonal protein (either whole or some part thereof) is the sine qua non of the PCNs, with the exception of a nonsecretory form of MM that comprises less than 1% of cases. The monoclonal protein (monoclonal immunoglobulin, paraprotein, M-protein) often has detrimental effects across multiple organ systems and is responsible for a significant amount of the morbidity seen with the more advanced forms of MM. In all cases, the monoclonal protein (M spike observed with protein electrophoresis) can serve as a surrogate marker for disease burden.

The PCNs encompass a spectrum of disease states that range from the relatively benign monoclonal gammopathy of undetermined significance (MGUS), marked only by the presence of a monoclonal protein in an asymptomatic individual, to clinically aggressive MM and plasma cell leukemia, in which tumor infiltration and monoclonal protein excess produce systemic complications resulting in significant morbidity and death.

Monoclonal Gammopathy of Undetermined Significance (MGUS)

MGUS is a benign monoclonal proliferation of plasma cells in the bone marrow that is often considered with PCNs because MGUS represents a precursor state for MM.[65] MGUS is usually detected when an elevated serum protein is found during routine laboratory testing. The diagnostic criteria for MGUS are listed in Box 34.5. Although the conversion of MGUS to overt MM is about 1% per year, a subset of patients with adverse risk factors has over a 60% chance of progression over a 20-year period. The serum M protein concentration, serum free light-chain ratio, and other markers can help assess the risk of conversion to MM or other PCN.

Plasma Cell (Multiple) Myeloma (MM)

Myeloma is a bone marrow-based disease with extramedullary extension to areas such as the bone or soft tissue. Strict criteria are used to establish the diagnosis of myeloma and smoldering myeloma based on the overall tumor burden (% plasma cells in the bone marrow), quantity of monoclonal protein in serum or urine, as well as the extent of systemic manifestations of disease such as such as hyper**c**alcemia, **r**enal failure, **a**nemia, or osteolytic **b**one lesions (CRAB criteria) (Box 34.5).[66] Extramedullary spread to bone, osteolytic lesions, and pathologic fractures are not uncommon in MM. Therefore imaging studies such as a skeletal survey or MRI of the pelvis and spine are a standard part of the diagnostic workup to establish the extent of disease and anticipate any potential serious complications (e.g., cord compression, fracture) that might need to be treated prophylactically.

Laboratory Findings

Overt involvement of the peripheral blood by circulating plasma cells is relatively rare until advanced or end-stage disease develops. Primary plasma cell leukemia and progression to secondary plasma cell leukemia are marked by the presence of 5% or more plasma cells on the peripheral blood film.[67] Primary plasma cell leukemia arises de novo and is a separate entity. Both forms of plasma cell leukemia are associated with a poor response to treatment and dismal prognosis.

BOX 34.5   Diagnostic Criteria for Plasma Cell Neoplasms

Monoclonal Gammopathy of Undetermined Significance (MGUS-Non IgM)

Both criteria must be met:
1. Serum monoclonal protein (non-IgM) <3 g/dL
2. Absence of end-organ damage (defined below)

Smoldering (Asymptomatic) Myeloma

Both criteria must be met:
1. Serum monoclonal protein (IgG or IgA) ≥3 g/dL or urine monoclonal protein ≥500 mg/24 h and/or clonal bone marrow plasma cells 10%–60%
2. Absence of myeloma defining events (defined below) or amyloidosis

Plasma Cell Myeloma

Clonal bone marrow plasma cells ≥10% or biopsy-proven extramedullary plasmacytoma

AND

At least one of the following myeloma-defining events:
1. Evidence of end-organ damage:
   Hypercalcemia*
   Renal insufficiency*
   Anemia*
   Osteolytic bone lesions (skeletal radiography/CT/ PET-CT)*
2. At least one of the following biomarkers of malignancy:
   Clonal bone marrow plasma cells ≥60%
   Involved:uninvolved† serum free light chain ratio ≥100
   More than one focal lesions on MRI

---

*CRAB features: hyper*C*alcemia, *R*enal failure, *A*nemia, or osteolytic *B*one lesions.

†Involved refers to the quantity of free light chain (kappa or lambda) produced by the plasma cell clone divided by the quantity of the uninvolved free light chain (kappa or lambda). For example, if the clone is producing excess kappa light chain, it is divided by the quantity of free lambda light chain. Healthy individuals have a kappa-to-lambda ratio of 0.26 to 1.65.

CT, Computed tomography; *FLC,* free light chain; *MRI,* magnetic resonance imaging; *PET,* positron emission tomography.

Modified from Rajkumar, S. V., Dimopoulos, M. A., Palumbo, A., et al. (2014). International Myeloma Working Group updated criteria for the diagnosis of multiple myeloma. *Lancet Oncol,* 15, e538–548.

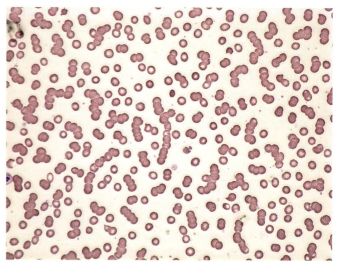

Figure 34.15 Plasma Cell (Multiple) Myeloma. Characteristic rouleaux formation of the red blood cells is the result of a high concentration of circulating immunoglobulins. (Peripheral blood, Wright-Giemsa stain, ×100.)

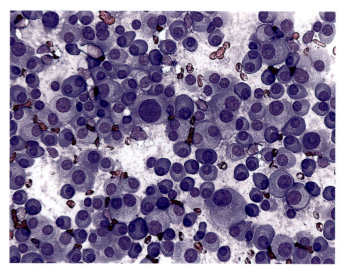

Figure 34.16 Plasma Cell (Multiple) Myeloma. Sheets of plasma cells can replace normal hematopoietic cells in bone marrow. Plasma cells are immature and have an aberrant appearance in this specimen. (Bone marrow aspirate smear, tetrachrome stain, ×500.)

The presence of rouleaux formation of the red blood cells in MM is de facto evidence for a circulating monoclonal protein (Figure 34.15). Bone marrow involvement with plasma cells in MM may be diffuse or focal (Figure 34.16). Caution should be undertaken when examining the bone marrow aspirate without a biopsy because a sampling error may miss the relevant plasma cell population, resulting in a false negative for presence of disease. The trephine biopsy may be more useful in detecting patchy clusters of plasma cells. Immunohistochemical stains for CD138 or kappa/lambda clonal excess may be useful in delineating malignant from reactive plasma cells. Malignant plasma cells in MM express high levels of CD38 and CD138 and low expression of the panleukocyte marker CD45; they may aberrantly express the NK cell-associated marker CD56. Immunophenotyping profiles are increasingly used in MM diagnosis and for quantifying minimal residual disease in patients following therapy.

Plasmacytoma

Solitary plasmacytoma of the bone represents a localized form of PCN without an accompanying monoclonal protein in serum or urine. Definitive diagnosis of this disorder relies on testing to ensure that the plasmacytoma is indeed localized to a single area and not a manifestation of underlying systemic disease. This distinction has therapeutic implications because plasmacytomas are generally treated with radiation therapy.

Waldenström Macroglobulinemia and Heavy Chain Disease

Like MM, Waldenström macroglobulinema (WM) and heavy chain disease are characterized by discrete secretory products. WM is a low-grade lymphoplasmacytic lymphoma (LPL) associated with aberrant secretion of IgM. High levels of IgM can result in hyperviscosity syndrome, requiring emergent plasmapheresis to alleviate symptoms. Extramedullary involvement includes nodal disease and hepatosplenomegaly. A distinct somatic mutation in the myeloid differentiation factor 88 *(MYD88)* gene, a member of the Toll-like receptor pathway, is found in over 90% of WM patients and has become a molecular marker for the disease. It is useful in differentiating WM from other lymphomas that may morphologically exhibit plasmacytic differentiation. Heavy chain disease is also a lymphoplasmacytic neoplasm. Symptoms are dependent on the immunoglobulin heavy chain involved, and as in myeloma, the monoclonal protein may result in significant damage to organs such as the kidney.

Treatment

Most patients with MGUS do not display the clinical manifestations seen in MM and, given the lack of symptoms, observation alone is the standard of care. This is also true for patients with a smoldering (asymptomatic) myeloma. Therapy is indicated for patients who are symptomatic. Successful treatment of MM relies on cytotoxic therapy designed to decrease the clonal plasma cell population and aggressive supportive measures to reverse systemic complications.

Historically, most MM patients were treated with the alkylating agent melphalan combined with the steroid prednisone. More recently, immunomodulatory agents (thalidomide/lenalidomide/pomalidomide), proteasome inhibitors (bortezomib/carfilzomib/ixazomib) and anti-CD38 monoclonal antibody (daratumumab) have radically changed the treatment paradigm for both "up-front" and relapsed refractory disease. Younger, "fit" patients may now receive varying combinations of the newer drugs with or without steroids as initial therapy for MM. These regimens have improved progression free and overall survival. Despite these treatment advances, myeloma for the most part remains an incurable disease whose course is marked by response to therapy followed by recurrence of disease. High-dose myeloablative therapy followed by rescue HSCT has been of some benefit in patients who can endure such aggressive therapy. In this population, melphalan is avoided because it has deleterious effects on the stem cells used as hematopoietic rescue. Sequential high-dose therapy (tandem autologous HSCT) has been investigated but found to benefit only a small group of patients who were initially resistant to the first round of high-dose therapy. The use of maintenance therapies over long periods to control minimal residual disease may be a more tolerable approach. In older patients who cannot handle a high-dose approach, melphalan combined with either bortezomib or lenalidomide has been found to improve treatment outcomes.[68]

Despite improvements in MM treatment, most patients with MM will eventually relapse. Generally, repeating the prior regimen immediately prior to relapse is not efficacious. Newer drugs have been introduced and found to have a role in treating relapsed disease. The second-generation proteasome inhibitor carfilzomib and the immunomodulatory agent pomalidomide have shown efficacy in patients with recurring disease and have been approved by the FDA for clinical use in these patients. Anti-CD38 antibody, daratumumab, or the anti-SLAMF7 monoclonal antibody have been found to benefit patients heavily treated with combination therapy in the past. Combinations of these newer drugs continue to be explored in ongoing clinical trials to identify optimal treatment regimens.[69] More recently, CAR-T cells directed against the B cell maturation antigen, BCMA, have been approved by the FDA for clinical use in patients relapsing after multiple prior therapies. Bispecific monoclonal antibodies targeting tumor BCMA and CD3 on the T cell are also being explored in clinical trials.[70]

SUMMARY

- Mature lymphoid neoplasms arise from malignant transformation of cells at various stages of development resulting from acquired genetic abnormalities that lead to abnormal changes in cell growth and differentiation patterns.
- Modern classification systems, such as that developed by the World Health Organization (WHO), are based on biological features and new molecular data to refine disease models and identify markers used in selecting therapy.
- Leukemias and lymphomas are related malignancies that share cells of origin but differ in clinical presentation. Leukemias primarily involve the peripheral blood and bone marrow, whereas lymphomas predominantly involve the spleen and lymph nodes. However, it is not uncommon for lymphoma cells to be found in the peripheral blood.
- Chronic lymphocytic leukemia (CLL), the most common leukemia in the Western world, is characterized by an accumulation of mature-appearing, functionally incompetent B lymphocytes that aberrantly express CD5. Clinical behavior and outcomes in CLL are largely related to the mutational status of the immunoglobulin heavy chain gene.
- Diffuse large B-cell lymphoma is the most common form of non-Hodgkin lymphoma. It is an aggressive disease that arises either de novo or from transformation of a more

- indolent form of leukemia or lymphoma. Circulating lymphoma cells can exhibit immature blastlike features.
- T-cell lymphomas are less common but more aggressive than B-cell lymphomas. Extranodal involvement including skin manifestations are frequently seen. Adult T-cell lymphoma and Sézary cells in peripheral blood have distinctive morphology, often including irregular nuclear shapes.
- Classic Hodgkin lymphoma has a bimodal age distribution with peaks in the 30s and again after age 50 years. It is characterized by painless lymphadenopathy and Reed-Sternberg cells in lymph node tissue. The cure rate, even in relapsed patients, is greater than 85%.
- Plasma cell (multiple) myeloma is a neoplasm in which proliferating malignant plasma cells in the bone marrow secrete monoclonal immunoglobulin and suppress normal hematopoiesis. Systemic manifestations include osteolytic lesions, hypercalcemia, anemia, and kidney failure. Circulating plasma cells are uncommon except in patients with end-stage disease or in primary plasma cell leukemia.

Now that you have completed this chapter, go back and read again the case study at the beginning and respond to the questions presented. Answers can be found in Appendix C.

REVIEW QUESTIONS

Answers can be found in Appendix C.

1. Non-Hodgkin lymphoma is typically diagnosed by:
   a. Imaging studies
   b. Excisional biopsy or fine needle aspiration
   c. Absolute lymphocyte count
   d. Blood film review

2. Which laboratory test is most suggestive of autoimmune hemolytic anemia in a patient with CLL?
   a. Direct antiglobulin test
   b. Hemoglobin
   c. Lymphocyte count
   d. Platelet count

3. What is the best test or method for determining if a clonal population of T cells is present in a specimen?
   a. Molecular diagnostic testing
   b. Flow cytometry for CD3, CD5, and CD7
   c. Immunohistochemical stain
   d. Karyotyping

4. A rise in the lymphocyte count from 4.1×10^9/L to 5.5×10^9/L in a patient with monoclonal B-cell lymphocytosis suggests:
   a. Acute lymphocyte leukemia
   b. Chronic lymphocytic leukemia
   c. Acute myelocytic leukemia
   d. A reactive condition

5. Which test is often used to differentiate CLL from mantle cell lymphoma?
   a. Annexin A staining
   b. Lymph node biopsy
   c. Immunohistochemistry for cyclin D1
   d. FISH for *BCL2* translocation

6. If not treated, which one of the following would generally be associated with the best outcome?
   a. Peripheral T-cell lymphoma
   b. Burkitt lymphoma
   c. Splenic marginal zone lymphoma
   d. Sézary syndrome

7. What do CLL and myeloma have in common?
   a. Osteolytic lesions
   b. Light chain restriction
   c. Cell of origin
   d. Immunophenotype

8. Which cell is clonal in Hodgkin lymphoma?
   a. Reed-Sternberg cell
   b. T cells
   c. B cells
   d. Histiocytes

9. In most cases the diagnosis of lymphoma relies on all of the following EXCEPT:
   a. Microscopic examination of affected lymph nodes
   b. Immunophenotyping
   c. Molecular analysis
   d. Peripheral blood examination and complete blood count

10. Which of the following is present in monoclonal gammopathy of underdetermined significance?
    a. Hypercalcemia
    b. Serum monoclonal protein
    c. Anemia
    d. Bone lesion

REFERENCES

1. Alaggio, R., Amador, C., Anagnostopoulos, I., et al. (2022). The 5th edition of the World Health Organization classification of haematolymphoid tumours: lymphoid neoplasms. *Leukemia, 36,* 1720–1748.
2. Swerdlow, S. H., Campo, E., Harris, N. L., et al. (2017). *WHO Classification of Tumours of Haematopoietic and Lymphoid Tissues.* (4 ed., Vol. 2). Lyon, France: International Agency for Research on Cancer (IARC).
3. Dave, B. J., Nelson, M., & Sanger, W. G. (2011). Lymphoma cytogenetics. *Clin Lab Med, 31*(4), 725–761.
4. Taylor, J., Xiao, W., & Abdel-Wahab, O. (2017). Diagnosis and classification of hematologic malignancies on the basis of genetics. *Blood, 130,* 410–423.
5. Hamblin, T. J., Davis, Z., Gardiner, A., et al. (1999). Unmutated Ig V(H) genes are associated with a more aggressive form of chronic lymphocytic leukemia. *Blood, 94,* 1848–1854.
6. Freedman, A. S., Friedberg, J. W., & Aster, J. C. (2023). Clinical presentation and initial evaluation of non-Hodgkin lymphoma. T. A. Lister, Editor. *UpToDate*: Waltham, MA. https://www.uptodate.com.
7. Akhtari, M., Milgrom, S. A., Pinnix, C. C., et al. (2018). Reclassifying patients with early-stage Hodgkin lymphoma based on functional radiographic markers at presentation. *Blood, 131,* 84–94.

8. Jain, H., Sengar, M., Nair, R., et al. (2015). Treatment results in advanced stage Hodgkin's lymphoma: a retrospective study. *J Postgrad Med, 61,* 88–91.
9. Wood, B. L., Arroz, M., Barnett, D., et al. (2007). 2006 Bethesda International Consensus recommendations on the immunophenotypic analysis of hematolymphoid neoplasia by flow cytometry: optimal reagents and reporting for the flow cytometric diagnosis of hematopoietic neoplasia. *Cytometry B Clin Cytom, 72*(Suppl. 1), S14–S22.
10. Jevremovic, D., & Olteanu, H. (2019). Flow cytometry applications in the diagnosis of T/NK-cell lymphoproliferative disorders. *Cytometry B Clin Cytom, 96,* 99–115.
11. Lister, T. A., Crowther, D., Sutcliffe, S. B., et al. (1989). Report of a committee convened to discuss the evaluation and staging of patients with Hodgkin's disease: Cotswolds meeting. *J Clin Oncol, 7,* 1630–1636.
12. Rosenberg, S. A. (1977). Validity of the Ann Arbor staging classification for the non-Hodgkin's lymphomas. *Cancer Treat Rep, 61,* 1023–1027.
13. Cheson, B. D., Fisher, R. I., Barrington, S. F., et al. (2014). Recommendations for initial evaluation, staging, and response assessment of Hodgkin and non-Hodgkin lymphoma: the Lugano classification. *J Clin Oncol, 32,* 3059–3068.

14. The International Non-Hodgkin's Lymphoma Prognostic Factors Project. (1993). A predictive model for aggressive non-Hodgkin's lymphoma. *N Engl J Med, 329*, 987–994.

15. Sehn, L. H., Berry, B., Chhanabhai, M., et al. (2007). The revised International Prognostic Index (R-IPI) is a better predictor of outcome than the standard IPI for patients with diffuse large B-cell lymphoma treated with R-CHOP. *Blood, 109*, 1857–1861.

16. SEER. (2023). Cancer Stat Facts: Leukemia — Chronic Lymphocytic Leukemia (CLL). National Cancer Institute. https://seer.cancer.gov/statfacts/html/clyl.html. Accessed April 30, 2023.

17. Hallek, M., Cheson, B. D., Catovsky, D., et al. (2018). iwCLL guidelines for diagnosis, indications for treatment, response assessment, and supportive management of CLL. *Blood, 131*, 2745–2760.

18. Oscier, D., Else, M., Matutes, E., et al. (2016). The morphology of CLL revisited: the clinical significance of prolymphocytes and correlations with prognostic/molecular markers in the LRF CLL4 trial. *Br J Haematol, 174*, 767–775.

19. Gulati, G. (2017). Feasibility of counting smudge cells as lymphocytes in differential leukocyte counts performed on blood smears of patients with established or suspected chronic lymphocytic leukemia/small lymphocytic lymphoma. *Lab Med, 48*, 137–147.

20. Marionneaux, S. M., Keohane, E. M., Lamanna, N., et al. (2021). Smudge cells in chronic lymphocytic leukemia: pathophysiology, laboratory considerations, and clinical significance. *Lab Med, 52*, 426–438.

21. Nowakowski, G. S., Hoyer, J. D., Shanafelt, T. D., et al. (2007). Using smudge cells on routine blood smears to predict clinical outcome in chronic lymphocytic leukemia: a universally available prognostic test. *Mayo Clin Proc, 82*, 449–453.

22. Matutes, E., & Polliack, A. (2000). Morphological and immunophenotypic features of chronic lymphocytic leukemia. *Rev Clin Exp Hematol, 4*, 22–47.

23. Wierda, W. G., Byrd, J. C., Abramson, J. S., et al. (2020). Chronic lymphocytic leukemia/small lymphocytic lymphoma, version 4.2020, NCCN Clinical Practice Guidelines in Oncology. *J Natl Compr Canc Netw, 18*, 185–217.

24. Rawstron, A. C., Bennett, F. L., O'Connor, S. J., et al. (2008). Monoclonal B-cell lymphocytosis and chronic lymphocytic leukemia. *N Engl J Med, 359*, 575–583.

25. Rai, K. R., Sawitsky, A., Cronkite, E. P., et al. (1975). Clinical staging of chronic lymphocytic leukemia. *Blood, 46*, 219–234.

26. Binet, J. L., Auquier, A., Dighiero, G., et al. (1981). A new prognostic classification of chronic lymphocytic leukemia derived from a multivariate survival analysis. *Cancer, 48*, 198–206.

27. Dohner, H., Stilgenbauer, S., Benner, A., et al. (2000). Genomic aberrations and survival in chronic lymphocytic leukemia. *N Engl J Med, 343*, 1910–1916.

28. Haferlach, C., Dicker, F., Weiss, T., et al. (2010). Toward a comprehensive prognostic scoring system in chronic lymphocytic leukemia based on a combination of genetic parameters. *Genes Chromosomes Cancer, 49*, 851–859.

29. Pflug, N., Bahlo, J., Shanafelt, T. D., et al. (2014). Development of a comprehensive prognostic index for patients with chronic lymphocytic leukemia. *Blood, 124*, 49–62.

30. Eksioglu-Demiralp, E., Alpdogan, O., Aktan, M., et al. (1996). Variable expression of CD49d antigen in B cell chronic lymphocytic leukemia is related to disease stages. *Leukemia, 10*, 1331–1339.

31. Rossi, D., Rasi, S., Fabbri, G., et al. (2012). Mutations of NOTCH1 are an independent predictor of survival in chronic lymphocytic leukemia. *Blood, 119*, 521–529.

32. Quesada, V., Conde, L., Villamor, N., et al. (2011). Exome sequencing identifies recurrent mutations of the splicing factor SF3B1 gene in chronic lymphocytic leukemia. *Nat Genet, 44*, 47–52.

33. Rossi, D., Fangazio, M., Rasi, S., et al. (2012). Disruption of BIRC3 associates with fludarabine chemorefractoriness in TP53 wild-type chronic lymphocytic leukemia. *Blood, 119*, 2854–2862.

34. Furman, R. R., Sharman, J. P., Coutre, S. E., et al. (2014). Idelalisib and rituximab in relapsed chronic lymphocytic leukemia. *N Engl J Med, 370*, 997–1007.

35. Roberts, A. W., Davids, M. S., Pagel, J. M., et al. (2016). Targeting BCL2 with venetoclax in relapsed chronic lymphocytic leukemia. *N Engl J Med, 374*, 311–322.

36. Brown, J. R. (2018). How I treat CLL patients with ibrutinib. *Blood, 131*, 379–386.

37. Maddocks, K., & Jones, J. A. (2016). Bruton tyrosine kinase inhibition in chronic lymphocytic leukemia. *Semin Oncol, 43*, 251–259.

38. Staber, P. B., Herling, M., Bellido, M., et al. (2019). Consensus criteria for diagnosis, staging, and treatment response assessment of T-cell prolymphocytic leukemia. *Blood, 134*, 1132–1143.

39. Grever, M. R., Abdel-Wahab, O., Andritsos, L. A., et al. (2017). Consensus guidelines for the diagnosis and management of patients with classic hairy cell leukemia. *Blood, 129*, 553–560.

40. Tiacci, E., Trifonov, V., Schiavoni, G., et al. (2011). BRAF mutations in hairy-cell leukemia. *N Engl J Med, 364*, 2305–2315.

41. Troussard, X., Maître, E., & Cornet, E. (2022). Hairy cell leukemia 2022: update on diagnosis, risk-stratification, and treatment. *Am J Hematol, 97*, 226–236.

42. Palmer, L., Briggs, C., McFadden, S., et al. (2015). ICSH recommendations for the standardization of nomenclature and grading of peripheral blood cell morphological features. *Int J Lab Hematol, 37*, 287–303.

43. WHO. (2022). Human T-lymphotropic virus type 1. World Health Organization. https://www.who.int/news-room/fact-sheets/detail/human-t-lymphotropic-virus-type-1. Accessed May 14, 2023.

44. Matsuoka, M., & Suzuki, R. (2022). Treatment and prognosis of adult T cell leukemia-lymphoma. A. G. Rosmarin, Editor. *UpToDate*: Waltham, MA. https://www.uptodate.com.

45. Jacobson, C., & LaCasce, A. (2014). How I treat Burkitt lymphoma in adults. *Blood, 124*, 2913–2920.

46. Tanaka, J. (2021). Recent advances in cellular therapy for malignant lymphoma. *Cytotherapy, 23*, 662–671.

47. Teras, L. R., DeSantis, C. E., Cerhan, J. R., et al. (2016). 2016 US lymphoid malignancy statistics by World Health Organization subtypes. *CA Cancer J Clin, 66*, 443–459.

48. Armitage, J. O., & Longo, D. L. (2022). Mantle-cell lymphoma. *N Engl J Med, 386*, 2495–2506.

49. Horn, H., Ziepert, M., Becher, C., et al. (2013). MYC status in concert with BCL2 and BCL6 expression predicts outcome in diffuse large B-cell lymphoma. *Blood, 121*, 2253–2263.

50. Sarkozy, C., Traverse-Glehen, A., & Coiffier, B. (2015). Double-hit and double-protein-expression lymphomas: aggressive and refractory lymphomas. *Lancet Oncol, 16*, e555–e567.

51. Alizadeh, A. A., Eisen, M. B., Davis, R. E., et al. (2000). Distinct types of diffuse large B-cell lymphoma identified by gene expression profiling. *Nature, 403*, 503–511.

52. Zucca, E., & Bertoni, F. (2016). The spectrum of MALT lymphoma at different sites: biological and therapeutic relevance. *Blood, 127*, 2082–2092.

53. Arcaini, L., Rossi, D., & Paulli, M. (2016). Splenic marginal zone lymphoma: from genetics to management. *Blood, 127*, 2072–2081.

54. Thieblemont, C., Molina, T., & Davi, F. (2016). Optimizing therapy for nodal marginal zone lymphoma. *Blood, 127,* 2064–2071.

55. Khan, N., Noor, S. J., & Horwitz, S. (2021). How we treat mycosis fungoides and Sézary syndrome. *Clin Adv Hematol Oncol, 19,* 573–581.

56. Hapgood, G., & Savage, K. J. (2015). The biology and management of systemic anaplastic large cell lymphoma. *Blood, 126,* 17–25.

57. Broccoli, A., & Zinzani, P. L. (2017). Peripheral T-cell lymphoma, not otherwise specified. *Blood, 129,* 1103–1112.

58. Brice, P., de Kerviler, E., & Friedberg, J. W. (2021). Classical Hodgkin lymphoma. *Lancet, 398,* 1518–1527.

59. van Nimwegen, F. A., Schaapveld, M., Cutter, D. J., et al. (2016). Radiation dose-response relationship for risk of coronary heart disease in survivors of Hodgkin lymphoma. *J Clin Oncol, 34,* 235–243.

60. Travis, L. B., Hill, D., Dores, G. M., et al. (2005). Cumulative absolute breast cancer risk for young women treated for Hodgkin lymphoma. *J Natl Cancer Inst, 97,* 1428–1437.

61. Koontz, M. Z., Horning, S. J., Balise, R., et al. (2013). Risk of therapy-related secondary leukemia in Hodgkin lymphoma: the Stanford University experience over three generations of clinical trials. *J Clin Oncol, 31,* 592–598.

62. Johnson, P., Federico, M., Kirkwood, A., et al. (2016). Adapted treatment guided by interim PET-CT scan in advanced Hodgkin's lymphoma. *N Engl J Med, 374,* 2419–2429.

63. Collins, G. P., Parker, A. N., Pocock, C., et al. (2014). Guideline on the management of primary resistant and relapsed classical Hodgkin lymphoma. *Br J Haematol, 164,* 39–52.

64. Younes, A., Bartlett, N. L., Leonard, J. P., et al. (2010). Brentuximab vedotin (SGN-35) for relapsed CD30-positive lymphomas. *N Engl J Med, 363,* 1812–1821.

65. Landgren, O. (2013). Monoclonal gammopathy of undetermined significance and smoldering multiple myeloma: biological insights and early treatment strategies. *Hematology Am Soc Hematol Educ Program, 2013,* 478–487.

66. Rajkumar, S. V., Dimopoulos, M. A., Palumbo, A., et al. (2014). International Myeloma Working Group updated criteria for the diagnosis of multiple myeloma. *Lancet Oncol, 15,* e538–e548.

67. Fernandez de Larrea, C., Kyle, R., Rosinol, L., et al. (2021). Primary plasma cell leukemia: consensus definition by the International Myeloma Working Group according to peripheral blood plasma cell percentage. *Blood Cancer J, 11,* 192.

68. Dispenzieri, A. (2016). Myeloma: management of the newly diagnosed high-risk patient. *Hematology Am Soc Hematol Educ Program, 2016,* 485–494.

69. Nooka, A. K., & Lonial, S. (2016). New targets and new agents in high-risk multiple myeloma. *Am Soc Clin Oncol Educ Book, 35,* e431–e441.

70. Dimopoulos, M. A., Moreau, P., Terpos, E., et al. (2021). Multiple myeloma: EHA-ESMO Clinical Practice Guidelines for diagnosis, treatment and follow-up. *Ann Oncol, 32,* 309–322.

Normal Hemostasis

*Jeanine M. Walenga and Kristen N. Krum**

OBJECTIVES

After completion of this chapter, the reader will be able to:

1. List the systems that interact to provide hemostasis.
2. Describe the properties of the vascular intima that initiate and regulate hemostasis and fibrinolysis.
3. List the hemostatic functions of tissue factor–bearing cells and blood cells, especially platelets.
4. Describe the relationships of platelets with von Willebrand factor and fibrinogen, and their impact on hemostasis.
5. Describe the nature, origin, and function of each of the tissue and plasma factors necessary for normal coagulation.
6. Explain the role of vitamin K in the production and function of the prothrombin group of plasma clotting factors.
7. Distinguish between coagulation pathway serine proteases and cofactors.
8. Describe six roles of thrombin in hemostasis.
9. Diagram fibrinogen structure, fibrin formation, fibrin polymerization, and fibrin cross-linking.
10. For each coagulation complex—extrinsic tenase, intrinsic tenase, and prothrombinase—identify the serine protease and the cofactor forming the complex, the type of cell involved, and the substrate(s) activated.
11. List the factors in order of reaction in the plasma-based extrinsic, intrinsic, and common pathways.
12. Describe the cell-based in vivo coagulation process and the role of tissue factor–bearing cells and platelets.
13. Show how tissue factor pathway inhibitor, the protein C pathway, and the serine protease inhibitor antithrombin function to regulate coagulation and prevent thrombosis.
14. Describe the fibrinolytic pathway, its regulators, and its products.

OUTLINE

Overview of Hemostasis
Vascular Intima in Hemostasis
  Anticoagulant Properties of Intact Vascular Intima
  Procoagulant Properties of Damaged Vascular Intima
  Fibrinolytic Properties of Vascular Intima
Platelets
Coagulation System
  Nomenclature of Procoagulants
  Classification and Function of Procoagulants
  The Coagulation System: Extrinsic, Intrinsic, and Common Pathways
  The Hemostatic System: Cell-Based Physiologic Coagulation

Coagulation Regulatory Mechanisms
  Protein C Regulatory System
  Antithrombin
  Tissue Factor Pathway Inhibitor
  Other Serine Protease Inhibitors
Fibrinolysis
  Plasminogen and Plasmin
  Plasminogen Activation
  Control of Fibrinolysis
  Fibrin Degradation Products and D-Dimer

*The authors extend appreciation to Margaret G. Fritsma and George A. Fritsma, whose work in prior editions provided the foundation for this chapter.

CASE STUDY

After studying the material in this chapter, the reader should be able to respond to the following case study. Answers can be found in Appendix C.

A pregnant woman developed a blood clot in her left leg (deep vein thrombosis [DVT]). Her mother reportedly had a history of thrombophlebitis. She had a brother who was diagnosed with DVT after a flight from Los Angeles to Sydney, Australia.

1. Is this hemostatic disorder typical of an acquired or an inherited condition?
2. Are these symptoms most likely caused by a deficiency of a procoagulant or an inhibitor?

Hemostasis is a complex physiologic process that keeps blood circulating in a fluid state until an injury occurs, then causes production of a blood clot to stop the bleeding, confines the blood clot to the site of injury, and finally dissolves the blood clot as the wound heals. When hemostasis systems are out of balance, either *hemorrhage* (uncontrolled bleeding) or *thrombosis* (pathologic clotting) can occur, which can be life-threatening. The absence of a single plasma procoagulant protein may cause the individual to experience lifelong *anatomic hemorrhage* and transfusion dependence. Conversely, absence of an anticoagulant protein allows coagulation to proceed unchecked and can result in *thrombosis*, including myocardial infarction, stroke, pulmonary embolism, and deep vein thrombosis.

Understanding the major systems of hemostasis—blood vessels, platelets, and plasma proteins—is essential to interpreting laboratory test results, along with being able to prevent, predict, diagnose, and manage hemostatic disease.

OVERVIEW OF HEMOSTASIS

Hemostasis involves the interaction of vasoconstriction, platelet adhesion and aggregation, and coagulation enzyme activation to stop bleeding. The coagulation system, similar to other humoral amplification mechanisms, is complex because it translates a diminutive physical or chemical stimulus into a profound lifesaving event.[1] The key cellular elements of hemostasis are the endothelial cells (ECs) of the vascular intima, extravascular tissue factor (TF)–bearing cells, and platelets. The plasma components include the coagulation and fibrinolytic proteins and their inhibitors.

Primary hemostasis (Table 35.1) refers to the role of blood vessels and platelets in the initial response to a vascular injury or to the commonplace desquamation of dying or damaged ECs. Blood vessels contract to seal the wound or reduce the blood flow (vasoconstriction). Platelets adhere to the damaged vessel wall by interactions with von Willebrand factor (VWF) and collagen. They subsequently become activated, which promotes secretion of the contents of their granules, aggregation with other platelets via fibrinogen, VWF, and fibronectin, and formation of a platelet plug. Vasoconstriction and platelet plug formation make up the initial, rapid, and short-lived response to vessel damage. However, to control major bleeding in the long term, the platelet plug must be reinforced by fibrin. Defects in primary hemostasis such as collagen abnormalities, thrombocytopenia, qualitative platelet disorders, or von Willebrand disease can cause debilitating, sometimes fatal, chronic bleeding.

Secondary hemostasis (see Table 35.1) describes the activation of a series of coagulation proteins in the plasma, mostly serine proteases, to form a fibrin clot. These proteins circulate as inactive zymogens (proenzymes), becoming activated during the process of coagulation and, in turn, form complexes that activate other zymogens. This pathway ultimately leads to the generation of thrombin, an enzyme that converts fibrinogen to fibrin. This allows for formation of a localized fibrin clot, which is stabilized by factor XIII. The final event of hemostasis is fibrinolysis, the gradual digestion and removal of the fibrin clot, which occurs as the injury heals.[2]

Although the various components of the coagulation system are divided between primary and secondary hemostasis for improved understanding and compartmentalization, they are associated with each other during early and late-stage hemostatic events. For example, platelets and vascular ECs, which are key components of primary hemostasis, secrete coagulation factors stored in their granules and Weibel-Palade bodies, respectively. In addition, platelets provide the essential cell membrane phospholipid on which coagulation complexes form. Conversely, coagulation proteins, particularly VWF and fibrinogen, are involved in platelet adhesion and aggregation, respectively. Throughout this chapter the vascular intima, platelets, coagulation factors, fibrinolysis proteins, and control proteins will be detailed, illustrating how they function to promote normal hemostasis.

VASCULAR INTIMA IN HEMOSTASIS

The vasculature consists of the blood vessels, including arteries, veins, and capillaries, carrying blood throughout the body. A blood vessel is structured into three layers: an inner layer (tunica intima), a middle layer (tunica media), and an outer layer (tunica adventitia or tunica externa). The tunica intima provides the interface between circulating blood and body tissues. This innermost lining of blood vessels is a monolayer of metabolically active ECs (Box 35.1 and Figure 35.1; refer also to Figure 11.9A).[3] ECs are complex and heterogeneous cells that are distributed throughout the body. They display unique structural and functional characteristics, depending on their

TABLE 35.1 **Primary and Secondary Hemostasis**		
Stage	**Primary Hemostasis**	**Secondary Hemostasis**
Activation	Desquamation and small injuries to blood vessels	Large injuries to blood vessels and surrounding tissues
Components	Vascular intima and platelets	Platelets and coagulation system
Timing	Rapid, short-lived response	Delayed, long-term response
Mechanism	Procoagulant substances exposed or released by damaged or activated endothelial cells	Tissue factor exposed on cell membranes

environment and physiologic requirements, not only in subsets of blood vessels such as arteries versus veins but also in the various tissues and organs of the body.[4,5] ECs play essential roles in immune response, vascular permeability, proliferation, and, of course, hemostasis.

ECs form a smooth, unbroken surface allowing for nonturbulent blood flow. The ECs are supported by a basement membrane and an elastin-rich internal elastic lamina. Arteries have an additional elastin-rich external lamina component. In all blood vessels, fibroblasts (important for maintenance, tissue metabolism, and structural framework) occupy the connective tissue layer, where they produce collagen. Smooth muscle cells present in the walls of all blood vessels, in much larger numbers in arteries than veins and only occasionally in capillaries, promote contraction when an injury occurs and primary hemostasis is initiated.

BOX 35.1 Vascular Intima of the Blood Vessel

Innermost Vascular Lining
Endothelial cells (endothelium)

Supporting the Endothelial Cells
Internal elastic lamina composed of elastin and collagen

Subendothelial Connective Tissue
Collagen and fibroblasts in veins
Collagen, fibroblasts, and smooth muscle cells in arteries

Anticoagulant Properties of Intact Vascular Intima

Intact vascular endothelium prevents thrombosis by numerous *anticoagulant* mechanisms, which are specified in Table 35.2 and see Figure 35.1. The first mechanism of intact ECs is their physical presence. ECs are rhomboid and contiguous, providing a smooth inner surface of the blood vessel promoting nonturbulent blood flow, which prevents activation of platelets and coagulation enzymes. ECs form a physical barrier, separating

TABLE 35.2 Anticoagulant Properties of Intact Vascular Endothelium

Endothelial Cell Structure/ Substance	Anticoagulant Property
Composed of rhomboid cells	Present a smooth, contiguous surface
Secrete prostacyclin	The eicosanoid platelet inhibitor
Secrete nitric oxide	A vascular "relaxing" factor
Secrete the glycosaminoglycan heparan sulfate	An anticoagulant that regulates thrombin generation
Secrete TFPI	A regulator of the extrinsic pathway of coagulation
Express the protein C receptor EPCR	An integral component of the protein C control system
Express cell membrane thrombomodulin	A protein C coagulation control system activator
Secrete TPA	Activates fibrinolysis

EPCR, Endothelial protein C receptor; *TFPI,* tissue factor pathway inhibitor; *TPA,* tissue plasminogen activator.

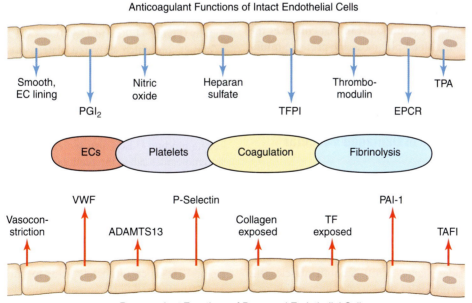

Figure 35.1 Hemostatic Properties of Endothelial Cells that Line the Inner Surface of All Blood Vessels. Depicted in this figure are the anticoagulant properties associated with normal intact endothelial cells (top) and the procoagulant properties associated with damaged endothelial cells (bottom) as they relate to the functions of the hemostatic system listed in the center. *ADAMTS13,* A disintegrin and metalloprotease with a thrombospondin type 1 motif, member 13; *ECs,* endothelial cells; *EPCR,* endothelial cell protein C receptor; *PAI-1,* plasminogen activator inhibitor-1; *PGI$_2$,* prostacyclin or prostaglandin I$_2$; *TAFI,* thrombin activatable fibrinolysis inhibitor; *TF,* tissue factor; *TFPI,* tissue factor pathway inhibitor; *TPA,* tissue plasminogen activator; *VWF,* von Willebrand factor.

platelets in blood from the collagen in the vascular intima that promotes platelet adhesion. The EC barrier also separates circulating procoagulant proteins from TF, present on underlying fibroblasts and smooth muscle cells, that activates coagulation. The ECs are covered with carbohydrates, known as a glycocalyx, consisting of proteoglycans and glycoproteins that have a negative charge. The negative charge repels cellular components, preventing binding to the adhesion molecules present on ECs.[6]

The second anticoagulant mechanism relates to the variety of substances synthesized and secreted by ECs. Prostacyclin (PGI$_2$) is synthesized through the eicosanoid pathway (Chapter 11) and prevents unnecessary or undesirable platelet activation in intact vessels by acting as an antagonist of thromboxane A$_2$ (TXA$_2$).[7,8] In addition, PGI$_2$ promotes vasodilation through a protein kinase A mechanism, leading to inhibition of the myosin light chain kinase with subsequent smooth muscle cell relaxation.[8] Nitric oxide is synthesized in ECs, vascular smooth muscle cells, neutrophils, and macrophages. Nitric oxide induces smooth muscle relaxation with subsequent vasodilation and inhibits platelet activation through a guanylate cyclase-dependent mechanism, while also being able to promote angiogenesis in healthy arterioles through vascular endothelial growth factor (VEGF) and basic fibroblast growth factor (bFGF).[8-10] An important EC-produced anticoagulant is tissue factor pathway inhibitor (TFPI), which controls activation of the TF pathway, also called the extrinsic coagulation pathway. TFPI limits the activation of the TF:VIIa:Xa complex, thereby limiting thrombin generation.

Finally, ECs synthesize and express on their surfaces two known inhibitors of thrombin function, thrombomodulin and heparan sulfate. Thrombomodulin promotes activation of the coagulation inhibitor protein C and subsequent anticoagulation. Heparan sulfate is a glycosaminoglycan that enhances the activity of antithrombin, a blood plasma serine protease inhibitor.[11] The pharmaceutical anticoagulant heparin, an important therapeutic agent used for many clinical indications, resembles EC heparan sulfate in both its structure and its inhibitory activity when bound to antithrombin.

Procoagulant Properties of Damaged Vascular Intima

Although the intact endothelium has anticoagulant properties, when damaged, the tunica intima (ECs and the subendothelial matrix) promotes coagulation through several *procoagulant* properties (Table 35.3 and see Figure 35.1). First, any harmful local stimulus, whether mechanical or chemical, induces vasoconstriction in arteries and arterioles where blood pressure is higher than on the venous side (Figure 11.9B). Smooth muscle cells contract, leading to narrowing of the vascular lumen, followed by decreased blood flow through the injured site. As veins and capillaries do not have as many smooth muscle cells to contribute to vasoconstriction, blood can escape into surrounding tissues, creating extravascular pressure on the blood vessel and causing compression, which effectively minimizes the escape of blood.

Second, the subendothelial connective tissues of arteries and veins are rich in collagen, a flexible, elastic structural protein. Upon injury to the vessel, collagen is exposed, leading

TABLE 35.3 Procoagulant Properties of Damaged Vascular Intima

Structure/Substance	Procoagulant Property
Smooth muscle cells in arterioles and arteries	Induce vasoconstriction
Exposed subendothelial collagen	Binds VWF; binds to and activates platelets
Damaged or activated ECs secrete VWF	Important for platelet binding to collagen at site of injury: platelet adhesion as a first line of defense against bleeding
Damaged or activated ECs secrete adhesion molecules: P-selectin, ICAMs, PECAMs	Promote platelet and leukocyte binding and activation at site of injury
Exposed smooth muscle cells and fibroblasts	Tissue factor exposed on cell membranes
ECs in inflammation	Tissue factor is induced by inflammation

ECs, Endothelial cells; *ICAMs,* intercellular adhesion molecules; *PECAMs,* platelet endothelial cell adhesion molecules; *VWF,* von Willebrand factor.

to binding of circulating VWF, which causes binding and activation of platelets (Figure 11.9B and 11.9C). Platelets subsequently bind to the collagen through their GPVI and $\alpha_2\beta_1$ receptors and adhere to the damaged area until new ECs grow. Throughout an individual's life span, connective tissue naturally degenerates, which leads to an increased tendency to bruise in the elderly.

Third, ECs secrete VWF from storage sites called Weibel-Palade bodies when activated by vasoactive agents such as thrombin. VWF is a large multimeric glycoprotein that acts as the necessary bridge that binds platelets to exposed subendothelial collagen in arterioles and arteries where blood flows rapidly (Figure 11.9C and 11.9D).[12] VWF has been described as a "carpet" on which activated platelets assemble. ADAMTS13, also secreted from ECs, serves an important function as it cleaves large VWF multimers into shorter chains that support normal platelet adhesion.

Fourth, on activation, ECs secrete and coat themselves with P-selectin, an adhesion molecule that promotes platelet and leukocyte binding.[13] ECs also secrete immunoglobulin-like adhesion molecules called intercellular adhesion molecules (ICAMs) and platelet EC adhesion molecules (PECAMs), which further promote platelet and leukocyte binding.[14]

Finally, subendothelial smooth muscle cells and fibroblasts support the constitutive membrane protein TF.[15] EC disruption exposes TF to circulating blood, promoting activation of the coagulation system through contact with plasma coagulation factor VII, which ultimately leads to fibrin formation (Figure 35.2). The formed fibrin surrounds the platelet plug, securing it to the damaged area such that the blood flow does not dislodge the platelet plug.

In arterioles and arteries, the larger VWF multimers form a fibrillar carpet on which the platelets assemble because of the high blood flow; a white clot consisting of essentially platelets, fibrin, and VWF is produced.[16] In veins, because of the slower blood flow, a bulky red clot is produced, consisting of mostly red blood cells and fibrin, with some platelets.[16]

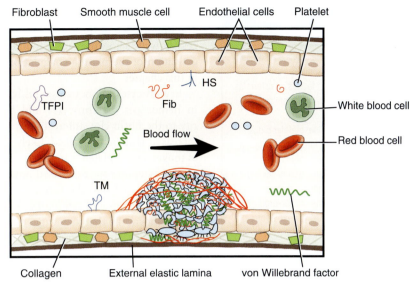

Figure 35.2 **Secondary Hemostasis.** Immediately after the initial response to vessel injury of platelet activation, adhesion, and aggregation (primary hemostasis), as detailed in Chapter 11 and Figure 11.9, the continued response of an injured blood vessel leads to the formation of a fibrin clot that stabilizes the initial platelet plug, as shown in this artist's rendering. Primary hemostasis requires interaction of platelets with subendothelial VWF and collagen. Secondary hemostasis requires exposure of TF from damaged endothelial cells and phospholipids from activated platelets that promotes activation of the coagulation cascade, thrombin generation, and fibrin formation that polymerizes around the platelet aggregate. *Fib,* Fibrinogen; *HS,* heparan sulfate; *TF,* tissue factor, *TFPI,* tissue factor pathway inhibitor (EC bound and soluble forms exist); *TM,* thrombomodulin (EC bound and soluble forms exist).

Fibrinolytic Properties of Vascular Intima

Through the secretion of tissue plasminogen activator (TPA), ECs support *fibrinolysis* (see Table 35.2 and see Figure 35.1), the breakdown of fibrin, leading to thrombus degradation and restoration of vessel patency. TPA activates fibrinolysis by converting plasminogen to the primary fibrinolytic enzyme plasmin, which gradually digests fibrin and restores blood flow. ECs also regulate fibrinolysis by providing inhibitors to prevent excessive plasmin generation. One of the fibrinolytic inhibitors secreted by ECs, as well as by other cells, is plasminogen activator inhibitor-1 (PAI-1).[17] Another inhibitor of plasmin generation is thrombin activatable fibrinolysis inhibitor (TAFI), which is activated by thrombin bound to EC membrane thrombomodulin.[18]

Although the significance of the tunica intima in hemostasis is well recognized, there are few valid laboratory methods to assess the integrity of ECs, smooth muscle cells, fibroblasts, and their collagen matrix.[19] Invasive blood vessel biopsies are not performed. Thus the diagnosis of blood vessel disorders is based on clinical symptoms, family history, and indirectly by laboratory tests that rule out platelet or coagulation disorders.

PLATELETS

Platelets are produced from the cytoplasm of bone marrow megakaryocytes.[20] Although platelets are only 2 to 3 μm in diameter on a fixed, stained peripheral blood film, they are complex, metabolically active cells that interact with their environment and initiate and control hemostasis.[21] Chapter 11 provides an in-depth description of platelet structure and function. An overview of the platelet functions critical in the initial stages of hemostatic control is given in this chapter.

Platelets serve as one of the body's first lines of defense against blood loss. At the time of injury, platelets adhere to the site of injury, aggregate, and secrete the contents of their granules (Table 35.4 and Figure 11.9).[22,23] *Adhesion* is the property by which platelets bind to nonplatelet surfaces such as subendothelial collagen and VWF. VWF links platelets to collagen through their GPIb/IX/V membrane receptors in areas of high shear stress such as arteries and arterioles.[24] In damaged veins and capillaries, platelets may bind directly to collagen via GPVI and $\alpha_2\beta_1$ receptors. The importance of platelet adhesion is underscored by bleeding disorders such as Bernard-Soulier syndrome (Chapter 37), in which the platelet GPIb/IX/V receptor is absent, and von Willebrand disease (Chapter 36), in which VWF is missing or defective.

Aggregation is the property by which platelets bind to one another. When platelets are activated, a change in the GPIIb/IIIa receptor allows binding of fibrinogen as well as VWF and fibronectin.[25] Fibrinogen binds to GPIIb/IIIa receptors on adjacent platelets and joins them together in the presence of ionized calcium (Ca^{2+}). Fibrinogen binding is essential for platelet aggregation as evidenced by bleeding and compromised aggregation in patients with afibrinogenemia or in patients who lack the GPIIb/IIIa receptor (Glanzmann thrombasthenia; Chapter 37).

Platelets *secrete* the contents of their α-granules and dense granules during adhesion and aggregation, with most secretion occurring late in the platelet activation process. Platelets secrete procoagulants (e.g., factor V, VWF, factor VIII, fibrinogen) as well as control proteins (e.g., protein S, TFPI, antithrombin, C1-inhibitor), along with Ca^{2+}, adenosine diphosphate (ADP) and other hemostatic molecules (Table 35.5).[26,27] Although these substances participate in thrombosis and hemostasis, the

TABLE 35.4   Platelet Function

Function	Mechanism of Action	Characteristics
Adhesion	Platelets roll and cling to nonplatelet surfaces	Reversible; seals endothelial gaps, some secretion of growth factors, in arterioles VWF is necessary for adhesion
Aggregation	Platelets adhere to each other	Irreversible; platelet plugs form, platelet contents are secreted, requires fibrinogen
Secretion	Platelets release the contents of their granules	Irreversible; occurs during aggregation, platelet contents are secreted, essential to coagulation

VWF, von Willebrand factor.

TABLE 35.5   Platelet Granule Contents

Platelet α-Granules (Large Molecules)	Platelet Dense Granules (Small Molecules)
Factors V, VIII, XI, prothrombin, fibrinogen	Adenosine diphosphate
VWF	Adenosine triphosphate
HMWK	Ionized calcium
Antithrombin, TFPI, protein S	Serotonin
C₁-inhibitor (control protein of the contact system)	Magnesium
Plasminogen	Potassium
PAI-1	Histamine
Platelet factor 4	
Platelet-derived growth factor, other growth factors	

HMWK, High-molecular-weight kininogen; *PAI-1,* plasminogen activator inhibitor-1; *TFPI,* tissue factor pathway inhibitor; *VWF,* von Willebrand factor.

role of platelets in inflammation, atherosclerosis, antimicrobial host defense, wound healing, angiogenesis, and malignancy has become increasingly appreciated as the function of platelets in the pathophysiology of these processes is being better defined.[27]

The platelet membrane consists of a *phospholipid bilayer.* During activation, ADP and Ca^{2+} activate phospholipase A_2, which converts platelet membrane phospholipids into arachidonic acid (Figure 11.12). Arachidonic acid is converted into the endoperoxides prostaglandin G_2 (PGG_2) and prostaglandin H_2 (PGH_2) by the cyclooxygenase enzyme-1 (COX-1). In the platelet, thromboxane synthetase converts these prostaglandins into TXA_2, which causes Ca^{2+} to be released from the dense tubules, thereby promoting platelet aggregation and vasoconstriction. Available Ca^{2+} (ionized calcium) is critical for normal platelet function because it is involved in helping with subsequent physical spreading of the platelet to cover the site of injury, along with promoting secretion of platelet granule content.[26,28]

The membrane of activated platelets is the key surface for coagulation enzyme-cofactor-substrate complex formation (see Figure 35.2), which is the foundation for secondary hemostasis to occur.[29] Platelets supply Ca^{2+}, the membrane phospholipid

phosphatidylserine, some procoagulant factors, and receptors. The importance of these substances in the blood clotting process, as well as how they serve to integrate platelet function with activation of the plasma coagulation system, will be described in this chapter.

Erythrocytes, monocytes, and lymphocytes also participate in hemostasis. Erythrocytes add bulk and structural integrity to the fibrin clot. Interestingly, those with anemia have an increased tendency to bleed, likely in part because of the lack of movement of platelets to the vessel wall (marginalization) by erythrocytes and the decreased number of erythrocytes able to be incorporated into the thrombus.[30] In inflammatory conditions, monocytes and lymphocytes, and possibly ECs, provide surface-borne TF that may trigger coagulation. Leukocytes also have a series of membrane integrins and selectins that bind adhesion molecules on platelets and other cells and help stimulate the production of inflammatory cytokines that promote the wound healing process and combat infection.[31]

COAGULATION SYSTEM

Nomenclature of Procoagulants

Plasma transports at least 16 procoagulants called *coagulation factors.* Nearly all are glycoproteins synthesized in the liver, although monocytes, ECs, and megakaryocytes produce a few (Table 35.6 and Figure 35.3). Eight are enzymes that circulate in an inactive form called *zymogens.* Others are cofactors that bind, stabilize, and enhance the activity of their respective enzymes. Fibrinogen is the substrate for the enzymatic action of thrombin, the primary enzyme of the coagulation system. In addition, there are plasma glycoproteins that act as control proteins that serve the important function of regulating the coagulation process to avoid unnecessary thrombin generation, fibrin formation, and blood clotting (see Figure 35.3). Reference intervals can be found after the Index at the end of the book.

Fibrinogen and prothrombin (factor II) were known in 1935; factors V and VII were identified in the period 1945 to 1950; and factors IX and X were described in the 1950s.[32] In 1958 the International Committee for the Standardization of the Nomenclature of the Blood Clotting Factors officially named the plasma procoagulants and cofactors using Roman numerals in the order of their initial description or discovery.[33] An additional convention adopted was the use of a lowercase *a* behind the Roman numeral to designate factors in their activated state—for instance, activated factor VII is VIIa.

There are multiple factors not usually identified by their Roman numerals. Factors I and II are customarily called fibrinogen and prothrombin, respectively, although occasionally they are identified by their numerals. The numeral III was given to tissue thromboplastin, a crude mixture of TF and phospholipid. Now that the precise structure of TF has been described, the numeral designation is seldom used. The numeral IV identified the plasma cation calcium (Ca^{2+}); however, calcium is referred to by its name or chemical symbol, not by its numeral. The numeral VI was assigned to a procoagulant that later was determined to be activated factor V; VI was withdrawn from

TABLE 35.6 Properties of the Plasma Procoagulants

Factor	Name	Function	Molecular Weight (Daltons)	Half-Life (hr)	Mean Plasma Concentration[†]
I*	Fibrinogen	Thrombin substrate, polymerizes to form fibrin	340,000	100–150	200–400 mg/dL
II*	Prothrombin	Serine protease	71,600	60	10 mg/dL
III*	Tissue factor	Cofactor	44,000	Insoluble	None
IV*	Ionized calcium	Mineral	40	NA	8–10 mg/dL
V		Cofactor	330,000	24	1 mg/dL
VII		Serine protease	50,000	6	0.05 mg/dL
VIII	Antihemophilic factor	Cofactor	260,000	12	0.01 mg/dL
VWF	von Willebrand factor	Factor VIII carrier and platelet adhesion	500,000–20,000,000	24	1 mg/dL
IX	Christmas factor	Serine protease	57,000	24	0.3 mg/dL
X	Stuart-Prower factor	Serine protease	58,800	48–52	1 mg/dL
XI		Serine protease	143,000	48–84	0.5 mg/dL
XII	Hageman factor	Serine protease	84,000	48–70	3 mg/dL
Prekallikrein	Fletcher factor, pre-K	Serine protease	85,000	35	35–50 µg/mL
High-molecular-weight kininogen	Fitzgerald factor, HMWK	Cofactor	120,000	156	5 mg/dL
XIII	Fibrin-stabilizing factor (FSF)	Transglutaminase, transamidase	320,000	150	2 mg/dL
Platelet factor 3	Phospholipids, phosphatidylserine, PF3	Assembly molecule	—	Released by platelets	—

*These factors are customarily identified by name rather than Roman numeral.
[†]Clinically, plasma concentration of all coagulation factors, except fibrinogen, can be given as percentage of normal (%) or units/dL, where the numeric value remains the same.

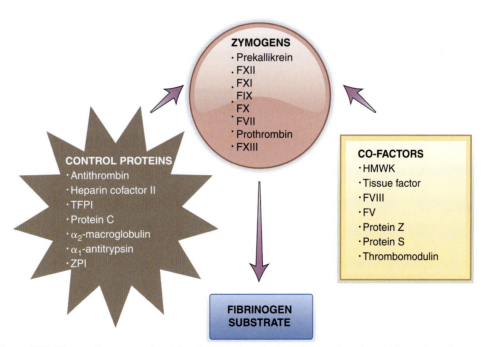

Figure 35.3 Plasma Components of the Coagulation System. Four categories of plasma-based components of the coagulation system of blood clotting include procoagulants (zymogens), cofactors, anticoagulants (regulatory or control proteins), and the final fibrinogen substrate. Throughout this chapter, figures will use the above-shaped symbols to aid in classifying each component: zymogens as *circles;* activated zymogens or serine proteases as hexagons (not shown here); cofactors as *rectangles;* control proteins as *stars;* other components as ovals. *HMWK,* High-molecular-weight kininogen; *TFPI,* tissue factor pathway inhibitor; *ZPI,* protein Z–dependent protease inhibitor.

the naming system and never reassigned. Although factor VIII is normally referred to as factor VIII, it was originally known as antihemophilic factor, which is a cofactor that circulates linked to a large carrier protein, VWF. Prekallikrein (pre-K), also called Fletcher factor, and high-molecular-weight kininogen (HMWK), also called Fitzgerald factor, have never received Roman numerals because they belong to the kallikrein and kinin systems, respectively, and their primary functions lie within these systems. Platelet phospholipids, particularly phosphatidylserine, are required for the coagulation process but were given no Roman numeral; instead they were once called collectively platelet factor 3.

Classification and Function of Procoagulants

The coagulation factors work together in a pathway in which one factor, when activated, activates the next factor in the sequence. The purpose is to generate the key enzyme, *thrombin,* which converts fibrinogen to fibrin, allowing for formation of a localized thrombus. The sequence of coagulation factor activation is shown in Figure 35.4.

The coagulation factors thrombin (FIIa), FVIIa, FIXa, FXa, FXIa, FXIIa, and pre-K are enzymes called *serine proteases* (Table 35.7).[34] Of note, while FXIII is also an enzyme, it is a transglutaminase. Serine proteases are proteolytic enzymes of the trypsin family.[35] Each member has a reactive seryl amino acid residue in its active site and acts on its substrate by hydrolyzing peptide bonds, thereby digesting the primary backbone. Small polypeptide fragments from each substrate are produced from this process.

Serine proteases are synthesized as inactive zymogens consisting of a single peptide chain. Activation occurs when the zymogen is cleaved at one or more specific sites by the action of another protease during the coagulation process.

In the coagulation pathway, there are multiple procoagulant *cofactors* that augment the enzymatic process. These cofactors participate in the formation of enzymatically active complexes with the serine proteases. The cofactor TF is located on membranes of fibroblasts and smooth muscle cells but also can be found on monocytes during inflammation and sepsis.[36] TF serves to initiate the coagulation pathway when there is vascular injury. Soluble plasma FV and FVIII, the other procoagulant cofactors, become activated and are then incorporated into procoagulant complexes of coagulation factors and other cofactors. Factors V and VIII are important for proper functioning of the coagulation system and normal thrombin generation. The cofactor HMWK functions in complex with FXIIa as a second means of activation of the coagulation pathway through the intrinsic pathway.

The remaining components of the coagulation pathway are fibrinogen, FXIII, phospholipids, ionized calcium, and VWF (Box 35.2). *Fibrinogen* is the ultimate substrate of the coagulation pathway. When hydrolyzed by thrombin, soluble fibrinogen is converted to the insoluble structural protein, *fibrin,* forming a more stable clot that is further stabilized by activated FXIII through cross-linking of the fibrin monomers.[37]

Ionized calcium (Ca^{2+}) is required for the previously stated coagulation complexes. These complexes assemble on platelet or cell membrane phospholipids, predominantly *phosphatidylserine.* Activated serine proteases bind to the negatively charged phospholipid surface through the positively charged calcium ions. This process serves to localize coagulation activation to the cell surface at the site of injury.

The molecular weights, plasma concentrations, and plasma half-lives of the procoagulant factors are given in Table 35.6.[38] These essential pieces of clinical information assist in the interpretation of laboratory tests, monitoring of anticoagulant

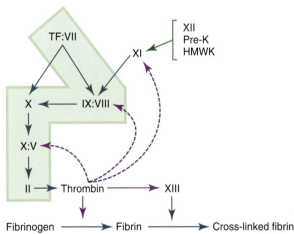

Figure 35.4 Simplified Coagulation Pathway. Exposed tissue factor *(TF)* activates factor VII, which activates FIX and FX. The IXa:VIIIa complex also activates FX, and the Xa:Va complex activates prothrombin (FII). The resulting thrombin cleaves fibrinogen to form fibrin and activates FXIII to stabilize the clot. Thrombin also activates factors V, VIII, XI, and platelets in a positive feedback loop. Exposure to negatively charged surfaces (e.g., bacterial cell membranes) activates the contact factors FXII, prekallikrein *(pre-K),* and high-molecular-weight kininogen *(HMWK),* which activate FXI.

TABLE 35.7	**Plasma Procoagulant Serine Proteases**		
Inactive Zymogen	**Active Protease**	**Cofactor**	**Substrate**
Prothrombin (II)	Thrombin (IIa)	—	Fibrinogen, V, VIII, XI, XIII
VII	VIIa	Tissue factor	IX, X
IX	IXa	VIIIa	X
X	Xa	Va	Prothrombin
XI	XIa	—	IX
XII	XIIa	High-molecular-weight kininogen	XI
Prekallikrein	Kallikrein	High-molecular-weight kininogen	XI

BOX 35.2	**Other Plasma Procoagulants**
Fibrinogen	
Factor XIII	
Phospholipids	
Calcium	
von Willebrand factor	

therapy, and design of effective replacement therapies in deficiency-related hemorrhagic diseases. It is of interest to note that fibrinogen, prothrombin, FVIII, and VWF are acute-phase reactants and their levels increase when there is inflammation as in trauma, pregnancy, infection, and stress.

Vitamin K–Dependent Prothrombin Group

Prothrombin (factor II), FVII, FIX, and FX, along with the regulatory proteins protein C, protein S, and protein Z, are dependent on vitamin K during synthesis to produce a functional structure (Table 35.8). These factors are named the *prothrombin group* because of their structural resemblance to prothrombin. All 7 proteins have 10 to 12 glutamic acid units near their amino terminal end. All are serine proteases when activated, except protein S and protein Z, which are cofactors.

Vitamin K is a quinone found in green leafy vegetables (Box 35.3); it is also produced by the intestinal organisms *Bacteroides fragilis* and *Escherichia coli*. Vitamin K is a coenzyme for the carboxylase that catalyzes an essential posttranslational modification of the prothrombin group proteins: γ-carboxylation of amino-terminal glutamic acids (Figure 35.5). Glutamic acid is modified to γ-carboxyglutamic acid when a second carboxyl group is added to the γ-carbon. With two ionized carboxyl groups, the γ-carboxyglutamic acids gain a net negative charge, which enables the binding of the positively charged ionized

calcium. As stated previously, it is the bound calcium that enables the vitamin K–dependent coagulation factors to bind to negatively charged phospholipids, localizing the coagulation process, as well as providing a platform for the formation of coagulation factor complexes.

In vitamin K deficiency or in the presence of the anticoagulant drug warfarin, a therapeutic inhibitor of vitamin K (Chapter 40), the vitamin K–dependent procoagulants are released from the liver without the second carboxyl group added to the γ carbon. These are called *des-γ-carboxyl proteins* or *proteins induced by vitamin K antagonists* (PIVKA factors). Because they lack the second carboxyl group, they cannot bind to Ca^{2+} and subsequently to phospholipids, so they cannot participate in the coagulation reaction.

Vitamin K–dependent procoagulants are essential for the assembly of three complexes in the coagulation pathway (Figure 35.6). These are the same coagulation complexes discussed

TABLE 35.8 Vitamin K–Dependent Coagulation Factors

Procoagulants	Regulatory Proteins
Prothrombin (II)	Protein C
VII	Protein S
IX	Protein Z
X	

BOX 35.3 Food Sources High in Vitamin K

Kale
Spinach
Turnip greens
Collards
Mustard greens
Swiss chard
Brussels sprouts
Broccoli
Asparagus
Cabbage
Green onions
Lettuce: Boston, romaine, or Bibb
Avocado
Cauliflower
Parsley, fresh

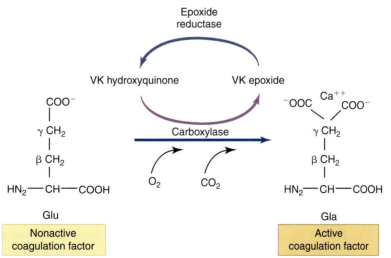

Figure 35.5 Posttranslational γ-Carboxylation of the Vitamin K–Dependent Coagulation Proteins. For coagulation factors II (prothrombin), VII, IX, and X, and control proteins C, S, and Z, vitamin K hydroxyquinone transfers a carboxyl *(COO–)* group to the γ carbon of glutamic acid *(Glu)*, creating γ-carboxyglutamic acid *(Gla)*. The negatively charged pocket formed by the two carboxyl groups attracts ionic calcium, which enables the molecule to bind to phosphatidylserine. Vitamin K hydroxyquinone is oxidized to vitamin K epoxide by carboxylase in the process of transferring the carboxyl group but is subsequently reduced to the hydroxyquinone form by epoxide reductase.

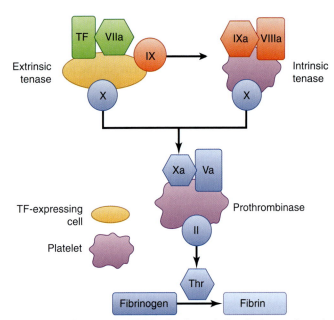

Figure 35.6 Complexes Within the Coagulation Pathway. Coagulation complexes form on tissue factor *(TF)*-bearing cells (TF:VIIa) and on platelet phospholipid membranes (IXa:VIIIa and Xa:Va). Each complex consists of a vitamin K–dependent serine protease coagulation factor, a cofactor, and Ca²⁺, bound to the cell membrane. Extrinsic tenase complex is FVIIa and TF on the membrane of a TF-bearing cell. This complex activates both FIX and FX. Intrinsic tenase complex, which is FIXa and its cofactor VIIIa on platelet membranes, activates FX also. Prothrombinase complex is FXa and its cofactor Va, bound to the surface of platelets. Prothrombinase cleaves prothrombin to the active enzyme thrombin *(Thr)*.

TABLE 35.9 Coagulation Complexes

Complex	Components	Activates
Extrinsic tenase	VIIa, tissue factor, phospholipid, and Ca²⁺	IX and X
Intrinsic tenase	IXa, VIIIa, phospholipid, and Ca²⁺	X
Prothrombinase	Xa, Va, phospholipid, and Ca²⁺	Prothrombin

TABLE 35.10 Hemostasis Cofactors

Cofactor	Function	Binds
Tissue factor	Procoagulant	VIIa
V	Procoagulant	Xa
VIII	Procoagulant	IXa
High-molecular-weight kininogen	Procoagulant	XIIa, prekallikrein
Thrombomodulin	Control (protein C)	Thrombin
	Antifibrinolytic (TAFI)	Thrombin
Protein S	Control	Protein C, TFPI
Protein Z	Control	ZPI

TAFI, Thrombin activatable fibrinolysis inhibitor; *TFPI,* tissue factor pathway inhibitor; *ZPI,* protein Z-dependent protease inhibitor.

earlier but described here in detail. The formation of these complexes is emphasized because of the critical role they play in thrombin generation and normal hemostasis.

Each complex is composed of a vitamin K–dependent serine protease, its nonenzyme cofactor, and Ca²⁺, which is bound to the negatively charged phospholipid membranes of activated platelets or TF-bearing cells. The initial complex, *extrinsic tenase,* comprises TF and FVIIa; it activates FIX and FX, which are components of the next two complexes (Table 35.9). *Intrinsic tenase complex* comprises FIXa and its cofactor FVIIIa; it also activates FX but much more efficiently than the TF:FVIIa extrinsic tenase complex. *Prothrombinase complex* comprises FXa and its cofactor FVa; it converts prothrombin to thrombin in a multistep hydrolytic process that releases thrombin and a peptide fragment called *prothrombin fragment 1+2* (F1+2). Prothrombin fragment 1+2 in plasma is thus a marker for thrombin generation.

Cofactors in Hemostasis

Procoagulant cofactors are TF, FV, FVIII, and HMWK. Cofactors of the coagulation control proteins are thrombomodulin, protein S, and protein Z (Table 35.10).[39] Thrombomodulin is also a cofactor in the control of fibrinolysis. Each cofactor binds to its particular serine protease, promoting stability and increased reactivity to the serine protease.

TF, a transmembrane receptor for FVII and FVIIa, is found on extravascular cells surrounding ECs, including fibroblasts

and smooth muscle cells. Vessel injury exposes blood to the subendothelial TF-bearing cells and leads to activation of coagulation through FVII. The activation of FVII is limited by the injury itself through the size and resulting amount of TF exposed. Of note, TF is expressed at high levels in cells of the brain, lung, placenta, heart, and kidney. These findings explain the significant tissue damage, morbidity, and mortality that can ensue after a bleed into these organs. In inflammatory conditions, including sepsis, monocytes and other cells express TF, initiating coagulation.[15,36]

Factors V and VIII are soluble plasma proteins. Factor V is a glycoprotein circulating in plasma and also present in platelet α-granules. During platelet activation and secretion, platelets release partially activated FV at the site of injury. Factor Va is a cofactor to FXa in the prothrombinase complex in coagulation. The prothrombinase complex accelerates thrombin generation more than 300,000-fold compared to FXa alone.[40] The initial small amount of thrombin generated activates the first amount of FV to FVa. As described in the "Protein C Regulatory System" section, thrombomodulin-bound thrombin activates protein C, which inactivates FVa to FVi. Therefore FV is both activated and then ultimately inactivated by the generation of thrombin, as is FVIII. Factor VIII is a cofactor to FIX, which together form the intrinsic tenase complex.

HMWK is produced by the liver and acts as a cofactor to FXIIa and pre-K in the *contact factor complex.* This complex of the coagulation pathway is a mechanism for activating coagulation via the intrinsic pathway in conditions in which foreign objects such as mechanical heart valves, bacterial membranes, or high levels of inflammation are present. Thus coagulation is initiated at the site of either the *extrinsic tenase* complex (FVIIa and TF) or the contact factor complex (FXIIa, pre-K, and HMWK).

Thrombomodulin, a transmembrane protein constitutively expressed by vascular ECs, is a thrombin cofactor in the protein C pathway. Together, thrombomodulin and thrombin activate protein C, a coagulation regulatory protein. In one of many examples of carefully regulated processes within the hemostatic system, once thrombin is bound to thrombomodulin, it loses its procoagulant ability to activate FV and FVIII, among other factors and, through activation of protein C, leads to destruction of FV and FVIII, thus suppressing further generation of thrombin—a negative feedback loop. Thrombin bound to thrombomodulin also activates TAFI, a fibrinolysis inhibitor.

Both protein S and protein Z are cofactors in the regulation and control of coagulation. Protein S is a cofactor to protein C as well as TFPI. Protein Z is a cofactor to Z-dependent protease inhibitor (ZPI). These cofactors will be discussed in detail in association with their hemostatic mechanisms described in this chapter.

Factor VIII and von Willebrand Factor

Factor VIII and VWF are key proteins for hemostasis as they are both critically involved in all protective mechanisms to avoid blood loss (i.e., platelets, vasculature, and blood coagulation leading to fibrin formation).

Factor VIII is produced by ECs.[41] Free FVIII is unstable in plasma, resulting in a significantly shortened half-life; however, when bound to VWF in circulation, its half-life increases to approximately 12 hours (Figure 35.7). Factor VIII deteriorates more rapidly than other coagulation factors in stored blood, decreasing to approximately 50% after 5 days in thawed component plasma.[42] During coagulation, FVIII is activated through cleavage from VWF by thrombin. Factor VIIIa subsequently binds to phospholipid on activated platelets, forming the intrinsic tenase complex with FIXa and Ca^{2+}. Like FVa, FVIIIa is also inactivated by protein C.

Factors VIII and IX are the only two plasma procoagulants whose production is governed by genes carried on the X chromosome.[43] Factor VIII is a cofactor, but its importance in hemostasis cannot be overstated, as evidenced by the severe bleeding and symptoms associated with hemophilia A and type 2N von Willebrand disease (Chapter 36).

VWF is a large multimeric glycoprotein that participates in platelet adhesion and transports the procoagulant FVIII. VWF is composed of multiple subunits of 240,000 Daltons each.[44] The subunits are produced by ECs and megakaryocytes, where they combine to form multimers that range from 500,000 to 20,000,000 Daltons.[45] VWF molecules are stored in α-granules in platelets and in Weibel-Palade bodies in ECs. ECs release ultralarge multimers of VWF into plasma, where they are normally degraded into smaller multimers by a VWF-cleaving protease, ADAMTS13 (*a d*isintegrin and *m*etalloprotease with a *t*hrombospondin type 1 motif, member *13*), in blood vessels with high shear stress.[46]

VWF has multiple binding sites for platelets, along with binding sites for collagen and FVIII (see Figure 35.7). Through its collagen binding site and primary platelet surface receptor, GPIb/IX/V, it is able to act as a bridge, binding platelets to exposed subendothelial collagen during platelet adhesion (Figure 11.9C). This is especially important in arteries and arterioles, where the flow of blood is faster and the collagen specific receptors on platelets are unable to bind to collagen directly. Through arginine-glycine-aspartic acid (RGD) sequences, VWF is also able to bind a second platelet receptor, GPIIb/IIIa, during platelet aggregation (Chapter 11).

The importance of VWF in hemostasis cannot be overstated as evidenced by the severe bleeding and symptoms associated with abnormalities in VWF molecular structure and concentration. von Willebrand disease, which is the most commonly inherited bleeding disorder, is associated with several described mutations (Chapter 36). Factor VIII deficiency, another common bleeding disorder, can be linked to von Willebrand disease because VWF is the carrier for FVIII.

Of note, levels of VWF vary by ABO blood type, with group O individuals having lower levels of VWF than the other blood group types.[47] In addition, VWF and factor VIII are both acute phase reactants with increased levels seen during pregnancy, trauma, bleeding, infection, and stress.

Factor XI and the Contact Factors

The *contact system* is a group of plasma proteins that responds to the presence of foreign material. The contact factors consist of factor XII, prekallikrein (pre-K; Fletcher factor), and HMWK (Fitzgerald factor). They are so named because they are activated by contact with negatively charged foreign surfaces such as stents, valve prostheses, and bacterial cell membranes. Upon activation, this system triggers blood coagulation via the intrinsic pathway. Additionally, it is responsible for the generation of proinflammatory products such as bradykinin, activation of the complement system, and plays a major role in the host-defense system.[48] This system is also called the plasma kallikrein-kinin system because it functions in inflammatory conditions.

Further to its contribution to the intrinsic coagulation pathway and fibrin clot formation, the contact system is involved with activation of fibrinolysis through FXIIa via a pre-K–mediated activation of plasminogen.[48,49] There is also suggestive evidence that FXI plays a role in the downregulation of fibrinolysis, which would help stabilize the formed blood clot.[48]

Factor XII and pre-K are zymogens that are activated to become serine proteases; HMWK is a nonenzymatic cofactor. Through coming into contact with a negatively charged surface, FXII becomes activated through autocatalytic conversion.[50,51] Activation by FXIIa transforms pre-K, a glycoprotein that circulates bound to HMWK, into its active form,

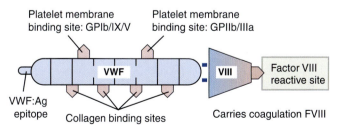

Figure 35.7 von Willebrand Factor *(VWF)*–Factor VIII Complex. VWF molecules of various lengths from 0.5 to 20 mDaltons are in blood circulation. Factor VIII circulates covalently bound to VWF. VWF provides three other active receptor sites: VWF binds to collagen; it binds to glycoprotein *(GP)* Ib/IX/V to support platelet adhesion; and it binds to GPIIb/IIIa to facilitate platelet aggregation. VWF:Ag epitope is the target of quantitative immunoassays.

kallikrein. Kallikrein is subsequently able to cleave HMWK to form bradykinin, which promotes inflammation and can cause vasodilation.

Factor XI is activated to FXIa in part by FXIIa but more significantly by thrombin during coagulation generated from TF:FVIIa activation (see Figure 35.4). Factor XIa activates FIX and the reaction proceeds as described previously for the coagulation pathway.

Factor XI–associated bleeding disorders are described in Chapter 36. Deficiencies of FXII, HMWK, or pre-K do not cause clinical bleeding disorders.[52] However, deficiencies do prolong laboratory tests and necessitate investigation. Factor XII is activated in vitro by negatively charged surfaces such as nonsiliconized glass, kaolin, or ellagic acid—used as test reagents for the partial thromboplastin time (PTT, activated PTT [APTT]) assay.

Thrombin

Thrombin is the main enzyme of the coagulation pathway with multiple key activities. The primary function of thrombin, however, is to cleave fibrinopeptides A and B (FPA and FPB) from the α and β chains of the fibrinogen molecule, triggering spontaneous fibrin polymerization and the beginning of the insoluble fibrin clot (Figure 35.8). FPA and FPB are measurable in plasma and serve as markers of thrombin activation.

Thrombin amplifies the coagulation pathway by activating cofactors V and VIII and FXI, providing a positive feedback mechanism that generates more thrombin (see Figure 35.4). Thrombin also activates FXIII, which forms covalent bonds between the D domains of the fibrin polymer to cross-link and ultimately stabilize the fibrin clot. In addition, thrombin initiates aggregation of platelets, which increases the platelet component of the thrombus.

Further, thrombin plays roles in both anticoagulation and antifibrinolysis. Through binding to thrombomodulin, thrombin activates the protein C pathway and TAFI. In the protein C pathway, it suppresses coagulation through degradation of FVa and FVIIIa. Thrombin activated TAFI leads to suppression of fibrinolysis.

Thrombin therefore plays a role in coagulation (fibrin formation), platelet activation, regulation of coagulation activation (protein C), and controlling fibrinolysis (TAFI). Because of its multiple autocatalytic functions, thrombin is the key protease of hemostasis.

Fibrinogen Structure and Fibrin Formation, Factor XIII

Fibrinogen is the primary substrate of thrombin; enzymatic action of thrombin leads to conversion of soluble fibrinogen to insoluble fibrin to produce a clot. Fibrinogen is also essential for platelet aggregation because it links activated platelets through their GPIIb/IIIa platelet fibrinogen receptor. Fibrinogen is a 340,000 Dalton glycoprotein synthesized in the liver. The normal plasma concentration of fibrinogen ranges from 200 to 400 mg/dL, the most concentrated of all the plasma procoagulants. Platelet α-granules absorb, transport, and release abundant fibrinogen.[53] Of note, fibrinogen is an acute phase reactant protein, meaning its level increases during inflammation, infection, and other stress conditions.

The fibrinogen molecule is a mirror image dimer, each half consisting of three nonidentical polypeptides, designated Aα, Bβ, and γ, united by several disulfide bonds (see Figure 35.8). The six N-terminals assemble to form a bulky central region called the E domain. The three carboxyl terminals on each outer end of the molecule assemble to form two D domains.[37]

Thrombin cleaves FPA and FPB from the protruding N-termini of each of the two α and β chains of fibrinogen, reducing the overall molecular weight by 10,000 Daltons. The cleaved fibrinogen is called fibrin monomer. The exposed fibrin monomer α and β chain ends (E domain) have an immediate affinity for portions of the D domain of neighboring monomers, spontaneously polymerizing to form fibrin polymers (Figure 35.9).

Factor XIII is a heterodimer whose α subunit is produced mostly by megakaryocytes and monocytes, and whose β subunit is produced in the liver.[54] The two subunits become joined in the plasma to form FXIII. After activation by thrombin, FXIIIa covalently cross-links fibrin polymers to form a more stable insoluble fibrin clot. Factor XIIIa is a transglutaminase that catalyzes the formation of covalent bonds between the carboxyl terminals of γ chains from adjacent D domains in the fibrin polymer (see Figure 35.9). These bonds link the ε-amino acid of lysine moieties and the γ-amide group of glutamine units. Multiple cross-links form to provide an insoluble meshwork of fibrin polymers linked by their D domains, providing physical strength to the fibrin clot. Factor XIIIa reacts with other plasma and cellular structural proteins and is essential to wound healing and tissue integrity.

Cross-linking of fibrin polymers by FXIIIa covalently incorporates fibronectin, a plasma protein involved in cell adhesion,

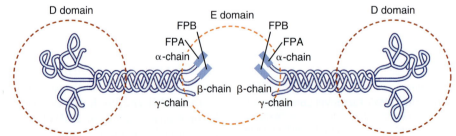

Figure 35.8 **Structure of Fibrinogen.** Fibrinogen has three domains. The central E domain and two terminal D domain nodules at the carboxyl ends of the molecule. The D and E domains are joined together by supercoiled α-helix regions. This trinodular structure comprises three pairs of disulfide-bonded polypeptides, two each of the Aα, Bβ, and γ chains. *FPA,* Fibrinopeptide A; *FPB,* fibrinopeptide B.

and α_2-antiplasmin that renders the fibrin mesh resistant to fibrinolysis. Plasminogen, the primary serine protease of the fibrinolytic system, also becomes covalently bound via lysine moieties on fibrin, as does TPA, a serine protease that ultimately hydrolyzes and activates bound plasminogen to initiate fibrinolysis, thus breaking down the clot.

The Coagulation System: Extrinsic, Intrinsic, and Common Pathways

In the past, two coagulation pathways were described, both of which activated FX at the start of a common pathway leading to thrombin generation (Figure 35.10). The pathways were characterized as cascades in that as one enzyme became activated, it in turn activated the next enzyme in sequence.

At that time, coagulation experts identified the activation of FXII as the primary step in coagulation because this factor could be found in blood, whereas TF could not. Consequently, the reaction system that begins with FXII and culminates in fibrin polymerization has been called the *intrinsic pathway*. The coagulation factors of the intrinsic pathway, in order of reaction, are XII, pre-K, HMWK, XI, IX, VIII, X, V, prothrombin (II), and fibrinogen. The laboratory test that detects the absence of one or more of these factors is the PTT (Chapter 41).

We now know that the contact factors XII, pre-K, and HMWK do not play a significant role in in vivo or physiologic coagulation with trauma-type injuries, although their deficiencies prolong the in vitro laboratory tests of the intrinsic pathway—in particular, the PTT. The contact system establishes a connection between inflammation and coagulation activation. This system is complex and is shown only in abbreviated format in this chapter. Despite decades of research, understanding of the contact system is still ongoing.

The presence of TF, which activates FVIIa, has since proven to be the primary in vivo initiation mechanism for coagulation.

Because TF is not present in blood, the TF pathway has been called the *extrinsic pathway*. This pathway includes the factors VII, X, V, prothrombin, and fibrinogen. The test used to measure the integrity of the extrinsic pathway is the prothrombin time (PT) (Chapter 41).

The two pathways have in common FX and FV, prothrombin, and fibrinogen; this portion of the coagulation pathway is called the *common pathway*. These designations—intrinsic, extrinsic, and common—are used extensively to interpret in vitro laboratory testing of blood plasma and to identify factor deficiencies.

Although the coagulation system was originally designated a "cascade," it is not that simple. An important aspect of this process is the formation of factor-cofactor enzymatic complexes, which are crucial to facilitate the generation of thrombin. Coagulation is initiated on tissue-factor bearing cells (such as fibroblasts) with the formation of the *extrinsic tenase complex* TF:FVIIa:Ca^{2+}, which activates FIX and FX, producing enough thrombin to activate platelets, FV, FVIII, and FXI in a feedback loop. Coagulation is then propagated on the surface of the activated platelet with the formation of the *intrinsic tenase complex* (FIXa:FVIIIa:phospholipid:Ca^{2+}) and the *prothrombinase complex* (FXa:FVa:phospholipid:Ca^{2+}), ultimately generating a burst of thrombin at the site of injury. The thrombin generated subsequently leads to production of fibrin to stabilize the clot.

Factors VIII and FIX are not considered part of the extrinsic pathway, even though their activated forms are produced in small quantities by TF:FVIIa, because the PT assay fails to identify their absence or deficiency. The FIXa:FVIIIa complex in the intrinsic pathway, crucial to the activation of FX, is readily assessed by the PTT assay.

The PT and PTT assays are used in tandem to screen for any coagulation factor deficiency. Not surprisingly, they do not adequately describe the complex interdependent reactions that occur with all components of in vivo hemostasis.

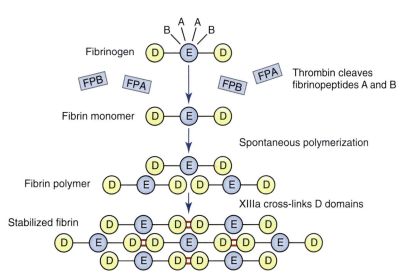

Figure 35.9 Formation of a Stabilized Fibrin Clot. Thrombin cleaves a small portion of the α and β chains in the central E domain node of fibrinogen, releasing free peptides, fibrinopeptide A *(FPA)* and fibrinopeptide B *(FPB)*. This forms fibrin monomer. Fibrin monomers spontaneously polymerize due to the affinity of thrombin-cleaved positively charged E domains for negatively charged D domains of other monomers. This forms the fibrin polymer. Factor XIIIa catalyzes the covalent cross-linking of γ chains of adjacent D domains *(double red line)* to form an insoluble stable fibrin clot.

The Hemostatic System: Cell-Based Physiologic Coagulation

An intricate combination of cellular and biochemical events function in harmony to keep blood liquid within the veins and arteries, to prevent blood loss from injuries by the formation of thrombi, and to reestablish blood flow during the healing process.[55] As noted earlier, the series of cascading proteolytic reactions in blood plasma, traditionally known as the extrinsic and intrinsic coagulation pathways, do not fully describe how coagulation occurs physiologically. These pathways are not distinct, independent, alternative mechanisms for generating thrombin but are actually *interdependent*. For example, a deficiency of FVII in the extrinsic pathway can cause significant bleeding, even when the intrinsic pathway is intact. Similarly, deficiencies of FVIII and FIX may cause severe bleeding, regardless of the presence of a normal extrinsic pathway.[56]

In addition to procoagulant and anticoagulant plasma proteins, normal physiologic coagulation requires the presence of two cell types for formation of coagulation complexes: cells that express TF (usually extravascular TF) and platelets (intravascular

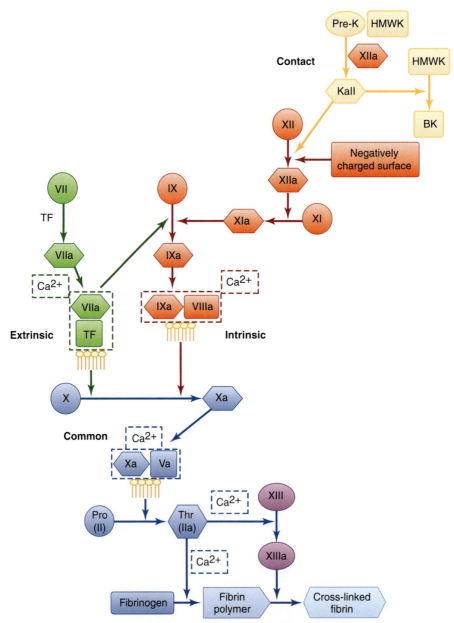

Figure 35.10 Plasma-Based Coagulation Cascade. The coagulation cascade consists of the contact system (simplified here) and the intrinsic, extrinsic, and common pathways. In the intrinsic pathway *(red)*, the contact factors FXII, prekallikrein *(pre-K)*, and high-molecular-weight kininogen *(HMWK)* are activated and proceed to activate factors XI, IX, VIII, X, and V and prothrombin *(Pro)*, which converts fibrinogen to fibrin. In the extrinsic pathway (green), tissue factor *(TF)* activates FVII, which activates FX, FV, and prothrombin, cleaving fibrinogen to fibrin. Both the intrinsic and extrinsic pathways converge with the activation of FX, so FX, FV, prothrombin *(Pro)*, and fibrinogen are called the common pathway *(blue)*. *Dashed boxes* indicate the coagulation factor complexes that assemble on phospholipid *(yellow symbol)*. These pathways are the basis of clinical coagulation laboratory tests. *BK,* Bradykinin; *Kall,* kallikrein; *Thr,* thrombin.

TF) (Figure 35.6 and Figure 35.11).[57] Operationally, coagulation can be described as occurring in two phases: *initiation,* which occurs on TF expressing cells and produces 3% to 5% of the total thrombin generated, and *propagation,* occurring on platelets, which produces 95% or more of the total thrombin.[58]

Initiation

In vivo, the principal mechanism for generating thrombin is begun by formation of the extrinsic tenase complex rather than the intrinsic pathway. The initiation phase refers to extrinsic tenase complex formation with the resulting generation of small amounts of FXa, FIXa, and thrombin (see Figure 35.11).

Damage to the endothelium allows blood, including platelets, to flow into the extravascular tissue, triggering a localized response. The magnitude of the response depends largely on the extent of the injury.

About 1% to 2% of FVIIa is present normally in blood in the activated form, but it is inert until bound to TF[59] and unaffected by TFPI and other inhibitors. Fibroblasts and other subendothelial cells provide TF, a cofactor to FVIIa. Upon injury, FVIIa binds to TF on the membrane of subendothelial cells, resulting in the formation of the extrinsic tenase complex TF:FVIIa.

TF:FVIIa activates low levels of both FIX and FX. A minute amount of thrombin is generated by membrane-bound FXa and FXa:FVa prothrombinase complexes. The initial minute amount of thrombin feeds back into the coagulation cascade to activate FV, FVIII, and FXI, which serves to amplify the production of more thrombin.[60]

Coagulation complexes bound to cell membranes are relatively protected from inactivation by most inhibitors. However, if FXa:FVa dissociates from the cell, it is rapidly inactivated by the protease inhibitors TFPI, antithrombin, and ZPI until a threshold of FXa:FVa activity is reached.

Even though the amount of thrombin generated in this phase is small, it is able to activate platelets, cofactors, and other procoagulant factors.[61] The low level of thrombin generated in the initiation phase (1) activates platelets through cleavage of protease activated receptors PAR-1 and PAR-4. It also (2) activates FV released from platelet α-granules. Through its interaction with FVIII (3), it is able to both activate FVIII and dissociate it from VWF. Thrombin also (4) activates FXI, the intrinsic accessory procoagulant that activates more FIX. Finally, through its main function, thrombin (5) splits FPA and FPB from fibrinogen and forms a preliminary fibrin network. Thus the initial platelet plug is formed.

Cleavage of fibrinopeptides from the fibrinogen molecule occurs at the end of the initiation phase and beginning of the propagation phase. In most clot-based coagulation assays, this is the visual endpoint of the assay.[37] It occurs with only 10 to 30 nmol/L of thrombin, or approximately 3% of the total thrombin generated.

Propagation

More than 95% of thrombin generation occurs during propagation. In this phase, the reactions occur on the surface of the activated platelet, which now has all the components needed for coagulation (see Figure 35.11). Large numbers of platelets adhere and aggregate at the site of injury, localizing the coagulation response.

Platelets are activated at the site of injury by both the low-level thrombin generated in the initiation phase and by adhering to exposed collagen. Platelets partially activated by *co*llagen *a*nd *t*hrombin are referred to as COAT platelets (Chapter 11).[62] These partially activated COAT platelets have a higher level of procoagulant activity than platelets exposed to collagen alone. They also provide a surface for formation and amplification of intrinsic tenase and prothrombinase complexes.

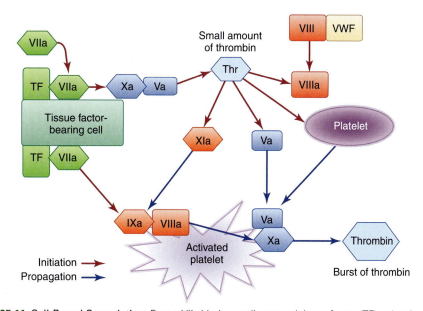

Figure 35.11 Cell-Based Coagulation. Factor VIIa binds to cell-exposed tissue factor *(TF)* and activates both FX and FIX. Cell-bound FXa combines with FVa and generates a small amount of thrombin *(Thr),* which activates platelets, FV, FVIII, and FXI and begins fibrin formation. Factor IXa, activated by both TF:VIIa and FXIa, combines with FVIIIa on the platelet surface to activate FX, which binds with FVa to form the prothrombinase complex (Xa:Va) and produces a burst of thrombin. *VWF,* von Willebrand factor.

The cofactors Va and VIIIa, activated by thrombin in the initiation phase, bind to platelet membranes and become receptors for FXa and FIXa. Factor IXa generated in the initiation phase binds to FVIIIa on the platelet membrane to form the intrinsic tenase complex FIXa:FVIIIa. More FIXa is also generated by platelet-bound FXIa. This intrinsic tenase complex activates FX at a 50- to 100-fold higher rate than the extrinsic tenase complex.[57] Factor Xa binds to FVa to form the prothrombinase complex, which activates prothrombin and generates a burst of thrombin. Thrombin both cleaves fibrinogen into fibrin to form a clot and activates FXIII that stabilizes the fibrin clot. In addition, thrombin binds to thrombomodulin activating the protein C control pathway, along with activating TAFI to inhibit fibrinolysis.

Because coagulation depends on the presence of both TF-bearing cells and activated platelets, clotting is localized to the site of injury. In addition, both protease inhibitors and intact endothelium prevent clotting from spreading to other parts of the body.

It may be helpful operationally to think of the extrinsic or TF pathway as occurring on the TF-bearing cell and the intrinsic pathway (minus FXII, HMWK, and pre-K) as occurring on the platelet surface. However, these are not separate and redundant pathways; they are interdependent and occur in parallel until a clot is formed at the site of injury, causing blood flow to cease, and the entire process is terminated by control mechanisms.

Both platelets and TF-bearing cells are essential for physiologic coagulation. In addition, deficiencies of any of the key proteins of coagulation complex formation and activity (FVII, FIX, FVIII, FX, FV, or prothrombin) compromise thrombin generation and can manifest as significant bleeding disorders.

COAGULATION REGULATORY MECHANISMS

Inhibitors, known as *control proteins,* and their cofactors regulate both the serine proteases and their associated cofactors in the coagulation system. They also provide feedback loops to maintain a complex and delicate balance between abnormal thrombosis and bleeding. These inhibitors are natural anticoagulants that function to slow the activation of procoagulants and suppress thrombin production. They ensure that coagulation is localized and does not become a systemic response by preventing excessive clot formation. The principal regulators are activated protein C with cofactor protein S, antithrombin, and TFPI. Acquired or inherited deficiencies of these proteins may be associated with increased incidence of venous thromboembolic disease because, with a deficiency, the hemostatic balance is shifted toward increased thrombin generation and coagulation, rather than normal termination of the activated pathway. Figure 35.12 illustrates coagulation mechanism regulatory points. Characteristics of these and other coagulation regulatory proteins are summarized in Table 35.11.

Protein C Regulatory System

During coagulation, thrombin cleaves fibrinogen, generating a fibrin clot, and activates factors V, VIII, and XI, propagating more thrombin generation. In intact normal vessels, where

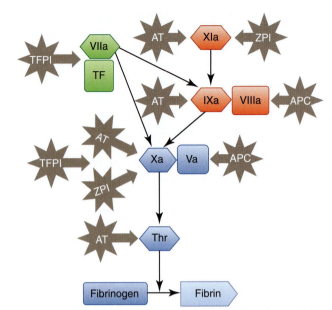

Figure 35.12 Coagulation Pathway Showing Regulatory Points. *APC,* Activated protein C; *AT,* antithrombin; *TFPI,* tissue factor pathway inhibitor; *Thr,* thrombin; *ZPI,* protein Z-dependent protease inhibitor.

coagulation would be inappropriate, thrombin avidly binds the EC membrane protein thrombomodulin and triggers an essential coagulation regulatory system called the protein C system.[63] The protein C system revises thrombin's function from a procoagulant enzyme to an anticoagulant.

Endothelial cell protein C receptor (EPCR) is a transmembrane protein that binds protein C adjacent to the thrombomodulin-thrombin complex. EPCR augments the action of thrombin-thrombomodulin at least five-fold in activating protein C to the serine protease activated protein C (APC) (Figure 35.13).[64,65] The APC dissociates from EPCR and binds its cofactor, free plasma protein S. The stabilized APC–protein S complex hydrolyzes and inactivates FVa and FVIIIa, resulting in a slowing or blocking of thrombin generation.

Protein S, the cofactor that binds and stabilizes APC, is synthesized in the liver and circulates in the plasma in two forms. About 40% of protein S is free, but 60% is covalently bound to the complement control protein C4b-binding protein (C4bBP).[66] Bound protein S cannot participate in the protein C anticoagulant pathway; only free plasma protein S can serve as the APC cofactor. Protein S-C4bBP binding is of particular interest in inflammatory conditions because C4bBP is an acute-phase reactant. When the plasma C4bBP level increases, additional protein S is bound and free protein S levels become proportionally decreased, which may increase the risk of thrombosis.

Chronic acquired or inherited protein C or protein S deficiency or mutations of protein C, protein S, or FV compromise the normal function of the protein C pathway to downregulate FVa and FVIIIa and are associated with venous thromboembolic disease (Chapter 39). Underscoring the importance of the protein C regulatory system, neonates who completely lack protein C can have a massive thrombotic condition called purpura fulminans and die in infancy unless treated with protein C replacement and therapeutic anticoagulation.[67]

TABLE 35.11 Coagulation Regulatory Proteins

Name	Function	Molecular Mass (Daltons)	Half-Life (hr)	Mean Plasma Concentration
Tissue factor pathway inhibitor	With Xa, binds TF:VIIa	33,000	Unknown	60–80 ng/mL
Thrombomodulin	EC surface receptor for thrombin	450,000	Does not circulate, although soluble truncated forms can be measured	Levels of soluble thrombomodulin increase with vascular disease
Protein C	Serine protease	62,000	7–9	2–6 µg/mL
Protein S	Cofactor	75,000	Unknown	20–25 µg/mL
Antithrombin	Serpin	58,000	68	24–40 mg/dL
Heparin cofactor II	Serpin	65,000	60	30–70 µg/mL
Protein Z-dependent protease inhibitor	Serpin	72,000	Unknown	1.5 µg/mL
Protein C inhibitor	Serpin	57,000	23	2–8 µg/mL
α_1-Protease inhibitor (α_1-antitrypsin)	Serpin	60,000	Unknown	250 mg/dL
α_2-Macroglobulin	Serpin	725,000	60	150–400 mg/dL

EC, Endothelial cell; *Serpin,* serine protease inhibitor; *TF,* tissue factor.

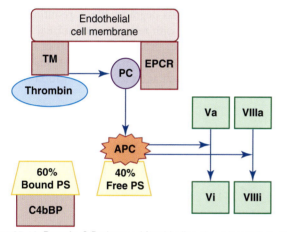

Figure 35.13 Protein C Pathway. After binding thrombomodulin *(TM),* thrombin activates protein C *(PC),* bound by endothelial cell protein C receptor *(EPCR).* Free protein S *(PS;* not bound to C4b binding protein [*C4bBP*]) binds and stabilizes activated protein C *(APC).* The APC–protein S complex digests and inactivates factors Va (*Vi*) and VIIIa (*VIIIi*).

Antithrombin

Antithrombin (AT) was the first of the coagulation regulatory proteins to be identified as a cause of thrombosis when deficient and the first to be assayed routinely in the clinical hemostasis laboratory.[68] AT is a serine protease inhibitor (serpin) that binds and neutralizes serine proteases. It is the main inhibitor of thrombin (FIIa) and FXa, along with FIXa, FXIa, FXIIa, pre-K, and plasmin.[69]

AT inhibition of the previously mentioned factors occurs normally in a slow rate; however, it can be significantly enhanced by the addition of a glycosaminoglycan such as heparin. *Heparin cofactor II* (HC II) is an inhibitor related to AT that primarily targets thrombin and similarly requires heparin.[70] Heparin is a member of the glycosaminoglycan family of carbohydrates. It is a heterogeneous mixture of variably sulfated disaccharide units that link together to form chains of varying length, molecular weight, and sulfation. Physiologically, glycosaminoglycans are available from endothelium-associated mast cell granules as

heparin or as heparan sulfate located in the glycocalyx of ECs.[69] Heparin is also available as a therapeutic anticoagulant drug.

The activity of AT is amplified 2000-fold by binding to heparin.[70] Heparin induces a conformational change in the AT molecule that allows binding of activated coagulation factors, which causes them to be inactivated. The inhibition of thrombin, FX, and other serine proteases by AT depends on the length of the heparin chain; for thrombin, only the longer heparin chains are able to bind both AT and thrombin to produce inhibition of thrombin. Thrombin inhibition via AT binding is illustrated in Figure 35.14.

When AT covalently binds thrombin, an inactive *thrombin-antithrombin complex* (TAT) is formed, which is then released from the heparin molecule. Laboratory measurement of TAT is used as an indicator of thrombin generation.

Tissue Factor Pathway Inhibitor

TFPI is a Kunitz-type (referring to its chemical structure) serine protease inhibitor and is the principal regulator of the TF pathway. The Kunitz-2 structural domain binds to and inhibits FXa, and the Kunitz-1 domain binds to and inhibits the TF:FVIIa complex.[71] TFPI is synthesized primarily by ECs and is also expressed by platelets upon activation.[71] In the initiation of coagulation, FVIIa and TF combine to activate FIX and FX. TFPI inhibits coagulation in a two-step process by first binding and inactivating FXa. The TFPI:FXa complex then binds to TF:FVIIa, forming a quaternary complex and preventing further activation of FX and FIX (Figure 35.15).[72,73] Alternatively, TFPI may bind to FXa in the TF:FVIIa:FXa complex. TFPI provides feedback inhibition because it is not actively engaged until coagulation is initiated and FX is activated.

Protein S, the cofactor of APC, is also a cofactor of TFPI and enhances FXa inhibition by TFPI 10-fold.[74] Because of the inhibitory action of TFPI, the TF:FVIIa:FXa reaction is short lived. Once TFPI shuts down the extrinsic tenase complex and FXa, additional FXa and FIXa production shifts to the intrinsic pathway.[61] Propagation of coagulation occurs as FX is activated by the FIXa:FVIII complex and more FIX is activated by FXIa.

Other Serine Protease Inhibitors

Other members of the serpin family include ZPI, protein C inhibitor, α_1-protease inhibitor (α_1-antitrypsin), α_2-macroglobulin, and α_2-antiplasmin, and PAI-1.[69]

Z-dependent protease inhibitor (ZPI), in the presence of its cofactor protein Z, is a potent inhibitor of FXa.[75,76] ZPI covalently binds protein Z and FXa in a complex with Ca^{2+} and phospholipid. Protein Z is a vitamin K–dependent plasma glycoprotein that is synthesized in the liver. Although protein Z has a structure similar to that of the other vitamin K–dependent proteins (FII, FVII, FIX, FX, and protein C), it lacks an activation site and, like protein S, is nonproteolytic. Protein Z increases the ability of ZPI to inhibit FXa 2000-fold.[77] ZPI also inhibits FXIa in a separate reaction that does not require protein Z, phospholipid, or Ca^{2+}. The inhibition of FXIa is accelerated two-fold by the presence of heparin.

Protein C inhibitor is a nonspecific, heparin-binding serpin that inhibits a variety of proteases, including APC, thrombin, FXa, FXIa, and urokinase.[77] It is found in plasma and also in many other body fluids and organs. Depending on its target, it can function as an anticoagulant (inhibits thrombin), as a procoagulant (inhibits thrombin-thrombomodulin and APC), or as a fibrinolytic inhibitor.

The serpins α_1-protease inhibitor and α_2-macroglobulin are able to inhibit serine proteases reversibly. See Table 35.12 and the "Fibrinolysis" section for details on α_2-antiplasmin and PAI-1.

FIBRINOLYSIS

Fibrinolysis, the final stage of hemostatic activation, is the systematic, accelerating hydrolysis of fibrin by plasmin. To concentrate and localize fibrinolysis to the site of injury where the clot has formed, fibrinolytic proteins become incorporated into the fibrin clot as it is forming.

Several hours after fibrin polymerization and cross-linking (thrombus formation) and in response to inflammation and coagulation, the fibrinolytic process is activated. Two activators of fibrinolysis, TPA and urokinase plasminogen activator (UPA), are released from ECs. These convert fibrin-bound plasminogen into the principal enzyme of the fibrinolytic system, *plasmin* (Figure 35.16; Table 35.12). Similar to the steps in the coagulation system, there is a delicate balance between the activators and inhibitors in this system.

The fibrinolytic process degrades fibrin, resulting in dissolution of the thrombus, with restoration of normal blood flow during the vascular repair process. Fibrinolysis of the fibrinogen molecule also occurs, which may reduce plasma fibrinogen levels affecting clot growth and platelet aggregation within the thrombus.

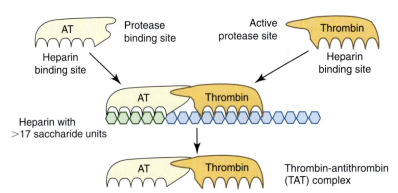

Figure 35.14 Mechanism of Antithrombin to Control Coagulation Activation. Glycosaminoglycans *(GAGs)* such as heparan sulfate and therapeutic heparin potentiate the antithrombin-thrombin reaction. When antithrombin *(AT)* binds the GAG, it is sterically modified, allowing AT to covalently bind thrombin, which inactivates the active enzymatic site of thrombin. Inhibition of thrombin requires that it simultaneously binds both AT and the GAG. Thrombin and AT, covalently bound, release the GAG and form measurable plasma thrombin-antithrombin *(TAT)* complexes. Inhibition of factor Xa is accomplished on shorter GAG chains (<17 saccharide units; 5 minimum) because FXa binds only to the AT molecule when AT is in complex with the GAG.

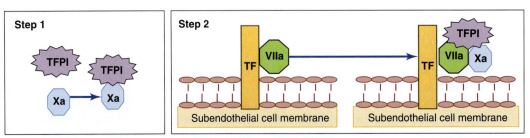

Figure 35.15 Tissue Factor Pathway Inhibitor *(TFPI)*. TFPI binds the complex of tissue factor *(TF)*:VIIa:Xa in a factor Xa-dependent mechanism. In **Step 1**, TFPI first binds to FXa and inactivates it. In **Step 2**, The TFPI:Xa complex then binds and inactivates the cell bound TF:VIIa complex, preventing more activation of FXa. Alternatively, TFPI may bind directly to FXa and FVIIa in the TF:VIIa:Xa complex.

TABLE 35.12   Proteins of the Fibrinolysis Pathway

Name	Function	Molecular Mass (Daltons)	Half-Life	Mean Plasma Concentration
Plasminogen	Active form is the plasma serine protease plasmin, digests fibrinogen and fibrin	92,000	24–26 hr	15–21 mg/dL
Tissue plasminogen activator (TPA)	Serine protease secreted by vascular ECs, activates plasminogen	68,000	Unknown	4–7 µg/dL
Urokinase plasminogen activator (UPA)	Serine protease secreted by renal ECs, activates plasminogen	54,000	Unknown	2–4 ng/mL
Plasminogen activator inhibitor-1 (PAI-1)	Serpin secreted by endothelium, inhibits TPA	52,000	1 hr	14–28 mg/dL
α₂-Antiplasmin	Serpin, inhibits free plasmin	51,000	Unknown	7 mg/dL
Thrombin activatable fibrinolysis inhibitor (TAFI)	Suppresses fibrinolysis by removing fibrin C-terminal lysine binding sites blocking TPA and plasminogen binding	55,000	8–10 min	5 µg/mL

EC, Endothelial cells; *serpin,* serine protease inhibitor.

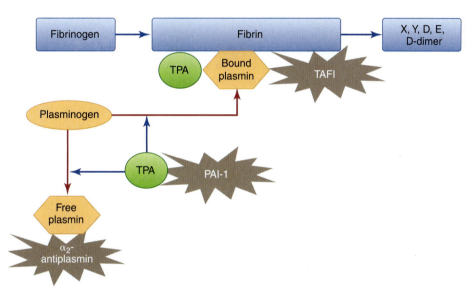

Figure 35.16 Fibrinolysis Pathway and Inhibitors. Plasminogen and tissue plasminogen activator *(TPA)* are bound to fibrin during coagulation. TPA converts bound plasminogen to plasmin, which slowly digests fibrin to form fibrin degradation products (FDPs) X, Y, D, E, and D-D *(D-dimer).* D-dimer is produced from cross-linked fibrin. Free plasmin is neutralized by α₂-antiplasmin. TPA is neutralized by plasminogen activator inhibitor-1 *(PAI-1).* Thrombin activatable fibrinolysis inhibitor *(TAFI)* inhibits fibrinolysis by cleaving lysine residues on fibrin, preventing the binding of plasminogen, plasmin, and TPA.

Excessive fibrinolysis can cause bleeding as a result of fibrinogen consumption as well as premature clot lysis before wound healing has been established. On the other hand, inadequate fibrinolysis can lead to clot extension and unwanted thrombosis.

Plasminogen and Plasmin

Plasminogen is a 92,000-Dalton plasma zymogen produced by the liver.[78,79] It is a single-chain protein possessing five glycosylated loops termed kringles. The kringle structure enables plasminogen, along with activators TPA and UPA, to bind the lysine moieties on the fibrin molecule during the polymerization process (Figure 35.17). This fibrin-binding step is essential to fibrinolysis.

Fibrin-bound plasminogen becomes converted into a two-chain active plasmin molecule when cleaved between arginine at position 561 and valine at position 562 by neighboring fibrin-bound TPA or UPA. Plasmin is a serine protease

that systematically digests fibrin polymer by the hydrolysis of arginine-related and lysine-related peptide bonds.[80] As fibrin becomes digested, the exposed carboxy-terminal lysine residues bind additional plasminogen and TPA, which further accelerates clot digestion.[81,82] There is also evidence that FXIa, FXIIa, and kallikrein produce an alternative mechanism of plasminogen activation.[78]

Bound plasmin digests clots and restores blood vessel patency (blood flow). Its localization to fibrin through lysine binding prevents systemic activity. However, free plasmin can be found in the circulation and is capable of digesting plasma fibrinogen, FV, FVIII, and fibronectin. Plasma α₂-antiplasmin rapidly binds and inactivates any free plasmin. A condition known as *primary fibrinolysis* occurs when free plasmin circulates unchecked, breaking down fibrinogen and formed fibrin clots, causing a potentially fatal hemorrhagic outcome.

Plasminogen Activation

Tissue Plasminogen Activator

ECs secrete TPA, which hydrolyzes fibrin-bound plasminogen and converts it to plasmin, thus initiating fibrinolysis. TPA, with two glycosylated kringle regions, forms covalent lysine bonds with fibrin during polymerization. Ultimately, TPA localizes at the surface of the thrombus with plasminogen (see Figure 35.17), where it begins the digestion process by converting plasminogen to plasmin. Circulating TPA is bound to inhibitors such as PAI-1, which results in clearance of the TPA from circulation. Synthetic recombinant TPAs, which mimic natural TPA, are a family of "clot-busting" drugs used to dissolve life- or limb-threatening clots that form in venous and arterial thrombotic disease.

Urokinase Plasminogen Activator

Urinary tract epithelial cells, monocytes, and macrophages secrete another intrinsic plasminogen activator called urokinase plasminogen activator. UPA circulates in plasma at a concentration of 2 to 4 ng/mL and becomes incorporated into the mix of fibrin-bound plasminogen and TPA at the time of thrombus formation (see Figure 35.17). UPA also converts plasminogen to plasmin. However, because it has only one kringle region, UPA does not bind firmly to fibrin and tends to have a lower affinity to plasminogen than TPA, thus having a relatively minor physiologic effect. Purified UPA preparations called urokinases are used therapeutically to dissolve thrombi in patients with myocardial infarction, stroke, and deep vein thrombosis.

Control of Fibrinolysis

The regulation of fibrinolytic activity via plasmin is as equally important as the regulation of thrombin generation on the coagulation side of hemostasis. The control proteins of the fibrinolytic system and their function are depicted in Table 35.12 and Figure 35.16.

Plasminogen Activator Inhibitor-1

PAI-1 is a single-chain glycoprotein serine protease inhibitor that is produced by ECs and several other cells.[17,83] PAI-1 is the principal inhibitor of plasminogen activation and rapidly inactivates both TPA and UPA, preventing them from converting plasminogen to the active fibrinolytic enzyme plasmin. There are two distinct pools of PAI-1, plasma and platelets, both of which are important for fibrinolytic activity. PAI-1 is usually present in excess of the TPA concentration in plasma and circulating TPA normally becomes bound to PAI-1. Only at times of EC activation, such as after trauma, does the level of TPA secretion exceed that of PAI-1 to initiate fibrinolysis. Of note, binding of TPA to fibrin protects TPA from PAI-1 inhibition.[84]

Plasma PAI-1 levels vary widely. PAI-1 deficiency has been associated with chronic mild bleeding caused by increased fibrinolysis. PAI-1 is an acute phase reactant and is increased in many conditions, including metabolic syndrome, obesity, atherosclerosis, sepsis, and stroke.[83] Increased PAI-1 levels correlate with reduced fibrinolytic activity and increased risk of thrombosis.

PAI-2, similar to PAI-1 but coming from the placenta, also binds to TPA and UPA, inhibiting their function and thus preventing fibrinolysis. PAI-2 occurs at high levels during pregnancy, and deficiencies of PAI-2 lead to poor outcomes in pregnancy.[85]

α₂-Antiplasmin

α_2-Antiplasmin (AP) is synthesized in the liver and is the primary inhibitor of free plasmin. AP is a serine protease inhibitor with the unique characteristic of both N- and C-terminal

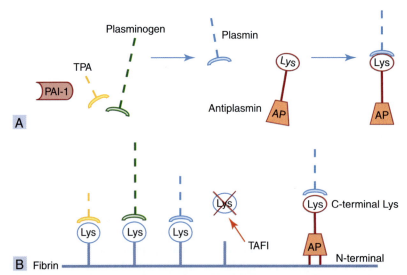

Figure 35.17 Schematic Diagram of the Action of Fibrinolytic Proteins. (**A**, *top*), Tissue plasminogen activator *(TPA)* activates plasminogen to the serine protease, plasmin. TPA is inhibited by plasminogen activator inhibitor-1 *(PAI-1)*. α_2-Antiplasmin *(AP)* rapidly inactivates free plasmin. (**B**, *bottom*), Fibrinolytic proteins TPA, plasminogen, and plasmin bind to C-terminal lysine residues *(Lys)* of fibrin during clotting. Thrombin activatable fibrinolysis inhibitor *(TAFI)* inhibits fibrinolysis by removing the C-terminal Lys from fibrin, thereby reducing binding of fibrinolytic proteins. AP N-terminus is bound to fibrin by factor XIIIa cross-linking. The AP C-terminus Lys competes with fibrin C-terminus Lys to bind plasmin, which will inactivate it.

extensions.[86] During thrombus formation, the N-terminus of AP is covalently linked to fibrin by FXIIIa (see Figure 35.17).[69] The C-terminal contains lysine, which is capable of reacting with the lysine-binding kringles of plasmin. Free plasmin can bind either to fibrin, where it is protected from AP because its lysine-binding site is occupied, or to the C-terminus of AP, which rapidly and irreversibly inactivates it. Thus AP, with its C-terminal lysine, slows fibrinolysis by competing with lysine residues in fibrin for plasminogen binding and also by binding directly to and inactivating plasmin when in circulation.

The therapeutic lysine analogs, tranexamic acid and ε-aminocaproic acid are antifibrinolytic agents through their affinity for kringles in plasminogen and TPA. Both inhibit the proteolytic activity of plasmin, thereby reducing clinical bleeding caused by excess fibrinolysis.

Thrombin Activatable Fibrinolysis Inhibitor

TAFI is a plasma procarboxypeptidase synthesized in the liver that becomes activated by the thrombin-thrombomodulin complex (the same complex of the protein C pathway). Activated TAFI functions as an antifibrinolytic enzyme by cleaving exposed carboxy-terminal lysine residues from partially degraded fibrin. This prevents TPA and plasminogen binding to fibrin, thus blocking the formation of plasmin (see Figure 35.17).[87] In coagulation factor-deficient states, such as hemophilia, decreased thrombin production may reduce the activation of TAFI, resulting in increased fibrinolysis that contributes to more bleeding. Conversely, in thrombotic disorders, increased thrombin generation may increase the activation of TAFI, resulting in decreased fibrinolysis, which may contribute to

further thrombosis. TAFI may also play a role in regulating inflammation and wound healing.[88]

Fibrin Degradation Products and D-Dimer

Fibrinogen and fibrin are cleaved by plasmin, leading to the production of a series of identifiable fragments or degradation products: X, Y, D, E, and D-D (Figure 35.18).[89] Several of these fragments inhibit hemostasis and contribute to hemorrhage by preventing platelet activation and by hindering fibrin polymerization as they compete for fibrinogen binding sites. Fragment X, from fibrinogen digestion, is the central E domain, with the two D domains (D-E-D) of fibrinogen, minus some peptides cleaved by plasmin. Fragment Y (D-E), also from fibrinogen digestion, is formed after cleavage of one D domain from fragment X. Eventually these fragments are further digested to individual D and E domains.

Fragments X, Y, D, and E are also produced by digestion of fibrin by plasmin. Elevated levels of these fragments indicate plasmin activity, nonspecific to fibrin or fibrinogen. In addition, however, other types of fragment variations are produced from the breakdown of the conjoined fibrin monomers. The *D-dimer* fragment is a specific product of digestion of cross-linked fibrin only. The D-D fragment, called D-dimer, is composed of two D domains from separate fibrin molecules (not fibrinogen) cross-linked by the action of FXIIIa. Thus D-dimer is generated by thrombin, FXIIIa, *and* plasmin activity, and is a marker of thrombosis *and* fibrinolysis.[90] Assessing D-dimer levels is an important diagnostic tool in identifying disseminated intravascular coagulation and ruling out venous thromboembolism and pulmonary embolism.[91]

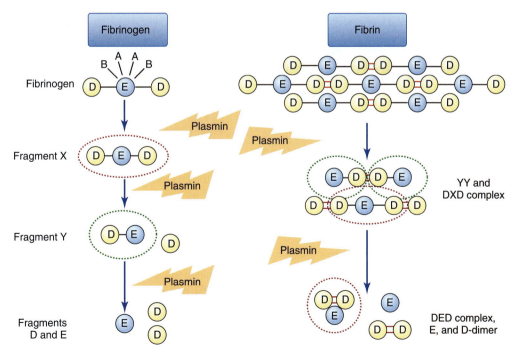

Figure 35.18 Fibrinolysis: Degradation of Fibrinogen and Fibrin by Plasmin. Plasmin systematically degrades fibrinogen and fibrin by cleaving off small peptides and digesting D-E domains. From fibrinogen, fragment X consists of a central E domain with two D domains (D-E-D); further cleavage produces fragment Y (D-E), with eventual degradation to D and E domains. From cross-linked, stabilized fibrin (note *double red line* on the D domains), plasmin digestion produces fragment complexes from one or more monomers. D-dimer consists of two D domains from adjacent monomers that have been cross-linked by factor XIIIa in the process of fibrin formation.

SUMMARY

- The tunica intima, platelets, tissue factor (TF)–bearing cells, and coagulation and fibrinolytic proteins interact to maintain hemostasis.
- Intact tunica intima prevents coagulation through synthesis of prostacyclin, nitric oxide, tissue factor pathway inhibitor (TFPI), thrombomodulin, and heparan sulfate.
- Damaged intima promotes coagulation by vasoconstriction, exposure of TF and collagen, and secretion of von Willebrand factor (VWF) and other adhesion molecules.
- Platelets function in primary and secondary hemostasis through adhesion, aggregation, secretion of granular contents, and exposure of phosphatidylserine on activation.
- Platelets adhere to collagen through VWF and aggregate through fibrinogen binding.
- Most coagulation factors are synthesized in the liver.
- The plasma factors of the prothrombin group (prothrombin; factors VII, IX, and X; protein C; protein S; and protein Z) require vitamin K in their production.
- Plasma coagulation factors include trypsinlike enzymes called serine proteases and cofactors that stabilize the proteases with the exception of factor XIIIa, which is a transglutaminase.
- The extrinsic pathway of coagulation consists of the membrane receptor TF and coagulation factors VII, X, V, II, and fibrinogen. Prothrombin time (PT) is a screening test for these factors.
- The intrinsic pathway factors are XII, prekallikrein (pre-K), high-molecular-weight kininogen (HMWK), XI, IX, VIII, X, V, II, and fibrinogen. Partial thromboplastin time (PTT, APTT) is a screening test for these factors.
- Coagulation factors in the extrinsic pathway and the intrinsic pathway, combined with ionized calcium and platelet phospholipid, form complexes that enhance the enzymatic activity.
- In vivo, coagulation is initiated on TF-bearing cells. TF:VIIa activates factors IX and X, generating enough thrombin to activate platelets and factors V, VIII, and XI. The latter step acts to amplify the generation of a larger amount of thrombin. Coagulation proceeds on activated platelet phospholipid membranes with the formation of IXa:VIIIa and Xa:Va complexes, which produce a burst of thrombin that cleaves fibrinogen to fibrin.
- Activation of coagulation pathways ultimately produces thrombin, which converts fibrinogen to a fibrin monomer. Thrombin also activates platelets and factors V, VIII, XI, and XIII, and binds to thrombomodulin to activate protein C and thrombin activatable fibrinolysis inhibitor (TAFI).
- Fibrinogen is cleaved by thrombin to form a fibrin monomer first; then it becomes a fibrin polymer, and finally, when acted on by factor XIIIa, results in cross-linked fibrin.
- The coagulation pathway is regulated by activated protein C (APC), TFPI, and the serpins, including antithrombin and protein Z–dependent protease inhibitor (ZPI). These control proteins prevent excessive thrombin generation and thus thrombosis, and confine clotting to the site of injury.
- The fibrinolytic pathway digests the thrombus. Plasminogen is converted to plasmin mostly by tissue plasminogen activator (TPA). Plasmin degrades fibrin to fragments X, Y, D, and E, and D-dimer. Control proteins are plasminogen activator inhibitor (PAI)-1, α_2-antiplasmin, and TAFI. Plasmin will also digest fibrinogen.

Now that you have completed this chapter, go back and read again the case study at the beginning and respond to the questions presented.

REVIEW QUESTIONS

Answers can be found in Appendix C.

1. What intimal cell synthesizes and stores von Willebrand factor (VWF)?
   a. Smooth muscle cell
   b. Endothelial cell
   c. Fibroblast
   d. Platelet

2. What subendothelial structural protein triggers coagulation through activation of factor VII?
   a. Thrombomodulin
   b. Nitric oxide
   c. Tissue factor
   d. Thrombin

3. What coagulation plasma protein should be assayed when platelets fail to aggregate properly?
   a. Factor VIII
   b. Fibrinogen
   c. Thrombin
   d. Factor X

4. What is the primary role of vitamin K for the prothrombin group factors?
   a. Provides a surface on which the proteolytic reactions of the factors occur
   b. Protects them from inappropriate activation by compounds such as thrombin
   c. Accelerates the binding of the serine proteases and their cofactors
   d. Carboxylates the factors to allow calcium binding

5. What is the source of prothrombin fragment F1+2?
   a. Plasmin proteolysis of fibrin polymer
   b. Thrombin proteolysis of fibrinogen
   c. Proteolysis of prothrombin by factor Xa
   d. Plasmin proteolysis of cross-linked fibrin

6. What serine protease forms a complex with factor VIIIa, and what is the substrate of this complex?
   a. Factor VIIa, factor X
   b. Factor Va, prothrombin
   c. Factor Xa, prothrombin
   d. Factor IXa, factor X

7. What protein secreted by endothelial cells activates fibrinolysis?
   a. Plasminogen
   b. TPA
   c. PAI-1
   d. TAFI

8. What two regulatory proteins form a complex that digests activated factors V and VIII?
   a. TFPI and Xa
   b. Antithrombin and protein C
   c. APC and protein S
   d. Thrombomodulin and plasmin

9. What are the primary roles of VWF?
   a. Inhibit excess coagulation and activate protein C
   b. Activate plasmin and promote lysis of fibrinogen
   c. Mediate platelet adhesion and serve as a carrier molecule for factor VIII
   d. Mediate platelet aggregation via the GPIIb/IIIa receptor

10. Most coagulation factors are synthesized in:
    a. The liver
    b. Monocytes
    c. Endothelial cells
    d. Megakaryocytes

11. The events involved in secondary hemostasis:
    a. Lead to the formation of a stable fibrin clot
    b. Usually occur independently of primary hemostasis
    c. Occur in a random fashion
    d. Are the first line of defense against blood loss

12. Which of the following coagulation factors is activated by thrombin and mediates the stabilization of the fibrin clot?
    a. Tissue factor
    b. Factor VII
    c. Factor IX
    d. Factor XIII

13. Which of the following endogenous plasma inhibitors is (are) important for the control of excessive thrombin generation?
    a. AT, TFPI
    b. Platelet factor 4
    c. TAT, F1+2
    d. a and b

REFERENCES

1. Aird, W. C. (2003). Hemostasis and irreducible complexity. *J Thromb Haemost, 1*, 227–230.
2. Collen, D., & Lijnen, H. R. (2004). Tissue-type plasminogen activator: a historical perspective and personal account. *J Thromb Haemost, 2*, 541–546.
3. Ruggeri, Z. M. (2003). Von Willebrand factor, platelets and endothelial cell interactions. *J Thromb Haemost, 1*, 1335–1342.
4. Aird, W. C. (2007). Phenotypic heterogeneity of the endothelium: structure, function, and mechanisms. *Circ Res, 100,* 158–173.
5. Aird, W. C. (2007). Phenotypic heterogeneity of the endothelium: representative vascular beds. *Circ Res, 100*, 174–190.
6. Kazmi, R. S., Boyce, S., & Lwaleed, B. A. (2015). Homeostasis of hemostasis: the role of endothelium. *Semin Thromb Hemost, 41*, 549–555.
7. Mitchell, J. A., Ferhana, A., Bailey, L., et al. (2008). Role of nitric oxide and prostacyclin as vasoactive hormones released by the endothelium. *Exp Physiol, 93*, 141–147.
8. Neubauer, K., & Zieger, B. (2021). Endothelial cells and coagulation. *Cell and Tissue Research, 387*, 391–398.
9. Looft-Wilson, R. C., Billaud, M., Johnstone, S. R., et al. (2012). Interaction between nitric oxide signaling and gap junctions: effects on vascular function. *Biochim Biophys Acta, 1818*(8), 1895–1902.
10. Moncada, S. P., Palmer, R. M. J., & Higgs, A. J. (1991). Nitric oxide: physiology, pathophysiology and pharmacology. *Pharmacol Rev, 43*, 109–142.
11. Huntington, J. A. (2003). Mechanisms of glycosaminoglycan activation of the serpins in hemostasis. *J Thromb Haemost, 1*, 1535–1549.
12. Furlan, M. (1996). Von Willebrand factor: molecular size and functional activity. *Ann Hematol, 72*(6), 341–348.
13. Bevilacqua, M. P., & Nelson, R. M. (1993). Selectins. *J Clin Invest, 91*, 379–387.
14. Kansas, G. S. (1996). Selectins and their ligands: current concepts and controversies. *Blood, 88*, 3259–3287.
15. Mackman, N., Tilley, R. A., & Key, N. S. (2007). Role of the extrinsic pathway of blood coagulation in hemostasis and thrombosis. *Arterioscler Thromb Vasc Biol, 27*, 1687–1693.
16. Chernysh, I. N., Nagaswami, C., Kosolapova, S., et al. (2020). The distinctive structure and composition of arterial and venous thrombi and pulmonary emboli. *Nature Research Scientific Reports, 10*, 5112–5124.
17. Dellas, C., & Loskutoff, D. J. (2005). Historical analysis of PAI-1 from its discovery to its potential role in cell motility and disease. *Thromb Haemost, 93*, 631–640.
18. Foley, J. H., Kim, P. Y., Mutch, N. J., et al. (2013). Insights into thrombin activatable fibrinolysis inhibitor function and regulation. *J Thromb Haemost, 11*(Suppl. 1), 306–315.
19. Polgar, J., Matuskova, J., & Wagner, D. D. (2005). The P-selectin, tissue factor, coagulation triad. *J Thromb Haemost, 3*, 1590–1596.
20. Bordé, E. C., & Vainchenker, W. (2012). Platelet production: cellular and molecular regulation. In Marder, V. J., Aird, W. C., Bennett, J. S., et al. (Eds.), *Hemostasis and Thrombosis: Basic Principles and Clinical Practice.* (6th ed., pp. 349–364). Philadelphia: Lippincott.
21. Fritsma, G. A. (1988). Platelet production and structure. In Corriveau, D. M., & Fritsma, G. A. (Eds.), *Hemostasis and Thrombosis in the Clinical Laboratory.* (pp. 206–228). Philadelphia: Lippincott.
22. Bennett, J. S. (2012). Overview of megakaryocyte and platelet biology. In Marder, V. J., Aird, W. C., Bennett, J. S., et al. (Eds.), *Hemostasis and Thrombosis: Basic Principles and Clinical Practice.* (6th ed., pp. 341–348). Philadelphia: Lippincott.
23. Abrams, C. S., & Brass, L. F. (2012). Platelet signal transduction. In Marder, V. J., Aird, W. C., Bennett, J. S., et al. (Eds.), *Hemostasis and Thrombosis: Basic Principles and Clinical Practice.* (6th ed., pp. 449–461). Philadelphia: Lippincott.

24. Berndt, M. C., & Andrews, R. K. (2012). Major platelet glycoproteins. GP Ib/IX/V. In Marder, V. J., Aird, W. C., Bennett, J. S., et al. (Eds.), *Hemostasis and Thrombosis: Basic Principles and Clinical Practice.* (6th ed., pp. 382–385). Philadelphia: Lippincott.

25. Ye, F., & Ginsberg, M. H. (2012). Major platelet glycoproteins. Integrin α2b β3 (GP IIb/IIIa). In Marder, V. J., Aird, W. C., Bennett, J. S., et al. (Eds.), *Hemostasis and Thrombosis: Basic Principles and Clinical Practice.* (6th ed., pp. 386–392). Philadelphia: Lippincott.

26. Sang, Y., Roest, M., de Laat, B., et al. (2021). Interplay between platelets and coagulation. *Blood Rev, 46,* 100733–100744.

27. Blair, P., & Flaumenhaft, R. (2009). Platelet α–granules: basic biology and clinical correlates. *Blood Rev, 23*(4), 177–189.

28. Rao, A. K. (2013). Inherited platelet function disorders: overview and disorders of granules, secretion, and signal transduction. *Hematol Oncol Clin North Am, 27,* 585–611.

29. Walsh, P. N. (2012). Role of platelets in blood coagulation. In Marder, V. J., Aird, W. C., Bennett, J. S., et al. (Eds.), *Hemostasis and Thrombosis: Basic Principles and Clinical Practice.* (6th ed., pp. 468–474). Philadelphia: Lippincott.

30. Alamin, A. A. (2021). The role of red blood cells in hemostasis. *Semin Thromb Hemost, 47,* 26–31.

31. Zarbock, A., Polanowska-Grabowska, R. K., & Ley, K. (2007). Platelet-neutrophil-interactions: linking hemostasis and inflammation. *Blood Rev, 21,* 99–111.

32. Onundarson, P. T., Palsson, R., Witt, D. M., et al. (2021). Replacement of traditional prothrombin time monitoring with the new FIIX prothrombin time increases the efficacy of warfarin without increasing bleeding. *Thrombosis J, 19,* 72–82.

33. Sherry, S. (1990). The founding of the International Society on Thrombosis and Haemostasis: how it came about. *Thromb Haemost, 64,* 188–191.

34. Saito, H. (1996). Normal hemostatic mechanisms. In Ratnoff, O. D., & Forbes, C. D. (Eds.), *Disorders of Hemostasis.* (3rd ed., pp. 23–52). Philadelphia: Saunders.

35. Coughlin, S. R. (2005). Protease-activated receptors in hemostasis, thrombosis and vascular biology. *J Thromb Haemost, 3,* 1800–1814.

36. Kretz, C. A., Vaezzadeh, N., & Gross, P. L. (2010). Tissue factor and thrombosis models. *Arterioscler Thromb Vasc Biol, 30,* 900–908.

37. Mosesson, M. W. (2005). Fibrinogen and fibrin structure and functions. *J Thromb Haemost, 3,* 1894–1904.

38. Greenberg, D. L., & Davie, E. W. (2006). The blood coagulation factors: their complementary DNAs, genes, and expression. In Colman, R. W., Marder, V. J., Clowes, A. M., et al. (Eds.), *Hemostasis and Thrombosis: Basic Principles and Clinical Practice.* (5th ed., pp. 21–58). Philadelphia: Lippincott.

39. Lane, D. A., Philippou, H., & Huntington, J. A. (2005). Directing thrombin. *Blood, 106,* 2605–2612.

40. Mann, K. G., Saulius, B., & Brummel, K. (2003). The dynamics of thrombin formation. *Arterioscler Thromb Vasc Biol, 23,* 17–25.

41. Shahani, T., Lavend'homme, R., Luttun, A., et al. (2010). Activation of human endothelial cells from specific vascular beds induces the release of a FVIII storage pool. *Blood, 115*(23), 4902–4909.

42. Scott, E., Puca, K., Heraly, J., et al. (2009). Evaluation and comparison of coagulation factor activity in fresh-frozen plasma and 24-hour plasma at thaw and after 120 hours of 1-6° C storage. *Transfusion, 49*(8), 1584–1591.

43. Jacquemin, M., De Maeyer, M., D'Oiron, R., et al. (2003). Molecular mechanisms of mild and moderate hemophilia A. *J Thromb Haemost, 1,* 456–463.

44. Sadler, J. E. (1991). Von Willebrand factor. *J Biol Chem, 266,* 22777–22780.

45. Blann, A. D. (2006). Plasma von Willebrand factor, thrombosis, and the endothelium: the first 30 years. *Thromb Haemost, 95,* 49–55.

46. Tsai, H. M. (2006). ADAMTS13 and microvascular thrombosis. *Expert Rev Cardiovasc Ther, 4,* 813–825.

47. Gill, J. C., Endres-Brooks, J., Bauer, P. J., et al. (1987). The effect of ABO group on the diagnosis of von Willebrand disease. *Blood, 69,* 1691–1695.

48. Wu, Y. (2015). Contact pathway of coagulation and inflammation. *Thrombosis J, 13,* 17–26.

49. Didiasovaa, M., Wujaka, L., Schaeferb, L., et al. (2018). Factor XII in coagulation, inflammation and beyond. *Cell Signal, 51,* 257–265.

50. Tillman, B. F., Gruber, A., McCarty, O. J. T., et al. (2018). Plasma contact factors as therapeutic targets. *Blood Rev, 32*(6), 433–448.

51. Weidmann, H., Heikaus, L., Long, A. T., et al. (2017). The plasma contact system, a protease cascade at the nexus of inflammation, coagulation, and immunity. *BBA – Molecular Cell Research, 1864,* 2118–2127.

52. Roberts, H. R., & Escobar, M. A. (2013). Less common congenital disorders of hemostasis. In Kitchens, C. S., Konkle, B. A., Kessler, C. M., et al. (Eds.), *Consultative Hemostasis and Thrombosis.* (2nd ed., pp. 60–78). Philadelphia: Saunders.

53. Harrison, P., Wilborn, B., Devilli, N., et al. (1989). Uptake of plasma fibrinogen into the alpha granules of human megakaryocytes and platelets. *J Clin Invest, 84,* 1320–1324.

54. Lorand, L. (2005). Factor XIII and the clotting of fibrinogen: from basic research to medicine. *J Thromb Haemost, 3,* 1337–1348.

55. Corriveau, D. M. (1988). Major elements of hemostasis. In Corriveau, D. M., & Fritsma, G. A. (Eds.), *Hemostasis and Thrombosis in the Clinical Laboratory.* (pp. 1–33). Philadelphia: Lippincott.

56. Monroe, D. M., & Hoffman, M. (2006). What does it take to make the perfect clot? *Arterioscler Thromb Vasc Biol, 26,* 41–48.

57. Hoffman, M. (2003). Remodeling the blood coagulation cascade. *J Thromb Thrombolysis, 16,* 17–20.

58. Mann, K. G., Brummel, K., & Butenas, S. (2003). What is all that thrombin for? *J Thromb Haemost, 1,* 1504–1514.

59. Morrissey, J. H., Macik, B. G., Neuenschwander, P. F., et al. (1993). Quantitation of activated factor VII levels in plasma using a tissue factor mutant selectively deficient in promoting factor VII activation. *Blood, 81,* 734–744.

60. Hoffman, M., & Monroe, D. M. (2007). Coagulation 2006: a modern view of hemostasis. *Hematol Oncol Clin North Am, 21,* 1–11.

61. Golino, P. (2002). The inhibitors of the tissue factor: factor VII pathway. *Thromb Res, 106,* V257–V265.

62. Hoffman, M., & Cichon, L. J. H. (2013). Practical coagulation for the blood banker. *Transfusion, 53,* 1594–1602.

63. Dahlback, B. (1995). The protein C anticoagulant system: inherited defects as basis for venous thrombosis. *Thromb Res, 77,* 1–43.

64. Taylor, F. B., Jr., Peer, G. T., Lockhart, M. S., et al. (2001). Endothelial cell protein C receptor plays an important role in protein C activation in vivo. *Blood, 97,* 1685–1688.

65. Van Hinsbergh, V. W. M. (2012). Endothelium-role in regulation of coagulation and inflammation. *Semin Immunopathol, 34,* 93–106.

66. Griffin, J. H., Gruber, A., & Fernandez, J. A. (1992). Reevaluation of total free, free, and bound protein S and C4b-binding protein levels in plasma anticoagulated with citrate or hirudin. *Blood, 79,* 3203–3211.

67. Price, V. E., Ledingham, D. L., Krumpel, A., et al. (2011). Diagnosis and management of neonatal purpura fulminans. *Semin Fetal Neonatal Med, 16*, 318–322.

68. de Moerloose, P., Bounameaux, H. R., & Mannucci, P. M. (1998). Screening test for thrombophilic patients: which tests, for which patient, by whom, when, and why? *Semin Thromb Hemost, 24*, 321–327.

69. Rau, J. C., Beaulieu, L. M., Huntington, J. A., et al. (2007). Serpins in thrombosis, hemostasis and fibrinolysis. *J Thromb Haemost, 5*(Suppl. 1), 102–115.

70. Bock, S. (2013). Antithrombin and the serpin family. In Marder, V. J., Aird, W. C., Bennett, J. S., et al. (Eds.), *Hemostasis and Thrombosis: Basic Principles and Clinical Practice.* (6th ed., pp. 286–299). Philadelphia: Lippincott.

71. Broze, G. J., Jr., & Girard, T. J. (2013). Tissue factor pathway inhibitor: structure-function. *Front Biosci, 17*, 262–280.

72. Lwaleed, B. A., & Bass, P. S. (2006). Tissue factor pathway inhibitor: structure, biology, and involvement in disease. *J Pathol, 208*, 327–339.

73. Monroe, D. M., & Key, N. S. (2007). The tissue factor-factor VIIa complex: procoagulant activity, regulation, and multitasking. *J Thromb Haemost, 5*, 1097–1105.

74. Hakeng, T. M., & Rosing, J. (2009). Protein S as cofactor for TFPI. *Arterioscler Thromb Vasc Biol, 29*, 2015–2020.

75. Corral, J., Gonzalez-Conejero, R., Hernandez-Espinosa, D., et al. (2007). Protein Z/Z-dependent protease inhibitor (PZ/ZPI) anticoagulant system and thrombosis. *Br J Haematol, 137*(2), 99–108.

76. Broze, G. J., Jr. (2001). Protein Z-dependent regulation of coagulation. *Thromb Haemost, 86*, 8–13.

77. Chung, D. W., Xu, W., & Davie, E. W. (2013). The blood coagulation factors and inhibitors: their primary structure, complementary DNAs, genes, and expression. In Marder, V. J., Aird, W. C., Bennett, J. S., et al. (Eds.), *Hemostasis and Thrombosis: Basic Principles and Clinical Practice.* (6th ed., pp. 110–145). Philadelphia: Lippincott.

78. Mutch, N. J., & Booth, N. A. (2013). Plasminogen activation and regulation of fibrinolysis. In Marder, V. J., Aird, W. C., Bennett, J. S., et al. (Eds.), *Hemostasis and Thrombosis: Basic Principles and Clinical Practice.* (6th ed., pp. 314–333). Philadelphia: Lippincott.

79. Bennett, B., & Ogston, D. (1996). Fibrinolytic bleeding syndromes. In Ratnoff, O. D., & Forbes, C. D. (Eds.), *Disorders of Hemostasis.* (3rd ed., pp. 296–322). Philadelphia: Saunders.

80. Kolev, K., & Machovich, R. (2003). Molecular and cellular modulation of fibrinolysis. *Thromb Haemost, 89*, 610–621.

81. Fay, W. P., Garg, N., & Sunkar, M. (2007). Vascular functions of the plasminogen activation system. *Arterioscler Thromb Vasc Biol, 27*, 1231–1237.

82. Esmon, C. T., & Esmon, N. L. (2013). Regulatory mechanisms in hemostasis. In Hoffman, R., Benz, E. J., Silberstein, L. E., et al. (Eds.), *Hematology: Basic Principles and Practice.* (6th ed., pp. 1842–1846). Philadelphia: Elsevier.

83. Cesari, M., Pahor, M., & Incalzi, R. A. (2010). Plasminogen activator inhibitor-1 (PAI-1): a key factor linking fibrinolysis and age-related subclinical and clinical conditions. *Cardiovasc Ther, 28*, 72–91.

84. Weisel, J. W., & Dempfle, C. (2013). Fibrinogen structure and function. In Marder, V. J., Aird, W. C., Bennett, J. S., et al. (Eds.), *Hemostasis and Thrombosis: Basic Principles and Clinical Practice.* (6th ed., pp. 254–271). Philadelphia: Lippincott.

85. Chapin, J. C., & Hajjar, K. A. (2015). Fibrinolysis and the control of blood coagulation. *Blood Rev, 29*(1), 17–24.

86. Coughlin, P. B. (2005). Antiplasmin: the forgotten serpin? *FEBS J, 272*, 4852–4857.

87. Bouma, B. N., & Meijers, J. C. M. (2003). Thrombin-activatable fibrinolysis inhibitor (TAFI, plasma procarboxypeptidase B, procarboxypeptidase R, procarboxypeptidase U). *J Thromb Haemost, 1*, 1566–1574.

88. Bouma, B. N., & Mosnier, L. O. (2003/2004). Thrombin activatable fibrinolysis inhibitor (TAFI) at the interface between coagulation and fibrinolysis. *Pathophysiol Haemost Thromb, 33*, 375–381.

89. Lowe, G. D. (2005). Circulating inflammatory markers and risks of cardiovascular and non-cardiovascular disease. *J Thromb Haemost, 3*, 1618–1627.

90. Adam, S. S., Key, N. S., & Greenberg, C. S. (2009). D-dimer antigen: current concepts and future prospects. *Blood, 113*, 2878–2887.

91. Geersing, G. J., Janssen, K. J. M., Oudega, R., et al. (2009). Excluding venous thromboembolism using point of care D-dimer tests in outpatients: a diagnostic meta-analysis. *BMJ, 339*, b2990.

36

Hemorrhagic Disorders and Laboratory Assessment

Mayukh Kanti Sarkar and George A. Fritsma

OBJECTIVES

After completion of this chapter, the reader will be able to:

1. Distinguish among the causes of localized versus generalized, anatomic versus mucocutaneous, and acquired versus congenital bleeding.
2. List and interpret laboratory tests to differentiate among acquired hemorrhagic disorders of trauma, liver disease, vitamin K deficiency, and kidney failure.
3. Discuss the laboratory monitoring of therapy for acquired hemorrhagic disorders.
4. Interpret laboratory assay results to diagnose, subtype, and monitor the treatment of von Willebrand disease.

5. Use the results of laboratory tests to identify and monitor the treatment of congenital single coagulation factor deficiencies such as deficiencies of factors VIII, IX, and XI.
6. Explain the principle and rationale for the use of each laboratory test for the detection and monitoring of hemorrhagic disorders.
7. Given clinical history and laboratory test results for patients with hemorrhagic disorders, suggest a diagnosis that is consistent with the information provided.

OUTLINE

Bleeding Symptoms
  Localized Versus Generalized Hemorrhage
  Mucocutaneous Versus Anatomic Hemorrhage
  Acquired Versus Congenital Bleeding Disorders
Acquired Coagulopathies
  Trauma-Induced Coagulopathy
  Liver Disease Coagulopathy
  Chronic Renal Failure and Hemorrhage
  Vitamin K Deficiency and Hemorrhage
  Auto-Anti-Factor VIII Inhibitor and Acquired
    Hemophilia A

  Additional Factor Inhibitors
  Acquired von Willebrand Disease
  Disseminated Intravascular Coagulation
Congenital Coagulopathies
  von Willebrand Disease
  Hemophilia A (Factor VIII Deficiency)
  Hemophilia B (Factor IX Deficiency)
  Hemophilia C (Rosenthal Syndrome, Factor XI
    Deficiency)
  Other Congenital Single-Factor Deficiencies

CASE STUDY

After studying the material in this chapter, the reader should be able to respond to the following case study. Answers can be found in Appendix C.

A 55-year-old male came to the emergency department with epistaxis (uncontrolled nosebleed). He reported that he has "bleeder's disease" and has had multiple episodes of inflammatory hemarthroses (joint bleeding). Physical examination revealed swollen, immobilized knees; mild jaundice; and an enlarged liver and spleen. CBC results indicated that the patient was anemic and had thrombocytopenia with a PLT count of 74,400/μL The PT was 18 seconds, and the PTT was 43 seconds. Reference intervals can be found after the Index at the end of the book.

1. What is the most likely diagnosis?
2. What treatment does the patient need?

BLEEDING SYMPTOMS

Though most bleeding occurs as the result of an injury, bleeding may take the form of easy or spontaneous bruising, internal bleeds, or hemorrhage. *Hemorrhage* is excessive bleeding that requires medical or physical intervention. Bleeding may be *local* or *general, mucocutaneous* or *anatomic, acquired* or *congenital*. If congenital, bleeding may result from *primary* (platelet-related)

or *secondary* (coagulation factor-related) hemostasis disorders or from unregulated *fibrinolysis,* in which clots are rapidly metabolized. Congenital hemorrhage may be provoked or spontaneous.

Except in emergent situations, the provider reviews the health record; conducts a comprehensive interview to document the patient's history, including a bleeding assessment tool (BAT), which documents epistaxis, bruising, gastrointestinal bleeding, menorrhagia, and up to 10 additional symptoms; and conducts a physical examination to establish the probable cause of a bleeding event or a patient's bleeding tendency before ordering diagnostic laboratory tests.[1] In most instances, the hemostasis laboratory contributes substantially to the diagnosis, provided that the provider judiciously selects laboratory tests on the basis of well-defined indications.[2]

Localized Versus Generalized Hemorrhage

Bleeding from a single location usually indicates injury, infection, tumor, or an isolated blood vessel defect and is called *localized bleeding* or localized hemorrhage. An example of localized bleeding is an inadequately cauterized or ineffectively sutured surgical site or an abnormal tangle of blood vessels in the capillary bed known as an arteriovenous malformation (AVM). Except for AVMs, localized bleeding seldom implies a blood vessel defect.

In contrast, a qualitative platelet defect, a reduced platelet count (thrombocytopenia), and a coagulation factor deficiency cause *generalized* and not localized bleeding. Bleeding from multiple sites, spontaneous and recurring bleeds, or a hemorrhage that requires physical intervention is generalized bleeding. Generalized bleeding is potential evidence for a disorder of *primary hemostasis,* such as a blood vessel or platelet defect, or thrombocytopenia (Chapters 37 and 38), or *secondary hemostasis,* characterized by single or multiple coagulation factor deficiencies or uncontrolled fibrinolysis (Chapter 35).

Mucocutaneous Versus Anatomic Hemorrhage

Generalized bleeding may exhibit either a mucocutaneous (in skin or at body orifices) or an anatomic (in muscles, central nervous system, joints, deep tissue) pattern. *Mucocutaneous* bleeding into the skin may appear as *petechiae,* red pinpoint spots (Figure 38.1A); *purpura,* purple skin lesions greater than 3 mm diameter (Figure 38.1B); or *ecchymoses* (bruises) greater than 1 cm, typically seen after trauma (Figure 38.1C).[3] The unprovoked presence of more than one such lesion may indicate a disorder of primary hemostasis. Other symptoms of a primary hemostasis defect include bleeding from the gums, epistaxis (uncontrolled nosebleed), hematemesis (vomiting of blood), blood in the urine or stool, and menorrhagia (profuse menstrual flow). Although nosebleeds are common and mostly innocuous, especially in children, they suggest a primary hemostatic defect when they occur repeatedly, last longer than 10 minutes, involve both nostrils, or require physical intervention or blood products.

Mucocutaneous hemorrhage is most likely to be associated with thrombocytopenia (platelet count less than 20,000/μL) (Chapter 38), qualitative platelet disorders, vascular disorders such as scurvy or telangiectasia (Chapter 37), or von Willebrand disease (VWD). A thorough patient history and physical examination may distinguish between mucocutaneous and anatomic bleeding; this distinction helps direct investigative laboratory testing and subsequent treatment.

Anatomic hemorrhage is seen in acquired or congenital defects in secondary hemostasis such as plasma coagulation factor deficiencies (coagulopathies).[4] Examples of anatomic bleeding include recurrent or excessive bleeding after minor trauma, dental extraction, or a surgical procedure. In such cases, hemorrhage may immediately follow a primary event, but it is often delayed or recurs minutes or hours after the event. Anatomic bleeding

episodes may even be spontaneous. Many anatomic bleeds are internal, such as bleeds into joints, body cavities, muscles, or the central nervous system, and may have few initially discernible signs. Joint bleeds (hemarthroses) cause swelling and acute pain. They may not be immediately perceived as hemorrhages, although patients with hemophilia who have experienced joint bleeds usually recognize the symptoms at their onset. Recurrent hemarthroses cause inflammation that may culminate in permanent cartilage damage that immobilizes the joint. Bleeds into muscle or fat may cause nerve compression and subsequent temporary or permanent loss of function.[5] When bleeding involves body cavities, it causes symptoms related to the affected organ. Bleeding into the central nervous system, for instance, may cause headaches, confusion, seizures, and coma, and is managed as a medical emergency. Bleeds into the kidney may present as hematuria and may be associated with acute renal failure.

Hemostasis laboratory testing is essential whenever a mucocutaneous or anatomic bleed is detected. Box 36.1 lists generalized symptoms that suggest a hemorrhagic disorder. Besides a complete blood count that includes a platelet count, laboratory directors offer the prothrombin time (PT), partial

---

BOX 36.1 Generalized Bleeding Signs Heralding a Possible Hemostatic Defect

Purpura—recurrent, chronic bruising in multiple locations; called petechiae when <3 mm, purpura when 3 mm to 1 cm, and ecchymoses when >1 cm in diameter
Epistaxis—nosebleeds that are recurrent, bleed from both nostrils, last longer than 10 minutes, or require physical intervention
Recurrent or excessive bleeding from trauma, surgery, or dental extraction
Bleeding into body cavities, muscles, fatty tissues, joints, or central nervous system
Simultaneous bleeding from several sites
Menorrhagia (menstrual hemorrhage)
Bleeding that is delayed or recurrent
Bleeding that is inappropriately brisk
Bleeding for no apparent reason
Hematemesis (vomiting of blood)

TABLE 36.1 Primary (Initial, First-Level) Assays for a Generalized Hemostatic Disorder

Assay	Assesses
Hemoglobin, hematocrit; reticulocyte count	Anemia associated with chronic bleeding or a hemolytic anemia; bone marrow response
Platelet count	Thrombocytopenia or thrombocytosis
Prothrombin time (PT)	Clotting time prolonged in FII (prothrombin), FV, FVII, and FX deficiency
Partial thromboplastin time (PTT, APTT)	Clotting time prolonged in all factor deficiencies except FVII and FXIII
Thrombin time (TT)	Followup (reflex) assay, prolonged by unfractionated heparin therapy, dysfibrinogenemia, hypofibrinogenemia, and afibrinogenemia
Quantitative fibrinogen assay	Reduced in dysfibrinogenemia, hypofibrinogenemia, and afibrinogenemia
Viscoelastometry	Global whole blood assay measures clotting time, clot strength, fibrinogen, and platelet function; Thromboelastograph, ROTEM, Quantra

F, Factor.

thromboplastin time (PTT, also known as activated partial thromboplastin time [APTT]), and fibrinogen assay (Table 36.1).[6] The thrombin time (TT) (also known as thrombin clotting time [TCT]) is occasionally used as a reflex assay or internal control. Some laboratory practitioners add viscoelastometry (VET), employing one of several near-patient whole blood coagulometers such as TEG, Quantra, or ROTEM (Chapter 42). VET is a global near-patient hemostasis testing method that reports clot onset, clot dynamics, clot strength, and fibrinolysis in 15 to 30 minutes. VET results require interpretation by experienced practitioners.[7]

Acquired Versus Congenital Bleeding Disorders

Liver disease, kidney failure, chronic infections, autoimmune disorders, obstetric complications, anemia, dietary deficiencies such as vitamin C or vitamin K deficiency, blunt or penetrating trauma, and inflammatory disorders all may be associated with *acquired* bleeding. If a patient's bleeding episodes begin early in childhood, are not associated with some disease or physical trauma, and are duplicated in relatives, they are probably *congenital*.

When an adult patient seeks treatment of generalized hemorrhage, the provider first looks for an underlying condition, disease, drug effect, or event and records a personal and family history (Box 36.2). The important elements of patient history are age, sex, current or past pregnancy, a chronic disorder such as diabetes or cancer, trauma, and exposure to drugs (including prescription drugs, over-the-counter nutritional supplements, drugs of abuse, and excessive alcohol [as in alcohol addiction]). The provider determines the trigger, location, and volume of bleeding and then orders a set of initial hemostasis laboratory assays (see Table 36.1). These tests take on clinical significance when the history and physical examination (employing a BAT) have already established the existence of abnormal bleeding. Because of their propensity to generate false-positive results in the absence of indications, hemostatic laboratory tests are ineffective when employed indiscriminately as population screens of healthy individuals (Chapter 3).[8]

Congenital hemorrhagic disorders are uncommon, occurring in fewer than 1 per 100 people, and are usually diagnosed in infancy or during the first years of life.[9] There may be first-degree relatives with similar symptoms. Congenital bleeding disorders lead to recurrent hemorrhages that may be spontaneous or may occur after minor injury or in unexpected locations, such as joints, body cavities, retinal veins and arteries, or the central nervous system. Patients with mild congenital hemorrhagic disorders may have no symptoms until they reach adulthood or experience some physical challenge, such as trauma, dental extraction, or a surgical procedure. The most common congenital deficiencies are VWD, factor VIII (FVIII) deficiency (hemophilia A), factor IX (FIX) deficiency (hemophilia B), and thrombocytopenia or platelet function disorders (Chapters 37 and 38). Inherited deficiencies of fibrinogen, prothrombin, FV, FVII, FX, FXI, and FXIII are rare.

ACQUIRED COAGULOPATHIES

We begin with the acquired coagulopathies because more patients have acquired bleeding disorders due to trauma, drug exposure, or disease rather than inherited coagulopathies. Disorders commonly associated with bleeding are liver disease, vitamin K deficiency, and renal failure. In all cases, laboratory test results are necessary to confirm the diagnosis and guide the management of acquired hemorrhagic events.[10]

Trauma-Induced Coagulopathy

In North America, unintentional injury is the leading cause of death among individuals aged 1 to 45 years. The total rises when statisticians include self-inflicted, felonious, and combat injuries. In the United States alone, trauma caused 214,000 deaths in 2015, or 63 per 100,000 residents.[11] Severe neurologic displacement (head or neck injury) accounts for 50% of trauma deaths, with most deaths occurring before the patient arrives at the hospital; however, of initial survivors, 20,000 die of hemorrhage or thrombosis within 48 hours.

Trauma-induced coagulopathy (TIC) accounts for most instances of fatal hemorrhage, yet 3000 to 4000 hemorrhage-related deaths can be prevented through coagulopathy management.[12] *Coagulopathy* is defined as any single or multiple coagulation factor or platelet deficiency, and TIC is triggered by the combination of injury-related acute inflammation, hypothermia, acidosis, and hypoperfusion (poor distribution of blood to tissues and release of tissue fluid to the vasculature associated with low blood pressure), all of which are elements of systemic shock. Systemic shock triggers the massive release of inflammatory cytokines and endothelial cell and platelet von Willebrand factor (VWF) leading to acute consumption of the enzyme ADAMTS13 (*a d*isintegrin *a*nd *m*etalloprotease with a *t*hrombo*s*pondin type 1 motif, member *13*), also called VWF cleaving protease. As ADAMTS13 stores are depleted, there is a related rise in undigested ultralarge VWF multimers that trigger thrombotic microangiopathy (Chapter 38).[13,14] Shock also leads to tissue factor release, coagulation factor activation, coagulation control protein C and antithrombin activation, and hyperfibrinolysis.[15] Major surgery, ruptured aortic aneurysm, gastrointestinal bleeding, esophageal varices, and postpartum hemorrhage are some clinical conditions where TIC can occur.

Trauma centers publish and maintain *massive transfusion protocols* (MTPs) for TIC management.[16] Massive hemorrhage is defined as blood loss exceeding total blood volume within 24 hours, loss of 50% of blood volume within a 3-hour period, blood loss exceeding 150 mL/min, or blood loss that necessitates transfusion.[17] An MTP is triggered when the emergency medical team encounters an otherwise healthy trauma victim whose systolic blood pressure is less than 90 mm Hg, pulse is more rapid than 120 beats/min, pH is less than 7.25, hematocrit is less than

---

BOX 36.2   Indications for Congenital Bleeding Disorders

Relatives with similar bleeding symptoms
Onset of bleeding in infancy or childhood
Excessive bleeding from umbilical cord or circumcision wound
Repeated hemorrhages in childhood or adulthood
Chronic petechiae, purpura, or ecchymoses
Bleeding into joints, central nervous system, muscles, fatty tissue, peritoneum

32%, hemoglobin is less than 10 g/dL, urine output is diminished, and PT is prolonged to more than 1.5 times the mean of the reference interval or generates an international normalized ratio (INR) of 1.5 or greater. In addition, near-patient VET can indicate with minimal delay prolonged clotting time, poor clot strength, and hyperfibrinolysis. The limits vary by institution; however, many or all of these points are employed in formal MTP prediction scoring systems.[18] Further, the Assessment of Blood Consumption (ABC) score assesses 1 point each for up to four nonlaboratory parameters: wound penetrating mechanism, positive Focused Assessment Sonography with Trauma (FAST) examination, arrival systolic blood pressure of 90 mm Hg or less, and arrival heart rate of ≥120 beats/min. Any two of the four clinical parameters activate the MTP.

Trauma center MTPs specify that unmatched thawed group AB or group A plasma be warmed and administered to the victim en route or immediately on hospital arrival.[19] Clinicians continue by administering warmed low titer group O whole blood or equal volumes (1:1:1) of warmed red blood cells (RBCs), plasma, and single (random) donor platelet concentrate, approximating the makeup of whole blood.[20] Though RBCs are essential for their oxygen-carrying capacity, their administration need not exceed the volumes of the other components.[21] In most instances, providers administer pheresis platelet concentrate preparations that provide the equivalent of four to six random platelet concentrate preparations; consequently, the practical component ratio is actually 6:6:1, with 1 representing pheresis platelet concentrate.[22]

Plasma is a key component of TIC management. Donor services separate and freeze plasma within 24 hours of collection, officially naming the product FP-24. From time-honored habit, laboratory practitioners and providers are inclined to call the product fresh frozen plasma (FFP), though the term no longer fits the product.[23] FP-24 may be subsequently thawed and stored at 1° C to 6° C for up to 5 days, a product officially named *thawed plasma*.[24] Trauma centers and mobile emergency services maintain an inventory of group A or AB thawed plasma ready for emergency administration. Activities of VWF, FV, and FVIII decline to approximately 60% after 5 days of refrigerator storage, so thawed plasma may require supplementation with factor concentrates, especially in patients with VWD or hemophilia.[25,26]

Most trauma center MTPs now specify that when components other than whole blood are used, platelet concentrate be administered as a standard component in equal proportion with RBCs and plasma, though some stipulate that platelet concentrates be administered only when the platelet count is less than 50,000/µL. Platelet concentrate inventories are limited and costly to manage, but concentrate contributes to positive outcomes because platelets slow microvascular bleeding.[27] Platelet concentrate therapy is generally ineffective when the patient has immune thrombocytopenia, thrombotic thrombocytopenic purpura (TTP), or heparin-induced thrombocytopenia (Chapter 38). In these conditions, therapeutic platelets are rapidly consumed and their administration may therefore be contraindicated, although they may provide temporary rescue in emergent situations.[28]

To reduce the risk of *transfusion-associated circulatory overload* (TACO) and *transfusion-related acute lung injury* (TRALI), improve patient outcomes, and conserve resources, transfusion service directors may employ other types of concentrates to augment or even replace blood component administration in TIC.[29] Activated prothrombin complex concentrates (APCCs) such as Autoplex T (Nabi Biopharmaceuticals) or factor eight inhibitor bypassing activity (FEIBA, Takeda) may be used at a dosage of 50 IU/kg every 12 hours not to exceed 200 IU/kg in 24 hours.[30] The dose-response relationship of Autoplex T or FEIBA varies among recipients and because both contain activated coagulation factors, their use, especially an overdose, may risk disseminated intravascular coagulation (DIC). Nonactivated prothrombin complex concentrates (PCCs) such as four-factor concentrate Kcentra (Behring) are safer and may also be employed. Kcentra was approved by the US Food and Drug Administration (FDA) in 2013 to treat hemorrhage in warfarin overdose, so its use in TIC is off label (meaning it is not FDA cleared for use in TIC).[31,32]

PCCs, either activated or nonactivated, may be used in conjunction with the antifibrinolytic lysine analogue tranexamic acid (TXA) (Cyklokapron, Pharmacia).[33,34] First FDA cleared in 1986 to prevent bleeding in hemophilic patients about to undergo invasive procedures, TXA is effective and commonly employed for TIC, though this too is an off-label application.

Human plasma-derived fibrinogen concentrates (RiaSTAP, Behring; Fibryga, Octapharma) are distributed as a single-dose vial containing approximately 1 g of lyophilized fibrinogen concentrate.[35] Fibrinogen concentrate is indicated when there is microvascular bleeding and the fibrinogen concentration is less than 150 mg/dL. In postpartum hemorrhage, plunging fibrinogen levels are of particular concern because they signal the risk of major blood loss. Alternatively, a 15- to 20-mL unit of cryoprecipitate (CRYO) provides 150 to 250 mg fibrinogen, 80 to 150 IU FVIII, 50 to 75 IU FXIII, and 100 to 150 IU of VWF.[36] Use of CRYO represents a theoretical risk of viral transmission, but because the risk of TACO induced by CRYO is lower than the risk of TACO associated with plasma use, the latter is contraindicated.[37] Though a typical fibrinogen reference interval is 220 to 500 mg/dL, in postpartum hemorrhage, a fibrinogen lower limit of 150 mg/dL is maintained, though some recommend 200 mg/dL.[38] Postpartum hemorrhage may also be managed with TXA.[39] VWF and FVIII concentrates are also indicated when the patient has a preexisting deficiency.[40]

Recombinant activated coagulation factor VII (rFVIIa) was FDA cleared in 1999 for treating hemophilia A or B when anti-FVIII or anti-FIX inhibitors are present, respectively; its often-used application in the treatment of TIC is off label. An rFVIIa dosage of 30 µg/kg is rapidly effective in halting microvascular hemorrhage in nonhemophilic trauma victims, and rFVIIa does not cause DIC.[41] However, studies found a possible link between off label rFVIIa use and arterial and venous thrombosis in patients with existing thrombotic risk factors.[42,43]

Laboratory directors monitor the effectiveness of all TIC therapy. A skilled operator employing VET may monitor the effects of plasma, CRYO, platelet concentrate, PCC, APCC, four-factor

PCC, TXA, and rFVIIa.[44,45] VET instruments include Quantra (HemoSonics), ROTEM (TEM, Werfen), Sonoclot (Sienco), and Thromboelastograph 5000 or Thromboelastograph 6s (TEG, Haemonetics). Fibrinogen concentrate or CRYO efficacy may be measured using VET or the fibrinogen assay. Laboratory directors further advise surgeons and emergency department providers to monitor the effectiveness of all TIC therapy indirectly by checking for the correction of platelet count, PT, and PTT to within their respective reference intervals. Platelet aggregometry may be used to measure posttherapy platelet function, and coagulation factor assays are valuable as follow-ups to PT and PTT to determine whether the target activity of 30 IU/dL has been met for each factor. Although PT, PTT, platelet count, and platelet function assays are accepted approaches, VET provides immediate feedback and may be more sensitive to small physiologic improvements.

The TIC victim who survives the first 24 hours often becomes prothrombotic partly due to the loss of control proteins antithrombin and protein C and partly because hyperfibrinolysis turns to hypofibrinolysis. Often, thrombosis is first discovered clinically; however, VET may provide an indication of hypofibrinolysis or increased clot strength. Most providers prescribe therapeutic low-molecular-weight heparin to control for the risk of thrombosis.[26]

Liver Disease Coagulopathy

The bleeding associated with liver disease may be localized or generalized, mucocutaneous or anatomic. Enlarged and collateral esophageal vessels called *esophageal varices* are a complication of chronic alcoholic cirrhosis; hemorrhaging from varices is localized bleeding, not a coagulopathy, though often fatal. Mucocutaneous bleeding occurs in liver disease-associated thrombocytopenia, often accompanied by decreased platelet function. Anatomic bleeding is the consequence of procoagulant dysfunction and deficiency.

The liver produces nearly all the plasma coagulation factors and regulatory proteins.[46] Hepatitis, cirrhosis, obstructive jaundice, cancer, poisoning, and congenital disorders of bilirubin metabolism may suppress the biosynthetic function of hepatocytes, reducing either the concentrations or the activities of the plasma coagulation factors to less than hemostatic levels (below 30 IU/dL).[47]

Liver disease alters the production of the vitamin K-dependent factors FII (prothrombin), FVII, FIX, and FX and control proteins C (PC), S (PS), and Z (PZ). In liver disease, these seven factors are produced in their *des-γ-carboxyl* (proteins induced by vitamin K antagonists, PIVKA) forms, which associate with reduced thrombin activity (Chapter 35). At the onset of liver disease, FVII, which has the shortest plasma half-life at 6 hours, is the first coagulation factor to exhibit decreased activity. Because the PT is particularly sensitive to FVII activity, it is characteristically prolonged in mild liver disease, serving as a sensitive early marker.[48] Additionally, vitamin K may become deficient when the diet is limited. Vitamin K deficiency independent of liver disease produces a similar effect on the PT.

Declining coagulation FV activity is a more specific marker of liver disease than deficient FII, FVII, FIX, or FX because FV is non-vitamin K dependent and is not affected by dietary vitamin K deficiency. The FV activity assay, performed in conjunction with the FVII assay (Chapter 41), may be used to distinguish liver disease from vitamin K deficiency.

Fibrinogen is an acute phase reactant that becomes elevated in early or mild liver disease. A moderately or severely diseased liver produces fibrinogen that is coated with excessive sialic acid, a condition called *dysfibrinogenemia,* in which the fibrinogen functions poorly. Dysfibrinogenemia causes generalized mucocutaneous bleeding associated with a prolonged thrombin clotting time and an exceptionally prolonged reptilase clotting time.[49] In end-stage liver disease, the fibrinogen level may fall to less than 100 mg/dL, a mark of liver failure.[50]

VWF, FVIII, and FXIII are acute phase reactants that may be unaffected or elevated in mild to moderate liver disease.[51] In contrast to the other coagulation factors, VWF is produced from endothelial cells and megakaryocytes (not liver) and is stored in endothelial cells and platelets.[52]

Moderate thrombocytopenia occurs in one-third of patients with liver disease.[53] Platelet counts of less than 150,000/μL may result from sequestration and shortened platelet survival associated with portal hypertension and resultant hepatosplenomegaly.[54] In alcoholism-related hepatic cirrhosis, acute alcohol toxicity also suppresses platelet production. Platelet aggregation and secretion properties are often suppressed; this is reflected in reduced platelet aggregometry and lumiaggregometry results and reduced VET clot strength (Chapter 41). Occasionally, platelets are hyperreactive. Although debatable, aggregometry may be used to predict bleeding and thrombosis risk.[55]

Chronic or compensated DIC (Chapter 39) is a significant complication of liver disease that is caused by decreased liver production of regulatory proteins antithrombin, PC, or PS, and by the release of activated procoagulants from degenerating liver cells. The failing liver cannot clear activated coagulation factors. In primary or metastatic liver cancer, hepatocytes may also produce nonspecific procoagulant substances that trigger chronic DIC, leading to ischemic complications.

In acute, uncompensated DIC, PT and PTT are prolonged, the fibrinogen level is reduced to less than 100 mg/dL, and D-dimer levels are significantly increased.[56] If DIC is chronic and compensated, the only indicative test result may be the markedly elevated D-dimer assay result, a hallmark of unregulated coagulation and fibrinolysis. Although DIC can be resolved only by removing its underlying cause, its hemostatic deficiencies may be corrected when the need is urgent by administering RBCs, plasma, activated or nonactivated PCC, TXA, platelet concentrates, or antithrombin concentrates, which include synthetic ATryn (rEVO Biologics) and plasma-derived Thrombate III (Grifols).[57,58]

PT, PTT, fibrinogen concentration, platelet count, and D-dimer concentration are used to characterize the hemostatic abnormalities in liver disease (Table 36.2). Assays for FV and FVII may be used in combination to differentiate liver disease from vitamin K deficiency. Both factors are decreased in liver disease, but FV levels remain within the reference interval in diet-related vitamin K deficiency.

TABLE 36.2 Hemostasis Laboratory Tests in Liver Disease

Assay	Interpretation
Fibrinogen	>400 mg/dL (elevated) in early mild liver disease; <200 mg/dL in advanced liver disease with dysfibrinogenemia/hypofibrinogenemia
Thrombin time (TT)	Prolonged in dysfibrinogenemia, hypofibrinogenemia, elevated fibrin degradation products, and unfractionated heparin therapy
Reptilase time	Prolonged in hypofibrinogenemia, significantly prolonged in dysfibrinogenemia; unaffected by heparin; assay rarely used
Prothrombin time (PT)	Prolonged, even in mild liver disease because of des-γ-carboxyl factors replacing normal FII (prothrombin), FVII, and FX
Partial thromboplastin time (PTT, APTT)	Mildly prolonged in advanced liver disease because of des-γ-carboxyl FII (prothrombin), FIX, FX, and possible DIC
Factor V assay	FV is reduced in liver disease but is unaffected by VK deficiency; FV level helps distinguish liver disease from VK deficiency
Platelet count	Mild thrombocytopenia, <150,000/μL
Platelet aggregometry	Mild suppression of platelet aggregation and secretion in response to most agonists
Quantitative D-dimer	>240 ng/mL or >500 ng/mL FEU

DIC, Disseminated intravascular coagulation; *F,* factor; *FEU,* fibrinogen equivalent unit; *VK,* vitamin K.

Plasminogen deficiency and an elevated D-dimer confirm pathologic fibrinolysis. The specialized *reptilase time* test (Chapter 41) may be useful to confirm dysfibrinogenemia. This test duplicates the TT test except that venom of the reptile *Bothrops atrox* (common lancehead viper) is substituted for the thrombin reagent. The *Bothrops* venom triggers fibrin polymerization by cleaving fibrinopeptide A, but not fibrinopeptide B (Chapter 35), from the fibrinogen molecule. The subsequent polymerization is slowed by structural defects, which prolong the time interval to clot formation. The reptilase time test is unaffected by standard unfractionated heparin therapy and can be used to assess fibrinogen function even when there is heparin in the specimen.

Oral or intravenous vitamin K therapy may correct the bleeding associated with nonfunctional des-γ-carboxyl FII (prothrombin), FVII, FIX, and FX; however, the therapeutic effect of vitamin K in liver disease is short-lived compared with its effect in dietary vitamin K deficiency because of the liver's impaired biosynthetic ability. In severe liver disease, plasma transfusion provides most of the coagulation factors in hemostatic concentrations. VWF, FV, and FVIII are not stable in stored products, and thus their levels may remain reduced with treatment. In addition, because of its small concentration and the short half-life of FVII, plasma is unlikely to return the PT to within the reference interval.

A unit of plasma provides a volume of 200 to 280 mL. The typical adult plasma dose for liver disease is 2 units, but the dose varies widely, depending on the indication and the ability of the

patient's cardiac and renal system to rapidly excrete excess fluid. TACO is likely to occur when 30 mL/kg has been administered, but it may occur with even smaller volumes in patients with compromised cardiac or kidney function.

If the fibrinogen level is less than 50 mg/dL, spontaneous bleeding is imminent, and fibrinogen concentrate or CRYO may be selected for therapy. Plasma and CRYO present a theoretical risk of virus transmission, as do other untreated single-donor human-source blood products, and allergic transfusion reactions are more common with plasma-containing products. Other therapeutic options for patients with liver disease-related bleeding are platelet concentrates, PCC, antithrombin concentrate, rFVIIa, and TXA.

Chronic Renal Failure and Hemorrhage

Chronic renal failure of any cause is often associated with *platelet dysfunction* and mild to moderate mucocutaneous bleeding.[59] Platelet adhesion to blood vessels and platelet aggregation are suppressed, perhaps because guanidinosuccinic acid or phenolic compounds coat the platelets.[60] Anemia and thrombocytopenia contribute to bleeding. Dialysis, RBC transfusions, or erythropoietin therapy (epoetin alfa [Procrit, Janssen Pharmaceuticals]) may correct these disorders.[61]

Hemostasis activation syndromes that deposit fibrin in the renal microvasculature reduce glomerular function. Examples are DIC, hemolytic uremic syndrome, and thrombotic thrombocytopenic purpura. Although these are thrombotic disorders, they invariably cause thrombocytopenia, which may lead to mucocutaneous bleeding. Fibrin also may be deposited in renal transplant rejection and in the glomerulonephritis syndrome of systemic lupus erythematosus.

Laboratory tests for bleeding in renal disease provide only modest information with little predictive or management value. The bleeding time test may be prolonged, but it is too unreliable to provide an accurate diagnosis or to assist in monitoring treatment.[62] Platelet aggregometry is nonpredictive.[63] The PT and PTT are expected to be normal.

Management of renal failure-related bleeding typically focuses on the severity of the hemorrhage without reliance on laboratory test results. Renal dialysis temporarily activates platelets and may ultimately improve platelet function, particularly when anemia is well controlled.[64,65] Desmopressin acetate (1-desamino-8-D arginine vasopressin [DDAVP]) (Stimate, Behring) may be administered intravenously or intranasally to increase the plasma concentration of VWF high-molecular-weight multimers. VWF aids platelet adhesion and aggregation.[66] Patients with renal failure should avoid aspirin, clopidogrel, prasugrel, ticagrelor, or other platelet inhibitors because these drugs increase the risk of hemorrhage.

Nephrotic syndrome is a state of increased glomerular permeability associated with a variety of conditions, such as chronic glomerulonephritis, diabetic glomerulosclerosis, systemic lupus erythematosus, amyloidosis, and renal vein thrombosis.[67] In nephrotic syndrome, low-molecular-weight proteins are lost through the glomerulus into the glomerular filtrate and the urine. FII (prothrombin), FVII, FIX, FX, and FXII have been detected in the urine, as have the coagulation regulatory proteins antithrombin and protein C. In 25% of cases, loss of regulatory proteins supersedes loss of procoagulants and leads to a tendency toward venous thrombosis.

Vitamin K Deficiency and Hemorrhage

Vitamin K, required for normal function of the vitamin K-dependent group of coagulation factors, is ubiquitous in foods, especially green leafy vegetables, and the daily requirement is small, so pure dietary deficiency is rare. Body stores are limited, however, and become exhausted when the usual diet is interrupted, as when patients are provided only parenteral (intravenous) nutrition for an extended period or when people embark on fad diets.[68] Also, because vitamin K is fat soluble and requires bile salts for absorption, biliary duct obstruction (atresia), fat malabsorption, and chronic diarrhea may become associated with vitamin K deficiency. Broad-spectrum antibiotics that disrupt normal gut flora may cause a slight reduction because they destroy bacteria that produce vitamin K.[69]

Because of their sterile intestines and the minimal concentration of vitamin K in human milk, newborns are constitutionally vitamin K deficient.[70] Hemorrhagic disease of the newborn was common in the United States before routine administration of vitamin K to infants was legislated in the 1960s, but it still occurs in developing countries. The activity levels of FII (prothrombin), FVII, FIX, and FX are lower in normal newborns than in adults (Chapter 43), and premature infants have even lower concentrations of these factors. Breastfeeding prolongs the deficiency because passively acquired maternal antibodies delay the establishment of gut flora.

The γ-carboxylation cycle of coagulation factors is interrupted by coumarin-type oral anticoagulants such as warfarin that disrupt the vitamin K epoxide reductase and vitamin K quinone reductase reactions (Figure 35.5).[71] In this situation, the liver releases dysfunctional des-γ-carboxyl FII (prothrombin), FVII, FIX, and FX and PC, PS, and PZ. Therapeutic overdose or accidental or felonious administration of warfarin-containing rat poisons may result in moderate to severe hemorrhage because of the deficiency of functional K-dependent factors. The effect of brodifacoum, or "superwarfarin," often used as a rodenticide, lasts for weeks to months, and treatment of poisoning with this substance requires repeated administration of vitamin K, with followup PT monitoring.[72]

A prolonged PT with or without a prolonged PTT supports the clinical suspicion of vitamin K deficiency. In PT and PTT mixing studies, if commercial platelet-free normal plasma (NP) (CRYOcheck Pooled Normal Plasma, Precision BioLogic) is combined with patient plasma, the mixture yields "corrected" PT and PTT results, which indicate that factor deficiencies caused the initially prolonged PT and (perhaps) PTT. Single-factor assays will detect low FVII (a common finding because of the short half-life of FVII), followed in sequence by decreases in FIX, FX, and FII (prothrombin), depending on the progression of the deficiency.

The standard therapy for vitamin K deficiency is oral or, in an emergency, intravenous vitamin K. Synthesis of functional vitamin K-dependent coagulation factors requires at least 3 hours,

so in the case of severe bleeding, the provider may administer plasma or four-factor PCC.[73] The most responsive assay for monitoring the efficacy of plasma or four-factor PCC is VET, but the patient's recovery may be monitored indirectly using the PT/INR.

Auto-Anti-Factor VIII Inhibitor and Acquired Hemophilia A

Acquired autoantibodies that specifically inhibit FII (prothrombin), FV, FVIII, FIX, FXIII, and VWF have been described in nonhemophilic patients.[74] Auto-anti-FVIII is the most common. Patients who develop an autoantibody to FVIII, which is diagnostic of acquired hemophilia A (AHA), are often older than 60 years of age and have no apparent underlying disease. AHA is occasionally associated with rheumatoid arthritis, inflammatory bowel disease, systemic lupus erythematosus, or lymphoproliferative disease. Pregnancy can trigger AHA 2 to 5 months after delivery. AHA has an incidence of 1 per 1 million per year. Patients experience sudden and severe anatomic bleeding that may include bleeding in the gastrointestinal or genitourinary tract.[75] AHA, even when treated, remains fatal in at least 20% of cases. Autoantibodies to procoagulants other than FVIII are less common but create similar symptoms.

The PT and PTT are recommended for any patient with sudden onset of anatomic hemorrhage that resembles AHA. In the presence of an FVIII inhibitor, PTT is likely prolonged, whereas PT is likely normal. A factor assay may reveal FVIII activity to be less than 40 IU/dL but activity is often undetectable.

Clot-based mixing studies (Chapter 41) confirm the presence of the inhibitor. PTT prolongation may be corrected initially by the addition of NP to the test specimen in a 1:1 ratio, but PTT again becomes prolonged after incubation of the 1:1 NP-patient plasma mixture at 37° C for 2 hours. The return of prolongation after incubation occurs because FVIII autoantibodies are often of the immunoglobulin G4 isotype, which are time and temperature dependent. Consequently, the inhibitor effect may be evident only after the patient's inhibitor is allowed to interact with the FVIII in the NP for 2 hours at 37° C before testing. Approximately 15% of inhibitors, called high-avidity inhibitors, may immediately prolong the PTT; in this case, an incubated mixing study is unnecessary.

FVIII neutralization by an autoantibody appears nonlinear using in vitro assays. Although there is early rapid loss of FVIII activity, residual activity remains, which indicates that the reaction has reached equilibrium. This is called type II kinetics (Figure 36.1). In contrast, alloantibodies to FVIII, which develop in 30% of patients with congenital hemophilia A in response to FVIII concentrate therapy, exhibit type I kinetics. In type I kinetics, there is linear in vitro neutralization of FVIII activity over 2 hours, which results in complete inactivation. In type I kinetics, in vitro measurement is relatively reliable, whereas in type II kinetics, the assay of inhibitor activity is semiquantitative.[76]

The Nijmegen-Bethesda assay (NBA) is employed to quantitate auto-anti-FVIII inhibitor levels (Chapter 41). The NBA is ordinarily employed to measure FVIII inhibitors in hemophilia A patients with alloantibodies to FVIII. Results of the NBA assay help the provider choose the proper therapy to control

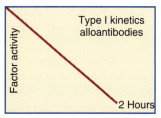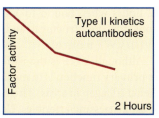

Figure 36.1 Factor Inhibitors Assayed Using Clot-Based Assays. In type I linear kinetics, the inhibitor fully inactivates the coagulation factor in vitro. This is typical of alloantibodies such as factor VIII inhibitors that develop in patients with severe hemophilia A. In type II kinetics, the inhibitor and coagulation factor reach equilibrium. This is typical of autoantibodies such as the factor VIII inhibitor in acquired hemophilia A. Because of the type II kinetics, the Nijmegen-Bethesda assay is considered a semiquantitative measure in acquired hemophilia, although the results are commonly used to distinguish low-titer from high-titer autoantibodies.

AHA bleeding. Repeat assays are used to follow the response to immunosuppressive therapy but are not needed for management of the bleeding symptoms.

Emicizumab (Hemlibra, Genentech) is an FVIII-mimetic monoclonal antibody that effectively treats congenital hemophilia A patients with inhibitors and is showing promise for the treatment of AHA, particularly for patients with high titer inhibitors.[77] Further advantages may include reduced adverse effects and ease of administration compared with standard care. Laboratory monitoring of FVIII in patients under treatment with this type of agent will require preassessment of the sensitivity of the assay. Chromogenic assays may detect monoclonal antibody therapy, whereas clot-based assays may be insensitive to the monoclonal antibody, depending on the reagents.

Obizur (Takeda) is a recombinant porcine FVIII that is the standard of care for replacement therapy for AHA.[78] To control acute bleeding, activated PCC or rFVIIa, which bypass the coagulation FVIII inhibitor, are used. Patients whose inhibitor titers are less than 5 Nijmegen-Bethesda units (NBUs) may respond to administration of desmopressin or FVIII concentrates, but close monitoring of their response with serial FVIII activity assays is warranted. Once bleeding is controlled, immune tolerance induction (ITI) by a defined treatment protocol may reduce the inhibitor titer. Plasma exchange may also be used in severe cases, but the response is less reliable than that of ITI.[79]

Additional Factor Inhibitors

Anti-prothrombin (FII) antibodies prolong the PT. These inhibitors develop as *lupus anticoagulant* variants with prothrombin specificity in approximately 30% of lupus anticoagulant patients.[80,81] Similar to all lupus anticoagulant variants, anti-prothrombin antibodies are typically associated with thrombosis, although a few patients experience bleeding.[82] Findings of reduced prothrombin activity by clot-based assay, anti-prothrombin antibodies via immunoassay, and a positive clot-based lupus anticoagulant test profile confirm the diagnosis. It is rare to detect anti-prothrombin antibodies that are not associated with lupus anticoagulant.

FXIII inhibitors are extremely rare but cause life-threatening bleeding. They may arise spontaneously or in association with

autoimmune or lymphoproliferative disorders. Auto-anti-FXIII has been documented in patients receiving isoniazid treatment for tuberculosis.[83,84]

Autoantibodies to FV may arise spontaneously in autoimmune disorders and after exposure to bovine thrombin in fibrin glue.[85,86] Fibrin glue-generated autoantibodies have largely disappeared since 2008, when manufacturers began to use plasma-derived human thrombin in place of bovine thrombin (VISTASEAL, Grifols).

Auto-anti-FX antibodies are rare; however, FX deficiency in amyloidosis may result from what seems to be an absorptive mechanism.[87,88] In many cases of acquired inhibitors, mixing studies show uncorrected prolongation without incubation (immediate mixing study), and inhibitor titers may be determined using the NBA.

Acquired von Willebrand Disease

Acquired VWD, with symptoms similar to congenital VWD, has been described in hypothyroidism; benign monoclonal gammopathies; Wilms tumor; intestinal angiodysplasia; congenital heart disease; pesticide exposure; uremia; lupus erythematosus; and autoimmune, lymphoproliferative, and myeloproliferative disorders.[89,90] The pathogenesis of acquired VWD may involve decreased VWF production; adsorption of VWF to abnormal cell surfaces, as seen in association with lymphoproliferative disorders, aortic stenosis, and Wilms tumor; or, in less than 2% of cases, a specific VWF autoantibody.[91]

Acquired VWD manifests with moderate to severe mucocutaneous bleeding and may be suspected in any patient with recent onset of bleeding who has no hemorrhage-related medical history.[92] Although PT is unaffected, PTT may be moderately prolonged if VWF reduction is severe enough to reduce FVIII to less than 40 IU/dL because VWF serves as the FVIII carrier molecule. As in congenital VWD, the diagnosis is based on a finding of diminished VWF activity and diminished VWF antigen by immunoassay. It may be difficult to differentiate between mild, previously asymptomatic congenital VWD and acquired VWD.[93]

If the patient requires treatment for bleeding, desmopressin or a plasma-derived FVIII/VWF concentrate such as Humate-P (Behring), Wilate (Octapharma), or Alphanate (Grifols) is effective at controlling the symptoms. CRYO is no longer recommended for treatment of VWD because it does not undergo viral inactivation.

Disseminated Intravascular Coagulation

DIC, although characteristically identified through its hemorrhagic symptoms, is classified as a thrombotic disorder and is described in Chapter 39.

CONGENITAL COAGULOPATHIES

von Willebrand Disease

VWD, first described by Finnish professor Erik von Willebrand in 1926, is the most prevalent inherited mucocutaneous bleeding disorder. Nearly 600 autosomal dominant and a few recessive germline mutations, many with incomplete penetrance, may cause VWD, as these mutations produce quantitative (type 1) or qualitative (functional, type 2) VWF deficiencies.[94] Both quantitative and functional abnormalities decrease platelet adhesion to injured vessel walls, impairing primary hemostasis. When solely defined by laboratory assays as VWF deficiency, VWD is reputed to affect approximately 1% of the global population. However, when defined by the number of patients who experience bleeds serious enough to seek medical assistance, prevalence is 1 in 20,000.[95] The prevalence of VWD in females who report menorrhagia is 24%.[96]

von Willebrand Factor Biology and Function

VWF is a *multimeric* glycoprotein whose molecular mass ranges from 500,000 to 20,000,000 Daltons, the largest molecule in human plasma. Its plasma concentration is 0.5 to 1.0 mg/dL, but a great deal more is readily available on demand from storage organelles. VWF is synthesized in the endoplasmic reticulum of endothelial cells and stored in their cytoplasmic Weibel-Palade bodies. It is also synthesized in megakaryocytes and stored in platelet α-granules. Weibel-Palade bodies (Figure 36.2) and platelet α-granules release VWF in response to a variety of therapeutic, hemostatic, and inflammatory stimuli.[97]

The *VWF* gene consists of 52 exons spanning 178 kilobase (kb) pairs on chromosome 12.[98] The translated protein is a monomer of 2813 amino acids composed of four structural domains, A through D. The monomers become glycosylated, then form dimers and oligomers that migrate to the storage organelles, where they polymerize to form ultralarge VWF (ULVWF) multimers. At the time of storage, a propeptide is cleaved from the end of domain D so that the mature monomers, already polymerized, consist of 2050 amino acids.[99] VWD mutations may occur anywhere on the *VWF* gene.[100]

Epitopes located along the structural domains of the VWF monomer support its various functions. Domain A supports binding sites for collagen and platelet glycoprotein (GP) Ib/IX/V. Domain C provides a site that binds platelet receptor GPIIb/IIIa, integrin designation $\alpha_{IIb}\beta_3$, and domain D provides the carrier site for FVIII (Figure 36.3). On release from intracellular stores, a percentage of VWF multimers complexes with FVIII. VWF protects FVIII from proteolysis, prolonging its plasma half-life from 2 to 4 hours when free to 8 to 12 hours when bound to VWF. Table 36.3 lists the designations for the structural and functional components of the FVIII/VWF molecule.

Although VWF is the FVIII carrier molecule (Figure 35.7), its primary function is to mediate platelet adhesion to subendothelial collagen in areas of high flow rate and high shear force, as in capillaries and arterioles. Upon injury or inflammatory stimulus, ULVWF strands are released to the plasma, where they circulate, attach to exposed subendothelial collagen, or remain attached to endothelial cells via P-selectin and other adhesion molecules. Whether bound or free in plasma, they bind platelet receptor GPIb, a subunit of GPIb/IX/V (Figure 11.9).

ADAMTS13 cleaves the linear ULVWF multimers, yielding multimers of various masses, including the functional high-molecular-weight VWF (HMW-VWF). The ADAMTS13 cleavage function also appears to modulate acute inflammation, stroke, and myocardial infarction. When HMW-VWF binds GPIb/IX/V, platelets become activated and express a

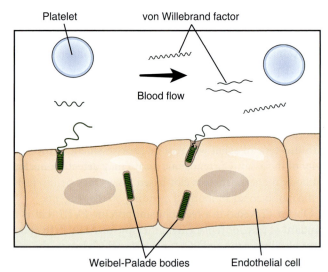

Figure 36.2 von Willebrand Factor. VWF is stored in endothelial cell Weibel-Palade bodies and platelet α-granules. On demand, the Weibel-Palade bodies and α-granules fuse with their respective plasma membranes and release VWF into the bloodstream. The ultralarge multimers of VWF are uncoiled in response to the shear forces of the blood flow, where they will be cleaved by the enzyme ADAMTS13 into high- and low-molecular-weight multimers.

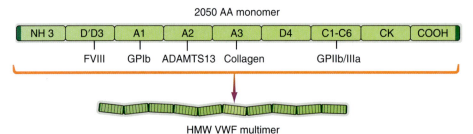

Figure 36.3 von Willebrand Factor Monomer. The *VWF* gene, located on the p arm of chromosome 12, spans 178 kb and is the template for the VWF prepropeptide of 2813 amino acids *(AA)*. Entering storage, a signal sequence of 22 AA and a propeptide of 741 AA are cleaved, leaving the mature monomer of 2050 AA, diagrammed here. The monomer consists of 12 subunits within the 4 domains (A–D) that support the active sites at the locations indicated on the diagram. The monomers polymerize to form multimers of various lengths that reach a molecular weight up to 20 million Daltons. *ADAMTS13, a disintegrin and metalloprotease with a thrombospondin type 1 motif, member 13; FVIII,* factor VIII; *GP,* glycoprotein; *HMW VWF,* high-molecular-weight von Willebrand factor; *kb,* kilobases.

TABLE 36.3 Nomenclature of Factor VIII/von Willebrand Factor Complex

Designation	Meaning
FVIII/VWF	Customary designation for the combination of FVIII and VWF
FVIII	Procoagulant FVIII, transported on VWF. In the coagulation cascade, FVIII binds activated FIX to form the complex FVIIIa-FIXa, which digests and activates FX. FVIII deficiency is called *hemophilia A.*
VWF:Ag	Epitope that is the antigenic target for the VWF immunoassay
VWF:Ac	VWF platelet-binding activity (assays in Table 36.5)
FVIII:C	FVIII coagulant activity as measured in a clot-based factor assay

F, Factor; *VWF,* von Willebrand factor.

second VWF binding site, GPIIb/IIIa ($\alpha_{IIb}\beta_3$). This receptor binds arginine-glycine-aspartic acid (arginylglycylaspartic acid [RGD]) sequences that are richly distributed in VWF and fibrinogen molecules, mediating irreversible platelet-to-platelet aggregation. The adhesion and aggregation sequences are essential to normal primary and secondary hemostasis.

von Willebrand Disease Pathophysiology

Quantitative or qualitative VWF deficiencies reduce *platelet adhesion,* which leads to *mucocutaneous hemorrhage* of varying severity: epistaxis, ecchymosis, menorrhagia, gastrointestinal bleeding, hematemesis, and surgical bleeding. Symptoms vary over time and within kindreds because VWF production and release are susceptible to a variety of physiologic influences. In addition, severe quantitative VWF deficiency creates FVIII deficiency because of its inability to protect unbound FVIII from proteolysis. Many individuals have VWF levels in the intermediate range of 30 to 50 IU/dL and maintain an FVIII level sufficient for competent coagulation. Unless they experience bleeding, these individuals are termed "Low VWF"; if bleeding is present, the VWD diagnosis is appropriate. When FVIII levels decrease to less than 30 IU/dL, anatomic bleeding typically accompanies the mucocutaneous VWD bleeding pattern.

von Willebrand Disease Types and Subtypes

Type 1. Type 1 VWD is a quantitative VWF deficiency caused by one of several autosomal dominant frameshifts, nonsense mutations, or missense mutations that may occur anywhere in the *VWF* gene. Type 1 comprises 40% to 70% of VWD cases.[99] The plasma concentrations of all VWF multimers and FVIII are variably, albeit proportionally, reduced (Figure 36.4). There is mild to moderate systemic bleeding, often after a hemostatic challenge such as dental extraction or surgery. In females menorrhagia, which predicts postpartum hemorrhage, is a common symptom. However, because mucocutaneous bleeding symptoms occur in people without VWD to varying degrees, diagnosis requires scrupulous laboratory testing.[100]

Subtype 1C. A VWD type I variant, termed subtype 1C, is a quantitative VWF deficiency in which the VWF secretion rate is near normal, but its plasma half-life is reduced from the anticipated 8 to 12 hours to 1 to 3 hours. Subtype 1C comprises

15% of all type 1 VWD diagnoses. Among other mutations, 1C includes *p.Arg1205His* (called VWF Vincenza). Subtype 1C VWD may be mischaracterized as type 3 VWD. Diagnosis depends on molecular testing.

Type 2. Type 2 VWD encompasses four qualitative VWF deficiencies. VWF concentrations may be normal or moderately decreased, but VWF function is consistently reduced. Laboratory testing is essential to identifying and confirming type 2 subtypes because the diagnosis affects treatment choices.

Subtype 2A. Of all patients with type 2 VWD, 10% to 20% have subtype 2A, which arises from well-characterized autosomal dominant point mutations in the VWF A2 and D1 structural domains (Table 36.4). These mutations render VWF susceptible to increased proteolysis by ADAMTS13, which leads to a predominance of low-molecular-weight VWF multimers (LMW-VWF) (see Figure 36.4). The smaller multimers support less effective platelet adhesion than high- or intermediate-molecular weight multimers. Patients with subtype 2A VWD have normal or slightly reduced VWF antigen levels as measured by immunoassay, with moderate to markedly reduced VWF activity because of the loss of the HMW-VWF molecules.

Subtype 2B. In subtype 2B VWD, identified in less than 5% of all VWD patients, a mutation within the A1 domain, *p.Pro1266Ile,* raises the affinity of VWF for the GIb unit of platelet GPIb/IX/V, its customary binding site; these are hence gain-of-function mutations. HMW-VWF multimers spontaneously bind resting platelets. The abnormal HMW-VWF multimers are consequently unavailable for normal platelet adhesion as they are cleared with the bound platelets. The electrophoretic multimer pattern is characterized by lack of HMW-VWF multimers, but intermediate-molecular-weight multimers may still be present (see Figure 36.4). Subtype 2B VWD may be identified phenotypically using the *ristocetin-induced platelet agglutination (RIPA) assay* (Chapter 41) that employs reduced ristocetin concentration and confirmed by molecular diagnosis. Moderate thrombocytopenia may also exist, caused by chronic platelet activation because multimer-coated platelets indiscriminately bind the endothelium and become cleared.

A platelet membrane mutation that raises GPIb affinity for normal HMW-VWF multimers creates a clinically similar disorder called *platelet-type VWD* (PT-VWD) or *pseudo-VWD.* In this instance, the large multimers also are lost from the plasma, and platelets become adhesive as in subtype 2B VWD. Pseudo-VWD may be the more appropriate name, though seldom used because this is not a true form of VWD. The prevalence of PT-VWD is approximately 10% of patients diagnosed with subtype 2B VWD. Both clinically and by phenotypic laboratory assays, the two entities are indistinguishable; the diagnosis requires molecular testing. Further, platelet-type VWD is often mistaken for immune thrombocytopenia.

Subtype 2M. Subtype 2M VWD describes a qualitative VWF variant that possesses poor platelet receptor binding despite generating a normal multimeric distribution pattern in electrophoresis. The distinguishing feature of subtype 2M that separates it from type 1 is a discrepancy between VWF concentration and its activity as measured using one of the VWF activity assays described in "First-Level Phenotypic

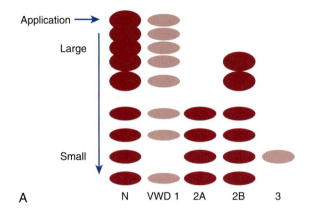

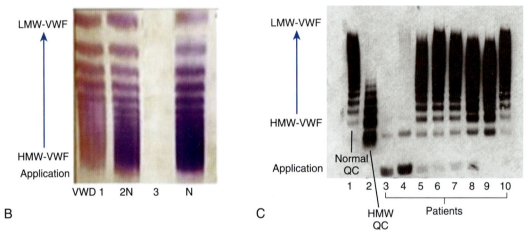

Figure 36.4 von Willebrand Factor Multimers. (A), Schematic of von Willebrand factor *(VWF)* multimer analysis by polyacrylamide gel electrophoresis (PAGE) shows diminished concentration but normal ratios in von Willebrand disease *(VWD)* type 1 (also subtype 2M), absence of large and intermediate multimers in subtype 2A, absence of large multimers in subtype 2B, and absence of all multimers in type 3. (B), Photograph of PAGE analysis illustrating VWD type 1, type 2N with normal multimer distribution, type 3 with no multimers, and a normal patient. (C), Photograph of PAGE analysis illustrating type 3 VWD in lanes 3 and 4 and ultralarge multimers characteristic of ADAMTS13 deficiency in lanes 8 and 9. *HMW,* High-molecular-weight; *LMW,* low-molecular-weight; *N,* normal; *QC,* quality control. (B modified from Skornova, I., Simurda, T., Stasko, J., et al. [2021]. Multimer analysis of von Willebrand factor in von Willebrand disease with a Hydrasys semi-automatic analyzer—single-center experience. *Diagnostics, 20,* 2153.)

TABLE 36.4	**von Willebrand Factor Mutation Locations and Pathology**		
Type	**Autosomal Dominant or Recessive**	**Mutation Domain**	**Biological Effect**
1C	Dominant	Propeptide	Shortened VWF half-life
2A	Dominant	A2	Impaired VWF secretion and increased sensitivity to ADAMTS13
	Dominant	CK	Impaired VWF dimerization
	Dominant	D3	Intracellular retention of VWF with reduced ADAMTS13 proteolysis
	Recessive	Propeptide, D2	Defective multimer assembly
2B	Dominant	A1	Increased GP1b binding
2M	Dominant	A1, A3	Defective collagen or GP1b binding
2N	Recessive	D'-D3	Reduced FVIII binding
3	Recessive	All	Mostly nonsense mutations; VWF not produced

ADAMTS13, a disintegrin and metalloproteinase with a thrombospondin type 1 motif, member 13; FVIII, coagulation factor VIII; GP1b, glycoprotein 1b platelet receptor; VWF, von Willebrand factor.

von Willebrand Disease Laboratory Diagnostic Profile" and "Second-Level Phenotypic von Willebrand Disease Laboratory Diagnostic Profile," despite a normal multimeric pattern. Subtype 2M is often incorrectly identified as type 1 or subtype 2A. It may be that the 10% to 20% prevalence data for subtype 2A and the 40% to 70% rate for type 1 are artificially elevated by misdiagnosed subtype 2M cases.

Subtype 2N (Normandy variant; autosomal hemophilia). One of several mutations in VWF domains D2, D', and D3 impairs the protein's FVIII binding site function. This condition, present in less than 5% of VWD patients, results in FVIII deficiency despite normal VWF concentration and activity, and a normal multimeric pattern (see Figure 36.4). The disorder is also known as autosomal hemophilia because its clinical symptoms are indistinguishable from the symptoms of hemophilia except that it affects both males and females. Subtype 2N is suspected when a girl or woman is diagnosed with hemophilia after experiencing anatomic bleeding, and is also suspected when a boy or man misdiagnosed with hemophilia A fails to respond to FVIII concentrate therapy. The poor therapeutic response occurs because free FVIII has a plasma half-life of 2 to 4 hours. Confirm VWD subtype 2N using the VWF:FVIII binding (VWF:FVIIIB) immunoassay available from specialized reference laboratories and confirm when necessary with molecular testing. In the US, the VWF:FVIIIB assay is labeled Research Use Only.

Type 3. Nonsense mutations or deletions within the *VWF* gene may occur anywhere on the gene. They produce severe mucocutaneous and anatomic hemorrhage in compound heterozygotes or, in consanguinity, homozygotes. This is the rarest form of VWD, where the VWF concentration measured by immunoassay or by activity assay is less than 10% (see Figure 36.4). FVIII is proportionally diminished, or absent, and primary and secondary hemostasis is impaired.

First-Level Phenotypic von Willebrand Disease Laboratory Diagnostic Profile

Definitive diagnosis of VWD requires a personal and family history of mucocutaneous bleeding. The provider applies a BAT when the pretest clinical suspicion is low. Diagnosis then involves laboratory demonstration of reduced VWF concentration (antigen) and platelet-binding activity (function) (Table 36.5). The provider orders a complete blood count to rule out anemia and thrombocytopenia as the cause of mucocutaneous bleeding and a PT and PTT, which assess the coagulation cascade to rule out a coagulopathy other than VWD. Owing to their poor predictive values, current guidelines recommend against the bleeding time test (Chapter 41) and the PFA-100 platelet function analyzer (Chapter 42).

The first-level VWD test profile, which is performed before associated assays are considered, consists of three assays: VWF concentration by immunoassay (VWF antigen [VWF:Ag]), FVIII:C activity, and VWF:Ac platelet-binding activity (including VWF:CB, VWF:GPIbM, VWF:GPIbR, or VWF:RCo). For a diagnosis of VWD, the VWF:Ag assay provides the most precise information of these assays. Figure 36.5 presents an algorithm for using this battery of laboratory tests to identify VWD and determine the subtypes. Expected test results for each VWD subtype are given in Table 36.6.

The *quantitative VWF:Ag* assay may employ enzyme immunoassay methodology, the traditional reference method that is typically batched and performed manually. Newer technical developments include automated latex immunoassay methodology (LIA), such as the STA-Liatest (Stago), or the chemiluminescence immunoassay (CLIA), such as the HemosIL AcuStar VWF:Ag (Werfen). The CLIA method has a 7% coefficient of variation and a lower limit of detection of 0.2 IU/dL.[101,102]

Another first-level profile component is the chromogenic substrate-based or clot-based *coagulation FVIII assay.* FVIII

TABLE 36.5	**von Willebrand Factor Assays***
VWF:Ag	Enzyme immunoassay, LIA, or CLIA quantitates VWF. VWF:Ag is the most reproducible of VWF assays and is used to monitor treatment.
FVIII:C	Clot-based or chromogenic factor VIII activity assay
VWF:Ac	VWF activity; commercial synonym for VWF:GP1bM.
VWF:RCo	Quantitative ristocetin cofactor (RCo) activity, also called VWF activity. VWF activity is measured by the ability of ristocetin to cause agglutination of reagent platelets by the patient's VWF.
VWF:CB	Collagen binding (CB) assay. Large VWF multimers bind immobilized target collagen. Measures platelet and collagen binding properties.
VWF:GPIbR	Platelet-free activity assay. Ristocetin-triggered binding of patient VWF to recombinant glycoprotein Ib (GPIb) on synthetic particles, detected by LIA or CLIA.
VWF:GPIbM	Platelet-free and ristocetin-free activity assay. Recombinant gain-of-function GPIb on synthetic particles binds patient VWF A1 domain. Reaction is detected by LIA.
RIPA	Ristocetin-induced platelet aggregometry. Followup assay that uses ristocetin and patient's own platelets, in contrast to VWF:RCo, which uses reagent platelets. This assay is modified by using low ristocetin concentrations to identify VWD subtype 2B, in which VWF multimers exhibit increased avidity for the platelet receptor site. This method is also called the ristocetin response curve.
VWF:FVIIIB	Immunoassay measures factor VIII binding to VWF.

*Platelet binding activity (functional) assay results are compared with VWF:Ag to distinguish qualitative from quantitative VWF deficiency. Most VWF activity assays are sensitive to the presence of high-molecular-weight VWF multimers, which are the most active multimers in platelet binding.

Ag, Antigen; *CLIA,* chemiluminescence immunoassay; *LIA,* latex immunoassay; *VWD,* von Willebrand disease; *VWF,* von Willebrand factor.

assay results are expected to parallel VWF:Ag and VWF:Ac platelet binding activity results in VWD types 1 and 3 and may parallel VWF:Ag in subtypes 2A, 2B, and 2M but are markedly reduced in VWD subtype 2N. When FVIII activity is less than 40 IU/dL, the PTT may be prolonged.

Competing methods exist for measuring *VWF:Ac plateletbinding activity* (function), the third component of the firstlevel profile. The *ristocetin cofactor* (VWF:RCo) assay has been employed since 1977.[103] Ristocetin is a glycopeptide antibiotic that was introduced in 1956 but withdrawn in 1960 when it was found to cause thrombocytopenia. Now used as a reagent, ristocetin is pipetted to an aliquot of patient plasma where it "unfolds" the VWF molecule and reduces repelling negative charges, enabling HMW-VWF multimers to bind platelet membrane GPIb.[104] The VWF:RCo assay employs formalinized reagent platelets and measures platelet agglutination, yielding a quantitative measure of VWF platelet adhesion function.[105] Because ristocetin avidity varies from lot to lot and the VWF:RCo assay is performed on a variety of aggregometers and coagulometers, poor reproducibility of the assay is observed. International proficiency surveys consistently reveal VWF:RCo assays to have an

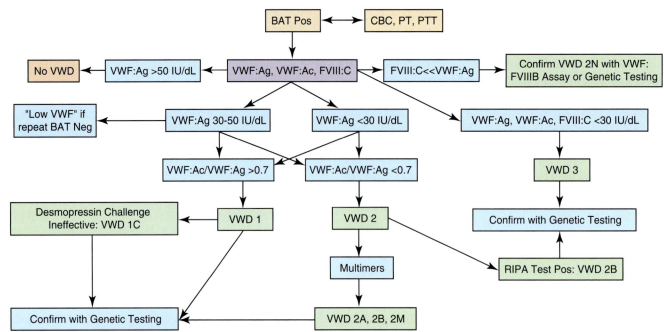

Figure 36.5 Algorithmic Laboratory Diagnosis Approach for von Willebrand Disease. With a clinical suspicion of von Willebrand disease *(VWD)*, the provider completes a bleeding assessment tool *(BAT)*, prothrombin time *(PT)*, partial thromboplastin time *(PTT)*, and complete blood count *(CBC)*. The primary VWD profile includes the VWF:Ag quantitative assay, a FVIII:C activity assay, and a VWF:Ac platelet binding assay (Table 36.5). If the VWF:Ag level is greater than 50 IU/dL, VWD is not indicated. If the VWF:Ag is between 30 and 50 IU/dL and bleeding is present, suspect VWD. If the VWF:Ag is between 30 and 50 IU/dL and no bleeding is present (original or repeat BAT negative), these individuals are termed "Low VWF." If the VWF:Ag level exceeds 50 IU/dL but the FVIII:C activity level is below 30 IU/dL, suspect VWD type 2N and confirm with the VWF:FVIII binding assay *(VWF:FVIIIB)*. If the VWF:Ag level is less than 30 IU/dL, VWD is likely. If the VWF:Ag, VWF:Ac, and FVIII:C levels are less than 30 IU/dL, suspect VWF type 3. If the VWF:Ac/VWF:Ag ratio is 0.7 or greater, suspect VWD type 1; continue with the desmopressin challenge assay to rule in or rule out VWD subtype 1C. If the VWF:Ac/VWF:Ag ratio is less than 0.7, suspect VWD type 2. The low-dose ristocetin-induced platelet aggregation *(RIPA)* or ristocetin response curve is employed to identify VWD subtype 2B. Multimeric analysis is used to identify and categorize subtypes 2A, 2B, and 2M. Genetic testing with next-generation sequencing is employed to confirm the phenotypic diagnosis for VWD subtypes 1C, 2B, 2M, and type 3. *<<*, much less than; *FVIII:C*, clotting activity of factor VIII; *Pos*, positive; *VWF:Ac*, von Willebrand factor platelet binding activity; *VWF:Ag*, von Willebrand factor antigen.

TABLE 36.6   von Willebrand Disease Detection and Classification: Phenotypic Laboratory Results*

Laboratory Test	Type 1	Subtype 2A	Subtype 2B	Subtype 2M	Subtype 2N	Type 3
VWF:Ac tests: VWF:RCo, VWF:CB, VWF:GPIbR, or VWF:GPIbM	Low	Low	Low	Low	Normal	Very low or absent
VWF:Ag	Low	Normal to slightly decreased	Normal to slightly decreased	Normal	Normal	Very low or absent
VWF:Ac/VWF:Ag ratio†	>0.7	≤0.7	≤0.7	≤0.7	>0.7	N/A
Platelet count	Normal	Normal	Decreased	Normal	Normal	Normal
Partial thromboplastin time (PTT, APTT)	Normal to slightly prolonged	Normal	Normal	Normal to slightly prolonged	Normal to slightly prolonged	Prolonged
RIPA	Decreased	Decreased	Increased	Decreased	Normal	Absent
Factor VIII:C	Slightly low	Normal	Normal	Normal	Low	<10 units/dL
VWF multimers	Normal pattern	Large and intermediate forms absent	Large forms absent	Normal pattern	Normal pattern	All forms absent

*Results vary over time and within affected kindred.
†Limits are locally established.
Ac, Activity; *Ag,* antigen; *CB,* collagen binding; *GP,* glycoprotein; *N/A,* not applicable; *RCo,* ristocetin cofactor; *RIPA,* ristocetin-induced platelet aggregometry; *VWF,* von Willebrand factor.

interlaboratory coefficient of variation of 30% or higher and a lower detection limit of only 6% to 12%.[106]

VWF:Ac platelet-binding activity may be measured using the ristocetin-triggered nonplatelet recombinant GPIb-based LIA and CLIA method such as HemosIL AcuStar *VWF:GPIbR* (Werfen).[107] VWF:GPIbR uses recombinant GPIb fragments tethered to microparticles that bind the A1 domain of HMW-VWF in the presence of ristocetin, eliminating the use of preserved whole platelets.[108] In the United States, the VWF:GP1bR assay is labeled Research Use Only.

The *VWF:GPIbM* assay employs a gain-of-function high-affinity recombinant GPIb target protein that resembles the GPIb of PT-VWD (pseudo-VWD) platelets. GPIb-coated microparticles bind the A1 domain of HMW-VWF without the need for ristocetin. This assay has been commercialized as an LIA (Innovance VWF Ac, Siemens), and it offers a VWF lower detection limit of 2 IU/dL and coefficient of variation of 5%.[109] The VWF:GPIbR and VWF:GPIbM methods are rapidly replacing VWF:RCo as they offer superior analytic sensitivity, specificity, and precision.[110] The VWF:GP1bM assay is FDA-approved.

When the ratio of the VWF:RCo, VWF:GPIbR, or VWF:GPIbM assay value to the VWF:Ag concentration, for instance VWF:GPIbM/VWF:Ag is less than 0.7 (ratio limit is generated from reference interval studies by individual laboratories), the laboratory professional infers type 2 VWD.[111]

Second-Level Phenotypic von Willebrand Disease Laboratory Diagnostic Profile

Followup tests are necessary to confirm subtype 1C and type 2 VWD and to differentiate type 2 subtypes. The following assays are performed after results of the first-level test profile are obtained. This two-step approach saves time and expense.

The low-dose *ristocetin induced platelet agglutination (RIPA)* assay, also called the *ristocetin response curve,* has been used in the past to identify subtype 2B. The low-dose RIPA test is performed on the patient's platelet-rich plasma, as opposed to a preserved platelet suspension used in the VWF:RCo assay, and requires a platelet aggregometer. In subtype 2B, the patient's platelets, theoretically coated with avid VWF multimers, agglutinate in response to less than 0.5 mg/mL ristocetin. In comparison, normal platelets agglutinate only at ristocetin concentrations greater than 0.5 mg/mL, and platelets from a patient with subtype 2A may not agglutinate at all.

VWF *multimer analysis* by sodium dodecyl sulfate-polyacrylamide gel electrophoresis is a technically demanding, second-level confirmatory procedure that helps establish VWD type 2 and differentiates between VWD subtypes 2A, 2B, and perhaps 2M. Although both subtypes 2A and 2B lack high-molecular-weight multimers, intermediate multimers are presumed to be present in the electrophoretic pattern of subtype 2B VWD samples but are absent from the pattern of a patient with subtype 2A VWD. In subtype 2M, the multimeric pattern appears to be normal despite the reduced platelet-binding activity (function) to VWF:Ag concentration ratio. Multimer analysis is available from specialized reference laboratories for differentiation of VWD type 2 subtypes. Targeted molecular testing is rapidly replacing the RIPA and multimeric analysis because type 2B variants may be identified in exon 28.

To test for VWD subtype 1C, the provider employs a *desmopressin challenge* (described subsequently in "von Willebrand Disease Treatment") with baseline and 1- and 4-hour postinfusion VWF:Ag assays to confirm increased VWF release from internal stores.[112]

The VWF *collagen binding assay* (VWF:CB) is available from several hemostasis specialty reference laboratories.[113] VWF:CB may serve as an alternative assay for platelet binding.[114] Whereas the other VWF functional assays focus on platelet binding, VWF:CB detects reduced platelet binding plus reduced binding to subendothelial collagen. The solid-phase target is composed of biological reagent collagen type 1, collagen type 3, or a combination of type 1 and 3 collagen. Adding VWF:CB activity to the VWD diagnostic profile may further reduce the need for VWF multimer analysis, as it detects a possible collagen binding defect.[115,116]

Aside from the VWF diagnostic tests described in this section, the provider periodically orders a complete blood count on VWD patients to test for thrombocytopenia and anemia associated with iron or folate deficiency.

von Willebrand Disease Genetic Testing

Table 36.6 lists the expected phenotypic test results for several VWD types and subtypes. In addition, *VWF* gene sequencing has identified nearly 600 disease-related mutations, 80% of which are missense mutations. The mutations associated with types 2 and 3 VWD are well characterized, and many tertiary care facility laboratories and reference laboratories offer sequencing that confirms or updates the phenotypic diagnosis (see Table 36.4 and Figure 36.5). However, the molecular basis of type 1 VWD is multifactorial, reflecting genetic factors within and even outside of the *VWF* gene.[117]

Because acquired VWD may mimic any one of the VWD types and subtypes, results of phenotypic profiles seldom help to differentiate it from the inherited condition. Review of the clinical history with emphasis on age at onset of bleeding, comorbid conditions, and family history may signal acquired disease rather than the congenital form.[118]

von Willebrand Disease Diagnostic Pitfalls

Varying genetic penetrance, ABO blood group, smoking, inflammation, hormones, and physical stress affect VWF concentration and platelet-binding activity.[119] VWF levels rise with age. Approximately 45% of patients, especially patients with moderately low levels at diagnosis, may achieve near-normal levels as they age.

VWF concentration and activity become reduced if the specimen is stored at refrigerator temperatures for several hours before testing, resulting in increased false-positive results especially when tested off site.[120] VWF activity rises when the phlebotomist allows the tourniquet to remain tied for more than one minute in preparation for venipuncture. VWF activity rises substantially in acute inflammation such as occurs postoperatively, after trauma or during an infection. Physical stress such as cold, exertion, or a child's crying or struggling during venipuncture causes VWF activity to rise. VWD patients experience fluctuation in disease severity over time, and the clinical manifestations of the disease vary from person to person within kindred, despite the assumption that everyone in the family possesses the same mutation. When the clinical presentation indicates VWD, the VWD laboratory assay profile should be repeated at least once or until the results are conclusive. Conversely, when the provider suspects VWD based on symptoms, it may be necessary to repeat a previously negative VWD profile.[121]

In 2021 the American Society for Hematology (ASH), International Society on Thrombosis and Haemostasis (ISTH), National Hemophilia Foundation (NHF), and World Federation of Hemophilia (WFH) established guidelines for VWD diagnosis. The panel recommends the diagnosis of type 1 VWD when the VWF level is below 30 IU/dL in all circumstances and below 50 IU/dL for patients with abnormal bleeding based on the results of VWF:Ag or a reliable measure of platelet-dependent VWF activity such as VWF:GPIbM. The 50 IU/dL represents the lower reference limit for many facilities, but laboratories employ their locally computed limit when it is below 50 IU/dL. The limits apply regardless of ABO group. VWF mutations are detected in 75% to 82% of patients with VWF levels below 30 IU/dL, whereas patients with VWF levels of 30 to 50 IU/dL possess VWF mutations 44% to 60% of the time. The panel recommends that laboratories perform VWD diagnostic testing only when patients are at a baseline state of health.

The panel further suggests that laboratories employ a platelet-dependent VWF:Ac/VWF:Ag ratio limit of 0.7 (not 0.5 as previously recommended) to identify type 2A, 2B, or 2M VWD in following up a positive first-level profile. Some patients with mucocutaneous bleeding may have both normal VWF:Ag and platelet-dependent VWF activity levels with a VWF:Ac/VWF:Ag ratio of 0.7 or lower, indicating a possible type 2 defect.

Restrictive laboratory assay profiles and inappropriate testing such as the bleeding time test or PFA-100 may miss documentable VWD. Rheumatoid factor and heterophile antibodies interfere to cause false-positive results. Occasionally, laboratory scientists and providers may diagnose hemophilia A in patients with VWD type 3 in the absence of a VWF primary profile. Moderate VWD may fail to appear until early adulthood, leading to a false diagnosis of acquired VWD.

In a well-managed facility, laboratory professionals and providers communicate regularly with all medical staff members who are challenged with VWD diagnosis and management including nurses, pharmacists, emergency department and primary care providers, internists, surgeons, gynecologists, and hematologists. Laboratory professionals ensure that providers who manage VWD patients are aware of the effects of estrogen levels, inflammation, physical stress, and specimen management on VWF activity and that they understand the strengths and limitations of VWF laboratory assay profiles, the proper interpretation of assay results, and the availability of confirmatory assays.

von Willebrand Disease Treatment

Mild mucocutaneous bleeding may resolve with physical measures such as limb elevation, pressure, and application of ice packs (the athlete's acronym is *PRICE*—*p*rotection, *r*est, *i*ce, *c*ompression, and *e*levation).[122]

In type 1 and type 2 VWD, excluding subtype 2B, intravenous, subcutaneous, or intranasal *desmopressin* is the most widely used therapy, as it raises VWF levels 2 to 4 times baseline within 30 to 60 minutes of administration.[123] Therapeutic dosages are monitored using periodic VWF:Ag assays. Desmopressin requires a supply of endogenous VWF, so it is not effective in type 3 VWD. After 2 to 3 days of treatment, VWF stores become exhausted (a condition termed *tachyphylaxis*) and therapy becomes ineffective. Desmopressin is contraindicated in type 2B VWD because the release of enhanced platelet GPIb receptor affinity VWF leads to increased platelet binding and thrombocytopenia. Desmopressin provides minor VWF increases in subtypes 2A and 2M VWD but may not provide a sufficient increase for efficacy during invasive procedures.

The provider may require a *desmopressin challenge,* employing VWF:Ag assays performed at baseline and at 1 and 4 hours after administration to determine if desmopressin treatment will provide a beneficial effect for the patient. The VWF level is expected to double the baseline and remain higher than 50 IU/dL for at least 4 hours.[124] In type 1C VWD, desmopressin is cleared prematurely, so levels may drop to baseline within 2 to 4 hours. Most type 1 VWD patients with levels greater than 30 IU/dL respond readily and so may not require this test.

Desmopressin is an antidiuretic, so prolonged usage may cause hyponatremia and fluid overload. Fluid restriction and electrolyte monitoring is recommended. Desmopressin is not recommended for use in patients with active cardiovascular disease, seizure disorders, females with preeclampsia, children younger than 2 years, or patients with type 1C VWD in situations that require a sustained response.

As not every patient responds predictably, VWF:Ag may reveal an inadequate response to desmopressin or may indicate the need to augment treatment with an agent that targets other hemostatic mechanisms. Common supplementation agents are estrogen, antifibrinolytics, or VWF concentrate, especially when the patient is being prepared for an invasive procedure.

The lysine analogues ε-*aminocaproic acid* (EACA) (Amicar, Akorn Pharmaceuticals) and *tranexamic acid* (TXA) (Pfizer) are used alone or in conjunction with desmopressin to help control bleeding as they block plasminogen binding sites and thus slow fibrinolysis.[125] The antifibrinolytics are administered orally, intravenously, topically, or as mouthwash when used in dental procedures.

In females with VWD, hormonal contraceptives *(estrogen)* and levonorgestrel intrauterine devices decrease menstrual blood loss.[126] TXA is substituted for females who hope to become pregnant.

During pregnancy, females undergo physiologic changes that support a procoagulant state.[127] In type 1 VWD, VWF and FVIII levels rise during the second and third trimesters to 2 to 3 times their baseline level and remain elevated for up to 12 weeks postpartum. In type 2 VWD, VWF:Ag and FVIII levels may rise, but platelet-binding activity remains diminished, and in type 3 VWD, VWF and FVIII remain low. Given the variability, VWF platelet-binding activity (VWF:GPIbM), VWF:Ag, and FVIII assay are performed periodically, especially during the third trimester and the postpartum period.[128]

Postpartum hemorrhage occurs in 50% of females with VWD, even when therapy raises VWF levels to 200 IU/dL, suggesting that females with VWD may need supratherapeutic levels in the postpartum setting.[129] TXA decreases the risk of postpartum hemorrhage and is continued for 7 to 15 days.[130]

For patients whose VWF levels do not respond to desmopressin, antifibrinolytics, or estrogen therapy, *VWF concentrates* may be necessary. Providers may consider prophylaxis for VWF, similar to hemophilia, instead of on-demand therapy to reduce bleeding episodes and hospitalization.[131] For treatment of type 3 VWD and subtype 2B, three commercially prepared human plasma-derived high-purity preparations are available that provide a mixture of VWF and FVIII (Humate-P, Alphanate, and Wilate).[132] VWF:Ag assays are essential to determine whether the dosage produces the target level and to follow its degradation between doses.[133] Once infused, in addition to the exogenous FVIII in the concentrate, the therapeutic VWF stabilizes endogenous FVIII, leading to accumulation. Thus it is necessary to monitor for elevated FVIII activity, which creates a thrombosis risk. For VWD subtype 2N, the provider begins with a DDAVP challenge. If ineffective, purified plasma-derived FVIII with VWF, such as Humate-P, Alphanate, or Wilate should be used, as pure synthetic FVIII is ineffective.

Vonvendi (Takeda), is a recombinant VWF that provides no accompanying FVIII.[134] The initial Vonvendi dose is 40 to 80 IU/kg body weight every 8 to 24 hours, adjusted to the extent of continued bleeding or the target VWF:Ag concentration. If the baseline FVIII concentration is less than 40 IU/dL, providers give recombinant FVIII that is free of VWF within 10 minutes of completing the Vonvendi infusion at a ratio of 1.3:1.

Recombinant and affinity-purified FVIII concentrates contain no VWF and cannot be used to treat VWD. CRYO and plasma are less desirable alternatives because of the risk of virus transmission, and the necessary plasma volume per dose may cause TACO.

Therapy for bleeding secondary to acquired VWD follows the same principles as delineated previously plus treatment of the primary disease, if applicable. Therapeutic recommendations for VWD are summarized in Table 36.7.

Hemophilia A (Factor VIII Deficiency)

The hemophilias are congenital single-factor deficiencies marked by anatomic bleeding. Second to VWD in prevalence among congenital bleeding disorders, hemophilias occur in 1 in 8000 individuals, mostly males. Of those affected, 85% have FVIII deficiency, 14% have FIX deficiency, and 1% have FXI deficiency or deficiency of one of the other coagulation factors, such as FII (prothrombin), FV, FVII, FX, or FXIII. Congenital deficiency of FVIII is called *classic hemophilia* or *hemophilia A*.

Factor VIII Structure and Function

FVIII is a two-chain, 285,000-Dalton protein translated from the X chromosome.[135] When the coagulation cascade is activated, thrombin cleaves plasma FVIII and releases a large polypeptide called the *B domain* that dissociates from the molecule. This leaves behind a calcium-dependent heterodimer, FVIIIa, which detaches from its VWF carrier molecule to bind phosphatidyl serine and FIXa. The FVIIIa/FIXa complex, called the *tenase complex,* cleaves and activates coagulation FX at a rate 10,000 times faster than free FIXa can cleave FX alone (Chapter 35). Consequently, FVIII deficiency significantly slows production of thrombin by the coagulation pathway and leads to hemorrhage (Figure 36.6). FVIII deteriorates in storage. Donor blood collected in standard citrate-dextrose-phosphate preservative provides 30 IU/dL FVIII activity, or approximately 50 IU/dL in leukodepleted donor blood, after 28 days of storage.[136]

Hemophilia A Genetics

The *F8* gene spans 186 kb of the X chromosome and is the site of approximately 2000 deletions, inversions, stop codons, and nonsense and missense mutations. Most of these mutations result in quantitative disorders in which the FVIII coagulant activity and antigen concentration match but in rare cases, low activity is seen despite near-normal antigen concentration.[137] The latter cases are due to qualitative or structural FVIII

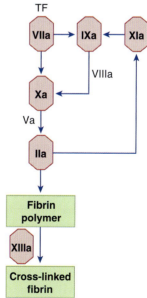

Figure 36.6 Factor Deficiencies That Cause Bleeding Disorders. The coagulation factors whose absence is related to hemorrhage are depicted in this simplified diagram of the mechanism of the coagulation cascade. *TF*, Tissue factor.

TABLE 36.7	**Therapeutic Strategies in von Willebrand Disease**	
Type	**Primary Approach**	**Other Options**
1	Estrogen, desmopressin, EACA, or TXA	VWF concentrate
2A	Estrogen, desmopressin, EACA, or TXA	VWF concentrate
2B	FVIII/VWF concentrate	EACA
2M	Estrogen, desmopressin, EACA, or TXA	VWF concentrate
2N	DDAVP challenge	VWF concentrate with FVIII
3	VWF concentrate	Platelet transfusions

EACA, ε-Aminocaproic acid; *FVIII,* factor VIII; *TXA,* tranexamic acid; *VWF,* von Willebrand factor.

abnormalities traditionally known as cross-reacting material-positive disorders.[138]

Male hemizygotes, whose sole X chromosome contains an *F8* gene mutation, experience anatomic bleeding, but female heterozygotes, who are carriers, typically do not. When a female carrier has children with an unaffected male the chances of inheritance of hemophilia A are a 25% chance of a normal daughter, 25% chance of a carrier daughter, 25% chance of a normal son, and 25% chance of a hemophilic son. All sons of males with hemophilia A and noncarrier females are normal, whereas all daughters are obligate carriers of the disease. In addition, approximately 30% of newly diagnosed cases arise because of spontaneous germline mutations in individuals who have no family history of hemophilia A.[139] Rarely, the symptoms of hemophilia A may be seen in females. This phenomenon could be due to true homozygosity or double heterozygosity, such as in the female offspring of a hemophilic father and a carrier mother. Other possibilities include a spontaneous germline mutation in the otherwise normal allele of a heterozygous female or a disproportional inactivation of the X chromosome with the normal gene, termed *extreme lyonization*. Finally, VWD of the Normandy (2N) subtype may mimic hemophilia A in males and females.

Hemophilia A Clinical Manifestations

Hemophilia A causes *anatomic bleeds* with deep muscle and joint hemorrhages; hematomas; wound oozing after trauma or surgery; and bleeding into the central nervous system, peritoneum, gastrointestinal tract, and kidneys. Acute joint bleeds (hemarthroses) are exquisitely painful and cause temporary immobilization. Over time, recurrent joint bleeds cause inflammation and eventual permanent loss of mobility, whereas bleeding into muscles may cause nerve compression injury, with first temporary and then lasting disability. Cranial bleeds lead to severe, debilitating, and durable neurologic symptoms, such as loss of memory, paralysis, seizures, and coma, and may be rapidly fatal. Bleeding may begin immediately after a triggering event or may become manifest after a delay of several hours. Some bleeding seems to be spontaneous.

The diagnosis of hemophilia A can be made soon after the birth of an infant to a mother who has a family history of hemophilia. In the absence of a family history, abnormal bleeding in the neonatal period, which may appear as easy bruising, bleeding from the umbilical stump, postcircumcision bleeding, hematuria, or intracranial bleeding, is suspicious for hemophilia. Severe hemophilia usually is diagnosed in the first year of life, whereas mild hemophilia may not become apparent until a triggering event such as trauma, surgery, or dental extraction occurs in late childhood, adolescence, or adulthood.

The laboratory diagnosis of coagulopathies in the newborn or older infant is complicated by the requirement for a non-hemolyzed specimen of at least 2 mL from tiny veins and by the predictably low newborn level of some coagulation factors. Medical laboratory practitioners expect PT and PTT to be prolonged because of physiologically low levels of FII (prothrombin), FVII, FIX, and FX, even in full-term infants (Chapter 43). However, healthy infant FVIII levels are close to adult levels, even in infants who are born prematurely; this allows skillful laboratory staff to provide the correct diagnosis of hemophilia A using a FVIII activity assay.

The severity of hemophilia A symptoms is inversely proportional to FVIII activity. Laboratory professionals classify an activity level of less than 1 IU/dL as severe, associated with spontaneous or exaggerated bleeding in the neonatal period. Activity levels of 1 to 5 IU/dL are seen in moderate hemophilia, which is usually diagnosed in early childhood after symptoms become apparent. In mild hemophilia, with activity levels of 5 to 40 IU/dL, hemorrhage follows significant trauma and becomes a risk factor mainly in surgery or dental extractions. Patients with mild hemophilia may go for long periods without symptoms.

As a result of frequent bleeds, hemophilia patients often experience debilitating and progressive musculoskeletal lesions and deformities and neurologic deficiencies following intracranial hemorrhage. In addition, other chronic disease effects, such as limited productivity, low self-esteem, poverty, drug dependency, and depression, are common problems. Before the advent of sterilized and recombinant factor concentrates, chronic hepatitis often resulted from repeated exposure to blood products. Of hemophilia patients treated before 1984, 70% are human immunodeficiency virus (HIV) positive or have died from acquired immunodeficiency syndrome.[140]

Hemophilia A Laboratory Diagnosis

The laboratory workup for a suspected congenital single coagulation factor deficiency starts with the PT, PTT, and fibrinogen assay and continues with specific two-stage chromogenic or one-stage clot-based factor assays (Chapter 41) based on the results of the initial tests. Before the provider initiates laboratory testing, however, a history of the patient's hemorrhagic symptoms and those of the patient's first-degree relatives is recorded, when available. In hemophilia A and B, PT and fibrinogen are likely to be normal and the PTT is likely to be prolonged, provided that the PTT reagent is sensitive to FVIII and FIX deficiencies at or less than the 40 IU/dL plasma activity level. Table 36.8 lists the expected results for each clot-based first-level assay for any single-factor deficiency associated with bleeding, including

TABLE 36.8 Results of Clot-Based Assays in Congenital Single-Factor Deficiencies*

Deficient Coagulation Factor	PT	PTT	Follow-up Test
Fibrinogen	Prolonged	Prolonged	Fibrinogen assay
Prothrombin	Prolonged	Prolonged	Prothrombin, V, VII, X assays
V	Prolonged	Prolonged	Prothrombin, V, VII, X assays
VII	Prolonged	Normal	VII assay
VIII	Normal	Prolonged	VIII, IX, XI assays
IX	Normal	Prolonged	VIII, IX, XI assays
X	Prolonged	Prolonged	Prothrombin, V, VII, X assays
XI	Normal	Prolonged	VIII, IX, XI assays
XIII	Normal	Normal	XIII quantitative assay

*Results are valid when the patient is not being treated with coagulation factors or anticoagulants. Results may vary in response to reagent sensitivities.
PT, Prothrombin time; *PTT,* partial thromboplastin time.

deficiencies of fibrinogen, FII (prothrombin), FV, FVII, FVIII, FIX, FX, FXI, and FXIII. Deficiencies of contact factors (FXII, high-molecular-weight kininogen, and prekallikrein) have no relationship to bleeding, and these factors are not listed in Table 36.8. Though important for diagnosis, factor assays are mostly used to monitor hemophilia therapy.

Approximately 90% of female carriers of hemophilia A are detected by measuring the ratio of FVIII activity to VWF:Ag concentration. This ratio is effective because VWF production is unaffected by FVIII deficiency. Using a ratio rather than an FVIII assay value alone normalizes for some of the physiologic variables that affect FVIII activity and VWF:Ag assays, such as estrogen levels, inflammation, physical stress, and exercise.

The laboratory professional establishes a reference interval for the FVIII to VWF:Ag ratio using plasmas from at least 30 females who are not carriers. If the ratio of the individual being tested is below the lower limit of the interval, the person under study is likely to be a carrier. These results may be influenced by excessive lyonization, variation in VWF production, and analytic variables; consequently, if carrier status is suspected and the FVIII to VWF:Ag ratio is greater than the lower limit of the reference interval, genetic testing may be necessary to detect one of the many polymorphisms associated with FVIII deficiency.[141]

Traditional Hemophilia A Therapy

Similar to patients with VWD, many patients with mild to moderate hemophilia can increase their FVIII activity using self-administration of desmopressin acetate, which may be administered in combination with an antifibrinolytic such as EACA or TXA under provider supervision. If these approaches are unsuccessful, as in severe hemophilia, the patient turns to coagulation factor concentrates.

Human plasma-derived FVIII (pdFVIII) concentrates are available worldwide. Products include Alphanate, Hemofil M (Takeda), Humate-P, and Wilate. These are collected from healthy plasmapheresis donors and are prepared using chemical fractionation, immunoaffinity column separation, pasteurization, and solvent-detergent sterilization.[142] All pdFVIII concentrates undergo viral inactivation and since 1985, none has transmitted lipid-envelope viruses such as HIV, hepatitis B virus, or hepatitis C virus. The pdFVIII concentrates, however, may transmit nonlipid viruses such as parvovirus B19 and hepatitis A virus. Alphanate, Humate-P, and Wilate contain VWF, fibrinogen, and noncoagulant proteins in addition to FVIII and may be used to treat VWD. Human plasma-derived factor concentrates have traditionally been employed for *on-demand* therapy rather than for *prophylactic* therapy.[143]

The goal of on-demand hemophilia A treatment is to raise the patient's FVIII activity to hemostatic levels whenever the patient suspects or experiences a bleed or anticipates a hemostatic challenge such as tooth extraction or surgery. The target activity level, typically 80 to 100 IU/dL, depends on the nature of the bleed or the anticipated bleeding risks of the procedure and should be maintained until the threat is resolved. In the case of a bleed into muscles, joints, or fatty tissue, the sooner the target factor level is reached, the less painful the episode and

the less likely the patient is to experience inflammation or nerve damage. Because FVIII has a half-life of 8 to 12 hours, twice-daily infusions may be required. The second and subsequent administrations employ half the initial dose.

In industrialized countries, hemophilia therapy relies mostly on recombinant FVIII (rFVIII). The first rFVIII products such as Recombinate (Takeda) employed human or animal serum and albumin in their manufacturing process, thus presenting a theoretical risk of viral disease transmission. Manufacturers now provide rFVIII products free of all human protein, such as Advate (Takeda) and Kovaltry (Bayer). Additionally, deleting the large central B domain shortens rFVIII molecules in the hope of rendering the molecule less immunogenic. The B-domain-deleted (BDD-rFVIII) preparations are ReFacto (Genetics Institute), which is produced using Chinese hamster ovary (CHO) cells grown in human albumin, and Xyntha (Wyeth), produced using CHO cells grown in synthetic, albumin-free culture medium.[144]

Because of the availability of rFVIII in industrialized nations, at least 70% of concentrate-dependent hemophilia patients use prophylactic regimens, administering approximately three infusions per week to maintain their FVIII activity at hemostatic levels.[145] The prophylactic approach conserves downstream resources and promotes better health by ameliorating the short- and long-term adverse effects of repeated hemorrhages.[146]

The first extended half-life (EHL) rFVIII preparation was Eloctate (Sanofi Genzyme), a BDD-rFVIII fused with the Fc portion of human immunoglobulin G1 (BDD-rFVIIIFc), which was released in 2014. The Fc fragment binds macrophage membrane Fc receptors, extending the plasma half-life to nearly 20 hours and reducing the infusion frequency to once every 4 to 5 days.[147] Also available are Adynovate (Takeda), Jivi (Bayer), and Esperoct (Novo Nordisk), all of which are rFVIII covalently conjugated with polyethylene glycol (PEG) (i.e., "PEGylated," "glycopegylated"). PEGylation is used in many drug applications; it extends the rFVIII half-life to approximately 20 hours and reduces the infusion rate to approximately twice weekly. Afstyla (Behring) is a full-length rFVIII that binds VWF with greater avidity than two-chain rFVIII formulations, resulting in an extended half-life of 22 hours. The pharmacokinetics of EHL rFVIII formulations are limited by their "dominant partner," VWF, whose half-life of 12 to 15 hours limits their ultimate plasma life span.[148]

When hematologists treat hemophilia, they base FVIII concentrate dosage calculations on the definition of an international unit (IU) of FVIII activity, which is the mean activity level present in 1 mL of NP and is synonymous with 100 IU/dL. They further calculate the desired increase after FVIII concentrate infusion by subtracting the patient's preinfusion factor activity from the target activity level, often 80 to 100 IU/dL.

The desired increase is multiplied by the patient's plasma volume to compute the dosage. The patient's plasma volume may be estimated from blood volume and hematocrit.[149] The blood volume is approximately 65 mL/kg of body weight, and the plasma volume is the "plasmacrit": (100% − hematocrit %) × blood volume. The FVIII concentrate dose may be computed using the following formulas:

$$\text{Plasma volume} = \text{weight in kilograms} \times 65 \text{ mL/kg} \times$$
$$(1 - \text{hematocrit})$$

$$\text{FVIII concentrate dose} = \text{plasma volume} \times$$
$$(\text{target FVIII level} - \text{initial FVIII level})$$

These formulas may also be used for VWF concentrates to treat VWD; however, in all cases of hemophilia or VWD therapy, the formula in the product package insert takes precedence. Hematologists avoid treatment overdose, as a relationship exists between elevated FVIII or VWF and venous thrombosis.[150,151] FVIII pharmacokinetics vary by patient age and condition, so regardless of the concentrate formulation and dose, laboratory monitoring and close clinical observation are essential to predict administration frequency and achieve therapeutic efficacy. The time-honored one-stage clot-based assay is being replaced by two-stage chromogenic substrate FVIII assay methods that employ a bovine factor X substrate that is unaffected by FVIII inhibitors or concentrates with structural modifications. In addition to superior limit of detection and coefficient of variation characteristics, chromogenic substrate assays more accurately measure most BDD-rFVIII and EHL-rFVIII formulations.[152]

Contemporary Hemophilia A Therapy

Emicizumab, available since 2017, and Mim8 (Novo Nordisk, in phase 3 trials) are FVIII mimetics, bispecific antibodies that bypass FVIII by binding FX and FIXa. Emicizumab is administered by subcutaneous injection weekly (1.5 mg/kg), every 2 weeks (3 mg/kg), or every 4 weeks (6 mg/kg) and is effective in hemophilia patients with anti-FVIII inhibitors. Less than 1% of patients treated with emicizumab have developed neutralizing alloantibodies to the treatment.[153]

The one-stage clot-based FVIII assay may be modified by diluting the plasma specimen 1:8 and employing an FVIII-depleted emicizumab calibrator and control (r2 Diagnostics) to monitor patients treated with emicizumab. Bovine-origin chromogenic substrate assays with FVIII calibrators, insensitive to emicizumab, are used to directly measure FVIII levels and to assay FVIII inhibitors using the Nijmegen-Bethesda assay.[154]

In 2019 and 2020 the European Association for Haemophilia and Allied Disorders surveyed providers who were caring for 3420 patients with severe hemophilia. The survey revealed that emicizumab was used for 100% of inhibitor patients and 88% of noninhibitor patients with no major adverse events. In 73% of inhibitor patients, the annual bleed rate was zero.[155] In industrialized countries, emicizumab is rapidly replacing factor concentrates.[156]

Fitusiran (Sanofi) is a small interfering RNA (siRNA) product administered once monthly by injection that reduces antithrombin levels by suppressing antithrombin RNA translation, thereby enhancing thrombin generation and restoring hemostasis in patients with hemophilia with or without inhibitors. In phase 3 trials, fitusiran was shown to reduce annual bleeds in severe hemophilia A and B by 90% compared with on-demand therapy. Additional dosage, efficacy, and safety studies are in progress to mitigate the risk of overdose thrombosis.[157]

Valoctocogene roxaparvovec (Roctavian, BioMarin Pharmaceutical) is a gene transfer therapy for adults with severe hemophilia A that was FDA approved in 2023. Approval was based on a phase 3 study with 134 participants who recorded an 85% reduction in annual bleed rate over 110 weeks. The mean annual FVIII infusion rate decreased by 98% from baseline, and the mean FVIII activity at 2 years was 23 IU/dL by chromogenic assay.[158] No participants developed FVIII inhibitors, malignancy, or thromboembolic events. As with many gene transfer methods, participants experienced a short-lived mild to moderate rise in liver enzymes, with no long-lasting clinical sequelae. Other adverse events were headache, arthralgia, nausea, and fatigue.[159]

Hemophilia A and Factor VIII Inhibitors

Alloantibody inhibitors of FVIII arise in response to concentrate therapy in 30% of patients with severe hemophilia and 3% of patients with moderate hemophilia.[160] The provider suspects the presence of an inhibitor when bleeding persists or when the plasma FVIII activity fails to rise to the target level after appropriately dosed concentrate administration. Most FVIII inhibitors are immunoglobulin G4, non-complement-fixing, warm-reacting antibodies. It is impossible to predict which patients are likely to develop inhibitors based on genetics, demographics, or the type of concentrate used.[161]

The FVIII assay is the first step in inhibitor detection. If FVIII activity exceeds 30 IU/dL, no inhibitor is present (conservative laboratory directors use 40 IU/dL as the limit). If the level is under the limit, the laboratory practitioner proceeds to clot-based mixing studies (Chapter 41). When plasma from the bleeding patient produces a prolonged PTT, it is mixed 1:1 with NP and incubated 2 hours at 37° C. The PTT of the incubated mixture is measured. If no inhibitor is present, the incubated mixture should produce a PTT result within 10% of the incubated NP PTT. If an inhibitor is present, however, the FVIII from the NP is partially neutralized and the PTT of the mixture remains prolonged or "uncorrected," presumptive evidence for the inhibitor. Laboratory directors may use alternative correction limits.

If mixing studies and the therapeutic results suggest the presence of an FVIII inhibitor, the Nijmegen-Bethesda assay may be used to quantitate the inhibitor (Chapter 41). NP, providing 100 IU/dL factor activity, is mixed at increasing dilutions (decreasing concentrations) in a series of tubes with undiluted patient plasma. Bovine-based chromogenic FVIII assays are performed on each mixture. The operator then computes the results of the various dilutions and expresses the titer as NBUs; 1 NBU is the reciprocal of the dilution that caused neutralization of 50% of the NP FVIII. The same assay is employed to measure FVIII inhibitors in acquired hemophilia. Although the complex kinetics of autoantibodies diminishes the accuracy of the results in acquired hemophilia, the Nijmegen-Bethesda assay adequately monitors therapy.[162]

Hemophilia patients with inhibitors are classified as *low* or *high responders*. Low responders generate inhibitor levels of 5 NBUs or less, and their inhibitor titers do not increase significantly after FVIII administration. High responders generate inhibitor levels that exceed 5 NBUs, and their NBU score further rises in response to therapy.

Each hemophilia patient with an inhibitor requires an individualized treatment plan to control bleeding. Emicizumab is the preferred treatment for hemophilia patients with inhibitors, as it bypasses the need for FVIII. Fitusiran and valoctocogene roxaparvovec are likely to join emicizumab for this purpose as they come online.

In the absence of emicizumab, low responders may respond to and be maintained using large FVIII concentrate doses. High responders may be treated with APCC (Autoplex T or FEIBA) or rFVIIa, both of which generate thrombin despite the presence of FVIII inhibitors. APCC is not used in combination with emicizumab, as it may induce thrombotic microangiopathy.[163] To prevent the risk of DIC, APCC dosage is limited to a maximum of 200 IU/kg/day. rFVIIa has not been shown to induce DIC.

For hemophilia A patients with inhibitor titers up to 40 NBUs, immune tolerance induction using repeated frequent FVIII administration may permanently reduce the antibody response through the formation of antiidiotypic antibodies.[164]

Hemophilia B (Factor IX Deficiency)

Hemophilia B, also called *Christmas disease*, comprises approximately 14% of hemophilia cases in the United States, although its incidence in India nearly equals that of hemophilia A. *Hemophilia B* is caused by deficiency of FIX, one of the vitamin K-dependent serine proteases. FIX is a substrate for both FXIa and FVIIa because it is cleaved by either protease to form dimeric FIXa. Subsequently, FIXa complexes with FVIIIa to cleave and activate its substrate, FX. FIX deficiency reduces thrombin production (see Figure 36.6) and causes anatomic bleeding that is indistinguishable from bleeding in hemophilia A. It also is a sex-linked, markedly heterogeneous disorder involving numerous separate mutations resulting in a range of mild to severe bleeding manifestations. Phenotypic determination of female carrier status is less successful in hemophilia B than in hemophilia A because of the large number of FIX mutations and the lack of a linked molecule such as VWF that can be used as a normalization index. DNA analysis may be used to establish carrier status when hemophilia B has been diagnosed and its specific mutation identified in a relative.[165]

The laboratory is essential to the diagnosis of hemophilia B. PTT typically is prolonged, whereas PT, fibrinogen assay, and TT are normal. If the clinical symptoms suggest hemophilia B, the chromogenic or clot-based FIX assay is performed, even if the PTT is within its reference interval because the PTT reagent may be insensitive to FIX deficiencies at the level of 30 IU/dL.

Immunine (Takeda) and Mononine (Behring) are human plasma-derived, immunopurified FIX concentrates. When applied to on-demand therapy, dosing is calculated the same way as for FVIII concentrates in hemophilia A except that the calculated initial dose is doubled to compensate for FIX distribution into the extravascular space. Repeat doses of FIX are given every 24 hours, reflecting the half-life of the factor. The second and subsequent doses, if needed, are half the initial dose, provided that factor assays determine that the target level

of FIX was achieved. It is necessary to monitor therapy with recurring laboratory assays because FIX pharmacokinetics are idiosyncratic.

BeneFix (Pfizer) is a recombinant FIX concentrate (rFIX) grown in CHO cells in the absence of human or animal protein. The abundance of rFIX concentrates supports prophylactic administration at a rate of 2 to 3 infusions per week. Extended half-life preparations include the Fc-fusion Alprolix (rFIX-Fc, Sanofi Genzyme), pegylated Rebinyn (Novo Nordisk), and albumin-fusion Idelvion (Behring). These preparations may extend prophylactic factor administration to as seldom as once every 2 weeks.

FIX therapy may be measured using the one-stage clot assay; however, chromogenic assays with improved accuracy, low-level sensitivity, and higher reproducibility are recommended.[166,167]

FIX inhibitors arise in 3% of hemophilia B patients, bind avidly with FIX, and may be detected using the Nijmegen-Bethesda assay. Bleeding in patients with inhibitors is treated as in patients with FVIII inhibitors using APCC or rFVIIa (but not emicizumab) and immune tolerance induction.

Etranacogene dezaparvovec (Hemgenix, Behring) is an adenoassociated virus vector-based gene therapy (AAV) that was FDA approved in 2022.[168,169] Hemgenix employs a FIX gain-of-function variant, FIX Padua, with activity levels 8 times normal FIX, which is inserted into a specialized AAV, AAV8.

Fitusiran, now in phase 3 trials, may be used to treat both hemophilia A and B, with or without inhibitors.

Hemophilia C (Rosenthal Syndrome, Factor XI Deficiency)

FXI deficiency is an autosomal recessive hemophilia with mild to moderate bleeding (see Figure 36.6).[170] More than 190 disease-causing mutations, including 66% missense mutations, result in a prevalence of 1 in 1 million unselected individuals. A founder effect (single ancestral mutation source) concentrates two mutations, *p.Glu117X* and *p.Phe283Leu*, in Ashkenazi and Iraqi Jews, so that 1 in 450 experiences homozygous or compound heterozygous FXI deficiency. Specific allele concentrations are also found in isolated French and English populations. The frequency and severity of bleeding episodes do not correlate with FXI levels, and laboratory monitoring of treatment serves little purpose after the diagnosis is established. The PTT is prolonged, and the PT is normal. In many cases, hemorrhage occurs only at the time of surgery, childbirth, or trauma. The provider treats first with antifibrinolytics TXA or EACA. If these are ineffective, plasma infusions may be employed during bleeds and times of hemostatic challenge. A human plasma-derived FXI concentrate, Hemoleven (LFB), is available in Canada and Europe.[171]

Other Congenital Single-Factor Deficiencies

The remaining congenital single-factor deficiencies listed in Table 36.9 are rare, are caused by autosomal recessive mutations, and are often associated with consanguinity. PT, PTT, and TT may be employed to distinguish among these disorders, as shown in Table 36.8 (see Figure 36.6). In addition, immunoassays may be performed to distinguish among the more prevalent quantitative and the less prevalent qualitative abnormalities. In

TABLE 36.9   Rare Congenital Single-Factor Deficiencies

Deficiency	Factor Levels	Symptoms	Therapy
Afibrinogenemia	No measurable fibrinogen	Severe anatomic bleeding	Fibrinogen concentrate or CRYO to reach >150 mg/dL
Hypofibrinogenemia	Fibrinogen activity assay <220 mg/dL	Moderate systemic bleeding	Fibrinogen concentrate or CRYO to reach >150 mg/dL
Dysfibrinogenemia	Fibrinogen activity assay <220 mg/dL	Mild systemic bleeding	Treat cause such as liver disease
Prothrombin (FII) deficiency	FII <30 IU/dL	Mild systemic bleeding	PCC or plasma to raise FII to 75 IU/dL
FV deficiency	FV <30 IU/dL	Mild systemic bleeding	Platelet concentrate or plasma to raise FV to 75 IU/dL
FVII deficiency	FVII <30 IU/dL	Moderate to severe anatomic bleeding	rFVIIa, PCC, 4-factor PCC to raise FVII to 75 IU/dL
FX deficiency	FX <30 IU/dL	Severe anatomic bleeding	PCC or plasma to raise FX to 75 IU/dL
FXI deficiency	FXI <50 IU/dL	Variable anatomic bleeding	Plasma to raise FXI to 75 IU/dL
FXIII deficiency	FXIII <1 IU/dL	Moderate to severe systemic bleeding, poor wound healing	Plasma or CRYO every 3 weeks

CRYO, Cryoprecipitate; *F,* factor; *PCC,* prothrombin complex concentrate.

qualitative disorders, often called *dysproteinemias,* the bleeding symptoms may be more severe than in quantitative deficiencies, but the risk of inhibitor formation is theoretically smaller. The clot-based measurement of FII (prothrombin) and FX may be replaced by more reproducible chromogenic substrate assays. Fibrinogen is usually measured using the Clauss clot-based assay (Chapter 41), a modification of the TT test, but it also may be measured by turbidimetry or immunoassay (Chapter 42).

Factor V Deficiency

Because platelets transport about 20% of circulating factor V, the platelet function in factor V deficiency may be diminished, which is reflected in abnormal platelet function test results. Both PT and PTT are prolonged. Because of the concentration of FV in platelet α-granules, platelet concentrate is an effective form of therapy for FV deficiency. A combined FV and FVIII deficiency may be caused by a genetic defect traced to chromosome 18 that affects transport of both factors by a common protein in the Golgi apparatus.[172]

Factor VII Deficiency

FVII deficiency causes moderate to severe anatomic hemorrhage.[173] The bleeding does not necessarily reflect the FVII activity level. The half-life of FVII is approximately 6 hours, which affects the frequency of therapy. rFVIIa at 30 µg/mL and nonactivated four-factor PCC preparations are effective and may provide a target FVII level of 10 to 30 IU/dL. Many FVII deficiencies are dysproteinemias. PT but not PTT is prolonged in FVII deficiency.

Factor X Deficiency

FX deficiency causes moderate to severe anatomic hemorrhage that may be treated with FX concentrate Coadex (Bio Products Laboratory), plasma, or nonactivated PCC to produce therapeutic levels of 10 to 40 IU/dL.[174] The half-life of FX is 24 to 40 hours. Acquired FX deficiency has been described in amyloidosis, in paraproteinemia, and in association with antifungal drug therapy. The hemorrhagic symptoms may be life-threatening. Both PT and PTT are prolonged in FX deficiency. In the specialized *Russell viper venom time* test (not to be confused with the *dilute* Russell viper venom test), which activates the

coagulation mechanism at the level of FX, clotting time is prolonged in deficiencies of FX, FV, prothrombin, and fibrinogen. The venom used is harvested from the Russell viper, the most dangerous snake in Asia. This test may be useful in distinguishing a FVII deficiency, which does not prolong the Russell viper venom clotting time, from deficiencies in the common pathway, although specific factor assays are the standard approach.

Factor XIII Deficiency

Plasma FXIII is a tetramer of paired α and β monomers. The intracellular form is a homodimer (two α chains) and is stored in platelets, monocytes, placenta, prostate, and uterus. The α chain contains the active enzyme site, and the β chain is a binding and stabilizing portion. FXIII deficiency occurs in three forms related to the affected chain, as shown in Table 36.10.

Inherited FXIII deficiency is an *autosomal recessive* disorder that affects both sexes in all races. The frequency is estimated at 0.5 in 1 million. *Acquired* FXIII deficiency may occur in association with chronic DIC, Crohn disease, leukemias, ulcerative colitis, and sepsis. In these cases, the FXIII level decreases to 50% of normal, not low enough to create symptoms, although occasionally acquired FXIII deficiencies produce low enough levels to cause mild bleeding. *Acquired FXIII inhibitors* have been described in patients treated with isoniazid, penicillin, valproate, and phenytoin.[175] These drugs may cause complete absence of FXIII.

FXIII activity levels lower than 5% result in hemorrhage. In congenital FXIII deficiency, bleeding is evident in infants, with seepage at the umbilical stump.[176] In adults, bleeding is slow but progressive, accompanied by poor wound healing and slowly resolving hematomas. Recurrent spontaneous abortion and posttraumatic hemorrhage are common. Acquired FXIII inhibitors cause severe bleeding that does not respond to therapy.

TABLE 36.10   Factor XIII Deficiency

Deficiency	Incidence	FXIII Activity	β-Protein	α-Protein
Type I	Rare	Absent	Absent	Absent
Type II	Infrequent	Absent	Normal	Low
Type III	Rare	Low	Absent	Low

Patients with FXIII deficiency have a normal PT and PTT despite anatomic bleeds and poor wound healing. They form weak (non-cross-linked) clots that dissolve within 2 hours when suspended in a 5-molar urea solution, a traditional FXIII screening assay. To confirm FXIII deficiency, factor activity may be measured accurately using a chromogenic substrate assay such as the Berichrom FXIII assay (Siemens) (Chapter 41).

Deficiency of Fibrinolytic Inhibitors

Finally, autosomal inherited deficiencies of the *fibrinolytic* regulatory proteins *α₂-antiplasmin* and *plasminogen activator inhibitor-1* have been reported to cause moderate to severe bleeding. These conditions cause an excess of fibrinolytic activity that leads to poor clot stability with resulting bleeding. Both are rare and may be diagnosed using chromogenic substrate assays.

SUMMARY

- Hemorrhage is classified as localized versus generalized, acquired versus congenital, and anatomic versus mucocutaneous (systemic).
- Acquired hemorrhagic disorders that are diagnosed in the hemostasis laboratory include thrombocytopenia of various etiologies (Chapters 37 and 38), the acute coagulopathy of trauma shock, anemia, liver and renal disease, vitamin K deficiency, acquired hemophilia, acquired von Willebrand disease (VWD), and disseminated intravascular coagulation.
- VWD is the most common congenital bleeding disorder, and the diagnosis and classification of the type and subtypes

require a series of clinical laboratory assays that include von Willebrand factor (VWF) concentration, VWF platelet-binding activity, and factor VIII coagulant activity.
- The hemophilias are congenital single-factor deficiencies that cause moderate to severe anatomic hemorrhage. The most common hemophilias are hemophilias A, B, and C. The clinical laboratory plays a key role in diagnosis, classification, and treatment monitoring in hemophilia.

Now that you have completed this chapter, go back, and read again the case study at the beginning and respond to the questions presented. Answers can be found in Appendix C.

REVIEW QUESTIONS

Answers can be found in Appendix C.

1. What is the most common acquired bleeding disorder?
   a. Trauma-induced coagulopathy
   b. Vitamin K deficiency
   c. Liver disease
   d. VWD
2. Which is a typical form of anatomic bleeding?
   a. Epistaxis
   b. Menorrhagia
   c. Hematemesis
   d. Central nervous system bleed
3. What factor becomes deficient early in liver disease, and what assay does its deficiency prolong?
   a. Prothrombin deficiency; PT
   b. FVII deficiency; PT
   c. FVIII deficiency; PTT
   d. FIX deficiency; PTT
4. Which of the following congenital conditions causes an isolated prolonged thrombin time?
   a. FVII deficiency
   b. Prothrombin deficiency
   c. Hypofibrinogenemia
   d. FXII deficiency
5. In what type or subtype of VWD is the RIPA test result positive when ristocetin is used at a concentration of less than 0.5 mg/mL?
   a. Subtype 2A
   b. Subtype 2B
   c. Subtype 2N
   d. Type 3

6. What is the typical treatment for vitamin K deficiency when the patient is bleeding?
   a. Vitamin K and plasma
   b. Vitamin K and four-factor PCC
   c. Vitamin K and platelet concentrate
   d. Vitamin K and FVIII concentrate
7. If a patient has anatomic bleeding and poor wound healing, but the PT, PTT, platelet count, and platelet functional assay results are normal, what factor deficiency is possible?
   a. Fibrinogen
   b. Prothrombin
   c. FXII
   d. FXIII
8. What therapy may be used for a young hemophilic male who is bleeding and who has a high FVIII inhibitor titer?
   a. Plasma
   b. Emicizumab
   c. Cryoprecipitate
   d. FVIII concentrate
9. What is the most prevalent form of VWD?
   a. Type 1
   b. Type 2A
   c. Type 2B
   d. Type 3
10. Which of the following assays is used to distinguish vitamin K deficiency from liver disease?
    a. PT
    b. Protein C assay
    c. FV assay
    d. FVII assay

11. Mucocutaneous hemorrhage is typical of:
   a. Acquired hemorrhagic disorders
   b. Localized hemorrhagic disorders
   c. Defects in primary hemostasis
   d. Defects in fibrinolysis

REFERENCES

1. Gresele, P., Orsini, S., Noris, P., et al. (2020). Validation of the ISTH/SSC bleeding assessment tool for inherited platelet disorders: a communication from the Platelet Physiology SSC. *J Thromb Haemost, 18,* 732–739.

2. Cunningham, J. M., & Kessler, C. M. (2019). A systematic approach to the bleeding patient: correlation of clinical symptoms and signs with laboratory testing. In Kitchens, C. S., Kessler, C. M., Konkle, B. A., et al. (Eds.), *Consultative Hemostasis and Thrombosis.* (4th ed., pp. 17–38). St. Louis: Elsevier-Saunders.

3. Kitchens, C. S. (2019). Purpura and other hematovascular disorders. In Kitchens, C. S., Kessler, C. M., Konkle, B. A., et al. (Eds.), *Consultative Hemostasis and Thrombosis.* (4th ed., pp. 167–179). St. Louis: Elsevier-Saunders.

4. Weiss, A. E. (1988). Acquired coagulation disorders. In Corriveau, D. M., & Fritsma, G. A. (Eds.), *Hemostasis and Thrombosis in the Clinical Laboratory.* (pp. 169–205). Philadelphia: Lippincott.

5. Vanderhave, K. L., Caird, M. S., Hake, M., et al. (2012). Musculoskeletal care of the hemophiliac patient. *J Am Acad Orthop Surg, 20,* 553–563.

6. Adcock, D. M. (2012). Coagulation assays and anticoagulant monitoring. *Hematology. Am Soc Hematol Educ Program,* 460–465.

7. Wikkelsø, A., Wetterslev, J., Møller, A. M., et al. (2017). Thromboelastography (TEG) or rotational thromboelastometry (ROTEM) to monitor haemostatic treatment in bleeding patients: a systematic review with meta-analysis and trial sequential analysis. *Anaesthesia, 72,* 519–531.

8. Ambaglio, C., Zane, F., Russo, M. C., et al. (2021). Preoperative bleeding risk assessment with ISTH-BAT and laboratory tests in patients undergoing elective surgery: a prospective cohort study. *Haemophilia, 27,* 717–723.

9. Napolitano, M., & Kessler, C. M. (2019). Hemophilia A and B. In Kitchens, C. S., Kessler, C. M., Konkle, B. A., et al. (Eds.), *Consultative Hemostasis and Thrombosis.* (4th ed., pp. 39–58). St. Louis: Elsevier-Saunders.

10. Kitchens, C. S. (2019). Consultative process. In Kitchens, C. S., Kessler, C. M., Konkle, B. A., et al. (Eds.), *Consultative Hemostasis and Thrombosis.* (4th ed., pp. 2–16). St. Louis: Elsevier-Saunders.

11. Centers for Disease Control and Prevention, National Center for Injury Prevention and Control. *Web-based Injury Statistics Query and Reporting System (WISQARS).* www.cdc.gov/injury/wisqars/index. Accessed April 2, 2022.

12. Balvers, K., van Dieren, S., Baksaas-Aasen, K., et al. (2017). Targeted action for curing trauma-induced coagulopathy (TACTIC) collaborators. Combined effect of therapeutic strategies for bleeding injury on early survival, transfusion needs and correction of coagulopathy. *Br J Surg, 104,* 222–229.

13. Kumar, M., Cao, W., McDaniel, J. K., et al. (2017). Plasma ADAMTS13 activity and von Willebrand factor antigen and activity in patients with subarachnoid haemorrhage. *Thromb Haemost, 117,* 691–699.

14. Russell, R. T., McDaniel, J. K., Cao, W., et al. (2018). Low plasma ADAMTS13 activity is associated with coagulopathy, endothelial cell damage and mortality after severe paediatric trauma. *Thromb Haemost 118,* 676–687.

15. Hayakawa, M. (2017). Pathophysiology of trauma-induced coagulopathy: disseminated intravascular coagulation with the fibrinolytic phenotype. *J Intensive Care, 5,* 14. https://doi.org/10.1186/s40560-016-0200-1.

16. Frelitz, A. J. (2016). Impacts of updated transfusion guidelines on a small hospital blood bank in a Chicago suburb. *Clin Lab Sci, 29,* 16–20.

17. Savage, S. A., Sumislawski, J. J., Zarzaur, B. L., et al. (2015). The new metric to define large-volume hemorrhage: results of a prospective study of the critical administration threshold. *J Trauma Acute Care Surg, 78,* 224–229.

18. Cantle, P. M., & Cotton, B. A. (2017). Prediction of massive transfusion in trauma. *Crit Care Clin, 33,* 71–84.

19. Novak, D. J., Bai, Y., Cooke, R. K., et al. (2015). Making thawed universal donor plasma available rapidly for massively bleeding trauma patients: experience from the Pragmatic, Randomized Optimal Platelets and Plasma Ratios (PROPPR) trial. *Transfusion, 55,* 1331–1339.

20. Yonge, J. D., & Schreiber, M. A. (2016). The pragmatic randomized optimal platelet and plasma ratios trial: what does it mean for remote damage control resuscitation? *Transfusion, 56 (Suppl. 2),* S149–S156.

21. Carson, J. L., Guyatt, G., Heddle, N. M., et al. (2016). Clinical practice guidelines from the AABB: red blood cell transfusion thresholds and storage. *JAMA, 316 (19),* 2025–2035.

22. Nguyen, M., Pirracchio, R., Kornblith, L. Z., et al. (2020). Dynamic impact of transfusion ratios on outcomes in severely injured patients: targeted machine learning analysis of the Pragmatic, Randomized Optimal Platelet and Plasma Ratios randomized clinical trial. *Trauma Acute Care Surg, 89,* 505–513.

23. Dumont, L. J., Cancelas, J. A., & Maes, L. A. (2015). The bioequivalence of frozen plasma prepared from whole blood held overnight at room temperature compared to fresh-frozen plasma prepared within eight hours of collection. *Transfusion, 55,* 476–484.

24. Benjamin, R. J., & McLaughlin, L. S. (2012). Plasma components: properties, differences, and uses. *Transfusion, 52 (Suppl. 1),* 9S–19S.

25. Tholpady, A., Monson, J., Radovancevic, R., et al. (2013). Analysis of prolonged storage on coagulation factor (F) V, FVII, and FVIII in thawed plasma: is it time to extend the expiration date beyond 5 days? *Transfusion, 53,* 645–650.

26. Moore, E. E., Moore, H. B., Kornblith, L. Z., et. al. (2021). Trauma-induced coagulopathy. *Nat Rev Dis Primers 7,* 30. https://doi.org/10.1038/s41572-021-00264-3.

27. Chang, R., Cardenas, J. C., Wade, C. E., et al. (2016). Advances in the understanding of trauma-induced coagulopathy. *Blood, 128,* 1043–1049.

28. American Association of Blood Banks, American Red Cross, America's Blood Centers, Armed Service Blood Program. (2021). *Circular of Information for the Use of Human Blood and Blood Components.* https://www.aabb.org/news-resources/resources/circular-of-information. Accessed April 2, 2022.

29. Bulle, E. B., Klanderman, R. B., Pendergrast, J., et al. (2022). The recipe for TACO: a narrative review on the pathophysiology and potential mitigation strategies of transfusion-associated circulatory overload. *Blood Rev, 52.* https://doi.org/10.1016/j.blre.2021.100891.

30. Hunt, A. R., Coffeen, S. N., Shiltz, D. L., et al. (2021). Factor VIII inhibitor bypassing activity (FEIBA) reversal for apixaban and rivaroxaban in patients with acute intracranial and nonintracranial hemorrhage. *Ann Pharmacother, 55,* 1455–1466.

31. Kao, T. W., Lee, Y. C., & Chang, H. T. (2021). Prothrombin complex concentrate for trauma induced coagulopathy: a systematic review and meta-analysis. *J Acute Med, 11,* 81–89.

32. Weber, B. J., & Kjelland, C. B. (2012). The use of tranexamic acid for trauma patients? *Can J Emerg Med, 14,* 53–56.

33. CRASH-2 trial collaborators. (2010). Effects of tranexamic acid on death, vascular occlusive events, and blood transfusion in trauma patients with significant haemorrhage (CRASH-2): a randomised, placebo-controlled trial. *Lancet, 376,* 23–32.

34. Maegele, M. (2016). Coagulation factor concentrate-based therapy for remote damage control resuscitation (RDCR): a reasonable alternative? *Transfusion, 56 (Suppl. 2),* S157–S165.

35. Whyte, C. S., Rastogi, A., Ferguson, E., et al. (2022). The efficacy of fibrinogen concentrates in relation to cryoprecipitate in restoring clot integrity and stability against lysis. *Int J Mol Sci, 23.* https://doi.org/10.3390/ijms23062944.

36. Winearls, J., Campbell, D., Hurn, C., et al. (2016). Fibrinogen in traumatic haemorrhage: a narrative review. *Injury, 48,* 230–242.

37. Seto, S., Itakura, A., Okagaki, R., et al. (2017). An algorithm for the management of coagulopathy from postpartum hemorrhage, using fibrinogen concentrate as first-line therapy. *Int J Obstet Anesth, 32,* 11–16.

38. Wikkelsø, A., Lunde, J., Johansen, M., et al. (2013). Fibrinogen concentrate in bleeding patients. *Cochrane Database Syst Rev, 8,* https://doi.org/10.1002/14651858.CD008864.pub2.

39. WOMAN Trial Collaborators. (2017). Effect of early tranexamic acid administration on mortality, hysterectomy, and other morbidities in women with post-partum haemorrhage (WOMAN): an international, randomised, double-blind, placebo-controlled trial. *Lancet, 389,* 2105–2116.

40. Tosetto, A., & Castaman, G. (2015). How I treat type 2 variant forms of von Willebrand disease. *Blood, 125,* 907–914.

41. Dutton, R. P., Parr, M., Tortella, B. J., et al. CONTROL Study Group. (2011). Recombinant activated factor VII safety in trauma patients: results from the CONTROL trial. *J Trauma, 71,* 12–19.

42. Levi, M., Peters, M., & Buller, H. R. (2005). Efficacy and safety of recombinant factor VIIa for treatment of severe bleeding: a systematic review. Crit *Care Med, 33,* 883–890.

43. Tatoulis, J., Theodore, S., Meswani, M., et al. (2009). Safe use of recombinant activated factor VIIa for recalcitrant postoperative haemorrhage in cardiac surgery. *Interact Cardiovasc Thorac Surg, 9,* 459–462.

44. da Luz, L. T., Nascimento, B., & Rizoli, S. (2013). Thrombelastography (TEG): practical considerations on its clinical use in trauma resuscitation. *Scand J Trauma Resusc Emerg Med, 21.* https://doi.org/10.1186/1757-7241-21-29.

45. Veigas, P. V., Callum, J., Rizoli, S., et al. (2016). A systematic review on the rotational thromboelastometry (ROTEM) values for the diagnosis of coagulopathy, prediction and guidance of blood transfusion and prediction of mortality in trauma patients. *Scand J Trauma Resusc Emerg Med, 24.* https://doi.org/10.1186/s13049-016-0308-2.

46. Lawson, J. W., & Kitchens, C. S. (2019). Understanding and managing the coagulopathy of liver disease. In Kitchens, C. S., Kessler, C. M., Konkle, B. A., et al. (Eds.), *Consultative Hemostasis and Thrombosis.* (4th ed., pp. 695–720). St. Louis: Elsevier-Saunders.

47. Allison, M. G., Shanholtz, C. B., & Sachdeva, A. (2016). Hematological issues in liver disease. *Crit Care Clin, 32,* 385–396.

48. Driever, E. G., & Lisman, T. (2022). Effects of inflammation on hemostasis in acutely ill patients with liver disease. *Semin Thromb Hemost, 48 (5),* 596–606.

49. Skornova, I., Simurda, T., Stasko J., et al. (2021). Use of fibrinogen determination methods in differential diagnosis of hypofibrinogenemia and dysfibrinogenemia. *Clin Lab, 67,* 1028–1034.

50. Shao, Z., Zhao, Y., Feng, L., et al. (2015). Association between plasma fibrinogen levels and mortality in acute-on-chronic hepatitis B liver failure. *Dis Markers.* https://doi.org/10.1155/2015/468596.

51. Hugenholtz, G. C., Adelmeijer, J., Meijers, J. C., et al. (2013). An unbalance between von Willebrand factor and ADAMTS13 in acute liver failure: implications for hemostasis and clinical outcome. *Hepatology, 58,* 752–761.

52. Groeneveld, D. J., Poole L. G., & Luyendyk, J. P. (2021). Targeting von Willebrand factor in liver diseases: a novel therapeutic strategy? *J Thromb Haemost, 19,* 1390–1408.

53. Fouad, Y. M. (2013). Chronic hepatitis C-associated thrombocytopenia: aetiology and management. *Trop Gastroenterol, 34,* 58–67.

54. Stravitz, R. T., Ellerbe, C., Durkalski, V., et al. (2016). Thrombocytopenia is associated with multi-organ system failure in patients with acute liver failure. *Clin Gastroenterol Hepatol, 14,* 613–620.

55. Lisman, T., & Porte, R. J. (2012). Platelet function in patients with cirrhosis. *J Hepatol, 56,* 993–994; author reply 994–995.

56. Bates, S. M. (2012). D-dimer assays in diagnosis and management of thrombotic and bleeding disorders. *Semin Thromb Hemost, 38,* 673–682.

57. Cai, K., Osheroff, W. P., Buczynski, G., et al. (2014). Characterization of Thrombate III, a pasteurized and nanofiltered therapeutic human antithrombin concentrate. *Biologicals, 42,* 133–138.

58. Wiedermann, C. J., & Kaneider, N. C. (2006). A systematic review of antithrombin concentrate use in patients with disseminated intravascular coagulation of severe sepsis. *Blood Coagul Fibrinolysis, 17,* 521–526.

59. Lambert, M. P. (2016). Platelets in liver and renal disease. *Hematology. Am Soc Hematol Educ Program,* 251–255.

60. Cohen, B. D. (2007). Premature aging in uremia. *Mol Cell Biochem, 298,* 195–198.

61. Galbusera, M., Remuzzi, G., & Boccardo, P. (2009). Treatment of bleeding in dialysis patients. *Semin Dial, 22,* 279–286.

62. Thomas, S., Katbab, H., & abu Fanas, S. H. (2010). Do preoperative cutaneous bleeding time tests predict the outcome of intraoral surgical bleeding? *Int Dent J, 60,* 305–310.

63. Showalter, J., Nguyen, N. D., Baba, S., et al. (2017). Platelet aggregometry cannot identify uremic platelet dysfunction in heart failure patients prior to cardiac surgery. *J Clin Lab Anal, 31.* https://doi.org/10.1002/jcla.22084.

64. Knehtl, M., Ponikvar, R., & Buturovic-Ponikvar, J. (2013). Platelet-related hemostasis before and after hemodialysis with five different anticoagulation methods. *Int J Artif Organs, 36,* 717–724.

65. Daugirdas, J. T., & Bernardo, A. A. (2012). Hemodialysis effect on platelet count and function and hemodialysis-associated thrombocytopenia. *Kidney Int, 82,* 147–157.

66. Heida, J. E., Gansevoort, R. T., & Meijer, E. (2021). Acid-base homeostasis during vasopressin V2 receptor antagonist treatment in autosomal dominant polycystic kidney disease patients. *Kidney Int Rep, 6,* 839–841.

67. Khanna, R. (2011). Clinical presentation and management of glomerular diseases: hematuria, nephritic and nephrotic syndrome. *Mo Med, 108,* 33–36.

68. DiNicolantonio, J. J., Bhutani, J., & O'Keefe, J. H. (2015). The health benefits of vitamin K. *Open Heart.* https://doi.org/10.1136/openhrt-2015-000300.

69. Murphy, M. C., & Klein, H. G. (2019). Blood component and pharmacologic therapy for hemostatic disorders. In Kitchens, C. S., Kessler, C. M., Konkle, B. A., et al. (Eds.), *Consultative Hemostasis and Thrombosis.* (4th ed., pp. 540–572). St. Louis: Elsevier-Saunders.

70. Burke, C. W. (2013). Vitamin K deficiency bleeding: overview and considerations. *J Pediatr Health Care, 27,* 215–221.

71. Streiff, M. B. (2019). Prevention and treatment of venous thromboembolism. In Kitchens, C. S., Kessler, C. M., Konkle, B. A., et al. (Eds.), *Consultative Hemostasis and Thrombosis.* (4th ed., pp. 39–58). St. Louis: Elsevier-Saunders.

72. Wright, E., Hafner, J. W., & Podolej, G. (2021). Severe vitamin K-dependent coagulopathy from rodenticide-contaminated synthetic cannabinoids: emergency department presentations. *West J Emerg Med, 22,* 1014–1019.

73. Martin, D. T., Barton, C. A., Dodgion, C., et al. (2016). Emergent reversal of vitamin K antagonists: addressing all the factors. *Am J Surg, 211,* 919–925.

74. Kershaw, G., & Favaloro, E. J. (2012). Laboratory identification of factor inhibitors: an update. *Pathology, 44,* 293–302.

75. Franchini, M., Vaglio, S., Marano, G., et al. (2017). Acquired hemophilia A: a review of recent data and new therapeutic options. *Hematology, 22,* 514–520.

76. Boylan, B., Niemeyer, G. P., Werner, B., et al. (2021). Evaluation of anti-factor VIII antibody levels in patients with haemophilia A receiving immune tolerance induction therapy or bypassing agents. *Haemophilia, 27,* e40–e50.

77. Knoebl, P., & Sperr, W. R. (2021). Emicizumab for the treatment of acquired hemophilia A. *Blood, 137,* 410–419.

78. Kruse-Jarres R., St-Louis, J., Greist, A., et al. (2015). Efficacy and safety of OBI-1, antihaemophilic factor VIII (recombinant), porcine sequence, in subjects with acquired haemophilia A. *Haemophilia, 21*(2), 162–170.

79. Shetty, S., Bhave, M., & Ghosh, K. (2011). Acquired hemophilia A: diagnosis, aetiology, clinical spectrum and treatment options. *Autoimmun Rev, 10,* 311–316.

80. Fareed, J., Paterson, C. A., & Crean, S. M. (2011). A multicenter pilot study to estimate the prevalence of bovine and human coagulation antibodies in the general US population. *Clin Appl Thromb Hemost, 17,* 164–170.

81. Bertolaccini, M. L., & Sanna, G. (2016). Recent advances in understanding antiphospholipid syndrome. *F1000Res, 5,* 2908. https://doi.org/10.12688/f1000research.9717.1.

82. Sreedharanunni, S., Ahluwalia, J., Kumar, N., et al. (2017). Lupus anticoagulant-hypoprothrombinemia syndrome: a rare cause of intracranial bleeding. *Blood Coagul Fibrinolysis, 28,* 416–418.

83. Franchini, M., Frattini, F., Crestani, S., et al. (2013). Acquired FXIII inhibitors: a systematic review. *J Thromb Thrombolysis, 36,* 109–114.

84. Tone, K. J., James, T. E., Fergusson, D. A., et al. (2016). Acquired factor XIII inhibitor in hospitalized and perioperative patients: a systematic review of case reports and case series. *Transfus Med Rev, 30,* 123–131.

85. Matsumoto, T., Nogami, K., & Shima, M. (2014). Coagulation function and mechanisms in various clinical phenotypes of patients with acquired factor V inhibitors. *J Thromb Haemost, 12,* 1503–1512.

86. Minkowitz, H., Navarro-Puerto, J., Lakshman, S., et al. (2019). Prospective, randomized, phase II, non-inferiority study to evaluate the safety and efficacy of topical thrombin (human) Grifols as adjunct to hemostasis during vascular, hepatic, soft tissue, and spinal open surgery. *J Am Coll Surg, 229,* 497–507.

87. Almasri, H., Almeer, A., Awouda, S., et al. (2021). Cardiac amyloidosis presenting with pre-excitation syndrome, heart failure, and severe factor X deficiency as part of systemic amyloid light-chain amyloidosis—a fatal combination. *Am J Case Rep, 22.* https://doi.org/10.12659/AJCR.933398.

88. Broze, G. J. (2014). An acquired, calcium-dependent, factor X inhibitor. *Blood Cells Mol Dis, 52,* 116–120.

89. Federici, A. B. (2011). Acquired von Willebrand syndrome associated with hypothyroidism: a mild bleeding disorder to be further investigated. *Semin Thromb Hemost, 37,* 35–40.

90. Go, A. S., Mozaffarian, D., Roger, V. L., et al. (2014). Heart disease and stroke statistics—2014 update: a report from the American Heart Association. *Circulation, 129,* 399–410.

91. Horiuchi, H., Doman, T., Kokame, K., et al. (2019). Acquired von Willebrand syndrome associated with cardiovascular diseases. *J Atheroscler Thromb, 26,* 303–314.

92. Tiede, A. (2012). Diagnosis and treatment of acquired von Willebrand syndrome. *Thromb Res, 130 (Suppl. 2),* S2–S6.

93. Franchini, M., & Lippi, G. (2007). Acquired von Willebrand syndrome: an update. *Am J Hematol, 82,* 368–375.

94. Connell, N. T., Flood, V. H., Brignardello-Peterson, R., et al. (2021). ASH ISTH NHF WFH 2021 guidelines on the management of von Willebrand disease. *Blood Adv, 5,* 301–325.

95. Favaloro, E. J., Pasalic, L., & Curnow, J. (2016). Laboratory tests used to help diagnose von Willebrand disease: an update. *Pathology, 48,* 303–318.

96. Sanigorska, A., Chaplin, S., Holland, M., et al. (2022). The lived experience of women with a bleeding disorder: a systematic review. *Res Pract Thromb Haemost, 6.* https://doi.org/10.1002/rth2.12652.

97. Naß, J., Terglane, J., & Gerke, V. (2021). Weibel Palade bodies: unique secretory organelles of endothelial cells that control blood vessel homeostasis. *Front Cell Dev Biol,* https://doi.org/10.3389/fcell.2021.813995.

98. Zolkova, J., Sokol, J., Simurda, T., et al. (2020). Genetic background of von Willebrand disease: history, current state, and future perspectives, *Semin Thromb Hemost, 46,* 484–500.

99. Samuelson-Bannow, B. T., & Konkle, B. A. (2019). Von Willebrand disease. In Kitchens, C. S., Kessler, C. M., Konkle, B. A., et al. (Eds.), *Consultative Hemostasis and Thrombosis.* (4th ed., pp. 93–107). St. Louis: Elsevier-Saunders.

100. Favaloro, E. J. (2020). Classification of von Willebrand disease in the context of modern contemporary von Willebrand factor testing methodologies. *Res Pract Thromb Haemost, 4,* 952–957.

101. Favaloro, E. J., & Mohammed, S. (2016). Evaluation of a von Willebrand factor three test panel and chemiluminescent-based assay system for identification of, and therapy monitoring in, von Willebrand disease. *Thromb Res, 141,* 202–211.

102. Verfaillie, C. J., De Witte, E., & Devreese, K. M. J. (2013). Validation of a new panel of automated chemiluminescence assays for von Willebrand factor antigen and activity in the screening for von Willebrand disease. *Int J Lab Hematol, 35,* 555–565.

103. Just, S. (2017). Laboratory testing for von Willebrand disease: the past, present, and future state of play for von Willebrand factor assays that measure platelet binding activity, with or without ristocetin. *Semin Thromb Hemost, 43*, 75–91.

104. Romansky, M. J., Limson, B. M., & Hawkins, J. E. (1956–57). Ristocetin; a new antibiotic-laboratory and clinical studies; preliminary report. *Antibiot Annu, 706*, 706–715.

105. Favaloro, E. J. (2014). Diagnosing von Willebrand disease: a short history of laboratory milestones and innovations, plus current status, challenges, and solutions. *Semin Thromb Hemost, 40*, 551–570.

106. James, A. H., Eikenboom, J., & Federici, A. B. (2016). State of the art: von Willebrand disease. *Haemophilia, 22 (Suppl. 5)*, 54–59.

107. Patzke, J., Budde, U., Huber, A., et al. (2014). Performance evaluation and multicenter study of a von Willebrand factor activity assay based on GPIb binding in the absence of ristocetin. *Blood Coagul Fibrinolysis, 25*, 860–870.

108. Sharma, R., & Haberichter S. J. (2019). New advances in the diagnosis of von Willebrand disease. *Hematology. Am Soc Hematol Educ Program*, 596–600.

109. Favaloro, E. J. (2022). Commentary on the ASH, ISTH, NHF, WFH 2021 guidelines on the diagnosis of VWD: reflections based on recent contemporary test data. *Blood Adv, 6*, 416–419.

110. Weyand, A. C., & Flood, V. H. (2021). Von Willebrand disease; current status of diagnosis and management. *Hematol Oncol Clin N Am, 35*, 1085–1101.

111. James, P. D., Connell, N. T., Ameer, B., et al. (2021). ASH, ISTH, NHF, WFH 2021 guidelines on the diagnosis of von Willebrand disease. *Blood Adv, 5*, 280–300.

112. Haberichter, S. L., Castaman, G., Budde, U., et al. (2008). Identification of type 1 von Willebrand disease patients with reduced von Willebrand factor survival by assay of the VWF propeptide in the European study: molecular and clinical markers for the diagnosis and management of type 1 VWD (MCMDM-1VWD). *Blood, 111*, 4979–4985.

113. Favaloro, E. J. (2017). Utility of the von Willebrand factor collagen-binding assay in the diagnosis of von Willebrand disease. *Am J Hematol, 92*, 114–118.

114. Flood, V. H., Gill, J. C., Friedman, K. D., et al. (2013). Collagen binding provides a sensitive screen for variant von Willebrand disease. *Clin Chem, 59*, 684–691.

115. Flood, V. H., Schlauderaff, A. C., Haberichter, S. L., et al. (2015). Crucial role for the VWF A1 domain in binding to type IV collagen. *Blood, 125*, 2297–2304.

116. Ferhat-Hamida, M. Y., Boukerb, H., & Hariti, G. (2015). Contribution of the collagen binding activity (VWF:CB) in the range of tests for the diagnosis and classification of von Willebrand disease. *Ann Biol Clin, 73*, 461–468.

117. Zolkova, J., Sokol, J., Simurda, T., et al. (2020). Genetic background of von Willebrand disease: history, current state, and future perspectives. *Semin Thromb Hemost, 46*, 484–500.

118. Swystun, L. L., & Lillicrap, D. (2018). Genetic regulation of plasma von Willebrand factor levels in health and disease. *J Thromb Haemost, 16*, 2375–2390.

119. DiGiandomenico, S., Christopherson, P. A., Haberichter, S. L., et al. (2021). Laboratory variability in the diagnosis of type 2 VWD variants. *J Thromb Haemost, 19*, 131–138.

120. Jaffray, J., Staber, J. M., & Malvar, J. (2020). Laboratory misdiagnosis of von Willebrand disease in post-menarchal females: a multi-center study. *Am J Hematol, 95*, 1022–1029.

121. Bucciarelli, P., Siboni, S. M., Stufano, F., et al. (2015). Predictors of von Willebrand disease diagnosis in individuals with borderline von Willebrand factor plasma levels. *J Thromb Haemost, 13*, 228–236.

122. Norton, C. (2016). How to use PRICE treatment for soft tissue injuries. *Nurs Stand, 30*, 48–52.

123. Heijdra, J. M., Cnossen, M. H., & Leebeek, F. W. G. (2017). Current and emerging options for the management of inherited von Willebrand disease. *Drug, 77*, 1531–1547.

124. Sreeraman, S., McKinlay, S., Li, A., et al. (2022). Efficacy of parenteral formulations of desmopressin in the treatment of bleeding disorders: A systematic review. *Thromb Res, 213*, 16–26.

125. Kouides, P. A. (2017). Antifibrinolytic therapy for preventing VWD-related postpartum hemorrhage: indications and limitations. *Blood Adv, 1*, 699–702.

126. Bofill-Rodriguez, M., Lethaby, A., & Jordan, V. (2020). Progestogen-releasing intrauterine systems for heavy menstrual bleeding. *Cochrane Database Syst Rev, 6*, CD002126.

127. Stanciakova, L., Dobrotova, M., Holly, P., et al. (2022). How can secondary thromboprophylaxis in high-risk pregnant patients be improved? *Clin Appl Thromb Hemost*. https://doi.org/10.1177/10760296211070004.

128. Leebeek, F. W. G., Duvekot, J., & Kruip, M. J. H. A. (2020). How I manage pregnancy in carriers of hemophilia and patients with von Willebrand disease. *Blood, 136*, 2143–2150.

129. Stoof, S. C., van Steenbergen, H. W., Zwagemaker, A., et al. (2015). Primary postpartum haemorrhage in women with von Willebrand disease or carriership of haemophilia despite specialised care: a retrospective survey. *Haemophilia, 21*, 505–512.

130. Castaman, G., & James, P. D. (2019). Pregnancy and delivery in women with von Willebrand disease. *Eur J Haematol, 103*, 73–79.

131. Peyvandi, F., Castaman, G., Gresele, P., et al. (2019). A phase III study comparing secondary long-term prophylaxis versus on-demand treatment with VWF/FVIII concentrates in severe inherited von Willebrand disease. *Blood Transfus, 17*, 391–398.

132. Berntorp, E., & Windyga, J. (2009). European Wilate Study Group: Treatment and prevention of acute bleedings in von Willebrand disease—efficacy and safety of Wilate, a new generation von Willebrand factor/FVIII concentrate. *Haemophilia, 15*, 122–130.

133. Batle, J., López-Fernández, M. F., Fraga, E. L., et al. (2009). Von Willebrand factor/ FVIII concentrates in the treatment of von Willebrand disease. *Blood Coagul Fibrinolysis, 20*, 89–100.

134. Leebeek, F. W. G., Peyvandi, F., Escobar, M., et al. (2022). Recombinant von Willebrand factor prophylaxis in patients with severe von Willebrand disease: phase 3 study results. *Blood, 140*, 89–98.

135. Borràs, N., Castillo-González, D., Comes, N., et al. (2022). Molecular study of a large cohort of 109 haemophilia patients from Cuba using a gene panel with next generation sequencing-based technology. *Haemophilia, 28*, 125–137.

136. Li, D. Y., Zhang, H. W., Feng, Q. Z., et al. (2015). Impacts of leukocyte filtration and irradiation on coagulation factors in fresh frozen plasma. *Exp Ther Med, 9*, 598–602.

137. Childers, K. C., Peters, S. C., & Spiegel, Jr., P. C. (2022). Structural insights into blood coagulation factor VIII: procoagulant complexes, membrane binding, and antibody inhibition. *J Thromb Haemost, 20*, 1957–1970.

138. Weiss, A. E. (1988). The hemophilias. In Corriveau, D. M., & Fritsma, G. A. (Eds.), *Hemostasis and Thrombosis in the Clinical Laboratory*. (pp. 128–168) Philadelphia: Lippincott.

139. Tomeo, F., Mariz, S., Brunetta, A. L., et al. (2021). Haemophilia, state of the art and new therapeutic opportunities, a regulatory perspective. *Br J Clin Pharmacol, 87*, 4183–4196.

140. Evatt, B. L. (2006). The tragic history of AIDS in the hemophilia population, 1982-1984. *J Thromb Haemost, 4*, 2295–2301.

141. Labarque, V., Perinparajah, V., Bouskill, V., et al. (2017). Utility of factor VIII and factor VIII to von Willebrand factor ratio in identifying 277 unselected carriers of hemophilia A. *Am J Hematol, 92*, E94–E96.

142. D'Amici, G. M., Blasi, B., D'Alessandro, A., et al. (2011). Plasma-derived clotting factor VIII: heterogeneity evaluation in the quest for potential inhibitory-antibody stimulating factors. *Electrophoresis, 32*, 2941–2950.

143. Ghosh, K., & Ghosh, K. (2021). Overcoming the challenges of treating hemophilia in resource-limited nations: a focus on medication access and adherence. *Expert Rev Hematol, 14*, 721–730.

144. Kessler, C. M., Gill, J. C., White, G. C., et al. (2005). B-domain deleted recombinant FVIII preparations are bioequivalent to a monoclonal antibody purified plasma-derived FVIII concentrate: a randomized, three-way crossover study. *Haemophilia, 11*, 84–91.

145. Gringeri, A., Lundin, V., von Mackensen, S., et al. (2009). Primary and secondary prophylaxis in children with haemophilia A reduces bleeding frequency and arthropathy development compared to on demand treatment: a 10-year, randomized clinical trial. *J Thromb Haemost, 7*, 780–786.

146. Konkle, B. A., Huston, H., & Nakaya-Fletcher, S. (2017). Hemophilia A. In Adam, M. P., Mirzaa, G. M., Pagon, R. A., et al. (Eds.), *GeneReviews*. Seattle, WA: University of Washington, Seattle.

147. Sommer, J. M., Moore, N., McGuffie-Valentine, B., et al. (2014). Comparative field study evaluating the activity of recombinant factor VIII Fc fusion protein in plasma samples at clinical haemostasis laboratories. *Haemophilia, 20*, 294–300.

148. Pipe, S. W., Montgomery, R. R., Pratt, K. P., et al. (2016). Life in the shadow of a dominant partner: the FVIII-VWF association and its clinical implications for hemophilia A. *Blood, 128*, 2007–2016.

149. Marques, M. B., & Fritsma, G. A. (2015). *Quick Guide to Coagulation Testing*. (3rd ed., p. 89). Washington, DC: American Association for Clinical Chemistry Press.

150. Girolami, A., Cosi, E., Tasinato, V., et al. (2016). Pulmonary embolism in congenital bleeding disorders: intriguing discrepancies among different clotting factors deficiencies. *Blood Coagul Fibrinolysis, 27*, 517–525.

151. Rietveld, I. M., Lijfering, W. M., le Cessie, S., et al. (2018). High levels of coagulation factors and venous thrombosis risk: strongest association for factor VIII and von Willebrand factor. *J Thromb Haemost, 17*, 99–109.

152. Ovanesov, M. V., Jackson, J. W., Golding, B., et al. (2021). Considerations on activity assay discrepancies in factor VIII and factor IX products. *J Thromb Haemost, 19*, 2102–2111.

153. Valsecchi, C., Gobbi, M., Beeg, M., et al. (2020). Characterization of the neutralizing anti-emicizumab antibody in a patient with hemophilia A and inhibitor. *J Thromb Haemost, 19*, 711–718.

154. Lowe, A., Kitchen, S., Jennings, I., et al. (2020). Effects of emicizumab on APTT, FVIII assays and FVIII inhibitor assays using different reagents: results of a UK NEQAS proficiency testing exercise. *Haemophilia, 26*, 1087–1091.

155. Krumb, E., Fijnvandraat, K., Makris, M., et al. (2021). Adoption of emicizumab (Hemlibra) for hemophilia A in Europe: data from the 2020 European Association for Haemophilia and Allied Disorders survey. *Haemophilia, 27*, 736–743.

156. Ellsworth, P., & Ma, A. (2021). Factor-mimetic and rebalancing therapies in hemophilia A and B: the end of factor concentrates? *Hematology. Am Soc Hematol Educ Program, 10*, 219–225.

157. Croteau, S. E., Wang, M., & Wheeler, A. P. (2021). 2021 clinical trials update: innovations in hemophilia therapy. *Am J Hematol, 96*, 128–144.

158. Rosen, S., Tiefenbacher, S., Robinson, M., et al. (2020). Activity of transgene-produced B-domain–deleted factor VIII in human plasma following AAV5 gene therapy. *Blood, 136*, 2524–2534.

159. George, L. A., Monahan, P. E., Eyster, M. E., et al. (2021). Multiyear factor VIII expression after AAV gene transfer for hemophilia A. *N Engl J Med, 385*, 1961–1973.

160. Franchini, M., Lippi, G., & Favaloro, E. J. (2012). Acquired inhibitors of coagulation factors: part II. *Semin Thromb Hemost, 38*, 447–453.

161. Favaloro, E. J., Meijer, P., Jennings, I., et al. (2013). Problems and solutions in laboratory testing for hemophilia. *Semin Thromb Hemost, 39*, 816–833.

162. Douglas, C., Quinton, T., Cabanban, E., et al. (2018). Standardized kit for a chromogenic modified Nijmegen-Bethesda assay: repeatability, reproducibility, and analytical sensitivity. *Blood, 132 (Suppl. 1)*. https://doi.org/10.1182/blood-2018-99-119491.

163. Ettingshausen, E. C., & Sidonio, Jr., R. F. (2021). Design of an international investigator-initiated study on MOdern Treatment of Inhibitor-positiVe pATiEnts with haemophilia A (MOTIVATE). *Ther Adv Hematol, 12*. https://doi.org/10.1177/20406207211032452.

164. Ter Avest, P. C., Fischer, K., Gouw, S. C., et al. (2010). Successful low dose immune tolerance induction in severe haemophilia A with inhibitors below 40 Bethesda IU. *Haemophilia, 16*, 71–79.

165. Bastida, J. M., González-Porras, J. R., Jiménez, C., et al. (2017). Application of a molecular diagnostic algorithm for haemophilia A and B using next-generation sequencing of entire F8, F9 and VWF genes. *Thromb Haemost, 117*, 66–74.

166. Jeanpierre, E., Pouplard, C., Lasne, D., et al. (2020). Factor VIII and IX assays for post-infusion monitoring in hemophilia patients: Guidelines from the French BIMHO group (GFHT). *Eur J Haematol, 105*, 103–115.

167. Kitchen, S., Tiefenbacher, S., & Gosselin, R. (2017). Factor activity assays for monitoring extended half-life FVIII and FIX replacement therapies. *Semin Thromb Hemost, 43*, 331–337.

168. Heo, Y. A. (2023). Etranacogene dezaparvovec: first approval. *Drugs 83*, 347–352.

169. Chowdary, P., Shapiro, S., Makris, M., et al. (2022). Phase 1-2 trial of AAVS3 gene therapy in patients with hemophilia B. *N Engl J Med, 387*, 237–352.

170. Asselta, R., Paraboschi, E. M., Rimoldi, V., et al. (2017). Exploring the global landscape of genetic variation in coagulation factor XI deficiency. *Blood, 130(4)*, e1–e6.

171. Bauduer, F., de Raucourt, E., Boyer-Neumann, C., et al. (2015). Factor XI replacement for inherited factor XI deficiency in routine clinical practice: results of the HEMOLEVEN prospective 3-year postmarketing study. *Haemophilia, 21*, 481–489.

172. Nichols, W. C., Seligsohn, U., Zivelin, A., et al. (1997). Linkage of combined factors V and VIII deficiency to chromosome 18q by homozygosity mapping. *J Clin Invest, 99*, 596–601.

173. Mariani, G., & Bernardi, F. (2009). Factor VII deficiency. *Semin Thromb Hemost, 35*, 400–406.

174. Menegatti, M., & Peyvandi, F. (2009). Factor X deficiency. *Semin Thromb Hemost, 35*, 407–415.

175. Franchini, M., Frattini, F., Crestani, S., et al. (2013). Acquired FXIII inhibitors: a systematic review. *J Thromb Thrombolysis, 36*, 109–114.

176. Mangla, A., Hamad, H., & Kumar, A. (2022). Factor XIII deficiency. In StatPearls. Treasure Island (FL). StatPearls Publishing. https://www.ncbi.nlm.nih.gov/books/NBK557467. Accessed January 4, 2023.

37

Qualitative Disorders of Platelets and Vasculature

*Walter P. Jeske and Phillip J. DeChristopher**

OBJECTIVES

After completion of this chapter, the reader will be able to:

1. Identify the most common type of hereditary platelet defect.
2. Differentiate hereditary platelet defects based on their underlying mechanism (adhesion, secretion, aggregation).
3. Distinguish among the following types of inherited platelet disorders: membrane receptor abnormalities, secretion disorders, and storage pool deficiency.
4. Describe the defect in each of the following hereditary disorders: storage pool disease, gray platelet syndrome, Glanzmann thrombasthenia, and Bernard-Soulier syndrome.
5. Contrast Glanzmann thrombasthenia and Bernard-Soulier syndrome.
6. Identify platelet disorders that are associated with giant platelets.
7. Identify platelet disorders that have storage pool defects.
8. List common causes leading to acquired platelet defects.
9. Discuss the four mechanisms of action of common antiplatelet drugs and list representative drugs for each.
10. Describe the impact of inherited disorders of receptors and signaling pathways on platelet function.
11. Explain the effects of paraproteins on platelet function.
12. Recognize the clinical presentation of patients with dysfunctional platelets.
13. Given results of laboratory tests used to diagnose platelet disorders, interpret and correlate the tests to determine the specific platelet disorder.
14. Discuss the platelet defects associated with myeloproliferative neoplasms, uremia, and liver disease.
15. Recognize conditions associated with acquired vascular disorders.
16. Describe the known hereditary vascular disorders.

OUTLINE

Qualitative Platelet Disorders: Inherited Defects
Disorders of Platelet Aggregation (Glycoprotein IIb/IIIa Function)
Disorders of Platelet Adhesion (Glycoprotein Ib/IX/V Function)
Inherited Giant Platelet Syndromes
Disorders of Platelet Secretion
Disorders of Receptors and Signaling Pathways

Qualitative Platelet Disorders: Acquired Defects
Drug-Induced Defects
Medical Conditions That Affect Platelet Function
Other Causes of Platelet Function Defects
Hyperaggregable Platelets
Vascular Disorders
Inherited Vascular Disorders
Acquired Vascular Disorders

CASE STUDY

After studying the material in this chapter, the reader should be able to respond to the following case study. Answers can be found in Appendix C.

A 19-year-old woman with a chief complaint of easy bruising, occasional mild nosebleeds, and heavy menstrual periods was examined by the provider. At the time of her examination, she had a few small bruises on her arms and legs, but no other findings. Initial laboratory data revealed PT and PTT within reference intervals. A CBC, including PLT and morphology, yielded results within reference intervals. Reference intervals can be found after the index at the end of the book.

A detailed history revealed that the patient's bleeding problems occurred most frequently after aspirin ingestion. Her mother and one of her brothers also had some of the same symptoms. Blood was drawn for platelet function studies. Platelet aggregation tests indicated that although the response to ristocetin and adenosine diphosphate were near normal, arachidonic acid-induced aggregation was absent, epinephrine induced only primary aggregation, and collagen-induced aggregation was decreased (but a near-normal aggregation response could be obtained with a high collagen concentration). Spontaneous aggregation was not observed.

1. What are three possible explanations for the test results?
2. Given the bleeding history in the patient's family, which of the three above explanations seems most likely?

A test for adenosine triphosphate (ATP) release from platelets was performed by the lumiaggregation assay using the luciferin-luciferase reagent (Chapter 41). The result of this test showed a marked decrease in the amount of ATP released when platelets were stimulated with thrombin.

3. Based on the ATP release test results, what is the likely cause of the patient's bleeding symptoms?

---

*The authors extend appreciation to Larry D. Brace, whose work in prior editions provided the foundation for this chapter.

Clinical manifestations of bleeding disorders can be divided into two broad, rather poorly defined groups: (1) *superficial bleeding* (e.g., petechiae, epistaxis, or gingival bleeding), usually associated with a platelet defect or vascular disorder, and (2) *deep tissue bleeding* (e.g., hematomas or hemarthrosis), usually associated with plasma clotting factor deficiencies.[1] This chapter focuses on qualitative platelet defects and vascular disorders; quantitative platelet disorders, i.e., specific thrombocytopenia disorders, are detailed in Chapter 38. Bleeding problems resulting from defects in the coagulation mechanism are described in Chapter 36.

QUALITATIVE PLATELET DISORDERS: INHERITED DEFECTS

Excessive bruising and superficial (mucocutaneous) bleeding in a patient whose platelet count is normal suggest an acquired or a congenital disorder of *platelet function*. Decades ago, the first major improvements in the understanding of these *qualitative* platelet disorders occurred following the widespread development of automated cell counters and test methods for measuring platelet activities. This chapter discusses the individual qualitative platelet disorders, grouped by the mechanism underlying the defect, as summarized in Box 37.1.

Many of the platelet function disorders are associated with defects in platelet structure. Figure 37.1 illustrates the relationship between defects in platelet surface and intracellular components responsible for specific platelet disorders.[2]

Congenital disorders that result from abnormalities of each of the major phases of platelet function (adhesion, secretion,

---

BOX 37.1   Inherited and Acquired Qualitative Platelet Abnormalities

Aggregation defects
  Glanzmann thrombasthenia
  Hereditary afibrinogenemia
  Acquired von Willebrand disease
  Acquired uremia
  Drug-induced membrane modifications
Adhesion defects
  Bernard-Soulier syndrome
  von Willebrand disease
  Acquired with:
    Myeloproliferative neoplasms
    Dysproteinemias
    Cardiopulmonary bypass surgery
    Chronic liver disease
Platelet secretion defects
  Storage pool diseases (e.g., gray platelet syndrome)
  Thromboxane pathway disorders
  Drug inhibition of the prostaglandin pathways
  Drug inhibition of platelet phosphodiesterase activity
Disorders of platelet membrane components
  Defects in receptors
  Defects in calcium mobilization
  Changes in membrane phospholipid distribution
Hyperactive prothrombotic platelets

---

and aggregation) have been described. Inherited platelet disorders are a heterogeneous group of often rare diseases caused by molecular anomalies in genes that are relevant to platelet formation and/or function. Table 37.1 lists the currently known underlying genetic mutations found to be associated with some of the more common inherited platelet function defects. Major improvements in the knowledge of these disorders have come from whole genome sequencing. The details of this expanding scope of diseases is beyond the scope of this chapter but are documented in recent reviews on the subject.[3,4]

Disorders of Platelet Aggregation (Glycoprotein IIb/IIIa Function)

Glanzmann Thrombasthenia

Glanzmann thrombasthenia (GT) is an autosomal recessive disorder most frequently seen in populations with a high degree of consanguinity. Heterozygotes are clinically normal, whereas homozygotes have serious bleeding problems. GT manifests clinically in the neonatal period or infancy, occasionally with bleeding after circumcision and frequently with epistaxis and gingival bleeding. Hemorrhagic manifestations, which can occur with varying severity, include petechiae, purpura (Figure 38.1), epistaxis, hemarthrosis, menorrhagia, gastrointestinal bleeding, and hematuria. The severity of the bleeding episodes seems to decrease with age.[5,6]

The biochemical lesion responsible for the disorder is a deficiency or abnormality of the platelet membrane glycoprotein (GP) IIb/IIIa (integrin $\alpha_{IIb}\beta_3$) complex (Chapter 11). This membrane receptor is capable of binding fibrinogen, von Willebrand factor (VWF), fibronectin, and other adhesive ligands. Binding of fibrinogen to the GPIIb/IIIa complex mediates normal platelet aggregation responses. Failure of such binding results in a profound defect in hemostatic platelet plug formation and the serious bleeding characteristic of thrombasthenia.[7-9]

Typically the platelets of homozygous individuals lack surface-expressed GPIIb/IIIa, whereas the GPIIb/IIIa content of platelets from heterozygotes has been found to be 50% to 60% of normal.[7,10] Historically, patients with GT have been designated as type 1 or type 2. Patients with type 2 disease have more GPIIb/IIIa complexes (10% to 20% of normal) than patients with type 1 disease (0% to 5% of normal), although there is considerable variability within each subdivision.[11,12] Additionally, patients with type 2 disease are less affected by abnormal clot formation and fibrinogen binding.

More than 70 mutations, distributed widely over the *ITGA2B* and *ITGB3* genes present on chromosome 17,[13] are known to give rise to GT.[14-16] Gene defects that impair production of either protein of the GPIIb/IIIa receptor complex lead to absence of the complex on the platelet surface. Defects that interfere with or prevent complex formation or affect complex stability have the same effect. Rarely, thrombocytopenia and large platelets (5 to 8 μm in diameter) may be seen with some of the mutations in these genes (see Table 37.1; also Table 38.1). The integrin component α_{IIb} is synthesized in megakaryocytes as pro-α_{IIb}, which complexes with the β_3 unit in the endoplasmic reticulum. This complex is transported to the Golgi body, where α_{IIb} is cleaved to heavy and light chains to form the complete complex. Uncomplexed α_{IIb} and β_3 are not processed in the Golgi body.

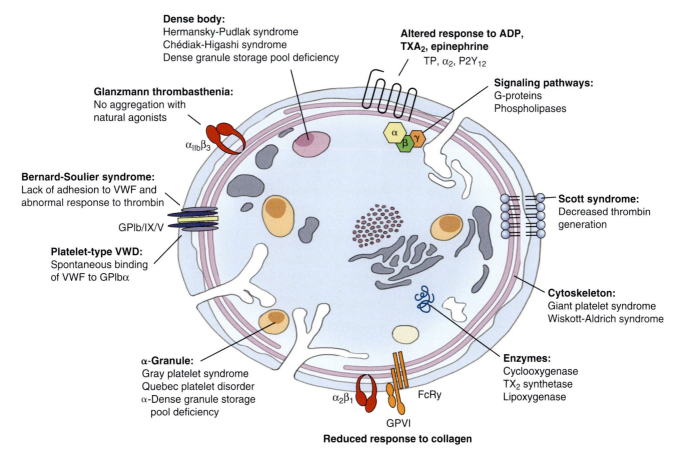

Figure 37.1 Illustration of the Primary Disorders Associated With Defects of the Surface and Intracellular Components of Platelets.

Both proteins of the GPIIb/IIIa complex must be produced and assembled into a complex to be expressed on the platelet surface.

Numerous variants of GT have been described in which α_{IIb} and β_3 are produced, form a complex, and are processed normally, but one or more functions of the complex (e.g., fibrinogen binding or signal transduction) are abnormal. As expected, bleeding in these patients ranges from mild to severe.

The β_3 unit of the $\alpha_{IIb}\beta_3$ integrin is also a component of the vitronectin receptor, $\alpha_V\beta_3$, found on endothelial cells, osteoclasts, fibroblasts, monocytes, and activated B lymphocytes, where it acts as a receptor for a variety of adhesive protein ligands. Patients who have β_3 gene defects that result in the absence of the $\alpha_{IIb}\beta_3$ integrin also lack the vitronectin receptor. These patients do not seem to have a more severe form of GT.[17,18] The vitronectin receptor is thought to play a role in vascularization, but to date, there is no evidence for abnormal blood vessel development in individuals lacking the vitronectin receptor. It also is unclear whether platelet vitronectin receptors play a significant role in normal platelet function.[14]

Rarely, a thrombasthenia-like state can be acquired.[19] This can result from the development of autoantibodies against GPIIb/IIIa in patients with solid cancers or multiple myeloma, with other autoimmune diseases, following organ transplantation, or with genetic defects in signaling molecules involved in GPIIb/IIIa activation such as kindlin-3 or calcium and diacylglycerol-regulated guanine nucleotide exchange factor-1. A thrombasthenia-like state also can be induced in individuals with otherwise normal platelet function by a variety of therapeutic antiplatelet drugs.[6,9]

Laboratory features. The typical laboratory features of GT include a normal platelet count, normal platelet morphology, and a lack of platelet aggregation in response to all platelet-activating agents (including adenosine diphosphate [ADP], collagen, thrombin, and epinephrine).[7,9] Stimulation with strong agonists (e.g., thrombin) induce the release/secretion reaction, even in the absence of aggregation. Ristocetin-induced binding of VWF to platelets and the resulting platelet agglutination are normal.

It has been shown that the release of platelet procoagulant substances is diminished in patients with GT.[10,20] When normal platelets are activated, procoagulant microvesicles are shed from the platelet surface; coagulation factors assemble on these microvesicle surfaces during activation of the coagulation system. In patients with GT, markedly fewer microvesicles are produced. Additionally, prothrombin binds directly to GPIIb/IIIa.[21] Because this complex is missing on platelets from patients with GT, significantly less thrombin is generated in response to tissue factor activation. In general, GT platelets are activated by thrombin to a lesser degree than normal platelets.[22-25]

Treatment. Thrombasthenia is one of the few forms of platelet dysfunction in which hemorrhage can be severe and disabling. Treatment of bleeding episodes in patients with GT requires the transfusion of normal platelets. It may be necessary to infuse more donor platelets than expected to control bleeding, as the defective platelets may interfere with the normal transfused platelets.[26,27] As the use of repeated transfusions in patients with GT may result in human leukocyte antigen (HLA)

TABLE 37.1	**Genomic Defects Causing Inherited Platelet Function Disorders**			
Disorder	**Gene**	**Chromosome Location**	**Autosomal Inheritance**	**Pathophysiology**
Aggregation Defects				
Glanzmann thrombasthenia	*ITGA2B*	17q21.31	Recessive	Severe bleeding tendency; defective GPIIb/IIIa; impaired fibrinogen-mediated aggregation
	ITGB3	17q21.32		
Adhesion Defects				
Bernard-Soulier syndrome	*GP1BA*	17p13.2	Recessive	Moderate to severe thrombocytopenia and giant platelets; defective GPIb/IX/V receptor; impaired adhesion to VWF
	GP1BB	22q11.21		
	GP9	3q21.3		
Platelet-type von Willebrand disease	*GPIBA*	17p13.2	Dominant	Defective GPIb/IX/V receptor; gain-of-function interaction between VWF and GPIbα
Platelet Granule Defects				
Gray platelet syndrome	*NBEAL2*	3p21.31	Recessive	Selective defective development of α-granules; moderate to severe bleeding tendency
	GFI1B		Dominant	
Quebec platelet syndrome	*PLAU*	10p22.2	Recessive	α-granule protein defect; increased storage of urokinase plasminogen activator
Hermansky-Pudlak syndrome	Multiple genes: *HPS1, AP3B1, HPS3 to HPS9*	Multiple different locations	All mutations recessive	Defective development of dense granules
Chédiak-Higashi syndrome	*LYST*	1q42.3	Recessive	Giant granules
Receptor and Signaling Defects				
ADP receptor defect	*P2RY12*	3q25.1	Recessive	Abnormal response to ADP; disaggregation with high-dose ADP
TXA$_2$ receptor defect	*TBXA2R*	19p13.3	Recessive	Abnormal response to TXA$_2$
GPVI defect	*GP6*	19q13.4	Recessive	Impaired response to collagen

ADP, Adenosine diphosphate; *GP,* glycoprotein; *TXA$_2$,* thromboxane A$_2$; *VWF,* von Willebrand factor.
Adapted from Al-Huniti, A., & Kahr, W. H. A. (2020). Inherited platelet disorders: diagnosis and management. *Transfus Med Rev, 34,* 277–285 and Palma-Barqueros, V., Revella, N., Sanchez, A., et al. (2021). Inherited platelet disorders: an updated overview. *Int J Mol Sci, 4521,* 1–31.

alloimmunization, it is recommended that patients with GT who are bleeding receive prestorage, leukocyte-reduced apheresis platelets or HLA-matched donor platelets.

In general, patients with GT should avoid the use of anticoagulants and antiplatelet agents such as aspirin and nonsteroidal anti-inflammatory drugs (NSAIDs) to reduce bleeding risk. A variety of treatments have been used successfully to control or prevent bleeding, alone or in combination with platelet transfusion. Largely, the site of hemorrhage determines the therapeutic approach.

Hormonal therapy (norethindrone acetate) has been used to control menorrhagia. Menorrhagia at the onset of menses is uniformly severe and can be a life-threatening condition, which has led some to suggest that birth control pills be started before menarche. Antifibrinolytic therapy (aminocaproic acid or tranexamic acid) can be used to control gingival hemorrhage or excessive bleeding after tooth extraction.[12] Recombinant factor VIIa (rFVIIa; NovoSeven) is used to treat surgical and nonsurgical bleeding in patients with GT who are refractory to platelet transfusions, with or without isoantibodies to GPIIb/IIIa.[28] rFVIIa is thought to enhance a burst of thrombin generation after activating factor X (FX) to FXa at the wound site by stimulating tissue factor-independent thrombin generation and fibrin formation.[29]

Disorders of Platelet Adhesion (Glycoprotein Ib/IX/V Function)

Bernard-Soulier Syndrome

Bernard-Soulier syndrome (BSS) is a rare autosomal recessive disorder of platelet adhesion that usually manifests in infancy or childhood, with hemorrhage characteristic of defective platelet function including ecchymoses, epistaxis, and gingival bleeding. Hemarthroses and expanding hematomas are rarely seen. Platelets from patients with BSS either lack the GPIb/IX/V complex or express a GPIb/IX/V complex with abnormal function, leading to an inability of platelets to bind to VWF and adhere to exposed subendothelium (Chapters 11 and 36). This defect in adhesion demonstrates the importance of initial platelet attachment for *primary hemostasis.* In many respects, this disorder resembles the defect seen in von Willebrand disease (VWD). In contrast to VWD, however, this abnormality cannot be corrected by the addition of normal plasma or cryoprecipitate, consistent with a defect that resides in platelets.

Heterozygotes who have about 50% of normal levels of GPIb, GPV, and GPIX have normal or near-normal platelet function. Homozygotes have enlarged platelets, thrombocytopenia, and usually decreased platelet survival, which lead to a moderate to severe bleeding disorder. Platelet counts generally range from 40,000/μL to near normal.[30] Although not typically categorized as an inherited giant platelet syndrome, large and giant platelets are associated with BSS. On peripheral blood films, platelets typically are 5 to 8 μm in diameter (normal diameter 2 to 3 μm), but they can be as large as 20 μm (Figure 37.2). Viewed by electron microscopy, BSS platelets contain a larger number of cytoplasmic vacuoles and membrane complexes, and megakaryocytes exhibit an irregular demarcation membrane system.[31]

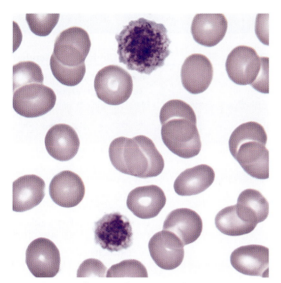

Figure 37.2 Bernard-Soulier Syndrome. Note the giant platelets. (Peripheral blood, Wright-Giemsa stain, ×1000.). (Modified from Carr, J. H., & Rodak, B. F. [2009]. *Clinical Hematology Atlas*. [3rd ed.] Philadelphia, PA: Saunders/Elsevier.)

The GPIb/IX/V complex consists of four glycoproteins: GPIbα, GPIbβ, GPIX, and GPV, present in the ratio of 2:2:2:1. Synthesis of three proteins, GPIbα, GPIbβ, and GPIX, is required for surface expression of the complex. The most frequent forms of BSS involve defects in GPIbα synthesis or expression. GPIbα is essential for normal function because it contains binding sites for VWF and thrombin. Defects in the GPIbβ and GPIX genes also are known to result in BSS.[32–34] Missense, frameshift, and nonsense mutations all have been reported.[35,36]

Variants. Several unusual variants of BSS have been described in which the surface expression of the GPIb/IX/V complex is normal, but its functionality is impaired. Mutations that affect binding domains impair interactions between elements of the complex, or they result in truncation of a specific protein in the complex, resulting in complexes that fail to bind VWF or do so poorly.[33] In rare circumstances, an antibody to GPIb/V can cause a Bernard-Soulier-like syndrome (pseudo-BSS).

Several gain-of-function mutations in the GPIb/IX/V complex can result in *platelet-type VWD (pseudo-VWD)*.[37–39] Such mutations result in spontaneous binding of plasma VWF to the mutated GPIb/IX/V complex. As a consequence, platelets and large VWF multimers with their associated factor VIII are removed from the circulation, resulting in thrombocytopenia and reduced factor VIII clotting activity.

Laboratory features. BSS platelets have normal aggregation responses to ADP, epinephrine, collagen, and arachidonic acid but do not respond to ristocetin and have diminished response to thrombin.[7] The lack of response to ristocetin is due to the inability of BSS platelets to bind VWF as a result of the lack of GPIb/IX/V complexes.

Treatment. Antiplatelet therapy should be avoided in all cases. Antifibrinolytic therapy may be useful to treat mucosal bleeding. There is no specific treatment for more severe bleeding associated with BSS. Platelet transfusions are the therapy of choice. To minimize the risk of alloimmunization prestorage, leukoreduced platelets should be used.[7] Other treatments that have been used include desmopressin acetate (DDAVP) and, more recently, rFVIIa.

Inherited Giant Platelet Syndromes

In addition to BSS, there are several other inherited syndromes in which patients exhibit *large platelets* (5 to 8 μm diameter) and *thrombocytopenia* (Table 37.2). With few exceptions, thrombocytopenia tends to be mild and bleeding tendency, if present, is also mild. In addition, the platelet ultrastructure is generally normal (Chapter 11). The exceptions include the *May-Hegglin anomaly* (Figure 38.2), in which there is an abnormal microtubule distribution, and *Epstein syndrome*, in which platelets are spherical and have a prominent surface-connected canalicular system. For most of these syndromes, the cause of the large platelets and thrombocytopenia remain to be determined. See Saito and colleagues[40] for a more complete discussion of these syndromes.

Disorders of Platelet Secretion

Platelet secretion is one of the primary functions of activated platelets in the hemostatic process. For instance, platelet-secreted ADP plays a major role in platelet activation, recruitment, aggregation, and growth of the hemostatic plug. Platelet secretion defects have been identified as related to a deficiency of granules, lack of packaging substances into the granules, or inability of the granules to release their substances. Defects of *dense granules* or *α-granules* are grouped under the heading of *storage pool disorders* (Box 37.2).

Storage pool and *release reaction defects* are the most common of the hereditary platelet function defects. Patients with these disorders present with mucocutaneous hemorrhage and hematuria, epistaxis, and easy and spontaneous bruising. Petechiae are less common than in other qualitative platelet disorders. Hemorrhage is rarely severe but may be exacerbated by ingestion of aspirin or other antiplatelet agents. In most of these disorders, the platelet count is normal. Platelet aggregation abnormalities are usually seen but vary depending on the disorder.[7,14,41]

Dense Granule Deficiency

Platelet-dense granules contain serotonin, nucleotides (e.g., ADP and adenosine triphosphate [ATP]), calcium, and pyrophosphate (Chapter 11). The inheritance of dense granule deficiency does not follow a single mode, and it is likely that a variety of genetic abnormalities leads to the development of this storage pool disorder. Dense granule deficiencies can be subdivided into deficiency states associated with albinism and deficiency states in otherwise healthy individuals (without albinism).

In the platelets of individuals without albinism with dense granule deficiency (Figure 37.3), there is evidence for the presence of dense granule membranes in normal to near-normal numbers, which suggests that the disorder arises from an inability to package the dense granule contents.[42,43] For example, serotonin accumulates in normal dense granules by an active uptake mechanism in which plasma serotonin is transported

TABLE 37.2   Inherited Giant Platelet Syndromes

Disease	Inheritance	Platelet Count (×10⁹/L)	Bleeding	Bleeding Site	Other Clinical Characteristics
Giant platelets with velocardiofacial syndrome	Autosomal recessive	100–200	None reported		Velopharyngeal insufficiency, conotruncal heart disease
Giant platelets with abnormal surface glycoproteins and mitral valve insufficiency	Autosomal recessive	50–60	Mild	Ecchymoses, epistaxis	Mitral valve insufficiency
Familial macrothrombocytopenia with GPIV abnormality	Autosomal dominant	45–normal	Mild		Defective GPIV glycosylation
Montreal platelet syndrome		5–40		Significant bruising	Low calpain activity; defective regulation of binding sites for adhesive proteins
May-Hegglin anomaly	Autosomal dominant	60–100	Mild		Döhle bodylike neutrophil inclusions
Fechtner syndrome	Autosomal dominant	30–90			Deafness, cataracts, nephritis
Sebastian syndrome	Autosomal dominant	40–120	Mild	Epistaxis, possible postoperative hemorrhage	Neutrophil inclusions
Hereditary macrothrombocytopenia	Autosomal dominant	50–120	Mild	Gingival bleeding, epistaxis, easy bruising, menorrhagia	High-frequency hearing loss
Epstein syndrome	Autosomal dominant	30–60	Mild	Epistaxis, GI bleeding, female genital tract	Nephritis, high-frequency hearing loss, proteinuria
Mediterranean macrothrombocytopenia		89–290			Stomatocytes in peripheral blood

GI, Gastrointestinal; *GP,* glycoprotein.

BOX 37.2   Platelet Storage Pool Disorders

Dense granule deficiencies
  Hermansky-Pudlak syndrome
  Chédiak-Higashi syndrome
  Wiskott-Aldrich syndrome
  Thrombocytopenia-absent radius (TAR) syndrome
α-Granule deficiencies
  Gray platelet syndrome

---

by a specific carrier-mediated system across the plasma membrane into the cytoplasm, and a second carrier-mediated system in the dense granule membrane transports serotonin from the cytoplasm to the interior of the dense granules.[44] In addition to serotonin transport mechanisms, a nucleotide transporter, MRP4 (ABCC4), that is highly expressed in platelets and dense granules has been identified. It would be expected that mutations in the genes for these transporters could affect accumulation of contents in dense granules.[45]

As an isolated abnormality, dense granule deficiency does not typically result in a serious hemorrhagic problem. Bleeding is usually mild and most often is limited to easy bruising.

The impact of dense granule deficiency is observed in platelet aggregation tests. The contents of these granules are extruded when platelet activation is induced. In the platelet function tests, addition of arachidonic acid to platelet-rich plasma fails to induce an aggregation response from platelets with dense granule deficiency (Chapter 41). Epinephrine and low-dose ADP induce only a primary wave of aggregation. Responses to low concentrations of collagen are decreased or absent, but a high concentration of collagen may induce a near-normal aggregation response.[14,44] This aggregation pattern, which is nearly identical to the pattern observed in patients taking aspirin (discussed in "Thromboxane Pathway Disorders: Aspirin-Like Effects"), is caused by the lack of ADP secretion.

In addition to occurring as an isolated problem, dense granule deficiency is found in association with several disorders described in the following.

Hermansky-Pudlak syndrome. Hermansky-Pudlak syndrome is an autosomal recessive disorder that is characterized by tyrosinase-positive oculocutaneous albinism, defective lysosomal function in a variety of cell types, ceroid-like pigment deposition in the cells of the reticuloendothelial system, and a profound platelet-dense granule deficiency.[46] Patients with this syndrome also have increased risk of progressive interstitial pulmonary fibrosis. Multiple mutations responsible for Hermansky-Pudlak syndrome have been mapped to chromosome 19. Mutations in more than 10 genes involved in intracellular vesicular trafficking, and the biogenesis of organelles can give rise to Hermansky-Pudlak syndrome.[47]

Although most bleeding episodes in Hermansky-Pudlak syndrome are not severe, life-threatening bleeding has been reported.[48] For patients undergoing extensive surgery or who experience prolonged bleeding, both red blood cell (RBC) and platelet transfusions are required. Thrombin-soaked absorbable gelatin sponge (Gelfoam) can be used to treat skin wounds that fail to spontaneously clot. Oral contraceptives can limit the

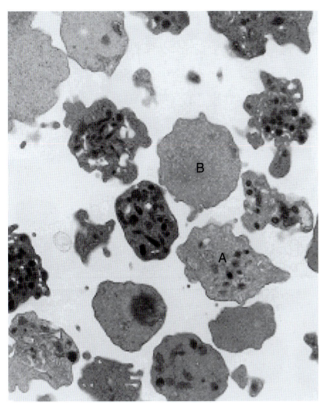

Figure 37.3 Storage Pool Disorder. Electron micrograph of platelets from a patient with storage pool disorder shows platelets with a normal distribution of dense granules *(A)* and platelets with a marked decrease of dense granules *(B)*. (From Barone, I., Meccariello, G., Cazzato, L., et al. [2013]. Management of platelet storage pool disease during pregnancy with recombinant factor VIIa. *Eur J Obstet Gynecol Reprod Biol,* 170, 576–577.)

duration of menstrual periods. A unique morphologic abnormality consisting of marked dilation and tortuosity of the surface-connecting tubular system (the "Swiss cheese" platelet) has been described in the platelets of four families with Hermansky-Pudlak syndrome.[20,49]

Chédiak-Higashi syndrome. Chédiak-Higashi syndrome is a rare autosomal recessive disorder that is characterized by partial oculocutaneous albinism, frequent pyogenic bacterial infections, giant lysosomal granules in cells of hematologic (Figure 26.2) and nonhematologic origin, platelet-dense granule deficiency, and hemorrhage. The disorder is accompanied by severe immunologic defects and progressive neurologic dysfunction in patients who survive to adulthood.

The gene for the Chédiak-Higashi syndrome protein is located on chromosome 1 (1q42.3). A number of nonsense and frameshift mutations result in a truncated Chédiak-Higashi syndrome protein that gives rise to a disorder of generalized cellular dysfunction involving fusion of cytoplasmic granules.

In 85% of patients with Chédiak-Higashi syndrome, the disorder progresses to an accelerated phase that is marked by lymphocytic proliferation in the liver, spleen, and marrow, with macrophage accumulation in tissues. During this stage, pancytopenia worsens, leading to hemorrhage and ever-increasing susceptibility to infection; the result is death at an early age. Initially, bleeding is increased because of dense granule

deficiency and consequent defective platelet function. During the accelerated phase, however, thrombocytopenia contributes to a prolonged bleeding tendency. Bleeding episodes vary from mild to moderate but worsen as the platelet count decreases.[20]

Wiskott-Aldrich syndrome. Wiskott-Aldrich syndrome (WAS) is a rare X-linked disease that is caused by mutations in the *WAS* gene on the short arm of the X chromosome Xp11.23 that encodes for a 502-amino acid protein, the Wiskott-Aldrich syndrome protein (WASp), that is found exclusively in hematopoietic cells. WASp plays a crucial role in actin cytoskeleton remodeling. Disease severity associated with *WAS* gene mutations ranges from the classic form of WAS with autoimmunity and/or malignancy to a milder form with isolated thrombocytopenia (X-linked thrombocytopenia (Chapter 38), to X-linked neutropenia. Approximately 50% of patients with *WAS* gene mutations have the WAS phenotype, and the other half have the X-linked thrombocytopenia phenotype. *WAS* gene mutations causing X-linked neutropenia are very rare.[50] Homozygous mutations of the *WIPF1* gene on chromosome 2 that encodes WASp-interacting protein (WIP), a cytoplasmic protein required to stabilize WASp, can also cause a WAS phenotype.[51]

The classic form of WAS, alternatively called *eczema-thrombocytopenia immunodeficiency syndrome*, is characterized by susceptibility to infections associated with immune dysfunction such as recurrent bacterial, viral, and fungal infections; thrombocytopenia; and severe eczema. Thrombocytopenia is present at birth, but the full expression of WAS develops over the first 2 years of life. Individuals with this disorder lack the ability to make antipolysaccharide antibodies, which results in a propensity for pneumococcal sepsis. Patients with classic WAS tend to develop autoimmune disorders, lymphoma, or other malignancies, often leading to early death. Bleeding episodes are typically moderate to severe. In WAS, a combination of ineffective thrombocytopoiesis and increased platelet sequestration and destruction accounts for the thrombocytopenia. As with all X-linked recessive disorders, it is found primarily in males.[10,20,33,52]

Wiskott-Aldrich platelets are also structurally abnormal. The number of dense granules is decreased, and the platelets are small (*microthrombocytes*), a feature of diagnostic importance. Other than in WAS, small platelets are seen only in association with TORCH (*t*oxoplasma, *o*ther agents, *r*ubella virus, *c*ytomegalovirus, *h*erpesvirus) infections. Diminished levels of stored adenine nucleotides are reflected in the lack of dense granules observed on transmission electron micrographs (see Figure 37.3). In laboratory testing, the platelet aggregation pattern in WAS is typical of a storage pool deficiency. The platelets show a decreased aggregation response to ADP, collagen, and epinephrine and lack a secondary wave of aggregation in response to these agonists (Chapter 41). The response to thrombin is normal, however.[20]

The most effective treatment for the thrombocytopenia in WAS seems to be splenectomy, which would be consistent with a mechanism of peripheral destruction of platelets. Platelet transfusions may be needed to treat hemorrhagic episodes. Bone marrow transplantation has been attempted, with some success.[20,53]

Thrombocytopenia-absent radii syndrome. Thrombocytopenia-absent radius (TAR) syndrome is a rare autosomal recessive disorder that is characterized by the congenital absence of the radial bones (the most pronounced skeletal abnormality), numerous cardiac and other skeletal abnormalities, and thrombocytopenia (90% of cases) (Chapter 38). Platelets have structural defects in dense granules, with corresponding abnormal aggregation responses. Marrow megakaryocytes may be decreased in number, immature, or normal.[54]

α-Granule Deficiency

Platelet α-granules contain proteins (Chapter 11) produced by the megakaryocyte (e.g., platelet-derived growth factor, thrombospondin, and platelet factor 4) or present in plasma and taken up by platelets and transported to α-granules for storage (e.g., albumin, immunoglobulin G [IgG], and fibrinogen). There are 50 to 80 α-granules per platelet, which are primarily responsible for the granular appearance of platelets on stained blood films.

Gray platelet syndrome. Gray platelet syndrome is a rare disorder, first described in 1971, that is characterized by the specific absence of morphologically recognizable α-granules in platelets.[55] This storage pool disorder is inherited in an autosomal recessive fashion. Clinically, gray platelet syndrome is characterized by lifelong mild bleeding tendencies, moderate thrombocytopenia, fibrosis of the marrow, and large platelets whose gray appearance on a Wright-stained blood film (Figure 37.4) is the source of the name of this disorder.[7,55] Mutations in region 3p21.31 involving the gene *NBEAL2*, crucial for the development of α-granules, have been identified.[56,57]

In electron photomicrographs, gray platelets appear to have virtually no α-granules, although they do contain vacuoles and small α-granule precursors that stain positive for VWF and fibrinogen. Other types of granules are present in normal numbers. The membranes of the vacuoles and the α-granule precursors contain P-selectin (CD62) and GPIIb/IIIa, which can be translocated to the cell membrane on platelet stimulation with thrombin. This suggests that these structures are α-granules that cannot store the typical α-granule proteins. This is supported by the observation that in gray platelet syndrome, the plasma levels of platelet factor 4 and β-thromboglobulin are increased; the proteins normally contained in α-granules are produced, but storage in those granules is not possible. Most patients develop early onset myelofibrosis, which may be attributed to the inability of megakaryocytes to store newly synthesized platelet-derived growth factors.[43]

Treatment of severe bleeding episodes may require platelet transfusions. Cryoprecipitate has been used to control bleeding. Desmopressin acetate was found to decrease bleeding and has been used as successful prophylaxis during dental extraction procedures. Some believe that desmopressin acetate should be the initial therapy of choice.[7,43,58,59]

Other Storage Pool Disorders

A rare disorder in which both α-granules and dense granules are deficient is known as *α-dense storage pool deficiency*. This

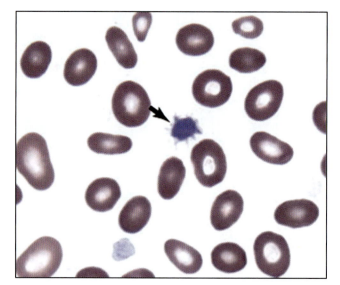

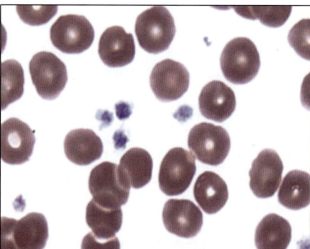

Figure 37.4 Gray Platelet Syndrome. Blood films showing platelets from a patient with gray platelet syndrome *(top)* and, for comparison, a healthy individual *(bottom)*. In gray platelet syndrome, note the large platelet with projections *(arrow)* and the large pale platelet lacking the usual fine purple α-granules *(lower part of top blood film)*. (Peripheral blood, Wright-Giemsa stain, ×1000.) (From Pozdnyakova, O. [2013]. Gray platelet syndrome. In *Hematopathology: A Volume in the High Yield Pathology Series.* Philadelphia, PA: Saunders/Elsevier.)

condition seems to be inherited in an autosomal dominant manner. Other membrane abnormalities also have been described.[33]

Quebec platelet disorder is an autosomal dominant bleeding disorder that results from a deficiency of multimerin (a multimeric protein that is stored complexed with factor V in α-granules). Even though α-granule structure is maintained, many α-granule proteins show signs of protease-related degradation. Thrombocytopenia may be present, although it is not a consistent feature.[33]

Thromboxane Pathway Disorders: Aspirin-Like Effects

Platelet secretion requires the activation of several biochemical pathways. One such pathway leads to thromboxane formation (Chapter 11). A series of phospholipases catalyze the release of arachidonic acid and several other compounds from membrane phospholipids. Arachidonic acid is converted to intermediate prostaglandins by cyclooxygenase and to thromboxane A_2 by thromboxane synthase (Figure 11.12). Thromboxane A_2 and other substances generated during platelet activation cause mobilization of ionic calcium from internal stores into the cytoplasm, initiating a cascade of events resulting in granule secretion and aggregation of platelets in response to stimulation by epinephrine, ADP, and low concentrations of collagen.[5,20,60,61]

Several acquired or congenital disorders of platelet secretion can be traced to structural and functional modifications of *arachidonic acid pathway enzymes*. Inhibition of cyclooxygenase occurs following ingestion of drugs such as aspirin and ibuprofen. As a result, the amount of thromboxane A_2 produced from arachidonic acid depends on the degree of inhibition.

Hereditary absence or abnormalities of the components of the thromboxane pathway are termed *aspirin-like defects* because the clinical and laboratory manifestations resemble those that follow aspirin ingestion. Platelet aggregation responses are similar to those in dense granule storage pool disorders. In contrast to storage pool disorders, however, ultrastructure and granular contents are normal. Deficiencies of the enzymes *cyclooxygenase* and *thromboxane synthase* are well documented, and dysfunction or deficiency of *thromboxane receptors* is known.[43]

Disorders of Receptors and Signaling Pathways
Collagen Receptors
The $\alpha_2\beta_1$ (GPIa/IIa) integrin is one of the collagen receptors in the platelet membrane. A deficiency of this receptor results in a lack of an aggregation response to collagen, inability of platelets to adhere to collagen, and a lifelong mild bleeding disorder in the affected individual.[62] A deficiency in another collagen receptor, GPVI, has also been reported; patients exhibit mild bleeding. Platelet function studies show a failure to aggregate in response to collagen, and impaired adhesion to collagen.[63] A family with gray platelet syndrome combined with defective collagen adhesion has been described. Affected members of the family were found to have a severe deficiency of the GPVI collagen receptor.[64]

Adenosine Diphosphate Receptors
Platelets contain at least three receptors for ADP. $P2X_1$ is linked to an ion channel that facilitates calcium ion influx. $P2Y_1$ and $P2Y_{12}$ are members of the seven-transmembrane domain family of G protein-linked receptors (Chapter 11). $P2Y_1$ is thought to mediate calcium mobilization and shape change in response to ADP. Polymorphisms in the $P2Y_1$ gene have been identified that may affect platelet reactivity to ADP.[65]

$P2Y_{12}$ is thought to be responsible for macroscopic platelet aggregation and is coupled to adenylate cyclase through a G-inhibitory (G_i) protein complex.[66] Patients with an *inherited deficiency of the $P2Y_{12}$ receptor* exhibit decreased platelet aggregation in response to ADP but normal platelet shape change and calcium mobilization.[67–69] Bleeding problems seem to be relatively mild in these patients. The only treatment for severe bleeding is platelet transfusion.

Other Receptors
Congenital defects of the *α2-adrenergic (epinephrine) receptor* associated with decreased platelet activation and aggregation in response to epinephrine are known. *PAR receptor* defects have been described in one family.[33]

Calcium Mobilization Defects
Calcium mobilization defects represent a heterogeneous group of disorders in which all elements of the thromboxane pathway are normal, but *insufficient calcium is released* from the dense tubular system, and the concentration of ionic calcium in the cytoplasm never reaches levels high enough to support secretion. Such defects result from *abnormal G protein subunits and phospholipase C isoenzymes*.[20,70,71]

Scott Syndrome
In the membrane of normal resting platelets, phosphatidylserine and phosphatidylethanolamine are restricted to the inner leaflet of the plasma membrane, and phosphatidylcholine is expressed on the outer leaflet. This asymmetry is maintained by the enzyme aminophospholipid translocase.[72] When platelets are activated, the asymmetry is lost, and phosphatidylserine and phosphatidylethanolamine flip to the outer leaflet, providing binding sites for vitamin K-dependent clotting factors and facilitating the assembly of clotting factor complexes. The phospholipid flip is mediated by a calcium-dependent enzyme, *scramblase*.[73]

Scott syndrome is a very rare autosomal recessive disorder (*ANO6* gene) in which platelets are unable to transport phosphatidylserine and phosphatidylethanolamine from the inner leaflet to the outer leaflet of the plasma membrane. As a result, while platelet adhesion, aggregation, secretion, and final platelet plug formation occur normally, clotting factor complexes do not assemble on the activated platelet surface, and thrombin generation is absent or much reduced. Because lack of thrombin generation leads to inadequate fibrin formation, the platelet plug is not stabilized, and a bleeding disorder results.[74,75]

Stormorken Syndrome
Stormorken syndrome is an autosomal dominant disorder characterized by a mild bleeding tendency due to platelet dysfunction, thrombocytopenia, anemia, functional asplenia, and other disorders. Stormorken syndrome is a condition in which platelets are always in an "activated" state and *express phosphatidylserine* on the outer leaflet of the membrane without prior activation. This syndrome results from autosomal dominant mutations in the *STIM1* or *ORAI1* genes on chromosome 11p15, which codes for a Ca^{2+} sensor in the endoplasmic reticulum.[76]

QUALITATIVE PLATELET DISORDERS: ACQUIRED DEFECTS

In contrast to inherited disorders of platelet function, which are rare, acquired disorders of platelet function are commonly encountered. The most frequent cause of acquired platelet dysfunction is drug ingestion. Therapeutic drugs have been developed to inhibit platelet function. Other drugs and certain agents developed for various nonplatelet targets have an identified antiplatelet side effect. The agents discussed here are summarized in Table 37.3, and the actions of the main therapeutic agents are illustrated in Figure 37.5.

Drug-Induced Defects

Drugs That Inhibit the Prostaglandin Pathway

Acetylsalicylic acid (*aspirin*) and other drugs that inhibit the platelet prostaglandin synthesis pathway are the most common cause of acquired platelet dysfunction. A single 200-mg dose of aspirin can irreversibly acetylate 90% of the platelet cyclooxygenase-1 (COX-1) (Figure 11.12). In platelets, the acetylated COX-1 enzyme is completely inactive. Because platelets lack a nucleus and cannot synthesize new enzymes, the inhibitory effect is maintained for the circulatory life span of the platelet (7 to 10 days).

Some patients have, or develop, *aspirin resistance*, a condition in which treated patients do not exhibit the desired clinical antiplatelet effect.[77] A number of mechanisms related to aspirin dosing, intrinsic variability of platelet function, and drug formulation may contribute to the interindividual differences in response to a single dose of aspirin.[78,79] Patients who do not respond well to aspirin have been shown to have worse cardiovascular outcomes than patients who respond well.[80] VerifyNow (Werfen) is one test system that provides measurement of a patient's antiplatelet response to aspirin (Chapter 42).

Individuals with a known hemostatic defect, such as a storage pool deficiency, thrombocytopenia, a vascular disorder, or VWD, may experience a marked increase in bleeding tendency after aspirin ingestion. Such individuals are advised to avoid the use of aspirin and related agents.[20]

Many drugs act as competitive, reversible inhibitors of cyclooxygenase, and as the blood concentration of the drug decreases, platelet function is recovered. This group of drugs includes ibuprofen and related compounds, such as ketoprofen, fenoprofen, naproxen, and sulfinpyrazone. In contrast to aspirin, most of these agents have little effect on platelet function tests (Chapter 41). Except for their potential to irritate the gastric mucosa, these drugs have not been reported to cause clinically important bleeding.[5,8,20,81] Interestingly, ingesting ibuprofen within 2 hours of aspirin appears to limit the antithrombotic actions of aspirin by blocking the acetylation site for aspirin on COX-1.

TABLE 37.3	Antiplatelet Drugs
Target	**Drug**
COX-1 (irreversible)	Aspirin
COX-1 (reversible)	Naproxen
	Sulfinpyrazone
	Ibuprofen (and like drugs)
ADP P2Y$_{12}$ (irreversible)	Clopidogrel
	Prasugrel
ADP P2Y$_{12}$ (reversible)	Ticagrelor
	Cangrelor
Thrombin PAR-1	Vorapaxar
GPIIb/IIIa	Abciximab
	Eptifibatide
	Tirofiban
Phosphodiesterase	Dipyridamole
	Aggrenox

ADP, Adenosine diphosphate; *COX-1,* cyclooxygenase-1; *GP,* glycoprotein; *PAR,* protease-activated receptor.

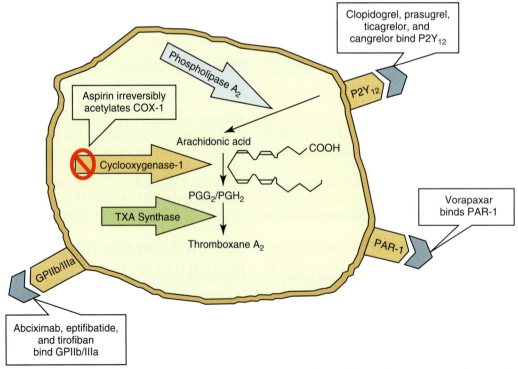

Figure 37.5 The Four Mechanisms of Common Antiplatelet Drugs. Aspirin irreversibly acetylates and inactivates cyclooxygenase-1. Clopidogrel (irreversible), prasugrel (irreversible), ticagrelor (reversible), and cangrelor (reversible) bind the adenosine diphosphate receptor P2Y$_{12}$. Abciximab (irreversible), eptifibatide (reversible), and tirofiban (reversible) block the fibrinogen binding site of the glycoprotein IIb/IIIa receptor. Vorapaxar blocks the thrombin binding site on the PAR-1 receptor. *COX-1,* Cyclooxygenase-1; *GP,* glycoprotein; *PGG$_2$,* prostaglandin G$_2$; *PGH$_2$,* prostaglandin H$_2$; *TXA,* thromboxane.

Ibuprofen and related NSAIDs should be avoided near the time of aspirin ingestion.[82]

Drugs That Inhibit Membrane Function

Many drugs interact with platelet membrane receptors and cause a clinically significant platelet function defect that may lead to hemorrhage. Some of these drugs are useful antiplatelet agents, whereas for other drugs, their effects on the platelet membrane are an adverse side effect.[60]

P2Y₁₂ (adenosine diphosphate) receptor inhibitors. The *thienopyridine* derivatives ticlopidine, clopidogrel, and prasugrel; the *nucleoside* ticagrelor; and the *nucleotide* mimetic cangrelor are antiplatelet agents that bind to the P2Y$_{12}$ platelet receptor.[67] These drugs inhibit stimulus-response coupling between those receptors and fibrinogen binding to GPIIb/IIIa. As a consequence, platelet activation and aggregation induced by ADP are markedly inhibited, and responses to other aggregating agents, such as collagen, are reduced.[67] Recovery of platelet function following cessation of treatment with an irreversible thienopyridine (clopidogrel) is 50% of normal at 3 days and complete at 7 to 10 days.[83] Both ticagrelor and cangrelor are reversible inhibitors of the P2Y$_{12}$ receptor.

In contrast to the immediate effect of aspirin, the effect of these agents that interact with the platelet membrane does not reach a steady state for 3 to 5 days, although a steady state can be reached sooner with a loading dose. These drugs are used to prevent myocardial infarction in patients with arterial occlusive disease, to reduce the risk of thrombotic stroke in patients with cerebrovascular disease, for stroke and myocardial infarction prophylaxis, and for patients who are intolerant of aspirin. As prophylactic agents, they have been shown to be as efficacious as aspirin. P2Y$_{12}$ inhibitors and aspirin are often used in combination to prevent arterial thrombosis, primarily based on the synergistic action of these two drugs, which inhibit platelet function by different mechanisms. This therapeutic approach is called *dual-antiplatelet therapy* (DAT).

Clopidogrel (Plavix) is a prodrug that requires conversion to the active drug by the 2C19 isoform of the P450 enzyme (CYP2C19) in the liver. The clinical effectiveness varies from patient to patient based on the extent of metabolism to the active drug. CYP2C19*1/*1 (wild type) represents two normal functioning alleles and normal metabolism of clopidogrel to the active drug.

Hypofunctional alleles are CYP2C19*2 to CYP2C19*10, whereas CYP2C19*17 is a hyperfunctional allele. Patients with one of the mutations resulting in decreased activity (e.g., CYP2C19*1/*2) are considered intermediate metabolizers. In these patients, the usual dose of clopidogrel does not achieve the degree of platelet inhibition desired, and these individuals remain at increased risk for thromboembolic events.[84] Patients who have two hypofunctional alleles (e.g., CYP2C19*2/*2, CYP2C19*2/*3) are poor metabolizers and do not derive significant benefit from clopidogrel therapy. Approximately 25% of individuals have one or two hypofunctional alleles of CYP2C19 and are considered *clopidogrel resistant*. The VerifyNow test system can measure a patient's antiplatelet response to clopidogrel and other ADP receptor inhibitor drugs (Chapter 42).

In contrast, patients with a CYP2C19*17 allele are rapid metabolizers and convert clopidogrel to the active drug at a faster rate. The resultant increased blood level of the active drug causes an increased risk of bleeding.[85] Individuals with one normal allele and one *17 allele (*1/*17) are considered to be rapid metabolizers, and those who are *17/*17 are ultrarapid metabolizers. Individuals with one hypofunctional and one hyperfunctional allele (e.g., *2/*17) have normal to intermediate clopidogrel metabolism. A variety of molecular methods are available to test for the most common alleles of CYP2C19. Although the US Food and Drug Administration (FDA) has recommended pharmacogenetic testing for these alleles, it is not common practice due to cost.

Clopidogrel has more effect on platelet function tests than aspirin, although there is little difference in the risk of clinical bleeding.[86] *Ticlopidine*, a thienopyridine that is structurally similar to clopidogrel, can produce major side effects in some patients, including long-lasting neutropenia, aplastic anemia, thrombocytopenia, gastrointestinal distress, and diarrhea. Clopidogrel has fewer of these side effects; however, vigilance is needed.

Prasugrel (Effient) is a third-generation thienopyridine derivative with the same mechanism of action as clopidogrel.[87] It is also a prodrug, but it is metabolized to the active drug by carboxylesterase-2 and several enzymes of the cytochrome P450 system, including CYP3A4 and CYP2B6. Because it is activated by several enzymes, mutations that result in decreased function of one or more of these enzymes have less impact on active drug levels, and the response is more uniform than with clopidogrel. Pharmacogenetic testing for mutations affecting prasugrel activation is not recommended.

Ticagrelor (Brilinta) is a nucleoside analog inhibitor of the P2Y$_{12}$ receptor.[87] Although its antiplatelet effect is similar, ticagrelor differs from prasugrel and clopidogrel in two key ways. First, it is not a prodrug and therefore does not require bioactivation. Because it is rapidly absorbed, its antiplatelet effect is predictable and achieved in a short period. Second, ticagrelor binds reversibly to the P2Y$_{12}$ (ADP) receptor. Therefore, unlike clopidogrel and prasugrel, whose effects are irreversible, platelet function returns quite rapidly with cessation of ticagrelor. However, this shorter half-life (7 to 9 hours) necessitates twice-daily dosing and may result in compliance issues with some patients.

Cangrelor (Kengreal) is a reversible nucleotide mimetic P2Y$_{12}$ inhibitor that, similar to ticagrelor, does not undergo metabolic activation.[88] Cangrelor is unique among the P2Y$_{12}$ inhibitors in that it is administered intravenously. Cangrelor is approved for use as an adjunct treatment for reducing the risk of myocardial infarction, repeat coronary intervention, and stent thrombosis in patients undergoing percutaneous coronary intervention. Owing to its rapid onset (minutes) and offset of action (60 to 90 minutes), cangrelor may be useful as bridge therapy in patients who need to discontinue thienopyridine therapy before surgery.[89]

Glycoprotein IIb/IIIa (αIIbβ3) receptor inhibitors. Another target for antiplatelet agents to reduce cardiovascular thrombotic risk is the platelet membrane GPIIb/IIIa ($\alpha_{IIb}\beta_3$) receptor.

Interference with the ability of this receptor to bind fibrinogen inhibits platelet aggregation stimulated in response to all of the usual platelet aggregating agents. Results of platelet function studies on platelets from patients receiving therapeutic doses of these drugs essentially mimic those of a mild form of GT.

Two different types of GPIIb/IIIa receptor inhibitors have been developed. The first is the mouse/human chimeric monoclonal antibody 7E3, *abciximab* (ReoPro), which, by binding to the GPIIb/IIIa receptor, prevents the binding of fibrinogen and limits platelet aggregation. Production of abciximab has been discontinued, and the drug is no longer available in the United States. The second type of agent in this class targets a site within the GPIIb/IIIa receptor that recognizes the arginine-glycine-aspartic acid (RGD) sequence found in fibrinogen and other adhesive proteins. These agents bind to the RGD recognition site, prevent the binding of fibrinogen, and consequently prevent platelet aggregation. *Tirofiban* (Aggrastat) is a nonpeptide RGD mimetic, and *eptifibatide* (Integrilin) is a cyclic heptapeptide that is also an RGD mimetic.

The goal of therapy with these drugs is to induce a controlled thrombasthenia-like state. These agents are primarily used in patients undergoing percutaneous coronary intervention and are administered concurrently with heparin and other antiplatelet agents.[90] The use of these agents is limited by their short half-lives and the need to administer them by constant intravenous infusion. There have been attempts to make an orally active agent of this type, but none has yet been approved for use.

PAR-1 antagonists. Thrombin activates platelets via G-protein-linked receptors called *protease-activated receptors* (PARs). There are three distinct PARs on human platelets (PAR-1, PAR-2, PAR-4). Thrombin activates platelets by cleaving a portion of the N-terminus of the receptor. The newly exposed N-terminus interacts with the transmembrane domains of the receptor and acts as a tethered ligand. *Vorapaxar* (Zontivity) inhibits thrombin-induced platelet aggregation by blocking the ligand-binding site on PAR-1. Its long half-life makes it essentially irreversible. Vorapaxar is used as secondary prevention in combination with low-dose aspirin and clopidogrel in patients with a history of myocardial infarction or peripheral artery disease. Patients with a history of stroke or transient ischemic attack should not be treated with vorapaxar due to an increased risk of bleeding.[91,92]

Other Drugs That Inhibit Platelet Function

Dipyridamole. The classic antiplatelet drug dipyridamole (Persantine) is an inhibitor of platelet phosphodiesterase, the enzyme responsible for converting cyclic adenosine monophosphate (cAMP) to AMP. Inhibition of phosphodiesterase leads to the accumulation of cAMP in the cytoplasm, and elevation of cytoplasmic cAMP is inhibitory to platelet function (Figure 11.12). Dipyridamole alone does not inhibit platelet aggregation in response to the usual platelet agonists, but it promotes inhibition by agents that stimulate cAMP formation, such as prostacyclin, stable analogues of prostacyclin, and nitric oxide. Dipyridamole is used in combination with aspirin to reduce the risk of stroke in patients with a history of transient ischemic attack or thrombotic stroke;

Aggrenox is a drug that combines both dipyridamole and aspirin in one tablet. Dipyridamole is used in combination with the anticoagulant warfarin to prevent clot formation after heart valve replacement.

Antibiotics. Antibiotics are well known for their ability to interfere with platelet function. Most of the drugs with this effect contain a β-lactam ring of either the penicillin or the cephalosporin families of medicines. While these drugs can inhibit platelet function tests, this effect is seen primarily in patients receiving large parenteral doses. The antiplatelet effect is thus a concern largely for hospitalized patients.

One postulated mechanism for the antiplatelet effect of antibiotics is that they associate with the platelet membrane via a lipophilic reaction and block receptor-agonist interactions or stimulus-response coupling between receptors and fibrinogen binding to GPIIb/IIIa. They also may inhibit calcium influx in response to thrombin stimulation, reducing the ability of thrombin to activate platelets. Although these drugs may prolong the in vitro aggregation response to certain agonists, their association with a hemostatic defect severe enough to cause clinical hemorrhage is uncertain and is likely not predicted by laboratory test results.[2,8,61,93]

Nitrofurantoin is a non-β-lactam antibiotic that may inhibit platelet aggregation when high concentrations are present in the blood. This drug is not known to cause clinical bleeding.[93]

Dextrans. Dextrans are partially hydrolyzed, branched-chain polysaccharides of glucose that are used as plasma expanders. The two most commonly used are dextran 70 (molecular mass of 70,000 Daltons) and dextran 40 (molecular mass of 40,000 Daltons, also known as low-molecular-weight dextran). Although dextrans can inhibit platelet aggregation and impair platelet procoagulant activity when given as an intravenous infusion, these drugs have no effect on in vitro platelet function when added directly to platelet-rich plasma. There does not seem to be any increased risk of hemorrhage associated with the use of these agents, but their efficacy in preventing postoperative pulmonary embolism is equal to that of low-dose subcutaneous heparin.[5,52,93] Because of these effects, dextrans have been extensively used as antithrombotic agents in hospitalized patients.

Hydroxyethyl starch. Hydroxyethyl starch, or hetastarch, is a synthetic glucose polymer with a mean molecular mass up to 450,000 Daltons that is used as a plasma expander. It has effects similar to those of the dextrans. The mechanism of action of plasma expander drugs has not been elucidated but is presumed to involve interaction with the platelet membrane.[5,52]

Diverse agents. Nitroglycerin, nitroprusside, propranolol, and isosorbide dinitrate are used to regulate cardiovascular function. These drugs, of diverse chemical structure and function, are known to inhibit platelet function, decreasing platelet secretion and aggregation. The mechanisms by which they induce platelet dysfunction, however, are largely unknown.

Patients taking phenothiazine or tricyclic antidepressants may have decreased platelet secretion and aggregation responses, but these effects are not associated with an increased risk for hemorrhage. Local and general anesthetics may impair in vitro aggregation responses. The same is true of antihistamines.

Some radiographic contrast agents are known to inhibit platelet function.[93] Treatment of B-cell malignancies with some Bruton tyrosine kinase (BTK) inhibitors, such as ibrutinib (Imbruvica), has been associated with mild bleeding.[94] Such bleeding results from BTK inhibitor-induced inhibition of platelet activation mediated through FcγIIa, GPVI, and CLEC-2 receptors.[94]

Medical Conditions That Affect Platelet Function
Myeloproliferative Neoplasms

Chronic myeloproliferative neoplasms (MPNs) include polycythemia vera, chronic myeloid (myelogenous) leukemia (CML), essential thrombocythemia (ET), and myelofibrosis with myeloid metaplasia (Chapter 32). Hemorrhagic complications occur in about one-third, thrombosis occurs in another third and, although it is uncommon, both develop in some patients. These complications are serious causes of morbidity and mortality in affected patients.

Although the occurrence of hemorrhage or thrombosis in patients with MPNs is largely unpredictable, certain patterns have emerged. Hemorrhage and thrombosis are less common in CML than in the other MPNs. Bleeding seems to be more common in myelofibrosis with myeloid metaplasia, but thrombosis is more common in the other MPNs.

In patients with these disorders, thrombosis may occur in unusual sites, including the mesenteric, hepatic, and portal circulations. Patients with ET may develop digital artery thrombosis and ischemia of the fingers and toes, occlusions of the microvasculature of the heart, and cerebrovascular occlusions that result in neurologic symptoms.[93]

Platelet dysfunction is a common finding in patients with these disorders and has been postulated as a contributing cause to the observed bleeding and/or thrombosis.[95] This hypothesis is supported by the observation that bleeding is usually mucocutaneous in nature, and thrombosis may be arterial or venous. A variety of platelet function defects have been described in patients with MPNs, but their clinical importance is uncertain. Platelets have been reported to have abnormal shapes, decreased procoagulant activity, a decreased number of secretory granules, and shortened survival. The risk of thrombosis or hemorrhage correlates poorly with platelet count elevation, so the role of iatrogenic platelet cytoreduction (by apheresis), although often requested, remains unclear.

The most common functional abnormalities are decreased aggregation and secretion in response to epinephrine, ADP, and collagen. Possible causes of the platelet dysfunction include loss of platelet surface membrane α-adrenergic (epinephrine) receptors, impaired release of arachidonic acid from membrane phospholipids in response to stimulation by agonists, impaired oxidation of arachidonic acid by the cyclooxygenase and lipoxygenase pathways, a decrease in the contents of dense granules and α-granules, and loss of a variety of platelet membrane receptors for adhesion and activation. There seems to be no correlation between a given MPN and the type of platelet dysfunction observed, with the exception that most patients with ET lack an in vitro platelet aggregation response to epinephrine, an observation that may be helpful in the differential diagnosis.[5,8,93,96]

Multiple Myeloma and Waldenström Macroglobulinemia

Platelet function can be inhibited by myeloma proteins, as observed in approximately one-third of patients with IgA myeloma or Waldenström macroglobulinemia, a much smaller percentage of patients with IgG multiple myeloma, and only occasionally in patients with monoclonal gammopathy of undetermined significance.

Abnormalities in platelet aggregation, secretion, and procoagulant activity correlate with the concentration of the plasma paraprotein and are likely due to coating of the platelet membrane with the paraprotein. Under these conditions, platelet adhesion and activation receptor functions are inhibited; the paraprotein coating also inhibits assembly of clotting factors on the platelet surface and likely interferes with fibrin polymerization. High concentrations of paraprotein can cause severe hemorrhagic manifestations as a result of hyperviscosity, platelet dysfunction, complications of amyloidosis (e.g., acquired factor X deficiency), and in rare instances, presence of a circulating heparin-like anticoagulant or fibrinolysis.[10,93]

While almost all patients with malignant paraprotein disorders have clinically significant bleeding, there is poor correlation between abnormal results on laboratory tests (e.g., prothrombin time [PT], activated partial thromboplastin time [PTT, APTT]), and evidence of clinical bleeding. Treatment for the bleeding complications of these disorders is primarily reduction in the level of the paraprotein by effective chemotherapy, sometimes supplemented by therapeutic plasma exchange, which is only temporarily effective. Longer-term treatment is usually chemotherapy or stem cell transplantation, with curative intent for the underlying plasma cell malignancy.[96,97]

Liver Disease

Moderate to severe liver disease is associated with a variety of hemostatic abnormalities, including reduction in clotting proteins, reduction of proteins in the natural anticoagulant pathways, dysfibrinogenemia, and excessive fibrinolysis (Chapter 36). Mild to moderate thrombocytopenia is seen in approximately one-third of patients with chronic liver disease in association with hypersplenism (secondary to portal hypertension) or as a result of alcohol toxicity.[7,93]

Abnormal platelet function test results seen in patients with chronic liver disease include reduced platelet adhesion, abnormal platelet aggregation (in response to ADP, epinephrine, and thrombin), abnormal phospholipid availability, and reduced procoagulant activity. An acquired storage pool deficiency also has been suggested. While the abnormal platelet function in these patients may respond to infusion of desmopressin acetate, it is unclear whether desmopressin acetate also prevents bleeding in these patients or simply corrects an abnormal laboratory test result.

The severe bleeding associated with end-stage liver disease has many causes, such as markedly decreased or negligible coagulation factor production, excessive fibrinolysis, dysfibrinogenemia, thrombocytopenia due to acquired thrombopoietin deficiency, splenic sequestration secondary to portal hypertension, and occasionally, disseminated intravascular coagulation (DIC; Chapter 39). Upper gastrointestinal tract bleeding (e.g., from esophageal or gastric varices) is a relatively common complication of cirrhosis, particularly alcoholic cirrhosis but occurs as a complication of end-stage liver disease of any etiology.[5,20,98,99]

In chronic alcoholic cirrhosis, thrombocytopenia and platelet abnormalities may result from the direct toxic effects of alcohol on bone marrow megakaryocytes. Chronic, periodic, and even acute alcohol consumption may result in a transient decrease in platelet function; however, the inhibitory effect seems to be more pronounced when alcohol is consumed in excess. The impaired platelet function is associated partly with inhibition of thromboxane synthesis.

Uremia

Uremia due to kidney failure is associated with abnormal platelet function that can lead to clinically significant bleeding in some patients.[60,62] In uremia, guanidinosuccinic acid (GSA) is present in the circulation in higher than normal levels as a result of inhibition of the urea cycle. Because GSA is a nitric oxide (NO) donor, NO is present in the circulation at higher than normal levels. NO diffuses into platelets; activates soluble guanylate cyclase; and inhibits platelet adhesion, activation, and aggregation.[100] GSA is dialyzable, and dialysis (peritoneal dialysis or hemodialysis) is usually effective in correcting, albeit temporarily, the abnormal platelet function characteristic of uremia.

Platelet aggregation pattern abnormalities are not uniform, and any combination of defects may be seen. There is evidence of a defective release reaction, such as lack of secondary ADP-induced aggregation, and subnormal platelet procoagulant activity. Anemia is an independent cause of prolonged bleeding, and the severity of anemia in uremic patients correlates with the severity of renal failure. Treatment with recombinant erythropoietin has some efficacy in patients with end-stage renal disease.

Bleeding in uremic patients is seen more often with concurrent use of drugs that interfere with platelet function or in association with heparin use in hemodialysis. Platelet concentrates have been used with limited success to treat severe hemorrhagic episodes in patients with uremia. Other therapies that may be effective in uremic bleeding include a means to increase fibrinogen levels such as with cryoprecipitate, DDAVP to increase FVIII:von Willebrand factor multimers, and conjugated estrogen by a mechanism yet to be determined.

Afibrinogenemia

Afibrinogenemia, a rare inherited disorder, has been documented in more than 150 families. Although it is not truly a platelet function disorder, platelets do not exhibit normal function in the absence or near-absence of fibrinogen. Abnormal results in platelet retention and adhesion are also documented. In addition, results of all clot-based tests (e.g., PT, APTT, thrombin time [TT], whole blood clotting) are abnormal. Addition of fibrinogen to samples or transfusion of fibrinogen concentrates into the patient results in correction of the abnormal test results.[101]

A high incidence of hemorrhagic manifestations is found in patients with afibrinogenemia (or severe hypofibrinogenemia).

Bleeding is the cause of death in about one-third of such patients. Cryoprecipitate or fibrinogen concentrate (RiaSTAP) can be used to treat bleeding episodes. Some patients develop antibodies to fibrinogen, and this treatment then becomes ineffective.[101]

Other Medical Conditions

Acquired platelet function defects are seen occasionally in patients with autoimmune disorders, including systemic lupus erythematosus, rheumatoid arthritis, scleroderma, and the immune thrombocytopenias such as immune thrombocytopenic purpura.[96]

Other Causes of Platelet Function Defects
Cardiopulmonary Bypass Surgery

The use of cardiopulmonary bypass (CPB) (heart-lung machine) *extracorporeal blood circulation* during cardiac surgery induces thrombocytopenia and a severe platelet function defect that assumes major importance in relation to postsurgical bleeding.[93] The functional defect likely results from platelet activation and fragmentation in the extracorporeal circuit subsequent to adherence and aggregation of platelets to fibrinogen (adsorbed onto the surfaces of the bypass circuit material), mechanical trauma and shear stresses, use of blood conservation devices (RBC salvage and saline suspension), bypass pump-priming solutions during surgery, hypothermia, complement activation, and exposure of platelets to the blood-air interface in bubble oxygenators.[102]

Some degree of platelet degranulation typically is found after cardiac surgery using CPB, which indicates that platelet activation and secretion have occurred during the operation. Platelet membrane fragments, or microparticles (extracellular microvesicles), are found in the blood of these surgical patients, providing additional evidence of the severe mechanical stress encountered by platelets during extracorporeal procedures.

The severity of the platelet function defect closely correlates with the length of time on the bypass circuit. Normal platelet function returns in about 1 hour after an uncomplicated surgical procedure, although the platelet count does not normalize for several days. Thrombocytopenia caused by hemodilution, accumulation of platelets on the artificial surfaces of the bypass circuits, sequestration or removal of damaged platelets by the liver and mononuclear phagocyte system, and consumption associated with normal hemostatic processes after surgery are multifactorial causes of defective platelet function.[93]

Other Potential Causes

Purified fibrin degradation products (Chapter 35) can induce platelet dysfunction in vitro. The pathophysiologic relevance of this observation is uncertain because the concentrations of fibrin degradation products required are unlikely to be reached in vivo.

Patients with DIC (Chapter 39) may have reduced platelet function as a result of in vivo stimulation by thrombin and other agonists, resulting in release of granule contents. This has been called *acquired storage pool disease*; however, the term *exhausted platelets* may be more appropriate.[103]

Hyperaggregable Platelets

Patients with a variety of disorders associated with thrombosis or increased risk for thrombosis, including hyperlipidemia, diabetes mellitus, peripheral arterial occlusive disease, acute arterial occlusion, myocardial infarction, and stroke, have been reported to have increased platelet reactivity. Platelets from these patients tend to aggregate at lower concentrations of aggregating agents than platelets from individuals without these conditions.

Sticky platelet syndrome is an autosomal-dominant, thrombophilic disorder that is associated with venous and arterial thromboembolic events.[104] The disorder is characterized by hyperaggregable platelets in response to ADP, epinephrine, or both. In these patients, venous and/or arterial thrombotic events are often associated with emotional stress. Prophylactic treatment of these patients with low-dose aspirin reverses clinical symptoms and normalizes hyperaggregable responses to aggregating agents in laboratory tests.

Spontaneous platelet aggregation, an in vitro phenomenon in which platelets aggregate in response to stirring only (first step in the test system before addition of an agonist; Chapter 41), is an indicator of abnormally increased platelet reactivity and often accompanies increased sensitivity to platelet agonists. The presence of spontaneous aggregation by itself is considered consistent with the presence of a hyperaggregable state. Because participation of platelets is necessary for the development of arterial thrombosis, the presence of hyperaggregable platelets is often an indication that an antiplatelet agent should be used as part of a therapeutic or prophylactic regimen for arterial thrombosis.[105,106]

VASCULAR DISORDERS

The pathophysiology of bleeding abnormalities associated with disorders of vessels and their supporting tissues is obscure. Laboratory studies of platelets and blood coagulation usually yield normal results. The diagnosis is often based on medical history and by ruling out other sources of bleeding disorders. The usual clinical sign is the tendency to bruise easily or to bleed spontaneously, especially from mucosal surfaces. Vascular disorders are summarized in Box 37.3.

Inherited Vascular Disorders

Hereditary Hemorrhagic Telangiectasia (Osler-Weber-Rendu Syndrome)

The mode of inheritance of hereditary hemorrhagic telangiectasia is autosomal dominant. The vascular defect of this disorder

---

BOX 37.3 Vascular Disorders

Hereditary vascular disorders
  Hereditary hemorrhagic telangiectasia (Osler-Weber-Rendu syndrome)
  Hemangioma-thrombocytopenia syndrome (Kasabach-Merritt syndrome)
  Ehlers-Danlos syndrome and other genetic disorders
Acquired vascular disorders
  Allergic purpura (Henoch-Schönlein purpura)
  Paraproteinemia and amyloidosis
  Senile purpura
  Drug-induced vascular purpuras

---

is characterized by thin-walled blood vessels with a discontinuous endothelium, inadequate smooth muscle, and inadequate or missing elastin in the surrounding stroma. Telangiectasias are dilated superficial blood vessels that create small, focal red lesions that occur throughout the body but are most obvious on the face, lips, tongue, conjunctiva, nasal mucosa, fingers, toes, trunk, and under the tongue. The lesions blanch when pressure is applied. The disorder usually manifests by puberty and progresses throughout life.

Telangiectasias are fragile and prone to rupture. Epistaxis is an almost universal finding, and symptoms usually worsen with age. The age at which nosebleeds begin is a good gauge of the severity of the disorder. Although the oral cavity, gastrointestinal tract, and urogenital tract are common sites of bleeding, bleeding can occur in virtually every organ.[107]

The diagnosis of hereditary hemorrhagic telangiectasia is based on the characteristic skin or mucous membrane lesions, a history of repeated hemorrhage, and a family history of a similar disorder.

Patients with hereditary hemorrhagic telangiectasia do well despite the lack of specific therapy and the seriousness of their hemorrhagic manifestations.[108] There are several other disorders and conditions in which telangiectasias are present, including cherry-red hemangiomas (common in older men and women), ataxia-telangiectasia (Louis-Bar syndrome), and chronic actinic telangiectasia; they also are seen in association with chronic liver disease and pregnancy.

Hemangioma-Thrombocytopenia Syndrome (Kasabach-Merritt Syndrome)

Kasabach and Merritt originally described the association of a giant cavernous hemangioma (vascular tumor), thrombocytopenia, and a bleeding tendency. The hemangiomas are visceral or subcutaneous but rarely both. External hemangiomas may become engorged with blood and resemble hematomas. Kasabach-Merritt syndrome is a rare consumptive coagulopathy associated with specific vascular tumors, kaposiform hemangioendothelioma, and tufted angioma. Its manifestations include acute or chronic DIC (Chapter 39), sequestration of platelets in the hemangiomas, and resultant microangiopathic hemolytic anemia. A hereditary basis for this syndrome has not been established, but the condition is present at birth. Several treatment modalities are available for the angiomas and the associated coagulopathy ranging from corticosteroid therapy to surgery, but none is completely effective. The mortality rate is 30%.[109]

Ehlers-Danlos Syndrome and Other Genetic Disorders

Ehlers-Danlos syndrome is transmitted as an autosomal dominant, recessive, or X-linked trait. It is manifested by hyperextensible skin, hypermobile joints, joint laxity, fragile tissues, and a bleeding tendency, primarily subcutaneous hematoma formation. Thirteen distinct subtypes of the disorder are recognized.[110] The severity of bleeding ranges from easy bruising to arterial rupture. The disorder generally can be ascribed to defects in collagen production, structure, or cross-linking, with resulting inadequacy of the connective tissues. Platelet abnormalities have been reported in some patients.

Other inherited vascular disorders include pseudoxanthoma elasticum (calcium and other mineral accumulation in the elastic fibers of the skin, eyes, and blood vessels) and homocystinuria, which are autosomal recessive disorders, and Marfan syndrome and osteogenesis imperfecta, which are autosomal dominant disorders.

Acquired Vascular Disorders

Allergic Purpura (Henoch-Schönlein Purpura)

The term *allergic purpura* or *anaphylactoid purpura* generally is applied to a group of nonthrombocytopenic purpuras characterized by apparently allergic manifestations including skin rash and edema. Allergic purpura has been associated with certain foods and drugs, cold, insect bites, and vaccinations. *Henoch-Schönlein purpura* is an acute IgA-mediated disorder with widespread generalized vasculitis involving the skin, joints, kidneys, gastrointestinal tract and, less commonly, the lungs. The purpuric skin lesions are frequently confused with the hemorrhagic rash of immune thrombocytopenic purpura.[52]

General evidence implicates autoimmune microvascular injury, but the pathophysiology of the disorder is unclear. The vasculitis is mediated by immune complexes containing IgA antibodies. It has been suggested that allergic purpura may represent autoimmunity to components of the vessel wall.

Henoch-Schönlein purpura is primarily a disease of children, occurring most commonly in children 3 to 7 years of age. It is relatively uncommon among children younger than age 2 or adults older than age 20. Twice as many boys as girls are affected. The onset of the disease is sudden, often following an upper respiratory tract infection. The infectious organism may damage the endothelial lining of blood vessels, which results in vasculitis.

Malaise, headache, fever, and rash may be the presenting symptoms. The delay in the appearance of the skin rash often poses a difficult problem in differential diagnosis. The skin lesions are urticarial and gradually become pinkish, then red, and finally hemorrhagic. The appearance of the lesions may be very rapid and accompanied by itching. The lesions have been described as "palpable purpura," in contrast to the perfectly flat lesions of thrombocytopenia and most other forms of vascular purpura. These lesions are most commonly found on the feet, elbows, knees, buttocks, and chest. Ultimately, a brownish-red eruption is seen. Petechiae also may be present.

As the disease progresses, abdominal pain, polyarthralgia, headaches, and renal disease may develop. Renal lesions are present in 60% of patients during the second to third week of the disorder. Proteinuria and hematuria are commonly present.[7] The platelet count is normal. Tests of blood coagulation usually yield normal results in patients with allergic purpura. Anemia generally is not present unless the hemorrhagic manifestations have been severe. The white blood cell count and the erythrocyte sedimentation rate are usually elevated. The disease must be distinguished from other forms of nonthrombocytopenic purpura. Numerous infectious diseases that may be associated with purpura also are included in the differential diagnosis.

In the pediatric age group, the average duration of the initial episode is about 4 weeks. Relapses are frequent, usually after a period of apparent well-being. Except for patients in whom chronic renal disease develops, the prognosis is usually good. Occasionally, death from renal failure has occurred. Management is directed primarily at symptomatic relief because there currently is no effective treatment. Corticosteroids sometimes have been helpful in alleviating symptoms. Most patients recover without treatment.

Amyloidosis

Amyloid is a fibrous protein consisting of rigid, linear, nonbranching, aggregated fibrils approximately 7.5 to 10 nm wide and of indefinite length. Amyloid is deposited extracellularly and may lead to damage of normal tissues. Various proteins can serve as subunits of the fibril, including monoclonal light chains (λ more frequently than κ). Amyloidosis, the deposition of abnormal quantities of amyloid protein in tissues, may be primary or secondary and localized or systemic. Purpura, hemorrhage, and thrombosis may be a part of the clinical presentation of patients with amyloidosis. Thrombosis and hemorrhage have been ascribed to amyloid deposition in the vascular wall and surrounding tissues. Platelet function has been shown to be abnormal in a few cases, and in rare cases, patients may have thrombocytopenia. Current treatments (including chemotherapy and other targeted therapies) for most forms of amyloidosis are not effective because none reverse the buildup of amyloid proteins from tissues and organs. Chemotherapy with allogeneic stem cell transplantation has had some success treating the early stages of light-chain amyloidosis.[109]

Senile Purpura

Senile purpura occurs more commonly in elderly men than in women and is due to a lack of collagen support for small blood vessels and loss of subcutaneous fat and elastic fibers. The incidence increases with advancing age. The blotches are flattened (Figure 38.1), are about 1 to 10 mm in diameter, do not blanch with pressure, and resolve slowly, often leaving a brown stain in the skin (age spots). The lesions are limited mostly to the extensor surfaces of the forearms and backs of the hands and occasionally occur on the face and neck. With the exception of increased capillary fragility, results of laboratory tests are normal, and no other bleeding manifestations are present.

Drug-Induced Vascular Purpuras

Purpura associated with drug-induced vasculitis occurs in the presence of functionally adequate platelets. A variety of drugs are known to cause vascular purpura, including aspirin, warfarin, barbiturates, diuretics, digoxin, methyldopa, and several antibiotics. Sulfonamides and iodides have been implicated most frequently. The lesions vary from a few petechiae to massive, generalized petechial eruptions. Mechanisms include development of antibodies to vessel wall components, development of immune complexes, and changes in vessel wall permeability. As soon as the disorder is recognized, the offending drug should be discontinued. No other treatment is necessary.

SUMMARY

- Inherited qualitative platelet disorders can cause bleeding ranging from mild to severe.
- Glanzmann thrombasthenia is caused by the lack of expression of glycoprotein (GP) IIb/IIIa complexes on the platelet surface. This complex is known as the platelet aggregation receptor, and its absence is associated with a severe bleeding disorder.
- Bernard-Soulier syndrome is caused by the lack of expression of GPIb/IX/V complexes on the platelet surface. This receptor complex is responsible for platelet adhesion, and its absence results in a severe bleeding disorder.
- Disorders of platelet secretion are related to deficiency of α-granules or dense granules (storage pool disorders), lack of packaging substances into the granules, or inability of the granules to release their substances. Platelet dysfunction and bleeding symptoms associated with these disorders are generally mild.
- Aspirin-like effects result from defects in elements of the arachidonic acid metabolic pathway. Platelet dysfunction mimics that seen after aspirin ingestion.
- Inherited deficiencies of several of the receptors for platelet activating substances have been documented, and bleeding symptoms of varying severity are associated with these deficiencies.

- Drugs are the most common cause of acquired platelet dysfunction, and aspirin is the most frequent culprit. New classes of antiplatelet agents with mechanisms different from aspirin, including adenosine diphosphate receptor antagonists, PAR-1 inhibitors, GPIIb/IIIa inhibitors, and thromboxane inhibitors, are available.
- A variety of medical conditions can result in platelet dysfunction, including hematologic malignancies, liver disease, and kidney disease.
- Mechanical devices, such as the cardiopulmonary bypass machine used in cardiac surgery, are a known cause of acquired platelet disorders.
- Vascular disorders that result in bleeding are uncommon. A few well-recognized inherited disorders, such as Ehlers-Danlos syndrome and hereditary hemorrhagic telangiectasia (Rendu-Osler-Weber syndrome), can result in substantial blood loss.
- Acquired vascular disorders are much more common than inherited vascular disorders; causes include the effects of aging, drugs, and allergic reactions.

Now that you have completed this chapter, go back and read again the case study at the beginning and respond to the questions presented. Answers can be found in Appendix C.

REVIEW QUESTIONS

Answers can be found in Appendix C.

1. The clinical presentation of platelet-related bleeding may include all of the following EXCEPT:
   a. Bruising
   b. Nosebleeds
   c. Gastrointestinal bleeding
   d. Bleeding into the joints (hemarthroses)

2. Glanzmann thrombasthenia results from a defect in:
   a. α-granule fusion
   b. Loss of GPIb expression
   c. Loss of GPIIb/IIIa expression
   d. Defective microtubule formation

3. Ristocetin-induced platelet aggregation can be used in the diagnosis of which of the following?
   a. Bernard-Soulier syndrome
   b. Chédiak-Higashi syndrome
   c. Wiskott-Aldrich syndrome
   d. Storage pool disorder

4. Which of the following is the most common of the hereditary platelet function defects?
   a. Glanzmann thrombasthenia
   b. Bernard-Soulier syndrome
   c. Storage pool defects
   d. Multiple myeloma

5. A reduction in thrombin generation in patients with Scott syndrome results from:
   a. Defective granule secretion
   b. Altered platelet aggregation
   c. Altered expression of phospholipids on the platelet membrane
   d. Deficiency of vitamin K-dependent clotting factors

6. The impaired platelet function in myeloproliferative neoplasms may result from:
   a. Abnormally shaped platelets
   b. Extended platelet life span
   c. Increased procoagulant activity
   d. Decreased numbers of α-granules and dense granules

7. The platelet defect associated with increased levels of paraproteins is:
   a. Impaired membrane activation owing to protein coating
   b. Hypercoagulability owing to antibody binding and membrane activation
   c. Impaired aggregation because the hyperviscous plasma prevents platelet-endothelium interaction
   d. Hypercoagulability because the increased proteins bring platelets closer together, which leads to inappropriate aggregation

8. In uremia, platelet function is impaired by higher than normal levels of:
   a. Urea
   b. Uric acid
   c. Creatinine
   d. Nitric oxide

9. Thrombocytopenia associated with the use of cardiopulmonary bypass is NOT caused by:
   a. Anti-GPIIb/IIIa antibodies
   b. Hemodilution
   c. Platelet binding to bypass circuitry
   d. Platelet consumption associated with normal postsurgical hemostatic activity

10. Aspirin inhibits platelet function by:
    a. Blocking synthesis of thromboxane A_2
    b. Reducing levels of ionized calcium
    c. Triggering PGI_2 synthesis
    d. Inhibiting the release of ADP stored in platelet α-granules

11. A mechanism of antiplatelet drugs targeting GPIIb/IIIa function is:
    a. Interference with platelet adhesion to the subendothelium by blockage of the collagen binding site
    b. Inhibition of transcription of the GPIIb/IIIa gene
    c. Direct binding to GPIIb/IIIa
    d. Interference with platelet secretion

12. Which is a congenital vascular disorder?
    a. Senile purpura
    b. Ehlers-Danlos syndrome
    c. Henoch-Schönlein purpura
    d. Waldenström macroglobulinemia

REFERENCES

1. Triplett, D. A. (1978). How to evaluate platelet function. *Lab Med Pract Phys*, July-Aug, 37–43.
2. Al-Huniti, A., & Kahr, W. H. A. (2020). Inherited platelet disorders: diagnosis and management. *Transfus Med Rev, 34*, 277–285.
3. Palma-Barqueros, V., Revilla, N., Sanchez, A., et al. (2021). Inherited platelet disorders: an updated review. *Int J Med Sci, 22*, 4521.
4. Noris, P., & Pecci, A. (2017). Hereditary thrombocytopenias: a growing list of disorders. *Hematology Am Soc Hematol Educ Program*, 385–399.
5. Nurden, P., & Nurden, A. T. (2008). Congenital disorders associated with platelet dysfunctions. *Thromb Haemost, 99*, 253–263.
6. George, J. N., & Shattil, S. J. (1991). The clinical importance of acquired abnormalities of platelet function. *N Engl J Med, 324*, 27–39.
7. Caen, J. P. (1989). Glanzmann's thrombasthenia. *Baillieres Clin Haematol, 2*, 609–623.
8. Sivapalaratnam, S., Rao, A. K., Ouwehand, W., et al. (2021). Inherited platelet disorders. In Kaushansky, K., Prchal, J. T., Burns, L. J., et al. (Eds.), *Williams Hematology*. (10th ed., Chapter 119). New York: McGraw-Hill.
9. Nurden, P., Stritt, S., Favier, R., Nurden, A. T. (2021). Inherited platelet diseases with normal platelet count: phenotypes, genotypes and diagnostic strategy. *Haematologica, 106*, 337–350.
10. Rapaport, S. I. (1987). *Introduction to Hematology*. (2nd ed.). Philadelphia: Lippincott.
11. Meyer, M., Kirchmaier, C. M., Schirmer, A., et al. (1991). Acquired disorder of platelet function associated with autoantibodies against membrane glycoprotein IIb-IIIa complex: 1. Glycoprotein analysis. *Thromb Haemost, 65*, 491–496.
12. Tarantino, M. D., Corrigan, J. J., Jr., Glasser, L., et al. (1991). A variant form of thrombasthenia. *Am J Dis Child, 145*, 1053–1057.
13. Friedlander, M., Brooks, P. C., Shaffer, R. W., et al. (1995). Definition of two angiogenic pathways by distinct a_v integrins. *Science, 270*, 1500–1502.
14. Bennett, J. S., & Rao, A. K. (2013). Inherited disorders of platelet function. In Marder, V. J., Aird, W. C., Bennett, J. S., et al. (Eds.), *Hemostasis and Thrombosis: Basic Principles and Clinical Practice*. (6th ed., pp. 805–819). Philadelphia: Lippincott Williams & Wilkins.
15. Nurden, A. T. (2005). Qualitative disorders of platelets and megakaryocytes. *J Thromb Haemost, 3*, 1773–1782.
16. Nurden, A. T., Fiore, M., Nurden, P., et al. (2011). Glanzmann thrombasthenia: a review of *ITGA2B* and *ITGB3* defects with emphasis on variants, phenotypic variability, and mouse models. *Blood, 118*, 5996–6005.
17. Coller, B. S., Cheresh, D. A., Asch, E., et al. (1991). Platelet vitronectin receptor expression differentiates Iraqi-Jewish from Arab patients with Glanzmann thrombasthenia in Israel. *Blood, 77*, 75–83.
18. French, D. L. (1998). The molecular genetics of Glanzmann's thrombasthenia. *Platelets, 9*, 5–20.
19. Nurden, A. T. (2019). Acquired Glanzmann thrombasthenia: from antibodies to anti-platelet drugs. *Blood Rev, 36*, 10–22.
20. Corriveau, D. M., & Fritsma, G. A. (1988). *Hemostasis and Thrombosis in the Clinical Laboratory*. Philadelphia: Lippincott.
21. Rosa, J. P., Artcanuthurry, V., Grelac, F., et al. (1997). Reassessment of protein tyrosine phosphorylation in thrombasthenic platelets: evidence that phosphorylation of cortactin and a 64 kD protein is dependent on thrombin activation and integrin $\alpha_{IIb}\beta_3$. *Thromb Haemost, 89*, 4385–4392.
22. Byzova, T. V., & Plow, E. F. (1997). Networking in the hemostatic system: integrin $\alpha_{IIb}\beta_3$ binds prothrombin and influences its activation. *J Biol Chem, 272*, 27183–27188.
23. Gemmell, C. H., Sefton, M. V., & Yeo, E. L. (1993). Platelet-derived microparticle formation involves glycoprotein IIb-IIIa: inhibition by RGDs and a Glanzmann's thrombasthenia defect. *J Biol Chem, 268*, 14586–14589.
24. Reverter, J. C., Beguin, S., Kessels, H., et al. (1996). Inhibition of platelet-mediated tissue factor-induced thrombin generation by the mouse/human chimeric 7E3 antibody: potential implications for the effect of c7E3 Fab treatment on acute thrombosis and clinical restenosis. *J Clin Invest, 98*, 863–874.
25. Caen, J. P. (1972). Glanzmann's thrombasthenia. *Clin Hematol, 1*, 383–392.
26. George, J. N., Caen, J. P., & Nurden, A. T. (1990). Glanzmann's thrombasthenia: the spectrum of clinical disease. *Blood, 75*, 1383–1395.
27. Jennings, L. K., Wang, W. C., Jackson, C. W., et al. (1991). Hemostasis in Glanzmann's thrombasthenia (GT): GT platelets interfere with the aggregation of normal platelets. *Am J Pediatr Hematol Oncol, 13*, 84–90.

28. Lisman, T., Adelmaier, J., Heijnen, H. F. G., et al. (2004). Recombinant factor VIIa restores aggregation of $\alpha_{IIb}\beta_3$-deficient platelets via tissue factor-independent fibrin generation. *Blood, 103,* 1720–1727.

29. Poon, M. C., d'Oiron, R., Von Depka, M., et al. (2004). International Data Collection on Recombinant Factor VIIa and Congenital Platelet Disorders Study Group. Prophylactic and therapeutic recombinant factor VIIa administration to patients with Glanzmann's thrombasthenia: results of an international survey. *J Thromb Haemost, 2,* 1096–1103.

30. Geddis, A. E., & Kaushansky, K. (2004). Inherited thrombocytopenias: toward a better molecular understanding of disorders of platelet production. *Curr Opin Pediatr, 16,* 15–24.

31. Nurden, P., & Nurden, A. (1996). Giant platelets, megakaryocytes and the expression of glycoprotein Ib-IX complexes. *C R Acad Sci III, 319,* 717–726.

32. Clementson, K. J. (1997). Platelet GPIb-V-IX complex. *Thromb Haemost, 78,* 266–270.

33. Liang, M., Soomro, A., Tasneem, S., et al. (2020). Enhancer-gene rewiring in the pathogenesis of Quebec platelet disorder. *Blood, 136*(23), 2679–2690.

34. Lopez, J. A., Andrews, R. K., Afshar-Kharghan, V., et al. (1998). Bernard-Soulier syndrome. *Blood, 91,* 4397–4418.

35. Savoia, A., Pastore, A., De Rocco, D., et al. (2011). Clinical and genetic aspects of Bernard-Soulier syndrome: searching for genotype/phenotype correlations. *Haematologica, 96,* 417–423.

36. Sumitha, E., Jayandharan, G. R., David, S., et al. (2011). Molecular basis of Bernard-Soulier syndrome in 27 patients from India. *J Thromb Haemost, 9,* 1590.

37. Takahashi, H., Murata, M., Moriki, T., et al. (1995). Substitution of Val for Met at residue 239 of platelet glycoprotein Ib alpha in Japanese patients with platelet-type von Willebrand disease. *Blood, 85,* 727–733.

38. Matsubara, Y., Murata, M., Sugita, K., et al. (2003). Identification of a novel point mutation in platelet glycoprotein Iba, Gly to Ser at residue 233, in a Japanese family with platelet-type von Willebrand disease. *J Thromb Haemost, 1,* 2198–2205.

39. Othman, M., Elbatarny, H. S., Notley, C., et al. (2004). Identification and functional characterization of a novel 27 bp deletion in the macroglycopeptide-coding region of the GPIba gene resulting in platelet-type von Willebrand disease. *Blood, 104,* Abstract 1023.

40. Saito, H., Matshushita, T., Yamamoto, K., et al. (2005). Giant platelet syndrome. *Hematology, 10*(Suppl 1), 41–46.

41. Pati, H., & Saraya, A. K. (1986). Platelet storage pool disease. *Indian J Med Res, 84,* 617–620.

42. Weiss, H. J., Lages, B., Vicic, W., et al. (1993). Heterogeneous abnormalities of platelet dense granule ultrastructure in 20 patients with congenital storage pool deficiency. *Br J Haematol, 83,* 282–295.

43. Rand, M. L., & Israels, S. J. (2023). Molecular basis of platelet function. In Hoffman, R., Benz, E. J., Jr. Silberstein, L. E., et al. (Eds.), *Hematology: Basic Principles and Practice.* (8th ed., pp.1950–1967). Philadelphia: Elsevier.

44. Abrams, C. S., & Brass, L. F. (2013). Platelet signal transduction. In Marder, V. J., Aird, W. C., Bennett, J. S., et al. (Eds.), *Hemostasis and Thrombosis: Basic Principles and Clinical Practice.* (6th ed., pp. 449–461). Philadelphia: Lippincott.

45. Jedlitschky, G., Tirwschmann, K., Lubenow, L. E., et al. (2004). The nucleotide transporter MRP4 (ABCC4) is highly expressed in human platelets and present in dense granules, indicating a role in mediator storage. *Blood, 104,* 3603–3610.

46. Li, W., Hao, C. J., Hao, Z. H., et al. (2022). New insights into the pathogenesis of Hermansky-Pudlak syndrome. *Pigment Cell Melanoma Res, 35,* 290–302.

47. Dell'Angellica, E. C., Aguilar, R. C., Wolins, N., et al. (2000). Molecular characterization of the protein encoded by the Hermansky-Pudlak syndrome type 1 gene. *J Biol Chem, 275,* 1300–1306.

48. Obeng-Tuudah, D., Hussein, B. A., Hakim, A., et al. (2021). The presentation and outcomes of Hermansky-Pudlak syndrome in obstetrics and gynecological settings: a systemic review. *Int J Glynecol Obstet, 154,* 412–426.

49. White, J. G. (1987). Inherited abnormalities of the platelet membrane and secretory granules. *Hum Pathol, 18,* 123–139.

50. Villa, A., Notarangelo, L., Macchi, P., et al. (1995). X-linked thrombocytopenia and Wiskott-Aldrich syndrome are allelic diseases with mutations in the *WASP* gene. *Nat Genet, 9,* 414.

51. Lanzi, G., Moratto, D., Vairo, D., et al. (2012). A novel primary human immunodeficiency due to deficiency in the WASP-interacting protein WIP. *J Exp Med, 209,* 29–34.

52. Quick, A. J. (1966). *Hemorrhagic Diseases and Thrombosis.* (2nd ed.). Philadelphia: Lea & Febiger.

53. Pai, S.-Y., & Notarangelo, L. D. (2023). Congenital disorders of lymphocytic function. In Hoffman, R., Benz, E. J., Jr. Silberstein, L. E., et al. (Eds.), *Hematology: Basic Principles and Practice.* (8th ed., pp. 736–749). Philadelphia: Elsevier.

54. Halpern, D., Pavord, S., & Myers, B. (2021). A case series review of patients with thrombocytopenia and absent-radii syndrome (TARS) and their management in pregnancy. *Platelets, 32*(8), 1124–1125.

55. Raccuglia, G. (1971). Gray platelet syndrome: a variety of qualitative platelet disorder. *Am J Med, 51,* 818–828.

56. Collins, J. H., Mayer, L., & Lopez, J. A. G. (2023). Immune dysregulation, autoimmunity, and granule defects in gray platelet syndrome. *J Thromb Haemost, 21*(6), 1409–1419.

57. Bottega, R., Nicchia, E., Alfano, C., et al. (2017). Gray platelet syndrome: novel mutations of the *NBESL2* gene. *Am J Hematol, 92*(2), E20–E22.

58. Berrebi, A., Klepfish, A., Varon, D., et al. (1988). Gray platelet syndrome in the elderly. *Am J Hematol, 28,* 270–272.

59. Pfueller, S. L., Howard, M. A., White, J. G., et al. (1987). Shortening of the bleeding time by 1-deamino-8-arginine vasopressin (DDAVP) in the absence of platelet von Willebrand factor in gray platelet syndrome. *Thromb Haemost, 58,* 1060–1063.

60. Brace, L. D., Venton, D. L., & Le Breton, G. C. (1985). Thromboxane A_2/prostaglandin H_2 mobilizes calcium in human blood platelets. *Am J Physiol, 249,* H1–H7.

61. Moake, J. L., & Funicella, T. (1983). Common bleeding problems. *Clin Symp, 35,* 1–32.

62. Nieuwenhuis, H. K., Sakariassen, K. S., Houdijk, W. P. M., et al. (1986). Deficiency of platelet membrane glycoprotein Ia associated with a decreased platelet adhesion to subendothelium: a defect in platelet spreading. *Blood, 68,* 692–695.

63. Moroi, M., Jung, S. M., Okuma, M., et al. (1989). A patient with platelets deficient in glycoprotein VI that lack both collagen-induced aggregation and adhesion. *J Clin Invest, 84,* 1440–1445.

64. Nurden, P., Jandrot-Perrus, M., Combrie, R., et al. (2004). Severe deficiency of glycoprotein VI in a patient with gray platelet syndrome. *Blood, 104,* 107–114.

65. Hetherington, S. L., Singh, R. K., Lodwick, D., et al. (2005). Dimorphism in the P2Y1 ADP receptor gene is associated with increased platelet activation response to ADP. *Arterioscler Thromb Vasc Biol, 25,* 252–257.

66. Cattaneo, M. (2003). Inherited platelet-based bleeding disorders. *J Thromb Haemost, 1,* 1628–1636.

67. Daniel, J. L., Dangelmaier, C., Jin, J., et al. (1998). Molecular basis for ADP-induced platelet activation: I. Evidence for three distinct ADP receptors on human platelets. *J Biol Chem, 273,* 2024–2029.

68. Nurden, P., Savi, P., Heilmann, E., et al. (1995). An inherited bleeding disorder linked to a defective interaction between ADP and its receptor on platelets. *J Clin Invest, 95,* 1612–1622.

69. Cattaneo, M., Zighetti, M. L., Lombardi, R., et al. (2003). Molecular basis of defective signal transduction in the platelet P2Y12 receptor of a patient with congenital bleeding. *Proc Natl Acad Sci USA, 100,* 1978–1983.

70. Rao, A. K. (1998). Congenital disorders of platelet function: disorders of signal transduction and secretion. *Am J Med Sci, 316,* 69–76.

71. Rao, A. K. (2003). Inherited defects in platelet signaling mechanisms. *J Thromb Haemost, 1,* 671–681.

72. Zhou, Q., Sims, P. J., & Wiedmer, T. (1998). Expression of proteins controlling transbilayer movement of plasma membrane phospholipids in B lymphocytes from a patient with Scott syndrome. *Blood, 92,* 1707–1712.

73. Zwall, R. F. A., Comfurius, P., & Bevers, E. M. (2004). Scott syndrome, a bleeding disorder caused by defective scrambling of membrane phospholipids. *Biochim Biophys Acta, 1636* (2–3), 119–128.

74. Zwaal, R. F., Comfurius, P., & Bevers, E. M. (2004). Scott syndrome, a bleeding disorder caused by a defective scrambling of membrane phospholipids. *Biochim Biophys Acta, 1636,* 119–128.

75. Sims, P., & Wiedmer, T. (2001). Unraveling the mysteries of phospholipid scrambling. *Thromb Haemost, 86,* 266–275.

76. Borsani, O., Piga, D., Costa, S., et al. (2018). Stormorken syndrome caused by a p.R304W *STIM1* mutation: the first Italian patient and a review of the literature. *Front Neurol, 9,* 859.

77. Van Oosterom, N., Barras, M., Cottrell, N., et al. (2022). Platelet function assays for the diagnosis of aspirin resistance. *Platelets, 33,* 329–338.

78. Le Quellec, S., Bordet, J. C., Negrier, C., et al. (2016). Comparison of current platelet functional tests for the assessment of aspirin and clopidogrel response. *Thromb Haemost, 116,* 638–650.

79. Bhatt, D. L., Grosser, T., Dong, J. F., et al. (2017). Enteric coating and aspirin nonresponsiveness in patients with type 2 diabetes mellitus. *J Am Coll Cardiol, 69,* 603–612.

80. Eikelboom, J. W., Hirsh, J., Weitz, J., et al. (2002). Aspirin resistant thromboxane biosynthesis and the risk of myocardial infarction, stroke, or cardiovascular death in patients at high risk for cardiovascular events. *Circulation, 105,* 1650–1655.

81. Green, D. (1988). Diagnosis and management of bleeding disorders. *Compr Ther, 14,* 31–36.

82. Catella-Lawson, F., Reilly, M. P., Kapoor, S. C., et al. (2001). Cyclooxygenase inhibitors and the antiplatelet effects of aspirin. *New Eng J Med, 345,* 1809–1817.

83. Schleinitz, M. D., & Heidenreich, P. A. (2005). A cost-effectiveness analysis of combination antiplatelet therapy of high-risk acute coronary syndromes: clopidogrel plus aspirin versus aspirin alone. *Ann Intern Med, 142,* 251–259.

84. Mao, L., Jian, C., Changzhi, L., et al. (2013). Cytochrome CYP2C19 polymorphism and risk of adverse clinical events in clopidogrel-treated patients: a meta-analysis based on 23,035 subjects. *Arch Cardiovasc Dis, 106,* 517–527.

85. Sibbing, D., Koch, W., Gebhard, D., et al. (2010). Cytochrome 2C19*17 allelic variant, platelet aggregation, bleeding events, and stent thrombosis in clopidogrel-treated patients with coronary stent placement. *Circulation, 121,* 512–518.

86. Wilhite, D. B., Comerota, A. J., Schmieder, F. A., et al. (2003). Managing PAD with multiple platelet inhibitors: the effect of combination therapy on bleeding time. *J Vasc Surg, 38,* 710–713.

87. Danielak, D., Karazniewicz-Lada, M., & Glowka, F. (2018). Ticagrelor in modern cardiology – an up-to-date review of most important aspects of ticagrelor pharmacotherapy. *Exp Opin Pharamcother, 19,* 103–112.

88. Sible, A. M., & Nawarskas, J. J. (2017). Cangrelor: a new route for P2Y$_{12}$ inhibition. *Cardiology in Review, 25,* 133–139.

89. Angiolillo, D. J., Firstenberg, M. S., & Price, M. J. (2012). Bridging antiplatelet therapy with cangrelor in patients undergoing cardiac surgery: a randomized controlled study. *JAMA, 307,* 265–274.

90. Capodanno, D., Milluzzo, R. P., & Angiolillo, D. J. (2019). Intravenous antiplatelet therapies (glycoprotein IIb/IIIa receptor inhibitors and cangrelor) in percutaneous coronary intervention: from pharmacology to indications for clinical use. *Ther Adv Cardiovasc Dis, 13,* 1–21.

91. Ungar, L., Rodriguez, F., & Mahaffey, K. W. (2016). Vorapaxar: emerging evidence and clinical questions in a new era of PAR-1 inhibition. *Coron Artery Dis, 27,* 604–615.

92. Gupta, R., Lin, M., Mehta, A., et al. (2021). Protease-activated receptor antagonist for reducing cardiovascular events – a review on vorapaxar. *Curr Probl Cardiol,* https://doi.org/10.1016/j.cpcardiol.2021.101035.

93. Gross, P. L., & López, J. A. (2023). Acquired disorders of platelet function. In Hoffman, R., Benz, E. J., Jr., & Silberstein L. E., et al. (Eds.), *Hematology: Basic Principles and Practice.* (8th ed., pp. 2007–2019). Philadelphia: Elsevier.

94. von Hundelshausen, P., & Siess, W. (2021). Bleeding by Bruton tyrosine kinase-inhibitors: dependency on drug type and disease. *Cancers, 13,* 1103.

95. Oyarzún, C. P., & Heller, P. G. (2019). Platelets as mediators of thromboinflammation in chronic myeloproliferative neoplasms. *Front Immunol, 10,* Article 1373.

96. Swart, S. S., Pearson, D., Wood, J. K., et al. (1984). Functional significance of the platelet alpha$_2$-adrenoreceptor: studies in patients with myeloproliferative disorders. *Thromb Res, 33,* 531–541.

97. Coppola, A., Tufano, A., DiCapua, M., et al. (2011). Bleeding and thrombosis in multiple myeloma and related plasma cell disorders. *Semin Thromb Hemost, 37*(8), 929–945.

98. Bick, R. L., & Scates, S. M. (1992). Qualitative platelet defects. *Lab Med, 23,* 95–103.

99. Haut, M. J., & Cowan, D. H. (1974). The effect of ethanol on hemostatic properties of human blood platelets. *Am J Med, 56,* 22–33.

100. Baaten, C. C., Schröer, J. R., Floege, J., et al. (2022). Platelet abnormalities in CKD and their implications for antiplatelet therapy. *CJASN, 17,* 155–170.

101. Casini, A., Neerman-Arbez, M., & deMoerloose, P. (2020). Heterogeneity of congenital afibrinogenemia, from epidemiology to clinical consequences and management. *Blood Rev, 48,* 100793.

102. Aquiccimarro, E., Jiritano, F., Serraino, G. F., et al. (2021). Quantitative and qualitative platelet derangements in cardiac surgery and extracorporeal life support. *J Clin Med, 10,* 615.

103. Pareti, F. I., Capitanio, A., Mannucci, L., et al. (1980). Acquired dysfunction due to circulation of exhausted platelets. *Am J Med, 69,* 235–240.

104. Moncada, B., Ruiz-Arguelles, G. J., & Castillo-Martinez, C. (2013). The sticky platelet syndrome. *Hematology, 18,* 230–232.

105. O'Donnell, M., Shatzel, J. J., Olson, S. R., et al. (2018). Arterial thrombosis in unusual sites: a practical review. *Eur J Haematol, 101,* 728–736.

106. Helgason, C. M., Hoff, J. A., Kondos, G. T., et al. (1993). Platelet aggregation in patients with atrial fibrillation taking aspirin or warfarin. *Stroke, 24,* 1458–1461.

107. Hayward, C. P. M., & Ma, A. D. (2023). Evaluation of the patient with suspected bleeding disorders. In Hoffman, R., Benz, E. J., Jr., Silberstein, L. E., et al. (Eds.) *Hematology: Basic Principles and Practice.* (8th ed., pp. 1988–1995). Philadelphia: Elsevier.

108. Maceyko, R. F., & Camisa, C. (1991). Kasabach-Merritt syndrome. *Pediatr Dermatol, 8,* 133–136.

109. Gertz, M. A., Buadi, F. K., Lacy, M. Q., et al. (2023). Immunoglobulin light chain amyloidosis (primary amyloidosis). In Hoffman, R., Benz, E. J., Jr., Silberstein, L. E., et al. (Eds.), *Hematology: Basic Principles and Practice.* (8th ed., pp. 1553–1566). Philadelphia: Elsevier.

110. Scicluna, K., Formosa, M. M., Farrugia, R., et al. (2022). Hypermobile Ehlers-Danlos syndrome: a review and a critical appraisal of published genetic research to date. *Clin Genet, 101*(1), 20–31.

38

Quantitative Disorders of Platelets: Thrombocytopenia and Thrombocytosis

Phillip J. DeChristopher and Walter P. Jeske*

OBJECTIVES

After completion of this chapter, the reader will be able to:

1. Define thrombocytopenia and thrombocytosis, and state their associated platelet counts.
2. Compare and contrast the clinical symptoms of platelet disorders and clotting factor deficiencies.
3. Explain the common pathophysiologic processes leading to thrombocytopenia.
4. List the unique diagnostic features of at least four disorders associated with congenital hypoplasia of the bone marrow and describe their inheritance patterns.
5. List possible causes of neonatal thrombocytopenia.
6. Differentiate between acute and chronic immune thrombocytopenia.
7. Describe the immunologic and nonimmunologic mechanisms by which drugs may induce thrombocytopenia.
8. Differentiate between neonatal alloimmune thrombocytopenia and neonatal autoimmune thrombocytopenia.
9. List mechanisms leading to nonimmune platelet destruction.
10. Differentiate thrombotic thrombocytopenic purpura, hemolytic uremic syndrome, and atypical hemolytic uremic syndrome based on laboratory findings and pathophysiology.
11. Describe how abnormalities in platelet distribution and dilution can contribute to the development of thrombocytopenia.
12. List pathologies associated with thrombocytosis.
13. Given clinical history and laboratory test results for patients with thrombocytopenia or thrombocytosis, suggest a diagnosis that is consistent with the information provided.

OUTLINE

Thrombocytopenia: Decrease in Circulating Platelets
  Decreased Platelet Production
  Increased Platelet Destruction
  Abnormalities in Distribution or Dilution

Thrombocytosis: Increase in Circulating Platelets
  Reactive Thrombocytosis
  Thrombocytosis Associated With Myeloproliferative Disorders

CASE STUDY

After studying the material in this chapter, the reader should be able to respond to the following case study. Answers can be found in Appendix C.

A 73-year-old Hispanic female who had four children in the remote past was hospitalized in the medical intensive care unit with end-stage liver disease secondary to cirrhosis secondary to chronic hepatitis B infection. Her clinical course was complicated by recurrent massive abdominal ascites, episodes of spontaneous bacterial peritonitis, disseminated intravascular coagulation, respiratory failure (she was intubated and ventilator dependent), and worsening renal failure (thought to be secondary to hepatorenal syndrome). Her PLTs, which averaged in the low 20s $\times 10^3/\mu L$, were not associated with spontaneous bleeding.

Reference intervals can be found after the Index at the end of the book. She was not on any medications that affect platelet function. Wanting to start hemodialysis, her provider requested the interventional radiology department to place a central line. The interventional radiologist insisted on a preprocedure PLT of at least $50 \times 10^3/\mu L$ before line placement. Despite platelet transfusions during the last 3 days, repeat platelet counts the next day remained at baseline.

1. What is the most likely cause of the patient's thrombocytopenia?
2. What laboratory tests should be ordered next?
3. One provider suggested that "specialized platelets" (e.g., crossmatched or HLA-matched components) might work better. Is this suggestion true?

*The authors extend appreciation to Larry D. Brace, whose work in prior editions provided the foundation for this chapter.

Bleeding disorders resulting from platelet abnormalities, whether quantitative, which will be discussed in this chapter, or qualitative (Chapter 37), usually manifest as bleeding into the skin, mucous membranes, or both (*mucocutaneous bleeding*). Common presenting symptoms include petechiae, purpura, ecchymoses, epistaxis, and gingival bleeding. Similar findings also are seen in patients with vascular disorders, but vascular disorders (e.g., Ehlers-Danlos syndrome, hereditary hemorrhagic telangiectasia) (Chapter 37) are relatively rare. In contrast, deep tissue bleeding, such as hematoma and hemarthrosis, is associated with clotting factor deficiencies (Chapter 36).

THROMBOCYTOPENIA: DECREASE IN CIRCULATING PLATELETS

Although the reference interval for the platelet count varies among laboratories, it is generally considered to be approximately 150,000 to 450,000/μL (150 to 450 × 10⁹/L). Thrombocytopenia (platelet count less than 100,000/μL) is the most common cause of clinically important bleeding. True thrombocytopenia has to be differentiated from the thrombocytopenia artifact that can result from poorly prepared blood films or automated cell counts when platelet clumping (Figure 14.2) or platelet satellitosis (Figure 14.1) is present (Chapters 13 and 14).

Small vessel bleeding in the skin attributed to thrombocytopenia manifests as hemorrhages of different sizes (Figure 38.1). *Petechiae* are small pinpoint hemorrhages about 1 mm in diameter, *purpura* are about 3 mm in diameter and generally round, and *ecchymoses* are 1 cm or larger and usually irregular in shape. Ecchymosis corresponds with the lay term *bruise*. Other conditions such as defective platelet function, vascular fragility, and trauma contribute to the hemorrhagic state.

The severity of clinical bleeding varies and often is not closely correlated with the platelet count. It is unusual for clinically significant bleeding to occur when the platelet count is greater than 50,000/μL, but the risk increases progressively as the platelet count decreases from 50,000/μL. In general, patients with platelet counts <10,000/μL are considered to be at high risk for severe spontaneous bleeding. The primary pathophysiologic processes that result in thrombocytopenia are decreased platelet production, increased platelet destruction, and abnormal platelet distribution (sequestration).

Decreased Platelet Production

Abnormalities in platelet production can result from a lack of adequate megakaryocytes in the bone marrow (*megakaryocyte hypoplasia*) or ineffective platelet production (*thrombopoiesis*). Chapter 11 reviews platelet production. Factors causing decreased platelet production can be congenital or acquired. Box 38.1 categorizes these disorders.

Congenital Types of Impaired Platelet Production

It is increasingly apparent that most inherited thrombocytopenias can be linked to specific chromosomal abnormalities or specific genetic defects. Table 38.1 lists inherited

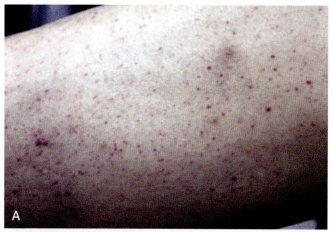
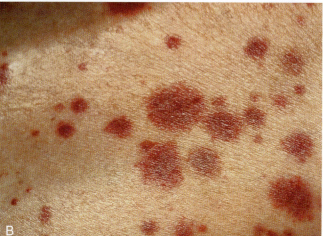
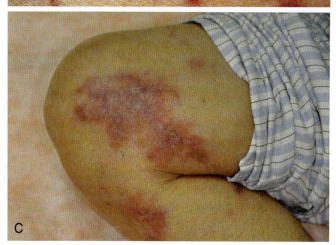

Figure 38.1 Patterns of Systemic (Mucocutaneous) Hemorrhage. The various presentations of systemic bleeding include **(A)** petechiae, **(B)** purpura, and **(C)** ecchymoses. (A from Abrams, C. S. [2015]. Thrombocytopenia. In Goldman L., & Schafer, A. I. [Eds.], *Goldman-Cecil Medicine* [25th ed.]. Philadelphia, PA: Elsevier; B from Piette, W. W. [2017]. Purpura: mechanism and differential diagnosis. In Bolognia, J. L., Schaffer, J. V., & Cerroni, L. [Eds.], *Dermatology* [4th ed., Vol. 22, pp. 357–367]. St. Louis: Elsevier; C from Yang, T.-H., Chen, W.-Y., & Tsai, H.-H. [2016]. Periarticular ecchymosis-like plaques and nodules. *J Am Acad Dermatol, 75*[1], e1–e2.)

BOX 38.1   Classification of Thrombocytopenias: Impaired or Decreased Production of Platelets

Congenital
May-Hegglin anomaly
Bernard-Soulier syndrome
Fechtner syndrome
Sebastian syndrome
Epstein syndrome
Montreal platelet syndrome
Fanconi anemia
Wiskott-Aldrich syndrome
Thrombocytopenia with absent radius (TAR) syndrome
Congenital amegakaryocytic thrombocytopenia
Autosomal dominant and X-linked thrombocytopenia

Acquired
Viral or bacterial infections
Drug induced

Neonatal
Alloimmune
Autoimmune
Infection
Inflammatory entities (e.g., acute bowel disorders such as spontaneous intestinal perforation or necrotizing enterocolitis [of varying degrees])
Perinatal asphyxia
Chronic fetal hypoxia (e.g., pregnancy-induced hypertension and gestational diabetes)

TABLE 38.1   Classification of Inherited Thrombocytopenias

Disease	Occurrence*	Spontaneous Bleeding	Gene; Chromosomal Location	Platelet Size†	Features
X-Linked					
Wiskott-Aldrich syndrome	R	Yes	*WAS;* Xp11.23	Small	Severe immunodeficiency; death in infancy
GATA1-related diseases	ER	Yes	*GATA1;* Xp11.23	Large	Hemolytic anemia; possible congenital dyserythropoietic anemia
FLNA-related (filamin A) thrombocytopenia	ER	Yes	*FLNA;* Xq28	Large	Periventricular nodular heterotopia
Autosomal Recessive					
Thrombocytopenia with absent radii	R	Yes	*RBM8A;* 1q21.1	Normal	Bilateral radial aplasia and/or other malformations; reduced megakaryocytes; platelet count normalizes into adulthood
Bernard-Soulier syndrome; biallelic	R	Yes	*GP1BA;* 17p13.2	Large	Mucosal bleeding; cutaneous bleeding; epistaxis; menorrhagia
Congenital megakaryocytic thrombocytopenia	VR	Yes	*MPL;* 1p34.1	Normal	Bone marrow aplasia in infancy; defects in thrombopoietin production and reactivity
Gray platelet syndrome	ER	Yes	*NBEAL2;* 3p21.31	Giant	Increased risk of developing myelofibrosis and splenomegaly
Thrombocytopenia associated with lipid accumulation	ER	No	*ABCG5, ABCG8;* 2p21	Large	Anemia; tendon xanthomas; atherosclerosis
Autosomal Dominant					
MYH9-related disease	R	No	*MYH9;* 22q12–13	Large	Presenile cataracts; nephropathy; progressive hearing loss
Paris-Trousseau thrombocytopenia	R	Yes	Large deletion; 11q23.3	Large	Cardiac, facial defects, developmental delays
Bernard-Soulier syndrome; monoallelic	VR	No	*GP1BB;* 22q11.21 *GP9;* 3q21.3	Large	—
Familial platelet disorder/predisposition to AML	ER	No	*RUNX1;* 21q22.12	Normal	High risk of leukemia or myelodysplastic syndrome
ANKRD26-related thrombocytopenia	ER	No	*ANKRD26;* 10p12.1	Normal	Risk of leukemia
ITGA2B/ITGB3-related thrombocytopenia	ER	No	*ITGA2B;* 17q21.31 *ITGB3;* 17q21.32	Large	—
TUBB1-related thrombocytopenia	ER	No	*TUBB1;* 20q13.3	Giant	Platelet aggregation and megakaryocytes morphologically normal
CYYCS-related thrombocytopenia	ER	No	*CYCS;* 7p15.3	Normal	—
Congenital thrombocytopenia with radioulnar bone fusion	ER	Yes	*HOXA11;* 7p15.2	Normal	Possible evolution into aplastic anemia

*Occurrence in families: *R,* rare, ~100 families; *VR,* very rare, ~ 50 families; *ER,* extremely rare, ≤ 10 families.
†Platelet size: normal, 1.5–3 μm; small, <1.5 μm; large, ~6 μm; giant, 5–8 μm or larger.
AML, Acute myelogenous leukemia.

thrombocytopenias associated with specific gene and chromosomal abnormalities, the mode of inheritance, and associated features.

Megakaryocytic hypoplasia is seen in a wide variety of congenital disorders, including Fanconi anemia (pancytopenia), thrombocytopenia with absent radius (TAR) syndrome, May-Hegglin anomaly, Wiskott-Aldrich syndrome, Bernard-Soulier syndrome, and other less common disorders. Although thrombocytopenia is a feature of Bernard-Soulier syndrome and Wiskott-Aldrich syndrome, the primary abnormality in these disorders is a qualitative platelet defect, and so these disorders are discussed in Chapter 37.

May-Hegglin anomaly. The exact incidence of this rare autosomal dominant disorder is unknown. May-Hegglin anomaly is characterized by abnormally enlarged (20 µm in diameter) or misshapen platelets on the peripheral blood film, and Döhle-like bodies are present in neutrophils (Figure 38.2) and occasionally in monocytes. Thrombocytopenia of varying degrees is present in about one-third to one-half of affected patients. Platelet function in response to platelet-activating agents is usually normal. In some patients, the number of megakaryocytes is increased, and their ultrastructure is abnormal. Mutations in the *MYH9* gene that encodes for nonmuscle myosin heavy chain (a cytoskeletal protein in platelets) have been reported.[1] This mutation may be responsible for the abnormal size of platelets in this disorder. Most patients are asymptomatic unless severe thrombocytopenia is present. In severe cases with clinical bleeding, transfusion with platelets may be necessary. Recent work has suggested that bleeding in patients with *MYH9* mutations may not result solely from abnormal platelet function, but may also result from impaired endothelial release of von Willebrand factor (VWF).[2]

Three other disorders involving mutations of the *MYH9* gene have been reported: Sebastian syndrome, Fechtner syndrome, and Epstein syndrome.[3] Sebastian syndrome is inherited as an autosomal dominant disorder characterized by large platelets, thrombocytopenia, and granulocytic inclusions. Similar abnormalities are observed in Fechtner syndrome and are accompanied by deafness, cataracts, and nephritis. In Epstein syndrome, large platelets are associated with deafness, ocular problems, and glomerular nephritis.[4] These disorders are discussed in more detail in Chapter 37.

Thrombocytopenia with absent radius syndrome. TAR syndrome is a rare autosomal recessive disorder characterized by severe neonatal thrombocytopenia and congenital absence or extreme hypoplasia of the radial bones of the forearms with absent, short, or malformed ulnae and other orthopedic abnormalities. TAR syndrome is associated with a mutation in the *RBM8A* gene located on the long arm of chromosome 1 or a 200-kb deletion involving the *RBM8A* gene (1q21.1). In addition to bone abnormalities, up to 90% of patients may have cardiac lesions or transient leukemoid reactions with elevated white blood cell (WBC) counts (sometimes with counts >100,000/µL).[5] Platelet counts are usually 10,000 to 30,000/µL during the first 2 years of infancy. Interestingly, platelet counts usually increase over time, with normal levels usually achieved by the time these children reach school age.

Fanconi anemia. This disorder is also associated with thrombocytopenia and other abnormalities, including bony abnormalities, abnormalities of visceral organs, and pancytopenia. Chapter 19 on bone marrow failure contains a more detailed description.

Congenital amegakaryocytic thrombocytopenia. This an autosomal recessive disorder reflecting bone marrow failure.[6] Affected infants usually have platelet counts ≤20,000/µL at birth, petechiae, and evidence of bleeding at or shortly after birth, with frequent physical anomalies. About half of infants develop aplastic anemia in the first year of life, and there are reports of myelodysplasia and leukemia later in childhood. Allogeneic stem cell transplantation is the only curative treatment for infants with clinically severe disease or aplasia.[7] A number of missense, nonsense, and splice site mutations in the *MPL* gene on chromosome 1 (1p34.1), resulting in complete loss of thrombopoietin receptor function, a reduction in megakaryocyte progenitors, and high circulating thrombopoietin levels, have been identified.[8]

Autosomal dominant thrombocytopenia. This disorder has been mapped to mutations in the *ANKRD26* gene on the short arm of chromosome 10 (10p12.1). Mutations in this gene lead to incomplete megakaryocyte differentiation and resultant thrombocytopenia. Platelet morphology and size are usually normal. Recent discovery of *ANKRD26* mutations in 21 of 210 thrombocytopenic pedigrees suggests that *ANKRD26* mutations may be a relatively common cause of autosomal dominant thrombocytopenia.[9] Bleeding in these patients is usually absent or mild, and platelet function is usually normal.[10]

X-linked thrombocytopenia. This disorder can result from mutations in the *WAS* (Wiskott-Aldrich syndrome) gene on the X chromosome (Xp11.23) or mutations in the *GATA1* gene, also on the X chromosome at Xp11.[11-14] X-linked thrombocytopenias range from mild conditions with small platelets and absent

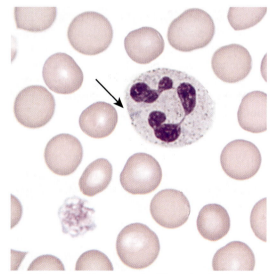

Figure 38.2 May-Hegglin Anomaly. Note the Döhle body *(arrow)* in the segmented neutrophil and the giant platelet. (Peripheral blood, Wright-Giemsa stain, ×1000.) (From Carr, J. H., & Rodak, B. F. [2013]. *Clinical Hematology Atlas* [4th ed.]. Philadelphia: Saunders.)

or mild bleeding to conditions with large platelets and severe bleeding.

Neonatal Thrombocytopenia

Thrombocytopenia (platelet count <150,000/μL) is evident in 1% to 5% of infants within 72 hours of birth. The causes of neonatal thrombocytopenia are numerous as illustrated in Table 38.2. Only a minority of these patients have immunologic disorders or coagulopathy causing thrombocytopenia.

TORCH (*t*oxoplasmosis, *o*ther [*Treponema pallidum,* varicella-zoster virus, parvovirus B19], *r*ubella, *c*ytomegalovirus [CMV], *h*erpes) syndrome infections are common causes of neonatal thrombocytopenia. Such infections cause thrombocytopenia with characteristically small platelets (*microthrombocytes,* seen only in TORCH and Wiskott-Aldrich syndrome). CMV is the most common infectious agent causing congenital thrombocytopenia, with an overall incidence of 0.5% to 1% of all births.[15] As only 10% to 15% of infected infants have symptomatic disease,[16] the incidence of significant neonatal thrombocytopenia caused by CMV is likely higher at about 1 in 1000

infants. Although the mechanism of thrombocytopenia is not well understood, reports suggest that CMV inhibits megakaryocytes and their precursors, which results in impaired platelet production.[17] About 1 in 1000 to 1 in 3000 infants are affected by congenital toxoplasmosis. About 40% of such infants develop thrombocytopenia.[18] Although persistent thrombocytopenia is a prominent feature in infants with congenital rubella syndrome, it is now rare in countries with organized immunization programs.[19,20] Though thrombocytopenia is fairly common in women with human immunodeficiency virus (HIV), due to either HIV disease progression or antiretroviral therapy, thrombocytopenia is rare in HIV-infected neonates of these women.[21]

Maternal ingestion of chlorothiazide diuretics or the oral hypoglycemic medication tolbutamide (both sulfonamides) can have a direct cytotoxic effect on the fetal marrow megakaryocytes. Bone marrow examination reveals a marked decrease or absence of megakaryocytes. Thrombocytopenia, which may be severe with platelet counts of 70,000/μL and sometimes lower, develops gradually, with recovery usually occurring within a few weeks after birth.[22,23]

Although infectious agents and certain drugs are well-known causes of neonatal thrombocytopenia, the most common cause is impaired platelet production. Most patients are preterm neonates born after pregnancies complicated by placental insufficiency or fetal hypoxia (preeclampsia and intrauterine growth restriction). These neonates have early onset thrombocytopenia and impaired megakaryopoiesis despite increased levels of thrombopoietin.

Increased platelet consumption or sequestration (discussed in detail in "Abnormalities in Distribution or Dilution") is another mechanism of neonatal thrombocytopenia, accounting for 2% to 25% of cases. Of these, 15% to 20% result from transplacental passage of maternal alloantibodies and autoantibodies. Another 10% to 15% of cases are due to disseminated intravascular coagulation (DIC), usually in very ill infants, particularly those with perinatal asphyxia or infections. Other causes of neonatal thrombocytopenia include thrombosis, platelet activation, platelet binding at inflammatory sites such as in necrotizing enterocolitis, and splenic sequestration.

In addition to the above-described acquired causes of neonatal thrombocytopenia, inherited thrombocytopenic syndromes are becoming recognized as causes of neonatal thrombocytopenia. Although considered rare, they may be more common than once believed.

Acquired Types of Impaired Platelet Production

Drug-induced hypoplasia of bone marrow. A wide array of chemotherapeutic agents used for the treatment of hematologic and nonhematologic malignancies suppress bone marrow megakaryocyte production and the production of other hematopoietic cells. Examples include the commonly used agents methotrexate, busulfan, cytosine arabinoside, cyclophosphamide, and cisplatin. Because the resulting thrombocytopenia may lead to hemorrhage, close monitoring of platelet counts is mandatory. Drug-induced thrombocytopenia is often the dose-limiting factor for many chemotherapeutic agents.

TABLE 38.2 Fetal and Neonatal Thrombocytopenias

Cause	Fetal	TIMING Neonatal <72 h After Birth	Neonatal >72 h After Birth
Increased Platelet Destruction			
Alloimmune	X	X	
Maternal autoimmune conditions (ITP, SLE)		X	
Platelet Activation/Consumption			
Necrotizing enterocolitis			X
Thrombosis (aortic, renal, or other vein)		X	
Decreased Platelet Production			
Aneuploidy (trisomy 13, 18, or 21, or triploidy)	X		
Bone marrow replacement (congenital leukemia)		X	
Uteroplacental vascular insufficiency (preeclampsia, IUGR)	X	X	
Miscellaneous			
Perinatal asphyxia		X	
Congenital infections (TORCH)	X	X	X
Perinatal infection (*Escherichia coli,* group B streptococcus, *Haemophilus influenzae*)		X	
Wiskott-Aldrich syndrome (congenital X-linked)			X
Kasabach-Merritt syndrome (congenital hemangioendothelioma)		X	X

ITP, Immune thrombocytopenic purpura; *IUGR,* intrauterine growth restriction; *SLE,* systemic lupus erythematosus; *TORCH,* *t*oxoplasmosis, *o*ther, *r*ubella, *c*ytomegalovirus, *h*erpes simplex virus.

Recombinant interleukin-11 has been approved for treatment of chemotherapy-induced thrombocytopenia, and thrombopoietin or its analogs may prove to be useful for this purpose.[24–26] Zidovudine (Retrovir, GlaxoSmithKline), previously used to treat HIV infections and now largely supplanted by modern antiretroviral medications, was known to cause myelotoxicity and severe thrombocytopenia.[27]

Several drugs specifically affect megakaryocytopoiesis without significantly affecting other hematopoietic cells. Anagrelide, for example, inhibits megakaryocyte colony development (Chapter 11)[28] and is therefore useful for treating thrombocytosis in patients with essential thrombocythemia and other myeloproliferative disorders.[29]

Long-term ingestion of ethanol (months to years) may result in persistent, severe thrombocytopenia. Although the mechanism is unknown, studies indicate that alcohol can inhibit megakaryocytopoiesis in some individuals. Mild thrombocytopenia is a common finding in alcoholic patients, but other causes unrelated to ethanol use, such as portal hypertension, splenomegaly, and folic acid deficiency, can also contribute. The platelet count usually returns to normal within a few weeks of alcohol withdrawal, but thrombocytopenia may persist for longer periods. A transient rebound thrombocytosis may develop when alcohol ingestion is stopped.[30]

Interferon therapy commonly causes mild to moderate thrombocytopenia, although under certain circumstances the thrombocytopenia can be severe and life-threatening. Interferon-α and interferon-γ inhibit stem cell differentiation and proliferation in the bone marrow (Chapter 5), but the mechanism of action is unclear.[31,32]

Thrombocytopenia presumably caused by megakaryocyte suppression has been reported following the administration of large doses of estrogen or estrogenic drugs such as diethylstilbestrol. Certain antibacterial agents (e.g., chloramphenicol), tranquilizers, and anticonvulsants also have been associated with thrombocytopenia caused by bone marrow suppression.[33,34]

Ineffective thrombopoiesis. Thrombocytopenia is a typical feature of the megaloblastic anemias (pernicious anemia, folic acid deficiency, and vitamin B_{12} deficiency). Quantitative studies indicate that as with erythrocyte production in these disorders, platelet production is ineffective. Although the bone marrow generally contains an increased number of megakaryocytes, the total number of platelets released into the circulation is decreased. Thrombocytopenia is caused by impaired DNA synthesis, and the bone marrow may contain grossly abnormal megakaryocytes with deformed, dumbbell-shaped nuclei, sometimes in large numbers. Stained peripheral blood films reveal large platelets that may have a decreased survival time and may have abnormal function. Thrombocytopenia is usually mild, and there is evidence of increased platelet destruction. Patients typically respond to vitamin replacement within 1 to 2 weeks.[23,35–37]

Infectious conditions, such as with viruses, are known to cause thrombocytopenia by acting on megakaryocytes or circulating platelets, either directly or in the form of viral antigen-antibody complexes. Live measles vaccine can cause degenerative vacuolization of megakaryocytes 6 to 8 days after vaccination. Some viruses interact readily with platelets by means of specific platelet receptors. Other viruses associated with thrombocytopenia include CMV, varicella-zoster virus, rubella virus, Epstein-Barr virus (causing infectious mononucleosis), and some serotypes of dengue virus that cause Thai hemorrhagic fever.[11]

Certain bacterial infections are commonly associated with the development of thrombocytopenia. This may be the result of toxins of bacterial origin, direct interactions between bacteria and platelets in the circulation, or extensive damage to the endothelium as in meningococcemia. Many cases of thrombocytopenia in childhood result from bacterial infection. Purpura may occur in many infectious diseases in the absence of thrombocytopenia, presumably because of vascular damage (Chapter 37).[11,38]

Infiltration of the bone marrow by malignant cells can result in a progressive decrease in bone marrow megakaryocytes as the abnormal cells replace normal marrow elements and a subsequent thrombocytopenia develops. Inhibitors of thrombopoiesis may be produced by these abnormal cells and may contribute to the thrombocytopenia. Associated conditions include myeloma, lymphoma, metastatic cancer, and myelofibrosis.[23,35,39]

Increased Platelet Destruction

Thrombocytopenia resulting from increased platelet destruction can be separated into two categories: increased platelet destruction caused by *immunologic* responses and increased destruction caused by *nonimmune* mechanisms (Box 38.2). Regardless of the process, increased production is required to maintain a normal platelet count, and thrombocytopenia develops only

---

BOX 38.2 Classification of Thrombocytopenias: Increased Platelet Destruction

Immune

Acute and chronic ITP
Drug induced: immunologic
Heparin-induced thrombocytopenia
Neonatal alloimmune thrombocytopenia
Neonatal autoimmune thrombocytopenia
Posttransfusion purpura
Secondary autoimmune thrombocytopenia

Nonimmune

Gestational thrombocytopenia (in pregnancy, preeclampsia, and HELLP syndrome)
HIV infection
Hemolytic disease of the newborn
Thrombotic microangiopathies (including TTP, HUS, aHUS)
Disseminated intravascular coagulation (consumption)
Bacterial infection, other infections/sepsis
Drug induced
Mechanical (including extracorporeal circulation)

aHUS, Atypical hemolytic uremic syndrome; *HELLP,* **h**emolysis, **e**levated **l**iver enzymes, and **l**ow **p**latelet count; *HIV,* human immunodeficiency virus; *HUS,* hemolytic uremic syndrome; *ITP,* immune thrombocytopenic purpura; *TTP,* thrombotic thrombocytopenic purpura.

when production capacity is no longer adequate to compensate for the increased rate of destruction.

Immune Mechanisms of Platelet Destruction

Immune thrombocytopenic purpura. The term *idiopathic thrombocytopenic purpura* (ITP) was used previously to describe cases of thrombocytopenia arising without apparent cause or underlying disease state. Although the acronym for the disorder remains the same, the word *idiopathic* has been replaced by *immune*, following the realization that acute and chronic ITP are immunologically mediated.

Acute immune thrombocytopenic purpura. Primarily a disorder of children, acute ITP may be seen occasionally in adults.[40] The incidence of acute ITP is estimated to be 4 in 100,000 children, with a peak frequency in children between 2 and 5 years of age without sex predilection.[41] The disorder is characterized by abrupt onset, sometimes over a few hours, of bruising, petechiae, and mucosal (e.g., epistaxis) or urinary tract bleeding in a previously healthy child.

In 60% to 80% of patients with acute ITP, there is a history of infection, usually viral (such as rubella, rubeola, chickenpox, and nonspecific respiratory tract infection), occurring 2 to 21 days before ITP onset. Acute ITP also may occur after immunization with live vaccine. When specified, the type of vaccination includes MMR (measles, mumps, rubella), DTP (diphtheria, tetanus, pertussis), and other vaccines such as polio, hepatitis A, hepatitis B, chickenpox, or smallpox. The observation that acute ITP often follows a viral illness or vaccination suggests that some children produce antibodies and immune complexes against viral antigens and that the thrombocytopenia, which often occurs 1 to 3 weeks later, may result from the binding of these antibodies or immune complexes to the platelet surface, targeting them for destruction.

The diagnosis of acute ITP in a child with severe thrombocytopenia almost always can be made without a bone marrow examination (Chapter 15). If the child has recent onset of bleeding signs and symptoms, otherwise normal results on complete blood count (for all RBC and WBC parameters and cell morphology), and normal findings on physical examination (except for signs of bleeding), there is a high likelihood that the child has ITP. In addition, if the bleeding symptoms develop suddenly and there is no family history of hemorrhagic abnormalities or thrombocytopenia, the diagnosis of ITP is almost certain. Currently there is no specific test that is diagnostic of ITP.

In mild cases of acute ITP, patients may have only scattered petechiae. In most cases of acute ITP, however, patients develop fairly extensive petechiae and some ecchymoses, and may experience hematuria, epistaxis, or both. About 3% to 4% of acute ITP cases are considered severe, with platelet counts <10,000/μL and noncutaneous bleeding such as gastrointestinal bleeding, hematuria, mucous membrane bleeding, and retinal hemorrhage.[42] Usually the severity of bleeding is correlated with the degree of thrombocytopenia.[43] In patients with severe disease, there is an increased risk for intracranial hemorrhage, which is the primary complication that contributes to the overall approximate 0.6% mortality rate for patients with acute ITP.[41]

Acute ITP usually is self-limited, with most patients recovering with or without treatment in about 3 weeks, although recovery may take up to 6 months for some. In about 10% to 15% of children initially thought to have acute ITP, the thrombocytopenia persists for 6 months or longer, and these children are reclassified as having chronic ITP.[41] In a small fraction of children, recurrent episodes of acute ITP occur after complete recovery from the first episode.[44]

In acute ITP, treatment for all but the most severely thrombocytopenic and hemorrhagic patients is contraindicated. When treatment is necessary, a good response to intravenous immunoglobulin (IVIG), corticosteroids, or both usually can be obtained, and splenectomy is rarely required.[40,41] Treatment with corticosteroids, IVIG, or anti-D immunoglobulin is mandatory in children with ITP who are experiencing active hemorrhage.

Chronic immune thrombocytopenic purpura. ITP can begin insidiously with platelet counts that are variably decreased and sometimes normal for periods. This is called chronic ITP. The differences between *acute* and *chronic* ITP are summarized in Table 38.3.

Most cases of chronic ITP are in patients between the ages of 20 and 50 years, although it can occur at any age. The overall incidence of chronic ITP ranges from 1 to 3 cases per 100,000 people per year.[45] Females with this disorder outnumber males 2 to 3:1, with the highest incidence in females between 20 and 40 years of age.

Chronic ITP initially manifests as a few scattered petechiae or other minor bleeding manifestations. Occasionally a bruising

TABLE 38.3   Differentiation of Acute and Chronic Immune Thrombocytopenic Purpura

Characteristic	Acute ITP	Chronic ITP
Age at onset	2–6 y	20–50 y
Sex predilection	None	Female over male, 3:1
Prior infection	Common	Unusual
Onset of bleeding	Sudden	Gradual
Platelet count	<20,000/μL	30,000–80,000/μL
Duration	2–6 weeks	Months to years
Spontaneous remission	90% of patients	Uncommon
Seasonal pattern	Higher incidence in winter and spring	None
Therapy		
Steroids	70% response rate	30% response rate
Splenectomy	Rarely required	<45 y, 90% response rate >45 y, 40% response rate

ITP, Immune thrombocytopenic purpura.
Data from Triplett, D. A. (Ed.). (1978). *Platelet Function: Laboratory Evaluation and Clinical Application.* Chicago: American Society of Clinical Pathologists; Quick, A. J. (1966). *Hemorrhagic Diseases and Thrombosis* (2nd ed.). Philadelphia: Lea & Febiger; and Arnold, D. M., Zeller, M. P., Smith, J. W., & Nazy, I. (2018). Diseases of platelet number: immune thrombocytopenia, neonatal alloimmune thrombocytopenia and posttransfusion purpura. In Hoffman, R., Benz, E. J., & Silberstein, L. E., et al. (Eds.), *Hematology: Basic Principles and Practice.* (7th ed., pp. 1944–1954). Philadelphia: Elsevier.

tendency, menorrhagia, or recurrent epistaxis may be present for months or years before diagnosis. In chronic ITP, there is typically a fluctuating clinical course, with episodes of bleeding that last a few days or weeks. Spontaneous remissions are uncommon and usually incomplete.[43] Platelet counts range from 5000/μL to 75,000/μL and are generally higher than counts in patients with acute ITP.

Platelet destruction in chronic ITP results from the binding of autoantibodies to platelets, which leads to enhanced platelet removal from the circulation by reticuloendothelial (RE) cells, primarily in the spleen. Autoantibodies that recognize platelet surface glycoproteins (GPs) such as GPIIb and GPIIIa ($\alpha_{IIb}\beta_3$), GPIa/IIa, and others occur in 50% to 60% of patients with ITP.[46,47] Because megakaryocytes also express GPIIb/IIIa and GPIb/IX on their membranes, these cells are also targets of the antibodies, leading to impaired megakaryocytopoiesis.[48] T cell-mediated destruction of platelets may also play a role.[49]

Platelet turnover studies have shown impaired platelet production in ITP. Overall, the life span of the platelet is shortened from the normal 7 to 10 days to a few hours. The rapidity with which platelets are removed from the circulation correlates with the degree of thrombocytopenia. If plasma from a patient with ITP is transfused into the circulation of a normal recipient, the recipient develops thrombocytopenia.[50] The thrombocytopenia-producing factor in the plasma of the ITP patient is an immunoglobulin G (IgG) antibody that can be removed from serum by adsorption with normal human platelets.

The only abnormalities in the peripheral blood of patients with ITP are related to platelets. In most cases, platelets number between 30,000/μL and 80,000/μL. Patients with chronic ITP undergo periods of remission and exacerbation, however, and their platelet counts may range from near normal to less than 20,000/μL. Morphologically, platelets appear normal, although larger in diameter than usual (Figure 38.3). This is reflected in an increased mean platelet volume as measured by electronic cell counters.

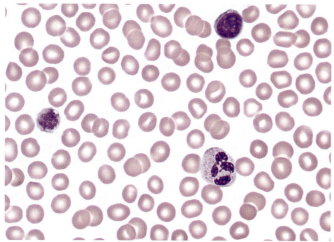

Figure 38.3 Blood Cell Morphology in Immune Thrombocytopenic Purpura. Note scarce platelets and increased platelet size but normal red blood cell and white blood cell morphology. (Peripheral blood, Wright-Giemsa stain, ×500.)

The marrow typically is characterized by megakaryocytic hyperplasia. Megakaryocytes are increased in size, and young forms with a single nucleus, smooth contour, and diminished cytoplasm are common. In the absence of bleeding, infection, or other underlying disorder, erythrocyte and leukocyte precursors are normal in number and morphology. Laboratory tests of platelet function show abnormal results. Although platelet-associated IgG levels are increased in most patients,[11,22,43] such testing for IgG platelet antibodies is neither sensitive nor specific for ITP and therefore is not diagnostically useful for any form of ITP.[42,43]

The initial treatment of chronic ITP depends on the urgency for increasing the platelet count. In the absence of additional risk factors, ITP patients with platelet counts >30,000/μL should not be treated, as their mortality rate is equal to that of the general population. If additional risk factors such as old age, coagulation defects, recent surgery, trauma, or uncontrolled hypertension are present, the platelet count should be maintained at 50,000/μL or higher. In patients in whom the need is considered urgent, IVIG remains the treatment of choice, often in combination with prednisone. About 70% to 90% of patients respond to this therapy with an increase in platelet count and a decrease in hemorrhagic episodes. Although reported response rates vary widely, about 50% of patients have a long-term beneficial effect from corticosteroid treatment.[51]

If the response to IVIG and corticosteroids is inadequate or no response is obtained, therapy can be supplemented with anti-D immunoglobulin.[51,52] For patients in whom prednisone is ineffective, intravenous rituximab can be tried. Responses to rituximab are usually seen within 3 to 4 weeks. In patients who are refractory to all medical therapies, splenectomy may become necessary. Splenectomy removes the primary site of platelet phagocytosis, and it removes the major site of autoantibody production. Splenectomy is an effective treatment for adult chronic ITP, with 88% of patients showing improvement and 66% having a complete and lasting response.[53]

Eltrombopag and other thrombopoietin receptor agonists in combination with other immunosuppressive drugs such as high-dose dexamethasone and rituximab are other suggested therapies.[54] In the most severe refractory cases, immunosuppressive (chemotherapeutic) agents such as azathioprine given alone or with steroids may be necessary. In such patients, platelet transfusions may be of transient benefit in treating severe hemorrhagic episodes but should not be given routinely.[43] IVIG given alone or just before platelet transfusion also may be beneficial.[40,43]

Chronic ITP occurring in association with HIV infection, hemophilia, or pregnancy presents special problems in diagnosis and therapy. Unexplained thrombocytopenia in otherwise healthy members of high-risk populations may be an early manifestation of acquired immunodeficiency syndrome (AIDS).[39,43]

Immunologic drug-induced thrombocytopenia. Many drugs can induce acute thrombocytopenia (Box 38.3). Drug-dependent antibodies typically develop after 1 to 2 weeks of exposure to a new drug. Drug-induced immune-mediated thrombocytopenia can be divided into several types based on

BOX 38.3   Common Drugs Causing Drug-Induced Immune Thrombocytopenia

Analgesics
Salicylates
Acetaminophen metabolites
Ibuprofen
Naproxen metabolites

Antibiotics
Cephalothin
Ceftriaxone
Penicillin
Streptomycin
Aminosalicylic acid
Rifampin
Sulfa drugs and sulfonamides
Furosemide
Trimethoprim-sulfamethoxazole
Chlorothiazide
Sulfisoxazole

Alkaloids
Quinidine
Quinine

Oral Hypoglycemics
Chlorpropamide
Tolbutamide

Sedatives and Anticonvulsants
Phenytoin
Haloperidol
Chlorpromazine
Diphenylhydantoin
Meprobamate
Phenobarbital
Carbamazepine

Heavy Metals
Gold
Mercury
Bismuth
Organic arsenicals

Miscellaneous
Simvastatin
Tirofiban
Vancomycin
Carbamazepine
Ranitidine
Chloroquine
Valproic acid

Data from Arnold, D. M., Nazi, I., Warkentin, T. E., et al. (2013). Approach to the diagnosis and management of drug-induced immune thrombocytopenia. *Transf Med Rev, 27*, 137–145; and Reese, J. A., Li, X., Hauben, M., et al. (2010). Identifying drugs that cause acute thrombocytopenia: an analysis using 3 distinct methods. *Blood, 116*, 2127–2133.

the mechanisms underlying the interaction of the antibody with the drug and platelets. The common mechanisms are depicted in Figure 38.4 and are discussed in the following paragraphs.

Drug-dependent antibodies. One mechanism of drug-dependent antibodies recognized for more than 100 years is typified by quinidine- and quinine-induced thrombocytopenia (Figure 38.4B). Antibodies induced by drugs of this type interact with platelets only in the presence of the drug. Many drugs can induce such antibodies, but quinine, quinidine, and sulfonamide derivatives do so more often than other drugs. When antibody production has begun, the platelet count falls rapidly and often may be <10,000/μL. Patients may have abrupt onset of bleeding symptoms. If this type of drug-induced thrombocytopenia develops in a pregnant woman, both the woman and her fetus may be affected.

The antibodies responsible for drug-dependent thrombocytopenia bind directly to platelets by their Fab regions. The Fab portion of the antibody binds to a platelet membrane constituent, usually the GPIb/IX/V complex or the GPIIb/IIIa complex, only in the presence of drug.[55,56] The mechanism by which the drug promotes binding of a drug-dependent antibody to a specific target on the platelet membrane without covalently linking to the target or the antibody remains to be determined. Because the Fc portion of the immunoglobulin is not involved in binding

to platelets, it is still available to bind the Fc receptors on phagocytic cells (Figure 38.4A). This situation may contribute to the rapid onset and relatively severe nature of thrombocytopenia. Most drug-induced platelet antibodies are of the IgG class, but in rare instances, IgM antibodies are involved.[49]

A similar pattern is seen with the antiplatelet agents tirofiban and eptifibatide, although with these drugs thrombocytopenia tends to occur within several hours of exposure. When these drugs bind to platelet GPIIb/IIIa, they create structural changes that result in neoepitopes to which antibodies are targeted (see Figure 38.4B). Thrombocytopenia results as the antibody bound platelets are removed from circulation.

Hapten-induced antibodies. Drug-induced thrombocytopenia can also result from the induction of hapten-dependent antibodies. Some drug molecules are too small by themselves to trigger an immune response, but they may act as a hapten and combine with a larger carrier molecule (usually a plasma protein or protein constituent of the platelet membrane) to form a complex that can act as a complete antigen.[49] Penicillin, penicillin chemical cousins, cephalosporins, and sulfonamide-containing medications are among the offending agents causing drug-induced thrombocytopenia by this mechanism. Drug-induced thrombocytopenia of this type is often severe, with an initial platelet count of <10,000/μL and sometimes <1000/μL. The number of bone marrow megakaryocytes is usually normal to elevated.[49] Bleeding is often severe and rapid in onset, and hemorrhagic blisters in the mouth may be prominent.

Drug-induced autoantibodies. Drug-induced autoantibodies represent a third mechanism of drug-induced thrombocytopenia. In this case the drugs stimulate the formation of an autoantibody that binds to a specific platelet membrane glycoprotein with no requirement for the presence of free drug. Gold salts, procainamide, and levodopa are examples of such drugs (see Figure 38.4B). The precise mechanism by which these drugs induce autoantibodies against platelets is not known with certainty.

Immune complex-induced thrombocytopenia. Heparin-induced thrombocytopenia (HIT) is a good example of immune complex-induced thrombocytopenia, the fourth mechanism of drug-induced thrombocytopenia (see Figure 38.4B). Binding of therapeutic heparin to platelet factor 4 (PF4), a protein released from activated platelets, causes a conformational change in PF4, resulting in the exposure of neoepitopes on PF4. The Fab portion of IgG binds to the PF4 neoepitope. The free Fc portion of the IgG binds with the platelet FcγIIa receptor. Platelets are activated by occupancy of their FcγIIa receptor,[57,58] leading to the release of procoagulant platelet microparticles and aggregation. This activation of platelets leads to their consumption and thrombocytopenia. Thrombocytopenia, typically beginning 5 to 14 days after heparin exposure, is usually mild to moderate, with platelet counts only rarely <15,000/μL. Paradoxically, patients with HIT rarely bleed but have a high risk of thrombosis that can be life-threatening. HIT is discussed in more detail in Chapter 39.

A condition similar to HIT, known as *vaccine-induced thrombotic thrombocytopenia* (VITT), has been observed in a small fraction of patients receiving either the Oxford-AstraZeneca or the Johnson & Johnson vaccines against severe

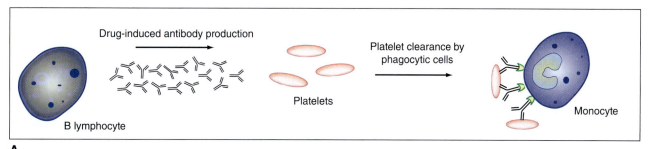

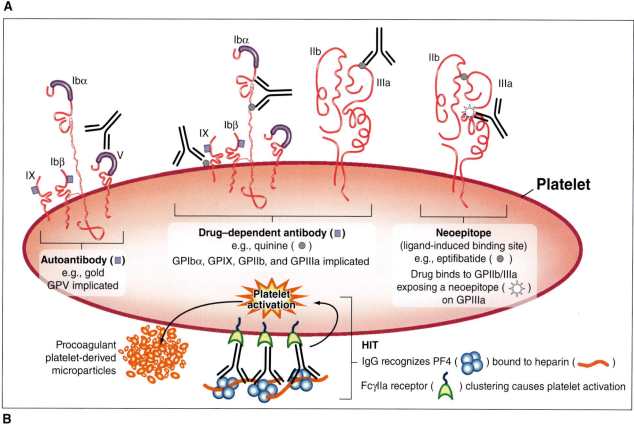

Figure 38.4 Mechanisms of Drug-Induced Thrombocytopenia. Certain drugs stimulate the production of immunoglobulins that bind a platelet membrane antigen or antigen and drug combination. **(A)**, Monocyte/macrophage Fc receptors bind the Fc portion of the immunoglobulin bound to the platelet resulting in platelet removal. **(B)**, Mechanisms of four specific drugs are depicted. *GP*, Glycoprotein; *HIT*, heparin-induced thrombocytopenia; *IgG*, immunoglobulin G; *PF4*, platelet factor 4. (Modified from Warkentin, T. E. [2018]. Thrombocytopenia caused by platelet destruction, hypersplenism, or hemodilution. In Hoffman, R., Benz, E. J., & Silberstein, L. E., et al. [Eds.], *Hematology: Basic Principles and Practice* [7th ed., pp. 1955–1972]. Philadelphia: Elsevier.)

acute respiratory syndrome coronavirus 2 (SARS-CoV-2), the virus responsible for coronavirus disease 2019 (COVID-19).[59] In affected patients, thrombocytopenia and thrombosis appear 7 to 10 days following vaccination.[60] Similar to HIT, antibodies capable of activating platelets via the FcγIIa receptor are generated against an epitope on PF4.[61] These patients, however, have not had recent exposure to heparin. It remains unclear why HIT and SARS-CoV-2 vaccine-induced antibodies develop only in some individuals and why specific patient cohorts are at risk of the thrombotic clinical course.

Treatment of patients with drug-induced thrombocytopenia. Identification of the offending drug, drug discontinuation, and substitution with another suitable therapeutic agent is the first approach to patient management. However, this can be difficult to accomplish. In patients taking multiple drugs, it is not always easy to determine which of the drugs is at fault for causing thrombocytopenia. Under these conditions, identifying the causative agent may be a trial-and-error procedure in which the most likely drugs are eliminated one at a time. In addition, even if the patient is taking only one agent, there may not be a suitable replacement, or a prolonged period may be required for the alternative drug to become effective. Furthermore, laboratory testing to identify specific drugs involved is beyond the capabilities of most clinical laboratories and is usually performed by reference laboratories, chiefly by flow cytometry-based test methods.

Although drugs usually are cleared from the circulation rapidly, dissociation of drug-antibody complexes may require longer periods, perhaps 1 to 2 weeks.[11] In some cases, such as those caused by gold salts, thrombocytopenia may persist for months.

Platelet transfusions may be administered to patients with life-threatening bleeds, but platelet transfusions in severe but not life-threatening bleeding should be individualized. Although the transfused platelets are destroyed rapidly, they may function to halt bleeding effectively before they are destroyed. In addition, high-dose IVIG may be used and is generally an effective treatment for most drug-induced immune thrombocytopenias.

Neonatal immune-mediated thrombocytopenia. There are two types of neonatal thrombocytopenia. The immune system of the mother is key to the pathophysiology.

Neonatal alloimmune thrombocytopenia. Neonatal alloimmune thrombocytopenia (NAIT) develops when the mother lacks a platelet-specific antigen that the fetus has inherited from the father. Fetal platelet antigens, which are inherited as codominant genes, may pass from the fetal to the maternal circulation as early as the 14th week of gestation.[62] If the mother is exposed to a fetal antigen she lacks, she may make antibodies to that foreign paternal-fetal antigen. These IgG antibodies cross the placenta, attach to the antigen-bearing fetal platelets, and result in thrombocytopenia in the fetus. In this regard, the pathophysiology of NAIT is analogous to that of hemolytic disease of the newborn. The mother of the fetus with NAIT is usually asymptomatic.

The most common cause (approximately 80%) of NAIT in White neonates is the HPA-1a antigen expressed on GPIIIa of the surface membrane GPIIb/IIIa complex. HPA-5b, which is found on the GPIa, accounts for 10% to 15% of cases. The antigen HPA-3a is present on GPIIb and is an important cause of neonatal thrombocytopenia in Asians. Platelet antigen HPA-4 accounts for the disorder in a few affected neonates.

Clinically severe thrombocytopenia as a result of NAIT occurs in 1 in 1000 live births and, in contrast to hemolytic disease of the fetus and newborn, commonly affects the first pregnancy in an at-risk couple.[63] With the first pregnancy, about 50% of neonates born to mothers lacking a specific platelet antigen are affected, whereas with subsequent pregnancies, the risk may increase to 75% to 97%.[63] The incidence of intracranial hemorrhage or death or both in affected offspring is about 25%, with about half of intracranial hemorrhages occurring in utero in the second trimester.

Affected infants may appear normal at birth but soon manifest scattered petechiae and purpuric hemorrhages. In many infants with NAIT, serious hemorrhage does not develop, but the risks are directly associated with the degree of thrombocytopenia. Infants may recover over a 1- to 2-week period as the level of passively transferred antibody decreases.[11,41] In symptomatic cases, platelet levels are usually <30,000/µL and may decrease even further in the first few hours after birth; however, in these circumstances, affected neonates must be followed in a neonatal intensive care setting for serial assessment of platelet counts and indicated interventional therapies.

The diagnosis of NAIT is one of exclusion of other causes of neonatal thrombocytopenia, including neonatal bacterial infection, maternal ITP, and maternal ingestion of drugs known to be associated with drug-induced thrombocytopenia. The presence of thrombocytopenia in a neonate with an appropriate HPA-negative mother or a history of the disorder in a sibling is strong presumptive evidence in favor of the diagnosis. Confirmation requires platelet typing of both parents and testing for evidence of a maternal antibody directed at paternal platelets.[40]

In situations in which suspicion of NAIT is high or there is a history of NAIT in a first pregnancy, it may be necessary to test or treat the fetus to prevent intracranial hemorrhage in utero. Fetal genotypes now can be determined at 15 to 16 weeks of gestation using polymerase chain reaction methods on cells obtained by chorionic villus sampling or amniocentesis.[64]

Serial cordocentesis and intrauterine platelet transfusion of fetuses has been largely abandoned because of high complication rates, including causing labor. In cases in which the fetal postnatal platelet counts do not increase with IVIG therapy, washed maternal platelets, if available, have been transfused into the fetus with good results.[65] Antenatal treatment of the mother with high-dose corticosteroids to decrease maternal antibody production is not recommended because of potential fetal toxicity.

In situations in which the diagnosis of NAIT is known or highly suspected, delivery by cesarean section (at 36 to 37 weeks' gestation ensuring fetal lung maturity) is recommended to avoid fetal trauma associated with vaginal delivery. After delivery, the affected infant may be treated with transfusion of the appropriate antigen-negative platelets. Whereas prompt transfusion of HPA-compatible platelets (such as washed, irradiated maternal platelets) are preferred, the extended time required for preparation often precludes their use. In severely thrombocytopenic preterm or bleeding neonates with NAIT, transfusion with random platelets is the treatment of choice. Although destined to have a suboptimal in vivo survival, such transfused platelets are hemostatically active and reduce the risk of bleeding.[66] IVIG can be used alone or in combination with platelet transfusion but should not be used as the sole treatment in a bleeding infant because response to this therapy usually takes 1 to 3 days.[63]

Neonatal autoimmune thrombocytopenia. Women very uncommonly (0.083 per 1000 pregnancies) develop chronic ITP during pregnancy[67]; however, if a pregnant woman does develop ITP, it remits after delivery. For women with a history of ITP, relapse is relatively common during pregnancy if the ITP had been in complete or partial remission. This has been attributed to the facilitation of RE phagocytosis by the high estrogen levels in pregnant women.

Neonatal autoimmune thrombocytopenia results from the passive transplacental transfer of maternal ITP autoantibodies. Less commonly, maternal autoantibodies associated with a collagen vascular disease such as systemic lupus erythematosus are transferred transplacentally. Corticosteroids are the primary treatment for pregnant women with ITP and at the dosages used, there is a low incidence of adverse fetal side effects.[68]

Neonatal autoimmune thrombocytopenia develops in about 10% of infants of pregnant women with autoimmune thrombocytopenia, and intracranial hemorrhage occurs in 1% or fewer infants. It is no longer recommended that high-risk infants be delivered by cesarean section to avoid the trauma of vaginal delivery and accompanying risk of hemorrhage in the infant, regardless of maternal platelet count.[69]

Affected newborns may have normal to decreased platelet counts at birth and demonstrate a progressive decrease in the platelet count for about 1 week postpartum (but possibly several months) before the platelet count begins to increase. It has been speculated that the falling platelet count is associated with maturation of the infant's RE system and accelerated removal of antibody-coated platelets by cells of the RE system.

Although treatment is not required in most cases, severely thrombocytopenic infants generally respond quickly to IVIG treatment. If an infant develops hemorrhagic symptoms, risks should be clinically stratified, and medical therapies (such as platelet transfusion, IVIG treatment, or corticosteroid therapy) should be started immediately.[40]

Posttransfusion purpura. Posttransfusion purpura (PTP) is a rare disorder that typically develops about 1 week after transfusion of platelet-containing blood components, including whole blood, fresh or frozen plasma, and washed RBCs. PTP is manifested by rapid onset of severe thrombocytopenia and moderate to severe hemorrhage that may be life-threatening. The recipient's plasma is found to contain alloantibodies to antigens on the platelets or platelet membranes of the transfused blood componet, directed against one or more platelet-specific antigens that the recipient lacks.

The mechanism by which the recipient's own platelets are destroyed is unclear, but it evidently requires stimulation of platelet autoantibodies, which also target recipient antigen-negative platelets. In more than 90% of cases, the primary alloantibody is directed against the HPA-1a antigen; in most of the remaining cases, the antibodies are directed against HPA-1b or other epitopes on GPIIb/IIIa.[40] Involvement of other alloantigens, such as HPA-3a, HPA-4, and HPA-5b, has also been reported. Most patients with PTP are multiparous middle-aged women, and almost all patients have a history of blood transfusion. PTP seems to be exceedingly rare in men who have never been transfused and in women who have never been pregnant or never been transfused.[63] PTP seems to require prior exposure to foreign platelet antigens and behaves in many respects like an anamnestic immune response.

No clinical trials have been conducted on the treatment of PTP, primarily because of the small number of cases. Therapeutic plasma exchange (TPE) has been used with some success in the past, but the treatment of choice is now IVIG. Many patients with PTP respond to a 2-day course of IVIG, generally initiated within the first 2 to 3 days of presentation, although a second course occasionally is necessary.[70] IVIG also is much easier to administer, and the response rates are higher than with TPE. Corticosteroid therapy is not particularly efficacious when used alone but may be beneficial in combination with other, more effective treatments.[37] If PTP is untreated or treatment is ineffective, mortality rates may approach 10%.[70] In addition, untreated or unresponsive patients who happen to survive have a protracted clinical course, with thrombocytopenia typically lasting 3 weeks but in some cases up to 4 months.

Secondary thrombocytopenia, presumed to be immune mediated. Severe thrombocytopenia has been identified in patients receiving biologic response modifiers such as

interferons, colony-stimulating factors, and interleukin-2.[71-73] Thrombocytopenia associated with use of these substances is reversible and, at least for interferon, may be immune mediated because increased levels of platelet-associated IgG have been measured. Immune thrombocytopenia develops in about 5% to 10% of patients with chronic lymphocytic leukemia and in a smaller percentage of patients with other lymphoproliferative disorders.[74,75] Thrombocytopenia is noted in 14% to 26% of patients with systemic lupus erythematosus.[76] In such secondary situations, the clinical picture and the response to therapeutic interventions are similar to that of ITP in that the bone marrow has a larger than normal number of megakaryocytes, and an increased level of platelet-associated IgG is often found.[39]

Parasitic infections also are known to cause thrombocytopenia. Malaria is the most studied disease in this group. The onset of thrombocytopenia corresponds to the first appearance of antimalarial antibodies, a decrease in serum complement, and a decrease in control of the parasitemia. There is evidence for the adsorption of microbial antigens to the platelet surface and subsequent antibody binding via the Fab terminus. Immune destruction of platelets seems to be the most likely mechanism for the thrombocytopenia.[77]

Nonimmune Mechanisms of Platelet Destruction

Nonimmune platelet destruction may result from activation of the coagulation process, platelet consumption by endovascular injury without measurable depletion of coagulation factors, or exposure of platelets to nonendothelial surfaces.[39] Many of these disorders are classified as *thrombotic microangiopathies* (TMAs), a broad group of disorders characterized by the presence of thrombocytopenia, clot formation within the arterioles and capillaries, and microangiopathic hemolytic anemia (MAHA). Although hemolytic uremic syndrome (HUS) and thrombotic thrombocytopenic purpura (TTP) are the most commonly known TMAs, TMA can occur secondary to a large number of clinical conditions (Box 38.4).

BOX 38.4 Thrombotic Microangiopathies in Association With Various Conditions

Thrombotic thrombocytopenic purpura (TTP) (classical TM)
Hemolytic uremic syndrome (HUS) (classical TM)
    Shiga toxin-associated HUS (such as *Escherichia coli* O157:H7)
    Atypical HUS (aHUS)
Drug-associated (e.g., clopidogrel, ticlopidine)
Transplant-associated (solid organ or stem cell)
Malignancy-associated
Pregnancy-associated
    HELLP syndrome
    Preeclampsia/eclampsia
Disseminated intravascular coagulation (DIC)
Catastrophic antiphospholipid syndrome (CAPS)
Connective tissue/autoimmune disorders (e.g., systemic lupus erythematosus)
HIV disease
Secondary immune-mediated (ITP-like) associated with COVID-19
Malignant hypertension

COVID-19, Coronavirus disease 2019; *HELLP,* **h**emolysis, **e**levated **l**iver enzymes, and **l**ow **p**latelet count; *HIV,* human immunodeficiency virus; *ITP,* immune thrombocytopenic purpura; *TM,* thrombotic microangiopathy.

Thrombocytopenia in pregnancy and preeclampsia. Incidental thrombocytopenia of pregnancy, also known as pregnancy-associated thrombocytopenia and gestational thrombocytopenia, is a benign physiologic condition that is the most common cause of thrombocytopenia in pregnancy and requires no evaluation or treatment.[78] Random platelet counts in pregnant and postpartum women are slightly higher than normal, but about 5% of pregnant women develop a mild thrombocytopenia (100,000/μL to 150,000/μL),[79] with 98% of them having platelet counts >70,000/μL. They are healthy, have no prior history of thrombocytopenia, and do not seem to be at increased risk for bleeding or for delivery of infants with neonatal thrombocytopenia. The cause of this type of thrombocytopenia is unknown. Maternal platelet counts return to normal within several weeks of delivery. Such women could experience recurrence in subsequent pregnancies.

Approximately 20% of cases of thrombocytopenia of pregnancy are associated with hypertensive disorders. These disorders include preeclampsia, preeclampsia-eclampsia, preeclampsia with chronic hypertension, chronic hypertension, and gestational hypertension. Preeclampsia complicates about 2% to 4% of pregnancies and typically occurs at about 20 weeks of gestation.[80] The disorder is characterized by the onset of hypertension and proteinuria and may include abdominal pain, headache, blurred vision, or mental function disturbances. Thrombocytopenia occurs in approximately 20% of patients with preeclampsia,[81] with 40% to 50% of these patients progressing to preeclampsia with severe features (severe hypertension, central nervous system symptoms, pulmonary edema, renal insufficiency) or eclampsia (hypertension, proteinuria, and seizures).[82]

Some patients with preeclampsia have a condition known as the *HELLP syndrome* (**h**emolysis, **e**levated **l**iver enzymes, and **l**ow **p**latelet count). HELLP syndrome affects an estimated 4% to 12% of women with severe preeclampsia[43,83] and seems to be associated with higher rates of maternal and fetal complications. This disorder is difficult to differentiate from TTP, complement-mediated TMAs, HUS, and DIC.[84] Therefore appropriate clinical differential diagnostic considerations are required (see Box 38.4).

Development of thrombocytopenia in these patients is thought to be due to increased platelet destruction. Though the mechanism of platelet destruction remains unclear, some evidence (elevated D-dimer) suggests that these patients have an underlying low-grade DIC.[85] Elevated platelet-associated immunoglobulin is commonly found in these patients, which indicates immune involvement.[86] It had been suggested that platelet activation contributes to the development of preeclampsia because low-dose aspirin therapy was shown to prevent preeclampsia in high-risk patients.[87,88] It has also been shown that aspirin therapy more effectively reduces the risk of preterm preeclampsia compared with term preeclampsia, with the beneficial effect dependent on both the daily dose of aspirin (>100 mg) and the time of therapy initiation (<16 weeks' gestation).[89]

The best treatment of preeclampsia is delivery of the infant whenever possible. After delivery, thrombocytopenia usually resolves in a few days. In cases in which delivery is less advisable (e.g., the fetus is too premature), bed rest and aggressive treatment of the hypertension helps to increase the platelet count in some patients.

As discussed previously, ITP is a relatively common disorder in women of childbearing age, and pregnancy does nothing to ameliorate the symptoms of this disorder. ITP should be part of the differential diagnosis of thrombocytopenia in a pregnant woman. There is little or no correlation between the level of maternal autoantibodies and the fetal platelet count. Other causes of thrombocytopenia during pregnancy include HIV infection, systemic lupus erythematosus, antiphospholipid syndromes, TTP, and HUS. Of all women who develop TTP, 10% to 25% present with the disease during pregnancy or in the postpartum period, and TTP tends to recur in subsequent pregnancies.[90-92] TPE is the treatment of choice to prevent maternal or fetal mortality, which can be 90% or greater without such treatment.

Hemolytic disease of the newborn. Thrombocytopenia, usually moderate in degree, occurs commonly in infants with hemolytic disease of the newborn. Although the erythrocyte destruction characteristic of this disorder is antibody mediated, the antigens against which the antibodies are directed are not expressed on platelets. Platelets may be destroyed as a result of their interaction with products of RBC breakdown, rather than their direct participation in an immunologic reaction.[39]

Thrombotic thrombocytopenic purpura. TTP is characterized by the triad of MAHA (Chapter 22), thrombocytopenia, and neurologic abnormalities (Table 38.4). In addition, fever and renal dysfunction (forming a pentad) classically may be present; however, MAHA and thrombocytopenia are the most common clinical findings. Additional symptoms, including diarrhea, anorexia, nausea, weakness, and fatigue, are present in most patients at the time of diagnosis. The prevalence of TTP has been estimated at approximately 10 cases per 1 million people with an annual incidence of approximately 1 new case per 1 million people.[93,94] About twice as many women as men are affected, and it is most common in women 30 to 40 years of age.[37,95] About half of the patients who develop TTP have a history of a viral-like illness several days before the onset of TTP, although there is no proof that such incidences are causal.

There are at least four types of TTP. In most patients, TTP occurs as a single acute episode. Second, recurrent TTP occurs in 11% to 28% of TTP patients.[96,97] Third, certain types of drugs can induce TTP. The primary agents involved are the thienopyridine agents ticlopidine (Ticlid) and clopidogrel (Plavix), which are used to inhibit platelet function (Chapter 37). Ticlopidine seems to cause TTP in about 0.025% of patients, whereas the incidence of clopidogrel-induced TTP is approximately 4 times less.[94] These common types of TTP generally result from autoantibodies that remove or block the function of ADAMTS13 (***a** **d**isintegrin **a**nd **m**etalloprotease with a **t**hrombo**s**pondin type 1 motif, member **13***), an important enzyme that cleaves high-molecular-weight multimers of VWF.

Finally, rarely, patients experience chronic relapsing TTP in which episodes occur at intervals of approximately 3 months starting in infancy.[98,99] This form of TTP, known as

TABLE 38.4 Attributes of Thrombotic Thrombocytopenic Purpura (TTP) in its Various Forms

Clinical Presentation	Causes / Pathophysiology	Diagnosis	Treatment
Acute TTP: Single episode Recurrent episodes (e.g., associated with viral infections such as HIV)	De novo or acquired autoantibodies to ADAMTS13 that remove or inhibit enzyme function; result in UL-VWF multimers, platelet microthrombi, widespread thrombotic-ischemic organ damage	Classic pentad (all may not be present): Thrombocytopenia Severe MAHA Fever Neurologic symptoms Renal function abnormalities Diagnostic aids: ADAMTS13 functional tests and immunoassays Immunoassays to detect antibodies to ADAMTS13 PLASMIC clinical score*	Caplacizumab, given early and in combination with TPE with plasma replacement Corticosteroids Immunosuppressants such as rituximab Individualized treatment of known viral diseases
Drug-induced or drug-associated TTP	Likely drug-induced, auto-antibody-associated	MAHA and thrombocytopenia	Stop the offending drug Short courses of TPE
Congenital TTP	Numerous ADAMTS13 mutations affecting enzyme levels and activity	Tends to be chronic, relapsing MAHA and thrombocytopenia Onset from infancy to adulthood Frequency <1:1000	Prophylactic plasma transfusions for symptomatic episodes
Chronic, relapsing TTP (USS)	Rare autosomal recessive disorder with near complete absence of ADAMTS13 enzyme activity Episodes often triggered by stressors such as viral infections, pregnancy, alcohol abuse, drugs, etc.	MAHA and thrombocytopenia	Consistent plasma replacement either as simple plasma transfusion or via TPE every 2 to 3 weeks

*Patients are assigned 1 point each for *P*latelet count <30,000/μL, hemo*L*ysis (measured in terms of reticulocyte count, haptoglobin, or indirect bilirubin), lack of *A*ctive cancer, no history of solid organ or *S*tem cell transplant, *m*ean red cell volume (*M*CV) <90 fL, *I*nternational normalized ratio <1.5, and *C*reatinine <2 mg/dL.
*ADAMTS13, A d*isintegrin *a*nd *m*etalloprotease with a *t*hrombo*s*pondin type 1 motif, member *13*; *HIV*, human immunodeficiency virus; *MAHA*, microangiopathic hemolytic anemia; *TPE*, therapeutic plasma exchange; *UL-VWF*, ultra-large von Willebrand factor; *USS*, Upshaw-Shulman syndrome.

Upshaw-Shulman syndrome (USS), is hereditary and congenital. It is associated with an autosomal recessive gene mutation that leads to ADAMTS13 dysfunction. Familial chronic relapsing TTP is characterized by recurrent episodes of thrombocytopenia with or without ischemic organ damage due to platelet microthrombi. TTP usually develops only when clinical conditions with increased VWF levels (e.g., infection) occur. In this type of TTP, ADAMTS13 activity is nearly completely deficient.[100,101]

Thrombotic thrombocytopenic purpura and thrombosis. Thrombi composed of platelets and VWF, but very little fibrin or fibrinogen, are found in the end arterioles and capillaries of patients with TTP.[102] As these platelet-VWF thrombi are deposited, thrombocytopenia develops (<30,000/μL). The degree of thrombocytopenia is directly related to the extent of microvascular platelet aggregation. RBCs flowing under arterial pressure are fragmented when they encounter the strands of these thrombi, which give rise to the peripheral blood findings of schistocytosis.

Hemolysis is usually quite severe, and most patients have less than 10 g/dL hemoglobin. Examination of the peripheral blood film reveals a marked decrease in platelets, RBC polychromasia, and schistocytes, a triad of features characteristic of MAHAs

(Figure 38.5). Nucleated RBC precursors and other laboratory evidence of intravascular hemolysis may also be present. Bone marrow examination reveals erythroid hyperplasia and a normal to increased number of megakaryocytes. The partial thromboplastin time, prothrombin time, fibrinogen, fibrin degradation products, and D-dimer test results are usually normal and are useful in differentiating TTP from DIC (Chapters 39 and 41).

The thrombotic lesions, deposited in the vasculature of all organs, give rise to the other characteristic manifestations of TTP. Symptoms depend on the severity of ischemia in each organ. Neurologic manifestations range from headache to paresthesia, to combativeness and coma. Visual disturbances may be of neurologic origin or may be due to thrombi in the choroid capillaries of the retina or hemorrhage into the vitreous. Renal dysfunction, present in more than half of patients,[96,97] is characterized by proteinuria and hematuria. Overwhelming renal damage with anuria and fulminant uremia usually does not occur, which distinguishes TTP from HUS and aHUS.[11] Abdominal pain is occasionally present as a result of occlusion of the mesenteric microcirculation, and gastrointestinal bleeding commonly occurs in severely thrombocytopenic patients.

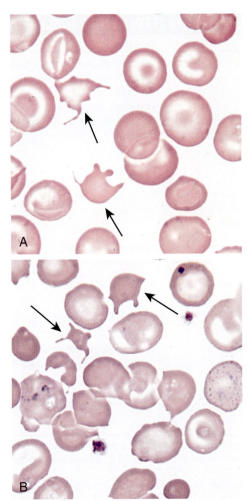

Figure 38.5 Blood Cell Morphology in Microangiopathic Hemolytic Anemia. Abundant schistocytes *(arrows)* reflect the platelet-rich clots in the microvasculature that occur with **(A)** thrombotic thrombocytopenic purpura and **(B)** hemolytic uremic syndrome. These conditions manifest with similar blood morphologies. (Peripheral blood; Wright-Giemsa stain, ×1000.) (From Carr, J. H., & Rodak, B. F. [2013]. *Clinical Hematology Atlas* [4th ed.]. Philadelphia: Saunders.)

Thrombotic thrombocytopenic purpura and role of ADAMTS13. The development of TTP is, in most cases, directly related to the accumulation of ultralarge von Willebrand factor (UL-VWF) multimers in the plasma. In normal plasma, the UL-VWF multimers are rapidly cleaved into the smaller VWF multimers by the VWF-cleaving protease ADAMTS13 (Figure 38.6). This zinc-containing metalloprotease seems to be more effective when VWF multimers are partially unfolded by high shear stress (Chapter 36 and Figures 36.2 and 36.4C).[103,104] Loss of ADAMTS13 activity results in an accumulation of the higher molecular weight (ultralarge) VWF multimers. The UL-VWF multimers are more effective than the normal plasma VWF multimers at binding platelet GPIb/IX or GPIIb/IIIa complexes under fluid shear stresses[98] and will bind spontaneously to platelets to form platelet aggregates within the arterial and capillary vasculature (see Figure 38.6).

Functional tests and immunoassays have been developed that measure ADAMTS13,[105] but they are commonly performed only in reference laboratories. Inhibitors of ADAMTS13, typically autoantibodies, can also be quantitated. A recent study reported that both the anti-ADAMTS13 IgG antibody level and ADAMTS13 antigen level correlate with outcome in patients with immune-mediated TTP.[106]

In patients with TTP, UL-VWF multimers tend to be present in the plasma at the beginning of the episode. These UL-VWF multimers disappear as the TTP episode progresses and the thrombocytopenia worsens. If the patient survives an episode of TTP and does not experience a relapse, the plasma VWF multimers are usually normal after recovery. If UL-VWF multimers are found in the plasma after recovery, however, it is likely that the patient will have recurrent episodes of TTP. Recurrences of TTP are monitored by serial hematologic testing (e.g., CBCs).

Thrombotic thrombocytopenic purpura treatment. As TTP is a life-threatening condition, treatment decisions must be made immediately, often before test results are available. Clinical prediction tools are useful for determining the pre-ADAMTS13-test probability of having TTP.[107,108]

The PLASMIC Score uses seven variables to predict TTP associated with severe ADAMTS13 deficiency. Patients are assigned 1 point each for **P**latelet count <30,000/μL, hemo**L**ysis (measured in terms of reticulocyte count, haptoglobin, or indirect bilirubin), lack of **A**ctive cancer, no history of **S**olid organ or **S**tem cell transplant, **m**ean red cell volume (**MCV**) <90 fL, **I**nternational normalized ratio <1.5, and **C**reatinine <2 mg/dL. Patients with TTP have a median PLASMIC Score of 7. In contrast, lower scores were found with rheumatologic disorders (median = 5), drug-associated TMA (median = 4), DIC (median = 4), and HUS/atypical HUS (median = 5). Three categories of risk for TTP are defined: low risk for scores 0 to 4, intermediate risk for a score of 5, and high risk for scores 6 to 7. A high PLASMIC Score correlates with TTP and severe ADAMTS13 deficiency and predicts a high rate of response to TPE therapy.[109]

Prophylactic plasma infusion is the most commonly used treatment of congenital TTP caused by a mutation in ADAMTS13,[102] with higher plasma doses being administered to treat acute events. The most effective and first-line recommended treatment for acquired TTP resulting from the presence of anti-ADAMTS13 is TPE using plasma replacement.[110] Thawed plasma (stored up to 5 days at 1°–6° C) retains ADAMTS13 levels after thawing and storage. Either of these plasma-replacement approaches may produce dramatic effects within a few hours.

TPE and replacement or infusion of plasma is effective for two reasons. First, some of the UL-VWF multimers are removed by apheresis, and plasma (simple transfusion or exchange) supplies the deficient ADAMTS13 protease, which is able to degrade the UL-VWF multimers in the blood of the patient.

Current recommendations are that all patients with TTP are treated with high-dose corticosteroids in addition to undergoing TPE. TPE typically is continued daily, with serial assessments of hemolysis and platelet counts. If the patient does not respond early to TPE and steroids, additional immunosuppressive treatments such as vincristine, azathioprine, and rituximab

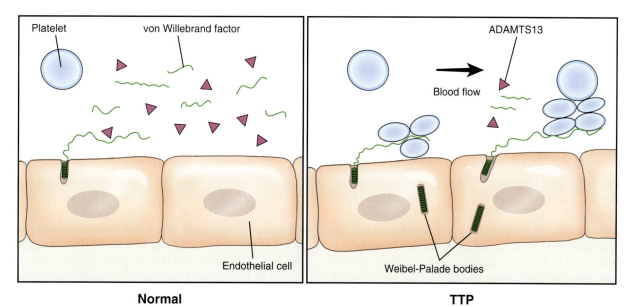

Figure 38.6 Mechanism for Thrombotic Thrombocytopenic Purpura. Ultralarge (UL) strings of von Willebrand factor (VWF), released from endothelial cells, are normally digested by the VWF-cleaving protease ADAMTS13 into smaller strings (multimers). In thrombotic thrombocytopenic purpura, the absence or dysfunction of ADAMTS13 allows the UL-VWF multimers to remain in circulation. UL-VWF multimers are more effective than the smaller multimers at binding platelets. Platelet aggregates form that block blood flow in the arterial and capillary vasculature. *ADAMTS13, a d*isintegrin *a*nd *m*etalloprotease with a *t*hrombo*s*pondin type 1 motif, member *13*; *TTP*, thrombotic thrombocytopenic purpura.

TABLE 38.5 Differentiation of Thrombotic Thrombocytopenic Purpura, Hemolytic Uremic Syndrome, and Disseminated Intravascular Coagulation

	TTP	HUS	DIC
Cause	Loss of ADAMTS13 function	Shiga toxin-induced renal endothelial damage	Inappropriate thrombin generation
CNS symptoms	+++	+/–	+/–
Renal impairment	+/–	+++	+/–
Hemolysis	+++	++	+
Thrombocytopenia	+++	++	+++
Coagulopathy	–	–	+++
Treatment	Plasma exchange	Supportive (fluids, renal support, transfusion)	Treat underlying cause; supportive coagulation

*ADAMTS13, a d*isintegrin *a*nd *m*etalloprotease with a *t*hrombo*s*pondin type 1 motif, member *13*; *CNS*, central nervous system; *DIC*, disseminated intravascular coagulation; *HUS*, hemolytic uremic syndrome; *TTP*, thrombotic thrombocytopenic purpura.

need to be considered before splenectomy. Platelet transfusions should be avoided unless intracranial bleeding or other serious hemorrhagic problems arise.[43]

A recombinant ADAMTS13 (rADAMTS13) is being developed as treatment for hereditary TTP. In a rat model mimicking acquired TTP, administration of rADAMTS13 prevented the full development of TTP-like symptoms (thrombocytopenia, hemolytic anemia, and VWF-rich thrombi in the kidneys and brain).[111] Analysis of plasma from treated animals confirmed the degradation of the UL-VWF multimers. A rADAMTS13 (TAK-755, Takeda Pharmaceuticals) has been tested in a phase I trial in patients with hereditary TTP, where it was found to be well tolerated and active in terms of cleavage of large VWF multimers.[112] Caplacizumab (Cablivi, Sanofi) is an anti-VWF humanized immunoglobulin fragment that inhibits interaction between VWF multimers and platelets.[113] Caplacizumab is indicated for treatment of acquired TTP in combination with plasma exchange and immunosuppressive therapy.

Before 1990, TTP was fatal in more than 90% of patients. With the means for rapid diagnosis and the advent of TPE as well as new therapies on the horizon, now 80% of patients who are treated early are expected to survive. The presence of UL-VWF multimers in patient samples after complete remission is significantly associated with one or more relapses on follow-up[114]; assessment may prove useful for the long-term management of TTP.

Hemolytic uremic syndrome. Clinically, HUS resembles TTP except that it is found predominantly in children 6 months to 4 years of age and is self-limiting (Table 38.5).[115] HUS is more common than TTP, with an annual incidence estimated at 2 to 6 per 100,000.[102] Approximately 90% of cases of HUS are caused by *Shigella dysenteriae* serotypes or enterohemorrhagic *Escherichia coli* OH serotypes, particularly O157:H7.[116] These organisms can sometimes but not always be cultured from stool specimens. The bloody diarrhea typical of childhood HUS is caused by colonization of the large intestine with the offending organism, which causes erosive damage to the colonic mucosa.

S. dysenteriae produces Shiga toxin, and enterohemorrhagic *E. coli* produces either Shiga-like toxin-1 (SLT-1) or SLT-2. The toxins enter the bloodstream and attach to renal glomerular capillary endothelial cells, which become damaged and swollen and release UL-VWF multimers.[116,117] This process leads to formation of hyaline thrombi in the renal vasculature and the development of renal failure, mild to moderate thrombocytopenia, and MAHA. Renal insufficiency is reflected in elevated blood urea nitrogen and creatinine levels. The urine nearly always contains RBCs, protein, and casts. The hemolytic process is demonstrated by a hemoglobin level of <10 g/dL, elevated reticulocyte count, and presence of schistocytosis in the peripheral blood.

The extent of renal involvement correlates with the rate of recovery. In more severely affected children, renal dialysis may be needed. The mortality rate associated with HUS in children is much lower than that for TTP, but there is often residual renal dysfunction that may lead to renal hypertension and some degree of chronic kidney injury. Because HUS in children is essentially an infectious disorder, it affects boys and girls equally and is often found in geographic clusters of cases rather than in random distribution.

The adult form of HUS is associated most often with exposure to immunosuppressive agents, chemotherapeutic agents, or both, but it also may occur during the postpartum period. Usually the symptoms of HUS do not appear until weeks or months after exposure to the offending agent.[118] This disorder most likely results from direct renal arterial endothelial damage caused by the drug or one of its metabolites. The damage to endothelial cells results in release of VWF (including UL-VWF multimers), turbulent blood flow in the arterial system with increased shear stresses on platelets, and VWF-mediated platelet aggregation in the renal arterial system. The renal impairment in adults seems to be more severe than that in childhood HUS, and dialysis is often required. The cause of HUS associated with pregnancy or oral contraceptive use is unclear, but it may be related to development of an autoantibody to endothelial cells. In outbreaks of HUS associated with consumption of *E. coli*-contaminated water, both children and adults have developed HUS.

Differentiating the adult form of HUS from TTP may be difficult. The lack of neurologic symptoms, the presence of renal dysfunction, and the absence of other organ involvement suggest HUS. Also, in HUS, thrombocytopenia tends to be mild to moderate (platelet consumption occurs primarily in the kidneys), whereas thrombocytopenia is usually severe in TTP. Similarly, fragmentation of RBCs and the resultant anemia tend to be milder than that observed in TTP because RBCs are being fragmented primarily in the kidneys. In some cases of HUS, other organs become involved, and the differentiation between HUS and TTP becomes less clear. Because on initial presentation it is difficult or impossible to differentiate adult-acquired TTP from adult HUS, the TPE therapy needs to be started urgently on a precautionary basis until the differential diagnosis is better established using ADAMTS13 assays.

Atypical hemolytic uremic syndrome. Although HUS and atypical HUS (aHUS) exhibit the same clinical signs and symptoms, each disease results from a distinct mechanism of action. Similar to HUS, aHUS is a life-threatening disease. However, in contrast to HUS, aHUS is not associated with an infection. aHUS is an extremely rare, progressive disease that is associated with defects in the regulation of *complement activation*.[119] Numerous mutations in complement regulatory proteins have been identified. Of these, mutations in factor H that impair the control of the complement alternative pathway appear to be the most common. Although endothelial cells, RBCs, and platelets can be activated by complement, the role of each of these cell types in mediating the clinical phenotype is unclear. Eculizumab (Soliris, Alexion) is a humanized monoclonal antibody that acts as a C5 terminal complement inhibitor that is approved as treatment for patients with aHUS.

Disseminated intravascular coagulation. A common cause of destructive thrombocytopenia is activation of the coagulation cascade (by a variety of agents or conditions), resulting in a consumptive coagulopathy that entraps platelets in intravascular fibrin clots. This disorder is discussed here briefly and described in more detail in Chapter 39. DIC has many similarities to TTP, including MAHA and deposition of thrombi in the arterial circulation of most organs (see Table 38.5). In DIC, the thrombi are composed primarily of fibrinogen (red clots), whereas in TTP, the thrombi are composed primarily of platelets and VWF (white clots).

Acute DIC has rapid platelet consumption and results in severe thrombocytopenia. In addition, levels of factor V, factor VIII, and fibrinogen are decreased as a result of thrombin generation. The test for D-dimer (a breakdown product of stabilized fibrin) almost always yields positive results. This form of DIC is life-threatening and must be treated immediately.

In chronic DIC, there is an ongoing, low-grade consumptive coagulopathy. Clotting factors may be slightly reduced or normal, and compensatory thrombocytopoiesis results in a moderately low to normal platelet count.[37] D-dimer may not be elevated or may be slightly or moderately increased. Chronic DIC is not generally life-threatening, and treatment usually is not urgent. Chronic DIC should be followed closely, however, because partly compensated DIC states can progress into the life-threatening acute form.

Chronic DIC, similar to all forms of DIC, is virtually always caused by some underlying condition, which can remain clinically elusive. If that condition can be corrected, the DIC usually resolves without further treatment.

Purpura fulminans. Purpura fulminans is a unique and devastating thrombotic disorder, often acute and fatal. It manifests as large irregular areas of blue-black cutaneous bleeding that rapidly progress to necrosis of superficial skin and deeper soft tissues.

Occurring most commonly in neonates and children,[120] purpura fulminans can be the presenting feature of acute sepsis resulting from bacterial infections with *Neisseria meningitidis*, *Streptococcus pneumoniae*, group A and B streptococci, and, less commonly, *Haemophilus influenzae* or *Staphylococcus aureus*. In sepsis, there is widespread activation of the systemic inflammatory response as well as the coagulation and complement pathways, which leads to increased bleeding. In the neonatal setting, purpura fulminans may be associated with congenital or acquired deficiency or dysfunction of the coagulation control factor protein C (PC), which promotes thrombosis. The principal laboratory features of purpura fulminans mirror those of DIC, including prolongation of coagulation times, thrombocytopenia, hypofibrinogenemia, and increased fibrin degradation products.

Although rare, the same clinical manifestations can occur in adults with sepsis, in whom a consistent feature is profound abnormalities in hemostasis.[121,122] Because of its rapid progression to multiorgan thrombotic injury, purpura fulminans is a hematologic emergency requiring urgent intervention. In addition to full supportive care and urgent broad-spectrum antimicrobial therapies, purpura fulminans with DIC requires plasma and platelet transfusions to replenish the consumptive coagulopathy. Without effective treatment, superficial and deep soft tissues (from full-thickness skin surface down to the bone) become gangrenous, requiring amputation. When microvascular necrosis extends to the visceral organs (lungs, kidneys, adrenals), mortality is high, and morbidity is severe in survivors.

In neonates or small children with any degree of heritable PC deficiency, replacement therapy with a human-derived PC concentrate (Ceprotin, Baxalta) is safe and effective. Intravenous dosing, however, may be required for long periods before the condition resolves. Children with more severe heritable forms have ongoing risks of purpura fulminans and require long-term antithrombotic therapy with PC replacement alone or in combination with warfarin or low-molecular-weight heparin.

Nonimmune drug-induced thrombocytopenia. A few drugs directly interact with platelets to cause thrombocytopenia in a nonimmune manner. Ristocetin, an antibiotic no longer in clinical use, facilitates the interaction of VWF with platelet membrane GPIb and leads to platelet agglutination and thrombocytopenia. Hematin, used for the treatment of acute intermittent porphyria, may give rise to a transient thrombocytopenia that seems to be the result of stimulation of platelet secretion and aggregation. Protamine sulfate and bleomycin may induce thrombocytopenia by a similar mechanism.[49]

Mechanical platelet destruction. Thrombocytopenia often follows surgery involving extracorporeal circulatory devices such as cardiopulmonary bypass (CPB) (heart-lung machine) circuits, use of various ventricular assist devices for patients with heart failure, and use of extracorporeal membrane oxygenation (ECMO) to assist patients with temporary pulmonary injuries. This is a consequence of platelet activation and damage caused by the pump circuitry. The most pronounced effects occur with

CPB use. Platelet count and function return to normal several days after removing the device.[43]

Abnormalities in Distribution or Dilution

A common clinical cause of thrombocytopenia is an abnormal distribution of platelets (*sequestration*) (Box 38.5). The normal spleen sequesters approximately one-third of the total platelet mass. Mild thrombocytopenia may be present in any form or etiology of hypersplenism. The total body platelet mass is often normal in these disorders, but numerous platelets are sequestered in the enlarged spleen, and consequently, the venous blood platelet count is low. Common disorders that cause splenomegaly include end-stage liver diseases causing hepatic cirrhosis and portal hypertension. Other diseases that are associated with splenomegaly include Hodgkin lymphoma, non-Hodgkin lymphoma, sarcoidosis, leukemias (such as chronic myeloid leukemia and hairy cell leukemia), and Gaucher disease.

Lowering the body temperature to less than 25° C, as is commonly done in cardiovascular surgery, results in a transient but mild thrombocytopenia secondary to platelet sequestration in the spleen and liver. An associated transient defect in platelet function also occurs with hypothermia. Platelet count and function return to baseline values on return to normal body temperature.[32] A second cause of thrombocytopenia associated with cardiac surgery is the dilution effect on platelet count resulting from asanguinous crystalloids used to prime the extracorporeal circuit.

The administration of massive amounts of stored whole blood may produce a transient thrombocytopenia. Stored blood contains platelets whose viability is severely impaired by the effects of storage and temperature. Under these conditions, the dead or damaged platelets are rapidly sequestered by the patient's RE system. Since contemporary transfusion therapy more commonly provides ad hoc component therapy as necessary, this situation is less commonly encountered.

Finally, mild thrombocytopenia may be encountered in patients with chronic renal failure, severe iron deficiency, megaloblastic anemia, postcompression sickness, and chronic hypoxia.

THROMBOCYTOSIS: INCREASE IN CIRCULATING PLATELETS

Thrombocytosis is defined as an abnormally high platelet count, typically >450,000/µL. This disorder often arises from an acquired condition (Box 38.6). However, there is a rare

---

BOX 38.5 Classification of Thrombocytopenias: Platelet Sequestration

Distribution
  Splenic sequestration (associated with hypersplenism, chronic liver disease)
  Kasabach-Merritt syndrome
  Hypothermia
  Massive blood transfusion
Dilution
  Extracorporeal circulation

BOX 38.6   Clinical States Resulting in Thrombocytosis

Conditions Associated With Reactive Thrombocytosis

Blood loss and surgery
Postsplenectomy
Iron deficiency anemia
Reactive thrombocytosis (such as infection or infection plus surgery)
Stress (including trauma and postoperative)
Rebound after myelosuppressive chemotherapy

Myeloproliferative Disorders Associated With Thrombocytosis

Polycythemia vera
Chronic myeloid [myelogenous] leukemia
Chronic myelomonocytic leukemia
Myelodysplastic syndrome variants (such as myelodysplasia with del[5q])
Primary myelofibrosis
Essential thrombocythemia

Adapted from Schafer, A. I. (2004). Thrombocytosis. *N Engl J Med*, *350*, 1211–1219; and Harrison, C. N., Bareford, D., Butt, N., et al. (2010). Guideline for investigation and management of adults and children presenting with a thrombocytosis. *Br J Haematol, 149*, 352–375.

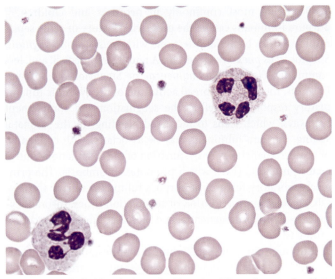

Figure 38.7 Cell Morphology in Reactive Thrombocytosis. Note the increased number of platelets but reasonably normal platelet morphology, characteristic of reactive thrombocytosis. (Peripheral blood, Wright-Giemsa stain, ×1000.)

condition of familial thrombocytosis associated with mutations of either the thrombopoietin or the thrombopoietin receptor genes.

Conditions that can cause elevated platelet counts are secondary to inflammation, trauma, or other underlying and seemingly unrelated conditions. The term *reactive thrombocytosis* is used to describe this type of thrombocytosis. A second category of thrombocytosis is associated with clonal *myeloproliferative disorders* such as polycythemia vera, chronic myeloid leukemia, and myelofibrosis with myeloid metaplasia, primary myelofibrosis or other myeloproliferative diseases. Marked and persistent elevation in the platelet count is a hallmark of these conditions, and platelet counts often exceed 1 million/μL. In the myeloproliferative disorder known as essential thrombocythemia (ET) (discussed subsequently in "Essential Thrombocythemia"), platelet counts may reach levels of several million.[37,123,124]

Reactive Thrombocytosis

Platelet counts between 450,000/μL and 800,000/μL with no change in platelet function can result from acute blood loss, splenectomy, childbirth, tissue necrosis secondary to surgery, chronic inflammatory disease, infection, exercise, iron deficiency anemia, hemolytic anemia, renal disorders, and various malignancies. Occasionally, patients present with a platelet count of 1 to 2 million/μL (Figure 38.7; compare with normal platelet count in Figure 1.1).

In reactive thrombocytosis, platelet production remains responsive to normal regulatory stimuli (e.g., thrombopoietin, a glycoprotein hormone that is produced chiefly in the liver parenchyma and secondarily in the kidney), and morphologically normal platelets are produced at a moderately increased rate.

This is in contrast to ET, which is characterized by unregulated or autonomous production of platelets of variable size.[123,124]

Examination of the bone marrow from patients with reactive thrombocytosis reveals a normal to increased number of megakaryocytes that are normal in morphology. Results of platelet aggregation tests usually reveal normal platelet function in response to various agents.

Reactive thrombocytosis is not associated with thrombosis, hemorrhage, or abnormal thrombopoietin levels. It seldom produces symptoms per se and disappears when the underlying disorder is brought under control.[123,124]

Reactive Thrombocytosis Associated With Hemorrhage or Surgery

After acute hemorrhage, the platelet count may be low for 2 to 6 days (if no platelet transfusion given) but typically rebounds to elevated levels for several days before returning to the prehemorrhage level. A similar pattern of thrombocytopenia and thrombocytosis is seen after major surgical procedures associated with significant blood loss. In both cases, the platelet count typically returns to normal 10 to 16 days after blood loss.

Postsplenectomy Thrombocytosis

The spleen normally sequesters about one-third of the circulating platelet mass. After splenectomy, there is normally an initial increase in the platelet count of approximately 30% to 50%. For unknown reasons, in postsplenectomy thrombocytosis, the platelet count can reach or exceed 1 million/μL, which far exceeds levels that could result from rebalancing the circulating platelet pool incorporating the splenic platelet pool. Unlike after blood loss from hemorrhage or surgery, the platelet count reaches a maximum 1 to 3 weeks after splenectomy and remains elevated for 1 to 3 months. In some patients who undergo splenectomy for treatment of anemias (e.g., autoimmune hemolytic anemia), the platelet count can remain elevated for several years.

Thrombocytosis Associated With Iron Deficiency Anemia

Iron deficiency anemia secondary to chronic blood loss is associated with reactive thrombocytosis.[125] Although the mechanism underlying the role of iron in thrombopoiesis is unknown, data suggest that low iron levels lead to a diversion of megakaryocytic-erythroid progenitors toward a megakaryocyte lineage commitment.[126] Additionally, treatment of the iron deficiency with iron replacement results in a normalization of the platelet count in thrombocytopenic patients, but it has also been reported to induce thrombocytopenia in patients with normal platelet counts.

Thrombocytosis Associated With Inflammation and Disease

Similar to elevations in C-reactive protein, fibrinogen, VWF, and other acute phase reactants, thrombocytosis may be an indication of inflammation. Thrombocytosis may be found in patients with rheumatoid arthritis, where the presence of thrombocytosis can be correlated with activation of the inflammatory process.

An elevated platelet count also may be early evidence of malignancies such as Hodgkin lymphoma and various carcinomas. Thrombocytosis may be found in patients with rheumatic fever, osteomyelitis, ulcerative colitis, and acute infections.

Kawasaki syndrome, a rare disorder caused by inflammation of small and medium-sized arteries, is of unknown etiology, although an infectious etiology is suspected. It affects infants and young children, with boys more likely than girls to develop the disease. The highest incidence is found in individuals of Japanese descent, although all ethnic groups can be affected. The initial acute febrile stage lasts 2 weeks or longer, with a fever of 40° C or higher, and is unresponsive to antibiotic therapy. The longer the fever continues, the higher the risk of cardiovascular complications. The subacute phase lasts an additional week to 10 days, during which the platelet count usually is elevated, with counts of 2 million/μL reported, and C-reactive protein and other proinflammatory markers are elevated. The higher the platelet count, the higher the risk of cardiovascular complications (coronary artery thrombosis and aneurysms). The treatment for Kawasaki syndrome is antiplatelet agents, such as aspirin and, importantly, IVIG.

Exercise-Induced Thrombocytosis

Strenuous exercise is a well-known cause of relative thrombocytosis and likely is due to the release of platelets from the splenic pool, hemoconcentration by transfer of plasma water to the extravascular compartment, or both. Normally the platelet count returns to its preexercise baseline level 30 minutes after completion of exercise.

Rebound Thrombocytosis

Thrombocytosis often follows the thrombocytopenia caused by marrow suppressive therapy or other conditions. Rebound thrombocytosis usually peaks 10 to 17 days after withdrawal

of the offending drug (e.g., alcohol or methotrexate) or after institution of therapy for the underlying condition with which thrombocytopenia is associated (e.g., vitamin B_{12} deficiency).[43]

Thrombocytosis Associated With Myeloproliferative Disorders

Primary or autonomous thrombocytosis is a typical finding in four chronic myeloproliferative disorders: polycythemia vera, chronic myeloid leukemia, myelofibrosis with myeloid metaplasia (primary myelofibrosis), and ET. Depending on the duration and stage of the myeloproliferative disorder at the time of diagnosis, it may be difficult to differentiate among these diseases. Chapter 32 provides a more complete description of these disorders. In the other types of myeloproliferative disorders, the platelet count seldom reaches the extreme values characteristic of ET. However, diagnosis of ET should not be based on platelet count alone and should take into account physical examination findings, history, and other laboratory data.[37,124]

Essential Thrombocythemia (ET)

Essential or primary thrombocythemia is a chronic myeloproliferative neoplasm characterized by persistent marked elevation of peripheral blood platelet counts (Figure 38.8) and uncontrolled proliferation of marrow megakaryocytes.

In contrast to other myeloproliferative disorders, the other marrow cell lines are not impacted in patients with ET. There is evidence that ET is caused by a clonal proliferation of a single abnormal pluripotent stem cell that eventually crowds out normal stem cells. As with most myeloproliferative disorders, ET is an acquired condition that is prevalent in middle-aged and older patients and affects equal numbers of men and women.

Clinical manifestations of essential thrombocythemia. Patients with ET present with hemorrhage, platelet dysfunction,

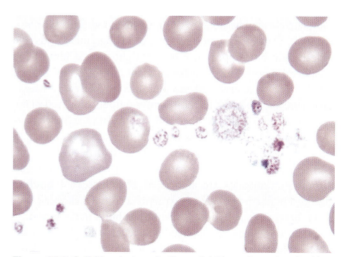

Figure 38.8 Cell Morphology in Essential Thrombocythemia. Note the increased number of platelets and wide variation in platelet size, characteristic of essential thrombocythemia. Red blood cell and white blood cell morphology is characteristically normal. (Peripheral blood, Wright-Giemsa stain, ×1000.) (From Carr, J. H., & Rodak, B. F. [2013]. *Clinical Hematology Atlas* [4th ed.]. Philadelphia: Saunders.)

and thrombosis. The degree of thrombocytosis has not been found to reliably predict hemorrhagic or thrombotic events. There is no specific clinical sign, symptom, or laboratory test that establishes the diagnosis of ET. It is a diagnosis of exclusion, made by ruling out the other myeloproliferative disorders and systemic illnesses that produce reactive thrombocytosis.

Thrombosis in the microvasculature is relatively common in ET, with an incidence at the time of diagnosis of 10% to 20%.[127,128] This thrombosis can lead to digital pain, digital gangrene, or erythromelalgia (throbbing, aching, and burning sensation in the extremities, particularly in the palms and soles).[122] The symptoms of erythromelalgia can be explained by arteriolar inflammation and occlusive thrombosis mediated by platelets. It can be relieved for several days by a single dose of aspirin.[129]

Thrombosis of large veins and arteries also may occur in ET. The arteries most commonly involved are those in the legs, the coronary arteries, and the renal arteries, but involvement of the mesenteric, subclavian, and carotid arteries is not uncommon. Neurologic complications are relatively common. Venous thrombosis may involve the large veins of the legs and pelvis, hepatic veins, or splenic veins.[130] The primary cause of death of patients with ET is attributed to a combination of advanced age and high incidence of cardiovascular thrombosis.[131]

In ET, hemorrhagic episodes occur less often than thrombotic episodes. The hemorrhagic manifestations of ET are mucocutaneous in nature, with gastrointestinal tract bleeding occurring most often. Other sites of bleeding include the mucous membranes of the nose and mouth, the urinary tract, and the skin. Bleeding symptoms may be aggravated by aspirin use. Occasionally a patient has a paradoxical combination of thromboembolic (clotting) and hemorrhagic episodes in association with ET. A patient with ET who has had a thrombotic event may have a hemorrhagic event later.[132]

Clinical laboratory findings. Platelet size is heterogeneous, and platelets may be notably clumped on blood films (see Figure 38.8). Platelets may be agranular or hypogranular and have a clear, light blue appearance on a Wright-stained film of the peripheral blood. The presence of giant and bizarrely shaped platelets is characteristic of myeloproliferative diseases. Megakaryocyte fragments or nuclei are commonly encountered in the peripheral blood. The number and volume of megakaryocytes are increased in the bone marrow, and they are predominantly large, show some cellular atypia, and tend to form clusters.

The platelets of some patients who have experienced thrombotic episodes are associated with increased binding affinity for fibrinogen. These patients also have elevated levels of thromboxane B_2 and β-thromboglobulin in the blood.[133] These findings suggest enhanced platelet activation and a possible explanation for the thrombotic tendencies of patients with ET.

The bleeding manifestations may be related to a variety of qualitative abnormalities in the platelets, including deficiencies in epinephrine receptors and ultrastructural defects in granules, mitochondria, and microfilaments. Often the platelets are functionally defective when tested in vitro. Platelet aggregation is usually absent in response to epinephrine and may be decreased with adenosine diphosphate but is usually normal with collagen. Lack of an epinephrine response may help to differentiate ET from reactive thrombocytosis because this response is usually normal in reactive thrombocytosis but absent in most cases of ET. Platelet adhesion also may be decreased in ET.[124]

Treatment of essential thrombocythemia. There is no cure for ET. Treatment is administered only to control symptoms and reduce the risk of complications from blood clots and bleeding. However, if symptoms become severe, hydroxyurea is a commonly prescribed drug. A variety of myelosuppressive agents (e.g., melphalan, busulfan) have also been used when treatment of ET is necessary due to thrombosis or bleeding.[123] In patients with life-threatening hemorrhage or thrombosis associated with extremely high platelet counts, therapeutic plateletpheresis may be used to rapidly reduce, albeit temporarily, the elevated platelet counts. In these situations, other agents are added for longer-term control of the platelet count.[134]

Pegylated interferon-α (Intron A, Merck; Pegasys, Genentech) has been used to treat ET, with approximately 60% of treated patients achieving complete remission; however, a significant percentage of patients given the drug cannot tolerate the dosages required.[135] Another agent that is useful for the treatment of ET is anagrelide (Agrylin, Shire). This drug acts by inhibiting megakaryocyte maturation and platelet release.[136] In one large study, anagrelide decreased the platelet count in 93% of patients.[137,138] Many patients cannot tolerate anagrelide, however, and in these patients other, more traditional agents such as low-dose aspirin, busulfan, and hydroxyurea can be more effective.

Approximately one-quarter of patients with ET have a mutation in the Janus-associated kinases (JAK1 and JAK2). ET patients with JAK-positive mutations are treated with ruxolitinib (Jakafi, Incyte). This drug is a kinase inhibitor that modulates the signaling of a number of cytokines and growth factors important for hematopoiesis.

The role of lowering platelet counts as a prophylactic treatment in this disease has not been established because the risks from exposure to mutagenic alkylating agents used to decrease the platelet count may be greater than the risk of thrombosis or hemorrhage. Recent guidelines and consensus recommendations for both diagnosis and treatment of ET depend on risk stratification, so patient treatment is best individualized based on the clinical course and comorbidities with the goal of reducing risk of hemorrhage and thrombosis.

In patients with ET, there is a low incidence of transformation to acute leukemia or fatal thrombotic or hemorrhagic complications. Therapy to prevent thrombotic complications seems to be effective in preventing morbidity but does not seem to improve overall survival, at least in high-risk patients.

- Thrombocytopenia manifests as small vessel bleeding in the skin and is the most common cause of clinically significant bleeding.
- Thrombocytopenia can result from decreased platelet production or increased destruction or abnormal distribution of platelets.
- Decreased production of platelets can be attributed to megakaryocyte hypoplasia, ineffective thrombopoiesis, or inclusion of abnormal cells within the marrow.
- A large number of congenital disorders associated with thrombocytopenia, such as May-Hegglin anomaly, have been identified.
- Neonatal thrombocytopenia can be caused by disorders of platelet production or increased destruction with origins in either the mother or the neonate.
- Patients experiencing increased platelet destruction become thrombocytopenic only when the rate of platelet production can no longer increase enough to compensate.
- Pathologic destruction of platelets can be caused by both immunologic and nonimmunologic mechanisms.
- Acute immune thrombocytopenic purpura (ITP) commonly occurs in children after a viral illness and usually resolves spontaneously. Chronic ITP is more commonly seen in women and requires treatment if the platelet count decreases to less than 30,000/μL.
- Treatment of drug-induced thrombocytopenia must begin with identification of the causative drug and discontinuation of its use.
- Thrombotic thrombocytopenic purpura (TTP) manifests with the classic triad of symptoms that includes microangiopathic hemolytic anemia, thrombocytopenia, and neurologic abnormalities.
- The nonimmune mechanism of TTP is often associated with dysfunction of the enzyme ADAMTS13 (*a d*isintegrin *a*nd *m*etalloprotease with a *t*hrombo*s*pondin type 1 motif, member *13*); measurements of ADAMTS13 activity or the presence of an inhibitor to ADAMTS13 aid in the diagnosis of TTP.
- The hallmark signs of hemolytic uremic syndrome (HUS) of renal dysfunction, mild thrombocytopenia, mild anemia, and presentation in children, can aid in differentiating HUS from TTP.
- A common cause of destructive thrombocytopenia is activation of the coagulation cascade that causes disseminated intravascular coagulation (DIC); DIC (red clots) can be differentiated from TTP (white clots) by the type of clots formed and the coagulation laboratory test abnormalities in DIC.
- Abnormal distribution of platelets is commonly caused by splenic sequestration, although there are other causes.
- Reactive thrombocytosis is secondary to inflammation, trauma, or a variety of underlying conditions; platelet counts are increased for a limited time.
- Thrombocytosis in myeloproliferative disorders is marked and persistent with the most extremely elevated platelet counts found in essential thrombocythemia.

Now that you have completed this chapter, go back and read again the case study at the beginning and respond to the questions presented. Answers can be found in Appendix C.

Answers can be found in Appendix C.

1. Patients with TTP:
   a. Present with a triad of symptoms, including hemolytic anemia, neurologic symptoms, and thrombocytosis
   b. Require treatment with an ADAMTS13 inhibitor
   c. Develop thrombi due to accumulation of high-molecular-weight VWF multimers
   d. Exhibit thrombocytopenia due to the development of anti-VWF antibodies
2. Which of the following is NOT a hallmark of ITP?
   a. Petechiae
   b. Thrombocytopenia
   c. Large overactive platelets
   d. Megakaryocyte hypoplasia
3. The specific antigen most commonly responsible for the development of NAIT in White patients is:
   a. HPA-3a
   b. HPA-1a
   c. GPIb
   d. Lewis antigen a

4. A 2-year-old child with an unexpected platelet count of 15,000/μL and a recent history of a viral infection most likely has:
   a. HIT
   b. NAIT
   c. Acute ITP
   d. Chronic ITP
5. Which drug causes a reduction in platelet count by inhibiting megakaryocyte maturation?
   a. Gold salts
   b. Tirofiban
   c. Anagrelide
   d. Quinidine
6. Platelet abnormalities often result in:
   a. Musculoskeletal bleeding
   b. Mucosal bleeding
   c. Hemarthroses
   d. None of the above

7. When a drug acts as a hapten to induce thrombocytopenia, an antibody forms against which of the following?
   a. Typically unexposed new platelet antigens
   b. The combination of the drug and the platelet membrane protein to which it is bound
   c. The drug alone in the plasma, but the immune complex then binds to the platelet membrane
   d. The drug alone, but only when it is bound to the platelet membrane

8. In contrast to acute ITP, the chronic form of the disease:
   a. Develops following a severe infection
   b. Is associated with a sudden onset of bleeding
   c. Occurs primarily in males
   d. Rarely remits spontaneously

9. Neonatal autoimmune thrombocytopenia occurs when:
   a. The mother lacks a platelet antigen that the infant possesses, and she builds antibodies, which cross the placenta, to that antigen
   b. The infant develops an autoimmune process such as ITP secondary to in utero infection
   c. The infant develops an autoimmune disease such as lupus erythematosus before birth

   d. The mother has an autoimmune antibody to her own platelets, which crosses the placenta and reacts with the infant's platelets

10. HUS in children is associated with:
    a. Diarrhea caused by *Shigella* species
    b. Meningitis caused by *Haemophilus* species
    c. Pneumonia caused by *Mycoplasma* species
    d. Pneumonia caused by respiratory viruses

11. Treatment with an anticomplement agent such as eculizumab is first-line therapy for:
    a. Hereditary TTP
    b. HUS
    c. ITP
    d. Atypical HUS

12. Which of the following statements regarding thrombocytosis is NOT true?
    a. Thrombocytosis can be associated with hemorrhage and thrombosis.
    b. Affected patients have platelet counts in excess of 450,000/μL.
    c. Primary thrombocytosis resulting from essential thrombocythemia is self-correcting.
    d. Thrombocytosis can be congenital or acquired.

REFERENCES

1. Kelley, M. J., Jawien, W., Ortel, T. L., et al. (2000). Mutations of *MYH9*, encoding for non-muscle myosin heavy chain A, in May Hegglin anomaly. *Nat Genet, 26*, 106–108.
2. Cao, Y., Sun, Y., Deng, Y., et al. (2022). Defective VWF secretion due to expression of *MYH9*-RD E1841K mutant in endothelial cells disrupts hemostasis. *Blood, 6*, 4537–4552.
3. The May Hegglin/Fechtner Syndrome Consortium. (2000). Mutations in *MHY9* result in May-Hegglin anomaly, and Fechtner and Sebastian syndromes. *Nat Genet, 26*, 103–105.
4. Mhawech, P., & Saleem, A. (2000). Inherited giant platelet disorders: classification and literature review. *Am J Clin Pathol, 113*, 176–190.
5. Hall, J. G. (1987). Thrombocytopenia and absent radius (TAR) syndrome. *J Med Genet, 24*, 79–83.
6. Freedman, M. H., & Doyle, J. J. (1999). Inherited bone marrow failure syndromes. In Lilleyman, J. S., Hann, I. M., & Branchette, V. S. (Eds.), *Pediatric Hematology.* (pp. 23–49). London: Churchill Livingstone.
7. Lackner, A., Basu, M., Bierings, M., et al. (2000). Haematopoietic stem cell transplantation for amegakaryocytic thrombocytopenia. *Br J Haematol, 109*, 773–775.
8. Germeshausen, M., & Ballmaier, M. (2021). CAMT-MPL: congenital amegakaryocytic thrombocytopenia caused by *MPL* mutations – heterogeneity of a monogenic disorder – a comprehensive analysis of 56 patients. *Haematologica, 106*, 2439–2448.
9. Balduini, C. L., Savoia, A., & Seri, M. (2013). Inherited thrombocytopenias frequently diagnosed in adults. *J Thromb Haemost, 11*, 1006–1019.
10. Stormorken, H., Hellum, B., Egeland, T., et al. (1991). X-linked thrombocytopenia and thrombocytopathia: attenuated Wiskott-Aldrich syndrome: functional and morphological studies of platelets and lymphocytes. *Thromb Haemost, 65*, 300–305.
11. Michaelson, A. D. (2019). Part IV: The clinical approach to disorders of platelet number and function. In Michaelson, A. D., Cattaneo, M., Frelinger, A., et al. (Eds.), *Platelets.* (4th ed., pp. 701–920). Philadelphia: Elsevier.
12. Candotti, F. (2018). Clinical manifestations and pathophysiological mechanisms of the Wiskott-Aldrich syndrome. *J Clin Immunol, 38*, 13–27.
13. Mehaffey, M. G., Newton, A. L., Gandhi, M. J., et al. (2001). X-linked thrombocytopenia caused by a novel mutation of *GATA-1*. *Blood, 98*, 2681–2688.
14. Freson, K. K., Devriendt, G., Matthijs, G., et al. (2001). Platelet characteristics in patients with X-linked macrothrombocytopenia because of a novel *GATA-1* mutation. *Blood, 98*, 85–92.
15. Nicloux, M., Peterman, L., Parodi, M., et al. (2020). Outcome and management of newborns with congenital cytomegalovirus infection. *Arch Pediatr, 27*(3), 160–165.
16. Brown, H. L., & Abernathy, M. P. (1998). Cytomegalovirus infection. *Semin Perinatol, 22*, 260–266.
17. Crapnell, K. E. D., Zanfani, A., Chaudhuri, J. L., et al. (2000). In vitro infection of megakaryocytes and their precursors by human cytomegalovirus. *Blood, 95*, 487–493.
18. Dubey, J. P., Murata, F. H. A., Cerqueria-Cezar, C. K., et al. (2021). Congenital toxoplasmosis in humans: an update of worldwide rate of congenital infections. *Parasitology, 148*, 1406–1416.
19. Sullivan, E. M., Burgess, M. A., & Forrest, J. M. (1999). The epidemiology of rubella and congenital rubella in Australia, 1992–1997. *Commun Dis Intell, 23*, 209–214.
20. Yazigi, A., De Pecoulas, A. E., Vauloup-Fellous, C., et al. (2017). Fetal and neonatal abnormalities due to congenital rubella syndrome: a review of literature. *J Matern Fetal Neonatal Med, 30*, 274–278.
21. Tovo, P. A., de-Martino, M., Gabiano, C., et al. (1992). Prognostic factors and survival in children with perinatal HIV-1 infection. The Italian Register for HIV Infections in Children. *Lancet, 339*, 1249–1253.

22. Lordkipanidze, M., Hvas, A. M., & Harrison, P. (2019). Clinical tests of platelet function. In Michelson, A. D., Cattaneo, M., Frelinger, A. L., et al. (Eds.), *Platelets*. (4th ed., pp. 593–626). Philadelphia: Elsevier.

23. Brown, B. A. (1993). *Hematology: Principles and Procedures*. (6th ed.). Philadelphia: Lea & Febiger.

24. Aster, R. (2019). Drug-induced thrombocytopenia. In Michelson, A. D., Cattaneo, M., Frelinger, A., et al. (Eds.), *Platelets*. (4th ed., pp. 725–739). Philadelphia: Elsevier.

25. Kuter, D. J. (2022). Treatment of chemotherapy-induced thrombocytopenia in patients with non-hematologic malignancies. *Haematologica, 107*, 1243–1263.

26. Basser, R. L., Underhill, C., Davis, M. D., et al. (2000). Enhancement of platelet recovery after myelosuppressive chemotherapy by recombinant human megakaryocyte growth and development factor in patients with advanced cancer. *J Clin Oncol, 18*, 2852–2861.

27. Koch, M. A., Volberding, P. A., Lagakos, S. W., et al. (1992). Toxic effects of zidovudine in asymptomatic human immunodeficiency virus-infected individuals with CD4+ cell counts of 0.5×10^9/L or less: detailed and updated results from Protocol 019 of the AIDS Clinical Trials Group. *Arch Intern Med, 152*, 2286–2292.

28. Birgegard, G. (2016). The use of anagrelide in myeloproliferative neoplasms, with focus on essential thrombasthenia. *Curr Hematol Malig Rep, 11*, 348–355.

29. Rippel, N., Tremblay, D., Zubizarreta, N., et al. (2022). Anagrelide for platelet-directed cytoreduction in polycythemia vera: insights into utility and safety outcomes from a large multi-center database. *Leuk Res, 119*, 106903.

30. Silczuk, A., & Habrat, B. (2020). Alcohol-induced thrombocytopenia: current review. *Alcohol, 86*, 9–16.

31. Yamane, A., Nakamura, T., Suzuki, H., et al. (2008). Interferon-alpha 2b-induced thrombocytopenia is caused by inhibition of platelet production but not proliferation and endomitosis in human megakaryocytes. *Blood, 112*, 542–550.

32. Sata, M., Yano, Y., Yoshiyama, Y., et al. (1997). Mechanisms of thrombocytopenia induced by interferon therapy for chronic hepatitis B. *J Gastroenterol, 32*, 206–221.

33. Gross, P. L., & Lopez, J. A. (2023). Acquired disorders of platelet function. In Hoffman, R., Benz, E. J., Silberstein, L. E., et al. (Eds.), *Hematology: Basic Principles and Practice*. (8th ed., pp. 2007–2019). Elsevier: Philadelphia.

34. Buoli, M., Serati, M., Botturi, A., & Altamura, A. C. (2018). The risk of thrombocytopenia during valproic acid therapy: a critical summary of available clinical data. *Drugs R D, 18*, 1–5.

35. Mansuri, B., & Thekdi, K. P. (2017). A prospective study on morphological alteration of megakaryocytes amongst megaloblastic anemia cases along with their clinic-hematological manifestations. *Int J Res Med Sci, 5*, 4127–4132.

36. Taghizadeh, M. (2009). Megaloblastic anemias. In Harmening, D. M. (Ed.), *Clinical Hematology and Fundamentals of Hemostasis*. (5th ed., pp. 138–154). Philadelphia: Davis.

37. Corriveau, D. M., & Fritsma, G. A. (Eds.). (1988). *Hemostasis and Thrombosis in the Clinical Laboratory*. Philadelphia: Lippincott.

38. Quick, A. J. (1966). *Hemorrhagic Diseases and Thrombosis*. (2nd ed.). Philadelphia: Lea & Febiger.

39. Davis, G. L. (1998). Quantitative and qualitative disorders of platelets. In Steine-Martin, E. A., Lotspeich-Steininger, C., & Koepke, J. A. (Eds.), *Clinical Hematology: Principle, Procedures, Correlations*. (2nd ed., pp. 717–734). Philadelphia: Lippincott.

40. Zeller, B., Rajantie, J., Hedlund-Treutiger, I., et al. (2005). Childhood idiopathic thrombocytopenic purpura in Nordic countries: epidemiology and predictors of chronic disease. *Acta Paediatr, 94*, 1708–1784.

41. Neunert, C. E., Buchanan, G. R., Imback, P., et al. (2008). Severe hemorrhage in children with newly diagnosed immune thrombocytopenic purpura. *Blood, 112*, 4003–4008.

42. Lui, X.-G., Hou, Y., Hou, X. (2023). How we treat primary immune thrombocytopenia in adults. *J Hematol Oncol, 16*(4), 1–20.

43. Despotovic, J. M., & Bussel J. B. (2019). Immune thrombocytopenia (ITP). In Michelson, A. D., Cattaneo, M., Frelinger, A. L., et al. (Eds.), *Platelets*. (4th ed., pp. 707–724). Philadelphia: Elsevier.

44. Schulze, H., & Gaedicke, G. (2011). Immune thrombocytopenia in children and adults: what's the same, what's different? (Editorial and Perspective). *Haematologica, 96*, 1739–1741.

45. Terrell, D. R., Beebe, L. A., Vesely, S. K., et al. (2010). The incidence of immune thrombocytopenic purpura in children and adults: a critical review of published reports. *Am J Hematol, 8*, 174–180.

46. Kunicki, T. J., & Newman, P. J. (1992). The molecular immunology of human platelet proteins. *Blood, 80*, 1386–1404.

47. McMillan, R. (2000). Autoantibodies and autoantigens in chronic immune thrombocytopenic purpura. *Semin Hematol, 37*, 239–248.

48. Khodadi, E., Asnafi, A. A., Shahrabi, S., et al. (2016). Bone marrow niche in immune thrombocytopenia: a focus on megakaryopoiesis. *Ann Hematol, 95*, 1765–1776.

49. Olsson, B., Andersson, P., Jernas, M., et al. (2003). T-cell–mediated cytotoxicity toward platelets in chronic idiopathic thrombocytopenic purpura. *Nat Med, 9*, 1123–1124.

50. Harrington, W. J., Minnich, V., Hollingsworth, J. W., et al. (1951). Demonstration of a thrombocytopenic factor in the blood of patients with thrombocytopenic purpura. *J Lab Clin Med, 38*, 1–10.

51. Wei, Y., Ji, X., Wang, Y., et al. (2016). High-dose dexamethasone vs prednisone for treatment of adult immune thrombocytopenia: a prospective multicenter randomized trial. *Blood, 127*, 296–302.

52. Zhu, X. L., Feng, R., Huang, Q. S., et al. (2022). Prednisone plus IVIG compared with prednisone or IVIG alone for immune thrombocytopenia in pregnancy: a national retrospective cohort study. *Ther Adv Hematol, 12*, 1–13.

53. Kojouri, K., Vesely, S. K., Terrell, D. R., et al. (2004). Splenectomy for adult patients with idiopathic thrombocytopenic purpura. *Blood, 104*, 2623–2634.

54. Miltiadous, O., Hou, M., & Bussel, H. B. (2020). Identifying and treating refractory ITP: difficulty in diagnosis and role of combination therapy. *Blood, 135*, 472–490.

55. Bougie, D. W., Wilker, P. R., & Aster, R. H. (2006). Patients with quinine-induced immune thrombocytopenia have both "drug-dependent" and "drug-specific" antibodies. *Blood, 108*, 922–927.

56. Pfueller, S. L., Bilsont, R. A., Logan, D., et al. (1988). Heterogeneity of drug-dependent platelet antigens and their antibodies in quinine- and quinidine-induced thrombocytopenia: involvement of glycoproteins Ib, IIb, IIIa, and IX. *Blood, 11*, 190–198.

57. Greinacher, A. (2015). Clinical practice. Heparin-induced thrombocytopenia. *N Eng J Med, 373*, 252–261.

58. McKenzie, S. E., & Sachais, B. S. (2014). Advances in the pathophysiology and treatment of heparin-induced thrombocytopenia. *Curr Opin Hematol, 21*, 380–387.

59. Klok, F. A., Pai, M., Huisman, M. V., et al. (2022). Vaccine-induced immune thrombotic thrombocytopenia. *Lancet Haematol, 9*, e73–e80.

60. Schultz, N. H., Sorvoll, I. H., Michelsen, A. E., et al. (2021). Thrombosis and thrombocytopenia after ChAdOx1 nCoV-19 vaccination. *N Eng J Med, 384*, 2124–2130.

61. Huynh, A., Kelton, J. G., Arnold, D. M., et al. (2021). Antibody epitopes in vaccine-induced immune thrombotic thrombocytopenia. *Nature, 596*, 565–569.

62. Gruel, Y., Boizard, B., Daffos, F., et al. (1986). Determination of platelet antigens and glycoproteins in the human fetus. *Blood, 68*, 488–492.

63. Risson, D. C., Davies, M. W., & Williams, B. A. (2012). Review of neonatal alloimmune thrombocytopenia. *J Paediatr Child Health, 48*, 816–822.

64. Peterson, J. A., McFarland, J. G., Curtis, B. R., et al. (2013). Neonatal alloimmune thrombocytopenia: pathogenesis, diagnosis and management. *Br J Haematol, 116*, 3–14.

65. Strong, N. K., & Eddleman, K. A. (2013). Diagnosis and management of neonatal alloimmune thrombocytopenia in pregnancy. *Clin Lab Med, 33*, 311–325.

66. Bussel, J. B., & Pramiani, A. (2008). Fetal and neonatal alloimmune thrombocytopenia: progress and ongoing debates. *Blood Rev, 22*, 33–52.

67. Care, A., Pavord, S., Knight, M., et al. (2017). Severe primary autoimmune thrombocytopenia in pregnancy: a national cohort study. *BJOG, 125*, 604–612.

68. Sun, D., Shehata, N., Ye, X. Y., et al. (2016). Corticosteroids compared with intravenous immunoglobulin for the treatment of immune thrombocytopenia in pregnancy. *Blood, 128*, 1329–1335.

69. Clerc, J. M. (1989). Neonatal thrombocytopenia. *Clin Lab Sci, 2*, 42–47.

70. Hawkins, J., Aster, R. H., & Curtis, B. R. (2019). Post-transfusion purpura: current perspectives. *J Blood Med, 10*, 405–415.

71. McLaughlin, P., Talpaz, M., Quesada, J. R., et al. (1985). Immune thrombocytopenia following α-interferon therapy in patients with cancer. *JAMA, 254*, 1353–1354.

72. Li, Y., Guo, R., Wang, L., et al. (2019). G-CSF administration results in thrombocytopenia by inhibiting the differentiation of hematopoietic progenitors into megakaryocytes. *Biochem Pharmacol, 169*, 113624.

73. Paciucci, P. A., Mandeli, J., Oleksowicz, L., et al. (1990). Thrombocytopenia during immunotherapy with interleukin-2 by constant infusion. *Am J Med, 89*, 308–312.

74. Fattizzo, B., & Barcellini, W. (2020). Autoimmune cytopenias in chronic lymphocytic leukemia: focus on molecular aspects. *Front Oncol, 9*, 1435.

75. Carey, R. W., McGinnis, A., Jacobson, B. M., et al. (1976). Idiopathic thrombocytopenic purpura complicating chronic lymphocytic leukemia: management with sequential splenectomy and chemotherapy. *Arch Intern Med, 136*, 62–66.

76. Galanopoulos, N., Christoforidou, A., & Bezirgiannidou, Z. (2017). Lupus thrombocytopenia: pathogenesis and therapeutic implications. *Mediterr J Rheumatol, 28*, 20–26.

77. Coelho, H., Lopes, S., Pimentel, J., et al. (2013). Thrombocytopenia in *Plasmodium vivax* malaria is related to platelets phagocytosis. *PLOS One, 8*, e63410.

78. Cines, D. B., & Levine, L. D. (2017). Thrombocytopenia in pregnancy. *Blood, 130*, 2271–2277.

79. Palta, A., & Dhiman, P. (2016). Thrombocytopenia in pregnancy. *J Obstet Gynaecol, 36*, 146–152.

80. Magee, L. A., Nicolaides, K. H., & von Dadelszen, P. (2022). Preeclampsia. *N Eng J Med, 386*, 1817–1832.

81. Habas, E., Rayani, A., & Ganterie, R. (2013). Thrombocytopenia in hypertensive disease of pregnancy. *J Obstet Gynaelcol India, 63*, 96–100.

82. Gibson, W., Hunter, D., Neame, P. B., et al. (1982). Thrombocytopenia in preeclampsia and eclampsia. *Semin Thromb Hemost, 8*, 234–247.

83. Martin, J. N., Jr., Blake, P. G., Perry, K. G., Jr., et al. (1991). The natural history of HELLP syndrome: patterns of disease progression and regression. *Am J Obstet Gynecol, 164*, 1500–1509.

84. Adorno, M., Maher-Griffiths, C., & Abadie, H. (2022). HELLP syndrome. *Crit Care Nurs Clin N Am, 34*, 277–288.

85. Trofatter, K. F., Jr., Howell, M. L., Greenberg, C. S., et al. (1989). Use of the fibrin D-dimer in screening for coagulation abnormalities in preeclampsia. *Obstet Gynecol, 73*, 435–440.

86. Burrows, R. F., Hunter, D. J. S., Andrew, M., et al. (1987). A prospective study investigating the mechanism of thrombocytopenia in preeclampsia. *Obstet Gynecol, 70*, 334–338.

87. Benigni, A., Gregorini, G., Frusca, T., et al. (1989). Effect of low-dose aspirin on fetal and maternal generation of thromboxane by platelets in women at risk for pregnancy-induced hypertension. *N Engl J Med, 321*, 357–362.

88. Askie, L. M., Duley, L., Henderson-Smart, D. J., et al. (2007). Antiplatelet agents for prevention of pre-eclampsia: a meta-analysis of individual patient data. PARIS Collaborative Group. *Lancet, 369*, 1791–1798.

89. Roberge, S., Bujold, E., & Nicolaides, K. H. (2018). Aspirin for the prevention of preterm and term preeclampsia: systemic review and metaanalysis. *Am J Obstet Gynecol, 218*, 287–291.

90. Ezra, Y., Rose, M., & Eldor, A. (1996). Therapy and prevention of thrombotic thrombocytopenic purpura during pregnancy: a clinical study of 16 pregnancies. *Am J Hematol, 51*, 1–6.

91. Dashe, J. S., Ramin, S. M., & Cunningham, F. G. (1998). The long-term consequences of thrombotic microangiopathy (thrombotic thrombocytopenic purpura and hemolytic uremic syndrome) in pregnancy. *Obstet Gynecol, 91*, 662–668.

92. Sika, P., Chopra, S., Aggarwal, N., et al. (2013). Thrombotic thrombocytopenic purpura in the first trimester of pregnancy. *Asian J Transfus Sci, 7*(1), 79–80.

93. Mariotte, E., Azoulay, E., Glaicier, L., et al. (2016). Epidemiology and pathophysiology of adulthood-onset thrombotic microangiopathy with severe ADAMTS13 deficiency (thrombotic thrombocytopenia purpura): a cross-sectional analysis of the French national registry for thrombotic microangiopathy. *Lancet Haematol, 3*(5), e237–e245.

94. Joly, B. S., Coppa, P., & Veyradier, A. (2017). Thrombotic thrombocytopenic purpura. *Blood, 129*, 2836–2846.

95. Tsai, H. M. (2019). Thrombotic thrombocytopenic purpura and hemolytic uremic syndrome. In Michelson, A. D., Cattaneo, M., Frelinger, A., et al. (Eds.), *Platelets.* (4th ed, pp. 769–794). Philadelphia: Elsevier.

96. Bell, W. R., Braine, H. G., Ness, P. M., et al. (1991). Improved survival in thrombotic thrombocytopenic purpura–hemolytic uremic syndrome: clinical experience in 108 patients. *N Engl J Med, 325*, 398–403.

97. Rock, G. A., Shumak, K. H., Buskard, N. A., et al. (1991). Comparison of plasma exchange with plasma infusion in the treatment of thrombotic thrombocytopenic purpura. *N Engl J Med, 325*, 393–397.

98. Moake, J. L., Turner, N. A., Stathopoulos, N. A., et al. (1986). Involvement of large plasma von Willebrand factor (VWF) multimers and unusually large VWF forms derived from endothelial cells in shear-stress induced platelet aggregation. *J Clin Invest, 78,* 1456–1461.

99. Furlan, M., Robles, R., Solenthaler, M., et al. (1997). Deficient activity of von Willebrand factor-cleaving protease in chronic relapsing thrombotic thrombocytopenic purpura. *Blood, 89,* 3097–3103.

100. Tsai, H. M., & Lian, E. C. Y. (1998). Antibodies to von Willebrand factor-cleaving protease in acute thrombotic thrombocytopenic purpura. *N Engl J Med, 339,* 1585–1594.

101. Furlan, M., & Lammle, B. (1999). von Willebrand factor in thrombotic thrombocytopenic purpura. *Thromb Haemost, 82,* 592–600.

102. Saha, M., McDaniel, J. K., & Zheng, X. L. (2017). Thrombotic thrombocytopenic purpura: pathogenesis, diagnosis and potential novel therapeutics. *J Thromb Haemost, 15,* 1889–1900.

103. Furlan, M., Robles, R., & Lammle, B. (1996). Partial purification and characterization of a protease from human plasma cleaving von Willebrand factor to fragments produced by in vivo proteolysis. *Blood, 87,* 4223–4234.

104. Tsai, H. M. (1996). Physiologic cleaving of von Willebrand factor by a plasma protease is dependent on its conformation and requires calcium ion. *Blood, 87,* 4235–4244.

105. Nakashima, M. O., Zhang, X., Rogers, H. J., et al. (2016). Validation of a panel of ADAMTS13 assays for diagnosis of thrombotic thrombocytopenic purpura: activity, functional inhibitor, and autoantibody test. *Int J Lab Hematol, 38,* 550–559.

106. Alwan, F., Vendramin, C., Vanhoorelbeke, K., et al. (2017). Presenting ADAMTS13 antibody and antigen levels predict prognosis in immune-mediated thrombotic thrombocytopenic purpura. *Blood, 130,* 466–471.

107. Coppo, P., Schwarzinger, M., Buffet, M., et al. (2010). Predictive features of severe acquired ADAMTS13 deficiency in idiopathic thrombotic microangiopathies: the French TMA reference center experience. *PLoS One, 5,* e10208.

108. Bendapudi, P. K., Hurwitz, S., Fry, A., et al. (2017). Derivation and external validation of the PLASMIC score for rapid assessment of adults with thrombotic microangiopathies: a cohort study. *Lancet Haematol, 4(4),* e157–e164.

109. Li, A., Khalighi, P. R., Wu, Q., et al. (2018). External validation of the PLASMIC score: a clinical prediction tool for thrombotic thrombocytopenic purpura diagnosis and treatment. *J Thromb Haemost 16,* 164–169.

110. Coppo, P. (2017). Treatment of autoimmune thrombotic thrombocytopenic purpura in the more severe forms. *Transfus Apher Sci, 56,* 52–56.

111. Tersteeg, C., Schiviz, A., De Meyer, S. F., et al. (2015). Potential for recombinant ADAMTS13 as an effective therapy for acquired thrombotic thrombocytopenic purpura. *Arterioscler Thromb Vasc Biol, 35,* 2336–2342.

112. Scully, M., Knobl, P., Kentourche, K., et al. (2017). Recombinant ADAMTS13: first-in-human pharmacokinetics and safety in congenital thrombotic thrombocytopenic purpura. *Blood, 130,* 2055–2063.

113. Scully, M., Cataland, S. R., Peyvandi, F., et al. (2019). Caplacizumab treatment for acquired thrombotic thrombocytopenic purpura. *N Eng J Med, 380,* 335–346.

114. Di Pasquale, I., Budde, U., Tona, F., et al. (2019). Link between von Willebrand factor multimers, relapses and coronary microcirculation in patients with thrombotic thrombocytopenic purpura in remission. *Thromb Res, 173,* 42–47.

115. Jokiranta, T. S. (2017). HUS and atypical HUS. *Blood, 129,* 2847–2856.

116. Hua, Y., Chromek, M., Frykman, A., et al. (2021). Whole-genome characterization of hemolytic uremic syndrome-causing Shiga toxin-producing *Escherichia coli* in Sweden. *Virulence, 12,* 1296–1305.

117. Joseph, A., Cointe, A., Kurkdjian, P. M., et al. (2020). Shiga toxin-associated hemolytic uremic syndrome: a narrative review. *Toxins, 12(2),* 67.

118. Hirata, C., Kenzaka, T., & Akita, H. (2020). Late onset of hemolytic uremic syndrome after the appearance of prodromal gastrointestinal tract symptoms. *Clin Case Rep, 8,* 1910–1913.

119. Yoshida, Y., Kato, H., Ikeda, Y., et al. (2019). Pathogenesis of atypical hemolytic uremic syndrome. *J Atheroscler Thromb, 26,* 99–110.

120. Colling, M. E., & Bendapudi, K. (2018). Purpura fulminans: mechanism and management of dysregulated hemostasis. *Transfus Med Rev, 32,* 69–76.

121. Francis, R. B. (1990). Acquired purpura fulminans. *Semin Thromb Hemost, 16,* 310–325.

122. Lerolle, N., Carlotti, A., Melican, K., et al. (2013). Assessment of the interplay between blood and skin vascular abnormalities in adult purpura fulminans. *Am J Respir Crit Care Med, 188(6),* 684–692.

123. Tefferi, A., & Pardanani, A. (2019). Essential thrombasthenia. *N Eng J Med, 381,* 2135–2144.

124. Bleeker, J. S., & Hogan, W. J. (2011). Thrombocytosis: diagnostic evaluation, thrombotic risk stratification and risk-based management strategies. *Thrombosis, Article ID 536062,* 1–16.

125. Dan, K. (2005). Thrombocytosis in iron deficiency anemia. *Intern Med, 44,* 1025–1026.

126. Xavier-Ferrucia, J., Scanlon, V., Li, X., et al. (2019). Low iron promotes megakaryocytic commitment of megakaryocytic-erythroid progenitors in humans and mice. *Blood, 134,* 1547–1557.

127. Scherber, R., Dueck, A. C., Johansson, P., et al. (2011). The myeloproliferative neoplasm symptom assessment form (MPN-SAF): international prospective validation and reliability trial in 402 patients. *Blood, 118,* 401–408.

128. Szuber, N., Mudireddy, M., Nicolosi, M., et al. (2019). 3023 Mayo Clinic patients with myeloproliferative neoplasms: risk-stratified comparison of survival and outcomes data among disease subgroups. *Mayo Clin Proc, 94,* 599–610.

129. Michiels, J. J., & Ten Cate, F. J. (1992). Erythromelalgia in thrombocythemia of various myeloproliferative disorders. *Am J Hematol, 39,* 131–136.

130. Marcellino, B. K., Mascarenhas, J., Iancu-Rubin, C., et al. (2023). Essential thrombocythemia. In Hoffman, R., Benz, E. J., Silberstein, L. E., et al. (Eds.), *Hematology: Basic Principles and Practice.* (8th ed., pp. 1169–1192). Philadelphia: Elsevier.

131. Lekovic, D., Gotic, M., Sefer, D., et al. (2015). Predictors of survival and cause of death in patients with essential thrombocythemia. *Eur J Haematol, 95,* 461–466.

132. Martin, K. (2017). Risk factors for and management of MPN-associated bleeding and thrombosis. *Curr Hematol Malig Rep, 12,* 389–396.

133. Michiels, J. J., Berneman, Z., Schroyens, W., et al. (2006). The paradox of platelet activation and impaired function: platelet-von Willebrand factor interactions, and the etiology of thrombotic and hemorrhagic manifestations in essential thrombocythemia and polycythemia vera. *Semin Thromb Hemost, 32,* 589–604.

134. Jiang, H., Jin, Y., Shang, Y., et al. (2021). Therapeutic plateletpheresis in patients with thrombocytosis: gender, hemoglobin before apheresis significantly affect collection efficiency. *Front Med, 8*, 762419.

135. Bewersdorf, J. P., Giri, S., Wang, R., et al. (2021). Interferon alpha therapy in essential thrombocythemia and polycythemia vera – a systematic review and meta-analysis. *Leukemia, 35*, 1643–1660.

136. Thiele, J., Kvasnicka, H. M., & Schmitt-Graeff, A. (2006). Effects of anagrelide on megakaryopoiesis and platelet production. *Semin Thromb Hemost, 32*, 352–361.

137. Harrison, C. N., Campbell, P. J., Buck, G., et al. (2005). Hydroxyurea compared with anagrelide in high-risk essential thrombocythemia. *N Eng J Med, 353*, 33–45.

138. Gisslinger, H., Gotic, M., Holowiecki, J., et al. (2013). Anagrelide compared to hydroxyurea in WHO-classified essential thrombocythemia: the ANAHYDRET study, a randomized controlled trial. *Blood, 121*, 1720–1728.

39

Thrombotic Disorders and Laboratory Assessment

Mayukh Kanti Sarkar, George A. Fritsma, and Jeanine M. Walenga

OBJECTIVES

After completion of this chapter, the reader will be able to:

1. List the causes and pathology of thrombosis.
2. Describe the prevalence of thrombotic disease in developed countries.
3. Define thrombophilia.
4. Differentiate between acquired and congenital thrombosis risk factors.
5. List the thrombosis risk factors that are assayed in the clinical laboratory.
6. Distinguish between venous and arterial thrombosis.
7. List the prevalence of the heritable risk factors in various ancestry groups.
8. Describe a clot-based lupus anticoagulant (LAC) test profile with diagnostic validity.
9. Describe anticardiolipin antibody and anti-β_2-glycoprotein I antibody assays.
10. Interpret the results of LAC, anticardiolipin, and anti-β_2-glycoprotein I antibody assays.
11. Diagram the protein C and protein S coagulation control pathway.
12. Describe the thrombotic relevance of assays for antithrombin, protein C and protein S, activated protein C resistance, factor V Leiden, and the prothrombin G20210A.
13. Describe the ability of the lipoprotein (a) and fibrinogen assays to assess arterial thrombotic risk.
14. Describe the causes and pathophysiology of disseminated intravascular coagulation (DIC).
15. Describe the assays comprising a primary test profile, and list advanced assays, for diagnosis and management of DIC.
16. Demonstrate the validity of quantitative D-dimer assays for DIC and venous thromboembolic disease.
17. Describe the pathophysiology, and clinical and laboratory diagnosis, of heparin-induced thrombocytopenia (HIT).
18. Distinguish primary HIT enzyme immunoassay assays from confirmatory platelet activation assays.
19. Diagram the mechanism of thromboinflammation.
20. Describe laboratory assays for thromboinflammation.
21. Given clinical history and laboratory test results for patients with thrombophilia, suggest a diagnosis that is consistent with the information provided.

OUTLINE

Thrombosis Risk Testing Developments
Thrombosis Etiology and Prevalence
    Thrombosis Etiology
    Thrombosis Prevalence
Thrombosis Risk Factors
    Acquired Thrombosis Risk Factors
    Congenital Thrombosis Risk Factors
    Thrombosis Double Hit
Laboratory Evaluation of Thrombophilia
    Antiphospholipid Antibodies
    Activated Protein C Resistance and Factor V Leiden Mutation
    Prothrombin G20210A
    Antithrombin
    Protein C Control Pathway
Arterial Thrombosis Predictors
    Lipoprotein (a)
    C-Reactive Protein
    Brain Natriuretic Peptide
    Fibrinogen Activity
    Factor VIII

Venous Thromboembolic Disease Diagnosis
    Deep Venous Thrombosis Symptoms
    Pulmonary Embolism Symptoms
    Deep Venous Thrombosis and Pulmonary Embolism Diagnostic Tests: D-Dimer
Disseminated Intravascular Coagulation
    Causes of Disseminated Intravascular Coagulation
    Pathophysiology of Disseminated Intravascular Coagulation
    Symptoms of Disseminated Intravascular Coagulation
    Laboratory Diagnosis of Disseminated Intravascular Coagulation
    Disseminated Intravascular Coagulation Treatment
Heparin-Induced Thrombocytopenia
    Pathophysiology of Heparin-Induced Thrombocytopenia
    Laboratory Diagnosis of Heparin-Induced Thrombocytopenia
    Therapy for Heparin-Induced Thrombocytopenia
Thromboinflammation
Thrombosis Risk Testing Future

CASE STUDY

After studying the material in this chapter, the reader should be able to respond to the following case study. Answers can be found in Appendix C.

A 42-year-old female with no significant medical history developed sudden onset of shortness of breath and chest pain. She was taken to an emergency department, where a pulmonary embolism was diagnosed using computed tomography. The emergency department provider initiated intravenous heparin therapy. After admission, the pulmonologist ordered a thrombosis risk assay profile.

1. For what conditions can the patient be tested while in the hospital?
2. List acquired thrombosis risk factors that could account for the pulmonary embolism.
3. How does a thrombosis risk factor affect laboratory management, therapy, and lifestyle?

THROMBOSIS RISK TESTING DEVELOPMENTS

Before 1992, medical laboratory professionals performed assays to detect only three inherited venous thrombosis risk factors: deficiencies of the coagulation control factors antithrombin (AT), protein C (PC), and protein S (PS).[1] These three deficiencies taken together appear in 0.9% of the unselected population and account for an increased risk of a first *venous thromboembolism* (VTE), but they had no apparent relationship to *arterial thrombosis*.[2] Since the report by Dahlbäck and colleagues[3] of activated protein C (APC) resistance in 1993 and the characterization by Bertina and colleagues[4] of the factor V Leiden (FVL) mutation as its cause in 1994, efforts devoted to thrombosis risk prediction and evaluation have led to the list of current assays that includes AT, PC, PS, APC resistance, FVL mutation, prothrombin G20210A mutation, lupus anticoagulant (LAC), and antiphospholipid (APL) antibodies. The quantitative D-dimer assay is instrumental in ruling out VTE and helps detect and monitor disseminated intravascular coagulation (DIC).[5]

THROMBOSIS ETIOLOGY AND PREVALENCE

Thrombosis Etiology

Thrombosis is the inappropriate formation of a *platelet* or *fibrin* clot that obstructs a blood vessel. Thrombosis is a multifaceted disorder resulting from circulatory stasis and abnormalities in the coagulation system, coagulation control mechanisms, platelet function, the endothelium, or inflammatory cytokines. Thrombotic obstructions cause *ischemia* (loss of blood supply) and *necrosis* (tissue death).[6]

Thrombophilia (previously called *hypercoagulability*) is the predisposition to thrombosis secondary to a congenital or acquired condition. Known causes of thrombophilia include the following:

- Physical, chemical, or biological events related to chronic or acute inflammation that release prothrombotic mediators from damaged blood vessels or suppress blood vessel production of normal antithrombotic substances
- Uncontrolled platelet activation
- Uncontrolled blood coagulation system activation
- Blood coagulation control protein deficiencies
- Uncontrolled suppression of fibrinolysis

Thrombosis Prevalence

From 2000 to 2010 the US death rate attributable to venous and arterial thrombotic disease declined 31%, and the number of thrombosis-related deaths declined by 17% per year. Yet in 2010 thrombosis accounted for one of every four deaths in the United States.[7] Of these, 25% of initial thrombotic events were fatal, and many fatal thromboses remained undiagnosed before autopsy.[8]

Prevalence of Venous Thromboembolic Disease

The annual incidence of VTE in the United States is estimated to be 104 to 183 per 100,000 among individuals of European descent and is more prevalent in females of childbearing age.[9,10] The most prevalent VTE is *deep venous thrombosis* (DVT), caused by clots that form in the iliac, popliteal, and femoral veins of the calves and upper legs.[11] Large occlusive thrombi may also form, although less often, in the veins of the upper extremities, liver, spleen, intestines, brain, and kidneys. Thrombosis symptoms include localized pain, the sensation of heat, erythema (redness), and edema.

Fragments of thrombi, called *emboli*, may separate from the proximal end of a venous thrombus. Emboli that move swiftly through the right chambers of the heart and lodge in the arterial pulmonary vasculature, causing ischemia and necrosis of lung tissue, are called *pulmonary emboli* (PEs).[12] Nearly 95% of PEs arise from thrombi in the deep leg and calf veins. Of the 250,000 US residents per year who experience PE, 10% to 15% die within 3 months. Since 2008 the death rates for PE have begun to climb back again at an average of 0.6% per year.[13] Many PE cases remain undiagnosed because of the ambiguity of the symptoms, which may resemble those of acute coronary syndrome (ACS), pleurisy, or pneumonia. PE has been nicknamed the great masquerader.

VTE risk factors parallel the risk factors for ACS, peripheral artery disease, and stroke. Advancing age, obesity, recent surgery or trauma, immobilization and hospitalization, hypertension, hypercholesterolemia, smoking, diabetes mellitus, and metabolic syndrome increase the risk of thrombotic disorders. The pathophysiology begins with chronic inflammation, thrombophilia, and endothelial cell (EC) injury. Coagulation system imbalances, such as inappropriate activation, gain of coagulation factor function, inadequate control of thrombin generation, or suppressed fibrinolysis, are the resulting VTE mechanisms. Chronic medical conditions resulting from malignancy; chronic heart, lung, or renal disease; rheumatological or gastrointestinal problems; or respiratory problems such as asthma or obstructive sleep apnea are often implicated in VTE.[14] Cancers associated with VTE include gastric, pancreatic, lung, gynecologic, and testicular cancers as well as lymphoma and acute leukemia. Predilection for DVT versus PE has a familial distribution.

Prevalence of Arterial Thrombosis

In 2016, the worldwide age-adjusted cardiovascular disease death rate was 278 per 100 000, a total of 17.6 million. Approximately 80% of acute myocardial infarctions and 85% of strokes are caused by thrombi that block coronary arteries or carotid end arteries of the vertebrobasilar system, respectively.[15] Transient ischemic attacks and peripheral arterial occlusions are more frequent than strokes and coronary artery disease and, although not fatal, represent substantial morbidity. Recent studies also suggest that coronavirus disease 2019 (COVID-19) may be an independent risk factor for arterial thrombosis.[16]

One important mechanism for arterial thrombosis is the well-described vessel wall unstable atherosclerotic plaque. Activated platelets, monocytes, and macrophages embed fatty plaque within the endothelial lining, suppressing the normal release of anti-thrombotic molecules such as nitric oxide and exposing prothrombotic substances such as tissue factor (Chapter 35). Small plaques rupture, occluding arteries and releasing mediators that trigger thrombotic events. The mediators activate platelets (Chapter 11), which combine with von Willebrand factor (VWF) to form arterial platelet plugs—the "white thrombi" that cause arterial ischemia and necrosis of surrounding tissue.

The hemostasis-related lesions we associate with arterial thrombosis are blood vessel wall destruction and platelet activation. Often these are inseparable. Researchers continue to examine new thrombosis markers that capture pathologic events in platelets and ECs before a thrombotic event occurs.[17]

THROMBOSIS RISK FACTORS

Acquired Thrombosis Risk Factors

Throughout life, we acquire a legion of habits and circumstances that either help maintain or damage our hemostasis system. Their variety and interplay make it difficult to pinpoint the factors that contribute to thrombosis or to determine which have the greatest influence. These factors seem to contribute to venous and arterial thrombosis in varying degrees. Table 39.1 lists the nondisease, *lifestyle risk factors* implicated in thrombosis.[18]

In addition to life events, several *conditions and diseases* have thrombotic risk components. Some of these are listed in Table 39.2, along with the laboratory's diagnostic contribution.[19]

Together, transient and chronic APL antibodies such as LAC and anti-β_2-glycoprotein I (anti-β_2-GPI) autoantibodies may be detected in 1% to 4% of the healthy population. The frequency of the specific type of APL antibody, anticardiolipin (ACL) antibodies, was found to be between 0.1% and 10% higher in healthy adults compared with younger patients, and similar trends were observed when adults with chronic illness were compared with a healthy adult population.[20] Chronic APL antibodies confer a risk of venous or arterial thrombosis, a condition known as antiphospholipid syndrome (APS). Chronic APL antibodies often accompany autoimmune connective tissue disorders, such as lupus erythematosus. Some appear in patients without any apparent primary disorder.

Malignancies often are implicated in venous thrombosis. One mechanism is tumor production of tissue factor analogs that trigger chronic low-grade DIC. In addition, venous and arterial stasis and inflammatory effects increase the risk of thrombosis. Migratory thrombophlebitis, or Trousseau syndrome, is a sign of occult adenocarcinoma such as cancer of the pancreas or colon.[21]

Myeloproliferative neoplasms such as essential thrombocythemia and polycythemia vera (Chapter 32) may trigger thrombosis, probably through platelet hyperactivity. A cardinal sign of acute promyelocytic leukemia (Chapter 31) is DIC secondary to the release of procoagulant granule contents from malignant promyelocytes. DIC may intensify during therapy at the time of vigorous cell lysis because of increased thrombin generation.[22] Paroxysmal

TABLE 39.1	Nondisease (Lifestyle) Factors That Contribute to Thrombosis		
Risk Factor	**Comment**	**Contribution to Thrombosis**	**Laboratory Diagnosis**
Age	Thrombosis after age 50	Risk doubles each decade after 50	
Immobilization	Sedentary, distance driving, air travel, restriction to wheelchair or bed, obesity	Slowed blood flow raises thrombosis risk	
Lipid metabolism imbalance	Hyperlipidemia, hypercholesterolemia, dyslipidemia, elevated triglycerides, decreased HDL-C, elevated LDL-C	Moderate arterial thrombosis association with LDL-C elevation and hypercholesterolemia, may be congenital	Lipid profile: TC, HDL-C, LDL-C, triglycerides
Oral contraceptive use	Formulated with progesterone	4× to 6× increased risk	
Pregnancy		3× to 5× increased risk	
Hormone replacement therapy		2× to 4× increased risk	
Femoral or tibial fracture		80% incidence of thrombosis if not treated with antithrombotic	
Hip, knee, gynecologic, prostate surgery		50% incidence of thrombosis if not treated with antithrombotic	
Smoking		Depends on degree	CRP
Inflammation	Chronic	Arterial thrombosis	CRP
Central venous catheter	Endothelial injury and activation	33% of children with central venous catheters develop venous thrombosis	

CRP, C-reactive protein; *HDL-C,* high-density lipoprotein cholesterol; *LDL-C,* low-density lipoprotein cholesterol; *TC,* total cholesterol.

TABLE 39.2 Diseases With Thrombotic Risk Components

Disease	Examples or Effects	Contribution to Thrombosis	Laboratory Diagnosis
Antiphospholipid syndrome	Chronic antiphospholipid antibody often secondary to autoimmune disorders	When chronic, 1.6× to 3.2× increased risk of stroke, myocardial infarction, recurrent spontaneous abortion, venous thrombosis	PTT mixing studies, lupus anticoagulant profile, anticardiolipin antibody, and anti-β_2-glycoprotein 1 immunoassays
Myeloproliferative neoplasms	Essential thrombocythemia, polycythemia vera, chronic myelogenous leukemia	Increased risk as a result of plasma viscosity, platelet activation	Platelet counts and platelet aggregometry
Hepatic disease	Diminished production of most coagulation control proteins	Increased risk as a result of deranged coagulation pathways, excess thrombin production, reduced fibrinolysis	Protein C, protein S, and antithrombin assays, factor assays, DIC profile
Cancer, adenocarcinoma	Trousseau syndrome, low-grade chronic DIC	20× increased risk of thrombosis; 10%–20% of people with idiopathic venous thrombosis have cancer	DIC profile: platelet count, D-dimer, PTT, PT, fibrinogen, blood film examination
Leukemia	Acute promyelocytic leukemia, acute monocytic leukemia	Increased risk for chronic DIC	DIC profile: platelet count, D-dimer, PTT, PT, fibrinogen, blood film examination
Paroxysmal nocturnal hemoglobinuria	Platelet-related thrombosis	Increased risk for DVT, PE, DIC	Flow cytometry phenotyping for CD55 and CD59; DIC profile: platelet count, D-dimer, PTT, PT, fibrinogen, blood film examination
Chronic inflammation	Diabetes, cancer, infection, autoimmune disorder, obesity, smoking		Fibrinogen, CRP, urinary 11-dehydrothromboxane B_2
Thromboinflammation	Retrovirus infection	Release of VWF, tissue factor, cytokines from endothelium	ADAMTS13:VWF ratio

ADAMTS13, **a** **d**isintegrin **a**nd **m**etalloproteinase with a **t**hrombo**s**pondin type 1 motif, member **13**; *CRP*, C-reactive protein; *DIC*, disseminated intravascular coagulation; *DVT*, deep venous thrombosis; *PE*, pulmonary embolism; *PT*, prothrombin time; *PTT*, partial thromboplastin time; *VWF*, von Willebrand factor.

nocturnal hemoglobinuria (Chapter 21) is caused by a stem cell mutation that modifies membrane-anchored platelet activation suppressors. Venous or arterial thromboses occur in at least 30% to 45% of paroxysmal nocturnal hemoglobinuria cases.[23]

Chronic inflammatory diseases cause thrombosis through a variety of mechanisms, such as fibrinogen and factor VIII (FVIII) elevation, suppressed fibrinolysis, promotion of atherosclerotic plaque formation, and reduced free PS activity secondary to increased C4b-binding protein (C4bBP) levels. Diabetes mellitus is a particularly dangerous chronic inflammatory condition that raises the risk of cardiovascular disease fivefold.[24]

Conditions associated with venous stasis, such as congestive heart failure, are also risk factors for venous thrombosis. Untreated atrial fibrillation increases the risk of ischemic stroke caused by clot formation in the right atrium and embolization to the brain.[25]

Nephrotic syndrome creates protein imbalances that lead to thrombosis through loss of plasma proteins such as antithrombin (AT). Nephrotic syndrome may also be associated with hemorrhage (Chapter 36).[26] However, it has been recently reported that there is no significant correlation between loss of AT activity and nephrotic syndrome in adults, but in pediatric patients with nephrotic syndrome, a qualitative deficiency of AT exists that may be corrected by therapeutic interventions.[27]

Congenital Thrombosis Risk Factors

Providers suspect congenital thrombophilia when a thrombotic event occurs in young adults; occurs in unusual sites such as the mesenteric, renal, or axillary veins; is recurrent; or occurs in a patient with a family history of thrombosis (Table 39.3). Because thrombosis is multifactorial, however, even patients with congenital thrombophilia

are most likely to experience thrombotic events because of a combination of constitutional and acquired conditions.[28]

The AT activity assay (previously called the antithrombin III or AT III assay) has been available since 1972, and protein C (PC) and protein S (PS) activity assays became available in the mid-1980s. In the 1990s the APC resistance assay and its confirmatory FVL mutation molecular assay plus the prothrombin G20210A mutation molecular assay became available. More recently developed tests include assays for polymorphisms in FVIII and FXI genes, dysfibrinogenemia, plasminogen deficiency, plasma tissue plasminogen activator (TPA), and plasma plasminogen activator inhibitor-1 (PAI-1).[29]

APC resistance is found in 3% to 8% of individuals of Northern European ancestry. APC resistance extends to Arab and Hispanic populations, but the mutation is nearly absent from African and East Asian populations.[30] APC resistance may exist in the absence of the FVL mutation and is occasionally acquired in pregnancy or in association with oral contraceptive therapy.[31,32]

The FVL gene mutation is the most common inherited thrombosis risk factor, and the prothrombin G20210A gene mutation is the second most common inherited thrombophilia in patients with a personal and family history of DVT.[33] Altogether, PC, PS, and AT deficiencies are found in only 0.2% to 1.0% of the world population. Homocysteinemia, once thought to be an important risk factor, has been found to have a limited association with increased risks of venous or arterial thrombosis.[34,35]

Thrombosis Double Hit

Thrombosis often is associated with a combination of genetic defect, disease, and lifestyle influences. Just because someone

TABLE 39.3 Predisposing Congenital Factors and Thrombosis Risk

| Risk Factor | Function | Thrombosis Relative Risk | PREVALENCE | | Laboratory Assays |
			Unselected Population	≥1 Thrombotic Event	
Antithrombin (AT) deficiency	AT, enhanced by heparin, inhibits FIIa (thrombin) and FXa	Heterozygous: 10× to 20× Homozygous: 100%, rarely reported	1 in 2–5000	1%–1.8%	Clot-based and chromogenic AT activity assays, AT concentration by immunoassay
Protein C (PC) deficiency	Activated PC is a serine protease that hydrolyzes FVa and FVIIIa, requires PS as a stabilizing cofactor	Heterozygous: 2× to 5× Homozygous: 100%, neonatal purpura fulminans	1 in 300	2.5%–5%	Clot-based and chromogenic PC activity assays, PC concentration by immunoassay
Free protein S (PS) deficiency	PS is a stabilizing cofactor for APC, 40% free, 60% circulates bound to C4bBP	Heterozygous: 1.6× to 11.5× Homozygous: 100% but rarely reported, neonatal purpura fulminans	Unknown	2.8%–5%	Clot-based free PS activity assays, PS concentration by free and total immunoassays
APC resistance	FV Leiden (R506Q) mutation gain of function renders FV resistant to APC	Heterozygous: 3× Homozygous: 18×	3%–8% of individuals of Northern European ancestry, uncommon in individuals of Asian and African ancestry	20%–25%	PTT-based APC resistance test and confirmatory molecular assay
Prothrombin G20210A	Mutation in prothrombin gene untranslated 3′ promoter region; moderate prothrombin activity elevation	Heterozygous: 1.6× to 11.5×	2%–3% of individuals of Northern European ancestry, less common in individuals of Asian and African ancestry	4%–8%	Molecular assay only; phenotypic assay provides no specificity
Hyperfibrinogenemia	Associated with arterial thrombosis	Acute phase reactant			Clauss fibrinogen clotting assay, immunoassay, nephelometric assay

APC, Activated protein C; *C4bBP,* complement component C4b-binding protein; *F,* coagulation factor; *PTT,* partial thromboplastin time.

possesses AT, PC, or PS deficiency does not mean that thrombosis is inevitable. Many heterozygotes experience no thrombotic event during their lifetime, whereas others experience clotting only when two or more risk factors converge. To illustrate, a female who is heterozygous for the FVL mutation has a 35-fold increase in thrombosis risk when using oral contraceptives.

LABORATORY EVALUATION OF THROMBOPHILIA

When the provider suspects thrombophilia, it is appropriate to assess all clinically significant risk factors. It is the accumulation of factors that determines the patient's risk of thrombosis.[36] Table 39.4 summarizes the clinically useful thrombosis risk assays and indicates those that can be relied on for accurate results during the acute inflammation that occurs immediately after a thrombotic event or while the patient is on anticoagulant therapy.

Experts discourage thrombosis risk testing immediately after a thrombotic event. The presence of a documented risk factor does not revise acute thrombosis therapy. Further, antithrombotic therapy and ongoing or recent thrombotic events interfere with the interpretation of clot-based AT, PC, PS, APC resistance, fibrinogen, and LAC testing results. These assays should be performed at least 14 days after anticoagulant therapy is discontinued. Connors writes, "Most patients with venous thromboembolism do not require thrombophilia testing, since the results will not affect management. Testing may be considered in younger patients with weak provoking factors, a strong family history, or recurrence at a young age."[37]

Antiphospholipid Antibodies

APL antibodies comprise a family of immunoglobulins that bind protein-phospholipid complexes.[38] APL antibodies include LACs, detected by clot-based profiles, and ACL and anti-β_2-GPI antibodies, detected by immunoassay. Chronic autoimmune APL antibodies are associated with APS, which is characterized by transient ischemic attacks, strokes, coronary and peripheral artery disease, venous thromboembolism, and recurrent pregnancy complications including pregnancy loss.[39]

APL antibodies arise as immunoglobulin M (IgM) or IgG isotypes. Because they may bind a variety of protein-phospholipid complexes, they are sometimes called nonspecific inhibitors. Their name implies that they were once thought to directly bind phospholipids; however, their target antigens are actually the proteins that assemble on anionic phospholipid surfaces. The plasma protein most often bound by APL antibodies is β_2-GPI, although annexin V and prothrombin are sometimes implicated as APL antibody targets. APL antibodies probably develop in response to newly formed protein-phospholipid complexes, and laboratory scientists continue to investigate how they cause thrombosis.[40–42]

Clinical Consequences of Antiphospholipid Antibodies

APL antibodies are present in 1% to 2% of unselected individuals of both sexes and all races and 5% to 15% of individuals

TABLE 39.4	**Thrombophilia Laboratory Test Profile**	
Assay	**Reference Interval**	**Comments**
APC resistance	Ratio ≥1.8	Clot-based screen employs PTT with FV-depleted plasma.
FV Leiden mutation*	Wild type	Molecular assay performed as followup to APC resistance ratio when it is <1.8.
Prothrombin G20210A*	Wild type	Molecular assay. There is no phenotypic assay for prothrombin G20210A.
LAC profile	Negative for LAC	Perform a minimum of two clot-based assays. Primary assays are based on DRVVT and PTT. Both include phospholipid neutralization follow-up test.
ACL antibody*	IgG: <12 GPL IgM: <10 MPL	Immunoassay for immunoglobulins of APL family. ACL depends on β_2-GPI in reaction mix.
Anti-β_2-GPI antibody*	IgG: <20 G units IgM: <20 M units	Immunoassay for an immunoglobulin of APL family. β_2-GPI is the key phospholipid-binding protein in the APL family.
AT activity	78%–126%	Serine protease inhibitor suppresses FIIa (thrombin) and FXa. When consistently below the reference interval, follow up with AT antigen assay.
PC activity	70%–140%	Activated PC digests FVIIIa and FVa. When consistently below reference interval, follow up with PC antigen assay.
PS activity	65%–140%	PC cofactor. When consistently below the reference interval, follow up with total and free PS antigen assay, C4b-binding protein assay.
Fibrinogen	220–498 mg/dL	Clot-based assay. Chronic elevation may be associated with arterial thrombosis.

*These measurements are valid during active thrombosis or anticoagulant therapy. All other measurements must be performed 14 days after anticoagulant therapy is discontinued.

ACL, Anticardiolipin; *APC,* activated protein C; *APL,* antiphospholipid antibody; *AT,* antithrombin; *β_2-GPI,* β_2-glycoprotein I; *DRVVT,* dilute Russell viper venom time; *F,* coagulation factor; *GPL,* IgG antiphospholipid antibody unit; *Ig,* immunoglobulin; *LAC,* lupus anticoagulant; *MPL,* IgM antiphospholipid antibody unit; *PC,* protein C; *PS,* protein S; *PTT,* partial thromboplastin time.

with recurrent venous or arterial thrombotic disease.[43] Most APL antibodies arise in response to a bacterial, viral, fungal, or parasitic infection or to treatment with one of a variety of drugs (Box 39.1) and disappear within 12 weeks. These are transient alloimmune APL antibodies with no clinical consequences. Nevertheless, the provider must follow up any positive APL antibody result to determine persistence. A relationship may exist between APL antibody and C-reactive protein (CRP), both of which may be associated with elevated thrombotic risk, and consequently, many laboratory directors add the CRP assay to their APL antibody test profile.[44,45]

Autoimmune APL antibodies are part of the family of autoantibodies that arise in collagen vascular diseases; 50% of patients with systemic lupus erythematosus have autoimmune APL antibodies. Autoimmune APL antibodies are also detected in patients with rheumatoid arthritis, scleroderma, and Sjögren syndrome but may arise spontaneously, which is termed *primary APS*. Autoimmune APL antibodies may persist, and 30% are associated with arterial and venous thrombosis. Chronic presence of an autoimmune APL antibody not associated with

a known underlying autoimmune disorder confers a 1.8- to 3.2-fold increased risk of thrombosis.[46]

A rare condition associated with APL antibody production is *catastrophic APS.* Due to widespread clotting over a short period (usually within a week), multiorgan failure occurs. Catastrophic APS is a medical emergency with a high mortality risk.

Detection and Confirmation of Antiphospholipid Antibodies

Providers suspect APS in patients with unexplained venous or arterial thrombosis, thrombocytopenia, or recurrent fetal loss.[47] Specialized clinical hemostasis laboratories offer APL antibody detection profiles that include clot-based assays for LAC and immunoassays for ACL and anti-β_2-GPI antibodies. Occasionally an LAC is suspected because of an unexplained prolonged PTT that does not correct in mixing studies (Figure 39.1).[48]

The mixing study (Chapter 41) is a first step in the LAC laboratory workup to establish the presence of an LAC because it can differentiate an LAC from a factor deficiency. In addition to the LAC, the mixing study is sensitive to other factor inhibitors such as anti-FVIII inhibitors.

Lupus Anticoagulant Test Profile

Clot-based assays with reduced reagent phospholipid concentrations are sensitive to LAC. There are two commonly used test systems, and both are required for an LAC profile. The need for two parallel assay systems arises from the multiplicity of LAC reaction characteristics: a confirmed positive result in one system is conclusive despite a negative result in the other. The two most commonly recommended test systems are the

BOX 39.1	**Agents Known to Induce Antiphospholipid Antibodies**
Various antibiotics	Procainamide
Phenothiazine	Phenytoin
Hydralazine	Cocaine
Quinine and quinidine	Elevated estrogens
Calcium channel blockers	

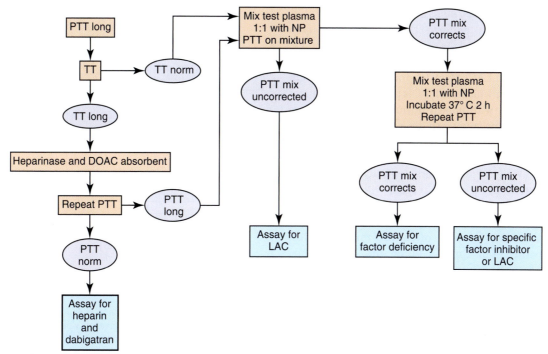

Figure 39.1 Mixing Study Employing a Partial Thromboplastin Time *(PTT)* Reagent With Intermediate Lupus Anticoagulant *(LAC)* Sensitivity. Beginning at the top left, when the PTT result exceeds the upper limit of the PTT reference interval, perform a thrombin time *(TT)* to detect unfractionated heparin (inpatient) or dabigatran (outpatient). If the TT exceeds the TT reference interval, presume that heparin or dabigatran is present. Treat an aliquot of the specimen with heparinase and another with a direct oral anticoagulant *(DOAC)* absorbent and repeat the PTT. If the new PTT is normal, assay the original sample for heparin and dabigatran. If the PTT remains prolonged, proceed by mixing the patient plasma with normal plasma *(NP)* and perform a PTT on the mixture. If the PTT remains prolonged (uncorrected) compared to the NP, proceed to assay for LAC. If the PTT mixture corrects, prepare a new 1:1 mix and incubate at 37° C for 2 hours and repeat the PTT, comparing the result with incubated NP. If the incubated PTT shows a correction, assay for a factor deficiency. If the incubated PTT remains prolonged, assay for a specific inhibitor such as anti-factor VIII or LAC (Figures 39.2 and 39.3). In 15% of cases, temperature-dependent LAC may be detected after incubation.

dilute Russell viper venom time (DRVVT) and the silica-based PTT, also called the silica clot time (SCT), both formulated with low-phospholipid concentrations designed to be LAC sensitive.[49] The time-honored dilute thromboplastin time (DTT), also named the tissue thromboplastin inhibitor assay, is used in many institutions and available from specialty laboratories and coagulation reagent distributors.[50] As illustrated in Figure 39.2, the PTT initiates coagulation at the level of FXII; DRVVT, at FX; and DTT, at FVII.

The 2020 International Society on Thrombosis and Haemostasis (ISTH) guidelines for LAC detection[49] require the following sequence:

1. Prolonged phospholipid-dependent clot formation using an initial (primary) assay such as a low-phospholipid PTT or DRVVT, often called the PTT or DRVVT *screen.*
2. Failure to correct the prolonged clot time when mixing with normal platelet-poor plasma and repeating the test.[51]
3. Shortening or correction of the prolonged initial assay result by addition of a reagent formulated with excess phospholipids, often called the PTT or DRVVT *confirm.*
4. Exclusion of other coagulopathies.

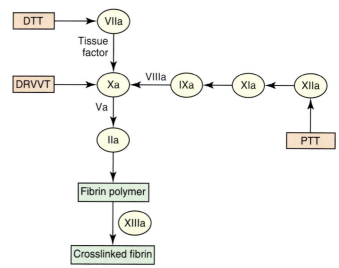

Figure 39.2 Simplified Coagulation Pathway Illustrating the Activation Points of the Lupus Anticoagulant (LAC) Assays. The dilute Russell viper venom time *(DRVVT)* assay, regarded as the most reliable LAC detection method, activates factor X. LAC-sensitive partial thromboplastin time *(PTT)* assay activates factor XII. The dilute thromboplastin time *(DTT)* test activates factor VII.

Performing the clot-based lupus anticoagulant test profile.
Laboratory practitioners perform the LAC profile upon provider request, often to find the cause for adverse thrombotic or obstetric events, or when an isolated prolonged PTT raises the presumption of an LAC. Many laboratory protocols begin with a mixing study in which the PTT is performed on patient plasma combined 1:1 with pooled normal plasma (NP) (see Figure 39.1). The mixing study includes a second step that uses a 2-hour, 37° C incubation because most specific inhibitors such as anti-FVIII and 15% of LACs require incubation to enhance their avidity. Practitioners typically perform the initial mixing study using a PTT reagent with intermediate LAC sensitivity.[52]

The mixing study includes a means for detecting unfractionated heparin (UFH), most often the thrombin clotting time or thrombin time (TT) or the chromogenic anti-FXa heparin assay. The practitioner may add heparinase (Hepzyme, Siemens) to the specimen to neutralize heparin, although this may be unnecessary because many LAC detection reagents provide heparin-neutralizing polybrene. Contamination from the direct oral anticoagulant (DOAC) dabigatran can similarly interfere with the PTT-based mixing study; a DOAC absorbent is available for its neutralization. Mixing studies based on a prothrombin time (PT), a DRVVT, or an LAC-sensitive PTT reagent seldom require 37° C incubation.

The NP that is mixed 1:1 with patient plasma is expected to shorten a prolonged PTT. Each laboratory director decides what degree of PTT shortening constitutes correction. Many define correction as a mixture result within 10% of the NP result; others define correction as return to a value within the PTT reference interval.

In performing mixing studies, the laboratory professional employs only platelet-poor plasma, which is plasma centrifuged so that it has a platelet count of less than 10,000/μL (Chapter 41). The use of platelet-poor plasma avoids LAC neutralization by platelet membrane phospholipids. Platelet membrane fragments that form during freezing and thawing can likewise neutralize LAC and lead to a false-negative LAC result.

Performing clot-based lupus anticoagulant tests.
Following a mixing study whose lack of correction suggests the presence of an LAC, the practitioner performs LAC-specific testing. Most LAC protocols begin with the DRVVT, considered the more specific of the LAC assays (Figure 39.3). If the DRVVT primary (screen) reagent-patient plasma result exceeds the upper limit of the DRVVT reference interval, LAC is presumed. The practitioner then confirms LAC by mixing an aliquot of the patient specimen with the DRVVT high-phospholipid confirmatory reagent, comparing the result in seconds to the DRVVT primary reagent patient plasma result. The reagent phospholipid neutralizes LAC and shortens the DRVVT. If the primary reagent result is prolonged over the DRVVT confirm reagent result (primary/confirm ratio) by a predetermined ratio or more, typically 1.2, LAC is confirmed.[53]

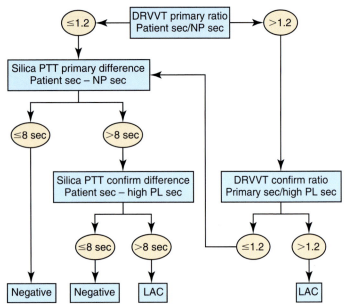

Figure 39.3 Lupus Anticoagulant *(LAC)* Algorithm. When LAC is suspected, perform the dilute Russell viper venom *(DRVVT) primary* (screen) assay, comparing the patient DRVVT result with the pooled normal plasma *(NP)* DRVVT result. If the ratio of patient to NP DRVVT in seconds is greater than 1.2, mix patient plasma 1:1 with high-phospholipid *(PL)* DRVVT *confirm* reagent and perform a new DRVVT assay. If the primary patient DRVVT result exceeds the DRVVT confirm patient plasma result by greater than 1.2, LAC is confirmed. If the ratio is 1.2 or less or if the primary DRVVT ratio was 1.2 or less, proceed to silica-based partial thromboplastin *(PTT)* primary and confirm assays. Compare the primary patient silica-based PTT to the NP result. If the difference is 8 seconds or less, no LAC is present. If the difference is greater than 8 seconds, mix the patient plasma with high-PL silica-based PTT confirm reagent and perform a new PTT. If the primary patient PTT exceeds the patient PTT confirm by more than 8 seconds, LAC is confirmed; if 8 seconds or less, LAC is not present.

If the DRVVT primary/confirm ratio is less than 1.2, the practitioner turns to the silica-based low-phospholipid LAC-sensitive PTT, using the same steps used for the DRVVT. In this instance, the difference between the primary (screen) and confirmatory reagent may be expressed as a ratio or in seconds; typically, a difference of 8 seconds is the threshold used to confirm an LAC.[53,54]

Numerous modifications to this algorithm exist. Many laboratory directors prefer to begin with the silica-based low-phospholipid PTT assay, and others include an intermediate NP mixing study step. Some incorporate the DTT. The 1.2 ratio and the 8-second difference are examples; each institution may choose to establish its own reference interval and threshold ratio or difference.

Some laboratory directors choose to normalize DRVVT or PTT-based ratios using the mean of the reference interval (MRI) or the NP value. The formula for normalization using the MRI is:

$$\text{Normalized ratio} = \frac{\text{Primary mix result in seconds}/\text{MRI}}{\text{Confirm mix results in seconds}/\text{MRI}} = \frac{\text{Primary ratio}}{\text{Confirm ratio}}$$

This formula is applied to both the DRVVT and the PTT-based assays. Because they are clot based, assays for LAC are affected by anticoagulant therapy, including oral anticoagulants, current thrombosis, and factor deficiencies.

Anticardiolipin Antibody Immunoassay

LAC and ACL antibodies coexist in 60% of cases, and both may be found in APS. The ACL test is an immunoassay that is not affected by anticoagulant therapy, current thrombosis, or factor deficiencies.[55] Evidence supports that antibodies directed at cardiolipin are mainly associated with infection, whereas patients with APS have β_2-GPI bound to cardiolipin as the antigenic target. Better-performing assays for anticardiolipin antibodies incorporate a complex of cardiolipin-β_2-GPI.

The manufacturer coats microplate wells with bovine heart cardiolipin and blocks (fills open receptor sites) with bovine serum. A solution containing β_2-GPI is then added. The laboratory practitioner pipettes test sera or plasmas to the wells alongside calibrators and controls (Figure 39.4).[56] ACL antibodies bind the solid-phase cardiolipin-β_2-GPI target complex and cannot be washed from the wells. The practitioner adds enzyme-labeled anti-human IgM or IgG conjugate after washing, followed by a color- or fluorophore-generating substrate. A color or fluorescence change indicates the presence of ACL, and intensities of the patient and control sample wells are compared with the calibrator curve wells. Results are expressed using GPL or MPL units, where 1 unit is equivalent to 1 μg/mL of an affinity-purified standard IgG or IgM sample.

Anti-β_2-Glycoprotein 1 Immunoassay

The practitioner performs IgM and IgG anti-β_2-GPI immunoassays as a part of the APS profile that includes the ACL assay. An anti-β_2-GPI result of greater than 20 IgG or IgM anti-β_2-GPI units correlates with thrombosis more closely than the presence of ACL antibodies.[57] Alternative newer detection techniques that can be run on automated coagulation analyzers using chemiluminescent fluorescent techniques or multiplex flow immunoassay methods are easier to use, apply consistent protocols, and show fewer interlaboratory and interoperator variations for APL detection assays.[58] Any positive ACL or anti-β_2-GPI assay repeated on a new specimen collected after 12 weeks distinguishes a transient alloantibody from a chronic autoantibody.

Antiphosphatidylserine and Antiprothrombin Immunoassays

For cases in which an APL antibody is suspected but the routine LAC, ACL, and β_2-GPI assay results are negative, the provider may wish to order antiphosphatidylserine and antiprothrombin immunoassays to detect APL antibodies specific for phosphatidylserine or prothrombin.[59] Antiphosphatidylserine and antiprothrombin assays are available from specialty reference laboratories.

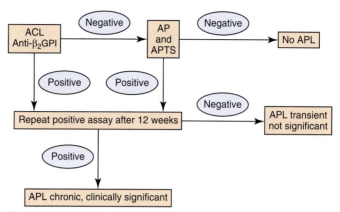

Figure 39.4 Antiphospholipid Antibody *(APL)* Immunoassay Algorithm. If APL is suspected, perform an anticardiolipin *(ACL)* or anti-β_2-glycoprotein I *(anti-β_2-GPI)* immunoassay. If either is positive, confirm chronicity using a new specimen collected at least 12 weeks later. If negative, perform an immunoassay to detect an antiprothrombin *(AP)* or antiphosphatidylserine *(APTS)* antibody. If positive, repeat after 12 weeks.

Activated Protein C Resistance and Factor V Leiden Mutation

Clinical Importance of Activated Protein C Resistance

When stabilized by PS, APC hydrolyzes activated factors V and VIII (FVa and FVIIIa). A mutation in the FV gene substitutes glutamine for arginine at position 506 of the FV molecule *(F5R506Q)*.[60,61] The arginine molecule is the normal cleavage site for APC, so the substitution slows or resists APC hydrolysis. The resistant FVa remains active (a gain of function) and raises thrombin activation, leading to thrombosis. The *F5R506Q* mutation is named for the city in The Netherlands in which Bertina first described it, Leiden (FVL mutation, also called APC resistance). Between 3% and 8% individuals of Northern European ancestry possess the FVL mutation (see Table 39.4).[62,63] Owing to its prevalence and the associated 3-fold higher thrombosis risk (18-fold higher for homozygotes), most acute care hemostasis laboratory directors provide APC resistance detection to screen for FVL.[64]

Activated Protein C Resistance Clot-Based Assay

In the APC resistance clot-based assay, patient plasma is mixed 1:4 with FV-depleted plasma.[65] PTT reagent is added to two aliquots of the mixture and incubated for 3 minutes (Figure 39.5). A solution of calcium chloride is pipetted into one mixture, and the clot formation is timed. A solution of calcium chloride *with APC* is added to the second mixture, and clotting is timed. The interval to clot formation of the second aliquot is expected to be at least 1.8 times longer than the time to clot formation of the first, increased by the presence of APC, so the expected ratio of PTT results between the two assays is 1.8 or greater. In APC resistance, the ratio is less than 1.8.

FV-depleted plasma compensates for potential factor deficiencies and for oral anticoagulant therapy by providing normal

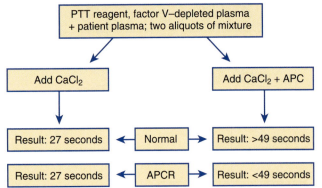

Figure 39.5 Activated Protein C Resistance Ratio *(APCR)* Measurement. Patient plasma is mixed 1:4 with factor V–depleted plasma and partial thromboplastin time *(PTT)* reagent. Two aliquots of this mixture are tested: one aliquot is mixed with calcium chloride *(CaCl₂)* alone, and the other aliquot is mixed with CaCl₂ plus activated protein C *(APC)*. The reaction in the mixture with the APC should be prolonged to at least 1.8 times longer than the mixture without APC. The results in seconds are examples. A ratio of 1.8 or less implies APC resistance.

coagulation factors. The laboratory professional uses only platelet-poor plasma in the APC resistance test to prevent loss of sensitivity caused by the release of FV, abundant in platelet α-granules. APC resistance reagent test kits contain polybrene or heparinase to neutralize UFH. LAC, however, affects the test system adversely.[66] If LAC is present, the molecular test for FVL is indicated.[67]

A similar clot-based assay for APC resistance, using the Russell viper venom reagent instead of the PTT reagent, is also available.

Factor V Leiden Mutation Assay

Most laboratories confirm the APC resistance diagnosis using the molecular FVL mutation test. Some laboratories omit the APC resistance test and directly measure FVL by molecular genetic testing. Determination of zygosity is necessary to predict the risk for thrombosis and establish a treatment regimen.

Prothrombin G20210A

A guanine-to-adenine mutation at base 20210 of the 3′ untranslated region of the prothrombin (FII) gene has been associated with mildly elevated plasma prothrombin levels, averaging 130%.[68] The increased risk of thrombosis in individuals with the mutation seems to be related to the elevated prothrombin activity.[69] The prevalence of this mutation among individuals with familial thrombosis is 5% to 18%, whereas prevalence worldwide is 0.3% to 2.4%.[70] The risk of venous thrombosis in heterozygotes is two to five times the baseline risk.[71] Although the mutation may cause a slight prothrombin elevation, a phenotypic prothrombin activity assay is of little diagnostic value because there is considerable overlap between normal prothrombin levels and prothrombin levels in people with the mutation.[72] Diagnosis of the prothrombin G20210A mutation requires molecular genetic testing.

Antithrombin

AT is a serine protease inhibitor (SERPIN) that neutralizes FII (thrombin), FIXa, FXa, FXIa, and FXIIa, all the coagulation system serine proteases except FVIIa (Chapter 35). AT activity is enhanced through binding to exogenous heparan sulfate found on EC surfaces. AT activity is enhanced 1000-fold by therapeutic UFH and 400-fold by low-molecular-weight heparin (LMWH) and pentasaccharide (fondaparinux) therapeutics (Figure 35.14). AT was the first of the plasma coagulation control proteins to be identified and the first to be assayed routinely in the clinical hemostasis laboratory. Other members of the SERPIN family are heparin cofactor II, α₂-macroglobulin, α₂-antiplasmin, and α₁-antitrypsin. Hemostasis specialty laboratories or reference laboratories provide assays for all the SERPINs.

Antithrombin Deficiency

Adult AT levels are reached by 3 months of age and remain steady in young adulthood except during periods of physiologic challenge. The plasma biologic half-life is 72 hours, and AT activity decreases with age.[73]

AT deficiency is defined as AT activity levels less than 70% of normal or antigen concentration less than 22 mg/dL. AT becomes depleted in liver disease and nephrotic syndrome; with prolonged heparin and L-asparaginase therapy; with the use of oral contraceptives; and in DIC. Hereditary AT deficiency occurs in 1 in 2000 to 1 in 5000 of the general population and accounts for about 1.2% of recurrent venous thromboembolic disease cases.[74,75] About 90% of congenital AT deficiency cases are quantitative, reflected in the antigen level; the rest are caused by mutations that create structural abnormalities in the *protease-binding* site or the *heparin-binding* site. Qualitative deficiency mutations only slightly reduce AT production, but the molecules are nonfunctional, as reflected in diminished activity assay results.[76] Elevated AT levels appear to have no clinical consequence.

Severe AT deficiency causing thrombosis may be treated with an AT concentrate (Thrombate III, Grifols; or synthetic antithrombin alfa, ATryn, LFB Biotechnologies).[77]

Antithrombin Activity Assay

Laboratory practitioners test for AT deficiency using a FIIa (thrombin) clot-based or FXa-based chromogenic functional assay.[78] Laboratory professionals perform the assays using automated coagulation analyzers, placing the reagents at designated spots within the analyzer. The analyzer is preprogrammed to mix all reagents and patient plasma to give a result. In the chromogenic substrate method, the analyzer mixes test plasma with a solution of heparin and FXa (Figure 39.6) and incubates the mixture at 37° C for several minutes. During incubation, the heparin-activated plasma AT irreversibly binds a proportion of the reagent FXa. Residual FXa hydrolyzes a chromogenic substrate, added as a second reagent. The degree of hydrolysis, measurable by colored end product intensity, is inversely proportional to the activity of test plasma AT.[79] The chromogenic substrate test detects

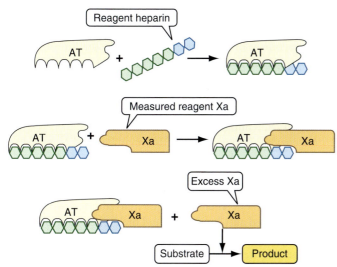

Figure 39.6 Chromogenic Antithrombin *(AT)* Functional Assay. Patient plasma is pipetted into a reagent consisting of heparin, a measured concentration of activated coagulation factor X *(Xa)*, and a chromogenic substrate specific to factor Xa. Patient AT is activated by heparin and binds factor Xa. Excess factor Xa hydrolyzes the substrate and produces a yellow product, paranitroaniline. The intensity of paranitroaniline color is inversely proportional to AT activity.

quantitative and qualitative AT deficiencies and detects mutations affecting the proteolytic site but not the heparin binding site. The clot-based assay has been available since 1972 and remains valid. Clot-based AT assays are affected by and therefore detect mutations in both the proteolytic and the heparin binding sites.

Antithrombin Antigen Assay

AT concentration is measured with a turbidometric microparticle immunoassay using a suspension of latex microbeads coated with antibody to AT. In the absence of AT, the wavelength of incident monochromatic light exceeds the latex microparticle diameter, so the light passes through unabsorbed. In the presence of AT, the particles form larger aggregates. The AT concentration is directly proportional to the rate of light absorption change.[80] The turbidometric immunoassay allows for a convenient application to high-throughput analyzers. Sandwich-type enzyme-linked immunosorbent assays are also available.

AT antigen levels are deficient in quantitative but are normal or slightly reduced in qualitative deficiencies. Warfarin therapy may raise the AT level and mask a mild deficiency. AT activity remains decreased for 10 to 14 days after a period of acute inflammation such as a thrombotic event or surgery, so the assay should not be used to establish a congenital deficiency during this period.

Heparin Resistance and the Antithrombin Assay

AT may become depleted during prolonged or intense UFH therapy, especially if the patient has a congenital deficiency. In this instance, because UFH requires AT to express its anticoagulant effect, UFH therapy at routine dosages fails to fully protect the patient. The decreased anticoagulant effect of UFH is observed in UFH monitoring assays such as the PTT, ACT, and chromogenic anti-Xa heparin assay (Chapter 40). This circumstance is known as *heparin resistance*. In such cases, an AT assay is necessary to confirm deficiency. Severe AT deficiency causing heparin resistance may be treated with plasma transfusion or an AT concentrate.

Protein C Control Pathway

Thrombin is an essential coagulation factor because it cleaves fibrinogen; activates platelets; and activates FV, FVIII, FXI, and FXIII. In the intact vessel, where clotting is unexpected, thrombin binds EC membrane thrombomodulin and becomes, paradoxically, an anticoagulant. The thrombin-thrombomodulin complex cleaves and activates PC (Chapter 35). The resultant APC binds free plasma PS.[81] The stabilized APC-PS complex, simultaneously bound to the endothelial PC receptor, hydrolyzes FVa and FVIIIa to reduce thrombin production, an essential coagulation control mechanism (Figure 35.13). Recurrent venous thrombosis is the consequence of PC or PS deficiency.[82,83] PS, the cofactor that binds and stabilizes APC, circulates either free or covalently bound to the complement binding protein *C4bBP*. Bound PS cannot participate in the PC anticoagulant pathway; only free plasma PS is available to serve as the APC cofactor. When acute phase reactant C4bBP level rises, binding additional PS, free PS levels become proportionally decreased.

Protein C and Protein S Deficiency

PC or PS deficiency is defined as activity or concentration levels less than 65% of normal. Heterozygous PC deficiency leads to a 2- to 5-fold increased risk and heterozygous PS deficiency leads to a 1.6- to 11.5-fold increased risk of recurrent DVTs and PEs. PS deficiency also has been implicated in transient ischemic attacks and strokes, particularly in young individuals.

Control proteins PC and PS (and PZ) and coagulation FII (prothrombin), FVII, FIX, and FX are vitamin K dependent. Because the half-life of PC is 6 hours, its level decreases as rapidly as that of FVII at the onset of warfarin therapy (an oral anticoagulant that reduces the vitamin K-dependent factors). In heterozygous PC deficiency, PC activity may drop to less than 65% more rapidly than the coagulation factor activities reach low therapeutic levels (less than 30%). Consequently, in early warfarin therapy, a patient may experience *warfarin-induced skin necrosis,* a condition in which the anticoagulant therapy paradoxically brings on thrombosis within the dermal vessels. This complication is suspected when the patient develops painful necrotic lesions that are preceded by severe itching, called pruritus. The necrosis may require surgical debridement. To avoid this risk, hematologists recommend coadministration of UFH, LMWH, or fondaparinux with warfarin until a satisfactory and stable international normalized ratio is reached (Chapter 40).[84]

PC and PS activity levels remain less than normal for 10 to 14 days after warfarin therapy is discontinued. Similarly, for several days after acute inflammation caused by a thrombotic event or surgery, these proteins can be diminished, even if warfarin has not been used. Their activities are depressed in pregnancy, liver or renal disease, vitamin K deficiency, and DIC, and with oral contraceptive use. PC and PS assays therefore cannot be used to identify a congenital deficiency when they are employed within 14 days after an acute inflammatory event or after the cessation of warfarin therapy; during pregnancy; or in the presence of DIC, liver disease, renal disease, vitamin K deficiency, or oral contraceptive use.[85]

Homozygous PC or PS deficiency results in neonatal purpura fulminans, a condition that is rapidly fatal when untreated (Chapter 38). Treatment includes PC concentrate and lifelong anticoagulant therapy.[86]

Protein C Assays

Clot-based or chromogenic functional assays detect both quantitative and qualitative PC deficiencies. For the chromogenic assay, the patient's plasma is mixed with Protac (Pentapharm), derived from the venom of the southern copperhead snake *Agkistrodon contortrix,* which activates PC. A substrate is added, which is hydrolyzed by the recently generated APC. The hydrolysis is reflected in the intensity of colored product, which is proportional to PC activity (Figure 39.7). The assay detects abnormalities that affect the molecule's *proteolytic* properties (active serine protease site) but misses abnormalities that affect the PC *phospholipid binding site* or PS *binding site*. In cases in which the PC chromogenic assay and immunoassay generate normal results but the clinical condition continues to indicate a possible PC deficiency, a clot-based assay may detect abnormalities at these additional sites on the molecule.

The clot-based PC assay is based on the ability of APC to prolong the PTT. The patient plasma is mixed with PC-depleted NP to ensure normal levels of all coagulation factors except PC. PTT reagent mixed with Protac and a heparin neutralizer is added, followed by calcium chloride, and the interval to clot formation is measured. Prolongation is proportional to PC activity. Interferences include therapeutic heparin concentrations greater than 1 IU/mL, which consume the heparin neutralizer, prolong the PTT, and lead to overestimation of

PC. APC resistance (FVL mutation), LAC, and the presence of therapeutic direct thrombin inhibitors (such as bivalirudin, argatroban, or dabigatran) or direct factor Xa inhibitors (such as apixaban, rivaroxaban, or edoxaban) may falsely prolong the PTT and falsely increase the PC activity level in clot-based assays, but not in chromogenic or antigenic assays.[87] Therapeutic use of the oral anticoagulant warfarin decreases PC activity and antigenic levels.

An enzyme immunoassay (EIA) may be used to measure PC antigen when the activity is low. Microtiter plates coated with rabbit anti-human PC antibody are used to capture test plasma PC, and the concentration of antigen is measured by color development after the sequential addition of peroxidase-conjugated anti-human PC and orthophenylene diamine substrate. The PC antigen concentration assay is available from specialty reference laboratories. The assay detects most acquired deficiencies and quantitative congenital deficiencies (type 1 deficiency), but it may return normal or near-normal levels in qualitative congenital abnormalities (type 2 deficiency).

Protein S Assays

PS deficiency may be detected using a clot-based functional assay. No chromogenic assay is available in the United States. In one method, the laboratory practitioner mixes the patient's plasma with PS-depleted NP to ensure normal levels of all factors other than PS. APC and Russell viper venom are added in a buffer that contains a heparin neutralizer, followed by calcium chloride. The interval to clot formation is proportional to PS activity (Figure 39.8).

Assay interferences include therapeutic heparin levels greater than 1 IU/mL that consume reagent heparin neutralizer and lead to overestimation of PS activity.[87] APC resistance (FVL mutation), LAC, and the presence of therapeutic direct thrombin inhibitors (such as bivalirudin, argatroban, or dabigatran) or direct factor Xa inhibitors (such as apixaban, rivaroxaban, or edoxaban) may prolong the clot time and falsely raise the activity levels in clot-based PS assays, but not in antigenic assays.[87] Therapeutic use of the oral anticoagulant warfarin decreases PS activity and antigenic levels.

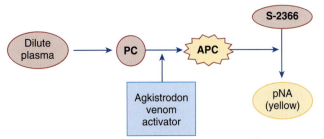

Figure 39.7 Chromogenic Protein C *(PC)* Assay. Patient plasma is pipetted into a reagent composed of *Agkistrodon contortrix* venom activator and chromogenic substrate S-2366 specific to activated protein C *(APC)*. The APC hydrolyzes the substrate to produce paranitroaniline *(pNA)*, a yellow product. The intensity of color is proportional to APC activity.

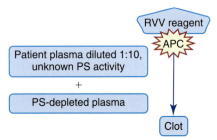

Figure 39.8 Clot-Based Protein S *(PS)* Assay. Patient plasma is diluted and pipetted into PS-depleted plasma. A second reagent is composed of Russell viper venom *(RVV)*, which activates clotting at the level of factor X, and activated protein C *(APC)*. The patient PS binds the reagent APC to prolong the clotting time. Clotting time is proportional to PS activity.

Coagulation FVII activation may occur during prolonged refrigeration of plasma at 4° C to 10° C, which may cause underestimation of PS activity by the same mechanism that causes a false effect in PT-based coagulation factor assays such as FV or FX assays.[88]

When there is a low activity level, EIAs are employed to measure both total and free PS antigen. These assays detect most quantitative congenital deficiencies and aid in the diagnosis of qualitative congenital deficiencies characterized by normal antigen but decreased PS activity. In a third form of PS deficiency, the PS activity and the concentration of free PS antigen are reduced, but not total antigen (Table 39.5). In this form, the plasma C4bBP, an acute phase reactant, is elevated, proportionally reducing the concentration of free PS. The concentration of plasma C4bBP, measured by immunoassay, helps classify this third PS deficiency type.

ARTERIAL THROMBOSIS PREDICTORS

Arterial thrombotic disease, including peripheral vascular occlusion, acute myocardial infarction (heart attack), and cerebrovascular ischemia (ischemic stroke), arises from atherosclerotic plaque. Eruption of unstable plaque mediates platelet-driven thrombosis formation. The traditional predictors of arterial thrombosis risk are elevated total cholesterol (TC) and low-density lipoprotein cholesterol (LDL-C), or an elevated ratio of TC to high-density lipoprotein cholesterol (HDL-C) (TC:HDL-C) secondary to HDL-C deficiency. One-third of primary cardiovascular and cerebrovascular events occur in patients whose lipid profiles are normal, however, and half of people with proven lipid risk factors never experience an arterial thrombotic event.

Researchers have sought additional arterial thrombosis predictors by performing prospective randomized studies of lipoprotein subtypes and markers of inflammation. Additional research investigations relevant to hemostasis encompass studies on fibrinolytic pathway components, in particular elevated PAI-1 and thrombin activatable fibrinolysis inhibitor; fibrinogen, FVIII, and VWF, which become elevated with inflammation; and activated platelets. Patients with arterial thrombosis are customarily treated with statins to reduce hyperlipidemia, with antiinflammatories, and antiplatelet drugs.

Lipoprotein (a)

Lipoprotein "little a" (Lp[a]) is an LDL that predicts arterial thrombosis. The plasma level is measured by EIA.[89]

C-Reactive Protein

CRP is an acute phase reactant whose plasma concentration rises 1000-fold 6 to 8 hours after the onset of an inflammatory event such as an infection, trauma, or surgery. Using a high-sensitivity assay, chronic plasma CRP concentrations that remain at 1.5 mg/L or greater indicate systemic low-grade inflammation.[90,91] Consequently, CRP is a clinical measure employed to predict cardiovascular or cerebrovascular disease.[92]

Brain Natriuretic Peptide

BNP is a misnomer for a hormone secreted from cardiomyocytes in response to hypertension and hypervolemia that leads to vasodilation, diuresis, and natriuresis. The pro-BNP immunoassay is employed to predict, detect, and monitor the progress of congestive heart failure.[93]

Fibrinogen Activity

Laboratory professionals measure fibrinogen using immunoassay, nephelometry, or the clot-based Clauss method to detect dysfibrinogenemia, hypofibrinogenemia, or afibrinogenemia (Chapter 41).[94] The same assays may be used to detect chronic hyperfibrinogenemia, which correlates with risk of stroke and myocardial infarction.[95,96] A correlation also exists between fibrinogen and TC (Figure 39.9). In contrast, low normal fibrinogen levels are associated with low risk of cardiovascular events, even in people with high TC levels. Fibrinogen becomes integrated into atherothrombotic lesions and contributes to their thrombotic potential.

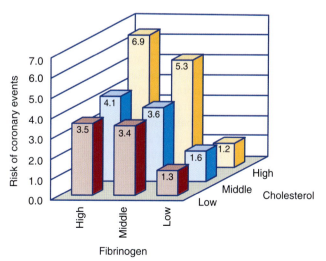

Figure 39.9 Coronary Thrombosis Risk Prediction by Fibrinogen and Cholesterol Concentrations. Fibrinogen and total cholesterol synergistically predict coronary risk. Tertiles of fibrinogen concentration are shown in relation to tertiles of total cholesterol concentration with the relative risk of coronary events indicated for each combination.

TABLE 39.5 Anticipated Protein S Test Results in Qualitative and Quantitative Deficiencies				
Type of PS Deficiency	PS Activity	PS Free Antigen	PS Total Antigen	C4bBP
I Quantitative	<65%	<65%	<65%	Normal
II Qualitative	<65%	>65%	>65%	Normal
III Inflammation	<65%	<65%	>65%	Elevated

C4bBP, C4b-binding protein; *PS*, protein S.

Although hyperfibrinogenemia predicts arterial thrombosis, use of the fibrinogen assay for this purpose is limited. There are no independent therapeutic regimens that specifically lower fibrinogen, and no clinical trials suggest that fibrinogen reduction reverses the odds of thrombosis. Further, the various fibrinogen assay methods await harmonization. Nevertheless, some providers use fibrinogen and FVIII levels to decide on antithrombotic therapy. Meanwhile, statin therapy, smoking cessation, and exercise lower fibrinogen levels alongside LDL-C and TC levels, and the assay results parallel those for the other members of the risk prediction profile.

Factor VIII

FVIII assays are designed to detect FVIII deficiency; they are now also being used to detect elevated levels. While the one-stage clot-based assay lacks accuracy at levels greater than the upper limit of the reference interval, typically 150 U/dL, the two-stage chromogenic assay offers linearity to 200 U/dL.[97] Similar to fibrinogen, coagulation FVIII is an acute phase reactant; consequently, an isolated case of elevated FVIII may relate to acute inflammation and provide little thrombosis risk predictive value. However, chronically elevated FVIII, similar to chronic hyperfibrinogenemia, may predict both arterial and venous thrombosis.

VENOUS THROMBOEMBOLIC DISEASE DIAGNOSIS

VTE, which includes DVT and PE, is the third most common thrombotic disease, just after ACS and stroke. In 2017 more than 300,000 hospital admissions were in response to suspected PE with a mortality rate of 3%, with many deaths occurring within minutes of initial symptoms.[98] DVT and PE present specific diagnostic challenges that are addressed through the D-dimer assay.[99]

Deep Venous Thrombosis Symptoms

The cardinal symptoms for DVT are edema, erythema, pain, and the sensation of heat. Depending on clot location, symptoms may involve the entire leg, calf, or ankle and foot. Often, the affected individual first misidentifies DVT as a muscle strain, also known as a charley horse; however, with DVT, the symptoms persist and grow over several days.

When symptoms are ambiguous, the provider may apply the Wells DVT scoring system.[100] One point each is scored for cancer, paralysis or recent plaster cast of lower extremities, bed rest for longer than 3 days or surgery within the previous 4 weeks, pain on palpation of deep veins, swelling of the entire leg, diameter of the affected calf exceeding that of the unaffected calf by 3 cm or more, pitting edema, and dilated superficial veins. Two points are deducted for a compelling alternative diagnosis. A score of zero eliminates the diagnosis of DVT, 1 or 2 points signals intermediate or equivocal pretest probability, and 3 or more points signal a high probability of DVT. The differential diagnosis for DVT includes superficial thrombophlebitis, ruptured Baker cyst, cellulitis, venous insufficiency, varicose veins, erythema nodosum, or postphlebitic syndrome.

Pulmonary Embolism Symptoms

Owing to the diagnostic predisposition toward acute coronary syndrome, providers are cautioned to maintain a heightened suspicion for PE. PE symptoms include dyspnea, shortness of breath, syncope, transient cyanosis, tachycardia, pleuritic pain, and distended neck veins. Providers apply the Wells PE scoring system (separate from the Wells DVT scoring system).[101] Wells criteria include current signs and symptoms of DVT, pulse greater than 100 beats/minute, immobilization or surgery within previous 4 weeks, prior PE or DVT, hemoptysis, or cancer. Simplified Wells criteria for the Wells PE scoring system have been proposed as well for its ease of use and when combined with age-adjusted D-dimer testing, it is thought to safely rule out PE in patients.[102] Other clinical scoring systems exist; all report one of two categories: PE likely or PE unlikely.

Deep Venous Thrombosis and Pulmonary Embolism Diagnostic Tests: D-Dimer

Using a clinical scoring system, high DVT or PE pretest probability triggers noninvasive imaging tests. Ultrasonography is effective for most DVT cases, whereas multislice or spiral chest computed tomography angiography is the reference method for PE. Computed tomography scan readily distinguishes PE from pneumonia, pleurisy, and ACS, supporting the differential diagnosis.

For low or intermediate pretest probability scores, the plasma *D-dimer* assay is chosen over imaging for its robust sensitivity and negative predictive index. The D-dimer is "promiscuous," meaning that it rises in response to all acute inflammatory conditions, especially ACS, congestive heart failure, pneumonia, sepsis, cancer, surgery, or pregnancy.[103] For this reason, the D-dimer cannot be employed to rule in DVT or PE; however, a normal D-dimer reliably rules out either condition without the need for imaging when the pretest probability score is low. If the D-dimer is negative, the provider considers alternative diagnoses.

The plasma D-dimer assay is reported in *D-dimer units* (DDUs) or *fibrinogen equivalent units* (FEUs), depending on the nature of the monoclonal antibody employed in the selected kit. One manufacturer's automated D-dimer monoclonal antibody binds a form of D-dimer that is cross linked through FDP "E" fragments (the D-E-D unit), yielding a molecular weight of 340,000 Daltons. The automated D-dimer assays of a competing manufacturer's monoclonal antibody detects D-D fragments of 170,000 Daltons (Figure 35.18). Consequently, the typical FEU decision limit is 500 ng/mL, whereas the DDU limit is often 240 ng/mL. In general, FEU results are about 1.7 times greater than DDU results; however, small differences exist in monoclonal antibody specificity, and thus laboratory directors establish local limits and discourage a simple multiplying conversion between reporting methods. While maintaining DDU and FEU distinctions, individual laboratory directors may choose to express results in milligrams per milliliter, milligrams per deciliter, or other units, a historical circumstance that demands ongoing communication between the laboratory practitioner and provider and establishes a need for harmonization.[104,105]

Further, D-dimer levels rise with advancing age, moving providers to request that the laboratory supply age-adjusted limits for patients older than 50. When reporting in FEUs, age adjustment relies on multiplication of age by 10 FEUs in nanograms per milliliter; thus the limit at age 60 would be 600 ng/mL FEUs, 700 ng/mL at age 70, and so on.[106] Using this strategy can minimize imaging studies to a large extent, with potential annual cost savings estimated to be greater than $80 million.[107] Laboratory directors who select a kit that reports in DDUs may choose to use age times 5 DDUs in ng/mL, thus 300 and 350 DDUs in ng/mL for ages 60 and 70, respectively. This approach is discouraged because age-related limit studies were performed using FEUs and it was found that a precise doubling relationship does not exist.[108,109]

DISSEMINATED INTRAVASCULAR COAGULATION

DIC, also called *defibrinating syndrome* or *consumption coagulopathy*, is generalized and uncontrolled hemostasis activation secondary to a systemic disorder. DIC is the Black Death of the Middle Ages, and it involves all hemostatic systems: vascular intima, platelets, leukocytes, coagulation pathways, coagulation control pathways, and fibrinolysis. DIC is microangiopathic, a condition in which fibrin microthrombi form in and occlude small vessels where they consume platelets, coagulation factors, coagulation control proteins, and fibrinolytic enzymes. Microangiopathic pathology produces schistocytes (Figure 16.1) visible on peripheral blood films. Fibrin degradation products (FDPs), including D-dimer, become elevated and interfere with normal fibrin formation as they coat platelets and fibrin.[110] This combination of events sets loose a series of toxic and inflammatory processes with secretion of the proinflammatory cytokines tumor necrosis factor-α (TNF-α), interleukin-1β (IL-1β), and IL-6.[111]

DIC may be *acute and uncompensated,* with deficiencies of multiple hemostasis components, or *chronic,* with slightly reduced, normal, or even elevated clotting factor levels. In chronic DIC, liver coagulation factor production and bone marrow platelet production incompletely compensate for consumption. Although DIC is a thrombotic process, the thrombi that form are small and ineffective, so systemic hemorrhage is often the first or most apparent symptom. Acute DIC is fatal in 25% to 50% of cases, depending on the cause, and requires immediate medical intervention. Diagnosis of DIC relies heavily on the hemostasis laboratory, and medical laboratory professionals often perform a DIC profile under emergent circumstances.

Causes of Disseminated Intravascular Coagulation

Any disorder that contributes hemostatic molecules or promotes their endogenous secretion may cause DIC. Listing and classifying all the causes of DIC is impractical, but the major triggering mechanisms and examples of each are listed in Table 39.6.

Chronic DIC may be associated with tissue necrosis, liver disease, renal disease, chronic inflammation, vascular prostheses, vascular tumors, and adenocarcinoma. The malignancies most associated with DIC are pancreatic, prostatic, ovarian, and lung cancers; multiple myeloma; acute promyelocytic leukemia; and myeloproliferative neoplasms. Trousseau syndrome, first described in 1865, is a term for tumor-induced chronic DIC that generates DVT and migrating subepithelial thromboses causing ecchymosis and purpura fulminans.[112] Trousseau syndrome is difficult to manage and may be the first symptom of previously undocumented adenocarcinoma.

The more acutely ill the patient, the more dangerous the pathology of DIC. Acute DIC is seen in association with obstetric emergencies, intravascular hemolysis, septicemia, viremia, burns, acute inflammation, crush injuries, dissecting aortic aneurysms, and cardiac disorders.

Pathophysiology of Disseminated Intravascular Coagulation

Tissue damage, endothelial damage, endothelial exposure to bacterial products, and exposure of blood to the subendothelium releases tissue factor, triggering the extrinsic pathway at the level of FVII and activating platelets. Exposure to TNF-α, IL-1β, hemolysis, and cell necrosis triggers activation of FXII and the intrinsic pathway. The osmotic imbalance of shock and endothelial exposure to TNF-α and IL-6 trigger the release of TPA, activating plasminogen. Although extrinsic coagulation pathway activation dominates, these events occur simultaneously and once triggered, DIC proceeds in a predictable sequence. *Circulating thrombin* becomes the primary culprit because it further activates platelets and coagulation factors, leading to fibrin formation (Chapter 35). Thrombin further activates fibrinolysis, resulting in expression of free plasmin.

Thrombin cleaves fibrinogen, producing fibrin monomers. In normal hemostasis, fibrin monomers spontaneously polymerize to form an insoluble gel that binds plasmin during its formation (Figure 35.9). The polymer becomes strengthened through FXIII-mediated cross linking. In DIC, a percentage of fibrin monomers fail to polymerize and circulate in plasma as soluble fibrin monomers. The monomers coat platelets and coagulation proteins, creating an anticoagulant effect that prolongs the TT, PT, and PTT assays.

Thrombin, soluble fibrin monomers, fibrin polymer, and cross-linked fibrin all activate plasminogen to form active plasmin. Normally, plasmin functions locally to digest only the solid fibrin clot to which it is bound (Chapter 35). In DIC, as a result of antiplasmin consumption, plasmin circulates in the plasma and

TABLE 39.6 Disseminated Intravascular Coagulation-Associated Conditions by Mechanism

Mechanism That Induces DIC	Examples of Conditions
Tissue factor is released into circulation through endothelial cell damage or monocyte activation	Physical trauma: crush or brain injuries, surgery Degradation of muscle; rhabdomyolysis Tissue ischemia; myocardial infarction Thermal injuries: burns or cold Adenocarcinoma Acute inflammation
Exposure of subendothelial tissue factor during vasodilatation	Hypovolemic and hemorrhagic shock Malignant hypertension Asphyxia and hypoxia Heatstroke Vasculitis
Endotoxins that activate cytokines	Bacterial, protozoal, fungal, and viral infections, septicemia* Toxic shock syndrome
Circulating immune complexes	HIT with thrombosis Drugs that trigger an immune response Acute hemolytic transfusion reactions Allergic reactions and anaphylaxis Bacterial and viral infections* Graft rejection
Particulate matter from tissue injury	Eclampsia, preeclampsia, HELLP syndrome* Retained dead fetus or missed abortion* Amniotic fluid embolism* Abruptio placentae* Rupture of uterus* Tubal pregnancy* Fat embolism
Infusion of activated clotting factors	Activated prothrombin complex concentrate therapy
Secretion of proteolytic enzymes	Acute promyelocytic or myelomonocytic leukemia Bacterial, protozoal, fungal, and viral infections*
Toxins that trigger coagulation	Snake or spider envenomation Pancreatitis
Thrombotic disease or thrombogenic conditions	Thrombotic thrombocytopenic purpura, hemolytic uremic syndrome Pregnancy, postpartum period, estrogen therapy DVT, PE Coagulation control system deficiencies Purpura fulminans, skin necrosis Thromboinflammation, retrovirus infection such as SARS-CoV2* Sepsis*
Severe hypoxia or acidosis	Trauma-induced coagulopathy Chronic inflammation Diabetes mellitus
Platelet activation	Vascular surgery, coronary artery bypass surgery Thrombocytosis, thrombocythemia, polycythemia Vascular tumors Vascular prostheses Aortic aneurysm

*Most common causes of DIC.
DIC, Disseminated intravascular coagulation; *DVT,* deep venous thrombosis; *HELLP,* **H**emolysis, **e**levated **l**iver enzymes, and **l**ow **p**latelet count; *HIT,* heparin-induced thrombocytopenia; *PE,* pulmonary embolism; *SARS-CoV2,* severe acute respiratory syndrome coronavirus 2.

digests all forms of fibrinogen and fibrin by the process termed *plasmin-mediated fibrinolysis.*[113] Consequently, FDPs labeled X, Y, D, and E and D-dimer are detectable in the plasma in concentrations exceeding 20,000 ng/mL (Figure 35.18). D-dimer arises from cross-linked fibrin polymer, whereas the other FDPs may be produced from fibrinogen or fibrin monomers or polymers.

Platelets become enmeshed in the fibrin polymer or are exposed to thrombin. Both events trigger platelet activation, which further drives coagulation and is reflected in moderate thrombocytopenia. Concurrently, coagulation pathway control is lost as PC, PS, and AT are consumed. These events lead to blood clotting. As DIC progresses, however, all hemostatic proteins become consumed. This consumption, combined with circulating plasmin, loss of control, and thrombocytopenia contributes to a consequential hemorrhagic outcome.

Free plasmin digests FV, FVIII, FIX, and FXI as well as other plasma proteins. Thrombin and plasmin also may trigger the complement pathway, which leads to hemolysis, and activation of the kinin system, which results in inflammation, hypotension, and shock.

During fibrinolytic therapy, in late-phase cardiopulmonary bypass surgery, liver disease, transplant surgery, trauma, and amyloidosis, plasminogen sometimes becomes activated independent of the coagulation pathway. This rare condition, called systemic fibrinolysis or *primary fibrinolysis,* is reflected in an elevated D-dimer and prolonged PT and PTT, while the platelet count remains normal.[114] Systemic fibrinolytic therapy has been proposed for COVID-19 patients who experience thrombotic complications, albeit with reservations because of the rapidly evolving nature of DIC in these patients.[115,116]

Symptoms of Disseminated Intravascular Coagulation

The symptoms signaling DIC often are masked by the symptoms of the underlying disorder and may be chronic, acute, or even fulminant. Ischemia of major organ microvasculature produces symptoms of organ dysfunction such as renal function impairment, acute respiratory distress syndrome, and central nervous system manifestations such as sudden vision loss or seizures. Skin, bone, and bone marrow necrosis may be seen. Purpura and ecchymoses leading to purpura fulminans (Chapter 38) are seen in meningococcemia, chickenpox, and spirochete infections.

Laboratory Diagnosis of Disseminated Intravascular Coagulation

DIC is foremost a clinical diagnosis that requires speedy laboratory confirmation (Chapter 41). Periodic laboratory testing can be used to follow the clinical progression of DIC. The initial laboratory profile includes a platelet count, blood film examination (Chapters 13 and 14), PT, PTT, TT, fibrinogen assay, and D-dimer. Table 39.7 lists anticipated DIC laboratory results.[117] Prolonged PT and PTT reflect coagulation factor consumption in 50% to 75% of cases. Fibrinogen may decrease in DIC, but because fibrinogen levels rise in inflammation, the fibrinogen concentration alone provides little reliable diagnostic information. The platelet count and peripheral blood film platelet estimate confirm thrombocytopenia in 90% of cases,

TABLE 39.7 Anticipated Results of Disseminated Intravascular Coagulation Primary Laboratory Profile

Test	Reference Interval	Typical Value in DIC
Platelet count	150,000–450,000/μL	<150,000/μL
Peripheral blood film examination	Normal RBC morphology, normal RBC indices	Schistocytes (MAHA) are present in 50% of DIC cases; leukocytosis is common
PT	11–14 seconds	>14 seconds
PTT	25–35 seconds	>35 seconds
TT, reptilase time	Normal, e.g., <20 seconds	Prolonged, e.g., >20 seconds. Fibrinogen levels <80 mg/dL, elevated FDPs, and soluble fibrin monomer all prolong TT and reptilase time
D-dimer	0–240 ng/mL DDU or 0–500 ng/mL FEU	>240 ng/mL DDU or >500 ng/mL FEU, often 10,000–20,000 ng/mL
Fibrinogen	220–498 mg/dL	<220 mg/dL, often higher, because fibrinogen is an acute phase reactant

DDU, D-dimer units; *DIC,* disseminated intravascular coagulation; *FDP,* fibrin degradation product; *FEU,* fibrinogen equivalent units; *MAHA,* microangiopathic hemolytic anemia; *PT,* prothrombin time; *PTT,* partial thromboplastin time; *RBC,* red blood cell; *TT,* thrombin time.

TABLE 39.8 Specialized Laboratory Assays That Assist in the Diagnosis of Disseminated Intravascular Coagulation

Assay	Value in DIC	Comments
Protein C, protein S, and AT activity assays	<50%	Also use to monitor AT concentrate therapy
Plasminogen, TPA, PAI-1	Decreased	May be useful for evaluating systemic fibrinolysis; specimen management protocol must be strictly observed
Factor assays: II (prothrombin), V, VIII, X	<30%	FV and FVIII rise in inflammation; assays may give misleading results

AT, Antithrombin; *DIC,* disseminated intravascular coagulation; *F,* coagulation factor; *PAI-1,* plasminogen activator inhibitor-1; *TPA,* tissue plasminogen activator.

Tests of the fibrinolytic pathway include chromogenic plasminogen activity assay and TPA and PAI-1 immunoassays.[122] These tests are seldom offered in the acute care hemostasis laboratory because they require meticulous specimen management, but they may help in the diagnosis of primary fibrinolysis.

Differential Diagnosis of Disseminated Intravascular Coagulation

Hemostasis laboratory assays cannot distinguish DIC from severe liver disease. Whereas in DIC, coagulation factors and controls, platelets, and the components of fibrinolysis are consumed, in advanced liver disease their production is diminished. In liver disease, D-dimers rise in response to inflammation and diminished hepatic clearance. A DIC scoring system can be used as a predictor of outcome of critically ill patients. The provider must base the diagnosis and management on history, symptoms, liver enzyme assays, and the DIC score.[123]

Dilutional coagulopathy may occasionally resemble DIC, prolonging the PT, PTT, and TT and reducing the platelet count. Treatment of severe hemorrhage with plasma, cryoprecipitate, red blood cells, and platelet concentrate causes dilutional coagulopathy. The provider distinguishes DIC from dilutional coagulopathy on the basis of recent history. In shock secondary to trauma, hypotension, acidosis, and hypothermia lead to DIC, which may coexist with dilutional coagulopathy.[124]

Obstetric complications preeclampsia, eclampsia, acute fatty liver of pregnancy, and HELLP (**h**emolysis, **e**levated **l**iver function tests, and **l**ow **p**latelets) syndrome all may mimic DIC laboratory results and must be resolved on the basis of history and symptoms. Resolution in all these cases calls for early delivery of the fetus and placenta.[125,126]

Thrombotic thrombocytopenic purpura (TTP) and its sibling, hemolytic uremic syndrome (HUS) (Chapter 38), both platelet activation-based microangiopathic thrombosis disorders, may resemble DIC in symptoms and laboratory results. In both TTP and HUS disorders, however, the PT, PTT, and TT remain relatively normal, while the platelet count drops to as low as 40,000 to 50,000/μL.[127] Clinically, DIC arises from an

though the platelet count remains at 30,000 to 40,000/μL. The presence of schistocytes, denoting microangiopathic hemolytic anemia, helps establish the diagnosis of DIC in 50% of cases.[118]

The D-dimer reference limit is typically 240 DDU ng/mL or 500 FEU ng/mL, depending on the D-dimer configuration as described earlier in "Deep Venous Thrombosis and Pulmonary Embolism Diagnostic Tests: D-Dimer." In 85% of DIC cases, D-dimer levels reach 10,000 to 20,000 ng/mL. A normal D-dimer assay result rules out DIC but is dependent on the D-dimer assay used.[119] D-dimer concentrations are typically elevated in VTE, inflammation, sickle cell crisis, pregnancy, and renal disease, so an abnormal result alone cannot be used to definitively diagnose DIC. The PT, PTT, TT, fibrinogen assay, platelet count, and blood film examination must be performed alongside the D-dimer to rule out other disorders.

Specialized Laboratory Tests for Disseminated Intravascular Coagulation

Table 39.8 lists specialized laboratory tests that may be used to further diagnose and classify DIC.[120] Results consistent with DIC and clinical comments are included. Many of these tests are available in acute care facilities, but they are not routinely applied to the diagnosis of DIC. Others are available only in tertiary care facilities and specialized hemostasis reference laboratories.

PC, PS, and AT are consumed in DIC, and their assay may contribute to the diagnosis. When plasma or AT concentrate is used to treat DIC, the AT assay is used to establish the necessity for therapy and monitor its effect.[121] Factor assays may clarify PT and PTT results.

existing condition, whereas TTP and HUS arise in individuals with no identifiable primary disorder.

Disseminated Intravascular Coagulation Treatment

To arrest DIC the provider must diagnose and treat the underlying disorder. Surgery, antiinflammatory agents, antibiotics, or obstetric procedures as appropriate may normalize hemostasis without requiring efforts to directly correct the coagulopathy. Supportive therapy, such as maintenance of fluid and electrolyte balance, always accompanies medical and surgical management.

In acute DIC, where ischemic multiorgan dysfunction and bleeding threaten the life of the patient, heroic measures are necessary. Treatment involves therapies that slow the clotting process and therapies that replace missing platelets and coagulation factors.

UFH may be used for its antithrombotic properties to stop the uncontrolled activation of the coagulation cascade.[128] Because UFH aggravates bleeding, careful dosing, observation, and support are required. Periodic chromogenic anti-FXa heparin assays are necessary to control UFH dosage because in DIC the PTT is ineffective for monitoring heparin therapy.

Plasma provides all the necessary coagulation factors and replaces blood volume lost during acute DIC hemorrhage. Prothrombin complex concentrate (Proplex T complex, Baxter; or Kcentra, Behring), fibrinogen concentrate (RiaSTAP, Behring), and FVIII concentrate (ADVATE, Baxter) may be used in place of plasma, particularly if there is concern for transfusion-associated circulatory overload. Periodic fibrinogen, PT, PTT, and TT assays are necessary to confirm the effectiveness of these therapeutics.[129] Platelet transfusions are necessary when thrombocytopenia is severe. Platelet counts are used to monitor the effectiveness of platelet concentrate and platelet consumption (Chapters 13 and 14). Red blood cells are administered as necessary to treat the resulting anemia. Antifibrinolytic therapy is contraindicated except in proven systemic fibrinolysis.

HEPARIN-INDUCED THROMBOCYTOPENIA

Heparin-induced thrombocytopenia (HIT) is the consequence of an immune response to UFH (standard intravenous heparin) and LMWH that is reflected in a reduced platelet count.[130] HIT may progress to venous and arterial thrombosis. The incidence of HIT as a response to UFH therapy is 0.5% to 5%. The risk for HIT in patients treated with LMWH therapy following major surgery is 1% to 10% the risk of its occurrence in response to UFH.[131] Risk levels depend on the current clinical condition, medical or surgical history, obstetric events, and the patient's general health. The incidence of HIT also relates to duration and dosage of heparin therapy, though there are published cases in which HIT follows a single dose or even the incidental use of heparin to flush a line.[132] Arterial and venous thromboembolic complications include DVT, PE, myocardial infarction, thrombotic stroke, limb ischemia, vein graft occlusion, and injection site skin lesions.[133] Mortality among patients with thrombosis rises to 30%, and up to 20% of patients who survive require amputation.[134] HIT diagnosis and treatment is complex, as 30% of patients who are receiving heparin develop mild thrombocytopenia with no additional consequence. Nevertheless, HIT must be considered with a high

index of suspicion in the clinical management of patients exposed to UFH and LMWH because of its grave outcomes.[135]

Pathophysiology of Heparin-Induced Thrombocytopenia

HIT involves platelet activation, inflammation, and thrombosis.[136] HIT antibodies are specific for *platelet factor 4* (PF4) *complexed with heparin* (UFH or LMWH).[137] PF4 is a positively charged tetrameric protein stored in platelet α-granules. When exposed, the charged amino acids on the PF4 protein bind negatively charged heparin to form the H:PF4 complex.[138] H:PF4 is a hapten that triggers immune production of IgG isotype anti-H:PF4 antibodies that bind the H:PF4, targeting a neoepitope on PF4 that is expressed with heparin binding. The Fc portion of the resultant IgG:H:PF4 immune complex binds platelet FcγIIa receptors, activating platelets and releasing additional PF4, initiating a cycle of platelet activation that generates procoagulant platelet microparticles (Figure 39.10).[139] Sustained platelet activation contributes to platelet clearance and a hypercoagulable state, resulting in thrombocytopenia and HIT-associated thrombosis.[140]

HIT antibodies also recognize PF4 bound to cell membranes.[141] For instance, the EC glycosaminoglycan heparan sulfate binds PF4, forming an H:PF4-like complex recognized by HIT antibodies. The reaction triggers an inflammatory state in which ECs, macrophages, monocytes, and neutrophils release tissue factor, PAI-1, and cytokines.[142] Inflammatory adhesion molecules promote additional platelet and monocyte binding.[143] The interrelationships of platelets, leukocytes, the endothelium, and inflammatory cytokines determine the clinical expression of HIT and may provide loci for thrombus formation.[144-146]

Laboratory Diagnosis of Heparin-Induced Thrombocytopenia

Early diagnosis of HIT demands a comprehensive interpretation of clinical and laboratory information.

Platelet Counts and Clinical Scoring for Heparin-Induced Thrombocytopenia

Surveillance for HIT begins with consecutive platelet counts, at least once every 48 hours during and after heparin therapy.[147] Hematologists customarily define HIT-related thrombocytopenia as a 30% to 50% drop in platelet count from the preheparin level.[148] The resultant platelet count may remain within the reference interval, though in most cases, the count falls to less than 150,000/μL, the lower limit of the reference interval, or even less than 100,000/μL. Patients with HIT rarely experience bleeding. In de novo HIT, the count begins to fall 5 to 10 days after heparin therapy is initiated, but if the patient has had heparin less than 120 days before the current therapy, thrombocytopenia may appear within hours. Delayed HIT may appear up to 30 days after discontinuation of therapy.

Thrombosis, which occurs in 30% of heparin-treated patients with thrombocytopenia, is a significant HIT signal. Patients with thrombocytopenia but without thrombosis at discharge from the hospital continue with a 50% risk of thrombosis within 30 days after the initial fall of the platelet count.

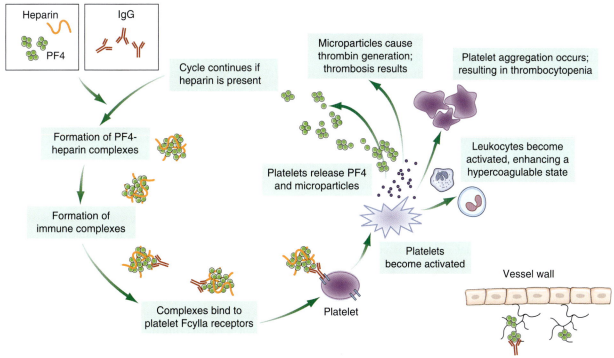

Figure 39.10 Heparin-Induced Thrombocytopenia With Thrombosis. The antibody IgG binds the heparin-platelet factor 4 *(PF4)* complex in plasma or on the platelet membrane. The Fc portion of the antibody binds monocyte or platelet Fc receptors, causing cellular activation. The activated platelets release procoagulant microparticles and aggregate to form platelet thrombi in the arterial or venous circulation. Platelet activation releases additional PF4 from granular stores, contributing to continuation of the cycle if heparin is present.

TABLE 39.9 4Ts Scoring System: Laboratory and Clinical Pretest Probability of Heparin-Induced Thrombocytopenia*

Indicator	SCORE		
	2	**1**	**0**
Acute thrombocytopenia	>50% decrease in platelet count to nadir of ≥20,000/μL	30%–50% decrease in platelet count, >50% if directly resulting from surgery, or to nadir of 10,000–19,000/μL	<30% decrease in platelet count or to nadir of <10,000/μL
Timing of platelet count decrease, thrombosis, or other sequelae of HIT (first day of heparin therapy is day 0)	Onset of decrease on days 5–10 or onset of decrease on day 1 if previous heparin exposure within past 5–30 days	Apparent decrease on days 5–10 but unclear due to missing platelet counts; or decrease after day 10; or decrease on day 1 if previous heparin exposure within past 31–100 days	Decrease at ≤4 days without recent heparin exposure
Thrombosis, skin lesions, acute system reaction	Proven new thrombosis or skin necrosis; acute systemic reaction after heparin exposure	Progressive, recurrent, or suspected thrombosis; erythematous skin lesions	None
Other causes for thrombocytopenia	No explanation for platelet count decrease is evident	Possible other cause is evident	Probable other cause is evident

*Maximum pretest probability score is 8; a score of 6–8 indicates high probability of HIT; 4–5, intermediate probability; 0–3, low probability. *HIT*, Heparin-induced thrombocytopenia.
From Crowther, M. A., Cook, D. J., Albert, M., et al. (2010). Canadian Critical Care Trials Group: the 4Ts scoring system for heparin-induced thrombocytopenia in medical-surgical intensive care unit patients. *J Crit Care, 25*, 287–293.

Providers employ platelet counts and thrombosis in the 4Ts clinical scoring system to evaluate the initial likelihood of HIT (Table 39.9).[149] Best practices dictate that scoring is performed prior to specialized HIT testing. There are many causes of thrombocytopenia in hospitalized patients; scoring improves diagnosis and management while preserving resources and reducing patient risk. The 4Ts system generates low, intermediate, and high probability scores.[150] Low scores provide reliable negative

predictive value, whereas intermediate or high 4T scores make it necessary to employ advanced laboratory methods.

The HIT Expert Probability (HEP) score is an alternative tool that further evaluates thrombosis and other causes of thrombocytopenia.[151] A separate scoring system for patients who have undergone cardiac surgery in which the cardiopulmonary bypass machine was used assesses the timing and extent of platelet count recovery during the postoperative period.[152]

Enzyme Immunoassays for Heparin-Induced Thrombocytopenia

Providers assess specialized HIT assay results with reference to the clinical context to avoid false-positive conclusions that lead to expensive alternative anticoagulants with increased bleeding risk.[153] Providers, laboratorians, and pharmacists meet to develop comprehensive diagnostic and treatment algorithms that rely on scoring systems to enhance diagnostic accuracy and effective therapy.[154] After scoring, HIT testing begins with EIA methods, available within many acute care facility laboratories, to determine whether antibodies to the H:PF4 complex are present.[155] Though unnecessary when the pretest score is low, the combination of a low pretest score and negative EIA HIT assay rules out HIT.

HIT EIAs employ solid-phase antigen targets surrogate to the H:PF4 complex.[156] Both manual and automated assays are available. EIAs are sensitive and prone to a high false-positive rate and must be confirmed using more specific followup platelet-based functional assays (confirmatory platelet activation assays for HIT). Though the anti-H:PF4 antibodies detectable by EIA are a critical part of the HIT mechanism, without platelet interaction, they fail to trigger thrombosis. Nonthrombotic anti-H:PF4 antibodies are the source for EIA false-positive results.

The LIFECODES PF4 IgG (Immucor GTI) kit illustrates EIA technology.[157] Patient plasma or serum is incubated in microtiter plate wells coated with a solid-phase complex of purified PF4 and polysulfonate, a heparin surrogate (Figure 39.11). Anti-H:PF4 antibodies bind the polysulfonate:PF4 complex. Enzyme-conjugated anti-human IgG antibodies attach to the bound antibodies, and a substrate chromophore is added. Manual EIA

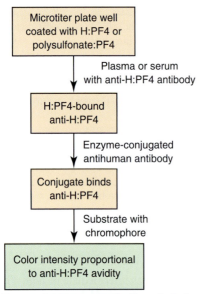

Figure 39.11 Enzyme Immunoassay for Heparin-Induced Thrombocytopenia (HIT). The solid-phase target antigen is a complex of platelet factor 4 and heparin or a heparin surrogate. Antiheparin/platelet factor 4 *(anti-H:PF4)* antibody in the patient plasma or serum binds the H:PF4 target and is bound in turn by enzyme-labeled anti-human antibody. The bound enzyme catalyzes the release of a chromophore from the anti-human antibody substrate; intensity of the chromophore color is proportional to the level of anti-H:PF4 antibody.

technology requires two intermediate washing phases and two 1-hour incubation phases. The operator employs a plate reader to record the resultant color intensity of each well as semiquantitative absorbance or optical density units that are proportional to HIT antibody concentration and avidity. Manufacturers may provide a positive decision point in absorbance or optical density units, or local operators may establish their own. Besides initial testing after clinical scoring, EIA methodology is used to monitor HIT patient progress during therapy.

Operators may follow up positive EIA results with a confirmatory step. Buffers with a high concentration of heparin, typically 100 units/mL, are used to displace or block solid-phase PF4. The EIA is repeated from the beginning with the high heparin buffer; a negative outcome confirms the heparin-dependent nature of the HIT antibody. It remains necessary to reflex to a functional assay.

Confirmatory Platelet Activation Assays for Heparin-Induced Thrombocytopenia

Positive EIA results are confirmed in a reflex-testing algorithm using a platelet function test, typically the washed platelet ^{14}C-serotonin release assay (SRA), available from a handful of high-quality specialized laboratories that possess isotope licenses.[158] Light transmittance platelet aggregometry using washed donor platelet-rich plasma was once an alternative that avoided radioactive labeling; however, the SRA offers superior sensitivity and is universally considered the reference assay (Figure 39.12).[159,160]

The SRA demonstrates the ability of the anti-H:PF4 HIT antibody to activate platelets in the presence of heparin. The operator obtains fresh platelet concentrate from a donor whose platelets demonstrated consistent reactivity in this assay. The platelets are washed in two special Tyrode buffers and labeled with ^{14}C-serotonin. Heparin and patient serum are added to the suspension, and platelet activation is reported by measurable ^{14}C-serotonin release, confirming HIT.

The operator continues to a high-concentration heparin confirmatory step similar to the EIA confirmatory step. Excess heparin does not allow for the conformation of the H:PF4 complexes that are recognized as an antigenic target by the HIT antibody. Thus there is no binding of the antibodies to platelets and no platelet activation occurs. A negative response confirms the heparin-dependent nature of the HIT antibody.

Rapid Turnaround Assays for Heparin-Induced Thrombocytopenia

Because of their manual format and lengthy incubations, EIAs are batched and performed once a day, necessitating a 24-hour turnaround time.[161] The SRA is a send out whose turnaround time may be 2 to 3 days. As HIT is an emergent diagnosis, providers make initial decisions to replace heparin therapy based solely on platelet count and the 4Ts (or other) scoring system, relying on advanced laboratory assays for subsequent confirmation.

A 30-minute turnaround latex-based HemosIL HIT-Ab(PF4-H) chemiluminescent assay from Werfen has been approved for North American and European markets. HemosIL HIT-Ab is

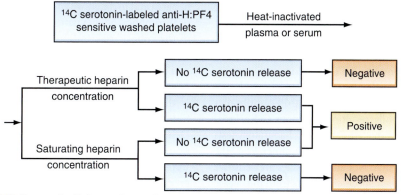

Figure 39.12 Serotonin Release Assay for Heparin-Induced Thrombocytopenia (HIT). Donor platelets proven to be antiheparin/platelet factor 4 *(anti-H:PF4)* antibody sensitive are washed and labeled with ^{14}C-serotonin, then suspended in albumin-free Tyrode buffer. Heat-inactivated patient plasma or serum is added. Heparin is added to two aliquots in therapeutic (0.1 to 0.4 units/dL) and saturating (100 units/dL) concentrations, respectively. Release of radioactive serotonin in the therapeutic aliquot compared to no release from the saturating aliquot confirms HIT. This pattern demonstrates H:PF4 antibody binding to and activating platelets in a heparin-dependent manner. Any platelet activation with saturating concentrations of heparin likely is due to nonspecific antiplatelet antibodies.

adapted to Werfen automated coagulometers.[162] Manufacturers continue to develop rapid turnaround assays that can generate clinical efficacy statistics similar to or somewhat more favorable than manual EIA methods and may be used in conjunction with a scoring system to rule out HIT.[163]

Several point-of-care rapid turnaround immunoassays for HIT diagnosis are available. Specificity among these assays compared to the laboratory functional assays can vary considerably.[148]

Therapy for Heparin-Induced Thrombocytopenia

When the provider is convinced of HIT, heparin therapy is stopped immediately. If needed, anticoagulant therapy is continued with a nonheparin drug. Effective alternatives are fondaparinux (Arixtra), argatroban, and bivalirudin (Angiomax), discussed in Chapter 40.[164,165] Though considered safe, these alternatives have a higher rate of serious bleeding that should be considered as part of the HIT therapeutic decision. DOAC therapy portends new and potentially safer alternatives, particularly for the nonacute HIT patient.[166]

THROMBOINFLAMMATION

Retroviruses such as the severe acute respiratory syndrome coronavirus-2 (SARS-CoV2), the cause of the 2020–2023 COVID-19 pandemic, have opened a new chapter in the field of thrombosis. Infections caused by these viruses have a clear association with inflammation and hemostatic activation mechanisms, resulting in potentially life-threatening thrombosis. The term *thromboinflammation* is now a part or our clinical vocabulary.

Coronaviruses such as SARS-CoV2 attack ECs via their angiotensin-converting enzyme-2 (ACE-2) receptors. Through endocytosis, ECs internalize the virus, triggering endothelial dysfunction, which includes reduction of EC barrier properties (Chapter 35) and secretion of ultra-large VWF multimers leading to plasma ADAMTS13 (*a d*isintegrin *a*nd *m*etalloproteinase

with a *t*hrombo*s*pondin type 1 motif, member *13*) consumption. These events trigger thrombotic microangiopathy-like conditions (Chapters 22 and 38) that cause symptomatic pulmonary, renal, cardiac, hepatic, pancreatic, and neurologic damage, potentially culminating in DIC.[167] In addition to endothelial injury, the infection is likely to stimulate the kallikrein-bradykinin system (linked to the intrinsic coagulation pathway) and raise ACE-2 levels, also driving coagulation and inflammation, notably in young patients.[168] Activation of the inflammatory cascade, or "cytokine storm," exacerbates endothelial dysfunction and explains at least some of the various outcomes of viral infections and postviral sequelae such as venous thromboembolic disease and long COVID.[169]

In addition to endothelial injury, infection activates platelets and the coagulation cascade through subendothelial tissue factor and collagen exposure.[170] Platelets aggregate by binding fibrinogen and VWF, whereupon they bind and activate neutrophils, monocytes, and T lymphocytes. The aggregates induce tissue factor expression on ECs and monocytes, which further contribute to morbidity and mortality.

Laboratory markers of thromboinflammation include the plasma appearance of platelet-secreted P-selectin, elevated fibrinogen and D-dimers, elevated CRP, and elevated TNF-α and IL-1β. Perhaps the most effective marker is the ADAMTS13 level, often expressed as the VWF:ADAMTS13 ratio. These join other inflammation markers including EC adhesion molecules, neutrophil extracellular traps, complement activation markers, and elevated eicosanoid synthesis pathway products such as urinary 11-dehydrothromboxane B_2. Reduced albumin within the microcirculation decreases oncotic pressure, causing tissue edema that exacerbates the thromboinflammatory state.[171]

Due to the morbidity and mortality of COVID-19 and its family of coronavirus diseases, medical scientists and providers rapidly elucidated their pathology. Continued research will uncover more specifics, which will be used to identify effective laboratory testing and treatment regimens.

Among the COVID-19 vaccines released in 2020 and 2021, the adeno-associated virus vector (AAV) vaccines were associated with a rare, occasionally fatal side effect, *vaccine-induced immune thrombotic thrombocytopenia* (VITT).[172] Greinacher and colleagues[173] described a mechanism resembling HIT where vaccine components form antigenic complexes (haptens) with platelet membrane PF4, generating avid anti-PF4 antibodies. The anti-PF4 antibodies activate platelets and neutrophils, resulting in venous and arterial thrombosis, bleeding, and, if untreated, acute DIC. Laboratory testing includes platelet count, PT, PTT, fibrinogen, D-dimer, PF4 HIT antibody immunoassay, and SRA. Not all HIT assays are sensitive to VITT antibodies because their specificity differs from the classic HIT antibody.[174] Management includes anticoagulation and intravenous immune globulin (IVIG). Expert groups provide guidelines; however, recommendations continue to evolve.[175]

THROMBOSIS RISK TESTING FUTURE

Before Dahlbäck described APC resistance in 1993, the typical hemostasis laboratory existed only to monitor warfarin and heparin and to diagnose and monitor the treatment of hemophilia or thrombocytopenia patients. Suddenly in 1994, with the advent of thrombosis risk testing for acquired and congenital clotting disorders in veins and arteries, hemostasis moved to center stage.

Laboratory personnel who specialize in hemostasis could now assess risk, diagnose, and monitor treatment for a variety of thrombotic disorders whose resolution required a combination of laboratory and clinical science in close communication. Deficiencies of AT, PC, and PS, APC resistance, FV Leiden mutation, prothrombin 20210 mutation, HIT, and DIC, conditions that were lost causes in 1992, are now managed successfully through precise laboratory assays directing pinpoint therapies.

The near future will connect thrombophilia and thrombosis risk testing with chronic and acute inflammation, EC analyses, molecular diagnostics, high-throughput human genome studies, and cytokine libraries. The laboratory contribution will continue to make inroads into arterial disease and platelet hyperactivity and reduce the burden of chronic disease.

SUMMARY

- Thrombosis is the most prevalent condition in developed countries and accounts for most illnesses and premature death.
- Thrombosis may be arterial, causing peripheral artery disease, heart disease, and stroke, or venous, causing deep venous thrombosis and pulmonary emboli.
- Most thrombosis occurs as a result of disease, lifestyle habits, and aging, but many thrombotic disorders are related to congenital risk factors.
- Thrombosis risk profiles may be offered to providers for screening purposes in high-risk populations.
- The main hemostasis predictors of arterial thrombotic disease are elevated C-reactive protein, fibrinogen, and individual coagulation factors.
- The main hemostasis predictors of venous thromboembolic disease are antiphospholipid antibodies; antithrombin (AT), protein C (PC), and protein S (PS) deficiencies; factor V Leiden (FVL) mutation; and prothrombin G20210A.
- Antiphospholipid antibody testing requires a series of essential hemostasis laboratory assays including clot-based tests and immunoassays.
- AT may be assayed using clot-based techniques, chromogenic substrate, and enzyme immunoassay analyses.

- Tests for evaluating the protein C pathway include PC and PS activity and concentration, activated protein C resistance, FVL mutation assay, and C4b-binding protein (C4bBP).
- The molecular test for the prothrombin G20210A mutation predicts the risk of venous thrombosis.
- Disseminated intravascular coagulation (DIC) is a clinical diagnosis that requires laboratory confirmation using a series of assays in an acute care facility.
- The quantitative D-dimer assay may be used to rule out venous thromboembolic disease and to diagnose and monitor DIC.
- Heparin-induced thrombocytopenia (HIT) is often associated with thrombosis; diagnosis of HIT requires high-complexity laboratory assays.
- Thromboinflammation illustrates the relationship among damaged endothelium, platelets, the coagulation pathway, complement, and inflammatory cytokines. Laboratory assays are essential to management and include ADAMTS13 (*a d*isintegrin *a*nd *m*etalloproteinase with a *th*rombo*s*pondin type 1 motif, member *13*), von Willebrand factor (VWF), D-dimer, and inflammatory markers.

Now that you have completed this chapter, go back and read again the case study at the beginning and respond to the questions presented. Answers can be found in Appendix C.

REVIEW QUESTIONS

Answers are found in Appendix C.

1. What is the prevalence of venous thrombosis in the United States?
   a. 0.01
   b. 1 in 1000
   c. 10% to 15%
   d. 500,000 cases per year

2. What is thrombophilia?
   a. Predisposition to thrombosis secondary to a congenital or acquired disorder
   b. Inappropriate triggering of the plasma coagulation system
   c. A condition in which clots form uncontrollably
   d. Inadequate fibrinolysis

3. What acquired thrombosis risk factor is assessed in the hemostasis laboratory?
   a. Smoking
   b. Immobilization
   c. Obesity
   d. Lupus anticoagulant

4. Trousseau syndrome, a low-grade chronic DIC, is often associated with what type of disorder?
   a. Renal disease
   b. Hepatic disease
   c. Adenocarcinoma
   d. Chronic inflammation

5. What is the most common heritable thrombosis risk factor in Northern European ancestry individuals?
   a. APC resistance (factor V Leiden mutation)
   b. Prothrombin G20210A mutation
   c. Antithrombin deficiency
   d. Protein S deficiency

6. In most LAC profiles, what test is primary (performed first) because it detects LAC with the least interference?
   a. Low-phospholipid PTT
   b. DRVVT
   c. KCT
   d. PT

7. A patient with venous thrombosis is tested for protein S deficiency. The protein S activity, antigen, and free antigen all are less than 65%, and the C4bBP level is normal. What type of deficiency is likely?
   a. Type I
   b. Type II
   c. Type III
   d. No deficiency is indicated because the reference interval is lower than 65%

8. An elevated level of what fibrinolytic system assay is associated with arterial thrombotic risk?
   a. PAI-1
   b. TPA
   c. Factor VIIa
   d. Factor XIII

9. What test may be used to confirm the presence of LAC?
   a. PT
   b. Bethesda titer
   c. Antinuclear antibody
   d. DRVVT using high-phospholipid reagent

10. What molecular test may be used to confirm APC resistance?
    a. Prothrombin G20210A mutation
    b. MTHFR 1298 polymorphism
    c. MTHFR 677 polymorphism
    d. Factor V Leiden mutation

11. What therapeutic agent may occasionally cause DIC?
    a. Factor VIII
    b. Factor VIIa
    c. Antithrombin concentrate
    d. Activated prothrombin complex concentrate

12. Which is not a fibrinolysis control protein?
    a. Thrombin-activatable fibrinolysis inhibitor
    b. Plasminogen activator inhibitor-1
    c. α_2-Antiplasmin
    d. D-dimer

13. What is the most important application of the quantitative D-dimer test?
    a. Diagnose primary fibrinolysis
    b. Diagnose liver and renal disease
    c. Rule out deep venous thrombosis
    d. Diagnose acute myocardial infarction

14. What is the first laboratory assay necessary to detect heparin-induced thrombocytopenia?
    a. Platelet count
    b. H:PF4 immunoassay
    c. Quick turnaround test
    d. Serotonin release assay

15. What assay appears to be the most useful in diagnosis and treatment monitoring in thromboinflammation?
    a. Prostacyclin
    b. C-reactive protein
    c. Brain natriuretic peptide
    d. ADAMTS13:VWF ratio

REFERENCES

1. Francis, J. L. (1998). Laboratory investigation of hypercoagulability. *Semin Thromb Hemost, 24*, 111–126.
2. De Minno, M. N. D., Ambrosino, P., Ageno, W., et al. (2015). Natural anticoagulants deficiency and the risk of venous thromboembolism: a meta-analysis of observational studies. *Thromb Res, 135*, 923–932.
3. Dahlbäck, B., Carlsson, M., & Svensson, P. J. (1993). Familial thrombophilia due to a previously unrecognized mechanism characterized by poor anticoagulant response to activated protein C: prediction of a cofactor to activated protein C. *Proc Natl Acad Sci U S A, 90*, 1004–1008.
4. Bertina, R. M., Koeleman, B. P. C., Koster, T., et al. (1994). Mutation in blood coagulation factor V associated with resistance to activated protein C. *Nature, 369*, 64–67.
5. Freed, J., & Bauer, K. A. (2019). Thrombophilia: clinical and laboratory assessment and management. In Kitchens, C. S., Kessler, C. M., Konkle, B. A., et al (Eds.), *Consultative Hemostasis and Thrombosis*. (4th ed., pp. 242–265). Philadelphia: Elsevier.
6. Yamaguchi, T., Wada, H., Miyazaki, S., et al. (2016). Fibrin-related markers for diagnosing acute-, subclinical-, and pre-venous thromboembolism in patients with major orthopedic surgery. *Int J Hematol, 103*, 560–566.
7. Wendelboe, A. M., & Raskob, G. E. (2016). Global burden of thrombosis – epidemiological aspects. *Circ Res, 118*, 1340–1347.
8. Mozaffarian, D., Benjamin, E. J., Go, A. S., et al. (2015). Heart disease and stroke statistics – 2015 update: a report from the American Heart Association. *Circulation, 131*, e29–e322.
9. Heit, J. A., Spencer, F. A., & White, R. H. (2016). The epidemiology of venous thromboembolism. *J Thromb Thrombolysis, 41*, 3–14.

10. Kalaitzopoulos, D. R., Panagopoulos, A., Samant, S., et al. (2022). Management of venous thromboembolism in pregnancy. *Thromb Res, 211*, 106–113.

11. Olaf, M., & Cooney, R. (2017). Deep venous thrombosis. *Emerg Med Clin North Am, 35*, 743–770.

12. Giordano, N. J., Jansson, P. S., Young, M. N., et al. (2017). Epidemiology, pathophysiology, stratification, and natural history of pulmonary embolism. *Tech Vasc Interv Radiol, 20*, 135–140.

13. Martin, K. A., Molsberry, R., Cuttica, M. J., et al. (2020). Time trends in pulmonary embolism mortality rates in the United States, 1999-2018. *JAHA*. https://doi.org/10.1161/JAHA.120.016784.

14. McLendon, K., Goyal, A., & Attia, M. (2022). Deep vein thrombosis risk factors. In: *StatPearls [Internet]*. Available from: https://www.ncbi.nlm.nih.gov/books/NBK470215/.

15. Benjamin, E. J., Muntner, P., Alonso, A., et al. (2019). American Heart Association Council on Epidemiology and Prevention Statistics Committee and Stroke Statistics Subcommittee. Heart disease and stroke statistics-2019 update: a report from the American Heart Association. *Circulation, 139*, e56-e528.

16. Glober, N., Stewart, L., Seo, J., *et al.* (2021). Incidence and characteristics of arterial thromboemboli in patients with COVID-19. *Thrombosis J*, https://doi.org/10.1186/s12959-021-00357-9.

17. Wang, M., Hao, H., Leeper, N. J., et al. (2018). Thrombotic regulation from the endothelial cell perspectives. *Arterioscl Thromb Vasc Biol, 38*, e90–e95.

18. Office of the Surgeon General. (2008). *The Surgeon General's Call to Action to Prevent Deep Vein Thrombosis and Pulmonary Embolism*. Rockville, MD: Office of the Surgeon General. http://www.ncbi.nlm.nih.gov/books/NBK44178/. Accessed August 17, 2022.

19. Previtali, E., Bucciarelli, P., Passamonti, S. M., et al. (2011). Risk factors for venous and arterial thrombosis. *Blood Transfus, 9*, 120–138.

20. Wysokinska, E., & Ortel, T. L. (2019). Antiphospholipid syndrome. In Kitchens, C. S., Kessler, C. M., Konkle, B. A., et al. (Eds.), *Consultative Hemostasis and Thrombosis*. (4th ed., pp. 374–395). Philadelphia: Saunders.

21. Connolly, G. C., & Khorana, A. A. (2019). Thrombosis and Cancer. In Kitchens, C. S., Kessler, C. M., Konkle, B. A., et al. (Eds.), *Consultative Hemostasis and Thrombosis*. (4th ed., pp. 430–447). Philadelphia: Saunders.

22. Mandernach, M. W., & Kitchens, C. S. (2019). Disseminated intravascular coagulation. In Kitchens, C. S., Kessler, C. M., Konkle, B. A., et al. (Eds.), *Consultative Hemostasis and Thrombosis* (4th ed., pp. 207–225). Philadelphia: Saunders.

23. Gris, J. C., Chea, M., Guillotin, F., et al. (2021). Thrombosis and paroxysmal nocturnal haemoglobinuria. *Thromb Update*. https://doi.org/10.1186/s12959-022-00407-w.

24. Joseph, J. J., Deedwania, P., Acharya, T., et al. (2022). Comprehensive management of cardiovascular risk factors for adults with type 2 diabetes: a scientific statement from the American Heart Association. *Circulation, 145*, e722–e759.

25. Kim, Y. H., & Roh, S. Y. (2016). The mechanism of and preventive therapy for stroke in patients with atrial fibrillation. *J Stroke, 18*, 129–137.

26. Loscalzo, J. (2013). Venous thrombosis in the nephrotic syndrome. *N Engl J Med, 368*, 956–958.

27. Abdelghani, E., Waller, A. P., Wolfgang, K. J., et al. (2021). Limited role of antithrombin deficiency in hypercoagulopathy associated with nephrotic syndrome. *Blood, 138* (Suppl 1), 294.

28. Middeldorp, S. (2016). Inherited thrombophilia: a double-edged sword. *Hematology Am Soc Hematol Educ Program, 1*, 1–9.

29. Martin-Fernandez, L., Gavidia-Bovadilla, G., Corrales, I., et al. (2017). Next generation sequencing to dissect the genetic architecture of *KNG1* and *F11* loci using factor XI levels as an intermediate phenotype of thrombosis. *PLoS One*. https://doi.org/10.1371/journal.pone.0176301.

30. Zakai, N. A., & McClure, L. A. (2011). Racial differences in venous thromboembolism. *J Thromb Haemost, 9*, 1877–1882.

31. Mohammed, S., & Favaloro, E. J. (2017). Laboratory testing for activated protein C resistance (APCR). *Methods Mol Biol, 1646*, 137–143.

32. Sedano-Balbás, S., Lyons, M., Cleary, B., et al. (2011). Acquired activated protein C resistance, thrombophilia and adverse pregnancy outcomes: a study performed in an Irish cohort of pregnant women. *J Pregnancy, 2011*, 1–9.

33. Evaluation of Genomic Applications in Practice and Prevention (EGAPP) Working Group. (2011). Recommendations from the EGAPP working group: routine testing for Factor V Leiden (R506Q) and prothrombin (20210G.A) mutations in adults with a history of idiopathic venous thromboembolism and their adult family members. *Genet Med, 13*, 67–76.

34. Romero, M. O., Cannegieter, S. C., den Heijer, M., et al. (2018). Hyperhomocysteinemia and risk of first venous thrombosis: the influence of (unmeasured) confounding factors. *Am J Epidemiol, 187*, 1392–1400.

35. Moll, S. (2019). Nonarteriosclerotic disorders of the arterial system. In Kitchens, C. S., Kessler, C. M., Konkle, B. A., et al. (Eds.), *Consultative Hemostasis and Thrombosis*. (4th ed., pp. 415–429). Philadelphia: Saunders.

36. Campello, E., Spiezia, L., Adamo, A., et al. (2019). Thrombophilia, risk factors and prevention. *Expert Rev Hematol, 12*, 147–158.

37. Connors, J. M. (2017). Thrombophilia testing and venous thrombosis. *N Engl J Med, 377*, 1177–1187.

38. Bustamante, J. G., Goyal, A., & Singhal, M. (2022). Antiphospholipid syndrome. In: *StatPearls [Internet]*. Available from: https://www.ncbi.nlm.nih.gov/books/NBK430980/.

39. Chaturvedi, S., & McCrae, K. R. (2017). Diagnosis and management of the antiphospholipid syndrome. *Blood Rev, 31*, 406–417.

40. Negrini, S., Pappalardo, F., Murdaca, G., et al. (2017). The antiphospholipid syndrome: from pathophysiology to treatment. *Clin Exp Med, 17*, 257–267.

41. Radic, M., & Pattanaik, D. (2018). Cellular and molecular mechanisms of anti-phospholipid syndrome. *Front Immunol, 9*, 1–11.

42. Bradacova, P., Slavik, L., Ulehlova, J., et al. (2021). Current promising biomarkers and methods in the diagnostics of antiphospholipid syndrome: a review. *Biomedicines, 9*, 1–15.

43. Chaturvedi, S., & McCrae, K. R. (2015). The antiphospholipid syndrome: still an enigma. *Hematology Am Soc Hematol Educ Program, 2015*, 53–60.

44. Gavris, C. M., Moga, S., Dima, L., et al. (2017). Predictive role of hs-C-reactive protein and platelet activation markers for recurrent thrombosis in patients with antiphospholipid syndrome. *Arc Balkan Med Union, 52*, 162–165.

45. Devreese, K. M. J., Verfaillie, C. J., Bisschop, F. D., et al. (2015). Interference of C-reactive protein with clotting times. *Clin Chem Lab Med, 53*(5), e141–e145.

46. Marques, M. B., & Fritsma, G. A. (2015). *Quick Guide to Hemostasis* (3rd ed.). Washington, DC: AACC Press.

47. Vandevelde, A., & Devreese, K. M. J. (2022). Laboratory diagnosis of antiphospholipid syndrome: Insights and hindrances. *J Clin Med, 11*, 1–26.

48. Favaloro E. J., Kershaw, G., Mohammed, S., et al. (2019). How to optimize activated partial thromboplastin time (APTT) testing: solutions to establishing and verifying normal reference intervals and assessing APTT reagents for sensitivity to heparin, lupus anticoagulant, and clotting factors. *Semin Thromb Hemost, 45*, 22–35.

49. Devreese, K. M. J., de Groot, P. G., de Laat, B., et al. (2020). Guidance from the scientific and standardization committee for lupus anticoagulant/antiphospholipid antibodies of the International Society on Thrombosis and Haemostasis: update of the guidelines for lupus anticoagulant detection and interpretation. *J Thromb Haemost, 18*, 2828–2839.

50. Yao, K., Zhang, L., Zhou, H., et al. (2017). Plasma antiphospholipid antibodies effects on activated partial thromboplastin time assays. *Am J Med Sci, 354*, 22–26.

51. Favaloro, E. (2020). Mixing studies for lupus anticoagulant: mostly yes, sometimes no. *Clin Chem Lab Med, 58*, 487–491.

52. Moore, G. W., Culhane, A. P., Daw, C. R., et al. (2016). Mixing test specific cut-off is more sensitive at detecting lupus anticoagulants than index of circulating anticoagulant. *Thromb Res, 139*, 98–101.

53. Smith, L. (2017). Laboratory diagnosis of the lupus anticoagulant. *Clin Lab Sci, 30*, 7–14.

54. Tripodi, A., & Chantarangkul, V. (2017). Lupus anticoagulant testing: activated partial thromboplastin time (APTT) and silica clotting time (SCT). *Methods Mol Biol, 1646*, 177–183.

55. Willis, R., Papalardo, E., & Nigel Harris, E. (2017). Solid phase immunoassay for the detection of anticardiolipin antibodies. *Methods Mol Biol, 1646*, 185–199.

56. Devreese, K. M. J., Ortel, T. L., Pengo, V., et al. (2018). Subcommittee on lupus anticoagulant/antiphospholipid antibodies. Laboratory criteria for antiphospholipid syndrome: communication from the SSC of the ISTH. *J Thromb Haemost, 218*, 809–813.

57. Willis, R., Papalardo, E., & Nigel Harris, E. (2017). Solid phase immunoassay for the detection of anti-β_2 glycoprotein I antibodies. *Methods Mol Biol, 1646*, 201–215.

58. Devreese, K. M. J. (2020). Testing for antiphospholipid antibodies: advances and best practices. *Int J Lab Hematol, 42* (Suppl. 1), 49–58.

59. Shi, H., Zheng, H., Yin, Y. F., et al. (2018). Antiphosphatidylserine/prothrombin antibodies (aPS/PT) as potential diagnostic markers and risk predictors of venous thrombosis and obstetric complications in antiphospholipid syndrome. *Clin Chem Lab Med, 56*, 614–624.

60. Dahlbäck, B., & Villoutreix, B. O. (2005). Regulation of blood coagulation by the protein C anticoagulant pathway: novel insights into structure-function relationships and molecular recognition. *Arterioscl Thromb Vasc Biol, 25*, 1311–1320.

61. Dean, E., & Favaoloro, E. J. (2020). The changing face of activated protein C resistance testing-a 10 year retrospective. *Ann Blood, 5*, 1–7.

62. Segers, K., Dahlbäck, B., & Nicolaes, G. A. (2007). Coagulation factor V and thrombophilia: background and mechanisms. *Thromb Haemost, 98*, 530–542.

63. Bouaziz-Borgi, L., Nguyen, P., Hezard, N., et al. (2007). A case control study of deep venous thrombosis in relation to factor V G1691A (Leiden) and A4070G (HR2 haplotype) polymorphisms. *Exp Mol Pathol, 83*, 480–483.

64. Anderson, J. M., & Weitz, J. I. (2023). Hypercoagulable states. In Hoffman, R., Benz, E. J., Silberstein. L. E., et al. (Eds.), *Hematology: basic principles and practice.* (8th ed., pp. 2167–2178). Philadelphia: Elsevier.

65. Johnson, N. V., Khor, B., & Van Cott, E. M. (2012). Advances in laboratory testing for thrombophilia. *Am J Hematol, 87*(Suppl. 1), S108–S112.

66. Moore, G. W., Chege, T., Culhane, A. P., et al. (2015). Maximising the diagnostic potential of APTT-based screening assays for activated protein C resistance. *Int J Lab Hematol, 37*, 844–852.

67. Moore, G. W., Van Cott, E. M., Cutler, J. A., et al. (2019). Recommendations for clinical laboratory testing of activated protein C resistance; communication from the SSC to the ISTH. *J Thromb Haemost, 17*, 1555–1561.

68. Poort, S. R., Rosendaal, F. R., Reitsma, P. Y., et al. (1996). A common genetic variation in the 3'-untranslated region of the prothrombin gene is associated with elevated plasma prothrombin levels and an increase in venous thrombosis. *Blood, 88*, 3698–3703.

69. Dziadosz, M., & Baxi, L. V. (2016). Global prevalence of prothrombin gene mutation G20210A and implications in women's health: a systematic review. *Blood Coagul Fibrinolysis, 27*, 481–489.

70. Naeem, M. A., Anwar, M., Ali, W., et al. (2006). Prevalence of prothrombin gene mutation (G-A 20210 A) in general population: a pilot study. *Clin Appl Thromb Hemost, 12*, 223–226.

71. Kujovich, J. L. (2021). Prothrombin thrombophilia. In Adam, M. P., Everman, D. B., Mirzaa, G. M., et al., (Eds.) *Gene Reviews* [Internet]. University of Washington, Seattle, 1993–2022.

72. Danckwardt, S., Hartmann, K., Gehring, N. H., et al. (2006). 3' end processing of the prothrombin mRNA in thrombophilia. *Acta Haematol, 115*, 192–197.

73. Cooper, P. C., Coath, F., Daly, M. E., et al. (2011). The phenotypic and genetic assessment of antithrombin deficiency. *Int J Lab Hematol, 33*, 227–237.

74. Di Minno, M. N., Dentali, F., Lupoli, R., et al. (2014). Mild antithrombin deficiency and risk of recurrent venous thromboembolism: a prospective cohort study. *Circulation, 129*, 497–503.

75. Croles, F. N., Borjas-Howard, J., Nasserinejad, K., et al. (2018). Risk of venous thrombosis in antithrombin deficiency: a systematic review and Bayesian meta-analysis. *Semin Thromb Hemost, 44*, 315–326.

76. Bravo-Perez, C., Moreno-Barrio, M. E., Vicente, V., et al. (2020). Antithrombin deficiency as a still underdiagnosed thrombophilia: a primer for internists. *Polish Arch Int Med, 130*, 868–877.

77. Cai, K., Osheroff, W. P., Buczynski, G., et al. (2014). Characterization of Thrombate III®, a pasteurized and nanofiltered therapeutic human antithrombin concentrate. *Biologicals, 42*, 133–138.

78. Van Cott, E. M., Orlando, C., Moore, G. W., et al. (2020). Recommendations for clinical laboratory testing for antithrombin deficiency; communication from the SSC of the ISTH. *J Thromb Haemost, 18*, 17–22.

79. Gausman, J. N., & Marlar, R. A. (2017). Assessment of hereditary thrombophilia: performance of antithrombin (AT) testing. *Methods Mol Biol, 1646*, 161–167.

80. Antovic, J., Söderström, J., Karlman, B., et al. (2001). Evaluation of a new immunoturbidimetric test (liatest antithrombin III) for determination of antithrombin antigen. *Clin Lab Haematol, 23*, 313–316.

81. Folsom, A. R., Nena, A., Wang, L., et al. (2022). Protein C, antithrombin, and venous thromboembolism incidence. *Arterioscl Thromb Vasc Biol, 22*, 1018–1022.

82. Huang, X., Xu, F., Assa, C. R., et al. (2018). Recurrent pulmonary embolism associated with deep vein thrombosis diagnosed as protein S deficiency owing to a novel mutation in PROS1: a case report. *Medicine, 97*, 1–4.

83. Gausman, J. M., & Marlar, R. A. (2017). Assessment of hereditary thrombophilia: performance of protein C (PC) testing. *Methods Mol Biol, 1646*, 145–151.

84. Cooper, P. C., Pavlova, A., Moore, G. W., et al. (2020). Recommendations for clinical laboratory testing for protein C deficiency, for the subcommittee on plasma coagulation inhibitors of the ISTH. *J Thromb Haemost, 18*, 271–277.

85. Marlar, R. A., Gausman, J. N., Tsuda, H., et al. (2021). Recommendations for clinical laboratory testing for protein S deficiency: communication from the SSC committee plasma coagulation inhibitors of the ISTH. *J Thromb Haemost, 19*, 68–74.

86. Manco-Johnson, M. J., Bomgaars, L., Palascak, J., et al. (2016). Efficacy and safety of protein C concentrate to treat purpura fulminans and thromboembolic events in severe congenital protein C deficiency. *Thromb Haemost, 116*, 58–68.

87. Siriez, R., Dogne, J. M., Gosselin, R., et al. (2021). Comprehensive review of the impact of direct oral anticoagulants on thrombophiliia diagnostic tests: practical recommendations for the laboratory. *Int J Lab Hematol, 43*, 7–20.

88. Ens, G. E., & Newlin, F. (1995). Spurious protein S deficiency as a result of elevated factor VII levels. *Clin Hemost Rev, 9*, 18.

89. Rigamonti, F., Carbone, F., Montecucco, F., et al. (2018). Serum lipoprotein (a) predicts acute coronary syndromes in patients with severe carotid stenosis. *Eur J Clin Invest, 48*. doi:10.1111/eci.12888.

90. Sproston, N. R., & Ashworth, J. J. (2018). Role of C-reactive protein at sites of inflammation and infection. *Front Immunol, 9*, 1–11.

91. Yousuf, O., Mohanty, B. D., Martin, S. S., et al. (2013). High-sensitivity C-reactive protein and cardiovascular disease: a resolute belief or an elusive link? *J Am Coll Cardiol, 62*, 397–408.

92. Fonseca, F. A. H., & de Oleivera-Izar, M. C. (2016). High-sensitivity C-reactive protein and cardiovascular disease across countries and ethnicities. *Clinics (Sao Paulo), 71*, 235–242.

93. Nadar, S. K., & Shaikh, M. M. (2019). Biomarkers in routine heart failure clinical care. *Card Fail Rev, 5*, 50–56.

94. Surma, S., & Banach, M. (2022). Fibrinogen and atherosclerotic cardiovascular diseases—review of literature and clinical studies. *Int J Mol Sci.* doi: 10.3390/ijms23010193.

95. Swarowska, M., Janowska, A., Polczak, A., et al. (2014). The sustained increase of plasma fibrinogen during ischemic stroke predicts worse outcome independently of baseline fibrinogen level. *Inflammation, 37*, 1142–1147.

96. Shojaie, M., Pourahmad, M., Eshraghian, A., et al. (2009). Fibrinogen as a risk factor for premature myocardial infarction in Iranian patients: a case control study. *Vasc Health Risk Manag, 5*, 673–676.

97. Quinton, T., Fraser, J., Black, K. M., Sadeghi-Khomami, A. (2020). Cryocheck chromogenic factor VIII: a new kit for the detection of FVIII:C activity. Poster presented at the *Thrombosis and Hemostasis Summit of North America* (THSNA) annual meeting, October 27–30.

98. Gupta, A., Ray, J. R., Streiff, M. B., et al. (2020). Mortality and associated comorbidities among patients hospitalized for deep vein thrombosis and pulmonary embolism in the United States: results from a nationally representative database. *Blood, 20*, 39–40.

99. Huisman, M. V., & Klok, F. A. (2013). Diagnostic management of acute deep vein thrombosis and pulmonary embolism. *J Thromb Haemost, 11*, 412–422.

100. Wells, P. S., Anderson, D. R., Bormanis, J., et al. (1997). Value of assessment of pretest probability of deep-vein thrombosis in clinical management. *Lancet, 350*, 1795–1798.

101. Wells, P. S., Anderson, D. R., Rodger, M., et al. (2000). Derivation of a simple clinical model to categorize patients' probability of pulmonary embolism: increasing the models utility with the Simplired D-dimer. *Thromb Haemost, 83*, 416–420.

102. Es, N. V., Kraaijpoel, N., Klok, F. A., et al. (2017). The original and simplified Wells rules and age-adjusted D-dimer testing to rule out pulmonary embolism: an individual patient data meta-analysis. *J Thromb Haemost, 15*, 678–684.

103. Johnson, E. D., Schell, J. C., & Rodgers, G. M. (2019). The D-dimer assay. *Am J Hematol, 94*, 833–839.

104. Tripodi, A. (2011). D-dimer testing in laboratory practice. *Clin Chem, 57*, 1256–1262.

105. Favaloro, E. J., & Dean, E. (2021). Variability in D-dimer reporting revisited. *Pathology, 53*, 538–540.

106. Righini, M., Van Es, J., Den Exter, P. L., et al. (2014). Age-adjusted D-dimer cutoff levels to rule out pulmonary embolism: the ADJUST-PE study. *JAMA, 311*, 1117–1124.

107. Robert-Ebadi, H., Robin, P., Hugli, O., et al. (2021). Impact of the age-adjusted D-dimer cutoff to exclude pulmonary embolism: a multinational prospective real-life study (the RELAX-PE study). *Circulation, 143*, 1828–1830.

108. Khoury, J. D., Adcock, D. M., Chan, F., et al. (2010). Increases in quantitative D-dimer levels correlate with progressive disease better than circulating tumor cell counts in patients with refractory prostate cancer. *Am J Clin Pathol, 134*, 964–969.

109. Madoiwa, S., Kitajima, I., Ohmori, T., et al. (2013). Distinct reactivity of the commercially available monoclonal antibodies of D-dimer and plasma FDP testing to the molecular variants of fibrin degradation products. *Thromb Res, 132*, 457–464.

110. Levi, M., Feinstein, D. I., Colman, R. W., et al. (2013). Consumptive thrombohemorrhagic disorders. In Marder, V. J., Aird, W. C., Bennett, J. S., et al. (Eds.), *Hemostasis and Thrombosis: Basic Principles and Clinical Practice.* (6th ed., pp. 1178–1196). Philadelphia: Lippincott Williams & Wilkins.

111. Popescu, N. I., Lupu, C., & Lupu, F. (2022). Disseminated intravascular coagulation and its immune mechanisms. *Blood, 139*, 1973–1986.

112. Trousseau, A. (1865). Phlegmasia alba dolens: Clinique Medicale de L'Hotel Dieu de Paris. *The New Sydenham Society, 3*, 94.

113. Singh, N., Pati, H. P., Tyagi, S., et al. (2017). Evaluation of the diagnostic performance of fibrin monomer in comparison to D-dimer in patients with overt and nonovert disseminated intravascular coagulation. *Clin Appl Thromb Hemost, 23*, 460–465.

114. Franchini, M., Zaffanello, M., & Mannucci, P. M. (2021). Bleeding disorders in primary fibrinolysis. *Int J Mol Sci.* https://doi.org/10.3390/ijms22137027.

115. Whyte, C. S., Morrow, G. B., Mitchell, J. L. et al. (2020). Fibrinolytic abnormalities in acute respiratory distress syndrome (ARDS) and versatility of thrombolytic drugs to treat COVID-19. *J Thromb Haemost, 18*, 1548–1555.

116. Asakura, H., & Ogawa, H. (2020). Perspective on fibrinolytic therapy in COVID-19: the potential of inhalation therapy against suppressed-fibrinolytic-type DIC. *J Intensive Care, 8*, 1–4.

117. Favaloro, E. J. (2010). Laboratory testing in disseminated intravascular coagulation. *Semin Thromb Hemost, 36*, 458–467.

118. Sawamura, A., Hayakawa, M., Gando, S., et al. (2009). Disseminated intravascular coagulation with a fibrinolytic phenotype at an early phase of trauma predicts mortality. *Thromb Res, 124*, 608–613.

119. Drolz, A., Horvatits, T., Rutter, K., et al. (2015). Disseminated intravascular coagulation score predicts mortality in critically ill patients with liver cirrhosis. *Crit Care, 19*, P377.

120. Longstaff, C. (2018). Measuring fibrinolysis: from research to routine diagnostic assays. *J Thromb Haemost, 16*, 652–662.

121. Wiedermann, C. J. (2018). Antithrombin concentrate use in disseminated intravascular coagulation of sepsis: meta-analyses revisited. *J Thromb Haemost, 16*, 455–457.

122. Levi, M., de Jonge, E., & van der Poll, T. (2006). Plasma and plasma components in the management of disseminated intravascular coagulation. *Best Pract Res Clin Haematol, 19*, 127–142.

123. Grafeneder, J., Buchtele, N., Egger, D., et al. (2022). Disseminated intravascular coagulation score predicts mortality in patients with liver disease and low fibrinogen level. *Thromb Haemost.* doi: 10.1055/a-1925-2300.

124. Thachil, J. (2016). Disseminated intravascular coagulation: a practical approach. *Anesthesiol, 125*, 230–236.

125. Haram, K., Mortensen, J. H., Mastrolia, S. A., et al. (2017). Disseminated intravascular coagulation in the HELLP syndrome: how much do we really know? *J Matern Fetal Neonatal Med, 30*, 779–788.

126. Ben-Ari, Z., Osman, E., Hutton, R. A., et al. (1999). Disseminated intravascular coagulation in liver cirrhosis: fact or fiction? *AM J Gastroenterol, 94*, 2977–2982.

127. Kappler, S., Ronan-Bentle, S., & Graham, A. (2017). Thrombotic microangiopathies (TTP, HUS, HELLP). *Hematol Oncol Clin North Am, 31*, 1081–1103.

128. Iba, T., Levi, M., Thachil, J., & Levy, J. H. (2022). Disseminated intravascular coagulation: the past, present, and future considerations. *Semin Thromb Hemost.* https://doi.org/10.1055/s-0042-1756300.

129. Junqueira, D. R., Zorzela, L. M., & Perini, E. (2017). Unfractionated heparin versus low molecular weight heparins for avoiding heparin-induced thrombocytopenia in postoperative patients. *Cochrane Database Syst Rev, 4*, CD007557. https://doi.org/10.1002/14651858.CD007557.pub3.

130. Salter, B. S., Weiner, M. M., Trinh, M. A., et al. (2016). Heparin-induced thrombocytopenia: a comprehensive clinical review. *J Am Coll Cardiol, 67*, 2519–2532.

131. Lovecchio, F. (2014). Heparin-induced thrombocytopenia. *Clin Toxicol (Phila), 52*, 579–583.

132. Warkentin, T. E. (2016). Clinical picture of heparin-induced thrombocytopenia (HIT) and its differentiation from non-HIT thrombocytopenia. *Thromb Haemost, 116*, 813–822.

133. Levy, J. H., & Hursting, M. J. (2007). Heparin-induced thrombocytopenia, a prothrombotic disease. *Hematol Oncol Clin North Am, 21*, 65–88.

134. Smith, B. W., Joseph, J. R., & Park, P. (2017). Heparin-induced thrombocytopenia presenting as unilateral lower limb paralysis following lumbar spine surgery: case report. *J Neurosurg Spine, 26*, 594–597.

135. Warkentin, T. E. (2019). Heparin-induced thrombocytopenia. In Kitchens, C. S., Kessler, C. M., Konkle, B. A., et al. (Eds.), *Consultative Hemostasis and Thrombosis.* (4th ed., pp. 491–527). Philadelphia: Saunders.

136. Staibano, P., Arnold, D. M., Bowdish, D. M., et al. (2017). The unique immunological features of heparin-induced thrombocytopenia. *Br J Haematol, 177*, 198–207.

137. Warkentin, T. E., & Greinacher, A. (2013). Heparin-induced thrombocytopenia. In Marder, V. J., Aird, W. C., Bennett, J. S., et al. (Eds.), *Hemostasis and Thrombosis: Basic Principles and Clinical Practice.* (6th ed., pp. 1293–1307). Philadelphia: Lippincott Williams & Wilkins.

138. Warkentin, T. E., Hayward, C. P., Boshkov, L. K., et al. (1994). Sera from patients with heparin-induced thrombocytopenia generate platelet-derived microparticles with procoagulant activity: an explanation for the thrombotic complications of heparin-induced thrombocytopenia. *Blood, 84*, 3691–3699.

139. Tutwiler, V., Madeeva, D., Ahn, H. S., et al. (2016). Platelet transactivation by monocyte promotes thrombosis in heparin-induced thrombocytopenia. *Blood, 127*, 464–472.

140. Madeeva, D., Cines, D. B., Poncz, M., et al. (2016). Role of monocytes and endothelial cells in heparin-induced thrombocytopenia. *Thromb Haemost, 116*, 806–812.

141. Rauova, L., Hirsch, J. D., Greene, T. K., et al. (2010). Monocyte bound PF4 in the pathogenesis of heparin-induced thrombocytopenia. *Blood, 116*, 5021–5031.

142. Khairy, M., Lasne, D., Amelot, A., et al. (2004). Polymorphonuclear leukocyte and monocyte activation induced by plasma from patients with heparin-induced thrombocytopenia in whole blood. *Thromb Haemost, 92*, 1411–1419.

143. Walenga, J. M., Jeske, W. P., & Messmore, H. L. (2000). Mechanisms of venous and arterial thrombosis in heparin-induced thrombocytopenia. *J Thromb Thrombolysis, 10*, S13–S20.

144. Walenga, J. M., Jeske, W. P., Prechel, M. M., et al. (2004). Newer insights on the mechanism of heparin-induced thrombocytopenia. *Semin Thromb Hemost, 30*(Suppl. 1), 57–67.

145. Poncz, M. (2005). Mechanistic basis of heparin-induced thrombocytopenia. *Semin Thorac Cardiovasc Surg, 17*, 73–79.

146. Kuter, D. J., Konkle, B. A., Hamza, T. H., et al. (2017). Clinical outcomes in a cohort of patients with heparin-induced thrombocytopenia. *Am J Hematol, 92*, 730–738.

147. Warkentin, T. E., & Greinacher, A. (2016). Management of heparin-induced thrombocytopenia. *Curr Opin Hematol, 23*, 462–470.

148. Linkins, L. A., Bates, S. M., Lee A. Y. Y., et al. (2015). Combination of 4Ts score and PF4/H-PaGIA for diagnosis and management of heparin-induced thrombocytopenia. *Blood, 126*, 597–603.

149. Crowther, M., Cook, D., Guyatt, G., et al. (2014). Heparin-induced thrombocytopenia in the critically ill: interpreting the 4Ts test in a randomized trial. *J Crit Care, 29*, 470.e7–e15.

150. Cuker, A., Arepally, G., Crowther, M. A., et al. (2010). The HIT expert probability (HEP) score: a novel pre-test probability model for heparin-induced thrombocytopenia based on broad expert opinion. *J Thromb Haemost, 8*, 2642–2650.

151. Demma, L. J., Winkler, A. M., & Levy, J. H. (2011). A diagnosis of heparin-induced thrombocytopenia with combined clinical and laboratory methods in cardiothoracic surgical intensive care unit patients. *Anesth Analg, 113*, 697–702.

152. Nagler, M., & Bakchoul, T. (2016). Clinical and laboratory tests for the diagnosis of heparin-induced thrombocytopenia. *Thromb Haemost, 116*, 823–834.

153. Minet, V., Dogné, J. M., & Mullier, F. (2017). Functional assays in the diagnosis of heparin-induced thrombocytopenia: a review. *Molecules*. https://doi.org/10.3390/molecules22040617.

154. Sylvester, K. W., Fanikos, J., & Anger, K. E. (2013). Impact of an immunoglobulin G-specific enzyme-linked immunosorbent assay on the management of heparin-induced thrombocytopenia. *Pharmacotherapy, 33*, 1191–1198.

155. Vianello, F., Sambado, L., Scarparo, P., et al. (2015). Comparison of three different immunoassays in the diagnosis of heparin-induced thrombocytopenia. *Clin Chem Lab Med, 53*, 257–263.

156. Bakchoul, T., Giptner, A., Bein, G., et al. (2011). Performance characteristic of two commercially available IgG-specific immunoassays in the assessment of heparin-induced thrombocytopenia (HIT). *Thromb Res, 127*, 345–348.

157. Warkentin, T. E., Arnold, D. M., Nazi, I., et al. (2015). The platelet serotonin-release assay. *Am J Hematol, 90*, 564–572.

158. Vitale, M., Tazzari, P., Ricci, F., et al. (2001). Comparison between different laboratory tests for the detection and prevention of heparin-induced thrombocytopenia. *Cytometry, 46*, 290–295.

159. Brace, L. D. (1992). Testing for heparin-induced thrombocytopenia by platelet aggregometry. *Clin Lab Sci, 5*, 80–81.

160. Tan, C. W., Ward, C. M., & Morel-Kopp, M. C. (2012). Evaluating heparin-induced thrombocytopenia: the old and the new. *Semin Thromb Hemost, 38*, 135–143.

161. Cuker, A., Gimotty, P. A., Crowther, M. A., et al. (2002). Predictive value of the 4Ts scoring system for heparin-induced thrombocytopenia: a systematic review and meta-analysis. *Blood, 120*, 4160–4167.

162. Sun, L., Gimotty, P. A., Lakshmanan, S., et al. (2016). Diagnostic accuracy of rapid immunoassays for heparin-induced thrombocytopenia. a systematic review and meta-analysis. *Thromb Haemost, 115*, 1044–1055.

163. Warkentin, T. E., Pai, M., Sheppard, J. I., et al. (2011). Fondaparinux treatment of acute heparin-induced thrombocytopenia confirmed by the serotonin-release assay: a 30-month, 16-patient case series. *J Thromb Haemost, 9*, 2389–2396.

164. Chanas, T., Palkimas, S., Maitland, H. S., et al. (2019). Evaluation of the use of argatroban or bivalirudin for the management of suspected heparin-induced thrombocytopenia in the setting of continuous renal replacement therapy. *Clin Med Insights: Trauma Intensive Med, 10*, 1–7.

165. Barlow, A., Barlow, B., Reinaker, T., et al. (2019). Potential role of direct oral anticoagulants in the management of heparin-induced thrombocytopenia. *Pharmacotherapy, 39*, 837–853.

166. Carre, J., Guerineau, H., Le Beller, C., et al. (2021). Direct oral anticoagulants as successful treatment of heparin-induced thrombocytopenia: a Parisian retrospective case series. *Front Med, 8*, 1–7.

167. Palazzuoli, A., Giustozzi, M., Ruocco, G., et al. (2021). Thromboembolic complications in COVID-19: from clinical scenario to laboratory evidence. *Life (Basel), 11*(5), 395.

168. Oxley, T. J., Mocco, J., Majidi, S., et al. (2020). Large-vessel stroke as a presenting feature of COVID-19 in the young. *N Engl J Med*. doi: 10.1056/NEJMc2009787.

169. Mehta, P., McAuley, D. F., Brown, M., et al. (2020). COVID-19: consider cytokine storm syndromes and immunosuppression. *Lancet*. doi: 10.1016/S0140-6736(20)30628-0.

170. Manne, B. K., Denorme, F., Middleton, E. A., et al. (2020). Platelet gene expression and function in patients with COVID-19. *Blood*. doi: 10.1182/blood.202000721.

171. Ahmadi, S., Firoozi, D., Dehghani, M., et al. (2022). Evaluation of nutritional status of intensive care unit COVID-19 patients based on the nutritional risk screening 2002 score. *Int J Clin Pract*. doi: 10.1155/2022/2448161.

172. Warkentin, T. E., & Cuker, A. (2022). COVID-19: vaccine-induced immune thrombotic thrombocytopenia (VITT). M. Crowther, & J. S. Tirnauer, Editors. *UpToDate*: Waltham, MA. https://www.uptodate.com.

173. Greinacher, A., Selleng, K., Palankar, R., et al. (2021). Insights in ChAdOx1 nCoV-19 vaccine-induced immune thrombotic thrombocytopenia. *Blood, 138*, 2256–2268.

174. Favaloro, E. J., Clifford, J., Leitinger, E., et al. (2022). Assessment of immunological anti-platelet factor 4 antibodies for vaccine-induced thrombotic thrombocytopenia (VITT) in a large Australian cohort: a multicenter study comprising 1284 patients. *J Thromb Haemost*. doi: 10.1111/jth.15881.

175. Paez-Alacron, M. E., & Greinacher, A. (2022). Vaccine-induced immune thrombotic thrombocytopenia (VITT) – update on diagnosis and management considering different resources: Comment. *J Thromb Haemost, 20*, 2707–2708.

40

Antithrombotic Therapies and Laboratory Assessment

Mayukh Kanti Sarkar and George A. Fritsma

OBJECTIVES

After completion of this chapter, the reader will be able to:

1. List and describe indications for antithrombotic therapy.
2. Distinguish between anticoagulant and antiplatelet therapy.
3. Diagram and describe the functional mechanism of each anticoagulant and antiplatelet therapeutic drug.
4. Monitor warfarin therapy using the prothrombin time, international normalized ratio, and the chromogenic factor X assay.
5. Monitor unfractionated heparin therapy using the partial thromboplastin time and the chromogenic anti-Xa heparin assay.
6. Monitor low-molecular-weight heparin and fondaparinux therapy using the chromogenic anti-Xa heparin assay.
7. Assess the direct oral anti-Xa anticoagulants rivaroxaban, apixaban, and edoxaban using the chromogenic anti-Xa assay.
8. Assess the direct thrombin inhibitor anticoagulants oral dabigatran and intravenous argatroban or bivalirudin using the ecarin chromogenic assay or plasma-diluted thrombin time.
9. Assess the therapeutic activity of intravenous platelet glycoprotein IIb/IIIa inhibitors eptifibatide and tirofiban.
10. Assess the therapeutic activity of oral platelet inhibitors aspirin, clopidogrel, prasugrel, and ticagrelor.
11. Monitor the effects of fibrinolytic therapy.

OUTLINE

Thrombosis and Antithrombotic Therapy
Warfarin
  Warfarin Action
  Warfarin Prophylaxis and Therapy
  Monitoring Warfarin Therapy
  Reversing Warfarin Therapy
Unfractionated Heparin
  Heparin Action
  Heparin Therapy
  Monitoring Heparin Therapy
  Limitations of Heparin Therapy Monitoring Using the PTT
  Reversing Heparin Therapy
Low-Molecular-Weight Heparin
  LMWH Action
  LMWH Therapy
  Laboratory Assessment of LMWH Therapy
Fondaparinux

Direct Anti-Xa Oral Anticoagulants
  Anti-Xa DOAC Action
  Anti-Xa DOAC Therapy
  Reversing Anti-Xa DOAC Therapy
  Laboratory Assessment of Anti-Xa DOACs
Direct Thrombin Inhibitors
  Oral Dabigatran
  Intravenous Direct Thrombin Inhibitors
Switching Anticoagulants and Periprocedural Management
Antiplatelet Therapy
  Parenteral Antiplatelet Therapeutic Drugs
  Oral Antiplatelet Therapeutic Drugs
  Laboratory Assessment of Oral Antiplatelet Therapeutic Drugs
Fibrinolytic Therapy
Future of Antithrombotic Therapy

CASE STUDY

After studying the material in this chapter, the reader should be able to respond to the following case study:

A 71-year-old woman with atrial fibrillation has taken 5 mg/day of warfarin for 8 years. Her monthly INR has been consistently within the target therapeutic range. Reference intervals can be found after the Index at the end of the book.

Recently, however, her INR was 6.5 and for several days, she had noticed that her gums bled after she brushed her teeth.

1. What could cause this change in the INR result?
2. What should be done about her INR result and symptoms?

THROMBOSIS AND ANTITHROMBOTIC THERAPY

Thrombosis, described in Chapter 39, is the pathologic presence of thrombi (blood clots) in veins or arteries that obstruct blood flow and cause tissue ischemia and necrosis. *Antithrombotic* therapeutic drugs have been employed to prevent and treat thrombosis since intravenous heparin was first approved by the US Food and Drug Administration (FDA) in 1935.[1] Antithrombotics include anticoagulants, which regulate coagulation and reduce thrombin formation, and antiplatelet therapeutics, which diminish platelet activation. *Fibrinolytic* drugs are employed to disperse or reduce clots obstructing veins and arteries.

Antithrombotic drugs include the pre-1990 therapeutics heparin, warfarin, and aspirin; heparin derivatives and antiplatelet therapeutics that joined clinical care in the 1990s; and the direct oral anticoagulants (DOACs) that entered clinical practice in 2010.[2] Table 40.1 provides a list of antithrombotics with their indications.

Venous thromboembolic disease (VTE, venous thromboembolic events) includes superficial thrombosis, deep vein thrombosis (DVT), and pulmonary embolism (PE). Providers treat VTE and reduce reocclusion (blood clot return) from the established blood clot with high *therapeutic* doses of intravenous standard unfractionated heparin (UFH), subcutaneous low-molecular-weight heparin (LMWH), subcutaneous synthetic pentasaccharide (fondaparinux), the oral vitamin K antagonist (VKA) warfarin, or a DOAC. Providers also employ these anticoagulant drugs *prophylactically* using lower dosages to prevent ischemic strokes associated with nonvalvular atrial fibrillation (AF), to prevent VTE with a provoking factor such as total hip and total knee replacement surgery, in orthopedic repair surgery, and to prevent thrombosis in patients with chronic inflammation and immobilization. Anticoagulants are used at higher than therapeutic doses (supratherapeutic dose) to prevent thrombosis during interventional and surgical procedures.

One of two intravenous direct thrombin inhibitors (DTIs), argatroban or bivalirudin, is substituted for UFH in patients who have developed heparin-induced thrombocytopenia (HIT) with thrombosis, a devastating arterial and venous thrombotic side effect of UFH therapy (Chapter 39).

Arterial thrombosis includes acute myocardial infarction (AMI), ischemic cerebrovascular accident (CVA, stroke), transient ischemic attack (TIA), and peripheral arterial occlusion (PAO) or peripheral artery disease (PAD). These disorders are managed with UFH, LMWH, fondaparinux, warfarin, and the antiplatelet therapeutic drugs aspirin, clopidogrel, prasugrel, and ticagrelor. Patients who have had a thrombotic event often take aspirin at less than 100 mg/day to prevent recurrence. A single aspirin tablet reduces morbidity and mortality when taken within minutes of the acute onset of stroke or cardiac symptoms of coronary artery blockage. The intravenous platelet glycoprotein IIb/IIIa inhibitor (GPI) pharmaceutical drugs eptifibatide and tirofiban are used to prevent thrombosis during percutaneous coronary intervention (PCI, cardiac catheterization) for angioplasty or stent implantation.

Thrombolytic therapy using fibrinolytic drugs may be used to resolve DVT, PE, PAO, AMI, and stroke, particularly when used within 4 hours after onset of clinical symptoms.[3] Thrombolytic therapy employs recombinant forms of tissue plasminogen activator (TPA), alteplase and tenecteplase. Thrombolytic therapy raises the risk of hemorrhage, particularly intracranial hemorrhage. The PT, PTT, fibrinogen assay, D-dimer, and viscoelastometry may be used to estimate thrombolytic efficacy and safety.[4]

Many lives have been saved through the judicious use of antithrombotic therapy, and countless more people have been spared thrombotic reocclusion through long-term antithrombotic therapy. However, all current antithrombotics and fibrinolytics present a bleeding risk because their effective dose ranges are narrow.[5] Overdose leads to emergency department visits for uncontrolled bleeding in outpatients, yet inadequate dosages are associated with reocclusion. Dosages and half-lives differ among the antithrombotic drugs because of variations in formulation and patient metabolism.[6]

Because of these risks, laboratory monitoring or assessment of antithrombotic therapy is important. Hemostasis laboratory professionals perform countless *prothrombin time* (PT), *partial thromboplastin time* (PTT/APTT), and *chromogenic anti-Xa* assays to assess anticoagulant therapy on a scheduled basis. Adjustment of antithrombotic drug dosages in response to laboratory outcomes is an essential aspect of patient health care. Although anticoagulant therapy assessment may seem routine, vigilance is critical for effective treatment and patient safety.[7]

The antiplatelet therapeutic drugs aspirin, clopidogrel, prasugrel, and ticagrelor, as well as LMWH, fondaparinux, and the DOACs, have fixed dose-response characteristics and require only on-demand *assessment* (not scheduled monitoring) when a clinical issue arises. However, these antiplatelet drugs and all antithrombotic drugs require assessment of activity in patients with the conditions listed in Box 40.1.

WARFARIN

Warfarin Action

As detailed in Chapter 35, the procoagulant factors II (prothrombin), VII, IX, and X depend on vitamin K for normal production, as do coagulation control proteins C, S, and Z. Vitamin K is responsible for the γ-carboxylation of a series of 12 to 18 glutamic acids near each molecule's N-terminus (amino terminus), a posttranslational modification that enables them to bind ionic calcium (Ca^{2+}) and cell membrane phospholipids, especially phosphatidylserine (Figure 35.5). Vitamin K is concentrated in green tea, avocados, and green leafy vegetables and is produced by gut flora; its absence results in the production of nonfunctional des-γ *carboxyl* forms of factors II, VII, IX, and X and proteins C, S, and Z.

Warfarin sodium (warfarin, 4-hydroxycoumarin) is a member of the coumarin pharmaceutical family and is the formulation of coumarin most often used in North America.[8] Another coumarin is dicoumarol (3,3′-methylenebis-[4-hydroxycoumarin]), the original anticoagulant extracted from moldy sweet clover, described in 1940, and used to this day in modified form as a rodenticide.[9] As rodents grew resistant to dicoumarol, manufacturers switched to

TABLE 40.1 Antithrombotic Therapeutic Drugs

Antithrombotic Drug	Indication	Mode of Action	Half-Life	Measurement	Reversal	FDA Approval
Oral Anticoagulants						
Warfarin	*Prophylaxis*: reduce postsurgical thrombosis risk, reduce risk of AF-related stroke, including mechanical heart valve or LAC *Therapy*: reduce risk of post-VTE reocclusion	Vitamin K antagonist	5 days	Monitor PT/INR; CFX	Vitamin K, 4-factor PCC, rFVIIa	1954
DOACs	*Prophylaxis*: reduce postsurgical thrombosis risk, reduce risk of NVAF-related stroke *Therapy*: reduce risk of post-VTE reocclusion	Rivaroxaban, apixaban, edoxaban: direct FXa inhibition; Dabigatran: direct thrombin inhibition	10–18 hr when the CrCl is normal	Rivaroxaban, apixaban, edoxaban: chromogenic anti-Xa Dabigatran: ecarin chromogenic assay, dilute thrombin time	Rivaroxaban, apixaban: andexanet alfa Dabigatran: idarucizumab	See Table 40.4
Heparin and Heparin Derivatives						
Unfractionated heparin (UFH)	Reduce risk of post-VTE and AMI reocclusion; intraoperative anticoagulation	IV; AT activation, inhibits thrombin and FXa	1–2 hr	Monitor PTT, ACT, chromogenic anti-Xa heparin assay	Protamine sulfate	1935
Low-molecular-weight heparins (LMWHs)	*Prophylaxis*: reduce risk of thrombosis after surgery, in medical conditions *Therapy*: reduce reocclusion risk after AMI, DVT/PE	SC; AT activation, inhibits FXa	3–5 hr	Chromogenic anti-Xa	Protamine sulfate (partial)	1993
Fondaparinux			12–17 hr	Chromogenic anti-Xa	Discontinue therapy	2001
Intravenous Direct Thrombin Inhibitors						
Argatroban	Anticoagulation in HIT	Directly bind and inhibit thrombin	50 min	PTT, ECA	Discontinue therapy	1997
Bivalirudin			25 min			2000
Antiplatelet Therapeutic Drugs						
Aspirin	Prevent AMI reocclusion	Oral, platelet COX inhibitor	7–10 days, related to platelet turnover	VerifyNow Aspirin, AspirinWorks, platelet aggregometry	Discontinue therapy	1900
Clopidogrel	Prevent AMI reocclusion	Oral, binds platelet $P2Y_{12}$ receptor	6–7 hr	Platelet aggregometry, VerifyNow		1998
Prasugrel						2013
Ticagrelor						2011
Eptifibatide	Maintain vascular patency during PCI and cardiac bypass surgery	IV, binds platelet GPIIb/IIIa receptor	2.5 hr	Platelet aggregometry		2001
Tirofiban						1999

ACT, Activated clotting time test; *AF*, atrial fibrillation; *AMI*, acute myocardial infarction; *AT*, antithrombin; *CFX*, chromogenic factor X activity; *COX*, cyclooxygenase; *CrCl*, creatinine clearance; *DOAC*, direct oral anticoagulants; *DVT*, deep vein thrombosis; *ECA*, ecarin chromogenic assay; *FDA*, US Food and Drug Administration; *FXa*, coagulation factor Xa; *HIT*, heparin-induced thrombocytopenia; *INR*, international normalized ratio; *IV*, intravenous; *LAC*, lupus anticoagulant; *NVAF*, nonvalvular atrial fibrillation; *PCC*, prothrombin complex concentrate; *PCI*, percutaneous coronary intervention; *PE*, pulmonary embolism; *PT*, prothrombin time; *PTT*, partial thromboplastin time; *rFVIIa*, recombinant activated factor VII; *SC*, subcutaneous; *VTE*, venous thromboembolic events.

CrCl, Creatinine clearance; *DIC,* disseminated intravascular coagulation.

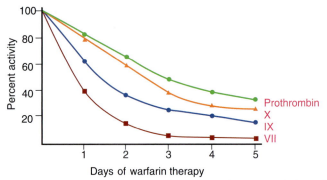

Figure 40.1 The Anticoagulant Effect of Warfarin at Initiation of Therapy. Factor (F) VII activity decreases to 50% of normal 6 hours after warfarin therapy is begun, prolonging the FVIIa-sensitive prothrombin time (PT) to near the therapeutic international normalized ratio (INR) of 2 to 3. The half-lives of FII (prothrombin), FIX, and FX are longer than that of FVII; FII activity requires at least 3 days to decline by 50%. The patient gains full anticoagulation effects approximately 5 days after the start of warfarin therapy.

brodifacoum ("superwarfarin"). From long habit, health care practitioners use the trade name "Coumadin" for warfarin, although Bristol-Myers Squibb discontinued Coumadin distribution in 2020 as generic warfarin captured the market.

Warfarin is a VKA that suppresses γ-carboxylation of glutamic acid by slowing the activity of the enzyme *vitamin K epoxide reductase* (VKORC1). During warfarin therapy, the activities of factors II, VII, IX, and X and proteins C, S, and Z become reduced as the nonfunctional des-carboxyl proteins are produced in their place. In the past, these were named "proteins induced by vitamin K antagonists" (PIVKA) factors. The des-carboxyl proteins bind few calcium ions and assemble weakly on phospholipid surfaces, causing reduced catalysis of their procoagulant substrates with resulting decrease in thrombin generation and clot formation.

Warfarin Prophylaxis and Therapy

Health care providers prefer the DOACs over warfarin for most prophylactic and therapeutic applications; however, warfarin remains the recommended oral anticoagulant for stroke prevention in patients with mechanical heart valves, AF with mitral valve stenosis, and antiphospholipid syndrome.[10] Data from a 2022 observational, retrospective study infer an association of warfarin with poorer clinical outcomes in aortic stenosis relative to DOAC therapy. This may further influence health care providers toward DOACs once a prospective randomized control trial is able to establish causality.[11] Considering the higher cost of DOACs, warfarin will predominate in underresourced locations.

Providers often start oral warfarin therapy at a fixed dosage of 5 or 10 mg per day for 2 or 3 consecutive days, often choosing 10 mg for patients who lack comorbidities, present few potential pharmaceutical interactions, and have high vitamin K intake.

Conversely, many providers choose *clinical dosing algorithms* for initial warfarin therapy. Algorithms provide dosage

recommendations based on age, sex, body mass index (BMI), potential pharmaceutical interactions, and liver disease. For instance, the effective dosage decreases with age and increases with BMI. Algorithms may also adjust for the presence of polymorphisms in genes of the cytochrome P 450 2 C9 (CYP2C9), CYP3A4, and VKORC1 enzyme metabolic pathways. Although clinical dosing algorithms that include genetic dose adjustments may yield improved time in the therapeutic range, published guidelines do not require polymorphism-based dose adjustment.

Warfarin resistance may render the patient unresponsive to typical warfarin dosages. Some patients require dosages of 20 mg/day or higher to achieve anticoagulation. Warfarin resistance has been traced to up to 26 mutations of the VKORC1 enzyme pathway.[12]

Providers begin monitoring warfarin anticoagulation at day 3 or 4 of therapy. The activity of each of the vitamin K-dependent coagulation factors begins to decline immediately but at different rates (Figure 40.1), and it takes about 5 days for all the factors to reach therapeutic levels. Table 40.2 lists the plasma half-life, plasma concentration, and minimum effective percentage of normal activity for the coagulation factors.

Control protein activities also become reduced on warfarin onset, especially the activity of protein C, which has a 6-hour half-life, so for the first 2 or 3 days of therapy, the patient paradoxically incurs the risk of thrombosis. A condition called *warfarin-induced skin necrosis,* a severe thrombotic reaction requiring dead tissue debridement, occurs if a large loading dose of warfarin is used. This can greatly reduce the level of protein C, particularly if the patient has a naturally low protein C level.[13] Today, loading doses of warfarin are avoided where possible. Alternatively, UFH or LMWH can be administered simultaneously with warfarin to prevent clotting during the first few days of warfarin therapy in a process called *bridging.*

Warfarin is contraindicated during pregnancy because it causes birth defects but may be prescribed during breastfeeding. When anticoagulation is desired during pregnancy—for instance, in women who possess a thrombosis risk factor—LMWH or fondaparinux is prescribed.

TABLE 40.2 Functional Properties of the Coagulation Factors

Factor	Half-Life	Plasma Level*	Hemostatic Level†
Fibrinogen	4 d	260 mg/dL	50 mg/dL
Prothrombin	60 hr	100 µg/mL	20 U/dL
V	16 hr	7 µg/mL	25 U/dL
VII	6 hr	0.5 µg/mL	20 U/dL
VIII	12 hr	0.2 µg/mL	30 U/dL
IX	24 hr	5 µg/mL	30 U/dL
X	30 hr	10 µg/mL	25 U/dL
XI	2–3 d	5 µg/mL	25 U/dL
XIII	7–10 d	30 µg/mL	2–3 U/dL
von Willebrand factor	30 hr	6 µg/mL	50 U/dL

*Butenas, S., & Mann, K. G. (2002). Blood Coagulation. *Biochemistry, 67*, 3–12.

†Minimum effective level; reference intervals typically range 80–120 U/dL. Levels given in units per deciliter per current guidelines can be converted to previously used % using the same numeric value.

d, Days; *hr*, hours.

Monitoring Warfarin Therapy

The PT/INR

The PT effectively monitors warfarin therapy because it is sensitive to reductions of factors II, VII, and X (Figure 40.2) (Chapter 41). The PT reagent is named *thromboplastin* and consists of tissue factor, phospholipid, and ionic calcium. It triggers the coagulation pathway at the level of factor VII. Owing to the 6-hour half-life of factor VII, the PT begins to prolong within 6 to 8 hours of warfarin ingestion; however, anticoagulation becomes therapeutic only when the activities of factors II and X decrease to less than 50% of normal, after approximately 5 days.

The first specimen for PT testing is collected and assayed on day 3 or 4 after warfarin therapy is initiated; subsequent PTs are performed daily until at least two consecutive results are within the target therapeutic range. Monitoring continues every 4 to 6 weeks, or up to 12-week intervals in patients with stable dosage levels, until the completion of therapy.[14] Therapy is typically continued for 6 months after a thrombotic event but can be lifelong. Monitoring is performed more frequently if there is a dietary change, a dosage change, when another medication is being started or stopped, or when the patient's medical condition changes. Because the therapeutic range is narrow, diligent monitoring is essential for successful therapy. Underanticoagulation incurs the danger of thrombotic reocclusion; overdose raises the risk of hemorrhage. Health care facilities offer anticoagulation clinics that specialize in near-patient warfarin monitoring; at-home monitoring devices are also available.

The medical laboratory professional reports PT results to the nearest tenth of a second and provides the PT reference interval (RI) in seconds for comparison. In view of inherent variations among thromboplastin reagents and to accomplish interlaboratory harmonization, all laboratories report the *international normalized*

ratio (INR) for patients who have reached a stable response to warfarin therapy. The INR has been validated only for stable warfarin monitoring. Laboratory practitioners use the following formula:[15]

$$INR = \left(PT_{patient}/PT_{normal}\right)^{ISI}$$

where $PT_{patient}$ is the PT of the patient in seconds, PT_{normal} is the geometric mean of the PT RI in seconds, and *ISI* is the international sensitivity index of the thromboplastin applied as an exponent.

Thromboplastin producers generate the ISI value by performing a regression analysis comparing the results of their respective thromboplastins with the results of the international reference thromboplastin (World Health Organization [WHO] human brain thromboplastin or equivalent) on the same plasma specimens. For this analysis, 50 or more warfarin plasma specimens and 10 or more normal specimens are used. Most manufacturers provide ISIs for a variety of coagulation instruments because each coagulometer may respond differently to their thromboplastins; for instance, some coagulometers rely on photometric detection of plasma changes, whereas others use an electromechanical system (Chapter 42), which affects sensitivity of clot endpoint detection. Most thromboplastin reagents have ISIs near 1.0, matching the ISI of the WHO's thromboplastin.

Automated coagulometers "request" the reagent ISI from the operator, or obtain it electronically from a reagent vial label bar code and compute the INR for each assay result. Although INRs are meant to be computed only for patients in whom the warfarin response has stabilized, they typically are reported for all patients, even those who are not taking warfarin. During the first 5 days of warfarin therapy (and for any patient not receiving warfarin), the astute medical laboratory practitioner and provider ignore the INR as unreliable and interpret the PT results in seconds, comparing it with the RI.

Warfarin INR Therapeutic Range

The provider adjusts the warfarin dosage to achieve the desired INR of 2 to 3, or 2.5 to 3.5 if the patient has a mechanical heart valve. INRs over 5 are associated with increased risk of hemorrhage and require immediate "read-back" communication with a member of the health care team.[16] Dosage adjustments are made conservatively because the INR requires 4 to 7 days to stabilize, but an elevated INR accompanied by hemorrhage is a medical emergency.[17]

Chromogenic Factor X Assay

The chromogenic coagulation factor X assay (CFX; not to be confused with the chromogenic anti-Xa heparin assay), recently available from Hyphen Biomed, has been recommended as an alternative to the PT/INR system. The CFX assay may be used to circumvent coagulation testing challenges when the PT is compromised by a lupus anticoagulant, a factor inhibitor, dual anticoagulation, or a coagulopathy.[18]

The CFX may eliminate the necessity for harmonization (as described earlier for INR).[19] The therapeutic range is typically 20% to 40% of normal factor X activity; however, individual laboratories must determine their own range by comparison of CFX values with the INR in a study of randomly selected

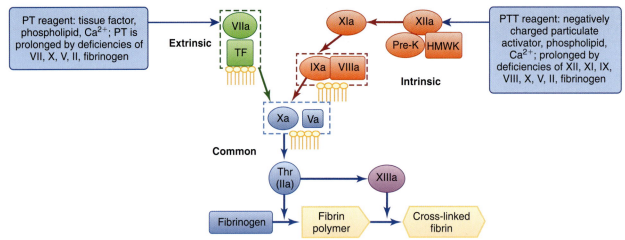

Figure 40.2 The Prothrombin Time *(PT)* and Partial Thromboplastin Time *(PTT)* Tests. The PT reagent activates the extrinsic coagulation pathway, beginning with factor (F) VII. The PT is prolonged by deficiencies of FVII, FX, FV, and FII (prothrombin), and fibrinogen when the fibrinogen concentration is less than 100 mg/dL. The PT is prolonged in warfarin therapy because it responds to the reduced FVII, FX, and prothrombin activities. The PTT reagent activates the intrinsic coagulation pathway through FXII, in association with prekallikrein *(pre-K)* and high-molecular-weight kininogen *(HMWK)*. The PTT is prolonged by deficiencies of pre-K; HMWK; FXII, FXI, FIX, FVIII, FX, FV, and prothrombin; and fibrinogen when the fibrinogen concentration is less than 100 mg/dL. The PTT is prolonged in unfractionated heparin (UFH) therapy because UFH activates the plasma control protein antithrombin (AT), which neutralizes the serine proteases FXIIa, FXIa, FXa, FIXa, and FIIa (thrombin). The PTT is also prolonged by the lupus anticoagulant. *TF*, Tissue factor.

specimens from stable warfarin patients.[20] The assay is mostly performed in specialized reference laboratories and it is not currently approved by the FDA.

Diet and Pharmaceutical Interference on Warfarin Activity

Dietary vitamin K decreases warfarin's effectiveness and reduces the INR. Green vegetables are a source of vitamin K, but vitamin K also is concentrated in green tea, cauliflower, liver, avocados, parenteral nutrition formulations, multivitamins, red wine, over-the-counter nutrition drinks, and over-the-counter dietary supplements. A patient on warfarin therapy is counseled to maintain a regular balanced diet, avoid supplements, and follow dietary changes or dietary supplement changes, with additional PT/INR levels and dosage adjustments when indicated.[21]

Warfarin is metabolized in the mitochondrial cytochrome P450 2 (CYP2C9) pathway of hepatocytes—the "disposal system" for at least 80 pharmaceuticals. Theoretically, parallel therapy with any pharmaceutical metabolized through the CYP2C9 pathway may unpredictably reduce or enhance the effects of warfarin because of competition for sites within the pathway. Examples include but are not limited to amiodarone, azole antifungals, phenytoin, rifampicin, sulfamethoxazole, statins, metronidazole, and cimetidine. Any therapeutic change must be followed with additional PT/INR assays and dosage adjustments.[22]

Reversing Warfarin Therapy

Table 40.3 provides recommendations for warfarin overdose reversal based on the INR and evidence of bleeding. Reversal requires oral or intravenous vitamin K and, if bleeding is severe, a means for substituting active coagulation factors such as four-factor prothrombin complex concentrate (Kcentra), recombinant

TABLE 40.3   Recommendations for Reversal of Warfarin Overdose Based on INR and Bleeding

Bleeding	INR	Intervention
No significant bleeding	3–5	Reduce dosage or omit one dose, monitor INR frequently
	5–9	Omit warfarin, monitor INR frequently, consider oral vitamin K (≤5 mg) if high risk for bleeding (surgery)
	>9	Stop warfarin, give 5–10 mg oral vitamin K, monitor INR frequently
Serious bleeding	Any INR	Stop warfarin, give 10 mg vitamin K by intravenous push (may repeat every 12 hr); give 4-factor PCC, rFVIIa, or plasma
Life-threatening bleeding	Any INR	Same as for serious bleeding, except stronger indication for 4-factor PCC, rFVIIa, or plasma

INR, International normalized ratio; *PCC*, prothrombin complex concentrate. *rFVIIa*, recombinant activated factor VIIa.

activated factor VII (rFVIIa, NovoSeven), three-factor nonactivated prothrombin complex concentrate (Profilnine), activated prothrombin complex concentrate (FEIBA), or, as a last resort, plasma. The effects of reversal are assessed through clinical observation and repeated PT/INR assays.[23]

It is important to note that before prescribing reversal of warfarin based on an elevated INR, the laboratory professional should ensure that there is no preanalytical error during sample collection. Contamination of sample and resulting erroneous prolongation of INR is not uncommon.

UNFRACTIONATED HEPARIN

Heparin Action

Standard UFH, often simply called *heparin,* was first used in 1935. It is a mixture of sulfated glycosaminoglycans (polysaccharides) extracted from porcine mucosa. The polysaccharides are linear chains that vary in length, chemical structure, and sulfation pattern. The molecular weights of the components within UFH range from 3000 to 30,000 Daltons (average 15,000 Daltons). Approximately one-third of its molecules support somewhere on their length a series of 5 sugar units (a pentasaccharide) arranged in a specific sequence that avidly binds plasma antithrombin. The mixture of polysaccharide chains provides additional binding sites for antithrombin and many other plasma proteins, but none that produce the high-affinity binding as this specific pentasaccharide sequence.[24]

The catalytic anticoagulant action of UFH is indirect, relying on liver-produced plasma antithrombin (AT, antithrombin III, ATIII). Heparin-bound AT undergoes a steric change *(allostery),* exposing an anticoagulant site that covalently binds and inactivates the coagulation pathway serine proteases, factors IIa (thrombin), IXa, Xa, XIa, and XIIa (Chapter 35). Principal among these is heparin's inhibition of thrombin and FXa. Laboratory practitioners call activated AT a serine protease inhibitor *(SERPIN),* and the protease-binding reaction yields, among other products, the measurable inactive plasma complex thrombin-antithrombin (TAT) (Figure 35.14). When UFH binds AT, the combination increases by 1000-fold the rate of inhibition of the serine proteases without heparin present.

Inactivation of thrombin requires binding of thrombin to both AT and UFH. Factor Xa, in contrast, becomes inactivated only through binding to the sterically modified AT. Factor Xa itself does not require binding to UFH and can be inhibited by the short pentasaccharide chain within UFH. The longer heparin chains support the inhibition of thrombin through a "bridging" *(approximation)* mechanism. If the UFH molecule exceeds approximately 17 linear saccharide units, thrombin assembles on the UFH molecule near the bound, activated AT. Bridging drives the thrombin inhibition reaction at a rate four times that of FXa inhibition.

Individual patient UFH dose responses diverge because numerous plasma and cellular proteins bind UFH at varying rates. Consequently, laboratory monitoring is essential.[25]

Heparin Therapy

The health care provider administers UFH intravenously to treat VTE, to provide initial treatment of AMI, to prevent reocclusion after stent placement, and to maintain vascular patency with extracorporeal cardiac support such as during cardiac surgery using the cardiopulmonary bypass (CPB) pump or in patients provided extracorporeal membrane oxygenation (ECMO) life support.

For VTE treatment, therapy begins with an intravenous bolus of 5000 to 10,000 units, followed by continuous infusion at approximately 1300 units/hr, adjusted to patient weight. During cardiac surgery, use of ECMO, and during interventional cardiology procedures, UFH doses that are higher than a treatment dose are used. UFH therapy is discontinued when the acute clinical state has resolved, after the procedure, or after surgery. If necessary, the patient is switched to an oral anticoagulant to reduce the risk of reocclusion.[26]

Monitoring Heparin Therapy

In response to its inherent pharmacologic variations and narrow therapeutic range, laboratory professionals diligently monitor UFH therapy using the PTT or the chromogenic anti-Xa heparin assay. For PTT monitoring, blood is collected and assayed before therapy is begun to ensure that the baseline PTT is normal. A prolonged baseline PTT may indicate an underlying coagulopathy or the presence of lupus anticoagulant. In this case, the laboratory employs the chromogenic anti-Xa heparin assay.[27]

A second PTT (or anti-Xa) specimen is collected a minimum of 4 to 6 hours but not longer than 24 hours after the initial UFH bolus. The PTT becomes prolonged within minutes of UFH administration, reflecting the immediate anticoagulant effect of intravenous UFH. The result for the second specimen should fall within the target *therapeutic range* (discussed in the following section), which is established by the laboratory practitioner and reported with the result. The provider adjusts the infusion (drip) rate to ensure that the PTT result remains within the target range. PTT measurement is subsequently repeated every 24 hours, and the dosage is repeatedly readjusted until UFH anticoagulation is complete.

The provider also requests that the laboratory monitors the platelet count daily. A 40% or greater reduction in the platelet count, even within the RI, is presumptive evidence for HIT. (Review the discussion of the *4T* and the *HIT Expert Probability* scores in Chapter 39). If HIT is suspected and thrombosis is present, UFH therapy is immediately discontinued and replaced with intravenous DTI therapy. If thrombosis has not developed, fondaparinux or a DOAC can be administered.

Determining the PTT Therapeutic Range for Heparin Therapy

The hemostasis quality assurance (QA) specialist establishes and communicates a PTT therapeutic range to monitor and manage UFH therapy. The QA specialist collects 20 to 30 plasma specimens (larger facilities may require 100) from patients being infused with UFH at all levels of anticoagulation, ensuring that fewer than 10% of the specimens are collected from the same patient, and measures PTT for all.[28] The specimens must be from patients who are not receiving simultaneous warfarin therapy; that is, their PT results must be within their RI and INR below 1.3. The QA specialist also performs PTTs on specimens from a minimum of 10 normal healthy nonanticoagulated subjects. A chromogenic anti-Xa heparin assay is performed on aliquots of all study specimens, and the paired results are displayed on a linear graph (Figure 40.3). The range in seconds of PTT results that corresponds to 0.3 to 0.7 chromogenic anti-Xa heparin units/mL is the therapeutic range.[29] This therapeutic range method, known as the ex vivo or *Brill-Edwards method,* is required by laboratory certification agencies. The UFH therapeutic range is communicated to the pharmacy and all inpatient facility units.

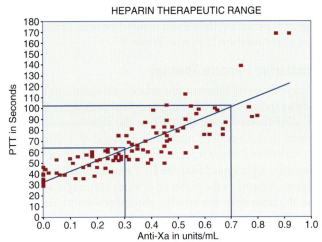

HEPARIN THERAPEUTIC RANGE

Figure 40.3 Heparin Therapeutic Range. Laboratory practitioners establish the partial thromboplastin time *(PTT)* therapeutic range for unfractionated heparin (UFH) by collecting specimens from 20 to 30 patients receiving UFH at representative dosages who have normal prothrombin times and at least 10 individuals not receiving heparin. PTT and chromogenic anti-factor Xa heparin assays are performed on all specimens, and a linear graph of paired results is prepared with PTT on the vertical scale. The PTT range in seconds is correlated with the chromogenic anti-factor Xa therapeutic range of 0.3 to 0.7 units/mL or the prophylactic range of 0.1 to 0.4 units/mL.

Other therapeutic range approaches are discouraged. For instance, experts once recommended a PTT therapeutic range of 1.5 to 2.5 times the mean of the RI. This approach, however, consistently results in inadequate anticoagulation, which raises the risk of a secondary thrombotic event. The practice of developing a therapeutic range by "spiking" normal plasma with measured volumes of heparin is prohibited because the curve that is generated tends to flatten at higher concentrations and does not represent the clinical condition.[30]

Clinical Practice of Heparin Therapy Monitoring Using the PTT

The medical laboratory practitioner reports the PTT results, the RI, and the UFH therapeutic range to the provider. Because reagent sensitivity varies among producers and among individual producers' reagent lots, the provider must evaluate PTT results in relationship to the institution's published therapeutic range and RI. No system analogous to the INR exists for normalizing PTT results because reagents and patient responses are inconsistent.[31]

Limitations of Heparin Therapy Monitoring Using the PTT

Several conditions render the patient unresponsive to UFH therapy, a circumstance called *heparin resistance.*[32] These conditions may affect heparin's anticoagulation efficacy and may interfere with the PTT. Inflammation is typically accompanied by fibrinogen levels raised to greater than 500 mg/dL and factor VIII activities of greater than 190 units/dL. Both elevations render the PTT less sensitive to heparin's effects, though the therapeutic effect may be unchanged. Further, in many patients, AT activity becomes depleted because of prolonged UFH therapy

or an underlying deficiency secondary to chronic inflammation. In this instance, the PTT result remains below the therapeutic range, becoming only modestly prolonged despite ever-increasing UFH dosages.

The provider may reduce inflammation with steroids, aspirin, or other nonsteroidal antiinflammatory pharmaceuticals and may administer AT concentrate. In the interim, however, it is necessary to use the chromogenic anti-Xa heparin assay, which is unaffected by coagulopathy, elevated procoagulant activity, or the presence of warfarin. Because the chromogenic anti-Xa heparin assay depends on patient AT to display the activity of UFH (in line with the mechanism of UFH), it is reduced in AT deficiency like the PTT.[33]

Platelets in whole blood specimens release *platelet factor 4* (PF4), a heparin-neutralizing protein (Chapter 11). In specimens from patients receiving UFH therapy, the PTT begins to shorten, masking the effect of UFH, as early as 1 hour after collection because of ex vivo PF4 release. For all UFH assays, it is imperative that patient specimens are centrifuged and the platelet-poor plasma is removed from the cells within 1 hour of collection (Chapter 41).[34]

Hypofibrinogenemia, factor deficiencies, and the presence of lupus anticoagulant, fibrin degradation products, or paraproteins falsely prolong the PTT independent of UFH levels. Here too the chromogenic anti-Xa assay is preferred for UFH monitoring.

Monitoring Heparin Using the Chromogenic Anti-Xa Assay

As a result of fewer interferences and improved assay stability, the chromogenic anti-Xa heparin assay is preferred over the PTT in routine clinical use. Its stability leads to fewer dosage adjustments and reductions in red cell transfusions.[35]

Conversely, the PTT provides a global impression of anticoagulation status, which some providers prefer, particularly for high-risk patients. Further, the chromogenic anti-Xa heparin assay reflects only the changes in AT-FXa binding, whereas the PTT responds to all plasma-based heparin activities. Some facilities offer the anti-Xa heparin assay for routine UFH monitoring but offer the PTT on physician request. Refer to "Measuring LMWH Therapy" further in this chapter for a description of the chromogenic anti-Xa heparin assay mechanism.

Monitoring Heparin Therapy Using The ACT and Viscoelastometry

The activated clotting time (ACT) is a near-patient test employed to monitor supratherapeutic UFH dosages (higher than therapeutic dosages) that yield plasma levels of 1 to 2 units/mL, exceeding PTT and anti-Xa analytical range limits.[36] Surgeons and cardiologists employ these high UFH dosages with use of the CPB pump, during ECMO life support, and during PCI.[37]

The ACT assay is performed using freshly collected whole blood immediately mixed with kaolin or celite activator and measured for clot formation by electromagnetic, optical, or biochemical changes on a dedicated instrument (Chapter 42). The median of the ACT RI is 98 seconds. Heparin is administered to yield results of 200 to 240 seconds during PCI or 480 to 600 seconds during cardiac surgery.[38]

Near-patient viscoelastometry (VET) instruments use freshly collected whole blood mixed with activators and immediately record coagulation activation over 5 to 10 minutes. They provide an initial clotting time that reflects the ACT. In a second step, some VET instruments can approximate heparin concentration by comparing maximum clot amplitude numbers with and without a heparin neutralizer such as heparinase or polybrene added to the patient's whole blood.[39,40]

Reversing Heparin Therapy

When the CPB pump in cardiac surgery is discontinued, supratherapeutic UFH anticoagulation is quickly reversed. *Protamine sulfate* (in Europe, protamine chloride), a synthetic cationic protein that mimics a salmon sperm extract, binds UFH and neutralizes it at a ratio of 100 units of UFH per milligram protamine.[41] The surgeon or anesthetist administers protamine sulfate slowly by intravenous push, targeting baseline (nonheparin) median ACT or VET results as their indication of reversal.

Protamine sulfate also may be employed to reverse a UFH overdose or bleeding in UFH-aspirin coadministration. Patients are monitored for several hours post-UFH reversal, because UFH stored in tissues reappears in the plasma. Protamine sulfate may cause a delayed form of HIT; consequently, platelet counts for patients who have received protamine sulfate are routinely monitored.[42]

LOW-MOLECULAR-WEIGHT HEPARIN

LMWH Action

The first LMWH, enoxaparin (Sanofi-Aventis), was approved for thrombosis prophylaxis in the United States and Canada in 1990, soon followed by tinzaparin (Leo Pharma) and dalteparin (Pfizer).[43] LMWH is prepared from UFH by chemical or enzymatic fractionation, cleaving the long polysaccharide chains to yield a product with a mean molecular weight of 4500 to 5000 Daltons, about one-third the mass of UFH.

LMWH possesses the same AT-binding pentasaccharide sequence as UFH. The FXa neutralization response is unchanged from that of UFH because this reaction does not rely on FXa bridging to long heparin polysaccharide chains (Figure 40.4). However, the shorter polysaccharide chains of LMWH support less TAT bridging with a resulting reduction in thrombin inhibition activity compared to UFH. LMWH provides similar clinical efficacy to UFH for controlling thrombosis in the clinical indications where it has been FDA cleared.

LMWH Therapy

LMWH is administered by subcutaneous injection once or twice a day using premeasured syringes at selected dosages—for instance, 30 mg subcutaneously every 12 hours or 40 mg subcutaneously once daily. Prophylactic applications provide coverage during or after general and orthopedic surgery and trauma, typically for 14 days from the time of the event. LMWH also is used to treat VTE and, along with fondaparinux, is moderately effective in controlling the progression of coronavirus disease 2019 (COVID-19) thromboinflammation. LMWH or fondaparinux is indicated during pregnancy for women at risk of VTE,

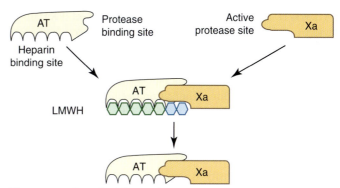

Figure 40.4 The Anti-Factor Xa Mechanism of Action of Low-Molecular-Weight Heparin (LMWH). Antithrombin (AT) molecules bind a pentasaccharide region on heparin polysaccharide chains, producing an allosteric change that activates AT, facilitating factor (F) Xa binding. The LMWH molecule is too short to support a FIIa (thrombin)-AT reaction. Figure 35.14 shows the mechanism for the longer chains of unfractionated heparin that inhibit thrombin. The activated AT binds FXa independently of the bridging phenomenon required for thrombin, producing an AT-FXa complex that inhibits FXa activity.

whereas warfarin is contraindicated, and DOAC administration in pregnancy requires further clinical investigation.[44]

The advantages of LMWH over UFH include home therapy; a half-life of 3 to 5 hours compared with 60 to 90 minutes for UFH; increased bioavailability after subcutaneous injection; less plasma protein binding, resulting in a more predictable dose response; and lower bleeding risk. The predictable dose response and safety of LMWH treatment eliminates the need for periodic laboratory monitoring, though measurement is required for the conditions listed in Box 40.1.[45]

Protamine sulfate may be used to reverse LMWH-associated bleeding, an uncommon event. In contrast to its effect on UFH, protamine reversal of LMWH is only partially effective. The incomplete neutralization is reflected in the results of the chromogenic anti-Xa heparin assay.

To avoid HIT (Chapter 39), LMWH or other anticoagulants are used in place of UFH where possible.[46] LMWH reduces the risk of HIT by 90% compared with UFH in patients who have never received heparin. However, LMWH may cross react with previously formed antibodies against the heparin-PF4 epitope in patients previously treated with heparin. Consequently, LMWH is contraindicated in patients who developed HIT after UFH therapy.

Laboratory Assessment of LMWH Therapy

The kidneys alone clear LMWH, so it accumulates in patients with renal insufficiency. Laboratory measurement of LMWH therapy is necessary when the creatinine clearance is less than 30 mL/min or the serum creatinine is greater than 4 mg/dL. During LMWH therapy, creatinine assays are performed periodically to document kidney function and avoid the risk of LMWH accumulation in plasma. LMWH therapy in children, in adults weighing less than 50 kg, in adults weighing more than 150 kg, and during pregnancy also require measurement because of fluid compartment imbalances or unstable coagulation (see Box 40.1).

LMWH selectively catalyzes the inhibition of FXa more avidly than the inhibition of thrombin; thus its effects cannot be measured using the PTT. For LMWH the chromogenic anti-Xa assay is the assay of choice.

The phlebotomist collects a blood specimen 4 hours after subcutaneous injection. The chromogenic anti-Xa heparin assay employs a reagent that provides a fixed concentration of FXa and a substrate specific to FXa but no AT (Figure 40.5). Heparin forms a complex with reagent FXa and patient AT; a measured excess of FXa digests the substrate, yielding a colored product whose intensity is inversely proportional to heparin concentration. Because the assay depends on patient AT, results are reduced in AT deficiency.[47]

To prepare a calibration curve, the laboratory practitioner obtains LMWH calibrators from the assay manufacturer, then computes and prepares dilutions that "bracket" the RI and the therapeutic range. If the chromogenic anti-factor Xa heparin assay is to be used to monitor UFH and LMWH, a single "hybrid" standard curve may be prepared.[48] The prophylactic range for LMWH is 0.2 to 0.5 unit/mL, and the therapeutic range is 0.5 to 1.2 units/mL (given twice daily) or 1.0 to 2.0 units/mL (given once daily).[49]

Other FXa inhibitor drugs, such as fondaparinux, rivaroxaban, apixaban, and edoxaban, are measured using the chromogenic anti-Xa assay based on separate standard curves using calibrators of the target pharmaceutical.

FONDAPARINUX

Fondaparinux (Arixtra) (GlaxoSmithKline) is a synthetic formulation of the active *pentasaccharide* sequence in UFH and LMWH (Figure 40.6). Unlike UFH or LMWH, fondaparinux has a uniform molecular structure, not a mixture of polysaccharide units. This pentasaccharide sequence is specific in the type, number, and placement of saccharide units. Sulfate groups placement and number are managed to produce the highest affinity to AT. Because of its short chain length, fondaparinux inhibits only factor Xa through AT, whose activity rises 400-fold when bound. It does not inhibit thrombin or other serine proteases. Compared with LMWH, fondaparinux offers a reduced major bleeding risk and a longer half-life of 17 to 21 hours. It is equivalent in clinical efficacy and reproducible dose response to LMWH and is administered subcutaneously once daily.[50]

Fondaparinux is approved for the prophylaxis and treatment of DVT and PE. It is widely prescribed for the prevention of VTE in postoperative adults undergoing hip and knee orthopedic surgery and abdominal surgery, and in immobilized patients due to acute illness who are at high risk for VTE. The use of fondaparinux continues to be explored for use in other conditions.

The recommended fondaparinux prophylaxis dosage is 2.5 mg for up to 10 days after abdominal surgery and 10 to 14 days for patients after hip fracture surgery or total hip or knee replacement surgery. When applied as post-VTE therapy or in COVID-19, the dosage is administered for up to 9 days and is weight based: patients less than 50 kg receive 5 mg, patients 50 to 100 kg receive 7.5 mg, and patients over 100 kg receive 10 mg.

Fondaparinux and DOACs offer similar efficacy profiles when used as alternatives to UFH in patients with HIT who are clinically stable.[51] Fondaparinux is FDA cleared for prevention of VTE after orthopedic and abdominal surgery and for treatment of acute VTE events, but its use is contraindicated in patients with creatinine clearance values of less than 30 mL/min.

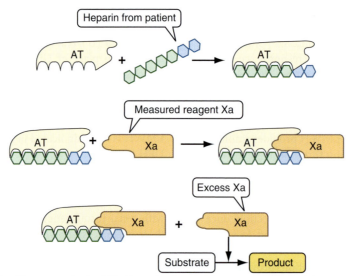

Figure 40.5 The Chromogenic Anti-Xa Heparin Assay. Therapeutic heparin (plasma specimen) binds patient antithrombin (AT), and the complex binds reagent factor (F) Xa. The assay protocol provides for a measured excess of reagent FXa. Factor Xa not bound to the complex digests its substrate to produce a colored product. The color intensity of the product is inversely proportional to plasma heparin. This assay is used for unfractionated heparin (UFH), low-molecular-weight heparin (LMWH), fondaparinux, and the anti-FXa direct-acting oral anticoagulants (DOACs). Calibrator curves for UFH, LMWH, or UFH/LMWH hybrid, fondaparinux, or the individual DOACs are prepared using calibrators specific to the therapeutic drug being measured.

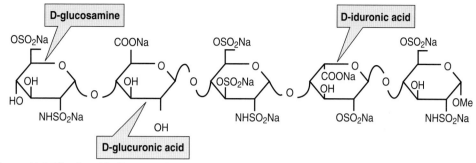

Figure 40.6 The Specific Pentasaccharide Sequence Synthesized to Produce Fondaparinux. The illustrated pentasaccharide sequence of heparin (glucosamine, glucuronic acid, glucosamine, iduronic acid, and glucosamine with associated sulfate groups at the defined positions) allows for the highest affinity binding of antithrombin (AT) to heparin. This is the minimum sequence of saccharide units, necessarily composed of the illustrated saccharide units of the shown specific chemical structures, that binds to AT with highest affinity and produces an anti-factor Xa activity. (From Turpie, A. G. G. [2002]. Pentasaccharides. *Semin Hematol, 39,* 159–171.)

Owing to its favorable safety and efficacy profile, providers seldom order fondaparinux assays. The chromogenic anti-Xa heparin assay is used, however, to measure fondaparinux therapy in children, adults weighing less than 50 kg or more than 150 kg, patients receiving treatment for more than 7 days, and pregnant women, and whenever there is a therapy-related question.

Blood is collected 4 hours after injection, and the target range is 0.2 to 0.4 mg/L for a 2.5-mg dose and 0.5 to 1.5 mg/L for a 7.5-mg dose. The operator prepares a calibration curve using fondaparinux—not UFH, LMWH, or a hybrid calibrator—because concentrations are expressed in mg/L, not units/mL. The PTT is not sensitive to the effect of fondaparinux because, although fondaparinux reacts with AT to inhibit FXa, it does not inhibit thrombin or factors IXa, XIa, or XIIa.

In the event of bleeding associated with fondaparinux overdose, protamine sulfate is ineffective. Recombinant factor VIIa may partially reverse the anticoagulant effect of fondaparinux.[52]

DIRECT ANTI-XA ORAL ANTICOAGULANTS

Anti-Xa DOAC Action

The anti-Xa DOACs, rivaroxaban (Xarelto) (Janssen), apixaban (Eliquis) (Bristol-Myers Squibb), and edoxaban (Savaysa) (Daiichi Sankyo), directly and stoichiometrically inhibit coagulation FXa, whether it is free, clot bound, or bound to FIXa (Table 40.4). They do not require AT to exert their anticoagulant activity.[53]

Anti-Xa DOAC Therapy

As established by results of several clinical trials, the direct acting anti-Xa DOACs possess efficacy and safety characteristics equivalent to or better than UFH, LMWH, or warfarin.[54] Rivaroxaban, apixaban, and edoxaban are approved by the US FDA, Health Canada, and the European Medicines Agency for prevention of secondary thrombosis subsequent to VTE, VTE prophylaxis in patients who are undergoing total knee or total hip replacement surgery, and prevention of ischemic stroke in patients with chronic nonvalvular atrial fibrillation.[55] DOACs may be used in patients with HIT who have become clinically

stable.[56] Efforts to determine the efficacy and safety of DOACs in pregnancy or post AMI therapy are ongoing.[57]

The anti-Xa DOACs possess half-lives of 10 to 18 hours and are cleared through the kidney, except for apixaban—70% of apixaban is cleared by the liver. When DOACs are prescribed, periodic kidney function tests are necessary. DOAC that is not eliminated is metabolized by the CYP450 enzyme 3A4 and the P-glycoprotein (P-gp) transport system. Drugs administered concomitantly with the DOAC that use the same metabolic pathways can raise or lower the plasma concentration of the DOAC as both drugs compete for the same pathways.

Reversing Anti-Xa DOAC Therapy

Although FXa inhibitor DOACs have a low bleeding risk, clinically relevant bleeds do occur with their use. A general corrective measure is to administer a prothrombin complex concentrate (PCC). By adding high levels of coagulation factors to the blood, the PCC quickly overcomes the inhibitory effect of the DOAC.

A more specific reversal agent is andexanet alfa (Andexxa) (AstraZeneca), a modified recombinant FXa protein that serves as a decoy for the natural FXa. DOAC that binds to andexanet is unavailable to bind to natural FXa. The noninhibited FXa remains available to generate thrombin. The andexanet-bound DOAC is eliminated from circulation, effectively removing the anticoagulant activity. Andexanet does not reverse thrombin inhibitor DOACs.

The American College of Cardiology recommends four-factor PCC (Kcentra) (Behring) to reverse bleeding associated with apixaban or rivaroxaban overdose at a 50-units/kg single treatment cost of approximately US$14,500. Andexanet is dosed at either 400 mg at 30mg/minute, followed by 4 mg/minute over 120 minutes or 800 mg at 30 mg/minute, followed by 8 mg/minute for up to 120 minutes, depending on the rivaroxaban or apixaban dose and time since last dose[58]

When there is uncertainty of whether a DOAC is onboard or which type of DOAC may be onboard, the laboratory director offers a urine chemistry strip (DOAC Dipstick) (Doasense) to distinguish between the oral direct anti-Xa anticoagulants and the oral DTI, dabigatran (Pradaxa, described in a subsequent

TABLE 40.4   Comparison of the Direct Oral Anticoagulants

Generic Name	Dabigatran	Rivaroxaban	Apixaban	Edoxaban
Trade Name	Pradaxa	Xarelto	Eliquis	Savaysa
Indication	Stroke prophylaxis in NVAF; after major surgery; VTE treatment			
FDA Approval	2010	2011	2012	2015
Function	DTI	Direct FXa inhibitor	Direct FXa inhibitor	Direct FXa inhibitor
Dosage	75 or 150 mg capsule	15 or 20 mg	10, then 2.5 or 5 mg*	15, 30, or 60 mg
Daily schedule	Twice	Once†	Twice	Once
Half-life	10–18 hr when kidney function is normal			
Laboratory assay	Dilute TT, ECA	Chromogenic anti-FXa assay validated to UFH; for hybrid anti-FXa assays, only the UFH calibrator is used to validate the assay; provides a qualitative measurement		
Kidney function	Normal function required	Normal function required	70% liver excretion	Normal function required
Food effect	No	Take with food	No	No
Drug interactions	P-gp modulators; drugs that impair hemostasis; antacids	CYP3A4 and P-gp modulators; drugs that impair hemostasis	CYP3A4 and P-gp modulators; drugs that impair hemostasis	CYP3A4 (minimal) and P-gp modulators; drugs that impair hemostasis
Reversal	Idarucizumab	Andexanet	Andexanet	Andexanet

*Seven days' loading dose of 10 mg twice a day, then 2.5 or 5 mg.
†For VTE, use 3-week loading period of twice daily.
CYP3A4, A liver cytochrome P450 enzyme; *DTI,* direct thrombin inhibitor; *DOAC,* direct oral anticoagulant; *ECA,* ecarin chromogenic assay; *F,* factor; *FDA,* US Food and Drug Administration; *LMWH,* low-molecular-weight heparin; *NVAF,* nonvalvular atrial fibrillation; *P-gp,* P-glycoprotein; *TT,* thrombin time; *UFH,* unfractionated heparin; *VTE,* venous thromboembolic events, including deep venous thrombosis (DVT) and pulmonary embolism (PE).

section). The DOAC Dipstick is currently approved for use in Canada and Northern Europe.[59]

Laboratory Assessment of Anti-Xa DOACs

Anti-factor Xa DOACs are prescribed without the requirement for laboratory monitoring; however, Box 40.1 lists the indications for DOAC measurement.[60] Rivaroxaban prolongs the PT in a reagent-dependent manner, edoxaban to a lesser degree, and apixaban has no effect on the PT.[61] Attempts to correlate PT results with dosage have revealed variability among individual DOAC responses and among PT reagents, rendering the PT invalid.[62] The PTT is insensitive to anti-Xa DOAC activity.

The amount of anti-Xa DOAC in the bloodstream may be *estimated* using the chromogenic anti-Xa heparin assay validated with UFH calibrators and controls, and may be *quantitated* using the chromogenic anti-Xa heparin assay based on anticoagulant-specific calibrators and controls.[63] Manufacturers offer calibrators and controls dedicated to chromogenic anti-factor Xa assays for rivaroxaban, apixaban, and edoxaban. Pending FDA kit approval, these are available for laboratory directors to offer as laboratory-developed tests with empirically determined therapeutic ranges.[64]

Anti-Xa DOACs interfere with clot-based coagulation assays, as does heparin. Factor assay results are falsely decreased. Tests for lupus anticoagulant, protein C, protein S, and AT yield false-positive lupus anticoagulant results and falsely increased AT, protein C, and protein S. Immunoassays and chromogenic substrate assays for these hemostatic proteins are unaffected.

If preferred, tablet-form products, DOAC-Remove (5 Diagnostics) and DOAC-Stop (DiaPharma), are available to pretreat patient plasma. These products deplete rivaroxaban, apixaban, and edoxaban, and the DTI dabigatran at one tablet per milliliter test plasma. Treated specimens are reported to yield PT and PTT results equivalent to the same specimen without a DOAC. The DOAC removers absorb up to an estimated 2000 ng/mL of any DOAC in less than 5 minutes and do not appear to interfere with warfarin or heparin measurements.[65] DOAC removal agents await FDA approval.

DIRECT THROMBIN INHIBITORS

Oral Dabigatran

Oral dabigatran etexilate (Pradaxa) (Boehringer Ingelheim) is a DOAC prodrug that is converted in vivo to active dabigatran, a DTI that binds both free and clot-bound thrombin (see Table 40.4). Dabigatran does not require AT as a cofactor; thus, like the anti-Xa DOACs, dabigatran is a direct-acting anticoagulant. Dabigatran is the first oral anticoagulant since warfarin; it was approved by the FDA in 2010.

Dabigatran's efficacy and safety match those of LMWH and warfarin, and it has limited clinically significant food interactions. It is cleared by the kidneys, has a half-life of 10 to 18 hours, and is not metabolized by liver cytochrome enzymes. However, it relies on the P-gp transport system for metabolism, which leads to drug interactions with unexpected raising or lowering of the DOAC plasma concentration if multiple drugs share the same metabolic pathway.[66]

Like the anti-Xa DOACS, dabigatran is approved for VTE prophylaxis and therapy and for stroke prevention in nonvalvular atrial fibrillation. In renal disease, dosing is adjusted as the half-life may be prolonged to as much as 60 hours. Dabigatran's activity is reversed within 30 minutes, as shown in laboratory assays, by idarucizumab (Praxbind), a monoclonal antibody specific for this anticoagulant.[67]

Oral Dabigatran Laboratory Assessment

Dabigatran, like all DOACs, is prescribed without the need for periodic monitoring. Measurement becomes necessary when one of the indications listed in Box 40.1 apply. Dabigatran prolongs the thrombin clotting time (TT, TCT), PTT, and elevates the ecarin chromogenic assay (ECA). The standard TT is exceptionally sensitive and is convenient for ruling out the presence of dabigatran; a normal TT definitively indicates that no DTI is present. A prolonged TT may indicate that dabigatran is present, but the concentration cannot be determined. The PTT generates a "curvilinear" response to dabigatran and is unreliable at low levels. There is considerable variability in sensitivity to dabigatran among PTT reagents.[68]

The ECA provides a precise, accurate linear response to dabigatran, with an analytical range of 18 to 470 ng/mL. Ecarin is a snake venom that activates prothrombin to form meizothrombin, an intermediate form of thrombin. Meizothrombin acts on its reagent substrate, producing a color whose intensity is proportional to the dabigatran plasma concentration.[69] The ECA can be adapted to all coagulometers.

Further, a modification of the TT is the plasma-diluted thrombin time (Hemoclot Direct Thrombin Inhibitor Assay, Hyphen Biomed).[70] Patient plasma is diluted with normal human plasma, and the TT is performed using standard assay technique. The assay provides linearity and analytical sensitivity data equivalent to those of the ECA. The ECA and the plasma-diluted thrombin time, both of which are performed on citrated plasma, await FDA approval. Meanwhile, as health care practitioners may request patient assessment, laboratory directors can perform what is defined as a laboratory-developed test using the available reagents, calibrators, and controls.[71]

Any clot-based coagulation assay, such as PT, PTT, factor assay, or lupus anticoagulant profile, is prolonged by dabigatran, leading to invalid test results. Dabigatran, like the direct anti-Xa DOACs, may be removed by in vitro plasma treatment with a DOAC absorbent before testing.

Intravenous Direct Thrombin Inhibitors

Providers order periodic platelet counts during UFH therapy because acquired thrombocytopenia is an indicator for HIT (Chapter 39). If the *4T* or *HIT Expert Probability* score indicates a strong likelihood, HIT patients are characteristically switched to one of the approved intravenous DTIs, argatroban or bivalirudin. Warfarin, which initially lowers proteins C and S activity, is prothrombotic for the first 5 days of treatment and is contraindicated.[72] Fondaparinux and the DOACs have been used off-label safely but await the results of prospective clinical trials for full adoption. LMWH cross reacts with existing heparin-PF4 (HIT) antibodies, and nascent LMWH may also trigger HIT at a frequency that is 10% of UFH-triggered HIT.

Like oral dabigatran, the intravenous DTIs rapidly bind and inactivate free and clot-bound thrombin (Figure 40.7).[73] In a patient with HIT, if UFH is discontinued without followup argatroban or bivalirudin, the thrombosis risk remains at 50% for 30 days after heparin is discontinued.[74,75]

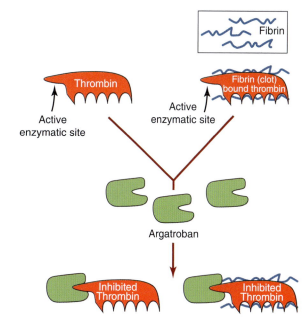

Enzymatic activity of thrombin inhibited

Figure 40.7 The Mechanism of Action of Direct Thrombin Inhibitors (DTIs). The thrombin inhibitor argatroban binds directly to and inhibits the active site of free and fibrin/clot-bound thrombin (factor IIa). Antithrombin is not involved in this reaction. Bivalirudin and dabigatran directly inhibit thrombin by interacting at the same site but with their own specific binding characteristics.

Argatroban

Argatroban (Mitsubishi) is a nonprotein L-arginine synthetic derivative that was FDA approved in 1997 for prophylaxis and treatment of thrombosis associated with HIT and for anticoagulation during PCI for patients with HIT.[76] Argatroban is a potent and highly specific inhibitor of thrombin with a quick onset and a quick offset of anticoagulant activity, beneficial characteristics for HIT thrombosis management. Off-label applications include use as an anticoagulant during cardiac surgery using CPB in patients with HIT, renal replacement therapy (dialysis) with or without HIT, and in heparin resistance.[77]

Owing to its 50-minute half-life, argatroban is administered by continuous infusion. The provider initiates infusion at 2 µg/kg per minute or in hepatic disease at 0.5 µg/kg per minute. During PCI, a bolus of 350 µg/kg is given over 3 to 5 minutes, followed by infusion at 25 µg/kg per minute. Argatroban is cleared by the liver and excreted in stool; thus dosages must be reduced in liver disease, though not in kidney disease.

On average, argatroban reduces the risk of reocclusion by 60% and confers a 7% significant bleeding risk; however, reocclusion and bleeding risks depend on the underlying condition of the patient and meticulous management. There is no direct reversal agent for argatroban, but on discontinuance, the anticoagulant effect clears in 2 to 4 hours.[78]

Bivalirudin

Bivalirudin (Angiomax) (The Medicines Company) is a synthetic 20-amino acid oligopeptide analog of the active site of hirudin, an anticoagulant produced in the saliva of the medicinal leech *Hirudo medicinalis*.[79] It is a potent and highly specific inhibitor of thrombin. The FDA originally cleared bivalirudin in 2000 for use as an anticoagulant in patients with unstable angina undergoing PCI.[80] Bivalirudin is used off-label as an anticoagulant in any patient with HIT, including during CPB surgery.

For PCI, cardiologists provide an intravenous bolus dose of 0.75 mg/kg bivalirudin, followed by an infusion of 1.75 mg/kg per hour for the duration of the procedure.[81] After 4 hours, an additional intravenous infusion may be given at a rate of 0.2 mg/kg per hour for up to 20 hours. The risk of reocclusion is similar to that of argatroban, but the risk of major bleeds is somewhat less.[82] The dosage must be decreased in patients with renal disease because bivalirudin is eliminated through the kidneys.[83]

There is no reversal agent for bivalirudin. However, in patients with normal renal function, the short half-life of 25 minutes allows for simple discontinuance of the infusion to reverse the anticoagulant effect.

Monitoring Argatroban and Bivalirudin

Argatroban and bivalirudin are monitored to ensure that they are maintained within the therapeutic range. Both prolong the thrombin time, PT, PTT, and ACT. For nonsurgical therapy, distributors recommend assaying either DTI with the PTT using the target therapeutic range of 1.5 to 3 times the initial baseline but not longer than 100 seconds. Blood is collected 2 hours after initiation of intravenous therapy for argatroban and 4 hours after bivalirudin initiation, and the dosage is adjusted to achieve a PTT within the therapeutic range.

Patients who require cardiovascular intervention for severe disease progression may have an underlying diagnosis of HIT. In these situations, argatroban or bivalirudin is substituted for UFH, which is normally used in the procedures. The point-of-care ACT is used to monitor the higher anticoagulation dosages used for interventional cardiology procedures. The target ACT for bivalirudin and argatroban is 300 to 450 seconds, with a median normal value of 98 seconds. The high doses used in cardiac surgery are also monitored by ACT, with a target value of 400 seconds or higher. Anticoagulation monitoring using VET also can be performed. Because these high-risk clinical procedures using DTI anticoagulation are not frequently performed, standardized anticoagulation dosing and monitoring protocols are still being refined and often are empirically determined by the health care provider in communication with the drug manufacturer.

When the baseline PTT or ACT is prolonged by lupus anticoagulant, factor inhibitors, or factor deficiencies, the ECA provides a reliable alternative assay for DTI monitoring.[84]

Clot-based coagulation assays are prolonged by argatroban and bivalirudin, leading to invalid results. Factor assays and fibrinogen levels are falsely low, and clot-based protein C and protein S levels are falsely elevated in the presence of a DTI.

SWITCHING ANTICOAGULANTS AND PERIPROCEDURAL MANAGEMENT

When clinical conditions improve, patients under anticoagulation who require long-term treatment need to transition to an oral formulation of anticoagulant. The following represent the

various transitioning scenarios depending on the anticoagulant. All situations demand attention to detail as risk of bleeding and thrombosis associate with all anticoagulant use.

The most common and long-standing anticoagulant switch is transitioning a patient from intravenous UFH to warfarin. In patients with active clotting, a crossover or *bridging* period, in which both anticoagulants are administered, is necessary because of the 5 days required to achieve full warfarin anticoagulation. During this period, UFH is monitored by the PTT and warfarin is simultaneously monitored by the PT/INR. There is no issue with monitoring because UFH and warfarin are not detected by the other assay at these dosages. UFH is continued until a therapeutic INR is achieved for two continuous days. If a DOAC is chosen over warfarin, there is no need for a bridging period with monitoring.

For patients with HIT, providers discontinue argatroban or bivalirudin treatment when the platelet count rises to the baseline or greater than 100,000/μL, signaling that HIT is resolved. For outpatients, if desired, providers switch to a DOAC, whose anticoagulant effect is immediate, and no further laboratory assessment is required.[85] If warfarin is chosen, the intravenous DTI is continued for 5 days to ensure anticoagulation coverage while warfarin achieves full anticoagulation. Transition from argatroban or bivalirudin to warfarin requires periodic monitoring of both anticoagulants using PTT and PT/INR, respectively. The DTIs, which are monitored using the PTT, also prolong the PT and raise the INR, so it is possible to record INR values of 6 or higher during the combined treatment period.[86] In this case, the INR elevation is an artifact that does not signal increased bleeding risk. Providers ensure that the INR has reached the therapeutic range of 2 to 3 before the DTI is discontinued using special protocols.[87] The CFX assay may be an effective alternative for monitoring warfarin dosage during the crossover period.

Surgeons observe *periprocedural* management of anticoagulants based on their assessment of thrombotic and bleeding risk, weighing both the procedural and patient condition risks. DOAC and warfarin therapy may be continued during minor procedures such as cataract surgery and most dental procedures. DOAC therapy is interrupted for procedures associated with moderate to high bleeding risk. The urine chemistry strip DOAC Dipstick assay may be useful to determine whether DOAC anticoagulation is sufficiently low before the procedure. DOAC therapy may be continued when thrombosis risk is moderate to high. Because of its long half-life, warfarin therapy is interrupted beginning 5 days before a moderate to high bleeding risk procedure. If the risk of thrombosis is moderate or high, LMWH is substituted until warfarin therapy is resumed.[88]

Catheter ablation is often used to manage atrial fibrillation. Because the thrombosis risk is high, supratherapeutic UFH is employed during the ablation procedure. Current studies support continuing warfarin or DOAC therapy while adding supratherapeutic UFH. Although supratherapeutic UFH activity has been traditionally monitored by the ACT, the ACT is unreliable in the presence of warfarin or a DOAC. The current recommendation is to employ weight-based UFH dosage to avoid the risk of overdose.[89] When an anti-Xa agent such as rivaroxaban or apixaban overlaps with UFH, the chromogenic anti-Xa heparin assay result should reflect both anticoagulants. If the provider desires to approximate the effects of both anticoagulants, the PTT may provide an estimate of the UFH activity.

ANTIPLATELET THERAPY

Although aspirin has been used medicinally since 1900, its antiplatelet effect and role in reducing the risk of *arterial thrombosis* were first appreciated in the 1990s when the cardiology community undertook clinical trials that established aspirin's ability to reduce secondary reocclusion in heart disease.[90] Chapter 37 provides a detailed description of aspirin, other antiplatelet pharmaceutical drugs, and their effect on platelet function.

Parenteral Antiplatelet Therapeutic Drugs

The parenteral glycoprotein IIb/IIIa inhibitors (GPIs) tirofiban and eptifibatide fill $\alpha_{IIb}\beta_3$ receptor sites and block fibrinogen or von Willebrand factor binding, reducing platelet aggregation (Figure 37.5).[91]

Cardiologists administer a GPI together with UFH by intravenous infusion to maintain vascular patency during PCI for angioplasty and intracoronary stent placement.[92] Before GPI infusion, providers determine the PT, PTT, ACT, hemoglobin, hematocrit, and platelet count to detect any hemostatic or hematologic abnormality. During infusion, UFH dosing is adjusted to maintain the ACT within the specified UFH supratherapeutic range. Platelet counts are performed at 2 hours, 4 hours, and 24 hours after the initial bolus of UFH. If the platelet count drops by 25% or more, UFH and GPI are discontinued, and the platelet count is monitored daily until it returns to baseline.[93] If desired, GPI efficacy may be measured using VET-based platelet function estimation.[94,95]

Eptifibatide (Integrilin) (Millennium) is an 832-Dalton heptapeptide GPI coadministered with aspirin and UFH for the management of acute cardiac ischemia. An intravenous bolus of 180 μg/kg is given upon initial diagnosis, and a continuous intravenous drip of 2 μg/kg per minute is continued for up to 96 hours after the initial bolus, including throughout cardiac catheterization.

Tirofiban hydrochloride (Aggrastat) (Medicure) is a 495-Dalton nonprotein GPI coadministered with aspirin and UFH. It is administered intravenously at an initial rate of 0.4 μg/kg per minute for 30 minutes and then continued at 0.1 μg/kg per minute throughout cardiac catheterization and for 12 to 24 hours after catheterization. Tirofiban is excreted through the kidney, so the dosage is halved when the creatinine clearance is less than 30 mL/min.

Oral Antiplatelet Therapeutic Drugs

The most prescribed oral antiplatelet drugs are aspirin, clopidogrel (Plavix) (Sanofi-Aventis), prasugrel (Effient) (Daiichi Sankyo), and ticagrelor (Brilinta) (AstraZeneca) (Figure 37.5).[96] The thienopyridines clopidogrel and prasugrel and the purine analog ticagrelor occupy the platelet membrane adenosine diphosphate (ADP) receptor $P2Y_{12}$, suppressing the normal platelet aggregation and secretion response to ADP.[97]

Aspirin can be given alone or in combination with clopidogrel, prasugrel, or ticagrelor. Combination therapy is called *dual antiplatelet therapy*. Aspirin given alone is prescribed at 81 or 325 mg/day to prevent secondary thrombotic events in patients with stable or unstable angina, AMI, transient cerebral ischemia, peripheral vascular disease, or stroke.[98] If the patient can tolerate aspirin, it is often prescribed at up to 100 mg/day in combination with one of the three oral antiplatelet therapeutics. Aspirin is recommended for primary thrombosis prophylaxis based on a benefit-to-risk ratio.[99]

Clopidogrel is prescribed at 75 mg/day. Clopidogrel is a prodrug, and patients have varying dose responses. Patients who possess a variant of the CYP2C19 liver enzyme responsible for activating clopidogrel, detected through molecular diagnostic techniques, may not get the full therapeutic effect. This raises the need for platelet function assays and dosage adjustment.[100]

Prasugrel is an oral prodrug that is converted in the liver via several cytochrome P450 pathways to an active metabolite whose elimination half-life is about 7 hours. Treatment begins with a single 60-mg oral loading dose and continues at 10 mg/day, or 5 mg/day for patients who weigh less than 60 kg. Up to 14% of patients may not achieve the full effect of prasugrel because of a genetic variant of the CYP2C19 liver activation enzyme. In addition, prasugrel dosage is affected by pharmaceutical interactions. Prasugrel carries a higher risk of bleeding than clopidogrel and may be associated with an increased risk of solid tumors. Platelet function assays may be used to assess the antiplatelet effect of prasugrel.[101]

Ticagrelor is a prodrug whose main active metabolite is formed via the CYP3A4 liver enzyme. It is provided in 90-mg tablets. Therapy is begun with 180 mg taken with 325 mg of aspirin, followed by 90 mg of ticagrelor twice a day and aspirin once a day. Ticagrelor reaches full effectiveness in 1.5 hours and maintains a steady state for at least 8 hours. Ticagrelor is susceptible to pharmaceutical interactions, and platelet function assays may be used to assess the antiplatelet effect of ticagrelor.

Laboratory Assessment of Oral Antiplatelet Therapeutic Drugs

Several investigations confirm that 10% to 20% of people who are taking aspirin generate an inadequate response as measured by arachidonic acid-triggered platelet aggregometry. Inadequate response has been termed *aspirin resistance*.[102] Likewise, the response to clopidogrel, prasugrel, or ticagrelor, as measured by ADP-triggered aggregometry, varies markedly among patients. Aggregometry results may be used to adjust dosage.[103] Prasugrel and ticagrelor generate less interpatient variation than aspirin or clopidogrel. Aggregometry (Chapter 41) is the reference method; however, several rapid assays are available.[104]

The near-patient VerifyNow system uses light transmittance aggregometry to test for responses to aspirin, clopidogrel, prasugrel, and ticagrelor (Chapter 42). For each assay, a cartridge provides the necessary agonist and a suspension of fibrinogen-coated beads. VerifyNow Aspirin uses arachidonic acid as its agonist and VerifyNow $P2Y_{12}$ (PRU test) uses ADP. The QA specialist establishes RI and therapeutic target limits for each assay. Results that are outside the therapeutic target range indicate possible treatment failure and the need to revise dosage or change to a new antiplatelet therapeutic drug. The VerifyNow assays are FDA approved.

The PlateletWorks assay determines the percent platelet aggregation in whole blood.[105] Fresh whole blood is transferred to a plain EDTA (lavender closure) tube, plus an EDTA tube coated with the agonists ADP or collagen. The practitioner performs platelet counts on the EDTA-only tube (baseline) and the agonist-treated EDTA tubes using an electronic cell counter. The differences, expressed as percentages, indicate the degree of platelet aggregation triggered by each agonist. An expected response for patients under antiplatelet therapy is a 40% to 60% reduction from baseline.

The PFA-100 system is a device for measuring platelet function via premade cartridges that house a small aperture (Chapter 42). The first cartridge is impregnated with collagen and epinephrine, and the second cartridge is impregnated with collagen and ADP. The operator pipettes 800 μL whole blood per cartridge and places each cartridge in turn on the instrument. The specimen passes through the aperture until activation by the agonist causes occlusion, generating a parameter called closure time. The PFA-100 tests for aspirin. A closure time that is shorter than the anticipated therapeutic range for aspirin indicates resistance. The PFA-100 is also used to reach a presumptive diagnosis for platelet function deficiency or von Willebrand disease. The Innovance PFA-200, available in Europe, adds a third cartridge that detects platelet $P2Y_{12}$-receptor blocking efficacy of $P2Y_{12}$-receptor antagonists clopidogrel, prasugrel, and ticagrelor.[106]

Viscoelastometry (VET; Chapter 42) derives a platelet function expression from the maximum clot amplitude parameter that also may be used to assess platelet response to aspirin, GPIs, or $P2Y_{12}$ antagonists.[107] Haemonetics TEG offers a "platelet mapping" test kit that provides a direct assessment of platelet function.

The AspirinWorks immunoassay measures a urine metabolite of platelet eicosanoid synthesis, 11-dehydrothromboxane B2 (Chapter 11). Hepatocyte 11-hydroxythromboxane dehydrogenase acts upon platelet-derived plasma thromboxane B_2, the product of eicosanoid synthesis and the stable analogue of thromboxane A2, to produce water-soluble 11-dehydrothromboxane B2.[108] The urine concentration of the metabolite is sufficient for measurement without extraction and, because platelets are a major source, reflects platelet activity within the previous 12 hours. Urine levels of 11-dehydrothromboxane B2 are frequently elevated in atherosclerosis; after stroke, transient ischemic attack, or intracerebral hemorrhage; and in atrial fibrillation. Levels of the metabolite are decreased in patients receiving aspirin therapy, even in those with atherosclerosis, AMI, and atrial fibrillation, but appear to remain normal in patients who are aspirin resistant. Aspirin resistance is associated with increased risk of stroke and AMI.[109]

FIBRINOLYTIC THERAPY

Endothelial cells secrete tissue plasminogen activator (TPA, Chapter 35), which binds to fibrin, where it converts adjacent fibrin-bound plasminogen to plasmin, the key enzyme responsible for physiologic fibrinolysis. Free TPA in plasma is neutralized by endothelial cell–secreted plasminogen activator inhibitor (PAI-1), preventing systemic plasminogen activation that would result in fibrinogen degradation. PAI-1 is stored in platelets and released during platelet activation.

In 1987, a recombinant TPA analogue (rTPA), alteplase (Activase) (Genentech) was FDA approved for the treatment of AMI, where it was able to recanalize coronary arteries, a breakthrough in AMI management that is now commonplace for patients who are unable to access timely PCI.[110] Alteplase was subsequently cleared for management of acute ischemic stroke and acute massive PE. Ischemic stroke management is the current leading alteplase indication.

In 2000, tenecteplase (TNKase) (Genentech) was FDA cleared for AMI treatment. A genetically modified variant of alteplase, tenecteplase takes less time to prepare and can be administered as a bolus, whereas alteplase requires an intravenous pump.[111] For these reasons, many stroke centers switched from approved alteplase to off-label tenecteplase during the COVID-19 pandemic.[112] Meanwhile, clinical trials comparing tenecteplase with alteplase efficacy and safety in ischemic stroke are in progress.[113]

Cardiologists who manage PCI prefer that the incoming AMI patient not receive fibrinolysis before the procedure unless they are delayed more than 90 minutes from the start of symptoms as fibrinolytic therapy raises the risk of periprocedural hemorrhage.[114] The key fibrinolysis risks are intracranial and subarachnoid hemorrhage; consequently, alteplase and tenecteplase are contraindicated in patients with internal bleeding, recent cranial or spinal surgery or head trauma, a bleeding disorder or uncontrolled hypertension.

To initiate fibrinolysis for ischemic stroke, the neurologist first orders and interprets an MRI scan to exclude intracranial hemorrhage as the cause. The intervention begins within 4 hours after symptom onset, although fibrinolysis has provided incremental improvement of symptoms when administered beyond the 4-hour limit.[115] Dosages are provided by the manufacturer and are weight based. Total alteplase dosage may not exceed 90 mg and tenecteplase may not exceed 50 mg. Stroke unit providers monitor the patient throughout administration for signs of bleeding and for hypertension and hypotension. Case reports indicate the antifibrinolytic agent tranexamic acid may effectively stop fibrinolytic therapy–induced bleeding.[116]

Before fibrinolytic therapy, the neurologist orders a baseline PT, PTT, and complete blood cell count to assess the risk of bleeding related to thrombocytopenia, anemia, coagulopathy, or the presence of warfarin or heparin therapy. The assays are repeated after therapy. Fibrinogen, D-dimer, and VET assays may be added to the posttreatment laboratory tests to rule out excessive activation of the fibrinolytic system (primary fibrinolysis) or disseminated intravascular coagulation (DIC). Fibrinogen becomes reduced by 4% to 15%. In patients without recent use of anticoagulants, fibrinolytic therapy may be initiated before the availability of hemostasis laboratory results but is discontinued if the pretreatment INR exceeds 1.7 or the PTT is prolonged. Laboratory test results should normalize within 12 hours of discontinuation of fibrinolytic therapy. Fibrinolytic therapy is followed with anticoagulation.

FUTURE OF ANTITHROMBOTIC THERAPY

Antithrombotic therapy, unchanged for more than 50 years at its onset, has seen marked improvements with the recent introduction of LMWHs, DOACs, DTIs, antiplatelet agents, and fibrinolytic therapy. Health care providers appreciate the current range of pharmaceutical options, and patient management has greatly benefited.

It is likely that there will be further changes between 2025 and 2030. The currently available antithrombotic drugs continue to be evaluated in clinical trials to identify additional clinical indications. Several DOACs in development or awaiting clearance are likely to continue to replace warfarin, LMWH, and fondaparinux. Some antithrombotic drugs under current study inhibit factors other than thrombin or FXa. Interest is being directed at the inhibition of FXIa and FXIIa. Because FXI deficiency is asymptomatic or associated with mild bleeding and FXII deficiency is asymptomatic, DOACs specific for these factors may provide a desirable safety profile.[117] Likewise, a series of new and emerging antiplatelet therapeutics and dual antiplatelet combinations will augment the time-honored aspirin tablet.[118] New fibrinolytic therapeutics, including desmoteplase, currently in phase 3 trials, offer improved efficacy up to 9 hours from the start of symptoms and an improved safety profile.[119]

The contributions of the clinical laboratory will reflect these changes. The movement will intensify from the PT and PTT to the chromogenic anti-Xa heparin assay, the CFX and other chromogenic assays, plasma dilute thrombin time, the ecarin chromogenic assay, and next-generation molecular assays. Platelet activation and antagonist efficacy measurement will grow in convenience and take advantage of flow cytometry, immunoassays, mass spectrometry, and rapid molecular assays.

▌ S U M M A R Y

- Warfarin was first used as an oral anticoagulant in 1952. It protects against venous thromboembolic events (VTE), but it has a narrow therapeutic range, and an overdose causes hemorrhage. Warfarin therapy is monitored by the prothrombin time (PT) assay and reported as an international normalized ratio (INR). PT measurement is available in central clinical laboratories and on portable point-of-care instrumentation. Anticoagulation clinics are available to facilitate warfarin monitoring and provide patient education and support.
- Unfractionated heparin (UFH) was first used as an intravenous anticoagulant in 1935. It provides immediate coagulation control. Its therapeutic effect is monitored using the partial thromboplastin time (PTT), which requires the laboratory practitioner to develop a therapeutic range in seconds calibrated to the chromogenic anti-Xa heparin assay. PTT results are subject to several interferences. The anti-Xa heparin assay also can be used to monitor UFH. Supratherapeutic doses of UFH are used during percutaneous coronary intervention (PCI) or cardiac surgery that requires extracorporeal circulation. In these acute settings, UFH is monitored by the activated clotting time (ACT) or viscoelastometry for their near-patient capabilities and sensitivity to high heparin doses.
- Low-molecular-weight heparin (LMWH) and fondaparinux are used as substitutes for UFH and are administered subcutaneously for both prophylaxis and treatment of established blood clots. Both provide near-complete bioavailability, predictable dose response, longer half-lives than UFH, and low risk of bleeding. LMWH and fondaparinux therapy require laboratory measurement only in patients with renal insufficiency, pregnant women, obese patients, children, and underweight adults using the chromogenic anti-Xa heparin assay.
- Rivaroxaban, apixaban, and edoxaban are direct oral anticoagulants (DOACs) that inhibit factor Xa and require little laboratory assessment. New measurement techniques include the chromogenic anti-Xa assays using rivaroxaban, apixaban, and edoxaban calibrators and controls.
- Dabigatran is another DOAC that functions by inhibiting thrombin and requires laboratory measurement for specific indications. Dabigatran may be measured using the ecarin chromogenic assay (ECA) or the plasma-diluted thrombin time.
- The intravenous direct thrombin inhibitors (DTIs) argatroban and bivalirudin directly bind thrombin and are substituted for heparin in patients with heparin-induced thrombocytopenia with thrombosis (HIT). Intravenous DTI therapy is monitored using the PTT or ECT. These pharmaceuticals affect the PT results, which must be considered when bridging to warfarin therapy, and other clot-based assays. At higher doses, as used during coronary intervention or cardiac surgery, argatroban and bivalirudin are monitored by the ACT.
- The intravenous antiplatelet pharmaceuticals eptifibatide and tirofiban are used during coronary interventional procedures to maintain vascular patency. Because they may cause thrombocytopenia, the platelet count is monitored periodically. Their efficacy may be monitored using platelet aggregometry or viscoelastometry.
- The oral antiplatelet therapeutic drugs aspirin, clopidogrel, prasugrel, and ticagrelor are prescribed after arterial thrombotic events to prevent secondary reocclusion. Patient responses to these therapies vary. Response variation is detected using platelet aggregometry, the VerifyNow system, viscoelastometry, PlateletWorks, the PFA-100, or the AspirinWorks assay.
- TPA analogs alteplase and tenecteplase are employed to accelerate fibrinolysis in acute myocardial infarction (AMI), ischemic stroke, and massive pulmonary embolism (PE). Laboratory assays are necessary to measure parallel anticoagulation and assess the risk of DIC.

Now that you have completed this chapter, go back and read again the case study at the beginning and respond to the questions presented. Answers can be found in Appendix C.

REVIEW QUESTIONS

Answers can be found in Appendix C.

1. What is the PT/INR therapeutic range for warfarin therapy when a patient with an atrial fibrillation has a mechanical heart valve?
   a. 1 to 2
   b. 2 to 3
   c. 2.5 to 3.5
   d. Warfarin is not indicated for patients with mechanical heart valves.

2. Monitoring of a patient taking warfarin showed that her anticoagulation results remained stable over a period of about 7 months. The frequency of her visits to the laboratory began to decrease, so the period between testing averaged 12 weeks. This new testing interval is:
   a. Standard in all cases
   b. Unnecessary, because warfarin monitoring is discontinued after 3 months of stable results
   c. Too long even for a patient with previously stable test results; 4 weeks is the standard
   d. Acceptable if the patient performs self-monitoring daily using an approved home testing instrument and reports unacceptable results promptly to her provider

3. What is the greatest advantage of point-of-care PT testing?
   a. It permits self-dosing of warfarin
   b. Inexpensive
   c. Short turnaround
   d. It is accurate

4. You collect a citrated whole blood specimen to monitor UFH therapy. What is the longest it may stand before the plasma must be separated from the cells?
   a. 1 hour
   b. 4 hours
   c. 24 hours
   d. Indefinitely

5. What test is used to monitor supratherapeutic UFH during an interventional cardiology procedure?
   a. PT
   b. PTT
   c. Bleeding time
   d. ACT

6. What test has been used most often to monitor UFH therapy in the central laboratory?
   a. PT
   b. PTT
   c. ACT
   d. Chromogenic anti-factor Xa heparin assay

7. What test is used most often to monitor LMWH therapy in the central laboratory?
   a. PT
   b. PTT
   c. ACT
   d. Chromogenic anti-factor Xa heparin assay

8. What is an advantage of LMWH therapy over UFH therapy?
   a. It is cheaper.
   b. It causes no bleeding.
   c. It has a predictable dose response.
   d. There is no risk of HIT.

9. In what situation is an intravenous DTI used?
   a. DVT
   b. HIT
   c. Any situation in which warfarin could be used
   d. Uncomplicated AMI

10. What test may be used to monitor intravenous DTI therapy when PTT results are unreliable?
    a. PT
    b. Ecarin clotting assay
    c. Chromogenic FX assay
    d. Reptilase clotting time

11. What is the reference method for detecting aspirin or clopidogrel resistance?
    a. Platelet aggregometry
    b. AspirinWorks
    c. VerifyNow
    d. PFA-100

12. What is the name of the measurable urinary platelet activation metabolite used to monitor aspirin resistance?
    a. 11-dehydrothromboxane B_2
    b. Arachidonic acid
    c. Thromboxane A_2
    d. Cyclooxygenase

13. Which is an intravenous antiplatelet pharmaceutical used during an interventional cardiology procedure?
    a. Eptifibatide
    b. Ticagrelor
    c. Prasugrel
    d. Clopidogrel

14. Which of the following is a DOAC?
    a. Argatroban
    b. Fondaparinux
    c. Bivalirudin
    d. Rivaroxaban

REFERENCES

1. Galanaud, J. P., Laroche, J. P., & Righini, M. (2013). The history and historical treatments of deep vein thrombosis. *J Thromb Haemost, 11,* 402–411.

2. Handin, R. I. (2016). The history of antithrombotic therapy: the discovery of heparin, the vitamin K antagonists, and the utility of aspirin. *Hematol Oncol Clin North Am, 30,* 987–993.

3. Mair, G., von Kummer, R., Adami, A., et al. (2017). Arterial obstruction on computed tomographic or magnetic resonance

angiography and response to intravenous thrombolytics in ischemic stroke. *Stroke, 48,* 353–360.

4. Kumar, M., & Cucchiara, B. (2019). Hematologic interventions for acute central nervous system disease. In Kitchens, C. S., Kessler, C. M., Konkle, B. A., et al. (Eds.), *Consultative Hemostasis and Thrombosis.* (4th ed., pp. 778–801). Philadelphia: Elsevier.

5. Whitlock, R. P., Sun, J. C., Fremes, S. E., et al. (2012). Antithrombotic and thrombolytic therapy for valvular disease: antithrombotic therapy and prevention of thrombosis. American College of Chest Physicians Evidence-Based Clinical Practice Guidelines (9th edition). *Chest, 141,* e576S–e600S.

6. Crowther, M. (2019). Parenteral antithrombotic agents. In Kitchens, C. S., Kessler, C. M., Konkle, B. A., et al. (Eds.), *Consultative Hemostasis and Thrombosis.* (4th ed., pp. 529–539). Philadelphia: Elsevier.

7. Quintenz, A. (2022). More than cost: The true impact of errors. Medical Laboratory Observer. https://www.mlo-online.com/management/qa-qc/article/21264175/more-than-cost-the-true-impact-of-errors.

8. Ageno, W., Gallus, A. S., Wittkowsky, A., et al. (2012). Oral anticoagulant therapy: antithrombotic therapy and prevention of thrombosis. American College of Chest Physicians Evidence-Based Clinical Practice Guidelines (9th edition). *Chest, 141,* e44S–e88S.

9. Duxbury, B. M., & Poller, L. (2001). The oral anticoagulant saga: past, present, and future. *Clin Appl Thromb Hemost, 7,* 269–275.

10. Fahmi, A. M., Elewa, H., & Jilany, H. E. (2022). Warfarin dosing strategies evolution and its progress in the era of precision medicine, a narrative review. *Int J Clinical Pharmacy, 44,* 599–607.

11. Hariri, E. H., Kassis, N., Badwan, O. Z., et al. (2022). Impact of oral anticoagulation on progression and long-term outcomes of mild or moderate aortic stenosis. Letter. *J Am Coll Cardiol, 80,* 181–163.

12. Oldenburg, J., Müller, C. R., Rost, S., et al. (2014). Comparative genetics of warfarin resistance. *Hamostaseologie, 34,* 143–159.

13. Zhang, L., Truong, K., Chan, L., et al. (2022). Warfarin-induced skin necrosis after the use of an anticoagulation reversal agent. *Australas J Dermatol, 63,* e159–e161.

14. Schulman, S., Parpia, S., Stewart, C., et al. (2011). Warfarin dose assessment every 4 weeks versus every 12 weeks in patients with stable international normalized ratios: a randomized trial. *Ann Intern Med, 155,* 653–659.

15. Poller, L., Keown, M., Chauhan, N., et al. (2005). European Concerted Action on Anticoagulation. A multicentre calibration study of WHO international reference preparations for thromboplastin, rabbit (RBT/90) and human (rTF/95). *J Clin Pathol, 58,* 667–669.

16. Korn, D., McMurtry, M. S., George-Phillips, K., et al. (2017). Critical international normalized ratio results after hours: to call or not to call? *Can Fam Physician, 63,* e170–e176.

17. Lippi, G., Adcock, D., Simundic, A., et al. (2017). Critical laboratory values in hemostasis: toward consensus. *Ann Med, 49,* 455–461.

18. McGlasson, D. L., Romick, B. G., & Rubal, B. J. (2008). Comparison of a chromogenic factor X assay with INR for monitoring oral anticoagulation therapy. *Blood Coagul Fibrinolysis, 19,* 513–517.

19. Greenmyer, J. R., Niaz, T., Kohorst, M. A., et al. (2021). Chromogenic factor X assay for monitoring warfarin anticoagulation in a child with a prosthetic mitral valve. *Case Reports Mayo Clin Proc Innov Qual Outcomes, 5,* 811–816.

20. McGlasson, D. L. (2019). The chromogenic factor X assay. DiaPharma. https://diapharma.com/clot-club-cfx/.

21. Amiri, S. V., Sidelmann, J. J., & Bor, M. V. (2022). Does vitamin K supplementation improve vitamin K antagonist therapy? A case report and update of the literature. *J Cardiol Cases, 25,* 359–362.

22. Cavallari, L. H., & Limdi, N. A. (2009). Warfarin pharmacogenomics. *Curr Opin Mol Ther, 11,* 243–251.

23. Koehl, K. E., Panos, N. G., Peksa, G. D., et al. (2022). Clinical outcomes after 4F-PCC for warfarin-associated ICH and baseline GCS less than or equal to 8. *Am J Emerg Med, 26,* 59–62.

24. Crowther, M. A. (2019). Parenteral antithrombotic agents. In Kitchens, C. S., Kessler, C. M., Konkle, B. A., et al. (Eds.), *Consultative Hemostasis and Thrombosis.* (4th ed., pp. 529–539). Philadelphia: Elsevier.

25. Garcia, D. A., Baglin, T. P., Weitz, J. I., et al. (2012). Parenteral anticoagulants: antithrombotic therapy and prevention of thrombosis. American College of Chest Physicians Evidence-Based Clinical Practice Guidelines (9th edition). *Chest, 141,* e24S–e43S.

26. Cuker, A. (2012). Unfractionated heparin for the treatment of venous thromboembolism: best practices and areas of uncertainty. *Semin Thromb Hemost, 38,* 593–599.

27. Lenahan, J. G., Frye, S., Jr., & Phillips, G. E. (1966). Use of the activated partial thromboplastin time in the control of heparin administration. *Clin Chem, 12,* 263–268.

28. Marlar, R. A., & Gausman, J. (2013). The optimum number and type of plasma samples necessary for an accurate activated partial thromboplastin time-based heparin therapeutic range. *Arch Pathol Lab Med, 137,* 77–82.

29. Brill-Edwards, P., Ginsberg, J. S., Johnston, M., et al. (1993). Establishing a therapeutic interval for heparin therapy. *Ann Intern Med, 119,* 104–109.

30. Eikelboom, J. W., & Hirsh, J. (2006). Monitoring unfractionated heparin with the aPTT: time for a fresh look. *Thromb Haemost, 96,* 547–552.

31. Tripodi, A., & van den Besselaar, A. (2009). Laboratory monitoring of anticoagulation: where do we stand? *Semin Thromb Hemost, 35,* 34–41.

32. Bahabri, A., Moffat, K. A., Carlino, S. A., et al. (2022). Mixing study to diagnose heparin-resistance caused by functional antithrombin deficiency. *Int J Lab Hematol, 44(5),* e227–e229.

33. Knapik, P., Cieśla, D., Przybylski, R., et al. (2012). The influence of heparin resistance on postoperative complications in patients undergoing coronary surgery. *Med Sci Monit, 18,* 105–111.

34. Adcock, D. M., Kressin, D. C., & Marlar, R. A. (1998). The effect of time and temperature variables on routine coagulation tests. *Blood Coagul Fibrinolysis, 9,* 463–470.

35. Belk, K. W., Laposata, M., & Craver, C. (2016). A comparison of red blood cell transfusion utilization between anti-activated factor X and activated partial thromboplastin monitoring in patients receiving unfractionated heparin. *J Thromb Haemost, 14,* 2148–2157.

36. Horton, S., & Augustin, S. (2013). Activated clotting time (ACT). *Methods Mol Biol, 992,* 155–167.

37. Slight, R. D., Buell, R., Nzewi, O. C., et al. (2008). A comparison of activated coagulation time–based techniques for anticoagulation during cardiac surgery with cardiopulmonary bypass. *J Cardiothorac Vasc Anesth, 22,* 47–52.

38. Ojito, J. W., Hannan, R. L., Burgos, M. M., et al. (2012). Comparison of point-of-care activated clotting time systems

utilized in a single pediatric institution. *J Extra Corpor Technol, 44*, 15–20.

39. Faraoni, D., & DiNardo, J. A. (2021). Viscoelastic hemostatic assays: update on technology and clinical applications. *Am J Hematol, 96*, 1331–1337.

40. Jackson, G. N. B., Ashpole, K. J., & Yentis, S. M. (2009). The TEG vs the ROTEM thromboelastography/thromboelastometry systems. *Anaesthesia, 64*, 212–215.

41. Choi, J. H., Chun, K. J., Jung, S. M., et al. (2022). Safety and efficacy of immediate heparin reversal with protamine after complex percutaneous coronary intervention. *BMC Cardiovasc Disord, 22*, 207–214.

42. Bakchoul, T., Zoliner, H., Amiral, J., et al. (2013). Anti-protamine-heparin antibodies: incidence, clinical relevance, and pathogenesis. *Blood, 121*, 2821–2827.

43. Solari, F., & Varacello, M. (2022). Low molecular weight heparin (LMWH). In: StatPearls [Internet]. StatPearls Publishing, Treasure Island, Florida. https://www.statpearls.com/point-of-care/24433.

44. Westendorf, J. B., Tittl, L., Bistervels, I., et al. (2020). Safety of direct oral anticoagulant exposure during pregnancy: a retrospective cohort study. *Lancet Haematol, 7*, e884–e891.

45. Douketis, J. D., Spyropoulos, A. C., Spencer, F. A., et al. (2012). Perioperative management of antithrombotic therapy: antithrombotic therapy and prevention of thrombosis. American College of Chest Physicians Evidence-Based Clinical Practice Guidelines (9th edition). *Chest, 141*, e326S–e350S.

46. Cuker, A. (2012). Current and emerging therapeutics for heparin-induced thrombocytopenia. *Semin Thromb Hemost, 38*, 31–37.

47. McGlasson, D. L., Kaczor, D. A., Krasuski, R. A., et al. (2005). Effects of pre-analytical variables on the anti-activated factor X chromogenic assay when monitoring unfractionated heparin and low molecular weight heparin anticoagulation. *Blood Coagul Fibrinolysis, 16*, 173–176.

48. McGlasson, D. L. (2005). Using a single calibration curve with the anti-Xa chromogenic assay for monitoring heparin anticoagulation. *Lab Med, 36*, 297–299.

49. Centeno, E. H., Militello, M., & Gomes, M. P. (2019). Anti-Xa assays: what is their role today in antithrombotic therapy? *Cleveland Clin J Med, 86*, 417–425.

50. Khan, M. Y., Ponde, C. K., Kumar, V., et al. (2022). Fondaparinux: a cornerstone drug in acute coronary syndromes. *World J Cardiol, 14*, 40–53.

51. Nilius, H., Kaufmann, I. J., Cuker, A., et al. (2021). Comparative effectiveness and safety of anticoagulants for the treatment of heparin-induced thrombocytopenia. *Am J Hematol, 96*, 805–815.

52. Frontera, J. A., Lewin, J. J., Rabinstein, A. A., et al. (2016). Guideline for reversal of antithrombotics in intracranial hemorrhage: a statement for healthcare professionals from the Neurocritical Care Society and Society of Critical Care Medicine. *Neurocrit Care, 24*, 6-46.

53. Gómez-Outes, A., Suárez-Gea, M. L., Lecumberri, R., et al. (2015). Direct-acting oral anticoagulants: pharmacology, indications, management, and future perspectives *Eur J Haematol, 95*, 389–404.

54. Cohen, A. T., Hamilton, M., Mitchell, S. A., et al. (2015). Comparison of the novel oral anticoagulants apixaban, dabigatran, edoxaban, and rivaroxaban in the initial and long-term treatment and prevention of venous

thromboembolism: systematic review and network meta-analysis. *PLoS One, 10*, e0144856.

55. Chen, A., Stecker, E., & Warden, B. A. (2020). Direct oral anticoagulant use: a practical guide to common clinical challenges. *J Am Heart Assoc, 9*, e017559.

56. Cuker, A., Arepally, G. M., Chong, B. H., et al. (2018). American Society of Hematology 2018 guidelines for management of venous thromboembolism: heparin-induced thrombocytopenia. *Blood Adv, 2*, 3360–3392.

57. Schulman, S., & Spencer, F. A. (2010). Antithrombotic drugs in coronary artery disease: risk benefit ratio and bleeding. *J Thromb Haemost, 8*, 641–650.

58. Demchuk, A. M., Yue, P., Zotova, E., et al. (2021). Hemostatic efficacy and anti-FXa (factor Xa) reversal with andexanet alfa in intracranial hemorrhage: ANNEXA-4 substudy trial. *Stroke, 52*, 2096–2105.

59. Merrelaar A. E., Bögl, M. S., Buchtele, N., et al. (2022). Performance of a qualitative point-of-care strip test to detect DOAC exposure at the emergency department: a cohort-type cross-sectional diagnostic accuracy study. *Thromb Haemost, 122*, 1723–1731.

60. Baglin, T., Hillarp, A., Tripodi, A., et al. (2013). Measuring oral direct inhibitors of thrombin and factor Xa: a recommendation from the Subcommittee on Control of Anticoagulation of the Scientific and Standardization Committee of the International Society on Thrombosis and Haemostasis. *J Thromb Haemost, 11*, 756–760.

61. Tripodi, A. (2013). Which test to use to measure the anticoagulant effect of rivaroxaban: the prothrombin time test. *J Thromb Haemost, 11*, 576–578.

62. Ten Cate, H., Henskens, Y. M. C., & Lance, M. D. (2017). Practical guidance on the use of laboratory testing in the management of bleeding in patients receiving direct oral anticoagulants. *Vasc Health Risk Manag, 13*, 457–467.

63. Samama, M. M. (2013). Which test to use to measure the anticoagulant effect of rivaroxaban: the anti-factor Xa assay. *J Thromb Haemost, 11*, 579–580.

64. Douxfils, J., Adcock, D. M., Bates, S. M., et al. (2021). 2021 update of the International Council for Standardization in Haematology recommendations for laboratory measurement of direct oral anticoagulants. *Thromb Haemost, 120*, 1008–1020.

65. Exner, T., Michalopoulos, N., Pearce, J., et al. (2018). Simple method for removing DOACs from plasma samples. *Thromb Res, 163*, 117–122.

66. Celikyurt, I., Meier, C. R., Kühne, M., et al. (2017). Safety and interactions of direct oral anticoagulants with antiarrhythmic drugs. *Drug Saf, 40*, 1091–1098.

67. Nalezinski, S. (2022). Methods to correct drug-induced coagulopathy in bleeding emergencies: a comparative review. *Lab Med, 53*, 336–343.

68. Harenberg, J., Giese, C., Marx, S., et al. (2012). Determination of dabigatran in human plasma samples. *Semin Thromb Hemost, 38*, 16–22.

69. Gosselin, R. C., Dwyre, D. M., & Dager, W. E. (2013). Measuring dabigatran concentrations using a chromogenic ecarin clotting time assay. *Ann Pharmacother, 47*, 1635–1640.

70. Avecilla, S. T., Ferrell, C., Chandler, W. L., et al. (2012). Plasma-diluted thrombin time to measure dabigatran concentrations during dabigatran etexilate therapy. *Am J Clin Pathol, 137*, 572–574.

71. Antovic, J. P., Skeppholm, M., Eintrei, J., et al. (2013). How to monitor dabigatran when needed: comparison of coagulation laboratory methods and dabigatran concentrations in plasma. *J Thromb Haemost, 11*(Suppl. 2), Abstract AS 02-3.

72. Srinivasan, A. F., Rice, I. L., Bartholomew, J. R., et al. (2004). Warfarin-induced skin necrosis and venous limb gangrene in the setting of heparin-induced thrombocytopenia. *Arch Intern Med, 164,* 66–70.

73. Grouzi, E. (2014). Update on argatroban for the prophylaxis and treatment of heparin-induced thrombocytopenia type II. *J Blood Med, 5,* 131–141.

74. Shantsila, E., Lip, G. Y., & Chong, B. H. (2009). Heparin-induced thrombocytopenia. A contemporary clinical approach to diagnosis and management. *Chest, 135,* 1651–1654.

75. Prechel, M., & Walenga, J. M. (2008). The laboratory diagnosis and clinical management of patients with heparin-induced thrombocytopenia: an update. *Semin Thromb Hemost, 34,* 86–96.

76. Bachler, M., Asmis, L. M., & Koscielny, J. (2022). Thromboprophylaxis with argatroban in critically ill patients with sepsis: a review. *Blood Coagul Fibrinolysis, 33,* 239–246.

77. Mahat, K. C., Sedhai, Y. R., & Krishnan, P. (2022). Argatroban. In: StatPearls [Internet]. StatPearls Publishing, Treasure Island, Florida.

78. Grouzi, E. (2014). Update on argatroban for the prophylaxis and treatment of heparin-induced thrombocytopenia type II. *J Blood Med, 5,* 131–141.

79. Chia, S., Van Cott, E. M., Raffel, O. C., et al. (2009). Comparison of activated clotting times obtained using Hemochron and Medtronic analyzers in patients receiving anti-thrombin therapy during cardiac catheterization. *Thromb Haemost, 101,* 535–540.

80. Joseph, L., Casanegra, A. I., Dhariwal, M., et al. (2014). Bivalirudin for the treatment of patients with confirmed or suspected heparin-induced thrombocytopenia. *J Thromb Haemost, 12,* 1044–1053.

81. Qaderdan, K., Vos, G. A., McAndrew, T., et al. (2017). Outcomes in elderly and young patients with ST-segment elevation myocardial infarction undergoing primary percutaneous coronary intervention with bivalirudin versus heparin: pooled analysis from the EUROMAX and HORIZONS-AMI trials. *Am Heart J, 194,* 73–82.

82. Li, S., Lv, D., Liu, C., et al. (2021). Practicability of bivalirudin plus glycoprotein IIb/IIIa inhibitors in patients undergoing percutaneous coronary intervention: a meta-analysis. *Clin Appl Thromb Hemost, 27,* doi: 10.1177/10760296211055165.

83. Zeng, X., Lincoff, A. M., Schulz-Schüpke, S., et al. (2018). Efficacy and safety of bivalirudin in coronary artery disease patients with mild to moderate chronic kidney disease: meta-analysis. *J Cardiol, 71,* 494–504.

84. Hvas, A. M., Favaloro, E. J., & Hellfritzsch, M. (2021). Heparin-induced thrombocytopenia: pathophysiology, diagnosis and treatment. *Expert Rev Hematol, 14,* 335–346.

85. Cirbus, K., Simone, P., & Austin Szwak, J. (2022). Rivaroxaban and apixaban for the treatment of suspected or confirmed heparin-induced thrombocytopenia. *J Clin Pharm Ther, 47,* 112–118.

86. Walenga, J. M., Fasanella, A. R., Iqbal, O., et al. (1999). Coagulation laboratory testing in patients treated with argatroban. *Semin Thromb Hemost, 25*(Suppl 1), 61–66.

87. Bartholomew, J. R., & Hursting, M. J. (2005). Transitioning from argatroban to warfarin in heparin-induced thrombocytopenia: an analysis of outcomes in patients with elevated international normalized ratio (INR). *J Thromb Thrombolysis, 19,* 183–188.

88. Spyropoulos, A. C., Al-Badri, A., Sherwood, M. W., et al. (2016). Periprocedural management of patients receiving a vitamin K antagonist or a direct oral anticoagulant requiring an elective procedure or surgery. *J Thromb Haemost, 14,* 875–885.

89. Hardy, M., Douxfils, J., Dincq, A. S., et al. (2022). Uninterrupted DOACs approach for catheter ablation of atrial fibrillation: do DOACs levels matter? *Front Cardiovasc Med.* doi: 10.3389/fcvm.2022.864899.

90. Brener, S. J., Mehran, R., Lansky, A. J., et al. (2016). Pretreatment with aspirin in acute coronary syndromes: lessons from the ACUITY and HORIZONS-AMI trials. *Eur Heart J Acute Cardiovasc Care, 5,* 449–454.

91. Rigattieri, S., Lettieri, C., Tiberti, G., et al. (2022). Primary percutaneous coronary intervention with high-bolus dose tirofiban: the FASTER (Favorite Approach to Safe and Effective Treatment for Early Reperfusion) multicenter registry. *J Interv Cardiol, 29.* doi: 10.1155/2022/9609970.

92. Rubboli, A., & Patti, G. (2018). What is the role for glycoprotein IIb/IIIa inhibitor use in the catheterisation laboratory in the current era? *Curr Vasc Pharmacol, 16,* 451–458.

93. Dézsi, D. A., Bokori, G., Faluközy, J., et al. (2016). Eptifibatide-induced thrombocytopenia leading to acute stent thrombosis. *J Thromb Thrombolysis, 41,* 522–524.

94. Gibbs, N. M. (2009). Point-of-care assessment of antiplatelet agents in the perioperative period: a review. *Anaesth Intensive Care, 37,* 354–369.

95. Corliss, B. M., Polifka, A. J., Harris, N. S., et al. (2018). Laboratory assessments of therapeutic platelet inhibition in endovascular neurosurgery: comparing results of the VerifyNow P2Y12 assay to thromboelastography with platelet mapping. *J Neurosurg, 129,* 1160–1165.

96. Winter, M. P., Grove, E. L., De Caterina, R., et al. (2017). Advocating cardiovascular precision medicine with P2Y12 receptor inhibitors. *Eur Heart J Cardiovasc Pharmacother, 3,* 221–234.

97. Yan, L., Zhou, Y., Yu, Z., et al. (2022). P2Y12 inhibitor pretreatment in patients with non ST-segment elevation acute coronary syndrome: a meta-analysis. *Medicine (Baltimore), 101,* e29824.

98. Giustino, G., Baber, U., Sartori, S., et al. (2015). Duration of dual antiplatelet therapy after drug-eluting stent implantation: a systematic review and meta-analysis of randomized controlled trials. *J Am Coll Cardiol, 65,* 1298–1310.

99. Kim, K., Hennekens, C. H., Martinez, L., et al. (2021). Primary care providers should prescribe aspirin to prevent cardiovascular disease based on benefit-risk ratio, not age. *Fam Med Community Health, 9,* e001475.

100. Flechtenmacher, N., Kämmerer, F., Dittmer, R., et al. (2015). Clopidogrel resistance in neurovascular stenting: correlations between light transmission aggregometry, VerifyNow, and the Multiplate. *Am J Neuroradiol, 36,* 1953–1958.

101. Alexopoulos, D., Xanthopoulou, I., Perperis, A., et al. (2013). Factors affecting residual platelet aggregation in prasugrel treated patients. *Curr Pharm Des, 19,* 5121–5126.

102. Piechota, W., Krzesiński, P., Piotrowicz, K., et al. (2022). Urine 11-dehydro-thromboxane B2 in aspirin-naive males with metabolic syndrome. *Clin Med, 11,* 3471.

103. Nakahara, H., Sarker, T., Dean, C. L., et al. (2022). A sticky situation: variable agreement between platelet function tests used to assess anti-platelet therapy response. *Front Cardiovasc Med, 9,* 899594.

104. Mueller, T., Dieplinger, B., Poelz, W., et al. (2009). Utility of the PFA-100 instrument and the novel Multiplate analyzer for the assessment of aspirin and clopidogrel effects on platelet function in patients with cardiovascular disease. *Clin Appl Thromb Hemost, 15*, 652–659.

105. Khan, H., Jain, S., Gallant, R. C., et al. (2021). Plateletworks as a point-of-care test for ASA non-sensitivity. *J Pers Med, 11*, 813–826.

106. Favaloro, E. J., Mohammed, S., Vong, R., et al. (2022). Harmonizing platelet function analyzer testing and reporting in a large laboratory network. *Int J Lab Hematol*, doi: 10.1111/ijlh.13907.

107. Cheng, D., Zhao, S., & Hao, Y. (2020). Net platelet clot strength of thromboelastography platelet mapping assay for the identification of high on-treatment platelet reactivity in post-PCI patients. *Biosci Repul, 40*, BSR20201346.

108. McGlasson, D. L., Chen, M., & Fritsma, G. A. (2005). Urinary 11-dehydrothromboxane B2 levels in healthy individuals following a single dose response to two concentrations of aspirin. *J Clin Ligand Assay, 28*, 147–150.

109. Tran, H. A., Anand, S. S., Hankey, G. J., et al. (2006). Aspirin resistance. *Thromb Res, 120*, 337–346.

110. Collen, D., & Lijnen, H. R. (2004). Tissue-type plasminogen activator: a historical perspective and personal account. *J Thromb Haemost, 2*, 541–546.

111. Warach, S. J., & Saver, J. L. (2020). Stroke thrombolysis with tenecteplase to reduce emergency department spread of coronavirus disease 2019 and shortages of alteplase. *JAMA Neurol, 77*, 1203–1204.

112. Berge, E., Whiteley, W., Audebert, H., et al. (2021). European Stroke Organisation (ESO) guidelines on intravenous thrombolysis for acute ischaemic stroke. *Eur Stroke J, 6*, I–LXII.

113. Menon, B. K., Buck, B. H., Singh, N., et al. (2022). Intravenous tenecteplase compared with alteplase for acute ischaemic stroke in Canada (AcT): a pragmatic, multicentre, open-label, registry-linked, randomised, controlled, non-inferiority trial. *Lancet*, doi: 10.1016/S0140-6736(22)01054-6.

114. Walters, D., & Mahmud, E. (2021). Thrombolytic therapy for ST-elevation myocardial infarction presenting to non-percutaneous coronary intervention centers during the COVID-19 crisis. *Curr Cardiol Rep, 23*, 152.

115. Idowu, A. O., Sanusi, A. A., Balogun, S. A., et al. (2022). Outcome of delayed administration of alteplase in a resource-poor area: a case report. *Cureus, 14*, e25996.

116. Hailu, K., Ragoonanan, D., & Davis, H. (2022). Tranexamic acid for treatment of symptomatic hemorrhagic conversion following administration of tenecteplase for acute ischemic stroke. *Am J Emergency Med*. doi: 10.1016/j.ajem.2022.06.022.

117. Matafonov, A., Leung, P. Y., Gailani, A. E., et al. (2014). Factor XII inhibition reduces thrombus formation in a primate thrombosis model. *Blood, 123*, 1739–1746.

118. Ponchia, P. I., Ahmed, R., Farag, M., et al. (2023). Antiplatelet therapy in end-stage renal disease patients on maintenance dialysis: a state-of-the-art review. *Cardiovasc Drugs Ther, 37*, 975–987.

119. Piechowski-Jozwiak, B., Abidi, E., El Nekidy, W. S., et al. (2021). Clinical pharmacokinetics and pharmacodynamics of desmoteplase. *Eur J Drug Metab Pharmacokinet, 47*, 165–176.

41

Laboratory Evaluation of Hemostasis

Mayukh Kanti Sarkar and George A. Fritsma

OBJECTIVES

After completion of this chapter, the reader will be able to:

1. Recognize the proper collection and transport of hemostasis blood specimens.
2. Reject hemostasis blood specimens due to clots, short draws, or hemolysis.
3. Recognize proper hemostasis blood specimen preparation for analysis.
4. Describe the principles of light transmittance and impedance platelet aggregometry.
5. Apply appropriate platelet function tests in a variety of conditions and interpret their results.
6. Describe how plasma markers of platelet activation are analyzed.
7. Describe the principle of, appropriately select, and correctly interpret the results of clot-based coagulation tests, including prothrombin time, partial thromboplastin time, and thrombin time.
8. Interpret clot-based assay results collectively to reach presumptive diagnoses, and then recommend confirmatory tests.
9. Interpret partial thromboplastin time mixing studies to detect factor deficiencies, lupus anticoagulants, and specific factor inhibitors.
10. Describe the principle of, select, and correctly interpret coagulation factor assays.
11. Describe the principle of and correctly interpret Nijmegen-Bethesda assays for coagulation factor inhibitors.
12. Describe the principle of, select, and correctly interpret tests of fibrinolysis, including D-dimer, plasminogen, plasminogen activator, and plasminogen activator inhibitor.
13. Interpret global coagulation assays: viscoelastometry and thrombin generation assays.
14. Describe the use of high-throughput genomic sequencing to detect coagulopathies and platelet abnormalities.

OUTLINE

Hemostasis Laboratory Testing
Hemostasis Specimen Collection
  Patient Management
  Materials for Hemostasis Blood Specimen Collection
  Specimen Collection Procedures
Hemostasis Specimen Management
  Hemostasis Specimen Transport and Storage
  Preparation of Hemostasis Specimens
Platelet Function Tests
  Bleeding Time Test
  Platelet Aggregometry
  von Willebrand Factor Activity Assays
  Heparin-Induced Thrombocytopenia Assays
Platelet Activation Markers
Clot-Based Screening Tests for Coagulation Disorders
  Prothrombin Time
  Partial Thromboplastin Time
  Partial Thromboplastin Time Mixing Studies
  Thrombin Time
  Venom Activated Assays

Coagulation Factor Assays
  Fibrinogen Assay
  Single-Factor Assays Using Partial Thromboplastin Time
  Factor Assays Using Chromogenic Substrate Technique
  Nijmegen-Bethesda Assay for Anti-Factor VIII Inhibitor
  Single-Factor Assays Using the Prothrombin Time
  Factor XIII Assay
Fibrinolysis Assays
  D-Dimer and Fibrin Degradation Products
  Plasminogen
  Tissue Plasminogen Activator
  Plasminogen Activator Inhibitor-1
Viscoelastometry and Global Coagulation Assays
  TEG and ROTEM
  Quantra
  Thrombin Generation Assays
Genetic Testing for Hemostatic Disorders

HEMOSTASIS LABORATORY TESTING

This chapter describes the techniques that underlie clinical hemostasis laboratory testing. Included are the techniques for specimen collection and management, platelet function tests, routine clot-based assays, factor assays, and assays to identify defects in coagulation control and fibrinolysis. Refer to the respective chapters devoted to assays specific to bleeding disorders (Chapter 36), platelet defects (Chapters 37 and 38), thrombotic disorders (Chapter 39), and antithrombotic drug monitoring (Chapter 40).

For diagnostic purposes, it is important to obtain results from assays that provide information on the *function* of platelets, coagulation factors, control proteins, and fibrinolytic components. Quantitative immunoassays are often essential but may not provide sufficient information for a diagnosis as they do not detect functionality of the hemostatic parameter.

HEMOSTASIS SPECIMEN COLLECTION

Medical laboratory practitioners, phlebotomists, patient care technicians, nurses, and physicians who collect and manage hemostasis blood specimens must adhere closely to published protocols to ensure assay validity. Principles of venipuncture for clinical laboratory specimen collection are provided in Chapter E2. For hemostasis tests, however, additional precautions are required beyond these general principles because hemostatic proteins are not stable and platelets are prone to activation. Blood specimen collection and management are the most vulnerable stages of the hemostasis blood testing process because every stage is manual and thus fraught with error. The laboratory or nursing supervisor is responsible for the up-to-date validity of specimen collection and management protocols and ensures that personnel employ approved techniques.[1]

Most hemostasis procedures are performed on platelet-poor plasma (PPP), which is plasma whose platelet count is less than 10,000/μL, prepared from venous whole blood collected by venipuncture. At the moment of collection, blood is mixed with sodium citrate anticoagulant and is maintained as well-mixed whole blood for assays that require whole blood such as platelet function tests and viscoelastometry or centrifuged to provide platelet-rich plasma (PRP), which is plasma with a platelet count of approximately 200,000/μL, for light transmittance platelet aggregometry or centrifuged to provide PPP for clot-based assays.

Patient Management

The medical laboratory practitioner, pharmacist, nurse, and physician shoulder substantial responsibility for preparing a patient for hemostasis testing. A diligent bleeding and thrombosis risk assessment is performed to aid in determining a diagnosis as well as bleeding risk at time of blood collection. The provider asks about family clotting and bleeding history; blood group (people with group O blood have a higher prevalence of von Willebrand disease [VWD]); pregnancy, which can be associated with a prothrombotic state; and liver or kidney disease, leukemia, anemia, and malnutrition, all of which can be associated with increased bleeding risk. Bleeding and clotting characteristics are assessed next, including location, frequency, volume, and whether events are spontaneous or follow an injury or a surgical or dental procedure.

Of equal importance is a 2-week drug history including, in particular, anticoagulants (blood thinners); antiplatelet drugs, especially aspirin (ASA) and nonsteroidal antiinflammatory drugs (NSAIDs); and contraceptives and hormone replacement therapy, which are prothrombotic.[2,3] The patient is also asked about over-the-counter remedies and dietary supplements, such as garlic, vitamin K, ginger, and St. John's wort, as most can cause platelet dysfunction and bleeding. The patient is instructed to discontinue nonprescription drugs at least 1 week before blood collection. Anticoagulants such as warfarin or direct oral anticoagulants (DOACs) and antiplatelet drugs such as ASA or clopidogrel are continued when the purpose is to assess their efficacy.

Lastly, the provider examines the patient for evidence of bleeding, bruising, and swelling. Standardized *bleeding assessment tools* (BATs) may be employed to enhance bleeding history accuracy.[4] Patients need to fast under only arranged circumstances but are advised to avoid caffeine and exercise for 2 hours and smoking for 30 minutes before collection. Patients should be inactive for 5 minutes before collection.[5]

Blood collectors manage patients using standard protocols for identification, cleansing, tourniquet use, and venipuncture (Chapter E2).[6] If there is a reason to anticipate excessive bleeding, for instance, if the patient has multiple bruises, mentions a tendency to bleed, or possesses a high-risk BAT score, the phlebotomist should extend the time for observing the venipuncture site from the usual 1 minute to 5 minutes and should apply a pressure bandage before dismissing the patient.[7]

Materials for Hemostasis Blood Specimen Collection

Needle Selection

The blood collector fits a 20- or 21-gauge, thin-walled, double-point needle to an adapter for standard evacuated tube collection. In the case of small, scarred, or fragile veins, the collector may fit a 23-gauge Luer adapter needle. To facilitate a difficult draw, a butterfly or winged needle infusion tube fitted to a syringe is used. This technique enables the collector to reduce and control the negative collection pressure on the blood.[8] A further advantage of the syringe technique is that it can be used to avoid platelet activation that is aggravated with the evacuated tube collection technique. The syringe technique is the preferred collection method for platelet function testing.

The needle bore should be large enough to prevent hemolysis and to prevent activation of platelets and procoagulants (Table 41.1). Needles are equipped with safety devices that prevent accidental needlestick injury following specimen collection.

Hemostasis Specimen Collection Tubes

Most hemostasis specimens are collected in plastic blue closure (blue top, blue stopper) sterile evacuated blood collection tubes containing a measured volume of buffered sodium citrate anticoagulant.[9] Siliconized (plastic-coated) glass tubes are available, but their use is declining because of concern for potential breakage, with consequent risk of exposure to bloodborne pathogens. Tubes of uncoated soda-lime glass are unsuitable for hemostatic testing because the glass preactivates the coagulation factors.[10]

Anticoagulants for Hemostasis Specimens

Sodium citrate. The anticoagulant used for most hemostasis testing is buffered 0.105 to 0.109 M (3.2%) sodium citrate. Sodium citrate binds calcium ions to prevent coagulation, and the buffer stabilizes specimen pH as long as the tube closure remains in place.[11]

Upon collection, the anticoagulant solution mixes with blood to produce a 9:1 ratio, that is, 9 parts whole blood to 1 part anticoagulant. In most cases, 0.3 mL of anticoagulant mixes with 2.7 mL of whole blood, or 0.2 mL of anticoagulant mixes with 1.8 mL of whole blood, the volumes in the most commonly used evacuated plastic collection tubes, but any volume is valid provided that the 9:1 ratio is maintained. The ratio yields a final citrate concentration of 10.5 to 10.9 mM of anticoagulant in whole blood.[12]

Sodium citrate volume adjustment for elevated hematocrit. The 9:1 blood-to-anticoagulant ratio is effective, provided that the patient's hematocrit is 55% or below. In polycythemia, the decrease in plasma volume relative to whole blood unacceptably raises the anticoagulant-to-plasma ratio, which causes falsely prolonged results for clot-based coagulation tests. The phlebotomist must prepare specially marked tubes with relatively reduced anticoagulant volumes for collection of blood from a patient whose hematocrit is known to be 55% or higher. The amount of anticoagulant may be computed by using the following formula:

$$C = \left(1.85 \times 10^{-3}\right)\left(100 - HCT\right)V$$

where C is the volume of sodium citrate in milliliters, V is total volume of whole blood plus sodium citrate solution in milliliters, and HCT is the hematocrit in percent.

For example, to collect 3 mL of blood/anticoagulant mixture from a patient who has a hematocrit of 65%, the sodium citrate volume is calculated as follows:

$$C = \left(1.85 \times 10^{-3}\right)(100 - 65) \times 3.0\,\text{mL}$$
$$C = \left(1.85 \times 10^{-3}\right)(35) \times 3.0\,\text{mL}$$
$$C = 0.19\,\text{mL of sodium citrate}$$

Laboratory practitioners remove the stopper from a 3-mL blue closure collection tube and pipette and discard 0.11 mL from the 0.3 mL of anticoagulant, leaving 0.19 mL. They collect blood in a syringe and transfer 2.81 (2.8) mL of blood to the tube, replace the stopper, and immediately mix by gently inverting at least three times. Alternatively, practitioners can prepare for collection of 10 mL of blood and anticoagulant solution in a 12-mL centrifuge tube as follows:

$$C = \left(1.85 \times 10^{-3}\right)(100 - 65) \times 10.0\,\text{mL}$$
$$C = \left(1.85 \times 10^{-3}\right)(35) \times 10.0\,\text{mL}$$
$$C = 0.64\,\text{mL of sodium citrate}$$

In this instance, 0.64 mL of sodium citrate is pipetted into the tube, and 9.36 (9.4) mL of whole blood is transferred from the collection syringe.

This formula may be expressed as a nomogram as shown in Figure 41.1. A complete nomogram appears in Clinical and Laboratory Standards Institute (CLSI) Standard GP41. No evidence exists suggesting a need for increasing the volume of anticoagulant for specimens from patients with anemia, even when the hematocrit is less than 20%.

Other anticoagulants for hemostasis specimens. Laboratory practitioners do not use ethylenediaminetetraacetic acid (EDTA) (lavender closure tube) anticoagulated specimens for clot-based coagulation testing because EDTA irreversibly chelates calcium ions.[13] Calcium ion chelation with citrate, on the other hand, is reversed with the addition of calcium chloride as one of the assay reagents.

EDTA is the anticoagulant used to collect specimens for complete blood counts, including platelet counts. To produce accurate platelet counts in cases of platelet satellitism or platelet clumping (Figures 14.1 and 14.2), sodium citrate or heparin (green closure tubes) can substitute for specimens collected in EDTA. Heparinized specimens have not been validated for plasma coagulation testing.

TABLE 41.1 Hemostasis Specimen Collection Needle Selection	
Application	**Preferred Needle Gauge and Length**
Adult with good veins	20- or 21-gauge, thin-walled, 1.0 or 1.25 inches long
Child or adult with small, fragile, or hardened veins	23-gauge, winged-needle set; collect with small evacuated tubes or syringe
Transfer of blood from syringe to tube	19-gauge safety transfer unit; slowly inject through tube closure

EDTA may be required for specimens used for molecular diagnostic testing, such as testing for the factor V Leiden mutation. Likewise, acid citrate dextrose (ACD) (yellow closure) and dipotassium EDTA (K_2EDTA) (white closure) gel tubes may be used for molecular diagnosis, as specified by institutional protocol.

Citrate theophylline adenosine dipyridamole (CTAD) (blue closure) tubes suppress in vitro platelet or coagulation activation for specialty assays such as the platelet activation marker platelet factor 4 (PF4) or the coagulation activation marker thrombin-antithrombin complex.

Specimen Collection Procedures

Venipuncture

The blood collector adheres strictly to standard venipuncture procedures, with additional precautions for hemostasis

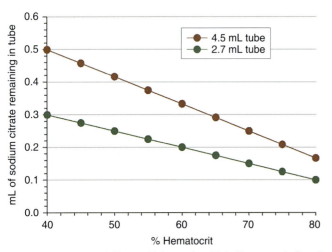

Figure 41.1 Adjusted Citrate Volume for High Hematocrit Specimens. This graph is used for determining the volume of sodium citrate anticoagulant to add to the hemostasis blood collection tube when the patient's hematocrit is 55% or more. Illustration is provided for the typical blood collection tubes: 2.7 mL blood with 0.3 mL citrate for a normal hematocrit and 4.5 mL blood with 0.5 mL citrate for a normal hematocrit.

specimen collection and evacuated tube or syringe collection. Specialized hemostasis laboratories may employ trained collectors to ensure specimen integrity.[14]

The blood collector consults an "order of draw" chart. If a series of evacuated tubes is to be filled from a single venipuncture site, the routine or special hemostasis specimen must be collected first or immediately after a *nonadditive* tube, such as a blood culture tube.[15,16] The hemostasis tube may not immediately follow a tube that contains heparin, EDTA, sodium fluoride (gray closure), or clot-promoting silica particles that are contained in plastic red closure or serum separator (gold or red-gray closure with gel) tubes. These additives may transfer to the hemostasis specimen and invalidate hemostasis test results. Other nonadditive tubes include red closure glass (but not plastic) tubes and clear closure plastic tubes. If nonadditive tubes are unavailable, the phlebotomist may use and discard a preliminary blue closure tube when following an additive tube.

Table 41.2 lists collection errors to avoid for all hemostasis specimens. Evacuated tubes are designed so that the negative internal pressure collects the correct volume of blood. Collection tube manufacturers indicate the allowable range of collection volume error in package inserts and provide a minimum volume indication on each tube. In most cases, the volume of blood collected must be within 90% of the calibrated volume. A *short draw*, that is, a specimen with a smaller volume than the minimum specified by the manufacturer, generates erroneously prolonged clot-based coagulation test results because the excess anticoagulant relative to blood volume adversely neutralizes test reagent calcium.[17] Short-draw specimens are discarded, and a fresh specimen is collected. The smaller the collection tube, the narrower the tolerance for short draws.

When collecting a specimen using a butterfly set, the blood collector compensates for the internal volume of the tubing, which is typically 12 inches long and contains approximately 0.5 mL of air, by first collecting and discarding a nonadditive tube or a blue closure tube. This step ensures that the needle set tubing is filled with fresh patient blood before the hemostasis specimen is collected and avoids an inadvertent short draw.[18]

TABLE 41.2	Hemostasis Specimen Collection and Management Errors That Require Specimen Rejection	
Error	**Comments**
Short draw	Whole blood volume less than 90% of required volume or less than manufacturer-specified minimum. PT and PTT are falsely prolonged.
Specimen clot	Each specimen is inspected visually before centrifugation or during analysis; even a small clot interferes with hemostasis test results.
Visible hemolysis	Pink or red plasma indicates in vitro activation of platelets and coagulation; unpredictable hemostasis test interference. Hemolysis interferes with optical endpoint coagulometer results.
Lipemia or icterus	Optical instruments may fail to measure clots in cloudy or highly colored specimens. Interferes with chromogenic substrate methods. The laboratory practitioner must employ an electromechanical detection method instrument.
Tourniquet application >2 minutes	Blood stasis activates endothelial cells and elevates the concentration of VWF and fibrinogen, falsely shortening clot-based test results.
Specimen storage at 1°–6° C	Storage at refrigerator temperatures causes precipitation of large VWF multimers, activation of coagulation factor VII, activation of platelets, and loss of platelet integrity.
Specimen storage at >25° C	Storage at above standard room temperature causes coagulation factors V and VIII to deteriorate.

PT, Prothrombin time; *PTT*, partial thromboplastin time; *VWF*, von Willebrand factor.

When collecting by syringe, the collector replaces the Luer adapter needle or butterfly needle with a Luer adapter-equipped large-bore safe transfer device and gently transfers the specimen from the syringe into evacuated tubes, using the same order of tube fill as for standard evacuated tube collection.

Clotted specimens are useless for hemostasis testing, even if the clot is small. A few seconds after collection, the blood collector must gently invert the specimen end over end at least three times to mix the blood with the anticoagulant to prevent clot formation. Excessive specimen agitation, called "cocktail shaking," causes hemolysis (red blood cell [RBC] rupture), procoagulant activation, and platelet activation. The medical laboratory practitioner visually examines the specimen for clots just before centrifugation and testing. Many coagulometers are equipped to detect the presence of clots. Clotted specimens are discarded, and a new specimen is collected.

Blood specimens for hemostatic testing must be collected using atraumatic technique. Excess needle manipulation may promote the release of connective tissue procoagulants that contaminate the specimen by activating clotting factors; hemolysis is another potential contaminant from a traumatic needlestick. Consequently, time to clot test results from specimens collected during a traumatic venipuncture may be falsely shortened and unreliable.[19]

During blood collection, the phlebotomist must remove the tourniquet, which slows venous flow, within 2 minutes of its application to avoid stasis.[20] Stasis results in endothelial cell activation and hemoconcentration with the local accumulation of coagulation factors V, VII, VIII, XII, and von Willebrand factor (VWF), which may falsely shorten clot-based coagulation test results.

Specimen Collection From Vascular Access Devices

Although CLSI Standard GP41 discourages the practice, specimens may of necessity be collected from heparin or saline locks, ports in intravenous (IV) lines, peripherally inserted central catheters (PICC tubes), central venous catheters, or dialysis catheters. Vascular access device management requires strict adherence to protocol to ensure sterility, prevent emboli, and prevent damage to the device. Blood collectors must be proficient and must recognize the signs of complications and take appropriate action. Institutional protocol may limit vascular access device blood collection to physicians and nurses.

Before blood is collected for hemostasis testing, the line must be flushed with 5 mL of saline, and the first 5 mL of blood, or six times the volume of the blood collection tube, must be collected and discarded. The blood collector *must not flush with heparin.* Blood is collected into a syringe and transferred to an evacuated tube using a safety transfer device.[21]

Though the practice is discouraged, nurses and phlebotomists may collect blood specimens while starting IV lines. Although a necessary convenience for the patient, IV cannulas are notorious for causing hemolysis. Once the site is flushed and before the IV drip is started, the phlebotomist or nurse collects the specimen via syringe, exerting minimal negative pressure. The test results from visibly hemolyzed specimens are

unreliable, as they can negatively or positively bias coagulation test parameters, and hence the specimen must be recollected.[22]

Specimen Collection Using Capillary Puncture

Point-of-care coagulometers, typically used in an anticoagulation clinic where warfarin monitoring takes place, generate prothrombin time (PT)/international normalized ratio (INR) results from a specimen consisting of 10 to 50 µL of whole blood. These instruments are designed to test either anticoagulated venous whole blood or capillary (fingerstick) blood. They are a significant convenience to patients and to anticoagulation clinics,[23] and some are designed for patient self-testing and pediatric or neonatal testing. Laboratory practitioners are often charged with training nurses, pharmacists, and patients in proper capillary puncture technique.[24]

Capillary specimen skin punctures are made using sterile spring-loaded lancets designed to produce an incision of standard depth and width while avoiding injury. The collector or patient cleanses the third (middle) or fourth (ring) finger and activates the device so that it produces a puncture that is just off center of the fingertip and perpendicular to the fingerprint lines. After wiping away the first drop of blood, which is likely to be contaminated by connective tissue procoagulants, the blood collector places the collection device adjacent to the free-flowing blood and allows the device to fill by capillary action and gravity. The collector then presses a gauze pad to the wound and instructs the patient to maintain pressure until bleeding ceases. Next, the collector wipes excess blood from the outside of the collection device and introduces it to the coagulometer to complete the assay.

The key to accurate capillary PT/INR measurement is a free-flowing puncture. Often it is necessary for the collector to warm the patient's hand to increase blood flow to the fingertips. Blood collection device distributors provide dry, disposable warming devices for this purpose. The collector avoids squeezing ("milking") the finger because this raises the concentration of tissue fluid relative to plasma and blood cells.[25]

HEMOSTASIS SPECIMEN MANAGEMENT

Hemostasis Specimen Transport and Storage

On the list of errors to avoid for hemostasis specimens at time of collection are specimen storage conditions (see Table 41.2). Further, proper specimen transport and long-term storage conditions are critical to maintain specimen integrity. Table 41.3 provides detailed information, including stability time interval and temperature, for hemostasis specimens.

Sodium citrate-anticoagulated whole blood specimens are placed in a rack and allowed to stand in a vertical position with the closure intact and uppermost. Maintaining the blood collection tube seal minimizes CO_2 diffusion, which otherwise allows the pH to rise, falsely prolonging the commonly ordered coagulation tests, PT and partial thromboplastin time (PTT).[26] Specimens are maintained at ambient temperature, 15° to 25° C, never at refrigerator temperatures or on ice. Storage at 1° to 6° C activates factor VII, activates platelets, and precipitates large VWF multimers.[27,28] Specimens are never stored or transported

TABLE 41.3 Hemostasis Specimen Storage Times and Temperatures

Application	Temperature	Specimen Stability
PT with no UFH	15°–25° C	Test within 24 h, maintain upright and sealed
PTT with no UFH	15°–25° C	Test within 4 h, maintain upright and sealed
PTT for monitoring UFH	15°–25° C	Centrifuge to separate plasma within 1 h, test within 4 h
PT when UFH is present	15°–25° C	Centrifuge to separate plasma within 1 h, test within 4 h
Factor assays	15°–25° C	Test within 4 h, maintain upright and sealed
Optical platelet aggregometry using PRP	15°–25° C	Wait 30 minutes after centrifugation, test within 4 h of collection
Whole blood aggregometry	15°–25° C	Test within 4 h of collection, maintain upright and sealed
Storage in household freezer	–20° C	2 weeks
Storage for 6 months	–70° C	6 months or indefinite

PRP, Platelet-rich plasma; *PT,* prothrombin time; *PTT,* partial thromboplastin time, *UFH,* unfractionated heparin.

at temperatures greater than 25° C because heat deteriorates coagulation factors V and VIII.

Specimens collected for PT may be held uncentrifuged or centrifuged at 15° to 25° C and tested within 24 hours of the time of collection.[29] Specimens collected for PTT and most other clot-based assays are also held uncentrifuged or centrifuged at 15° to 25° C, but they must be tested within 4 hours of time of collection. If a patient is receiving unfractionated heparin (UFH) therapy, PTT specimens must be centrifuged within 1 hour of the time of collection to avoid depletion of the heparin. Centrifuges that are used to prepare hemostasis specimens must maintain a temperature of 15° to 25° C.[30]

If any plasma-based hemostasis assay cannot be completed within the prescribed interval, the practitioner must centrifuge the specimen within 1 hour of collection. The practitioner immediately transfers the plasma by plastic pipette to a plastic freezer tube, taking care to avoid stirring up the buffy coat. Glass containers should never be used because glass stimulates the intrinsic coagulation pathway. The freezer tube is labeled, sealed, and frozen. It may be stored at –20° C for up to 2 weeks or at –70° C for long-term storage.[31,32] At the time the test is performed, the frozen specimen is thawed rapidly at 37° C, mixed, and tested within 1 hour of the time it is removed from the freezer. If it cannot be tested immediately, the specimen may be stored at 1° to 6° C for up to 2 hours after thawing.[33] To avoid cryoprecipitation of VWF, specimens may not be frozen and thawed more than once.

Preparation of Hemostasis Specimens
Whole Blood Specimens
Blood for whole blood platelet aggregometry, lumiaggregometry, or viscoelastometry is collected with 3.2% sodium citrate and held at 15° to 25° C until testing. Chilling destroys platelet activity and should be avoided. Aggregometry should be started immediately and must be completed within 4 hours of specimen collection for undiminished ex vivo platelet activity. The practitioner mixes the specimen by gentle inversion, checks for clots just before testing, and rejects specimens with clots. Most specimens for whole blood aggregometry are mixed 1:1 with normal saline before testing, although the specimen is tested undiluted if the platelet count is less than 100,000/μL.[34]

Platelet-Rich Plasma Specimens
Light-transmittance (optical) platelet aggregometers are designed to test PRP, plasma with a platelet count of 200,000 to 300,000/μL. Sodium citrate-anticoagulated blood is first checked visually for clots and then slow-centrifuged at a relative centrifugal force (RCF) of 50g for 30 minutes with the tube closure in place to maintain the pH. The supernatant PRP is transferred by plastic pipette to a clean plastic tube (never glass), and the tube is sealed and stored at 15° to 25° C (ambient temperature) until the test is begun. Specimens for PRP-based light-transmittance aggregometry must stand undisturbed for 30 minutes after centrifugation while the platelets regain responsiveness. Specimens must be tested within 4 hours of collection to avoid spontaneous in vitro platelet activation and loss of normal activity. To produce sufficient PRP, the original specimen must measure 9 to 12 mL of whole blood. Light-transmittance aggregometry is unreliable when the patient's whole blood platelet count is less than 100,000/μL.

Platelet-Poor Plasma Specimens
Clot-based plasma coagulation tests, chromogenic tests, and immunoassays require PPP, plasma with a platelet count of less than 10,000/μL.[35] Sodium citrate-anticoagulated whole blood is centrifuged at 1500g RCF for 15 minutes in a horizontal-head centrifuge to produce supernatant PPP. Alternatively, a HemoCue American StatSpin Express 4 angle-head centrifuge that generates 4400g RCF can produce PPP within 3 minutes. The advantage of the horizontal centrifuge head is that it produces a straight, level plasma-blood cell interface, making it possible for automated coagulometers to sample from the supernatant plasma of the blood collection tube (the "primary" tube). Angled centrifuge heads cause platelets to adhere to the side of the tube. If the "angle-spun" tube is allowed to stand, the adherent platelets drift back into the plasma and release granule contents. Each hemostasis laboratory manager establishes the correct centrifugation speed and times locally.

In the special hemostasis laboratory, the manager may choose a double-spin approach. The primary tube is centrifuged as described in the preceding paragraph and the plasma is transferred to a secondary plastic tube, which is labeled and centrifuged again. The double-spin approach may be used to produce PPP with a plasma platelet count of less than 5000/μL, which some laboratory directors prefer for lupus anticoagulant (LAC) testing and for freezing.

A plasma platelet count greater than 10,000/μL affects clot-based test results. Platelets become activated in vitro and release microparticles and the membrane phospholipid phosphatidylserine, which trigger plasma coagulation and interfere with LAC testing. Platelets also secrete fibrinogen, factors V and VIII and VWF (Chapter 11). These may desensitize PT and PTT assays and interfere with clot-based coagulation assays. In addition, platelets release PF4, a protein that binds and neutralizes therapeutic heparin in vitro, falsely shortening the PTT and interfering with heparin management.

The hemostasis laboratory manager arranges to perform PPP platelet counts on coagulation plasmas at regular intervals to ensure that they are consistently platelet poor. Many managers select 10 to 12 specimens from each centrifuge every 6 months, perform plasma platelet counts, and document that their samples remain appropriately platelet poor, even if the initial platelet count is elevated.

Laboratory practitioners inspect hemostasis plasmas for hemolysis (pink plasma from damaged RBCs), lipemia (cloudy, milky plasma from lipids), and icterus (golden yellow plasma from bilirubin) (see Table 41.2). Visible hemolysis implies platelet or coagulation pathway activation. Visibly hemolyzed specimens are rejected, and new specimens must be obtained. Lipemia and icterus may affect the endpoint results of optical coagulation instruments (Chapter 42). The hemostasis laboratory manager may choose to maintain a separate electromechanical endpoint coagulometer to substitute for the optical instrument for specimens too cloudy for optical determinations. Some optical instruments detect and compensate for hemolysis, lipemia, and icterus via spectrophotometric analysis.[36,37]

PLATELET FUNCTION TESTS

Platelet function tests are designed to detect qualitative (functional) platelet abnormalities in patients who are experiencing symptoms of mucocutaneous bleeding (Chapter 37). A platelet count is performed, and the blood film (Chapter 14) is reviewed before platelet function tests are begun because thrombocytopenia, a common cause of hemorrhage, should be ruled out.[38] Qualitative platelet abnormalities are suspected only when bleeding symptoms are present and the platelet count exceeds 50,000/μL.

Bleeding Time Test

The bleeding time test, first described by Duke in 1912 and modified by Ivy in 1941, is the original test of platelet function.[39,40] It is still used today, although infrequently. To perform the test, the phlebotomist uses a lancet to make a small, controlled puncture wound on the forearm and records the duration of bleeding, comparing the results with the reference interval of 2 to 9 minutes. In 1969 Mielke and colleagues[41] introduced a template to standardize the incision depth and applied a blood pressure cuff to the upper arm, inflated to 40 mm Hg, to standardize blood pressure. In 1976 a calibrated spring-loaded lancet (Surgicutt Bleeding Time Device) was developed.[42]

A prolonged bleeding time could theoretically signal VWD, a functional platelet disorder such as Glanzmann thrombasthenia, or a vascular disorder such as scurvy or vasculitis. Also, a prolonged bleeding time was thought to have a predictable result in therapy using aspirin and other NSAIDs.

Limitations of the bleeding time test that affect reliability of the results have led to its decreased use. The bleeding time is affected by the nonplatelet variables of intracapillary pressure, skin thickness at the puncture site, and size and depth of the wound, all of which interfere with accurate interpretation of the test results.[43] Accurate test results are also dependent on the operator. A series of studies in the 1990s revealed that the bleeding time test has inadequate predictive value of surgical bleeding.[44]

Platelet Aggregometry

Functional platelets adhere to subendothelial collagen, aggregate with one another, and secrete the contents of their α-granules and dense granules (Figure 41.2) (Chapter 11). Normal *adhesion* requires intact platelet membranes and functional plasma VWF. Normal *aggregation* requires that platelet membranes and platelet activation pathways are intact, that the plasma fibrinogen concentration is normal, and that normal *secretions* are released from platelet granules. Platelet adhesion, aggregation, and secretion are assessed using platelet aggregometry that can be detected by one of three different types of instruments, as will be described in the following sections. Platelet aggregometry is a high-complexity laboratory test requiring a skilled, experienced operator.

Light-Transmittance Platelet Aggregometry Using Platelet-Rich Plasma

PRP aggregometry is performed using a specialized photometer called a *light-transmittance aggregometer* distributed by Chrono-Log, Helena Laboratories, or BioData (Chapter 42).[45] After calibrating the instrument in accordance with manufacturer instructions, the operator pipettes the PRP to instrument-compatible cuvettes, usually 500 μL; drops in one clean plasticized stir bar per sample; places the cuvettes in incubation wells; and allows the samples to warm to 37° C for 5 minutes. The operator then transfers the first cuvette, containing specimen and stir bar, to the instrument's reaction well and starts the stirring device and the recording computer. The stirring device turns the stir bar at 800 to 1200 rpm, a gentle speed that keeps

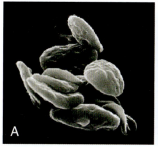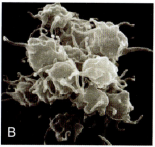

Figure 41.2 Scanning Electron Micrographs of Resting and Activated Platelets. **(A)**, Resting platelets. **(B)**, Activated platelets.

the platelets in suspension. The instrument directs focused light through the sample cuvette to a photodetector (Figure 41.3). As the PRP is stirred, the recorder tracing stabilizes to generate a baseline, near 0% light transmittance.

After a few seconds, the operator pipettes an agonist (platelet activator) (Table 41.4) directly into the specimen to trigger aggregation. In a normal specimen, after the agonist is added, the shape of the suspended platelets changes from discoid to spherical, followed by pseudopod extension (see Figure 41.2), and the intensity of light transmittance initially (and briefly) decreases, then increases in proportion to the degree of shape change. Percent light transmittance is monitored continuously and recorded (Figure 41.4). As platelet aggregates form, more light passes through the PRP, and the tracing begins to move toward 100% light transmittance. Platelet function deficiencies are reflected in diminished or absent aggregation; many laboratory directors choose 40% aggregation as the lower limit of normal.

An innovative 2019 study compared the established platelet aggregation testing on a dedicated optical platelet aggregometer instrument with performance of the same testing on a coagulation analyzer. Partial agreement has encouraged others to confirm the study in an attempt to find a method that simplifies and potentially automates platelet function testing.[46]

Whole Blood Platelet Aggregometry

In whole blood platelet aggregometry, platelet aggregation is measured by *electrical impedance*. Specimens are diluted 1:1 with normal saline and tested immediately.[47] The operator pipettes aliquots of the whole blood suspension to cuvettes and adds equal volumes of saline. Suspension volume may be 300 to 500 μL. The operator drops in one stir bar per cuvette and places the cuvettes in 37° C incubation wells for 5 minutes. The operator transfers the first cuvette to a reaction well, pipettes an agonist (see Table 41.4) directly into the specimen, and suspends a pair of low-voltage cartridge-mounted disposable direct current electrodes into the mixture (Figure 41.5).

As aggregation occurs, platelets adhere to the electrodes and one another, impeding the current. The rise in impedance, which is directly proportional to platelet aggregation, is amplified and recorded. A whole blood aggregometry tracing closely resembles a PRP-based light-transmittance aggregometry tracing (see Figure 41.4).

Platelet Lumiaggregometry

The Chrono-Log Model 700 Whole Blood/Optical Lumi-Aggregometer is used for the simultaneous measurement of platelet aggregation and the *secretion of adenosine triphosphate* (ATP) from dense granules of activated platelets.[48] The procedure for lumiaggregometry differs little from that for light-transmittance. The advantage of lumiaggregometry, however, is that its detection properties simplify the diagnosis of platelet dysfunction.[49,50] As platelet ATP is released, it oxidizes a firefly derived luciferin-luciferase reagent (Chrono-Lume from Chrono-Log) to generate chemiluminescence proportional to the ATP concentration.[51] A photodetector amplifies the luminescence, which is recorded as a second tracing on the aggregation report (Figure 41.6).[52]

To perform lumiaggregometry, the operator adds an ATP standard to the first sample, then adds luciferin-luciferase, and tests for full luminescence. The operator then adds luciferin-luciferase and an agonist to the second sample; the instrument monitors for aggregation and secretion simultaneously. Thrombin (or thrombin receptor-activating peptide [TRAP]) is typically the first agonist used because thrombin induces full secretion. The operator ordinarily begins with 1 unit/mL of thrombin to induce the release of 1 to 2 nM of ATP. The luminescence induced by thrombin is measured, recorded, and used for comparison with the luminescence produced by other agonists (Table 41.5). Normal secretion induced by agonists other than thrombin produces luminescence at a level of about 50% of that resulting from thrombin. Thrombin-induced secretion may

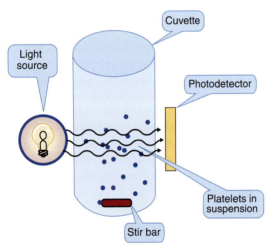

Figure 41.3 Platelet Function Testing Using an Optical Aggregometer. Platelets in a platelet-rich plasma specimen are maintained in suspension by a magnetic stir bar turning at 800 to 1200 rpm. As platelet aggregation proceeds, the platelets form large clumps that allow more light transmission through the specimen. (Courtesy Chrono-Log Corp., Havertown, PA.)

TABLE 41.4	Whole Blood and Light Transmittance Platelet Aggregometry Agonists and Their Target Mechanisms	
Agonist	**Typical Final Concentration**	**Platelet Membrane Receptors Targeted by the Agonist**
Thrombin	1 unit/mL	PAR1 and PAR4; GPIb and GPV
TRAP	10 μM, 50 μM, 100 μM	PAR1 and PAR4; GPIb and GPV
ADP	1–10 μM	$P2Y_1$, $P2Y_{12}$
Epinephrine	2–10 μg/mL [LTA only]	α_2-Adrenergic receptor
Collagen	5 μg/mL	GPIa/IIa, GPVI
Arachidonic acid	500 μM	TPα, TPβ
Ristocetin	1 mg/mL	GPIb/IX/V in association with von Willebrand factor

ADP, Adenosine diphosphate; *GP*, glycoprotein; *LTA*, light transmittance aggregometry; *PAR*, protease-activatable receptor; *P2Y*, platelet membrane ADP receptor; *TP*, thromboxane receptor; *TRAP*, thrombin receptor-activating peptide.

be diminished to less than 1 nM in storage pool deficiencies, but it is relatively unaffected by platelet membrane disorders or pathway enzyme deficiencies (Chapter 37).

Platelet Agonists in Aggregometry

Agonists used to activate platelets are thrombin or synthetic TRAP, adenosine diphosphate (ADP), epinephrine, collagen, arachidonic acid, and ristocetin. Table 41.4 lists representative agonists and the final reaction mixture concentrations used in light-transmittance aggregometry, whole blood aggregometry, and lumiaggregometry. Small volumes (2 to 5 μL) of concentrated agonist are used so that they have little dilutional effect in the reaction system. Table 41.5 lists representative normal results for whole blood impedance lumiaggregometry.[53]

Laboratory practitioners use these platelet agonists to test for abnormalities of specific membrane binding sites on platelets. Arachidonic acid is the agonist used to check for deficiencies in the eicosanoid synthesis pathway. Ristocetin is used to check for abnormalities of plasma VWF in VWD. Lumiaggregometry provides more definitive information for conditions where recording platelet secretion, in addition to platelet aggregation, is an important diagnostic factor.

Thrombin or thrombin receptor-activating peptide. This agonist cleaves two platelet membrane protease activatable receptors (PARs), PAR-1 and PAR-2, both members of the seven-transmembrane repeat receptor family. Thrombin or TRAP also cleaves glycoprotein (GP) 1b and GPV. Membrane-associated G proteins and both the eicosanoid and the diacylglycerol pathways trigger internal platelet activation (Chapter 11). Thrombin-induced activation results in full secretion and

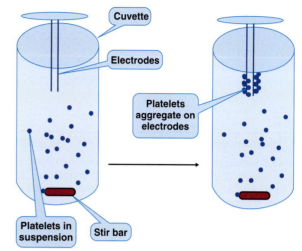

Figure 41.5 Platelet Function Testing Using a Whole Blood Platelet Aggregometer. Aggregating platelets form a layer on the electrodes. As the platelet layer grows with aggregated platelets, the electrical current is impeded. Impedance (in ohms) is proportional to aggregation, and a tracing is provided that resembles the tracing obtained using optical aggregometry. (Courtesy Chrono-Log Corp., Havertown, PA.)

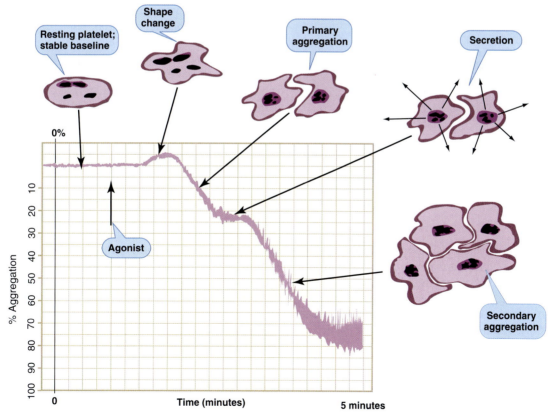

Figure 41.4 Platelet Aggregation Response. This optical aggregometry tracing shows the five phases of platelet aggregation: baseline at 0% aggregation, platelet shape change after addition of the agonist, primary aggregation, release of adenosine diphosphate and adenosine triphosphate from platelet granules, and second-wave aggregation that forms large platelet clumps. The percentage of platelet aggregation is measured by intensity of light transmittance through the test specimen. (Courtesy Chrono-Log Corp., Havertown, PA.)

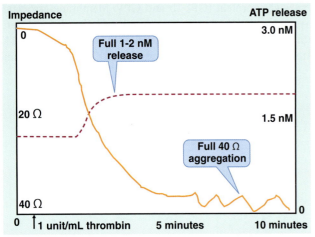

Figure 41.6 Lumiaggregometry Tracing of Normal Platelet Function. This tracing of platelet activity illustrates a monophasic aggregation curve with a superimposed secretion (release) reaction curve. Aggregation is measured in ohms *(Ω)* using the left y-axis scale; release is measured in nanomolars *(nM)* of adenosine triphosphate (ATP) based on luminescence using the right y-axis scale. Curve illustrates full aggregation and secretion response to 1 unit/mL of thrombin.

TABLE 41.5   Typical Whole Blood Platelet Impedance Lumiaggregometry Reference Intervals

Agonist	Final Concentration	Aggregation RI	ATP Secretion
Thrombin	1 unit/mL	Often causes clotting	1.0–2.0 nM
TRAP	10 µM, 50 µM, 100 µM	15–27 Ω	1.0–2.0 nM
Collagen	1 µg/mL	15–27 Ω	0.5–1.7 nM
	5 µg/mL	15–31 Ω	0.9–1.7 nM
ADP	5 µM	1–17 Ω	0.0–0.7 nM
	10 µM	6–24 Ω	0.4–1.7 nM
Arachidonic acid	500 µM	5–17 Ω	0.6–1.4 nM
Ristocetin	1 mg/mL	>10 Ω	Not recorded

ADP, Adenosine diphosphate; *ATP*, adenosine triphosphate; *RI*, reference interval; *TRAP*, thrombin receptor-activating peptide.

aggregation. The disadvantage of thrombin is that it often triggers coagulation (fibrin formation) simultaneously with aggregation, abolishing the value of the aggregation tracing. The use of TRAP avoids this pitfall. Reagent thrombin is stored dry at −20° or −70° C and is reconstituted with saline immediately before use. Leftover reconstituted thrombin may be divided into aliquots, frozen, and thawed for later use.

Adenosine diphosphate. This agonist binds platelet membrane receptors P2Y$_1$ and P2Y$_{12}$, also members of the seven-transmembrane repeat receptor family. ADP-induced platelet activation relies on the physiologic response of membrane-associated G protein and the eicosanoid synthesis pathway (Chapter 11). The end product of eicosanoid synthesis, thromboxane A$_2$, raises cytosolic free calcium, which mediates platelet activation and induces secretion of the ADP stored

in dense granules. The secreted ADP activates neighboring platelets.

In aggregometry systems that measure only aggregation and not luminescence, the operator adjusts the ADP concentration to between 1 µM and 10 µM to induce biphasic aggregation as shown in Figure 41.4. At ADP concentrations near 1 µM, platelets achieve only *primary aggregation* (no platelet secretion), followed by disaggregation. This is observed as an aggregometry recording line that deflects from the baseline for 1 to 2 minutes, then returns to baseline. Primary aggregation involves shape change with formation of microaggregates; both are reversible processes. *Secondary aggregation* is full platelet aggregation after release of platelet dense granule ADP. At agonist ADP concentrations near 10 µM, there is simultaneous irreversible shape change, secretion, and formation of aggregates, resulting in a monophasic curve with full deflection of the aggregometry tracing.

ADP concentrations between 1 µM and 10 µM induce the biphasic curve: primary aggregation followed by a brief flattening of the curve called the lag phase, platelet secretion, and then a secondary irreversible aggregation. Operators expend considerable effort to discover the ADP concentration that generates a biphasic curve with a visible lag phase, as the appropriate concentration varies among patients. This procedure enables operators to use aggregometry to distinguish between membrane-associated platelet defects and storage pool or release defects.

Lumiaggregometry provides a clearer and more reproducible measure of platelet secretion, rendering the quest for the biphasic curve unnecessary. Secretion in response to ADP at 5 µM is diminished in platelet membrane disorders, eicosanoid synthesis pathway enzyme deficiencies, or therapy with ASA or NSAIDs. Secretion is absent in storage pool deficiency when thrombin or TRAP is used as the agonist.

Reagent ADP is stored at −20° C or −70° C, reconstituted with saline, and used immediately after reconstitution. Leftover reconstituted ADP may be aliquoted and frozen for later use.

The thienopyridine antiplatelet drugs clopidogrel and prasugrel irreversibly occupy the ADP receptor P2Y$_{12}$, whereas the nucleoside ticagrelor is reversibly bound (Chapters 37 and 40). The P2Y$_{12}$ inhibitors suppress platelet aggregation and secretion responses to ADP.[54] Platelet aggregometry is employed to monitor response to these antiplatelet drugs.[55] The VerifyNow system (Werfen) offers a specific assay for monitoring the effect of the P2Y$_{12}$ inhibitors and is available in point-of-care settings (Chapter 42).

Epinephrine. This agonist binds platelet α-adrenergic receptors, identical to muscle receptors, and activates platelets through the same metabolic pathways as reagent ADP. The results of epinephrine-induced aggregation match those of ADP except that epinephrine cannot induce aggregation in storage pool disorder or eicosanoid synthesis pathway defects no matter how high its concentration. Epinephrine does not work in whole blood aggregometry. Epinephrine is stored at 1° to 6° C and reconstituted with distilled water immediately before it is used. Leftover reconstituted epinephrine may be aliquoted and frozen for later use.

Collagen. This agonist binds GPIa/IIa and GPVI, but it induces no primary aggregation. After a lag of 30 to 60 seconds, aggregation begins, and a monophasic curve develops. Aggregation induced by collagen at 5 μg/mL requires intact membrane receptors, functional membrane G proteins, and normal eicosanoid pathway function. Loss of collagen-induced aggregation may indicate a membrane abnormality, storage pool disorder, release defect, or the presence of aspirin. Collagen preparations vary; most laboratory managers purchase lyophilized fibrillar collagen preparations from the platelet aggregometer manufacturer such as Chrono-Par Collagen (Chrono-Log). Collagen is stored at 1° to 6° C and used without further dilution. Collagen may not be frozen.

Arachidonic acid. This agonist assesses the viability of the eicosanoid synthesis pathway. Free arachidonic acid agonist is added to induce a monophasic aggregometry curve with virtually no lag phase. Aggregation is independent of membrane integrity. Deficiencies in eicosanoid pathway enzymes, including deficient or inhibited cyclooxygenase, result in reduced aggregation and secretion. Arachidonic acid is readily oxidized and must be stored at −20° C or −70° C in the dark. The operator dilutes arachidonic acid with a solution of bovine albumin for immediate use. Aliquots of bovine albumin-dissolved arachidonic acid may be frozen for later use.

All NSAIDs inhibit *cyclooxygenase* (Chapters 37 and 40).[56] ASA permanently inhibits cyclooxygenase, whereas ibuprofen, indomethacin, and sulfinpyrazone temporarily inactivate it. NSAIDs limit or eliminate the aggregation and secretion responses to arachidonic acid and collagen. Platelet aggregometry is employed to monitor response to these antiplatelet drugs.[57] The VerifyNow system offers a specific assay for monitoring the effect of ASA and is available in point-of-care settings (Chapter 42).

von Willebrand Factor Activity Assays

VWF analysis requires a profile of quantitative and functional assays, including the chromogenic or clot-based coagulation factor VIII assay, the quantitative VWF antigen (VWF:Ag) immunoassay, and a VWF platelet-binding activity (VWF:Ac). These assays and several follow-up specialty assays are detailed in Chapter 36.

A direct platelet-binding function immunoassay, the REAADS VWF Activity assay and the collagen binding assay (VWF:CB) are available from DiaPharma. The former employs a monoclonal antibody specific for an active VWF epitope, and the latter mimics the collagen adhesion property of VWF. Both offer improved precision compared to the original platelet-binding activity assay, the ristocetin cofactor assay (VWF:RCo), performed on a platelet aggregometer. The assay for VWF:GP1bM, available from several manufacturers, is now widely ordered for its ability to detect VWF binding to the GPIb platelet receptor.

Heparin-Induced Thrombocytopenia Assays

The clinical manifestations and mechanism of heparin-induced thrombocytopenia (HIT) are described in Chapter 39. An immunoassay to determine the presence of PF4-heparin auto-antibodies is the first approach for the laboratory diagnosis of HIT; several assays are available.[58–61] Confirmation that HIT antibodies are functionally active is accomplished using the carbon-14 (^{14}C) serotonin release assay (SRA), a washed platelet assay that measures platelet activation and secretion induced by HIT antibodies in the presence of heparin.[62] SRA is the reference method for HIT, but the ^{14}C-SRA is confined to reference laboratories that possess a radioisotope license and have the skill and experience to perform the complex ^{14}C-SRA. Current attempts to develop a nonradioactive SRA include enzyme immunoassays and high-performance liquid chromatography to measure secreted serotonin and immunoassays to measure secreted PF4 or P-selectin.[63]

PLATELET ACTIVATION MARKERS

β-Thromboglobulin, P-selectin, PF4, and other soluble platelet release factors, when increased in circulating concentrations, reflect platelet activation and may accompany arterial thrombosis.[64] A β-thromboglobulin immunoassay is available from Hyphen BioMed, and measurement of β-thromboglobulin may be of diagnostic or prognostic significance.[65] Blood collectors employ CTAD tubes to prevent in vitro platelet activation.[66] Other platelet activation markers can be measured by specific immunoassays.

Thromboxane A_2, the active product of the eicosanoid pathway, has a half-life of 30 seconds, diffuses from the platelet, and spontaneously reduces to thromboxane B_2, a stable, measurable plasma metabolite (Chapter 11). Liver enzymes act on thromboxane B_2 to produce an array of soluble urine metabolites, including 11-dehydrothromboxane B_2, which is stable and measurable.[67] An immunoassay of urinary 11-dehydrothromboxane B_2, available from specialized reference laboratories, is employed to characterize in vivo platelet activation.[68] This assay is performed on random urine specimens with no special pretest preparation. Urinary 11-dehydrothromboxane B_2 assay also may be used to monitor aspirin therapy and to identify cases of aspirin therapy failure.[69,70]

CLOT-BASED SCREENING TESTS FOR COAGULATION DISORDERS

The Lee-White whole blood coagulation time test, described in 1913, was the first laboratory procedure designed to assess coagulation.[71] The Lee-White test is no longer used, but it was the first in vitro clot procedure that employed the principle that the time interval from the initiation of clotting to visible clot formation reflects the condition of the coagulation mechanism. A prolonged clotting time indicates a *coagulopathy,* a coagulation deficiency. A 1953 modification, the activated clotting time (ACT) test, uses a particulate clot activator in the test tube, which speeds the clotting process (Chapters 40 and 42). The ACT is still widely used as a near-patient assay to monitor UFH therapy in hypertherapeutic applications such as cardiac catheterization and coronary artery bypass graft surgery.

The standard clot-based coagulation *screening* tests, PT, PTT, fibrinogen assay, and thrombin time (TT) (or thrombin clotting time, TCT), use the clotting time principle of the Lee-White test.

Many *specialized* tests, such as coagulation factor assays, tests of fibrinogen, inhibitor assays, reptilase time Russell viper venom (RVV) time, and dilute RVV time (dRVVT), are also based on the relationship between time to clot formation and coagulation system function. Reference intervals for these tests can be found after the Index at the end of the book.

Prothrombin Time
Prothrombin Time Principle

PT reagents, often called thromboplastin or tissue thromboplastin, consist of recombinant or affinity-purified *tissue factor* suspended in *phospholipids* mixed with a buffered 0.025 M solution of *calcium chloride*.[72] A few thromboplastins are organic extracts of emulsified rabbit brain or lung suspended in calcium chloride. When mixed with citrated PPP, the PT reagent triggers fibrin polymerization by adding calcium ions and activating plasma factor VII (Figure 41.7). Calcium and phospholipids participate in the formation of the tissue factor-factor VIIa complex, the factor VIIIa-factor IXa complex, and the factor Va-factor Xa complex. The clot is detectable by optical or electromechanical sensors (Chapter 42).

Although analysis of the coagulation pathway would seem to imply that the PT would be prolonged in deficiencies of fibrinogen, prothrombin, and factors V, VII, and X, the procedure is most sensitive to factor VII deficiencies, moderately sensitive to factors V and X deficiencies, sensitive to severe fibrinogen and prothrombin deficiencies, and insensitive to deficiencies of factors VIII, IX, and XIII.[73] The PT is prolonged in patients with multiple factor deficiency disorders that include combined deficiencies of factors VII and X.

The PT is used most often to monitor the effects of therapy with the oral anticoagulant warfarin (Chapter 40). The PT has been proposed as a monitor of antifactor Xa DOACs, but the sensitivity and specificity vary with DOAC and the reagent preparation.

Prothrombin Time Procedure

The tissue factor-phospholipid-calcium chloride reagent is warmed to 37° C. An aliquot of test PPP, 50 μL or 100 μL, is transferred to the reaction vessel, which also is maintained at 37° C. The PPP aliquot is incubated at 37° C for at least 3 minutes but no more than 10 minutes. Incubation longer than 10 minutes causes a false prolongation of the test as coagulation factors begin to deteriorate or are affected by evaporation and pH change. Following the prewarm step, a premeasured volume of reagent, 100 μL or 200 μL, respectively, is speedily and directly added to the PPP aliquot, and a timer is simultaneously started. When the clot forms, the timer stops, and the elapsed time is recorded in seconds of time to clot. Most laboratory practitioners perform PT tests using semiautomated or automated instruments that strictly control temperature, pipetting, and interval timing (Chapter 42).

All reagents must be reconstituted with the correct diluents and volumes following manufacturer instructions. Reagents must be stored and shipped according to manufacturer instructions and never used after the expiration date.

Prothrombin Time Quality Control

The medical laboratory practitioner tests commercially prepared normal and prolonged control PPP specimens at the beginning of each 8-hour shift or with each change of reagent. Controls may be shipped frozen or lyophilized and are tested alongside patient specimens using the same protocol as for patient PPP testing. Frozen controls must be rapidly thawed at 37° C and mixed well. Lyophilized control materials are reconstituted with the supplied buffer using caution to ensure that no material is expelled during reconstitution, mixed well, and allowed to stand for 20 to 30 minutes following manufacturer specifications. Once prepared, controls are placed in temperature-controlled wells.

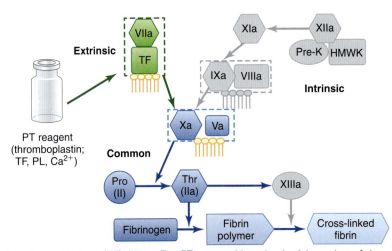

Figure 41.7 Prothrombin time (*PT*) Assay. The PT reagent (thromboplastin) consists of tissue factor (*TF*), phospholipid (*PL*), and ionized calcium (*Ca²⁺*). The reagent activates the extrinsic and common pathways of the coagulation mechanism, beginning with factor VII (*colored area in figure*). The PT is prolonged by deficiencies of factors VII, X, and V; prothrombin; and fibrinogen when fibrinogen is less than 100 mg/dL. The PT is prolonged in warfarin therapy because production of factor VII, factor X, and prothrombin is suppressed. *a*, Activated form of each factor; *HMWK*, high-molecular-weight kininogen; *Pre-K*, prekallikrein; *Pro*, prothrombin (II); *Thr*, thrombin.

The normal control result should be within the reference interval, and the prolonged control result should be within the therapeutic range for warfarin. If the control results fall within the stated limits provided in the laboratory protocol, the test results are considered valid. If the results fall outside the control limits, the reagents, controls, and equipment are checked; the problem is corrected; and the control and patient specimens are retested. The operator records all the actions taken. Control results are recorded and analyzed at regular intervals to maintain long-term validity of the PT.

Reporting Prothrombin Time Results and International Normalized Ratio

The medical laboratory practitioner reports PT results to the nearest tenth of a second, along with the PT reference interval. When the PT is used for warfarin monitoring, the INR, calculated from the PT result and detailed in Chapter 40, is employed to normalize results from laboratories around the world.[74] Laboratories typically report a combination of the PT and the INR as the PT/INR.

Prothrombin Time Reference Interval

The PT reference interval, computed from PT values of healthy individuals, varies from site to site, as it is dependent on the local population, type of thromboplastin used, type of instrument used, and pH and purity of the reagent diluent. Each center must establish its own interval for each new lot of reagents or at least once a year. This may be done by testing, over several days, a sample of at least 30 specimens from healthy donors of both sexes spanning the adult age range and computing the 95% confidence interval of the results. One example of a typical PT reference interval is 12.6 to 14.6 seconds, though the interval varies among facilities largely due to reagent differences.

The Prothrombin Time as a Diagnostic Assay

The PT is performed diagnostically when any coagulopathy is suspected. Acquired multiple deficiencies such as disseminated intravascular coagulation (DIC), liver disease, and vitamin K deficiency all affect factor VII activity and are detected through prolonged PT results. The PT is particularly sensitive to liver disease, in which factor VII levels rapidly diminish because the half-life of factor VII is only 6 hours (Chapter 36).

Vitamin K deficiency is seen in severe malnutrition, during use of broad-spectrum antibiotics that destroy gut flora, with parenteral nutrition, and in malabsorption syndromes. Vitamin K levels are low in newborns, in which bacterial colonization of the gut has not begun. Hemorrhage is likely in vitamin K deficiency, and the PT is the best indicator. To distinguish between vitamin K deficiency and liver disease, the laboratory practitioner determines factor V and factor VII levels. Both factor V and factor VII are reduced in liver disease, but only factor VII is reduced in vitamin K deficiency. Chapter 36 provides details regarding liver disease and vitamin K deficiency.

The PT is prolonged in congenital single-factor deficiencies of factors X, VII, or V, profound prothrombin deficiency, and fibrinogen deficiency when the fibrinogen level is 100 mg/dL or less. When the PT is prolonged, but the PTT and TT test results are normal, factor VII activity may be deficient. Any suspected single-factor deficiency is confirmed with a factor assay. The PT is not affected by factor VIII or IX deficiency because the concentration of tissue factor in the reagent is high, and those factors are bypassed in thrombin generation.

Minimal Effectiveness of Prothrombin Time as a Screening Tool

Preoperative PT screening of asymptomatic surgical patients to predict intraoperative hemorrhage is not supported by prevalence studies.[75] No clinical data support the use of the PT as a general screening test for individuals at low risk of bleeding, and the PT is not useful for establishing baseline values in warfarin therapy.[76] The diagnostic efficacy of the PT increases when used in the context of a bleeding indication.

Prothrombin Time Limitations

Specimen variations profoundly affect PT results (Table 41.6). The ratio of whole blood to anticoagulant is crucial so collection tubes must be filled to within tube manufacturers' specifications and not underfilled or overfilled. Anticoagulant volume must be adjusted when the hematocrit is greater than 55% to avoid false prolongation of the results. Specimens must be inverted at least three times immediately after collection to ensure good anticoagulation, but the mixing must be gentle. Practitioners must reject clotted and visibly hemolyzed specimens because they give unreliable results. Plasma lipemia or icterus may affect the results obtained with optical instrumentation.

Heparin may prolong the PT. If the patient is receiving therapeutic heparin, it should be noted on the order and commented on when the results are reported. The laboratory manager selects thromboplastin reagents that are maximally sensitive to

TABLE 41.6 Factors That Interfere With the Validity of Clot-Based Test Results	
Specimen Variation	**Solution**
Blood collection volume less than specified minimum	PT and PTT falsely prolonged; recollect specimen.
Hematocrit ≥55%	Adjust anticoagulant volume using formula or nomogram and recollect specimen using new anticoagulant volume.
Specimen clot	All results are affected unpredictably; recollect specimen.
Visible hemolysis	PT and PTT falsely shortened; recollect specimen.
Icterus or lipemia	Measure PT and PTT using a mechanical coagulometer.
UFH therapy	Use a reagent known to be insensitive to UFH or one that includes a UFH neutralizer such as polybrene.
Lupus anticoagulant	PT and PTT results invalid; use alternative methods, for instance, chromogenic assays.
Incorrect calibration, incorrect dilution of reagents	Correct analytical error and repeat assay.

PT, Prothrombin time; *PTT,* partial thromboplastin time; *UFH,* unfractionated heparin.

warfarin and relatively insensitive to heparin. Many reagent manufacturers incorporate polybrene (5-dimethyl-1,5-diazau-nde camethylene polymethobromide, or hexadimethrine bromide, Millipore Sigma) in their thromboplastin reagent to neutralize heparin. The medical laboratory practitioner may detect unexpected heparin by using the TT test.

LACs prolong some thromboplastins. LACs are members of the antiphospholipid antibody family (Chapter 39) and may partially neutralize PT reagent phospholipids. Warfarin is often prescribed to prevent thrombosis in patients with LACs, but the PT may be an unreliable monitor of warfarin therapy in such cases. Patients who have an LAC and are taking warfarin should be monitored using an alternative system such as a factor X assay, in particular, a chromogenic endpoint assay rather than a clot-based assay.[77–79] A recent study showed that the chromogenic factor X assay is useful for monitoring pediatric patients and patients with mitral valve defects who are on warfarin therapy.[80]

Chromogenic (color) endpoint assays are described in Chapter 42 (Figure 42.3). The chromogenic factor X assay is a two-stage assay (DiaPharma). In stage one, factor X is converted to factor Xa by the activator RVV in the presence of calcium. In stage two, activated factor X hydrolyzes the chromogenic substrate S-2765 (specific for factor Xa), which liberates the chromophore paranitroaniline (pNA). The color intensity from this reaction, read with a spectrophotometer at 405 nm, is directly proportional to the factor X activity in the patient sample.[81]

Partial Thromboplastin Time

Partial Thromboplastin Time Principle

The PTT (also called the activated partial thromboplastin time [APTT]) is employed to monitor the effects of UFH and to detect LAC and specific coagulation factor antibodies such as the antifactor VIII antibody.[82] The PTT is also prolonged in all congenital and acquired procoagulant deficiencies except for deficiencies of factors VII or XIII.[83]

The PTT reagent contains *phospholipid* (previously called partial thromboplastin or cephalin) and a *negatively charged particulate activator* such as silica, kaolin, ellagic acid, or celite in suspension. The phospholipid mixture, which was historically extracted from rabbit brain, is now produced synthetically. The activator provides a surface that mediates a conformational change in plasma factor XII that results in its activation (Figure 41.8). Factor XIIa forms a complex with two other plasma components: high-molecular-weight kininogen (Fitzgerald factor) and prekallikrein (Fletcher factor). These three plasma glycoproteins, termed *contact activation factors*, initiate in vitro clot formation through the intrinsic pathway but are not associated with bleeding when reduced. The complexed factor XIIa, a serine protease, activates factor XI (XIa), which activates factor IX (IXa) (Chapter 35).

Factor IXa forms a complex with factor VIIIa, reagent calcium, and reagent phospholipid. This complex catalyzes factor X. The resultant factor Xa forms a second complex with calcium, phospholipid, and factor Va, catalyzing the conversion of prothrombin to thrombin. Thrombin catalyzes the polymerization of fibrinogen and the formation of the fibrin clot, which is the endpoint of the PTT.

Most PTT reagents are designed so that the PTT is prolonged when the specimen has less than approximately 30% of factors VIII, IX, XI, or XII. Significant variability exists in factor sensitivities among different PTT reagents,[84] which must be carefully considered by laboratory managers when implementing a PTT reagent for clinical diagnostic purposes.

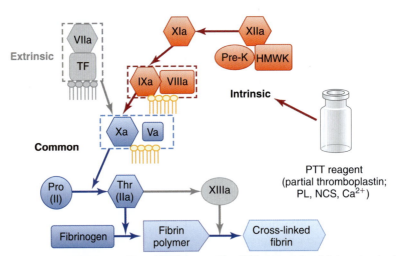

Figure 41.8 Partial Thromboplastin Time (*PTT*) Assay. The PTT reagent (partial thromboplastin) consists of phospholipid (*PL*), a negatively charged particulate activator (*NCS*), and ionized calcium (*Ca²⁺*). The reagent activates the intrinsic and common pathways of the coagulation mechanism through the contact factors XII, prekallikrein (*pre-K*), and high-molecular-weight kininogen (*HMWK*) (colored area in figure). The PTT is prolonged by deficiencies in pre-K; HMWK; factors XII, XI, IX, VIII, and X and prothrombin; and fibrinogen when less than 100 mg/dL. The PTT is prolonged in unfractionated heparin therapy because unfractionated heparin bound to antithrombin neutralizes thrombin (IIa), factor Xa, and other coagulation serine proteases. The PTT is prolonged in the presence of lupus anticoagulant because lupus anticoagulant neutralizes reagent phospholipids. *a*, Activated form of each factor; *Pro*, prothrombin (factor II); *TF*, tissue factor; *Thr*, thrombin.

Partial Thromboplastin Time Procedure

To initiate contact activation, 50 or 100 μL of warmed (37° C) reagent consisting of phospholipid and particulate activator is mixed with an equal volume of warmed PPP. The mixture is allowed to incubate for the exact manufacturer-specified time, usually 3 minutes. Next, 50 or 100 μL of warmed 0.025 M calcium chloride is forcibly added to the mixture, and a timer is started. When a fibrin clot forms, the timer stops, and the time to clot interval is recorded. Timing may be done with the same automated electromechanical or photooptical device as used for the PT. Results are reported to the nearest tenth of a second, along with the PTT reference interval.

Reagents and controls must be reconstituted with the correct diluents and volumes or thawed following manufacturer instructions. Reagents must be stored and shipped according to manufacturer instructions and never used after the expiration date. Specimen errors that affect the PT similarly affect the PTT (see Table 41.6).

Partial Thromboplastin Time Quality Control

The medical laboratory practitioner tests normal and prolonged control plasma specimens as done for the PT assay. Controls are run at the beginning of each 8-hour shift or with each new batch of reagent, but the laboratory director may require more frequent use of controls. Controls are tested using the protocol for patient plasma testing.

The normal control result should be within the reference interval, and the abnormal control result should be within the UFH therapeutic range (Chapter 40). If the control results fall within the stated limits in the laboratory protocol, the test results are considered valid. If the results fall outside the control limits, the reagents, control, and equipment are checked; the problem is corrected; and the control and patient specimens are retested. The operator records each control run and all the actions taken. Control results are recorded and analyzed at regular intervals to determine the long-term validity of results.

Partial Thromboplastin Time Reference Interval

The PTT reference interval varies from site to site as it is dependent on the local population, type of reagent, type of instrument, and pH and purity of the diluent. One medical center laboratory has established 25 to 35 seconds as its reference interval. This is typical, but each center must establish its own interval for each new lot of reagent or at least once a year. This may be done by testing a sample of 40 or more specimens from healthy donors of both sexes spanning the adult age range over several days and computing the 95% confidence interval of the results.

Monitoring Heparin Therapy With the Partial Thromboplastin Time

Since the early 1970s, the PTT has been the standard method for monitoring UFH, an anticoagulant used to treat patients with venous thrombosis, pulmonary embolism, myocardial infarction, and other thrombotic events.[85] The laboratory practitioner establishes a therapeutic range using the ex vivo Brill-Edwards curve and publishes it to all hospital units.[82] A typical therapeutic range is 60 to 100 seconds; however, the range varies widely and must be established locally.[86] The range must be reestablished with each change of PTT reagent, including each lot change and on instrument recalibration. Details on UFH monitoring and establishment of the PTT therapeutic range are provided in Chapter 40.

The Partial Thromboplastin Time as a Diagnostic Assay

The provider orders a PTT when a hemorrhagic disorder is suspected or when recurrent thrombosis or the presence of an autoimmune disorder points to the possibility of LAC.[87] The PTT result is prolonged when there is a deficiency of one or more of the following coagulation factors: prothrombin; factors V, VIII, IX, X, XI, or XII; or fibrinogen when the fibrinogen level is 100 mg/dL or less. The most common deficiencies that are reflected in an isolated prolonged PTT are deficiencies of factors VIII, IX, or XI—hemophilia A, hemophilia B, and Rosenthal syndrome, respectively (Chapter 36). Factor VII and factor XIII deficiencies have no effect on the PTT. Deficiencies of factor XII, prekallikrein, or high-molecular-weight kininogen prolong the PTT but are not associated with bleeding.

The PTT also is prolonged in the presence of a specific inhibitor, such as antifactor VIII or antifactor IX; a nonspecific inhibitor, such as LAC, an immunoglobulin with affinity for phospholipid-bound proteins; and interfering substances, such as fibrin degradation products (FDPs) or paraproteins, which are present in myeloma.

DIC prolongs PTT results because of consumption of multiple procoagulants, but a diagnosis of DIC must be confirmed using the D-dimer, platelet count, and erythrocyte morphology. Vitamin K deficiency results in diminished activities of procoagulant factors II (prothrombin), VII, IX, and X; the PTT eventually becomes prolonged when factor levels sufficiently decrease. Because factor VII deficiency does not affect the PTT and because it is the first coagulation factor whose activity becomes deficient, the PTT is less sensitive to vitamin K deficiency or warfarin therapy than the PT.

Partial Thromboplastin Time Mixing Studies
Lupus Anticoagulants

LACs are IgG immunoglobulins directed against a number of phospholipid-protein complexes.[88] Because they have a variety of target antigens, LACs are called nonspecific inhibitors. LACs prolong the phospholipid-dependent PTT reaction.

Most laboratories employ a moderate-phospholipid or high-phospholipid PTT reagent in their routine PTT assay, which is designed to monitor UFH therapy and detect coagulopathies. Laboratories use a second low-phospholipid PTT reagent such as PTT-LA (Diagnostica Stago), which is more sensitive to LAC, for LAC detection (Chapter 39).

Every acute care laboratory provides a means for the initial detection of LACs, as their presence signals a potential thrombotic risk.[89] Laboratory directors employ repeated LAC assays separated by a minimum 12-week interval to distinguish chronic from acute LACs as thrombotic risk is customarily associated with chronic LAC presence, although there is evidence that implicates transient LACs with thrombosis as well.

Together, chronic and transient LACs are found in 1% to 2% of randomly selected individuals.

Specific Factor Inhibitors

Specific factor inhibitors are IgG immunoglobulins directed against coagulation factors. Specific inhibitors arise in severe congenital factor deficiencies in response to factor concentrate treatment. Antifactor VIII, the most common of the specific inhibitors, is detected in 10% to 20% of patients with severe hemophilia A, and antifactor IX is detected in 1% to 3% of patients with factor IX deficiency. Autoantibodies to factor VIII occasionally arise in individuals without hemophilia, usually in young women, where they are associated with a postpartum bleeding syndrome, or in patients older than 60 with autoimmune disorders. The presence of these types of antibodies is called *acquired hemophilia* (Chapter 36). Alloantibodies and autoantibodies to factor VIII are associated with severe anatomic hemorrhage.

Detection of Lupus Anticoagulants, Other Inhibitors, and Factor Deficiencies

LAC testing is part of every thrombophilia profile and may be ordered when a provider confirms a primary thrombotic patient event (Chapter 39). An unexpectedly prolonged initial PTT may also trigger an LAC investigation. *PTT mixing studies* are necessary for the presumptive detection of LACs.[90] Mixing studies also distinguish LACs from specific inhibitors and factor deficiencies and should be available from all coagulation laboratories.[91]

When the PTT is prolonged beyond the upper limit of the reference interval, the laboratory practitioner first tests for UFH or a direct thrombin inhibitor such as dabigatran using the TT. A TT result that exceeds the upper limit of the TT reference interval is evidence for UFH or dabigatran therapy. UFH often prolongs the TT to 30 to 40 seconds. UFH may be neutralized in vitro using polybrene or heparinase (Hepzyme, Siemens); the treated sample may then be used for PTT mixing studies. Dabigatran may likewise be neutralized in vitro with a DOAC remover such as DOAC-Stop (a reagent for research use only; DiaPharma).

The anticoagulant-free or anticoagulant-neutralized patient plasma is then mixed 1:1 with reagent *platelet-poor normal plasma* (PNP) (Figure 39.1). Several manufacturers prepare and distribute PNP (for example, frozen CRYO*check* Normal Reference Plasma, Precision BioLogic). A repeat PTT is performed immediately on the 1:1 patient plasma-PNP mixture. If the mixture PTT corrects to within 10% of the PNP PTT (or to within the reference interval) and the patient is experiencing bleeding, the operator presumes there is a coagulation factor deficiency (coagulopathy).[92]

If the PTT of the initial or incubated mixture fails to correct and the patient is not bleeding, the laboratory practitioner suspects LAC and automatically orders an LAC profile as described in Chapter 39. LAC profiles are available from tertiary care facilities and specialty reference laboratories.

About 15% of LACs appear to be temperature dependent, and 85% of antifactor VIII inhibitors are temperature-dependent

IgG4 class antibodies, so an *incubated mix* becomes necessary. To avoid missing an elusive LAC diagnosis, if the immediate mix PTT corrects, a new 1:1 mixture is prepared and incubated 2 hours at 37° C. If the incubated mixture PTT fails to correct to within 10% of the incubated PNP PTT, an inhibitor may be present. The inhibitor could be an LAC, but if the patient is bleeding, a specific inhibitor such as antifactor VIII is suspected and a factor VIII activity assay is performed. Although antifactor IX and other inhibitors have been documented, antifactor VIII is the most common. The Nijmegen-Bethesda assay (NBA), discussed later in "Nijmegen-Bethesda Assay for Anti-Factor VIII Inhibitor," is used to confirm the presence of specific anticoagulation factor antibodies.

Thrombin Time

Thrombin Time Reagent and Principle

As described in Chapter 35, thrombin cleaves fibrinopeptides A and B from plasma fibrinogen to form a detectable fibrin polymer. This principle is followed in the TT, where commercially prepared bovine thrombin reagent at 5 National Institutes of Health (NIH) units/mL is used to initiate the reaction in patient plasma (Figure 41.9).[93]

Thrombin Time Procedure

Reagent thrombin is warmed to 37° C for a minimum of 3 minutes and a maximum of 10 minutes. Thrombin deteriorates during incubation and must be used within 10 minutes of the time incubation is begun. An aliquot of patient plasma, usually 100 μL, is also incubated at 37° C for a minimum of 3 minutes and a maximum of 10 minutes. The operator pipettes 200 μL of thrombin into the PPP aliquot, starts a timer, and records the interval to clot formation. Automated TT assays are available on

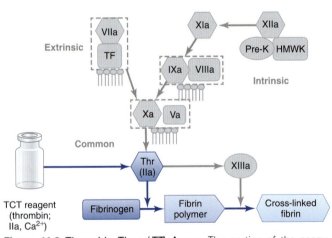

Figure 41.9 Thrombin Time (*TT*) Assay. The portion of the coagulation pathway evaluated in the TT is the same as the pathway evaluated in the reptilase time assay. The reagent activates the coagulation pathway at the level of thrombin and tests for the polymerization of fibrinogen (*colored area in figure*). The TT is prolonged by unfractionated heparin; direct thrombin inhibitors; fibrin degradation products; and dysfibrinogenemia, hypofibrinogenemia, and afibrinogenemia. The reptilase time is unaffected by heparin. *a,* Activated form of each factor; *HMWK,* high-molecular-weight kininogen; *Pre-K,* prekallikrein; *TF,* tissue factor; *Thr,* thrombin.

all coagulometers. Specimen errors that affect the PT and PTT likewise affect the TT (see Table 41.6).

Thrombin Time Quality Control

The medical laboratory practitioner tests a normal control sample and an abnormal control sample with each batch of TT assays and records the results. The normal control results should fall within the laboratory's reference interval. The abnormal control results should be prolonged to the range reached by the TT in moderate hypofibrinogenemia. If the results fall outside the laboratory's control limits, the reagents, control, and equipment are checked; the problem is corrected; and the control is retested. The actions taken to correct out-of-limit tests are recorded. Control results are analyzed at regular intervals (weekly is typical) to determine the longitudinal validity of the procedure.

Reporting of Thrombin Clotting Time Results and Clinical Utility

Although the TT reference interval is established locally, a typical TT reference interval is 15 to 20 seconds. The TT is prolonged when the fibrinogen level is less than 100 mg/dL (*hypofibrinogenemia*) or in the presence of antithrombotic materials such as FDPs, paraproteins, the DOAC dabigatran, or UFH. *Afibrinogenemia* (absence of fibrinogen) and *dysfibrinogenemia* (presence of fibrinogen that is biochemically abnormal and nonfunctional) also prolong the TT.

Before a prolonged TT may be considered as evidence of diminished or abnormal fibrinogen, the presence of antithrombotic substances, such as UFH, FDPs, or paraproteins, must be ruled out. The TT is part of the PTT mixing study protocol (Figure 39.1) and is used to determine whether dabigatran or UFH is present whenever the PTT is prolonged. The TT is not prolonged by factor XIII deficiency.

The TT provides binary (qualitative) evidence for dabigatran; if drug is present, the TT is markedly prolonged. A normal TT rules out dabigatran. A TT modification, the plasma-diluted TT, provides a quantitative measure of dabigatran when used with calibrators of specific drug concentrations.[94]

Venom Activated Assays

Reptilase Time

Reptilase is a thrombinlike enzyme, batroxobin, isolated from the snake venom of *Bothrops atrox* that catalyzes the conversion of fibrinogen to fibrin (Pefakit Reptilase Time; Pentapharm). In contrast to thrombin, this enzyme cleaves only fibrinopeptide A from the ends of the fibrinogen molecule, whereas thrombin cleaves both fibrinopeptides A and B.[95]

The specimen requirements, procedure, and quality assurance protocol are the same as those for the TT. The reagent is reconstituted with distilled water and is stable for 1 month when stored at 1° to 6° C. Reptilase time reagent may be fatal if it enters the bloodstream.

The reptilase time assay is insensitive to factor XIII deficiency and is unaffected by antithrombotic substances but is markedly prolonged in dysfibrinogenemia, so it is occasionally employed to rule out an antithrombotic in a patient who has a prolonged PTT. This renders the reptilase time test useful for detecting hypofibrinogenemia or dysfibrinogenemia in patients receiving antithrombotic therapy, and it may be used for workup in a bleeding patient in whom factors VIII, IX, and XI are normal. The reptilase time is prolonged in the presence of FDPs and paraproteins.

Russell Viper Venom Test

RVV from the *Daboia russelii* viper, which triggers coagulation at the level of factor X, was once used as an alternative to the PT. The assay was named the Stypven time, but is now obsolete. However, buffer-diluted RVV is prolonged by the LAC and the dilute RVV time is routinely employed to detect LAC, as described in Chapter 39.

COAGULATION FACTOR ASSAYS

Coagulation assays, described in "Clot-Based Screening Tests for Coagulation Disorders," are performed using traditional clotting endpoint assays that detect the functional capacity of the coagulation system. The specific coagulation factor assays discussed in this section are also measured using clot-based laboratory assays. However, modern improvements in coagulation laboratory techniques include the development of nonclot-based assays (Chapter 42). These assays use a chromogenic or color endpoint and are more specific than clot-based assays because there is less assay interference. In some cases, they eliminate an indirect measurement of the analyte by cumbersome techniques.

Chromogenic substrates are derived from basic enzymology. As the understanding of the molecular structures of the hemostatic serine proteases, their substrates, activators, and inhibitors became clearer, it was possible to synthesize oligopeptides that mimic the cleavage site of the natural substrate. Chromogenic substrates were initially developed in the 1970s, and development of chromogenic substrate assays for hemostasis began in the 1980s. These assays will be discussed in this section and in the "Fibrinolysis Assays" section where relevant.

Fibrinogen Assay

The clot-based method of Clauss, a modification of the TT, is the recommended procedure for estimating fibrinogen function.[96] The modifications that allow for quantitation of fibrinogen are dilution of the patient PPP and incorporation of a fibrinogen calibration curve.[97] There is an inverse relationship between the interval to clot formation and the concentration of functional fibrinogen. When the thrombin reagent is concentrated and the PPP is diluted, the relationship is linear, provided that the fibrinogen concentration is 100 to 480 mg/dL.

An attractive alternative to the Clauss method is the automated PT-derived fibrinogen assay. Some optical coagulometers (ACL TOP, Werfen) estimate fibrinogen by assessing reaction mixture turbidity while performing the PT assay.[98] This offers the convenience of a fibrinogen result with each PT.

Fibrinogen Assay Procedure

Clauss fibrinogen assay thrombin reagent. Laboratory managers choose commercially manufactured lyophilized bovine thrombin reagent such as HemosIL QFA, 100 NIH units/mL (Werfen).[99] The reagent is reconstituted according to manufacturer instructions and placed on the coagulometer.

Clauss fibrinogen assay calibration curve. The laboratory practitioner programs the coagulometer to generate a calibration curve at 6-month or shorter intervals, with each change of reagent lot number, with shift in control results, and following instrument maintenance. The instrument prepares 1:5, 1:10, 1:15, 1:20, and 1:40 dilutions using reconstituted fibrinogen calibration plasma (Helena Laboratories). An aliquot of each dilution, for instance 200 μL, is transferred to reaction cuvettes, warmed to 37° C, and tested by adding 100 μL of thrombin reagent. Time from addition of thrombin to clot formation is recorded, and the values in seconds are graphed against computed fibrinogen concentration (Figure 41.10). Because patient PPPs are diluted 1:10 before testing, the 1:10 calibration plasma dilution is assigned the same fibrinogen value as the undiluted reconstituted calibration plasma.

Clauss fibrinogen assay test protocol. The coagulometer prepares a 1:10 dilution of each patient and control PPP with Owren buffer. An aliquot of each of the diluted samples is warmed to 37° C in a cuvette for 3 minutes. After incubation, thrombin reagent is added; the timer starts and then stops when a clot forms. The interval in seconds is compared with the calibration curve, and results are reported in mg/dL.

If the clotting time of the patient PPP dilution is short, indicating a fibrinogen level greater than 480 mg/dL, the instrument prepares and assays a 1:20 Owren buffer dilution of the PPP, then multiplies the result by the dilution factor of 2. If the clotting time is prolonged, indicating less than 200 mg/dL of fibrinogen, the instrument employs a low concentration curve. Specimen errors that affect the PTT likewise affect the fibrinogen assay (see Table 41.6).

Fibrinogen Assay Quality Control

Normal and abnormal control samples are assayed with each batch of patient samples. The normal control results should fall within the laboratory's reference interval, and the abnormal control results should be near or less than 100 mg/dL. If either control result falls outside the control limits, the reagents, control, and equipment are checked; the problem is corrected; and the control is retested. The actions taken to correct out-of-limit tests are recorded.

Fibrinogen Assay Results and Clinical Utility

One institution's reference interval for fibrinogen concentration is 220 to 498 mg/dL, although each local institution prepares its own interval. *Hypofibrinogenemia*, a fibrinogen level of less than 220 mg/dL, may be congenital or may indicate DIC or severe liver disease. Conversely, early or moderate liver disease, pregnancy, and chronic inflammation may be accompanied by an increase in the fibrinogen level to greater than 498 mg/dL. *Congenital afibrinogenemia* is reflected in prolonged clotting times and is associated with variable anatomic hemorrhage. *Dysfibrinogenemia* may resemble hypofibrinogenemia by the Clauss method as abnormal fibrinogen species are hydrolyzed more slowly by thrombin than normal fibrinogen. Conversely, the PT-derived fibrinogen assay, though able to estimate hypofibrinogenemia and afibrinogenemia, usually returns normal results for afibrinogenemia.[100]

Fibrinogen Assay Limitations

Diluting the PPP minimizes the antithrombotic effects of dabigatran, UFH, FDPs, and paraproteins. UFH levels less than 0.6 units/mL and FDP levels less than 100 μg/dL do not affect the results of the assay provided that the fibrinogen concentration is 150 mg/dL or greater. Dabigatran and UFH levels greater than 0.6 units/mL and FDP levels greater than 100 μg/mL prolong the clotting time and give falsely lowered fibrinogen results.

The operator ensures that the thrombin reagent is pure and has not degenerated. Exposure to sunlight or oxidation results in rapid thrombin breakdown.

Single-Factor Assays Using Partial Thromboplastin Time

Principle of Single-Factor Assays Based on Partial Thromboplastin Time

If the PTT is prolonged and the PT is normal, and a normal TT indicates there is no antithrombotic therapy, a mixing study is the next step. If there is correction after the immediate and incubated mix, the operator suspects a congenital single-factor deficiency (Table 41.7).[101] Three factor deficiencies that give this reaction pattern and accompany anatomic hemorrhage are factor VIII deficiency (hemophilia A), factor IX deficiency (hemophilia B), and factor XI deficiency (Rosenthal syndrome) (Chapter 36).[102] These deficiencies are most often diagnosed in childhood using PTT-based single-factor assays. Factor assays are commonly performed on specimens from patients with previously identified single-factor deficiencies to regularly monitor prophylactic therapy or to document the efficacy of on-demand therapy during bleeds or invasive procedures.

Because hemophilia A is the most common single-factor deficiency disorder, the following discussion is confined to the factor VIII assay but may be generalized to factor IX or XI assays. The medical laboratory practitioner uses the PTT to determine

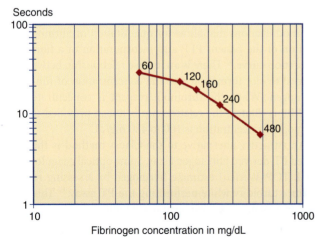

Figure 41.10 Fibrinogen Assay Calibration. This graph illustrates a calibration curve of fibrinogen concentration plotted against the clot times obtained from the fibrinogen assay, using log-log axes.

TABLE 41.7	Factor Assays Using Thrombin Time, Prothrombin Time, and Partial Thromboplastin Time Test Systems
Factor	**System**
Fibrinogen (I)	Clauss method; modified TT
Prothrombin (II)	Prothrombin time
Factor V	Prothrombin time
Factor VII	Prothrombin time
Factor VIII	Partial thromboplastin time
Factor IX	Partial thromboplastin time
Factor X	Prothrombin time
Factor XI	Partial thromboplastin time
Factor XIII	Chromogenic assay

TT, thrombin time.

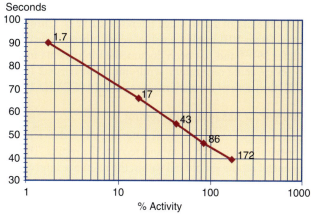

Figure 41.11 Factor VIII Assay Calibration. This graph illustrates a calibration curve of factor VIII concentration plotted against the clot times obtained from the factor VIII assay, using linear-log axes.

the activity of functional factor VIII by incorporating a commercially prepared factor VIII-*depleted* PPP in the test system (CRYO*check* Factor VIII Deficient Plasma, Precision BioLogic). Distributors collect plasma from normal donors and employ immunodepletion, relying on an anti-factor VIII antibody bound to a separatory column, to prepare factor VIII-depleted plasma.[103] Because immunodepletion may reduce VWF activity, some laboratory managers prefer factor-depleted plasma with added purified VWF (CRYO*check* Factor VIII Deficient Plasma with VWF, Precision BioLogic). *Factor-deficient plasmas* collected from donors with a known hemophilia condition (Congenital Factor VIII Deficient Plasma, George King Bio-Medical) can also be used for the factor assay.

In the PTT-based factor assay system, factor VIII-depleted PPP provides normal activity of all procoagulants except factor VIII. Tested alone, factor VIII-depleted PPP has a prolonged PTT but when normal PPP is added, the PTT reverts to normal. In contrast, a prolonged result for a mixture of patient PPP and factor VIII-depleted PPP implies that the patient PPP is factor VIII deficient. The clotting time interval for the mixture of patient PPP and factor VIII-depleted PPP is compared with a calibrated reference curve to estimate the level of factor VIII activity in the patient PPP. Alternatively, the chromogenic factor VIII assay, discussed in the next section, may be employed in place of the clot-based PTT factor assay.[104]

Factor VIII Assay Reference Curve

To prepare a reference curve for the factor VIII assay, the laboratory practitioner obtains reference plasma such as Precision BioLogic CRYO*check* Normal Reference Plasma and programs the coagulometer to prepare a series of dilutions with buffered saline.[105] Although laboratory protocols vary, most laboratory practitioners prepare a series of five dilutions, from 1:5 to 1:500. Most clinical laboratories use the preprogrammed software that is included with the coagulometer to generate a linear-log graph, where each dilution is mixed with reagent factor VIII-depleted plasma and tested using the PTT reagent system (Figure 41.11). The 1:10 dilution is assigned the factor VIII assay activity value found on the package insert. When patient PPP is tested, the time interval obtained is automatically entered on the vertical coordinate and converted to a percentage of factor VIII (factor

levels may also be given in units/dL where the numerical value is the same).

Factor VIII Assay Procedure

The coagulometer is programmed to prepare 1:10, 1:20, 1:40, and 1:80 or similar dilutions of each patient PPP and control specimen and then mixes each dilution with equal volumes of factor VIII-depleted plasma and PTT reagent. In most cases, 100 μL of PTT reagent is mixed with 100 μL each of patient PPP dilution and factor VIII-depleted plasma mixture. After incubation at 37° C for the manufacturer-specified time, typically 3 minutes, 100 μL of 0.025 M calcium chloride is dispensed and a timer starts. The interval in seconds for each dilution is entered into the curve and the factor VIII level is reported for each. Factor activity results for the 1:20, 1:40, and 1:80 dilutions are multiplied by 2, 4, and 8, respectively, to compensate for the dilutions. The results should match the results of the 1:10 dilution within 10%. If the results of the higher dilutions do not match the 1:10 dilution within 10%, they are considered *nonparallel.* In this situation, a factor VIII inhibitor or LAC may be present, and the assay cannot provide a reliable estimate of factor VIII activity.

Tests for factors IX and XI are performed using the same approach except that the appropriate factor-depleted plasma is substituted for factor VIII-depleted plasma. Tests for the contact factors XII, prekallikrein, and high-molecular-weight kininogen are seldom requested because deficiencies are not associated with bleeding disorders. Acquired and congenital contact factor deficiencies are relatively common, however, and cause PTT prolongation. Factor XII, prekallikrein, and high-molecular-weight kininogen assays are available from hemostasis reference laboratories, and they may be necessary to account for an unexplained prolonged PTT.

Expected Results and Clinical Utility of Single-Factor Assays

One facility's reference interval for factor VIII activity is 50 to 186 units/dL (%). Spontaneous hemophilia A and B bleeds occur at activity levels of 5 units/dL or less; however, the clot-based factor assay offers poor accuracy at less than 5 units/dL.[106]

Evaluation of patients with factor VIII levels below 5 units/dL requires the use of a low-range reference curve.[107] Chronically elevated factor VIII implies a risk of venous thrombotic disease (Chapter 39)[108] and has been documented in patients infected with severe acute respiratory syndrome coronavirus 2 (SARS-CoV2), the cause of coronavirus disease 2019 (COVID-19).[109]

Single-Factor Assay Quality Control

The laboratory practitioner tests a normal and a deficient control specimen with each assay and records the results. The normal control results should fall within the reference interval. The deficient control results should be in the range of 10 units/dL factor VIII activity or below. If either control result falls outside the control limits, the reagents, control, and equipment are checked; the problem is corrected; and the control is retested. The practitioner records all actions taken to correct out-of-limit tests. Control results are analyzed at regular intervals (weekly is typical) to determine the longitudinal validity of the procedure.

Limitations of Clot-Based Single-Factor Assays

Interlaboratory coefficients of variation for factor VIII assay proficiency testing surveys reach 80%, implying undesirable imprecision in the interpretation of therapeutic monitoring results from separate institutions. To reduce inherent variation, the medical laboratory practitioner uses commercial calibrated plasma to prepare the reference curve and selects reference dilutions that correspond to only the linear portion of the curve. In many facilities the curve is included in each test run, despite the expense.[105,110] The laboratory must assay three or more dilutions of patient PPP to check for inhibitors. The practitioner also selects a matching reagent-instrument system with a demonstrated internal day-to-day coefficient of variation of less than 5%. As with the PT, PTT, and TT, good specimen management is essential. Clotted, hemolyzed, icteric, or lipemic specimens are rejected because they give unreliable results. Reagents must be reconstituted with the correct diluents and volumes following manufacturer instructions. Reagents must be stored and shipped in accordance with manufacturer instructions and never used after the expiration date.

Clot-based assays do not accurately measure B-domain-deleted recombinant factor VIII (rFVIII) or the extended half-life rFVIII formulations, therapies that have been available since 2014.[111] Two-stage chromogenic substrate factor VIII and IX assay methods that employ noninterfering bovine substrates give an accurate measurement of these formulations, providing a superior limit of detection and coefficient of variation characteristics (Chapter 36).[112]

Factor Assays Using Chromogenic Substrate Technique

Chromogenic Factor VIII Assay

The chromogenic factor VIII assay (CRYO*check* Chromogenic Factor VIII, Precision Biologic) is less prone to interferences from therapeutics such as emicizumab (Chapter 36) and can be used on automated coagulometers.[113]

In the first stage of the assay, patient PPP is added to a reaction mixture that comprises calcium, phospholipids, purified human thrombin, and factor IXa, which is added to bovine factor X. The reaction mixture activates factor VIII (in the patient plasma), then the complex of factors VIIIa and IXa activates factor X. The amount of factor Xa is proportional to the amount of functional factor VIII present in the patient sample. In the second stage of the assay, the generated factor Xa is measured through cleavage of a factor Xa-specific chromogenic substrate. The substrate produces a yellow color, the intensity of which is directly proportional to the amount of factor VIII in the patient plasma. Color is measured spectrophotometrically by absorbance at 405 nm. Factor VIII levels are determined using a standard curve.[114]

Chromogenic Factor IX Assay

The chromogenic factor IX assay was developed following the same principle as the chromogenic factor VIII assay. This assay promises a more accurate factor IX measurement than the one-stage factor IX clot-based assay and has the advantage of quantitating the extended half-life factor IX concentrate therapies.[115]

The chromogenic factor IX assay (CRYO*check* Chromogenic Factor IX, Precision Biologic) may be applied to automated coagulometers. In the first stage of the assay, factor IX in the patient PPP is activated by factor XIa; activated factor IXa then activates factor X in the presence of factor VIIIa, calcium, and phospholipids. The second stage of the assay measures factor Xa using the same procedure as described above for the chromogenic factor VIII assay, where the intensity of color from the chromogenic substrate is directly proportional to factor IX activity.[116]

Nijmegen-Bethesda Assay for Antifactor VIII Inhibitor

The NBA confirms and quantifies antifactor VIII inhibitors, which are typically IgG4 class immunoglobulins.[117] Using the *traditional Bethesda titer,* before the Nijmegen upgrade, 200 μL of patient PPP is incubated with 200 μL of PNP for 2 hours at 37° C. A so-called control consisting of 200 μL of imidazole buffer at pH 7.4 mixed with 200 μL of PNP is incubated simultaneously. During incubation, antifactor VIII inhibitor from the patient PPP neutralizes a percentage of the PNP factor VIII activity (starting value of factor VIII activity is 100 units/dL). The percentage of factor VIII activity neutralized is proportional to the level of inhibitor activity. After incubation, residual factor VIII activity in the patient PPP-PNP mixture is measured using the factor VIII activity assay as described in the section on factor assays using the PTT.

The traditional Bethesda titer is expressed as a percentage of the control. If the patient PPP-PNP mixture retains 75% or more of the residual factor VIII activity of the control, presumably 75 units/dL or more, no factor VIII inhibitor is present. If the residual factor VIII level is 25% or less that of the control, 25 units/dL or less, the patient PPP factor VIII inhibitor level is titered using several dilutions of the patient specimen in PNP. The new dilutions are tested in the Bethesda assay to determine the level of antibody, where *1 Bethesda unit* (BU) of activity is the amount of antibody that leaves 50% residual factor VIII activity in the mixture.

A median 40% of patients with severe hemophilia are tested for inhibitors at US hemophilia centers using the Bethesda titer. The traditional method is characterized by a 32% false-positive rate, a 5% false-negative rate, and an interlaboratory coefficient of variation that exceeds 50%.[118] An important contributing factor to this imprecision is that patients are not cleared of therapeutic factor concentrate before the specimen is collected, a practice that would produce an optimal laboratory specimen but expose the patient to bleeding risk. Not only is the Bethesda titer affected by residual therapeutic plasma coagulation factor, but it is also affected by the coexistence of LAC, differences in inhibitor epitope specificity, and neutralizing versus non-neutralizing inhibitor kinetics.[119]

Refinements to the Bethesda titer were offered in 1995, whereupon the procedure was renamed the *Nijmegen-Bethesda assay*.[120] In 2012 the US Centers for Disease Control and Prevention expanded on these modifications to reduce NBA variability and improve specificity.[121] The 1995 and 2012 refinements combined are as follows:

- Include an inhibitor positive control in all NBA runs.
- Heat patient plasma at 56° C for 30 minutes and centrifuge to eliminate residual factor VIII.
- Serially dilute heated patient plasma in factor VIII-depleted plasma, not imidazole buffer, or alternatively, dilute in bovine serum albumin (BSA).
- Serially dilute unheated commercial 100 Nijmegen-Bethesda unit (NBU)/dL-positive PNP in factor VIII-deficient plasma or BSA.
- Incubate at 37° C for 2 hours, then perform the PTT-based factor VIII assay.
- Convert residual factor VIII activity to NBU/mL.

Only a few laboratories have made this full conversion. At the present time, 70% of US laboratories use a hybrid NBA that uses imidazole buffered saline diluent at pH 7.4, not the recommended factor VIII-deficient plasma, to reduce expense. For these laboratory managers, BSA may become an acceptable alternative.

Promising additional approaches are the fluorogenic and chromogenic NBA. Instead of employing the PTT, the operator adds a factor Xa fluorogenic or chromogenic substrate with a thrombin inhibitor and stopping buffer to measure factor Xa production as a surrogate to factor VIII activity. One fluorogenic or chromogenic Bethesda unit (CBU) equals the level of inhibitor per milliliter of patient PPP that inactivates 50% of factor VIII in 1 mL of PNP.[122]

Single-Factor Assays Using the Prothrombin Time

If the PTT and the PT are both prolonged, the TT is normal, and there is no ready explanation for the prolonged test results, such as liver disease, vitamin K deficiency, DIC, or warfarin therapy, the medical laboratory practitioner may suspect a congenital single-factor deficiency of the common pathway (Chapter 35). Three relatively rare factor deficiencies that give this reaction pattern and cause hemorrhage are prothrombin (factor II) deficiency, factor V deficiency, and factor X deficiency. If the PT is prolonged and all other test results are normal, factor VII deficiency is suspected (see Table 41.7). The next step is the

performance of a one-stage single-factor assay based on the PT. The principles and procedure described in "Single-Factor Assays Using Partial Thromboplastin Time" may be applied, except that the PT reagent replaces the PTT reagent in the test system and the PT protocol is followed. Factor II-depleted, factor V-depleted, factor VII-depleted, and factor X-depleted plasmas are available from in vitro diagnostics distributors.

Factor XIII Assay

Coagulation factor XIII is a transglutaminase that catalyzes covalent cross-linking bonds between the α and γ chains of fibrin polymer (Chapter 35).[123] Cross-linking strengthens the fibrin clot and renders it resistant to proteases. This is the final event in coagulation, and is essential for normal hemostasis and normal wound healing (Chapter 36),[124,125] but neither the PT nor the PTT is prolonged by factor XIII deficiency.

When a patient presents for treatment of bleeding and poor wound healing and the PTT, PT, platelet count, and fibrinogen level are normal, the laboratory practitioner may recommend a chromogenic factor XIII assay such as the Technochrom Factor XIII (DiaPharma) or the Berichrom Factor XIII (Siemens). Both of these assays are for research use only. In a representative assay, quantitation of factor XIII activity is based on the measurement of ammonia released during an in vitro transglutaminase reaction.[126] Plasma factor XIII is first activated by reagent thrombin. The resultant factor XIIIa then cross-links the fibrin amine substrate glycine ethyl ester to the glutamine residue of a peptide substrate, releasing ammonia. The concentration of ammonia is monitored in a glutamate dehydrogenase-catalyzed reaction that depends on NADPH, the reduced form of nicotinamide adenine dinucleotide phosphate. NADPH consumption is measured by the decrease of absorbance at 340 nm. The absorbance is inversely proportional to factor XIII activity. Several manufacturers also market immunoassays for factor XIII, which provide factor XIII concentration values but do not identify functional factor XIII abnormalities.

FIBRINOLYSIS ASSAYS

D-Dimer and Fibrin Degradation Products

During coagulation, fibrin polymers become cross-linked by factor XIIIa and simultaneously bind plasma plasminogen and tissue plasminogen activator (TPA) (Chapter 35). Over several hours, bound TPA activates nearby plasminogen to form plasmin. The bound plasmin cleaves fibrinogen and fibrin, yielding FDPs D, E, X, and Y and D-dimer (Figure 35.18). The FDPs are fragments of the original *fibrinogen* domains, and D-dimers are a subset of covalently linked D domains reflecting the cross-linking effects of factor XIIIa in the production of *fibrin*.[127]

FDP assays, including D-dimer, are convenient for detecting active fibrinolysis, which indirectly implies thrombosis. Normally, FDPs, including D-dimer, circulate at concentrations of less than 2 ng/mL. Fibrinolysis generates FDPs and D-dimer at concentrations greater than 200 ng/mL. Increased FDP and D-dimer concentrations are characteristic of *thrombotic* episodes associated with acute and chronic DIC, systemic fibrinolysis, deep vein thrombosis, pulmonary embolism, and stroke.[128–130] Elevated levels of FDPs, including D-dimer, however, are also detected in plasma after thrombolytic therapy, with severe infection, and with inflammatory disorders.[129–131]

Principle of Quantitative D-Dimer Assay

Plasma D-dimer immunoassays abound, and several diagnostics distributors offer automated quantitative immunoassays for plasma D-dimers that generate results within 30 minutes.[132] Microlatex particles in buffered saline are coated with monoclonal anti-D-dimer antibodies. The coated particles are agglutinated by patient plasma D-dimer; the resultant turbidity is measured using turbidometric or nephelometric technology (Chapter 42). Sensitivity varies, depending on the avidity of the monoclonal anti-D-dimer antibody and the detection method; however, most methods detect concentrations as low as 10 ng/mL. D-dimer results may be reported in D-dimer units (DDUs) or fibrinogen equivalent units (FEUs) depending on the monoclonal antibody target. D-dimer results and interpretation are discussed in Chapter 39.

Principle of Fibrin Degradation Product Assay

Although the FDP assay has largely been replaced by the automated quantitative D-dimer assay, FDPs may be detected using a qualitative immunoassay that identifies FDPs in serum and urine.[133] The FDP assay detects FDPs from plasmin degradation of both fibrinogen and fibrin.

One method, the Thrombo-Wellcotest (Thermo Fisher Scientific), is a manual slide agglutination method in which the practitioner mixes one drop of sample with one drop of latex suspension.[134] The polystyrene latex particles in buffered saline are coated with polyclonal antibodies specific for D and E fragments calibrated to detect FDPs at a concentration of 2 µg/mL or greater. Positive results have the appearance of visible agglutination. The assay usually is performed on urine or serum collected in special tubes that promote clotting and prevent in vitro fibrinolysis. Owing to inadequate sensitivity at low concentrations, qualitative FDP assays are confined to diagnosis and monitoring of DIC.

Plasminogen

Plasminogen, the inactive precursor of the trypsinlike proteolytic enzyme plasmin, is produced in the liver and circulates as a single-chain glycoprotein (Chapter 35). When bound to fibrin, plasminogen is converted to plasmin by the action of nearby TPA. Bound plasmin degrades fibrin, whereas a circulating inhibitor, α_2-antiplasmin, rapidly inactivates free plasmin. Plasmin is the central enzyme of the fibrinolytic pathway.

Excessive fibrinolysis, which occurs in trauma, acute inflammation, and pregnancy, is reflected in a radical increase in circulating plasmin that may be associated with hemorrhage.[135] Bone trauma, fractures, and surgical dissection of bone as in cardiac surgery, also increase fibrinolysis. *Hyperfibrinolysis* may be documented using viscoelastometry, discussed in the "Viscoelastometry and Global Coagulation Assays" section.

Conversely, *hypofibrinolysis* occurs when TPA or plasminogen levels become depleted or when excess secretion of plasminogen activator inhibitor-1 (PAI-1) suppresses TPA activity. These conditions are associated with *thrombosis*. Congenital plasminogen deficiencies associated with thrombosis in some families have been identified.[136] Acquired plasminogen deficiencies are seen in DIC, acute promyelocytic leukemia, hepatitis, and cancer.[137] Further, thrombolytic therapy used to treat life-threatening thrombotic events is ineffective when plasminogen activity is low.

Principle of Plasminogen Assay

Plasminogen is measured by a chromogenic substrate assay, not a clot-based assay. The assay mimics the natural enzymatic process whereby plasminogen is converted to active plasmin, which cleaves its substrate fibrinogen. To detect the generated plasmin in the assay, a chromogenic substrate is used in place of the natural substrate. The enzymatic active site of plasmin in the natural substrate, fibrinogen, is mirrored in the synthetic sequence of valine-leucine-lysine (Val-Leu-Lys). The chromophore pNA is covalently bound to the carboxyl terminus of this oligopeptide. The chromogenic substrate S-2251 for plasmin is thus composed of H-D-Val-Leu-Lys-pNA.

For the assay, streptokinase, derived from cultures of β-hemolytic streptococci, is the plasminogen activator. Streptokinase is added to patient PPP, where it binds and activates plasminogen to form plasmin. The resulting streptokinase-plasmin complex hydrolyzes a bond in the substrate S-2251, releasing the pNA (Figure 41.12). Free pNA produces a yellow color, the intensity of which is proportional to the plasminogen concentration. Results of patient specimens and controls read from a calibration curve are recorded. A typical plasminogen reference interval is 5 to 13.5 mg/dL. Several analogous chromogenic and fluorogenic substrates are suitable for plasminogen measurement.

Tissue Plasminogen Activator

The two physiologic plasminogen activators are TPA and urokinase.[138,139] TPA is synthesized in vascular endothelial cells and released into the circulation, where its half-life is approximately 3 minutes and its plasma concentration averages 5 ng/mL. Urokinase is produced in the kidney and vascular endothelial cells, has a half-life of approximately 7 minutes, and has a plasma concentration of 2 to 4 ng/mL. Both activators are serine proteases that form ternary complexes with bound plasminogen at the surface of fibrin, activating plasminogen to form plasmin, initiating thrombus degradation. The endothelial-secreted PAI-1 covalently inactivates both.

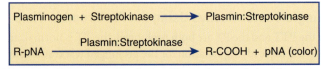

Figure 41.12 Plasminogen Assay. Plasma levels of plasminogen are quantitated using a chromogenic substrate method. Reagent streptokinase activates plasminogen to form plasmin. *R-pNA* designates a chromogenic substrate, where *R* indicates a peptide sequence specific to the enzyme being measured and *pNA* (paranitroaniline) is the chromophore. In the case of plasminogen, the R represents the peptide sequence valine-leucine-lysine (Val-Leu-Lys). Plasmin recognizes the Val-Leu-Lys amide sequence as its enzymatic cleavage site, releasing the pNA, which generates a yellow color.

Decreased TPA levels, which cause *impaired fibrinolysis,* may correlate with increased risk of myocardial infarction, stroke, or deep vein thrombosis.[140] TPA, the primary mediator of fibrinolysis, serves as the model for recombinant TPA (alteplase [Activase, Genentech]), the drug used in thrombolytic therapy to dissolve life-threatening thrombi.

Specimen Collection for Tissue Plasminogen Activator Assay

TPA activity exhibits diurnal variation and rises with exercise. Further, TPA is unstable in vitro because it rapidly binds PAI-1 after blood collection. For specimen collection, patients should be at rest, tourniquet application should be minimal, the phlebotomist should record the collection time, and immediate acidification of the specimen in acetate buffer is necessary.[141] Acidification may be accomplished using the Biopool Stabilyte acidified citrate tube (DiaPharma). Supernatant PPP may be frozen at −70° C until the assay is performed.

Principle of Tissue Plasminogen Activator Assay

To measure TPA *activity,* a chromogenic assay is used. A specified concentration of reagent plasminogen (Chromolyse TPA Activity, Diagnostica Stago) is added to the patient PPP. Plasma TPA activates the plasminogen and the resultant plasmin activity is measured using a chromogenic substrate specific for plasmin such as S-2251. The resulting color intensity is proportional to TPA activity (Figure 41.13). The system may incorporate soluble fibrin to increase TPA activity.

Plasma concentration of TPA *antigen* may be estimated by enzyme immunoassay. The reference interval upper limit for TPA activity is 1.1 units/mL, and the upper limit for TPA antigen concentration is 14 ng/mL.

Plasminogen Activator Inhibitor-1

PAI-1 is produced by vascular endothelial cells and hepatocytes, circulates in plasma bound to vitronectin at an average concentration of 10 ng/mL, and has diurnal variations.[142] An inactive form of PAI-1 is stored in high concentrations in platelets. PAI-1 inactivates free TPA by covalent binding.

Venous thrombosis is associated with *elevated* PAI-1 levels. PAI-1 may be a cardiovascular risk factor and a marker of senescence.[143,144] On the other hand, of the few reported cases of PAI-1 *deficiency,* associated hemorrhage apparently occurs only when a homozygous or compound heterozygous *SERPINE1*

mutation is detected causing complete PAI-1 deficiency.[145] Because the reference interval of PAI-1 activity starts at zero in most laboratories, the ability to discriminate between normal and low levels by phenotype alone is limited. The prevalence of complete PAI-1 deficiency is high in the Old Order Amish population of eastern and southern Indiana, implying a pathogenic founder variant.

Principle of Plasminogen Activator Inhibitor-1 Assay

For the PAI-1 assay, patients are to be at rest before blood collection. Drawn blood is collected into an acidified citrate tube (Stabilyte) to avoid in vitro release of platelet PAI-1; collection tubes are centrifuged immediately to prepare PPP.[146]

Several immunologic and chromogenic substrate methods are available for estimation of PAI-1 antigen and PAI-1 activity, respectively. One enzyme immunoassay for functional PAI-1 uses urokinase to bind PAI-1. The urokinase-PAI-1 complex is immobilized with solid-phase monoclonal anti-PAI-1 antibodies and is measured using monoclonal antiurokinase immunoglobulin as the detecting antibody.

Most chromogenic substrate kits for PAI-1 use an indirect measurement approach. Patient PPP is mixed with a measured amount of reagent TPA (Spectrolyse PAI-1 Activity Assay, BioMedica Diagnostics). Residual TPA is assayed in the plasminogen system as shown in Figure 41.14. The resulting color intensity is inversely proportional to plasma PAI-1 activity.

Total PAI-1 deficiency may be confirmed using the *serum PAI-1 assay.* In serum, platelet PAI-1 is expressed in excess. In true PAI-1 absence, no PAI-1 is detectable in serum.

VISCOELASTOMETRY AND GLOBAL COAGULATION ASSAYS

TEG and ROTEM

Thromboelastography and its more recent modification rotational thromboelastometry are two forms of viscoelastometry (VET). Thromboelastography had its beginning in the 1940s as one of the original quantitative whole blood clotting assays to assess the hemostatic status of patients. The TEG 5000 and TEG 6S Thromboelastograph Hemostasis Analyzers (Haemonetics) and the ROTEM (Werfen) are global *whole blood* analyzers that sense the viscoelastic properties of blood clotting under low shear stress conditions and activation by a specific reagent. The

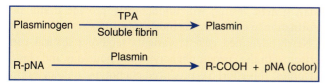

Figure 41.13 Tissue Plasminogen Activator *(TPA)* **Assay.** Plasma levels of TPA are quantitated using a chromogenic substrate method. To assay, plasma that contains TPA is added to plasminogen to produce plasmin. Plasmin activity is measured using the same chromogenic substrate as in the plasminogen assay illustrated in Figure 41.12. The intensity of color is proportional to TPA activity. *pNA,* Paranitroaniline; *R,* variable peptide sequence.

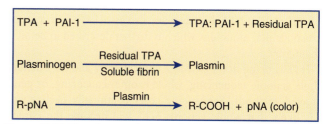

Figure 41.14 Plasminogen Activator Inhibitor-1 *(PAI-1)* **Assay.** Activity of PAI-1 is measured using a chromogenic substrate method. Plasma containing PAI-1 is added to reagent tissue plasminogen activator *(TPA)* of known concentration. The residual TPA is assayed, as shown in Figure 41.13. The intensity of color is inversely proportional to PAI-1 level. *pNA,* Paranitroaniline; *R,* variable peptide sequence.

instruments measure clotting time and the dynamics of clot formation and dissolution as affected by the kinetics of thrombin generation, platelet activation, fibrin generation, clot strength, clot stability, fibrinolysis and inhibitory effects on any of these aspects.[147] These coagulometers that are used mainly in liver surgery, cardiac surgery, and trauma are described in detail in Chapter 42. The TEG 6S and ROTEM Sigma are cartridge-based systems that improve precision as they reduce pipetting errors.[148]

Quantra

The Quantra coagulometer (Hemosonics/Diagnostica Stago) is an automated cartridge-based VET system approved for use in trauma and liver or cardiac surgery.[149] It uses ultrasound technology to send a pulse through the whole blood sample. It measures clot time, elasticity and fibrinolysis via sonic estimation of elasticity by resonance (SEER), also known as sonorheometry. The technology does not make direct contact with the patient blood sample.[150] Cartridge-based technology provides improved precision and accuracy.

Thrombin Generation Assays

Although the endpoint of clotting assays is based on thrombin generation followed by thrombin conversion of soluble fibrinogen to insoluble fibrin, the clotting time result of the PT and PTT may differ from the amount of thrombin formed. Assay systems that assess thrombin generation such as the Calibrated Automated Thrombogram (CAT, Diagnostica Stago) and the Technothrombin TGA (DiaPharma) are under investigation for their clinical utility. These systems measure the phased kinetics of thrombin generation from initiation and peak generation through downregulation and inactivation. Thrombin generation assays may help to better categorize the physiologic mechanisms of hemostasis and to better assess bleeding risk, thrombotic risk, and their modification by hemostatic or antithrombotic agents.

GENETIC TESTING FOR HEMOSTATIC DISORDERS

Since 2007, high-throughput sequencing (HTS) has become the reference approach to identifying the genetic variants that underlie platelet-related and coagulopathy-related bleeding disorders. Table 41.8 lists the genetic variants that have been definitively identified with coagulation disorders. Tables 37.1 and 38.1 list the identified genetic variants associated with platelet disorders. Thrombophilia disorders are also associated with numerous congenital mutations which is further described in detail in Chapter 39.

HTS is being developed as a clinical assay and may include whole genome sequencing, whole exome sequencing, or gene-targeted methods. Sequencing costs continually decline and it is likely that whole genome HTS will become the clinical standard, gradually replacing inherently imprecise phenotypic assays, such as time-honored platelet function testing, quantitative platelet activation immunoassays, and clot-based coagulation factor assays.

TABLE 41.8 Clinically Detectable Genetic Variants That Have Been Associated With Coagulopathies and Thrombosis

Variant	Disorder	Mode of Inheritance
Mutations Causing Familial Coagulopathies		
F2	Prothrombin deficiency	Autosomal recessive
F5	Factor V deficiency	Autosomal recessive
F7	Factor VII deficiency	Autosomal recessive
F8	Hemophilia A	X-linked recessive
F9	Hemophilia B	X-linked recessive
F10	Factor X deficiency	Autosomal recessive
F11	Factor XI deficiency	Autosomal recessive
F13A1, F13B	Factor XIII deficiency	Autosomal recessive
FG4		Autosomal dominant
FGB		Autosomal recessive
FGG	Fibrinogen deficiency	Autosomal recessive
LMAN1, MCFD2	Combined factor V and factor VIII deficiency	Autosomal recessive
KLKB1	Prekallikrein (Fletcher factor) deficiency	Autosomal recessive
KNG1	Kininogen (Fitzgerald factor) deficiency	Autosomal recessive
VWF	von Willebrand disease	Autosomal dominant
PLG	Plasminogen deficiency	Autosomal recessive
SERPINE1	Plasminogen activator inhibitor-1 deficiency	Autosomal recessive
GGCX	Multiple coagulation factor deficiency type 1	Autosomal recessive
VKORC1	Multiple coagulation factor deficiency type 2	Autosomal recessive
Mutations Causing Familial Thrombosis		
F2	Prothrombin 20210 mutation	Autosomal recessive
F5	Factor V Leiden mutation	Autosomal recessive
Numerous point mutations	Antithrombin deficiency	Autosomal recessive
Numerous point mutations	Protein C deficiency	Autosomal recessive
Numerous point mutations	Protein C deficiency	Autosomal recessive

Besides the currently known hemostatic variants, the extreme precision of HTS enables the detection of many additional variants for hemorrhagic and thrombotic disorders not currently named or identified by trivial nomenclature. As only 30% of thrombotic episodes can be associated with a known cause today, genetic testing will undoubtedly provide useful new information to aid future diagnostic measures.

Newly identified genetic variants require statistical comparison with the current phenotypic methodology and clinical outcomes. This effort has produced phenotypic ontologies (formal naming systems) such as the Human Phenotype Ontology, which is more precise than the *International Classification of Diseases-Tenth Revision* (ICD-10) system, leading to further platelet and coagulopathy disorder associations and consolidation of terminology.[151]

SUMMARY

- Proper specimen collection, transport, storage, and centrifugation ensure a valid hemostasis test result.
- Specimens that are short draws, clotted, or hemolyzed are rejected.
- Platelet function testing, including aggregometry, helps determine the cause of nonthrombocytopenic mucocutaneous bleeding.
- von Willebrand disease is diagnosed and monitored through judicious selection and performance of plasma- and platelet function-based laboratory tests.
- Plasma platelet factor 4 (PF4) and urinary 11-dehydro-thromboxane B_2 are used to assess platelet activation.
- Clot-based routine coagulation tests include prothrombin time, partial thromboplastin time, and thrombin clotting time.
- Mixing studies are employed in acute care facilities to differentiate factor deficiencies, lupus anticoagulants, and specific factor inhibitors.
- Clot-based coagulation factor assays detect and measure coagulation factor deficiencies.

- Chromogenic factor assays accurately measure coagulation factors in hemophilia patients receiving B-domain-deleted and extended half-life therapeutic factor concentrates.
- Nijmegen-Bethesda assay detects and measures coagulation factor inhibitors.
- Tests of fibrinolysis include assays for fibrin degradation products, D-dimer, plasminogen, tissue plasminogen activator, and plasminogen activator inhibitor-1.
- Viscoelastometry assesses whole blood hemostasis by measuring clotting time, clotting kinetics, maximum clot strength, and fibrinolysis.
- Thrombin generation assays may become common in future hemostasis laboratory testing.
- Next-generation cohort and whole genome sequencing is replacing less precise phenotypic methods to identify platelet function disorders, coagulopathies, and thrombophilic disorders caused by multiple mutations.

Now that you have completed this chapter, go back and read again the case study at the beginning and respond to the questions presented. Answers can be found in Appendix C.

REVIEW QUESTIONS

Answers can be found in Appendix C.

1. What happens if a coagulation specimen collection tube is underfilled?
   a. The specimen clots and is useless.
   b. The specimen is hemolyzed and is useless.
   c. Clot-based test results are falsely prolonged.
   d. Chromogenic test results are falsely decreased.
2. If you collect blood into a series of tubes, when in the sequence should the hemostasis (blue top) tube be filled?
   a. After a lavender top or green top tube
   b. First, or after a nonadditive tube
   c. After a serum separator tube
   d. Last
3. What is the effect of hemolysis on a hemostasis specimen?
   a. In vitro platelet and coagulation activation
   b. The specimen is icteric or lipemic
   c. Hemolysis has no effect
   d. The specimen is clotted
4. Except for platelet aggregometry, most coagulation testing must be performed on PPP, which is plasma with a platelet count less than:
   a. 1000/μL
   b. 10,000/μL
   c. 100,000/μL
   d. 1,000,000/μL
5. You wish to obtain a 5-mL specimen of whole blood/anti-coagulant mixture. The patient's hematocrit is 65%. What volume of anticoagulant should you use?
   a. 0.32 mL
   b. 0.5 mL
   c. 0.64 mL
   d. 0.68 mL

6. You perform whole blood lumiaggregometry on a specimen from a patient who reports easy bruising. Aggregation and secretion are diminished when the agonists ADP, arachidonic acid, and collagen are used. The agonist TRAP induces partial aggregation but negative secretion. What is the most likely platelet abnormality?
   a. Glanzmann thrombasthenia
   b. Aspirin-like syndrome
   c. ADP receptor anomaly
   d. Storage pool disorder
7. What is the reference assay for HIT?
   a. Enzyme immunoassay
   b. Serotonin release assay
   c. Platelet lumiaggregometry
   d. Washed platelet aggregation
8. What agonist is used in platelet aggregometry to detect VWD?
   a. Arachidonic acid
   b. Ristocetin
   c. Collagen
   d. ADP
9. Deficiency of which congenital single factor is likely when the PT result is prolonged and the PTT result is normal?
   a. Factor V
   b. Factor VII
   c. Factor VIII
   d. Prothrombin
10. A prolonged PT and a low factor VII level but a normal factor V level are characteristic of an acquired coagulopathy associated with which of the following?
    a. Vitamin K deficiency
    b. Thrombocytopenia
    c. Liver disease
    d. Hemophilia

11. The patient has deep vein thrombosis. The PTT is prolonged and is not corrected in an immediate mix of patient PPP with an equal part of PNP. What is the presumed condition?
    a. Factor VIII inhibitor
    b. Lupus anticoagulant
    c. Factor VIII deficiency
    d. Factor V Leiden mutation

12. What condition causes the most pronounced elevation in the result of the quantitative D-dimer assay?
    a. Deep vein thrombosis
    b. Fibrinogen deficiency
    c. Paraproteinemia
    d. DIC

13. What is the name given to the type of assay that uses a synthetic polypeptide substrate that releases a chromophore on digestion by its serine protease?
    a. Clot-based assay
    b. Molecular diagnostic assay
    c. Fluorescence immunoassay
    d. Chromogenic substrate assay

14. What component of the fibrinolytic process binds and neutralizes free plasmin?
    a. TPA
    b. PAI-1
    c. Urokinase
    d. α_2-Antiplasmin

15. What type of high-throughput genomic sequencing is likely to become a standard clinical assay?
    a. Human genotypic ontogeny
    b. Whole genome sequencing
    c. Whole exome sequencing
    d. Gene-targeted sequencing

REFERENCES

1. Clinical and Laboratory Standards Institute. (2008). *Collection, Transport, and Processing of Blood Specimens for Testing Plasma-Based Coagulation Assays: Approved Guideline.* (5th ed.). CLSI Document H21-A5. Wayne, PA: Clinical and Laboratory Standards Institute.
2. Magnette, A., Chatelain, M., Chatelain, B., et al. (2016). Pre-analytical issues in the haemostasis laboratory: guidance for the clinical laboratories. *Thromb J, 14,* 49–63.
3. Gosselin, R. C. (2021). Review of coagulation preanalytical variables with update on the effect of direct oral anticoagulants. *Int J Lab Hematol, 43* (Suppl 1), 109–116.
4. Elbaz, C., & Scholzberg, M. (2020). An illustrated review of bleeding assessment tools and common coagulation tests. *Res Pract Thromb Haemost, 4,* 761–773.
5. Guder, W. G., & Narayanan, S. (2015). *Pre-Examination Procedures in Laboratory Diagnostics: Preanalytical Aspects and Their Impact on the Quality of Medical Laboratory Results.* Berlin, Germany: DeGruyter.
6. Bennett, A., Fritsma, G. A., & Ernst, D. J. (2016). *Quick Guide to Blood Collection.* (2nd ed.). Washington, DC: AACC Press.
7. Tosetto, A., Castaman, G., & Rodeghiero, F. (2013). Bleeders, bleeding rates, and bleeding score. *J Thromb Haemost, 11* (Suppl 1), 142–150.
8. Strasinger, S. K., & DiLorenzo, M. S. (2003). *The Phlebotomy Workbook.* (2nd ed., pp. 135–162). Philadelphia: F. A. Davis.
9. Ernst, D. J. (2017). *Procedures for the Collection of Diagnostic Blood Specimens by Venipuncture: Approved Standard.* (7th ed.). CLSI Document GP41. Wayne, PA: Clinical and Laboratory Standards Institute.
10. Dubrovny, N. (2010). *Tubes and Additives for Venous Blood Specimen Collection: Approved Standard.* (6th ed.). CLSI Document. GP39. Wayne, PA: Clinical and Laboratory Standards Institute.
11. Adcock-Funk, D. M., Lippi, G., & Favaloro, E. J. (2012). Quality standards for sample processing, transportation, and storage in hemostasis testing. *Semin Thromb Hemost, 38,* 576–585.
12. van den Besselaar, A. M., Meeuwisse-Braun, J., Schaefer-van Mansfeld, H., et al. (1997). Influence of plasma volumetric errors on the prothrombin time ratio and international sensitivity index. *Blood Coagul Fibrinolysis, 8,* 431–435.
13. Lima-Oliveira, G., Salvagno, G. L., Danese, E., et al. (2015). Sodium citrate blood contamination by K2-ethylenediaminetetraacetic acid (EDTA): impact on routine coagulation testing. *Int J Lab Hematol, 37,* 403–409.
14. McCall, R., & Tankersley, C. (2023). *Phlebotomy Essentials.* (6th ed.). Philadelphia: Lippincott.
15. Kitchen, S., Adcock, D. M., Dauer, R., et al. (2021). International Council for Standardisation in Haematology (ICSH) recommendations for collection of blood samples for coagulation testing. *Int J Lab Hematol, 43,* 571–580.
16. Smock, K. J., Crist, R. A., Hansen, S. J., et al. (2010). Discard tubes are not necessary when drawing samples for specialized coagulation testing. *Blood Coagul Fibrinolysis, 21,* 279–282.
17. Lippi, G., Salvagno, G. L., Montagnara, M., et al. (2012). Quality standards for sample collection in coagulation testing. *Semin Thromb Hemost, 38,* 565–575.
18. Ernst, D. J. (2008). *Blood Specimen Collection FAQs.* Ramsey, IN: Center for Phlebotomy Education.
19. Marques, M., & Fritsma, G. A. (2015). *Quick Guide to Coagulation Testing.* (3rd ed.). Washington, DC: AACC Press.
20. Gosselin, R. C., & Marlar, R. A. (2019). Preanalytical variables in coagulation testing: setting the stage for accurate results. *Semin Thromb Hemost, 45,* 433–448.
21. Ernst, C., & Ernst, D. J. (2001). *Phlebotomy for Nurses and Nursing Personnel.* Ramsey, IN: Center for Phlebotomy Education.
22. Pan, L. L., Lee, C. H., Hung, K. C., et al. (2021). Differential impacts of hemolysis on coagulation parameters of blood samples. A STROBE-compliant article. *Medicine, 100,* e25798.
23. Vanderslice, N. C., & Rios, A. S. (2017). Advances in point-of-care coagulation analyzer technology. *Diagnostic Interventional Cardiology.* https://www.dicardiology.com/article/advances-point-care-coagulation-analyzer-technology. Accessed January 10, 2023.

24. Lijima, S., Baba, T., Ueno, D., Ohishi, A. (2014). International normalized ratio testing with point-of-care coagulometer in healthy term neonates. *BMC Pediatrics, 14,* 179–184.

25. Clinical and Laboratory Standards Institute. (2008). *Procedures and Devices for the Collection of Diagnostic Capillary Blood Specimens.* Approved Standard. CLSI Document GP42. Wayne, PA: Clinical and Laboratory Standards Institute.

26. McGraw, A., Hillarp, A., & Echeneguciia, M. (2010). Considerations in the laboratory assessment of haemostasis. *Haemophilia, 16* (Suppl 5), 74–78.

27. Sevenet, P. O., Kaczor, D. A., & Depasse, F. (2017). Factor VII deficiency: from basics to clinical laboratory diagnosis and patient management. *Clin Appl Thromb Hemost, 23,* 703–710.

28. National Heart, Lung, and Blood Institute. (2007). *The Diagnosis, Evaluation, and Management of Von Willebrand Disease.* NIH Publication No. 08-5832, Bethesda, MD: US Department of Health and Human Services, National Institutes of Health.

29. Toulon, P., Metge, S., & Hangard, M. (2017). Impact of different storage times at room temperature of unspun citrated blood samples on routine coagulation tests results. Results of a bicenter study and review of the literature. *Int J Lab Hem, 39,* 1–11.

30. Polack, B., Schved, J. F., & Boneu, B. (2001). Preanalytical recommendations of the 'Groupe d'Etude sur l'Hémostase et la Thrombose' (GEHT) for venous blood testing in hemostasis laboratories. *Haemostasis, 31,* 61–68.

31. Foshat, M., Bates, S., Russo, W., et al. (2015). Effect of freezing plasma at –20° C for 2 weeks on prothrombin time, activated partial thromboplastin time, dilute Russell viper venom time, activated protein C resistance, and D-dimer levels. *Clin Appl Thromb Hemost, 21,* 41–47.

32. Gosselin, R. C., Honeychurch, K., Kang, H. J., et al. (2015). Effects of storage and thawing conditions on coagulation testing. *Int J Lab Hem, 37,* 551–559.

33. Rimac, V., & Herak, D. C. (2017). Is it acceptable to use coagulation plasma samples stored at room temperature and 4° C for 24 hours for additional prothrombin time, activated partial thromboplastin time, fibrinogen, antithrombin, and D-dimer testing? *Int J Lab Hem, 39,* 1–7.

34. Dyszkiewicz-Korpanty, A. M., Frenkel, E. P., & Sarode, R. (2005). Approach to the assessment of platelet function: comparison between optical-based platelet-rich plasma and impedance-based whole blood platelet aggregation methods. *Clin Appl Thromb Hemost, 11,* 25–35.

35. Vandevelde, A., Chayoua, W., de Laat, B., et al. (2022). Added value of antiphosphatidylserine/prothrombin antibodies in the workup of thrombotic antiphospholipid syndrome: communication from the ISTH SSC Subcommittee on Lupus Anticoagulant/Antiphospholipid Antibodies. *J Thromb Haemost, 20,* 2136–2150.

36. Lippi, G., Plebani, M., & Favaloro, E. J. (2013). Interference in coagulation testing: focus on spurious hemolysis, icterus, and lipemia. *Semin Thromb Hemost, 39,* 258–266.

37. Mastella, A. K., de Carvalho, J., Stein, C., et al. (2021). Interference of icterus on plasma D-dimer levels measured using immunoturbidimetric assays. *Blood Coag Fibrinol, 32,* 162–163.

38. Palma-Barqueros, V., Revilla, N., Sanchez, A., et al. (2021). Inherited platelet disorders: an updated overview. *Int J Mol Sci, 22,* 4521.

39. Duke, W. W. (1912). The pathogenesis of purpura haemorrhagica with especial reference to the part played by the blood platelets. *Arch Intern Med, 10,* 445–469.

40. Ivy, A. C., Nelson, D., & Bucher, G. (1941). The standardization of certain factors in the cutaneous "venostasis" bleeding time technique. *J Lab Clin Med, 26,* 1812–1822.

41. Mielke, C. H., Jr., Kaneshiro, M. M., Maher, I. A., et al. (1969). The standardized normal Ivy bleeding time and its prolongation by aspirin. *Blood, 34,* 204–215.

42. Kumar, R., Ansell, J. E., Canoso, R. T., et al. (1978). Clinical trial of a new bleeding device. *Am J Clin Pathol, 70,* 642–645.

43. Finazzi, G., Budde, U., & Michiels, J. J. (1996). Bleeding time and platelet function in essential thrombocythemia and other myeloproliferative syndromes. *Leuk Lymphoma, 22* (Suppl 1), 71–78.

44. Lind, S. E. (1991). The bleeding time does not predict surgical bleeding. *Blood, 77,* 2547–2552.

45. Hvas, A.-M., & Favaloro, E. J. (2017). Platelet function analyzed by light transmission aggregometry. *Methods Mol Biol, 1646,* 321–331.

46. Stratmann, J., Karmal, L., Zwinge, B., et al. (2019). Platelet aggregation testing on a routine coagulation analyzer: a method comparison study. *Clinical Applied Thromb Hemost, 25,* 1–10.

47. Fritsma, G. A., & McGlasson, D. L. (2017). Whole blood platelet aggregometry. *Methods Mol Biol, 1646,* 333–347.

48. Fritsma, G. A. (2007). Platelet function testing: aggregometry and lumiaggregometry. *Clin Lab Sci, 20,* 32–37.

49. Vucenik, I., & Podczasy, J. J. (1998). Whole blood lumi-aggregation: evaluation of reagents. *Clinical Applied Thromb Hemost, 4,* 253–256.

50. Pai, M., Wang, G., Moffat, K. A., et al. (2011). Diagnostic usefulness of a lumi-aggregometer adenosine triphosphate release assay for the assessment of platelet function disorders. *Am J Clin Path, 136,* 350–358.

51. Goldenberg, S. J., Veriabo, N. J., & Soslau, G. (2001). A micromethod to measure platelet aggregation and ATP release by impedance. *Thromb Res, 103,* 57–61.

52. Mezzano, D., Harrison, P., Frelinger, A. L., et al. (2022). Expert opinion on the use of platelet secretion assay for the diagnosis of inherited platelet function disorders: communication from the ISTH SSC Subcommittee on Platelet Physiology. *J Thromb Haemost, 20,* 2127–2135.

53. Trampuš-Bakija, A., Jazbec, J., & Faganel-Kotnik, B. (2022). Platelet lumiaggregation testing: reference intervals and the effect of acetylsalicylic acid in healthy adults. *J Med Biochem, 39,* 422–427.

54. Kuliczkowski, W., Zurawska-Plaksej, E., Podolak-Dawidziak, M., et al. (2021). Platelet reactivity and response to aspirin and clopidogrel in patients with platelet count disorders. *Cardiol Res Practice, 2021,* 1–7.

55. Legrand, D., Barbato, E., Chenu, P., et al. (2015). The STIB score: a simple clinical test to predict clopidogrel resistance. *Acta Cardiol, 70,* 516–521.

56. Guirgis, M., Thompson, P., & Jansen, S. (2017). Review of aspirin and clopidogrel resistance in peripheral arterial disease. *J Vasc Surg, 66,* 1576–1586.

57. Raichand, S., Moore, D., Riley, R. D., et al. (2013). Protocol for a systematic review of the diagnostic and prognostic utility of tests currently available for the detection of aspirin resistance in patients with established cardiovascular or cerebrovascular disease. *Syst Rev, 26,* 2–16.

58. Nagler, M., & Cuker, A. (2017). Profile of Instrumentation Laboratory's HemosIL® AcuStar HIT-Ab(PF4-H) assay for diagnosis of heparin-induced thrombocytopenia. *Expert Rev Mol Diagn, 17,* 419–426.

59. Nazi, I., Arnold, D. M., Moore, J. C., et al. (2015). Pitfalls in the diagnosis of heparin-induced thrombocytopenia: a 6-year experience from a reference laboratory. *Am J Hematol, 90,* 629–633.

60. Warkentin, T. (2019). Heparin-induced thrombocytopenia. In Kitchens, C. S., Kessler, C. M., Konkle, B. A., et al. (Eds.), *Consultative Hemostasis and Thrombosis.* (4th ed., pp. 491–527). St. Louis: Elsevier.

61. Warkentin, T. E. (2019). Laboratory diagnosis of heparin induced thrombocytopenia. *Int J Lab Hematol, 41* (Suppl 1), 15–25.

62. Warkentin, T. E., Arnold, D. M., Nazi, I., et al. (2015). The platelet serotonin-release assay. *Am J Hematol, 90,* 564–572.

63. Harenberg, J., Huhle, G., Giese, C., et al. (2000). Determination of serotonin release from platelets by enzyme immunoassay in the diagnosis of heparin-induced thrombocytopenia. *Br J Haematol, 109,* 182–186.

64. Baidildinova, G., Nagy, M., Jurk, K., et al. (2021). Soluble platelet release factors as biomarkers for cardiovascular disease. *Thromb Haemost, 108,* 1–20.

65. Kubota, Y., Alonso, A., & Folsom, A. R. (2017). β-thromboglobulin and incident cardiovascular disease risk: the Atherosclerosis Risk in Communities study. *Thromb Res, 155,* 116–120.

66. Rand, M. L., Leung, R., & Packham, M. A. (2003). Platelet function assays. *Transfus Apher Sci, 28,* 307–317.

67. Fritsma, G. A., Ens, G. E., Alvord, M. A., et al. (2001). Monitoring the antiplatelet action of aspirin. *JAAPA, 14,* 57–62.

68. Wang, N., Vendrov, K. C., Simmons, B. P., et al. (2018). Urinary 11-dehydro-thromboxane B2 levels are associated with vascular inflammation and prognosis in atherosclerotic cardiovascular disease. *Prostaglandins Other Lipid Mediat, 134,* 24–31.

69. De Stefano, V., Rocca, B., Tosetto, A., et al. (2018). The aspirin regimens in essential thrombocythemia (ARES) phase II randomized trial design: implementation of the serum thromboxane B2 assay as an evaluation tool of different aspirin dosing regimens in the clinical setting. *Blood Cancer J, 8,* 49.

70. Cahill, K. N., Cui, J., Kothari, P., et al. (2019). Unique effect of aspirin therapy on biomarkers in aspirin-exacerbated respiratory disease. *Am J Resp Crit Care Med, 200,* 704–711.

71. Lee, R. I., & White, P. D. (1913). A clinical study of the coagulation time of blood. *Am J Med Sci, 243,* 279–285.

72. Clinical and Laboratory Standards Institute. (2008). *One-Stage Prothrombin Time (PT) Test and Activated Partial Thromboplastin Time (APTT) Test; Approved Guideline.* (2nd ed.). CLSI Document H47-A2. Wayne, PA: Clinical and Laboratory Standards Institute.

73. Mannucci, P. M., & Tripodi, A. (2012). Hemostatic defects in liver and renal dysfunction. *Am Soc Hematol Educ Program, 2012,* 168–173.

74. Poller, L. (1986). Laboratory control of anticoagulant therapy. *Semin Thromb Hemost, 12,* 13–19.

75. Capoor, M. N., Stonemetz, J. L., Baird, J. C., et al. (2015). Prothrombin time and activated partial thromboplastin time testing: a comparative effectiveness study in a million-patient sample. *PLoS ONE, 10* (8), e0133317.

76. McKinly, L., & Wrenn, K. (1993). Are baseline prothrombin time/partial thromboplastin time values necessary before instituting anticoagulation? *Ann Emerg Med, 22,* 697–702.

77. Baumann Kreuziger, L. M., Datta, Y. H., Johnson, A. D., et al. (2014). Monitoring anticoagulation in patients with an unreliable prothrombin time/international normalized ratio: factor II versus chromogenic factor X testing. *Blood Coagul Fibrinolysis, 25,* 232–236.

78. McGlasson, D. L. (2013). Monitoring coumadin-the original oral anticoagulant. *Clin Lab Sci, 26,* 43–47.

79. Garcia, D., & Erkan, D. (2018). Diagnosis and management of the antiphospholipid syndrome. *N Engl J Med, 378,* 2010–2021.

80. Greenmyer, J. R., Niaz, T., Kohorst, M. A., et al. (2021). Chromogenic factor X assay for monitoring warfarin anticoagulation in a child with a prosthetic mitral valve. *Mayo Clin Proc Innov Qual Outcomes, 5,* 811–816.

81. McGlasson, D., & Gosselin, R. C. (2020). Hemostasis: laboratory testing and instrumentation. In McKenzie, S. B., Landis-Piwowar, K., & Williams, L. (Eds.), *Clinical Laboratory Hematology.* (4th ed., pp. 866–903). New Jersey: Pearson.

82. Marlar, R. A., Clement, B., & Gausman, J. (2017). Activated partial thromboplastin time monitoring of unfractionated heparin therapy: issues and recommendations. *Semin Thromb Hemost, 43,* 253–260.

83. Tripodi, A., Lippi, G., & Plebani, M. (2016). How to report results of prothrombin and activated partial thromboplastin times. *Clin Chem Lab Med, 54,* 215–222.

84. Toulon, P., Eloit, Y., Smahi, M., et al. (2016). In vitro sensitivity of different activated partial thromboplastin time reagents to mild clotting factor deficiencies. *Int J Lab Hematol, 38,* 389–396.

85. Alsulaiman, D., Sylvester, K., Stevens, C., et al. (2016). Comparison of time to therapeutic aPTT in patients who received continuous unfractionated heparin after implementation of pharmacy-wide intervention alerts. *Hosp Pharm, 51,* 656–661.

86. Toulon, P., Smahi, M., & De Pooter, N. (2021). APTT therapeutic range for monitoring unfractionated heparin therapy. Significant impact of the anti-Xa reagent used for correlation. *J Thromb Haemost, 19,* 2002–2006.

87. Hayward, C. P. (2018). How I investigate for bleeding disorders. *Int J Lab Hematol, 40* (Suppl 1), 6–14.

88. Bustamante, J. G., Goyal, A., & Singhal, M. (2022). Antiphospholipid syndrome. In: *StatPearls.* https://www.ncbi.nlm.nih.gov/books/NBK430980. Accessed January 4, 2023.

89. Devreese, K. M. J., de Groot, P. G., de Laat, B., et al. (2020). Guidance from the Scientific and Standardization Committee for Lupus Anticoagulant/Antiphospholipid Antibodies of the International Society on Thrombosis and Haemostasis: update of the guidelines for lupus anticoagulant detection and interpretation. *J Thromb Haemost, 18,* 2828–2839.

90. Favaloro, E. (2020). Mixing studies for lupus anticoagulant: mostly yes, sometimes no. *Clin Chem Lab Med, 58,* 487–491.

91. Favaloro, E. J. (2020). Coagulation mixing studies: utility, algorithmic strategies and limitations for lupus anticoagulant testing or follow up of abnormal coagulation tests. *Am J Hematol, 95,* 117–128.

92. Tripodi, A. (2021). Diagnostic challenges on the laboratory detection of lupus anticoagulant. *Biomedicines, 9,* 844.

93. Ignjatovic, V. (2013). Thrombin clotting time. *Methods Mol Biol, 992,* 131–138.

94. Hasan, R. A., Pak, J., Kirk, C. J., et al. (2023). Monitoring direct thrombin inhibitors with calibrated diluted thrombin time vs activated partial thromboplastin time in pediatric patients. *Am J Clin Pathol, 159,* 60–68.

95. Karapetian, H. (2013). Reptilase time (RT). *Methods Mol Biol, 992,* 273–277.

96. Clinical and Laboratory Standards Institute. (2001). *Procedure for the Determination of Fibrinogen in Plasma: Approved Guideline.* (2nd ed.). CLSI Document H30-A2. Wayne, PA: Clinical and Laboratory Standards Institute.

97. Stang, L. J., & Mitchell, L. G. (2013). Fibrinogen. *Methods Mol Biol, 992*, 181–192.

98. van den Besselaar, A. M., Haas, F. J., van der Graaf, F., et al. (2009). Harmonization of fibrinogen assay results: study within the framework of the Dutch project 'Calibration 2000'. *Int J Lab Hematol, 31*, 513–520.

99. Lew, W. K., & Weaver, F. A. (2008). Clinical use of topical thrombin as a surgical hemostat. *Biologics, 2*, 593–599.

100. Miesbach, W., Schenk, J., Alesci, S., et al. (2010). Comparison of the fibrinogen Clauss assay and the fibrinogen PT derived method in patients with dysfibrinogenemia. *Thromb Res, 126*, e428–e433.

101. Losos, M., & Chen, J. (2022). Utility and interpretation of coagulation mixing studies. *J Clin Transl Pathol, 2*, 8–11.

102. James, P., Salomon, O., Mikovic, D., et al. (2014). Rare bleeding disorders—bleeding assessment tools, laboratory aspects and phenotype and therapy of FXI deficiency. *Haemophilia, 20* (Suppl 4), 71–75.

103. Takeyama, M., Nogami, K., Okuda, M., et al. (2008). Selective factor VIII and V inactivation by iminodiacetate ion exchange resin through metal ion adsorption. *Br J Haematol, 142*, 962–970.

104. Bowyer, A. E., & Gosselin, R. C. (2023). Factor VIII and factor IX activity measurements for hemophilia diagnosis and related treatments. *Semin Thromb Hemost, 49, 609–620.*

105. Lattes, S., Appert-Flory, A., Fischer, F., et al. (2011). Measurement of factor VIII activity using one-stage clotting assay: a calibration curve has not to be systematically included in each run. *Haemophilia, 17*, 139–142.

106. Castellone, D. D., & Adcock, D. M. (2017). Factor VIII activity and inhibitor assays in the diagnosis and treatment of hemophilia A. *Semin Thromb Hemost, 43*, 320–330.

107. Pikta, M., Laane, E., Vaide, I., et al. (2017). Modified assay for quantitation of low FVIII:C values. *Hemophilia, 23* (Suppl 2), 76.

108. Algahtani, F. H., & Stuckey, R. (2019). Case report: high factor VIII levels and arterial thrombosis: illustrative case and literature review. *Therapeutic Adv Hematol, 10*, 1–10.

109. El-Lateef, A. E., Alghamdi, S., Ebid, G., et al. (2022). Coagulation profile in COVID-19 patients and its relation to disease severity and overall survival: a single center study. *Br J Biomed Sci, 79*, 1–9.

110. van Moort, I., Meijer, P., Priem-Visser, D., et al. (2019). Analytical variation in factor VIII one-stage and chromogenic assays: experiences from the ECAT external quality assessment programme. *Haemophilia, 25*, 162–169.

111. Favaloro, E. J., & Lippi, G. (2017). Emerging treatments for hemophilia: patients and their treaters spoilt for choice, but laboratories face a difficult path? *Ann Transl Med, 5*, 101–103.

112. Ovanesov, M. V., Jackson, J. W., Golding, B., et al. (2021). Considerations on activity assay discrepancies in factor VIII and factor IX. *J Thromb Haemost, 19*, 2102–2111.

113. Kizilocak, H., Marquez-Casas, E., Brown, J., et al. (2021). Factor VIII level comparison in patients with severe hemophilia A on emicizumab with inhibitors with one stage, bovine and human chromogenic assays and the factor VIII equivalency of emicizumab using in vivo global hemostasis assays. *Blood, 138* (Suppl 1), 4234.

114. Mosher, K. A., & Adcock, D. M. (2014). Chromogenic factor VIII activity assay. *Am J Hematol, 89*, 781–783.

115. Kitchen, S. K., Tiefenbacher, S., & Gosselin, R. (2017). Factor activity assays for monitoring extended half-life FVIII and factor IX replacement therapies. *Semin Thromb Hemost, 43*, 331–337.

116. Marlar, R. A., Strandberg, K., Shima, M., & Adcock, D. M. (2020). Clinical utility and impact of the use of the chromogenic vs one stage factor assays in haemophilia A and B. *Eur J Haematol, 104*, 3–14.

117. Duncan, E., Collecutt, M., & Street, A. (2013). Nijmegen-Bethesda assay to measure factor VIII inhibitors. *Methods Mol Biol, 992*, 321–333.

118. Soucie, J. M., Miller, C. H., Kelly, F. M., et al. (2014). National surveillance for hemophilia inhibitors in the United States: summary report of an expert meeting. *Am J Hematol, 89*, 621–625.

119. Miller, C. H. (2018). Laboratory testing for factor VIII and IX inhibitors in haemophilia: a review. *Haemophilia, 24*, 186–197.

120. Verbruggen, B., Novakova, I., Wessels, H., et al. (1995). The Nijmegen modification of the Bethesda assay for factor VIII:C inhibitors: improved specificity and reliability. *Thromb Haemost, 73*, 247–251.

121. Miller, C. J., Platt, S. J., Rice, A. S., et al. (2012). Validation of Nijmegen-Bethesda assay modifications to allow inhibitor measurement during replacement therapy and facilitate inhibitor surveillance. *J Thromb Hemost, 10*, 1055–1061.

122. Miller, C. H., Rice, A. S., Boylan, B., et al. (2013). Hemophilia Inhibitor Research Study Investigators. Comparison of clot-based, chromogenic and fluorescence assays for measurement of factor VIII inhibitors in the US Hemophilia Inhibitor Research Study. *J Thromb Hemost, 11*, 1300–1309.

123. Malkhassian, D., Sabir, S., & Sharma, S. (2022). Physiology, Factor XIII. In *StatPearls*. Treasure Island, FL: StatPearls Publishing. https://www.ncbi.nlm.nih.gov/books/NBK538271. Accessed February 6, 2023.

124. Franchini, M., Frattini, F., Crestani, S., & Bonfanti, C. (2013). Acquired FXIII inhibitors: a systematic review. *J Thromb Thrombolysis, 36*, 109–114.

125. Mangla, A., Hamad, H., & Kumar, A. (2022). Factor XIII deficiency. In *StatPearls*. Treasure Island, FL: StatPearls Publishing. https://www.ncbi.nlm.nih.gov/books/NBK557467. Accessed January 4, 2023.

126. Durda, M. A., Wolberg, A. S., & Kerlin, B. A. (2018). State of the art in factor XIII laboratory assessment. *Transfus Apher Sci, 57*, 700–704.

127. Linkins, L. A., & Takach Lapner, S. (2017). Review of D-dimer testing: good, bad, and ugly. *Int J Lab Hematol, 39* (Suppl 1), 98–103.

128. Wannamethee, S. G., Whincup, P. H., Lennon, L., et al. (2012). Fibrin D-dimer, tissue-type plasminogen activator, von Willebrand factor, and risk of incident stroke in older men. *Stroke, 43*, 1206–1211.

129. Xu, H., Xie, J., Zhou, J., et al. (2021). Ability of plasma-based or serum-based assays of D-dimer for diagnosing periprosthetic joint infection: protocol for a prospective single-centre, parallel comparative study. *BMJ Open, 11*, e046442.

130. Logothetis, C. N., Weppelmann, T. A., Jordan, A., et al. (2021). D-dimer testing for the exclusion of pulmonary embolism among hospitalized patients with COVID-19. *JAMA Netw Open, 4*, e2128802.

131. Dong, J., Duan, X., Feng, R., et al. (2017). Diagnostic implication of fibrin degradation products and D-dimer in aortic dissection. *Sci Rep, 7*, 43957.

132. Pernod, G., Wu, H., de Maistre, E., et al. (2017). Validation of STA-Liatest D-Di assay for exclusion of pulmonary embolism according to the latest Clinical and Laboratory Standard Institute/Food and Drug Administration guideline. Results of a multicenter management study. *Blood Coagul Fibrinolysis, 28*, 254–260.

133. Drewinko, B., Surgeon, J., Cobb, P., et al. (1985). Comparative sensitivity of different methods to detect and quantify circulating fibrinogen/fibrin split products. *Am J Clin Pathol, 84,* 58–66.

134. Garvey, M. B., & Black, J. M. (1972). The detection of fibrinogen-fibrin degradation products by means of a new antibody-coated latex particle. *J Clin Pathol, 25,* 680–682.

135. Franchini, M., & Mannucci, P. M. (2018). Primary hyperfibrinolysis: facts and fancies. *Thromb Res, 166,* 71–75.

136. Shapiro, A. D., Nakar, C., Parker, J. M., et al. (2018). Plasminogen replacement therapy for the treatment of children and adults with congenital plasminogen deficiency. *Blood, 131,* 1301–1310.

137. Shapiro, A. D., Menegatti, M., Palla, R., et al. (2020). An international registry of patients with plasminogen deficiency (HISTORY). *Haematologica, 105,* 554–561.

138. Mutch, N. J., & Booth, N. A. (2013). Plasminogen activation and regulation of fibrinolysis. In Marder, V. J., Aird, W. C., Bennett, J. S., et al. (Eds.), *Hemostasis and Thrombosis: Basic Principles and Clinical Practice.* (6th ed., pp. 314–333). Philadelphia: Lippincott.

139. Jilani, T. N., & Siddiqui, A. H. (2022). Tissue plasminogen activator. In *StatPearls.* Treasure Island, FL: StatPearls Publishing, https://www.ncbi.nlm.nih.gov/books/NBK507917. Accessed February 6, 2023.

140. Prabhudesai, A., Shetty, S., Ghosh, K., et al. (2017). Dysfunctional fibrinolysis and cerebral venous thrombosis. *Blood Cells Mol Dis, 65,* 51–55.

141. Chandler, W. L., Schmer, G., & Stratton, J. R. (1989). Optimum conditions for the stabilization and measurement of tissue plasminogen activator activity in human plasma. *J Lab Clin Med, 113,* 362–371.

142. Boinska, J., Kozinski, M., Kasprzak, M., et al. (2022). Diurnal oscillations of fibrinolytic parameters in patients with acute myocardial infarction and their relation to platelet reactivity: preliminary insights. *J Clin Med, 11,* 7105.

143. D'Elia, J. A., Bayliss, G., Gleason, R. E., et al. (2016). Cardiovascular-renal complications and the possible role of plasminogen activator inhibitor: a review. *Clin Kidney J, 9,* 705–712.

144. Vaughan, D. E., Rai, R., Khan, S. S., et al. (2017). Plasminogen activator inhibitor-1 is a marker and a mediator of senescence. *Arterioscler Thromb Vasc Biol, 37,* 1446–1452.

145. Heiman, M., Gupta, S., Khan, S. S., et al. (2017). Complete plasminogen activator inhibitor 1 deficiency. In Pagon, R. A., Adam, M. P., Ardinger, H. H., et al. (Eds.), *GeneReviews®* [Internet]. Seattle, WA: University of Washington, Seattle; 1993–2017.

146. Nilsson, T. K., Boman, K., Jansson, J. H., et al. (2005). Comparison of soluble thrombomodulin, von Willebrand factor, tPA/PAI-1 complex, and high-sensitivity CRP concentrations in serum, EDTA plasma, citrated plasma, and acidified citrated plasma (Stabilyte) stored at -70 degrees C for 8-11 years. *Thromb Res, 116,* 249–254.

147. Whiting, D., & DiNardo, J. A. (2014). TEG and ROTEM: technology and clinical applications. *Am J Hematol, 89,* 228–232.

148. Faraoni, D., & DiNardo, J. A. (2021). Viscoelastic hemostatic assays: update on technology and clinical applications. *Am J Hematol, 96,* 1331–1337.

149. CAP Today. (2022). *FDA clears HemoSonics Quantra with QStat cartridge.* https://www.captodayonline.com/fda-clears-hemosonics-quantra-with-qstat-cartridge. Accessed February 6, 2023.

150. Volod, O., Bunch, C. M., Zackariya, N., et al. (2022). Viscoelastic hemostatic assays: a primer on legacy and new generation devices. *J Clin Med, 11,* 860.

151. Freson, K., & Turrot, E. (2017). High-throughput sequencing approaches for diagnosing hereditary bleeding and platelet disorders. *J Thromb Hemost, 15,* 1262–1272.

42

Hemostasis and Coagulation Instrumentation

Debra A. Hoppensteadt*

Debra A. Hoppensteadt*

OBJECTIVES

After completion of this chapter, the reader will be able to:

1. Describe methodologies in the hemostasis laboratory that were previously considered specialized but are now routinely available on clinical analyzers.
2. Identify the different assay endpoint detection techniques used for tests in the hemostasis laboratory.
3. Describe the advantages and disadvantages of each endpoint detection technique used in different assays.
4. Describe the differences among manual, semiautomated, and automated coagulation analyzers.
5. List common coagulation instrument flags that alert operators to specimen and instrument problems.
6. Identify characteristics that should be evaluated when selecting the appropriate coagulation analyzer for an individual laboratory setting.
7. Describe the different assays available for point-of-care coagulation testing.
8. Describe what is measured in global hemostasis assessment assays.
9. Define the similarities and differences between thromboelastography and rotational thromboelastometry.
10. State the advantages of using platelet function testing analyzers in the hemostasis laboratory and the capabilities of the different instrumentation.
11. Identify the role of flow cytometry in the hemostasis laboratory.
12. Describe the methods available for molecular testing in the clinical hemostasis laboratory and the analytes that can be measured using these techniques.
13. Develop a plan of action for the selection and evaluation of analyzers for the hemostasis laboratory.

OUTLINE

The Clinical Coagulation Laboratory
Historical Perspective
Assay Endpoint Detection Principles
Clot Endpoint
Chromogenic Endpoint
Immunologic Endpoint
Advantages and Disadvantages of Detection Methods
Coagulation Instrumentation and Technology Advancements
Improved Test Performance
Improved Specimen Management
Improved Reagent Handling
Quality Improvement Features

Selection of Coagulation Instrumentation
Currently Available Coagulation Instruments
Point-of-Care Coagulation Testing
Global Hemostasis Assessment
Platelet Function Testing
Platelet Aggregometers
Platelet Function Analyzers
Flow Cytometry
Molecular Genetic Testing in Coagulation

*The author extends appreciation to David L. McGlasson and Jo Ann Molnar, whose work in prior editions helped lay the foundation for this chapter.

CASE STUDY

After studying the material in this chapter, the reader should be able to respond to the following case study. Answers can be found in Appendix C.

A 65-year-old woman came to the hospital emergency department with swollen legs and shortness of breath. A chest x-ray and venogram were ordered. After reviewing the results, the physician made a diagnosis of deep vein thrombosis (DVT) and pulmonary embolism (PE). Shen was hospitalized and started on heparin. The following day, she was also given warfarin at 10 mg/day. On days 3 and 5 after starting warfarin, her blood was drawn for PT/INR. When the specimen arrived in the laboratory, it was centrifuged and was processed by an automated analyzer using photo-optical endpoint detection methodology. Results on day 3 were 20.7 sec/2.6 and results on day 5 were 7.3 sec/0.4 (flag).

Reference intervals and therapeutic target ranges can be found after the Index at the end of the book.

The laboratory's policy was to investigate all flagged results and retest all unusual coagulation results. On day 5, the PT/INR was repeated; similar values were obtained.

1. Should the operator report the test results as shown for day 5?
2. What action should the operator take to address the results of the specimen on day 5?
3. On day 5, would you expect this patient to be at risk for bleeding, based on these test results?

THE CLINICAL COAGULATION LABORATORY

The clinical coagulation laboratory is an ever-changing environment populated by automated analyzers that offer advances in specimen volume, test selection, and methodology.[1] For many years, the *routine* coagulation test menu consisted of only prothrombin time (PT) with the international normalized ratio (INR), partial thromboplastin time (PTT; also referred to as the activated partial thromboplastin time [APTT]), fibrinogen, and thrombin time assays (Chapter 41). Other tests, including all the newly identified hemostatic proteins, were considered *specialized,* and testing was performed in tertiary care institutions or reference laboratories employing medical laboratory scientists with high-level training.

With the introduction of new instrumentation and test methodologies, coagulation testing capabilities have expanded significantly, so many formerly specialized tests now can be performed routinely by general medical laboratory staff. New instrumentation has also made coagulation and expanded hemostasis testing more standardized, consistent, and cost effective.

Automation has not advanced, however, to the point of making coagulation testing foolproof or an exact science. Operators must develop expertise in correlating critical test results with the patient's diagnosis and when monitoring antithrombotic therapy. Selection and validation of assays and testing procedures, appropriate quality assurance practices, critical assessment of test results, and theoretical understanding of the hemostatic mechanisms are still required to ensure the accuracy and validity of test results so that health care providers can make an informed decision about patient care.

Historical Perspective

Laboratory assessment of blood clotting began in the 18th century with visual techniques. In 1780, Hewson, using a basin to collect the blood, determined that human blood clotted in 7 minutes. Scientists were also able to observe visible clot formation and turbidity of blood using the newly discovered microscope.[1,2]

Many advances in the assessment of blood clotting took place from 1822 to 1921 and included temperature control, detecting a clot as a resistance in the blood, and the use of different size glass tubes for visualizing clot formation. In the early 1900s, researchers monitored the length of time it took whole blood to clot in a glass tube while it was being tilted. A blood clot was defined as no spilling of the contents of the tube when the tube was tilted. This technique was the basis for the Lee-White clotting time test, the first means to standardize assessment of the coagulation system in a written procedure.

Plasma (usually platelet-poor plasma or plasma with a platelet count of less than 10,000/μL), anticoagulated with sodium citrate, came to replace whole blood in coagulation testing (Chapter 41). Except for a few specific coagulation tests (e.g., point-of-care testing, for which whole blood is still used), citrated plasma remains the specimen of choice for the largest volume of coagulation testing.

In 1920, Gram laid the groundwork for today's PT and PTT assays by adding calcium chloride to citrate anticoagulated plasma incubated at 37° C.[3] The assay endpoint was determined by the increasing viscosity of the plasma during fibrin monomer polymerization.

For many years, only the PT and PTT assays were performed in a clinical setting. Plasma and reagents were added to a glass tube held in a 37° C water bath, and clot formation was determined by visual inspection of the plasma as the tube was tilted while looking for the white strands of fibrin monomer formation. A stopwatch was used to determine the time to clot. This method is referred to as the *tilt-tube technique,* a simple and inexpensive technique that can still be found in use.

However, development of instrumentation for coagulation testing also occurred. In 1910, the first clot detection instrument, the "Koaguloviskosimeter," was developed by Kottman. This apparatus measured the change in the viscosity of blood as it clotted. This process generated a voltage change which, plotted against time, was the measure of clot formation. Using the principle of a change in viscosity as blood clots, Hartert developed the *thromboelastograph* (TEG; detailed in the "Global Hemostasis Assessment" section) in 1948. A related clot detection device based on sonar clot detection soon followed. Both devices are still in use today.[2]

In 1920, nephelometers were used for coagulation testing. These devices measure 90° light dispersion of a colloidal suspension. A change in light scatter measured over time determined the plasma clot formation.

The 1950s witnessed the development of the original instrument dedicated to coagulation assays, the *BBL Fibrometer.* This device detects a plasma clot by electromechanical technology. This advancement allowed laboratories to transition from manual methods to a semiautomated testing process. The Fibrometer became the mainstay instrument for clinical coagulation testing and remained so for many years. It can still be found in some coagulation laboratories, although it is no longer manufactured. Subsequent 20th-century innovations included other means to detect clots, the development of fully automated instrumentation, and enhancements with computerization and software innovations.

Today's hemostasis laboratory still employs clot-based assays for assessment of the coagulation cascade and single factors, but it has expanded. Additional testing options became necessary to quantitate the newly identified hemostatic proteins discovered in the late 20th century (Chapters 35 and 41).[4,5] The new analytes were first evaluated by clot-based tests, but improved accuracy was achieved turning to simple chemistry-type assays. The advent of a novel color endpoint methodology using synthetic substrates in place of the natural plasma protein substrate created test improvements that remain in place today. Early on, basic spectrophotometers were employed to read the optical density endpoints.

Further expansion of hemostatic testing led to the development of monoclonal antibodies for measurements of single proteins and other immunoassays for specific measurements. The detectors for these assays first used nephelometry as a means of determining the assay endpoint, or visual techniques were employed.

During the early period of hemostatic laboratory expansion multiple analyzers had to be purchased to offer clot-based, synthetic substrate-based, and immunoassay-based testing methods. Today's modern hemostasis clinical laboratory now incorporates all three endpoint mechanisms into one platform. Since 1990, instrument manufacturers have successfully applied multiple detectors to a single analyzer, which allows a laboratory to purchase and train the staff on only one instrument, providing both routine and specialized testing capabilities.[4,5]

Thus the clinical laboratory has grown and matured from the simple assessment of whole blood time to clot to highly advanced *multiprobe* instruments with robust accuracy and precision testing capabilities. These will be detailed in this chapter.

ASSAY ENDPOINT DETECTION PRINCIPLES

Instrument methodologies used for coagulation and hemostasis testing are classified into three groups based on the endpoint detection principle (Box 42.1).

Instruments for assessing coagulation function (*clot formation*), such as with the PT and PTT assays, apply detection principles that identify clot formation by either "observing" the clot (optical and nephelometric devices) or "sensing" the clot (mechanical and viscosity devices). Today, photo-optical detection is the most commonly employed endpoint to detect plasma clots.

In addition to the clotting assays, hemostasis laboratories now have the need to detect other assay endpoints. A second category of instrument uses a spectrophotometer type of detector. This determines endpoints of the *chromogenic* (colorimetric)

BOX 42.1 Endpoint Detection Principles Used in Coagulation Analyzers

Clot-Based Assays
Mechanical (physical)
Photo-optical (turbidometric)
Viscoelastic (physical)

Chromogenic Assays
Spectrophotometric

Immunoassays
Nephelometric
Spectrophotometric (light absorbance)
Chemiluminescent
Other

assays that assess the function of individual hemostatic proteins, such as antithrombin.

A third category of instrument commonly found in hemostasis laboratories today is one used to determine the endpoint of *immunoassays*. These assays indicate quantity and not function of the hemostatic parameter. Depending on the manufacturer of the assay, one of several assay endpoints can be used that will require a detector for light (color), agglutination of antigen-antibody complexes, fluorescence, chemiluminescence, or radiation.

Clot Endpoint
Mechanical Clot Endpoint Detection

Electromechanical clot detection systems measure a change in conductivity between two metal electrodes in plasma. The BBL Fibrometer was the first semiautomated instrument to be used routinely in the clinical coagulation laboratory. The probe of this instrument has one stationary and one moving electrode. During clotting, the moving electrode enters and leaves the plasma at regular intervals. When a clot forms, the fibrin strand conducts current between the electrodes, even when the moving electrode exits the solution. The current completes a circuit that stops the timer.[6,7]

Another mechanical clot detection method uses a magnetic sensor that monitors the movement of a steel ball within the test plasma. Two principles are used for this type of mechanical clot detection in routinely used coagulation instruments. In one system, an electromagnetic field detects the oscillation of a steel ball within the plasma-reagent solution.[3] As fibrin strands form, the viscosity starts to increase, slowing the movement (Figure 42.1). When the oscillation decreases to a predefined rate, the timer stops, indicating the clotting time of the plasma. This methodology is found on all Diagnostica Stago analyzers.

In the second system, a steel ball is positioned in an inclined well. The position of the ball is detected by a magnetic sensor. As the well rotates, the ball remains positioned on the incline. When fibrin forms, the ball is swept out of position. As it moves away from the sensor, there is a break in the circuit, which stops the timer. This technology can be found on AMAX and Destiny instruments distributed by Tcoag and on the original Hemochron ACT (activated clotting time test) instruments.

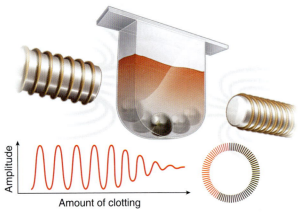

Figure 42.1 Electromechanical Clot Detection. In this example, a steel ball oscillates in an arc from one side of the cuvette holding patient plasma to the other. Movement is monitored continuously within a magnetic field. As the specimen clots, viscosity rises and movement of the steel ball is impeded. A timer is stopped when the variation in plasma viscosity, measured as amplitude, reaches a predetermined threshold, indicating the clotting time. (From Rodak, B. F., et al. [2013]. Hematology - E-Book: *Clinical Principles and Applications*, [4th ed]. Elsevier.)

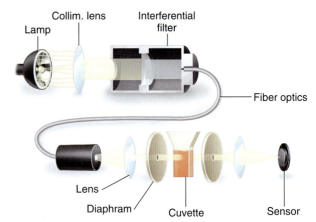

Figure 42.2 Photo-Optical (Turbidometric) Clot Detection. Polychromatic light is focused by a collimator lens (*Collim. lens*) and filtered to transmit a selected wavelength. Monochromatic light is transmitted by fiber optics and focused on the reaction cuvette, where the plasma specimen is held. As fibrin forms, opacity increases and the intensity of light reaching the sensor decreases. (From Rodak, B. F., et al. [2013]. Hematology - E-Book: *Clinical Principles and Applications*, [4th ed]. Elsevier.)

Photo-Optical Clot Endpoint Detection

Coagulation instruments often use a photo-optical (turbidometric) system that detects a change in light transmittance through plasma during the clotting process in which *turbidity* of the specimen increases. Light of a specified wavelength, typically a fixed wavelength between 500 and 600 nm, passes through plasma, and its intensity (optical density [OD]) is recorded by a photodetector over the period of clot formation (Figure 42.2).[8] The color and clarity of the specimen can affect the OD; therefore the pretest OD of each specimen is obtained to establish a baseline. Formation of fibrin strands causes light to scatter, allowing less light to fall on the photodetector, generating a decrease in OD (transmitted light), which becomes less as the clot becomes denser. When the OD decreases to a predetermined variance from baseline, the timer stops, indicating clot formation. Because the baseline OD is subtracted from the final OD, effects of lipemia and icterus are minimized.[9] Most of the automated and semiautomated coagulation instruments developed since 1970 use photo-optical clot detection.

Viscoelastic Clot Detection

The *viscoelastometry* (VET) technique used in the past to detect clot formation by an increase in blood viscosity linked with mechanical tension created by the clot is still used today. These instruments are dedicated for *whole blood* clotting assays. The assays on VET instrumentation are not high volume. But the benefit of these assays is that by their design, they provide a considerable amount of information about the entire blood clotting process not available by any other type of coagulation testing device. All coagulation instruments only detect the time to a final formed clot. In contrast, VET instruments provide information on the time to clot initiation, kinetics of clot formation, clot strength, fibrinolytic activity, and the individual contribution of platelets and fibrinogen.[10,11] VET instrumentation is detailed in the "Global Hemostasis Assessment" section.

Chromogenic Endpoint

Assays with a chromogenic endpoint are assays that apply basic enzymology. Enzymes are proteins that catalyze most of the chemical reactions in the body. The chemical compound upon which the enzyme exerts its catalytic activity is called a substrate. Proteolytic enzymes act on their natural substrates by hydrolyzing a peptide bond to give subunits of the substrate. A chromogenic assay uses a synthetic replica of the peptides of the natural substrate at the site of the proteolytic hydrolysis, or cleavage, by the enzyme (Figure 42.3).[12–16] The reaction of the assay mimics the specific enzyme-substrate reaction in the body.

Chromogenic (*synthetic substrate, amidolytic, colorimetric*) assays are simple chemical reactions that have a color (most often yellow) endpoint. Chromogenic methodology uses a synthetic small peptide (oligopeptide) substrate conjugated to a chromophore, usually paranitroaniline (pNA). Chromogenic analysis is a means for measuring the *activity* of a specific coagulation factor because it exploits the factor's enzymatic (protease) property.

For example, to quantitate thrombin, the synthetic substrate will consist of the amino acid sequence within fibrinogen corresponding to the active enzymatic site where thrombin acts. The hemostatic factor cleaves the chromogenic substrate at the site where the oligopeptide binds to the pNA, freeing the pNA. Free pNA is yellow, whereas bound pNA is clear. The OD of the solution is proportional to protease activity and is measured by a photodetector at 405 nm. Simple spectrophotometers can be used for endpoint detection.

Assays for hemostatic proteins are often available for both clot-based and chromogenic-based endpoints, such as for protein C. However, functional assays for certain hemostatic proteins, such as parameters of the fibrinolytic system, are only available on the chromogenic substrate platform. On the other hand, some analytes such as protein S are only available using

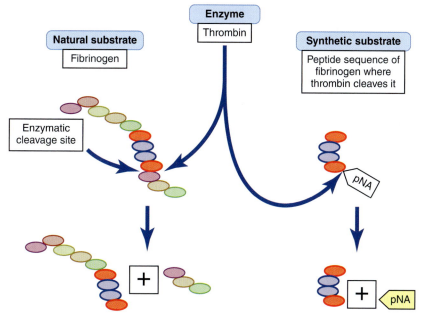

Figure 42.3 Chromogenic Substrate Assay. An illustration of the design of a chromogenic assay that uses a synthetic substrate. By mimicking the active enzymatic site on the natural substrate, the synthetic substrate provides for a specific and functional reaction of the enzyme-substrate combination. Many chromogenic assays use paranitroaniline (pNA) as the chromophore. This produces a yellow color after the enzyme cleaves it off the oligopepetide, signaling the assay endpoint.

clot-based technology. Chromogenic assays have become standard in clinical coagulation.

Examples of hemostatic assays using the chromogenic substrate principle are given in previous chapters (Figures 39.6, 41.12, 41.13, and 41.14). The activity of coagulation enzymes is measured by direct or indirect chromogenic methods:

- *Direct chromogenic assay:* OD is proportional to the activity of the analyte being measured. For instance, protein C activity is measured by a chromogenic substrate specific for activated protein C (Figure 39.7).
- *Indirect chromogenic assay:* The protein or analyte being measured inhibits a target enzyme. It is the target enzyme that has activity directed toward the chromogenic substrate. The greater the inhibition of the target enzyme, the less target enzyme there is available to react with the substrate. The change in OD is thus *inversely* proportional to the concentration or activity of the substance being measured. This principle is illustrated by heparin quantitation using the antifactor Xa assay (Figure 40.5).

Immunologic Endpoint
Nephelometric Endpoint Detection

Nephelometry is a modification of photo-optical endpoint detection in which 90° or forward-angle *light scatter*, rather than OD, is measured. A light-emitting diode produces incident light at approximately 600 nm, and a photodetector detects variations in light scatter at 90° (side scatter) and 180° (forward-angle scatter) (Figure 42.4).

The original use of nephelometry in the coagulation laboratory was an adaptation to measure the dynamics or kinetics of clot formation. As fibrin polymers form, side scatter and forward-angle light scatter increase.[17,18] The timer stops when

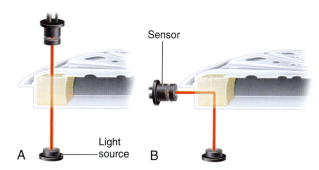

Figure 42.4 Nephelometric Clot Detection. **(A)**, For forward-angle light scatter detection, light from below passes through the patient plasma specimen in a cuvette *(yellow area)* to the detector above. **(B)**, For side scatter light detection, as fibrin polymerizes, light is deflected and is detected at a right angle from the original path. (From Rodak, B. F., et al. [2013]. Hematology - E-Book: *Clinical Principles and Applications*, [4th ed]. Elsevier.)

scatter reaches a predetermined intensity, and the time to clot interval is recorded. When continuous readings are taken throughout the clotting period, the entire clotting sequence is measured to completion, and a clot curve or "signature" is produced.

Nephelometry was the first technique applied to immunoassays, an application that can still be found today. As antigen-antibody complexes (immune complexes) are formed, they agglutinate and precipitate, and the resulting turbidity scatters the incident light.[17–20] In reactions in which the immune complexes are known to be too small for detection, the antibodies are first attached to microlatex particles.

Nephelometry is often used in today's high-volume, complex, automated coagulation instruments (coagulometers) that allow for multiple-assay coagulation profiles using both clot-based assays and immunoassays on one platform.

Light Absorbance Endpoint Detection

Immunologic assays are the most recently developed assays available for routine coagulation testing. These assays are based on antigen-antibody reactions. In slight contrast to the nephelometry principle that uses a light scatter endpoint, another common means to detect an endpoint in an immunoassay is to use *light absorbance*.

Latex microparticles are coated with antibodies directed against the selected analyte (antigen). Monochromatic light passes through the suspension of latex microparticles. When the wavelength is greater than the diameter of the particles, only a small amount of light is absorbed.[21] When the coated latex microparticles come into contact with their antigen, however, the antigen attaches to the antibody, causing the particles to agglutinate. As the diameter of the agglutinates increases relative to the wavelength of the monochromatic light beam, light is absorbed. The increase in light absorbance is proportional to the size of the agglutinates, which in turn is proportional to the antigen level.

Immunoassay technology became available on coagulometers in the 1990s and is used to measure a growing number of coagulation factors and proteins, such as D-dimer. These assays, which used to take hours to perform using traditional manual, time-consuming antigen-antibody detection methodologies (e.g., enzyme-linked immunosorbent assay [ELISA] or electrophoresis), now can be done in minutes on an automated analyzer.

ADVANTAGES AND DISADVANTAGES OF DETECTION METHODS

Operator expertise in performing quality testing and interpreting results is a key component of a professional hemostasis laboratory. Attention to technical issues is an important consideration in coagulation laboratory testing. Table 42.1 summarizes advantages and disadvantages of the different detection methodologies, which represent essential aspects of test result evaluation taken by the laboratory director.

Importantly, all coagulation tests that use clot-based endpoints need special considerations with result interpretation. There are many variables that affect coagulation function. It is important to always consider that the *integrity of the entire coagulation cascade* is relevant to the final test result, even if only one factor is being evaluated. Thus all clot-based assays are not highly specific. On the other hand, chromogenic or immunologic endpoint assays that do not rely on the coagulation cascade are single analyte specific.

Of particular interest to directors of hemostasis laboratories is that assays based on a chromogenic endpoint can play a useful role evaluating specimens from patients who have circulating inhibitors or who are on anticoagulant treatment. Clot-based assays will show effects of all substances that interfere in the coagulation cascade; thus routine PT/INR and PTT assays may

---

TABLE 42.1   Advantages and Disadvantages of Detection Systems of Hemostatic Analyzers

Endpoint Detection Method	Advantages	Disadvantages
Mechanical	Detects functional activity No interference from specimen lipemia or bilirubinemia Specimen and reagent volumes as small as 25 μL in some instruments Able to detect weak clots	Reliance on the integrity of the entire coagulation cascade Inability to observe graph of clot formation
Photo-optical	Detects functional activity Good precision Increased test menu flexibility and specimen quality information when multiple wavelengths are used Ability to observe graph of clot formation with some instrumentation	Interference from lipemia, hemolysis, bilirubinemia, and increased plasma proteins; has been addressed by some manufacturers with readings from multiple wavelengths May not detect short clotting times owing to long lag phase May not detect small weak clots that are translucent
Chromogenic	Detects functional activity Ability to measure proteins that do not clot More specific than clot-based assays Expanded test menu options Replaces clot-based assays affected by preanalytical variables	Limited by wavelength capabilities of some instruments May need large test volume to be cost effective
Immunologic	Ability to automate tests previously available only using manual, time-consuming methods Expanded test menu options	Does not detect functional activity Limited number of automated tests available Higher cost of instruments and reagents Need to have additional instruments in laboratories without automated coagulation analyzers that have random access capability
Nephelometric (for immunoassays)	Ability to measure antigen-antibody reactions for proteins in small concentrations	Does not detect functional activity Limited number of tests available Higher cost of reagents Need for special staff training

not provide accurate results. However, the specificity of chromogenic assays allows for targeted evaluation of the analyte in question. For chromogenic assays, the test is isolated to the specific chemical (enzymatic) reaction in question. For instance, patients on warfarin therapy who have a lupus anticoagulant cannot be monitored by the PT/INR because of interference from the circulating inhibitor. The chromogenic factor X assay is thus employed. In addition, heparin anticoagulation is more effectively monitored using the chromogenic antifactor Xa heparin assay rather than the PTT because of the nonheparin coagulation effects detected by the PTT.

Another important distinction between detection methods is that some assay endpoints reveal *functional* properties of the hemostatic protein, whereas other assay endpoints associate only with *quantitation* of the protein, with no information on functionality. Assays that use clot and chromogenic endpoints demonstrate the functional activity of the hemostatic protein because its mechanism of action is evaluated. Immunoassays, including those using nephelometry, do not demonstrate function of the hemostatic protein; these assays only quantitate that protein.

Clot detectors using photo-optical endpoint detection are commonplace and useful. However, test results can be confounded by icteric (bilirubinemia) or lipemic specimens, which erroneously prolong the clotting time because of a masking of the change in OD by the color or turbidity of the specimen. Many optical systems use multiple wavelengths that discriminate and filter out the effects of icterus and lipemia. Additionally, some of these coagulation instruments may be unable to use PT and PTT reagents manufactured with synthetic material because the high translucency of the reagents generates a plasma clot that is not detected by certain instruments.[22]

There are several important advantages of mechanical clot-based methods, as opposed to photo-optical clot-based methods. Test results are not affected by icteric or lipemic plasma. Mechanical methods, such as the movement of a steel ball in an electromagnetic field, also provide a sensitive endpoint able to detect weak clots, such as those formed in plasmas with low fibrinogen where clots are not stable.

Hemolysis, icterus, and lipemia interference in chromogenic assays is limited because of the dilution of the patient sample and the multiple wavelengths incorporated into the instrument for correction. New coagulation instrumentation is equipped with modules that detect these interfering substances and flag the specimens to prevent the reporting of erroneous results.[23–25]

COAGULATION INSTRUMENTATION AND TECHNOLOGY ADVANCEMENTS

Coagulometers are manual, semiautomated, or automated (Table 42.2). Manual and semiautomated coagulometers require that the operator delivers test plasma and reagents manually to the reaction cuvette and limit testing to one or two specimens at a time. Manual result recording and calculation of the results are also done. The use of manual and semiautomated coagulometers requires considerable operator time and expertise. These are relatively inexpensive instruments, and they are useful for low-volume clinical laboratories and research laboratories.

Significant advances have been made in the capability and flexibility of automated coagulation instrumentation. Current technology allows a "walkaway" environment. After specimens and reagents are loaded and the testing sequence is initiated, the operator can move on to perform other tasks. Fully automated analyzers provide pipetting systems that automatically transfer reagents and test plasma to reaction vessels and measure the endpoint without operator intervention. Multiple specimens can be tested simultaneously. Automated coagulometers are expensive, and laboratory staff require specialized training to operate and maintain them.

Regardless of technology, all automated and semiautomated analyzers offer better coagulation testing accuracy and precision than the manual methods. Clot endpoint detection methods have remained consistent through the years, but with the advent of chromogenic- and immunologic-based assays, other instrumentation needed to be brought into the coagulation laboratory. Multiple methodologies are now incorporated into single analyzers. From instruments that performed only clot-based assays, clinical laboratory instruments have been developed that

TABLE 42.2	Levels of Coagulation Instrumentation Automation	
Level	**Description**	**Examples**
Manual	All reagents and specimens are transferred manually to the instrument by the operator. Temperature is maintained by a water bath or heat block; external measurement by the operator may be required. Endpoint is determined visually by the operator. Timer is initiated and stopped by the operator. Data management is performed manually.	Tilt tube Wire loop
Semiautomated	All reagents and specimens are transferred manually to the instrument by the operator. Instrument usually contains an internal device for maintaining constant 37° C temperature. Analyzer may internally monitor temperature. Instrument has a mechanism to initiate a timing device automatically on addition of final reagent and a mechanism for detecting clot formation and stopping the timer. Data management is performed manually.	Fibrometer STart 4 Cascade M and M-4 BFT-II KC1 and KC4
Automated	All reagents are automatically pipetted by the instrument. Specimens may or may not be automatically pipetted. Analyzer contains monitoring devices to detect any mechanical malfunction. There is an internal mechanism to maintain and monitor a constant 37° C temperature throughout the testing sequence. Timers are initiated and clot formation is detected automatically. Data management is handled electronically.	ACL TOP STA-R Evolution STA Compact Sysmex CA-series BCS XP

perform both clot-based and chromogenic-based assays.[26–33] The most recent advancement has been the development of a single multiprobe instrument that performs clot, chromogenic, and immunologic assays on one platform.[29–33]

Many technical advances have greatly improved specimen, reagent, data management, and test performance, and have increased throughput, as will be detailed.

Improved Test Performance
Accuracy and Precision
In the days of visual methods, coagulation assays were performed in duplicate to reduce the coefficient of variation, which generally exceeded 20%. Semiautomated instruments improved upon precision, but the requirement for manual pipetting of plasma and reagents continued to necessitate duplicate testing. With the advent of fully automated instruments, precision improved to the extent that duplicate testing is no longer necessary, decreasing material and reagent costs. Assays are performed with confidence because coefficients of variation of less than 5% are typically achieved and even less than 1% for some tests (Jo Ann Molnar, personal communication, 2020).

Random Access Testing
Automated coagulometers provide random access testing. Through simple programming, a variety of tests can be run in any order on single or multiple specimens within a testing sequence. Previous automated analyzers were capable of running only one or two assays at a time, so batching was necessary. The disadvantage was that specimens with multiple orders had to be handled multiple times and *stat testing* (the highest priority, with results needed immediately to manage a medical emergency) could be challenging. For current automated analyzers, the ability to run multiple tests is limited only by the number of reagents that can be stored in the analyzer and the instrument's ability to simultaneously interweave tests that require different endpoint detection methodologies (clot, chromogenic, and/or immunologic). Random access benefits include improved turnaround times, reduced errors, and reduced labor costs.[28–32]

Improved Specimen Management
Primary Tube Sampling
A new design feature of today's coagulometers is sampling from the primary blood collection tube. After centrifugation, the blood collection tube, called the *primary tube,* is placed directly on the instrument without separating the plasma into a secondary tube. Instruments often accommodate multiple tube sizes. Significant time saving occurs as a result of elimination of the extra specimen preparation steps, and errors resulting from mislabeling of the aliquot tube are reduced.[28–32]

Closed-Tube Sampling
Closed-tube sampling of specimens has improved the safety and efficiency of coagulation testing. After centrifugation, the operator places the primary blood collection tube on the analyzer without removing the blue stopper. The cap is pierced by a needle with in the instrument that aspirates plasma. The specimen aspiration probe is incorporated with a sensor that recognizes the presence of liquid and stops at the optimized liquid level, between 4 and 250 μL. This allows aspiration of the specimen to occur without disturbing the cell layer. Crossover between specimens is eliminated by washing the needle between specimens with a rinse solution.[28–32]

Not only does closed-tube sampling save staff time, it also reduces the risk to the staff of specimen exposure through aerosols or spillage. An added advantage for stability of coagulation proteins is that closed-tube sampling promotes plasma pH stabilization. When closed-tube sampling is used as a measure of quality assurance, specimens are visually checked for clots after centrifugation by looking for the presence of fibrin strands. For example, if the assay result is a short clotting time or the corresponding coagulation tracing (available on some instruments) is abnormal, the staff rims the specimen with wooden sticks to determine if a clot was present (Jo Ann Molnar, personal communication, 2020).

Automatic Dilutions
Many instruments automatically perform multiple dilutions on patient specimens, calibrators, or controls, eliminating the need for the operator to perform this task manually. This reduces the potential for dilution errors. These conditions can be automatically programmed into the individual test setups on the analyzer.[28–32]

Improved Reagent Handling
Reduced Reagent and Specimen Volumes
Automated and semiautomated coagulometers now have the capability to perform tests on smaller specimen volumes. Traditionally, PT assays required 100 μL of patient plasma and 200 μL of thromboplastin/calcium chloride reagent. PTT was performed using 100 μL of plasma, 100 μL of activated partial thromboplastin, and 100 μL of calcium chloride. Modern analyzers can perform the same tests using half or even one-quarter the traditional volumes of reagents and patient specimen. This promotes the use of smaller specimen volumes, especially beneficial for pediatric patients and those from whom specimens are difficult to draw. Reagent costs are also reduced (Jo Ann Molnar, personal communication, 2020).

Open Reagent System
Laboratory directors want the flexibility of selecting reagents that best suit their needs and prefer not to be restricted in their choices by the analyzer being used. Recognizing that the ability to select reagents independent of the analyzer is a high priority, instrument manufacturers have responded by developing systems that provide optimal performance with the variety of coagulation test reagents available from themselves as well as alternative manufacturers, provided that the reagents are compatible with the instrument's methodology (Jo Ann Molnar, personal communication, 2020).

Reagent Tracking
Many automated instruments keep records of reagent lot numbers and expiration dates, which makes it easier for the laboratory to maintain reagent integrity and comply with regulatory

requirements. An additional feature on current instrumentation includes onboard monitoring of reagent volumes, with flagging systems to alert the operator when an insufficient volume of reagent is present in relation to the number of specimens programmed to be run. Reagent bar coding supports record keeping by tracking reagent properties and enabling the operator to load reagents onto the coagulometer without stopping specimen analysis.[26,30–33]

Quality Improvement Features

Expanded Computer Capabilities

The advanced coagulometers manufactured today use computer control to a lesser or greater extent. For the highly advanced coagulation analyzers, the computer circuitry incorporates internal data storage and retrieval systems. Hundreds of results can be stored, retrieved, and compiled into cumulative reports. Multiple calibration curves can be stored and accessed. Quality control files can be stored.[28–32]

These features serve to eliminate the time-consuming task of manually logging and graphing quality control values. Westgard rules can be applied and failures automatically flagged. Some analyzers feature automatic repeat testing when failures occur on the initial run. The quality control files can be reviewed or printed on a regular basis to meet regulatory requirements (Jo Ann Molnar, personal communication, 2020).

Computerization provides for programming flexibility of modern analyzers that has enhanced the opportunities to provide expanded test menus. Most advanced analyzers are preprogrammed with several routine test protocols ready for use. Specimen and reagent volumes, incubation times, and other testing parameters do not need to be determined by the operator but can be changed easily when necessary. Additional tests can be programmed into the analyzer by the user whenever needed, which allows for enhanced flexibility of the analyzer and reduces the need for laboratories to have multiple instruments.

Instrument interfacing to a laboratory information system (LIS) and bar coding capabilities have become a priority as facilities of all sizes endeavor to reduce dependence on manual record keeping. Bar coding is now found on patient specimen labels, reagents, and quality control material. The LIS computer system helps manage laboratory data by inputting, processing, and storing quality control and patient test result information. Bidirectional interfaces improve the efficiency through the ability of the instrument to send bar code information to the LIS and receive a response listing the tests that have been ordered. This eliminates the need for the operator to program each specimen and test. Additional features of the LIS are enhanced data integrity and improved laboratory operation with reduced staff time and effort.[28–32]

Flagging

Automated checks by the instrument ensure proper test performance and specimen quality.[28–33] Flags (alerts or alarms) can be related to analyzer function, material, test completion, quality control, maintenance, and LIS. A selection of common instrument flags is given in Box 42.2.

BOX 42.2 Warning Flags Available on Coagulometers

Instrument Malfunction Flags
Temperature error
Photo-optics error
Mechanical movement error
Probe not aspirating

Sample Quality Flags
Lipemia
Hemolysis
Icterus
Abnormal clot formation
No endpoint detected

When preset criteria have been exceeded, results are flagged, alerting the operator of a noncompliance issue. Particular specimen quality set points, such as the following, are important for valid coagulation test results:

- *Clotted specimen:* Will cause falsely shortened clotting time result because of premature activation of coagulation factors and platelets that generate FVIIa and thrombin.
- *Lipemia:* Can cause falsely prolonged clotting times on OD-sensing instruments because of interference with light transmittance.
- *Hemolysis:* Can cause falsely shortened clotting times because of premature activation of coagulation factors and platelets that generate FVIIa and thrombin.
- *Icterus (bilirubinemia):* Can interfere with OD-sensing instruments.
- *Abnormal clot formation:* Can lead to falsely elevated clotting times because of instrument inability to detect an endpoint.
- *No endpoint detected:* Indicates that the instrument was unable to detect clot formation; the specimen may need to be tested using an alternative type of instrument.

Reflex Testing

Reflex testing is the automatic ordering/performing of tests based on preset parameters or based on the results of prior tests. Instruments can make additional dilutions if the initial result is outside established linearity limits, or supplementary tests can be run automatically if clinically indicated by the initial test result. The first result does not wait for review and approval by the operator before followup action is initiated automatically by the instrument.[30–33]

Kinetics of Clot Formation

Graphing the kinetics of clot formation is provided on some analyzers, such as the ACL TOP from Werfen. The graph is generated by an algorithm used to convert multiple raw optical measurements collected over the course of the assay into a final result. In addition to determining the time to clot, this instrument smooths the raw data into a visible curve and uses the curve to check for clot formation integrity. Multiple checks are automatically performed to ensure an accurate and reproducible result. If the data do not meet all acceptability criteria, an error flag is generated. The clot curve is examined to troubleshoot

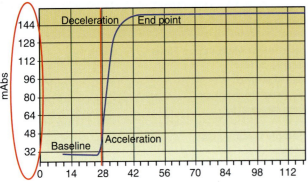

Figure 42.5 Clot Signature from the ACL TOP Coagulation Analyzer (Werfen). As the fibrinogen in the patient plasma specimen converts to fibrin and a solid clot, the change in light transmission through the specimen is recorded. The clot curve consists of baseline, acceleration phase, deceleration phase, and endpoint. The baseline is recorded before clotting occurs. Acceleration reflects clotting and is normally steep because clotting is rapid. The deceleration phase represents the later, decreasing rate of clot formation as the final available fibrinogen converts to fibrin. The endpoint is flat and stable, reflecting consumption of all fibrinogen. A key component in evaluating the clot curve is the absorbance (*mAbs*, milliabsorbance units), given on the *y*-axis, where a defined minimum identifies that a clot has developed. Absorbance plotted over time on the *x*-axis determines the time to clot endpoint of the test. Absorbance adjusts to compensate for baseline fibrinogen and interferences such as lipemia or icterus. (Clot Signature from the ACL TOP Family 50 Series Hemostasis Testing System. Courtesy Werfen, Bedford, MA.)

potential technical irregularities. The clot formation graph may also be used as a clot "signature" of the patient specimen that correlates with a disease state. Figure 42.5 shows an example of a typical clot curve.[30]

SELECTION OF COAGULATION INSTRUMENTATION

More than ever before, in today's clinical laboratory cost effectiveness, testing capabilities, and standardization are top priorities. Cost is not the only determining factor for hemostasis laboratory operation.

As an increasing number of tests become available, laboratories must determine which tests to incorporate to provide guidance to providers in diagnosis and treatment. Test selection has to include the decision to have a functional test or an immunoassay. If a functional test is selected, determine if a clot-based or a chromogenic-based test would be a more suitable fit. Identification of testing needs based on patient population should be the first step in the process. The decisions regarding which tests are the most appropriate for the clinical situations encountered by each laboratory should be made in conjunction with the medical staff. When that input has been obtained, the laboratory can determine the availability and cost of instruments that would meet those requirements.

An instrument should be matched to the anticipated workload. It may not be necessary to purchase a highly sophisticated analyzer capable of performing a large menu of tests if the setting is a smaller hospital laboratory with a low volume of orders for the less-routine tests. A batch analyzer with high throughput of the routine coagulation tests may be more appropriate for this

BOX 42.3   Selection Criteria for Hemostasis Instrumentation

Instrument cost
Consumables cost
Service availability and response time
Reliability and downtime
Maintenance requirements and time
Operator ease of use
Breadth of testing menu
Ability to add new testing protocols
Reagent lot to lot variation
Throughput for high-volume testing
Laboratory information systems (LIS) interface capabilities
Footprint (space the instrument occupies) and benchtop or floor model
Special requirements (water, power, waste drain)
Flexibility in using other manufacturers' reagents
Availability of a training program and continued training support

situation. The option to send out tests to a reference laboratory is always available.

Instrument selection criteria may include but are not limited to the items listed in Box 42.3. When the choices have been narrowed based on the most desirable criteria, consideration should be given to additional features. Table 42.3 summarizes some of the specialized features found on coagulation instrumentation. Because no instrument has all the desired features, prioritizing helps the laboratory focus on the capabilities that would be the most advantageous for them.

CURRENTLY AVAILABLE COAGULATION INSTRUMENTS

The heart of any clinical coagulation laboratory is the instrumentation that performs the high-volume tests of PT and PTT. Related clot-based assay availability and options for integrated chromogenic and immunoassays on the same platform are increasingly more common needs for the laboratory. Developments on today's coagulometers also address the increasing demand for improved efficacy of testing higher volumes, random access testing, and expanded test menus.

All analyzers perform routine testing quickly and efficiently. The challenges lie in determining which instruments should be considered for a particular laboratory setting and, when considering new instrumentation purchase, in developing an organized approach for instrument evaluation. Table 42.4 lists several of the clinical laboratory coagulation analyzers currently available, with key features highlighted by the manufacturer in the product information, which laboratory directors use for their initial decision making. Additional features not listed are PT/PTT specimen volumes, typically 50 μL or less, and capability to detect hemolysis and turbidity.[29-33]

The most recent development in hemostasis instrumentation is the ACL AcuStar (Werfen-IL) (Figure 42.6). By using state-of-the-art chemiluminescent technology, this instrument enhances accuracy and sensitivity of specialized hemostasis tests—tests that until now have required time-consuming manual processes and highly technical skills.[34] The AcuStar is fully automated with

TABLE 42.3   Specialized Features on Advanced Plasma Clot-Based Coagulometers

Instrument Feature	Comment
Random access	A variety of tests can be performed on a single specimen or multiple specimens in any order as determined by the operator.
Primary tube sampling	Plasma is directly aspirated from an open or a capped, centrifuged, blood collection tube by the analyzer.
Cap piercing	Analyzer aspirates plasma from the closed, centrifuged primary blood collection tube.
Bar coding	Reagents and specimens are identified with a bar code, eliminating manual information entry.
Bidirectional laboratory information system (LIS) interface	Analyzer queries the host computer via the LIS to determine which tests have been ordered. After verification results are sent from the analyzer to the host computer via the LIS.
Specimen and instrument flagging	Automated alerts indicate problems with specimen integrity or instrument malfunction.
Liquid level sensing	Operator is alerted when there is inadequate specimen or reagent volume for the number of tests ordered. An alert is also given when the instrument fails to aspirate the required specimen volume. Volume is verified each time a specimen or reagent is aspirated.
On-board quality control	Instrument stores and organizes quality control data; may include application of Westgard rules for flagging out-of-range results; instrument may transmit quality control data to the LIS.
Stat capabilities	Operator can interrupt a testing sequence to place a specimen next in line for testing.
On-board refrigeration of specimens and reagents	Refrigeration maintains the integrity of specimens and reagents throughout testing; allows reagents to be kept in the analyzer for extended periods reducing setup time.
On-board specimen storage capacity	Indicates the number of specimens that can be loaded at a time.
Reflex testing	Instrument can be programmed to perform repeat or additional testing under operator-defined circumstances.
Patient data storage	Test results can be stored for future retrieval; clot formation graphs may be included.
Throughput	Number of tests that can be processed within a specified interval, (usually number of tests per hour); depends on test mix and methodologies.
Total testing (dwell) time	Length of time from specimen placement in the analyzer until testing is completed; depends on the type and complexity of the procedure.
Graph of clot formation	Operator can visualize how the clot is formed over time.

continuous sample loading, self-contained onboard reagents, and a barcode reader. It has a 60 sample per hour throughput with rerun testing and result autovalidation features.

The current tests approved by the US Food and Drug Administration (FDA) on the AcuStar are immunoassays for D-dimer and heparin-induced thrombocytopenia (HIT) antibody. Future tests will include a panel for detection of antiphospholipid antibodies, screening and typing for von Willebrand disease (VWD), and an activity assay for *a d*isintegrin *a*nd *m*etalloprotease with a *t*hrombo*s*pondin type 1 motif, member *13* (ADAMTS13) to diagnose and monitor thrombotic thrombocytopenic purpura (TTP).

POINT-OF-CARE COAGULATION TESTING

Point-of-care (POC) instruments are typically handheld devices that permit near-patient testing during clinical procedures or surgeries, bedside testing for hospitalized patients, and self-testing for outpatients. In addition, these devices are used for testing in infants as the small specimen volume is an advantage. The instantaneous turnaround time of results, portability of the devices, and small specimen volume are conveniences appreciated by both providers and patients.

Table 42.5 summarizes the variety of POC devices and assays currently available.[29] Each device uses an individual patented technology and one of various endpoint detection techniques.[35–40] All devices are easy to use and provide test results quickly. Most devices, but not all, have a federal Clinical Laboratory Improvement Amendments (CLIA)-waived status. This means that because these devices only perform simple tests (not complex or moderately complex tests), they can be used outside of the clinical laboratory and performing the tests can be delegated to anyone (i.e., not limited only to certified laboratory scientists).

POC coagulation analyzers use whole blood specimens, eliminating the need for centrifugation, a time saver.[37] Most devices use capillary (fingerstick collection) whole blood, but some require anticoagulated whole blood (venipuncture collection).[29,39,40] Typically, a 10- to 50-μL whole blood specimen is transferred to a cartridge that contains the test reagents. After charging the cartridge with whole blood, it is immediately inserted into the POC test module.

POC coagulation testing has been in practice since 1966, with the introduction of the whole blood activated clotting time (ACT) assay used for heparin monitoring during cardiac surgery (Chapter 40).[39,40] The fast turnaround time of the ACT was necessary to allow for immediate heparin dosage changes, avoiding both bleeding and clotting in the patient and clotting of the extracorporeal cardiopulmonary bypass pump that serves as heart and lungs for the patient during the operation. At the conclusion of surgery, the high dose of heparin needed during the procedure is reversed with protamine. This reversal is also monitored with the ACT to ensure there is no residual heparin in the patient that can cause postoperative bleeding. The ACT is commonly used to this day in cardiac surgery and interventional cardiology.

A second common POC test is the PT/INR for monitoring the oral anticoagulant warfarin (Chapter 40).[29,35,37] Patients on warfarin therapy are required to be monitored monthly. In the outpatient setting, anticoagulation clinics can be high-volume users of POC testing. Having test results quickly available allows for dose adjustments at the same clinic visit and reduces patient wait time. Test devices for at-home use are also available.

The PTT has recently been developed for use on a limited number of POC devices, but this is not yet widely accepted.[29] The thrombin clotting time test and quantitation of fibrinogen levels would be beneficial as near-patient tests for trauma or surgical patient care. However, developing reliable POC adaptations of these traditional coagulation tests has proven to be challenging.[35–40]

Before a POC device is placed in service, laboratory scientists validate the results against the plasma-based assay performed in the central clinical laboratory, considered the reference coagulometer, method, and assay (Chapter 3). The whole blood ACT (never designed as a plasma-based assay) is validated in a different manner. In this instance, freshly collected patient specimens are immediately evaluated in a side-by-side comparison of the ACT device being validated and an established ACT device. Whole blood supplemented in vitro with heparin at varying concentrations is used to determine linearity.[40]

TABLE 42.4   Comparison of Available Clinical Coagulation Analyzers

Manufacturer and Instrument Name	Sample Handling System	Clot-Based Tests	Chromogenic Tests	Immunologic Tests	Methodologies Supported
Diagnostica Stago STA-R Max	Rack with continuous access	PT, PTT, TT, fibrinogen, reptilase, factors, protein C, protein S, lupus anticoagulant, DRVVT screen and confirm	Heparin (UFH, LMWH), protein C, AT, plasminogen, antiplasmin	D-dimer, VWF, total and free protein S, AT antigen	Mechanical clot detection; chromogenic; immunologic
Diagnostica Stago STA Max Compact	Continuous specimen access; primary tube	PT, PTT, TT, fibrinogen, reptilase, factors, protein C, protein S, lupus anticoagulant, DRVVT	Heparin (UFH, LMWH), protein C, AT, plasminogen, antiplasmin	D-dimer, VWF, total and free protein S, AT antigen	Mechanical clot detection
Helena Laboratories Cascade M-4	Manual	PT, PTT, fibrinogen, TT, FII, FV, FVII to FXII	None	None	Optical, turbidometric clot detection
Siemens BCS XP	10-tube specimen rack	PT, PTT, fibrinogen, TT, reptilase, factors, DRVVT screen and confirm, FV Leiden, protein C activity, protein S activity	Innovance AT, Berichrom AT, plasminogen, FVIII, antiplasmin, protein C, heparin	Innovance D-dimer	Optical clot detection; chromogenic; immunologic
Sysmex CA-620/660	10-tube specimen rack	PT, PTT, fibrinogen, TT, reptilase, protein C activity, factors	Innovance AT, Berichrom AT, protein C, heparin	Innovance D-dimer	Optical, turbidometric clot detection; chromogenic; immunologic
Sysmex CS-2500	10-tube sample rack × 5	PT, PTT, fibrinogen, TT, reptilase, factors, DRVVT screen and confirm, FV Leiden, protein C activity, protein S activity	Innovance AT, Berichrom AT, plasminogen, FVIII, antiplasmin, protein C, heparin	Innovance D-dimer	Optical, turbidometric clot detection; chromogenic; immunologic
Sysmex CS-5100	Rack	PT, PTT, fibrinogen, TT, reptilase, factors, DRVVT screen and confirm, FV Leiden, protein C activity, protein S activity	Innovance AT, Berichrom AT, plasminogen, FVIII, antiplasmin, protein C, heparin	Innovance D-dimer	Optical, turbidometric clot detection; chromogenic; immunologic
Werfen ACL TOP 350	Continuous rack loading	PT, PTT, fibrinogen, TT, factors, FVIII (with VWF)	Anti-FXa heparin, AT	D-dimer, D-dimer HS, HIT	LED optical clot detection; chromogenic; immunologic (turbidometric)
Werfen ACL TOP 550	Continuous rack loading	PT, PTT, fibrinogen, TT, factors, lupus (SCT and DRVVT), protein C, protein S, aPCR-V, FVIII (with VWF)	Anti-FXa heparin, protein C, AT, plasminogen, plasmin inhibitor	D-dimer, D-dimer HS, VWF, free protein S, FXIII antigen, homocysteine, HIT	LED optical clot detection; chromogenic; immunologic (turbidometric)
Werfen ACL TOP 750	Continuous rack loading	PT, PTT, fibrinogen, TT, factors, lupus (SCT and DRVVT), aPCR-V, protein C, protein S, FVIII (with VWF)	Anti-FXa heparin, protein C, AT, plasminogen, plasmin inhibitor	D-dimer, D-dimer HS, VWF, free protein S, FXIII antigen, homocysteine, HIT	LED optical clot detection; chromogenic; immunologic

Only US FDA-cleared tests are listed.

aPCR-V, Activated protein C resistance due to a mutation in the FV gene; *AT,* antithrombin; *DRVVT,* dilute Russell viper venom test; *F,* factor; *HIT,* heparin-induced thrombocytopenia; *HS,* high sensitivity; *LED,* light-emitting diode; *LMWH,* low molecular weight heparin; *PT,* prothrombin time; *PTT,* partial thromboplastin time; *SCT,* silica clotting test; *TT,* thrombin clotting time; *UFH,* unfractionated heparin; *VWF,* von Willebrand factor.

POC assays and the plasma-based central laboratory assays can show a weak correlation as a result of differences in instrumentation, reagents, and specimens. This knowledge is critical to apply to coagulation testing, and care must be taken to ensure that clinical decisions are accurate.[37] Typically, it is recommended to use one system for patient care and ease of comparing test results over time. For example, with warfarin monitoring, the POC device is used consistently, without switching between the central laboratory and POC. However,

any questionable result from a POC device is assessed using the central laboratory instrumentation and assay system, which provides the definitive value. In the case of warfarin monitoring, a POC-obtained INR that exceeds 6.0 or any unexpected INR change is also confirmed with a venipuncture blood specimen tested by the plasma-based assay in the central laboratory.

Nearly all POC devices have built-in quality control programs. The newer versions of POC devices include touch screen, wireless transmission of results in real time, and microblood volumes.[29]

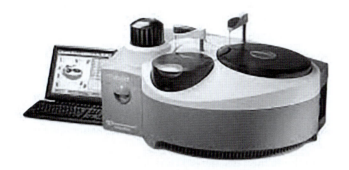

Figure 42.6 The ACL AcuStar (Werfen). The AcuStar is a fully automated instrument that performs highly sensitive immunoassays for hemostasis testing. It uses chemiluminescence endpoint detection to measure D-dimer and antibodies causing heparin-induced thrombocytopenia. (The ACL AcuStar Hemostasis Testing System. Courtesy Werfen, Bedford, MA.)

GLOBAL HEMOSTASIS ASSESSMENT

A technique that uses the *viscoelastic* property of blood clotting to evaluate the complete process of whole blood clotting was developed in 1948 and to this day, follows the same general format. The assay provides information on the entire kinetic process of whole blood clot formation. Not only is the singular clot endpoint determined as detected by today's coagulometers, but the initiation of thrombin generation, clot strength, contribution of fibrinogen, and fibrinolytic activity are also determined in one assay.[41–43] Furthermore, by using whole blood (not plasma) as the specimen, the contribution of platelets to the clotting process is measured. Additionally, the interactions of all blood cellular elements and blood proteins with coagulation factors in the clotting process can be observed.[41–43]

TABLE 42.5	Comparison of Point-of-Care Instruments for Coagulation Testing		
Manufacturer and Instrument	**Test**	**Specimen**	**Clot Detection Principle**
Abbott iSTAT	PT/INR, PTT, ACT	Venipuncture	Electrogenic
CoaguSense PT/INR Monitoring System	PT/INR	Fingerstick	Mechanical
Helena Actalyke Mini II	ACT	Venipuncture	2-point electromechanical
Helena Actalyke XL	ACT	Venipuncture	2-point electromechanical
Medtronic ACT Plus	ACT	Venipuncture	Mechanical
Medtronic HMS Plus	ACT, protamine titration	Venipuncture	Mechanical
Roche CoaguCheck XS	PT/INR	Venipuncture/fingerstick	Amperometric
Roche CoaguCheck XS Plus	PT/INR	Venipuncture/fingerstick	Amperometric
Roche CoaguCheck XS Pro	PT/INR	Venipuncture/fingerstick	Amperometric
Siemens Xprecia Stride	PT/INR	Fingerstick	Electrochemical with amperometric
Werfen GEM Hemochron 100	ACT	Venipuncture/fingerstick	Mechanical
Werfen Hemochron Signature Elite	PT/INR, PTT, ACT	Venipuncture/fingerstick	Mechanical

Only US FDA-cleared tests are listed.
ACT, Activated clotting time test; *INR,* international normalized ratio; *PT,* prothrombin time test; *PTT,* (activated) partial thromboplastin time test.

The VET technique assesses both bleeding and thrombosis risk. It is the only hemostatic assay that has the ability to indicate a hypercoagulable state. Results from VET assays define the global (entire) hemostatic status of patients. It has become particularly useful clinically for managing patients with hepatic disease, obstetrical disorders, trauma, and during liver transplantation or cardiac surgery. VET provides information that directs a health care provider to administer patient-specific products in terms of clotting factor or platelet replacement. In addition, VET results can be used to select anticoagulant, antiplatelet, or antifibrinolytic therapy as needed. Algorithms have been developed to aid in diagnosis and management. This practice has been shown to save both lives and cost.[41-43]

Devices are placed not only in the central laboratory but also POC in the operating room, emergency department, and trauma bays. Initial results are available within 10 to 20 minutes to aid in clinical decision making.

The original technology presents several challenges because results are operator dependent, training is required, attention to detail is required, and a level of skill is demanded to perform a quality assay. Result interpretation also requires skill, knowledge, and experience. However, new technical developments circumvent these issues. There are two instruments that offer VET testing: the original thromboelastograph (TEG) and a recent modification, the rotational thromboelastometry (ROTEM).

The TEG 5000 Thromboelastograph System (Haemonetics) uses either nonanticoagulated or citrated whole blood. The freshly collected specimen is pipetted into a cylindrical cup that oscillates by 4.75°. A stationary pin with a diameter 1 mm smaller than the cup's diameter is suspended by a torsion wire into the cup. Kaolin (or another activator) is added to trigger intrinsic pathway clotting. As the blood clots, fibrin links the pin to the cup and viscoelasticity changes are transmitted to the pin. The resulting pin torque generates an electrical signal from the torsion wire. The signal is plotted as a function of time to produce a TEG tracing. The tracing is analyzed to determine the *speed, strength,* and *stability* of clot formation and the downstream effect of fibrinolysis (Figure 42.7).[41-43] Through computerization, the trace furnishes real-time information about the evolving clot from platelet activation and initial fibrin formation through fibrin cross-linkage and fibrinolysis.[41] Two test channels are available on each instrument; manual pipetting is required. Assay kits are available for specific platelet function and other testing.

The new TEG 6s system (Haemonetics) is an easier platform to use which lends itself to trauma and surgical settings. The TEG 6s assesses clot viscoelasticity as in the TEG 5000 device, but the clotting endpoint is measured by resonance. A small amount of citrated or heparinized blood is automatically transferred to a microfluidic cartridge that contains reagents for multiple assays that can be performed simultaneously; manual pipetting of the specimen is not required. Blood is exposed to a fixed vibration (20 to 500 Hz) and light-emitting diode illumination detects vertical motion of the blood meniscus. Frequency is identified using a Fourier transformer, which is mathematically converted to a tracing that represents the same clot dynamics as for the TEG 5000.[44,45]

Similar to the TEG, the ROTEM *delta* (Werfen) uses a whole blood specimen and one of various coagulation activators manually pipetted into the cup. A suspended pin is immersed into the blood. The pin rotates (the cup is stationary) and, upon clot formation, the increased tension from fibrin binding the cup to the pin is detected by sensors. The tracing is recorded as the clot evolves over time. The recorded clot formation kinetics and measured parameters for the ROTEM are the same as for the TEG (see Figure 42.7). The TEG and ROTEM clot signatures and their parameters are directly compared in Table 42.6. Differences from the TEG system are that the ROTEM system is not sensitive to vibrations, and it has four test channels, a touch screen, and an automated manual pipettor. Differences between TEG and ROTEM also can be found in the quality control and instrument maintenance schedules.[46,47]

The ROTEM *sigma* (Werfen) is the newest version of the ROTEM. The same cup-and-pin technology is used as in its predecessor ROTEM *delta*, but the ROTEM *sigma* is designed to be

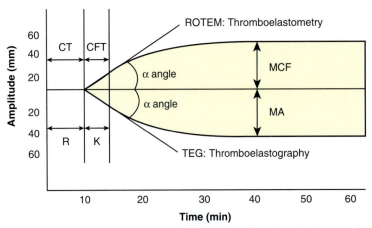

Figure 42.7 Clot Signature of Viscoelastometry (*VET*) Assays. The thromboelastograph *(TEG)* and the rotational thromboelastometry *(ROTEM)* instruments provide complete information on the dynamics of whole blood clot formation. TEG and ROTEM measured parameters from the kinetic reaction of clot formation are the same but are labeled differently, as shown in the diagram. Refer to Table 42.6 for explanation of the measured parameters.

a closed, fully automated system that includes a sample handler and reagent cartridges for several assays.[48]

Similar to TEG and ROTEM systems, the Quantra Hemostasis Analyzer (HemoSonics/Diagnostica Stago) measures the physical viscoelastic properties of whole blood clotting over time.[49] This whole blood analyzer has single-use disposable cartridges to perform whole blood tests. The device uses a patented high-frequency ultrasound technology based on sonic estimation of elasticity via resonance (SEER) or sonorheometry. Ultrasound pulses are sent to the whole blood sample, inducing a resonance and causing oscillation of the sample. As the blood clots, it increases in stiffness, resulting in an increase in oscillations. The clotting time and stiffness are measured from the evolving shear modulus, and transmitted data are extrapolated into final results similar to those given by the TEG and ROTEM.[49] Specified fibrinogen contribution and platelet contribution information is provided.

PLATELET FUNCTION TESTING

In addition to coagulation factor testing, clinical hemostasis laboratories have expanded their test menu to include assays that evaluate platelet function. The demand for rapid, cost-effective methods for the evaluation of platelet function has increased because of the need to monitor the efficacy of antiplatelet therapy such as aspirin, clopidogrel, and other ADP receptor antagonists used in patients with cardiovascular disorders (Chapters 37 and 40). In addition, preoperative evaluation of platelet function is important in hemostatic management, particularly if the patient has a history of bleeding or if the patient is on antiplatelet medication.[50]

Platelet function testing has been a challenge for the clinical laboratory because of the lack of reliable, accurate, and easy to perform assays. In addition, proper specimen procurement and handling for platelet function testing plays an important role in the reliability and accuracy of the test.

Platelet function historically has been assessed by the bleeding time test and platelet aggregation assays (Chapter 41). The bleeding time is highly dependent on the individual performing the test, and results can fail to correlate with intraoperative bleeding risk.[51–54] Thus the bleeding time test has been discontinued in most institutions. Platelet aggregometers are still in use, and several new devices are available to assess platelet function. The VET devices described in the previous section are another means of obtaining platelet function information.

Platelet Aggregometers

Classic platelet aggregometry using the light transmission principle was developed in 1962 by Born. This test system measures the increase in light transmission that occurs in direct proportion to platelet aggregation induced by various agonists (e.g., collagen, adenosine diphosphate [ADP], epinephrine) (Figures 41.3 and 41.4). The reduced amount of light able to be transmitted through a platelet-rich plasma (PRP) specimen is the baseline to compare with the increased light that is transmitted through a specimen with aggregated platelet clumps and clear plasma. Three test parameters are calculated for each specimen: maximum percentage aggregation, area under the curve, and velocity. Since its inception, platelet aggregation using PRP assays and *light transmission aggregation* (LTA) detection has been the primary means to assess platelet function.

In addition to LTA, platelet aggregation can be detected by impedance, luminescence, and light scatter. Platelet aggregation in whole blood uses the *impedance* principle. Upon activation, platelets become sticky and adhere to metal sensor wires (electrodes) (Figure 41.5).[55] The greater the platelet aggregate formation, the greater the impedance. The theoretical advantage of whole blood aggregometry is that it is a more physiologic test for measuring platelet aggregation in the presence of erythrocytes, leukocytes, and blood proteins. Incorporation of the *luminescence* detector and the luciferase reagent allows for the simultaneous assessment of platelet secretion and platelet aggregation (Figure 41.6).

Table 42.7 compares commonly used platelet aggregometers. The PAP-8E (BioData) is an eight-channel platelet aggregometer with a touch screen and on-screen procedure templates (Figure 42.8). It has a programmable pipette and an optional bar code scanner. The PAP-8E uses LTA and a small sample volume (225 μL). BioData also has a dedicated centrifuge for preparing the PRP specimen, the PDQ.[56] PRP can be

TABLE 42.6	Comparison of Clot Formation Kinetic Parameters Measured for the TEG and ROTEM		
Parameter*	**TEG**	**ROTEM**	**Comment**
Clot initiation or clotting time	R (reaction time)	CT (clotting time)	Time of initial clot formation. Initiation of thrombin generation.
Clot kinetics	K (clot formation time)	CFT (clot formation time)	A measure of the speed to reach a specific level of clot strength. Platelets, coagulation factors, thrombin generation, and fibrinogen contribute.
Angle (clot kinetics and clot strength)	α (angle in degrees)	α (angle in degrees)	Measure of the rate of clot formation; reflects the rate of fibrin formation and cross-linking. Thrombin-activated platelets, coagulation factors, fibrinogen, fibrin formation and polymerization, and FXIII contribute.
Clot strength	MA (maximum amplitude)	MCF (maximum clot firmness)	Measure of the strength of the clot. Platelets, fibrinogen, fibrin polymerization, and FXIII contribute.
Clot stability	Ly30 (clot lysis at 30 minutes as a ratio of MA)	CLI (clot lysis index)	Measure of the rate of amplitude reduction; clot stability/fibrinolysis.

*Refer to Figure 42.7 to visualize how the parameters are obtained.

TABLE 42.7	**Comparison of Platelet Aggregometers**		
Manufacturer	**BioData**	**Chrono-Log**	**Helena Laboratories**
Instrument	Platelet Aggregation Profiler (PAP-8E)	Whole Blood/Optical Lumi-Aggregation System (Model 700)	AggRAM
Detection	LTA	LTA; impedance; luminescence	LTA
Operation	Batch, random access	Batch, random access	Batch, random access
Reagents	Open reagent system, assay kits, reagents, controls, diluents, buffers	Open reagent system, assay kits, reference plasma, controls	Open reagent system
Specimen	PRP	Whole blood or PRP	PRP
Sample volume/test	225 µL	225 µL	225 µL
Model	Benchtop	Benchtop	Benchtop
Number of channels	8	2–4	4–8
Time required for maintenance	Weekly:15 min; Monthly: 30 min	30 min when optical calibration required	Daily: 15 min; Weekly: 15 min; Monthly: 1 hr

Only US FDA-cleared instruments are listed.
LTA, Light transmission aggregation; *PRP,* platelet-rich plasma.

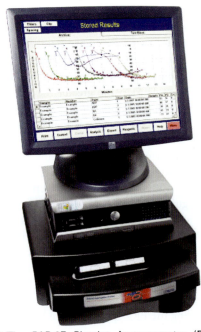

Figure 42.8 The PAP-8E Platelet Aggregometer (BioData). The PAP-8E is an eight-channel device that detects platelet aggregation by changes in light transmission through the platelet-rich plasma specimen; as platelets clump together, more light is able to pass through the cleared plasma. This instrument allows for the analysis of platelet function, measurement of ristocetin cofactor activity for detecting von Willebrand disease, identifying platelet function abnormalities such as heparin-induced thrombocytopenia, and monitoring antiplatelet therapy. (Courtesy BioData, Horsham, PA.)

prepared in 3 minutes, platelet-poor plasma can be prepared in 120 seconds, and platelet-free plasma can be prepared in 180 seconds, a time-saving improvement over the traditional centrifugation procedure.

Chrono-Log offers the Whole Blood/Optical Lumi-Aggregation System. The Model 700 aggregometer provides for platelet aggregation in whole blood or PRP while simultaneously measuring platelet secretion. Electrical impedance is used to detect whole blood aggregation, and optical density is used to detect platelet secretion by luminescence. The instrument can be configured as either a two- or four-channel aggregometer.[55] Either disposable or reusable electrodes can be used for impedance measurements. Chrono-Log instruments are also available with single and not the combined functions.

The AggRAM (Helena Laboratories) is a modular system for platelet aggregation and ristocetin cofactor testing using PRP. Its optics use a laser diode at a wavelength of 650 nm to enhance precision of the aggregation tracing.[57] The AggRAM has four channels capable of microvolume testing, customized result reporting, and internal quality control programs.

Platelet Function Analyzers
PFA-100

The PFA-100 Platelet Function Analyzer (Siemens) provides rapid results on quantitative and qualitative platelet abnormalities (Figure 42.9). Test cartridges contain membranes coated with collagen/epinephrine or collagen/ADP to stimulate platelet aggregation. Whole blood is aspirated under controlled flow conditions through a microscopic aperture in the membrane. The time required for a platelet plug to occlude the aperture is an indication of platelet function.[58] The PFA-100 detects von Willebrand disease and the efficacy of aspirin therapy.[59,60]

Verify Now

The Verify Now (Werfen) is an optical detection system that measures platelet aggregation by microbead agglutination (Figure 42.10). The system uses a disposable cartridge that contains lyophilized fibrinogen-coated beads and a platelet agonist specific for the test. Whole blood is dispensed from the blood collection tube directly into the device, with no blood handling or pipetting required by the operator. The instrument provides an aspirin assay using arachidonic acid as the test reagent and a $P2Y_{12}$ inhibitor assay (PRU test) using ADP as the test reagent for clopidogrel, prasugrel, and ticagrelor antiplatelet drugs.[61–65] Results, available in about 10 minutes, are used to determine if

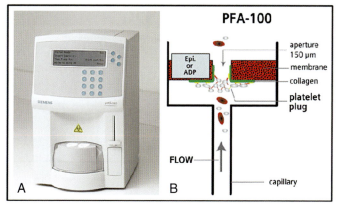

Figure 42.9 The Platelet Function Analyzer (PFA-100) (Siemens). **(A)**, The PFA-100 is an automated system that measures platelet function. **(B)**, The internal mechanics of the PFA-100 are shown. The induced high shear stress of whole blood flow simulates in vivo conditions; activators induce platelet adhesion and aggregation that close an aperture, signaling the assay endpoint. (Courtesy Siemens Medical Solutions USA, Inc.)

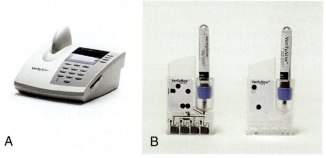

Figure 42.10 Verify Now (Werfen). The VerifyNow offers two tests to determine the level of antiplatelet therapy; one test is for aspirin and the second test is for P2Y$_{12}$ inhibitor drugs such as clopidogrel, prasugrel, and ticagrelor (PRU test). **(A)**, The device uses light transmission aggregometry (LTA) to detect microbead agglutination of fibrinogen-coated beads. **(B)**, A close-up of the reaction cartridge is shown. Sample preparation or pipetting is not required; the blood collection tube is placed directly into the reagent cartridge that is inserted into the device. (VerifyNow platelet-reactivity testing system. Courtesy Werfen, Bedford, MA.)

the antiplatelet therapy is within the therapeutic range. Drug dosing is modified if the platelet reactivity is too high (treatment is underdosed) or too low (treatment is over-dosed). This device can be placed in clinical laboratories or in surgical/procedure rooms for near-patient testing.

Plateletworks

The Plateletworks platelet function assay (Helena Laboratories) is a kit that can be run on any standard impedance cell counter found in the hematology laboratory (Chapter 13). Aggregation results are based on a platelet count before (high count) and after (lower count) platelet activation. Blood specimens are collected via venipuncture directly into tubes provided with the kit, which includes an ethylenediaminetetraacetic acid (EDTA) tube for the baseline specimen and tubes with different agonists to aggregate platelets. Testing requires 1 mL of whole blood for the baseline count and 1 mL whole blood for each additional agonist-containing reagent tube. Results can be obtained in 2 minutes. The Plateletworks platelet function

kit can be used for presurgical screening and to monitor antiplatelet therapy.[65]

Total Thrombus Formation Analyzer System

The Total Thrombus Formation Analyzer System (T-TAS 01, Diapharma) is an automated system for measuring thrombus formation. Single-use microchips evaluate platelet-specific (PL chip) and comprehensive (AR chip) thrombus formation.[66] The reaction takes place inside capillary channels of a microchip, where pressure differentials are measured. Using a small volume of benzylsulfonyl-D-Arg-Pro-4-amidinobenzylamide (BAPA) anticoagulated whole blood, platelets become activated by shear stress and specific activators, then adhere and aggregate to the walls of the microfluidic channels, causing occlusion of the blood flow. Sensors detect the change in pressure. The overall dynamics of thrombus formation and dissolution are quantified as area under the pressure-time curve. The T-TAS 01 evaluates a patient for bleeding. It is sensitive to acquired and hereditary dysfunction of primary platelet hemostasis as well as antiplatelet therapy. This device is only in use for research at this time.

Flow Cytometry

Flow cytometric assays are being developed for platelet function analysis. Flow cytometry offers several advantages over conventional platelet aggregation studies. Whole blood testing is performed, making for a more physiologic evaluation. Minimal specimen volumes are required (~5 μL/test), allowing for ease of testing pediatric and difficult-to-draw patients. The method is highly sensitive and able to capture platelet activity in patients with thrombocytopenia. In addition to the traditional platelet secretion and aggregation markers, flow cytometry can measure multiple platelet activation—dependent changes.[67-69] Platelet surface receptor upregulation, receptor activation, generation of cellular microparticles, and binding of platelets to leukocytes are some of the advanced measurements.[67-69] Flow cytometry assays are also available for the diagnosis of HIT.[70] At this time all platelet assays using flow cytometric analysis are laboratory-developed tests (LDTs).

MOLECULAR GENETIC TESTING IN COAGULATION

As our knowledge of the pathophysiology of hemostatic disorders improves, the genetic basis for many bleeding (Chapters 36, 37, and 38) and thrombotic (Chapter 39) defects is understood. With this knowledge, definitive diagnoses can be obtained through the use of molecular tests of the genome or proteome. Major advantages of molecular testing for hemostatic disorders are the high sensitivity and specificity of the assay format, as well as the lack of interference by anticoagulants or inhibitors that significantly hampers the clot-based coagulation assays.[71,72]

For thrombophilia, molecular testing is available for genetic mutations of factor V (FV Leiden), prothrombin (prothrombin G20210A), and methylene-tetrahydrofolate reductase (MTHFR). The American College of Medical Genetics and Genomics (ACMG) has recently recommended, however, that MTHFR testing should not be routinely performed for the

TABLE 42.8   Molecular Techniques for the Evaluation of a Hypercoagulable State

Assay	Accuracy	Throughput	Clinical Applications: GeneticMutations Detected
PCR/RFLP	Good	Limited	Factor V Leiden, prothrombin G20210A, MTHFR
PCR/ARMS	Excellent	Intermediate	Factor V Leiden, prothrombin G20210A, MTHFR
Light cycler	Excellent	Intermediate	Factor V Leiden, prothrombin G20210A, MTHFR
Array technology	Excellent	Very high	Factor V Leiden, prothrombin G20210A, MTHFR
Invader assays	Excellent	Limited	Factor V Leiden, prothrombin G20210A, MTHFR
Ligand-based technologies	Excellent	Very high	Factor V Leiden, prothrombin G20210A, MTHFR

ARMS, Amplification refractory mutation system; *MTHFR*, methylene-tetrahydrofolate reductase; *PCR*, polymerase chain reaction; *RFLP*, restriction fragment length polymorphism.

workup of patients with thrombophilia as the clinical relevance is not clear.[73]

For bleeding disorders, numerous inherited platelet abnormalities have been linked to specific genes or chromosomal locations (Tables 37.1 and 38.1). von Willebrand disease is a highly heterogeneous disease that can have alterations in von Willebrand factor (VWF) or in other genes involved in regulating the synthesis, processing, and secretion of VWF. The genetic mutations in factor VIII, factor IX, and other genes that cause hemophilia are being understood (Table 41.8).[72] Molecular testing for these disorders is now used to obtain a definitive diagnosis.

Many mutations that cause hemostatic disorders tend to be rare; therefore reference laboratories are most often used to perform the molecular testing. Clinical laboratories in medical centers, however, now can be equipped to perform molecular tests for higher volume orders such as for FV Leiden and the prothrombin mutation.

Several testing methods are available for the clinical laboratory (Table 42.8). The most common test methods are polymerase chain reaction (PCR)-based assays. PCR is accurate for the detection of both point mutations and single-nucleotide polymorphisms. FV Leiden, prothrombin G20210A, and MTHFR mutations are detectable by this method. A common method to analyze PCR products is restriction fragment-length polymorphism (RFLP) analysis. However, RFLP analysis is not a high-throughput method and is not suitable for high-volume laboratories.

Other methods for molecular testing in the clinical laboratory that are PCR based or not PCR based and do not require restriction digestion are also available.[71–74] A popular non–PCR-based method is the Invader assay, which uses allele-specific hybridization in a high-throughput format. In an effort to obtain rapid and reliable results, sequence-specific primers, allele-specific oligonucleotides, hybridization, rapid-cycle PCR using LightCycler instrumentation, and nanochips have been developed.

High-throughput sequencing (HTS) is available for the diagnosis of hereditary bleeding and platelet disorders. The traditional sequencing information used a low-throughput technique called Sanger sequencing. This technique was slow, expensive, and had a low sensitivity. HTS, on the other hand, allows for the sequencing of multiple DNAs in parallel, resulting in the sequencing of millions of DNA molecules at the same time. HTS can sequence an entire exome that can be used to identify variants or mutations in DNA and RNA. HTS has become the primary means of identifying genetic variants.[75] The complexity and size of the sequencing data require teams composed of clinicians, geneticists, and bioinformaticians.

The role of molecular diagnostics for the diagnosis of thrombophilia and bleeding disorders will continue to grow with the identification of new, clinically relevant genetic mutations and polymorphisms and identification of important combinations of mutations. Molecular testing will expand as it becomes more accessible. Beyond accuracy and throughput, cost and labor are to be considered when evaluating which test system a laboratory should choose. Molecular diagnostics is the future of hemostatic testing.[76]

SUMMARY

- Advances in endpoint detection methodologies have greatly expanded the testing capabilities available in the routine coagulation laboratory.
- Coagulation laboratory testing today includes clot-based assays, chromogenic/colorimetric-based assays, and immunologic assays.
- Endpoint detection methodologies used by modern coagulation analyzers include mechanical, photo-optical, viscoelastic, spectrophotometric, nephelometric, and chemiluminescent methods.

- Each method of endpoint detection has advantages and disadvantages that must be recognized and understood to ensure the validity of test results.
- Advanced technology used in semiautomated and automated analyzers has greatly improved coagulation testing accuracy and precision.
- Improved instrument precision and reduced reagent volume requirements have led to substantial cost savings in coagulation testing.

- Instrument manufacturers have incorporated many features that have enhanced efficiency, safety, and diagnostic capabilities in hemostasis testing.
- Coagulation analyzer flagging alert functions warn the operator when specimen or instrument conditions exist that might lead to invalid test results so that appropriate actions can be taken to ensure test accuracy.
- A systematic approach to the evaluation and selection of a new coagulation analyzer should be developed and followed to determine the best instrument for a specific laboratory setting.
- Coagulation testing has been incorporated into the arena of point-of-care testing, primarily to enhance the patient's and physician's ability to monitor anticoagulant therapy.

- Global (complete) hemostasis assessment is performed using whole blood and viscoelastography, evaluating the contribution of all blood components to the kinetic response of the clotting process.
- Several methods to evaluate platelet function are available for both general platelet function testing and antiplatelet drug monitoring.
- The role of molecular diagnostics has become an important diagnostic tool in hemostasis testing and will continue to grow as new mutations and polymorphisms associated with bleeding and clotting disorders are identified.

Now that you have completed this chapter, go back and read again the case study at the beginning and respond to the questions presented. Answers can be found in Appendix C.

REVIEW QUESTIONS

Answers can be found in Appendix C.

1. Which of the following includes the advances made in technology in the coagulation laboratory?
   a. Primary tube sampling
   b. Random access testing
   c. Reduced specimen and reagent volumes
   d. All of the above
2. Which of the following is considered to be an advantage of the mechanical endpoint detection methodology?
   a. It is not affected by lipemia in the test specimen.
   b. It has the ability to provide a graph of clot formation.
   c. It can incorporate multiple wavelengths into a single testing sequence.
   d. It can measure proteins that do not have fibrin formation as the endpoint.
3. What method of detection is used in both the TEG and ROTEM?
   a. Photo-optical
   b. Chromogenic endpoint
   c. Viscoelastic
   d. Immunologic
4. Which of the following is a feature of semiautomated coagulation testing analyzers?
   a. The temperature is maintained externally by a heat block or water bath
   b. Reagents and specimens usually are added manually by the operator
   c. Timers are automatically started as soon as the analyzer adds the specimen to the test cuvette
   d. The endpoint must be detected by the operator
5. When a specimen has been flagged as being icteric by an automated coagulation analyzer, which method would be most susceptible to erroneous results because of the interfering substance?
   a. Mechanical clot detection
   b. Immunologic antigen-antibody reaction detection
   c. Photo-optical clot detection
   d. Chromogenic endpoint detection

6. Which of the following newer techniques can be used for the measurement of platelet function testing in patients with thrombocytopenia and in pediatrics?
   a. PFA-100
   b. Flow cytometry
   c. Lumi-aggregation
   d. PAP-8E
7. All of the following are performance characteristics to consider in the selection of a coagulation analyzer except:
   a. Location of the manufacturer's home office
   b. Instrument footprint
   c. Ease of use for the operator
   d. Variety of tests the instrument can perform
8. Platelet function is measured by the PFA-100 using which of the following methods?
   a. Detecting the change in blood flow pressure along a small tube when a clot impairs blood flow
   b. Detecting the aggregation of latex beads coated with platelet activators
   c. Graphing the transmittance of light through platelet-rich plasma over time after addition of platelet activators
   d. Detecting the time it takes for a clot to form as blood flows through a small aperture in a tube coated with platelet activators
9. A clinical setting in which point-of-care testing is used in high volume is:
   a. To monitor patients receiving oral anticoagulant therapy
   b. To monitor patients taking platelet inhibitors such as aspirin
   c. To provide a baseline for all subsequent patient test result comparisons when the patient starts any kind of anticoagulant therapy
   d. To monitor obstetric patients at risk of fetal loss
10. Molecular testing can be used to diagnose patients with:
    a. von Willebrand disease
    b. Factor V Leiden
    c. Prothrombin mutation
    d. All the above

REFERENCES

1. McGlinchey, K. (2009). Sophistication in coagulation platforms. *Adv Med Lab Prof, 20,* 20–21.

2. Owen, C. A. (2002). History of blood coagulation. *JAMA, 87,* 1051–1052.

3. Bender, G. T. (1998). *Principles of Chemical Instrumentation: STA-R Operator's Manual.* (pp. 119–124). Parsippany, NJ: Diagnostica Stago.

4. Johns, C. S. (2007). Coagulation instrumentation. In Rodak, B. G., Fritsma, G. A., & Doig, K. (Eds.), *Hematology: Clinical Principles and Applications.* (3rd ed., pp. 714–728). St. Louis: Elsevier.

5. Gram, J., & Jespersen, J. (1999). Introduction to laboratory assays in haemostasis and thrombosis. In Jespersen, J., Bertina, R. M., & Haverkate, F. (Eds.), *Laboratory Techniques in Thrombosis—A Manual.* (2nd ed., pp. 1–7). Boston: Kluwer.

6. *BBL FibroSystem Manual.* (1992). Sparks, MD: BD Diagnostics Systems.

7. Tekkesin, N., & Kilinc, C. (2012). Optical and mechanical clot detection methodologies: a comparison study for routine coagulation testing. *J Clin Lab Anal, 16,* 125–129.

8. Bing, B., Christie, D. J., Gorman, R. T., et al. (2008). Comparison of optical clot detection for routine coagulation testing in a large volume clinical laboratory. *Blood Coagul & Fibrinoly, 19,* 569–575.

9. Aggarwal, S., Nayak, D. M., & Manohan, C. (2014). Clot endpoint detection. *Indian J Hematol Blood Transfus,* (Suppl. 1), 402–404.

10. Gurbal, P. A., Bliden, K. P., Tantry, U. S., et al. (2016). First report of the point-of-care TEG: a technical validation study on the TEG-6s system. *Platelets, 27,* 642–649.

11. Hobson, A. R., Agarwala, R. A., Swallow, K. D., et al. (2006). Thromboelastography: current clinical applications and its potential role in interventional cardiology. *Platelets, 17,* 509–518.

12. Lijnen, H. R. (1983). Chromogenic substrate assays: mechanism, specificity and application in blood coagulation and fibrinolysis. *Acta Clinica Belgica, 38,* 102–110.

13. Fareed, J., Bermes, E. W., Jr., & Walenga, J. (1984). Automation in coagulation testing. *J Clin Lab Auto, 4,* 415–425.

14. Fareed, J., & Walenga, J. (1983). Current trends in hemostatic testing. *Semin Thromb Hemost, 9,* 379–391.

15. Fareed, J., Bick, R. L., Squillaci, G., et al. (1983). Molecular markers of hemostatic disorders: implications in the diagnosis and therapeutic management of thrombotic and bleeding disorders. *Clin Chem, 29,* 1641–1658.

16. Lehman, C. M., & Thompson, C. (2007). Instrumentation for the coagulation laboratory. In Bennett, S. T., Lehman C. M., & Rodgers G. M. (Eds.) *Laboratory Hemostasis: A Practical Guide for Pathologists.* (pp. 41–55). Heidelberg: Springer.

17. *Behring Nephelometer 100 Operator's Manual.* (1995). Deerfield, IL: Dade Behring, Inc.

18. Hoffman, J. J., & Verhappen, M. A. (1988). Automated nephelometry of fibrinogen: analytical performance and observations during thrombolytic therapy. *Clin Chem, 34,* 2135–2140.

19. Song, J. (2022). Advances in laboratory assessment of thrombosis and hemostasis. *Blood Res, 57,* S93–S100.

20. Favaloro, E. J., & Lippi, G. (2019). Recent advances in mainstream hemostasis diagnostics and coagulation testing. *Semin Thromb Hemost, 45,* 228–246.

21. *STA Liatest D-Di.* (2005). Parsippany, NJ: Diagnostica Stago.

22. Allen, R., & Sheridan, B. (1999). Coagulation analyzers. Service above all. *CAP Today, 13*(1), 39–50.

23. Hedeland, Y., Gustafsson, C. M., Touza, Z., et al. (2020). Hemolysis interferences in 10 coagulation assays on instrumentation with viscosity-based, chromogenic, and turbidimetric clot detection. *Int J Lab Hematol, 42,* 341–349.

24. Jilma-Stohlawetz, P., Lysy, K., Belik, S., et al. (2019). Interference in specialized coagulation assays affecting the protein C pathway: effects of marked haemolysis, hyperbilirubinaemia and lipaemia on chromogenic and clotting tests on two coagulation platforms. *Int J Lab Hematol, 41,* 404–411.

25. Lippi, G., Plebani, M., & Favaloro, E. J. (2013). Interference in coagulation testing: focus on spurious hemolysis, icterus, and lipemia. *Semin Thromb Hemost, 39,* 258–266.

26. Favaloro, E., & Lippi, G. (2019). Mainstream hemostasis diagnostic and coagulation testing. *Sem Thromb Hemost, 45,* 228–246.

27. Scherer-Buric, P. A., Lesser, J., Nagel, D., et al. (2022). Performance testing of 4 automated coagulation analyzers in a university setting with focus on global coagulations assays. *Int J Lab Hematol, 44,* 643–653.

28. Aria, M., Erten, A., & Yalcin, O. (2019). Technology advances in blood coagulation measurements for point-of-care diagnostic testing. *Front Bioeng Biotechnol, 7,* 395–347.

29. CAP. (2022). Coagulation analyzers. *CAP Today.* (Jan. pp. 1–6).

30. *ACL TOP Family 50 series Brochure.* (2019). Bedford, MA: Werfen.

31. *STA Compact MAX Brochure.* (2016). Parsippany, NJ: Diagnostic Stago.

32. *STA-R MAX Brochure.* (2014). Parsippany, NJ: Diagnostic Stago.

33. Kim, H., Oh, A. C., Hong, Y. J., et al. (2021). Analytical performance and compatibility of three new coagulation analyzers. *Clin Lab, 67,* 125–133.

34. *ACL AcuStar Brochure.* (2021). Bedford, MA: Werfen.

35. Aria, M. M., Erten, A. E., & Yalcin, O. (2019). Technology advances in blood coagulation and measurements for point-of-care diagnostic testing. *Front in Bioeng and Biotech, 7,* 1–10.

36. Dabkowski, B. (2012). Coagulation analyzers-point of care, self-monitoring. *CAP Today.* (May, pp. 20–30).

37. Ansell, J., Zappe, S., Jiang, X., et al. (2019). A novel whole blood point-of-care coagulometer to measure the effect of direct oral anticoagulants and heparins. *Semin Thromb Hemost, 45,* 259–263.

38. Nadkami, S. K. (2019). Comprehensive coagulation profiling at the point-of-care using a novel laser-based approach. *Semin Thromb Hemost, 45,* 264–274.

39. Harris, L. F., Castro-Lopez, V., & Killard, A. S. (2013). Coagulation monitoring devices: past, present and future. *Trends Analy Chem, 50,* 85–95.

40. Toben, B., & Martin, M. (2020). Rapid assessment of coagulation at the point of care with hemochron signature elite. *J Near-Patient Testing & Technology, 19,* 116–121.

41. Hobson, A. R., Agarwal, R. A., Swallow, K. D., et al. (2006). Thromboelastography: current clinical applications and its potential role in interventional cardiology. *Platelets, 17,* 509–518.

42. Tscholl, D. W., Rossler, J., Said, S., et al. (2020). Situation awareness-oriented patient monitoring with visual patient technology: a qualitative review of the primary research. *Sensors, 20,* 2112.

43. Kelly, J. M., Rizoli, S., Veigas, P., et al. (2018). Using rotational thromboelastometry clot firmness at 5 minutes (ROTEM, EXTEM a5) to predict massive transfusion and in hospital mortality in trauma: a retrospective analysis of 1146 patients. *Anaesthesia, 73,* 1103–1109.

44. Gurbel, P. A., Bliden, K. P., Tantry, U. S., et al. (2016). First report of the point-of-care TEG: a technical evaluation study of the TEG6s system. *Platelets, 27,* 642–649.

45. Gill, M. (2017). The TEG 6s on shaky ground? a novel assessment of the TEG 6s performance under a challenging condition. *J Extra Corpor Technol, 4,* 26–29.

46. Ziegler, B., Voelckel, W., Zipperle, J., et al. (2019). Comparison between the new fully automated viscoelastic coagulation analyzers TEG 6s and ROTEM*sigma* in trauma patients: a prospective observational study. *Eur J Anaesthesiol, 36,* 834–842.

47. *ROTEMdelta Manual.* (2011). Munich, Germany: Tem Innovations GmbH.

48. Schenk, B., Gorlinger, K., Treml, B., et al. (2019). A comparison of the new ROTEM*sigma* with its predecessor the ROTEM*delta*. *Anaethesiology, 74,* 348–356.

49. *Quantra QPlus System Brochure.* (2022). Durham, NC: HemoSonics.

50. Harrison, P., & Mumford, A. (2009). Screening tests of platelet function: update on their appropriate uses for diagnostic testing. *Semin Thromb Hemost, 35,* 150–157.

51. Rodgers, R. P. C., & Levin, J. (1990). A critical reappraisal of the bleeding time. *Semin Thromb Hemost, 16,* 1–20.

52. Lind, D. E. (1991). The bleeding time does not predict surgical bleeding. *Blood, 77,* 2547–2552.

53. Gerwitz, A. S., Miller, M. L., & Keys, T. F. (1996). The clinical usefulness of the preoperative bleeding time. *Arch Pathol Lab Med, 120,* 353–356.

54. Peterson, P., Hayes, T. C., Arkin, C. F., et al. (1998). The preoperative bleeding time test lacks clinical benefit: College of American Pathologists' and American Society of Clinical Pathologists' position article. *Arch Surg, 133,* 134–139.

55. *Model 700 Aggregometer Product Information.* (2006). Havertown, PA: Chrono-Log Corporation.

56. *PAP-8E Product Information.* (2005). Horsham, PA: BioData Corporation.

57. *AggRAM Product Information.* (2005). Beaumont, TX: Helena Laboratories.

58. Kundu, S. K., Heilmann, E. F., Sio, R., et al. (1996). Characterization of an in vitro platelet function analyzer, PFA-100. *Clin Appl Thromb Hemost, 2,* 241–249.

59. Franchini, M. (2005). The platelet function analyzer (PFA-100): an update on its clinical use. *Clin Lab, 51,* 367–372.

60. Favaloro, E. J. (2008). Clinical utility of the PFA-100. *Semin Thromb Hemost, 34,* 709–733.

61. McKee, S. A., Sane, D. C., & Deliargyris, E. N. (2002). Aspirin resistance in cardiovascular disease: a review of prevalence, mechanisms, and clinical significance. *Thromb Haemost, 88,* 711–715.

62. Lordkipanidze, M., Pharand, C., Schampaert, E., et al. (2007). A comparison of six major platelet function tests to determine the prevalence of aspirin resistance in patients with stable coronary artery disease. *Eur Heart J, 28,* 1702–1708.

63. Dyskiewicz-Korpanty, D. M., Kim, A., Durner, J. D., et al. (2007). Comparison of a rapid platelet function assay-VerifyNow Aspirin-for the detection of aspirin resistance. *Thromb Res, 120,* 485–488.

64. McGlasson, D. L., & Fritsma, G. A. (2008). Comparison of four laboratory methods to assess aspirin sensitivity. *Blood Coagul Fibrinolysis, 19,* 120–123.

65. Hussein, H. M., Emiru, T., Georgiadis, A. L., et al. (2013). Assessment of platelet inhibition by point-of-care testing in neuroendovascular procedures. *Am J Neuroradiol, 34,* 700–706.

66. *T-TAS 100 Brochure.* (2021). West Chester, OH: DiaPharma.

67. Ramstrom, S., Sodergren, A. L., Tynngard, N., et al. (2016). Platelet function determined by flow cytometry: new perspectives? *Semin Thromb Hemost, 42,* 268–281.

68. van Asten, I., Schutgens, R. E., Baaij, M., et al. (2018). Cytometry based platelet function diagnostics. *Semin Thromb Hemost, 44,* 197–205.

69. Hayward, C. P. M., Moffat, K. A., Brunet, J., et al. (2019). Update on diagnostic testing on platelet disorders: what is practical and useful? *Internal J Lab Hematol, 41*(Suppl 1), 26–32.

70. Malicev, E. (2020). The use of flow cytometry in the diagnosis of heparin-induced thrombocytopenia (HIT). *Transfusion Medicine Reviews, 34,* 34–41.

71. Ballestros, E. (2006). Molecular diagnostics in coagulation. In Coleman, W. B., & Tsongalis, J. (Eds.), *Molecular Diagnostics for the Clinical Laboratorian.* (2nd ed., pp. 311–320). New York: Humana Press.

72. Perrotta, P. L., & Svensson, A. M. (2009). Molecular diagnostics in hemostatic disorders. *Clin Lab Med, 29,* 367–390.

73. Hickey, S. E., Curry, C. J., & Toriello, H. V. (2013). ACMG practice guideline: lack of evidence for MTHFR polymorphism testing. *Genet Med, 15,* 153–156.

74. Nagy, P. L., Schrijver, I., & Zehnder, J. L. (2004). Molecular diagnosis of hypercoagulable states. *Lab Med, 35,* 214–221.

75. Freson, K., & Turro, E. (2017). High-throughput sequencing approaches for diagnosing hereditary bleeding and platelet disorders. *J Thromb Haemost, 15,* 1262–1272.

76. Lee, A. I., & Connors, J. M. (2019). The next (gen) step in coagulation testing. *Blood, 134,* 2002–2003.

43

Hematology and Hemostasis in the Pediatric, Pregnant, Geriatric, and Transgender Populations

Brandy Gunsolus and Natasha Marie Savage*

OBJECTIVES

After completion of this chapter, the reader will be able to:

1. Describe the major differences in reference intervals for the complete blood count, reticulocyte count, and nucleated red blood cells in preterm and full-term neonates, infants, children, adults, and elderly adults.
2. Explain the cause of physiologic anemia of infancy and anemia of prematurity and the time frame in which it is expected.
3. Describe normal red blood cell and lymphocyte morphology in neonates.
4. Recognize and list factors affecting specimen collection that can have an impact on the interpretation of hematology values in neonates.
5. Compare the absolute lymphocyte count in children and adults.
6. Describe common anemias found in children and pregnant women including physiologic anemia of pregnancy.
7. Describe the general association between age and hemoglobin levels in elderly adults.
8. Explain the clinical significance of anemia in elderly adults.
9. Name the two most common anemias in elderly adults and their common causes.
10. Name hematologic neoplasms that are more common in elderly adults than in other age groups.
11. Compare the hemostatic systems of neonates, children, adults, pregnant women, and elderly adults, including the risk of bleeding and thrombosis.
12. Describe the impact of hormones, hormone replacement therapy, and gender-affirming hormone therapy on hematopoiesis and hemostasis.
13. Discuss issues impacting interpretation and reporting of hematology and hemostasis results and reference intervals in transgender populations.

OUTLINE

Pediatric Hematology and Hemostasis
    Hematopoiesis
    Pediatric Developmental Stages
    Gestational Age and Birth Weight
    Specimen Collection for the Neonate
    Anemia and Polycythemia in the Neonate
    Red Blood Cell Values in the Neonate
    Anemia in Infants and Children
    White Blood Cell Values in the Neonate
    Platelet Values in the Neonate
    Neonatal Hemostasis
Gestational Hematology and Hemostasis
    Anemia and Pregnancy
    Gestational Hemostasis

Geriatric Hematology and Hemostasis
    Aging and Hematopoiesis
    Hematologic Parameters in Elderly Adults
    Anemia and Elderly Adults
    Hematologic Neoplasia in Elderly Adults
    Geriatric Hemostasis
Transgender Populations
    Diversity in Transgender Populations
    Sex Hormone Effects on Hematopoiesis
    Hormone Therapy and Hematopoiesis
    Hematologic Parameters in Transgender Populations
    Hormone Therapy and Hemostasis
    Electronic Health Record Challenges

*The authors extend appreciation to Linda H. Goossen, whose work in prior editions provided the foundation of this chapter.

CASE STUDY

After studying this chapter, the reader should be able to respond to the following case study. Answers can be found in Appendix C.

A full-term neonate in no apparent distress had a complete blood count performed as part of a panel of testing for neonates born to mothers who received no prenatal care. Results were as follows. Reference intervals can be found after the Index at the end of the book.

WBC	18×10^9/L	HCT	55.5%
RBC	5.28×10^{12}/L	MCV	105.1 fL
HGB	18.5 g/dL		

WBC differential: 50% neutrophils and 50% lymphocytes.
RBC morphology: macrocytic RBCs with slight to moderate polychromasia; 7 NRBCs/100 WBCs.

1. Are the results for the hemoglobin and hematocrit within the reference intervals expected for a full-term neonate?
2. What is the significance of the elevated MCV and the NRBCs and polychromasia?
3. Comment on the WBC and differential count.

Hematology and hemostasis values are generally stable throughout adult life, but differences exist in pediatric, pregnant, geriatric, and transgender populations. This chapter focuses on the more significant differences.

PEDIATRIC HEMATOLOGY AND HEMOSTASIS

Infants and children are not simply small adults. Neonates or newborns (less than 28 days), infants (0 to 1 year), young children, and older children have significant hematologic differences from adults; thus it is inappropriate to use adult reference intervals for the assessment of pediatric blood values. Historically, pediatric reference intervals were inferentially established from adult data due to limitations in obtaining sufficient "normal" pediatric specimens. As technology has improved to require smaller volume specimens, pediatric reference intervals are now easier to determine, but challenges remain.

In the first few hours and days after birth, dramatic changes occur within the blood and bone marrow, allowing a wide fluctuation in hematologic laboratory results. Additionally, significant differences are seen between neonates born at term and preterm neonates. This section expands on neonatal hematopoiesis, discussed in detail in Chapter 5, and the changes in pediatric hematology reference intervals, morphologic features, and age-specific physiology.

Hematopoiesis
Prenatal Hematopoiesis
Hematopoiesis begins in the first weeks of embryonic development and proceeds systematically through three phases of development: *mesoblastic* (yolk sac), *hepatic* (liver), and *myeloid* (bone marrow). The first cells produced in the developing embryo are primitive erythroblasts that form in the yolk sac. These cells appear megaloblastic and circulate as large, nucleated cells, synthesizing embryonic hemoglobins. A second wave of yolk sac–derived erythroid progenitor cells, termed burst-forming units-erythroid, appear around 4 weeks and seed the fetal liver.[1,2]

By the second month of gestation, hematopoiesis ceases in the yolk sac and the liver becomes the center for hematopoiesis, reaching peak activity during the third and fourth gestational months. Megakaryocytes and myeloid precursors of each stage systematically make their appearance. During the fourth and fifth gestational months, the bone marrow emerges as a major site of blood cell production and by birth, becomes the primary site (Chapter 5).[1]

Hematopoiesis in the Neonate
At the time of birth, the bone marrow is fully active, being almost completely cellular, with all hematopoietic cell lineages undergoing cellular differentiation and proliferation. In addition to the mature cells in fetal blood, a significant number of circulating progenitor cells may be seen in cord blood. Newer practices of delayed cord clamping have identified both blood volume and iron level increases in the neonate.[1,3]

While it was previously thought that hematopoiesis ceases in the liver shortly after birth, newer evidence has identified hepatic hematopoiesis at low levels throughout childhood and into adult life. Other extramedullary hematopoiesis may be seen in times of stress or neoplasm in the spleen, lymph nodes, and paravertebral regions.[4]

Pediatric Developmental Stages
Pediatric hematologic values change markedly in the first weeks and months of life, and many variables influence the interpretation of what may be considered healthy at the time of birth. Thus it is important to provide age-appropriate pediatric hematology reference intervals that extend from neonatal life through adolescence. The pediatric population can be categorized with reference to three different developmental stages: the *neonatal period*, which represents the first 4 weeks of life; *infancy*, which incorporates up to 1 year of life; and *childhood*, which spans from age 1 to puberty (8 to 13 years). Pediatric reference intervals can be found after the Index at the end of the book.

Gestational Age and Birth Weight
Hematologic values obtained from full-term neonates generally do not correlate with preterm neonates, and laboratory values for preterm neonates differ from values for extremely low-birth-weight neonates. *Full-term* neonates are born between 39 weeks 0 days and 40 weeks 6 days of gestation. *Early term* neonates are born between 37 weeks 0 days to 38 weeks 6 days of gestation; *preterm* neonates are born before 37 weeks of gestation. *Late-term* neonates are born between 41 weeks 0 days and 41 week 6 days of gestation, and *postterm* neonates are born on or after 42 weeks 0 days of gestation.[5] Neonates can be further subcategorized by birth weight as 1) appropriate size for gestational age; 2) small for gestational age, including low-birth-weight neonates of 2500

g or less; 3) very low-birth-weight neonates of 1500 g or less; 4) extremely low-birth-weight micropreemies of 1000 g or less; and 5) large for gestational age or more than 4000 g in weight.[6]

Specimen Collection for the Neonate

Neonatal hematologic values are affected by the gestational age of the neonate, the birth weight, the age in hours after delivery, the presence of illness or clinical instability, and the level of life-sustaining support required. Other important variables to be considered when evaluating laboratory data include the site of specimen collection, collection technique including capillary versus venous puncture, and warming of the extremity of the collection site (Chapter E2), as well as timing of the collection, conditions that may have occurred during the course of labor, including issues with the umbilical vessels and/or placenta, and maternal drug use.[1]

Anemia and Polycythemia in the Neonate

Reference intervals for neonates can be found after the Index at the end of the book.

Anemia

Placenta-dependent oxygenation and predominance of fetal hemoglobin (Hb F) with a higher affinity for oxygen (Chapter 8) leads to physiologic fetal hypoxia. Tissue hypoxia and rapid fetal growth stimulate erythropoietin (EPO) production in utero leading to increased red blood cell (RBC) production.[7] This causes the RBC count, hemoglobin concentration, and hematocrit to be relatively increased in the late fetal gestational period.

At birth, the onset of breathing dramatically increases oxygenation, which leads to a drop in EPO levels resulting in a decline in RBC production.[8] As a result of this drop, a transient anemia typically develops by 4 to 6 weeks of life, called *physiologic anemia of infancy*.[8] With the EPO levels greatly reduced or undetectable, the RBC count, hemoglobin concentration, hematocrit, and reticulocyte count gradually decrease during the first 4 to 6 weeks of life. When the hemoglobin concentration decreases to approximately 11 g/dL, erythropoietic activity increases until it reaches adult levels by age 14 years.[1,3]

Preterm neonates often develop an *anemia of prematurity* with lower hemoglobin concentration and a sharper drop in hemoglobin during the first 4 to 6 weeks of life compared with term neonates.[9] Contributing to this anemia is an impaired production of EPO in response to hypoxia, the shorter life span of fetal RBCs, iron depletion, and frequent blood draws.[9] The life span of erythrocytes in full-term neonates is 60 to 70 days compared with 35 to 50 days for preterm neonates.[10] Preterm neonates are also more at risk of developing iron deficiency, as most of the maternal transfer of iron to the fetus occurs late in the third trimester.[10] Finally, many preterm neonates develop iatrogenic anemia from frequent blood collection. Preterm neonates may require a combination of transfusions, erythropoiesis-stimulating agent therapy, and/or iron supplementation until they can maintain their own erythropoiesis.[9]

Polycythemia

Neonatal polycythemia may develop in neonates born from hypertensive mothers, in recipient twins in twin-to-twin

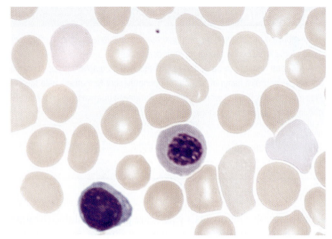

Figure 43.1 Peripheral Blood Film From a Healthy Neonate. Note the normal lymphocyte, macrocytes, polychromasia, and one nucleated red blood cell. (Peripheral blood, Wright-Giemsa stain, ×1000.)

transfusion syndrome, and in neonates with chromosomal abnormalities or delayed cord clamping. Delaying the umbilical cord clamping by 3 minutes has been shown to increase blood volume by as much as 30%.[8,11] More than 50% of neonates with neonatal polycythemia exhibit one or more organ dysfunctions due to polycythemia. Neonates who develop polycythemia outside of the above indications are typically either dehydrated or hypoglycemic from diabetic mothers.[8]

Red Blood Cell Values in the Neonate

Erythrocyte Morphology of the Neonate

Early normoblasts are megaloblastic, hypochromic, and irregularly shaped. During hepatic hematopoiesis, normoblasts are smaller than the megaloblasts of the yolk sac but are still macrocytic. Erythrocytes remain macrocytic from the first 11 weeks of gestation until day 5 of postnatal life.[3,8] The macrocytic RBC morphology gradually changes to the characteristic normocytic, normochromic morphology through the first weeks of life. Orthochromic normoblasts are often identified in the peripheral blood of full-term neonates on the first day of life but disappear within 3 to 4 days after birth. These nucleated RBCs (NRBCs) may persist longer in preterm neonates and are due to intrauterine and/or postnatal stress events such as hypoxia, fetal acidemia, meconium passage, and other perinatal complications.[12] Figure 43.1 depicts a blood film from a healthy neonate showing macrocytes and an NRBC. The average number of NRBCs ranges from 3 to 10 per 100 white blood cells (WBCs) in a healthy full-term neonate, whereas NRBCs can be up to 25 per 100 WBCs in a preterm neonate (Figure 43.2). The presence of NRBCs after 5 days of life is a potential indicator of critical illness in the neonate. Additionally, NRBCs >10 per 100 WBCs is associated with higher mortality.[12]

The erythrocytes of neonates show additional morphologic differences. The number of biconcave discs relative to stomatocytes is reduced in neonates (43% discs, 40% stomatocytes) compared with adults (78% discs, 18% stomatocytes).[13] In addition, increased numbers of burr cells, spherocytes, and other abnormally shaped erythrocytes are seen in neonates.

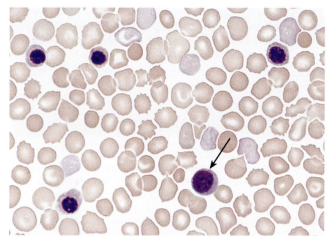

Figure 43.2 Peripheral Blood Film From a Premature Neonate. Note the normal lymphocyte *(arrow)*, four nucleated red blood cells, and increased polychromasia. (Peripheral blood, Wright-Giemsa stain, ×500.)

The number of these irregularly shaped RBCs is even higher in preterm neonates with an average of 40% biconcave discs, 30% stomatocytes, and 27% other RBC abnormal shapes.[13] Physiologic hyposplenism may contribute to this poikilocytosis.

Reticulocyte Count

Reticulocytosis occurs during gestation, decreasing from 90% reticulocytes at 12 weeks of gestation to 15% at 28 weeks of gestation to 4% to 6% at birth. Reticulocytosis decreases over the first several days of life to approximately 0.8% by the end of the first week of life. At 2 months, the number of reticulocytes increases slightly due to the resumption of EPO production, then falls until reaching approximately 1.5%, which is within the reference interval through adulthood.[1,14] The reticulocyte count of preterm neonates is usually higher than that of term neonates at birth; however, the count can vary dramatically depending on the extent of illness in the neonate.[15] Significant polychromasia can be seen on Wright-stained peripheral blood films of preterm neonates due to the higher reticulocyte counts (Figure 43.2).

Hemoglobin

Hemoglobin synthesis results from an orderly evolution of a series of embryonic, fetal, and adult hemoglobins. Chapter 8 provides an in-depth discussion of the ontogeny, structure, and types of hemoglobin. The concentration of hemoglobin fluctuates in the first few weeks and months after birth as a result of physiologic changes, maternal anemia, inherited hemoglobinopathies, other germline/constitutional abnormalities, dietary deficiencies related to feeding practices, the introduction of nonbreast milk or nonformula foods, and socioeconomic disparities.[6,16–18] The site of specimen collection, gestational age, and time of umbilical cord clamping can also influence hemoglobin levels in neonates.[1,11]

The reference interval for hemoglobin for a full-term neonate at birth is 16.5 to 21.5 g/dL; levels less than 14 g/dL are considered abnormal.[3] Hemoglobin values for a small preterm neonate can range from 6.8 to 22.1 g/dL; values less than 13.7 g/dL are considered abnormal.[19]

Hematocrit

The reference interval for the capillary hematocrit at birth for healthy full-term neonates is 48% to 68%.[1] Often neonates with increased hematocrits experience hyperviscosity of the blood causing problems in producing a high-quality peripheral blood film. The hematocrit usually increases by approximately 5% in the first 48 postnatal hours, followed by a slow decline through the first few months of life. Mean adult values of approximately 47% for men and 42% for women are achieved during adolescence.

Red Blood Cell Indices

RBC indices and the red cell distribution width (RDW) provide information that is helpful in determining the cause of anemia (Chapter 16).

Mean cell volume. The RBCs of neonates are markedly macrocytic at birth. The mean cell volume (MCV), which is the average volume of the RBCs, is 119 ± 9.4 fL for a full-term neonate at birth; however, a sharp decrease occurs during the first 24 hours of life.[1,3] The MCV continues to decrease to 90 ± 12 fL in months 3 to 4 of life.[3] The more premature the neonate, the higher the MCV. A neonate with an MCV of less than 94 fL should be evaluated for α-thalassemia or congenital iron deficiency.[3,10]

Mean cell hemoglobin. Mean cell hemoglobin (MCH), which is a measure of the average weight of hemoglobin in the RBCs, is typically 30 to 42 pg in healthy neonates and 27 to 41 pg in preterm neonates.[3,10]

Mean cell hemoglobin concentration. The mean cell hemoglobin concentration (MCHC), which is the average concentration of hemoglobin in each individual RBC, is approximately 33 g/dL and is the same for preterm neonates, full-term neonates, children, and adults. An elevated MCHC may indicate spherocytosis such as seen in hereditary spherocytosis.

Red cell distribution width. The RDW is the coefficient of variation of RBC volume and correlates with anisocytosis on the peripheral blood film. It is elevated in neonates with a reference interval as high as 18.0% in the first 30 days of life. After that, it gradually decreases and reaches the adult reference interval by 6 months.[3]

Anemia in Infants and Children

Nutritional deficiencies in infants and children can result in iron deficiency anemia and, rarely, in megaloblastic anemia (Chapters 17 and 18), particularly in low-birth-weight and preterm neonates.

Iron Deficiency Anemia

Iron deficiency anemia is the most common pediatric hematologic disorder and the most common cause of anemia in childhood.[3,20] Studies have shown that more than 50% of pregnant women, including in developed countries, are iron deficient thus increasing the likelihood of iron deficient neonates.[20,21] Iron deficiency anemia in pregnancy leads to intrauterine growth restriction, low birth weight, neonatal anemia, and, in severe cases, birth asphyxia.[20] The prevalence of iron deficiency in infants has decreased in the United States because of iron fortification of infant formula; however, the prevalence is still 13.5% in toddlers 1 to 2 years and 3.7% in children 3 to 5 years.[22] As iron is essential not only for hemoglobin production, but also for neuron metabolism, functioning, and myelination, iron deficient infants and young children are at risk of neurological deficits, including social, cognitive, and adaptive measures.[20] Chapter 17 provides an in-depth discussion of iron deficiency anemia.

Ancillary Tests for Anemia in Infants and Children

The differential diagnosis of anemia in infants and children relies on a variety of ancillary tests. The reference intervals for a number of these tests differ from those of adults. Haptoglobin levels are so low as to be undetectable in neonates, which makes it unreliable as a marker of neonatal hemolysis.[23] Transferrin levels are also lower in neonates, increasing rapidly after birth and reaching adult levels by 6 months.[23] Both serum ferritin and serum iron are high at birth, rise during the first month, then drop to their lowest levels between 6 months and 4 years, continuing to remain low through childhood.[3] Additional testing, if hemolytic anemia is a concern, includes the direct antiglobulin test in the neonate and ABO and Rh typing of both the mother and the neonate (Chapter 23), hemoglobin electrophoresis/high-performance liquid chromatography for a possible hemoglobinopathy or thalassemia (Chapters 24 and 25), peripheral blood film evaluation for erythrocyte membrane defects, and testing for glucose-6-phosphate dehydrogenase and pyruvate kinase deficiency (Chapter 21).[23]

White Blood Cell Values in the Neonate

Fluctuations in the number of WBCs are common at all ages but are greatest in neonates. Leukocytosis is typical at birth for full-term and preterm neonates, with a wide reference interval.[3,6] There is an excess of segmented neutrophils and bands and occasional metamyelocytes. The absolute neutrophil count rises within the first 8 to 12 hours after birth and then declines to relatively consistent levels.[3,24] Pediatric reference intervals for the WBC count and differential can be found after the Index at the end of the book.

Neutrophils

Term and preterm neonates have higher absolute neutrophil counts than older children who characteristically maintain a predominance of lymphocytes. Band forms are also higher for the first 3 to 4 days after birth (Table 43.1). Neonates whose mothers have undergone labor have higher counts than neonates delivered by cesarean section with no preceding maternal labor.[24]

At birth, preterm neonates exhibit a left shift, and the trend to lymphocyte predominance occurs later in infancy compared with full-term neonates. The neutrophil counts in premature neonates are similar to those of full-term neonates; however, very low-birth-weight neonates tend to have significantly lower counts compared with larger preterm neonates.[24]

Neutropenia. Neutropenia accompanied by bands and metamyelocytes is often associated with infection, particularly in preterm neonates. In determining the cause of the neutropenia,

TABLE 43.1   Neutrophil and Band Counts for Neonates During the First 2 Days of Life*

Age	Absolute Neutrophil Count (x 10⁹/L)	Absolute Band Count (x 10⁹/L)
Birth	3.5–6.0	1.3
12 h	8.0–15.0	1.3
24 h	7.0–13.0	1.3
36 h	5.0–9.0	0.7
48 h	3.5–5.2	0.7

*Reference intervals were obtained from the assessment of 3100 separate white blood cell counts obtained from 965 infants; 513 counts were from infants considered to be completely healthy at the time the count was obtained and for the preceding and subsequent 48 hours. There was no difference in the reference intervals when values were stratified by infant birth weight or gestational age.
h, Hours.
Adapted from Luchtman-Jones, L., & Wilson, D. B. (2001). The blood and hematopoietic system. In Martin, R. J., Fanaroff, A. A., & Walsh, M. C. (Eds.), *Fanaroff and Martin's Neonatal-Perinatal Medicine.* (9th ed., p. 1325). Philadelphia: Mosby.

conditions that decrease neutrophil production as well as those that cause increased neutrophil consumption should be considered (Chapter 26).[25] Other possible considerations include but are not limited to congenital neutropenia, medications, toxins, and autoimmune neutropenia.

Neutrophilia. As neutrophilia is essentially present at birth, using the absolute number of neutrophils as an indicator of infection in preterm and full-term neonates is often challenging. Neonatal sepsis affects an estimated 3 million neonates annually with greater than 10% mortality rate.[26] Morphologic changes that indicate infection include Döhle bodies, vacuoles, and toxic granulation. Vacuoles in isolation should not be considered as confirmation of toxic changes, as they may be seen during neutrophil degeneration. Döhle bodies and toxic granulation are more specific for true toxic changes associated with infection (Chapter 26).

Eosinophils and Basophils

The percentages of eosinophils and basophils remain consistent throughout infancy and childhood.

Lymphocytes

Lymphocytes constitute about 30% of the WBCs at birth and increase to 60% at 4 to 6 months. They decrease to 50% by 4 years, to 40% by 6 years, and then to 30% by 8 years and remain through adulthood.[27] Benign immature B cells (*hematogones*), although predominantly found in the bone marrow, can sometimes be seen in the peripheral blood of neonates.[28] These lymphocytes are primarily midstage B cells, vary in diameter from 10 to 20 μm, have scant cytoplasm, have condensed but homogeneous nuclear chromatin, and may have small indistinct nucleoli (Figures 43.3 and 43.4).[24,28] Although these lymphocytes may be similar in appearance to the malignant cells seen in acute lymphoblastic leukemia (ALL), these benign cells lack the aberrant antigen expression seen in ALL and thus can usually be differentiated from the lymphoblasts of infant ALL by immunophenotyping (Chapter 28).[28]

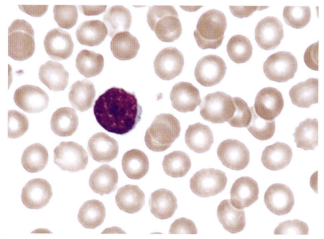

Figure 43.3 Peripheral Blood Film From a Healthy Neonate. Note the benign lymphocyte. (Peripheral blood, Wright-Giemsa stain, ×1000.)

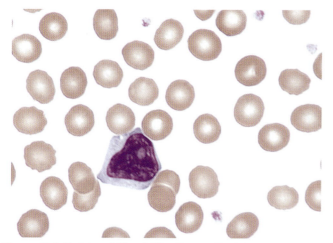

Figure 43.4 Peripheral Blood Film From a Healthy Neonate. Note the benign lymphocyte with visible nucleoli. (Peripheral blood, Wright-Giemsa stain, ×1000.)

ALL is the most common leukemia found in children, with a peak incidence in early childhood. It is characterized by the presence of lymphoblasts in peripheral blood and increased lymphoblasts in the bone marrow (Chapter 31).

Monocytes

The mean monocyte count of neonates is higher than adult values. At birth, the average proportion of monocytes is 6% and then increases to an average of 9% during the second and third weeks of life. It then decreases to an average of 5% and reaches the same as adult levels by 3 to 5 months.[1,10,24] Neonatal monocytes also have increased vacuolization of the cytoplasm and reduced expression of CD11b and CD14 compared with adult monocytes.[29]

Neonatal hematologic response to infection. The immune response of neonates is considered immature, with decreased responsiveness to antigens. While monocytes are critical in initial pathogen recognition, the monocytes of neonates have decreased expression of HLA-DR and CD80, resulting in poor antigen presentation.[29] Neonatal monocytes also produce a large amount of IL (interleukin)-6, which has an inhibitory effect

TABLE 43.2 Platelet Count Reference Intervals

Age	Platelet Count (× 10^9/L; mean ± 1 SD)
Preterm infants, 27–31 weeks	275 ± 60
Preterm infants, 32–36 weeks	290 ± 70
Term infants	310 ± 68
Healthy child/adult	300 ± 50

SD, Standard deviation.
Adapted from Oski, F. A., & Naiman, J. L. (1982). Normal blood values in the newborn period. In *Hematologic Problems in the Newborn*. Philadelphia: Saunders.

on neutrophil response, potentially accounting for reduced migration of neutrophils to inflammatory sites; however, the phagocytic response of these cells is the same as in adults.[29,30]

Because of the transient neutrophilia that occurs during the first 24 hours after birth, followed by a rapid decline, the neutrophil count is not a satisfactory index of infection in the neonate. Many providers use the band count and its derived immature-to-total neutrophil ratio as an indicator of sepsis in neonates.[26] However, repeat proficiency testing has shown high variability and low reproducibility in band counting. Thus the reliability of band counting as a determinant of infection is questionable.

Platelet Values in the Neonate

The platelet count ranges from 150 to 400 × 10^9/L for full-term and preterm neonates, comparable to adult values (Table 43.2). Thrombocytopenia of less than 100 × 10^9/L may be seen in high-risk neonates with sepsis or respiratory distress and neonates with trisomy syndromes.[10,24] Platelets in neonates have great variation in diameter and shape and are classically characterized as hypofunctional compared with adult platelets. Due to the volume of blood needed to carry out platelet function testing, studies are performed on cord blood-derived platelets if needed.[31] These studies have shown that cord blood-derived platelets have impaired calcium mobilization, impaired glycoprotein IIb/IIIa activation, impaired dense granule secretion, and impaired α-granule release compared with adult platelets.[31] However, as discussed in Chapters 41 and 42, PFA-100 closure times and viscoelastometry are superior platelet function tests and are particularly useful for small specimen volumes.

There are specific differences in megakaryocytes between neonates and adults (Table 43.3). These differences coupled with neonatal impaired regulation and mobilization of calcium may explain the neonatal platelet hypofunctionality.[31]

Neonatal Hemostasis
Specimen Collection and Management

Specimen collection and handling for hemostasis testing in neonates follow the principles described in Chapter 41. However, for this population, attention should be given to the collection procedure guidelines established for patients with very small vessels, capillary specimen collection by skin puncture, and procedures for heel puncture specimen collection described in Chapter E2.

TABLE 43.3   Differences Between Neonate and Adult Megakaryocytes

	Neonates	Adults
Megakaryocytes	Smaller size	Larger size
	Low ploidy	High ploidy
	Mature at low ploidy	Maturation increases with ploidy
Megakaryocyte progenitors	More abundant in blood	Sparse in blood
	Form large colonies	Form small colonies
	Highly proliferative	Less proliferative
	Highly sensitive to TPO	Less sensitive to TPO
TPO	High concentration	Low concentration
	Inhibits megakaryocyte polyploidization	Stimulates megakaryocyte polyploidization

TPO, Thrombopoietin.
Adapted from Tesfamariam, B. (2017). Distinct characteristics of neonatal platelet reactivity. *Pharmacol Res, 123*, 1–9.

Hemostatic Components

The physiology of the hemostasis system in infants and children is different from that in adults (Chapter 35) (reference intervals can be found after the Index at the end of the book). The vitamin K-dependent coagulation factors (factors II, VII, IX, and X) are about 30% of adult values at birth; they reach adult values after 2 to 6 months, although the mean values remain lower in children than in adults. Activity levels of factor XI, factor XII, prekallikrein, and high-molecular-weight kininogen are between 35% and 55% of adult values at birth, reaching adult values after 4 to 6 months.[32]

To counterbalance these reduced coagulation factor levels, neonates have high von Willebrand factor (VWF) activity in addition to very low levels of coagulation inhibitors.[32] However, preterm neonates do not have such balance and are very susceptible to bleeding and thrombosis, including but not limited to intracerebral hemorrhages and ischemic stroke.[32]

GESTATIONAL HEMATOLOGY AND HEMOSTASIS

Pregnancy brings about numerous physiologic changes in women to meet the needs of the developing fetus. These physiologic changes are largely beneficial to the mother and the baby but can sometimes cause problems. Expansion of the RBC mass and plasma volume are necessary to maintain the blood supply for the developing fetus. These changes can lead to a physiologic anemia as well as an iron deficiency anemia. The increase in uterine blood flow can also lead to hemorrhage at the time of delivery. Increases in levels of coagulation factors help to combat this but result in a hypercoagulable state and increase the risk for thromboembolic events. Recognizing and treating the hematologic and hemostatic disorders that occur during pregnancy can be difficult because of the scarcity of data available that are specific to the hematology and hemostasis of pregnancy. This section discusses the physiologic changes and related disorders that occur in the hematologic and hemostatic systems during pregnancy.

Anemia and Pregnancy

The most common hematologic complication during pregnancy is anemia. Several normal physiologic changes occur during pregnancy. The plasma volume expands 40% to 60% compared with the proportionally smaller increase in RBC mass of 20% to 50%, resulting in a physiologic (dilutional) anemia of pregnancy, which peaks at 32 weeks.[33] The increase in plasma volume and RBC mass supports amniotic fluid production, diminishes hemodynamic insults such as hemorrhage, improves oxygen binding capacity, and facilitates oxygen delivery to tissues.

Anemia of pregnancy is identified in the first and third trimesters if the hemoglobin is less than 11 g/dL or the hematocrit is less than 33% and in the second trimester if the hemoglobin is less than 10.5 g/dL or the hematocrit is less than 32%.[33] Physiologic anemia of pregnancy is normochromic and normocytic; therefore if a pregnant patient has microcytic hypochromic anemia, nonphysiologic causes must be considered.[33,34]

Anemia can also be caused by an undiagnosed hemoglobinopathy. Roughly 1 in 66 individuals has sickle cell trait in the United States, and this can lead to pregnancy-related morbidity and mortality.[35] The American College of Obstetricians and Gynecologists (ACOG) now recommends universal hemoglobinopathy testing, regardless of race or ethnicity, at the initial prenatal visit to identify individuals at increased risk for anemia and other complications.[36] Hemoglobinopathies are discussed in detail in Chapter 24.

Iron Deficiency Anemia

Iron deficiency comprises 75% of nonphysiologic gestational anemia.[33] If hemoglobin in a pregnant patient falls to less than 11 g/dL, testing for iron deficiency anemia should be initiated. In normal pregnancy, there is an increased requirement for iron; however, most pregnant patients do not have sufficient iron stores to maintain iron needs during pregnancy.[33,34] In addition to inadequate iron stores, poor diet or a diet rich in foods or nonfood substances (pica) that diminish iron absorption can contribute to the iron deficiency (Chapter 17).[37]

The risk of anemia increases with the progression of pregnancy. Minor complications from iron deficiency anemia include fatigue, pallor, lightheadedness, tachycardia, impaired lactation, preterm labor, and postpartum depression; postpartum depression can also be a severe complication.[34,38] Other severe complications that can develop due to iron deficiency anemia include placental abruption, postpartum hemorrhage, fetal growth restriction, shock, and stillbirth.[38]

Diagnosis of iron deficiency anemia in pregnancy. Diagnosis of iron deficiency anemia can be difficult because serum ferritin increases during the third trimester of pregnancy, and microcytosis can be masked by a physiologic increase of 5 to 10 fL in MCV.[33,34] Serum ferritin is an acute phase reactant and as such, begins to increase as early as 1 month before and through delivery, with a postpartum increase similar to that of C-reactive protein or IL-6, which does not reflect iron stores.[33] Chapter 17 includes additional information about the diagnosis and treatment of iron deficiency anemia.

Megaloblastic Anemia

At one time, megaloblastic anemia due to folate deficiency was the second most common anemia in pregnancy. Now with government mandated folate fortification programs, megaloblastic anemia is no longer a common occurrence.[33] However, pregnant women and those considering pregnancy should be aware that folate deficiency in early pregnancy increases the risk of neural tube defects such as spina bifida in the fetus, and folic acid supplementation is recommended before and during the first weeks of pregnancy by the US Centers for Disease Control and Prevention, the Institute of Medicine, and the US Preventive Services Task Force.[39] Chapter 18 has an in-depth discussion of folate and vitamin B_{12} and their role in megaloblastic anemia.

Hemoglobinopathies

Early screening of pregnant women for sickle cell anemia, thalassemia, and other hemoglobinopathies is critical for prenatal diagnosis and genetic counseling. Pregnant women with hemoglobinopathies and thalassemia (disease and trait) require additional medical care to address sequelae associated with the condition.[40–42]

Pregnant patients with sickle cell disease are at increased risk for maternal and fetal mortality.[40] Pregnant patients with sickle cell trait have higher risks of preeclampsia, spontaneous abortion, thromboembolism, and oligohydramnios (decreased amniotic fluid).[41] The most common risk to pregnant patients with thalassemia besides anemia is thromboembolism and ensuing complications.[42] The hemoglobinopathies and thalassemias are discussed in depth in Chapters 24 and 25.

Acute Blood Loss

Acute blood loss is now the second most common cause of anemia in pregnancy.[37] It is most commonly attributed to subchorionic hematomas, where the chorionic membrane partially detaches from the decidual membrane resulting in bleeding and subsequent hematoma.[43,44] The bleeding can occur between 8 and 33 weeks of gestation and occurs in as many as 48% of pregnancies. Bleeding can be either contained between the myometrium and the chorionic membrane or can result in vaginal bleeding, which can be severe resulting in the need for transfusion.[43,44]

Parasitic Infections

Organisms such as *Ancylostoma* (hookworm), *Trichuris trichiura* (whipworm), *Ascaris lumbricoides* (roundworm), and *Plasmodium* (malaria) are common causes of infections in less developed countries.[45] These infections often result in an anemia because of nutritional depletion, gastrointestinal bleeding, or hemolysis.[45,46] Coinfection with these organisms is common and leads to complex problems for pregnant women.

Gestational Hemostasis

Profound hemostatic changes occur during pregnancy. Normal pregnancy is a hypercoagulable state associated with significantly increased levels of coagulation factors and decreased levels of coagulation inhibitors. The hemostasis balance shifts toward enhanced coagulation which, on one hand, protects pregnant women from excessive bleeding and hemorrhage during delivery and in the postpartum period (puerperium), but on the other hand, predisposes them to thromboembolism. Thrombotic disorders are discussed in detail in Chapter 39.

Thrombophilia and Thrombosis in Pregnancy

Thrombotic processes have been described as an important pathogenic factor of severe obstetric conditions such as preeclampsia, intrauterine growth restriction, and placental abruption by influencing the placental perfusion. All of these contribute to maternal morbidity and mortality. Overall, there is 4- to 5-fold increased risk of thrombosis throughout pregnancy and the postpartum period.[47] The rates of both deep vein thrombosis and pulmonary embolism have increased over the last 20 years by 14%, with pulmonary embolism accounting for 11% of all pregnancy-related deaths in the United States over the same time frame.[47]

Venous thromboembolism. Virchow's triad of hypercoagulability, stasis, and endothelial damage underlies the pathogenesis of venous thromboembolism (VTE) in pregnancy.[48] The hypercoagulable state is created by an increase in levels of coagulation factors, including factors VII, VIII, IX, X, fibrinogen, and VWF; acquired resistance to activated protein C; decreased free protein S; and impaired fibrinolysis.[48] Diminished blood flow to the lower extremities creates stasis, and endothelial damage occurs during either vaginal or cesarean section delivery, creating the ideal environment for thrombosis.

Both inherited and acquired thrombophilia are implicated in the pathophysiologic processes associated with thrombotic damage of the placenta and are associated with increased risk of VTE. The prevalence of VTE during gestation and puerperium is increased in women with inherited thrombophilia states such as deficiencies of antithrombin, protein C, and protein S. Activated protein C resistance caused by homozygous factor V Leiden mutation (G1691A) is associated with higher risk, as is homozygous prothrombin (factor II) mutation (G20210A); heterozygosity for either conveys a much lower risk than homozygosity, but increased risk from the normal population still exists.[48]

Treatment of VTE is discussed in Chapter 40. Pregnancy, however, presents special treatment issues. The type of anticoagulant therapy used during pregnancy is an important decision that must balance risk and benefit to both the mother and the fetus. Dosing requirements for pregnant women may vary from those of nonpregnant adults. Dosing is often based on weight in pregnancy and may vary from the early months of pregnancy to near the time of delivery. Placental crossover of the anticoagulant has to be considered as well as whether the anticoagulant is detected in breast milk for mothers who will breastfeed. Certain anticoagulants such as warfarin are contraindicated in pregnancy due to teratogenic effects, and the newer drugs may not have sufficient data to be able to recommend dosing in the pregnant population. Women with a history of thrombosis who are on long-term anticoagulation before pregnancy should continue anticoagulation during and after pregnancy.

Antiphospholipid syndrome. Antiphospholipid syndrome (APS) is an autoimmune disorder and an acquired thrombophilic state that is characterized by the presence of at least one of the following: lupus anticoagulant, anticardiolipin antibodies, and/or anti-β_2-glycoprotein 1 antibodies.[49] Antiphospholipid antibodies have been found to inhibit trophoblast proliferation and implantation as well as embryo implantation, resulting in an increased risk of recurrent pregnancy loss.[49] Chapter 39 has additional information on APS.

Thrombocytopenia and Bleeding Disorders

Thrombocytopenia is defined as a platelet count of less than 150,000/μL and can be caused by either decreased production or increased destruction of platelets. Thrombocytopenia is common in pregnancy, affecting up to 10% of all pregnancies, and gestational thrombocytopenia accounts for approximately 75% of these cases.[50] Gestational thrombocytopenia occurs secondary to the physiologic changes that occur in pregnancy, such as the increase in blood volume, platelet activation, and increased platelet clearing. Most cases are mild, with platelet counts of 100,000 to 150,000/μL, do not require treatment, and are not associated with any adverse events for mother or baby.[50] The decreased count is most pronounced during the third trimester but rarely drops to less than 75,000/μL, and counts typically return to normal by 6 weeks postpartum.[50]

A drop in the platelet count below 50,000/μL eliminates gestational thrombocytopenia, and other conditions should be considered. The differential diagnosis of acute thrombocytopenia includes thrombotic thrombocytopenic purpura (TTP), immune thrombocytopenic purpura (ITP), HELLP (**h**emolysis, **e**levated **l**iver enzymes, and **l**ow **p**latelet count) syndrome, hemolytic uremic syndrome, and conditions resulting in disseminated intravascular coagulation (DIC).[50] These conditions are described in detail in Chapter 38. Table 43.4 summarizes the differential diagnosis of thrombocytopenia in pregnancy.

Immune thrombocytopenia. ITP is the second most common cause of thrombocytopenia after gestational thrombocytopenia and should be considered if the platelet count drops to less than 100,000/μL.[51] Complications include placental abruption, severe maternal bleeding, and neonatal thrombocytopenia as maternal antiplatelet antibodies can cross the placenta.[51]

Thrombotic thrombocytopenic purpura. TTP is a systemic disorder of microvascular thrombosis associated with a deficiency or an inhibition of activity of the enzyme ADAMTS13 (**a d**isintegrin **a**nd **m**etalloprotease with a **t**hrombo**s**pondin type 1 motif, member **13**), which degrades high-molecular-weight VWF. It is most often an acquired autoimmune disorder but has been found to be hereditary in nearly a third of pregnancy-related cases.[52] Pregnancy-associated TTP is most often postpartum in the first few days after a cesarean delivery (70% of cases) to first-time mothers (58% of cases) with an average maternal age of 29 years.[53] TTP does not cause fetal thrombocytopenia and typically causes fetal mortality only if it was preceded by another pregnancy-related complication, such as preeclampsia or obstetric hemorrhage.[53] Patients with TTP during pregnancy should be treated with emergent plasma exchange similar to other patients with TTP, guided by ADAMTS13 levels, and urgent delivery of the fetus when possible. Untreated TTP is associated with high maternal mortality.[52,53]

TABLE 43.4   Differential Diagnosis of Thrombocytopenia in Pregnancy

Pregnancy Related	Not Pregnancy Related
Acute fatty liver of pregnancy	Autoimmune diseases: APS, SLE
Gestational thrombocytopenia	Bone marrow dysfunction
HELLP syndrome	Disseminated intravascular coagulation
Preeclampsia/eclampsia	Drug-related causes: heparin
	Hemolytic uremic syndrome
	Hypersplenism
	Immune thrombocytopenic purpura
	Infections: HIV, HBV, HCV, sepsis
	Nutritional deficiencies: vitamin B_{12}, folate
	Pseudothrombocytopenia
	Thrombotic thrombocytopenic purpura
	von Willebrand disease type 2B

APS, Antiphospholipid syndrome; *HBV,* hepatitis B virus; *HCV,* hepatitis C virus; *HELLP, h*emolysis, *e*levated *l*iver enzymes, *l*ow *p*latelets; *HIV,* human immunodeficiency virus; *SLE,* systemic lupus erythematosus. Adapted from Ciobanu, A. (2016). Thrombocytopenia in pregnancy. *Maedica (Bucur), 11,* 55–60.

Preeclampsia and HELLP syndrome. Preeclampsia is the most common cause of pregnancy-related mortality worldwide, affecting 7% of all pregnancies, with greater than 70,000 maternal deaths and greater than 500,000 fetal deaths each year.[54] It is characterized by gestational hypertension and proteinuria after 20 weeks' gestation and is commonly responsible for thrombocytopenia in the second and third trimesters.[50,54] Hematologic complications include microangiopathic hemolytic anemia with fragmented RBCs (schistocytes) on the peripheral blood film and coagulation abnormalities. Uteroplacental ischemia is the primary driver of the hypertension and ensuing multiorgan failure pathology of preeclampsia.[54]

HELLP syndrome occurs in approximately 10% of pregnancies with preeclampsia. Risk factors include advanced maternal age ($\geq$35 years) and a prepregnancy comorbidity, such as chronic kidney disease, diabetes, or systemic lupus erythematosus.[55] Laboratory results include elevated lactate dehydrogenase $\geq$600 U/L, total bilirubin $\geq$1.2 mg/dL, aspartate aminotransferase $\geq$70 U/L, and platelets $\leq$100,000/μL.[56] Prompt delivery of the fetus, if possible, is the mainstay of treatment.[55,56]

GERIATRIC HEMATOLOGY AND HEMOSTASIS

In 2020 there were 56.1 million people in the United States 65 years and older, accounting for nearly 20% of the population.[57] As life expectancy and quality of life of elderly adults has improved dramatically in recent decades, the older population in 2060 is projected to number 95 million and represent more than a quarter of the total US population.[57] Before the coronavirus disease 2019 (COVID-19) pandemic in 2019, life expectancy in the United States was at an all-time high of 79 years. Since the pandemic, life expectancy fell to 76 years in 2021, a striking reminder of the cost of life due to COVID-19.[58]

Aging and Hematopoiesis

The aging process is associated with the functional decline of several organ systems, such as cardiovascular, renal, musculoskeletal, pulmonary, and bone marrow reserve. With aging, most cells have a decreased ability to divide, and some, such as nervous tissue, lose the ability to divide entirely.[59] Marrow cellularity begins at 80% to 100% in infancy, decreases to approximately 50% by 30 years, and continues to decline to as little as 20% by 65 years.[60] These changes are primarily due to a reduction in the volume of trabecular or spongy bone and the increase of fat in the marrow rather than a decrease in hematopoietic tissue.[60] Telomere shortening, which correlates with life span and aging, has been identified as critical in the stimulation of CD4 immune cells; however, more research is needed to determine its full association with hematopoiesis.[61]

Hematologic Parameters in Elderly Adults

In 1930 Wintrobe published hematologic reference intervals that are still in use today. These reference intervals were derived from healthy, young adults from Tulane Medical School and Sophie Newcomb Women's College.[62] While the publication was revolutionary for the field at the time, whether these reference intervals can be considered "normal" for elderly or diverse populations is a matter of speculation. Research is ongoing to establish appropriate age-adjusted hematologic reference intervals, but this has been challenging due to the high number of chronic morbidities that would exclude such individuals from conventional reference interval studies.[63]

The heterogeneity in the aging process and difficulty in separating the effects of age from the effects of pathologic diseases that accompany aging emphasize the importance of proper interpretation of hematologic data, which requires a complete understanding of the association between disease and older age. This section focuses on hematologic changes in elderly adults and discusses hematopathologic conditions seen in the geriatric population.

Red Blood Cells

Most RBC parameters for healthy elderly adults do not show significant deviations from parameters for younger adults, but physiological changes can be identified. There is a gradual decline in hemoglobin starting at middle age, with the mean level decreasing by about 1 g/dL during the sixth through eighth decades, which is more pronounced in men.[64] A similar decrease is seen in the RBC count. This is due to the decrease in androgen levels, such as testosterone, which stimulate erythropoiesis. Table 43.5 contains age-adjusted reference intervals for ages 50 to 100 years by decade in life.

White Blood Cells

In the absence of any underlying pathologic condition, there are no statistically significant differences between the WBC count and WBC differential for the geriatric population.

Immune response in elderly adults. Infectious diseases are an important cause of morbidity and mortality in elderly adults.

Aged adults are more susceptible to infection and take longer to recover from infection due to comorbid conditions or often multiple organ system involvement.[65] Additionally, there are delayed immune system responses and a gradual reduction in the body's ability to maintain physiologic homeostasis due to outside stressors, which is referred to as immunosenescence.[65] The thymus gradually atrophies with age, with less than 10% of activity by 70 years.[66] Certain acute and chronic infections can accelerate the thymus atrophy process. As a result, the number of naïve T cells decreases in elderly adults, increasing the dependence on memory T cells, which are pooled in secondary tissues.[66] This, accompanied by decreased expression of costimulatory receptor ligand molecules CD80 and CD86, gives an impaired response to mitogens and antigens as they help regulate T cell activation.[67] The CD80 and CD86 reduction was once thought to be a marker of Alzheimer disease; however, this has been disproven and is now believed to be part of immunosenescence.[68]

B lymphocyte precursor production in bone marrow significantly decreases with age, primarily due to reduced level of IL-7 needed for pro-B cell development and hematopoietic stem cell bias to produce a predominance of myeloid cells.[69,70] The reason for this bias is still unknown.

Monocytes and Macrophages

The aging process also affects macrophages and monocytes, including decreased toll-like receptor signaling and phagocytosis, contributing to immunosenescence and decreased immune response.[71]

Platelets

Platelets typically decline in advanced age; however, they also become hyperactive, leading to faster clot formation and increased risk of thrombosis.[72] This hyperactivity is thought to be due to changes in the RNA platelet transcriptome. Newer research has identified drastic platelet transcriptome changes due to cancer, chronic inflammation, and other comorbid conditions.[72-74]

Thrombocytopenia may be drug induced or secondary to marrow infiltration of metastatic cancer, lymphoma, or leukemia (Chapter 38). Essential thrombocythemia is a myeloproliferative neoplasm characterized by sustained proliferation of megakaryocytes, resulting in a platelet count of 450×10^9/L or greater (Chapter 32). Thrombocytosis can also be seen in chronic myeloid leukemia as well as other myeloproliferative neoplasms.

Anemia and Elderly Adults

Anemia is common in elderly adults, and its prevalence increases with age. The World Health Organization (WHO) defines anemia as hemoglobin less than 13 g/dL in men and less than 12 g/dL in women. Using the WHO definition of anemia, the Third National Health and Nutrition Examination Survey (NHANES III), a national study that samples clinical specimens, found the prevalence of anemia in the United States in individuals older than 65 years to be 11% in men

TABLE 43.5   Age-Adjusted Reference Intervals for Adults Ages 50 to 100 Years*

Parameter	Age Range (y)	Men		Women	
		Mean	Interval	Mean	Interval
RBC (× 10⁶/μL)	50–60	4.94	4.26–5.62	4.55	3.92–5.18
	60–70	4.84	4.16–5.57	4.56	3.95–5.22
	70–80	4.70	3.94–5.47	4.49	3.82–5.19
	80–90	4.54	3.69–5.40	4.40	3.66–5.15
	90–100	4.35	3.50–5.20	4.32	3.53–5.17
HGB (g/dL)	50–60	15.1	13.2–17.0	13.7	12.1–15.6
	60–70	14.9	13.0–16.9	13.7	12.0–15.5
	70–80	14.5	12.3–16.7	13.5	11.7–15.4
	80–90	14.1	11.5–16.6	13.3	11.2–15.4
	90–100	13.4	11.0–16.4	13.0	10.7–15.3
HCT (%)	50–60	43.8	38.7–49.4	40.3	35.6–45.7
	60–70	43.4	38.2–49.2	40.5	35.5–45.9
	70–80	42.3	36.0–48.7	40.0	34.4–45.7
	80–90	41.4	34.5–48.4	39.4	33.1–45.7
	90–100	39.7	32.4–47.7	38.8	32.4–46.6
MCV (fL)	50–60	88.6	80.8–97.0	88.5	81.0–96.7
	60–70	89.4	81.6–97.9	88.8	81.3–97.1
	70–80	90.1	82.3–98.7	89.1	81.5–97.4
	80–90	90.7	82.4–99.8	89.3	81.1–98.3
	90–100	91.0	82.0–100.0	89.4	80.6–98.6
MCH (pg)	50–60	30.6	28.0–33.5	30.1	27.6–32.8
	60–70	30.8	28.1–33.7	30.1	27.5–32.9
	70–80	30.9	28.2–33.8	30.1	27.6–33.0
	80–90	30.9	38.0–33.9	30.1	27.5–33.0
	90–100	30.9	27.8–34.3	30.1	27.1–33.0
MCHC (g/dL)	50–60	34.6	32.7–36.5	34.0	32.2–35.9
	60–70	34.4	32.5–36.4	33.9	32.1–35.7
	70–80	34.3	32.3–36.3	33.8	31.9–35.7
	80–90	34.0	31.9–36.2	33.7	31.7–35.7
	90–100	33.9	31.8–36.2	33.6	31.5–35.7
WBC (× 10³/μL)	50–60	6.63	4.00–10.99	6.26	3.76–10.41
	60–70	6.63	4.09–10.77	6.24	3.86–10.10
	70–80	6.59	4.09–10.58	6.35	3.96–10.18
	80–90	6.64	4.15–10.55	6.47	3.99–10.49
	90–100	6.16	3.70–10.05	6.51	4.12–9.13
PLT (× 10³/μL)	50–60	234	153–356	264	179–392
	60–70	225	145–349	258	171–384
	70–80	213	132–339	251	165–384
	80–90	208	127–340	246	156–388
	90–100	209	133–329	240	145–398

*Reference intervals were obtained from the assessment of 3,029,904 clinical specimens, with 566,775 specimens from individuals considered healthy at the time the count was obtained.

HCT, Hematocrit; *HGB,* hemoglobin concentration; *MCH,* mean cell hemoglobin; *MCHC,* mean cell hemoglobin concentration; *MCV,* mean cell volume; *PLT,* platelet count; *RBC,* red blood cell count; *WBC,* white blood cell count; *y,* years.

Adapted from Zierk, J., Krebs, A., Rauh, M., et al. (2020). Blood counts in adult and elderly individuals: defining the norms over eight decades of life. *Br J Haematol, 189,* 777–789.

and 10.2% in women.[75] Approximately one-third of cases of anemia in elderly adults are due to chronic kidney disease, and another third are due to nutritional deficiencies.[75,76] *Unexplained anemia of aging* accounts for the final third of cases.[76] However, due to associated high morbidity and mortality, anemia in the elderly should be investigated as likely due to gastrointestinal blood loss until diagnostics (e.g., colonoscopy) prove otherwise.[77]

Anemia of Inflammation

Anemia of inflammation, also known as anemia of chronic disease, often occurs with chronic inflammatory disorders (e.g., rheumatoid arthritis, vasculitis, hepatitis), chronic infections, congestive heart failure, and malignant diseases.[78] This is the most common form of anemia in hospitalized geriatric patients.[78] The pathogenesis involves iron-restricted erythropoiesis due to hepcidin-induced inhibition of iron absorption in the intestines and inhibition of iron mobilization from macrophages and hepatocytes triggered by inflammatory cytokines (Chapter 17).

Iron Deficiency Anemia

Iron deficiency anemia is a common cause of anemia in elderly patients. It not only affects erythrocytes but also the metabolic pathways of iron-dependent tissue enzymes. Hemoglobin synthesis is reduced, and even a minimal decrease can cause profound functional disabilities in an elderly patient.[77] The serum iron level decreases progressively with each decade of life, although elderly adults will usually still have serum iron levels within the adult reference interval.[77] Ferritin level, when no inflammatory condition is present, is the best marker for iron deficiency anemia outside of an iron stain on a well-prepared bone marrow aspirate smear.[77]

In industrialized nations, dietary deficiency of iron is rare because of the prevalence of iron fortification in grains and consumption of meats containing heme iron. Iron deficiency in elderly adults most often results from conditions leading to chronic gastrointestinal blood loss, including long-term use of nonsteroidal antiinflammatory medications, gastritis, peptic ulcer disease, gastroesophageal reflux disease with esophagitis, colon cancer, and angiodysplasia.[76–78]

Nutritional Deficiencies

Next to iron deficiency, vitamin B_{12} and folic acid deficiencies are the next most common causes of nutritional anemia in elderly patients.[79] As age increases, the incidence of polypharmacy, including agents that alter the absorption and metabolism of vitamin B_{12}, also increases. In less than 2% of patients, vitamin B_{12} or folic acid deficiencies are due to dietary causes; most deficiencies are due to malabsorption from long-term use of medications that interfere with vitamin B_{12} metabolic uptake, including but not limited to proton pump inhibitors, metformin, methotrexate, and H_2 receptor antagonists.[79]

Other nutritional causes of anemia include deficiencies in copper and selenium. Zinc supplements, commonly taken by elderly adults, reduce copper absorption, thus inhibiting hematopoietic stem cell maturation; selenium deficiency is typically found in elderly patients on total parenteral nutrition, which often provides insufficient selenium for the needs of elderly patients.[79]

Unexplained Anemia of Aging

Unexplained anemia of aging is not entirely unexplained but rather is likely multifactorial. Androgen deficiency and hypogonadism, undiagnosed myelodysplastic neoplasm, and chronic inflammation can reduce EPO levels resulting in anemia.[76,80] Hip fracture repairs and hip replacements leave patients with anemia with reduced bone marrow to make a full recovery.[76,81] All can result in ineffective erythropoiesis and hypoproliferative anemia in addition to potential undiagnosed nutritional deficiencies or endocrine disease. In some patients with anemia, molecular evaluation may reveal clonal cytopenia of undetermined significance.

Ineffective Erythropoiesis

Ineffective erythropoiesis has been attributed not only to maturation disorders such as vitamin B_{12} and folic acid deficiency but also to other hematologic conditions. The destruction of late-stage erythroid precursors in the bone marrow is the primary mechanism of ineffective erythropoiesis in myelodysplastic neoplasms, thalassemia, and sideroblastic anemias.[82] Additional information regarding sideroblastic anemia and megaloblastic anemia can be found in Chapters 17 and 18 respectively.

Hematologic Neoplasia in Elderly Adults

Although hematologic malignancies may occur at any age, certain disorders are more common in patients older than 50 years. A brief overview of these disorders is included in this chapter, with references to more detailed discussions.

The 2022 World Health Organization Classification of Haematolymphoid Tumours revised the 2016 classification, including the use of new defining cytogenetic and molecular abnormalities.[83,84] Table 43.6 identifies the most commonly mutated genes in elderly patients with leukemia and their frequency. In addition to the higher frequency of these mutations, multiple mutations are common.[85,86]

Most Common Hematologic Neoplasms

Myelodysplastic neoplasms. Myelodysplastic neoplasms are a common hematologic malignancy in elderly adults, with a median age at diagnosis of approximately 70 years and fewer than 10% of cases diagnosed in individuals younger than 50 years.[87] The overall incidence of myelodysplastic neoplasms is 4 cases per 100,000 individuals; however, for individuals older than 70 years, the incidence increases to 50 cases per 100,000.[87] Typical features include progressive cytopenias, dyspoiesis in one or more cell lines, and a subsequent increase in blasts in the peripheral blood and bone marrow. Chapter 33 provides a complete discussion of myelodysplastic neoplasms.

Myeloproliferative neoplasms. Myeloproliferative neoplasms (MPNs) are monoclonal proliferations of hematopoietic stem cells with overaccumulation of RBCs, WBCs, or platelets in various combinations. This includes disorders such as chronic myeloid leukemia, polycythemia vera (PV), essential thrombocythemia, primary myelofibrosis, chronic eosinophilic leukemia, chronic neutrophilic leukemia, and other unclassifiable MPNs. The incidence of MPNs increases from 11.1 per 100,000 in adults 50 to 54 years to 41.8 per 100,000 in adults 70 to 74 years and 70.7 per 100,000 in adults 85 years and older.[88] Chapter 32 provides a complete discussion of myeloproliferative neoplasms.

Chronic lymphocytic leukemia. Although all types of leukemia can occur in elderly adults, chronic lymphocytic leukemia (CLL) is the most common type found in this age group. CLL is a malignancy of B lymphocytes characterized by clonal lymphocytosis with an aberrant expression of surface antigens detected by immunophenotyping. Chapter 34 provides a complete discussion of CLL.

TABLE 43.6 Common Genetic Abnormalities in Myeloid Neoplasms With Overall Incidence versus Incidence in Elderly Adults

Mutated Gene	Overall Incidence (%)	Incidence in Elderly Adults ≥75 y (%)
TET2	4	42
DNMT3A	1	35
NPM1	3	32
SRSF2	2	25
ASXL1	10	21
RUNX1	7	19
FLT3-ITD	14	18
NRAS	7	17
IDH2	2	15
TP53	7	14
FLT3-TKD	2	12
IDH1	3	9

Data from Prassek, V. V., Rothenberg-Thurley, M., Sauerland, M.C., et al. (2018). Genetics of acute myeloid leukemia in the elderly: mutation spectrum and clinical impact in intensively treated patients aged 75 years or older. *Haematologica, 103*, 1853–1861; and Liu, M., Wang, F., Zhang, Y., et al. (2021).Gene mutation spectrum of patients with myelodysplastic syndrome and progression to acute myeloid leukemia. *Int J Hematol Oncol, 10*, IJH34.

Geriatric Hemostasis

Age-related changes occur in the vascular and hemostasis systems, including alterations in platelets, coagulation, and fibrinolytic factors. These changes contribute to the increased incidence of thrombosis in elderly adults. The overall rate of thrombosis is 1 per 1000 but is 5 per 1000 in adults 80 years and older.[89]

The aging process in healthy individuals brings increases of fibrinogen, factors V, VII, VIII, IX, and XIII, VWF, high-molecular-weight kininogen, and prekallikrein.[89] Fibrinogen, which has been implicated as a primary risk factor for thrombotic disorders including ischemic heart disease, increases with both age and other outside risk factors associated with increased age.[90,91] Increases in fibrinogen are also seen in women after menopause, with larger increases in women on hormone replacement therapy (HRT). Diabetes, malignancy, smoking, and other comorbidities all increase fibrinogen levels in both men and women, also increasing the thrombosis risk.[91] Elderly adults are also at increased risk of severe illness and respiratory failure; both also increase the risk of thrombosis.[89]

Fibrinolysis is impaired in elderly adults, primarily due to increased levels of plasminogen activator inhibitor-1 (PAI-1). PAI-1 controls fibrinolytic activity by inhibiting plasminogen activators, especially tissue plasminogen activator.[92] D-dimer levels increase with age due to increases in fractures, obesity, trauma, and inflammation.[93] The recent introduction of age-adjusted D-dimer cutoff values for exclusion of deep vein thrombosis (DVT) in elderly adults has potential for enhanced utility of the test. Patients without DVT are more efficiently ruled out using the age-adjusted cutoff values, resulting in reduced exposure of these patients to unnecessary radiologic diagnostic procedures.[93]

Platelet activity increases with age as evidenced by platelet aggregation studies in older patients with aggregation occurring at lower concentrations of ADP, arachidonic acid, collagen, and epinephrine.[72] Additionally, both platelet factor 4 and β-thromboglobulin, two substances released from activated platelets, are increased in elderly patients consistent with an enhanced prothrombotic state.[72]

Elderly adults are also prone to bleeding problems. Thrombosis experienced by elderly patients may necessitate antiplatelet or anticoagulation therapy, which can cause significant bleeding problems in older patients due at least in part to alterations in blood flow, particularly through the kidneys. Additionally, bleeding disorders such as acquired hemophilia A and acquired von Willebrand disease occur in elderly adults. The changing renal function, modification in immune regulation, and underlying disease processes in elderly adults can give rise to these bleeding disorders.[94]

TRANSGENDER POPULATIONS

According to the American Psychological Association, any individual whose behavior, gender expression, or gender identity does not match those traditionally associated with the sex they were assigned at birth falls under the umbrella of transgender.[95] A *transgender man (trans man, female to male)* has a male gender identity but was assigned female at birth. A *transgender woman (trans woman, male to female)* has a female gender identity but was assigned male at birth. *Nonbinary* is a subset of transgender individuals who do not identify with either a male or female gender. An individual who does not identify as transgender or nonbinary is referred to as a *cis man* or *cis woman*.[95]

A survey by the Pew Research Center in 2022 found that 1.6% of the US population identifies as either transgender or nonbinary.[96] Using an estimated US population of 300 million, there are approximately 4.8 million transgender and nonbinary individuals in the United States alone.

Diversity in Transgender Populations

Transgender men need health care specific to where they are in their transition.[95] A transgender man may have been on gender-affirming hormone therapy (GAHT) for a sufficient period of time to develop masculine features and have had a double mastectomy, also known as gender-affirming surgery or top surgery, but they will still need gynecologic care while they have ovaries, a uterus, cervix, and/or vagina. Some transgender men never have a hysterectomy and/or phalloplasty. Transgender women have similar needs as transgender men in obtaining equitable health care.[95] Not all transgender individuals choose to have gender-affirming surgery.[97]

Nonbinary individuals may choose to have GAHT for hormone suppression alone.[98] This is to suppress the secondary sex characteristics without hormonally transitioning to the opposite gender. Medical professionals should be aware that both transgender and nonbinary individuals may use hormones without the supervision of a health care provider or may utilize GAHT prescriptions differently than prescribed, which may affect the interpretation of laboratory results as further discussed in this chapter.[99]

Sex Hormone Effects on Hematopoiesis

As more research is performed on the cis and transgender populations, differences in hematopoiesis have been identified. Not only is this difference seen within the cis population but also within patients receiving hormone therapy, either as HRT or GAHT.[100,101]

Hormones inherently drive changes within hematopoiesis as can be seen with reference interval differences from childhood through puberty (reference intervals can be found after the Index at the end of the book). Both estrogen and testosterone aid in regulating immune responses as well as driving the differentiation and maturation of hematopoietic stem cells.[101,102]

Estrogens have been shown to promote hematopoietic stem cell activity, particularly in response to blood loss during menstruation.[103] Estradiol stimulates the maturation of multipotent progenitors, in addition to expanding erythroid differentiation.[104] Additionally, estrogens have been linked to bone marrow microenvironment remodeling, although the mechanism is still unknown.[105] Women have lower relapse rates following hematopoietic stem cell transplantation; thus with the link between estrogens and hematopoietic stem cell activity, some current research protocols include estrogens as part of posttransplant therapy to improve regeneration.[106]

Once estrogen levels drop following menopause, stem cell hematopoiesis also decreases.[103] While women have a somewhat sudden shift in sex hormones during menopause, men experience a gradual decrease in testosterone over their life span. It has been well documented that both endogenous and exogenous testosterone, increase erythropoiesis, although the exact mechanism is still unknown.[101,107]

Hormone Therapy and Hematopoiesis

HRT may be prescribed for cis men or women. Estrogen may be prescribed for contraception, menstrual disorders, or as HRT to aid in relieving menopausal symptoms, including bone loss, hot flashes, and night sweats.[108,109] Testosterone HRT aids in relieving hypogonadal symptoms, including difficulty concentrating, fatigue, impotence, and reduced muscle mass.[110]

Estrogen replacement therapy has been demonstrated to have positive effects on bone regeneration and bone strengthening, thereby reducing risk for fracture.[101,106] In addition, it has been found to augment hematopoietic stem cells and bone marrow stromal cell proliferation.[101]

Long-term testosterone therapy, both as HRT and GAHT, is a known cause of secondary polycythemia.[111] Individuals on testosterone therapy for more than 12 months may see increases in RBC count, hemoglobin, and hematocrit of up to 20%.[112,113] While major adverse clinical events, such as myocardial infarction, are common in polycythemia vera (PV), there is little evidence that such risks occur in testosterone therapy-induced secondary polycythemia.[111,112] Long-term testosterone therapy does make it difficult to differentiate PV from secondary polycythemia. The presence of either *JAK2* V617F or *JAK2* exon 12 mutation confirms PV (Chapter 32); however, differentiating between unmutated *JAK2* PV and secondary polycythemia in a patient on long-term testosterone therapy can be challenging.[114] Nevertheless, unmutated *JAK2* PV is exceedingly rare.

Hematologic Parameters in Transgender Populations

Identifying hematologic reference intervals for transgender populations is challenging. Studies have identified that cis reference intervals are not reliable for transgender populations, even if they are flipped to the opposite sex.[115,116] Studies have attempted to obtain reference intervals for this population; however, each has fallen short for a variety of reasons, including lack of participating transgender individuals in each needed reference interval category and that nearly all studies have been retrospective analyses performed using different laboratory equipment and even different testing methodology.[115–118]

Additional research is needed to determine reference intervals for transgender men on GAHT for less than 6 months, for 6 to 12 months, and for greater than 12 months (stable); who began transition before menopause; who began transition after menopause; and who have had gender-affirming surgery. Additional research is needed to determine reference intervals for transgender women on GAHT for less than 6 months; for 6 to 12 months; for greater than 12 months (stable); and for those who have had gender-affirming surgery. Research is also needed for both transgender men and women who began transition during prepuberty or during any of the Tanner[119] stages of puberty. Finally, nonbinary individuals who receive hormonal suppression therapy but do not transition to the opposite gender also need reference intervals. Establishing appropriate reference intervals for these diverse populations would give providers the ability to accurately interpret laboratory test results to provide optimal and equitable patient care.

In the studies that have been performed, some hematologic differences have been observed. Table 43.7 lists transgender hematologic reference intervals that have been published to date.

Hormone Therapy and Hemostasis

Long-term estrogen therapy in cis women has been shown to have a twofold increased risk of venous thrombosis, with higher risk in women taking oral therapy versus transdermal therapy.[108] Besides venous thrombosis, estrogen therapy has been linked to arterial thrombosis and other thromboses at unusual sites.[109] Arterial thrombosis risk is higher in transgender women taking GAHT than in cis women.[120] Estrogen therapy increases thromboses by increasing VWF, fibrinogen, and factors II, VII, VIII, and X.[109] Additionally, an increased risk in cardiovascular events is seen in cis women who take HRT past 60 years, and transgender women have a 2.6 times incidence of cardiovascular death.[108,120] Due to these risks, current guidelines recommend tapering off estrogen therapy after age 60[108]; however, this is not always possible for transgender women, especially those who begin transition later in life.

While cis men taking long-term testosterone therapy were once thought to have increased thrombotic risk, that theory has since been disproven.[101,120] However, transgender men on long-term testosterone GAHT have a higher risk of ischemic heart disease and stroke than both cis men and women.[97] More research has been done in this area with estrogen therapy compared with testosterone therapy; therefore more risks may be determined with further research.[120]

TABLE 43.7   Transgender Hematologic Reference Intervals Published to Date*

Cohort	Parameter	Transgender Reference Interval	Cis Reference Interval
Transgender men (testosterone GAHT)	WBC ($\times 10^3/\mu L$)	3.8–12.8	4.0–10.3
	RBC ($\times 10^6/\mu L$)	4.3–6.0	4.5–5.9
	HGB (g/dL)	12.8–17.4	13.1–17.9
	HCT (%)	39–51	39–51
	MCV (fL)	79–97	81.5–98.5
	MCHC (g/dL)	31.5–35.0	32.1–36.3
	PLT ($\times 10^3/\mu L$)	181–415	150–400
	RDW (%)	11.9–15.2	10.3–14.5
Transgender women (estrogen GAHT)	WBC ($\times 10^3/\mu L$)	4.4–12.8	4.0–10.3
	RBC ($\times 10^6/\mu L$)	3.7–5.3	3.9–5.1
	HGB (g/dL)	11.6–15.7	11.7–15.5
	HCT (%)	35.0–47.0	35.5–46.0
	MCV (fL)	83.4–98.6	81.5–98.5
	MCHC (g/dL)	31.5–35.9	32.1–36.3
	PLT ($\times 10^3/\mu L$)	150–443	150–400
	RDW (%)	11.5–14.7	10.3–14.5

*Reference intervals were obtained from the assessment of 79 transgender/nonbinary men on stable testosterone therapy for a minimum of 12 months and 93 transgender/nonbinary women on stable estrogen therapy for a minimum of 12 months.
GAHT, Gender-affirming hormone therapy; *HCT,* hematocrit; *HGB,* hemoglobin concentration; *MCHC,* mean cell hemoglobin concentration; *MCV,* mean cell volume; *PLT,* platelet count; *RBC,* red blood cell count; *RDW,* red cell distribution width; *WBC,* white blood cell count.
Adapted from Greene, D. N., McPherson, G. W., Rongitsch, J., et al. (2019). Hematology reference intervals for transgender adults on stable hormone therapy. *Clin Chim Acta, 492,* 84–90.

Electronic Health Record Challenges

Electronic health records (EHRs) will require improvement over current systems as more providers and health care facilities work to provide more equitable and consistent care of transgender patients. These software programs were designed to collect and report data based on the binary recording of sex as male or female. Therefore much of the patient medical record is tied to sex, including laboratory reference intervals, pharmacy dosing, state reporting, quality indicators, and more. This is because research investigations from which these data were derived were designed in such a manner. Future work is needed to incorporate the expanded populations. Some EHRs have added preferred pronouns; this change makes the experience better for patients but does not indicate which laboratory reference interval should be used because such intervals have not yet been established.[121] Other EHRs may restrict test availability based on a patient's sex, which would then not allow a provider to order a Pap smear on a transgender man or a prostate-specific antigen test on a transgender woman if the patient has retained the applicable organs.[122] EHR vendors, providers, and health care facilities should work together, with input from the transgender community, to improve the interoperability and inclusivity of both transgender and nonbinary patients within the medical record.

SUMMARY

- Neonatal hematology parameters change over the first few days, weeks, and months of life. Laboratory results must be assessed considering gestational age, birth weight, and developmental differences between preterm neonates, full-term neonates, and older infants.
- The erythrocytes of neonates are markedly macrocytic at birth, with increased polychromasia. A condition known as physiologic anemia of infancy occurs after the first 4 to 6 weeks of life. Neonates born prematurely also experience a decrease in hemoglobin concentration, which is termed physiologic anemia of prematurity.
- Iron deficiency is the most common cause of anemia in children.
- Fluctuations in the number of white blood cells are common at all ages but are greatest in infants. Leukocytosis is typical in healthy full-term and preterm neonates at birth. There is an increase in segmented neutrophils, bands, and occasional metamyelocytes, with no evidence of disease.
- Sepsis in neonates is a common cause of morbidity, particularly in premature and low-birth-weight infants. Defective B cell response against polysaccharide agents and abnormal cytokine release by neutrophils and monocytes have been implicated.
- Although hemostatic values are different in infants and children from those in adults, this population is not at increased risk of bleeding or thrombosis.
- The most common hematologic complication during pregnancy is anemia. Physiologic anemia of pregnancy is caused by expansion of the plasma volume compared to the RBC volume.
- The increased need for iron during pregnancy for maternal RBC production, for the placenta and the fetus, and to

recover from blood loss often results in iron deficiency anemia in the mother.

- Megaloblastic anemia due to folate deficiency has become an uncommon cause of nutritional anemia in pregnancy due to government-mandated folate fortification of foods. Low folate levels in early pregnancy, however, increases the risk of neural tube defects in the fetus.
- Normal pregnancy is considered to be a hypercoagulable state with significantly increased concentrations of some coagulation proteins and decreased levels of coagulation inhibitors.
- Thrombocytopenia is common in pregnancy, occurring in approximately 10% of all pregnancies.
- There is a gradual decline in hemoglobin starting at middle age, and the mean level decreases by about 1 g/dL during the sixth through eighth decades.
- Although anemia is common in elderly patients, it is not a normal occurrence in the aging process. The cause of anemia may be multifactorial in elderly patients.
- Iron deficiency anemia and anemia of inflammation are common anemias seen in elderly adults.
- Immunosenescence refers to the adverse changes in the immune system associated with aging.

- Elderly adults experience an increased frequency of hematologic malignancies, such as myelodysplastic neoplasms, myeloproliferative neoplasms, and chronic lymphocytic leukemia.
- Elderly adults are at an increased risk of thrombosis associated with age-related changes in the vascular and hemostatic systems.
- The transgender population is diverse, and more research is needed to establish reference intervals for this population at various stages of transition; more research is also needed to study the long-term effects of hormone therapy on hematopoiesis and hemostasis.
- Electronic health record vendors, providers, and health care facilities should work together, with input from the transgender community, to improve the interoperability and inclusivity of both transgender and nonbinary patients within the medical record.

Now that you have completed this chapter, go back and read again the case study at the beginning and respond to the questions presented. Answers can be found in Appendix C.

REVIEW QUESTIONS

Answers can be found in Appendix C.

1. The CBC results for children (aged 3 to 12 years) differ from those of adults chiefly in what respect?
   a. NRBCs are present
   b. Polychromasia is present
   c. Platelet count is lower
   d. Absolute lymphocyte count is higher
2. Physiologic anemia of infancy results from:
   a. Iron deficiency caused by a milk-only diet during the early neonatal period
   b. Increased oxygenation of blood and decreased erythropoietin
   c. Replacement of active marrow with fat soon after birth
   d. Hb F and its diminished oxygen delivery to tissues
3. Morphologically, the hematogones in neonates are:
   a. Similar to those seen in megaloblastic anemia
   b. Easily confused with leukemic blasts
   c. Monocytoid in appearance
   d. Similar to adult lymphocytes
4. The most common cause of anemia in childhood is:
   a. Vitamin B_{12} deficiency
   b. Drug-related hemolysis
   c. Iron deficiency
   d. Folate deficiency
5. The physiologic anemia of pregnancy is a result of:
   a. A decrease of EPO response during pregnancy
   b. Inability of the pregnant woman to absorb dietary iron
   c. Increased hepcidin synthesis during gestation
   d. Increased plasma volume proportionally greater than the increase in RBC mass

6. A pregnant woman was seen in the emergency department with the following: decreased platelet count, proteinuria, fragmented RBCs, and increased liver enzymes. What is the most likely cause of these abnormalities?
   a. HELLP syndrome
   b. ITP
   c. Antiphospholipid syndrome (APS)
   d. DIC
7. Which of the following are common anemias in elderly adults?
   a. Megaloblastic anemia and hemolytic anemia
   b. Sideroblastic anemia and megaloblastic anemia
   c. Myelophthisic anemia and anemia of inflammation
   d. Iron deficiency anemia and anemia of inflammation
8. When iron deficiency is recognized in an elderly patient, the cause is usually:
   a. An iron-deficient diet
   b. Gastrointestinal bleeding
   c. Diminished absorption
   d. Impaired incorporation of iron into heme
9. Which one of the following conditions is least likely in an elderly patient?
   a. Acute lymphoblastic leukemia
   b. Polycythemia vera
   c. Myelodysplastic neoplasm
   d. Chronic lymphocytic leukemia

10. The hypercoagulable state in pregnancy is due to an increase in:
    a. Protein C, protein S, and plasmin activation
    b. VWF, fibrinogen, and other coagulation factors
    c. Red blood cell, white blood cell, and platelet counts
    d. Factors V and VIII with a decrease in VWF and fibrinogen

11. Which one of the following statements is TRUE about the transgender population?
    a. A transgender man was assigned male at birth.
    b. All transgender men are expected to have the same hematology reference intervals.
    c. Female hematology reference intervals can be reliably used for transgender women.
    d. The EHR needs improvement to provide better care for transgender patients.

REFERENCES

1. Chou, S. T. (2020). Development of the hematopoietic system. In Kliegman, R., St Geme, J. W., Blum, N. J., et al. (Eds.), *Nelson Textbook of Pediatrics*. (21st ed., pp. 2500–2505). Philadelphia: Elsevier.

2. Palis, J., & Koniski, A. (2018). Functional analysis of erythroid progenitors by colony-forming assays. *Methods Mol Biol, 1698*, 117–132.

3. Juul, S., & Christensen, R. (2018). Developmental hematology. In Gleason, C., & Juul, S. (Eds.), *Avery's Diseases of the Newborn*. (10th ed., pp. 1113–1120). Philadelphia: Elsevier.

4. Kim, C. (2010). Homeostatic and pathogenic extramedullary hematopoiesis. *J Blood Med, 1*, 13–19.

5. American College of Obstetricians and Gynecologists Committee on Obstetric Practice, Society for Maternal-Fetal Medicine. Definition of term pregnancy, Number 579 (Reaffirmed 2022). https://www.acog.org/clinical/clinical-guidance/committee-opinion/articles/2013/11/definition-of-term-pregnancy. Accessed April 8, 2023.

6. Pachter, L. (2020). Child health disparities. In Kliegman, R., St Geme, J. W., Blum, N. J., et al. (Eds.), *Nelson Textbook of Pediatrics*. (21st ed., pp. 9–21). Philadelphia: Elsevier.

7. Teramo, K. A., & Widness, J. A. (2009). Increased fetal plasma and amniotic fluid erythropoietin concentrations: markers of intrauterine hypoxia. *Neonatology, 95*, 105–116.

8. Proytcheva, M. A. (2009). Issues in neonatal cellular analysis. *Am J Clin Path, 131*, 560–573.

9. Saito-Benz, M., Flanagan, P., & Berry, M. J. (2020). Management of anaemia in pre-term infants. *Br J Haematol, 188*, 354–366.

10. Diaz-Miron, J., Miller, J., & Vogel, A. M. (2013). Neonatal hematology. *Semin Pediatr Surg, 22*(4), 199–204.

11. Angelo, A., Derbie, G., Demtse, A., et al. (2021). Umbilical cord blood hematological parameters reference interval for newborns from Addis Ababa, Ethiopia. *BMC Pediatr, 21*(1), 275.

12. Morton, S. U., Brettin, K., Feldman, H. A., et al. (2020). Association of nucleated red blood cell count with mortality among neonatal intensive care unit patients. *Pediatr Neonatol, 61*(6), 592–597.

13. Zipursky, A., Brown, E., Palko, J., et al. (1983). The erythrocyte differential count in newborn infants. *Am J Pediatr Hematol Oncol, 5*(1), 45–51.

14. Parodi, E., Romano, F., & Ramenghi, U. (2020). How we use reticulocyte parameters in workup and management of pediatric hematologic diseases. *Front Pediatr, 8*, 588617.

15. Yamada, M., Chishiki, M., Kanai, Y., et al. (2020). Neonatal reticulocyte count during the early postnatal period. *Pediatr Neonatol, 61*(5), 490–497.

16. Li, H., Xiao, J., Liao, M., et al. (2020). Anemia prevalence, severity and associated factors among children aged 6–71 months in rural Hunan Province, China: a community-based cross-sectional study. *BMC Public Health, 20*(1), 989.

17. Mohammed, S. H., Habtewold, T. D., & Esmaillzadeh, A. (2019). Household, maternal, and child related determinants of hemoglobin levels of Ethiopian children: hierarchical regression analysis. *BMC Pediatr, 19*(1), 113.

18. Heesemann, E., Mähler, C., Subramanyam, M. A., et al. (2021). Pregnancy anaemia, child health and development: a cohort study in rural India. *BMJ Open, 11*(11), e046802.

19. Kalteren, W. S., Mebius, M. J., Verhagen, E. A., et al. (2021). Neonatal hemoglobin levels in preterm infants are associated with early neurological functioning. *Neonatology, 118*(5), 593–599.

20. Abu-Ouf, N. M., & Jan, M. M. (2015). The impact of maternal iron deficiency and iron deficiency anemia on child's health. *Saudi Med J, 36*(2), 146–149.

21. Abbaspour, N., Hurrell, R., & Kelishadi, R. (2014). Review on iron and its importance for human health. *J Res Med Sci, 19*(2), 164–174.

22. Gupta, P., Perrine, C., Mei, Z., et al. (2016). Iron, anemia, and iron deficiency anemia among young children in the United States. *Nutrients, 8*(6), 330.

23. Nassin, M. L., Lapping-Carr, G., & De Jong, J. L. O. (2015). Anemia in the neonate: the differential diagnosis and treatment. *Pediatr Ann, 44*(7), e159–e163.

24. Christensen, R. D., Henry, E., Jopling, J., et al. (2009). The CBC: reference ranges for neonates. *Semin Perinatol, 33*(1), 3–11.

25. Dinauer, M. C. (2016). Primary immune deficiencies with defects in neutrophil function. *Hematology Am Soc Hematol Educ Program, 2016*(1), 43–50.

26. Hayes, R., Hartnett, J., Semova, G., et al. (2023). Neonatal sepsis definitions from randomised clinical trials. *Pediatr Res, 93*(5), 1141–1148.

27. Christensen, R. D., & Ohls, R. K. (2012). Anemia in the neonatal period. In Buonocore, G., Bracci, R., & Weingling, M. (Eds.), *Neonatology a Practical Approach to Neonatal Diseases*. (pp. 784–798). Milan: Springer-Verlag.

28. Aly, M. M., Mahfouz, R. Z., & Eltonsi, I. (2016). Hematogones detection in hematological malignancies and bone marrow transplantation. JSM *Bone Marrow Res, 1*(1), 1001.

29. Tsafaras, G. P., Ntontsi, P., & Xanthou, G. (2020). Advantages and limitations of the neonatal immune system. *Front Pediatr, 8*, https://doi.org/10.3389/fped.2020.00005.

30. Angelone, D. F., Wessels, M. R., Coughlin, M., et al. (2006). Innate immunity of the human newborn is polarized toward a high ratio of IL-6/TNF-α production in vitro and in vivo. *Pediatr Res, 60*(2), 205–209.

31. Tesfamariam, B. (2017). Distinct characteristics of neonatal platelet reactivity. *Pharmacol Res, 123*, 1–9.

32. Kenet, G., Barg, A. A., & Nowak-Göttl, U. (2022). New insights into neonatal hemostasis. *Thromb Update, 7*, 100103.

33. Al-Khaffaf, A., Frattini, F., Gaiardoni, R., et al. (2020). Diagnosis of anemia in pregnancy. *J Lab Precis Med*, 5, https://doi.org/10.21037/jlpm.2019.12.03.

34. Shah, T., Khaskheli, M. S., Ansari, S., et al. (2022). Gestational anemia and its effects on neonatal outcome, in the population of Hyderabad, Sindh, Pakistan. *Saudi J Biol Sci*, 29(1), 83–87.

35. Pecker, L. H., & Naik, R. P. (2018). The current state of sickle cell trait: implications for reproductive and genetic counseling. *Blood*, 132(22), 2331–2338.

36. The American College of Obstericians and Gynecologists (2022). Hemoglobinopathies in pregnancy: practice advisory. https://www.acog.org/clinical/clinical-guidance/practice-advisory/articles/2022/08/hemoglobinopathies-in-pregnancy. Accessed April 8, 2023.

37. American College of Obstetricians and Gynecologists' Committee on Practice Bulletins. (2021). Anemia in pregnancy: ACOG practice bulletin, number 233. *Obstet Gynecol, 138*(2), e55–e64.

38. Shi, H., Chen, L., Wang, Y., et al. (2022). Severity of anemia during pregnancy and adverse maternal and fetal outcomes. *JAMA Netw Open*, 5(2), e2147046.

39. Centers for Disease Control and Prevention. Folic acid recommendations. https://www.cdc.gov/ncbddd/folicacid/recommendations.html. Accessed March 23, 2023.

40. Smith-Whitley, K. (2019). Complications in pregnant women with sickle cell disease. *Hematology Am Soc Hematol Educ Program*, 2019(1), 359–366.

41. Kasparek, J., Burkhardt, T., Hoesli, I., et al. (2021). Pregnancy outcomes in women with a hemoglobinopathy trait: a multicenter, retrospective study. *Arch Gynecol Obstet*, 304(5), 1197–1203.

42. Petrakos, G., Andriopoulos, P., & Tsironi, M. (2016). Pregnancy in women with thalassemia: challenges and solutions. *Int J Women's Health*, 8, 441–451.

43. Yue, M., Ma, L., Cao, Y., et al. (2021). Application of a nomogram for predicting the risk of subchorionic hematoma in early pregnancy with in vitro fertilization-embryo transfer/frozen embryo transfer. *Front Endocrinol*, 12, 631097.

44. West, B. T., Kavoussi, P. K., Odenwald, K. C., et al. (2020). Factors associated with subchorionic hematoma formation in pregnancies achieved via assisted reproductive technologies. *J Assist Reprod Genet*, 37(2), 305–309.

45. Lee, A. I., & Okam, M. M. (2011). Anemia in pregnancy. *Hematol Oncol Clin North Am*, 25(2), 241–259.

46. Means, R. T. (2019). Anemias during pregnancy and the postpartum period. In Greer, J. P., Rodgers, G. M., Glader, B., et al. (Eds.), *Wintrobe's Clinical Hematology*. (14th ed., pp. 1025–1030). Philadelphia: Wolters Kluwer.

47. Abe, K., Kuklina, E. V., Hooper, W. C., et al. (2019). Venous thromboembolism as a cause of severe maternal morbidity and mortality in the United States. *Semin Perinatol*, 43(4), 200–204.

48. Devis, P., & Knuttinen, M. G. (2017). Deep venous thrombosis in pregnancy: incidence, pathogenesis and endovascular management. *Cardiovasc Diagn Ther*, 7(Suppl 3), S309–S319.

49. Garcia, D., & Erkan, D. (2018). Diagnosis and management of the antiphospholipid syndrome. *N Engl J Med*, 378(21), 2010–2021.

50. Ciobanu, A. M., Colibaba, S., Cimpoca, B., et al. (2016). Thrombocytopenia in pregnancy. *Maedica*, 11(1), 55–60.

51. Baucom, A. M., Kuller, J. A., & Dotters-Katz, S. (2019). Immune thrombocytopenic purpura in pregnancy. *Obstet Gynecol Surv*, 74(8), 490–496.

52. Soffer, M. D., Bendapudi, P. K., Roberts, D. J., et al. (2020). Congenital thrombotic thrombocytopenic purpura (TTP) with placental abruption despite maternal improvement: a case report. *BMC Pregnancy Childbirth*, 20(1), 365.

53. Gupta, M., Govindappagari, S., & Burwick, R. M. (2020). Pregnancy-associated atypical hemolytic uremic syndrome. *Obstet Gynecol*, 135(1), 46–58.

54. Rana, S., Lemoine, E., Granger, J. P., et al. (2019). Preeclampsia: pathophysiology, challenges, and perspectives. *Circ Res*, 124(7), 1094–1112.

55. Lisonkova, S., Muraca, G. M., Wang, L. Q., et al. (2021). Incidence and risk factors for severe preeclampsia, hemolysis, elevated liver enzymes, and low platelet count syndrome, and eclampsia at preterm and term gestation: a population-based study. *Am J Obstet Gynecol*, 225(5), 538.e1–538.e19.

56. Li, B., & Yang, H. (2022). Comparison of clinical features and pregnancy outcomes in early- and late-onset preeclampsia with HELLP syndrome: a 10-year retrospective study from a tertiary hospital and referral center in China. *BMC Pregnancy Childbirth*, 22(1), 186.

57. Vespa, J., Medina, L., & Armstrong, D. M. (2018, revised 2020). Demographic turning points for the United States: population projections for 2020 to 2060. U.S. Department of Commerce, U.S. Census Bureau. https://www.census.gov/content/dam/Census/library/publications/2020/demo/p25-1144.pdf. Accessed April 8, 2023.

58. Rabin, R. C. (Sept 1, 2022). U.S. life expectancy falls again in 'historic' setback. *The New York Times*. https://www.nytimes.com/2022/08/31/health/life-expectancy-covid-pandemic.html. Accessed April 8, 2023.

59. Tomasetti, C., Poling, J., Roberts, N. J., et al. (2019). Cell division rates decrease with age, providing a potential explanation for the age-dependent deceleration in cancer incidence. *Proc Nat Acad Sci*, 116(41), 20482–20488.

60. Longo, D. L. (2008). Bone marrow in aging: changes? yes; clinical malfunction? not so clear. *Blood*, 112(11), sci-1.

61. Lin, J., & Epel, E. (2022). Stress and telomere shortening: insights from cellular mechanisms. *Ageing Res Rev*, 73, 101507.

62. Fred, H. L. (2007). Maxwell Myer Wintrobe: new history and a new appreciation. *Tex Heart Inst J*, 34(3), 328–335.

63. Zierk, J., Krebs, A., Rauh, M., et al. (2020). Blood counts in adult and elderly individuals: defining the norms over eight decades of life. *Br J Haematol*, 189(4), 777–789.

64. Nilsson-Ehle, H., Jagenburg, R., Landahl, S., et al. (2000). Blood haemoglobin declines in the elderly: implications for reference intervals from age 70 to 88. *Eur J Haematol*, 65(5), 297–305.

65. Esme, M., Topeli, A., Yavuz, B. B., et al. (2019). Infections in the elderly critically-ill patients. *Front Med*, 6, 118.

66. Luo, M., Xu, L., Qian, Z., et al. (2021). Infection-associated thymic atrophy. *Front Immunol*, 12, 652538.

67. Trzupek, D., Dunstan, M., Cutler, A. J., et al. (2020). Discovery of CD80 and CD86 as recent activation markers on regulatory T cells by protein-RNA single-cell analysis. *Genome Med*, 12(1), 55.

68. Busse, S., Steiner, J., Alter, J., et al. (2015). Expression of HLA-DR, CD80, and CD86 in healthy aging and Alzheimer's disease. *J Alzheimers Dis*, 47(1), 177–184.

69. de Mol, J., Kuiper, J., Tsiantoulas, D., et al. (2021). The dynamics of B cell aging in health and disease. *Front Immunol*, 12, 733566.

70. Kikuchi, K., Lai, A. Y., Hsu, C.-L., et al. (2005). IL-7 receptor signaling is necessary for stage transition in adult B cell

development through up-regulation of EBF. *J Exp Med, 201*(8), 1197–1203.

71. De Maeyer, R. P. H., & Chambers, E. S. (2021). The impact of ageing on monocytes and macrophages. *Immunol Lett, 230,* 1–10.

72. Le Blanc, J., & Lordkipanidzé, M. (2019). Platelet function in aging. *Front Cardiovasc Med, 6,* 109.

73. Best, M. G., Vancura, A., & Wurdinger, T. (2017). Platelet RNA as a circulating biomarker trove for cancer diagnostics. *J Thromb Haemost, 15*(7), 1295–1306.

74. Clancy, L., & Freedman, J. E. (2015). The role of circulating platelet transcripts. *J Thromb Haemost, 13,* S33–S39.

75. Guralnik, J. M., Eisenstaedt, R. S., Ferrucci, L., et al. (2004). Prevalence of anemia in persons 65 years and older in the United States: evidence for a high rate of unexplained anemia. *Blood, 104*(8), 2263–2268.

76. Guralnik, J., Ershler, W., Artz, A., et al. (2022). Unexplained anemia of aging: etiology, health consequences, and diagnostic criteria. *J Am Geriatr Soc, 70*(3), 891–899.

77. Burton, J. K., Yates, L. C., Whyte, L., et al. (2020). New horizons in iron deficiency anaemia in older adults. *Age Ageing, 49*(3), 309–318.

78. Ganz, T. (2019). Anemia of inflammation. *N Engl J Med, 381*(12), 1148–1157.

79. Gadó, K., Khodier, M., Virág, A., et al. (2022). Anemia of geriatric patients. *Physiol Int, 109*(2), 119–134.

80. Tettamanti, M., Lucca, U., Gandini, F., et al. (2010). Prevalence, incidence and types of mild anemia in the elderly: the "health and anemia" population-based study. *Haematologica, 95*(11), 1849–1856.

81. Moon, T., Smith, A., Pak, T., et al. (2021). Preoperative anemia treatment with intravenous iron therapy in patients undergoing abdominal surgery: a systematic review. *Adv Ther, 38*(3), 1447–1469.

82. Cazzola, M. (2022). Ineffective erythropoiesis and its treatment. *Blood, 139*(16), 2460–2470.

83. Alaggio, R., Amador, C., Anagnostopoulos, I., et al. (2022). The 5th edition of the World Health Organization classification of haematolymphoid tumours: lymphoid neoplasms. *Leukemia, 36*(7), 1720–1748.

84. Khoury, J. D., Solary, E., Abla, O., et al. (2022). The 5th edition of the World Health Organization classification of haematolymphoid tumours: myeloid and histiocytic/dendritic neoplasms. *Leukemia, 36*(7), 1703–1719.

85. Liu, M., Wang, F., Zhang, Y., et al. (2021). Gene mutation spectrum of patients with myelodysplastic syndrome and progression to acute myeloid leukemia. *Int J Hematol Oncol, 10*(2), IJH34.

86. Prassek, V. V., Rothenberg-Thurley, M., Sauerland, M. C., et al. (2018). Genetics of acute myeloid leukemia in the elderly: mutation spectrum and clinical impact in intensively treated patients aged 75 years or older. *Haematologica, 103*(11), 1853–1861.

87. Fenaux, P., Haase, D., Santini, V., et al. (2021). Myelodysplastic syndromes: ESMO clinical practice guidelines for diagnosis, treatment and follow-up. *Ann Oncol, 32*(2), 142–156.

88. National Institutes of Health. (2022). Leukemia incidence rates by age at diagnosis, 2015-2019. www.seer.cancer.gov/statistics-network/explorer/application.html. Accessed April 8, 2023.

89. Gross, P. L., & Chan, N. C. (2020). Thromboembolism in older adults. *Front Med, 7,* 470016.

90. Favaloro, E. J., Franchini, M., & Lippi, G. (2014). Aging hemostasis: changes to laboratory markers of hemostasis as we age - a narrative review. *Semin Thromb Hemost, 40*(6), 621–633.

91. Kryczka, K. E., Kruk, M., Demkow, M., et al. (2021). Fibrinogen and a triad of thrombosis, inflammation, and the renin-angiotensin system in premature coronary artery disease in women: a new insight into sex-related differences in the pathogenesis of the disease. *Biomolecules, 11*(7), 1036.

92. Urano, T., Suzuki, Y., Iwaki, T., et al. (2019). Recognition of plasminogen activator inhibitor type 1 as the primary regulator of fibrinolysis. *Curr Drug Targets, 20*(16), 1695–1701.

93. Zhang, K., Zhu, Y., Tian, Y., et al. (2021). Role of a new age-adjusted D-dimer cutoff value for preoperative deep venous thrombosis exclusion in elderly patients with hip fractures. *J Orthop Surg Res, 16*(1), 649.

94. Kruse-Jarres, R. (2015). Acquired bleeding disorders in the elderly. *Hematology Am Soc Hematol Educ Program, 2015,* 231–236.

95. American Psychological Association. (2022). Understanding transgender people, gender identity and gender expression. https://www.apa.org/topics/lgbtq/transgender. Accessed April 8, 2023.

96. Brown, A. (2022). About 5% of young adults in the U.S. say their gender is different from their sex assigned at birth. Pew Research Center. https://www.pewresearch.org/fact-tank/2022/06/07/about-5-of-young-adults-in-the-u-s-say-their-gender-is-different-from-their-sex-assigned-at-birth/. Accessed October 13, 2022.

97. Swe, N. C., Ahmed, S., Eid, M., et al. (2022). The effects of gender-affirming hormone therapy on cardiovascular and skeletal health: a literature review. *Metabol Open, 13,* 100173.

98. Cocchetti, C., Ristori, J., Romani, A., et al. (2020). Hormonal treatment strategies tailored to non-binary transgender individuals. *J Clin Med, 9*(6), 1609.

99. Restar, A., Dusic, E. J., Garrison-Desany, H., et al. (2022). Gender affirming hormone therapy dosing behaviors among transgender and nonbinary adults. *Humanit Soc Sci Commun, 9*(1), 304.

100. Honigberg, M. C., Zekavat, S. M., Niroula, A., et al. (2021). Premature menopause, clonal hematopoiesis, and coronary artery disease in postmenopausal women. *Circulation, 143*(5), 410–423.

101. Lechner, J., & Gstraunthaler, G. (2019). Sex and sex hormones in tissue homeostasis. In. IntechOpen. https://doi.org/10.5772/intechopen.76177.

102. Quatrini, L., Ricci, B., Ciancaglini, C., et al. (2021). Regulation of the immune system development by glucocorticoids and sex hormones. *Front Immunol, 12,* 672853.

103. Bujko, K., Cymer, M., Adamiak, M., et al. (2019). An overview of novel unconventional mechanisms of hematopoietic development and regulators of hematopoiesis – a roadmap for future investigations. *Stem Cell Rev Rep, 15*(6), 785–794.

104. Fañanas-Baquero, S., Orman, I., Becerra Aparicio, F., et al. (2018). Estrogens enhance human hematopoietic stem cell engraftment in a xenogenic transplantation model. *Blood, 132*(Supplement 1), 2042–2042.

105. Sánchez-Aguilera, A., & Méndez-Ferrer, S. (2016). Regulation of hematopoietic progenitors by estrogens as a basis for new antileukemic strategies. *Mol Cell Oncol, 3*(1), e1009728.b.

106. Knewtson, K. E., Ohl, N. R., & Robinson, J. L. (2022). Estrogen signaling dictates musculoskeletal stem cell behavior: sex differences in tissue repair. *Tissue Eng Part B Rev, 28*(4), 789–812.

107. Dhindsa, S., Nargunan, V., Reddy, A., et al. (2020). Testosterone decreases erythropoietin stimulating agent use in men on hemodialysis. *Androg Clin Res Ther, 1*(1), 32–39.

108. Pinkerton, J. V. (2020). Hormone therapy for postmenopausal women. *N Engl J Med, 382*(5), 446–455.

109. Abou-Ismail, M. Y., Sridhar, D. C., & Nayak, L. (2020). Estrogen and thrombosis: a bench to bedside review. *Thromb Res, 192*, 40–51.

110. Moreau, K. L., Babcock, M. C., & Hildreth, K. L. (2020). Sex differences in vascular aging in response to testosterone. *Biol Sex Differ, 11*(1), 18.

111. White, J., Petrella, F., & Ory, J. (2022). Testosterone therapy and secondary erythrocytosis. *Int J Impot Res, 34*(7), 693–697.

112. Hudson, J., Cruickshank, M., Quinton, R., et al. (2022). Adverse cardiovascular events and mortality in men during testosterone treatment: an individual patient and aggregate data meta-analysis. *Lancet Healthy Longev, 3*(6), e381–e393.

113. Ederveen, E. G. T., Van Hunsel, F. P. A. M., Wondergem, M. J., et al. (2018). Severe secondary polycythemia in a female-to-male transgender patient while using lifelong hormonal therapy: a patient's perspective. *Drug Saf Case Rep, 5*(1), 6.

114. Gangat, N., Szuber, N., Pardanani, A., et al. (2021). JAK2 unmutated erythrocytosis: current diagnostic approach and therapeutic views. *Leukemia, 35*(8), 2166–2181.

115. Humble, R. M., Greene, D. N., Schmidt, R. L., et al. (2022). Reference intervals for clinical chemistry analytes for transgender men and women on stable hormone therapy. *J Appl Lab Med, 7*(5), 1131–1144.

116. Greene, D. N., McPherson, G. W., Rongitsch, J., et al. (2019). Hematology reference intervals for transgender adults on stable hormone therapy. *Clin Chim Acta, 492*, 84–90.

117. Cheung, A. S., Cook, T., Ginger, A., et al. (2022). Sex specific reference ranges and transgender care. *BMJ, 376*, e069874.

118. Cheung, A. S., Lim, H. Y., Cook, T., et al. (2021). Approach to interpreting common laboratory pathology tests in transgender individuals. *J Clin Endocrinol Metab, 106*(3), 893–901.

119. Miller, B. S., Sarafoglou, K., & Addo, O. Y. (2020). Development of Tanner stage-age adjusted CDC height curves for research and clinical applications. *J Endocr Soc, 4*(9), bvaa098.

120. Deloughery, T. G. (2022). Hematologic concerns in transgender patients. *Clin Adv Hematol Oncol, 20*(8), 516–523.

121. Kronk, C. A., Everhart, A. R., Ashley, F., et al. (2022). Transgender data collection in the electronic health record: current concepts and issues. *J Am Med Inform Assoc, 29*(2), 271–284.

122. Moseson, H., Zazanis, N., Goldberg, E., et al. (2020). The imperative for transgender and gender nonbinary inclusion. *Obstet Gynecol, 135*(5), 1059–1068.

INDEX

A

Abbott, 199b, 210–213, 211f
  hemoglobin determination, 210
  MAPSS, for WBC count, WBC differential, NRBC, platelet, and reticulocyte analysis, 210–213, 211f–212f
  RBC and platelet analysis, impedance for, 210
Abbott CELL-DYN Sapphire, 204t
Abetalipoproteinemia (ABL), 363
Abnormal cellular function, 623
Absolute reticulocyte count, 3, 189, 220
Absorbed ferritin, 131
Absorption
  of dietary iron
    ferritin absorption, 124, 125f
    heme absorption, 124, 125f
    ionic iron absorption, 125–126, 125f
  and disposition
    folate, impaired, 301
    vitamin B_{12}, 301–303
Acanthocytes, 100, 267t, 269f, 362–363
Accidental release measures, 881.e7
Accuracy, 22–23, 22f
  in coagulation instrumentation, 848
Acetylcholinesterase-derived megakaryocyte growth stimulating peptide, 163
Acetylsalicylic acid (aspirin), in platelets, 722
Achlorhydria, 306
Achromatic objective lens, 881.e28
Acid hydrolases, 48
Acidophilia, 80–81
Acid sphingomyelinase deficiency (ASMD), 473
ACL AcuStar (Werfen), 850–851, 853f
Ac platelet-binding activity, 697–699
Acquired aplastic anemia, 314–318
  clinical findings, 316
  etiology, 314b–315b, 315
  incidence, 314
  laboratory findings, 316–318, 317f–318f, 317t
  pathophysiology, 315–316
  treatment and prognosis, 318
Acquired coagulopathies, 688–693
  acquired hemophilia, 692–693
    management for, 693
  acquired von Willebrand disease, 693
  chronic renal failure and hemorrhage, 691–692
  disseminated intravascular coagulation. See Disseminated intravascular coagulation
  liver disease, 690–691
  trauma-induced coagulopathy, 688–690
  vitamin K deficiency and hemorrhage, 692
Acquired FXIII deficiency, 706
Acquired FXIII inhibitors, 706
Acquired hypoplasia, 738–739
Acquired iron overload, 287
Acquired pure red cell aplasia, 321–322
Acquired red blood cell membrane abnormalities, 363–368
  acquired stomatocytosis, 363
  paroxysmal nocturnal hemoglobinuria, 364–368
  spur cell anemia, 363
Acquired sideroblastic anemias, 286
Acquired stomatocytosis, 363
Acquired storage pool disease, 726

Acquired von Willebrand disease, 693
Acquisition and intracellular trafficking, iron, 129–131, 130f
Acrocyanosis, autoimmune hemolytic anemia and, 399
Actin, 166
Actin junctional complex, 101, 102f
Activated clotting time (ACT), in unfractionated heparin, 796–797
Activated partial thromboplastin time (APTT). See Partial thromboplastin time
Activated protein C (APC) resistance, 762, 764, 765t, 769–770, 770f
Activation, platelets, 169–171
  adhesion, 169, 170f
  aggregation, 169–170, 171f
  eicosanoid synthesis, 171–173, 173f
  G-proteins, 171, 172f
  inositol triphosphate-diacylglycerol pathway, 173
  markers, 821
  microparticles, 171
  pathways, 171–173
  secretion, 171, 172t
Active transport, plasma membrane, 49
  primary, 49
  secondary, 49
  vesicular, 49
Acute abdominal pain, sickle cell disease and, 418
Acute anemia, 418–419
  and sickle cell disease, 418–419
Acute basophilic leukemia (ABL), 574
Acute blood loss, 220
  during pregnancy, 869
Acute chest syndrome, 434
Acute erythroid leukemia, 575, 576f
Acute hemolysis, 331–332, 341
Acute hemolytic anemia, 370, 370b
Acute hemolytic transfusion reaction (AHTRs), 405
Acute leukemias, 566–582, 566f, 566b. See also Acute
  of ambiguous lineage, 577, 577b
  classification schemes for, 567–568, 567f
  cytochemical stains and interpretations, 577–579, 578t
  cytogenetics, 561, 561f–562f
  general characteristics of, 490, 491t
  introduction to, 567
  laboratory diagnosis of, 567, 568t
Acute leukemias of ambiguous lineage (ALALs), 577, 577b
Acute lymphoblastic leukemia (ALL), 4, 152, 568–570, 881.e39
  clinical presentation of, 568
  cytogenetics, 559, 559b
  diagnosis of, 568
  genetic and molecular findings of, 570
  immunophenotyping in, 569–570, 569t
  morphology of, 568, 569f
  prognosis of, 569, 569t
  Sudan Black B staining, 573, 574f
  WHO classification of, 568, 569t
Acute megakaryoblastic leukemia, 575, 577f
Acute monoblastic/monocytic leukemias, 574–575, 576f

Acute myeloid leukemia (AML), 4, 570–576, 881.e39
  acute basophilic leukemia, 574
  acute myelomonocytic leukemia, 574, 575f
  clinical presentation of, 570
  cytochemical stains and interpretations, 577–579, 578f, 578t
  cytogenetics, 559, 559b, 561, 562f
  defined by differentiation, 507–508, 509f–510f, 573–575, 574t
  with defining genetic abnormalities, 507, 508f–509f, 571–573
    with BCR::ABL1, 573
    with CBFB-MYH11, 571–572, 572f
    with CEBPA mutation, 573
    with DEK-NUP214, 573
    with MECOM rearrangement, 573
    with NPM1 mutation, 573
    with PML-RARA, 572–573, 572f
    with RBM15::MRTFA, 573
    with RUNX1::RUNX1T1, 571, 572f
  diagnosis of, 570
  esterases staining, 578–579, 579f
  Fanconi anemia and, 319
  flow cytometric analysis of, 506–510, 507f
  French-American-British (FAB) classification of, 573, 574t
  with KMT2A rearrangements, 573, 573f
  with maturation, 574, 575f
  with minimal differentiation, 573, 574f
  with myelodysplasia-related, 573
  myeloid neoplasms, secondary, 576
  myeloid sarcoma, 576
  risk categories of, 571
  WHO classification of, 570–571, 571t, 571b
  without maturation, 574, 575f
Acute myelomonocytic leukemia, 574, 575f
Acute promyelocytic leukemia, 763–764
Acute undifferentiated leukemias (AULs), 577
ADAMTS-13, 381
  and thrombotic thrombocytopenic purpura, 746–747
Adaptive immunity, 151
Additives in collection tubes, 881.e13
Adenine, 523–524
Adeno-associated virus vector (AAV) vaccines, 782
Adenocarcinoma, 764t
Adenosine deaminase deficiency (ADA-SCID), 466
Adenosine diphosphate (ADP), 168, 820
  pyruvate kinase deficiency and, 374
  receptors, 721
Adenosine triphosphate (ATP), 91, 96
  pyruvate kinase deficiency and, 374
  RBC membrane osmotic balance and permeability and, 104–105
  secretion of, platelet aggregation and, 818
Adhesion
  plasma membrane receptors for, 166–168, 167f, 168t
  platelets, 665
  vascular matrix bindings by platelets, 169, 170f
Adipocytes, 55
Adjacent cells, 49
ADP. See Adenosine diphosphate
α_2-adrenergic (epinephrine) receptor, 721

Note: Page numbers followed by "f" refer to illustrations; page numbers followed by "t" refer to tables; page numbers followed by "b" refer to boxes.

Adult hematopoietic tissue, 60–68
  bone marrow, 60–64, 62f–63f
  liver, 64, 64f
  lymph nodes, 66, 67f
  spleen, 64–66, 65f–66f
  thymus, 66–68, 67f–68f
Adult stem cells, 496
Adult T-cell leukemia/lymphoma (ATLL), 646–647, 647f
Advanced hematology procedures, 5–6
Adventitial reticular cells, 61–62
Adverse events, 9
Afferent lymphatic vessels, 66
Afibrinogenemia, 706t, 726
Aged adults. See Elderly adults
Agencies, quality assurance, 38
AggRAM, 856
Aggregation, platelet, 169–170, 171f, 665
Aggregometers, platelet, 855–856, 856f, 856t
Aging, hematopoiesis and, 871
Agnogenic myelofibrosis, 604
AG-NOR-banding, 554
Agonists, 165
  platelet aggregometry, 818t, 819–821
Agranular myeloid cells, 621f
Agranular neutrophil, promyelocyte or myelocyte devoid of, 621, 622f
Agranular promyelocytes, 621
Agranulocytosis, 476–477
AKT2 inhibitors, 425
Albumin, 337
Alcohol consumption, thrombocytopenia and, 739
Alder-Reilly anomaly (ARA), 475, 475f
Alkali denaturation test, 458
Alkaline hemoglobin electrophoresis, 421–422, 421f
Allergic purpura, 728
Allergic reactions, 881.e19
Alloantibodies, 393
Alloimmune antiphospholipid antibodies, 765–766
Alloimmune hemolytic anemias, 401–403
  hemolytic disease of the fetus and newborn, 401–403, 402t
  hemolytic transfusion reaction, 401
Alteplase (Activase) (Genentech), 804
Alternative (research) hypothesis, 19–20
American College of Obstetricians and Gynecologists (ACOG), 868
American Proficiency Institute, 38
American Society for Clinical Laboratory Science (ASCLS), 11
Aminolevulinate synthase, 112–113
Aminolevulinic acid (ALA), 286
Aminolevulinic acid synthase 2 (ALAS2), 284–285
Amplicon, 529
Amplification, by polymerase chain reaction
  DNA, 529–532, 530f
    detection of, 532–533
  RNA, 530–532, 531f
Amyloid, 246
Amyloidosis, 728
Anaerobic glycolysis, 96–98, 96b, 97f, 98t
  diversion pathways, 98–99
    hexose monophosphate, 97f, 98, 98t
    methemoglobin reductase, 97f, 98–99
    Rapoport-Luebering, 97f, 99
  first phase, 96, 98t
  second phase, 96, 98t
  third phase, 96–98, 98t
Anagrelide, 739
Analgesics, 423
Analysis of variance (ANOVA), 19–20, 24, 24t
Analytical phase, in Total Testing Process, 9
Analytical specificity, 28
Anaphase, 53
Anaplasma phagocytophilum, in neutrophils, 481

Anaplastic large cell lymphoma, 652, 652f
Anatomic (soft tissue) hemorrhage, 687
Andexanet alfa (Andexxa), 799
Anemia, 1–2
  aplastic, 314–321, 314b
    acquired, 314–318
      clinical findings, 316
      etiology, 314b–315b, 315
      incidence, 314
      laboratory findings, 316–318, 317f–318f, 317t
      pathophysiology, 315–316
      treatment and prognosis, 318
    inherited, 318–321
      dyskeratosis congenita, 319–320
      Fanconi, 318–319
      Shwachman-Bodian-Diamond syndrome, 320–321
  approach to evaluating, 266–271
    morphologic classification, 268–271, 270f
    pathophysiologic, 271, 272b
  caused by deficiency in folate and vitamin B₁₂, 298–300, 299f
  of chronic kidney disease, 324–325
  congenital dyserythropoietic, 300, 323–324, 323f
  definition of, 263, 276
  Diamond-Blackfan, 322–323, 323t
  differential diagnosis, 321, 321t–322t, 346–347, 347f
  in elderly adults. See Elderly adults; anemia in
  Fanconi, 318–319, 737
  general concepts in, 276–289
  hemolytic, 331, 331t
    alloimmune, 401–403
    autoimmune, 396–401, 398t
    bartonellosis and, 387–388
    caused by drugs and chemicals, 388
    caused by extensive burns, 388f
    caused by infectious agents, 384–388
    caused by venoms, 388
    chronic hereditary nonspherocytic, 371
    clostridial sepsis and, 387
    cold agglutinin disease, 399–400, 400f
    disseminated intravascular coagulation, 383
    exercise-induced hemoglobinuria, 384
    HELLP syndrome, 383
    hemolytic disease of the fetus and newborn, 397–399, 402t
    hemolytic transfusion reaction, 401
    hemolytic uremic syndrome, 382–383
    macroangiopathic, 383–384
    malaria and, 384–385
    microangiopathic hemolytic anemia (MAHAs), 380–383, 381b
    mixed-type autoimmune, 401
    nonimmune causes, 379–391, 380f, 380b
    paroxysmal cold hemoglobinuria, 400–401
    thrombotic thrombocytopenic purpura, 381–382, 382f
    traumatic cardiac hemolytic anemia, 383, 384f
    warm autoimmune, 397–399
  in infants and children, 865–866
    ancillary tests, 866
    iron deficiency anemia, 865–866
  of inflammation, 281–284
    in elderly adults, 872–873
    etiology, 281–283
    treatment of, 284
  iron deficiency, 276–281
    epidemiology of, 279
    etiology of, 276–277
      chronic blood loss, 277
      impaired absorption, 276–277
      inadequate intake, 276
      increased need, 276
    laboratory diagnosis of, 279–281

Anemia (Continued)
    diagnosis of iron deficiency in, 279–280, 280t
    screening for, 278f, 279
    specialized tests of, 280–281, 281f
  pathogenesis of, 277–278, 277f
    stage 1, 278
    stage 2, 277f, 278
    stage 3, 277f, 278
  thalassemia minor and, 459
  treatment and its effects, 281
  laboratory diagnosis of, 265–266
    bone marrow examination, 266
    complete blood count with red blood cell indices, 265
    other tests, 266
    peripheral blood film examination, 266
    reticulocyte count, 265–266, 265t
  laboratory findings, 342–346, 346t
  macrocytic, 268–270
    algorithm for preliminary investigation of, 309f
    nonmegaloblastic, 306–308
    pernicious, 303, 307f
  mechanisms of, 264–265
    blood loss and hemolysis, 264–265
    in chronic inflammatory conditions, 281, 283f
    ineffective and insufficient erythropoiesis, 264
  megaloblastic, 297
    caused by defects of DNA metabolism, 296–312
    differential diagnosis, 321t
    etiology of, 297–300, 297b
      defect in megaloblastic anemia caused by deficiency in folate and vitamin B₁₂, 298–300, 299f
      other causes of, 300
      physiologic roles of vitamin B₁₂ and folate, 297–298, 298f
    laboratory diagnosis of, 303–306
      screening tests, 303–305
      specific diagnostic tests, 305–306
    systemic manifestations of folate and vitamin B₁₂ deficiency, 300–301
    treatment of, 308
    vitamin deficiencies, causes of, 301–303
  microangiopathic hemolytic anemia (MAHAs), 380–383, 381b
    disseminated intravascular coagulation, 383
    HELLP syndrome, 383
    hemolytic uremic syndrome, 382–383
    thrombotic thrombocytopenic purpura, 381–382, 382f
  morphologic classification of, reticulocyte count and, 271, 271f, 272t
  myelophthisic, 324, 324f
  in neonates, 864
  nonimmune causes, 379–391, 380f, 380b
    babesiosis and, 386–387
      clinical findings, 387
      geographic distribution, 387
      laboratory findings and diagnosis, 387, 387f
    bartonellosis, 387–388
    clostridial sepsis, 387
    drugs and chemicals, 388
    extensive burns, 388, 388f
    infectious agents, 384–388
    malaria, 384–385
      clinical and laboratory findings, 385
      hemolytic anemia caused by, 384–388
      microscopic examination, 385, 385f
      pathogenesis, 384–385
      Plasmodium falciparum and, 385, 386f
      Plasmodium knowlesi and, 386f
      Plasmodium malariae and, 385, 386f

Anemia *(Continued)*
    Plasmodium ovale and, 385, 386f
    Plasmodium vivax and, 385, 385f
    prevalence, 384
    red blood cell injury, 388, 388f
    venoms, 388
  paroxysmal cold hemoglobinuria, 331–332
  pathophysiology, 364–365
  patient history and clinical findings, 263
  pernicious, 268–270
  physiologic adaptations in, 263–264, 264b
  pregnancy and, 868–869
    acute blood loss, 869
    hemoglobinopathies, 869
    iron deficiency anemia, 868
    megaloblastic anemia, 869
    parasitic infections, 869
  of prematurity, 864
  sickle cell, 412–427
  sideroblastic, 284–286, 285f, 285b
    in elderly adults, 873
    lead poisoning and, 286
    porphyrias, 284, 285t
Aneuploidy, 557
Angiotensin-converting enzyme-2 (ACE-2)
    receptor, 781
Anisocytosis, 267t
ANKRD26 mutations, 737
Ankyrin, 101
ANO6 gene (Scott syndrome), 721
Anterior medial surface of tibia, 246
Anterior superior iliac crest, 246
Antibiotics, for platelet function inhibition, 724
Antibodies
  assays, 306
  characteristics in DIIHA, 404
  drug-dependent, 404
  drug-independent, 404
Anticardiolipin (ACL) antibody, 763
  immunoassay, 769, 769f
Anticoagulants, 813–814, 881.e13, 881.e22
  activity
    in direct anti-xa oral anticoagulants,
      799–800, 800t
    in oral dabigatran, 800–801
  citrate theophylline adenosine dipyridamole,
    814
  EDTA, 813
  measurement of, 792b
  periprocedural management of, 802–803
  sodium citrate, 813
    volume adjustment for elevated hematocrits,
      813–814, 814f
  switching, 802–803
Anticoagulated aspirate smears, 250
Anti-factor VIII inhibitor, Nijmegen-Bethesda
    assay for, 830–831
Antigens, blood group, 102–103. *See also*
    Alloimmune hemolytic anemias
  hemolytic disease of fetus and newborn caused
    by other, 402–403
  used in flow cytometry, 504t
Antiglycolytic agent, 881.e13
Antimicrobial wipes, 881.e12
Antiparallel heterodimer, 103
Antiphosphatidylserine immunoassay, 769
Antiphospholipid antibodies, in thrombophilia,
    765–769
  clinical consequences of, 765–766, 766b
  detection and confirmation of, 766, 767f
Antiphospholipid syndrome (APS), 763, 764t
  during pregnancy, 869–870
  primary, 766
α_2-Antiplasmin, 680–681
Antiplatelet therapy, 790, 803–804
  laboratory assessment of, 803–804
  measurement of, clinical conditions that
    require, 792b

Antiplatelet therapy *(Continued)*
  oral, 803
  parenteral, 803
Antiports, plasma membrane, 49
Antiprothrombin (factor II), 693
Antiprothrombin immunoassay, 769
Antithrombin (AT), 677, 678f
  activity, 764
    assay, 770–771, 771f
  antigen assay, 771
  assay, 771
  deficiency, 765t, 770
Antithrombotic therapies, 789–810
  future of, 805
Anti-Xa DOACs, 799
Anti-β_2-glycoprotein 1 antibody, immunoassay,
    769
Aorta-gonad-mesonephros (AGM) region, 60
APC. *See* Activated protein C
Aperture diameter, 200
Aperture diaphragm, 881.e28
Apixaban, 800t
Aplastic anemia, 314–321, 314b
  acquired, 314–318
    clinical findings, 316
    etiology, 314b–315b, 315
    incidence, 314
    laboratory findings, 316–318, 317f–318f,
      317t
    pathophysiology, 315–316
    treatment and prognosis, 318
  differential diagnosis, 321, 321t–322t
  inherited, 318–321
    dyskeratosis congenita, 319–320
    Fanconi, 318–319
    Shwachman-Bodian-Diamond syndrome,
      320–321
Apoferritin, 131
Apoptosis, 54, 55f, 55t, 71
  chronic myelogenous leukemia and, 586, 592
  erythropoietin (EPO) and inhibition of, 88–89
  and evasion of apoptosis by erythroid
    progenitors and precursors, 88–89
  neutrophils, 481
    apoptotic nuclei, 481, 481f
    pyknotic nuclei, 481
  process, 88
  programmed cell death, 88
  reduced marrow transit time and, 89
Apoptosome, 54
Apoptotic nuclei, 481, 481f
Apoptotic protease-activating factor-1 (APAF-1), 54
Aquaporin-1, 104
Aquaporins, 48–49
Arachidonic acid, 171–172
  pathway enzymes, 721
  platelet aggregometry and, 821
Argatroban, 791t, 801
  monitoring, 802
Arithmetic mean, 21
Arterial thrombosis, 790
  disseminated intravascular coagulation and,
    775–778
  causes of, 775, 776t
    differential diagnosis of, 777–778
    laboratory diagnosis of, 776–778, 777t
    pathophysiology of, 775–776
    specialized laboratory tests for, 777, 777t
    treatment, 778
  predictors of, 773–774
    C-reactive protein, 773
    factor VIII, 774
    fibrinogen activity, 773–774, 773f
    lipoprotein (a), 773
  prevalence of, 762–763
Arteriole, 63f
Arteriovenous malformation (AVM), 687
Artery, splenic, 66

Asciminib, 591–592
Aspirate smear stains, 251, 251t
Aspiration, bone marrow, 246–249
  core biopsy procedure of, 247–249
  examination of, 251–255, 251t, 252b
  patient care of, 249
  preparation of, 246–247
Aspirin, 791t
  for oral antiplatelet therapeutic drugs, 803
  resistance, 803
Aspirin-like effects, 720–721
AspirinWorks immunoassay, for antiplatelet
    drugs, 804
Assay endpoint detection, principles of, 843–846,
    843b
  chromogenic endpoint, 844–845
  immunologic endpoint, 845–846
  light absorbance endpoint detection, 846
  mechanical clot end-point detection, 843, 844f
  nephelometric endpoint detection, 845–846,
    845f, 846t
  photo-optical clot endpoint detection, 844, 844f
  viscoelastic clot detection, 844
Assays. *See also* Laboratory diagnosis; Single-
    factor assays
  antibody, 306
  array-based, 542
  feasibility, 36
  fibrinogen, 5
  for folate, vitamin B_{12}, methylmalonic acid, and
    homocysteine, 305–306, 306b, 307f
  holotranscobalamin, 306
  Taqman, 534–535
Assembly, hemoglobin, 113f, 114
Associated disorders, membrane deformation
    and, 104
Asthma, 147
Autoantibodies, 393
  cold agglutinin disease and, 399–400
  warm autoimmune hemolytic anemia and,
    397–399
Autoantibody induction, RBC, 404
Auto-anti-factor VIII inhibitor, 692–693
Autocrine signaling, 49
Autohemolysis test, 358
Autoimmune antiphospholipid antibodies, 766
Autoimmune hemolytic anemia (AIHA), 396–401
  characteristics of, 398t
  cold agglutinin disease, 399–400, 400f
  mixed-type, 401
  paroxysmal cold hemoglobinuria, 400–401
  warm, 397–399
Autoimmune neutropenia, 478
Automated blood cell analysis, 198–224
  analyzer selection, 221–222
  clinical utility of, 219–221
    nucleated red blood cells, 221
    platelet analysis, 221
    red cell distribution width, 219–220, 220f
    reticulocyte analysis, 220–221
    traditional complete blood count, 219
  complete blood count parameters available on,
    199b
  general principles of, 199–203
    cytochemical and fluorescent staining,
      202–203
    electronic impedance, 199–201
    hemoglobin determination,
      spectrophotometry for, 203
    optical light scatter, 201f, 202
    radiofrequency conductivity, 201–202,
      201f–202f
  limitations and interferences, 216–219,
    217t–218t
    data suppression and flagging, 219
    hemoglobin determination, errors in,
      216–218
    impedance technology, limitations of, 216

Automated blood cell analysis *(Continued)*
  red blood cell agglutination, effects of, 218–219
  reticulocyte counting, errors in, 219
  specimen integrity and stability, 219
  spurious thrombocytopenia, 219
  principal analyzers, 203–216
    Abbott, 199b, 210–213, 211f
    Beckman Coulter, 203–207, 204t, 205f
    Siemens Healthineers, 213–216, 214f
    Sysmex, 207–210
    validation and calibration of, 216
Automated coagulometers, 847–848
Automated erythrocyte sedimentation rate, 191–192, 192t
Automated microscopic examination, peripheral blood film, 235
Automated reticulocyte count, 190
Automated slide making and staining, 228–229
Automatic dilutions, in coagulation instrumentation, 848
Automation, reticulocyte analysis, 220
Autophagic vacuolation, 480–481
Autosomal dominant thrombocytopenia, 737
Autosomal recessive disorder, 706
Avascular necrosis (AVN), 419
Average, 21
Axial light loss (ALL), 206
Azacitidine, 424
Azanucleosides, 628
Azure dust, 150
Azurophilic granules, 141

B
Babesiosis and, 386–387
  clinical findings, 387
  geographic distribution, 387
  laboratory findings and diagnosis, 387, 387f
Bacteria organisms, 481–482, 482f
Balanced reciprocal translocation, 559
Bands, 3, 101, 141–143
  chromosomes, 554, 555f–556f
  clinical utility of, 238b
  neutrophils, 141–143, 144f, 238b
Bartonellosis, 387–388
Basement membrane, 62
Basic fibroblast growth factor (bFGF), 664
Basopenia, 3
Basophilia, 3, 478
  diffuse, 268t
Basophilic normoblast, 83, 83f
Basophilic stippling, 268t, 269f, 286, 374
Basophils, 3, 139–140, 147–149
  development, 148
  functions, 148–149
  granules, 148–149, 149b
  hypogranular, 483, 483f
  immature, 148
  kinetics, 148
  mature, 148, 148f
  pediatric, 866
  quantitative abnormalities of, 478
BBL Fibrometer, 843
B cell neoplasms, mature, 512, 514f
BCL-2, 54
BCL11A gene, 410, 425, 450
Bcl-xL proteins, 162
BCR::ABL1 fusion protein, 588
BCR::ABL1-negative myeloproliferative neoplasms, 584–607
  diagnosis, 597
  disease progression, 596
  epigenetic modifiers, 596–597
  molecular pathophysiology of, 593–596, 594f–595f
  mutations in splicing factors, 597
  signal transduction genes, 597

BCR::ABL1-negative myeloproliferative neoplasms *(Continued)*
  transcription factors, 597
  treatment, 597–599
    combination therapies, 598
    JAK2 inhibitors, 598
    non-JAK inhibitors, 598–599
BCR::ABL1-positive myeloproliferative neoplasms, 584–592
  chronic myeloid leukemia, 584–592
    incidence, 584
    laboratory findings, 587–588
    molecular genetics, 585–586, 585f
    pathogenetic mechanism, 586, 586f
    peripheral blood and bone marrow, 587, 587f–588f, 588t
    Philadelphia chromosome, cytogenetics, 584–585
    progression, 588–589
    treatment, 589–592, 589f, 591f
BCR/ABL gene, 585, 585f
  imatinib and, 589, 589f, 591f
  non-, 585f
B domain, factor VIII, 701
Beckman Coulter, 203–207, 204t, 205f
  hemoglobin determination, 205
  VCS, for WBC differential, NRBC and reticulocyte analyses, 206–207, 206f–207f
Benign cells, 881.e40t
Benign immature B cells, 866
Benzylsulfonyl-D-Arg-Pro-4-amidinobenzylamide (BAPA), 857
Bernard-Soulier syndrome (BSS), 716–717, 717f, 737
  inherited. *See* Inherited giant platelet syndromes
  laboratory features, 717
  treatment, 717
  variants, 717
Bethesda titer, for anti-factor VIII inhibitor, 830
Betibeglogene autotemcel, 450
BFU-E. *See* Burst-forming unit-erythroid
Biallelic *TP53* inactivation, 624
Bilirubin, 304–305, 305b, 342
  degradation of hemoglobin, 333, 334b
  increase in hemolysis, 342
  laboratory testing for serum, 334b
  physiologic metabolism, 333–335, 333f
Bilirubin crystals, 881.e39, 881.e39f
Bilirubinemia, 346–347
  in specimen quality set point, 849
BinaxNOW, 372
Bioavailability, of dietary iron, 131
Biochemical qualitative screening tests, 372
Biohazards
  in blood and body fluids, 881.e8
  disposal containers, 881.e12
Biopsy, bone marrow, 246–249, 247f
  examination of, 251t, 252b
  imprints, 250–251
  patient care of, 249
  preparation of, 246–247, 247f
Biosynthesis
  globin, 114
  heme, 112–114, 113f
Birth weight, gestational age and, 863–864
2,3-Bisphosphoglycerate (2,3-BPG), 263–264
Bisphosphoglycerate mutase, 97f, 99
Bisphosphoglycerate phosphatase, 99
Bivalirudin, 791t, 801–802
Bland-Altman difference plot, 25, 27f
Blast phase, 588
Blebs, 104
Bleeding assessment tool (BAT), 686–687
Bleeding diathesis, 607
Bleeding disorders. *See* Hemorrhage
Bleeding time test, 33–34, 817
Blind loops, 303

Blocker bar, 202
Blood
  cells. *See* Cells
  collection. *See* Specimen collection
  loss. *See* Hemorrhage
Bloodborne pathogens, 881.e2, 881.e12
Blood cell analysis, automated, 198–224
Blood clot assessment, historical perspective of, 842–843
Blood count, blood cell analyzers, 204t
Blood culture, collection of blood for, 881.e22
Blood exchange transfusion, 423
Blood film examination, 5. *See also* Peripheral blood films
Blood group antigens, 102–103. *See also* Alloimmune hemolytic anemias
  in flow cytometry, 504t
  hemolytic disease of fetus and newborn caused by other, 402
Blood specimen collection, 881.e11–881.e25
  handling, 881.e22
  legal issues in phlebotomy, 881.e23
  physiologic factors affecting test results, 881.e12, 881.e13b
  quality assurance in, 881.e22
    anticoagulants and other additives, 881.e22
    collection of blood for blood culture, 881.e22
    collection procedures, 881.e22
    quality control and preventive maintenance, 881.e22, 881.e23b
    reasons for specimen rejection, 881.e22, 881.e23b
    requirements for quality specimen, 881.e22
    technical competence, 881.e22
  responsibility of phlebotomist in infection control, 881.e12
  safety, 881.e12
  skin puncture, 881.e20
    collection sites, 881.e20, 881.e20f
    equipment for, 881.e20, 881.e21f
    order of draw, 881.e21b
    precautions with, 881.e20
    procedure, 881.e12
  venipuncture, 881.e12
    in children, 881.e18
    complications encountered in, 881.e18
    equipment for, 881.e12
    inability to obtain blood specimen, 881.e19
    procedure, 881.e16
    selection of vein for routine, 881.e16
    in special situations, 881.e19
B lymphoblastic leukemia/lymphoma, 511, 512f, 570
  with *BCR::ABL1* fusion, 511
  BCR-ABL1-like, 511
  with *KMT2A* rearrangement, 511
B lymphocytes, 151, 152f
  development, 152
  functions, 153
Body fluids
  analysis in hematology laboratory, 881.e34–881.e50
  bronchoalveolar lavage specimens, 881.e46
  cell counts, 183, 183t, 881.e35
    automated methods, 881.e35
    manual methods, 881.e35
  cerebrospinal fluid, 881.e36
    cell counts of, 881.e37
    differential cell counts of, 881.e38, 881.e38f, 881.e39f
    gross examination of, 881.e36, 881.e38t
  differential counts, 881.e35
    automated methods, 881.e36
    manual methods, 881.e36
  preparing cytocentrifuge slides of, 881.e36, 881.e36f
  serous fluid, 881.e40, 881.e41f, 881.e44f
    differential cell counts of, 881.e41, 881.e42f, 881.e43f, 881.e44f

Body fluids *(Continued)*
  gross examination of, 881.e41
    transudates *vs.* exudates, 881.e40, 881.e41t
  synovial fluid, 881.e43, 881.e44f, 881.e46f
    crystals, 881.e44, 881.e45f
    differential cell counts of, 881.e43, 881.e44f
    gross examination of, 881.e43
Bomedemstat, 598–599
Bone marrow, 60–64, 62f–63f
  anatomy and architecture, 245, 246f
  aspiration, 246–249
    examination of, 251–255
    imprints, 251–255
    patient care, 249
    preparation of, 246–247
    procedure, 249, 250t
  biopsy, 246–249
    core biopsy specimen examination, 255–258, 255t, 256f–258f
    preparation of, 246–247
    sickle cell disease and, 418
  body iron status and, 132t, 133
  chronic eosinophilic leukemia and, 608–609
  chronic myelogenous leukemia and, 587, 587f–588f, 588t
  chronic neutrophilic leukemia and, 607
  circulation, 62–63
  definitive studies, 258, 258t
  essential thrombocythemia and, 599–600, 600f, 600t
  examination, 5–6, 244–261, 266
    for anemia, 305, 305f
    core biopsy, 247–249, 248f–249f
    hemolysis and, 346
    high-power (500x), 253–254, 253f–254f, 254t
    indications for, 245–246, 245t
    low-power (100x), 251–253, 252f
    reports, 258, 259f
  failure, 313–329
    aplastic anemia, 314–321, 314b
    chronic kidney disease and, 324–325
    Diamond-Blackfan anemia, 322–323, 323t
    myelophthisic anemia, 324, 324f
    pathophysiology of, 314
    to produce blood cells, 321t
    pure red cell aplasia, 321–323
  hematopoietically active, 61, 160f
  hypoplasia, 322t
  megakaryocytes, 737
  microenvironment of, 90, 90f
    hematopoietic, 55–56, 63–64
  polycythemia vera and, 602, 603f, 603t
  primary myelofibrosis and, 605, 606f, 606t
  red, 61, 62f, 246
  specimen collection sites, 246, 246f
  specimen preparation, 249–251
    anticoagulated aspirate smears, 250
    direct aspirate smears, 249–250
    histologic sections, 251
    imprints, 250–251
    marrow core biopsy and aspirate smear stains, 251, 251t
    particle smears, 250
  transplantation, 496
    for chronic myelogenous leukemia, 592
    for sickle cell disease, 425
Bone marrow failure syndrome, 365–366
Bone morphogenic protein (BMP), 127t
Bone morphogenic protein receptor (BMPR), 127t
Bothrops atrox, 691
Brain natriuretic peptide, 773
Breast tumor cells, 881.e40f
Brightfield illumination, 881.e29
Brill-Edwards curve, 31
Brodifacoum, 692
Bronchoalveolar lavage specimens, 881.e46
  differential cell counts of, 881.e46, 881.e47f

"Bronzed diabetes", 288
Bruise, 735, 735f
Bruton tyrosine kinase (BTK)
  deficiency, 466–467
  inhibitors, 724–725
BSS. *See* Bernard-Soulier syndrome
Budd-Chiari syndrome, 365, 599
Buffy coat smears, 250
Burkitt's lymphoma, 647–648, 648f
Burn circuits, 200
Burned, damaged, scarred, and occluded veins, 881.e19
Burns, 388, 388f
Burr cells, 267t, 269f
Burst-forming unit-erythroid (BFU-E), 72, 863

C

C4b-binding protein (C4bBP), 676
C4bBP. *See* C4b-binding protein
Cabot ring, 268t
Calcium
  mobilization defects, 721
  pyrophosphate dihydrate crystals, 881.e45
Calculations, manual cell counts, 180–181
  reticulocyte, 189
    corrected, 189
    production index, 189
Calibration, 216
  verification, 31
Calibrators, 23
Calmodulin, 104
Cancer. *See also* Neoplasms
  chemotherapy, 299, 299b
    drug-induced thrombocytopenia and, 738–739
  cytogenetics, 559–562
    leukemia, 559–561, 559b, 560f–562f
    solid tumors, 561–562, 562f
  lymphoid, flow cytometric analysis of, 510–513
  myeloid, flow cytometric analysis of, 506–510, 506f–507f
Cangrelor, 723
Capillary electrophoresis
  detection of amplified DNA, 532, 532f
  DNA sequencing by, 536–538, 540f
Capillary gel electrophoresis, 532, 532f
Capillary puncture, hemostasis blood specimen collection using, 815
Capillary zone electrophoresis (CZE), 456
Caplacizumab, 749
Carbohydrates, cell membrane, 45, 100–101
Carbon dioxide transport, 117, 118f
Carbon monoxide, 345
  and carboxyhemoglobin, 119
Carboxyhemoglobin, 119, 184b
Cardiopulmonary bypass (CPB), 726, 751
  scoring system for, 779
Cardiovascular diseases, 763
Carrión disease, 387–388
Cartilage cells, 881.e39, 881.e39f
Caspases, 54
Catabolism
  glucose, 98t
  heme, 333, 333f
Catastrophic antiphospholipid syndrome (CAPS), 766
Catheter ablation, 802–803
Catovsky-Matutes scoring for, 643b
CD2, 506
CD3, 506
CD4, 66–68, 316, 508
CD4+, 153–154
CD7, 506–508
CD8, 67–68
CD8+, 153–154, 316
CD10, 506

CD11b, 506–507
CD13, 506
CD14, 367, 508
CD15, 367, 507–510
CD16, 367
CD19, 506
CD22, 506
CD24, 367
CD25, 316
CD33, 506
CD34, 70, 162, 316, 505, 507, 508f, 511, 592, 605
CD38, 70, 505
CD41, 506
CD42, 162
CD45, 367, 505–507, 506f
CD55, 364–365, 367
CD56, 506
CD59, 364–365, 367
CD61, 212, 219
CD62, 162
CD64, 367, 506, 508
CD66b, 367
CD71, 506
CD117, 505, 507
CD163, 335–337
Cell adhesion moecules (CAMs), 52
CellaVision DC-1, 235
CellaVision DM9600, 235, 235f
Cell-based physiologic coagulation, 674–676, 675f
Cell communication and signal transduction, 49–52, 50f–51f
  cell adhesion moecules (CAMs), 52
  cell-to-cell signaling, 52
  cyclic adenosine monophosphate (cAMP), 49
  extracellular matrix (ECM), 52
  guanosine diphosphate (GDP), 52
  guanosine triphosphate (GTP), 52
  target cells, 49
Cell counts
  body fluids
    manual, 183
    performing, 881.e35
    preparing cytocentrifuge slides of, 881.e36, 881.e36f
  coulter (impedance) principle of, 199, 199f
  manual, 180–183
    calculations for, 180–181
    disposable blood cell count dilution systems, 183, 183f
    equipment for, 180, 180f
    with most common dilutions, 183t
    platelet, 181b
    principle, 180
    red blood cell, 183
    reticulocyte, 187–190
    white blood cell, 180
  point-of-care testing, 195
Cell counts on body fluids, 881.e35
Cell cycle, 52–54, 552
  regulation of, 53–54, 54t
  stages, 52–53, 53f
Cell-mediated response, 3
Cell processes, selected, 48–54
Cells, 1
  cluster of differentiation, 45
  cycle, 52–54, 552
    DNA replication and, 525–527, 526f
    proteins, 492
    regulation, 53–54, 53f
    stages, 52–53, 53f
  cytoplasm, 47–48
    centrosomes, 46t, 48
    endoplasmic reticulum, 45f, 46t, 47
    Golgi apparatus, 45f, 46t, 47
    intermediate filaments, 46t, 48
    lysosomes, 46t, 48
    microfilaments, 46t, 48

Cells (Continued)
   microtubules, 46t, 48
   mitochondria, 46t, 47–48, 47f
   ribosomes, 46t, 47
  death, by necrosis and apoptosis, 54, 55f, 55t, 88
  hematopoietic microenvironment, 55–56
  increased destruction of, 321t
  iron acquisition and intracellular trafficking,
    129–131, 130f
  membrane
   carbohydrates, 45
   proteins, 45
  nucleus, 44, 46–47, 46t
   chromatin, 46–47
   nuclear envelope, 47
   nucleoli, 47
   to-cytoplasm ratio, 81b
  organization, 44, 44f–45f, 46t
  plasma membrane, 44–45, 46t
  selected processes, 48–54
   cell communication and signal transduction,
    49–52, 50f–51f
   cell cycle and regulation, 52–54, 53f, 54t
   cell death by necrosis and apoptosis, 52–53,
    55f, 55t
   plasma membrane transport, 48–49, 48b
  sorting, 515
  structure and function, 43–58
Cell-to-cell signaling, 52
Cellular activity
  basophilic normoblast, 83, 83f
  erythrocyte, 86, 87f
  orthochromic normoblast, 84f, 85
  polychromatic erythrocyte, 85–86, 85f–86f, 86b
  polychromatic normoblast, 84, 84f
  pronormoblast, 82, 83f
Cellular iron acquisition, 129–131, 130f
Centers for Medicare and Medicaid Services, 38
Central dogma in genetics, 521–523
Centrosomes, 46t, 48
Cerebrospinal fluid (CSF), 881.e36, 881.e37f
  cell counts of, 881.e37
  differential cell counts of, 881.e38, 881.e38f,
   881.e39f
  gross examination of, 881.e36, 881.e38t
Certification, laboratory staff, 36
Charcot-Leyden crystal protein, 146
Checkpoint control proteins, 492
Chédiak-Higashi syndrome (CHS), 467, 467f, 719
Chelation therapy, 423
Chemical hazards, 881.e6
Chemistry, iron, 123
Chemokines, 73
Chemotherapy, 299, 299b
  drug-induced thrombocytopenia and, 738–739
  for leukocyte neoplasms, 494–495
Childhood myelodysplastic neoplasms, 626
  with increased blasts, 626
  with low blasts, 626
Childhood myelodysplastic neoplasm with
  increased blasts (cMDS-IB), 626
Childhood myelodysplastic neoplasm with low
  blasts (cMDS-LB), 626
Children. See also Neonates; Pediatric hematology
  and hemostasis
  acute leukemia in, 561, 561f–562f
  iron deficiency anemia in, 279
  sickle cell disease in, 423
  splenectomy in, 359
  venipuncture in, 881.e18
Chloride shift, 117
Chlorothiazide diuretics, maternal ingestion of,
  738
Cholesterol, 99–100
  crystals in synovial fluid, 881.e45
  esterified, 165
Choosing Wisely, 11, 13

Chorea acanthocytosis (ChAc), 363
Choroid plexus cells, 881.e38
Christmas disease. See Hemophilia
Chromatic aberrations, 881.e28
Chromatin, 46–47, 552
Chromogenic anti-Xa heparin assay, 31
Chromogenic (color) end point assays, 824
Chromogenic endpoint detection, 844–845, 845f,
  846t
Chromogenic factor IX assay, 830
Chromogenic factor VIII assay, 830
Chromogenic factor X assay, 824
  in unfractionated heparin, 796
  in warfarin therapy, 793–794
Chromogenic substrate assay, 832, 832f
Chromogenic substrates, 827
  factor assays using, 830
Chromosomal microarray (CMA), 542, 543f,
  562–563, 563f
Chromosomes
  abnormalities, 557–559
   inherited thrombocytopenia associated with,
    735–737
   numeric, 557, 558f
   structural, 558–559, 558f
  architecture, 552
  banding, 554, 555f–556f
  cytogenetics, 550–565
   analysis, 6, 552–556, 552t, 555f–556f
   cancer, 559–561, 559b, 560f–562f
   fluorescence in situ hybridization, 554–556,
    556f–557f
   metaphase analysis, 554
   nomenclature, 556–557, 557f
  identification, 553, 554f
  metaphase, 553
  microarray analysis, 562–563, 563f
  number, 553
  Philadelphia, 559–561, 584–585
  preparation and analysis techniques for,
   553–556, 555f–556f
  reasons for analysis of, 552, 552t
  size and type, 553, 554f
  structure, 552, 553f
Chronic anemia, 287
  in SCD, 419
Chronic blood loss, and iron deficiency anemia, 277
Chronic eosinophilic leukemia, 608–609
Chronic granulomatous disease (CGD), 469–470
Chronic hemolysis, 331–332, 341
Chronic hemolytic anemia, 418–419
Chronic hereditary nonspherocytic hemolytic
  anemia (CNSHA), 371
Chronic idiopathic myelofibrosis, 604
Chronic immune thrombocytopenic purpura,
  740–741, 741f
Chronic inflammation, thrombotic risk
  components of, 764t
Chronic leukemias
  general characteristics of, 490, 491t
  leukemoid reaction vs., 476, 477t
Chronic lymphocytic leukemia (CLL), 4, 642–644,
  873
  Catovsky-Matutes scoring for, 643b
  diagnosis, 643
  morphology of, 643, 643f
  staging and prognosis of, 643–644, 644t
  treatment for, 644
Chronic myelogenous leukemia (CML), 584–592,
  626–627
  cytogenetics, 560–561, 560f
  cytogenetics of Philadelphia chromosome and,
   584–585
  flow cytometric analysis of, 506–510
  incidence of, 584
  laboratory findings of, 587–588
  molecular genetics in, 585–586, 585f

Chronic myelogenous leukemia (CML)
  (Continued)
  pathogenetic mechanism of, 586, 586f
  peripheral blood and bone marrow, 587,
   587f–588f, 588t
  progression of, 588–589
  treatment of, 589–592, 589f, 591f
Chronic myelomonocytic leukemia (CMML), 626
Chronic neutrophilic leukemia (CNL), 607–608
  clinical presentation of, 607
  diagnosis of, 607–608
  incidence of, 607
  pathogenetic mechanism, 608
  peripheral blood and bone marrow, 607
  prognosis of, 608
  therapy for, 608
Chronic nonspherocytic hemolytic anemia
  (CNSHA), 369
Chronic renal disease, 324–325
Chronic renal failure, and hemorrhage, 691–692
Chrono-log, 856
Ciliated epithelial cells, 881.e47, 881.e47f
Circulating neutrophil pool (CNP), 144
Circulation, marrow, 62–63
Circumferential microtubules, 165–166
Cis mutations, 432
Cisternae, 47
Citrate, 881.e13
Citrate theophylline adenosine dipyridamole
  (CTAD), 814
Classic platelet aggregometry, 855
Classification of hemolytic disorders
  acquired hemolysis, 332
  intrinsic vs. extrinsic hemolysis, 332
  site and mechanism of hemolysis, 332–333
CLIMB trial, 450
Clinical and laboratory findings. See also
  Laboratory diagnosis
  acquired aplastic anemia, 316–318, 317f–318f,
   317t
  babesiosis, 386–387
  chronic myelogenous leukemia, 587–588
  cold agglutinin disease, 399–400
  dehydrated hereditary stomatocytosis, 362
  essential thrombocythemia, 754
  hemoglobin E, 429–430
  hemoglobin SC, 431
  hemolysis, 342
   tests of accelerated red blood cell
    destruction, 342–345
   tests of increased erythropoiesis, 345–346,
    346t
  hemolytic anemia, 342, 346t
  hemolytic disease of fetus and newborn, 403
  hereditary elliptocytosis, 360–361, 360f–361f
  hereditary hydrocytosis, 362, 362f
  hereditary ovalocytosis, 361
  hereditary spherocytosis, 355–357, 359, 359t
  hereditary xerocytosis, 362
  immune hemolytic anemia, 396, 397f
  malaria, 385
  mastocytosis, 611
  overhydrated hereditary stomatocytosis, 362,
   362f
  paroxysmal nocturnal hemoglobinuria,
   366–367, 366t, 367f
  polycythemia vera, 603
  pyruvate kinase deficiency, 373–374, 374f
  sickle cell disease, 416–419, 416b
  Southeast Asian ovalocytosis, 361
  unstable hemoglobin variants, 434
  α-thalassemia, 453
Clinical and Laboratory Standards Institute
  (CLSI), 38, 216, 881.e16
  specimen collection, 179–180
  "testing site neutrality", 193
Clinical bleeding, and platelet count, 735

Clinical coagulation laboratory, 842–843
Clinical dosing algorithms, 792
Clinical laboratory, Total Testing Process in, 9, 10f
Clonal cytopenia of unknown significance (CCUS), 619
Clonal hematopoiesis of indeterminate potential (CHIP), 619
Clopidogrel, 723, 791t
  for oral antiplatelet therapeutic drugs, 803
  platelet aggregometry and, 820
Closed-tube sampling, in coagulation instrumentation, 848
Clostridial sepsis, 387
Clot activators, 881.e13
Clot-based assays
  for acquired hemophilia detection, 693, 693f
  APC resistance, 769–770, 770f
Clot-based testing
  for coagulation disorders, 821–827
  lupus anticoagulant tests, 768–769, 768f
  partial thromboplastin time, 824–825
    as diagnostic assay, 825
    mixing studies for, 825–826
    monitoring heparin therapy with, 825
    principles for, 824, 824f
    procedure for, 825
    quality control for, 825
    reference interval for, 825
  platelet-poor plasma specimens, 816–817
  prothrombin time, 822–824
    as diagnostic assay, 823
    limitations of, 823–824, 823t
    minimal effectiveness of, as screening tool, 823
    principle for, 822
    procedure for, 822
    quality control for, 822–823
    reference interval, 823
    reporting of, 823
  thrombin time, 826–827
    procedure for, 826–827
    quality control for, 827
    reagent and principle for, 826, 826f
    reporting of, 827
  venom activated assays in, 827
    reptilase time, 827
    Russell viper venom test, 827
Clot endpoint detection, 843–844
Cloth laboratory coats, 881.e3
Clots
  formation
    abnormal, in specimen quality set points, 849
    kinetics of, 849–850, 850f, 855t
    in specimen quality set points, 849
Clustered regularly interspaced short palindromic repeats (CRISPR), 425–426
Cluster of differentiation, 45, 502–503, 504t
Coagulation, 5, 170
  cascade mechanism, hemorrhage and, 701f
  instrumentation, 841–861
    assay endpoint detection principles in, 843–846, 843b
      chromogenic endpoint, 844–845
      light absorbance endpoint detection, 846
      mechanical clot endpoint detection, 843, 844f
      nephelometric endpoint detection, 845–846, 845f, 846t
      photo-optical clot endpoint detection, 844, 844f
      viscoelastic clot detection, 844
    clinical coagulation laboratory in, 842–843
      blood clot assessment, historical perspective of, 842–843
      currently available, 850–851, 852t, 853f
      detection methods in, advantages and disadvantages, 846–847, 846t

Coagulation (Continued)
    global hemostasis assessment in, 853–855, 854f, 855t
    molecular coagulation testing in, 857–858, 858t
    platelet function testing in, 855–857
      flow cytometry, 857
      platelet aggregometers, 855–856, 856f, 856t
      platelet function analyzers, 856–857
    point-of-care coagulation testing in, 851–853, 852t
    selection of, 850, 850b, 851t
    technology advancements and, 847–850, 847t
      accuracy and precision in, 848
      clot formation, kinetics of, 849–850, 850f
      computer capabilities in, 849
      flagging in, 849, 849b
      quality improvement features, 849–850
      random access testing in, 848
      reagent handling in, 848–849
      reflex testing in, 849
      specimen management in, 848
      specimen quality set points in, 849
      test performance, 848
  regulatory mechanisms, 676–678, 676f, 677t
    antithrombin, 677, 678f
    protein C regulatory system, 676, 677f
    tissue factor pathway inhibitor, 677, 678f
Coagulation factor assays, 827–831
  fibrinogen assay, 827–828
    calibration curve, 828, 828f
    limitations of, 828
    procedure for, 827–828
    quality control for, 828
    reagent for, 827
    results and clinical utility of, 828
    test protocol for, 828
  Nijmegen-Bethesda assay, for anti-factor VIII inhibitor, 830–831
  single-factor assays, using the PTT, 828–831, 829t
    expected results and clinical utility of, 829–830
    limitations of, 830
    principle of, 828–829
    quality control for, 830
Coagulation screening assays, 827
Coagulation system, 666–676
  cell-based physiologic coagulation, 674–676, 675f
  common pathways, 673, 674f
  extrinsic pathways, 673, 674f
  factor VIII and von Willebrand factor, 671
  factor XI and contact factors, 671–672
  factor XIII, 672–673
  intrinsic pathways, 673, 674f
  plasma procoagulants. See Procoagulants
  procoagulant cofactors, 670, 670t
  thrombin, 672
  vitamin K-dependent prothrombin group, 669–670, 669f–670f, 669t–670t, 669b
Coagulation testing, 881.e17
Coagulopathies, 688
  acquired, 688–693
  congenital, 693–707
  liver disease, 690–691
Codocytes, 267t
Codons, 521–522
Coefficient of variation, 21
Coincidence correction, 200
Coincident passage loss, 200
Cold agglutinin disease (CAD), 399–400, 400f
Collagen
  platelet aggregometry and, 821
  in primary myelofibrosis, 604–605
  receptors, 721

Collagen binding assay, 699
Collection tubes, 881.e12
  additives in, 881.e13
    anticoagulants, 881.e13
    antiglycolytic agent, 881.e13
    clot activators, 881.e13
    separator gel, 881.e13
College of American Pathologists, 9, 38
Colloid osmotic hemolysis, 104–105
Colony-forming unit-erythroid (CFU-E), 72
Colony-forming units-granulocyte, erythrocyte, monocyte, and megakaryocyte (CFU-GEMM), 68
Colony-forming units-spleen (CFU-S), 68
Colony-stimulating factors (CSFs), 72
Combination therapies, 598
Common gamma chain deficiency, 465–466
Common lymphoid progenitor, 68
Common myeloid progenitor (CMP), 68, 160
Comparative genomic hybridization (aCGH), 542
Complement system, 144
Complete blood count (CBC), 4–5, 4b, 8b, 11, 13, 225–243, 344
  calibration, 23
  hemolysis and, 345–346
  megaloblastic anemia and, 304, 304f
  summarizing
    neutrophilia, 238b
    organization of results, 235
    platelet parameters, 240–241, 240f, 241b
    red blood cell parameters, 237–240, 238t, 239f
    relative vs. absolute white blood cell counts, 236, 237t
    results relative to reference intervals, 236
    summarizing, 235–241
    white blood cell parameters, 236–237, 236t
  thalassemia diagnosis and, 455
Composition/information on ingredients, 881.e7
Compound heterozygosity, 430–432, 431f
  hemoglobin SC, 431
Compound microscope, 881.e26, 881.e27, 881.e27f
Computation
  diagnostic efficacy, 35t
  of mean, 20–21
  of median, 21
  of mode, 21
  standard deviation, 21, 22f
  of variance, 21
Computer capabilities, in coagulation instrumentation, 849
Computerized algorithms, 200
Computerized cluster analysis, 215
Computer software, 203
Concentrate smears, bone marrow, 250
Concomitant cis mutations with hemoglobin S, 432
  hemoglobin C-Harlem, 432
  hemoglobin S-Antilles and S-Oman, 432, 433t
Condenser, microscope, 881.e28, 881.e29f
Confidence interval, 21, 30
Confirmatory platelet activation assays, for heparin-induced thrombocytopenia, 780, 781f
Congenital amegakaryocytic thrombocytopenia, 737
Congenital coagulopathies, 693–707
  hemophilia. See Hemophilia
  von Willebrand disease. See von Willebrand disease
Congenital dyserythropoietic anemia (CDA), 300, 323–324, 323f
Congenital erythropoietic porphyria (CEP), 285t
Congenital hemorrhagic disorders, 688, 688b
Congenital neutropenias, 467–468, 468t
Congenital toxoplasmosis, 738
Constant systematic error, 25
Consumption coagulopathy, 775

Contact-dependent or juxtacrine signaling, 49
Contact factors, 671–672
Contact system, 671
Contaminated sharps, 881.e2, 881.e3f, 881.e4f, 881.e12
Continuing education, laboratory staff, 38
Control proteins, 676
Controls, 31–32, 32f, 32t
Coordinated care, 14
Cords of Billroth, 65
Core biopsy, bone marrow. See Biopsy; bone marrow
Coronaviruses, 781. See also COVID-19 Pandemic
    arterial thrombosis and, 763
Corrected reticulocyte count, 189
Cosmo Biomedical MCDh, 230
Coumadin. See Warfarin
Coumarin, 790–792
COVID-19 pandemic, 742–743, 781, 830
    arterial thrombosis and, 763
    fondaparinux and, 798
    life expectancy in the United States, 870
    low molecular weight heparin for, 797
    systemic fibrinolytic therapy for, 776
    tenecteplase during, 804
    vaccines, 782
C-reactive protein (CRP), in arterial thrombosis predictors, 773
CRISPR-Cas9, 425–426, 426f
Cristae, 47–48
Critical illumination, 881.e29
Crizanlizumab, 425
Cryohydrocytosis, 362
Cryoprecipitate, 689
Crystals, in synovial fluid, 881.e44, 881.e45f
Cyanmethemoglobin, 2, 183
    procedure, 184f, 184b
Cycle sequencing, 536, 540f
Cyclic neutropenia, 468
Cyclin, 53–54, 54t
Cyclin-dependent kinases (CDKs), 53–54, 54t
Cyclooxygenase, pathway, 171–172
Cytocentrifuge slides, 881.e36, 881.e36f
Cytochemical staining, 202–203
Cytochemical stains, interpretations and, 577–579, 578f, 578t
    esterases, 578–579, 579f
    myeloperoxidase, 577–578, 578f
    Sudan Black B staining, 578, 578f
Cytochemistry, for WBC count, WBC differential, NRBCs and reticulocyte analysis, 213–216, 215f
Cytochrome, 98–99
Cytogenetics, 550–565, 550b–551b, 551f
    analysis
        reasons for, 552, 552t
        techniques for chromosome preparation and, 553–556, 555f–556f
    cancer, 559–562
        leukemia, 559–561, 559b, 560f–562f
        solid tumors, 561–562, 562f
    chromosomal microarray analysis, 562–563, 563f
    chromosome abnormalities and, 557–559
        numeric, 557, 558f
        structural, 558–559, 558f
    chromosome identification and, 553, 554f
    chromosome structure and, 552, 553f
    fluorescence in situ hybridization, 554–556, 556f–557f
    metaphase analysis, 554
    metaphase chromosomes and, 553
    myelodysplastic neoplasms, 627
    nomenclature, 556–557, 557f
Cytogenetics/cytogenomics. See also Genetics
    acute myeloid leukemias with defining genetic abnormalities in, 507, 508f–509f

Cytogenetics/cytogenomics (Continued)
    analysis, 6
        of Philadelphia chromosome, 584–585
Cytogenomic techniques, 6
Cytokines
    growth factors and, 70–72, 71f
    of megakaryocytopoiesis, 163, 163t
Cytokinesis, 53
Cytomegalovirus (CMV), and neonatal thrombocytopenia, 738
Cytoplasm, 47–48
    basophilic normoblast, 83, 83f
    bone marrow aspiration examination, 254f
    centrosomes, 46t, 48
    endoplasmic reticulum, 45f, 46t, 47
    erythrocyte, 86, 87f
    Golgi apparatus, 45f, 46t, 47
    intermediate filaments, 46t, 48
    lysosomes, 46t, 48
    microfilaments, 46t, 48
    microtubules, 46t, 48
    mitochondria, 46t, 47–48, 47f
    nucleus-to-cytoplasm ratio, 81b
    orthochromic normoblast, 84, 84f
    polychromatic erythrocyte, 85, 85f–86f
    polychromatic normoblast, 84, 84f
    pronormoblast, 81, 83f
    ribosomes, 46t, 47
Cytoplasmic trafficking of iron, 131
Cytoplasmic viscosity, 353
Cytosine, 523–524
Cytoskeletal proteins, 45, 102f, 103–104, 104t, 105f
Cytoskeleton, platelet, 165–166, 165f
Cytosol, 47
Cytosolic PCBP2, 125
Cytotoxic T lymphocytes, 154

D
Dabigatran, 800, 800t
    thrombin clotting time and, 827
Dacryocyte, 267t
Darkfield microscopy, 881.e31
Data Innovations North America, 38
Data suppression, 219
Dawn of neutrophilia, 141
Day-to-day variation, 25–26
DC detection system, for RBC analyses and platelet distribution, 207, 208f
D-dimer, 681, 681f, 874
D-dimer immunoassay, 5, 774–775, 832
    principle of, 832
D-dimer units (DDUs), 774–775
Death, cell, 54, 55f, 55t, 88
    erythrocyte, 90–91
Death receptor pathway, 54
Decay-accelerating factor (DAF), 103
Decitabine, 424
Deep tissue bleeding, 735
Deep venous thrombosis (DVT), 762, 874
    diagnostic tests, 774–775
    symptoms of, 774
Deferasirox, 423
Deferoxamine, 423
Defibrinating syndrome, 775
Deformability, RBC membrane, 99, 104
Dehydrated hereditary stomatocytosis (DHS), 362
    clinical and laboratory findings, 362
    pathophysiology, 362
Dehydrated stomatocytosis, 105
Delayed hemolytic transfusion reaction (DHTR), 401
Delta checks, 33
Demarcation system (DMS), 162
Dematin, 101

Dense granule deficiency, 717–720, 718b, 719f
    Chédiak-Higashi syndrome, 719
    α-Granule deficiency, 720, 720f
    Hermansky-Pudlak syndrome, 718–719
    Quebec platelet disorder, 720
    thrombocytopenia with absent radii syndrome (TAR), 720
    Wiskott-Aldrich syndrome (WAS), 719
Dense granules, 165f, 166, 166t, 717
    deficiencies, 717–720
        Chédiak-Higashi syndrome, 719
        Hermansky-Pudlak syndrome, 718–719
        thrombocytopenia with absent radii syndrome (TAR), 720
        Wiskott-Aldrich syndrome (WAS), 719
α-Dense storage pool deficiency, 720
Dense tubular system (DTS), 165, 165f
Deoxyribonucleic acid (DNA)
    amplification of, by polymerase chain reaction, 529, 530f
    antiparallel and complementary strands, 523, 524f
    cell cycle and, 52
    central dogma in genetics and, 521–523
    chromatin, 46
    chromosome structure and, 552
    circulating tumor, 544
    detection of amplified, 532–533
        capillary gel electrophoresis, 532, 532f
        DNA sequencing, 536–538, 540f
        restriction endonuclease methods, 533
    fluorescence in situ hybridization, 554–555
    isolated from clinical specimens, 527–528
    megakaryocytes and, 160
    in mitochondria, 47–48
    molecular diagnostic testing overview, 527, 528b
    at the molecular level, 523–524, 523f–525f
    necrosis and, 54
    nucleic acid isolation, 527–529
    nucleotide strands, 523, 523f
    repair genes, 494
    repair proteins, 492
    replication and the cell cycle, 525–527, 526f
    structure and function of, 521–527
    transcription and translation, 524–525
Deoxythymidine triphosphate (dTTP), 297–298
Deoxyuridine monophosphate (dUMP), 297–298
Depolarized side scatter (DSS), 210
Desmopressin, 700
Desquamation, 662
Des-γ-carboxyl proteins, 669
Dextrans, 724
Diabetes, bronzed, 288
Diagnostic efficacy assessment, 33–36, 35t
    computations, 35t
    effects of population incidence and odds ratios on, 34–36
Diamond-Blackfan anemia (DBA), 322–323, 323t
Diapedesis, 144
DIC. See Disseminated intravascular coagulation (DIC)
Dietary iron, 131
    in intestines, absorption of
        ferritin absorption, 124, 125f
        heme absorption, 124, 125f
        ionic iron absorption, 125–126, 125f
Differential cell counts
    bronchoalveolar lavage specimens, 881.e46, 881.e47f
    cerebrospinal fluid, 881.e38, 881.e38f, 881.e39f
    serous fluid, 881.e41, 881.e42f, 881.e43f, 881.e44f
    synovial fluid, 881.e43, 881.e44f
Differential diagnosis, 280t, 289. See also Laboratory diagnosis
    hemolytic anemia, 346–347, 347f, 348t
    hemolytic uremic syndrome, 383

Differential diagnosis (Continued)
 hereditary spherocytosis, 359, 359t
 iron overload, 280t, 289
 leukemia, 321, 321t–322t
 megaloblastic anemia, 321t
 pancytopenia, 321, 321t
 paroxysmal nocturnal hemoglobinuria, 321t
 thalassemia, 459
 thrombotic thrombocytopenic purpura, 383
Differential scatter technique, 213, 215f
Diffuse basophilia, 268t
Diffuse large B cell lymphoma, 649–650, 650f
DiGeorge syndrome, 466
Digital morphology analyzers, 235, 242
Digital polymerase chain reaction (ddPCR), 535, 538f
Dihydrofolate (DHF), 297–298
Dilutional anemia of pregnancy, 270, 270f, 272t
Dilutional coagulopathy, disseminated intravascular coagulation and, 777
Dilution systems, disposable blood cell count, 183, 183f
Dimorphic erythrocyte population, 620, 620f
Diphyllobothrium latum, 303
Dipyridamole, 724
Direct antiglobulin test (DAT), 266, 359, 396
Direct anti-xa oral anticoagulants, 799–800
 anti-Xa DOAC action, 799, 800t
 anti-Xa DOAC therapy, 799
 laboratory assessment of, 800
 reversing anti-Xa DOAC therapy, 799–800
Direct aspirate smears, 249–250
Direct chromogenic assay, 845
Direct current (DC) detection method, 201, 201f
Direct oral anticoagulants (DOACs), 768, 799, 800t
Direct reference interval determination, 30
Direct thrombin inhibitors (DTIs), 800–802
 intravenous, 801–802, 801f
Discontinuous replication, 527
Disequilibria, 104–105
Disintegrin and metalloproteinase with a thrombospondin type 1 motif, member 13 (ADAMTS-13), 381
Disposable blood cell count dilution systems, 183, 183f
Disposal consideration, 881.e7
Disseminated intravascular coagulation (DIC), 383, 693, 775–778
 causes of, 775, 776t
 differential diagnosis of, 777–778
 differentiation, 749t
 laboratory diagnosis of, 776–778, 777t
 and neonatal thrombocytopenia, 738
 pathophysiology of, 775–776
 periodic laboratory testing, 776–777
 scoring system, 777
 specialized laboratory tests for, 777, 777t
 treatment, 778
Divalent metal transporter 1 (DMT1), 125, 131, 338
Diversion pathways, glycolysis, 98–99
 hexose monophosphate, 97f, 98, 98t
 methemoglobin reductase, 97f, 98–99
 Rapoport-Luebering, 97f, 99
Division
 basophilic normoblast, 83, 83f
 erythrocyte, 86, 87f
 orthochromic normoblast, 84, 84f
 polychromatic erythrocyte, 85, 85f–86f
 polychromatic normoblast, 84, 84f
 pronormoblast, 81, 83f
DNA-based mutation detection, 372
DNA-based testing, 372
Documentation and reliability, 28
Döhle bodies, 480, 480f
Donath-Landsteiner antibody, 400
Down syndrome, 576

Drabkin reagent, 2
Drug adsorption and DIIHA, 403–404
Drug-dependent antibodies, 404
Drug-independent antibodies, 404
Drug-induced hypoplasia, 738–739
Drug-induced immune hemolytic anemia (DIIHA), 403–404
 antibody characteristics, 404
 mechanisms of, 403–404, 403f
 nonimmune drug-induced hemolysis and, 404
 treatment, 404
Drug-induced immune-mediated thrombocytopenia, 741–744, 742b, 743f
 drug-dependent antibodies, 742
 drug-induced autoantibodies, 742
 hapten-induced antibodies, 742
 treatment of, 743–744
Drug-induced vascular purpuras, 728
Drug-RBC membrane protein immunogenic complex, 404
Drying artifact, on red blood cells, 229, 229f
DTIs. See Direct thrombin inhibitors
Dual-antiplatelet therapy (DAT), 723
Duodenal cytochrome B (Dcytb), 125
Duplication, chromosome, 559
Dyserythropoiesis, 620, 620f
Dysfibrinogenemia, 706t
Dysfunctional endothelial nitric oxide synthase, 415–416
Dyshemoglobins, 118–119
 carboxyhemoglobin, 119
 methemoglobin, 118–119
 sulfhemoglobin, 119
Dyskeratosis congenita (DKC), 319–320
Dysmegakaryopoiesis, 622, 622f–623f
 morphologic evidence of, 623b
Dysmyelopoiesis, 620–622, 621f–622f, 621b
Dysproteinemias, 706

E
Early-acting multilineage growth factors, 72
Early-onset thrombocytopenia, 738, 738t
Early-term neonates, 863–864
ECA. See Ecarin chromogenic assay
Ecarin chromogenic assay (ECA), 801
Ecchymoses, 687, 735, 735f
Ecchymosis (Bruise), 881.e18
Echinocyte, 267t
Ecological information, 881.e7
ECPR. See Endothelial cell protein C receptor
Eculizumab, 367–368
Eczema thrombocytopenia immunodeficiency syndrome, 719
Edema, 881.e19
Edoxaban, 800, 800t
EDTA. See Ethylenediaminetetraacetic acid
Effective health care, 11
Effective hematology, and hemostasis testing, 11, 11t
Effective laboratory testing, 11
Efferent lymphatic vessels, 66
Efficient hematology, and hemostasis testing, 11–12
Efficient laboratory testing, 11
Effusion, 881.e40
Ehlers-Danlos syndrome, 727–728
Eicosanoid synthesis pathway, 171–173, 173f
Ektacytometry, 358
Elasticity, 353
Elderly adults. See also Geriatric hematology and hemostasis
 anemia in, 871–873
 anemia of inflammation, 872–873
 ineffective erythropoiesis, 873
 of inflammation, 872–873
 iron deficiency anemia, 873
 nutritional deficiencies, 873

Elderly adults (Continued)
 unexplained anemia of aging, 873
 hematologic neoplasia in, 873, 874t
 hematologic parameters of, 871
 monocytes and macrophages, 871
 platelets, 871
 red blood cells, 871, 872t
 white blood cells, 871
 hematology and hemostasis in, 870–874
 hematopoiesis and, 871
 hemostasis in, 874
 immune response in, 871
 ineffective erythropoiesis in, 873
 folic acid deficiency, 873
 vitamin B_{12} deficiency, 873
Electrical hazards, 881.e8
Electrical impedance, 199–201, 199f–200f
Electrical pulses, 206
Electromechanical clot detection systems, 843, 844f
Electronic health records (EHRs), 876
Electronic volume thresholds, 199
Elliptocytes, 267t
Elliptocytosis, 360
Eltrombopag, 741
EMA binding test, 358
Embden-Meyerhof pathway, 97f, 374
Emboli, 762
Emicizumab (Hemlibra, Genentech), 693, 704
Endocrine signaling, 49
Endocytosis, 49, 124, 165
Endomitosis, 160, 160b
Endoplasmic reticulum, 45f, 46t, 47
Endosomes, 48–49, 129
Endosteum, 62
Endothelial cell protein C receptor (EPCR), 676, 677f
Endothelial cells, 5, 61–62, 804
 function of, 662
 hemolytic uremic syndrome and, 382
 intact, 663f
 prostacyclin and, 664
 structural and functional characteristics of, 662–663
Endothelial nitric oxide synthase (eNOS), 415–416
Energy production, anaerobic glycolysis, 96–98, 96b, 97f, 98t
Enolase, 96–98
Enterocytes, 124
Enzymatic white blood cell defects, 470
Enzyme chromographic test (ECT) method, 372
Enzyme immunoassays, for heparin-induced thrombocytopenia, 780, 780f
Enzyme-linked receptors, 52
Enzymopathies, 368–374
 glucose-6-phosphate dehydrogenase, 97f, 98
 glucose-6-phosphate dehydrogenase deficiency, 368–373, 368f, 369t
 acute hemolytic anemia, 370, 370b
 chronic hereditary nonspherocytic hemolytic anemia, 371
 clinical manifestations, 370–371
 laboratory findings, 371–373
 hemolytic anemia, general tests for, 371
 tests for, 371–373, 372f
 neonatal hyperbilirubinemia, 370–371
 pathophysiology, 370
 treatment, 373
 pyrimidine 5′-nucleotidase type 1 (P5′NT-1) deficiency, 374
 pyruvate kinase deficiency, 373–374
 clinical manifestations, 373
 laboratory findings, 373–374, 374f
 pathophysiology, 373
 treatment, 374
Eosinopenia, 3
Eosinophilia, 3, 80–81, 147, 478

Eosinophils, 3, 139–140, 146–147, 229, 482–483
  bone marrow aspiration examination, 256, 257f
  development, 146
  functions, 146–147
  granules, 146, 147b
  kinetics, 146
  mature, 146, 147f
  metamyelocytes, 146
  myelocytes, 146
  pediatric, 866
  quantitative abnormalities of, 478
    eosinophilia, 478
  ruptured and smudged eosinophils, 482
  in serous fluids, 881.e39f, 881.e42
EPB41 mutations, 360
Ependymal cells, 881.e39f
Epidemiology
  of iron deficiency anemia, 279
  of thalassemias, 441
Epigenetics
  mechanisms, 492–493, 492t
  myelodysplastic neoplasms, 627
Epinephrine, 168
  platelet aggregometry and, 820
Epitopes, 3–4
Epoc device, 194, 195f
Epstein-Barr virus, 315
Epstein syndrome, 737
Eptifibatide, 791t, 803
Equation reference interval, 189
Equipments
  bone marrow aspiration and biopsy, 247
  manual cell counts, 180–183, 180f
Equitable health care, 12
Equitable hematology, and hemostasis testing, 12
Equitable laboratory testing services, 12
Erythroblastic islands (EBI), 90
Erythroblasts, 62, 63f, 284
Erythrocyte enzymopathies, 368–374
  assay, 6
  glucose-6-phosphate dehydrogenase deficiency,
    97f, 98, 368–373, 368f, 369t
    acute hemolytic anemia, 370, 370b
    chronic hereditary nonspherocytic hemolytic
      anemia, 371
    clinical manifestations, 370–371
    laboratory findings, 371–373
      hemolytic anemia, general tests for, 371
      tests for, 371–373, 372f
    neonatal hyperbilirubinemia, 370–371
    pathophysiology, 370
    treatment, 373
  pyrimidine 5′-nucleotidase type 1 (P5′NT-1)
    deficiency, 374
  pyruvate kinase deficiency, 373–374
    clinical manifestations, 373
    laboratory findings, 373–374, 374f
    pathophysiology, 373
    treatment, 374
Erythrocyte iron sensing and hepcidin production,
  127–128, 129f–130f
Erythrocytes, 1, 2f, 86, 87f
  abnormalities
    proteins, 45
  blood film examination, 5
  count, 1–2
    summarizing, 237–240, 238t, 239f
  dehydrated hereditary stomatocytosis, 362
    clinical and laboratory findings, 362
    pathophysiology, 362
  destruction, 330–378
    extrinsic defects, 379–391
    fragmentation hemolysis, 91
    intrinsic defects, 90–91, 352–378, 353f
    macrophage-mediated hemolysis, 91
  erythrokinetics, 86
    hypoxia, 87, 87b

Erythrocytes (Continued)
  erythropoiesis, 79–86
  hemoglobin, hematocrit, and red blood cell
    indices, 2
  hereditary elliptocytosis, 359–361
    clinical and laboratory findings, 360–361,
      360f–361f
    pathophysiology, 360
    treatment, 361
  hereditary ovalocytosis, 361
    clinical and laboratory findings, 361
    pathophysiology, 361
  hereditary spherocytosis (HS), 354t, 355–359
    additional tests, 357–358, 358f
    clinical and laboratory findings, 355–357
    complications, 358–359
    differential diagnosis, 359, 359t
    pathophysiology, 355, 356f
    treatment, 359, 359f
  inclusions, 268t
  indices, 187, 187t
    mean cell hemoglobin, 2, 187
    mean cell hemoglobin concentration, 2, 187
    mean cell volume, 2, 187
    moving average of, 32–33
  maturation
    criteria used in identification of erythroid
      precursors in, 80–81, 81f, 81b
    process, 79
    sequence, 81–86, 82f, 82t
    terminology, 79t
  membrane, 99–105
    abnormalities, 353–368
      abetalipoproteinemia, 363
      acquired, 363–368
      acquired red blood cell, 363–368
      acquired stomatocytosis, 363
      chorea acanthocytosis, 363
      cryohydrocytosis, 362
      familial pseudohyperkalemia, 362
      hereditary elliptocytosis, 359–361
      hereditary ovalocytosis, 361
      hereditary spherocytosis, 354t, 355–359
      hereditary with acanthocytes, 362–363
      McLeod syndrome, 363
      neuroacanthocytosis, 363
      paroxysmal nocturnal hemoglobinuria,
        364–368
      Rh deficiency syndrome, 362
      spur cell anemia, 363
    deformability, 99, 104, 353–368
    lipids, 99–101, 100f
    osmotic balance and permeability, 104–105
    proteins, 101–104, 102f, 103t
    structure and function, 95–108, 353–354
  metabolism, 95–108
    energy production through anaerobic
      glycolysis, 96–98, 96b, 97f, 98t
    glycolysis diversion pathways, 98–99
    hexose monophosphate, 97f, 98, 98t
    methemoglobin reductase, 97f, 98–99
    Rapoport-Luebering, 97f, 99
  microenvironment of bone marrow and, 90f
  microhematocrit, 184–186, 185f
  morphology, 1, 234
    classification of anemia based on mean cell
      volume, 268–271
    hereditary elliptocytosis, 360, 360f
  nucleus, 86, 87f
  overhydrated hereditary stomatocytosis, 361–362
    clinical and laboratory findings, 362, 362f
    pathophysiology, 361–362
  paroxysmal nocturnal hemoglobinuria, 315,
    321t, 331–332
  production and destruction, 78–94
  red cell distribution width (RDW), 2, 265
  reticulocytes, 3

Erythrocytes (Continued)
  sedimentation rate, 6, 190–192
    automated, 191–192
    disposable kits, 191, 193t
    factors affecting, 192t
    modified Westergren, 190, 191f
    reference interval, 190b
    sources of error and comments, 190b
    Wintrobe, 190–191
  values in the neonate, 864–865
    anemia and, 865–866
    hematocrit, 865
    hemoglobin, 865
    morphology, 864, 864f
    red blood cell indices, 865
    reticulocyte count, 865, 865f
Erythroferrone, 127–128, 127t
Erythroid hyperplasia, 621f
Erythroid lineage, 506
Erythroid precursors, 79, 80f, 621f
Erythroid progenitors, 79
Erythrokinetics, 86
  hypoxia, 87, 87b
Erythrophages, 881.e39
Erythrophagocytosis, 332
Erythropoiesis, 72, 79–86
  impaired, 283
  ineffective, 444, 873
    folic acid deficiency, 873
    insufficient and, 264
    vitamin B$_{12}$ deficiency, 873
  systemic regulation of, 115–116
  tests of increased, 345–346, 346t
Erythropoiesis-stimulating agents (ESAs), 324–325
Erythropoietic protoporphyria (EPP), 285–286,
  285t
Erythropoietin (EPO), 72, 87–90, 864
  early release of reticulocytes and, 88
  inhibition of apoptosis and, 88–89
  measurement of, 89
  in polycythemia vera, 593, 595f
  regulation of hemoglobin production and, 115
  therapeutic uses of, 89–90
Erythropoietin receptor (EPOR), 127t
ESCAPED trial, 423
Escherichia. coli, 382
Essential thrombocythemia (ET), 4, 599–601,
  753–754, 753f
  clinical laboratory findings, 754
  clinical manifestations of, 753–754
  clinical presentation of, 599
  diagnosis of, 599
  incidence of, 599
  pathogenetic mechanism of, 599
  peripheral blood and bone marrow, 599–600,
    600f, 600t
  prognosis of, 600–601
  treatment of, 600–601, 754
Esterases, 578–579, 579f
Estrogen replacement therapy, 875
Estrogens, 875
Ethylenediaminetetraacetic acid (EDTA), 179,
  881.e13
  anticoagulated aspirate smears and, 250
  dependent anti-platelet antibody, 219
  particle smears and, 250
  peripheral blood films and, 226
  white blood cell count, 181
Etiology
  acquired aplastic anemia, 314b–315b, 315
  acquired iron overload, 287
  of anemia of chronic inflammation, 281–283
  hemoglobin C, 428–429, 429f
  hemoglobin E, 429–430
  hereditary Iron Overload, 287
  iron deficiency anemia, 276–281
    impaired absorption, 276–277

Etiology *(Continued)*
  inadequate intake, 276
  increased need, 276
  iron overload, 287
    acquired, 287
    hereditary, 287
  megaloblastic anemia, 297–300, 297b
    defect in megaloblastic anemia caused by
      deficiency in folate and vitamin B$_{12}$,
      298–300, 299f
    other causes, 300
    physiologic roles of vitamin B$_{12}$ and folate,
      297–298, 298f
  sickle cell anemia, 414–416
  thrombosis, 762
Etranacogene dezaparvovec (Hemgenix, Behring),
  705
Euchromatin, 46–47
Evacuated tubes, 881.e13, 881.e14f
Evidence-based practice, 13
  in hematology and hemostasis laboratory, 13
Exercise-induced hemoglobinuria, 384
Exercise-induced thrombocytosis, 753
Exhausted platelets, 726
Exocytosis, 49
Exposure controls and personal protection, 881.e7
External quality assessment, 33
Extracellular ferritin, 131
Extracellular matrix (ECM), 52, 61–62
Extracorporeal membrane oxygenation (ECMO),
  751, 795
Extramedullary hematopoiesis, in primary
  myelofibrosis, 605
Extravascular cords, 62, 63f
Extravascular hemolysis, 91, 338–339, 338f
Extrinsic hemolytic conditions, 332
Extrinsic tenase, 670
Eyepieces, microscope, 881.e27
Eyewear, 881.e4

F

Facilitated diffusion, plasma membrane, 48–49
Factor V, 670
  deficiency, 706, 706t
  depleted plasma, 769–770
  Leiden mutation, 762, 769–770
    assay, 770
Factor Va, 670
Factor VII deficiency, 706, 706t
Factor VIII, 671
  in arterial thrombosis predictors, 774
  assay
    procedure for, 829
    reference curve for, 829, 829f
  structure and function of, 701
Factor X deficiency, 706, 706t
Factor XI, 671–672
  deficiency, 705, 706t
Factor XIII, 672–673
  assay, 831
  deficiency, 706–707, 706t
Factor XIII inhibitors, 693
Fainting (syncope), 881.e18
Familial pseudohyperkalemia, 362
Fanconi anemia, 318–319, 737
Fat cells, 55
Favism, 370
Feasibility, assay, 36
Fechtner syndrome, 737
Fedratinib, 598
Ferritin, 124, 131, 133–134
  absorption, 124, 125f
Ferrokinetics, impaired, 281–283
Ferroportin, 281–282
Ferrozine, 132
Fetal hemoglobin, drugs to increase, 424

Fetus. *See also* Neonates
  fetal thrombocytopenia, 738t
  hemolytic disease of, 401–403, 402t
  marrow megakaryocytes, 738
  thalassemias with increased levels of
    hemoglobin, 451
Fibrin
  degradation, 681, 681f
  formation, 672–673, 673f
Fibrinogen, 666
  activity, in arterial thrombosis predictors,
    773–774, 773f
  in elderly adults, 874
  structure, 672–673, 672f
Fibrinogen assay, 5, 827–828
  calibration curve, 828, 828f
  limitations of, 828
  procedure for, 827–828
  quality control for, 828
  reagent for, 827
  results and clinical utility of, 828
  test protocol for, 828
Fibrinogen equivalent units (FEUs), 774–775
Fibrinolysis, 678–681, 679f, 679t
  control of, 679f, 679t, 680–681
  disseminated intravascular coagulation and,
    383
  in elderly adults, 874
  plasmin, 679
  plasminogen, 679
    activation, 680
Fibrinolysis assays, 831–833
  D-dimer immunoassay, 831–832
  fibrin degradation product immunoassay,
    831–832
  plasminogen, 832
    chromogenic substrate, 832, 832f
  plasminogen activator inhibitor-1, 833
    principle of, 833, 833f
  tissue plasminogen activator assay, 832–833
    principle of, 833, 833f
    specimen collection for, 833
Fibrinolytic drugs, 790
Fibrinolytic inhibitors, deficiency of, 707
Fibrinolytic therapy, 804
Fibroblasts, 55
Fibronectin, 90
Field diaphragm, 881.e28
50x oil immersion objective examination of blood
  films, 231
Films, peripheral blood, 226–235
  drying of, 229
  examination of, 231–235
    10x objective, 231
    40x high-dry objective, 231, 232b
    50x oil immersion objective, 231, 232b
    100x oil immersion objective, 231–232
    for anemia, 267t
    automated microscopic, 235
    macroscopic, 231
    for malaria, 385, 385f
    microscopic, 231–235
    optimal assessment area, 232, 233f
  specimen collection for, 226–227, 226f
  staining of, 229–230
    automated, 228–229
    features of proper, 230, 231b
    manual technique, 229, 230f
    quick, 230
    types of, 227–229, 228f
    wedge, 227–228, 228f
Fire drills, 881.e6
Firefighting measures, 881.e7
Fire hazards, 881.e6, 881.e6t
Fire response plan, 881.e6
First-aid measures, 881.e7
Fish tapeworm, 303

Fitusiran (Sanofi), 704–705
Five-part differential, 202
Flagging, 219
  in automated assay performance, 849, 849b
Flat field lenses, 881.e28
Flippases, 100
Floppases, 100
Flow cytometers, 202
Flow cytometry, 501f, 502
  analysis of, 503–505
    data analysis, 505, 505f–506f
    gating in, 503–505
  in hematologic disorders, 500–518
    lymphoid neoplasms, 510–513
    myeloid neoplasms, 506–510, 506f–507f
  cell populations identified by, 505–506
    erythroid lineage, 506
    granulocytic lineage, 506
    lymphoid lineage, 506
    megakaryocytic lineage, 506
    monocytic lineage, 506
  cell sorting and, 515
  diagram of, 503, 504f
  hematological antigens used in, 504t
  hematologic malignancies, immunophenotyping
    of, 513–516, 515f
  immunophenotyping, 5–6
  lineage-associated markers in, 503t
  multicolor or multiparameter, 502
  in platelet function testing, 857
  principle and instrumentation of, 502–503
  specimen processing in, 502
FLT3, 72
Fluorescein-labeled proaerolysin variant (FLAER),
  367
Fluorescence flow cytometry, for WBC count,
  WBC differential, NRBCs, and reticulocyte
  analyses, 207–210, 209f
Fluorescence, in flow cytometry, 503, 504f
Fluorescence in situ hybridization (FISH),
  554–556, 556f–557f
Fluorescence resonance energy transfer (FRET),
  533
Fluorescence technology, 199
Fluorescent dyes, 203
Fluorescently labeled fragments, 537, 540f
Fluorescent microscope, 881.e31
Fluorescent platelet count (PLT-F), 209–210
Fluorescent spot test, 372
Fluorescent staining, 202–203
Foam cells, 473
Focus controls, microscope, 881.e28
Folate, 297–298, 298f
  assays for, 305–306, 307f
  defect in megaloblastic anemia caused by,
    298–300, 299f
  deficiency
    causes of, 301, 301b, 306b
    laboratory tests used to, 308t
    systemic manifestations of, 300–301
Folate deficiency, 366
Folded cells, 267t
Folic acid deficiency, in elderly adults, 873
Follicular lymphoma, 648, 648f
Fondaparinux, 791t, 798–799, 799f
Food-cobalamin malabsorption, 303
Foramina, 62–63
40x high-dry objective examination of blood films,
  231, 232b
Forward scatter (FSC), 207–209
4Ts scoring system, for heparin-induced
  thrombocytopenia, 779, 779t
FOXP3$^+$, 316
Fragmentation hemolysis, 91
Free cholesterol, 99
FREEDOM trial, 598
Free eosin, 229

Free methylene blue, 229
Free protein S (PS) deficiency, 765t
French-American-British (FAB) classification, 491–492, 623
Front-end load capability, 203
Fructose-bisphosphate aldolase, 96, 97f
Full-term infant, platelet count reference intervals for, 867t
Full-term neonate, 863–864
  hemoglobin for, reference interval, 865
Full-term neonates, 863–864
Functional iron deficiency (FID), 134, 134f, 220–221
Fungal organisms, 481–482, 482f

G

G1 checkpoint, 53
G1 (gap 1) stage, cell cycle, 52
G2 (gap 2) stage, cell cycle, 52
G6PD deficiency, 368–373
Gain-of-function mutation, 493
Gardos channel, 362
Gastric analysis, 306
Gastric bypass surgery, 266
Gating, 503–505
Gaucher cells, 471
Gaucher disease, 48, 470–473, 472t
Gaussian distribution, 30, 31f
Gelatinase granules, 141
Gender-affirming hormone therapy (GAHT), 874–875
Gene amplification, 493
Gene expression studies, 592
Gene function, 627
Genes, 522–523
Gene therapy, 425–427, 449–450
Genetic abnormalities, myelodysplastic neoplasms with, 623–624
  with biallelic TP53 inactivation, 624
  with low blasts and isolated 5q deletion, 623–624
  with low blasts and SF3B1 mutation, 624
Genetics
  acquired aplastic anemia and, 315
  acute lymphoblastic leukemia and, 570
  acute myeloid leukemia and, 571–573, 572f
  central dogma in, 521–523
  congenital dyserythropoietic anemia and, 323–324
  defects in, causing thalassemia, 443, 444f
  Diamond-Blackfan anemia and, 322–323
  dyskeratosis congenita and, 319–320
  Fanconi anemia, 319
  globin, 409–410
  of globin synthesis, 442, 442f
  hemoglobin, 410–411, 410t
  molecular, in chronic myelogenous leukemia, 585–586, 585f
  mutations
    cis, 432
    point, 522–523
  Shwachman-Bodian-Diamond syndrome, 320–321
  sickle cell anemia and, 412–413, 413f
Genetic testing, for hemostatic disorders, 834, 834t
Genome-editing technologies, 425, 427
Geometric mean, 21
Gerbich antigens, 360
Geriatric hematology and hemostasis
  anemia and, 871–873
    ineffective erythropoiesis, 873
    of inflammation, 872–873
    iron deficiency anemia, 873
    nutritional deficiencies, 873
    unexplained anemia of aging, 873
  hematopoiesis, 871

Geriatric hematology and hemostasis (Continued)
  hemostasis in, 874
  neoplasia in, 873, 874t
  parameters of, 871
    monocytes and macrophages, 871
    platelets, 871
    red blood cells, 871, 872t
    white blood cells, 871
Geriatric hematology and hemostasis, 870–874
Gestational age, birth weight and, 863–864
Gestational hematology and hemostasis, 868–870
  anemia and, 868–869
    acute blood loss, 869
    hemoglobinopathies, 869
    iron deficiency anemia, 868
    megaloblastic anemia, 869
    parasitic infections, 869
  hemostasis, 869–870
    thrombocytopenia and bleeding disorders, 870, 870t
    thrombophilia and thrombosis, 869–870
Gestation, hematopoiesis and, 863
Giant cell (temporal) arteritis, 190
Giant platelets, 221
Giant platelet syndromes, inherited, 717, 718t
Girdle syndrome, sickle cell disease and, 418
Givinostat, 598–599, 604
Glanzmann thrombasthenia, 714–716
  laboratory features of, 715
  treatment of, 715–716
Global coagulation assays, 833–834
  TEG and ROTEM, 833–834
  thrombin generation assays as, 834
Global hemostasis assessment, 853–855, 854f, 855t
Globin. See also Hemoglobin
  biosynthesis, 114
  chain synthesis, 268
  genetic structure, 409–410
  regulation, 114–115
  structure, 110–111, 110t, 111f
  synthesis of, genetics of, 442, 442f
Globin transcription factor-1 (GATA-1), 160, 160b
Gloves, 881.e3, 881.e5f, 881.e12
Glucose-6-phosphate dehydrogenase (G6PD), 97f, 98, 368–373, 368f, 369t
  acute hemolytic anemia, 370, 370b
  assay, 6
  chronic hereditary nonspherocytic hemolytic anemia, 371
  clinical manifestations, 370–371
  laboratory findings, 371–373
    hemolytic anemia, general tests for, 371
    tests for, 371–373, 372f
  neonatal hyperbilirubinemia, 370–371
  pathophysiology, 370
  treatment, 373
Glut1, 361–362
Glutathione reductase, 98
Glycation, 112
Glyceraldehyde-3-phosphate dehydrogenase, 96, 97f
Glycine, 112–113
Glycocalyx, 45, 165
Glycolipids, 100–101
Glycolysis, anaerobic, 96–98, 96b, 97f, 98t
  diversion pathways, 98–99
    hexose monophosphate, 97f, 98, 98t
    methemoglobin reductase, 97f, 98–99
    Rapoport-Luebering, 97f, 99
  first phase, 96, 98t
  second phase, 96, 98t
  third phase, 96–98, 98t
Glycoprotein C (GPC), 360
Glycoproteins, 165
Glycosylation, 101
Glycosylphosphatidylinositol (GPI), 364f

Golgi apparatus, 45f, 46f, 47, 254
GPI-anchored proteins, 364–365
GPI anchor, paroxysmal nocturnal hemoglobinuria and, 364
GP IIb/IIIa (α_{IIb}/β_3) receptor inhibitors, 723–724
G-protein coupled receptors, 52
G-proteins, 171, 172f
  inositol triphosphate-diacylglycerol activation pathway and, 173
α-Granule deficiency, 720, 720f
Granules, 229
  basophils, 148–149, 149b
  eosinophils, 146, 147b
  neutrophil, 139–140, 142b
  platelet, 165f, 166, 166t
  promyelocyte or myelocyte devoid of, 621, 622f
α-Granules, 717
  α-Granule deficiency, 720, 720f
Granulocyte-monocyte progenitor (GMP), 140–141
Granulocytes, 139–149, 578
  basophils, 3, 139–140, 147–149
    development, 148
    functions, 148–149
    granules, 148–149, 149b
    immature, 148
    kinetics, 148
    mature, 148, 148f
  eosinophils, 3, 139–140, 146–147
    development, 146
    functions, 146–147
    granules, 146, 147b
    kinetics, 146
    mature, 146, 147f
    metamyelocytes, 146
    myelocytes, 146
  mast cells, 149, 149f
  neutrophils, 3, 139–146
    development, 140–143, 141f
    functions, 144–146
    granules, 141, 142b
    kinetics, 143–144
    metamyelocytes, 141, 141f, 144f
    myeloblasts, 141, 141f
    myelocytes, 141, 142f–143f
    promyelocytes, 141, 141f, 143f
    segmented, 141–143, 145f
Granulocytic lineage, 506
Granulomas, 246
Granzyme B, 148–149
Gray platelet syndrome, 720, 720f
Growth factors
  hematopoietic, 70–72, 71f
  receptors, 56, 492
Guanine, 523–524
Guanosine diphosphate (GDP), 52
Guanosine triphosphate (GTP), 52

H

Hairy cell leukemia (HCL), 321t, 645–646, 645f
Hand-foot syndrome, 423
Hand hygiene, 881.e2, 881.e3f
Handling and storage, 881.e7
Hand washing, 881.e12
Haptocorrin, 301–303
Haptoglobin, 128, 335–337, 337f, 344–345
  hemopexin-methemalbumin system, 336f, 337
Harlem-C-Georgetown, 429
Hazard(s) identification, 881.e7
HCT. See Hematocrit
Health care, 13
Health care delivery systems, 8–9
Health care professionals, essential competencies for, 12–13
  evidence-based practice and patient-centered care, 13

Health care professionals, essential competencies for (Continued)
informatics and quality improvement processes, 13
interprofessional teamwork, 12–13
Health care quality
definition of, 9
six aims of, 9–12, 10t
effective hematology and hemostasis testing, 11, 11t
efficient hematology and hemostasis testing, 11–12
equitable hematology and hemostasis testing, 12
patient-centered hematology and hemostasis testing, 12
safe hematology and hemostasis testing, 9–11
timely hematology and hemostasis testing, 12
Health Professions Education: A Bridge to Quality, 12
Healthy, definition of, 263
Heavy chain disease, 656–657
Heinz bodies, 268t, 370, 434
HELLP syndrome, 383, 870
Helmet cell, 267t
Hemacytometers, 2, 180, 180f
procedure for, 181b, 182f
Hemangioma-thrombocytopenia syndrome, 727
Hematocrit (HCT), 2
elevated, sodium citrate volume adjustment for, 813–814, 814f
pediatric, 865
point-of-care testing, 194, 194f–195f
reticulocyte production index and, 189
rule of three, 186
Hematogone, 152, 152f
Hematologic malignancies
cellular processes perturbed in, 492, 492b
immunophenotyping of, 513–516, 515f
therapy for, general categories of, 494–497, 494b
Hematologic neoplasia, in elderly adults, 873, 874t
chronic lymphocytic leukemia, 873
myelodysplastic neoplasms, 873
myeloproliferative neoplasms, 873
Hematology
evidence-based practice in, 13
informatics in, 13
interprofessional teamwork in, 12–13
patient-centered care in, 13
quality improvement in, 13
Hematology laboratory, safety in, 881.e1–881.e10
occupational hazards, 881.e6
biohazards in blood and body fluids, 881.e8
chemical hazards, 881.e6
electrical hazards, 881.e8
fire hazards, 881.e6, 881.e6t
radioactive hazards, 881.e8
standard precautions, 881.e2
hepatitis B virus vaccination, 881.e5
housekeeping, 881.e5
laundry, 881.e5
Occupational Safety and Health Administration Standard, 881.e2
regulated medical waste management, 881.e6
training and documentation, 881.e6
Hematoma, 881.e18, 881.e18f
Hematopoiesis, 59–77
adult tissue, 60–68
bone marrow, 60–64, 62f–63f
liver, 64, 64f
lymph nodes, 66, 67f
spleen, 64–66, 65f–66f
thymus, 66–68, 67f–68f
aging and, 871

Hematopoiesis (Continued)
development, 59–60, 61f
hepatic phase, 60
medullary phase, 60
mesoblastic phase, 60
hormone therapy and, 875
ineffective, 299, 321t
lineage-specific, 72–73
erythropoiesis, 72
leukopoiesis, 72
megakaryocytopoiesis, 72–73
of neonate, 863
prenatal, 863
in primary myelofibrosis, 605
sex hormone effects on, 875
sites of, by age, 61f
stem cells and cytokines, 68–72
cytokines and growth factors, 70–72, 71f
stem cell cycle kinetics, 70, 70f
stem cell phenotypic and functional characterization, 70
stem cell theory, 68–70, 69f, 69t
therapeutic applications, 73, 73t–74t
Hematopoietically active bone marrow, 61
Hematopoietic inductive microenvironment, 69–70
Hematopoietic microenvironment, 55–56, 63–64
Hematopoietic stem and progenitor cells (HSPCs), 425
Hematopoietic stem cells (HSCs), 59, 68–69, 450
for aplastic anemias, 319–320
for chronic myelogenous leukemia, 589
for sickle cell disease, 423–424
Hematopoietic stem cell transplantation (HSCT), 448–450
for leukocyte neoplasms, 496–497, 497f
Heme. See also Hemoglobin
biosynthesis, 112–114, 113f
with bound iron, 128
metabolism disorders, 275–295
regulation, 114
structure, 110, 110f
Heme absorption, 124, 125f
Heme carrier protein 1 (HCP1), 124, 337
Heme, catabolism, 333, 333f
Heme regulatory gene-1 (HRG-1), 124
Hemochromatosis, 287t
protein, 127t, 287
Hemoconcentration, 881.e18
HemoCue, 184b, 185f
Hemoglobin, 2
Bart hydrops fetalis syndrome, 454
biosynthesis, 112–114
assembly, 113f, 114
globin, 114
heme, 112–114, 113f
ontogeny, 114, 115f, 115t
C, 428–429, 429f
crystal, 267t, 269f
C-Harlem, 429, 432
concentration, point-of-care testing, 194
content of reticulocytes, 132t, 134
C-thalassemia, 455
D, 430
degradation, 333, 334b
determination, 183–184
principle, 183–184
sources of error and comments, 184b
development, 410
dyshemoglobins, 118–119
carboxyhemoglobin, 119
methemoglobin, 118–119
sulfhemoglobin, 119
E, 429–430, 430f
E-thalassemia, 455
fragmentation hemolysis and salvage of, 335–338, 340b

Hemoglobin (Continued)
function, 116–118
carbon dioxide transport, 117, 118f
nitric oxide transport, 118
oxygen transport, 116–117, 116f–117f
G, 430
genetic mutations, 410–411, 410t
compound heterozygosity with hemoglobin S and, 430–432, 431f
glycation, 112, 345
H, 268t
disease, 453–454
with increased and decreased oxygen affinity, 434–435
induction agents, 449
M, 432–434
mean cell, 2
measurement, 119
metabolism, 109–121
O-Arab, 430
pediatric, 865
physiologic fragmentation hemolysis and salvage of, 335–338, 340b
production regulation, 114–116
reference interval for, 865
rule of three, 186
S, 412–428
compound heterozygosity with, 430–432, 431f
concomitant CIS mutations with, 432
Korle Bu, 432
S-Antilles, 432, 433t
SC, 431
crystal, 267t, 269f
SD, 432
SD-Punjab, 432
SG-Philadelphia, 432
SO-Arab, 432
solubility test, 420–421, 421f
S-Oman, 432, 433t
S-thalassemia, 454–455
structure, 110–112, 112f
complete molecule, 111–112, 111f–112f
globin, 110–111, 110t, 111f
heme, 110, 110f
unstable variants, 434
variants, 411, 412b–413b
assessment of normal and, 456–457, 456f–457f
geographic distribution of inherited, 414f
structural, thalassemia associated with, 454–455, 455t
unstable, 434
zygosity and, 411
Hemoglobin determination
Abbott, 210
Beckman Coulter, 205
errors in, 216–218
Siemens Healthineers, 213
spectrophotometry for, 203
Sysmex, 207
Hemoglobin distribution width (HDW), 213
Hemoglobinemia, 335, 340b
Hemoglobinopathies, 408–439, 409f
defined, 409
genetic mutations and, 410–411, 410t
global burden of, 435
hemoglobin C, 428–429, 429f
hemoglobin C-Harlem, 429
hemoglobin D and hemoglobin G, 430
hemoglobin development and, 410
hemoglobin E, 429–430, 430f
hemoglobin M, 432–434
hemoglobin O-Arab, 430
hemoglobin SC and hemoglobin SG-Philadelphia, 432
hemoglobin S, concomitant cis mutations with, 432, 433t

Hemoglobinopathies (Continued)
  hemoglobin S-Korle Bu, 432
  hemoglobins with increased and decreased
      oxygen affinity, 434–435
  hemoglobin S-β-thalassemia, 431
  nomenclature, 411–412
  pathophysiology, 411
  during pregnancy, 869
  sickle cell disease, 66, 412–427
    clinical features, 416–419, 416b
    course and prognosis, 427
    etiology and pathophysiology, 414–416
    geographic distribution of inherited
        hemoglobin variants and, 414–416,
        414f
    history of, 412–413
    incidence with malaria, 419–420
    inheritance pattern, 413, 413f
    irreversible, 415
    laboratory diagnosis, 420–422, 420f–421f
    malaria and, 419–420
    prevalence, 413–414
    reversible, 415
    trait, 427–428
    treatment, 422–427
  SO-Arab and SD-Punjab, 432
  structure of globin genes and, 409–410
  zygosity and, 411
Hemoglobinuria, 340, 366
  exercise-induced, 384
Hemogram. See Complete blood count
Hemojuvelin, 127t
Hemolysis, 331, 333–338, 366, 747, 881.e19
  acute, 331–332, 341
  bilirubin metabolism and, 333–335, 333f
  blood loss and, 264–265
  chronic, 331–332, 341
  classification of hemolytic disorders, 331–333,
      331t
  clinical features, 340–341
  clinical signs and symptoms, 341
    acute hemolysis, 341
    chronic hemolysis, 341
  differential diagnosis, 346–347, 347f, 348t
  extrinsic, 332
  fragmentation, 91, 332
    macrophage-mediated hemolysis vs., 339t
    pathologic, 339–340, 341f–344f
    plasma hemoglobin salvage, 335–338, 336f,
        340b
  inherited, 332
  intravascular, 91
  intrinsic, 332
  laboratory findings, 346
    tests of accelerated red blood cell
        destruction, 342–345
    tests of increased erythropoiesis, 345–346,
        346t
    laboratory tests to determine specific processes,
        346, 346t
  macrophage-mediated, 91
  nonimmune drug-induced, 404
  pathologic macrophage-mediated, 338–339,
      338f
  plasma hemoglobin salvage and fragmentation,
      335–338, 340b
  site and mechanism of, 332–333
  in specimen quality set points, 849
Hemolysis area (HA), 458–459
Hemolytic anemias, 220, 287, 301, 331, 331t
  alloimmune, 396–401
    hemolytic disease of the fetus and newborn,
        401–403, 402t
    hemolytic transfusion reaction, 401
  autoimmune, 396–401
    characteristics of, 398t
    cold agglutinin disease, 399–400, 400f

Hemolytic anemias (Continued)
    mixed-type, 401
    paroxysmal cold hemoglobinuria, 331–332,
        400–401
    warm, 397–399
  clinical features, 340–341
  differential diagnosis, 346–347, 347f
  general tests for, 371
  immune, 392–407, 393f–395f
    drug-induced, 403–404, 403f
    laboratory findings in, 396, 397f
    major mechanisms of, 396t
    overview of, 393–396, 394b
    pathophysiology, 393–396
  laboratory findings, 342, 346t
  macroangiopathic, 383–384
    exercise-induced hemoglobinuria, 384
    traumatic cardiac hemolytic anemia, 383,
        384f
  malaria and, 332
  microangiopathic, 380–383, 381b
    disseminated intravascular coagulation, 383
    HELLP syndrome, 383
    hemolytic uremic syndrome, 382–383
    thrombotic thrombocytopenic purpura,
        381–382, 382f
  nonimmune causes, 379–391, 380f, 380b
    babesiosis and, 386–387
      clinical findings, 387
      geographic distribution, 387
      laboratory findings and diagnosis, 387,
          387f
    bartonellosis, 387–388
    clostridial sepsis, 387
    drugs and chemicals, 388
    extensive burns, 388, 388f
    infectious agents, 384–388
    malaria, 384–385
      clinical and laboratory findings, 385
      hemolytic anemia caused by, 384–388
      microscopic examination, 385, 385f
      pathogenesis, 384–385
      Plasmodium falciparum and, 385, 386f
      Plasmodium knowlesi and, 385, 386f
      Plasmodium malariae and, 385, 386f
      Plasmodium ovale and, 385, 386f
      Plasmodium vivax and, 385, 385f
      prevalence, 384
    red blood cell injury, 388, 388f
    venoms, 388
  nonimmune causes, malaria, 332
  pathophysiology of, 364–365
Hemolytic crises, 358–359
Hemolytic disease of the fetus and newborn
    (HDFN), 401–403, 402t
Hemolytic jaundice, 340
Hemolytic transfusion reaction (HTR), 401
Hemolytic uremic syndrome (HUS), 382–383,
    749–750
  atypical, 750
  differentiation, 749t
Hemopexin, 128, 336f, 337
Hemophagocytic lymphohistiocytosis, 467
Hemophilia
  A, 701–705
    clinical manifestations, 702
    contemporary therapy, 704
    genetics, 701–702
    and inhibitors, 704–705
    laboratory diagnosis, 702–703, 702t
    traditional therapy, 703–704
  B, 705
  C, 705
Hemorrhage, 686
  acquired vs. congenital, 688, 688b
  anemia and, 263, 277
  bleeding time test, 33–34

Hemorrhage (Continued)
  chronic renal failure and, 691–692
  deep tissue bleeding, 735
  laboratory assessment and, 686–712
  localized vs. generalized, 687
  mucocutaneous vs. anatomic, 687–688, 687t
  nephrotic syndrome, 691–692
  from platelet abnormalities, 735
  reactive thrombocytosis associated with, 752
  reversal of warfarin overdose based on, 794t
  signs, hemostatic defect, 687b
  symptoms, 686–688, 735
  and thrombocytopenia, 735
  vitamin K deficiency and, 692
Hemorrhagic disease of the newborn, vitamin K
    deficiency, 692
Hemorrhagic thrombocythaemia, 599
Hemosiderin, 340, 345f
Hemostasis, 4, 661–685
  clot-based screening tests for coagulation
      disorders, 821–827
  coagulation factor assays for, 827–831
  cofactors in, 670–671
  disorders, genetic testing for, 834, 834t
  fibrinolysis assays, 831–833
  global coagulation assays for, 833–834
  hormone therapy and, 875
  instrumentation, 841–861, 850b
  laboratory evaluation of, 811–840
  laboratory tests, and liver disease, 691t
  overview of, 662
  platelet activation markers, 821
  primary, 662, 662t
  primary standards, 22–23
  secondary, 662, 662t
  vascular intima in, 662–665. See also Vascular
      intima
  viscoelastometry for, 833–834
Hemostasis laboratory
  evidence-based practice in, 13
  informatics in, 13
  interprofessional teamwork in, 12–13
  patient-centered care in, 13
  quality improvement in, 13
Hemostasis specimen collection, 812–815
  anticoagulants for, 813–814
    citrate theophylline adenosine dipyridamole,
        814
    EDTA, 813
    sodium citrate as, 813
  blood
    clotted, 815
    materials for, 813–814
      collection tubes for, 813
      needle selection in, 813, 813t
    procedure for, 814–815
      with butterfly set, 814
      with syringe, 815
      venipuncture and, 814–815
    short draw in, 814
    using capillary puncture, 815
    from vascular access devices, 815
  errors in, 814t
  heparinized, 813
  management of, 815–817
    preparation, 816–817
    transport and storage, 815–816
  patient management during, 812
  platelet function tests for, 817–821
  transport and storage of, 816t
Hemostasis testing
  effective hematology and, 11, 11t
  efficient hematology and, 11–12
  equitable hematology and, 12
  patient-centered hematology and, 12
  safe hematology and, 9–11
  timely hematology and, 12

Hemostatic system, cell-based physiologic coagulation, 674–676, 675f
Henoch-Schönlein purpura, 728
Heparin, 881.e13
Heparin action, 795
Heparin cofactor II (HC II), 677
Heparin-induced thrombocytopenia (HIT), 778–781
    assays, 821
    clinical scoring for, 778–779, 779t
    confirmatory platelet activation assays for, 780, 780f
    enzyme immunoassays for, 780, 780f
    pathophysiology of, 778, 779f
    platelet counts for, 778–779, 779t
    rapid turnaround assays for, 780–781
    therapy for, 781
Heparin resistance, 771
Hepatic disease, 764t
Hepatic function test, 266
Hepatic phase, of hematopoiesis, 60
Hepatitis B virus (HBV), 881.e12
    vaccination, 881.e5
Hepcidin, 125–127, 126f, 127t, 281–282
Hepcidin-ferroportin axis, 125
Hepcidin production
    erythrocyte iron sensing and, 127–128, 129f–130f
    liver iron sensing and, 126–127, 126f, 127t
Hephaestin, 126
Hereditary elliptocytosis (HE), 104, 359–361
    clinical and laboratory findings, 360–361, 360f–361f
    pathophysiology, 360
    treatment, 361
Hereditary hemochromatosis (HH), 287, 287t
Hereditary hemorrhagic telangiectasia, 727
Hereditary hydrocytosis, 354–355, 361–362
    clinical and laboratory findings, 362, 362f
    pathophysiology, 361–362
Hereditary iron overload, 287
Hereditary nonspherocytic hemolytic anemia, 98
Hereditary ovalocytosis, 361
    clinical and laboratory findings, 361
    pathophysiology, 361
Hereditary pyropoikilocytosis (HPP), 354–355
Hereditary red blood cell membrane abnormalities, 354–363, 355b
Hereditary sideroblastic anemias, 284–286, 286f
Hereditary spherocytosis (HS), 104, 354t, 355–359
    additional tests, 357–358, 358f
    clinical and laboratory findings, 355–357, 359, 359t
    complications, 358–359
    differential diagnosis, 359, 359t
    pathophysiology, 355, 356f
    treatment, 359, 359f
Hereditary xerocytosis (HX), 105, 354–355, 362
    clinical and laboratory findings, 362
    pathophysiology, 362
Hermansky-Pudlak syndrome, 718–719
Hetastarch, 724
Heterochromatin, 46–47
Heterozygosity, compound, 430–432, 431f
Hexokinase, glucose-6-phosphate isomerase, 96, 97f
Hexose monophosphate pathway, 97f, 98, 98t
High hyperdiploidy, 557
High-molecular-weight kininogen (HMWK), 670
High-performance liquid chromatography (HPLC), 421–422, 422f
    thalassemia and, 457, 457f
High-throughput sequencing (HTS), 834, 858
Histiocytes, 881.e47, 881.e47f
Histologic sections, bone marrow aspiration, 251
History, of laboratory hematology, 1–7
HIT. See Heparin-induced thrombocytopenia
HIT Expert Probability (HEP) score, 779

HLA-DR, 70, 505
Hodgkin lymphoma, 246, 653–655, 654f
Holotranscobalamin assay, 306
Homocysteine, assays for, 305, 307f
Homocysteinemia, 764
Homology directed repair (HDR), 426
HOPE trial, 425
Hormone replacement therapy (HRT), 875
Hormones, 875
    of megakaryocytopoiesis, 163, 163t
Hormone therapy
    and hematopoiesis, 875
    and hemostasis, 875
Housekeeping, 881.e5
    monocyte/macrophage functions, 151
Howell-Jolly bodies, 268t, 269f
H pattern, antecubital fossa, 881.e16, 881.e16f
Human granulocytic anaplasmosis (HGA), 481
Human immunodeficiency virus (HIV), 622–623, 738
    acquired aplastic anemia and, 315
    flow cytometry and, 514
    Pneumocystis jiroveci and, 881.e47, 881.e47f
Human monocytic ehrlichiosis (HME), 481
Human plasma-derived fibrinogen concentrates, 689
Humoral response, 3
100x oil immersion objective examination of blood films, 231–232
HUS. See Hemolytic uremic syndrome
Hyaline thrombi, 750
Hybridization probes, 533
Hydrodynamic focusing, 200, 503
Hydrophobic ligands, 49–50
Hydroxycarbamide therapy, 425
Hydroxyethyl starch, 724
Hydroxymethylbilane, 113–114
Hyperaggregable platelets, 727
Hypercoagulability, 762
Hypercoagulable state, molecular techniques for, 858t
Hyperdiploid cells, 557
Hyperfibrinogenemia, 765t
Hyperparathyroidism, 246
Hyperproliferation, 596
Hypersegmentation, neutrophil, 304, 475, 475f
Hypersplenism, 66
Hypertonic cryohemolysis test, 358
Hypochromic microcytes, 620
Hypodiploid cell, 557, 558f
Hypofibrinogenemia, 706t, 796
Hypoplasia, bone marrow, 322t
Hypoplastic MDS (h-MDS), 624
Hypovolemia, 418–419
Hypoxia, 87, 87b
    methemoglobinemia and, 118

I

Ibrutinib (Imbruvica), 724–725
Icterus, in specimen quality set points, 849
Identification, 881.e7
    chromosome, 553, 554f
Idiopathic thrombocytosis, 599
Immature basophils, 148, 148f
Immature granulocytes, Pelger Huet neutrophils and, 474–475
Immature platelet fraction (IPF), 240
Immature reticulocyte fraction (IRF), 3, 220
    anemia diagnosis and, 265
Immature T cells, 153
Immersion oil, 881.e30
Immune hemolytic anemia, 392–407, 393f–395f
    drug-induced, 403–404, 403f
    laboratory findings in, 396, 397f
    major mechanisms of, 396t
    overview of, 393–396, 394b
    pathophysiology, 393–396

Immune system
    acquired aplastic anemia and, 316
    basophils and, 148
    in elderly adults, 871
    eosinophils and, 144
    mast cells, 149
    monocyte/macrophage function and, 151
    neutrophils and, 144
Immune thrombocytopenia, during pregnancy, 870
Immune thrombocytopenic purpura, 740
    acute, 740
        chronic vs., 740, 740t
        diagnosis of, 740
        hemorrhage risk, 740
        incidence of, 740
        treatment of, 740
    chronic, 740–741, 741f
        acute vs., 740, 740t
        incidence of, 740
        peripheral blood abnormalities in, 741
        platelet destruction in, 741
        risk factors for, 741
        treatment of, 741
    drug-induced immune-mediated thrombocytopenia, 741–744, 742b, 743f
Immune tolerance induction (ITI), 693
Immunoassay technology, 846
Immunologic assays, 846
Immunologic endpoint detection, 845–846
Immunophenotyping, in acute lymphoblastic leukemia, 569–570, 569t
Immunosuppressive therapy, 628
Impaired fibrinolysis, 833
Impedance technology, 200–201
    limitations of, 216
Imprints, core biopsy, 250
Improving Diagnosis in Health Care, 8–9
Inclusions, erythrocytes, 268t
Incubated osmotic fragility test, 357
Independent expert laboratories, 23
Indices, red blood cell, 2
    complete blood count with, 265
    mean cell hemoglobin, 2
    mean cell hemoglobin concentration, 2
    mean cell volume, 2
Indirect antiglobulin test (IAT), 396
Indirect chromogenic assay, 845
Indirect reference interval determination, 30
Indirect transmission, 881.e12
Ineffective erythropoiesis, 264, 444, 873
    folic acid deficiency, 873
    insufficient and, 264
    vitamin B_{12} deficiency, 873
Ineffective hematopoiesis, 299, 321t
Ineffective thrombopoiesis, 735
Infection, 370
Infection control, responsibility of phlebotomist in, 881.e12
Infections
    associated with thrombocytopenia, 739
    babesiosis and, 386–387
        clinical findings, 387
        geographic distribution, 387
        laboratory findings and diagnosis, 387, 387f
    bartonellosis, 387–388
    clostridial sepsis, 387
    Epstein-Barr virus, 315
    hemolytic anemia caused by, 384–388
    malaria, 332
        clinical and laboratory findings, 385
        hemolytic anemia caused by, 384–388
        microscopic examination, 385, 385f
        pathogenesis, 384–385
        Plasmodium falciparum and, 385, 386f
        Plasmodium knowlesi and, 385, 386f
        Plasmodium malariae and, 385, 386f

Infections *(Continued)*
 Plasmodium ovale and, 385, 386f
 Plasmodium vivax and, 385, 385f
 prevalence, 384
 neonatal hematologic response to, 867
 sickle cell disease and, 418
Infectious disease load, pathogen detection and, 542
Infectious mononucleosis, 484
Infectious wastes, 881.e12
Inflammation, 597
 anemia of, 281–284
  etiology, 281–283
  laboratory diagnosis of, 283–284, 283f
  treatment of, 284
 chronic, thrombotic risk components of, 764t
 and disease, reactive thrombocytosis associated with, 753
Inflammation, platelets and, 173
Informatics, 13
 in hematology and hemostasis laboratory, 14
Information technology, 13
Inherited aplastic anemia, 318–321
 dyskeratosis congenita, 319–320
 Fanconi anemia, 318–319
 Shwachman-Bodian-Diamond syndrome, 320–321
Inherited FXIII deficiency, 706
Inherited giant platelet syndromes, 717, 718t
Inherited hemolytic conditions, 332
Inherited platelet disorders, 714, 716t
Inherited thrombocytopenia, 735–737
 associated with chromosomal abnormalities, 735–737
 Fanconi anemia, 737
 list of, 736t
 May-Hegglin anomaly, 737, 737f
 neonatal thrombocytopenia and, 738, 738t
 TAR syndrome, 737
Innate immunity, 151
Inositol triphosphate-diacylglycerol activation pathway, 173
Insertion, chromosome, 558, 558f
Institute of Medicine (IOM), 8–9
Insufficient erythropoiesis, 264
Integrins, 52, 144
Intercept, 25
Interferon therapy, thrombocytopenia by, 739
Interferon-α, 589
Interleukins (ILs), 71
Intermediate angle scatter (IAS) scatter, 210
Intermediate filaments, 46t, 48
Internal quality control, 31–33
Internal tandem duplication, 493
International Classification of Diseases-Tenth Revision (ICD-10) system, 834
International Consensus Classification (ICC), 623, 625t
International Council for Standardization in Haematology (ICSH), 216
International Normalized Ratio, 823
International Prognostic Scoring System (IPSS), 627
International sensitivity index (ISI), 793
International Society for Laboratory Hematology (ISLH), 203
Interphase, 53
Interprofessional teamwork, 12–13
 in hematology and hemostasis laboratory, 13
Interpupillary control, microscope, 881.e27
Interstitial deletion, 558, 558f
Intracellular acidosis, 263–264
Intracellular calcium pyrophosphate crystals, 881.e45f
Intracellular iron
 regulation, 131
 trafficking, 131
Intravascular hemolysis, 91, 332, 339–340, 341f–344f
Intravenous direct thrombin inhibitors, 801–802, 801f
Intravenous (IV) fluids, 417

Intravenous therapy, 881.e19
Intrinsic accessory pathway proteins. *See* Contact factors
Intrinsic factor, lack of, 303
Intrinsic hemolytic conditions, 332
Intrinsic tenase, 670
Ionic iron absorption, 125–126, 125f
Ionized calcium (Ca^{2+}), 668
Iron, 122–138
 chemistry, 123
 compartments, 123, 123t
 deficiency, 134, 134f, 279. *See also* Iron deficiency anemia
 dietary, 131
 kinetics, 124–131
  cellular, 129–131
  disorders, 275–295
  recycling, body iron and salvage, 128–129
  systemic body, 124–128, 124f
 laboratory assessment of body, 132–134, 132t
  ferritin, 133–134
  hemoglobin content of reticulocytes, 134
  percent transferrin saturation, 132–133
  Prussian blue staining, 133
  serum iron, 132
  soluble transferrin receptor, 134
  soluble transferrin receptor/log ferritin, 134
  Thomas plot, 134, 134f
  total iron-binding capacity, 132
  zinc protoporphyrin, 134
Iron deficiency anemia, 276–281
 in elderly adults, 873
 epidemiology of, 279
 etiology of, 276–277
  chronic blood loss, 277
  impaired absorption, 276–277
  inadequate intake, 276
  increased need, 276
 laboratory diagnosis of, 279–281
  specialized tests of, 280–281, 281f
 pathogenesis of, 277–278, 277f
  stage 1, 278
  stage 2, 277f, 278
  stage 3, 277f, 278
  treatment and its effects, 281
 pediatric, 865–866
 in pregnancy, 868
 reactive thrombocytosis associated with, 753
 thalassemia minor and, 459
Iron overload, 286–289
 differential diagnosis of, 280t, 289
 etiology of, 287
 laboratory diagnosis of, 288–289
  directed testing, 288
  directed testing for treatment, monitoring, and genetic counseling, 288–289
  routine testing, 288
 phenotype and epidemiology of, 288
 sickle cell disease and, 423
 treatment of, 289
Iron-sulfur clusters, 123, 123t
Irreversible sickle cells, 415
Ischemia, 762
iSED (Alcor Scientific), 191
Isochromosomes, 558, 558f
Isocitrate dehydrogenase 1 *(IDH1)*, 596–597
Isocitrate dehydrogenase 2 *(IDH2)*, 596–597
Isoelectric focusing (IEF), 422
Isolation, nucleic acid, 527–529
Isovolumetric sphering, 200
I-STAT instrument, 194, 194f

J

JAK2 inhibitors, 450, 598
JAK2 V617F mutation, 594, 598–599, 875
Jakitinib, 598

Janus kinase 2 (JAK2), 52
Jaundice, 370–371
 hemolytic, 340
 prehepatic, 340
Joint Commission, 38
Juvenile myelomonocytic leukemia (JMML), 609–610
 clinical presentation of, 609
 diagnosis of, 609
 peripheral blood and bone marrow, 609
 prognosis of, 609–610

K

Karyogram, 554
Karyotype, 554
Kasabach-Merritt syndrome, 727
Keratocyte, 267t
Kidneys
 chronic renal failure and hemorrhage, 691–692
 disease, chronic, 324–325
 renal peritubular interstitial cells, 72
Kinetics
 basophils, 148
 eosinophils, 146
 iron, 124–131
  cellular, 129–131
  recycling, body iron and salvage, 128–129
  systemic body, 124–128, 124f
 monocyte/macrophage, 150–151, 151f
 neutrophils, 143–144
KIT ligand, 72, 163
Kleihauer-Betke acid elution slide test, 458
Koaguloviskosimeter, 842
Koehler illumination, 881.e29
Kringles, 679
KRT232 inhibitor, 598–599
Kupffer cells, 64, 282

L

Laboratory diagnosis, 288–289. *See also* Assays; Clinical and laboratory findings; Differential diagnosis
 anemia of chronic inflammation, 283, 283f
 babesiosis, 387, 387f
 chronic eosinophilic leukemia, 609
 chronic myelogenous leukemia, 587–588
 chronic neutrophilic leukemia, 607–608
 directed testing for diagnosis, 288
 directed testing for treatment, monitoring, and genetic counseling, 288–289
 essential thrombocythemia, 599
 hemoglobin E, 430, 430f
 hemoglobin SC, 431
 iron deficiency anemia, 279–281
  diagnosis of iron deficiency in, 279–280, 280t
  screening for, 278f, 279
  specialized tests, 280–281, 281f
 iron overload, 288–289
  directed testing, 288
  directed testing for treatment, monitoring, and genetic counseling, 288–289
  routine testing, 288
 mastocytosis, 611–612
 megaloblastic anemia, 303–306
  screening tests, 303–305
  specific diagnostic tests, 305–306, 305f
 molecular methods, 527, 528b
 of polycythemia vera, 601–602, 602b
 routine testing, 288
 sickle cell disease, 420–422, 420f–421f
 of thalassemias, 455–459, 456t
 unstable hemoglobin variants, 434
 β-thalassemia minor, 452

Laboratory hematology
  additional procedures, 6
  advanced procedures, 5–6
  blood film examination in, 5
  body iron status, 132–134, 132t
  coagulation in, 5
  complete blood count in, 4–5, 4b
  endothelial cells in, 5
  history of, 1–7
  platelets in, 4
  quality assurance and quality control, 6–7
  red blood cells in, 1–3, 2f
  white blood cells in, 3–4
Laboratory Medicine Quality Improvement, 38
Laboratory safety, 7
Laboratory staff competence, 36–38
Laboratory testing services, 9
Lactate dehydrogenase, 96–98, 266, 345
  levels, 304–305, 305b
Lagging strand, DNA replication, 527
Laminar flow, 200
Langerhans cells, 246
Large granular lymphocytes (LGLs), 646
L-arginine, 424
Latent iron deficiency, 134, 134f
Late-term neonates, 863–864
Laundry, 881.e5
Leading strand, DNA replication, 527
Lead poisoning, 286
Lecithin cholesterol acyltransferase, 99–100
Lee-White whole-blood coagulation time test, 821
Left shift, band neutrophils, 3, 237, 238b
Lenalidomide, 628
Lentiviral vectors, 425
Leukemias, 4, 321, 321t, 490, 642–646
  acute. See Acute leukemias
  B lymphoblastic, 511, 512f
  chronic. See Chronic leukemias; Chronic
    lymphocytic leukemia; Chronic
    myelogenous leukemia
  chronic lymphocytic leukemia, 642–644, 643f,
    643b, 644t
  cytogenetics, 559–561, 559b
  defined, 567
  flow cytometric analysis of, 506–510
  hairy cell leukemia, 645–646, 645f
  large granular lymphocytes, 646
  large granular lymphocytic, 646
  minimal residual disease in, 535, 537f
  monoclonal B-cell lymphocytosis, 644
  small lymphocytic lymphoma, 642–644
  spleen in, 66
  thrombotic risk components of, 764t
  T lymphoblastic, 511, 513f
  T-prolymphocytic leukemia, 644–645, 645f
Leukemic stem cells, 492
Leukemic transformation, 607
Leukemogenesis, 492
Leukemoid reaction, 476, 477t
LeukoChek, 183f
Leukocyte adhesion disorder type I, 469
Leukocyte adhesion disorder type II, 469
Leukocyte adhesion disorder type III, 469
Leukocyte neoplasms, 489–499
  classification schemes of, 490f, 491–492
  general characteristics of, 490–491
  incidence, prevalence, and etiology of, 491
  molecular pathogenesis of, 492–494
    DNA repair genes, 494
    epigenetic mechanisms, 492–493, 492t
    hematologic malignancies, cellular processes
      perturbed in, 492, 492b
    oncogenes, 493, 494t
    tumor suppressor genes, 493–494, 494t
  therapy for, 494–497, 494b
    chemotherapy, 494–495
    hematopoietic stem cell transplantation,
      496–497, 497f

Leukocyte neoplasms (Continued)
    radiation, 495
    supportive, 495
    targeted, 495–496
Leukocyte number and function, congenital
    defects of, 465–470
  22q11.2 deletion syndrome, 466
  Bruton tyrosine kinase deficiency, 466–467
  Chédiak-Higashi syndrome, 467
  phagocyte number and/or function, congenital
    defects of, 467–470
  severe combined immune deficiency, 465–466
  Wiskott-Aldrich syndrome, 466
Leukocytes, 3
  adhesion disorders, 468–469
  counts, 3, 232b
    peripheral blood film examination, 232–234,
      233f
    relative vs. absolute, 237t
    summarizing, 236–237, 236t
    white blood cell differential, 232–234, 233f, 304
  development of, 139–158
  granulocytes, 140–149
    basophils, 3, 139–140, 147–149
    eosinophils, 3, 139–140
    mast cells, 149, 149f
    neutrophils, 3, 139–146
  lymphocytes, 3
    T, 64–65, 67–68
  mononuclear cells, 140
    lymphocytes, 151–154
    monocytes, 149–151
  morphologic abnormalities of, without
    associated immunodeficiency, 474–476
    Alder-Reilly anomaly, 475
    May-Hegglin anomaly, 475–476, 475f
    neutrophil hypersegmentation, 475, 475f
    Pelger-Huët anomaly, 474
    pseudo- or acquired Pelger-Huët anomaly,
      474–475
  in neonates
    eosinophils and basophils, 866
    lymphocytes, 866–867, 867f
  quantitative abnormalities of, 476–479, 476b, 477t
    basophils, 478
    eosinophils, 478
    lymphocytes, 479
    monocytes, 478–479
    neutrophils, 476–478
  storage artifacts in, 479
Leukocytosis, 3
Leukoerythroblastic picture, 476
Leukoerythroblastic reaction (LER), 476
Leukoerythroblastosis, 476
Leukopenia, 3
Leukopoiesis, 72
Levels of laboratory assay approval, 28, 29t
Levey-Jennings chart, 31, 32f
L-glutamine, 424
Licensure, laboratory staff, 38
Lifecodes PF4 IgG (Immucor GTI) kit, in enzyme
    immunoassays, 780
Ligands, 49–50, 165
Ligase, 527
Light absorbance end-point detection, 846, 846t
Light scatter
  for RBC and platelet analyses, 213, 215f
  signals, 210–212
  for WBC count, WBC differential, NRBCs and
    reticulocyte analysis, 213–216, 215f
Light transmission aggregation (LTA) detection, 855
Light transmittance platelet aggregometry, 780
  platelet-rich plasma for, 816
Lineage-specific hematopoiesis, 72–73
  erythropoiesis, 72
  leukopoiesis, 72
  megakaryocytopoiesis, 72–73
Linearity, 26–28, 28f

Linear regressions, 25, 27f
Lipemia, in specimen quality set points, 849
Lipids, RBC membrane, 100, 100f
Lipoprotein (a), in arterial thrombosis predictors,
    773
Liver, 64, 64f
  biopsy, Prussian blue staining and, 132t, 133
  pathophysiology, 64
Liver disease
  coagulopathy, 690–691
    disseminated intravascular coagulation, 693
    hemostasis laboratory tests, 691t
  platelet dysfunction in, 725–726
Liver iron sensing and hepcidin production,
    126–127, 126f, 127t
Liver sensing
  of circulating iron, 126f, 127, 128f
  of stored iron, 126f, 127
LMWH. See Low-molecular-weight heparin
Location
  basophilic normoblast, 83, 83f
  erythrocyte, 86, 87f
  orthochromic normoblast, 84, 84f
  polychromatic erythrocyte, 85, 85f–86f
  polychromatic normoblast, 84, 84f
  pronormoblast, 82
Long-term testosterone therapy, 875
Loss-of-function mutations, 493
Lot-to-lot comparisons, 29, 30t
Low-angle light scatter (LALS), 206
Lower limit of detection, 28
Lower median-angle light scatter (LMALS), 206
Low molecular weight heparin (LMWH), 791t,
    797–798
  action, 797, 797f
  laboratory assessment of, 797–798, 798f
  therapy, 797
Lumbar puncture, 881.e36, 881.e37f
Luminescence detector, 855
Lupus anticoagulants, 825–826
  profile, 766–769, 767f
    clot-based, 768
Lupus erythematosus cells, 881.e42, 881.e43f, 881.
    e44
Luspatercept, 598, 628
Lymphatic capillaries, 66
Lymph nodes, 66, 67f
  pathophysiology, 66
Lymphoblastic leukemia/lymphoma, flow
    cytometric analysis of, 510–513
Lymphoblasts, 490f, 491, 567, 881.e40f
Lymphocytes, 3, 151–154, 483–484, 881.e38, 881.e38f
  B, 151–152
    bone marrow aspiration examination, 257,
      257f
    development, 152–153, 152f–153f
    natural killer cells, 151
    pediatric, 866–867, 867f
    quantitative abnormalities of, 479
      lymphocytosis, 479
      lymphopenia, 479
    reactive lymphocytes, 483–484
    T, 64–65, 67–68, 151
Lymphocytopenia, 3
Lymphocytosis, 3, 479
Lymphoid lineage, 506
Lymphomas, 490
  Hodgkin, 246
Lymphopenia, 479
Lysosomal storage disorders (LSDs), 470–474
Lysosome membrane, 48
Lysosomes, 46t, 48, 165f, 166

M

Macroangiopathic hemolytic anemia, 383–384
  exercise-induced hemoglobinuria, 384
  traumatic cardiac hemolytic anemia, 383, 384f

Macrocytes
associated disease states, 267t
oval, 267t
Macrocytic anemias, 268–270
algorithm for preliminary investigation of, 309f
certain drugs, 297b
nonmegaloblastic, 306–308
Macrophage colony-stimulating factor (M-CSF), 149
Macrophages, 3–4, 61–62
in elderly adults, 871
functions, 151
kinetics, 150–151, 151f
mediated hemolysis, 91
-mediated hemolysis, 333–335, 335f
fragmentation hemolysis *vs.*, 338–339, 339t
pathologic, 338–339, 338f
in serous fluids, 881.e39
Macropinocytosis, 124
Major basic protein (MBP), 147
Major molecular response (MMR), 590
Malabsorption, 303
Malaria, 332
clinical and laboratory findings, 385
hemolytic anemia caused by, 384–388
microscopic examination, 385, 385f
pathogenesis, 384–385
Plasmodium falciparum and, 385, 386f
Plasmodium knowlesi and, 385, 386f
Plasmodium malariae and, 385, 386f
Plasmodium ovale and, 385, 386f
Plasmodium vivax and, 385, 385f
prevalence, 384
Malignant cells, in cerebrospinal fluid, 881.e39, 881.e42
Malignant lymphoma cell clusters, 256
Mantle cell lymphoma, 648–649, 649f
Manual cell counts, 180–183
body fluid, 183
calculations for, 180–183
disposable blood cell count dilution systems, 183, 183f
equipments for, 180, 180f
with most common dilutions, 183t
platelet, 182
principle, 180
red blood cell, 183
reticulocyte, 187–190
white blood cell, 181
Manual wedge technique, 227–228, 228f
Marginal zone lymphoma, 650–651, 651f
Marginated neutrophil pool (MNP), 144
Massive hemorrhage, 688–689
Massive transfusion protocols (MTPs), 688–689
Massive transfusion, trauma-induced coagulopathy, 688–689
Mast cells, 149, 149f
growth factor, 163
Mastectomy, 881.e19
Mastocytosis, 611–612
clinical presentation of, 611
diagnosis of, 611–612
incidence of, 611
pathogenetic mechanism, 612
prognosis of, 612
Matriptase-2, 127t
Matrix-assisted laser desorption/ionization-time of flight (MALDI-TOF) mass spectrometry, 544
Maturation, RBC
criteria used in identification of erythroid precursors in, 80–81, 81f, 81b
process, 79
sequence, 81–86, 82f, 82t
terminology, 79t
Mature basophils, 148, 148f
Mature eosinophils, 146

Mature lymphoid neoplasms, 510–513, 634–660, 635b
approach to diagnosis of, 637
Catovsky-Matutes scoring for, 643b
chromosome and gene abnormalities in, 636t
classification schemas based on cell differentiation, 635–637
clinical behavior of, 637b
clinical signs and symptoms of, 637
common immunophenotypes for, 640t
diagnostic procedure for, 637–641
anatomic pathology testing, 641
clinical laboratory testing, 637–641, 640f
imaging studies, 641
prognostic assessment, 642
staging system, 641–642, 642t, 644t
genetic abnormalities, 635, 636t
Hodgkin lymphoma, 653–655, 654f
immunologic diversity, 635
leukemias and, 642–646
monoclonal B-cell lymphocytosis (MBL), 644
non-Hodgkin lymphoma and, 646–653, 646b
T-prolymphocytic leukemia, 644–645, 645f
treatment of, 646
WHO classification of, 638b–639b
Mature red blood cells, 62
May-Hegglin anomaly (MHA), 475–476, 475f, 737, 737f
MCH. *See* Mean cell hemoglobin
MCHC. *See* Mean cell hemoglobin concentration
McLeod syndrome (MLS), 363
MCV. *See* Mean cell volume
MD Anderson Prognostic Scoring System (MDAPSS), 627
MDS. *See* Myelodysplastic syndromes
MDS/MPN with *SF3B1* mutation and thrombocytosis (MDS/MPN-*SF3B1*-T), 627
Mean cell hemoglobin (MCH), 2, 187, 237, 865
anemia diagnosis and, 265
megaloblastic anemia and, 304
Mean cell hemoglobin concentration (MCHC), 2, 187, 237, 865
anemia diagnosis and, 265
megaloblastic anemia and, 304
Mean cell volume (MCV), 2, 187, 237, 238t, 356–357, 865
anemia diagnosis and, 265
exercise-induced hemoglobinuria and, 384
hemolysis diagnosis and, 346
megaloblastic anemia and, 304
Mean, computation of, 20–21
Mean fluorescence intensity (MFI), 358
Mean peroxidase activity index (MPXI), 215
Mean platelet volume (MPV), 163, 221
Mechanical clot endpoint detection, 843, 844f, 846t
Median-angle light scatter (MALS), 206
Median, determination of, 21
Medical errors, 9
Medical laboratory professionals, 12–14
Medullary phase of hematopoiesis, 60
Megakaryoblasts, 161f, 162
acute megakaryoblastic leukemia, 575, 577f
Megakaryocytes, 60, 62, 63f, 160, 161f
bone marrow aspirate examination, 252–253, 252f, 256
differentiation and progenitors, 160, 161f
Megakaryocytic hypoplasia, 735
Megakaryocytic lineage, 506
Megakaryocytopoiesis, 72–73, 160–163
endomitosis, 160, 160b
hormones and cytokines of, 163, 163t
megakaryocyte differentiation and progenitors, 160, 161f
megakaryocyte membrane receptors and markers, 162, 163t
terminal megakaryocyte differentiation, 160–162, 161f, 162t
thrombocytopoiesis, 161f–162f, 162

Megaloblastic anemia, 268–270, 296b, 297
caused by defects of DNA metabolism, 296–312
differential diagnosis, 321t
in elderly adults, 873
etiology of, 297–300, 297b
defect in megaloblastic anemia caused by deficiency in folate and vitamin B_{12}, 298–300, 299f
other causes of, 300
physiologic roles of vitamin B_{12} and folate, 297–298, 298f
laboratory diagnosis of, 303–306
screening tests, 303–305
specific diagnostic tests, 305–306
in pregnancy, 869
systemic manifestations of folate and vitamin B_{12} deficiency, 301–303
treatment of, 308
vitamin deficiencies, causes of, 301–303
Megaloblastic crisis, 358–359
Megaloblastosis, causes of, 300
Membrane, 99–105
deformability, 99, 104, 353–368
lipids, 99–101, 100f
osmotic balance and permeability, 104–105
proteins, 45, 101–104, 102f, 103t
cytoskeletal, 102f, 103–104, 104t, 105f
transmembrane, 45, 101–103, 102f, 103t
structure and function, 95–108, 353–354
Membrane abnormalities, 353–368
abetalipoproteinemia, 363
acquired, 363–368
acquired red blood cell, 363–368
acquired stomatocytosis, 363
chorea acanthocytosis, 363
cryohydrocytosis, 362
familial pseudohyperkalemia, 362
hereditary elliptocytosis, 359–361
clinical and laboratory findings, 360–361, 360f–361f
pathophysiology, 360
treatment, 361
hereditary hydrocytosis, 354–355, 361–362
clinical and laboratory findings, 362, 362f
pathophysiology, 361–362
hereditary ovalocytosis, 361
clinical and laboratory findings, 361
pathophysiology, 361
hereditary red blood cell, 354–363, 355b
hereditary spherocytosis, 355–359
hereditary spherocytosis, 354t, 355–359
additional tests, 357–358, 358f
clinical and laboratory findings, 355–357, 359, 359t
complications, 358–359
differential diagnosis, 359, 359t
pathophysiology, 355, 356f
treatment, 359, 359f
hereditary with acanthocytes, 362–363
hereditary xerocytosis, 354–355, 362
clinical and laboratory findings, 362
pathophysiology, 362
McLeod syndrome, 363
neuroacanthocytosis, 363
paroxysmal cold hemoglobinuria, 331–332
paroxysmal nocturnal hemoglobinuria, 364–368
acquired aplastic anemia and, 315
differential diagnosis, 321t
Rh deficiency syndrome, 362
spur cell anemia, 363
structure and function and, 353–354
Membrane inhibitor of reactive lysis (MIRL), 103
Membrane proteins, 358
Membrane structure and function, 99–105
Mesenchymal cells, 61–62
Mesoblastic phase of hematopoiesis, 60
Mesothelial cells, in cerebrospinal fluid, 881.e42

Metabolism, erythrocytes, 95–108
    energy production through anaerobic
        glycolysis, 96–98, 96b, 97f, 98t
    erythrocyte membrane, 99–105
        deformability, 99, 104
        lipids, 99–101, 100f
        osmotic balance and permeability, 104–105
        proteins, 101–104, 102f, 103t
            cytoskeletal, 102f, 103–104, 104t, 105f
            transmembrane, 101–103, 102f, 103t
        structure and function, 95–108
    erythrocyte membrane structure and function,
        99–105
    glycolysis diversion pathways, 98–99
        hexose monophosphate, 97f, 98, 98t
        methemoglobin reductase, 97f, 98–99
        Rapoport-Luebering, 97f, 99
Metamyelocytes
    eosinophils, 146
    neutrophils, 141, 141f, 144f
Metaphase, 53
    analysis, 554
    checkpoint, 53
    chromosomes, 553
Metastatic tumors, 246
Methanol-free stain, 230
Methemoglobin, 118–119
    reductase pathway, 97f, 98–99
Methemoglobinemia, 118–119
Methylcobalamin, 297
Methylene blue, 242
Methylmalonic acid, 305–306, 306b, 307f
Microangiopathic hemolytic anemia (MAHA),
    380–383, 381b, 747, 748f, 776–777
    disseminated intravascular coagulation, 383
    HELLP syndrome, 383
    hemolytic uremic syndrome, 382–383
    thrombotic thrombocytopenic purpura,
        381–382, 382f
Micro Chromatic Detection for Haematology
    (MCDh), 230
Microcyte, 267t
Microcytic anemias, 268
Microfilaments, 46t, 48, 165–166, 165f
Microhematocrit, 184–186
    maximum packing time for, 185b
    principle, 184–186
    procedure, 185f, 185b
    sources of error and comments, 185b
Microscope(s), 881.e26
    basic troubleshooting, 881.e30
    care of, 881.e30
    component parts and their functions, 881.e27,
        881.e27f
    compound, 881.e26, 881.e27, 881.e27f
    darkfield microscopy, 881.e31
    examination of peripheral blood films,
        231–235
    fluorescent microscope, 881.e31
    immersion oil and types, 881.e30
    operating procedure with Koehler illumination,
        881.e29
    phase-contrast microscope, 881.e30
    polarized light microscope, 881.e31
    principles of, 881.e26
Microscopy, of malaria, 385, 385f
Microsomal triglyceride transfer protein (MTP)
    gene, 363
Microstrokes, 419
Microtubules, 46t, 48, 165–166, 165f
    circumferential, 165–166
Miller disc, 188f, 188b
Minimal residual disease in leukemia, 535, 537f
Mitochondria, 46t, 47–48, 47f
Mitogen-activated protein kinase (MAPK) stress
    response, 424
Mitosis, 53

Mixed phenotype acute leukemias (MPALs), 577
Mixed-type autoimmune hemolytic anemia,
    401
Mode, determination of, 21
Model 700 aggregometer, 856
Modified Westergren erythrocyte sedimentation
    rate, 190, 191f
Moist chamber, 181b
Molecular alterations, myelodysplastic neoplasms,
    627
Molecular coagulation testing, 857–858, 858t
Molecular diagnostics, in hematopathology,
    519–549, 520f–521f, 520b–522b
    amplification of nucleic acids by polymerase
        chain reaction, 529–532, 530f
        for amplifying DNA, 529, 530f
        reverse transcription for amplifying RNA,
            530–532, 531f
    chromosomal microarrays, 542, 543f
    current developments in, 542–545
    detection of amplified DNA, 532–533
        capillary gel electrophoresis, 532, 532f
        DNA sequencing, 536–538, 540f
        restriction endonuclease methods, 533
    diagnosis assays, 5
    next-generation sequencing, 538–542, 541f
    nucleic acid isolation, 527–529
    pathogen detection and infectious disease load,
        522b, 542
    real-time polymerase chain reaction, 533–536,
        533f
        digital polymerase chain reaction, 535,
            538f
        minimal residual disease in leukemia, 535,
            537f
        multiplex ligation-dependent probe
            amplification, 535, 539f
        mutation enrichment strategies, 535–536
        qualitative, 534–535, 534f
        quantitative, 535, 536f
    structure and function of DNA in, 521–527
        central dogma in genetics and, 521–523,
            522f
        DNA at molecular level and, 523–524,
            523f–525f
        DNA replication and the cell cycle, 525–527,
            526f
        transcription and translation in, 524–525
    testing overview, 527, 528b
Momelotinib, 598
MOMENTUM clinical trial, 598
Monochromatic light, 202
Monoclonal B-cell lymphocytosis (MBL), 644
Monoclonal gammopathy of undetermined
    significance (MGUS), 655
Monocyte distribution width (MDW), 206
Monocytes, 3–4, 149–151, 881.e38, 881.e38f
    acute monocytic leukemia, 574–575, 576f
    development, 149–150
    in elderly adults, 871
    functions, 151
    green-blue inclusions in, 482, 482f
    intracellular organisms in, 481–482
    kinetics, 150–151, 151f
    pediatric, 867
    quantitative abnormalities of, 478–479
        monocytopenia, 479
        monocytosis, 478, 478b
    secondary changes in, 479–482
Monocytic lineage, 506
Monocytopenia, 479
Monocytosis, 3–4, 478, 478b
Mononuclear cells, 140, 149–154
    lymphocytes, 3, 151–154
    monocytes, 3–4, 149–151
Mononucleosis, infectious, 484
Monophyletic theory, 68

Monosodium urate crystals, 881.e45, 881.e45f
Morphology, 1
    of acute lymphoblastic leukemia, 568, 569f
    chronic lymphocytic leukemia, 643, 643f
    classification of anemia based on mean cell
        volume, 268–271
    hereditary elliptocytosis, 360, 360f
    red blood cell, 234
Motility, defects of, 467
Moving average of red blood cell indices, 32–33
M pattern, antecubital fossa, 881.e16, 881.e16f
MPL gene mutation, 737
MPNs. See Myeloproliferative neoplasms
mRNA processing errors, 443
M (mitosis) stage, cell cycle, 53
Mucocutaneous hemorrhage, 687
Mucopolysaccharidoses, 470
Multiangle polarized scatter separation (MAPSS), for
    WBC count, WBC differential, NRBC, platelet,
    and reticulocyte analysis, 210–213, 211f–212f
Multiple myeloma, 246, 655–656, 656f, 725
Multiplex ligation-dependent probe amplification
    (MLPA), 535, 539f
Mycoplasma pneumoniae, 399
Mycosis fungoides (MF), 651–652, 652f
Myeloblasts, 141, 142f, 567
    acute monoblastic leukemias, 574–575, 576f
Myelocytes, 141, 141f
    eosinophils, 146
    neutrophils, 141, 143f
Myelodysplasia, acute myeloid leukemia with, 573
Myelodysplastic/myeloproliferative neoplasms,
    618–633, 873. See also Myeloproliferative
    neoplasms
    abnormal cellular function, 623
    childhood myelodysplastic neoplasms, 626
        with increased blasts, 626
        with low blasts, 626
    chronic myelomonocytic leukemia, 626
    classification of, 623, 626b
        French-American-British classification, 623
        International Consensus Classification, 623,
            625t
        World Health Organization classification,
            623, 624b
    cytogenetics, 627
    with defining genetic abnormalities, 623–624
        with biallelic TP53 inactivation, 624
        with low blasts and isolated 5q deletion,
            623–624
        with low blasts and SF3B1 mutation, 624
    epigenetics, 627
    etiology, 619–620
    future directions, 628
    MDS/MPN, not otherwise specified, 627
    molecular alterations, 627
    morphologically defined, 624–626
        with increased blasts, 626
        with low blasts, 624
        myelodysplastic neoplasm, hypoplastic, 624
    myelodysplastic/myeloproliferative neoplasms,
        626–627
        chronic myelomonocytic leukemia, 626
        classification of, 626b
        MDS/MPN, not otherwise specified, 627
        with neutrophilia, 626–627
        with SF3B1 mutation and thrombocytosis, 627
    with neutrophilia, 626–627
    peripheral blood and bone marrow,
        morphologic abnormalities in, 620–622
        dyserythropoiesis, 620, 620f
        dysmegakaryopoiesis, 622, 622f–623f
        dysmyelopoiesis, 620–622, 621f–622f, 621b
    prognosis, 627–628
    treatment, 628
Myelodysplastic/myeloproliferative neoplasm with
    neutrophilia (MDS/MPN-N), 626–627

Myelodysplastic neoplasm with biallelic *TP53* inactivation (MDS-biTP53), 624
Myelodysplastic neoplasm with increased blasts (MDS-IB), 626
Myelodysplastic neoplasm with low blasts (MDS-LB), 624
Myelodysplastic neoplasm with low blasts and isolated 5q deletion (MDS-5q), 623–624
Myelodysplastic syndromes (MDS), 300, 321t, 508–510, 511f, 619
Myelofibrosis, 598, 604–605
   with myeloid metaplasia, 604
   primary, 604–607
      collagen in, 604–605
      hematopoiesis and extramedullary hematopoiesis in, 605
      incidence and clinical presentation of, 605
      pathogenetic mechanism of, 605
      peripheral blood and bone marrow in, 605, 606f, 606t
      treatment and prognosis of, 605–607
Myeloid cells, 62, 63f, 621f
   nuclear ring in, 620, 622f
Myeloid-erythroid (ME) layer, concentrate smears, 250
Myeloid/lymphoid neoplasms, 610–611
Myeloid neoplasm post cytotoxic therapy (MN-pCT), 619–620
Myeloid neoplasms with germline predisposition, 620
Myeloid sarcoma, 576, 588
Myeloperoxidase (MPO)
   deficiency, 470
   stains and interpretations, 577–578, 578f
Myelophthisic anemia, 324, 324f
Myeloproliferative neoplasm-not otherwise specified, 610
   diagnosis, 610
   prognosis, 610
Myeloproliferative neoplasms (MPNs), 583–617, 725, 763–764, 764t, 873
   categories, 584
   chronic eosinophilic leukemia, 608–609
   chronic myelogenous leukemia (CML), 584–592
      cytogenetics of Philadelphia chromosome and, 584–585
      incidence of, 584
      laboratory findings of, 587–588
      molecular genetics in, 585–586, 585f
      pathogenetic mechanism of, 586, 586f
      peripheral blood and bone marrow, 587, 587f–588f, 588t
      progression of, 588–589
      treatment of, 589–592, 589f, 591f
   chronic neutrophilic leukemia, 607–608
   in elderly adults, 873
   essential thrombocythemia, 4, 599–601, 753–754
      clinical presentation of, 599
      diagnosis of, 599
      incidence of, 599
      pathogenetic mechanism of, 599
      peripheral blood and bone marrow, 599–600, 600f, 600t
      treatment and prognosis of, 600–601
   flow cytometric analysis of, 508–510
   juvenile myelomonocytic leukemia, 609–610
      clinical presentation of, 609
      diagnosis of, 609
      peripheral blood and bone marrow, 609
      prognosis of, 609–610
   mastocytosis, 611–612
   not otherwise specified, 610
      diagnosis, 610
      prognosis, 610
   polycythemia vera, 601–604

Myeloproliferative neoplasms (MPNs) *(Continued)*
      clinical presentation of, 602–603
      diagnosis of, 601–602, 602b
      incidence of, 601
      pathogenetic mechanism of, 594f–595f, 601
      peripheral blood and bone marrow, 602, 603f, 603t
      treatment and prognosis of, 603–604
   primary myelofibrosis, 604–607
      collagen in, 604–605
      hematopoiesis and extramedullary hematopoiesis in, 605
      incidence and clinical presentation of, 605
      pathogenetic mechanism of, 605
      peripheral blood and bone marrow in, 605, 606f, 606t
      treatment and prognosis of, 605–607
   thrombocytosis associated with, 753–754
MYH9 gene, mutations in, 737

N

NAM. *See* National Academy of Medicine
α-naphthyl acetate, 578–579
α-naphthyl butyrate esterase reaction, 579, 579f
National Academy of Medicine (NAM), 8–9, 14
Natural killer (NK) cells, 151
   development, 153
   functions, 154
Navitoclax, 598
Near-haploid cells, 557
Near-patient viscoelastometry (VET), 797
Neck, microscope, 881.e27
Necrosis, 54, 55f, 55t, 762
Needle
   bone marrow aspiration and biopsy, 247, 247f
   selection of, for hemostasis blood specimen collection, 813, 813t
   venipuncture, 881.e13, 881.e15f
Needle holders, venipuncture, 881.e13, 881.e15f
Neimann-Pick disease, 48
Neisseria meningitidis, 367–368
Neogenin (NEO), 126f, 127t
Neonatal alloimmune neutropenia, 477
Neonatal alloimmune thrombocytopenia, 744
Neonatal autoimmune thrombocytopenia, 744–745
Neonatal hyperbilirubinemia, 370–371
Neonatal purpura fulminans, 772
Neonatal thrombocytopenia, 738
   causes of, 738
   and fetal thrombocytopenia, classification of, 738t
Neonates. *See also* Children; Pediatric hematology and hemostasis
   anemia in, 864
   full-term
      hemoglobin for, reference interval, 865
      platelet count reference intervals for, 867t
   gestational age and birth weight in, 863–864
   hematologic response to infection, 867
   hemolytic disease of fetus and, 401–403, 402t
   hemostasis, 867–868
      bleeding and thrombosis, 868
      hemostatic components, 868
      specimen collection and management, 867
   mean monocyte count of, 867
   neonatal thrombocytopenia, 738
      causes of, 738
      and fetal thrombocytopenia, classification of, 738t
   platelet values in, 867, 867t–868t
   polycythemia in, 864
   postterm, 863–864
   preterm, 863–864
      hemoglobin values in, 865
      platelet count reference intervals for, 867t
   red blood cell values in, 864–865

Neonates *(Continued)*
      anemia, 865–866
      distribution width, 865
      erythrocyte morphology, 864–865, 864f
      hematocrit, 865
      hemoglobin, 865
      indices, 865
      mean cell hemoglobin, 865
      mean cell hemoglobin concentration, 865
      mean cell volume, 865
      reticulocyte count, 865, 865f
   sickle cell disease screening in, 422
   specimen collection for, 864
   white blood cell values in, 866–867
      eosinophils and basophils, 866
      lymphocytes, 866–867, 867f
Neoplasms. *See also* Cancer
   acute myeloid, flow cytometric analysis of, 506–510
   chronic myelogenous leukemia, 584–592
      cytogenetics, 560–561, 560f
      flow cytometric analysis of, 506–510
      incidence of, 584
      laboratory findings of, 587–588
      molecular genetics in, 585–586, 585f
      pathogenetic mechanism of, 586, 586f
      peripheral blood and bone marrow, 587, 587f–588f, 588t
      Philadelphia chromosome and, 584–585
      progression of, 588–589
      treatment of, 589–592, 589f, 591f
   chronic neutrophilic leukemia, 607–608
   essential thrombocythemia, 4, 599–601
      clinical presentation of, 599
      diagnosis of, 599
      incidence of, 599
      pathogenetic mechanism of, 599
      peripheral blood and bone marrow, 599–600, 600f, 600t
      treatment and prognosis of, 600–601
   leukocyte, 489–499
      classification schemes of, 490f, 491–492
      general characteristics of, 490–491
      incidence, prevalence, and etiology of, 491
      molecular pathogenesis of, 492–494
         DNA repair genes, 494
         epigenetic mechanisms, 492–493, 492t
         hematologic malignancies, cellular processes perturbed in, 492, 492b
         oncogenes, 493, 494t
         tumor suppressor genes, 493–494, 494t
      therapy for, 494–497, 494b
         chemotherapy, 494–495
         hematopoietic stem cell transplantation, 496–497, 497f
         radiation, 495
         supportive, 495
         targeted, 495–496
   mature lymphoid, 634–660, 635b
      approach to diagnosis of, 637
      Catovsky-Matutes scoring for, 643b
      classification schemas based on cell differentiation, 635–637
      clinical behavior of, 637b
      clinical signs and symptoms of, 637
      common immunophenotypes for, 640t
      diagnostic procedure for, 637–641
         anatomic pathology testing, 641
         clinical laboratory testing, 637–641, 640f
         imaging studies, 641
         prognostic evaluation, 642
         staging system, 641–642, 642t, 644t
      genetic abnormalities, 635, 636t
      Hodgkin lymphoma, 653–655, 654f
      immunologic diversity, 635
      leukemias and, 642–646

Neoplasms (Continued)
  monoclonal B-cell lymphocytosis (MBL), 644
  non-Hodgkin lymphoma, 646–653, 646b
  T-prolymphocytic leukemia, 644–645, 645f
  treatment of, 646
  WHO classification of, 638b–639b
myelodysplastic/myeloproliferative. See also Myeloproliferative neoplasms
myelodysplastic syndromes, 321t
myeloid/lymphoid neoplasms, 610–611
myeloproliferative, 583–617, 763–764, 764t
  chronic eosinophilic leukemia, 608–609
  chronic myelogenous leukemia (CML), 584–592
    cytogenetics of Philadelphia chromosome and, 584–585
    incidence of, 584
    laboratory findings of, 587–588
    molecular genetics in, 585–586, 585f
    pathogenetic mechanism of, 586, 586f
    peripheral blood and bone marrow, 587, 587f–588f, 588t
    progression of, 588–589
    treatment of, 589–592, 589f, 591f
  chronic neutrophilic leukemia, 607–608
  essential thrombocythemia, 4, 599–601
    clinical presentation of, 599
    diagnosis of, 599
    incidence of, 599
    pathogenetic mechanism of, 599
    peripheral blood and bone marrow, 599–600, 600f, 600t
    treatment and prognosis of, 600–601
  flow cytometric analysis of, 508–510
  mastocytosis, 611–612
  not otherwise specified, 610
  polycythemia vera, 601–604
    clinical presentation of, 602–603
    diagnosis of, 601–602, 602b
    incidence of, 601
    pathogenetic mechanism of, 594f–595f, 601
    peripheral blood and bone marrow, 602, 603f, 603t
    treatment and prognosis of, 603–604
  primary myelofibrosis, 604–607
    collagen in, 604–605
    hematopoiesis and extramedullary hematopoiesis in, 605
    incidence and clinical presentation of, 605
    pathogenetic mechanism of, 605
    peripheral blood and bone marrow in, 605, 606f, 606t
    treatment and prognosis of, 605–607
  secondary, myeloid, 576
Nephelometric endpoint detection, 845–846, 845f, 846t
Nephelometry, 845–846
Nephrotic syndrome, hemorrhage and, 691–692
Nerve damage, 881.e19
Neuroacanthocytosis, 363
Neutropenias, 3, 467–468, 476–478, 866
  acquired, 477
  autoimmune, 478
  congenital, 467–468, 468t
  cyclic, 468
  drug-induced, 477
  neonatal alloimmune, 477
Neutrophil extracellular traps (NETs), 146
Neutrophilia, 3, 468–469, 476, 476b, 866
Neutrophils, 3, 139–146, 145f, 881.e38, 881.e38f
  development, 140–143, 141f
  with Döhle Bodies, 480f
  functions, 144–146
  granules, 141, 142b
  green-blue inclusions in, 482, 482f

Neutrophils (Continued)
  hypersegmentation of, 304, 475, 475f
  intracellular organisms in, 481–482
    bacteria and fungal organisms, 481–482, 482f
  kinetics, 143–144
  metamyelocytes, 141, 144f, 256, 257f
  myeloblasts, 141
  myelocytes, 141, 143f, 256, 257f
  promyelocytes, 141
  pyknosis and apoptosis in, 481
    apoptotic nuclei, 481, 481f
    pyknotic nuclei, 481
  quantitative abnormalities in, 475, 475f
  quantitative abnormalities of, 476–478
    leukemoid reaction, 476
    leukoerythroblastic reaction, 476
    neutropenia, 476–478
    neutrophilia, 476
  secondary changes in, 479–482
  segmented, 141–143, 145f, 256, 257f
Neutrophil, vacuolation, 480–481
  autophagic vacuolation, 480–481
  toxic vacuoles, 480
Next-generation sequencing (NGS), 538–542, 541f
Niemann-Pick disease (NP), 470, 473–474, 473f
  acute neuronopathic form, 473
  nonneuronopathic form, 473
  NP type C, 473–474
Nijmegen-Bethesda assay, for anti-factor VIII inhibitor, 830–831
Nijmegen-Bethesda units (NBUs), 693
Nitric oxide (NO), 365
  transport, 118
Nitrofurantoin, 724
Nodal marginal zone lymphoma, 651
Nomenclature
  cytogenetic, 556–557, 557f
  hemoglobinopathies, 411–412
  procoagulants, 666–668, 667f, 667t
  transmembrane proteins, 101
Nonclonal or secondary acquired SAs, 286
Non-Hodgkin lymphoma, 646–653, 646b
  adult T-cell leukemia/lymphoma, 646–647, 647f
  anaplastic large cell lymphoma, 652, 652f
  Burkitt's lymphoma, 647–648, 648f
  diffuse large B cell lymphoma, 649–650, 650f
  follicular lymphoma, 648, 648f
  mantle cell lymphoma, 648–649, 649f
  marginal zone lymphoma, 650–651, 651f
  mycosis fungoides (MF)/Sézary syndrome, 651–652, 652f
  nodal marginal zone lymphoma, 651
  peripheral T cell lymphoma, not otherwise specified (PTCL,NOS), 653, 653f
Nonhomologous end joining (NHEJ), 426
Nonimmune causes of hemolytic anemia, 379–391, 380f, 380b
  babesiosis and, 386–387
    clinical findings, 387
    geographic distribution, 387
    laboratory findings and diagnosis, 387, 387f
  bartonellosis, 387–388
  clostridial sepsis, 387
  drugs and chemicals, 388
  extensive burns, 388f
  infectious agents, 384–388
  malaria, 332, 384–385
    clinical and laboratory findings, 385
    hemolytic anemia caused by, 384–388
    microscopic examination, 385, 385f
    pathogenesis, 384–385
    Plasmodium falciparum and, 385, 386f
    Plasmodium knowlesi and, 385, 386f
    Plasmodium malariae and, 385, 386f
    Plasmodium ovale and, 385, 386f

Nonimmune causes of hemolytic anemia (Continued)
    Plasmodium vivax and, 385, 385f
    prevalence, 384
  venoms, 388
Nonimmune drug-induced hemolysis, 404
Nonimmune drug-induced thrombocytopenia, 751
Nonmalignant leukocyte disorders, 464–488
  infectious mononucleosis, 484
  leukocyte number and function, congenital defects of, 465–470
    22q11.2 deletion syndrome, 466
    Bruton tyrosine kinase deficiency, 466–467
    Chédiak-Higashi syndrome, 467
    phagocyte number and/or function, congenital defects of, 467–470
    severe combined immune deficiency, 465–466
    Wiskott-Aldrich syndrome, 466
  primary immunodeficiency diseases, 465–470
  quantitative abnormalities of leukocytes, 476–479
  secondary morphologic changes, 479–484
    eosinophils and basophils, 482–483
    leukocytes, storage artifacts in, 479
    lymphocytes, 483–484
    neutrophils and monocytes, secondary changes in, 479–482
Nonmegaloblastic anemias, 270
Non-transfusion-dependent thalassemia (NTDT), 446, 450
Normocytic anemia, 270
NRBCs. See Nucleated red blood cells
Nuclear-cytoplasmic asynchrony, 299–300
Nuclear envelope, 47
Nuclear transcription factors, 492
Nucleated cells, 62
Nucleated red blood cells (NRBCs), 205f
  automated blood cell analysis, clinical utility of, 221
  blood cell analyzers, 204t
  cytochemistry and light scatter for, 213–216, 215f
  fluorescence flow cytometry for, 207–210, 209f
  MAPSS for, 210–213, 211f–212f
  volume, conductivity, scatter technology, 206–207, 206f–207f
Nucleic acid
  amplification of, by polymerase chain reaction, 529–532, 530f
  isolation, 527–529
  sequencing, 536–542
  stains, 3
Nucleolar organizer regions, 554
Nucleoli, 47
Nucleolus, cell, 46t
Nucleoside, 523
Nucleosome, 553
Nucleotide strands, 523, 523f
Nucleus, cell, 44, 46–47, 46t
  basophilic normoblast, 83, 83f
  chromatin, 46–47
  erythrocyte, 86, 87f
  nuclear envelope, 47
  nucleoli, 47
  orthochromic normoblast, 84, 84f
  polychromatic erythrocyte, 85, 85f–86f
  polychromatic normoblast, 83, 84f
  pronormoblast, 81, 83f
  to-cytoplasm ratio, 81b
Null hypothesis, 19–20
Numerical aperture (NA), 881.e28
Numeric chromosome abnormalities, 557, 558f
Nutritional deficiencies, in elderly adults, 873

O
Obesity, 881.e19
Obizur (Takeda), 693

Objective lenses, microscope, 881.e28, 881.e28f
Occupational hazards, 881.e6
    biohazards in blood and body fluids, 881.e8
    chemical hazards, 881.e6
    electrical hazards, 881.e8
    fire hazards, 881.e6, 881.e6t
    radioactive hazards, 881.e8
Occupational Safety and Health Administration
    (OSHA), 881.e2, 881.e12
    applicable safety practices required by, 881.e2
Odds ratios effects on diagnostic efficacy, 34–36
Okazaki fragments, 527
Oligoblastic leukemia, 619
Oncogenes, 493, 494t
100x oil immersion objective examination of
    blood films, 231–232
Ontogeny, hemoglobin, 114, 115f, 115t
Opacity, 206
Open reagent systems, in coagulation
    instrumentation, 848
Optical genome mapping (OGM), 544, 544f
Optical light scatter, 201f, 202
Optical tube, microscope, 881.e27
Organic anion transporter (OAT) proteins, 333f, 334
Orthochromic normoblast, 84–85, 84f
Orthogonal light (90°) scatter, 202
Osmoscan, 358
Osmosis, 48–49
Osmotic balance, of erythrocyte membrane,
    104–105
Osmotic fragility, 357
Osteoblasts, 55, 61–62, 254, 254f
Osteoclasts, 55, 61–62, 254
Outer coverings, 881.e2
Oval macrocytes, 267t, 620f
Ovalocytes, 269f
Overhydrated hereditary stomatocytosis (OHS),
    361–362
    clinical and laboratory findings, 362, 362f
    pathophysiology, 361–362
Overhydrated stomatocytosis, 105
Overlap neoplasm, 508–510
Overload, iron, 286–289
    etiology of, 287
    laboratory diagnosis of, 288–289
    sickle cell disease and, 423
    treatment of, 289
Oxalate bind calcium, 881.e13
Oxidant stress, 368
Oxidation, 370
Oxidative stress, 370
Oxygen affinity, hemoglobins with increased and
    decreased, 434–435
Oxygen transport, 116–117, 116f–117f
    dyshemoglobins and, 118–119
    sulfhemoglobin and, 119

P

P2Y$_{12}$ (ADP) receptor inhibitors, 723
Packed cell volume (PCV), 2, 184
Pacritinib, 598
Pancytopenia, 315–317, 317f, 317t
    differential diagnosis, 321, 321t–322t
PAP-8E, 855–856, 856f
Pappenheimer bodies, 268t
PAR-1 antagonists, 724
Paracrine signaling, 49
Parasites
    babesiosis and, 386–387
        clinical findings, 387
        geographic distribution, 387
        laboratory findings and diagnosis, 387, 387f
    infections, during pregnancy, 869
    malaria and, 332, 385
        clinical and laboratory findings, 385
        hemolytic anemia caused by, 384–388

Parasites (Continued)
        pathogenesis, 384–385
        Plasmodium falciparum and, 385, 386f
        Plasmodium knowlesi and, 385, 386f
        Plasmodium malariae and, 385, 386f
        Plasmodium ovale and, 385, 386f
        Plasmodium vivax and, 385, 385f
        prevalence, 384
    sickle cell disease and, 419–420
    stool analysis for, 306
Parcentric, 881.e30
Parenteral antiplatelet therapeutic drugs, 803
Parfocal, 881.e28
Paroxysmal cold hemoglobinuria (PCH),
    400–401
Paroxysmal nocturnal hemoglobinuria (PNH),
    331–332, 364–368, 763–764
    acquired aplastic anemia and, 315
    classification, 365–366, 366t
    clinical manifestations, 365, 365t
    differential diagnosis, 321
    flow cytometry and, 514–515, 515f
    hemolytic anemia, pathophysiology of, 364–365
    laboratory findings in, 366–367, 366t, 367f
    thrombotic risk component of, 764t
    treatment, 367–368
Parsaclisib, 598
Partial thromboplastin time (PTT), 5, 30, 824–825
    as diagnostic assay, 825
    mixing studies for, 825–826
        detection of, factor deficiencies and, 826
        lupus anticoagulants, 826
        specific factor inhibitors, 826
    monitoring heparin therapy with, 825
    principles for, 824, 824f
    procedure for, 825
    quality control for, 825
    reference interval for, 825
    single-factor assays using, 828–830
    for unfractionated heparin
        clinical practice of, 796
        limitations of, 796–797
        therapeutic range, 795–796, 796f
Partial voteout, 206
Particle smears of bone marrow aspirate, 250
Passive transport, plasma membrane, 48–49
Pathogen detection and infectious disease load,
    522b, 542
Pathogenetic mechanism, in chronic neutrophilic
    leukemia, 608
Pathologic fragmentation hemolysis, 339–340,
    341f–344f
Pathologic macrophage-mediated hemolysis,
    338–339, 338f
Pathophysiology
    acquired aplastic anemia, 315–316
    anemias, 271, 272b
    bone marrow failure, 314
    chronic myelogenous leukemia, 586, 586f
    dehydrated hereditary stomatocytosis, 362
    dyskeratosis congenita, 319–320
    essential thrombocythemia, 599
    Fanconi anemia, 319
    hemoglobin C, 428, 429f
    hemoglobin E, 429
    hemoglobinopathies, 411
    hemolytic anemia, 364–365
    hereditary elliptocytosis, 360
    hereditary hydrocytosis, 361–362
    hereditary ovalocytosis, 361
    hereditary spherocytosis, 355, 356f
    hereditary xerocytosis, 362
    immune hemolysis, 393–396, 394f–395f
    iron deficiency anemia, 277–278, 277f
    liver, 64
    lymph node, 66
    malaria, 384–385

Pathophysiology (Continued)
    overhydrated hereditary stomatocytosis,
        361–362
    polycythemia vera, 594f–595f, 601
    primary myelofibrosis, 605
    pyruvate kinase deficiency, 373
    Shwachman-Bodian-Diamond syndrome,
        320–321
    sickle cell anemia, 414–416
    Southeast Asian ovalocytosis, 361
    spleen, 65f, 66
    stage 1, 278
    stage 2, 277f, 278
    stage 3, 277f, 278
    thalassemia, 444–445, 445f
    thymus, 68
Patient-centered care, 13
    in hematology and hemostasis laboratory, 14
Patient-centered hematology, and hemostasis
    testing, 12
Patient-centered laboratory testing services, 12
Patient safety, 7
    definition of, 9
    in hematology and hemostasis testing, 8–17
PCH. See Paroxysmal cold hemoglobinuria
Pearson correlation coefficient, 24–25
Pearson marrow-pancreas syndrome (PMPS), 285
Pediatric hematology and hemostasis, 863–868
    developmental stages in, 863
    gestational age and birth weight in, 863–864
    hematopoiesis in, 863
    neonatal hemostasis, 867–868
        bleeding and thrombosis, 868
        hemostatic components, 868
        specimen collection and management, 867
    platelet values in the neonate, 867, 867t
    red blood cell values in the neonate, 864–865
        anemia, 865–866
        distribution width, 865
        erythrocyte morphology, 864–865, 864f
        hematocrit, 865
        hemoglobin, 865
        indices, 865
        mean cell hemoglobin, 865
        mean cell hemoglobin concentration, 865
        mean cell volume, 865
        reticulocyte count, 865, 865f
    specimen collection for the neonate, 864
    white blood cell values in, 866–867
        eosinophils and basophils, 866
        lymphocytes, 866–867, 867f
        monocytes, 867
Pediatric phlebotomy, 881.e18
Pelabresib, 598
Pelger-Huët anomaly (PHA), 474
    challenges associated with, 474
    pseudo- or acquired, 467
Pelger Huet neutrophils
    and immature granulocytes, 474–475
    pseudo- and true Pelger-Huët neutrophils, 475
Penicillin, 418
Pentasaccharide, 795
Pentose phosphate shunt, 97f, 98, 98t
Peptide epitopes, 102
Percent transferrin saturation, 132–133, 133f
Periarteriolar lymphatic sheath, 64–65
Periosteal arteries, 62–63
Peripheral blood
    and bone marrow, morphologic abnormalities
        in, 620–622
        dyserythropoiesis, 620, 620f
        dysmegakaryopoiesis, 622, 622f–623f
        dysmyelopoiesis, 620–622, 621f–622f, 621b
    chronic eosinophilic leukemia and, 608–609
    chronic myelogenous leukemia and, 587,
        587f–588f, 588t
    chronic neutrophilic leukemia and, 607

Peripheral blood (Continued)
  essential thrombocythemia and, 599–600, 600f, 600t
  polycythemia vera and, 602, 603f, 603t
  primary myelofibrosis and, 605, 606f, 606t
Peripheral blood films, 225–243, 360–361
  for anemia, 267t
  examination of, 231–235
    10x objective, 231
    40x high-dry objective, 231, 232b
    50x oil immersion objective, 231, 232b
    100x oil immersion objective, 231–232
    automated microscopic, 235
    macroscopic, 231
    for malaria, 385, 385f
    microscopic, 231–235
    optimal assessment area, 232, 233f
    performance of white blood cell differential, 232–234, 233f
    platelet estimate, 234–235
    red blood cell morphology, 234
  film preparation, 227–229, 228f
    automated slide making and staining, 228–229
    drying of films, 229
    manual wedge technique, 227–228, 228f
  specimen collection for, 226–227, 226f
  staining of, 228–229
    automated, 228–229
    features of proper, 230, 231b
    manual, 229, 230f
    quick, 230
    Wright (Wright-Giemsa), 229–230
  thalassemia diagnosis and, 455
Peripheral eosinophilia, in chronic eosinophilic leukemia, 608
Peripheral proteins, 103
Peripheral T cell lymphoma, not otherwise specified (PTCL,NOS), 653, 653f
Periprocedural management, of anticoagulants, 802–803
Permeability, of erythrocyte membrane, 104–105
Pernicious anemia, 268–270, 303, 307f
Peroxidase, 202–203
Peroxidase (PEROX) channel, 214, 215f
PERSIST-1 clinical trial, 598
Personal protective equipment (PPE), 7, 881.e2
Petechiae, 687, 735, 735f, 881.e19
PFA-100 Platelet Function Analyzer, 856, 857f
PFA-100 system, for antiplatelet drugs, 804
Phagocyte number, congenital defects of, 467–470
Phagocytes, congenital defects of, 467–470
Phagocytize, 3–4
Phagocytosis, 49, 145, 145b
Phagosomes, 48
Phase-contrast microscope, 881.e30
Phenotype and epidemiology, 288
Phenotypic assays, 372
Phenotypic mosaicism, 365
Philadelphia chromosomes, 511, 559–561, 584–585
Phlebotomist, responsibility in infection control, 881.e12
Phlebotomy. See also Specimen collection
  iron overload treatment, 289
  legal issues in, 881.e23
  for polycythemia vera treatment, 603–604
  trays, 881.e4
Phosphatidylcholine, 100
Phosphatidylethanolamine, 100
Phosphatidylinositol, 103
  glycan anchor biosynthesis, 103
Phosphatidylinositol N-acetylglucosaminyltransferase subunit A, 364–365

Phosphatidylserine, 99, 666
6-phosphofructokinase, 96
Phosphoglycerate mutase, 96–98
Phospholipase C, 173
Phospholipids, 99, 164–165
Phosphopyruvate hydratase, 96–98
Photo-optical clot endpoint detection, 844, 844f, 846t
Physical and chemical properties, 881.e7
Physiological adaptations in anemia, 263–264
Physiologic anemia
  of infancy, 864
  of pregnancy, 868
Physiologic fragmentation hemolysis, 332, 335–338
  macrophage-mediated hemolysis vs., 339t
  pathologic, 339–340, 341f–344f
  plasma hemoglobin salvage and, 335–338, 336f, 340b
Physiologic hemolysis, 331, 333–338
  acute, 331–332
  bilirubin metabolism and, 333–335, 333f
  chronic, 331–332
  classification of hemolytic disorders, 331–333, 331t
  clinical features, 340–341
  differential diagnosis, 346–347, 347f, 348t
  fragmentation, 332
    macrophage-mediated hemolysis vs., 339t
    pathologic, 339–340, 341f–344f
    plasma hemoglobin salvage, 335–338, 336f, 340b
  inherited, 332
  laboratory findings, 346
    tests of accelerated red blood cell destruction, 342–345
    tests of increased erythropoiesis, 345–346, 346t
  laboratory tests to determine specific processes, 346, 346t
  pathologic macrophage-mediated, 338–339, 338f
  plasma hemoglobin salvage and fragmentation, 335–338, 340b
Physiologic roles, of vitamin B$_{12}$ and folate, 297–298, 298f
Pica, 263
Piecemeal degranulation, 146–147
PIGA gene, 364–365
PIGA mutant, 365
Pinocytosis, 49
Placenta-dependent oxygenation, 864
Plan achromatic lens, 881.e28
Plan apochromatic lens, 881.e28
Plasma
  cells, 152, 258, 258f
  in disseminated intravascular coagulation, 778
  membrane, 44–45, 46t
    receptors for adhesion, 166–168, 167f, 168t
    transport. See Plasma membrane transport
  platelet-poor plasma specimens, 816–817
  platelet-rich
    light-transmittance platelet aggregometry, 817–818, 817f–819f
    plasma specimens, 816
  procoagulants. See Procoagulants
  trauma-induced coagulopathy, 689
Plasma cell lymphocyte, 152, 153f
Plasma cell neoplasms, 655–657
  diagnostic criteria for, 656b
  heavy chain disease, 656–657
  monoclonal gammopathy of undetermined significance, 655
  multiple myeloma, 655–656, 656f
  plasmacytoma, 656
  Waldenström macroglobulinemia, 656–657
Plasma cells, 152
Plasmacytoid lymphocytes, 152, 153f
Plasmacytoma, 656

Plasma hemoglobin, 342–344
Plasma kallikrein-kinin system, 671
Plasma membrane transport, 48–49, 48b
  active transport, 49
  facilitated diffusion, 48–49
  passive transport, 48–49
  phagocytosis, 49
  pinocytosis, 49
  receptor mediated endocytosis, 49
  simple diffusion, 48–49
  vesicular transport, 49
Plasmin, 679
Plasminogen, 679, 832
  chromogenic substrate, 832, 832f
Plasminogen activation, 680
Plasminogen activator inhibitor-1 (PAI-1), 680, 833, 833f
  principle of, 833
Plasminogen activator inhibitor-2 (PAI-2), 680
Plasminogen activator inhibitory type-1 (PAI-1), 874
Plasmodium falciparum, 369, 385, 386f
Plasmodium knowlesi, 385, 386f
Plasmodium malariae, 385, 386f
Plasmodium ovale, 385, 386f
Plasmodium vivax, 385, 385f
Platelet aggregometers, 855–856, 856f, 856t
Platelet aggregometry, 817–821, 817f–818f
  agonists, 818t, 819–821
  platelet lumiaggregometry, 818–819, 820f, 820t
  platelet-rich plasma specimens, 816
  using platelet-rich plasma, 817–818, 817f–819f
  whole-blood specimens for, 816, 818, 819f
Platelet analysis
  Abbott, 210
  automated blood cell analysis, clinical utility of, 221
  Beckman Coulter, 205–206
  light scatter for, 213, 215f
  MAPSS for, 210–213, 211f–212f
Platelet clumping, 219, 227f
Platelet destruction
  immune mechanisms of, 740–745
    drug-induced immune-mediated thrombocytopenia, 741–744, 742b, 743f
    immune thrombocytopenic purpura, 740
      acute, 740
      chronic, 740, 741f
  increased, 735, 739–751
    by immunologic responses, 739–740
  nonimmune mechanisms of, 745–751
    hemolytic disease of newborn, 746
    hypertensive disorders, 746
    idiopathic thrombocytopenic purpura (ITP), 740
    incidental thrombocytopenia of pregnancy, 746
    preeclampsia, 746
    thrombotic thrombocytopenic purpura, 746–749
Platelet distribution, DC detection system for, 207, 208f
Platelet distribution width (PDW), 240
Platelet factor 4 (PF4), 778, 796
  drug-induced thrombocytopenia and, 742
Platelet Function Analyzer (PFA-100), 856, 857f
Platelet function testing, 855–857
  flow cytometry, 857
  for hemostasis, 817–821
    bleeding time test, 817
    heparin-induced thrombocytopenia assays in, 821
    platelet aggregometry as, 817–821
    von Willebrand factor activity assays in, 821
  platelet aggregometers, 855–856, 856f, 856t
  platelet function analyzers, 856–857

Platelet granulation, abnormal, 622, 622f
Platelet production, impaired or decreased, 735–739
  acquired (drug-induced) hypoplasia, 738–739
  autosomal dominant thrombocytopenia, 737
  categories, 739–740
  congenital amegakaryocytic thrombocytopenia, 737
  ineffective thrombopoiesis, 735
  inherited thrombocytopenia/congenital hypoplasia, 735–737
    associated with chromosomal abnormalities, 735–737
    Fanconi anemia, 737
    list of, 736t
    May-Hegglin anomaly, 737, 737f
    neonatal thrombocytopenia and, 737f, 738
    TAR syndrome, 737
  neonatal thrombocytopenia, 738, 738t
  X-linked thrombocytopenia, 737–738
Platelets, 163–164, 665–666, 666t
  abnormalities
    bleeding disorders from, 735
    distribution or dilution of, 751
  activation, 169–171
    adhesion, 169, 170f
    aggregation, 169–170, 171f
    eicosanoid synthesis, 171–172, 173f
    G-proteins, 171, 172f
    inositol triphosphate-diacylglycerol pathway, 173
    markers, 821
    microparticles, 171
    pathways, 171–173
    secretion, 171, 172t
  concentrate, trauma-induced coagulopathy, 689
  consumption or sequestration, and neonatal thrombocytopenia, 738
  counts, 182, 227
    clinical bleeding and, 735
    for heparin-induced thrombocytopenia, 778–779, 779t
    point-of-care testing, 194–195
    procedure, 182b
    reference range for, 735
    summarizing, 240–241, 240f, 241b
  in elderly adults, 871
  estimate, 234b
  HELLP syndrome, 383
  impedance histograms for, 200, 201f
  and inflammation, 173
  megakaryocytopoiesis, 160–163
    endomitosis, 160, 160b
    hormones and cytokines of, 163, 163t
    megakaryocyte differentiation and progenitors, 160, 161f
    megakaryocyte membrane receptors and markers, 162, 163t
    terminal megakaryocyte differentiation, 160–162, 161f, 162t
    thrombocytopoiesis, 161f–162f, 162
  in neonate, 867, 867t–868t
  proteome, 174
  reticulated, 164, 164f
  satellitosis, 226
  shedding, 161f–162f, 162
  stress, 164, 164f
  ultrastructure, 164–169
    additional membrane receptors, 168–169
    cytoskeleton, 165–166, 165f
    dense tubular system, 165, 165f
    plasma membrane receptors for adhesion, 166–168, 167f, 168t
    platelet granules, 165f, 166, 166t
    resting plasma membrane, 164–165, 164f
    seven-transmembrane repeat receptors, 168, 169t
    surface-connected canalicular system, 165, 165f

"Platelet satellitosis", 182b
Platelet secretion disorders, 717–721
    dense granule deficiency, 717–720, 718b, 719f
    thromboxane pathway disorders, 720–721
PlateletWorks platelet function assay, 804, 857
Pluripotent hematopoietic stem cell, 68
Pneumatic tube system, 881.e4
Pneumococcal disease, and SCD, 423
Pneumocystis jiroveci, 881.e47, 881.e47f
PNH. See Paroxysmal nocturnal hemoglobinuria
Poikilocytosis, 267t
Point mutations, 493, 522–523
Point-of-care (POC) testing, 192–195
    cell and platelet counts, 195
    coagulation, 851–853, 852t
    hematocrit, 194, 194f–195f
    hemoglobin concentration, 194
Poisoning, lead, 286
Polarized light microscope, 881.e31
PolyA tail, 531–532
Polychromatic erythrocytes, 3, 85–86, 85f–86f
Polychromatic normoblast, 83–84, 84f
Polycythemia, 1–2, 864
Polycythemia vera (PV), 601–604, 875
    clinical presentation of, 602–603
    diagnosis of, 601–602, 602b
    incidence of, 601
    pathogenetic mechanism of, 594f–595f, 601
    peripheral blood and bone marrow, 602, 603f, 603t
    treatment and prognosis of, 603–604
Polymerase chain reaction (PCR), 529–532, 530f
    digital, 535, 538f
    pathogen detection and infectious disease load, 522b, 542
    real-time, 533–536, 533f
        digital polymerase chain reaction, 535, 538f
        minimal residual disease in leukemia, 535, 537f
        multiplex ligation-dependent probe amplification, 535, 539f
        mutation enrichment strategies, 535–536
        qualitative, 534–535, 534f
        quantitative, 535, 536f
        reverse transcription, 530–532, 531f
        single-sided, 537
        thalassemia diagnosis by, 457–458
Polymorphonuclear cells (PMNs), 139–140, 145f
Poly(rC) binding proteins (PCBP), 125, 131
Population incidence effects on diagnostic efficacy, 34–36
Porphobilinogen, 113–114
Porphyrias, 64, 284, 284f
Postanalytical phase, in Total Testing Process, 9
Postanalytical quality assurance, 20t, 38
Posterior superior iliac crest, 246, 246f
Postpartum hemorrhage, 701
Postpolycythemic myeloid metaplasia, 603
Postsplenectomy thrombocytosis, 752f
Postterm neonates, 863–864
Posttransfusion purpura (PTP), 745
Prasugrel, 723, 791t
    for oral antiplatelet therapeutic drugs, 803
    platelet aggregometry and, 820
Preanalytical phase, in Total Testing Process, 9
Preanalytical quality assurance, 19t, 38
Precision, 25–26
    in coagulation instrumentation, 848
Prediction interval, 21
Predominance of fetal hemoglobin (Hb F), 864
Preeclampsia, in pregnancy, 870
Prefibrotic myelofibrosis, diagnostic criteria for, 604

Pregnancy. See also Gestational hematology and hemostasis
  anemia and, 868–869
    acute blood loss, 869
    hemoglobinopathies, 869
    iron deficiency anemia, 868
    megaloblastic anemia, 869
    parasitic infections, 869
  thrombocytopenia during, 870, 870t
    hemolytic disease of newborn, 746
    idiopathic thrombocytopenic purpura (ITP), 740
    incidental thrombocytopenia of pregnancy, 746
    preeclampsia, 745b, 746
    thrombotic thrombocytopenic purpura, 746–749
Prehepatic jaundice, 340
Preleukemia, 619
Premature infant. See Preterm infant
Prematurity, anemia of, 864
Prenatal hematopoiesis, 863
Pre-T cells, 153
Preterm infant, platelet count reference intervals for, 867t
Preterm neonate, hemoglobin values in, 865
Primaquine, 388
Primary active transport, plasma membrane, 49
Primary fibrinolysis, 679, 776
Primary (azurophilic) granules, 141
Primary hemostasis, 687
Primary immunodeficiency diseases, 465–470
    congenital defects of phagocytes as, 467–470
    lysosomal storage diseases, 470–474
    morphologic abnormalities of leukocytes without associated immunodeficiency, 474–476
Primary myelofibrosis (PMF), 604–607
    collagen in, 604–605
    hematopoiesis and extramedullary hematopoiesis in, 605
    incidence and clinical presentation of, 605
    pathogenetic mechanism of, 605
    peripheral blood and bone marrow in, 605, 606f, 606t
    treatment and prognosis of, 605–607
Primary standards, 22–23
Primary structure, hemoglobin, 111–112
Primary thrombocythemia. See Essential thrombocythemia
Primary thrombocytosis, 599
Primary tube sampling, in coagulation instrumentation, 848
Proapoptotic Bak proteins, 162
Procoagulant cofactors, in hemostasis, 670, 670t
Procoagulants
    classification and function of, 668–673, 668f, 668b
    nomenclature of, 666–668, 667f, 667t
Proficiency systems, laboratory staff, 36
Promegakaryocyte, 161f, 162
Prometaphase, 53
    M (mitosis) stage, 53
Promonocytes, 149, 574–575, 576f
Promoters, 524–525
Promyelocytes, 141, 141f, 143f
Pronormoblast, 81–82, 83f
Prophase, 53
Proportional systematic error, 25
Prostacyclin, 168
Prostaglandin pathway, drugs inhibiting, 722–723
Protamine sulfate, for LMWH-associated bleeding, 797
Pro-T cells, 153
Proteinase K, 528

Proteins
  4.1, 101, 102f
  4.2, 101
  body iron and
    bone morphogenic, 127t
    hemochromatosis, 127t
    hemojuvelin, 127t
  C
    activity, 764
    assays, 772, 772f
    control pathway, 771–773
    deficiency, 765t, 771–772
    inhibitor, 678
    regulatory system, 676, 677f
  central dogma in genetics and, 521–523
  cytokine, 71
  induced by vitamin K antagonists (PIVKA), 669, 690, 792
  mutations that alter membrane transport, 355b
  organic anion transporter, 333f, 334
  RBC membrane, 45, 101–104, 102f, 103t
    cytoskeletal, 102f, 103–104, 104t, 105f
    transmembrane, 101–103, 102f, 103t
  S, 676–677
    activity, 764
    assays, 772–773, 772f, 773t
    deficiency, 771–772
Proteoglycans, 165
Proteome, platelets, 174
Prothrombin complex concentrate (PCC), 799
Prothrombin deficiency, 706t
Prothrombin fragment, 670
Prothrombin G20210A, 764, 765t, 770
Prothrombin time, 5, 822–824
  as diagnostic assay, 823
  international normalized ratio (PT/INR) in warfarin therapy, 793, 794f
  limitations of, 823–824, 823t
  minimal effectiveness of, as screening tool, 823
  principle for, 822
  procedure for, 822
  quality control for, 822–823
  reference interval, 823
  reporting of, 823
Protooncogene, overexpression of, 493
Prussian blue staining, 133, 255, 255f
Pseudo-Chédiak-Higashi granules, 467
Pseudodiploid cells, 557
Pseudo-Gaucher cells, 471–473
Pseudogout, 881.e45
Pseudoleukocytosis, 226
Pseudo- or acquired Pelger-Huët anomaly (PPHA), 474–475
PTT. See Partial thromboplastin time
Pulmonary embolism, 774–775
Pulmonary hypertension (PHT), 418
Pulse signals, 210
Pure erythroid leukemia, 575
Pure red cell aplasia (PRCA), 321–323
Purine, 523–524, 524f
Purpura, 687, 735, 735f
Purpura fulminans, 750–751, 775
Pyknosis, neutrophils, 481
  apoptotic nuclei, 481, 481f
  pyknotic nuclei, 481
Pyknotic nuclei, 481
Pyrimidine 5′-nucleotidase type 1 (P5′NT-1) deficiency, 374
Pyrimidines, 523–524, 524f
Pyroptosis, 620
Pyrosequencing, 537
Pyruvate kinase, 96–98, 97f
  deficiency, 373–374
    clinical manifestations, 373
    laboratory findings, 373–374, 374f
    pathophysiology, 373
    treatment, 374

Q
Qualitative platelet disorders, 714–721, 714b, 715f, 716t
  inherited giant platelet syndromes, 717, 718t
  platelet adhesion, 716–717
  platelet aggregation, 714–716
  platelet dysfunction, 721–727, 722f, 722t
    cardiopulmonary bypass surgery, 726
    drug-induced defects, 722–725
    hereditary afibrinogenemia, 726
    hyperaggregable platelets, 727
    liver disease, 725–726
    medical conditions, 726
    multiple myeloma and Waldenström macroglobulinemia, 725
    myeloproliferative neoplasms, 725
    uremia, 726
  platelet secretion, 717–721
    dense granule deficiency, 717–720, 718b, 719f
    thromboxane pathway disorders, 720–721
  receptors and signaling pathways, disorders of, 721
Qualitative real-time polymerase chain reaction, 534–535, 534f
Quality assessment, external, 33
Quality assurance, 6–7
  agencies addressing, 38
  assay feasibility and, 36
  assessing diagnostic efficacy in, 33–36, 34f, 35t
  components of, 19, 19t, 19b
  external quality assessment, 33
  in hematology and hemostasis testing, 18–42
  laboratory staff competence and, 36–38
  lot-to-lot comparisons, 29, 30t
  postanalytical, 20t, 38
  preanalytical, 19t, 38
  receiver operating characteristic curve, 36, 37f
  reference interval
    direct, 30
    indirect, 30
  statistical significance and expressions of central tendency and dispersion, 19–21
    coefficient of variation, 21
    mean in, 20–21
    median in, 21
    mode in, 21
    standard deviation in, 21, 22f
    statistical significance, 19–20, 20t
    variance in, 21
  therapeutic target range, 30
  validation, 21–28
    accuracy, 22–23
    analytical measurement range, 26–28
    analytical sensitivity, 28
    analytical specificity, 28
    documentation and reliability, 28
    levels of laboratory assay approval and, 28, 29t
    linearity, 26–28, 28f
    lower limit of detection, 28
    precision, 25–26
    statistical tests, 23–25
Quality Chasm Series, 8–9
Quality control, 6–7, 19
  controls, 31–32, 32f, 32t
  delta checks, 33
  for fibrinogen assay, 828
  internal, 31–33
  moving average of red blood cell indices, 32–33
  for partial thromboplastin time, 825
  for prothrombin time, 822–823
  for single-factor assays, using the PTT, 830
  for thrombin clotting time, 827
Quality improvement, 13
  in hematology and hemostasis laboratory, 14
Quality specimen, requirements for, 881.e22

Quantitative real-time polymerase chain reaction, 535, 536f
Quantra coagulometer, 834
Quaternary structure, hemoglobin, 112
Quebec platelet disorder, 720
Quick stains, 230

R
Radiation therapy, for leukocyte neoplasms, 495
Radioactive hazards, 881.e8
Radiofrequency conductivity, 201–202, 201f–202f
Random access testing, in coagulation instrumentation, 848
Rapid turnaround assays, for heparin-induced thrombocytopenia, 780–781
Rapoport-Luebering pathway, 97f, 99
RBC hemoglobin content histogram (RBC HC), 213
RBM8A gene, 737
Reactive lymphocytes, 153, 483–484
Reactive monocytes, 482, 482f
Reactive thrombocytosis, 752–753, 752f
  associated with hemorrhage or surgery, 752
  associated with inflammation and disease, 753
  associated with iron deficiency anemia, 753
READACRIT centrifuge, 185b, 187f
Reagent handling, in coagulation instrumentation, 848–849
Reagent tracking, in coagulation instrumentation, 848–849
Real-time polymerase chain reaction, 533–536, 533f
  digital polymerase chain reaction, 535, 538f
  minimal residual disease in leukemia, 535, 537f
  multiplex ligation-dependent probe amplification, 535, 539f
  mutation enrichment strategies, 535–536
  qualitative, 534–535, 534f
  quantitative, 535, 536f
Rebound thrombocytosis, 753
Receiver operating characteristic curve (ROC), 36, 37f
Receptor-mediated endocytosis, 49, 129
Receptors, 49–50
Recombinant activated coagulation factor VII (rFVIIa), 689
Recombinant interleukin-11, 738–739
Recombinant TPA analogue (rTPA), 804
Recycling, body iron and salvage, 128–129
Red blood cells. See Erythrocytes
  Abbott, 210
  agglutination, effects of, 218–219
  Beckman Coulter, 205–206
  DC detection system for, 207, 208f
  impedance histograms for, 200, 201f
  light scatter for, 213, 215f
  membrane, structure and function, 99–105
  oscilloscope display and histogram, 199–200, 200f
  survival, 345
Red cell distribution width (RDW), 2, 219–220, 220f, 265
  anemia diagnosis and, 265–266
  morphologic classification and, 271
  in red blood cell indices, 865
Reference intervals, 29–31, 31f, 236
  for globin synthesis, 442, 442t
Reference limit, 34
Reference methods, 23
Reflex testing, in automatic ordering/performing test, 849
Refractive index, 881.e30
Refractory anemia, 619
Regulated medical waste management, 881.e6

Regulation
  of body iron
    erythrocyte iron sensing and hepcidin
      production, 127–128, 129f–130f
    liver iron sensing and hepcidin production,
      126–127, 126f, 127t
    liver sensing of circulating iron, 126f, 127,
      128f
    liver sensing of stored iron, 126f, 127
    cellular iron, 129, 130f
    hemoglobin production, 114–116
    systemic body iron, 126–128, 126f, 127t,
      281–282
      erythrocyte iron sensing and hepcidin
        production, 127–128, 129f–130f
      liver iron sensing and hepcidin production,
        126–127, 126f, 127t
      liver sensing of circulating iron, 126f, 127, 128f
      liver sensing of stored iron, 126f, 127
Regulatory information, 881.e7
Reilly bodies, 475
Relaxed state, hemoglobin, 116, 117f
Reliability and documentation, 28
Renal insufficiency, 750
Renal iron salvage, 337–338
Renal peritubular interstitial cells, 72
Rendu-Osler-Weber syndrome, 727
Replication, DNA, 525–527, 526f
Reptilase time, 827
Respiratory burst, defects of, 469–470, 469t
Resting plasma membrane, 164–165, 164f
Restriction endonuclease methods, 533
Retic scatter absorption cytogram, 215–216
Reticular adventitial cells, 55, 61–62
Reticulated platelets, 164, 164f
Reticulocyte analysis
  automated blood cell analysis, clinical utility of,
    220–221
  cytochemistry and light scatter for, 213–216,
    215f
  fluorescence flow cytometry for, 207–210,
    209f
  MAPSS for, 210–213, 211f–212f
  volume, conductivity, scatter technology,
    206–207, 206f–207f
Reticulocytes, 3
  blood cell analyzers, 204t
  control, 189
  count, 187–190, 239
    absolute, 3, 189
    automated, 190
    corrected, 189
    equation reference interval, 189
    errors in, 219
    hemolysis and, 346
    Miller disc for, 188f, 188b
    in paroxysmal nocturnal hemoglobinuria,
      366
    pathophysiologic classification of, 271, 272b
    pediatric, 865, 865f
    principle of, 187–188, 188f
    procedure, 188b
    sources of error and comments, 188f, 188b,
      191f
  erythropoietin (EPO) and early release of, 88
  hemoglobin content of, 132t, 134, 220–221
  hemolysis and, 346
  production index, 189, 265
  shift, 88, 189
Reticulocytosis, 346–347, 373, 400
Retrogression, 61
Retroviruses, 781
Reverse transcription polymerase chain reaction,
  530–532, 531f
Reversible sickle cells, 415
Revised International Prognostic Scoring System
  (IPSS-R), 627

Revolving nosepiece, microscope, 881.e28
rFVIIa. See Recombinant activated coagulation
  factor VII
Rhabdomyolysis, 117
Rh-associated glycoprotein (RhAG), 361–362
Rh deficiency syndrome, 362
Rh system, 102–103
Ribonucleic acid (RNA), 3
  central dogma in genetics and, 521–523, 522f
  fluorescence in situ hybridization, 554–555
  isolated from clinical specimens, 528–529
  in mitochondria, 48
  necrosis and, 54
  nucleoli and, 47
  reverse transcription polymerase chain reaction
    for amplifying, 530–532, 531f
  ribosomes and, 47
  transcription and translation, 524–525
Ribosomes, 46t, 47
Ring chromosomes, 558, 558f
Ring sideroblasts, 284
Risk factors, thrombosis, 763–765
Ristocetin cofactor, 697–699
Ristocetin induced platelet agglutination (RIPA)
  assay, 699
Rivaroxaban, 800, 800t
Robertsonian translocation, 559, 559f
Ropeginterferon α-2b, 598–599
Rosenthal syndrome, 705
Rotated light scatter (RLSn), 206
Rotational thromboelastometry (ROTEM),
  833–834, 854, 854f
Rough endoplasmic reticulum (RER), 46t, 47
Routine cleaning, 881.e5
Routine venipuncture, vein selection for, 881.e16
Rule of three, 186
Ruptured eosinophils, 482
Rusfertide, 598–599
Russell viper venom test, 827
Ruxolitinib, 598

S
Safe health care, 9
Safe hematology and hemostasis testing, 9–11
Safety, 7
  laboratory safety, 7
  patient safety, 7
  personal protective equipment (PPE), 7
Safety Data Sheets (SDS), 881.e7
Safety shields, 881.e4f
Sanger DNA sequencing, 536–538, 540f, 858
Sarcoma, myeloid, 576
SARS-CoV-2 (COVID-19), 742–743
Satellitosis, 219
Saturation, transferrin, 132, 132t, 279–280
Scatter signals, 202
Schistocytes, 267t, 269f
Schistosoma haematobium, 279
Schizocyte, 267t
Scopio Labs X100, 235
Scott syndrome, 721
Scramblases, 100
Screening tests, 34. See also Laboratory diagnosis
Sea-blue histiocytes, 473
Sebastian syndrome, 737
Secondary active transport, plasma membrane, 49
Secondary hemostasis, 687
Secondary myeloid neoplasms, 576
Secondary structure, hemoglobin, 111–112
Secondary thrombocytopenia, 745
Secretory granule, 146
Secretory vesicle, 146
Sedimentation rate, erythrocytes, 6, 190–192
  automated, 191–192
  disposable kits, 191, 193t
  factors affecting, 192t

Sedimentation rate, erythrocytes (Continued)
  modified Westergren, 190, 191f
  reference interval, 190b
  sources of error and comments, 190b
  Wintrobe, 190–191
Segmented neutrophils, 256, 257f, 474
Seizures, 881.e19
Selectins, 144
Selective serotonin reuptake inhibitors, 423
Senescence, 91
Senile purpura, 728
Separator gel, 881.e13
Sepsis, clostridial, 387
Sequencing, DNA, 536–538, 540f
Serine proteases, 668, 668t
Serotonin release assay (SRA), for heparin-
  induced thrombocytopenia, 780, 781f
Serous fluid, 881.e40, 881.e41f, 881.e44f
  differential cell counts of, 881.e41, 881.e42f,
    881.e43f, 881.e44f
  gross examination of, 881.e41
  transudates vs. exudates, 881.e40, 881.e41t
Serum bilirubin, 334b
Serum ferritin, 283
  level, 132t, 133
Serum gastrin, 306
Serum haptoglobin, 266
Serum iron, 132, 132t
Seven-transmembrane repeat receptors, 168,
  169t
Severe acute respiratory syndrome coronavirus 2
  (SARS-CoV2), 781, 830
Severe combined immune deficiency (SCID),
  465–466
Sex hormone effects, on hematopoiesis, 875
Sézary syndrome, 651–652, 652f
SF3B1 mutation, 624
Shear force, 169
Shift, 220
Shift reticulocytes, 88, 189
Shift to the left, 479–480
Shigella, 382
Shock, 418–419
Shortened red blood cell life span, 283
Shwachman-Bodian-Diamond syndrome (SBDS),
  316, 320–321
Shwachman-Diamond syndrome (SDS), 468
Sickle cells, 66, 267t, 269f
  disease, 412–427
    clinical features, 416–419, 416b
    course and prognosis, 427
    dysfunctional endothelial nitric oxide
      synthase, 415–416
    etiology and pathophysiology, 414–416
    gene therapy, 425–427
    geographic distribution of inherited
      hemoglobin variants and, 414f
    history of, 412–413
    incidence with malaria, 419–420
    infection prevention, 423
    inheritance pattern, 413, 413f
    intracellular hydration, 415
    irreversible, 415
    laboratory diagnosis, 420–422, 420f–421f
    mutation, 414
    newer drug options, 424–425
    pain care, 423
    polymerization and sickling, 414–415
    prevalence, 413–414
    rapid detection and genotyping of, 422
    reversible, 415
    stem cell transplant, 423–424
    transfusions, 423
    treatment, 422–427
  hemoglobin SC disease and, 431
  malaria and, 419–420
  trait, 427–428

Side fluorescent light (SFL), 207–209
Sideroblastic anemias (SAs), 276, 284–286, 285f, 285b
  acquired sideroblastic anemias, 286
  in elderly adults, 873
  hereditary sideroblastic anemias, 284–286
  lead poisoning and, 286
  porphyrias, 284, 285t
Sideropenia, 280
Siderophages, 881.e39
Side scatter (SSC), 202, 207–209
Siemens ADVIA 2120i, 204t
Siemens Healthineers, 213–216, 214f
  cytochemistry and light scatter, for WBC count, WBC differential, NRBCs and reticulocyte analysis, 213–216, 215f
  hemoglobin determination, 213
  RBC and platelet analyses, light scatter for, 213, 215f
Siemens PFA-100 Platelet Function Analyzer, 856, 857f
Signaling receptors, 101
Signal transduction, 101
  pathways, 50, 586, 586f
  proteins, 492
Signet ring cells, 881.e42, 881.e42f
Silent carriers, 355–356
Silent carrier state
  of α-thalassemia, 452
  of β-thalassemia, 446–447
Simple diffusion, plasma membrane, 48–49
Simple microscope, 881.e27
Single-factor assays, using the PTT, 828–831, 829t
  expected results and clinical utility of, 829–830
  limitations of, 830
  principle of, 828–829
  quality control for, 830
Single-molecule real-time sequencing (SMRT), 544
Single nucleotide polymorphism array (SNP-A), 542
Single-sided PCR, 537
Sister chromatids, 52
Skin disinfection, solutions for, 881.e16
Skin puncture, 881.e20
  collection sites, 881.e20, 881.e20f
  equipment for, 881.e20, 881.e21f
  order of draw, 881.e21b
  precautions with, 881.e20
  procedure, 881.e12
    preparation of peripheral blood films, 881.e13
Small lymphocytic lymphoma (SLL), 642–644
Small-vessel bleeding in skin, 735
Smoldering leukemia, 619
Smooth endoplasmic reticulum (SER), 46t, 47
Smudged eosinophils, 482
Social determinants of health, 12
Sodium butyrate, 424
Sodium citrate, 227, 813
  volume adjustment for elevated hematocrits, 813–814, 814f
Sodium dodecyl sulfate-polyacrylamide gel electrophoresis (SDS-PAGE), 101, 101f, 358
Sodium lauryl sulfate (SLS), 119, 203
Sodium-potassium ATPase, 49
Solenoid, 553
Solid tumor cytogenetics, 561–562, 562f
Soluble fibrin monomers, 775–776
Soluble transferrin receptor, 132t, 134, 280, 281f
Soluble transferrin receptor/log ferritin (sTfR), 132t, 134
Sonic estimation of elasticity by resonance (SEER), 834
Sonorheometry, 834
Sons of mothers against decapentaplegic (SMAD) protein, 127t

Sorting, cell, 515
Southeast Asian ovalocytosis (SAO), 354–355, 361
  clinical and laboratory findings, 361
  pathophysiology, 361
Specimen collection, 179–180
  anticoagulants for, 813–814
    citrate theophylline adenosine dipyridamole, 814
    EDTA, 814
    sodium citrate as, 813
  blood
    clotted, 815
    materials for, 813–814
      collection tubes for, 813
      needle selection in, 813–814, 813t
    procedure for, 814–815
      with butterfly set, 814
      with syringe, 815
      venipuncture and, 814–815
    short draw in, 814
    using capillary puncture, 815
    from vascular access devices, 815
  bone marrow, 250
  errors in, 814t
  heparinized, 813
  patient management during, 812
  for peripheral blood films, 226–227, 226f
  platelet function tests for, 817–821
  sites, bone marrow, 246
  transport and storage of, 816t
Specimen integrity, 10–11, 219
Specimen management, 815–817
  nucleic acid isolation, 527–529
  preparation, 816–817
  transport and storage, 815–816
Specimen quality set points, 849
Specimen rejection, reasons for, 881.e22, 881.e23b
Spectrin stabilization, 103–104
Spectrophotometry, for hemoglobin determination, 203
S phase checkpoint, 53
Spheric aberrations, 881.e28
Spherocytes, 267t, 269f, 344, 357f, 359
Sphingolipidoses, 470–474, 472f
Sphingomyelin (SP), 100
Spinous process of vertebrae or ribs, 246
Spleen, 64–66, 65f–66f
  pathophysiology of, 65f, 66
Splenectomy, 66, 359, 359f
Splenic artery, 66
Splenic marginal zone lymphoma (SMZL), 650–651, 651f
Splenomegaly, 66
  in acute myeloid leukemia, 570
Spur cells, 267t
  anemia, 363
Spurious thrombocytopenia, 219
SRA. See Serotonin release assay
S (DNA synthesis) stage, cell cycle, 52
Stability and reactivity, 881.e7
Stage, microscope, 881.e28
Staining of peripheral blood films, 228–229
  automated, 228–229
  features of proper, 230, 231b
  manual technique, 229, 230f
  quick, 230
Standard deviation, 21, 22f
Standard precautions, 881.e2, 881.e12
  hepatitis B virus vaccination, 881.e5
  housekeeping, 881.e5
  laundry, 881.e5
  regulated medical waste management, 881.e6
  training and documentation, 881.e6
Stand, microscope, 881.e27
Statistical significance, 19–20, 20t
Stem cell factor, 163

Stem cells
  cycle kinetics, 70, 70f
  hematopoietic stem cell (HSC), 59, 68–69
    transplantation, 319
  phenotypic and functional characterization, 70
  theory, 68–70, 69f, 69t
  therapeutic applications, 73, 73t–74t
  transplantation, 319, 496–497
Stem cell transplant, 423–424
Sternum, 246
Stomatocytes, 267t, 269f
Stomatocytosis, acquired, 363
Stool analysis, for parasites, 306
Storage artifacts, in leukocytes, 479
Storage pool disorders, 717, 718b
Stormorken syndrome, 721
Stress, 220
Stromal cells, 56, 61–62
Structural chromosome abnormalities, 558–559, 558f
Student t-test, 19–20, 20t, 23–24, 24t
Succinyl coenzyme A, 112–113, 113f
Sudan Black B staining, 573, 574f, 578, 578f
Sulfhemoglobin, 119
Superficial veins of the antecubital fossa, 881.e16, 881.e16f
Superwarfarin, 692
Supravital staining, 454f, 456
Surface carbohydrates, 101
Surface-connected canalicular system (SCCS), 165, 165f
SUSTAIN clinical trial, 425
Symports, plasma membrane, 49
Synovial cells, 881.e44, 881.e45f
Synovial fluid, 881.e43, 881.e44f, 881.e46f
  crystals, 881.e44, 881.e45f
  differential cell counts of, 881.e43, 881.e44f
  gross examination of, 881.e43
Syringe, 881.e15
Sysmex, 207–210, 208f
  fluorescence flow cytometry, for WBC count, WBC differential, NRBCs, and reticulocyte analyses, 207–210, 209f–210f
  hemoglobin determination, 207
  RBC analyses and platelet distribution, DC detection system for, 207, 208f
Sysmex XN-3100, 204t
Systemic body iron kinetics, 124–128, 124f
  absorption, ionic, 125–126, 125f
  regulation, 126–128, 126f, 127t
  transport, 126
Systemic body iron regulation, 281–282
Systemic fibrinolysis, 776
Systemic fibrinolytic therapy, for COVID-19, 776
Systemic (mucocutaneous) hemorrhage, 735, 735f

T

TACO. See Transfusion-associated circulatory overload
Tapeworm, fish, 303
Taqman assays, 534–535
Taq polymerase, 529
Target cells, 49, 269f
Targeted therapy, for leukocyte neoplasms, 495–496
TAR syndrome, 737
  RBM8A gene mutation, 737
T cell
  neoplasms, mature, 512–513, 514f
  production of, 60
Teamwork, 13
Teardrop cells, 267t, 269f
TEG 5000 Thromboelastograph System, 854
Telomere biology disorders (TBDs), 319–320
Telophase, 53
10x objective examination of blood film, 231
Tenase complex, factor VIII, 701
Tenecteplase (TNKase) (Genentech), 804

Ten eleven translocation 2 (TET2), 596–597
Terminal megakaryocyte differentiation, 160–162, 161f, 162t
Tertiary structure, hemoglobin, 111–112
Tetramer, 112
Tetraploidy (4n), 557
Thalassemias, 332, 414f, 440–463
    categories of, 443
    definitions and history of, 441
    diagnosis of, 455–459
        alkali denaturation test in, 458
        assessment of hemolysis in, 456
        assessment of normal and variant hemoglobins in, 456–457, 456f–457f
        complete blood count with peripheral blood film review, 455
        differential, 459
        high performance liquid chromatography (HPLC), 457, 457f
        history and physical examination in, 455
        laboratory methods for, 455–459
        molecular genetic testing in, 457–458
        polymerase chain reaction and, 457–458
        reticulocyte count in, 456
        supravital staining in, 454f, 456
    epidemiology of, 441
    genetic defects causing, 443, 444f
    genetic designations in, 443t
    genetics of globin synthesis, 442, 442f, 442t
    hemoglobin C-, 455
    hemoglobin E-, 455
    hemoglobin Lepore, 451
    hemoglobin S-, 454–455
    hemoglobin S-β-, 431
    with increased levels of fetal hemoglobin, 451
    pathophysiology of, 444–445
    α-, 441, 452–454
        clinical syndromes of, 452–454, 453t
        mechanisms in, 445
        minor, 452–453
        silent carrier state, 452
    β-, 443
        caused by defects in the β-globin gene cluster, 451
        clinical syndromes of, 445–451, 447t
        intermedia, 450–451
        major, 447–450, 448f–449f
        mechanisms in, 444–445, 445f
        minor, 447, 447f
            screening for, 451–452
        pathophysiology of, 446f
        silent carrier state of, 446–447
    β-globin gene cluster, 445–452
Thawed plasma, 689
The Joint Commission (TJC), 9
Therapeutic range development, 29–31, 31f
Therapeutic target range, 30
Thermal sensitivity, 360–361
Thermocycler, 529
Thomas plot, 134, 134f
Three-part differential, 200
Thrombin, 168, 672, 819–820
    time, 5
Thrombin activatable fibrinolysis inhibitor, 681
Thrombinantithrombin complex (TAT), 677
Thrombin receptor-activating peptide, 819–820
Thrombin time, 826–827
    procedure for, 826–827
    quality control for, 827
    reagent and principle for, 826, 826f
    reporting of, 827
Thrombocytes, 4
Thrombocythemia, essential, 4, 599–601
    clinical presentation of, 599
    diagnosis of, 599
    incidence of, 599
    pathogenetic mechanism of, 599

Thrombocythemia, essential (Continued)
    peripheral blood and bone marrow, 599–600, 600f, 600t
    treatment and prognosis of, 600–601
Thrombocytopenia, 4, 221, 380, 735–751, 776
    with absent radii syndrome, 720
    alcohol consumption and, 739
    artifact, 735
    bacterial infections associated with, 739
    and bleeding, 735
    classification of
        increased platelet destruction, 739b
        platelet production, impaired or decreased, 735–739, 736b
        platelet sequestration, 751b
    inherited, 735–737
        associated with chromosomal abnormalities, 735–737
        Fanconi anemia, 737
        list of, 736t
        May-Hegglin anomaly, 737, 737f
        neonatal thrombocytopenia and, 738, 738t
        TAR syndrome, 737
    mechanical platelet destruction, 751
    neonatal, 738
        causes of, 738
        and fetal thrombocytopenia, classification of, 738t
    pathophysiologic processes in, 735
    in pregnancy, 870, 870t
        hemolytic disease of newborn, 746
        idiopathic thrombocytopenic purpura (ITP), 740
        incidental thrombocytopenia of pregnancy, 746
        preeclampsia, 745b, 746
        thrombotic thrombocytopenic purpura, 746–749
    systemic (mucocutaneous) hemorrhage, 735, 735f
    viruses associated with, 739
Thrombocytopoiesis, 161f–162f, 162
Thrombocytosis, 4, 751–754, 752b
    associated with myeloproliferative disorders, 753–754
    essential thrombocythemia, 753–754
    definition of, 751–752
    reactive, 752–753. See also Reactive thrombocytosis
Thromboelastography (TEG), 833–834, 842, 854, 854f
Thromboinflammation, 764t, 781–782
Thrombolytic therapy, 790
Thrombomodulin, 664, 670, 771
Thrombophilia, 762
    laboratory evaluation of, 765–773, 766t
        activated protein C resistance and factor V Leiden mutation, 769–770
        antiphospholipid antibodies, 765–769
        antithrombin, 770–771
        protein C control pathway, 771–773
        prothrombin G20210A, 770
    molecular diagnostics in, 857–858
    during pregnancy, 869–870
Thrombosis, 4, 778
    antithrombotic therapy and, 790
    arterial, 790
        disseminated intravascular coagulation and, 775–778
        causes of, 775, 776t
        differential diagnosis of, 777–778
        laboratory diagnosis of, 776–778, 777t
        pathophysiology of, 775–776
        specialized laboratory tests for, 777, 777t
        symptoms of, 776
        treatment, 778
    predictors of, 773–774
        C-reactive protein, 773

Thrombosis (Continued)
        factor VIII, 774
        fibrinogen activity, 773–774, 773f
        lipoprotein (a), 773
    prevalence of, 762–763
    etiology and prevalence of, 762–763
    in neonates, 868
    predictors, of arterial, 773–774
    in pregnancy, 869–870
    risk factors, 763–765
        acquired, 763–764, 763t
        congenital, 764, 765t
        double hit, 764–765
    risk testing
        developments, 762
        future, 782
Thrombotic disorders, 761–788
Thrombotic microangiopathies (TMAs), 234, 380, 745, 745b
Thrombotic thrombocytopenic purpura (TTP), 381–382, 382f, 745–749, 870
    ADAMTS13 and, 746, 748
    attributes of, 747t
    clinical monitoring of, 746
    differential diagnosis, 383
    differentiation, 749t
    mechanism for, 749f
    and thrombosis, 747
    treatment of, 748–749
Thromboxane A$_2$ (TXA$_2$), 168, 172–173
Thromboxane pathway disorders, 720–721
Thymine, 523–524
Thymus, 66–68, 67f–68f
    at birth, 67–68, 67f
    pathophysiology, 68
Ticagrelor, 723, 791t
    for oral antiplatelet therapeutic drugs, 803
Tilt-tube technique, 842
Timely hematology, and hemostasis testing, 12
Timely laboratory testing, 12
Tirofiban, 724, 791t
Tirofiban hydrochloride, 803
Tissue factor, 670
    pathway inhibitor, 677, 678f
Tissue plasminogen activator (TPA), 665, 678f, 680, 804, 832–833
    principle of, 833, 833f
    specimen collection for, 833
T lymphoblastic leukemia/lymphoma, 511, 513f
T lymphocytes, 64–65, 151–152
    development, 153
    functions, 153–154
    maturation of, 153, 154f
To Err Is Human, 8–9
Tolbutamide, cytotoxic effect of, 738
Tolerance, 151
Total iron-binding capacity (TIBC), 132, 132t, 133f
Total Symptom Score (TSS), 598
Total Testing Process, in clinical laboratory, 9, 10f
Total Thrombus Formation Analyzer System, 857
Total voteout, 206
Touch preparations, bone marrow, 250–251
Tourniquet, 881.e12
Towelettes, 881.e12
Toxic granulation, 480
Toxic methemoglobinemia, 118–119
Toxicological information, 881.e7
Toxic vacuoles, 480
TP53, 54
T-prolymphocytic leukemia (T-PLL), 644–645, 645f
    laboratory findings, 645
    treatment, 645
Trabeculae, 60–61
Trabecular veins, 65
Traditional complete blood count, 219

Training and documentation, 881.e6
Transcription activator-like effector nucleases (TALENS), 425
Transcription, DNA, 524–525
Transferrin, 113–114
    saturation, 132, 132t, 279–280
Transferrin receptor 1, 127t, 129
Transferrin receptor 2, 127t, 129
Transfusion-associated circulatory overload (TACO), 689
Transfusion-dependent thalassemia (TDT), 446
Transfusion-related acute lung injury (TRALI), 689
Transfusion-related hemosiderosis, 287
Transfusion therapy
    for SCD, 423
    for thalassemias, 448
Transgender populations, 874–876
    diversity in, 874
    electronic health records, 876
    hematologic parameters in, 875, 876t
    hormone therapy
        and hematopoiesis, 875
        and hemostasis, 875
    sex hormone effects on hematopoiesis, 875
Transient erythroblastopenia of childhood (TEC), 321–322
Translation errors, 443
Translations, DNA/RNA, 524–525
Translocations, chromosome, 559
Transmembrane proteins, 45, 101–103, 102f, 103t
    blood group antigens, 102
    GPI anchor and paroxysmal nocturnal hemoglobinuria, 103
    nomenclature, 101
Transport
    iron, 126
    mutations that alter membrane proteins in, 354–355, 355b
Transport information, 881.e7
Transudates, exudates vs., 881.e40, 881.e41t
Trauma-induced coagulopathy (TIC), 688–690
Traumatic cardiac hemolytic anemia, 383, 384f
Treatment-free remission, 592
Trichuris trichiura, 279
Triploidy (3n), 557, 558f
Trousseau syndrome, 775
True thrombocytopenia, 735
T-test, 19–20, 20t, 23–24, 24t
Tumor cells, 881.e43f
Tumor necrosis factor receptor 1 (TNFR1), 54
Tumor suppressor genes (TSGs), 493–494, 494t
Tumor suppressor proteins, 54
Tungsten-halogen light bulbs, 881.e29
Turnaround time, 12
22q11.2 deletion syndrome (22DS), 466
Two-dimensional distribution scattergram, 202, 202f
Type A, immersion oil, 881.e30
Type B, immersion oil, 881.e30
Type C, immersion oil, 881.e30
Tyrosine kinase inhibitor (TKI) therapy, 592

U
Ulcers, 419
Unconjugated bilirubin, 266
Unesterified cholesterol, 99
Unexplained anemia, of aging, 873
Unfractionated heparin (UFH), 791t, 795–797
    in disseminated intravascular coagulation, 778
    heparin action, 795
    LMWH action, 797, 797f
    monitoring, 795–796
        PTT therapeutic range, 795–796, 796f
        using activated clotting time, 796–797
        using chromogenic anti-Xa assay, 796

Unfractionated heparin (UFH) (Continued)
        using PTT, 796
        using viscoelastometry, 796–797
    reversing, 797
    therapy, 795
UniCel DxH 900 system, 203
Unifying theory in DIIHA, 404
Unstable hemoglobin variants, 434
Upper median-angle light scatter (UMALS), 206
Upshaw-Schülman syndrome, 381
Uremia, 726
Urinalysis, 266
Urine hemoglobin, 342–344
Urine hemosiderin, 342–344
Urobilinogen, 334–335, 335f, 342
Urokinase plasminogen activator, 680

V
Vaccine-induced immune thrombotic thrombocytopenia (VITT), 742–743, 782
Vacuolation, neutrophil, 480–481
Vacuoles, E1 enzyme, X-linked, autoinflammatory, somatic (VEXAS), 480–481
Validation, 21–28
    accuracy, 22–23
    analytical measurement range, 26–28
    analytical sensitivity, 28
    analytical specificity, 28
    documentation and reliability, 28
    levels of laboratory assay approval and, 28, 29t
    linearity, 26–28, 28f
    lower limit of detection, 28
    precision, 25–26
    statistical tests, 23–25
Valoctocogene roxaparvovec (Roctavian, BioMarin Pharmaceutical), 704
Variance, computation of, 21
Vascular access devices, hemostasis blood specimen collection from, 815
Vascular disorders, 727–728, 727b
    acquired, 728
    bleeding disorders vs., 735
    inherited, 727–728
Vascular intima
    damaged, procoagulant properties of, 664
    fibrinolytic properties of, 665
    functions of, 662–663
    in hemostasis, 662–665, 663b
    intact, anticoagulant properties of, 663–664, 663f, 665f
    and platelets, 665–666
Vasoconstriction and platelet plug formation, 662
Vasoocclusive crisis (VOC), 416–417, 417f
Velocardiofacial syndrome, 466
Venipuncture, 814–815, 881.e12
    in children, 881.e18
    complications encountered in, 881.e18
        allergic reactions, 881.e19
        ecchymosis (bruise), 881.e18
        fainting (syncope), 881.e18
        hematoma, 881.e18, 881.e18f
        hemoconcentration, 881.e18
        hemolysis, 881.e19
        nerve damage, 881.e19
        petechiae, 881.e19
        seizures, 881.e19
        vomiting, 881.e19
    equipment for, 881.e12
        collection tubes, 881.e12
        needle holders, 881.e13, 881.e15f
        needles, 881.e13, 881.e15f
        solutions for skin disinfection, 881.e16
        syringe, 881.e15
        tourniquet, 881.e12
        winged blood collection set (butterfly), 881.e15, 881.e15f

Venipuncture (Continued)
    inability to obtain blood specimen, 881.e19
        failure to draw blood, 881.e18f, 881.e19
        missing patient, 881.e20
        patient refusal, 881.e20
    order of draw for, 881.e17b
    procedure, 881.e16
        coagulation testing, 881.e17
    selection of vein for routine, 881.e16
    in special situations, 881.e19
        burned, damaged, scarred, and occluded veins, 881.e19
        edema, 881.e19
        intravenous therapy, 881.e19
        mastectomy, 881.e19
        obesity, 881.e19
Venom activated assays, 827
    reptilase time, 827
    Russell viper venom test, 827
Venoms, 388
Venous thromboembolic disease, 790
    diagnosis of, 774
    prevalence of, 762
Venous thromboembolism (VTE), in pregnancy, 869
    treatment of, 869
VerifyNow system, 722, 803–804, 856–857, 857f
Verotoxins, 382
Vertical anchorages, 104
Vesicles, 104
Vesicular transport, plasma membrane, 49
Viruses, Epstein-Barr, 315
Viscoelastic clot detection, 844
Viscoelastometry (VET), 804, 833–834
    assays, 854, 854f
    in unfractionated heparin, 796–797
Vital stains, 3
Vitamin B$_{12}$
    assays for, 305–306, 306b, 307f
    competition for, 303
    deficiency, 298–300, 299f
        causes of, 301–303, 302f
        in elderly adults, 873
        laboratory tests used to, 308t
        systemic manifestations of, 300–301
    failure to separate
        from haptocorrin, 303
        from proteins, 303
Vitamin C (ascorbic acid), 99
Vitamin deficiencies, causes of, 301–303
Vitamin K antagonist, 792
Vitamin K deficiency, 831
    hemorrhage and, 692
        detection of, 692
        hemorrhagic disease of the newborn, 692
        warfarin for, 692
Vitamin K-dependent prothrombin group, 669–670, 669f–670f, 669t–670t, 669b
Volume, conductivity, scatter (VCS) technology, 205f–207f, 206–207
Volume distribution histogram, 199–200
Volume/hemoglobin concentration (V/HC) cytogram, 213
Vomiting, 881.e19
von Willebrand disease, 693–701
    Ac platelet-binding activity, 697–699
    collagen binding assay, 699
    concentrates, 701
    diagnostic pitfalls in, 699–700
    genetic testing, 698t, 699
    laboratory diagnostic profile
        first-level phenotypic, 697–699, 697t
        second-level phenotypic, 699
    pathophysiology of, 695
    pregnancy and, 700
    ristocetin cofactor, 697–699

von Willebrand disease *(Continued)*
    subtype 1C, 695
    subtype 2A, 695
    subtype 2B, 695
    subtype 2M, 695–696
    subtype 2N, 696–697
    treatment for, 700–701, 701t
    type 1, 695, 696f
    type 2, 695
    type 3, 697
von Willebrand factor (VWF), 169, 662, 671, 671f, 737
    activity assays, 821
    molecular biology and function of, 694–695, 694f
    nomenclature of, 695t
    thrombotic thrombocytopenic purpura and, 381
Voting, 206
Voxelotor, 425
VWF-cleaving protease, 169

W

Waldenström macroglobulinemia, 656–657, 725
Warfarin, 692, 790–794, 791t
    action, 790–792
    inducing skin necrosis, 771, 792
    INR therapeutic range, 793
    monitoring, 793–794
        anticoagulants in, 795
        chromogenic factor X assay in, 793–794
        diet and pharmaceutical interference, 794
        PT/INR in, 793
    prophylaxis and therapy, 792, 792f, 793t
    reversing, 794, 794t
    for venous thromboembolism, 869
    as vitamin K antagonists, 792
Warfarin resistance, 792
Warfarin sodium (4-hydroxycoumarin, Coumadin), 790–792

Warm autoimmune hemolytic anemia (WAIHA), 397–399
WAS. *See* Wiskott-Aldrich syndrome
Wells scoring system
    in deep venous thrombosis, 774
    in pulmonary embolism, 774
Westergren method, 191
Westerman-Jensen needle, 247, 247f
Westgard rules, 31–32, 32t
White blood cell cytoplasm, uneven staining of, 621, 622f
White blood cells (WBCs), 139, 871. *See also* Leukocytes
    count
        cytochemistry and light scatter for, 213–216, 215f
        fluorescence flow cytometry for, 207–210, 209f
        MAPSS for, 210–213, 211f–212f
    differential
        Beckman Coulter, 205–206
        blood cell analyzers, 204t
        cytochemistry and light scatter for, 213–216, 215f
        fluorescence flow cytometry for, 207–210, 209f
        MAPSS for, 210–213, 211f–212f
        volume, conductivity, scatter technology, 206–207, 206f–207f
        impedance histograms for, 200, 201f
WHO Classification-Based Prognostic Scoring System (WPSS), 627
Whole-blood calibration, 216
Whole Blood/Optical Lumi-Aggregation System, 856
Whole-blood specimens, for platelet aggregometry, 816, 818, 819f
Winged blood collection set (butterfly), 881.e15, 881.e15f
Wintrobe erythrocyte sedimentation rate, 190–191
Wintrobe hematocrit tubes, 247

Wiskott-Aldrich syndrome (WAS), 466, 719, 737
Wiskott-Aldrich syndrome protein (WASP), 466
Within-day variation, 25–26
Women
    aplastic anemia in, 315
    HELLP syndrome in, 383
    iron deficiency anemia in, 279
World Health Organization (WHO)
    classification of myelodysplastic neoplasms, 623, 624b
    tumors of hematopoietic system, 584
Wright (Wright-Giemsa) stain, 1, 229–230
    automated slide stainers, 229–230, 230f
    manual technique, 229, 230f
    marrow smear dyes, 251

X

Xerocyte, 361
X-linked agammaglobulinemia, 466
X-linked erythropoietic protoporphyria (XLEPP), 285t
X-linked SCID, 465–466
X-linked sideroblastic anemia (XLSA), 284–285
X-linked thrombocytopenia, 737–738

Y

Yellow marrow, 61

Z

Z-dependent protease inhibitor (ZPI), 678
Zenker fixative, 247
Zidovudine, 738–739
Zinc finger nucleases (ZFNs), 425, 450
Zinc protoporphyrin, 132t, 134, 280, 281f
ZPI. *See* Z-dependent protease inhibitor
Zygosity, 411
Zymogens, 666, 667f

HEMATOLOGY/BODY FLUIDS/HEMOSTASIS REFERENCE INTERVALS

The following tables list typical reference intervals for common hematology, body fluid, and hemostasis laboratory assays. Unless otherwise noted, data for reference interval tables were compiled from multiple sources and may vary slightly from intervals listed within chapters. Some reference intervals are listed in common units and in the international system of units (SI units) in parentheses. Each laboratory must establish its particular intervals based on its instrumentation, methodology, and demographics of the population it serves.

HEMATOLOGY LABORATORY ASSAYS

Complete Blood Count Reference Intervals (Adult)

Assay	Units	Reference Intervals	Assay	Units	Reference Intervals
RBC, male	$\times10^6/\mu L$ ($\times10^{12}/L$)	4.20–6.00	RETIC	%	0.5–2.5
RBC, female	$\times10^6/\mu L$ ($\times10^{12}/L$)	3.80–5.20	NRBC	/100 WBC	0
HGB, male	g/dL (g/L)	13.5–18.0 (135–180)	WBC	$\times10^3/\mu L$ ($\times10^9/L$)	3.6–10.6
HGB, female	g/dL (g/L)	12.0–16.0 (120–160)	NEUT	%	50–70
HCT, male	% (L/L)	40–54 (0.40–0.54)	NEUT (ANC)	$\times10^3/\mu L$ ($\times10^9/L$)	1.7–7.5
			LYMPH	%	18–42
HCT, female	% (L/L)	36–47 (0.36–0.47)	LYMPH	$\times10^3/\mu L$ ($\times10^9/L$)	1.0–4.0
			MONO	%	2–11
MCV	fL	80–100	MONO	$\times10^3/\mu L$ ($\times10^9/L$)	0.1–1.0
MCH	pg	26–34	EO	%	1–3
MCHC	g/dL	32–36	EO	$\times10^3/\mu L$ ($\times10^9/L$)	0–0.3
RDW-CV	%	11.5–14.5	BASO	%	0–2
RDW-SD	fL	39–47	BASO	$\times10^3/\mu L$ ($\times10^9/L$)	0–0.2
RETIC	$\times10^3/\mu L$ ($\times10^9/L$)	20–115	PLT	$\times10^3/\mu L$ ($\times10^9/L$)	150–450
			MPV	fL	7.0–12.0

Reference Intervals for Other Commonly Ordered Assays (Adult)

Assay	Units	Reference Intervals	Assay	Units	Reference Intervals
ESR, male (Westergren)	mm 1 hour	0–15 (0–50 y) 0–20 (>50 y)	Serum ferritin, male	ng/mL	40–400
			Serum ferritin, female	ng/mL	12–160
ESR, female (Westergren)	mm 1 hour	0–20 (0–50 y) 0–30 (>50 y)	Serum vitamin B_{12}	pg/mL	200–900
			Serum folate	ng/mL	>4.0
Serum iron	$\mu g/dL$	50–160	RBC folate	ng/mL	>120
Total iron-binding capacity	$\mu g/dL$	250–400	Haptoglobin	mg/dL	30–200
Transferrin saturation	%	20–55	Free serum hemoglobin	mg/dL	0–10

Hemoglobin Fraction Reference Intervals

Fraction	Adult Reference Intervals (%)	Newborn Reference Intervals (%)
Hb A	>95	10–40
Hb F	0–2.0	60–90
Hb A_2	0–3.5	

BODY FLUIDS LABORATORY ASSAYS

Body Fluid Cell Count Reference Intervals

Fluid	Reference Intervals
Cerebrospinal fluid	RBC: 0/μL
	WBC: 0–30/μL (0 to 30 d)
	0–7/μL (31 d to 16 y)
	0–5/μL (16 y to adult)
Synovial fluid	WBC: 0–200/μL, less than 25% neutrophils
Serous fluid	Dependent on source; WBC usually less than 1000 total WBCs and less than 25% neutrophils

d, Days; *RBC,* red blood cell; *WBC,* white blood cell; *y,* years.

HEMOSTASIS LABORATORY ASSAYS

Coagulation Reference Intervals (Infants to Age 6 Months)

Assay	Day 1	Day 5	Day 30	Day 90	Day 120
PT (sec)	10.1–15.9	10.1–15.3	10.0–14.3	10.0–14.2	10.7–13.9
PTT (sec)	31.3–54.3	25.4–59.8	32.0–55.2	29.0–50.1	26.6–40.3
Thrombin time (sec)	19.0–28.3	18.0–29.2	19.4–29.2	20.5–29.7	19.7–30.3
Fibrinogen (mg/dL)	167–399	162–462	162–378	150–379	150–387
Factor VIII (%)	50–178	50–154	50–157	50–125	50–109
Factor IX (%)	15–91	15–91	21–81	21–113	36–136
VWF (%)	50–287	50–254	50–246	50–206	50–197
Antithrombin (%)	39–87	41–93	40–108	73–121	84–124
Protein C (%)	17–53	20–64	21–65	28–80	37–81
Protein S (%)	12–60	22–78	33–93	54–118	55–119

Andrew, M., Paes, B., & Johnston, M. (1990). Development of the hemostatic system in the neonate and young infant. *Am J Pediatr Hematol Oncol, 12,* 95–104.

Coagulation Reference Intervals (Pediatric Population Ages 7–17 Years)

Assay	7–9	10–11	12–13	14–15	16–17
PT (sec)	13.0–15.4	13.0–15.6	13.0–15.2	12.8–14.5	12.6–15.7
PTT (sec)	27–38	27–38	27–39	26–36	26–35
Factor VIII (%)	76–199	80–209	72–198	69–237	63–221
Factor IX (%)	70–133	72–149	73–152	80–161	86–176
VWF activity (%)	52–176	60–195	50–184	50–203	49–204
VWF antigen (%)	62–180	63–189	60–189	57–199	50–205

Flanders, M. M., Crist, R. A., Roberts, W. L., et al. (2005). Pediatric reference intervals for seven common coagulation assays. *Clin Chem, 51,* 1738–1742.

Bone Marrow Aspirate Reference Intervals (Adult)

WBC Differential	Reference Intervals (%)
Blasts	0–3
Promyelocytes	1–5
Myelocytes	6–17
Metamyelocytes	3–20
Band neutrophils	9–32
Segmented neutrophils	7–30
Eosinophils and precursors	0–3
Basophils and mast cells	0–1
Lymphocytes	5–18
Plasma cells	0–1
Monocytes	0–1
Histiocytes	0–1

Erythrocyte Series	Reference Intervals (%)
Pronormoblasts	0–1
Basophilic normoblasts	1–4
Polychromatophilic normoblasts	10–20
Orthochromic normoblasts	6–10

Other	Reference Intervals
M:E ratio	1.5–3.3:1
Megakaryocytes	2–10/lpf

Complete Blood Count Reference Intervals (Pediatric)*

Assay	Units	0–1 d	2–4 d	5–7 d	8–14 d	15–30 d	1–2 mo	3–5 mo	6–11 mo	1–3 y	4–7 y	8–13 y
RBC	$\times 10^6$/µL ($\times 10^{12}$/L)	4.10–6.10	4.36–5.96	4.20–5.80	4.00–5.60	3.20–5.00	3.40–5.00	3.65–5.05	3.60–5.20	3.40–5.20	4.00–5.20	4.00–5.40
HGB	g/dL (g/L)	16.5–21.5 (165–215)	16.4–20.8 (164–208)	15.2–20.4 (152–204)	15.0–19.6 (150–196)	12.2–18.0 (122–180)	10.6–16.4 (106–164)	10.4–16.0 (104–160)	10.4–15.6 (104–156)	9.6–15.6 (96–156)	10.2–15.2 (102–152)	12.0–15.0 (120–150)
HCT	%	48–68	48–68	50–64	46–62	38–53	32–50	35–51	35–51	34–48	36–46	35–49
MCV	fL	95–125	98–118	100–120	95–115	93–113	83–107	83–107	78–102	76–92	78–94	80–94
MCH	pg	30–42	30–42	30–42	30–42	28–40	27–37	25–35	23–31	23–31	23–31	26–32
MCHC	g/dL	30–34	30–34	30–34	30–34	30–34	31–37	32–36	32–36	32–36	32–36	32–36
RDW-CV	%	†	†	†	†	†	†	†	11.5–14.5	11.5–14.5	11.5–14.5	11.5–14.5
RETIC	%	1.8–5.8	1.3–4.7	0.2–1.4	0–1.0	0.2–1.0	0.8–2.8	0.5–1.5	0.5–1.5	0.5–1.5	0.5–1.5	0.5–1.5
RETIC	$\times 10^3$/µL ($\times 10^9$/L)	73.8–353.8	56.7–280.1	8.4–81.2	0.0–56.0	6.4–50.0	27.2–140.0	18.3–75.8	18.0–78.0	17.0–78.8	20–78.0	20–124.2
NRBC	/100 WBC	2–24	5–9	0–1	0	0	0	0	0	0	0	0
WBC	$\times 10^3$/µL ($\times 10^9$/L)	9.0–37.0	8.0–24.0	5.0–21.0	5.0–21.0	5.0–21.0	6.0–18.0	6.0–18.0	6.0–18.0	5.5–17.5	5.0–17.0	4.5–13.5
NEUT (ANC)	$\times 10^3$/µL ($\times 10^9$/L)	3.7–30.0	2.6–17.0	1.5–12.6	1.2–11.6	1.0–9.5	1.2–8.1	1.1–7.7	1.2–8.1	1.2–8.9	1.5–11.0	1.6–9.5
LYMPH	$\times 10^3$/µL ($\times 10^9$/L)	1.6–14.1	1.3–11.0	1.2–11.3	1.5–13.0	2.1–12.8	2.5–13.0	2.7–13.5	2.9–14.0	2.0–12.8	1.5–11.1	1.0–7.2
MONO	$\times 10^3$/µL ($\times 10^9$/L)	0.1–4.4	0.2–3.4	0.2–3.6	0.2–3.6	0.1–3.2	0.2–2.5	0.1–2.0	0.1–2.0	0.1–1.9	0.1–1.9	0.1–1.5
EO	$\times 10^3$/µL ($\times 10^9$/L)	0.0–1.5	0.0–1.2	0.0–1.3	0.0–1.1	0.0–1.1	0.0–0.7	0.0–0.7	0.0–0.7	0.0–0.7	0.0–0.7	0.0–0.5
BASO	$\times 10^3$/µL ($\times 10^9$/L)	0.0–0.7	0.0–0.5	0.0–0.4	0.0–0.4	0.0–0.4	0.0–0.4	0.0–0.4	0.0–0.4	0.0–0.4	0.0–0.3	0.0–0.3
PLT	$\times 10^3$/µL ($\times 10^9$/L)	150–450	150–450	150–450	150–450	150–450	150–450	150–450	150–450	150–450	150–450	150–450

*Pediatric reference intervals are from Riley Hospital for Children, Indiana University Health, Indianapolis, IN.

†The RDW is markedly elevated in newborns, with a range of 14.2% to 19.9% in the first few days of life, gradually decreasing until it reaches adult levels by 6 months of age.

ANC, Absolute neutrophil count (includes segmented neutrophils and bands); *BAND,* neutrophil bands; *BASO,* basophils; *d,* days; *EO,* eosinophils; *ESR,* erythrocyte sedimentation rate; *Hb,* hemoglobin fraction; *HCT,* hematocrit; *HGB,* hemoglobin concentration; *lpf,* low power field; *LYMPH,* lymphocytes; *MCH,* mean cell hemoglobin; *MCHC,* mean cell hemoglobin concentration; *MCV,* mean cell volume; *M:E,* myeloid:erythroid; *mo,* months; *MONO,* monocytes; *MPV,* mean platelet volume; *NEUT,* neutrophils; *NRBC,* nucleated red blood cells; *PLT,* platelets; *RBC,* red blood cell; *RDW-CV,* red cell distribution width, coefficient of variation; *RDW-SD,* red cell distribution width, standard deviation; *RETIC,* reticulocytes; *WBC,* white blood cell; *y,* years.